Ronald E. Goldstein's
Esthetics in Dentistry

THIRD EDITION

VOLUME 2

Esthetic Problems of Individual Teeth
Esthetic Challenges of Malocclusion
Esthetic Problems of Special Populations, Facial Considerations, and Supporting Structures
Problems of the Emergency and Failure
Chairside Procedures
Technical Advances and Proper Maintenance of Esthetic Restorations

Ronald E. Goldstein's
Esthetics in Dentistry

THIRD EDITION

VOLUME 2

Esthetic Problems of Individual Teeth
Esthetic Challenges of Malocclusion
Esthetic Problems of Special Populations, Facial Considerations, and Supporting Structures
Problems of the Emergency and Failure
Chairside Procedures
Technical Advances and Proper Maintenance of Esthetic Restorations

Edited by

Ronald E. Goldstein, DDS
Clinical Professor of Restorative Sciences at The Dental College of Georgia at Augusta University, Augusta, GA; Adjunct Clinical Professor of Prosthodontics, Boston University School of Dental Medicine, Boston; Adjunct Professor of Restorative Dentistry, University of Texas Health Science Center, San Antonio, TX; Former Visiting Professor of Oral and Maxillofacial Imaging and Continuing Education, University of Southern California, School of Dentistry, Los Angeles, CA; Private Practice, Atlanta, GA, USA

Stephen J. Chu, DMD, MSD, CDT
Adjunct Clinical Professor, Ashman Department of Periodontology and Implant Dentistry, Department of Prosthodontics, New York University College of Dentistry, New York, NY; Private Practice, New York, NY, USA

Ernesto A. Lee, DMD
Clinical Professor, University of Pennsylvania School of Dental Medicine, Philadelphia, PA; Former Director, Postdoctoral Periodontal Prosthesis Program, Penn Dental Medicine, University of Pennsylvania School of Medicine, Philadelphia, PA; Private Practice, Bryn Mawr, PA, USA

Christian F.J. Stappert, DDS, MS, PhD
Professor and Former Director of Postgraduate Prosthodontics, Department of Prosthodontics, University of Freiburg, Germany; Professor and Former Director of Periodontal Prosthodontics and Implant Dentistry, Department of Periodontics, University of Maryland School of Dentistry, Baltimore, MD, USA; Past Director of Aesthetics and Periodontal Prosthodontics, Department of Periodontology and Implant Dentistry, New York University College of Dentistry, New York, NY, USA; Private Practice, Zurich, Switzerland

WILEY Blackwell

This third edition first published 2018 © 2018 by John Wiley & Sons, Inc.

Edition History
1e 1976 Lippincott Williams & Wilkins; 2e 1998 B.C. Decker

All rights reserved. No part of this publication may be reproduced, stored in a retrieval system, or transmitted, in any form or by any means, electronic, mechanical, photocopying, recording or otherwise, except as permitted by law. Advice on how to obtain permission to reuse material from this title is available at http://www.wiley.com/go/permissions.

The right of Ronald E. Goldstein, Stephen J. Chu, Ernesto A. Lee and Christian F.J. Stappert to be identified as the authors of the editorial material in this work has been asserted in accordance with law.

Registered Office
John Wiley & Sons, Inc., 111 River Street, Hoboken, NJ 07030, USA

Editorial Office
111 River Street, Hoboken, NJ 07030, USA

For details of our global editorial offices, customer services, and more information about Wiley products visit us at www.wiley.com.

Wiley also publishes its books in a variety of electronic formats and by print-on-demand. Some content that appears in standard print versions of this book may not be available in other formats.

Limit of Liability/Disclaimer of Warranty

The contents of this work are intended to further general scientific research, understanding, and discussion only and are not intended and should not be relied upon as recommending or promoting scientific method, diagnosis, or treatment by physicians for any particular patient. In view of ongoing research, equipment modifications, changes in governmental regulations, and the constant flow of information relating to the use of medicines, equipment, and devices, the reader is urged to review and evaluate the information provided in the package insert or instructions for each medicine, equipment, or device for, among other things, any changes in the instructions or indication of usage and for added warnings and precautions. While the publisher and authors have used their best efforts in preparing this work, they make no representations or warranties with respect to the accuracy or completeness of the contents of this work and specifically disclaim all warranties, including without limitation any implied warranties of merchantability or fitness for a particular purpose. No warranty may be created or extended by sales representatives, written sales materials or promotional statements for this work. The fact that an organization, website, or product is referred to in this work as a citation and/or potential source of further information does not mean that the publisher and authors endorse the information or services the organization, website, or product may provide or recommendations it may make. This work is sold with the understanding that the publisher is not engaged in rendering professional services. The advice and strategies contained herein may not be suitable for your situation. You should consult with a specialist where appropriate. Further, readers should be aware that websites listed in this work may have changed or disappeared between when this work was written and when it is read. Neither the publisher nor authors shall be liable for any loss of profit or any other commercial damages, including but not limited to special, incidental, consequential, or other damages.

A catalogue record for this book is available from the Library of Congress and the British Library

ISBN 9781119272830

Cover images: (background) © Natapong Supalertsophon/Getty Images; (first inset image) courtesy of Jacinthe Paquette, DDS; (middle inset images) courtesy of Dr. James Fondriest; (fourth inset image) courtesy of Dentsply Sirona, Inc.
Cover design by Wiley

Set in 10/12 pt MinionPro by SPi Global, Pondicherry, India
Printed and bound in Singapore by Markono Print Media Pte Ltd

10 9 8 7 6 5 4 3 2 1

Contents

List of Contributors — ix
Contributors at Large — xvii
Preface to Third Edition — xix
Acknowledgments — xxi

VOLUME 1

PART I PRINCIPLES OF ESTHETICS 1

1. Concepts of Dental Esthetics — 3
   Ronald E. Goldstein and Gordon Patzer

2. Successful Management of Common Psychological Challenges — 25
   Shirley Brown

3. Esthetic Treatment Planning: Patient and Practice Management Skills in Esthetic Treatment Planning — 47
   Ronald E. Goldstein and Maurice A. Salama

4. Digital Smile Design: A Digital Tool for Esthetic Evaluation, Team Communication, and Patient Management — 85
   Christian Coachman, Marcelo Calamita, and Andrea Ricci

5. Esthetics in Dentistry Marketing — 113
   Roger P. Levin and Ronald E. Goldstein

6. Legal Considerations — 131
   Edwin J. Zinman

7. Practical Clinical Photography — 155
   Glenn D. Krieger

8. Creating Esthetic Restorations Through Special Effects — 185
   Ronald E. Goldstein, Jason J. Kim, Pinhas Adar, and Adam Mieleszko

9. Proportional Smile Design — 243
   Daniel H. Ward, Stephen J. Chu, and Christian F.J. Stappert

10. Understanding Color — 271
    Rade D. Paravina

PART 2 ESTHETIC TREATMENTS 295

11. Cosmetic Contouring — 297
    Ronald E. Goldstein

12. Bleaching Discolored Teeth — 325
    So Ran Kwon and Ronald E. Goldstein

13. Adhesion to Hard Tissue on Teeth — 355
    Roland Frankenberger, Uwe Blunck, and Lorenzo Breschi

14. Composite Resin Bonding — 375
    Ronald E. Goldstein and Marcos Vargas

15. Ceramic Veneers and
    Partial-Coverage Restorations 433
    Christian F.J. Stappert, Ronald E. Goldstein,
    Fransiskus A. Tjiptowidjojo,
    and Stephen J. Chu

16. Crown Restorations 499
    Kenneth A. Malament, Ronald E. Goldstein,
    Christian F.J. Stappert, Mo Taheri,
    and Thomas Sing

PART 3 ESTHETIC CHALLENGES OF MISSING TEETH 541

17. Replacing Missing Teeth with Fixed
    Partial Dentures 543
    Jacinthe M. Paquette, Jean C. Wu,
    Cherilyn G. Sheets, and Devin L. Stewart

VOLUME 2

PART 4 ESTHETIC PROBLEMS OF INDIVIDUAL TEETH 667

21. Management of Stained and Discolored Teeth 669
    Ronald E. Goldstein, Samantha Siranli,
    Van B. Haywood, and W. Frank Caughman

22. Abfraction, Abrasion, Attrition, and Erosion 693
    Ronald E. Goldstein, James W. Curtis Jr,
    Beverly A. Farley, Samantha Siranli,
    and Wendy A. Clark

23. Chipped, Fractured, or Endodontically
    Treated Teeth 721
    Ronald E. Goldstein, Daniel C.N. Chan,
    Michael L. Myers, and Gerald M. Barrack

24. Endodontics and Esthetic Dentistry 749
    John West, Noah Chivian, Donald E. Arens, and
    Asgeir Sigurdsson

18. Esthetic Removable Partial Dentures 581
    Carol A. Lefebvre, Roman M. Cibirka,
    and Ronald E. Goldstein

19. The Complete Denture 611
    Walter F. Turbyfill Jr

20. Implant Esthetics: Concepts,
    Surgical Procedures, and Materials 637
    Sonia Leziy and Brahm Miller

Appendices

Appendix A: Esthetic Evaluation Form A1
Appendix B: The Functional-Esthetic Analysis B1
Appendix C: Laboratory Checklist C1
Appendix D: Pincus Principles D1

Index i1

PART 5 ESTHETIC CHALLENGES OF MALOCCLUSION 809

25. Oral Habits 811
    Ronald E. Goldstein, James W. Curtis Jr,
    Beverly A. Farley, and Daria Molodtsova

26. Restorative Treatment of Diastema 841
    Barry D. Hammond, Kevin B. Frazier,
    Anabella Oquendo, and Ronald E. Goldstein

27. Restorative Treatment of Crowded Teeth 877
    Ronald E. Goldstein, Geoffrey W. Sheen,
    and Steven T. Hackman

28. Esthetics in Adult Orthodontics 897
    Eladio DeLeon Jr

29. Surgical Orthodontic Correction
    of Dentofacial Deformity 929
    John N. Kent, John P. Neary, John Oubre,
    and David A. Bulot

PART 6 ESTHETIC PROBLEMS OF SPECIAL POPULATIONS, FACIAL CONSIDERATIONS, AND SUPPORTING STRUCTURES 967

30. Pediatric Dentistry 969
    Claudia Caprioglio, Alberto Caprioglio, and Damaso Caprioglio

31. Geresthetics: Esthetic Dentistry for Older Adults 1015
    Linda C. Niessen, Ronald E. Goldstein, and Maha El-Sayed

32. Facial Considerations: An Orthodontic Perspective 1051
    David Sarver

33. Facial Considerations in Esthetic Restorations 1085
    Ronald E. Goldstein and Bruno P. Silva

34. Plastic Surgery Related to Esthetic Dentistry 1131
    Foad Nahai and Kristin A. Boehm

35. Cosmetic Adjuncts 1143
    Ronald E. Goldstein, Richard Davis, and Marvin Westmore

36. Esthetic Considerations in the Performing Arts 1153
    Ronald E. Goldstein and Daniel Materdomini

37. Periodontal Plastic Surgery 1181
    W. Peter Nordland and Laura M. Souza

PART 7 PROBLEMS OF THE EMERGENCY AND FAILURE 1213

38. Esthetic and Traumatic Emergencies 1215
    Ronald E. Goldstein and Shane N. White

39. Esthetic Failures 1235
    Ronald E. Goldstein, Azadeh Esfandiari, and Anna K. Schultz

PART 8 CHAIRSIDE PROCEDURES 1261

40. Tooth Preparation in Esthetic Dentistry 1263
    Ronald E. Goldstein, Ernesto A. Lee, and Wendy A. Clark

41. Impressions 1287
    Ronald E. Goldstein, John M. Powers, and Ernesto A. Lee

42. Esthetic Temporization 1311
    Ronald E. Goldstein and Pinhas Adar

43. The Esthetic Try-In 1331
    Ronald E. Goldstein and Carolina Arana

44. Cementation of Restorations 1355
    Stephen F. Rosenstiel and Ronald E. Goldstein

PART 9 TECHNICAL ADVANCES AND PROPER MAINTENANCE OF ESTHETIC RESTORATIONS 1367

45. Esthetic Principles in Constructing Ceramic Restorations 1369
    Robert D. Walter

46. Digital Impression Devices and CAD/CAM Systems 1387
    Nathan S. Birnbaum and Heidi B. Aaronson

47. Maintenance of Esthetic Restorations 1409
    Ronald E. Goldstein, Kimberly J. Nimmons, Anita H. Daniels, and Caren Barnes

Index i1

List of Contributors

Heidi B. Aaronson, DMD
Former Clinical Instructor
Tufts University School of Dental Medicine
Boston, MA;
Private Practice
Wellesley, MA
USA

Pinhas Adar, MDT, CDT
Adjunct Clinical Professor
Tufts University School of Dentistry
Adar International, Inc.
Atlanta, GA
USA

Carolina Arana, DMD, MPH
Private Practice
Decatur, GA
USA

Donald E. Arens, DDS, MSD (Deceased)
Former Professor Emeritus in Endodontics Indiana;
Indiana University School of Dentistry
Indianapolis, IN;
Former Visiting Professor of Endodontics
College of Dental Medicine
Nova SE University
Davie, FL
USA

Caren Barnes, RDH, BS, MS
Professor, Coordinator of Clinical Research
University of Nebraska Medical Center College
of Dentistry
Department of Dental Hygiene
Lincoln, NE
USA

Gerald M. Barrack, DDS
Private Practice
Ho-Ho-Kus, NJ
USA

Nathan S. Birnbaum, DDS
Associate Clinical Professor
Tufts University School of Dental Medicine
Boston, MA;
Private Practice
Medford, MA
USA

Uwe Blunck, DDS
Associate Professor
Department for Operative, Endodontic and
Preventive Dentistry
School of Dentistry
Charité-Universitaetsmedizin
Berlin
Germany

Kristin A. Boehm, MD, FACS
Assistant Clinical Professor Plastic & Reconstructive Surgery
Emory University School of Medicine
Atlanta, GA;
Private Practice
Atlanta, GA
USA

Lorenzo Breschi, DDS, PhD
Associate Professor
Department of Biomedical and Neuromotor Sciences
University of Bologna - Alma Mater Studiorum
Bologna
Italy

Shirley Brown, DMD, PhD
Rittenhouse Collaborative
Vector Group Consulting
Philadelphia, PA
USA

David A. Bulot, DDS, MD
Assistant Clinical Professor
LSU Oral and Maxillofacial Surgery
New Orleans, LA;
Private Practice
Baton Rouge, LA
USA

Marcelo Calamita, DDS, MS, PhD
Former Associate Professor of Prosthodontics at University Braz Cubas;
University of Guarulhos
São Paulo
Brazil

Alberto Caprioglio, DDS, MS
Associate Professor and Chairman
Department of Orthodontics
School of Dentistry
University of Insubria
Varese
Italy

Claudia Caprioglio, DDS, MS
Visiting Professor Department of Orthodontics
Pediatric Dentistry University of Pisa
Pisa
Italy

Damaso Caprioglio, MD, MS
Former Full Professor of Orthodontics
University of Parma School of Dentistry
Parma;
Lecturer in Ethics
University of Parma
Parma
Italy

W. Frank Caughman, DMD, MEd
Professor Emeritus
The Dental College of Georgia at Augusta University
Augusta, GA
USA

Daniel C.N. Chan, DMD, MS, DDS
Chair Department of Restorative Dentistry
School of Dentistry
University of Washington
Seattle, WA
USA

Noah Chivian, DDS
Clinical Professor
Department of Endodontics
Rutgers School of Dental Medicine
Newark, NJ;
Adjunct Professor of Endodontics
University of Pennsylvania
School of Dental Medicine
Philadelphia, PA
USA

Stephen J. Chu, DMD, MSD, CDT
Adjunct Clinical Professor
Ashman Department of Periodontology & Implant Dentistry
Department of Prosthodontics
New York University College of Dentistry, New York;
Private Practice
New York, NY
USA

Roman M. Cibirka, DDS, MS
Former Assistant Professor
Department of Rehabilitation
The Dental College of Georgia at Augusta University
Augusta, GA
USA

Wendy A. Clark, DDS, MS
Clinical Assistant Professor
Department of Prosthodontics
University of North Carolina School of Dentistry
Chapel Hill, NC
USA

Christian Coachman, DDS, CDT
Private Practice
São Paulo
Brazil

James W. Curtis Jr, DMD
Director
Dental Education
Palmetto Health Dental Center
Columbia, SC
USA

Anita H. Daniels, RDH
Adjunct Clinical Instructor
University of Miami
Department of Dental Implants
School of Medicine
Miami, FL
USA

Richard Davis
Professional Hair Stylist
Atlanta, GA
USA

List of Contributors

Eladio DeLeon Jr, DMD, MS
Goldstein Chair of Orthodontics
The Dental College of Georgia at Augusta University
Augusta, GA
USA

Maha El-Sayed, BDS, DMD, MS
Private Practice
Atlanta, GA
USA

Azadeh Esfandiari, DMD
Private Practice
Atlanta, GA
USA

Beverly A. Farley, DMD (Deceased)
Formerly in Private Practice
Irmo, SC
USA

Roland Frankenberger, DMD, PhD
Professor and Chair
Department of Operative Dentistry and Endodontics
Medical Center for Dentistry
University of Marburg
Marburg
Germany

Kevin B. Frazier, DMD, EDS
Professor
Oral Rehabilitation
The Dental College of Georgia at Augusta University
Augusta, GA
USA

Ronald E. Goldstein, DDS
Clinical Professor
Department of Restorative Sciences
The Dental College of Georgia at Augusta University
Augusta, GA;
Adjunct Clinical Professor of Prosthodontics
Boston University School of Dental Medicine
Boston;
Adjunct Professor of Restorative Dentistry
University of Texas Health Science Center
San Antonio, TX;
Former Visiting Professor of Oral and Maxillofacial Imaging and Continuing Education
University of Southern California
School of Dentistry
Los Angeles, CA;
Private Practice
Atlanta, GA
USA

Steven T. Hackman, DDS
Formerly, Department of Oral Rehabilitation
The Dental College of Georgia at Augusta University
Augusta, GA
USA

Barry D. Hammond, DMD
Associate Professor and Director of Dental Continuing Education
The Dental College of Georgia at Augusta University
Augusta, GA
USA

Van B. Haywood, DMD
Professor
Department of Oral Rehabilitation
The Dental College of Georgia at Augusta University
Augusta, GA
USA

John N. Kent, DDS
Former Boyd Professor and Head
Department of Oral and Maxillofacial Surgery
LSU School of Dentistry and LSU School of Medicine at Shreveport;
Professor Emeritus, LSUSD and LSUHSC
New Orleans, LA
USA

Jason J. Kim, CDT
Clinical Assistant Professor
New York University College of Dentistry
Oral Design Center
New York, NY
USA

Glenn D. Krieger, DDS, MS
Private Practice
Lewisville, TX
USA

So Ran Kwon, DDS, MS, PhD, MS
Associate Professor
Center for Dental Research
Loma Linda University School of Dentistry
Loma Linda, CA
USA

Ernesto A. Lee, DMD
Clinical Professor
University of Pennsylvania School of Dental Medicine;
Director
Postdoctoral Periodontal Prosthesis Program
Penn Dental Medicine;
Private Practice
Bryn Mawr, PA
USA

Carol A. Lefebvre, DDS, MS
Dean and Professor
Oral Rehabilitation and Oral Biology
The Dental College of Georgia at Augusta University
Augusta University
Augusta, GA
USA

Roger P. Levin, DDS
CEO/President
Levin Group Inc.
Owings Mills, MD
USA

Sonia Leziy, DDS
Associate Clinical Associate Professor
University of British Columbia
Vancouver
British Columbia;
Private Practice
Vancouver
Canada

Kenneth A. Malament, DDS, MScD
Clinical Professor
Tufts University
Medford, MA
USA

Daniel Materdomini, CDT
DaVinci Dental Studios
Beverly Hills, CA
USA

Adam Mieleszko, CDT
Technical instructor
New York University College of Dentistry
New York, NY
USA

Brahm Miller, DDS, MSc
Associate Clinical Professor and Sessional Lecturer
University of British Columbia
Vancouver, British Columbia;
Private Practice
Vancouver
Canada

Daria Molodtsova, MS
Moscow
Russia

Michael L. Myers, DMD
Professor
Department of Oral Rehabilitation
The Dental College of Georgia at Augusta University
Augusta, GA
USA

Foad Nahai, MD, FACS
Clinical Professor of Plastic Surgery
Emory University
Atlanta GA;
Private Practice
Atlanta, GA
USA

John P. Neary, MD, DDS
Assistant Professor and Chairman
Department of Oral and Maxillofacial Surgery
LSU Health Sciences Center-New Orleans
New Orleans, LA;
Assistant Professor
LSU Department of General Surgery
LSU Health Sciences Center-New Orleans,
New Orleans, LA;
Former Adjunct Professor
University of Leon
Department of Maxillofacial and Plastic Surgery
Leon, Nicaragua;
Former Clinical Assistant Professor
Case-Western University
Department of Oral and Maxillofacial Surgery
Cleveland, OH
USA

Linda C. Niessen, DMD, MPH, MPP
Dean
Nova Southeastern University
Fort Lauderdale, FL
USA

Kimberly J. Nimmons, RDH, BS
Clinical Specialist
Atlanta, GA
USA

W. Peter Nordland, DMD, MS
Associate Professor of Periodontics
Loma Linda University
Loma Linda, CA;
Private Practice
Newport Beach, CA
USA

Annabella Oquendo, DDS
Clinical Assistant Professor
Cariology and Comprehensive Care
New York University College of Dentistry
New York, NY
USA

John Oubre, DDS
Private Practice
Lafayette, LA
USA

List of Contributors

Jacinthe M. Paquette, DDS
Private Practice
Newport Beach, CA
USA

Rade D. Paravina, DDS, MS, PhD
Professor
Department of Restorative Dentistry and Prosthodontics;
Director
Houston Center for Biomaterials and Biomimetics;
Ralph C. Cooley Distinguished Professor
The University of Texas School of Dentistry at Houston
Houston, TX
USA

Gordon Patzer, PhD
Professor
Roosevelt University
Chicago, IL
USA

John M. Powers, PhD
Professor of Oral Biomaterials
Department of Restorative Dentistry and Biomaterials
UT Health Dental Branch
Houston, TX
USA

Andrea Ricci, DDS
Private Practice
Florence
Italy

Stephen F. Rosenstiel, BDS, MSD
Professor Emeritus
Ohio State University College of Dentistry
Columbus, OH
USA

Maurice A. Salama, DMD
Faculty
University of Pennsylvania
Philadelphia, PA;
Clinical Assistant Professor
Department of Periodontics
The Dental College of Georgia at Augusta University
Augusta, GA;
Visiting Professor of Periodontics at Nova Southeastern University
Fort Lauderdale, FL;
Private Practice
Atlanta, GA
USA

David Sarver, DMD, MS
Adjunct Professor
University of North Carolina
Department of Orthodontics
Chapel Hill, NC;
Clinical Professor
University of Alabama Department of Orthodontics
Birmingham, AL;
Private Practice
Birmingham, AL
USA

Anna K. Schultz, DMD
Private Practice
Atlanta, GA
USA

Geoffrey W. Sheen, DDS, MS
Department of Oral Rehabilitation
Dental College of Georgia
Augusta University
Augusta, GA
USA

Cherilyn G. Sheets, DDS
Clinical Professor
Department of Restorative Dentistry
University of Southern California
Ostrow School of Dentistry
Los Angeles, CA;
Private Practice
Newport Beach, CA
USA

Asgeir Sigurdsson, DDS, MS
Associate Professor and Chairman
Department of Endodontics
NYU College of Dentistry
New York, NY
USA

Bruno P. Silva, DMD, PhD
Clinical Assistant Professor
Department of Prosthodontics
University of Seville
School of Dentistry
Spain;
Private Practice
Seville
Spain

Thomas Sing, MDT
Visiting Lecturer
Postdoctoral Program for Prosthodontics
Tufts University
School of Dental Medicine
Boston, MA;
Visiting Lecturer
Harvard School of Dental Medicine
Boston, MA;
Private Practice
Boston, MA
USA

Samantha Siranli, DMD, PhD
Former Adjunct Faculty
Department of Oral Rehabilitation
The Dental College of Georgia
Augusta University
Augusta, GA;
Former Associate Professor of Prosthodontics
University of Pittsburgh
Pittsburgh, PA;
Private Practice
Washington, DC
USA

Laura M. Souza, DDS
Private Practice
San Diego, CA
USA

Christian F.J. Stappert, DDS, MS, PhD
Professor and Former Director of Postgraduate Prosthodontics
Department of Prosthodontics
University of Freiburg
Germany;
Professor and Former Director of Periodontal Prosthodontics and Implant Dentistry
Department of Periodontics
University of Maryland School of Dentistry
Baltimore, MD;
Past Director of Aesthetics and Periodontal Prosthodontics
Department of Periodontology and Implant Dentistry
New York University College of Dentistry
New York, NY
USA;
Private Practice
Zurich
Switzerland

Devin L. Stewart, DDS
Private Practice
San Luis Obispo
Los Angeles, CA;
Former Clinical Instructor
Removable Department
UCLA
Los Angeles, CA
USA

Mo Taheri, DMD
Clinical Instructor
Tufts University
Medford, MA
USA

Fransiskus A. Tjiptowidjojo, DDS, MS
Adjunct Instructor
University of Detroit Mercy School of Dentistry
Department of Restorative Dentistry
Detroit, MI
USA

Walter F. Turbyfill Jr, DMD
Private Practice
Columbia, SC
USA

Marcos Vargas, DDS, MS
Professor
Department of Family Dentistry
The University of Iowa
Iowa City, IA
USA

Robert D. Walter, DDS, MSD
Associate Professor
School of Dentistry
Loma Linda University
Loma Linda, CA
USA

Daniel H. Ward, DDS
Former Assistant Clinical Professor
Department of Restorative and Prosthetic Dentistry
College of Dentistry
The Ohio State University
Columbus OH;
Private Practice
Columbus, OH
USA

John West, DDS, MSD
Affiliate Associate Professor
Department of Endodontics
School of Dentistry
University of Washington
Seattle, WA
USA

Marvin Westmore
Professional Makeup Artist and Licensed Aesthetician
Hollywood, CA
USA

Shane N. White, BDentSc, MS, MA, PhD
Professor
UCLA School of Dentistry
Los Angeles, CA
USA

Jean C. Wu, DDS
Former Lecturer
Restorative Dentistry Department
University of Tennessee
Memphis, TN;
Private Practice
Newport Beach, CA
USA

Edwin J. Zinman, DDS, JD
Former Lecturer
Department of Periodontology
UCSF School of Dentistry
San Francisco CA;
Private Law Practice
San Francisco, CA
USA

Contributors at Large

Wendy A. Clark, DDS, MS
Clinical Assistant Professor
Department of Prosthodontics
University of North Carolina School of Dentistry
Chapel Hill, NC
USA

Nadia Esfandiari, DMD
Private Practice
Atlanta, GA
USA

David A. Garber, DMD
Clinical Professor
Department of Periodontics
The Dental College of Georgia at Augusta University
Augusta, GA;
Clinical Professor
Department of Prosthodontics
Louisiana State University Department of Restorative Dentistry
Baton Rouge, LA;
University of Texas in San Antonio
San Antonio, TX;
Private Practice
Atlanta, GA
USA

Cary E. Goldstein, DMD
Clinical Professor
Department of Restorative Sciences
The Dental College of Georgia at Augusta University
Augusta, GA;
Private Practice
Atlanta, GA
USA

Henry Salama, DMD
Former Director and Clinical Assistant Professor
Department of Periodontics
Implant Research Center
University of Pennsylvania
Philadelphia, PA;
Private Practice
Atlanta, GA
USA

Maurice A. Salama, DMD
Faculty
University of Pennsylvania
Philadelphia, PA;
Clinical Assistant Professor
Department of Periodontics
The Dental College of Georgia at Augusta University
Augusta, GA;
Visiting Professor of Periodontics at Nova Southeastern University
Fort Lauderdale, FL;
Private Practice
Atlanta, GA
USA

Preface to Third Edition

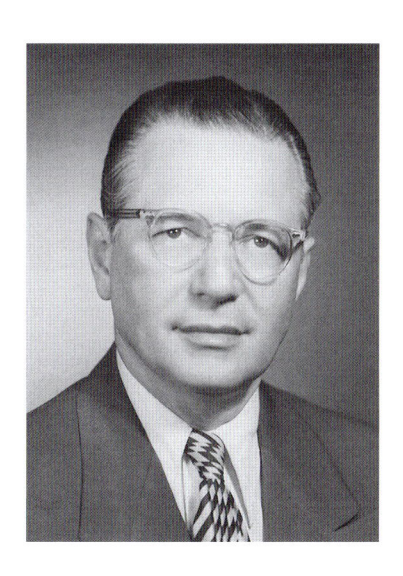

I owe so much of my career in esthetic dentistry to my first and most important mentor… my father, Dr Irving H. Goldstein, a great dentist, civic leader, and philanthropist. I learned so much watching him create the most beautiful smiles and only wish Dad had kept a photo library as I have done in my career. He taught me that being an average dentist was never an option… rather to always work to be the best, and at 84 years, I am still striving every day I practice.

I was first drawn to the study of esthetics a number of years before my 1969 article "The study of the need for esthetic dentistry" was published in the *Journal of Prosthetic Dentistry*. That article identified dentistry's lack of appreciation for the patients' appearances and their self-perception.

During the first half of the 1970s, I avidly pursued my study of esthetics, investigating every known aspect of dentofacial appearance. I became convinced of the huge untapped potential the field offered for improving patient outcomes and enhancing dental practice. Eventually, I was inspired to dedicate my professional career to promoting a comprehensive interdisciplinary approach to dentistry that united function and esthetics in total dentofacial harmony.

When the first edition of this text was published in 1976, the United States was in the midst of a celebration marking the 200th anniversary of our birth as a nation. It was an unprecedented national observance of the highly successful American Revolution. At the time, I considered the two events—both of considerable importance to me—distinct from one another. Since that time, however, I have come to recognize that, although the publishing of any textbook could never be considered in the same breath with the emergence of a nation, both events were indeed revolutionary.

Six decades ago, esthetics was considered, at best, a fortuitous by-product of a dental procedure—a bridesmaid, but certainly not a bride. In the years that have ensued, esthetics has taken its rightful place, along with functionality, as a bona fide objective of dental treatment. The revolution that has transpired has not only enhanced our knowledge of the field but also in methodology and technology. Today's patients are highly informed about the possibilities of esthetic dental restorations and fully expect that esthetics will be considered, from the inception of treatment to the final result.

Consumers know that dental esthetics play a key role in their sense of well-being, their acceptance by others, their success at work, in relationships, and their emotional stability. Informed by magazines, books, internet, and ongoing social media coverage, plus driven by the desire to live better lives, patients seek out dentists who can deliver superior esthetic services.

The ongoing effort to meet these demands with state-of-the-art and science treatment represents the continuation of that revolution. At the time this text book first appeared, I hoped that esthetics would eventually hold a preeminent position in our profession. That goal has been accomplished. Esthetics is recognized worldwide today as a basic principle of virtually all dental treatment.

We have been so fortunate in having over 75 world authorities helping to update the 47 chapters in two volumes. Virtually every phase of esthetic dentistry has now been included. It is my hope that, in some small way, this updated edition will serve to advance all aspects of the esthetic dental revolution and, in so doing, help patients and practitioners achieve even greater, more satisfying outcomes.

I feel so fortunate that three of the world's best known, talented, and respected academicians, clinicians, and teachers agreed to co-edit this third edition with me—Drs Steven Chu, Ernesto Lee, and Christian Stappert have continuingly contributed greatly in making the third edition more far-reaching into the high-tech worldwide revolution in esthetic dentistry.

Ronald E. Goldstein

Acknowledgments

So many people have worked on various aspects of this third edition that it would take far too much space to mention all of them. However, there were those who gave significant time to the project, and it is those people who I will attempt to thank at this time.

Most helpful in every way was the extraordinary 7-year effort of my personal editorial assistant, Annette Mathews. Annette's attention to detail and meticulous follow-through helped us greatly to complete this third edition. Despite the frustration of dealing with three different publishers, Annette helped coordinate with over 75 contributors, in addition to continuously proofreading the 47 chapters. I have had the pleasure of working with many individuals in my 60 years of practice, but none better than Annette. She wins the prize!

Others who assisted me on various aspects of the book were Daria Molodtsova, Candace Paetzhold, and Yhaira Grigsby.

My clinical office staff has always been generous with their help over the years. Those assistants who have been most helpful with this edition were Sondra Williams and Charlene Bennett.

It also takes a talented group of professionals for the day-to-day support necessary to sustain a lengthy project such as this text. I am most appreciative of the support from my long-time partners, David Garber and Maurice Salama. No one could ask for a more understanding and gifted friend than David. Maurice and Henry Salama have always been ready to lend a hand or help solve a dilemma as only they can. Wendy Clark, Nadia Esfandiari, and Maha El Sayed were particularly helpful during the writing and editing stages. Thanks also to Pinhas Adar, who has always been willing and available to help with technical or illustrative assistance. Thanks also to Zach Turner for his excellent illustrations throughout the text.

Last but not least, I must thank my busy but devoted family; my dentist sons Cary and Ken plus my dental daughter Cathy Goldstein Schwartz were particularly helpful in the second edition, and my physician son, Rick, managed to keep me healthy enough to complete the task.

I must pay the final tribute to my wife, Judy, who has continued to support and advise me throughout my career. She has put up with the tremendous hours over 60 years of writing articles and books and helped me through the good and bad times… fortunately more good than bad. My only promise to her was that this third edition of *Esthetics in Dentistry* will definitely be my last textbook as author or co-author.

Ronald E. Goldstein

PART 4
ESTHETIC PROBLEMS OF INDIVIDUAL TEETH

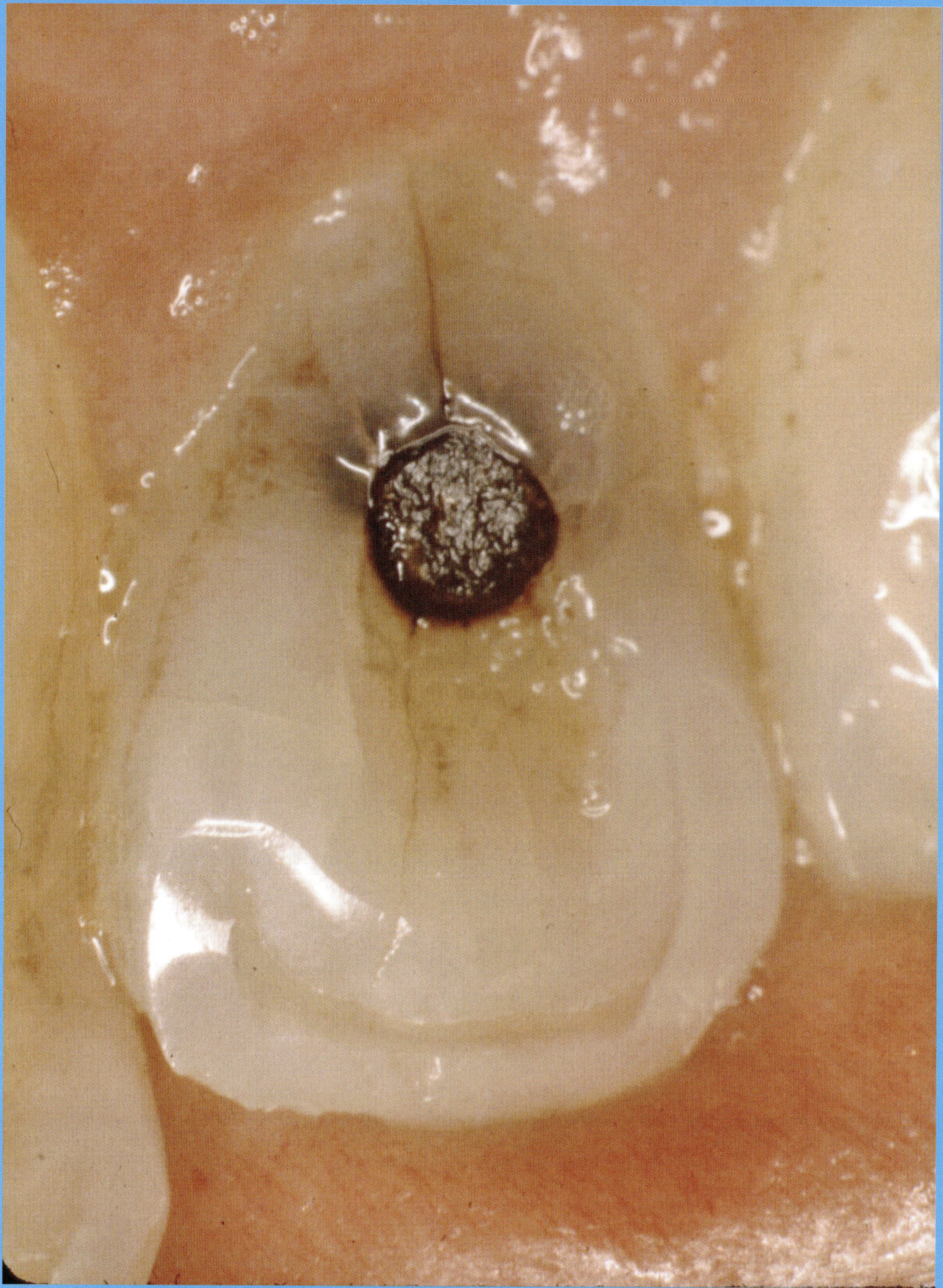

Chapter 21 Management of Stained and Discolored Teeth

Ronald E. Goldstein, DDS, Samantha Siranli, DMD, PhD,
Van B. Haywood, DMD, and W. Frank Caughman, DMD, MEd

Chapter Outline

Types of stains: causes and treatment options	670	Erythroblastosis fetalis, or hemolytic disease of newborns	682
Stains and discolorations caused by tooth defects	670	Hepatic–biliary disorders	682
Dental caries	670	Porphyria	682
Discolored deep grooves	670	Pulp injury	682
Stains caused by leakage around restorations	670	Internal resorption	682
Extrinsic stains	671	Stains of various medications	682
Nathoo classification and causes	671	Single dark teeth	682
Types of stains	674	Localized brown discoloration	682
Toothpastes that help maintain whiteness	676	Localized white discoloration	683
Matching color to individual patient	678	Tetracycline staining	683
Intrinsic stains	678	Treatment	687
Enamel hypoplasia	679	Bleaching	687
Amelogenesis imperfecta	679	Bleaching as a stepping-stone to veneers	687
Enamel hypocalcification	679	Bleaching and other restoration procedures	687
Dental fluorosis	679	Discoloration of composite resin restorations	689
Dentinogenesis imperfecta	680		
Blood-borne pigment	681		

Discoloration and staining is a topic of special interest to many dental patients; however, it has not received as much attention in the contemporary scientific literature. Much of the discussion about dental diseases and discolorations dates back to the middle of the last century, and the latest review on the topic was published in 2001 by Watts and Addy, being the only readily available review since 1975.[1] This only highlights the importance of dentists being able to answer the numerous questions that are posed by patients seeking whiter teeth.

Each year, millions of individuals change toothpaste, purchase ineffective preparations, and even change their dentists in their quest for "whiter teeth." Many an attractive smile is marred by some discoloration or stain, either on an individual tooth or on all teeth (Figure 21.1A and B). There are many causes and

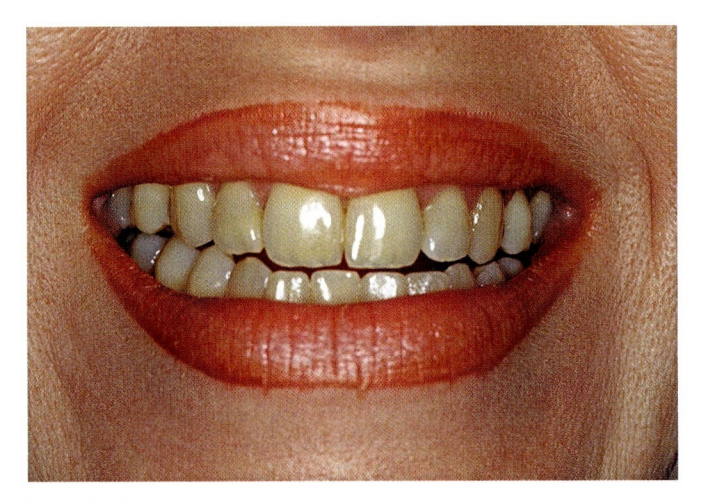

Figure 21.1 (A) The first line of defense for staining is bleaching.

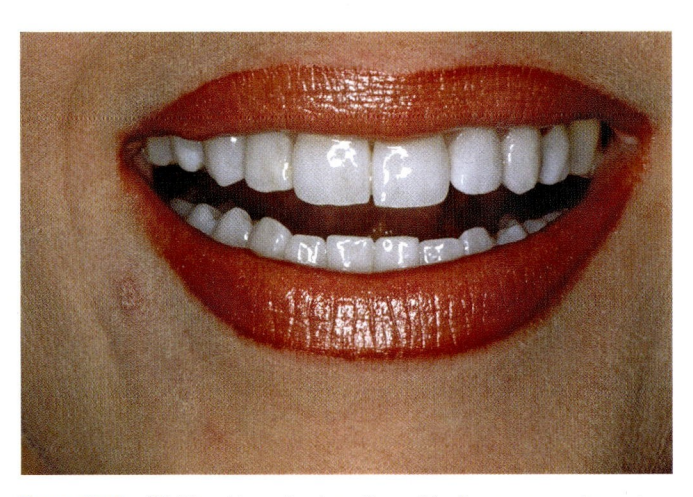

Figure 21.1 (B) Bleaching plus bonding with direct composite resin was done to improve this lady's smile.

corresponding treatments for these stains and discolorations. The dentist needs to be able to correctly diagnose the cause of discolorations, as it is crucial for a successful treatment outcome. Some treatments must be performed in the dental office, some can be performed at home by patient, and some are a combination of home and office treatments.

Types of stains: causes and treatment options

Generally, stains can be divided into extrinsic (located on the outside of the tooth) and intrinsic (located within the tooth). Moreover, extrinsic stains can become intrinsic over time. Hence, stains can originate from the outside in or from the inside out. The clinical appearance can be in a variety of colors. Table 21.1 provides a summary of tooth discoloration and associated conditions. Some examples of these different discolorations can be seen in Figures 21.2A and B, 21.3, and 21.4. In addition, the discoloration can be either of a generalized nature or specific to one tooth or one location on a tooth (Table 21.2).

A number of treatment options should be considered, in order of increasing aggressiveness (Table 21.3).

Stains and discolorations caused by tooth defects

Dental Caries

Dental caries is one of the chief causes of unsightly tooth stains. The progress of caries can be evaluated visually, tactually, and radiographically. In direct lighting, incipient lesions may appear as dull, chalky white areas where the enamel has been decalcified and has lost its translucency. Interproximal decay may be seen as a gray area deep to the marginal ridge of the affected surface. Recurrent decay may also be seen as a gray area adjacent to the margin of a defective restoration. Viewed with transillumination (Addent), proximal lesions on anterior teeth can be seen as shadows.

As the lesion progresses, the decalcified area becomes stained with food and bacterial debris. The discoloration can vary from light to dark brown (Figure 21.5). The degree of discoloration depends on how long the decay process has been active in the tooth. Therefore, the earlier the treatment, the smaller the chance of tooth staining. For this reason, radiographs should be taken, periodically, of all patients.

Discolored deep grooves

Diagnosis for decay is difficult in deep grooves. If there is a possibility, first use an air-abrasive or hard-tissue laser (Solea) to remove the organic pellicle and any caries present and then either fill or seal the tooth rather than merely watch the area.[2] Patients who complain about discolored grooves will be better served with a highly filled tinted or opaque sealant rather than a clear sealant through which the groove can be seen. In addition, clear sealants that were chemically cured may exhibit an amber or yellow discoloration over time and require replacement (Figure 21.6). Prior to the placement of a sealant, the grooves should be cleaned of organic matter.[3] The cleaning of grooves can be mechanically accomplished by use of a #1/4 round bur in a high-speed handpiece, hard-tissue laser or air abrasion. Placing 3% hydrogen peroxide in the grooves is a chemical option to debride the grooves.[4] If peroxide is used, the cessation of bubbling will indicate that the grooves are clean. A caries detection agent (Seek Caries Indicator, Ultradent Products), a laser (DIAGNOdent, KaVo; Cariescan), or a high-intensity light illuminator can all aid in detecting caries. A sealant should then be placed to prevent further staining. Some sealants have acetone water chasers to improve the bond to the enamel (UltraSeal, Ultradent Products).

Stains caused by leakage around restorations

Stains around restorations are usually the result of simple leaks (Figure 21.7A and B). These restorations should be replaced. Unfortunately, dentists tend to leave in amalgam and other restorations entirely too long, perhaps to satisfy the patient's desire for a "permanent restoration" or out of fear of the patient's displeasure at having to spend additional fees to replace restorations. Many patients arriving for examination have the same request: "Don't find anything." Most patients have as little desire

Table 21.1 Common Discolorations and Associated Causes

Tooth Discoloration	Associated Condition
Yellow	Aging
	Calcific metamorphosis
	Loss of vitality
	Tetracycline ingestion
	Amoxicillin syrup
	Stannous fluoride
	Imipenem for cystic fibrosis
	Amelogenesis imperfecta
Opaque	Fluorosis
	Sickle cell anemia
	Osteogenesis imperfecta
White	Fluorosis
	Chronic kidney failure
	Hypomineralization
Brown	Fluorosis
	Smoking
	Coffee
	Soy sauce
	Cola
	Tea
	Calcific metamorphosis
	Loss of vitality
	Chlorhexidine ingestion
	Iron
	Tetracycline ingestion
	Antitartar toothpaste
	Osteogenesis imperfecta
	Chlorhexidine glucamate (Hibitane) disinfectant
	Tannic acid
	Ochronosis
	Dental materials
Black	Occupational: glass blowers
	Betel nut chewers
	Pipe/cigar smokers
	Dental materials (pins)
	Caries
Blue	Tetracycline ingestion
	Osteogenesis imperfecta
Green	Hyperbilirubinemia
	Congenital biliary atresia
	Occupational: brass factory
	Marijuana smoking
	Nasmyth's membrane
Orange	Poor oral hygiene
	Chromic acid fumes
	Chromogenic bacteria
Red	Internal resorption
	Congenital erythropoietic porphyria
	Periapical granuloma in lepromatous leprosy
	Death
Gray	Tetracycline ingestion for cystic fibrosis
	Minocycline for acne in adults
	Dentinogenesis imperfecta
	Amalgam restorations
	Cyclosporine

to spend money for the replacement of dental restorations as they do to maintain cars, appliances, and other parts of their bodies (Figure 21.8).

Always make the patient aware of the limited life of restorations. Phillips has said, "leakage causes as much pain and pulpal inflammation as do the materials themselves."[5] Therefore, leakage should be avoided if at all possible, and if it occurs, the restorations must be replaced. In general, dentistry needs to change its philosophy and provide patients with functional esthetic restorations and be realistic when it comes to replacement.

One major advantage of composite resin restorations is the ability to easily see future microleakage. The brown stain signifies beginning microleakage that can be easily refinished or be treated with air abrasion and resealed with flowable or conventional composite resin restoration to extend the life of the original composite (Figure 21.9A–D).

Extrinsic stains

Extrinsic discoloration occurs after the completion of the fully eruption of a tooth and is defined as stains located on the outer surface of the tooth structure and caused by topical or extrinsic agents.

Nathoo classification and causes

The Nathoo classification system of extrinsic dental stain describes three categories as follows:[6]

- **Nathoo type 1 (N1):** N1-type colored material (chromogen) binds to the tooth surface. The color of the chromogen is similar to that of dental stains caused by tea, coffee, wine, chromogenic bacteria, and metals (Figure 21.10A–F).
- **Nathoo type 2 (N2):** N2-type colored material changes color after binding to the tooth. The stains actually are N1-type food stains that darken with time (Figure 21.10G).
- **Nathoo type 3 (N3):** N3-type colorless material or prechromogen binds to the tooth and undergoes a chemical reaction to cause a stain. N3-type stains are caused by carbohydrate-rich foods (e.g., apples, potatoes), stannous fluoride, and chlorhexidine (Figure 21.11A and B).

Certain factors predispose children and adults to extrinsic stains, including enamel defects, salivary dysfunction, and poor oral hygiene.[7] Microscopic pits, fissures, and defects in the outer surface of the enamel are susceptible to the accumulation of stain-producing food, beverages, tobacco, and other topical agents.

Since saliva plays a major role in the physical removal of food debris and dental plaque from the outer and interproximal tooth surfaces, diminished salivary output contributes to extrinsic discoloration. Decreased output may be caused by local disease (e.g., salivary obstructions and infections), systemic disease (e.g., Sjögren syndrome), head and neck radiation therapy for cancer, chemotherapy, and multiple medications (e.g., anticholinergics, antihypertensives, antipsychotics, antihistamines).

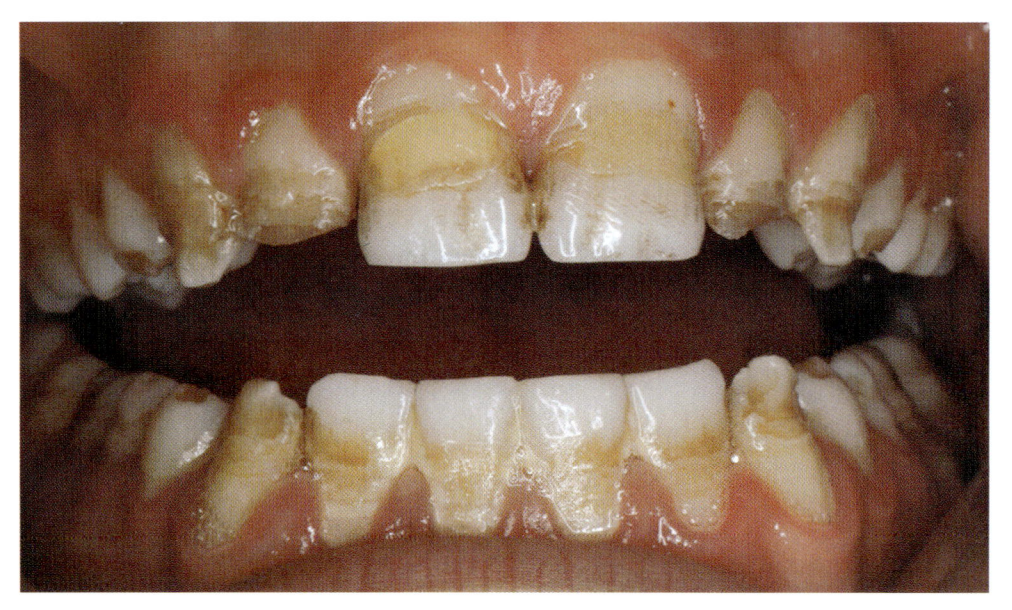

Figure 21.2 (A) An example of severe extrinsic stains, including discolored restorations.

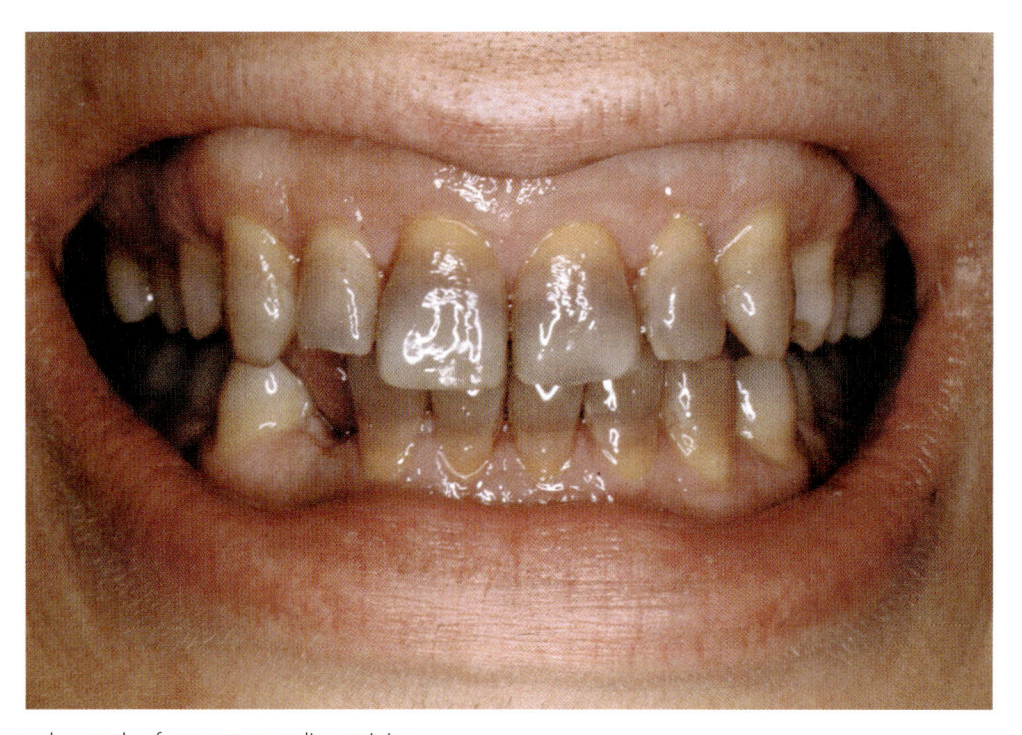

Figure 21.2 (B) A good example of severe tetracycline staining.

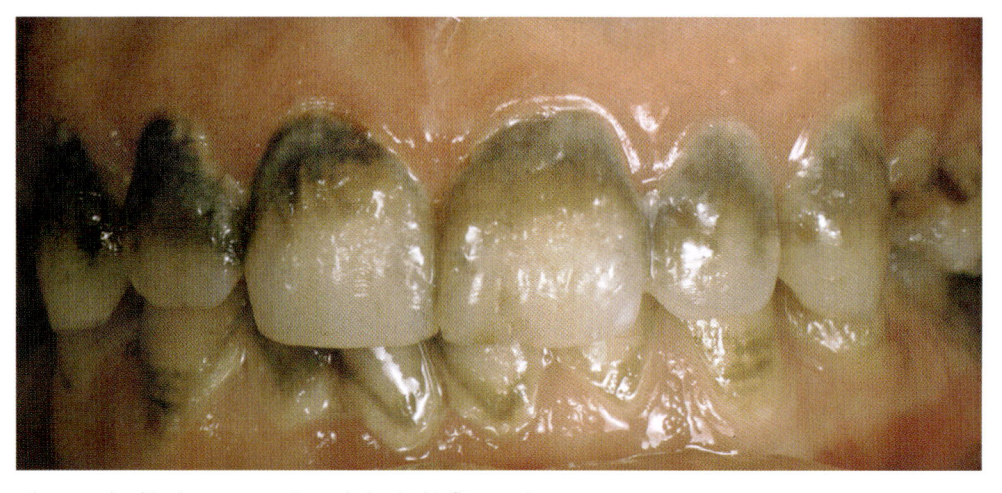

Figure 21.3 Total neglect resulted in the green stain and gingival inflammation.

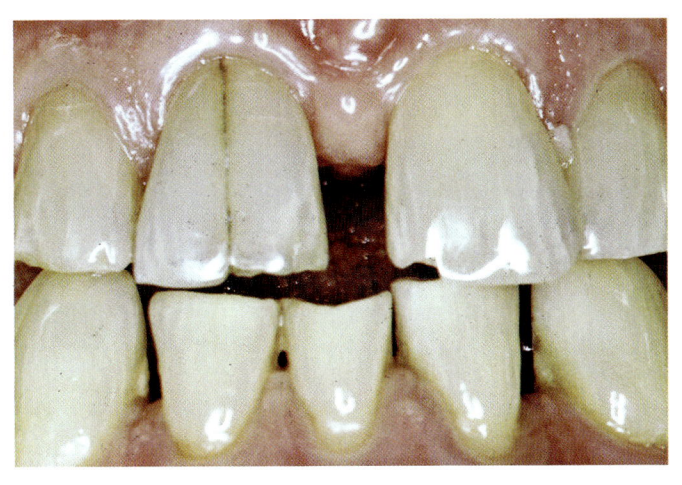

Figure 21.4 Staining can occur in tooth defects such as the vertical crack line on the central incisor, which can be difficult and almost impossible to remove by just polishing.

Table 21.2 Clinical Appearance and Causes of Discoloration

Clinical Presentation	Consideration
Single dark tooth (radiograph needed for diagnosis of pathology)	Vital: blood-borne pigments from trauma, calcific metamorphosis, internal resorption Nonvital: blood stains during endodontic therapy, remaining pulp material in chamber, restoration type (amalgam) or leaking, internal resorption
Generalized discoloration of all of the teeth	From smoking (extrinsic or intrinsic), chromogenic foods, drugs (tetracycline), diseases, aging, or genetically inherited
Localized discoloration to one tooth	White spots: surface or subsurface fluorosis, white surface demineralization Brown spots: fluorosis, formation defects
Localized discoloration to one area on all of the teeth	Chromogenic foods, chlorhexidine, smoking (extrinsic), often associated with plaque and poor oral hygiene
Discoloration associated with a restoration	Amalgam: show-through because of thin enamel, stained dentin Composite: staining of margins, staining beyond margins, complete discoloration of restoration
Discoloration associated with caries	Aproximal and occlusal stained additionally by food or saliva
Tooth defects: pitted, poorly formed	Facial, lingual, or incisal defects from fever or trauma during development, genetics (peg laterals or deep grooves)
Translucency: dark incisal	Finger test on lingual to determine translucency; may appear darker with bleaching due to loss of further color

The most common cause of extrinsic stains is poor oral hygiene.[7] The inability to remove stain-producing materials and/or the use of dentifrices with inadequate cleaning and polishing actions cause discolorations.

Table 21.3 Treatment Options for Stained Teeth

Treatment Options	Intrinsic	Extrinsic
Prophylaxis		✓
Air polisher		✓
Bleaching external with 10% or more CP	✓	✓
Bleaching external with 35% HP	✓	
Bleaching internal with 10% CP	✓	
Bleaching internal with 35% HP	✓	
Sealant or preventive resin	✓	
Macroabrasion: handpiece, burs, disks		✓
Microabrasion: rubber dam and acid		✓
Resurface and seal restoration		✓
Replace restoration	✓	✓
Replace portion of restoration (composite to mask over amalgam)	✓	✓
Veneer (partial or complete, composite or ceramic)	✓	
Crown (PFM, porcelain butt, all ceramic)	✓	

CP, carbamide peroxide; HP, hydrogen peroxide; PFM, porcelain fused to metal.

Extrinsic stains can be caused by various drugs, mouthwashes, foods, and drinks. A complete list of staining agents can be found in Table 21.2. Extrinsic discoloration was further classified as direct and indirect,[1] or metallic and nonmetallic.[1] Direct or nonmetallic staining occurs when the stain from a chemical compound gets incorporated into the acquired pellicle.[1] It is often associated with chromogens found in dietary sources, such as coffee, tobacco, red wine, and chromogenic bacteria. Indirect or metallic staining occurs by the means of metal salts and cationic antiseptics that stain the tooth's surface by a chemical reaction.[1] In either case, such superficial discoloration can be removed by tooth brushing, bleaching, or professional cleaning (Figures 21.11A and B and 21.15A and B). One extrinsic stain hard to remove occurs in microcracks. These microcracks can be caused by trauma, chewing ice, or even severe tooth grinding.

Prior to diagnosis of the stain or discoloration, a complete prophylaxis should be performed to remove minor surface staining. For instance, an air polisher can be used on the posterior occlusal surfaces to help diagnose whether the grooves are stained or carious. The diagnosis of occlusal decay is better done by visual means rather than by tactile sensation with an explorer. Proponents of the visual method explain that some grooves will not "stick" but will have decay, whereas others will stick mechanically due to their surface topography but will contain no decay.

Extrinsic stains can also be caused by the use of a mouth rinse containing chlorhexidine (refer to Figure 21.11A and B). This product is often prescribed to promote gingival health. The dark stain resulting from the product's use is a major disadvantage to an otherwise very beneficial product. There is an ongoing debate in the scientific literature regarding the mechanism of stain

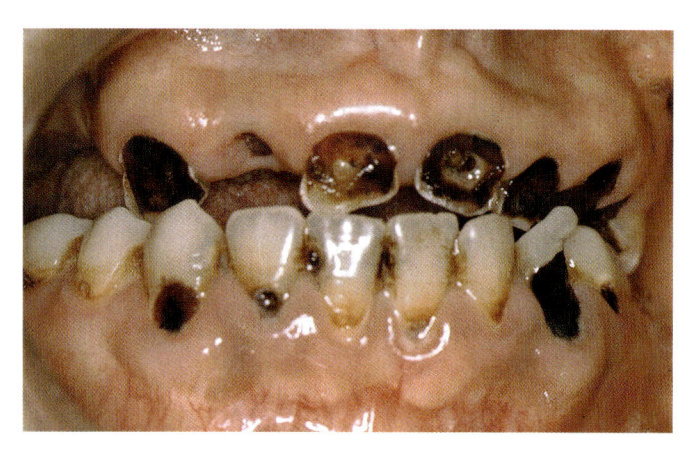

Figure 21.5 Dark brown advanced caries is the result of total neglect.

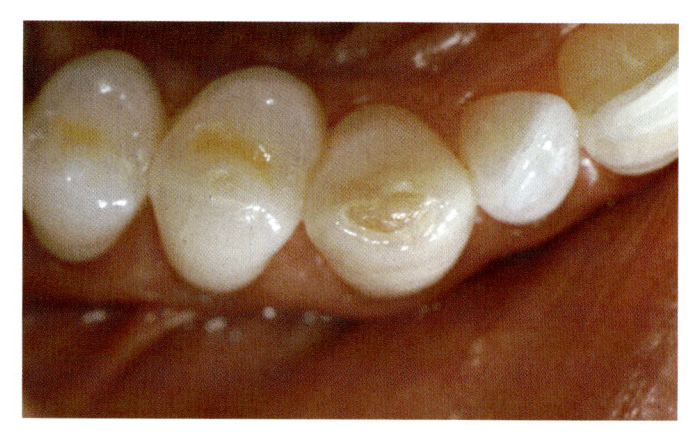

Figure 21.6 Some clear sealants that were chemically cured tend to yellow over time, becoming unesthetic.

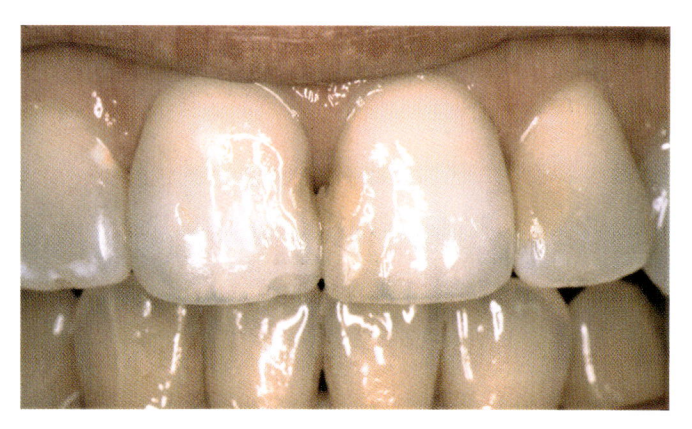

Figure 21.7 **(A)** Stains around restorations are usually a result of simple leaks around the margins of the old restoration.

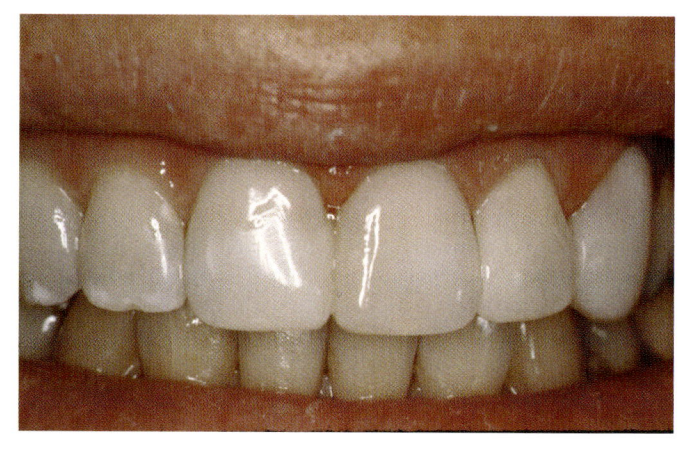

Figure 21.7 **(B)** Replacement with composite resin is usually the best solution.

formation by chlorhexidine and other mouthwashes.[1] Most in-vitro and in-vivo evidence supports the mechanism of precipitation of dietary chromogenic anions onto the areas of absorbed cations. Chlorhexidine and other antiseptics act by absorption into the enamel, and once absorbed they form complexes with other ions in the oral cavity, such as polyphenols, thus forming a stain.[4] Some patients are able to overcome this disadvantage by employing 10% carbamide peroxide in a bleaching tray periodically (Figure 21.11A and B). This approach is possible only if the patient is a reasonable candidate for bleaching or if their teeth are already as light as they can become. Otherwise, more frequent prophylaxis is required for esthetics.

Types of stains

Green stain

Green stain is most often found in children, in association with remnants of Nasmyth's membrane, the primary dental cuticle. It ranges in color from light- or yellowish-green to very dark green (Figure 21.12). It is most frequently seen on the cervical one-third to one-half of the labial surfaces of the maxillary incisors; however, it may cover the entire labial surface of the teeth involved. Green stain is composed of inorganic elements as well as decomposed hemoglobin and chromogenic bacteria and fungi; it is associated with poor oral hygiene. As the epithelial tags are often attached to surface irregularities in the enamel, the stain is quite tenacious and can be removed only with some difficulty by scaling and polishing. If left untreated, the remnants of the dental cuticle and the adherent stain will be abraded from the surface by frictional forces of mastication and muscle movement.

Orange stain

Orange stain appears as a thin, brick-red, orange, or yellow line on the cervical third of the teeth involved, usually the incisors (Figure 21.10A and B). Although rare, it is most frequently seen in children and is thought to be caused by chromogenic bacteria. It is easily removed by prophylactic procedures, but may return. A yellow or black stain can also be caused by the ingestion of iron over time.

Black line stain

Also known as black or brown stain, black line stain is a continuous thin band along the free gingival margin on the enamel surface that follows the crestal contour of the tooth on the lingual and proximal surfaces. It is seen in patients of all ages and has some predilection for female patients. The cause is thought to be chromogenic bacteria, coupled with the patient's natural tendency to form a mucinous plaque, for which the bacteria haven an affinity. Tobacco use and poor oral hygiene are not blamed for staining of this sort. However, the stain is more extensive if home care is inadequate. Scaling will remove the stain, but it tends to recur.

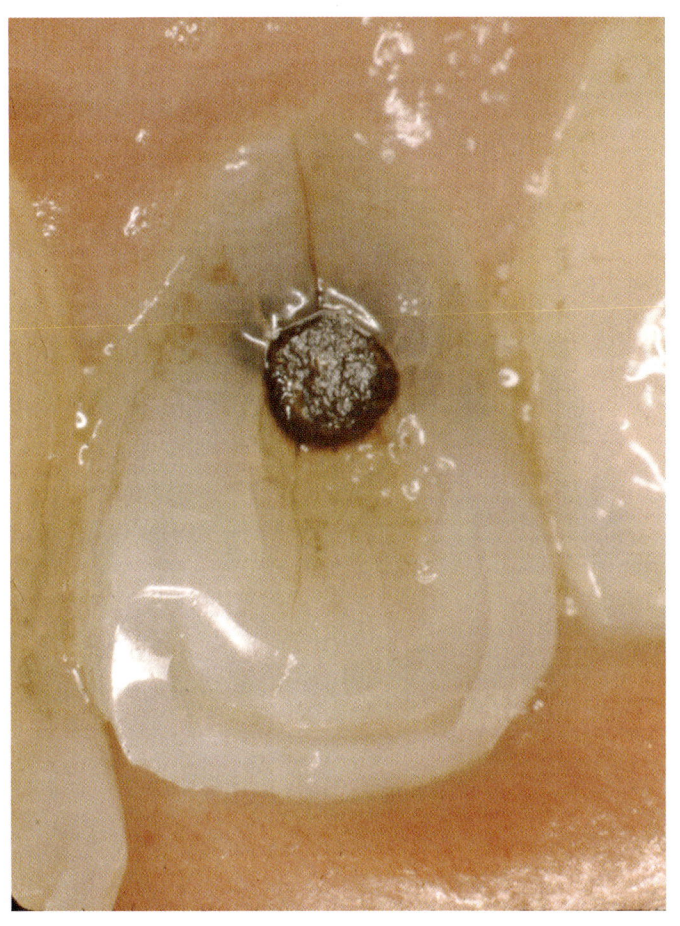

Figure 21.8 Too many patients leave their old amalgam restorations too long. Although the original restoration was done to protect the tooth, it now serves as the source of decay and microcracks.

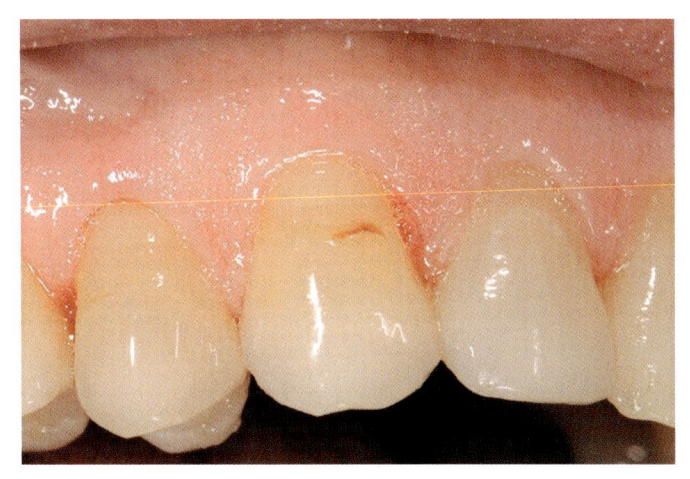

Figure 21.9 (A) The brown stain around this composite restoration is evidence of microleakage.

Tobacco stain

Discolorations are seen as a yellowish-brown to black diffuse plaque along the cervical one-third to one-half of the teeth, mainly on the lingual surfaces. It may also be deposited in the pits and fissures of the occlusal, facial, and lingual surfaces. It can be removed by scaling and polishing. Heavy deposits, especially from chewing tobacco, may penetrate the enamel surface and become intrinsic. Patients who smoke a great deal and tend to accumulate stain should be told to use the more abrasive tooth powders or pastes. Figure 21.10C shows permanent staining due to dipping snuff for 15 years. Discoloration in a 68-year-old man due to cigar smoke is shown in Figure 21.13.

Food stain

Certain foods can cause extrinsic staining. Developmental grooves, pits and fissures, and other acquired enamel defects can harbor dark stains. Patients who drink excessive amounts of coffee (Figure 21.14A and B) or tea often have stained teeth.

Metal stains

Metallic dusts from various industries or metals used in compounding medications tend to impart characteristic color to dental plaque. Iron yields a brown to greenish brown color; copper or brass yields green or bluish-green; nickel yields green; and cadmium yields yellow or golden brown. Unless the stain penetrates the enamel surface and becomes intrinsic, it can be removed by scaling or polishing.

Amalgam stain

One of the most common causes of stained teeth is amalgam restorations. There are two ways an amalgam may impart a stained appearance to the tooth: (1) show through and (2) penetration of corrosion products. Correct preparation and an opaque base or liner can prevent these.

If the cavity preparation necessitates leaving a thin labial or proximal wall supported by little dentin, the darkness of the amalgam metal may show through the relatively translucent

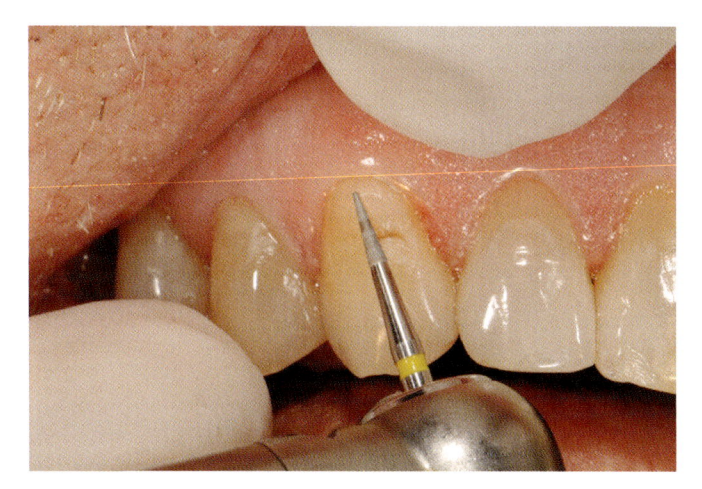

Figure 21.9 (B) The overlay technique makes it easy to refinish areas where stain later occurs either using a 30 blade carbide or 15 μm diamond (DET6EF Brasseler, USA).

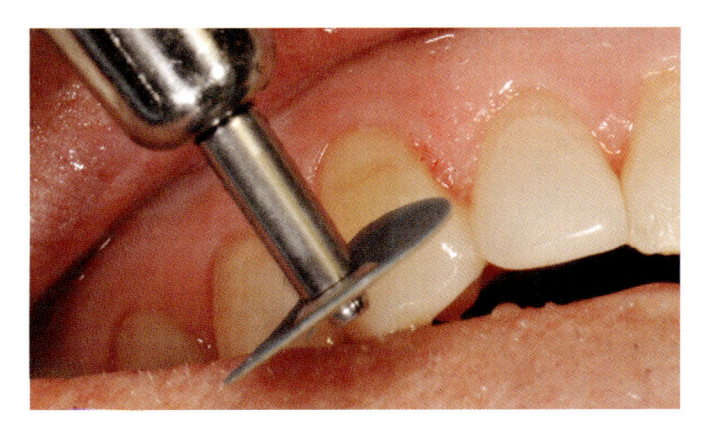

Figure 21.9 (C) Final polish can be with discs or impregnated cups or points.

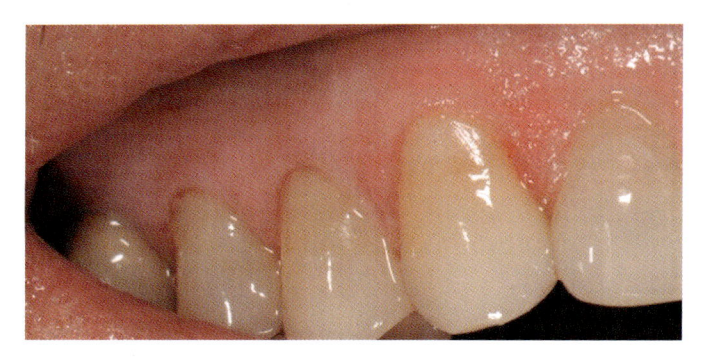

Figure 21.9 (D) The final result shows how the restoration can achieve years more life due to the ability to continue repolishing or repair as needed.

enamel. This may be unavoidable, owing to the extent of decay, but the possible consequences should be recognized.

After removing an old amalgam from a tooth, you may notice that the dentin has become severely discolored and even softened.

This greenish black pigment permeating the dentin is predominately corrosion products of tin. The mechanism of discoloration is a slow diffusion of metal ions into the dentin. These ions are liberated under the influence of galvanic currents within the restoration and sulfides that presumably originate from saliva. The use of a copal resin cavity varnish will prevent this discoloration. It has been shown that the carboxylic acid groups in the varnish react with the tin corrosion compounds, thus absorbing and retaining them. Therefore, the varnish works not by forming a "membrane" impermeable to the pigments, but by reacting to impede the diffusion of tin compounds. When amalgam stains become an esthetic problem, crowning may be necessary to completely mask teeth that are broken down (Figure 21.10D and E).

Toothpastes that help maintain whiteness

Once the dental officer has removed the extrinsic stains, the patient can use a toothpaste to maintain the whiteness of the teeth. There are a number of toothpastes on the market advertised for whitening, and patients are always seeking something

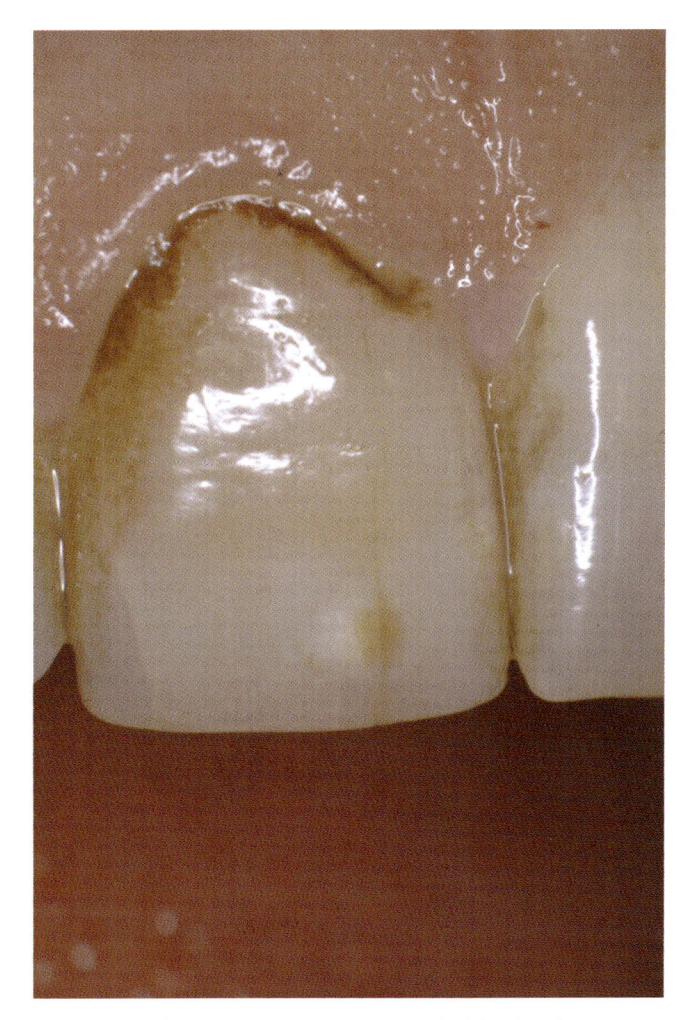

Figure 21.10 (A) Orange stain appears as a thick brick-red, orange, and yellow line on the cervical third of the teeth involved, usually the incisors, and is associated with poor oral hygiene and chromogenic foods.

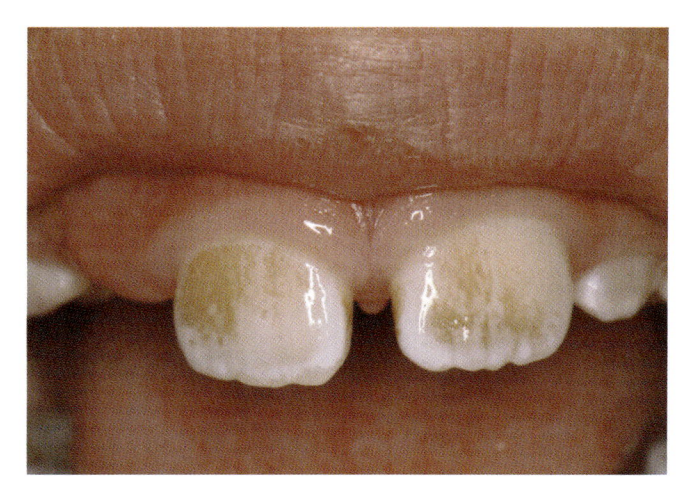

Figure 21.10 (B) Orange–brown stain may cover more of the facial area due to poor oral hygiene and ingestion of chromogenic foods.

that they can use at home to obtain whiter teeth. The US Food and Drug Administration allows any toothpaste that removes stains to make claims as a whitening toothpaste. However, the mechanism of action of the different toothpastes is generally divided into three categories:[8,9]

- **Abrasive toothpastes:** The original whitening toothpastes, commonly referred to as the "smoker's toothpaste," remove extrinsic stains by mechanical abrasion, which can make the tooth appear whiter. However, overuse of these toothpastes will eventually reduce enamel, causing the teeth to appear more yellow due to the show-through of the dentin. These toothpastes are not recommended, especially in persons who are already aggressive with their tooth brushing technique or use a hard toothbrush.

- **Chemical toothpastes:** Some toothpastes attempt to remove stains by changing the surface chemistry of the tooth so that plaque and tartar will not adhere. These types of "tartar control" toothpaste act much like Teflon on a frying pan, and if there is no plaque or tartar on the tooth, there is less substrate to be stained. One of the problems with this approach is that, in some patients, these types of toothpastes cause marked sensitivity. Another class of chemical toothpastes that have become popular since the advent of bleaching are those that contain peroxide. Many of these products also contain baking soda. Baking soda is a mild abrasive, but the peroxide acts by chemical means. The problem with the use of a peroxide dentifrice for whiter teeth is that the contact time on the tooth is too short to produce any noticeable whitening. However, a peroxide-containing toothpaste may be useful in color maintenance after the dentist has whitened the teeth.

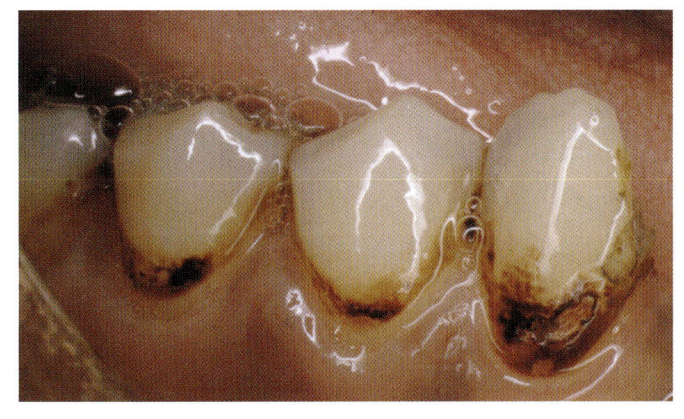

Figure 21.10 (C) Black tobacco stain from dipping snuff for 15 years.

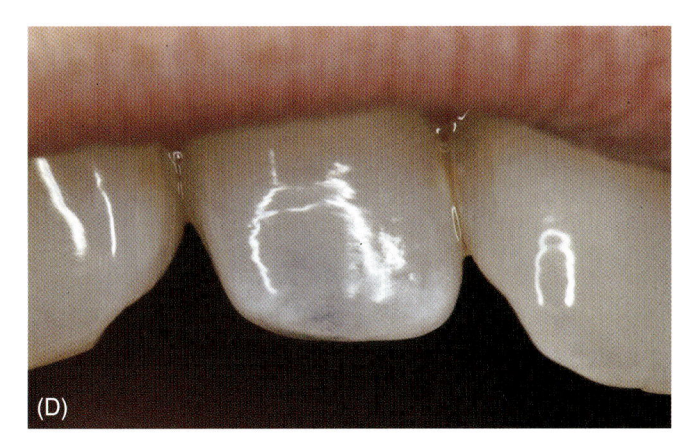

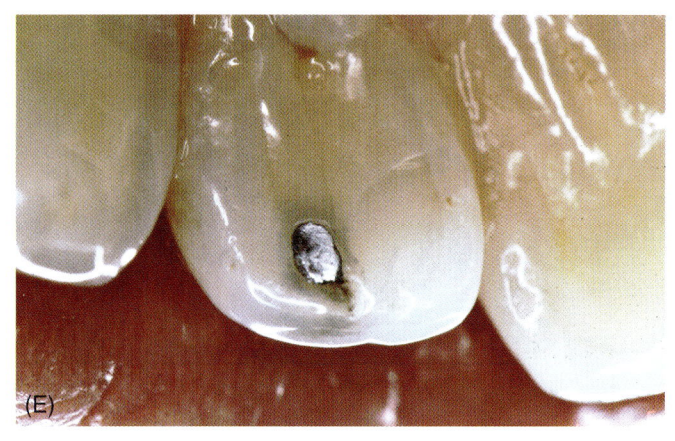

Figure 21.10 Gray stain on lateral incisor (D) is a result of an amalgam restoration on the lingual surface of the tooth (E).

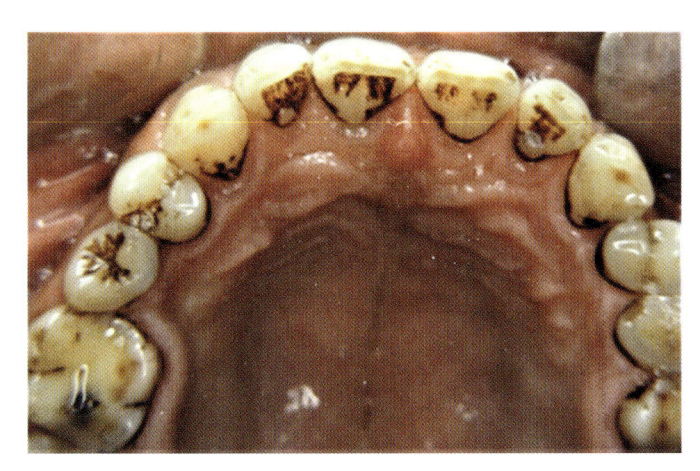

Figure 21.10 (F) Black stain from chewing betel nuts over time.

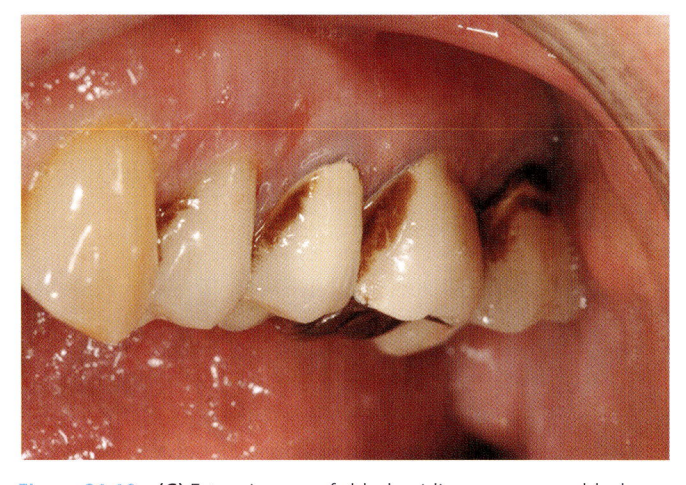

Figure 21.10 (G) Extensive use of chlorhexidine can cause a black stain on the teeth surface.

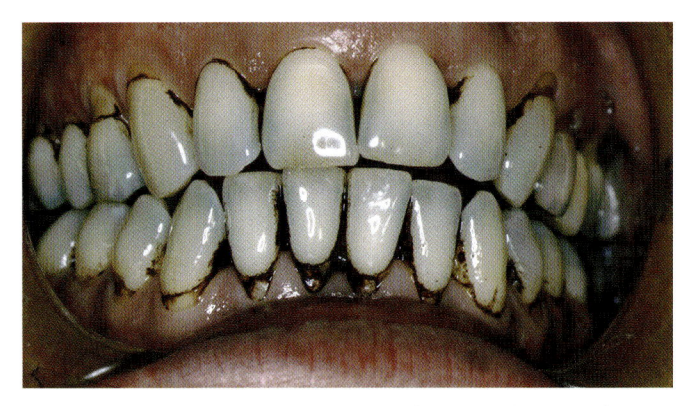

Figure 21.11 **(A)** Patient on regular use of chlorhexidine rinse for gingival treatment shows marked staining of teeth.

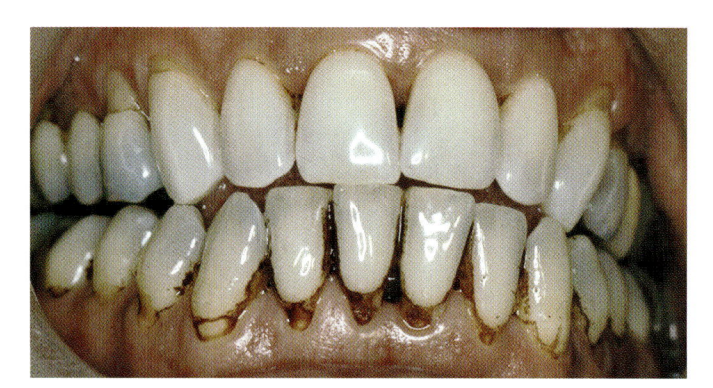

Figure 21.11 **(B)** Stains were removed, and the patient continued with chlorhexidine use while simultaneously bleaching the maxillary arch. After 3 months of treatment, there is markedly less staining on the maxillary teeth.

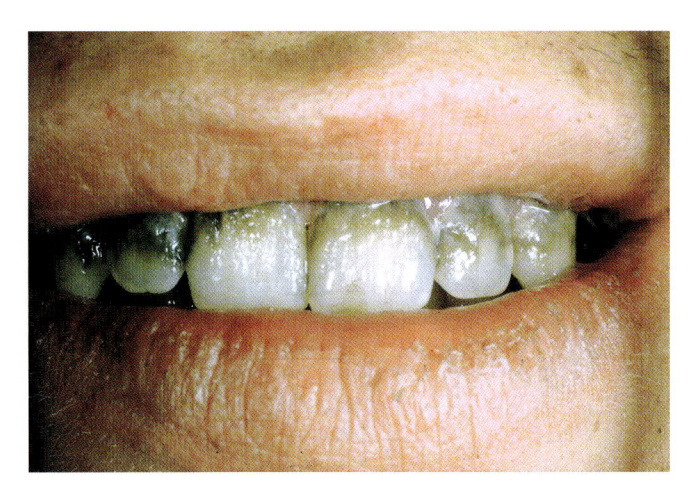

Figure 21.12 Green stain associated with poor oral hygiene and gingival inflammation.

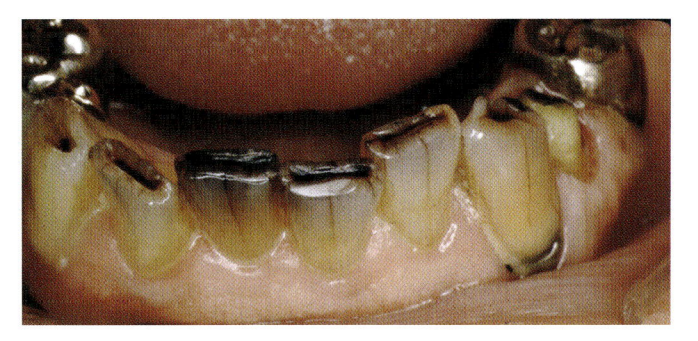

Figure 21.13 This 68-year-old man presented with black tobacco stain due to cigar smoking.

Matching color to individual patient

The color of make-up, lipstick, or clothes can also impact the perceived color of a patient's teeth. Just as certain colors of clothing make the complexion look either whiter or more tanned, so do certain redder colors of lipstick make the teeth appear whiter. In the same manner, a whiter complexion (or white makeup, as used by a circus clown) makes the teeth appear more yellow. Some patients may wish to consult with a color or makeup specialist to improve other aspects of their appearance than their teeth. Improvements in areas of the face and head will, in turn, have an impact on the color of the teeth. Although some experts feel the color of the teeth should closely match the color of the sclera (white part) of the eye for a natural appearance, Goldstein says many patients disagree. They ask for shades much whiter than the white parts of their eyes.[9–11]

Intrinsic stains

Several factors may be responsible for intrinsic or endogenous staining of the teeth. Congenital defects may result in the faulty deposition or calcification of enamel that allows the enamel rods to be penetrated by chromogenic substances. Trauma during the eruption of a developing tooth can cause hemorrhage within the pulp chamber, resulting in extravasations of blood into the dentinal tubules, with subsequent blood breakdown. Such stains would reflect the progressive degradation of the red blood cells. Systemic disease and medications can interrupt the normal sequence of dentinal and enamel formation and will be reflected in various stains. Endogenous stains can be said to be a form of vital staining. External materials can cause intrinsic stains when defects in the enamel surface allow chromogens to become embedded in the surface irregularities.

Intrinsic stains result from the change in structural composition or the thickness of hard dental tissues, which can be drug induced or associated with a health condition or injury.[1, 12] In addition, teeth defects that facilitate staining can be acquired throughout lifetime. For instance, tooth wear thins the enamel, making it more transparent and causing dentin to show and the tooth to appear darker.[1] Gingival recession also exposes dentine,

- **Cosmetic toothpastes:** Most of the whitening toothpastes should be classified as a cosmetic, in that they apply something to the surface of the tooth. Most whitening toothpastes contain titanium dioxide, which is essentially a "sticky white paint." This "paint" then adheres to the cracks and crevices on the tooth and to the embrasures, giving the illusion of whiter teeth. However, cosmetic toothpastes are only temporary and do not change the inherit tooth color.

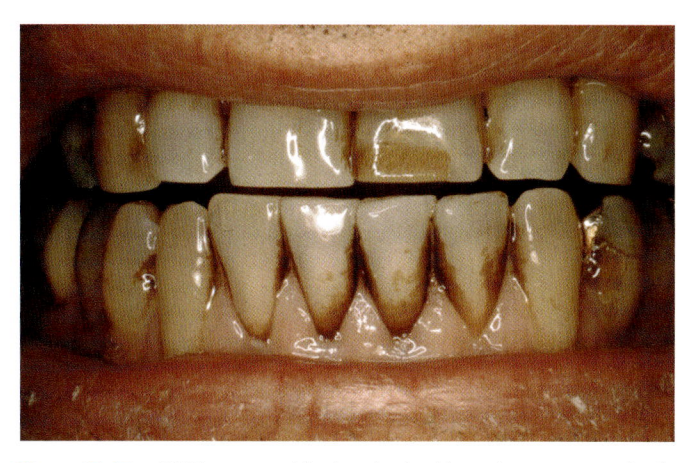

Figure 21.14 **(A)** The severe black stains in this patient are a result of drinking eight cups of coffee per day.

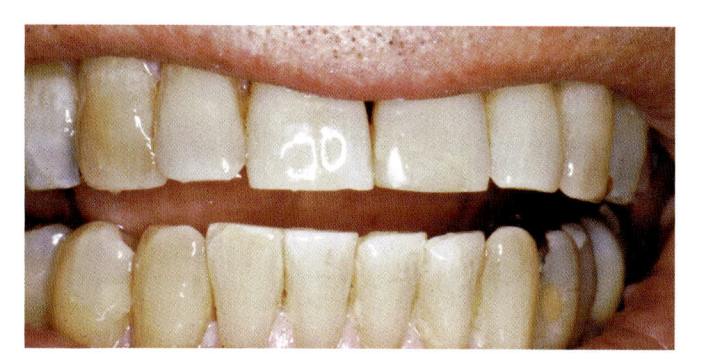

Figure 21.14 **(B)** Polishing with coarse pumice, the stains were removed and the patient was advised to severely reduce his coffee intake.

allowing the chromogens to enter the body of the tooth.[1] Some of the materials used in restorative dental treatment also have an effect on the color of teeth. For instance, root canal therapy can cause intrinsic stains if eugenol and phenolic compounds are employed. Also, amalgam restorations can cause staining of gray to black color, which is caused by the migration of tin into the tubules of dental tissues.[1] A complete list of drugs and health conditions causing intrinsic discoloration can be found in Table 21.1. These factors are well known to interfere with dental processes, causing discoloration as a consequence.[12]

Enamel hypoplasia

According to Bhaskar and coworkers,[13] enamel hypoplasia is a reduction in the thickness or amount of enamel formed and is not associated with the calcification process. It is a defect in which the tooth enamel is hard but thin and deficient in the amount. The etiology may be local, systemic, or hereditary.

In its mildest form, enamel hypoplasia is seen as horizontal grooves, or waves, on the labial surfaces of affected teeth. As it progresses, the grooves increase in depth, and there is often pitting and discoloration. Hypoplastic teeth may be grossly deformed. Hypoplasia is associated with systemic diseases that occur at the time of tooth development, affecting the teeth bilaterally and symmetrically. The incisors, cuspids, and first molars are most frequently involved. The regions of the teeth usually affected are the incisal and middle thirds of the central incisors, the incisal one-third of the lateral incisors, the tips of the cuspids, and the occlusal one-third of the first molars (Figure 21.15). When groups of teeth are affected, the hypoplasia can be attributed to severe and prolonged debilitating disease, chronic metabolic and/or endocrine abnormalities, or prolonged antibiotic therapy. However, if isolated teeth are affected, irradiation, trauma, or infection is usually the cause. Cosmetic contouring, microabrasion, bonding resins, veneering, or crowning can be used to treat hypoplastic defects.

Amelogenesis imperfecta

This is a form of enamel hypoplasia or agenesis, which is a heterogeneous genetic disorder that is characterized by defective enamel formation. It is inherited as an autosomal dominant, autosomal

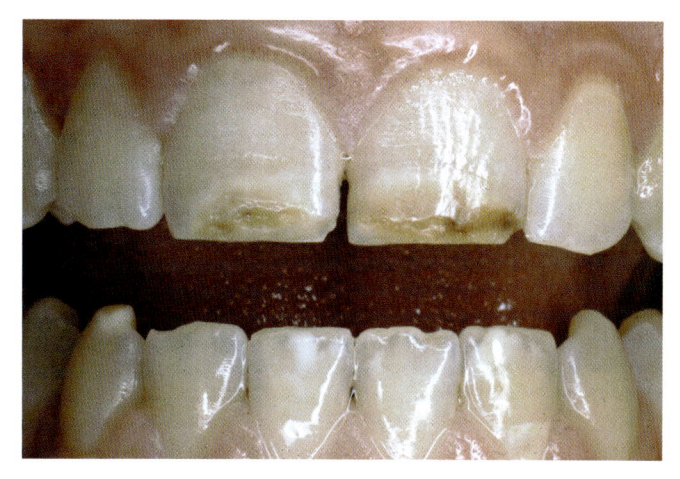

Figure 21.15 In enamel hypoplasia, the incisal and middle thirds of the central incisors are affected most frequently.

recessive, and X-linked disorder in which both the baby teeth and permanent teeth are affected. This developmental disorder causes the teeth to be covered with a thin, soft, abnormally formed enamel that appears yellowish brown and is easily damaged. The appearance may be similar to that shown in Figure 21.16. If the patient feels an esthetic need for treatment, either acid-etch bonding to the labial surface or full crowing can be done. Bleaching is difficult because the dentinal layer shows through, and it is usually painful because of the thinness of enamel.

Enamel hypocalcification

A condition of diminished calcification of the enamel, which is not associated with enamel thickness. It can occur locally as a white spot (Figure 21.17A and B) or systemically on several teeth (Figure 21.18A–D). Treatment can be cosmetic contouring, if the surface layer is not too deep, microabrasion, bonding, or porcelain veneers.

Dental fluorosis

Mottled enamel may be a developmental defect caused by the ingestion (during the period of enamel calcification) of water or foods containing excessive amounts of fluorine. The concentration of fluorine is believed to cause a metabolic alteration in the ameloblasts during enamel formation, which results in a defective matrix and improper calcification.[14] Fluorosis is classified as mild, moderate, or severe, depending on the amount of fluorides ingested during amelogenesis. Mild fluorosis is seen as flat gray or white flecks on the enamel surface. Most of all, the enamel surface is dull, unglazed, or chalky white in moderate fluorosis; there may also be pitting, with or without stains. Severe fluorosis causes marked tooth deformity; abnormally shaped crowns that show severe pitting and staining are also seen. Enamel opacities due to fluoride ingestion are poorly demarcated, and at the time of the eruption of affected teeth these opacities are not stained. In contrast, non-fluoride opacities are usually round or oval and well demarcated in the center of the enamel surface. Treatment usually consists of a series of bleaching treatments (see Chapter 11), composite resin bonding, porcelain veneers, and even crowning at times (Figure 21.19A, B and C).

Dentinogenesis imperfecta

This is a genetic disorder that is characterized by defective dentin, resulting in opalescent teeth. Like amelogenesis imperfecta, dentinogenesis imperfecta is dominant and not sex linked in which both the baby teeth and permanent teeth can be affected.

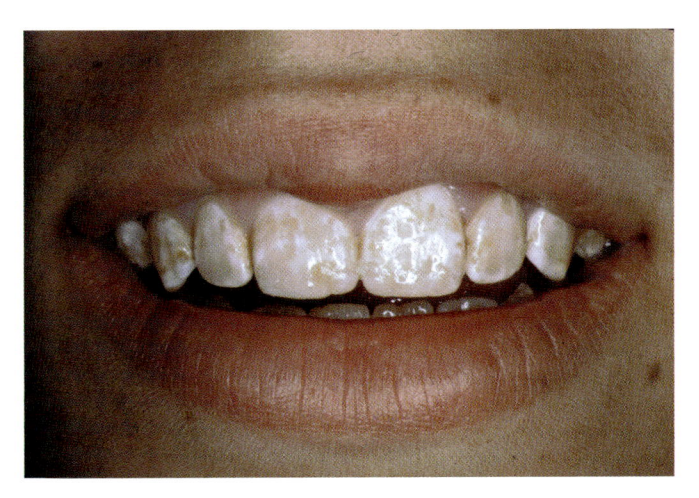

Figure 21.16 This patient presented with a case of moderate amelogenesis imperfecta in which the yellowish - brown enamel is thin, soft and easily damaged and sensitive.

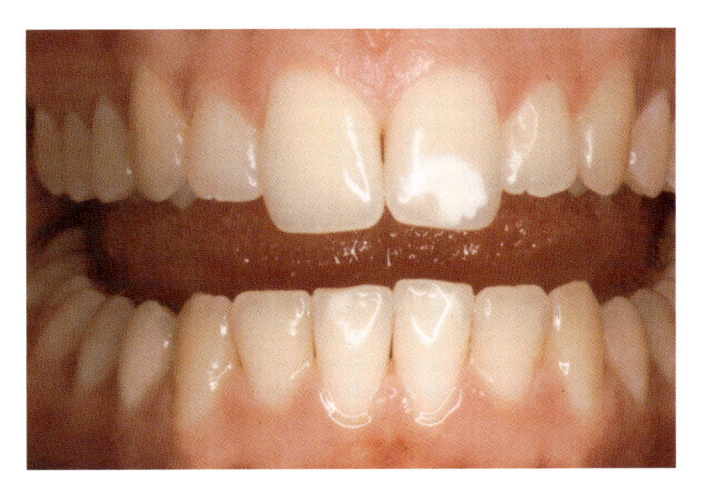

Figure 21.17 (A) This patient illustrates a good example of enamel hypocalcification on a single tooth.

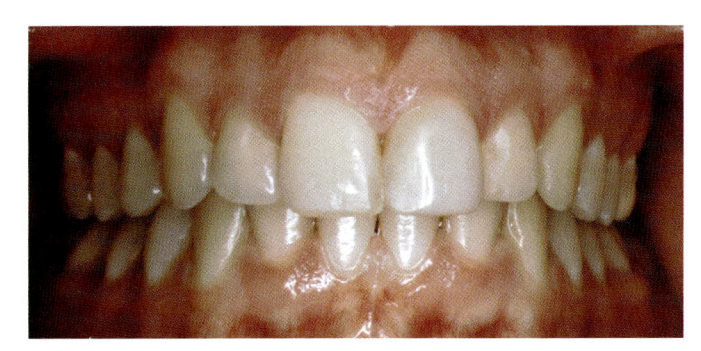

Figure 21.17 (B) Direct composite bonding was done to mask the localized white spot.

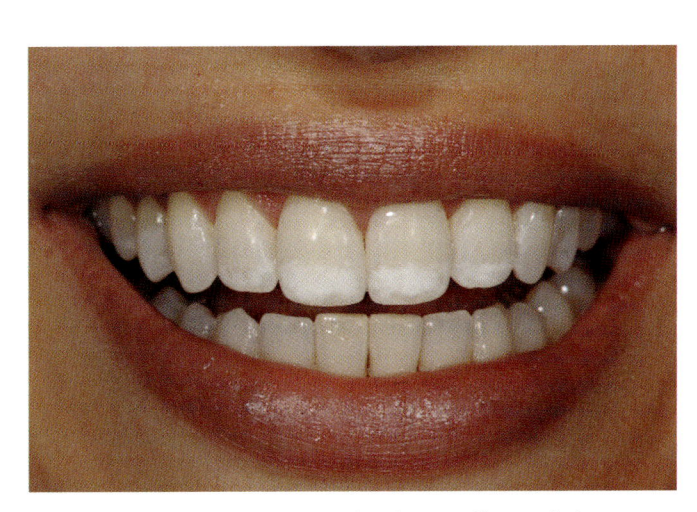

Figure 21.18 (A) Patient presented with enamel hypocalcification throughout her upper teeth.

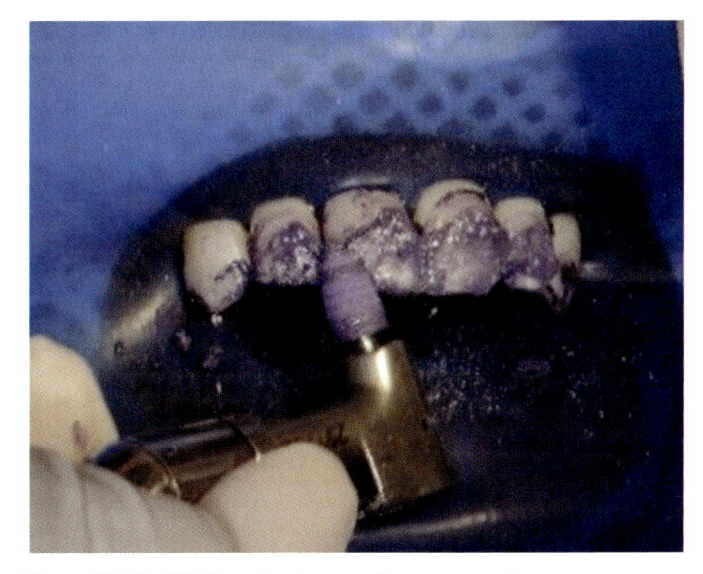

Figure 21.18 (B) Microabrasion was first attempted to remove as much of the white hypocalcification as possible.

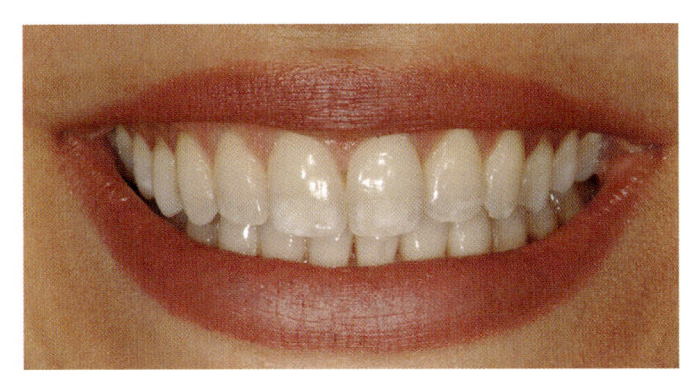

Figure 21.18 **(C)** Many of the white spots were diminished after the microabrasion.

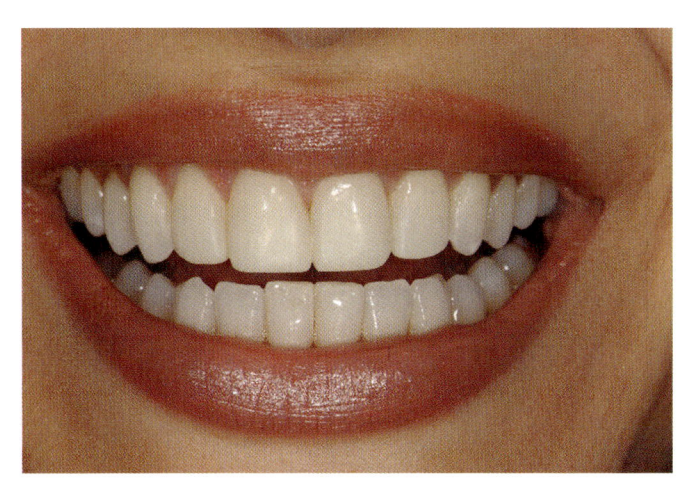

Figure 21.18 **(D)** Direct composite bonding masked the remainder of the white spots to produce a better-looking smile.

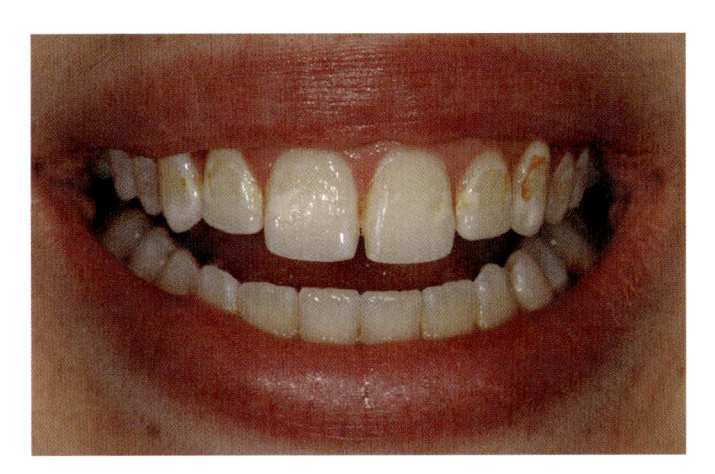

Figure 21.19 **(A)** This patient was embarrassed to smile due to her fluorosis staining.

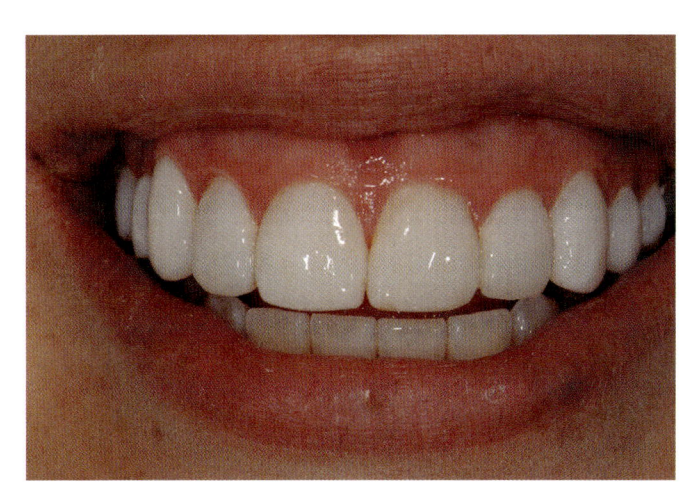

Figure 21.19 **(B)** Composite resin bonding was selected to mask the stain and improve her smile.

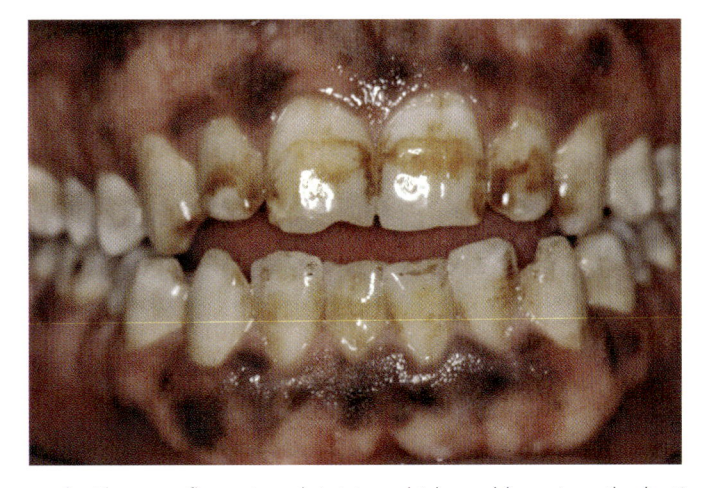

Figure 21.19 **(C)** This man was diagnosed with severe fluorosis and staining which would require orthodontics, bleaching and possibly bonding and veneers.

The dentin is stained gray, brownish-violet, or yellowish-brown and the pulp chamber and canal are usually greatly reduced in size and are sometimes undetectable on radiographs. Severe attrition is associated with the disease (Figure 21.20). The teeth appear opalescent.

Blood-borne pigment

Pigments circulating in the blood are transmitted to the dentin from the pulp capillaries. Although rare, some of these discolorations are worth noting.

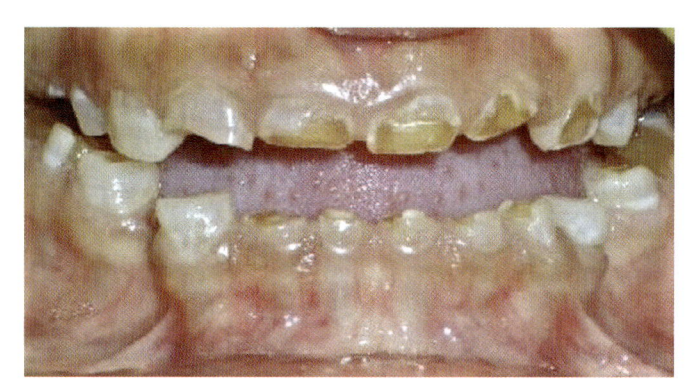

Figure 21.20 Severe attrition and yellowish-brown stained teeth are most frequently seen in dentinogenesis imperfecta.

Erythroblastosis fetalis, or hemolytic disease of newborns

This is due to incompatibility between Rh-negative red blood cells of the mother and Rh-positive ones of the fetus. Maternal antibodies destroy fetal blood cells, and the concentration of blood pigments circulating in the fetus's bloodstream increases. The primary dentition is markedly discolored—erupting teeth are bluish-black, greenish-blue, tan, or brown.

Hepatic–biliary disorders

Conditions such as intense, prolonged jaundice, cause bile pigments to be deposited into forming dental tissues, thus causing green or yellow discoloration of the teeth.

Porphyria

Abnormal metabolism or porphyrins may be congenital or secondary to infection. This disorder affects primary and secondary teeth, causing red or brown stains.

Pulp injury

Hemorrhage in the pulp chamber may allow red blood cells and blood pigments to penetrate the dentinal tubules and degenerate, causing discoloration of the crowns of teeth involved. Soon after the injury, the crown is pink; with time, the pink becomes orange, brown, or black, indicating the progressive breakdown of the blood.

Internal resorption

Chronic irritation or injury to the tooth induces a chronic granulomatous reacting in the pulp. Pressure from proliferating tissue on the dentin causes dentinal resorption in the crown or root of the affected tooth. When the resorption nears the enamel surface, a pinkish discoloration is seen.

Stains of various medications

Medicaments and materials used in dental procedures often induce staining. These include: silver amalgam, causing gray to black stain; silver nitrate, causing black or bluish-black discoloration; volatile oils, giving yellowish brown; iodine,

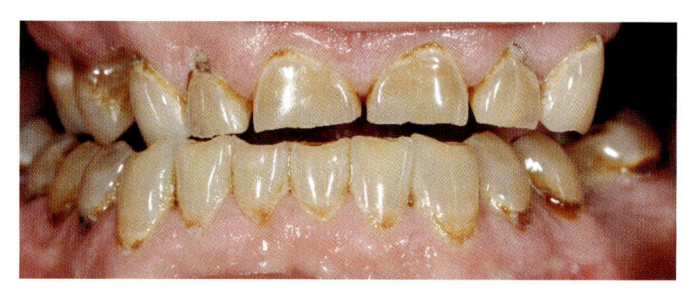

Figure 21.21 This patient illustrates a good example of tooth stains and decay associated with various medications that cause xerostomia.

leading to brown, orange, or yellow: aureomycin, causing yellow discoloration; root canal sealer containing silver, giving a black discoloration; and pins, leading to a blue-grayish stain (Figure 21.21).

Single dark teeth

A single tooth may become dark either from trauma, after completion of endodontic therapy, or from internal resorption. The first step in the treatment of this tooth is to take a radiograph to determine whether there is any periapical pathology and to pulp test the tooth for vitality.[15]

If the single dark tooth tests vital, there are two options for treatment. One option is when the patient wishes to lighten the other teeth as well. The other option is when the patient only wants to bleach the single tooth. If the patient wants to lighten all teeth, a conventional bleaching tray is fabricated, and carbamide peroxide is placed on all the teeth. When the unaffected teeth cease to lighten, treatment is continued by placing the material only on the darkened tooth until it matches the color of the other teeth.

If a single dark tooth does not test vital, the radiograph is negative for periapical pathology, and the patient has had no symptoms; the treatment can be the same as a single dark vital tooth without initiation of endodontic therapy. However, the patient should be informed that there is a chance that the tooth may need a root canal treatment should symptoms eventually occur.

Other situations for dark teeth occur after the tooth had received endodontic therapy. If the tooth has not been restored, or if the treating dentist is not certain that all of the remaining pulp material had been removed from the tooth, then some form of inside bleaching should be performed (Figure 21.22A–E).

Localized brown discoloration

Typically, a brown discoloration is associated with high fluoride ingestion.[16] The discoloration is generally localized to sporadic areas on the tooth. Usually, microabrasion is considered the primary treatment.[14] Microabrasion is the application of acid and pumice to selectively remove the enamel surface discolorations.[2] However, Nightguard vital bleaching has been shown to successfully remove brown discolorations.[17–19] It is estimated that 80% of these brown discolorations are amenable to bleaching with 10% carbamide peroxide.[20] More recent articles have shown removal of brown discoloration after 4–6 weeks of bleaching, with no return or need for additional treatment at seven years recall.[21]

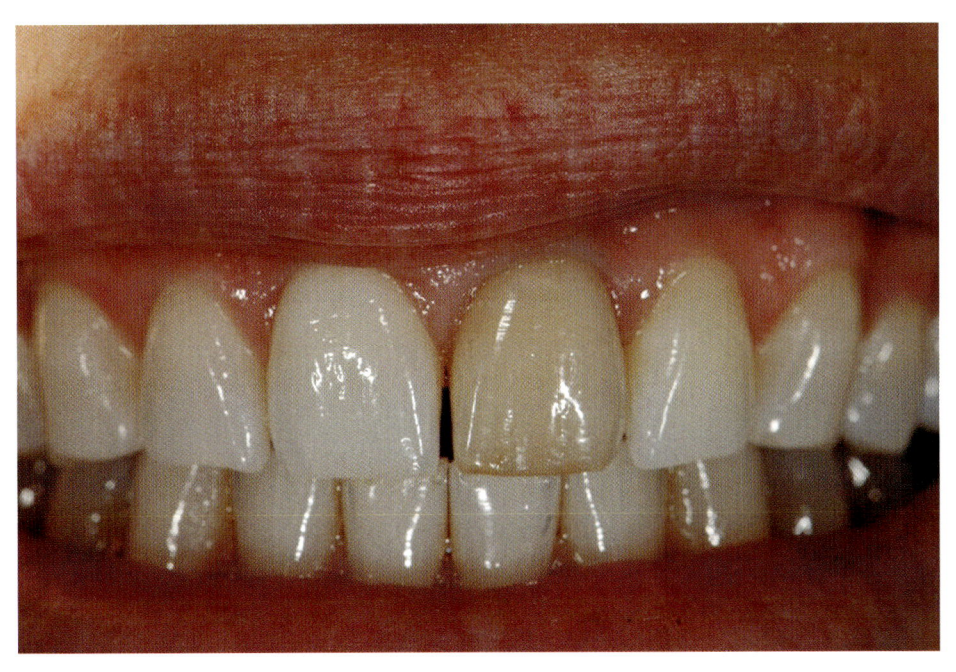

Figure 21.22 **(A)** This patient presented with a single dark tooth following endodontic treatment.

Certainly, attempting bleaching first avoids the removal of the fluoride-rich enamel layer, and microabrasion[22] or macroabrasion[23] can be attempted should bleaching not be successful.[24, 25] When time is of the utmost importance to the patient, a combination approach can be most effective (Figure 21.23A and B).

Localized white discoloration

As with brown discolorations, white discolorations are often associated with high fluoride ingestion, high fever, or other disturbances during enamel formation. Bleaching does not remove white spots and may occasionally make them lighter during treatment, but it does lighten the surrounding tooth so as to make the white spot less noticeable (Figure 21.24A and B).[26] During bleaching, the white spot may get whiter, but on termination of the bleaching, it generally turns to its original color. It is thought that these white spots are differently formed portions of enamel that respond differently to the bleaching material. Teeth with white spots undergoing bleaching often develop a "splotchy look" during the first or second week of bleaching. However, patients should be encouraged to continue through this stage, so that the darker portions of the teeth can "catch up." Often, malformed parts of enamel below the surface of the tooth contribute to this splotchy appearance. On termination of bleaching, the white spots return to their original color. Bleaching with 10% carbamide peroxide is still the first treatment of choice because it can lighten the other portions of the tooth, so that the white spot is no longer as noticeable.

Tetracycline staining

Tetracyclines lead to permanent tooth staining if ingested by an expectant mother or by a child during the developmental period of primary or secondary teeth. Tetracycline-/minocycline-induced discoloration is one of the most difficult stains to remove.

The ability of tetracycline to intrinsically stain teeth during odontogenesis has been well known for five decades.[5, 14, 27–29]

One of the side effects of tetracycline is incorporation into tissues that are calcifying at the time of their administration. They pass through the placenta and can have toxic effects on the developing fetus. Toxic effects on the developing fetus include dental discoloration, enamel hypoplasia, and a 40% depression of bone growth. They have the ability to chelate calcium ions and to be incorporated into teeth, cartilage, and bone, resulting in a discoloration of both primary and permanent dentitions.

The major factors impacting the amount of tetracycline deposition are dosage, duration of treatment, stage of tooth mineralization, activity of the mineralization process,[30] and the type of the specific drug.[1, 31] The discoloration, which is permanent, varies from yellow or gray to brown depending on the dose or the type of drug received in relation to body weight (Figure 21.25A and B). After tooth eruption and exposure to light, the fluorescent yellow discoloration gradually changes over a period of months to years to a non-fluorescent brown color.[32] The labial surfaces of yellow-stained anterior teeth will darken in time, while the palatal surfaces and buccal surfaces of posterior teeth will remain yellow.[33] The staining of the permanent teeth creates an esthetic and psychological concern for which patients may look for advice and treatment to improve their appearance.[34]

The drug diffuses into the tooth and binds irreversibly with calcium ions, forming a stable complex in the hydroxyapatite crystals located in dentin and enamel.[1, 31] In-office bleaching is a possible treatment method but is generally contraindicated due to the number of treatments required and the concurrent high fee and patient discomfort. With the advent of at-home bleaching, these tetracycline stains can be managed more easily.[35–37] Treatment times may vary from 2 months to 1 year (Figure 21.26A–C). Patients are seen monthly to replenish solutions and evaluate for continuing color change. Patients should

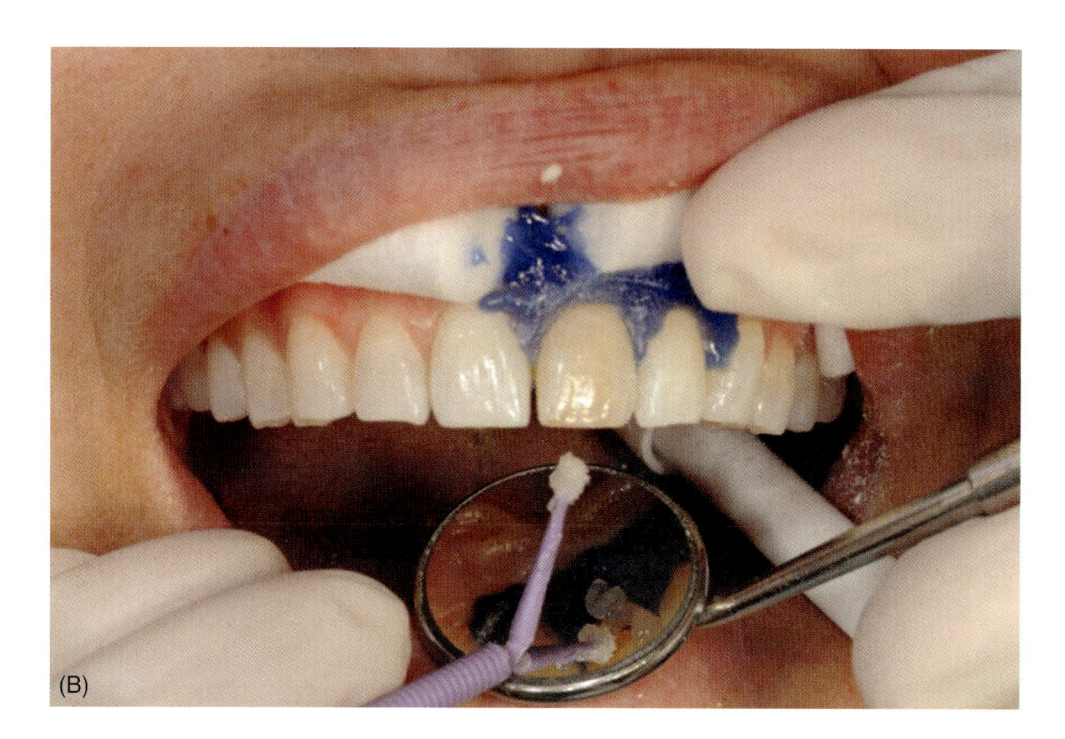

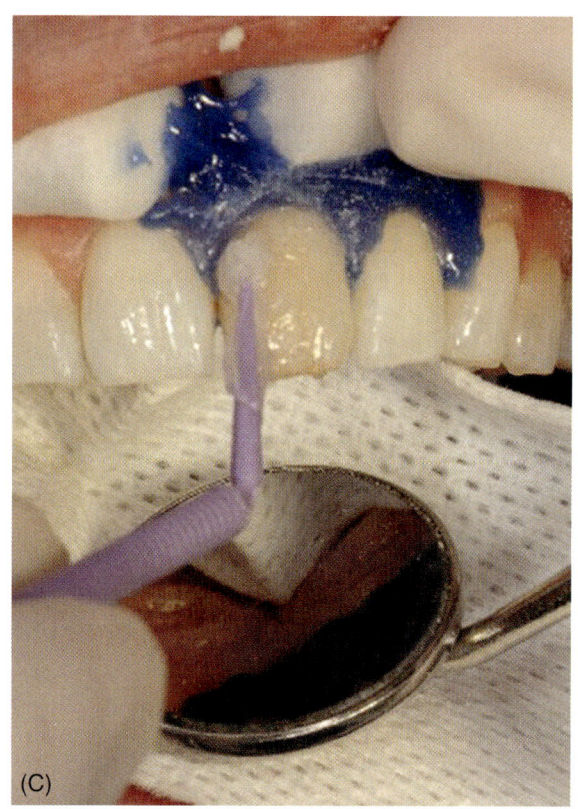

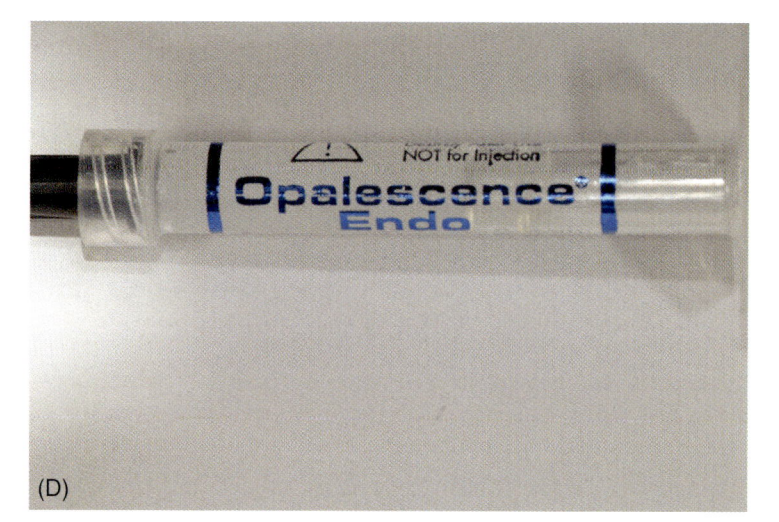

Figure 21.22 **(B–D)** An access opening was created, gutta percha sealed with glass ionomer base, and internal and external bleaching with 35% hydrogen peroxide (Opalescence Endo, Ultradent Products Inc.).

agree to a minimum of 2 months of nightly treatment before deciding to proceed to more aggressive treatment. Fees are generally the cost of a monthly office recall visit and additional material. Once lightening is observed, patients should continue treatment until a month has passed with no obvious color change.

Dark tetracycline stains located in the gingival third of the tooth or dark blue or gray stains have the least favorable prognosis. However, even in these situations, there can be some improvement. This improvement may be sufficient for a patient's esthetic demands. If not, bleaching for up to a year can be quite successful. However, compliance by the patient is necessary for success.

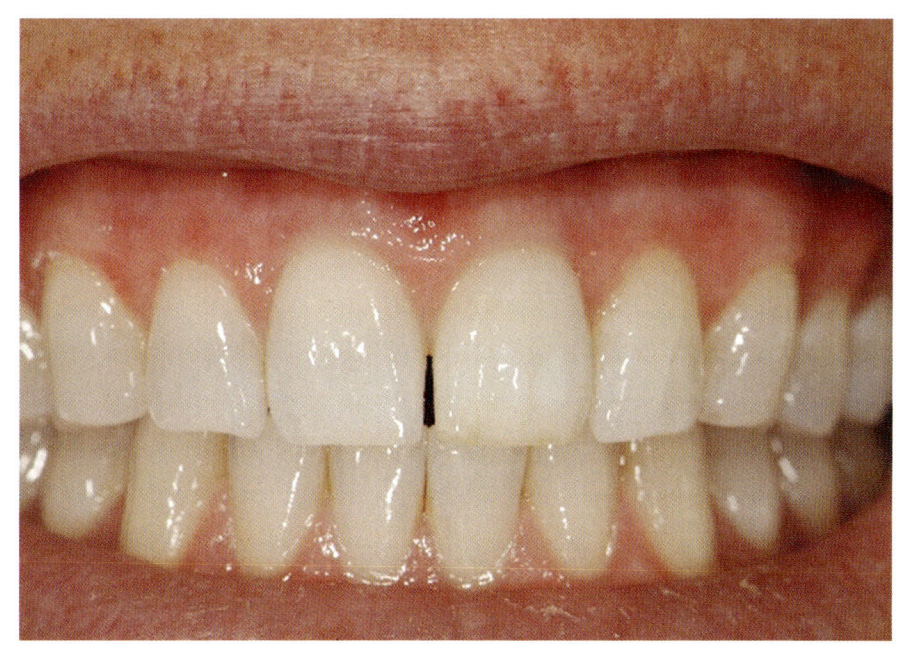

Figure 21.22 **(E)** Final result shows the matching of the single tooth to the rest of the teeth.

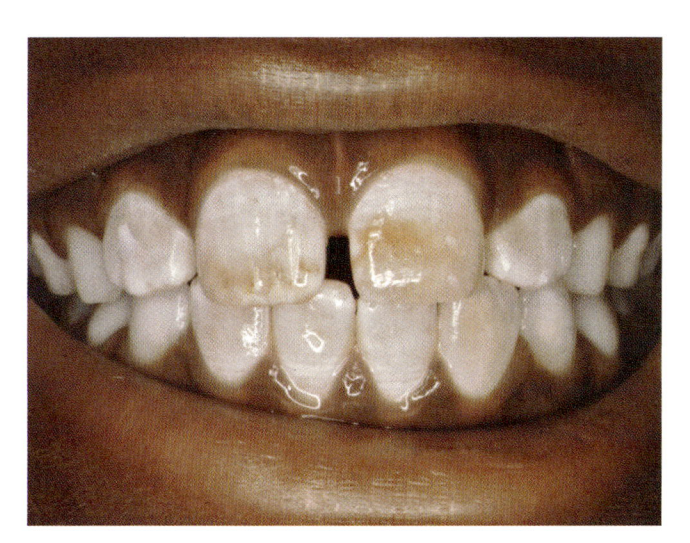

Figure 21.23 **(A)** Dark brown spots associated with high fluoride ingestion are present in this young boy.

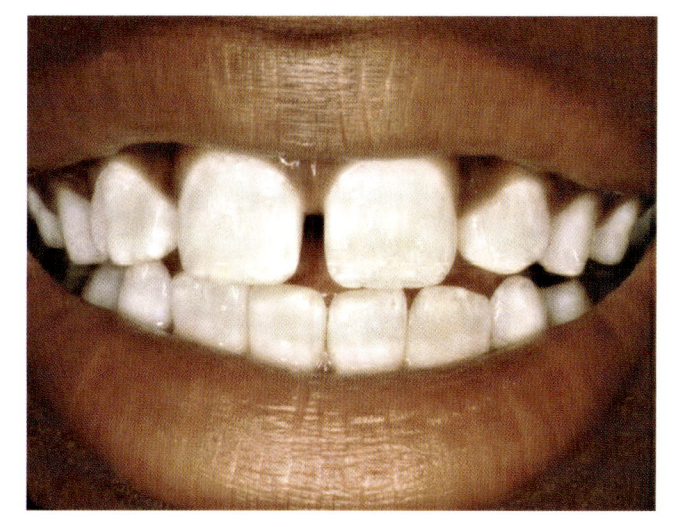

Figure 21.23 **(B)** Individual in-office bleaching was effective in eliminating the stain and producing a more pleasant smile.

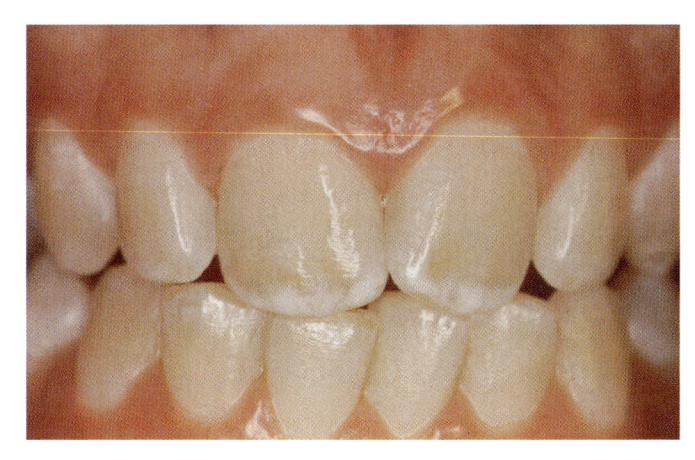

Figure 21.24 **(A)** White spots on the incisal edges are accentuated by the yellow of the teeth.

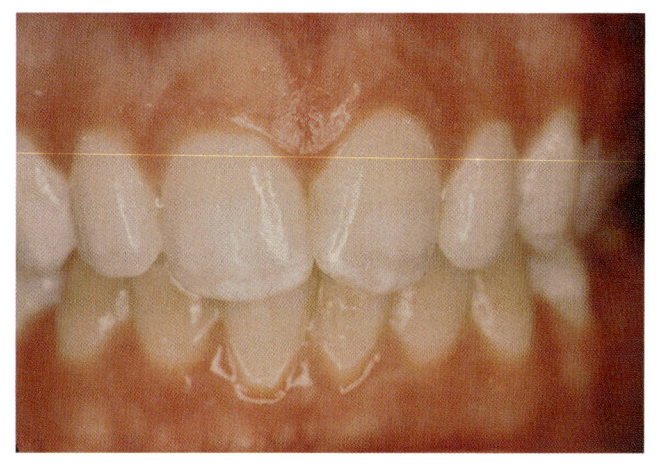

Figure 21.24 **(B)** After 5 weeks of nightly treatment with 10% carbamide peroxide, the white is less noticeable because the yellow has been removed.

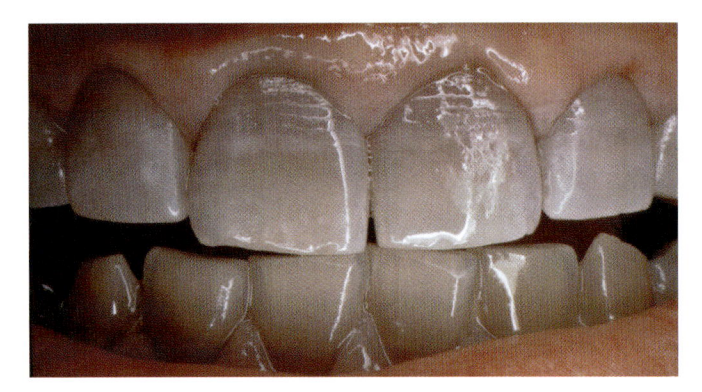

Figure 21.25 **(A)** This patient illustrates moderate tetracycline staining.

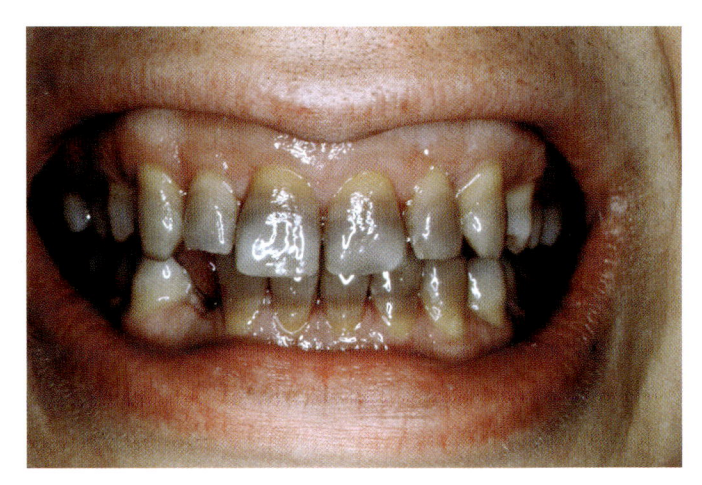

Figure 21.25 **(B)** This patient is a good example of severe tetracycline staining.

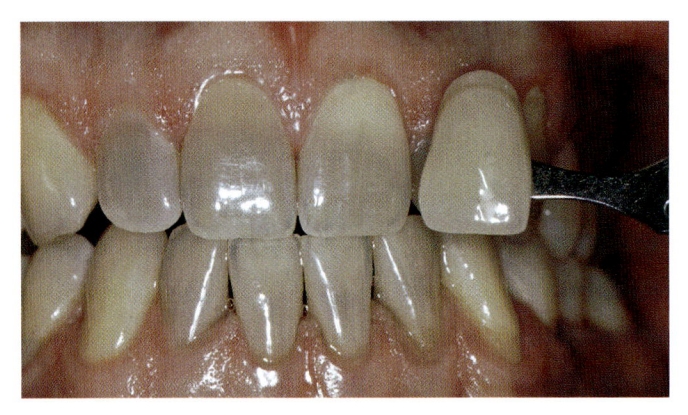

Figure 21.26 **(A)** Patient with moderately tetracycline-stained teeth is considering bleaching or veneers. Bleaching is initiated to either resolve the issue or provide a lighter base onto which the veneers can be placed.

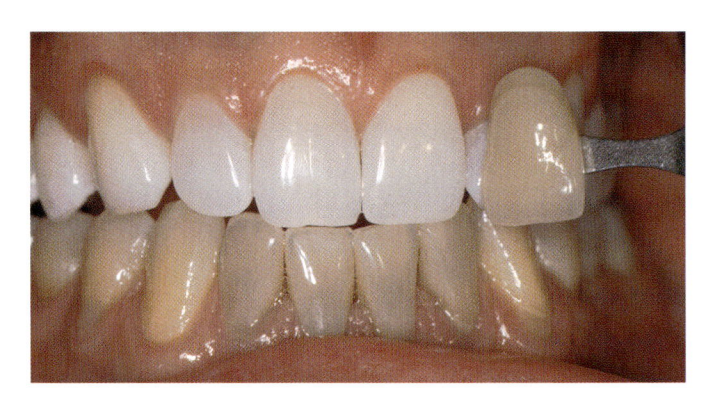

Figure 21.26 **(B)** Four months of bleaching of the maxillary arch using 10% carbamide peroxide produces a remarkable shade change.

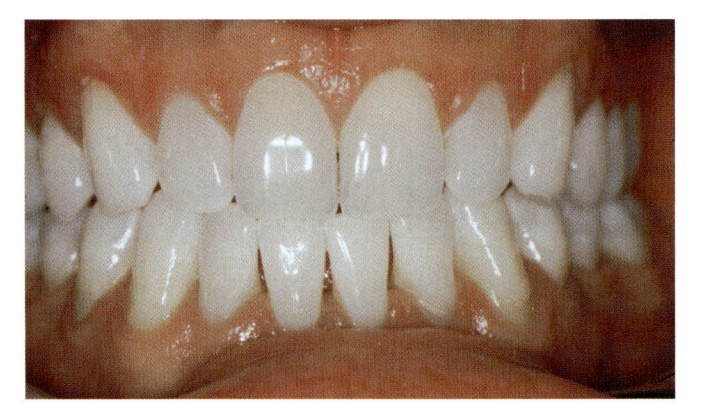

Figure 21.26 **(C)** The mandibular arch is subsequently lightened.

Patients with tetracycline staining often view the at-home bleaching regime similar to a weight loss or an exercise program. Application of the bleaching material at night becomes a regular part of their routine. There is no increase in side effects with this long-term bleaching since most side effects occur in the initial weeks of treatment. Two other therapies that are helpful in removing the spots are microabrasion and/or masking with composite resin bonding and porcelain veneers.

Treatment

Correction of defects caused by intrinsic staining depends on the amount of tooth structure affected. In mild forms of enamel hypoplasia, for example, simple procedures may be all that is necessary: superficial selective grinding and polishing of the affected surface or acid-etch and bonded composite resin restoration of the area. In more severe defects, such as systemic drug-induced discolorations and congenital defects, full crown coverage may be necessary to improve the appearance of the teeth.

Bleaching

Typically, bleaching with 20% carbamide peroxide in a custom-fitting tray easily treats discolorations due to aging, smoking, or chromogenic foods and beverages. Although these types of stains generally require only 2–6 weeks of bleaching treatment, some are more stubborn. Nicotine staining of long-term duration may require as long as 3 months of nightly treatment.[9] Tetracycline staining may take anywhere from 2 to 12 months of nightly treatment.[35] Patients must be counseled regarding realistic expectations for the outcomes of bleaching. Long-term treatment is best presented as one that is worthwhile but may not produce the desired results.[10]

Bleaching as a stepping-stone to veneers

Bleaching may not produce an acceptable result on all tetracycline-stained teeth, but it can provide the patient with a better idea of how their smile will appear with whiter teeth. Often, bleaching is the stepping-stone to veneers. Once the patient has seen what a little color change will do for their appearance, they are often more excited about completing the restorative process. Even when veneers are the ultimate goal, bleaching lightens the underlying tooth, decreasing the masking needs of restoration. If the tooth shade regresses after the placement of the veneers, the teeth can sometimes be rebleached through the lingual surfaces. However, it would be wise to use a more opaque shade of cement for the veneers.

Bleaching and other restoration procedures

Bleaching does not change the color of other restorations. In fact, existing restorations tend to appear darker as the adjacent teeth lighten. Patients should be informed of the possible need for replacement of restorations in the esthetic area should there be a color mismatch posttreatment. However, the color stability of restorations can also be a benefit to the clinician. Usually, crowns that match adjacent natural teeth are placed. Over time, the teeth may have darkened to the point where they no longer match the crowns. Rather than replace the otherwise acceptable crown with a darker shade crown, bleaching is the treatment of choice. In these instances, the patient can carefully bleach the teeth until the natural teeth return to the shade they were when the crowns were fabricated. To avoid overbleaching of the teeth, patients are instructed to apply the whitening solution for only 1–2 h a day until they see how responsive the natural teeth will be to the process. This avoids a color mismatch, where the teeth become lighter than the crowns from bleaching, which might require replacing the crowns with a lighter shade.

Tetracycline-stained teeth often require significant tooth reduction to provide the dentist and the laboratory technician an adequate space for the restorative material to mask the discoloration. Some suggest the use of an opaque resin to mask the discolorations prior to the cementation of the porcelain veneers.[12]

Lithium disilicate veneers

The masking of tetracycline staining with the use of lithium disilicate (e.max) is compared with feldspathic porcelain in Figure 21.27A, showing that masking can be achieved with less amount of tooth structure removal. However, it is still essential to take the stump shade of the prepared teeth for the ceramist to be able to visualize the amount of masking needed.

The 48-year-old man shown in Figure 21.27B presented to the office with tetracycline staining. He had a brown discoloration on his teeth, which represents a heavy ingestion of tetracycline compared with yellow or gray discolorations.

A wax-up (Figure 21.27C) was done with the ideal desired final contours of the veneers prior to prepping the teeth. Thus, additive wax-up can be done to evaluate whether veneered teeth can tolerate the additive porcelain material that would lead to

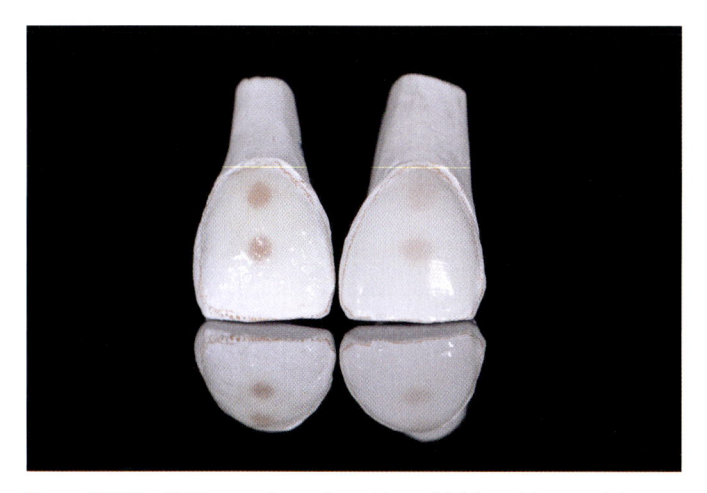

Figure 21.27 **(A)** Comparison of masking of feldspathic porcelain on the left versus lithium disilicate on the right with the same amount of porcelain thickness.

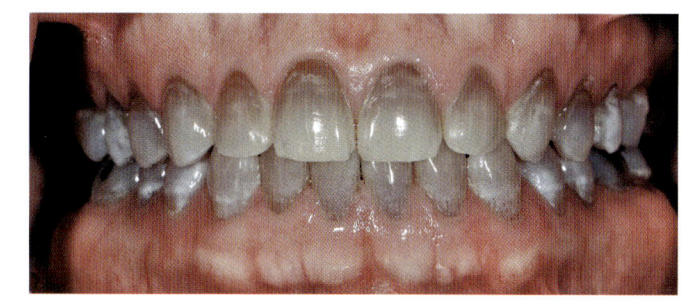

Figure 21.27 **(B)** This 48-year-old man presented to the office with tetracycline staining.

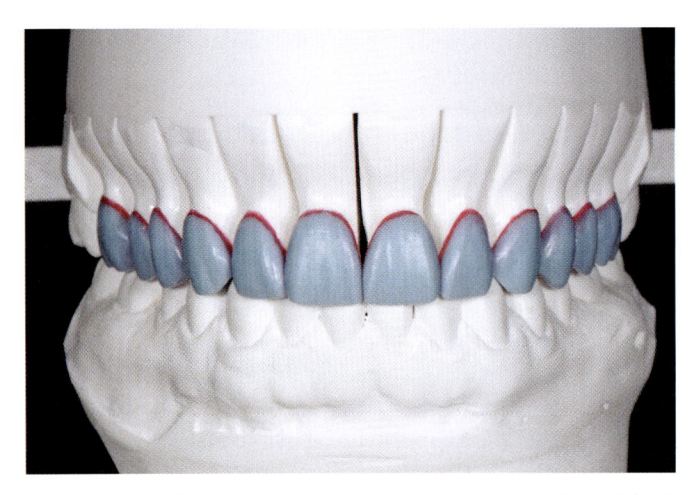

Figure 21.27 (C) A wax-up has been done with the ideal desired final contours of the veneers prior to tooth preparations.

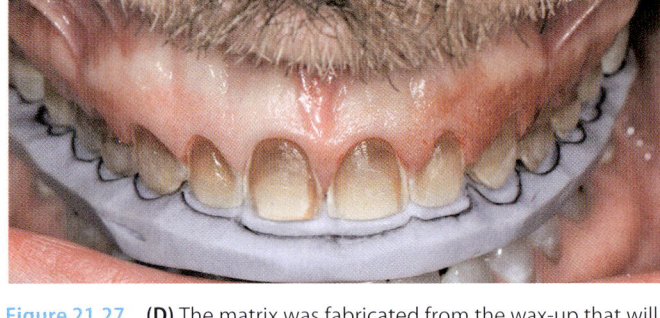

Figure 21.27 (D) The matrix was fabricated from the wax-up that will be utilized as the reduction guide at the time of the tooth preparation.

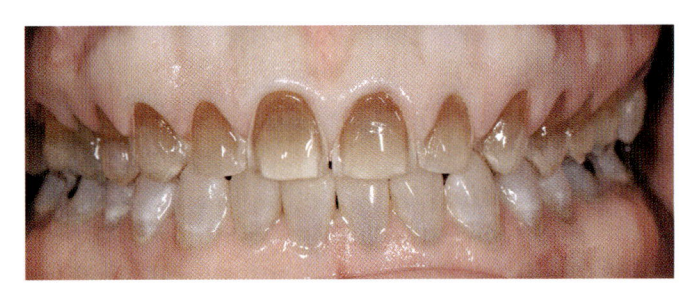

Figure 21.27 (E) The preparation of the teeth completed for the lithium disilicate veneers.

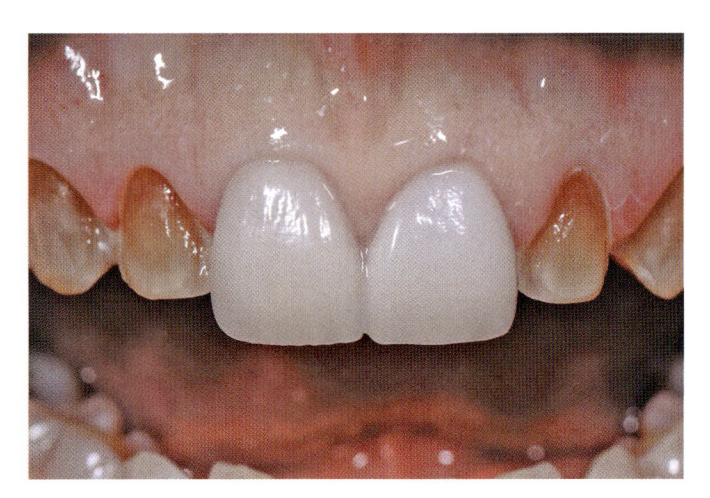

Figure 21.27 (F) The amount of masking of the tetracycline stain is portrayed with lithium disilicate veneers.

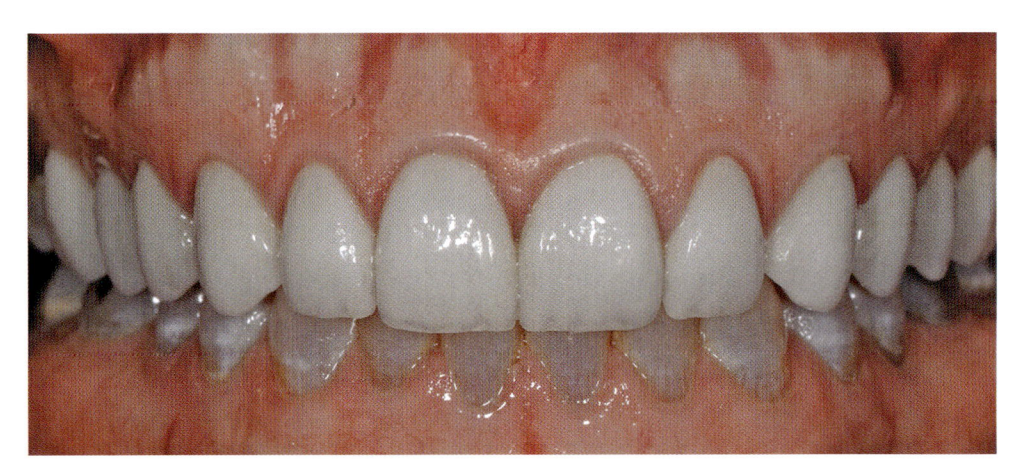

Figure 21.27 (G) The veneers were bonded with the recommended etching and bonding guidelines.

less tooth structure removal. The matrix was fabricated from the wax-up that would be utilized as the reduction guide at the time of teeth preparation (Figure 21.27D). The preparation of the teeth was completed for the lithium disilicate veneers (Figure 21.27E), the final impression was made, and the teeth were provisionalized with the direct provisional technique.

At the laboratory site, full contour wax-up was done prior to pressing the lithium disilicate porcelain. A 5% cutback was performed on the incisal edge for the layering (Figure 21.27F). The veneers were bonded with the recommended etching and bonding guidelines for lithium disilicate with the help of rubber dam isolation. (Figure 21.27G).

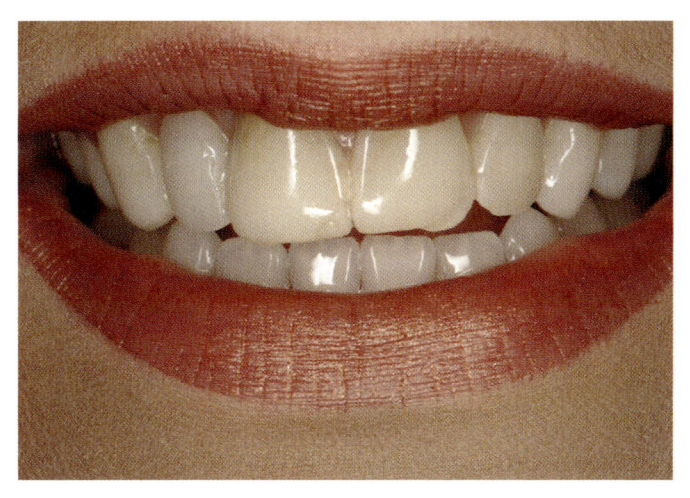

Figure 21.28 **(A)** This dentist was concerned about her aging composite resin veneers and wanted to have them rebonded for better esthetics.

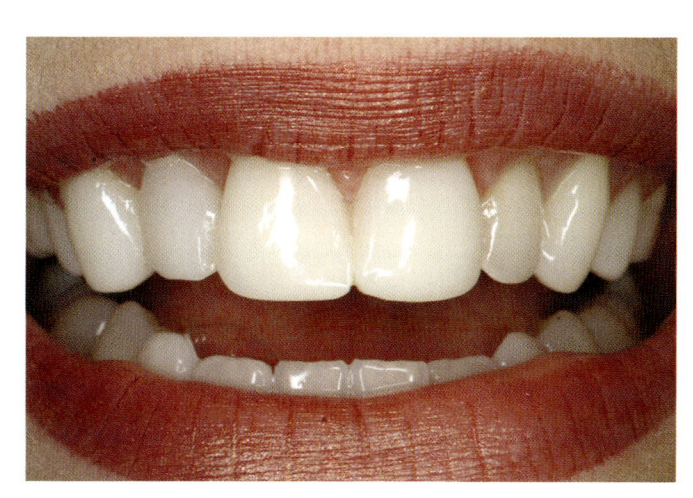

Figure 21.28 **(B)** Direct bonding with a microfilled composite was utilized for maximum polish.

Discoloration of composite resin restorations

Stains to composite resin restorations can occur in the body of composite, on the surface of the composite, or at the restoration margins. Bulk discoloration of chemically cured composites was common before the advent of light curing. Benzoyl peroxide, which is the chemical initiator in all chemically cured composites, is not color stable and will cause the restoration to darken over time. This phenomenon may necessitate the replacement of many otherwise serviceable restorations (Figure 21.28A and B). Darkening of light-cured composites is a result of extrinsic stains from food, drink, or oral habits. Orange stain can be the result of chromogenic bacteria. If these stains recur after thorough prophylaxis, refer the patient to an oral pathologist for culture, which will help determine a specific antibiotic to help prevent the recurrence of the bacteria. These stains can often be removed by merely repolishing the restoration. Care must be taken not to use certain aggressive cleaning devices during prophylaxis (i.e., Prophy-jet air polisher, Dentsply Professional) because these technologies can roughen the surface finish of composite restorations.[38]

It is not uncommon for staining to occur at the margins of composite restorations as the restorations age. If the staining is superficial, it can often be removed by bleaching, air abrasion, or the use of diamond or carbide finishing burs. After stain removal, the composite's margins should be etched for 15 s with 32–37% phosphoric acid, rinsed, and resealed with a bonding agent or surface sealant. When a marginal stain is not easily removed by conservative finishing techniques, the affected area should be mechanically removed because of the possible presence of recurrent decay. If, on penetration and exploration, the stain is found to be superficial, the restoration's margins can be repaired with fresh composite. If the stain is extensive, the entire restoration should be replaced. The postfinish application of a surface sealant (Fortify, Bisco, Optiguard, KerrDental) has been shown to improve the composite's marginal integrity over time and can provide a more esthetic restoration by sealing surface irregularities.

Discolorations around porcelain veneers

Marginal staining of porcelain veneers may necessitate the replacement of otherwise acceptable restorations. Marginal staining can result from any of these clinical situations, as follows:

- The cement line may become obvious after several years if a dual-cured or chemically cured composite luting agent was used instead of a more color-stable, light-cured resin cement. Also, unsightly margins may develop when extensive stains accumulate on improperly polished margins. However, the eventual esthetic failure of veneers may be due to advance marginal staining. The final potential cause of unsightly margins is marginal leakage. This occurs when the tooth–composite bond becomes compromised. Although the first two margin discolorations present only an esthetic concern, staining as a result of leakage may signal a problem with decay under the restoration. As stated earlier, Nightguard bleaching with 10% carbamide peroxide may be helpful as both a therapeutic and a diagnostic procedure. If the stain around the veneer is removed by the at-home bleaching, the margin can be refinished[39] and/or resealed and the veneer salvaged.

- Discoloration can be microleakage due to failure of the adhesive cement or an inadequate bond at virtually any part of the veneer. Because of the physiologic problems associated with maintaining an adequate bond in the cervical area, this leakage is most often seen associated with the cervical portion of the veneer. Treatment of this problem generally consists of replacement of the veneer. However, it is sometimes possible to repair the gingival aspect with composite resin (refer to Chapter 14). If this treatment option is selected, it is advisable to use abrasive technology with a metal strip to avoid any unnecessary trauma or injury to the remaining porcelain. Often, jet-black stain caused by chromogenic bacteria is found underneath the defective part of the veneer.

- Both vital and endodontically treated teeth under veneers may darken over time. Bleaching may be a conservative treatment for this condition. In this instance, the bleaching material is applied to the surface of the tray that contacts the lingual surface of the tooth. The bleaching of the underlying tooth may return the veneered tooth to an acceptable shade.

Esthetic considerations for facial composite restorations

There are several factors that should be kept in mind when esthetically restoring the Class V restoration.

- **Color match:** For most patients, the objective will be to correctly match the present tooth shade. If using composite resin, a microparticle restorative material is preferred rather than a hybrid composite since there will be usually no occlusal force with which to deal and the polishability of a microfilled composite will be of benefit to the patient. Generally, a slightly darker shade should be applied first at the cervical-most portion of the restoration, followed by either a blending body tone or translucent shade to help create a natural look to the tooth. If the patient is bleaching their teeth first, wait 2–3 weeks following termination of bleaching before appointing the patient for the restoration procedure.

- **Gingival seal:** Perhaps the most difficult procedure to accomplish is obtaining an effective gingival seal when bonding a Class V restoration. However, failure to obtain proper gingival adhesion will eventually result in either the restoration becoming debonded or subsequent microleakage can result in a gray–black stain that can, in time, be detected. Use of a rubber dam is the best way to avoid contamination. If a rubber dam is not used, then the placement of a gingival retraction cord 10–15 min prior to restoring the tooth may help prevent crevicular contamination.

- **Shape:** After color, the shape of the restoration becomes the most important element of an esthetic restoration. Using the overlay technique (see Chapter 14), be sure to slightly overbuild the restoration so that sufficient material remains to finish and polish the restoration. Both building up and contouring of the restoration should be accomplished by viewing the tooth not only from the facial aspect but also occlusally and laterally to best obtain the correct silhouette form.

Although the patient may tend to focus on specific discolorations or stains, it is important for the dentist to remain objective and view the stains in the context of the entire smile and face. In other words, will removal of the stain truly satisfy the patient's quest to look better, or will a more comprehensive approach not only improve the tooth color but also provide a smile that would better improve their self-image? The answer to this question may be found in esthetic computer imaging or even a Trial Smile. Actually showing your patient the difference in just removing the stains and changing the smile provides the truest form of informed consent.

Summary

The staining or discoloration of teeth can be indicative of a variety of clinical situations, ranging from severe systemic conditions that may be life threatening to the mere buildup of extensive stains as a result of oral habits. Therefore, the first step in the treatment of a patient whose chief complaint is stains or discolorations is the diagnosis of the cause of the discoloration. The diagnosis will dictate the appropriate treatment options from which to choose. It is incumbent on the dentist to select the most conservative treatment option for the specific stain, while preparing the patient for subsequent treatments should the selected one not be effective.

References

1. Watts A, Addy M. Tooth discoloration and staining: a review of the literature. *Br Dent J* 2001;190(6):309–316.
2. Mertz-Fairhurst EJ, Smith CD, Williams JE, et al. Cariostatic and ultraconservative sealed restorations: six-year results. *Quintessence Int* 1992;23:827–838.
3. Waggoner WF, Siegal M. Pit and fissure sealant application: updating the technique. *J Am Dent Assoc* 1996;127:351–361.
4. Addy M, Moran J, Griffiths A, Wills-Wood NJ. Extrinsic tooth discoloration by metals and chlorhexidine. Surface protein denaturation or dietary precipitation? *Br Dent J* 1985;159:281–285.
5. Schwachman H, Schuster A. The tetracyclines: applied pharmacology. *Pediatr Clin North Am* 1956;3:295–303.
6. Nathoo SA. The chemistry and mechanisms of extrinsic and intrinsic discoloration. *J Am Dent Assoc* 1997;128(Suppl):6S–10S.
7. Hattab FN, Qudeimat MA, al-Rimawi HS. Dental discoloration: an overview. *J Esthet Dent* 1999;11(6):291–310.
8. Frazier KB. An overview of tooth whitening procedures. *J Pract Hygiene* 1998;7:32–33.
9. Haywood VB. Achieving, maintaining, and recovering successful tooth bleaching. *J Esthet Dent* 1996;8(1):31–38.
10. Blankenau R, Goldstein RE, Haywood VB. The current status of vital tooth whitening techniques. *Compendium* 1999;20:781–794.
11. Haywood VB. Nightguard vital bleaching: current concepts and research. *J Am Dent Assoc* 1997;128:19S–25S.
12. Tredwin CJ, Scully C, Bagan-Sebastian J-V. Drug-induced disorders of teeth. *J Dent Res* 2005;84:596–602.
13. Parikh DR, Ganesh M, Bhasker V. Prevalence and characteristics of molar incisor hypomineralisation (MIH) in the child population residing in Gandhinagar, Gujarat. *Eur Arch Paediatr Dent* 2012;13(1):21–26.
14. Wallman IS, Hilton HB. Teeth pigmented by tetracycline. *Lancet* 1962;1:827–829.
15. Haywood VB, Heymann HO. Response of normal and tetracycline-stained teeth with pulp-size variation to Nightguard vital bleaching. *J Esthet Dent* 1994;6:109–114.
16. Trendley Dean H. Chronic endemic dental fluorosis. *JAMA* 1936;107:1269–1273.
17. Haywood VB, Heymann HO, Kusy RP, et al. Polishing porcelain veneers: an SEM and spectral reflectance analysis. *Dent Mater* 1988;4:116–121.

18. Levin LS. The dentition in the osteogenesis imperfect syndromes. *Clin Orthop* 1981;159:64–74.
19. Parkins FM, Furnish G, Bernstein M. Minocycline use discolors teeth. *J Am Dent Assoc* 1992;123:87–89.
20. Haywood VB. Whitening teeth by Nightguard vital bleaching. *Pract Rev Pediatr Dent* 1998;8(6):1.
21. Haywood VB, Leonard RH. Nightguard vital bleaching removes brown discoloration for 7 years: a case report. *Quintessence Int* 1998;29:450–451.
22. Croll TP. Enamel micro abrasion: the technique. *Quintessence Int* 1989;20:395–400.
23. Heymann HO, Sockwell CL, Haywood VB. Additional conservative esthetic procedures. In: CM Sturdevant, ed. *The Art and Science of Operative Dentistry*, 3rd edn. St. Louis, MO: CV Mosby; 1995:643–647.
24. Coll JA, Jackson P, Strassler HE. Comparison of enamel microabrasion techniques: Prema Compound versus a 12-fluted finishing bur. *J Esthet Dent* 1991;3:180–186.
25. Haywood VB. Bleaching and microabrasion options. *Esthet Dent Update* 1995;6:99–100.
26. Haywood VB. Nightguard vital bleaching: current information and research. *Esthet Dent Update* 1990;1(2):7–12.
27. Davies PA, Little K, Aherne W. Tetracyclines and yellow teeth. *Lancet* 1962;1:742–743.
28. Frankel MA, Hawes RR. Tetracyclines antibiotics and tooth discoloration. *J Oral Ther* 1964;1:147–155.
29. Madison JF. Tetracycline pigmentation of teeth. *Arch Dermatol* 1963;88:58–59.
30. Cohlan SQ. Tetracycline staining of teeth. *Teratology* 1977;15:127–129.
31. Pearson NL. Nothing to smile about: drug-induced tooth discoloration. *Can Pharm J* 2007;140(4):263–265.
32. Van Der Bijl P, Pitigoi-Aron G. Tetracyclines and calcified tissues. *Ann Dent* 1995;54:69–72.
33. Mello HS. The mechanism of tetracycline staining in primary and permanent teeth. *J Dent Child* 1967;34:478–487.
34. Scoop IW, Kazandjian G. Tetracycline-induced staining of teeth. *Postgrad Med* 1986;79:202–203.
35. Haywood VB. Bleaching tetracycline-stained teeth. *Esthet Dent Update* 1996;7(1):25–26.
36. Haywood VB. Extended bleaching of tetracycline-stained teeth: a case report. *Contemp Esthet Restor Pract* 1997;1(1):14–21.
37. Haywood VB, Leonard RH, Dickinson GL. Efficacy of six-months Nightguard vital bleaching of tetracycline-stained teeth. *J Esthet Dent* 1997;9(1):13–19.
38. Frazier KB. *Aesthetic Dentistry*. Stuttgart: Georg Thieme; 1998.
39. Haywood VB, Heymann HO, Kusy RP, et al. Polishing porcelain veneers: an SEM and spectral reflectance analysis. *Dent Mater* 1988;4:116–121.

Additional resources

Allen K, Agosto C, Estefan D. Using microabrasive material to remove fluorosis stains. *J Am Dent Assoc* 2004;135:319–323.
Ardu S, Stavridakis M, Krejci I. A minimally invasive treatment of severe dental fluorosis. *Quintessence Int* 2007;38:455–458.
Atkinson HF, Hartcourt JK. Tetracyclines in human dentine. *Nature* 1962;195:508–509.
Bagheri R, Burrow MF, Tyas M. Influence of food-simulating solutions and surface finish on susceptibility to staining of esthetic restorative materials. *J Dent* 2005;33:389–398.
Bevelander G, Rolle GK, Cohlan SG. The effect of the administration of tetracycline on the development of teeth. *J Dent Res* 1961;40:1020–1024.
Croll TP, Cavanaugh RR. Enamel color modification by controlled hydrochloric acid-pumice abrasion. I. Technique and examples. *Quintessence Int* 1986;17:81–87.
Croll TP. Enamel microabrasion for removal of superficial discoloration. *J Esthet Dent* 1989;1:14–20.
De Lacerda AJF, Da Silva Avila DM, Borges AB, et al. Adhesive systems as an alternative material for color masking of white spot lesions: do they work? *J Adhes Dent* 2016;18(1):43–50.
Hatai Y. Extreme masking: achieving predictable outcomes in challenging situations with lithium disilicate bonded restorations. *Int J Esthet Dent* 2014;9:206–220.
Haywood VB, Cordero R, Wright K. Brushing with a potassium nitrate dentifrice to reduce bleaching sensitivity. *J Clin Dent* 2005;16:17–22.
Heymann G, Grauer D. A contemporary review of white spot lesions in orthodontics. *J Esthet Restor Dent* 2013;25(2):85–95.
Levy SM, Broffitt B, Marshall TA. Associations between fluorosis of permanent incisors and fluoride intake from infant formula, other dietary sources, and dentifrice during early childhood. *J Am Dent Assoc* 2010;141:1190–1201
Schilichting LH, Stanley K, Magne M, Magne P. The non-vital discolored central incisor dilemma. *Int J Esthet Dent* 2015;10(4):548–562.
Strassler HE. Clinical case report: treatment of mild-to-moderate fluorosis with a minimally invasive treatment plan. *Compend Contin Educ Dent* 2010;31:54–58.
Strassler HE, Griffin A, Maggio M. Management of fluorosis using macro- and micro abrasion. *Dent Today* 2001;30:94–96.
Tong LS, Pang MK, Mok NY, et al. The effects of etching, micro abrasion, and bleaching on surface enamel. *J Dent Res* 1993;72:67–71.
Vogel RI. Intrinsic and extrinsic discoloration of the dentition. A review. *J Oral Med* 1975;30:99–104.
Wei SH, Ingram MI. Analysis of the amalgam tooth interface using the electron microprobe. *J Dent Res* 1969;48:317.
Zhang N, Chen C, Weir MD, et al. Antibacterial and protein-repellent orthodontic cement to combat biofilm and white spot lesions. *J Dent* 2015;43:1529–1538.

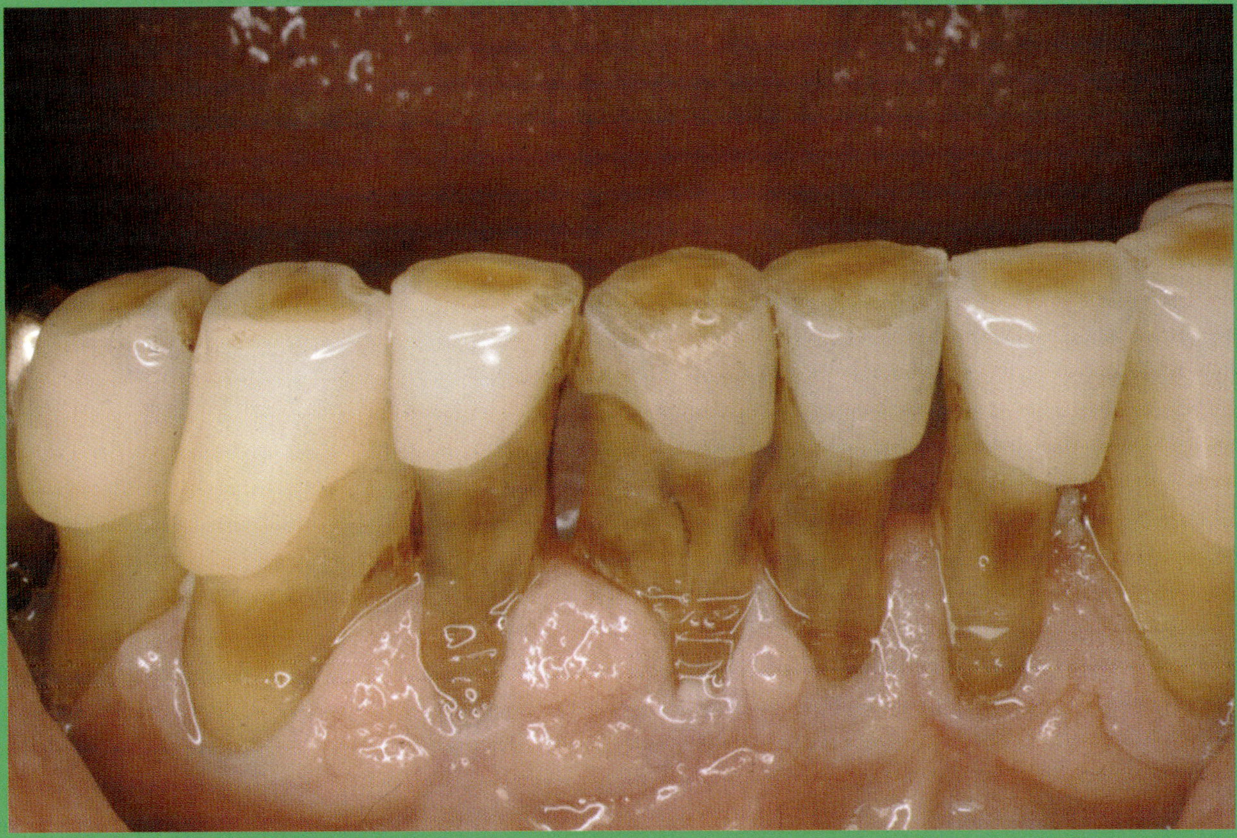

Chapter 22 Abfraction, Abrasion, Attrition, and Erosion

Ronald E. Goldstein, DDS, James W. Curtis Jr, DMD, Beverly A. Farley, DMD*, Samantha Siranli, DMD, PhD, and Wendy A. Clark, DDS, MS

Chapter Outline

Attrition	696	Abrasion	708
Bruxism	697	Erosion	709
Abfraction	704	Differential diagnosis	711
Restoration defect	707		

In contemporary life, cervical and occlusal tooth wear has become part of dentists' regular assessments, and providing information to patients about tooth wear is growing in importance. Throughout the years, the dental profession has held a variety of theories about the causes of tooth wear, including chemical wasting of the teeth, the effects of tooth brushing, and lateral forces. Tooth wear may present as abfraction, abrasion, attrition, and erosion.

During their lifetime, many people will experience the effects of one or more of these conditions. The stress of today's fast-paced lifestyle may lead to various habits that can directly cause or contribute to these problems. The etiologies of abfraction, abrasion, attrition, and erosion may be interrelated; therefore, multiple conditions may be seen in a single patient (Figure 22.1A–K).

A review of the literature frequently reveals confusion, controversy, and contradiction concerning the terminology and etiology related to the loss of tooth structure due to noncarious processes. For example, even though the term erosion is frequently used in the dental literature to denote loss of tooth structure due to chemical dissolution, the actual definition of erosion is the abrasive destruction of a material that occurs as a result of movement of liquid or gas, with or without solid particles, over the surface of the material. So possibly, the term "erosion" could be called "corrosion" more accurately, as it describes the chemical dissolution of teeth. However, in this text we will utilize the term "erosion" as it is commonly known in the profession.

Often, the lines between the chemical and physical forces that cause noncarious tooth structure loss are blurred. When the etiologic factors of more than one of these conditions are simultaneously present, the resultant loss of tooth structure will be accelerated or magnified. As an example, bulimics who brush their teeth immediately after regurgitation may increase the rate of enamel loss. This is due to the greater effect of abrasion on acid-etched enamel. In assessing these various conditions, the possibility of multifactorial etiology should always be kept in mind.[1]

* Deceased

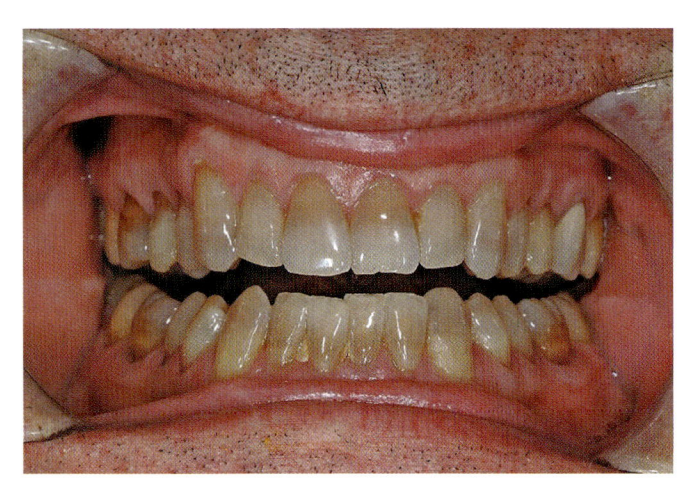

Figure 22.1 **(A)** This 48-year old male became concerned about his tetracycline stained teeth that had become darker but especially the tooth abrasion and erosion that had occurred over the years.

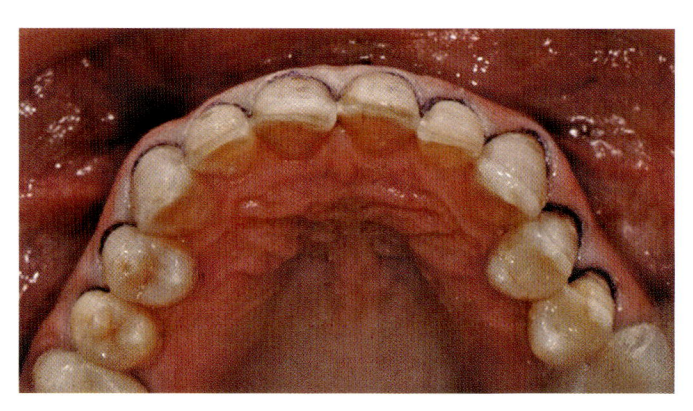

Figure 22.1 **(B)** The treatment plan called for porcelain veneers to solve both the labial defects plus the tetracycline stained teeth. Ten teeth were prepared for porcelain veneers plus one molar for a full all-ceramic crown.

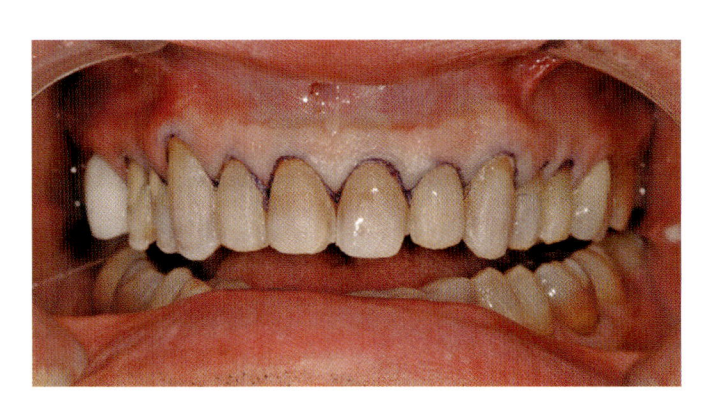

Figure 22.1 **(C)** Cotton retraction cord (Ultradent) displaced the gingival tissue to obtain an accurate vinyl polysiloxane impression. (Aquasil, Dentsplyl).

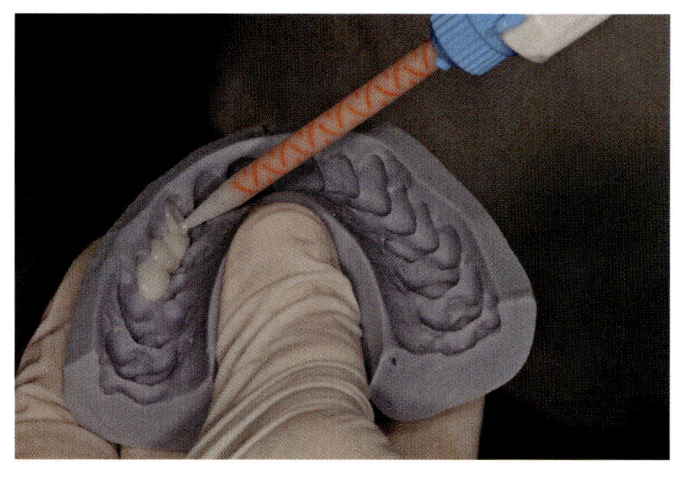

Figure 22.1 **(D)** A siltek matrix formed from the patient's waxed model is being loaded with temporary acrylic material (Luxatemp DMG) to make the interim veneers.

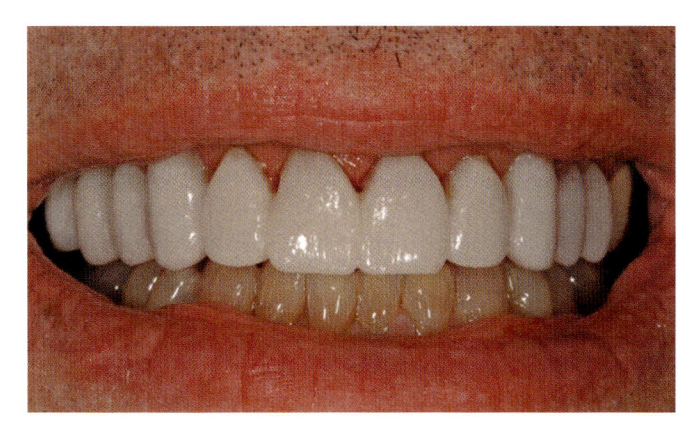

Figure 22.1 **(E)** The temporary veneers are bonded together for strength in the patient's chosen shade to act as both tooth protection and as a trial smile for shape and shade.

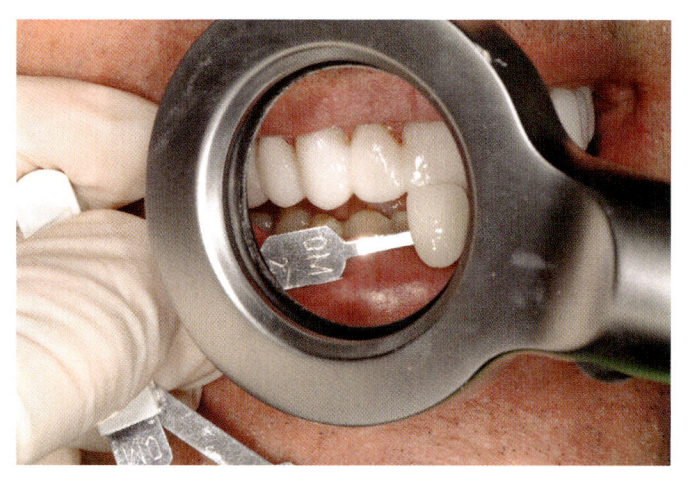

Figure 22.1 **(F)** A special color corrected light was utilized to verify shade. (AdDent).

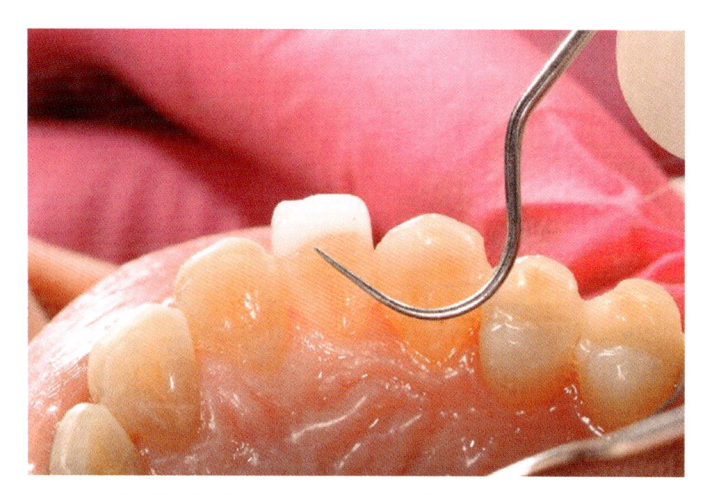

Figure 22.1 **(G)** The final veneers are first fitted individually one by one and then as a group.

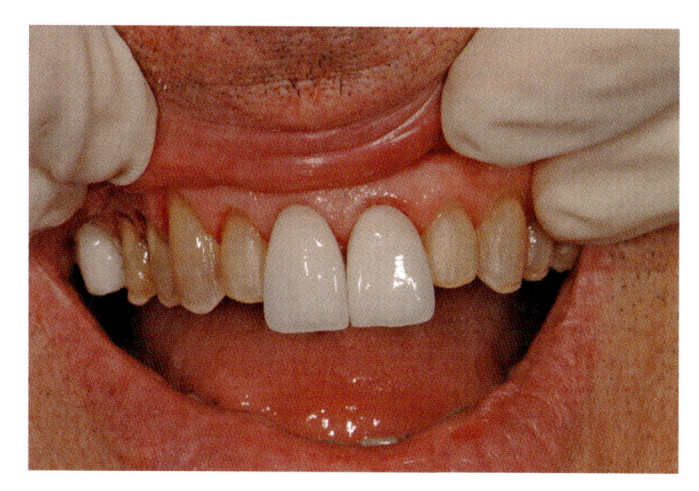

Figure 22.1 **(H)** The two central incisors are bonded to place first, followed by the lateral incisors and then the 2nd and 1st bicuspids. Finally, the cuspids are refitted and bonded.

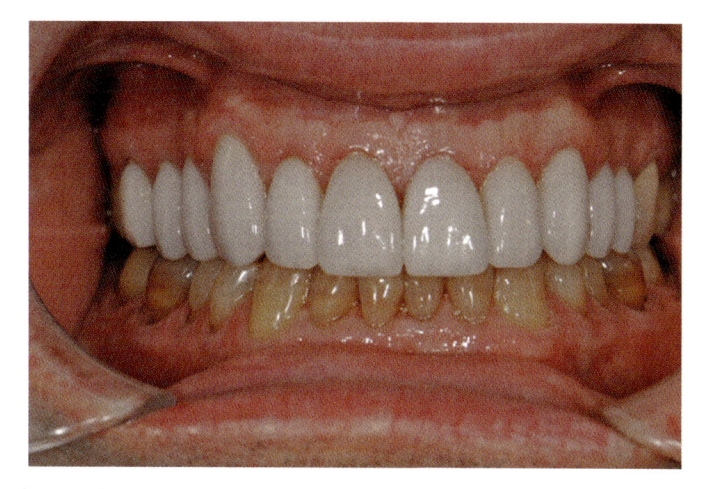

Figure 22.1 **(I)** The final restorations have all been cemented and any residual cement removed.

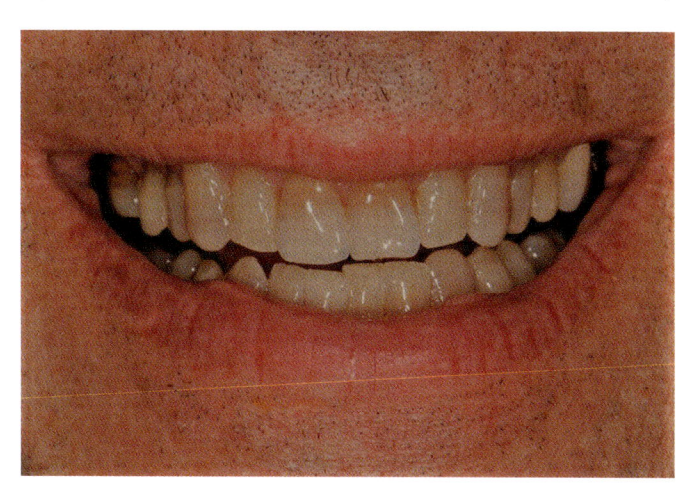

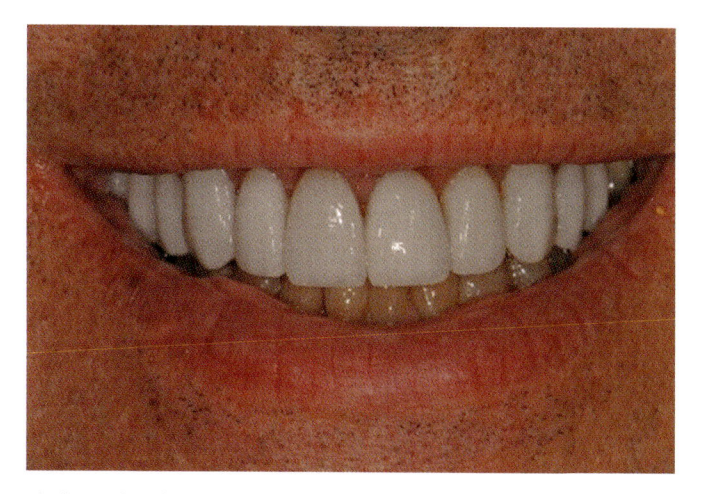

Figure 22.1 **(J–K)** The before and after smile showing good blocking the underlying discolored teeth. The patient did not feel he showed his lower discolored teeth much so he postponed veneers on these teeth. An alternative plan is in place to restore the mandibular cervical eroded defects with composite resin bonding.

It is important to recognize that wear of the dentition has been present since the origin of humankind. Young provides an extremely interesting summary of the literature relating to dental wear in the aboriginal populations of Australia and New Zealand.[2] The anthropologic studies of the University of Adelaide Dental School show the gamut of "development, progressive modification, and adaptability of the human occlusion to the demands of the environment before Western culture shock."[2] Through these studies, it was shown that human dentition was better able to withstand wear against the plaque-induced diseases that are primarily related to modern diets. In essence, these data support the fact that wear enhances the efficiency of teeth for the purposes for which they were intended: incising, shearing, crushing, and grinding foods. Begg wrote a series of articles on his analysis of prehistoric dentitions.[3-6] These articles provide insight into the orthodontic implications of dental wear as it relates to the preservation of dental arch integrity. Barrett determined that Australian aborigines with abrasive diets did not have significant malocclusion from a functional perspective.[7]

In 1958, Barrett noted that teeth in modern populations rarely exhibit the patterns of wear seen occurring in a natural fashion in aboriginal civilizations.[8] Herein lies part of the dilemma faced by the profession today. Radical changes in our environment and diet over the past few centuries have altered the extent and type of wear present in teeth.[9] These same dietary alterations have increased the prevalence of plaque-related dental diseases and the subsequent effects of such diseases.[10] Further compounding the picture are cultural shifts that have led to heightened awareness and the demand for esthetic dentistry.[11] Ultimately, as a profession, it is important that we recognize that anthropologic evidence related to tooth wear and the consequences of basic stomatognathic function on the longevity of teeth and restorations.

Attrition

Attrition is the loss of tooth structure by mechanical forces from opposing teeth. The wear from attrition may be seen on the occlusal surfaces of posterior teeth, the palatal surfaces of maxillary anterior teeth, and the labial surfaces of mandibular anterior teeth. The affected surfaces are usually hard, smooth, and shiny. However, the teeth may be sharp and jagged in certain cases. The areas of attrition may exhibit a yellowish-brown discoloration if the wear has penetrated the enamel. Wear may also occur interproximally, causing mesial drifting and broadening of proximal contacts.

Young mouths typically do not exhibit severe attrition. However, wear may be seen in the primary and mixed dentitions (Figure 22.2A). Numerous articles have reported on wear in children and adolescents.[12-19] As expected, increasing wear is seen with increasing age. This, as well as the fact that men exhibit more wear as they age, was demonstrated in a study of 586 subjects aged 45 and older[20] (Figure 22.2B-D).

It is well established that the most common cause of attrition is bruxism. Functional habits, such as chewing and swallowing, rarely result in tooth contact, and when contact does occur it

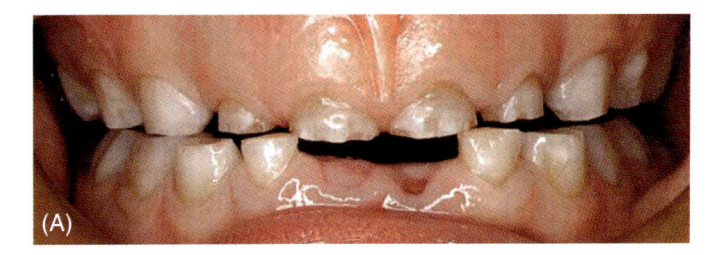

Figure 22.2 **(A)** This young girl demonstrated severe wear and attrition in her mixed dentition.

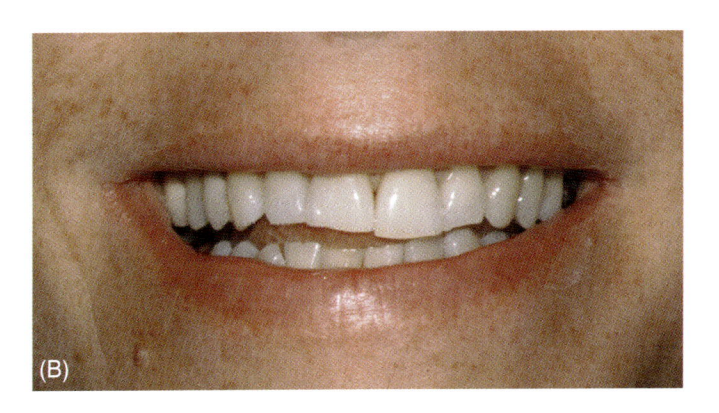

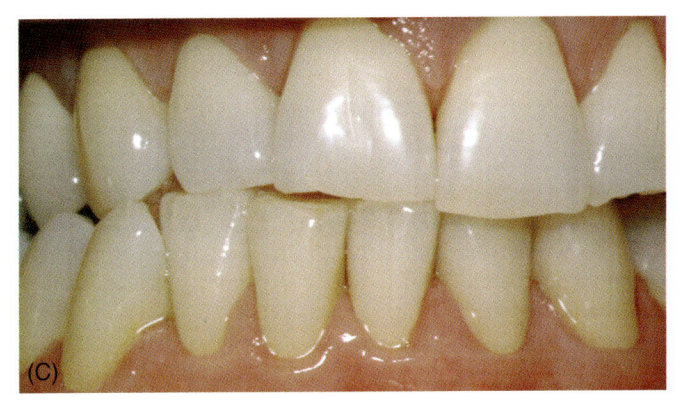

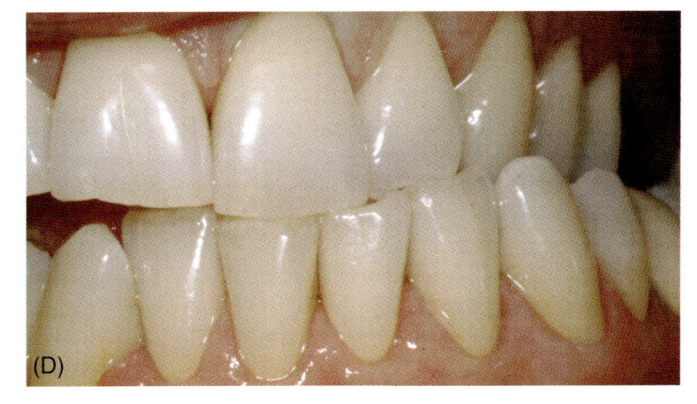

Figure 22.2 **(B–D)** It is so important for both hygienist and dentist to diagnose early bruxism habits as soon as possible to prevent from further tooth loss.

results in very little force. On the other hand, parafunctional habits, such as clenching and bruxism, result in significant forces on opposing teeth. This will be discussed at greater length in the bruxism section. There are numerous etiological factors that contribute to attrition. These include malocclusion, environmental factors, and genetic factors. Considering occlusion, we see greater wear in teeth that are in crossbite, both anteriorly and posteriorly. Environmentally, chronic exposure to dust and dirt can also cause increased wear in humans. This can occur in agricultural areas[21] or be associated with various industrial settings, such as cement factories.[22] Genetic factors should also be considered, such as dentinogenesis imperfecta, a disorder that affects the collagen protein causing deformities in dentin,[23–36] or amelogenesis imperfecta, which is a hypoplastic enamel. Both of these conditions make the teeth more susceptible to wear at an increased rate. When first examining a patient and diagnosing tooth wear, it is important to remember that the tooth wear may not be actively occurring at the time of exam. In other words, the current damage may be present from historical behaviors. It is important to monitor the progression of the tooth loss over time. This can be done by making casts and taking digital photographs of the teeth with wear, and repeating this process at different intervals. The same wear facets can be measured on the different casts to determine the continued activity of tooth wear. Likewise, if care is taken to replicate the same positioning in the photographs, one can visualize the progression of exposed dentin. To quantify the amount of tooth structure that has been lost due to wear, several authors have created indices. One of the most frequently cited is the tooth wear index published by Smith and Knight in 1984 (Table 22.1).[37]

Table 22.1 Smith and Knight's Tooth Wear Index

Score	Surface	Criterion
0	B/L/O/I	No loss of enamel surface characteristics
	Cervical	No change in contour
1	B/L/O/I	Loss of enamel surface characteristics
	Cervical	Minimal loss of contour
2	B/L/O	Loss of enamel exposing dentin for less than one-third of surface
	Incisal	Loss of enamel just exposing dentin
	Cervical	Defect less than 1 mm deep
3	B/L/O	Loss of enamel exposing dentin for more than one-third of surface
	Incisal	Loss of enamel and substantial loss of dentin, but not exposing the pulp
	Cervical	Defect 1–2 mm deep
4	B/L/O	Complete loss of enamel, pulp exposure, or exposure of secondary dentin
	Incisal	Pulp exposure or exposure of secondary dentin
	Cervical	Defect more than 2 mm deep, pulp exposure, or exposure of secondary dentin

Bruxism

Bruxism is a condition in which persons grind, gnash, or clench their teeth. This can include unconsciously clenching of the teeth during the day or clenching or grinding them at night (sleep bruxism).[122] Sleep bruxism is considered a sleep-related movement disorder. Mild bruxism may not require treatment, but bruxism can be frequent and severe enough to lead to jaw disorders, headaches, damaged teeth, and other problems. Bruxism can lead to extreme loss of occlusal and incisal tooth structure (Figures 22.3 and 22.4). For example, a young woman was treated for her defective restorations in 1968. Although she continued with routine maintenance appointments for a few years, she never accepted the advice to have a bite appliance constructed to treat her bruxism habit. Thirty-one years later, she returned with extremely worn dentition, as seen in Figure 22.4C–E. Crown lengthening and full crowns were necessary to restore this patient's smile (Figure 22.4 F and G).

Bruxism may also produce abfractions in the cervical regions.[38] It was suggested that bruxism and malocclusion generate occlusal forces on the tooth of sufficient duration and magnitude to cause tooth flexure, which is followed by lesion formation.[39,40] Patients suffering from bruxism may also experience symptoms of myofacial pain dysfunction syndrome or related disorders.[41,42] It is imperative to look closely at wear patterns in patients suspected of bruxism and evaluate for other signs and symptoms of occlusal dysfunction.

Owing to the gradual loss of tooth structure that most commonly occurs with bruxism, there is rarely loss of the vertical dimension of occlusion. This is due to the continued eruption of the teeth and their surrounding alveolar bone, as the teeth maintain their occlusal stops. The typical thought process would suggest that vertical dimension should be increased restoratively by opening the bite, thereby creating space for restorative materials to lengthen the worn teeth. This approach, however, may be ill advised. Often, the patient's posterior teeth are unworn and in occlusion. If this is the case, alternative treatment options, including orthodontic movement and crown lengthening, should be considered in conjunction with the prosthetic rehabilitation of the worn teeth.

When treating a patient with worn dentition, it is essential to first diagnose the cause and the type of wear, and whether restorative space is available. Turner proposed a classification system for occlusal wear in 1984, which has since become the standard for clinical and academic discussions regarding this topic. Three categories of wear patients are described:[43]

Category 1: excessive wear with loss of occlusal vertical dimension (OVD) (Figure 22.5A–K).

Category 2: excessive wear without loss of OVD but with space available.

Category 3: excessive wear without loss of OVD but with limited space.

First, one must establish if there has been a loss of OVD by clinical examination. If there has been a loss, the patient is assigned to the first category. For these patients, opening the vertical dimension of occlusion is indicated and will create the necessary space for restorative materials. If there has not been a

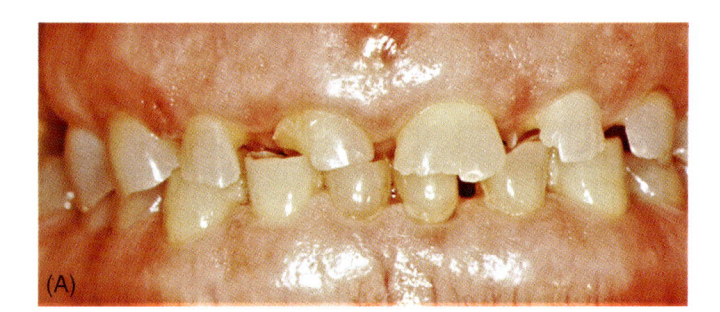

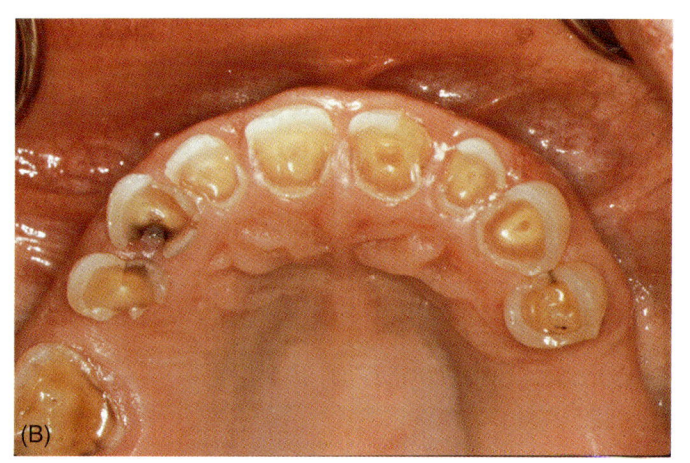

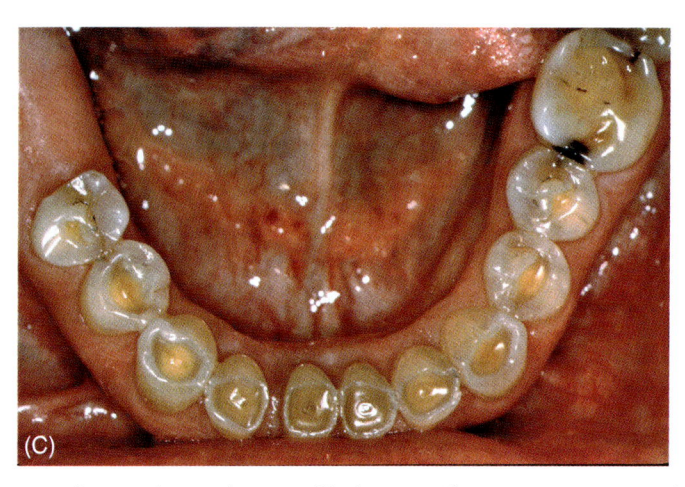

Figure 22.3 This case illustrates the severe damage that can be caused by bruxism. The patient is a 56-year-old man who reports that his wife tells him he grinds his teeth while sleeping. He is also a farmer and is exposed to dust for extended periods of time for much of the year. The combined bruxism and environmental factors have likely contributed to the extreme wear present. As is most commonly seen with cases in which the wear progresses slowly, there has been no discernible loss of vertical dimension, as evidenced by lip position and speech patterns. Note the traumatic occlusal relationship when the patient is in complete intercuspation **(A)**. Views of the severe wear of the maxillary and mandibular arches. Note the calcified, exposed pulp chambers and caries **(B and C)**.

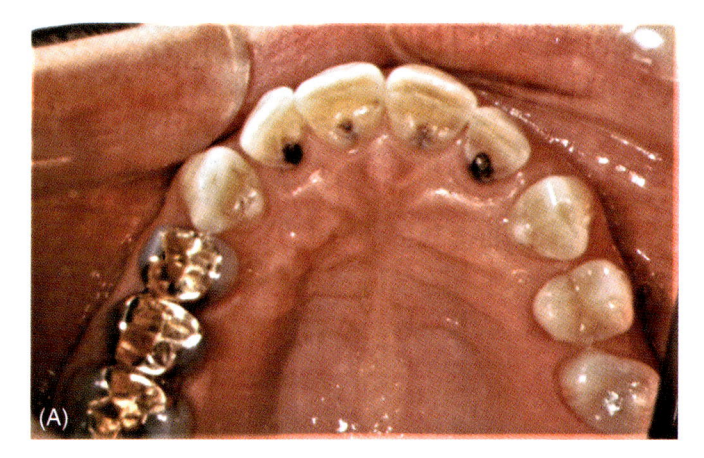

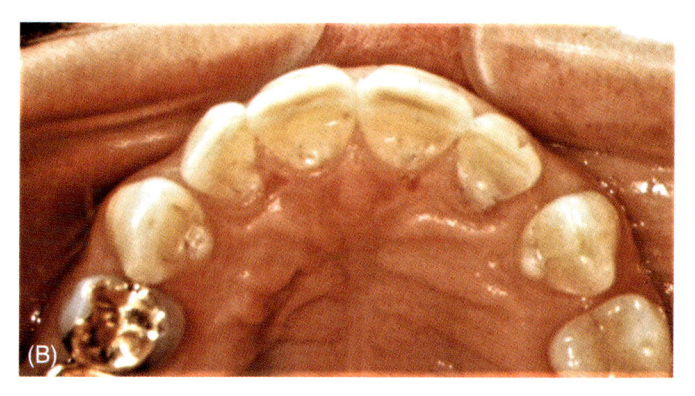

Figure 22.4 **(A, B)** This young woman's defective amalgam restorations were replaced in 1968 with tooth-colored restorations. At that time, and during the ensuing few years of maintenance recalls, she was advised to have a bite appliance constructed for her severe bruxism habit.

loss of OVD, one must determine whether space is available for restorative materials. This can be done by clinically evaluating the closest speaking space or by having the patient wear an occlusal splint made at the desired vertical opening. If it is determined that restorative space is unavailable, then space must be gained either with orthodontic intrusion or periodontal crown lengthening. Nel et al. described a variety of techniques that can be used in restoring wear from bruxism.[44]

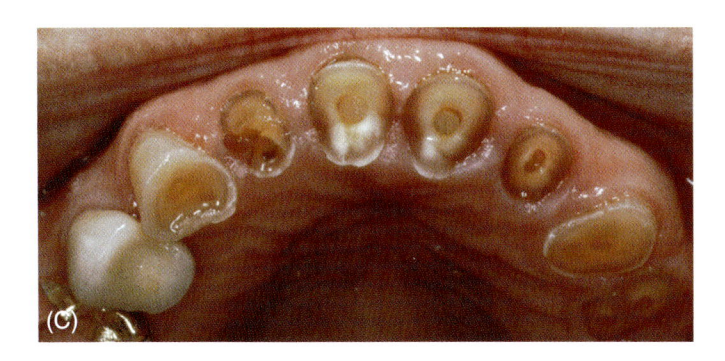

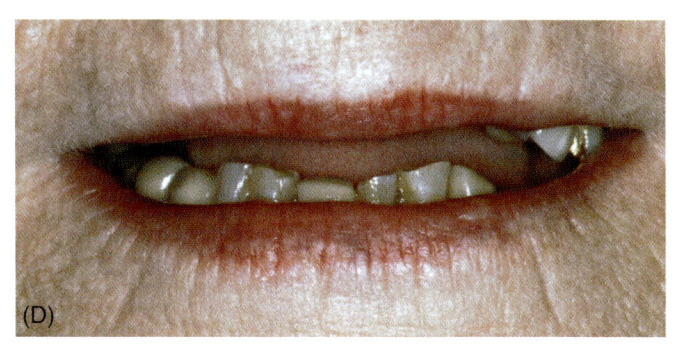

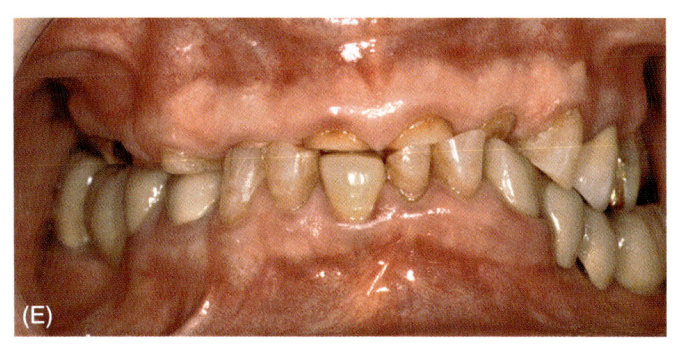

Figure 22.4 (C–E) She returned 31 years after her first appointment with an extremely worn dentition.

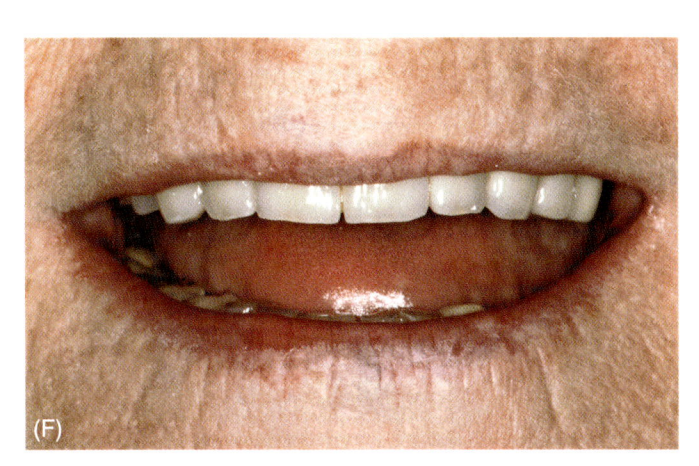

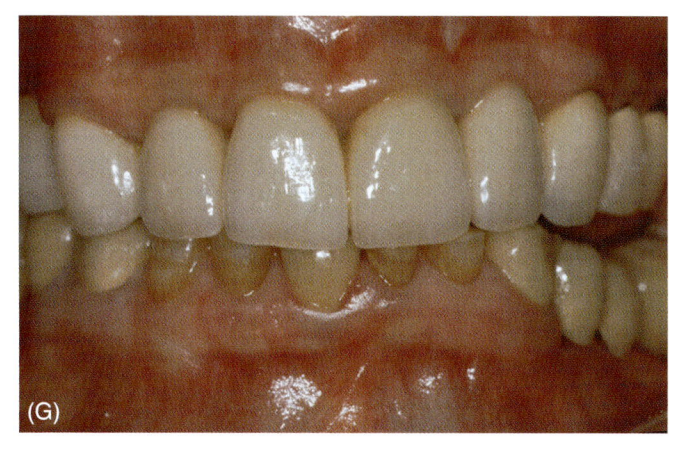

Figure 22.4 (F, G) Treatment consisted of crown lengthening and full crowns, which restored the patient's smile and her self-confidence. The lower left arch was treatment planned to replace the fixed bridge, but in unideal occlusion to occlude with the new maxillary restoration.

Once the patient's Turner classification has been identified, treatment planning can begin with a diagnostic wax-up. Dawson[45,46] recommends the following sequence:

1. Develop maxillary incisal edge position.
2. Develop mandibular incisal edge position.
3. Develop maxillary occlusal plane.
4. Develop mandibular posterior occlusal plane.

Following this sequence, you can determine from the diagnostic wax-up if the treatment will require orthodontics, esthetic and/or functional crown lengthening, as well the extent of the restorative rehabilitation. As you are beginning your diagnostic process with the maxillary incisal edge position, the patient's incisal display must be evaluated. As previously mentioned, the lost tooth structure is often compensated with continuous eruption of the tooth, along with its alveolar bone and gingival tissues. If this is the case, the incisal edge is often in the correct position, even though the teeth may be significantly worn down. The length needed to achieve esthetics in this situation needs to come from the gingival direction rather than the incisal. Osseous crown lengthening is frequently needed.

Orthodontically[47,48] repositioning the teeth should be the first treatment option when both functional and esthetic improvements can be achieved. Although patient motivation may not be easily obtained, the slow eruption or intrusion of anterior teeth combined with functional orthodontic intervention can many times result in the ideal solution to this problem. Therefore, it is wise to seek an orthodontic consultation before providing the patient with alternative treatment plans.

Turner Class I patients have the most straightforward treatment planning; teeth have excessive wear and there is also space

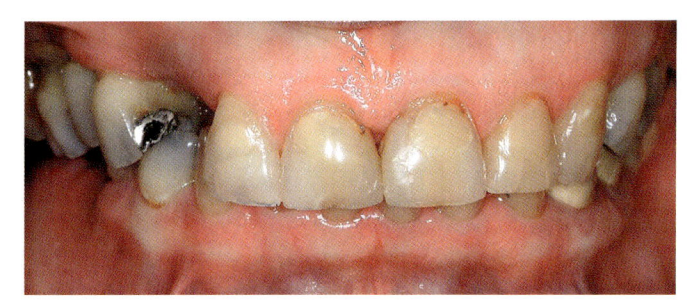

Figure 22.5 **(A)** The 56-year-old woman shown was not aware of her bruxism habit.

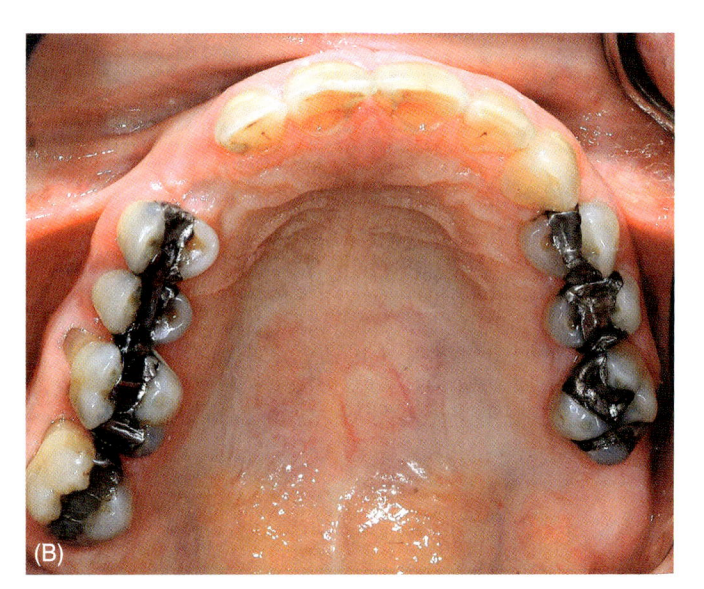

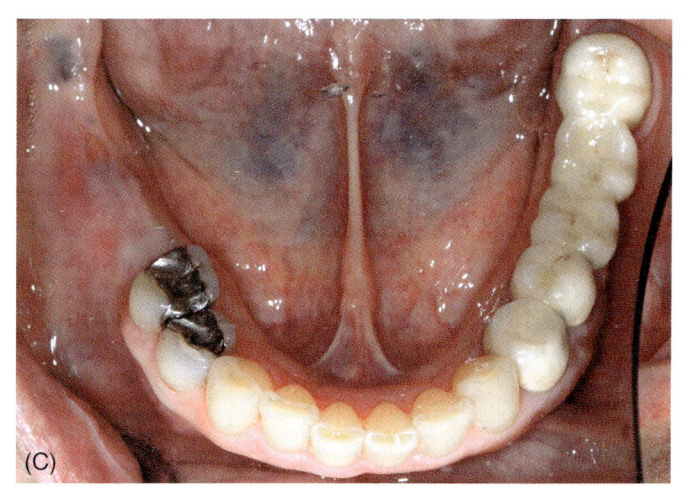

Figure 22.5 **(B, C)** The patient presented with severe wear on the lingual surfaces of teeth #8 and #9, moderate wear on the lingual and incisal surfaces of teeth #7, #10, and #11 as well as mandibular anterior teeth due to bruxism. Cupping areas were also detected on the occlusal surfaces of the teeth #4, #5, #12, #13, #28, and #29 probably due to combined effect of erosion and attrition.

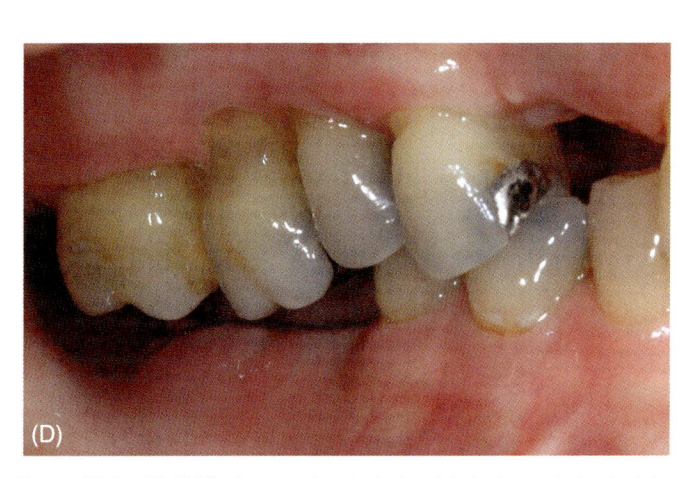

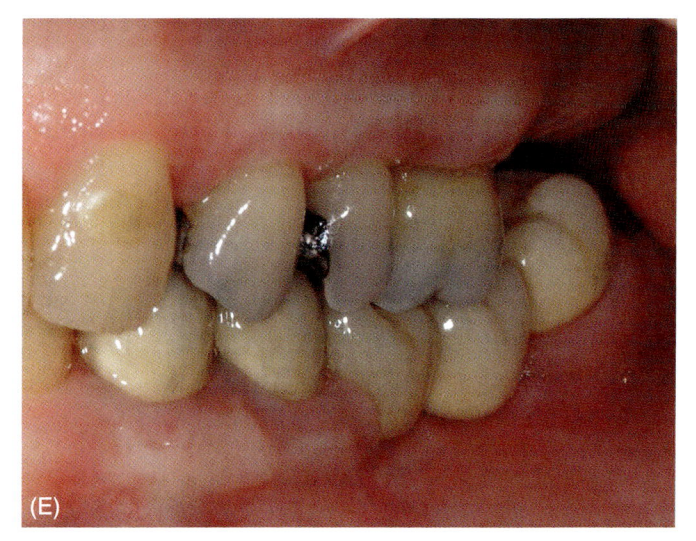

Figure 22.5 **(D, E)** The interocclusal relationship is shown in both right and left views.

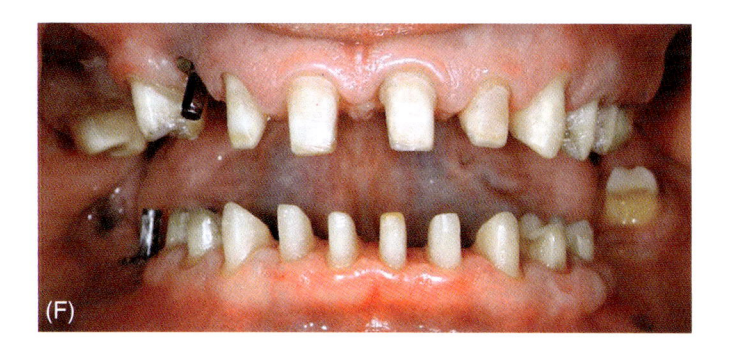

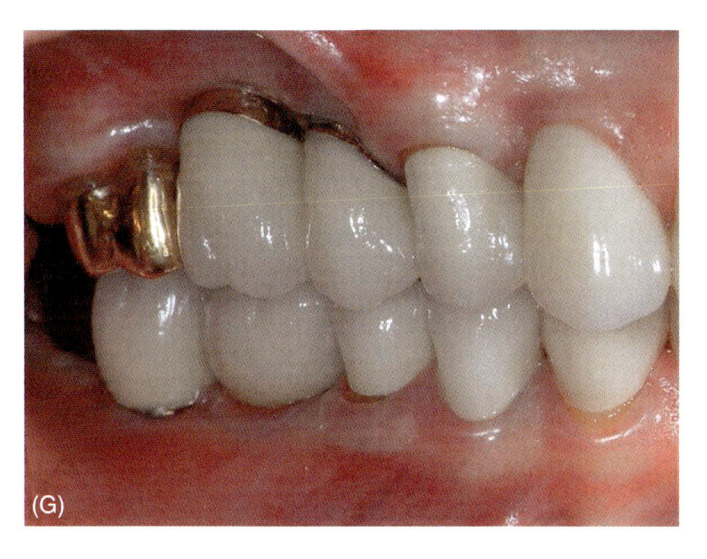

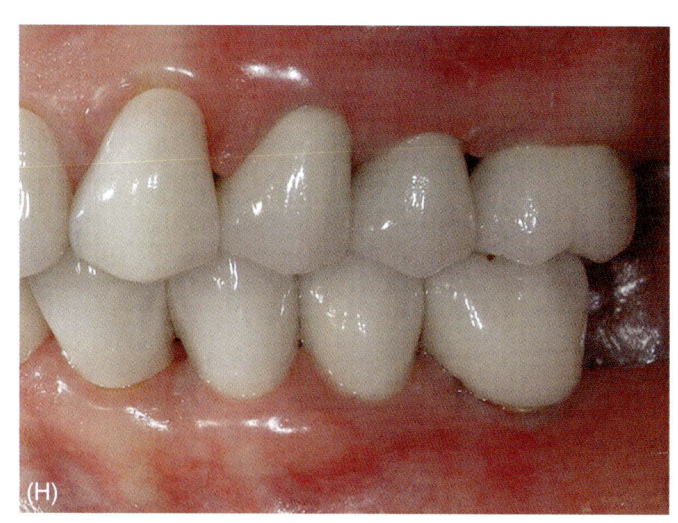

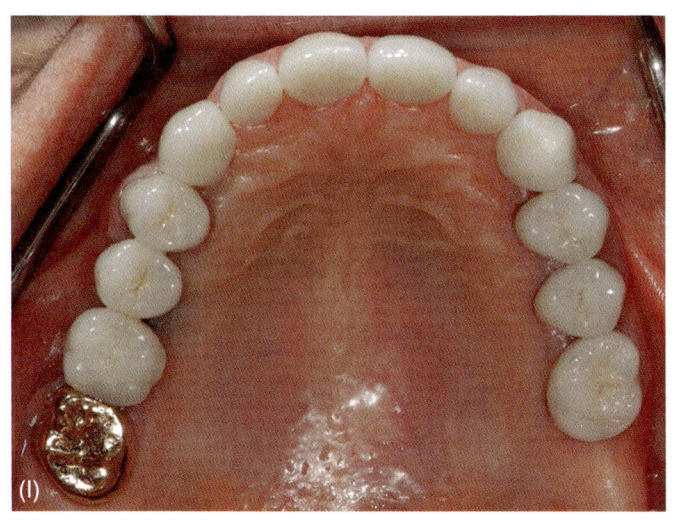

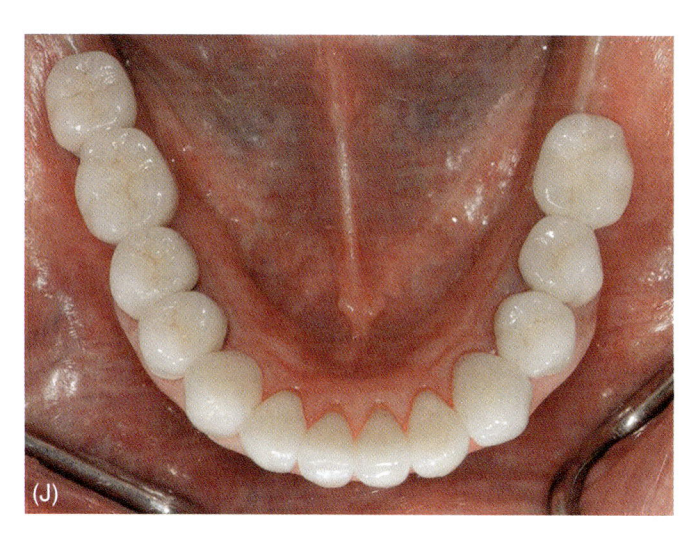

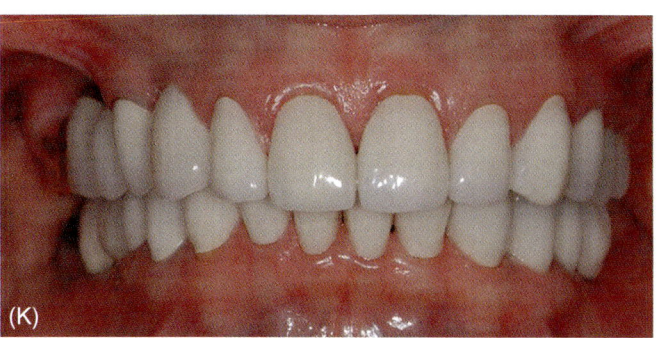

Chapter 22 Abfraction, Abrasion, Attrition, and Erosion

Figure 22.5 **(F–K)** Extraction of a supererupted tooth, surgical implant placement, crown lengthening, and full coverage crowns were necessary to restore this patient's smile as well as proper function.

available to restore the dentition. This type of patient typically presents with:

- posterior teeth missing and anterior teeth flared out;
- erosion on teeth that caused tooth wear at a rate that continuous eruption could not occur;
- genetic disorders such as dentinogenesis imperfecta or amelogenesis imperfecta.

With these patients, a new OVD should first be determined. In the literature, different methods have been discussed, including facial proportion method, phonetic evaluation (closest speaking space), Niswonger's freeway space evaluation, and transcutaneous electric neural stimulation.

Another method that has been discussed is utilization of an occlusal splint. With this technique, patients need to wear an acrylic appliance made to replicate the targeted amount of opening. This is typically worn for about three months as a way to evaluate whether the new OVD is acceptable. After determining the proper OVD, the diagnostic wax-up should be completed. Possible orthodontic treatment with an esthetic crown lengthening should be considered. Prosthetic rehabilitation should be completed as a final treatment following the provisionals being tested esthetically and functionally.

Clinical case study 22.1

A 56-year-old woman (shown in Figure 22.5A) was not aware of her bruxism habit. She presented with severe wear on the lingual surfaces of teeth #8 and #9 and moderate wear on the lingual and incisal surfaces of teeth #7, #10, and #11 and mandibular anterior teeth due to bruxism. Cupping areas were also detected on the occlusal surfaces of the teeth #4, #5, #12, #13, #28, and #29 probably due to combined effect of erosion and attrition (Figure 22.5B and C). The interocclusal relationship is shown in Figure 22.5D and E.

A functional occlusal analysis revealed a first centric occlusal contact between teeth #14–#18 and #19 with approximately 0.1 mm forward and 0.3 mm right lateral slide into maximum intercuspation. There was also a protrusive interference between teeth #14 and #17. This might have precipitated the grinding habit. Extraction of a supererupted tooth, surgical implant placement, crown lengthening, and full coverage crowns were necessary to esthetically restore this patient's smile and proper function (Figure 22.5 F–K).

Clinical case study 22.2

The treatment planning for Turner Class II patients tends to be more complex due to the continuous eruption that frequently takes place. Because of this, the tooth size is compromised but the OVD is maintained. Like Class I patients, the restorative OVD needs to be determined. Subsequently, the diagnostic wax-up will help determine whether to restore the worn dentition more apically or incisally. Again, both orthodontic treatment and esthetic crown lengthening should be considered, and provisional restorations must be used to verify esthetics and function before proceeding with final restorations. However, there are exceptions where palliative treatments may suffice (Figure 22.6A–C).

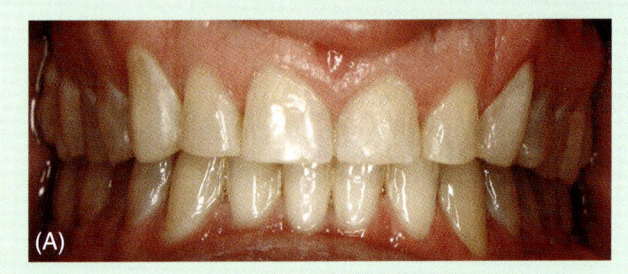

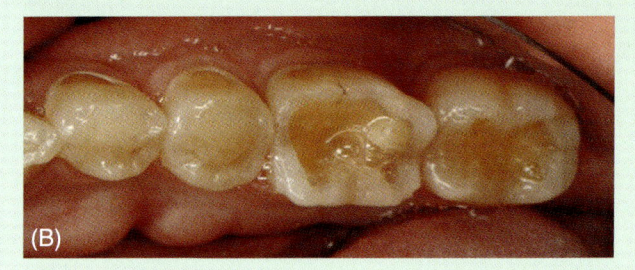

Figure 22.6 (A, B) Patient presented with moderate/severe attrition without loss of vertical dimension but with space available. Patient was not interested in esthetic improvement of the anterior teeth and nor was he complaining of any symptoms other than sensitivity in the posteriors.

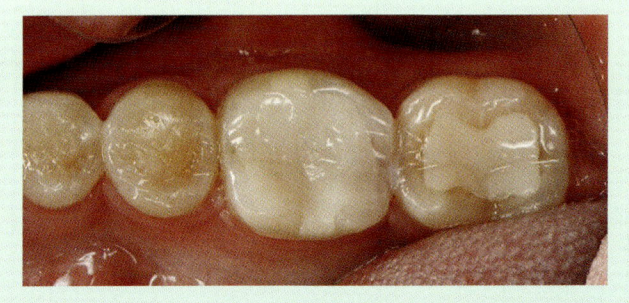

Figure 22.6 (C) The decision was made to a restore the excessive wear on the molars with composite resin bonding, and a bite guard was fabricated to help control his bruxism.

Clinical case study 22.3

In the case of a Turner Class III patient, there is no space available to restore the worn dentition. This type of patient typically presents with wear on the anterior teeth, with no signs of bruxism on the posterior teeth. These patients should be diagnosed immediately, and the OVD does not need to be opened. Depending on the incisal display and the need for restorative space, orthodontic intrusion and osseous crown lengthening also should be considered. Finally, the restorative rehabilitation should be completed after testing the new function and esthetics of the teeth with provisionals. An alternative treatment would be to alter opposing incisors in order to regain tooth length (Figure 22.7A–J).

In any bruxism/attrition patient, once the prosthetic rehabilitation is completed, an occlusal guard should be fabricated.

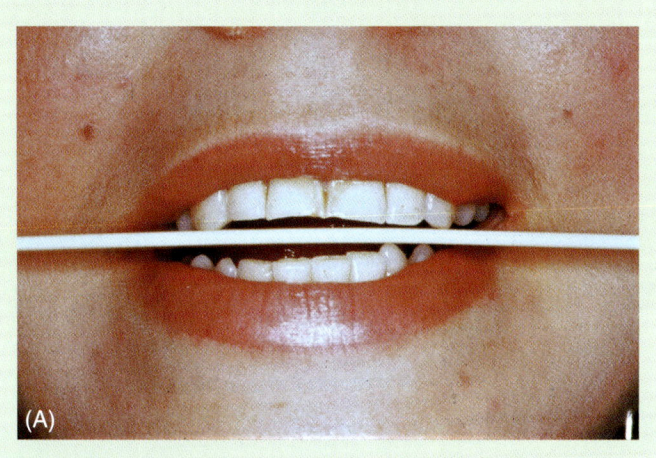

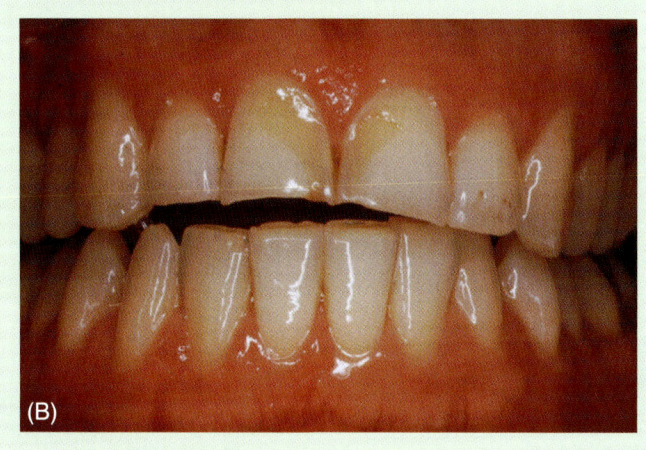

Figure 22.7 (A, B) This 23-year-old woman presented with advanced anterior incisal wear.

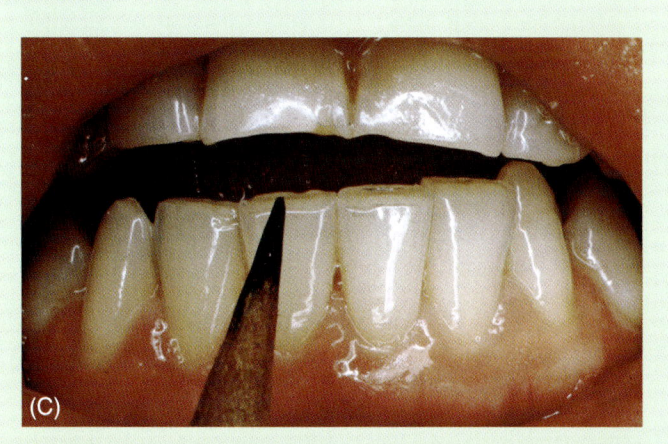

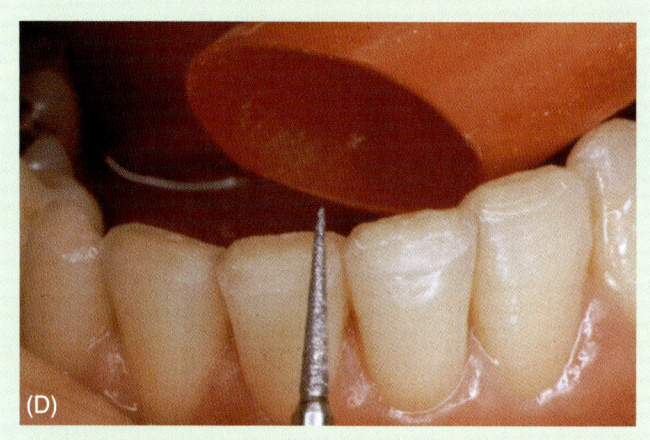

Figure 22.7 (C, D) The lower incisors were shortened and slightly beveled with a diamond bur.

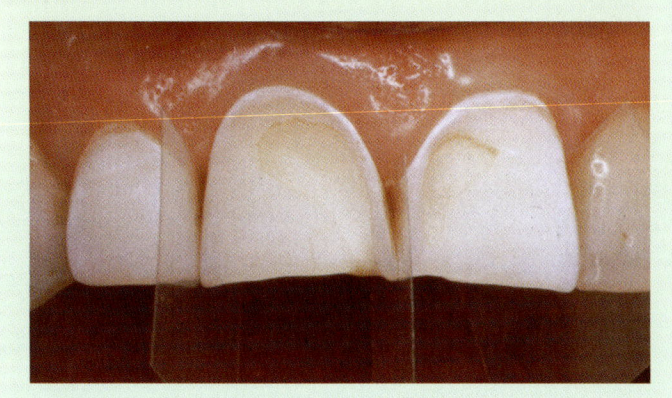

Figure 22.7 (E) The maxillary right lateral and central incisors were etched and veneered with composite resin to add length.

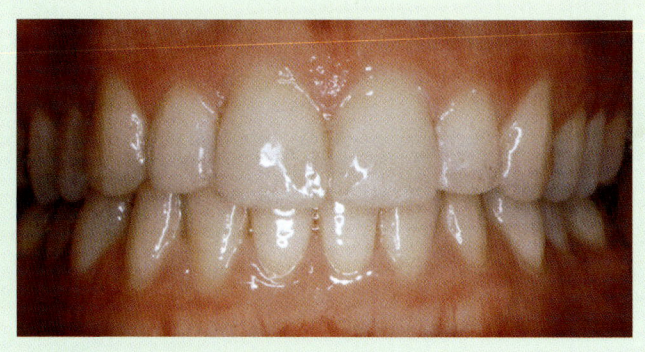

Figure 22.7 (F) The final result shows a younger-appearing incisal plane.

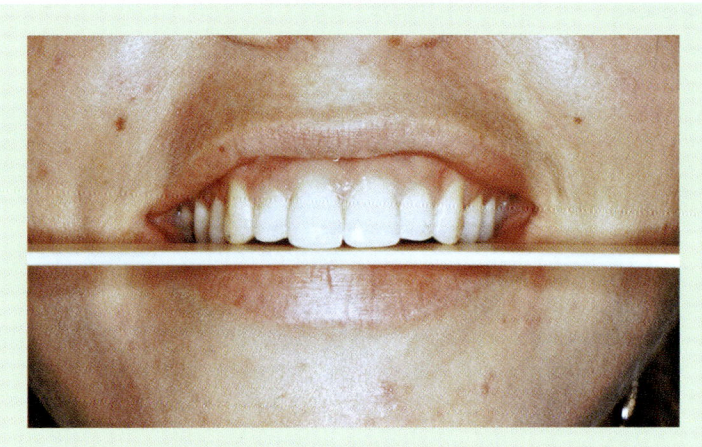

Figure 22.7 **(G)** Note the improvement of the smile line by comparing this figure with Figure 22.7A.

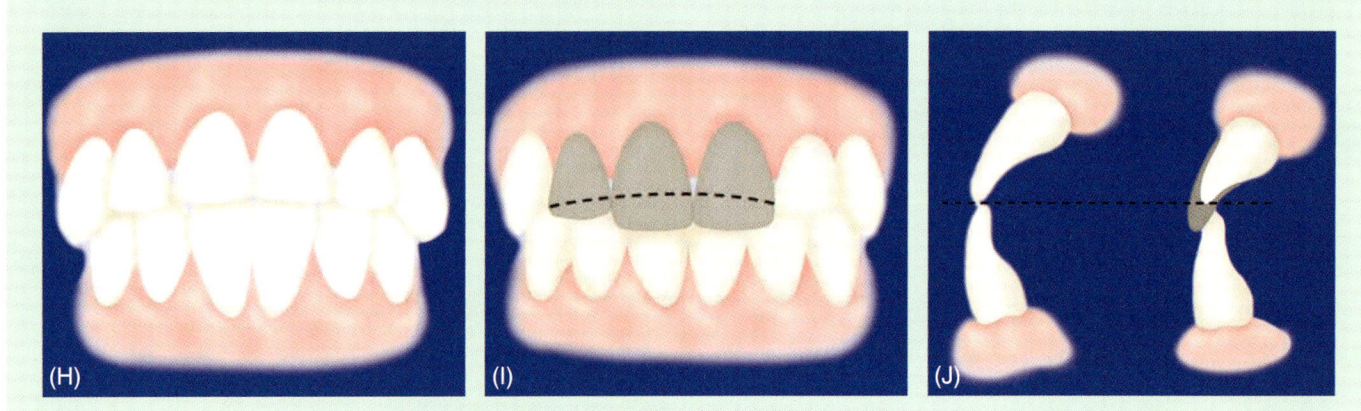

Figure 22.7 **(H–J)** These diagrams show how this procedure was accomplished. A balance was achieved by shortening and beveling the mandibular anteriors (J) to compensate for the lengthening of the maxillary incisal edges.

Abfraction

Abfraction, a type of noncarious cervical tooth loss, is a poorly understood condition. Other terms have also been suggested for this phenomenon, including noncarious cervical lesions (NCCLs) and stress erosion. Clinically, abfraction is represented by a wedge-shaped cervical lesion that results from repeated tooth flexure caused by occlusal loading (Figure 22.8). Although these lesions have been recognized for years, their etiology had been debated. Numerous hypotheses were put forward over time to explain the cause of these lesions. The most common theory was that of toothbrush abrasion occurring independently or in conjunction with erosion.[49] However, the sharp angles and frequent subgingival location of these cervical lesions cannot be adequately explained by any of the previous hypotheses. It was not until the early to mid-1980s that the concept of tensile stress as the etiology of these lesions came into the forefront.[50–52] Grippo originated the term abfraction to describe this pathologic loss of both enamel and dentin caused by biomechanical loading

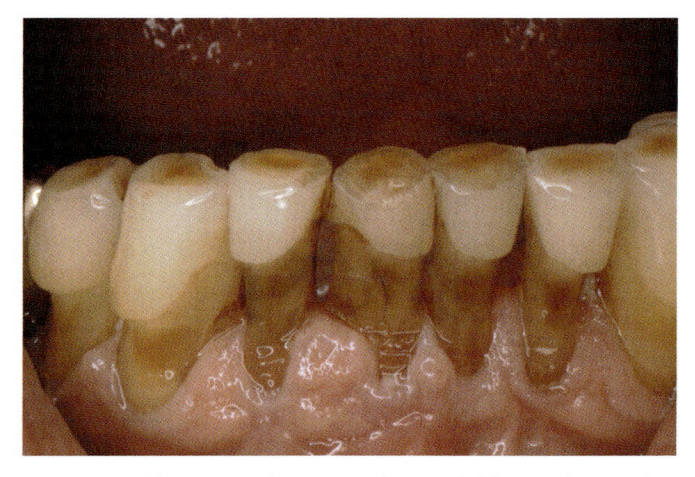

Figure 22.8 This patient shows typical signs of abfraction lesions due to his constant clenching and grinding.

forces. He stated that the forces could be static (such as those produced by swallowing and clenching) or cyclic (as in those generated during chewing action). The abfractive lesions were caused by flexure and ultimate material fatigue of susceptible teeth at locations away from the point of loading. The breakdown was dependent on the magnitude, duration, direction, frequency, and location of the forces. Sufficient experimental and clinical evidence has now been gathered to establish the primary etiology of these lesions as tensile stress of occlusal origin.[41,53–63] However, even in light of strong scientific evidence, this topic remains highly controversial.

An abfraction can be commonly found on any tooth that has an exceptionally heavy occlusal marking on an inclined plane. Abfractions are also found quite frequently on patients with slight anterior open bites for the same reason—guidance coming from the bicuspids, rather than the cuspid. The open bite is usually the result of an abnormal motor action of the tongue. If damaging lateral forces are not obvious during excursive motions, then one needs to evaluate the position and motion of the tongue. The hypothesis is basically simple and easily tested in any dental office. Abfractions are not generally found on teeth of calm, nonstressed individuals with a natural and ideal (noncrowded, nonortho) Class I occlusion. These individuals with a noncrowded natural Class I occlusion will normally have a good cuspid rise during lateral excursions. With cuspid rise, the loading forces of the excursive movement will be directed onto the cuspid. Abfractions are frequently found, however, on cases where malaligned cuspids cause initial lateral guidance forces to be exerted on the lingual incline of the buccal cusp of the first maxillary bicuspid (or whichever tooth bears the initial lateral guiding force of excursion). Dawson[45,46] described the requirements for a stable occlusion. These included: (1) having stable stops on all teeth when the condyles were in centric relation, (2) having anterior guidance in harmony with border movements of the envelope of function, and (3) disclusion of all posterior teeth in protrusive and excursive movements, including posterior teeth on the nonworking (balancing) and working side. If a tooth has an abfraction, the occlusal loading on the tooth can be tested in centric occlusion and in excursive movements with occlusal marking paper. There is a good chance that the tooth with the abfraction will have a heavy marking on one of the inclines of a cusp. This damaging lateral force produces stress lines in the tooth and results in tooth breakdown as described by Lee and Eakle.[50,64] McCoy[51,52] suggested that, to resolve the problem, the tooth needed to be reshaped. To prevent Class V abfractive restorations from falling out, however, one needs to treat the cause of the abfraction before restoring it.

As lateral and occlusal forces are generated during mastication and parafunction, flexure of the tooth occurs at the cervical fulcrum (Figure 22.9). This flexure concentrates tensile stresses that disrupt the chemical bonds of the crystalline structure of enamel and dentin. Small molecules then enter the microfractures and prevent the reformation of the chemical bonds. Loss of tooth structure ultimately occurs in the regions of concentrated stresses. After the initiation of these lesions, they may be accelerated by erosion and/or abrasion. In particular, if the lesion progresses so that dentin gets exposed, the tooth becomes highly susceptible to further mechanical and chemical wear. Thus, there are additional factors that accelerate the impact of abfraction, such as tooth brushing pressure that can enhance microfractures and reduced salivary flow and salivary quality due to xerostomia and aging that will increase the amount of food particles in contact with teeth, especially on the buccal side.[40,65]

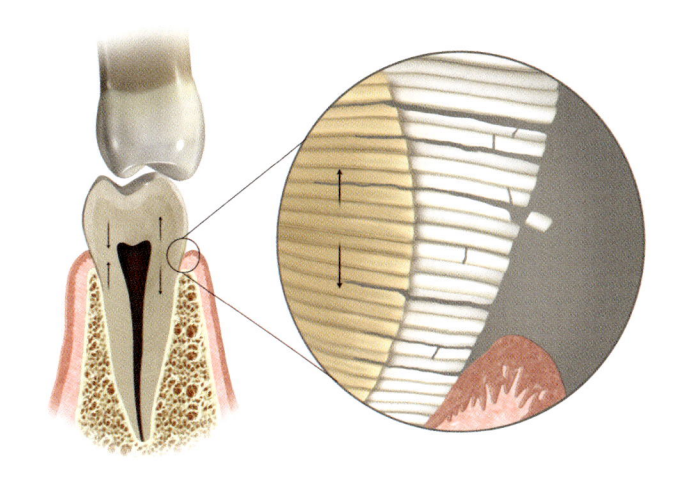

Figure 22.9 Model of tensile stress etiology of abfraction. Lateral forces create tension and compression in the cervical region, as indicated by arrows. Magnified section shows disruption of hydroxyapatite crystals of enamel and microfractures of dentin. When small molecules enter microcracks, reestablishment of chemical bonds is prevented. These areas are more susceptible to destruction from factors such as abrasion and chemical dissolution. *Source:* Reproduced with permission from Lee and Eakle.[64]

The concept of abfraction is supported only by studies conducted in vitro, where teeth were subjected to occlusal forces, while being stored in water.[39] These studies are unable to simulate the biomechanical dynamics of teeth and their supporting structures, as well as the changes that take place as teeth are exposed to the intraoral environment. The common findings of these studies suggest no differences in the location of the lesion with the direction of the forces applied, while clinically abfraction preferably occurs on the facial side rather than lingual. Furthermore, an applied force is never maintained in clinical situations. Hence, the results of in vitro studies should be interpreted with caution.

Some findings are consistent with the concept of abfraction and suggest tooth structure loss due to occlusal forces acting on the high stress cervical area. Indeed, cervical enamel is more brittle and vulnerable than occlusal enamel due to scalloping.[66] Human dentinoenamel junction (DEJ) scallop varies greatly between different tooth types, with larger and more pronounced scallops in teeth subjected to higher masticatory loads, such as molars, and anterior teeth having smaller scallops. Scalloping is the process taking place during tooth formation and is largely determined by the genetics of an individual. Thus, some people may have a stronger DEJ scallop, which provides more resistance to axial and nonaxial forces, while in others the DEJ may be more vulnerable to microcracking (Figure 22.10A–C).

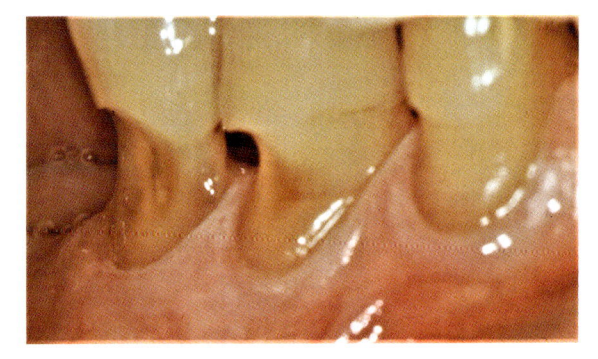

Figure 22.10 **(A)** The buccal surfaces of the mandibular teeth have lesions that possess components of both abfraction (sharp margins in the occlusal regions) and abrasion (concave geometry and gingival recession in the cervical regions).

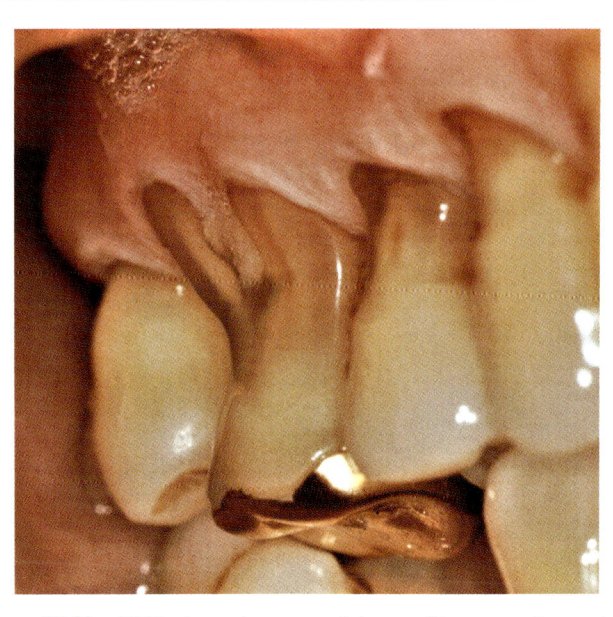

Figure 22.10 **(B)** The buccal aspects of the maxillary posterior teeth show smooth, concave configurations that are consistent with toothbrush abrasion and/or erosion.

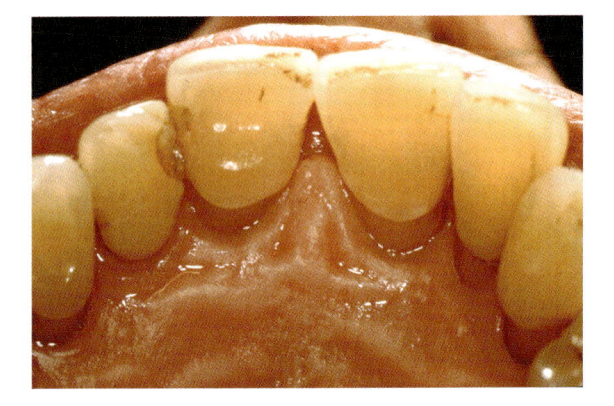

Figure 22.10 **(C)** The palatal cervical regions of the maxillary anterior teeth exhibit sharp, wedge-like lesions that are characteristic of abfraction. These areas would be difficult, if not impossible, to have resulted from toothbrush abrasion.

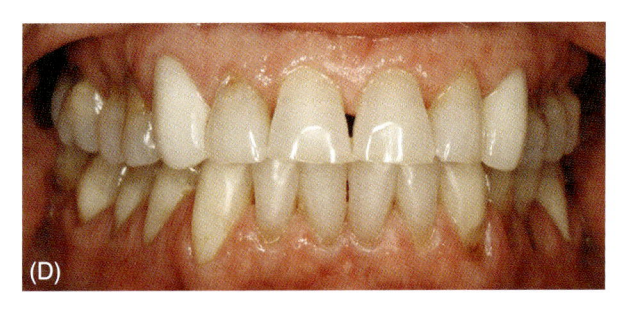

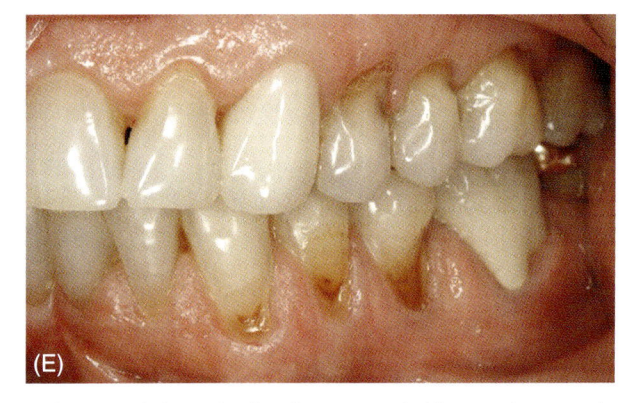

Figure 22.10 **(D, E)** This lady wanted to improve her smile because she was embarrassed about the discoloration and abfraction lesions in her teeth.

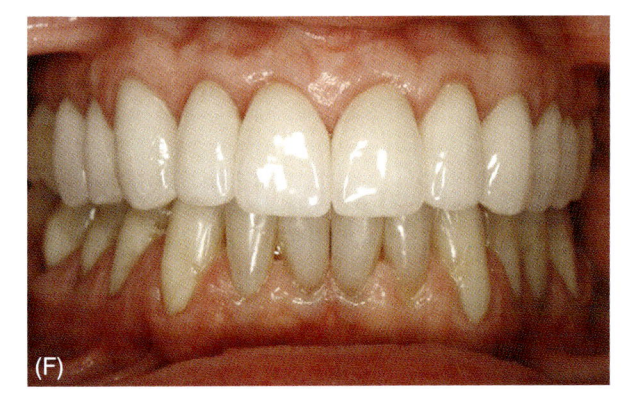

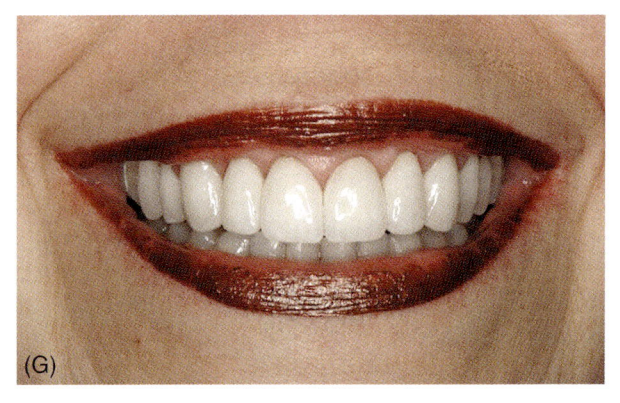

Figure 22.10 **(F, G)** All ceramic crowns and veneers were combined to restore the defects and improve the esthetics of her smile.

According to only a few clinical studies, cervical wear was related to erosion and abrasion rather than abfraction or occlusal loading.[36,39] These clinical studies were based on individual assessments and questionnaires. There is only one study that has investigated the progression of cervical lesions over time.[67] This 6-year longitudinal clinical study reported the results for 55 people with cervical wear, and the authors observed that both consumption of dietary acids and frequency of tooth brushing correlated to increased wear, suggesting synergistic effects of abfraction and abrasion or erosion.

From the clinical data combined, abfraction is unlikely to lead to cervical lesion formation independently. Instead, it may be a part of a more complex process that leads to the formation of v-shaped cervical lesions. It was suggested that mechanical microcracks on cementum and dentin may act as the initial contributor to the formation of cervical defects. Abfraction has a possibility of being the initial factor and the dominant progressive modifying factor in producing cervical lesions[68] (Figure 22.10D–G). Perhaps the best summary regarding causative factors was stated by Heymann in his excellent 2016 presentation on NCCLs at the annual meeting of the American Academy of Esthetic Dentistry.[69]

Restoration defect

When NCCLs are restored, there tends to be relatively high failure rates if the occlusal problems that initiated the lesions are not corrected. This is true for both bonded and nonbonded restorations.[47,62,70-77] Although not reported in the literature, some clinicians suspect that the occasional case of facial porcelain debonding in ceramo-metal crowns used to restore teeth with abfractions is caused by the same stresses that caused the original lesions. This apparently occurs when the facial crown margin has been placed at the same level as the apical aspect of the abfraction and the occlusal disharmony has not been corrected. Again, the key to restorative success for abfraction is control of the destructive occlusal forces that initially caused the lesions.

Glass ionomer cements (GICs), resin-modified GICs (RMGICs), a GIC/RMGIC liner/base laminated with a resin composite, resin composite in combination with a dentin bonding agent and microfilled composites, which are slightly more flexible than conventional hybrid composites, represent restorative options.[78] Problems with restoring cervical lesions include difficulty in obtaining moisture control, gaining access to subgingival margins, loss of retention, secondary caries, discoloration, and sensitivity.[78] Cervical restorations may also contribute to increased plaque accumulation, potentially leading to caries and periodontal disease.

In cases when the root surface gets exposed and the outcome is an elongated clinical crown, a soft tissue graft or coronally positioned flap are possible treatment options for improved esthetics.[79] Typically, if the loss of tooth structure is relatively deep, an advanced flap will provide the necessary thickness of healed tissue and serve as a tissue barrier against possible future breakdown from inflammation due to bacterial plaque or traumatic toothbrush/toothpaste abrasion.

To prolong the life of cervical restorations, the lateral stress issue needs to be addressed. Occlusal adjustment and/or occlusal splints can be used to reduce heavy contacts and bruxism, as well as nonaxial forces on teeth.[80]

Clinical case study 22.4

A 42-year-old man presented with a complaint related to the space between the maxillary left central and lateral incisors. He reported that the space had been present as long as he could remember, but it had increased over time. Although he was aware of the notching defect on the central incisor, he could not recall how long it had been present. The abfraction extended from the midfacial to the distolingual line angle. There was significant gingival recession, particularly on the distal aspect of the left central incisor that was accompanied by gingival inflammation and a probing defect of 4–5 mm. Further, there was a marked right shift of the dental midline and the solid contact between the maxillary and mandibular left central incisors in protrusion (Figure 22.11).

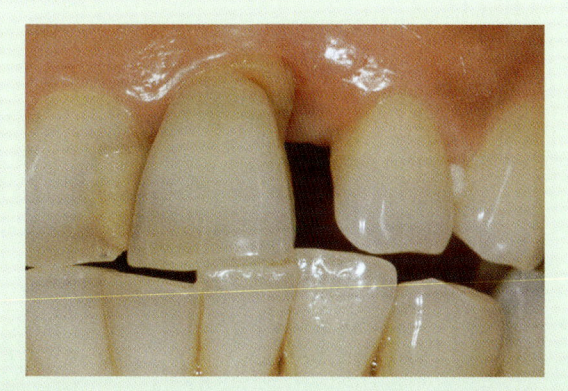

Figure 22.11 This 42-year-old man has a space between the left lateral and central incisors. It is easy to see that traumatic occlusion could have played a role in the development of the cervical lesion on the distolabial area.

Clinical case study 22.5

A 70-year-old man presented with an extreme loss of tooth structure owing to abfraction (Figure 22.12A). Figure 22.12B shows the severe nature of the abfractions on the palatal surfaces of all posterior teeth on the right side. Both molars had exposures of the pulp chambers due to abfractions. The pulp tissue in the second molar was clearly visible and vital, but the first molar was necrotic. Neither tooth was symptomatic. The maxillary left region was similarly involved. The mandibular arch also had generalized abfractions, but they were not as severe as those in the maxilla (Figure 22.12A and B).

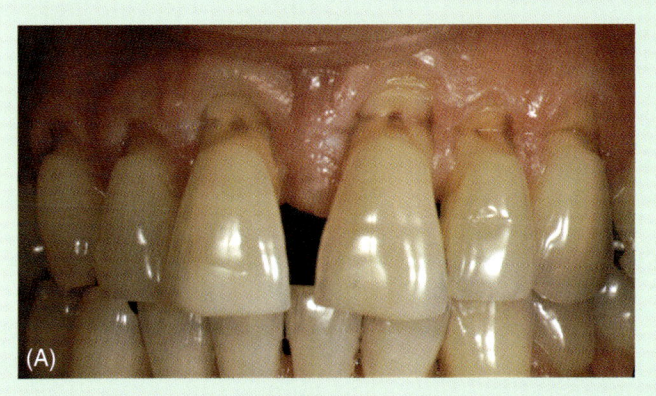

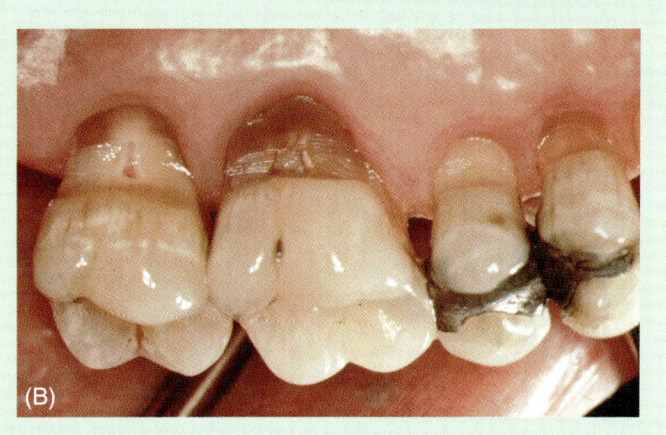

Figure 22.12 **(A, B)** These two photos are excellent examples of how extreme loss of tooth structure due to abfraction can exist and invade the pulp chamber without causing any symptoms.

Abrasion

The loss of tooth structure due to repeated mechanical contact with objects other than teeth is termed abrasion. Any object placed against the teeth can cause abrasion. If this tooth loss begins at the cemento-enamel junction, then progression of tooth loss can be rapid since enamel is very thin in this region of the tooth. Once past the enamel, abrasion quickly destroys the softer dentin and cementum structures. Evidence exists of various forms of abrasion in prehistoric populations.[81–85] A number of dental specimens recovered from the Sima de los Huesos Middle Pleistocene cave site in Spain exhibited a particular type of interproximal groove between the posterior teeth. The grooves were found only in adults and were apparently caused by the habitual probing of the interdental spaces with rigid objects (i.e., prehistoric toothpicks). Particles in the diet likely enhanced this abrasive phenomenon.[86] This same condition is seen in present-day societies. Other articles present information on various forms of tooth sharpening.[87,88]

Numerous oral habits cause abrasion; these are further discussed in Chapter 25. Examples of these habits include the localized occlusal defects in some pipe smokers who clench the pipe stem or individuals who chew on pens and pencils. Incisal notching is fairly common among seamstresses who hold pins or needles between the anterior teeth. Abrasion also can be produced by the clasps of partial dentures.[89] If teeth are worn on their occlusal surface and incisal surfaces by friction from the food bolus, this wear is termed "masticatory abrasion"[89] or "demastication." Masticatory abrasion also can occur on the facial and lingual aspects of teeth as coarse food is forced against these surfaces by the tongue, lips, and cheeks during mastication.[89] Abrasion can occur as a result of overzealous toothbrushing or improper use of dental floss. Toothbrush abrasion in particular has a characteristic appearance of a v-shaped lesion with horizontal striations from the bristles, as is most often seen on the canines and premolars. As a treatment modality, modification of the causative oral hygiene habit is important to prevent further progression. Existing defects caused by abrasion can be restored with composite resin or glass ionomers (Figure 22.13A and B). For severe abrasion that involves pulp of the tooth, root canal treatment may be needed.

The most conservative restoration of Class V defects is composite resin bonding. It generally requires little or no tooth reduction, thereby retaining as much tooth structure as possible to an already compromised tooth. A typical procedure can be seen in Figure 22.14, which shows a 45-year-old man with evidence of gingival and incisal abrasion, erosion, and abfraction. It is important to convey to patients that, by treating these types of defects as early as possible, less tooth structure is lost and more enamel is present to enable a stronger bonded restoration.

Figure 22.15A shows a 29-year-old woman who has abrasion and gingival recession confined to the anterior left segment, involving the canine and two incisors on that side. Closer examination revealed the smooth, rounded nature of the abraded areas (Figure 22.15B). Although she could not recall her specific age at the time, she reported that she was told by a hygienist that her brushing technique was improper when she was a teenager. She stated that she was instructed in brushing and flossing by this hygienist and had noted no progression of the recession since that time. For the past 8 years, she had been a patient in the same dental practice, and the clinical charting indicates that there had been no worsening of the problem. She had been informed about gingival surgery to correct the defects but has declined since she does not show her teeth when smiling.

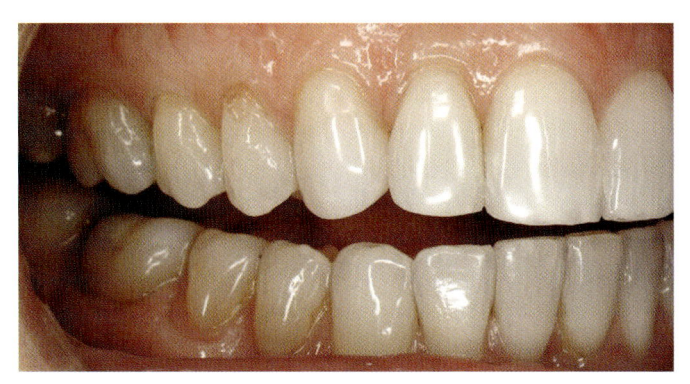

Figure 22.13 **(A)** This is an example of abrasion, most commonly seen in canines and premolars as a result of improper tooth brushing technique.

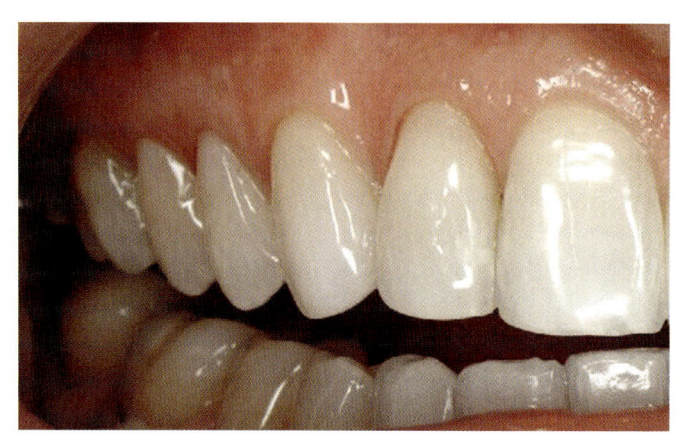

Figure 22.13 **(B)** The abrasion defect was restored using composite resin. It is important to educate the patient on proper tooth brushing technique to prevent further destruction.

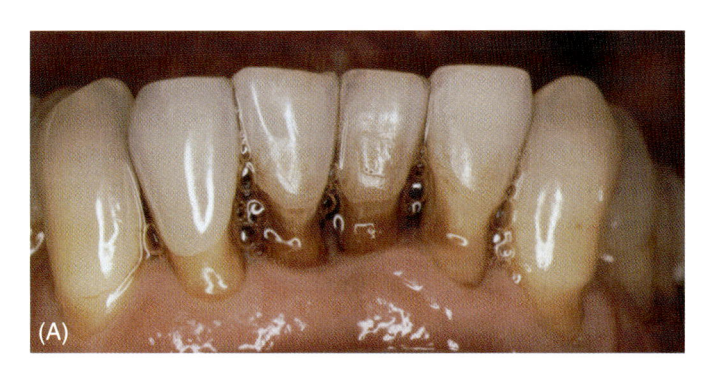

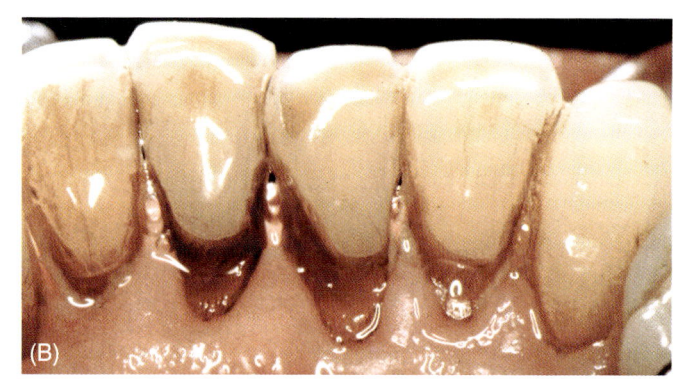

Figure 22.14 **(A, B)** This 45-year-old man shows extreme tooth loss due to combination lesions both gingivally and incisally of abrasion, erosion, and abfraction.

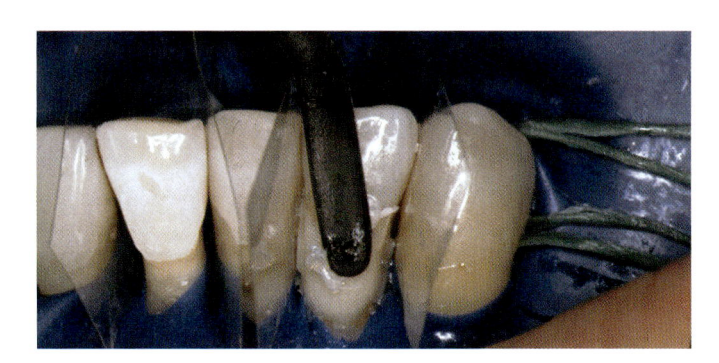

Figure 22.14 **(C)** A dentin/enamel bonding agent is applied, then a dentin/enamel resin, and finally an appropriate tooth-colored microfilled composite resin is placed using a Goldstein #3 composite instrument (Hu-Friedy, Chicago, IL).

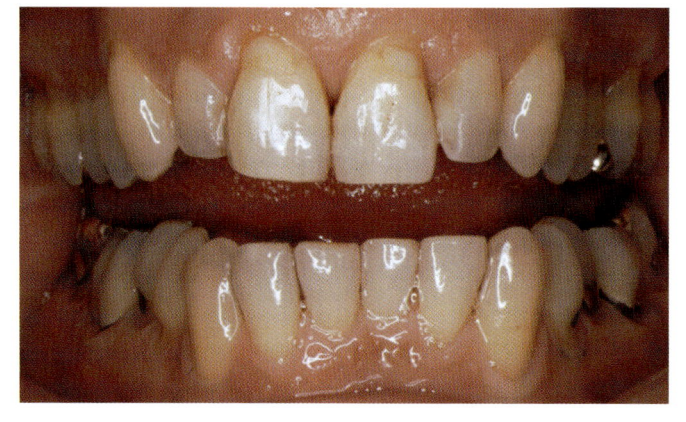

Figure 22.14 **(D)** Careful shade selection and attention to detail should produce an invisible margin. Warning: Research shows that ultrasonic scaling on teeth with Class V direct composite resin bonding may cause microleakage at the cervical margins.[123]

Erosion

Erosion is a perplexing and frustrating problem. It is defined as the noncarious loss of tooth structure due to chemical dissolution not related to acids produced by the dental plaque. Erosion can present as a solitary lesion or involve a significant number of teeth. In certain medical conditions, such as gastroesophageal reflux disease (GERD) and bulimia, the corrosive lesions have a characteristic pattern.[90-98]

There have been a number of theories regarding the etiology of erosion, and they suggest two categories: intrinsic and extrinsic causes.[89,99-104] Extrinsic causes include environmental, dietary, medication, and lifestyle factors. Chronic contact with acidic fumes in factories that produce or use acids has been cited as a

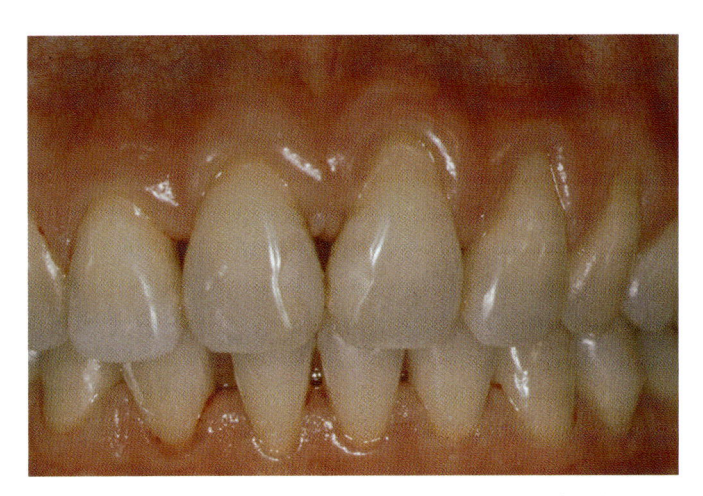

Figure 22.15 (A) A 29-year-old female with abrasion confined to the maxillary left canine and lateral and central incisors.

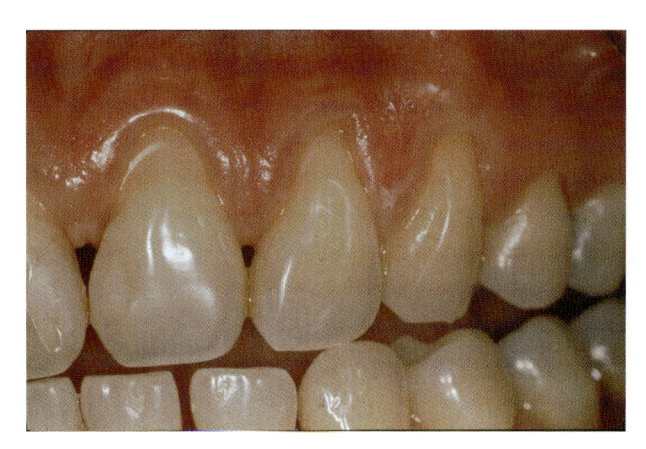

Figure 22.15 (B) Close examination reveals smooth, rounded, abraded areas that are suspected to be the result of improper brushing.

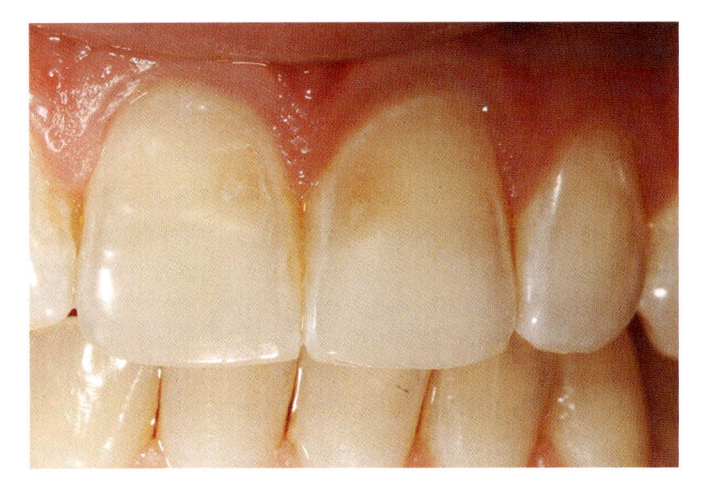

Figure 22.16 (A) This patient presented with erosion on her two central incisors but was not positive of the cause.

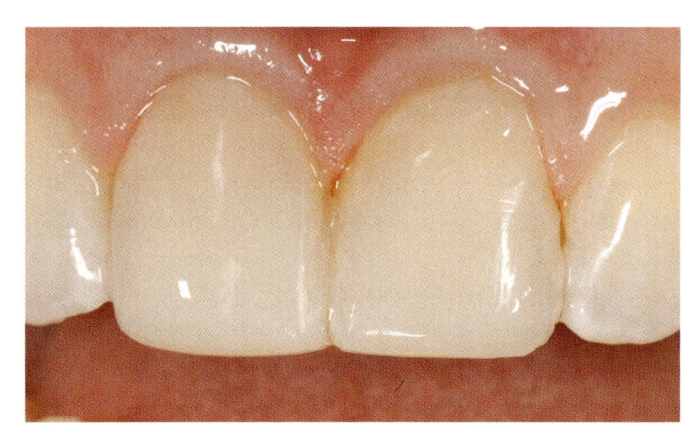

Figure 22.16 (B) The treatment of this patient consisted of direct bonding with composite resin.

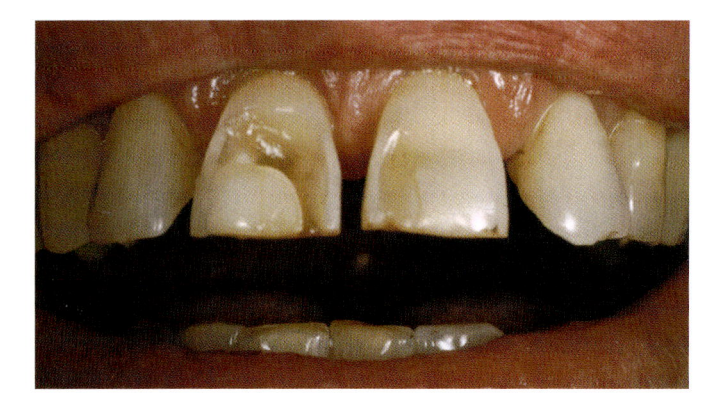

Figure 22.17 This patient had a habit of sucking lemons, which caused typical erosion patterns on her anterior upper teeth. But even after the dentist restored her tooth, she continued her habit, which caused more erosion.

notable cause of erosion.[83,105–108] Another environmental cause of erosion is prolonged swimming in pools with a low pH. Certain medications[109] and oral hygiene products have also been implicated in the development of dental erosion. It is well known that a drop in oral pH below 5.5 initiates demineralization. Salivary flow rates and the buffering capacity of saliva also affect demineralization. In addition, it has been postulated that extreme alkaline conditions promote chelation of calcium out of teeth.

Dietary factors receive widespread attention and likely affect the greatest number of people.[52] Wine has been shown to lead to erosion in wine makers,[110] wine tasters,[111] and wine merchants.[112] Carbonated soft drinks and other acidic beverages play a major role in the development of erosive lesions and dental caries.[113–118] Many patients are unaware of the damaging effects of these dietary factors (Figures 22.16 and 22.17). Tables 22.2 and 22.3 list the pH of foods and beverages that may be implicated in tooth erosion. Whether the causes are acidic foods or beverages, the frequency and time of consumption are major lifestyle factors that contribute to erosion. Before treatment, it is important to identify the destructive foods or beverages in the diet and counsel the patient on the harm that is occurring to their dentition as a result (Figure 22.18).

Treatment of these types of lesions should be done only when the causative problem is under control. Otherwise, restorations will have too short a lifespan, ending in esthetic failure. It is acceptable, however, to use provisional restorations during the corrective phase. During the corrective phase, measures should

Table 22.2 The pH Values of Acidic Beverages

Beverage	pH
Cranberry juice	2.3–2.5
Wine	2.3–3.8
Coffee	2.4–3.3
Sprite	2.6
Pepsi and Coke	2.7
Gatorade	3.3
Beer	4.0–5.0
Black Tea	4.2

Source: From Ren.[119]

Table 22.3 The pH Values of Acidic Foods

Food	pH
Lemons and limes	1.8–2.4
Pickles	2.5–3.0
Apples	2.9–3.5
Strawberries	3.0–4.2
Italian salad dressing	3.3
Tomatoes	3.7–4.7
Yogurt	3.8–4.2

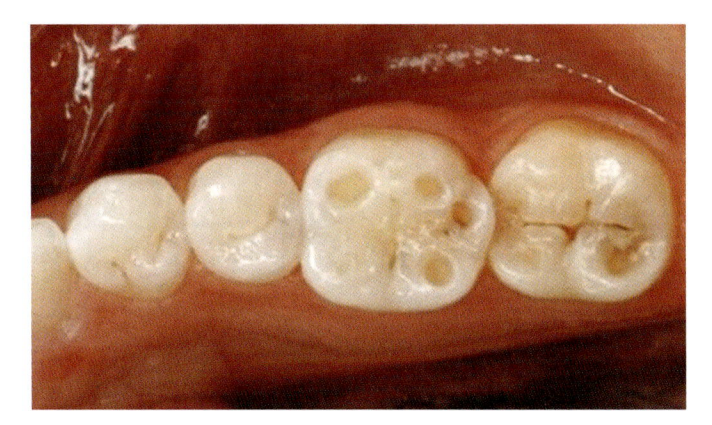

Figure 22.18 (A) This young lady presented with severe occlusal erosion.

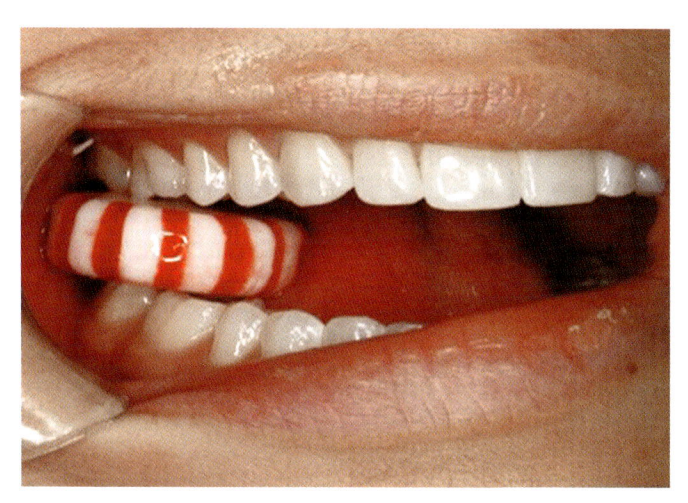

Figure 22.18 (B) When reviewing the patient's history, it was discovered that she had a habit of biting peppermint candy and holding it in place in between her posterior teeth while working at her desk.

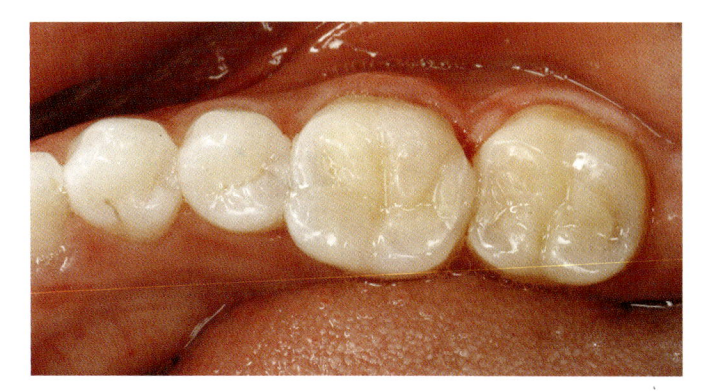

Figure 22.18 (C) The defects were prepared and restored using a microhybrid composite resin.

be taken to keep the patient comfortable (in the case of dentin hypersensitivity) and try to remineralize the teeth. The patient should drink plenty of water and modify their diet if deemed necessary. Products to promote remineralization should also be considered, such as RECALDENT (MI Paste and MI Paste Plus, GC America).

Differential diagnosis

Proper diagnosis is required to achieve successful treatment outcomes. As noted at the beginning of this chapter, patients may simultaneously have more than one of the conditions described. Thus, when occlusal or incisal changes are noted, the cervical regions of the teeth should also be closely examined. Likewise, the occlusal scheme should be fully evaluated for cervical notches or defects.

When evaluating a patient who has any of these lesions, it is necessary to correctly diagnose the condition and address the etiologic factors. Many patients with these conditions may be asymptomatic and/or unaware of them. In addition, they may have received "routine" dental care in the past and be surprised when these conditions are brought to their attention. In the case of bruxism, some patients are so surprised that they actually deny the problem. If this is the case, the best way to demonstrate to them that they have a bruxing problem is through visual images. A variety of means are available to illustrate the problem, including intraoral photographs, diagnostic study casts, surgical microscopes, and intraoral or extraoral video images. With the aid of even simple visual references, the patient can be shown the extent of the damage that has been done and how they are causing it.[120] Once the patient is convinced of the problem, the next step is attempting to determine when it is occurring. If it occurs primarily during waking hours, the patient may be able to control or correct the problem.[122] If not, you may need to construct a daytime appliance for the patient until the habit is controlled. Generally, this will consist of a removable acrylic appliance fabricated on the lower arch that will not inhibit speech. If it occurs during sleep, a nighttime appliance will be necessary to control bruxing and/or prevent further damage to the dentition.

Although some of the aforementioned mechanisms do act independently, many additive or synergistic combinations of mechanisms may occur simultaneously, sequentially, or alternatively, leading to the progression of Class V cervical lesions.[89] The possible combinations include attrition–abrasion (lateral stress due to tooth-to-tooth contact; e.g., in bruxism or clenching), abrasion–abrasion (friction from abrasive material in the area where stress concentration due to loading forces may wear tooth substance), erosion–abrasion (chemical dissolution on areas of excess stress concentration), attrition–erosion (chemical dissolution in the areas of tooth-to-tooth contact), and abrasion–erosion (action of an acid together with abrasive particles).[89] In such situations, enamel may be lost rapidly and extensively.

Clinical case study 22.6 Severe tooth erosion in a woman with history of bulimia

A 28-year-old woman had a severe bulimic condition over the course of many years (Figure 22.19A–C). After years of therapy and overcoming her illness, she desired to restore her smile. Since so much tooth structure had been eroded, it was necessary to place provisional restorations followed by crown lengthening (Figure 22.19D) and eventual replacement with the final ceramo-metal restorations (Figure 22.19E–G).

A key criterion when examining a suspected abfraction is the presence of lateral occlusal stresses during mastication or parafunctional movements. Thus, signs of attrition in the form of notable wear facets and/or loss of anterior guidance are highly probable when abfraction is present. The orientation of the long axis of the tooth in relation to occlusal loading should also be evaluated. The physical characteristics of abfraction are that of a sharp, angular defect, and these lesions may be located completely beneath the gingival margin. Abrasion in the cervical region can be usually distinguished from abfraction by the smooth, rounded nature of the lesion. Minimal to extreme gingival recession, with or without mucogingival defects, will likely accompany abrasion. Gingival recession may also be seen with abfraction, but it is not a hallmark of these defects.

A novel method of determining the progression of cervical lesions over time is to undertake a scratch test.[39] A number 12 scalpel blade is used to superficially scratch the tooth surface. Visual observation of the scratch will give an indication of the rate of the tooth structure loss. Loss of scratch definition or loss of the scratch altogether signifies active tooth structure loss. Another indicator of the factors contributing to lesion progression is the staining of teeth.[121] Stained teeth suggest that the acid erosion is inactive, whereas stain-free teeth suggest that the erosive process is taking place. The rationale behind this is that persistent acid exposure removes the outer layer of enamel or dentin, creating a stain-free surface.

Teeth that exhibit any kind of cervical lesion need to be monitored over time, and preventive measures should be taken to avoid interventive operation. These include educating the patient about proper toothbrushing technique to prevent excessive pressure and abrasion to the teeth. Dietary advice would include consuming acidic foods in moderation and, preferably, during meal times, or drinking using a straw to minimize contact between beverage and tooth surfaces to reduce dissolution of enamel. Patients should be discouraged from brushing their teeth immediately after consuming acids, but instead wait for at least 30 min, as studies have shown that the time needed for softened enamel and dentin to reharden after an erosive challenge ranges from 2 to 30 min. Fluoride treatments help to harden enamel surfaces and promotes remineralization.[121]

Dental practitioners should have a high level of suspicion when they see generalized lingual erosion of the maxillary anterior teeth. Bulimia or GERD will be the likely cause. It is important to carefully obtain a history that will allow proper diagnosis. Individuals with GERD will more readily provide information that will assist in the diagnosis. Patients who suffer from bulimia may be reluctant to reveal their condition and are sometimes outwardly defensive when questioned concerning the issues related to their eating disorder. Often, however, a dentist may be the first medical professional to recognize signs of bulimia and can be instrumental in initiating an appropriate referral to address the overall condition.

Dentists must be diligent when they examine patients. They must look beyond the routine of caries, periodontal diseases, and missing teeth and closely evaluate patients for the loss of tooth structure due to noncarious processes. When these conditions are found, dentists must take time to assess potentially interrelated conditions and perform a thorough clinical examination.

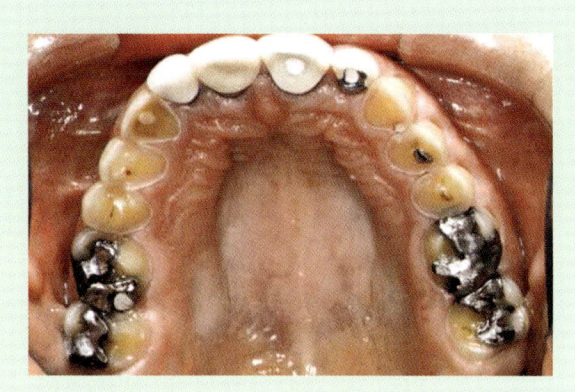

Chapter 22 Abfraction, Abrasion, Attrition, and Erosion

Figure 22.19 **(A)** Severe occlusal erosion in a woman with history of bulimia.

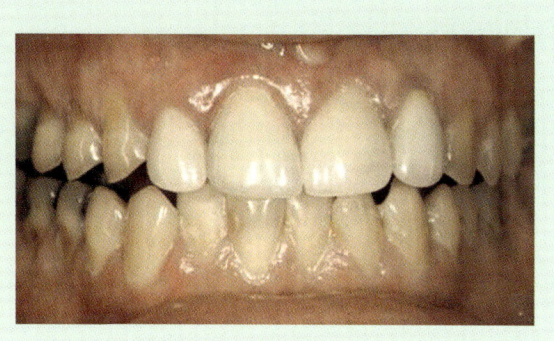

Figure 22.19 **(B)** Labial erosion also contributed to discoloration.

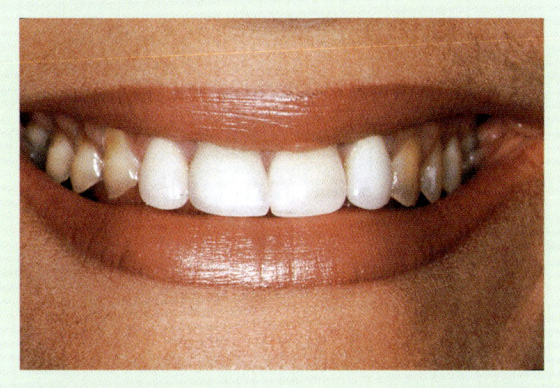

Figure 22.19 **(C)** Her smile demonstrated severe labial erosion on the posterior teeth.

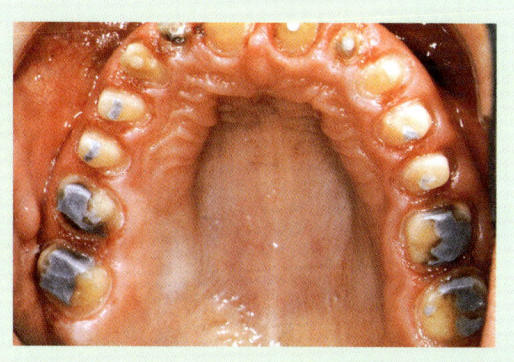

Figure 22.19 **(D)** Crown lengthening and buildups with composite resin were necessary before making the impressions for the final restorations.

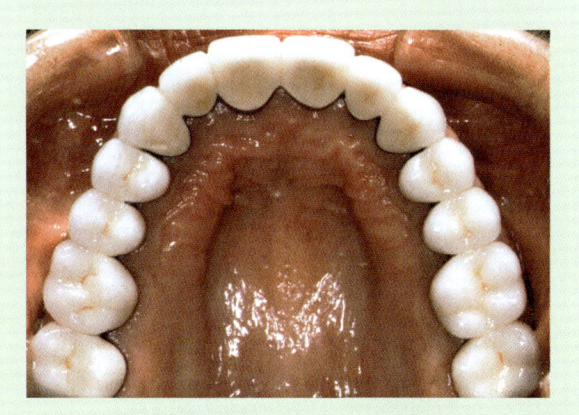

Figure 22.19 **(E)** The final splinted restorations were constructed using ceramo-metal.

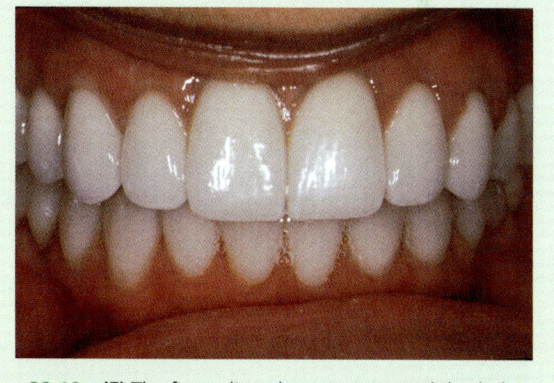

Figure 22.19 **(F)** The five splinted crowns restored this lady's smile. Note the lighter shade the patient selected.

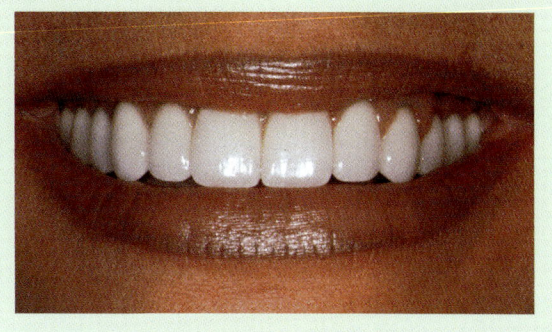

Figure 22.19 **(G)** The new, improved shapes and shade helped to achieve the smile the patient desired.

Discovering and helping to identify destructive habits, such as bruxism, needs to be a team effort. Frequently, the dental hygienist or assistant can be the observant individual who calls attention to a potential problem before it becomes an esthetic deformity. Team educational meetings are useful in teaching staff exactly what signs to observe. Knowing the correct anatomy of anterior and posterior teeth is of considerable value in being able to recognize even minor cusp or incisal edge changes that are a result of bruxism. Thus, the esthetics of the patient's smile not only depends on good oral hygiene but also becomes a shared team responsibility to keep it looking as good as possible throughout life.

References

1. Seow WK. Clinical diagnosis of enamel defects: pitfalls and practical guidelines. *Int Dent J* 1997;47:173–182.
2. Young WG. Anthropology, tooth wear, and occlusion ab origine. *J Dent Res* 1998;77:1860–1863.
3. Begg PR. Stone Age man's dentition. *Am J Orthod* 1954;40:298–312.
4. Begg PR. Stone Age man's dentition. *Am J Orthod* 1954;40:373–383.
5. Begg PR. Stone Age man's dentition. *Am J Orthod* 1954;40:462–475.
6. Begg PR. Stone Age man's dentition. *Am J Orthod* 1954;40:517–531.
7. Barrett MJ. Functioning occlusion. *Ann Aust Coll Dent Surg* 1969;2:68–80.
8. Barrett MJ. Dental observations on Australian aborigines. Continuously changing functional occlusion. *Aust Dent J.* 1958;58:39–52.
9. Langsjoen OM. Dental effects of diet and coca-leaf chewing on two prehistoric cultures of northern Chile. *Am J Phys Anthropol* 1996;101:475–489.
10. Kerr NW. Dental pain and suffering prior to the advent of modern dentistry. *Br Dent J* 1998;184:397–399.
11. Vallitu PK, Vallitu AS, Lassila VP. Dental aesthetics—a survey of attitudes in different groups of patients. *J Dent.* 1996;24:335–338.
12. Abreu Tabarini HS. Dental attrition of Mayan Tzu-tujil children—a study based on longitudinal materials. *Bull Tokyo Med Dent Univ* 1995;42:31–50.
13. Bartlett DW, Coward PY, Nikkah C, Wilson RF. The prevalence of tooth wear in a cluster sample of adolescent schoolchildren and its relationship with potential explanatory factors. *Br Dent J* 1998;184:125–129.
14. Hugoson A, Ekfeldt A, Koch G, Hallonsten AL. Incisal and occlusal tooth wear in children and adolescents in a Swedish population. *Acta Odontol Scand* 1996;54:263–270.
15. Millward A, Shaw L, Smith AJ, et al. The distribution and severity of tooth wear and the relationship between erosion and dietary constituents in a group of children. *Int J Paediatr Dent* 1994;4:151–157.
16. Milosevic A, Lennon MA, Fear SC. Risk factors associated with tooth wear in teenagers: a case control study. *Community Dent Health* 1997;14:143–147.
17. Nystrom M, Kononen M, Alaluusua S, et al. Development of horizontal tooth wear in maxillary anterior teeth from five to 18 years of age. *J Dent Res* 1990;69:1765–1770.
18. Silness J, Berge M, Johannessen G. Longitudinal study of incisal tooth wear in children and adolescents. *Eur J Oral Sci* 1995;103:90–94.
19. Silness J, Berge M, Johannessen G. Re-examination of incisal tooth wear in children and adolescents. *J Oral Rehabil* 1997;24:405–409.
20. Donachie MA, Walls AW. The tooth wear index: a flawed epidemiological tool in an aging population group. *Community Dent Oral Epidemiol* 1996;24:152–158.
21. Healy WB. Soils and dental research. *N Z Dent J* 1998;94:114.
22. Touminen M, Touminen R. Tooth surface loss among people exposed to cement and stone dust in the work environment in Tanzania. *Community Dent Health* 1991;8:233–238.
23. Bauer W, van den Hoven F, Diedrich P. Wear in the upper and lower incisors in relation to incisal and condylar guidance. *J Orofac Orthop* 1997;58:306–319.
24. Bishop KA, Briggs PF, Kelleher MG. Modern restorative management of advanced tooth-surface loss. *Prim Dent Care* 1994;1:20–23.
25. Da Silva AM, Oakley DA, Hemmings KW, et al. Psychosocial factors and tooth wear with a significant component of attrition. *Eur J Prosthodont Restor Dent* 1997;5:51–55.
26. Hudson JD, Goldstein GR, Georgescu M. Enamel wear caused by three different restorative materials. *J Prosthet Dent* 1995;74:647–654.
27. Jagger DC, Harrison A. An in vitro investigation into the wear effects of selected restorative materials on enamel. *J Oral Rehabil* 1995;22:275–281.
28. Jagger DC, Harrison A. An in vitro investigation into the wear effects of selected restorative materials on dentine. *J Oral Rehabil* 1995;22:349–354.
29. Kelleher M, Bishop K. The aetiology and clinical appearance of tooth wear. *Eur J Prosthodont Restor Dent* 1997;5:157–160.
30. Mair LH, Stolarski TA, Vowles RW, Lloyd CH. Wear: mechanisms, manifestations and measurement. Report of a workshop. *J Dent* 1996;24:141–148.
31. Mayhall JT, Kageyama I. A new, three-dimensional method for determining tooth wear. *Am J Phys Anthropol* 1997;103:463–469.
32. Richards LC, Miller SL. Relationships between age and dental attrition in Australian aboriginals. *Am J Phys Anthropol* 1991;84:159–164.
33. Ritchard A, Welsh AH, Donnelly C. The association between occlusion and attrition. *Aust Orthod J* 1992;12:138–142.
34. Shaw L. The epidemiology of tooth wear. *Eur J Prosthodont Restor Dent* 1997;5:153–156.
35. Smith BG, Robb ND. The prevalence of toothwear in 1007 dental patients. *J Oral Rehabil* 1996;23:232–239.
36. Kim JW, Simmer JP. Hereditary dentin defects. *J Dent Res* 2007;86:392–399.
37. Smith BG, Knight JK. A comparison of patterns of tooth wear with aetiological factors. *Br Dent J* 1984;157:16–19.
38. Khan F, Young WG, Daley TJ. Dental erosion and bruxism. A tooth wear analysis from south east Queensland. *Aust Dent J* 1998;43:117–127.
39. Michael JA, Townsend GC, Greenwood LF, Kaidonis JA. Abfraction: separating fact from fiction. *Aust Dent J* 2009;54:2–8.
40. Takehara T, Takano T, Akhter R, Morita M. Correlations of non-carious cervical lesions and occlusal factors determined by using pressure-detecting sheet. *J Dent* 2008;36(10):774–779.

41. Lavigne GJ, Rompre PH, Montplaisir JY. Sleep bruxism: validity of clinical research diagnostic criteria in a controlled polysomnographic study. *J Dent Res* 1996;75:546–552.
42. Tsolka P, Walter JD, Wilson RF, Preiskel HW. Occlusal variable, bruxism and temporomandibular disorders: a clinical and kinesiographic assessment. *J Oral Rehabil* 1995;22:849–856.
43. Turner KA, Missirlian DM. Restoration of the extremely worn dentition. *J Prosthet Dent* 1984;52(4):467–474.
44. Nel JC, Marais JT, van Vuuren PA. Various methods of achieving restoration of tooth structure loss due to bruxism. *J Esthet Dent* 1996;8:183–188.
45. Dawson PE. *Evaluation, Diagnosis, and Treatment of Occlusal Problems*. St. Louis, MO: CV Mosby; 1989.
46. Dawson PE. *Functional Occlusion: From TMJ to Smile Design*. St. Louis, MO: CV Mosby; 2007.
47. Douglas WH. Form, function and strength in the restored dentition. *Ann R Australas Coll Dent Surg* 1996;13:35–46.
48. Kokich VG. Esthetics and vertical tooth position: orthodontic possibilities. *Compend Cont Educ Dent* 1997;18:1225–1231.
49. Radentz WH, Barnes GP, Cutright DE. A survey of factors possibly associated with cervical abrasion of tooth surfaces. *J Periodontol* 1976;47:148–154.
50. Lee WC, Eakle WS. Possible role of tensile stress in the etiology of cervical erosive lesions of teeth. *J Prosthet Dent* 1984;52:374–380.
51. McCoy G. The etiology of gingival erosion. *J Oral Implantol* 1982;10:361–362.
52. McCoy G. On the longevity of teeth. *J Oral Implantol* 1983;11:248–267.
53. Bader JD, McClure F, Scurria MS, et al. Case–control study of non-carious cervical lesions. *Community Dent Oral Epidemiol* 1996;24:286–291.
54. Bevenius J, L'Estrange P, Karlsson S, Carlsson GE. Idiopathic cervical lesions: In vivo investigation by oral microendoscopy and scanning electron microscopy. A pilot study. *J Oral Rehabil* 1993;20:1–9.
55. Braem M, Lambrechts P, Vanherle G. Stress-induced cervical lesions. *J Prosthet Dent* 1992;67:718–722.
56. Dawid E, Meyer G, Schwartz P. The etiology of wedge-shaped defects: a morphological and function-oriented investigation. *J Gnathol* 1991;10:49–56.
57. Goel VK, Khera SC, Ralston JL, Chang KH. Stresses at the dentinoenamel junction of human teeth—a finite element investigation. *J Prosthet Dent* 1991;66:451–459.
58. Grippo JO. Abfractions: a new classification of hard tissue lesions of teeth. *J Esthet Dent* 1991;3:14–19.
59. Grippo JO. Bioengineering seeds of contemplation: a private practitioner's perspective. *Dent Mater* 1996;12:198–202.
60. Grippo JO, Simring M. Dental "erosion" revisited. *J Am Dent Assoc* 1991;122:41–47.
61. Levitch LC, Bader JD, Shugars DA, Heymann HO. Non-carious cervical lesions. *J Dent* 1994;22:195–207.
62. Powell LV, Johnson GH, Gordon GE. Factors associated with clinical success of cervical abrasion/erosion restorations. *Oper Dent* 1995;20:7–13.
63. Spranger H. Investigation into the genesis of angular lesions at the cervical region of teeth. *Quintessence Int* 1995;26:183–188.
64. Lee WC, Eakle WS. Stress-induced cervical lesions: review of advances in the past 10 years. *J Prosthet Dent* 1996;75:487–494.
65. McComb D, Erickson RL, Maxymiw WG, Wood RE. A clinical comparison of glass ionomer, resin-modified glass ionomer and resin composite restorations in the treatment of cervical caries in xerostomic head and neck radiation patients. *Oper Dent* 2002;27(5):430–437.
66. Brauer DS, Marshall GW, Marshall SJ. Variations in human DEJ scallop size with tooth type. *J Dent* 2010;38:597–601.
67. Lussi A, Schaffner M. Progression of and risk factors for dental erosion and wedge-shaped defects over a 6-year period. *Caries Res* 2000;34:182–187.
68. Hanaoka K, Nagao D, Mitusi K, et al. A biomechanical approach to the etiology and treatment of non-carious dental cervical lesions. *Bull Kanagawa Dent Coll* 1998;26(2):103–111.
69. Heymann HO. Etiology and treatment of non-carious cervical lesions: counterpoint. Presented at: *Point Counterpoint: The Controversies & Innovations in Esthetic Dentistry*, AEED 41st Annual Meeting, August 3–5, 2016, Monarch Beach Resort, Dana Point, CA.
70. Boghosian A. Clinical evaluation of a filled adhesive system in Class 5 restorations. *Compend Cont Educ Dent* 1996;17:750–757.
71. Grippo JO. Noncarious cervical lesions: the decision to ignore or restore. *J Esthet Dent* 1992;4(Suppl):55–64.
72. Heymann HO, Sturdevant JR, Bayne S, et al. Examining tooth flexure effects on cervical restorations: a two year clinical study. *J Am Dent Assoc* 1991;122:41–47.
73. Horsted-Bindslev P, Knudsen J, Baelum V. 3-year clinical evaluation of modified Gluma adhesive systems in cervical abrasion/erosion lesions. *Am J Dent* 1996;9:22–26.
74. Matis BA, Cochran M, Carlson T. Longevity of glass-ionomer restorative materials: results of a 10-year evaluation. *Quintessence Int* 1996;27:373–382.
75. Miller MB. Restoring class V lesions. Part 2: abfraction lesions. *Pract Periodont Aesthet Dent* 1997;9:505–506.
76. Neo J, Chew CL. Direct tooth-colored materials for noncarious lesions: a 3-year clinical report. *Quintessence Int* 1995;27:183–188.
77. Osborne-Smith KL, Burke FJ, Farlane TM, Wilson NH. Effect of restored and unrestored non-carious cervical lesions on the fracture resistance of previously restored maxillary premolar teeth. *J Dent* 1998;26:427–433.
78. Bartlett DW, Shah P. A critical review of non-carious cervical wear lesions and the role of abfraction, erosion and abrasion. *J Dent Res*. 2006;85:306–312.
79. Hempton TJ, Ovadia R, McManama JC, Bonacci FJ. Addressing cervical class V lesions. *Dimens Dent Hyg* 2010:8(3):48–51.
80. Carre C, Brunton PA. *A Study of Occlusal Factors in Relation to Restoration of Non-Carious Cervical Lesions with Resin Composite* [MPhil thesis]. University of Manchester; 2003.
81. Alexandersen V, Noren JG, Hoyer I, et al. Aspects of teeth from archeological sites in Sweden and Denmark. *Acta Odontol Scand* 1998;56:14–19.
82. Borrman H, Engstrom EU, Alexandersen V, et al. Dental conditions and temporomandibular joints in an early Mesolithic bog man. *Swed Dent J* 1996;20:1–14.
83. Chikte UM, Josie-Perez AM, Cohen TL. Industrial dental erosion—a case report. *J Dent Assoc S Afr* 1996;51:647–650.
84. Frayer DW. On the etiology of interproximal grooves. *Am J Phys Anthropol* 1991;85:299–304.
85. Villa G, Giacobini G. Subvertical grooves of interproximal facets in Neanderthal posterior teeth. *Am J Phys Anthropol* 1995;96:51–62.
86. Bermudez de Castro JM, Arsuaga JL, Perez PJ. Interproximal grooving in the Atapuerca-SH hominid dentitions. *Am J Phys Anthropol* 1997;102:369–376.
87. Murray CG, Sanson GD. Thegosis—a critical review. *Aust Dent J* 1998;43:192–198.
88. Ungar PS, Fennell KJ, Gordon K, Trinkaus E. Neanderthal incisor beveling. *J Hum Evol* 1997;32:407–421.

89. Grippo JO, Simring M, Schreiner S. Attrition, abrasion, corrosion and abfraction revisited. A new perspective on tooth surface lesions. *J Am Dent Assoc* 2004;135:1109–1118.
90. Bartlett DW, Evans DF, Smith BG. The relationship between gastro-oesophageal reflux disease and dental erosion. *J Oral Rehabil* 1996;23:289–297.
91. Bartlett DW, Smith BG. The dental impact of eating disorders. *Dent Update* 1994;21:404–407.
92. Bouquot JE, Seime RJ. Bulimia nervosa: dental perspectives. *Pract Periodont Aesthet Dent* 1997;9:655–663.
93. Evans RD, Briggs PF. Tooth-surface loss related to pregnancy-induced vomiting. *Prim Dent Care* 1994;1:24–26.
94. Nunn JH. Prevalence of dental erosion and the implications for oral health. *Eur J Oral Sci* 1996;104:156–161.
95. O'Sullivan EA, Curzon ME, Roberts GJ, et al. Gastroesophageal reflux in children and its relationship to erosion of primary and permanent teeth. *Eur J Oral Sci* 1998;106:765–769.
96. Ruffs JC, Koch MO, Perkins S. Bulimia: dentomedical complications. *Gen Dent* 1992;40:22–25.
97. Rytomaa I, Jarvinen V, Kanerva R, Heinonen OP. Bulimia and tooth erosion. *Acta Odontol Scand* 1998;56:36–40.
98. Yettram AL, Wright KWJ, Rickard HM. Finite element stress analysis of the crowns of normal and restored teeth. *J Dent Res* 1976;55:1004–1011.
99. Bartlett DW. The causes of dental erosion. *Oral Dis* 1997;3:209–211.
100. Grenby TH. Methods of assessing erosion and erosive potential. *Eur J Oral Sci* 1996;104:207–214.
101. Imfeld T. Dental erosion. Definition, classification and links. *Eur J Oral Sci* 1996;104:151–154.
102. Jarvinen VK, Rytomaa II, Heinonen OP. Risk factors in dental erosion. *J Dent Res* 1991;70:942–947.
103. Lussi A, Schaffner M, Hotz P, Suter P. Dental erosion in a population of Swiss adults. *Community Dent Oral Epidemiol* 1991;19:286–290.
104. Ten Cate JM, Imfeld T. Dental erosion, summary. *Eur J Oral Sci* 1996;104:241–244.
105. Chikte UM, Josie-Perez AM, Cohen TL. A rapid epidemiological assessment of dental erosion to assist in settling an industrial dispute. *J Dent Assoc S Afr* 1998;53:7–12.
106. Touminen M, Touminen R. Dental erosion and associated factors among factory workers exposed to inorganic acid fumes. *Proc Finn Dent Soc* 1991;87:359–364.
107. Touminen M, Touminen R. Tooth surface loss and associated factors among factory workers in Finland and Tanzania. *Community Dent Health* 1992;9:143–150.
108. Touminen ML, Touminen RJ, Fubusa F, Mgalula N. Tooth surface loss and exposure to organic and inorganic acid fumes in workplace air. *Community Dent Oral Epidemiol* 1991;19:217–220.
109. Lussi A, Portmann P, Burhop B. Erosion on abraded dental hard tissues by acid lozenges: an in situ study. *Clin Oral Investig* 1997;1:191–194.
110. Ferguson MM, Dunbar RJ, Smith JA, Wall JG. Enamel erosion related to winemaking. *Occup Med* 1996;46:159–162.
111. Wiktorsson AM, Zimmerman M, Angmar-Mansson B. Erosive tooth wear: prevalence and severity in Swedish winetasters. *Eur J Oral Sci* 1997;105:544–550.
112. Chaudhry SI, Harris JL, Challacombe SJ. Dental erosion in a wine merchant: an occupational hazard? *Br Dent J* 1997;182:226–228.
113. Al-Hiyasat AS, Saunders WP, Sharkey SW, Smith GM. The effect of a carbonated beverage on the wear of human enamel and dental ceramics. *J Prosthodont* 1998;7:2–12.
114. Gedalia I, Dakuar A, Shapira L, et al. Enamel softening with Coca-Cola and rehardening with milk or saliva. *Am J Dent* 1991;4:120–122.
115. Harrison JL, Roeder LB. Dental erosion caused by cola beverages. *Gen Dent* 1991;39:23–24.
116. Johansson AK, Johansson A, Birkhead D, et al. Dental erosion associated with soft-drink consumption in young Saudi men. *Acta Odontol Scand* 1997;55:390–397.
117. Lussi A, Jaeggi T, Jaeggi-Scharer S. Prediction of the erosive potential of some beverages. *Caries Res* 1995;29:349–354.
118. Touyz LZ. The acidity (pH) and buffering capacity of Canadian fruit juice and dental implications. *J Can Dent Assoc* 1994;60:454–448.
119. Ren Y-F. Dental erosion: etiology, diagnosis, and prevention. *RDH Mag* 2011;(August):75–84. http://rdhmag.com/etc/medialib/new-lib/rdh/site-images/volume-31/issue-8/1108RDH075-085.pdf (accessed October 11, 2017).
120. Cook DA. Using crayons to educate patients about front-tooth wear patterns. *J Am Dent Assoc* 1998;129:1149–1150.
121. Bartlett DW, Smith BGN. Definition, classification and clinical assessment of attrition, erosion and abrasion of enamel and dentine. In: Addy M, Embery G, Edgar WM, Orchardson R (Eds.), *Tooth Wear and Sensitivity: Clinical Advances in Restorative Dentistry*. London: Martin Dunitz; 2000:87–93.
122. Goldstein RE, Auclair Clark W. The clinical management of awake bruxism. *J Am Dent Assoc* 2017 Jun;148(6):387–391.
123. Goldstein RE, Lamba S, Lawson NC, Beck P, Oster RA, Burgess JO. Microleakage around Class V Composite Restorations after Ultrasonic Scaling and Sonic Toothbrushing around their Margin. *J Esthet Restor Dent* 2017 Jan-Feb;29(1): 41–48.

Additional resources

Abdullah A, Sherfudhin H, Omar R, Johansson A. Prevalence of occlusal tooth wear and its relationship to lateral and protrusive contact schemes in a young adult Indian population. *Acta Odontol Scand* 1994;52:191–197.

Abe S, Yamaguchi T, Rompre P.H., et al. Tooth wear in young subjects: a discriminator between sleep bruxers and controls? *Int J Prosthodont* 2009;22:342–350.

Ahmed SN, Donovan TE. Dental erosion: the unrecognized epidemic. *J Esthet Restor Dent* 2015;27(3):119–121.

Alghilan MA, Cook NB, Platt JA, et al. Susceptibility of restorations and adjacent enamel/dentine to erosion under different salivary flow conditions. *J Dent* 2015;43:1476–1482.

Al-Hiyasat AS, Saunders WP, Sharkey SW, et al. The abrasive effect of glazed, unglazed, and polished porcelain on the wear of human enamel, and the influence of carbonated soft drinks on the rate of wear. *Int J Prosthodont* 1997;10:269–282.

Al-Hiyasat AS, Saunders WP, Sharkey SW, et al. Investigation of human enamel wear against four dental ceramics and gold. *J Dent* 1998;26:487–495.

Altshuler BD. Eating disorder patients. Recognition and intervention. *J Dent Hyg* 1990;64:119–125.

Attin T, Koidl U, Buchalla W, et al. Correlations of microhardness and wear in differently eroded bovine dental enamel. *Arch Oral Biol* 1997;42:243–250.

Attin T, Zirkel C, Hellwig E. Brushing abrasion of eroded dentin after application of sodium fluoride solutions. *Caries Res* 1998;32:344–350.

Bartlett DW, Ricketts DN, Fisher NL. Management of the short clinical crown by indirect restorations. *Dent Update* 1997;24:431–436.

Becker W, Ochsenbein C, Becker BE. Crown lengthening: the periodontal–restorative connection. *Compend Cont Educ Dent* 1998;19:239–240, 242, 244–246.

Beckett H. Dental abrasion caused by a cobalt–chromium denture base. *Eur J Prosthodont Restor Dent* 1995;3:209–210.

Berge M, Johannessen G, Silness J. Relationship between alignment conditions of teeth in anterior segments and incisal wear. *J Oral Rehabil* 1996;23:717–721.

Bishop K, Bell M, Briggs P, Kelleher M. Restoration of a worn dentition using a double-veneer technique. *Br Dent J* 1996;180:26–29.

Bishop K, Kelleher M, Briggs P, Joshi R. Wear now? An update on the etiology of tooth wear. *Quintessence Int* 1997;28:305–313.

Blair FM, Thomason JM, Smith DG. The traumatic anterior overbite. *Dent Update* 1997;24:144–152.

Bohmer CJ, Klinkenberg-Knol EC, Niezen-de Boer MC, et al. Dental erosions and gastro-oesophageal reflux disease in institutionalized intellectually disabled individuals. *Oral Dis* 1997;3:272–275.

Bowles WH, Wilkinson MR, Wagner MJ, Woody RD. Abrasive particles in tobacco products: a possible factor in dental attrition. *J Am Dent Assoc* 1995;126:327–331.

Brady JM, Woody RD. Scanning microscopy of cervical erosion. *J Am Dent Assoc* 1977;94:726–729.

Briggs P, Bishop K. Fixed prostheses in the treatment of tooth wear. *Eur J Prosthodont Restor Dent* 1997;5:175–180.

Briggs PF, Bishop K, Djemal S. The clinical evolution of the "Dahl principle". *Br Dent J* 1997;183:171–176.

Brown S, Bonifazi DZ. An overview of anorexia and bulimia nervosa, and the impact of eating disorders on the oral cavity. *Compend Cont Educ Dent* 1993;14:1594, 1596–1602, 1604–1608.

Burke FJ, Whitehead SA, McCaughey AD. Contemporary concepts in the pathogenesis of the Class V non-carious lesion. *Dent Update* 1995;22:28–32.

Čalić A. Peterlin B. Epigenetics and bruxism: possible role of epigenetics in the etiology of bruxism. *Int J Prosthodont*. 2015;28(6):594–599.

Caneppele TM, Jeronymo RD, Di Nicolo R, et al. In vitro assessment of dentin erosion after immersion in acidic beverages: surface profile analysis and energy-dispersive X-ray fluorescence spectrometry study. *Braz Dent J* 2012;23:373–378.

Carlson-Mann LD. Recognition and management of occlusal disease from a hygienist's perspective. *Probe* 1996;30:196–197.

Darbar UR, Hemmings KW. Treatment of localized anterior toothwear with composite restorations at an increased occlusal vertical dimension. *Dent Update* 1997;24:72–75 [erratum: *Dent Update* 1997;24:157].

Donachie MA, Walls AW. Assessment of tooth wear in an ageing population. *J Dent* 1995;23:157–164.

Douglas WH. Considerations for modeling. *Dent Mater* 1996;12:203–207.

Evans RD. Orthodontics and the creation of localised inter-occlusal space in cases of anterior tooth wear. *Eur J Prosthodont Restor Dent* 1997;5:69–73.

Formicola V. Interproximal grooving: different appearances, different etiologies. *Am J Phys Anthropol* 1991;86:85–87.

Gladys S, Van Meerbeek B, Lambrechts P, Vanherle G. Marginal adaptation and retention of a glass-ionomer, resin-modified glass-ionomers and a polyacid-modified resin composite in cervical class-V lesions. *Dent Mater* 1998;14:294–306.

Goldstein RE. *Esthetics in Dentistry*. Philadelphia, PA: Lippincott; 1976:162–174.

Goldstein RE. Current concepts in esthetic treatment. In: *Proceedings of the Second International Prosthodontic Congress*, Los Angeles, CA. Chicago: Quintessence, 1979:310–312.

Goldstein RE. Esthetics in dentistry. *J Am Dent Assoc* 1982;104:301–302.

Goldstein RE. Diagnostic dilemma: to bond, laminate, or crown? *Int J Periodont Restor Dent* 1987;87(5):9–30.

Goldstein RE. Finishing of composites and laminates. *Dent Clin North Am* 1989;33:305–318.

Goldstein RE, Feinman RA, Garber DA. Esthetic considerations in the selection and use of restorative materials. *Dent Clin North Am* 1983;27:723–731.

Goldstein RE, Garber DA, Schwartz CG, Goldstein CE. Patient maintenance of esthetic restorations. *J Am Dent Assoc* 1992;123:61–66.

Goldstein RE, Garber DA, Goldstein CE, et al. The changing esthetic dental practice. *J Am Dent Assoc* 1994;125:1447–1457.

Gregory-Head B, Curtis DA. Erosion caused by gastroesophageal reflux: diagnostic considerations. *J Prosthodont* 1997;6:278–285.

Hacker CH, Wagner WC, Razzoog ME. An in vitro investigation of the wear of enamel on porcelain and gold in saliva. *J Prosthet Dent* 1996;75:14–17.

Haines DJ, Berry DC, Poole DFG. Behavior of tooth enamel under load. *J Dent Res* 1963;42:885–888.

Hasselkvist A, Johansson A, Johansson AK. A 4 year prospective longitudinal study of progression of dental erosion associated to lifestyle in 13–14 year-old Swedish adolescents. *J Dent* 2016;47:55–62.

Hazelton LR, Faine MP. Diagnosis and dental management of eating disorder patients. *Int J Prosthodont* 1996;9:65–73.

Hood JA. Biomechanics of the intact, prepared and restored tooth: some clinical implications. *Int Dent J* 1991;41:25–32.

Ichim I, Loughran J, Swain MV, Kieser J. Restoration of non-carious cervical lesions. Part 1. Modelling of restorative fracture. *Dent Mater* 2007;23:1553–1561.

Imfeld T. Prevention of progression of dental erosion by professional and individual prophylactic measures. *Eur J Oral Sci* 1996;104:215–220.

Irish JD, Turner CG II. Brief communication: first evidence of LSAMAT in non-native Americans: historic Senegalese from West Africa. *Am J Phys Anthropol* 1997;102:141–146.

Isacsson G, Bodin L, Selden A, Barregard L. Variability in the quantification of abrasion on the Bruxcore device. *J Orofac Pain* 1996;10:362–368.

Johansson A. A cross-cultural study of occlusal tooth wear. *Swed Dent J Suppl* 1992;86:1–59.

Jonsgar C, Hordvik PA, Berge ME, et al. Sleep bruxism in individuals with and without attrition-type tooth wear: an exploratory matched case–control electromyographic study. *J Dent* 2015;43:1504–1510.

Josephson CA. Restoration of mandibular incisors with advanced wear. *J Dent Assoc S Afr* 1992;47:419–420.

Kaidonis JA, Richards LC, Townsend GC, Tansley GD. Wear of human enamel: a quantitative in vitro assessment. *J Dent Res* 1998;77:1983–1990.

Kanzow P, Wegehaupt FJ, Attin T, Wiegand A. Etiology and pathogenesis of dental erosion. *Quintessence Int* 2016;47(4):275–278.

Khan F, Young WG, Shahabi S, Daley TJ. Dental cervical lesions associated with occlusal erosion and attrition. *Aust Dent J* 1999;44:176–186.

Kiliaridis S, Johansson A, Haraldson T, et al. Craniofacial morphology, occlusal traits, and bite force in persons with advanced occlusal tooth wear. *Am J Orthodont Dentofac Orthop* 1995;107:286–292.

Knight DJ, Leroux BG, Zhu C, et al. A longitudinal study of tooth wear in orthodontically treated patients. *Am J Orthod Dentofac Orthop* 1997;112:194–202.

Kwon E, Choi S, Cheong Y, et al. Scanning electron microscopy study of the effect of the brushing time on the human tooth dentin after exposure to acidic soft drinks. *J Nanosci Nanotechnol* 2012;12:5199–5204.

Lambrechts P, van Meerbeek B, Perdigao J, et al. Restorative therapy for erosive lesions. *Eur J Oral Sci* 1996;104:229–240.

Leinfelder KF, Yarnell G. Occlusion and restorative materials. *Dent Clin North Am* 1995;39:355–361.

Lobbezoo F, Ahlberg J, Glaros AG, et al. Bruxism defined and graded: an international consensus. *J Oral Rehabil* 2013;40:2–4.

Lussi A. Dental erosion clinical diagnosis and case history taking. *Eur J Oral Sci* 1996;104:191–198.

Lussi A, Jaeggi T. *Dental Erosion: Diagnosis, Risk Assessment, Prevention, Treatment*. London, UK: Quintessence Publishing; 2011:1–132.

Lyttle HA, Sidhu N, Smyth B. A study of the classification and treatment of noncarious cervical lesions by general practitioners. *J Prosthet Dent* 1998;79:342–346.

Magnusson T. Is snuff a potential risk factor in occlusal wear? *Swed Dent J* 1991;15:125–132.

McIntyre JM. Erosion. *Aust Prosthodont J* 1992;6:17–25.

Meurman JH, ten Cate JM. Pathogenesis and modifying factors of dental erosion. *Eur J Oral Sci* 1996;104:199–206.

Meyers, F. Khan. Restoration of the worn dentition. In: Khan F, Young WG (Eds.), *Toothwear: The ABC of the Worn Dentitions*. Chichester: Wiley-Blackwell; 2011:182–204.

Millward A, Shaw L, Smith AJ. Dental erosion in four-year-old children from differing socioeconomic backgrounds. *ASDC J Dent Child* 1994;61:263–266.

Milosevic A. Tooth wear: an aetiological and diagnostic problem. *Eur J Prosthodont Restor Dent* 1993;1:173–178.

Milosevic A. Toothwear: aetiology and presentation. *Dent Update* 1998;25:6–11.

Milosevic A. Burnside G. The survival of direct composite restorations in the management of severe tooth wear including attrition and erosion: a prospective 8-year study. *J Dent* 2016;44:13–19.

Milosevic A, Lo MS. Tooth wear in three ethnic groups in Sabah (northern Borneo). *Int Dent J* 1996;46:572–578.

Milosevic A, Brodie DA, Slade PD. Dental erosion, oral hygiene, and nutrition in eating disorders. *Int J Eat Disord* 1997;21:195–199.

Mixson JM, Spencer P, Moore DL, et al. Surface morphology and chemical characterization of abrasion/erosion lesions. *Am J Dent* 1995;8:5–9.

Morley J. The esthetics of anterior tooth aging. *Curr Opin Cosmet Dent* 1997;4:35–39.

Nemcovsky CE, Artzi Z. Erosion-abrasion lesions revisited. *Compend Cont Educ Dent* 1996;17:416–418.

Neo J, Chew CL, Yap A, Sidhu S. Clinical evaluation of tooth-colored materials in cervical lesions. *Am J Dent* 1996;9:15–18.

Nunn J, Shaw L, Smith A. Tooth wear—dental erosion. *Br Dent J* 1996;180:349–352.

Owens BM, Gallien GS. Noncarious dental "abfraction" lesions in an aging population. *Compend Cont Educ Dent* 1995;16:552–562.

Paesani DA. Tooth wear. In: Paesani DA (Ed.), *Bruxism: Theory and Practice*. London, UK: Quintessence Publishing; 2010.

Pintado MR, Anderson GC, DeLong R, Douglas WH. Variation in tooth wear in young adults over a two-year period. *J Prosthet Dent* 1997;77:313–320.

Piotrowski BT, Gillette WB, Hancock EB. Examining the prevalence and characteristics of abfractionlike cervical lesions in a population of US veterans. *J Am Dent Assoc* 2001;132:1694–1701.

Plavcam JM, Kelley J. Evaluating the "dual selection" hypothesis of canine reduction. *Am J Phys Anthropol* 1996;99:379–387.

Ponduri S, Macdonald E, Addy M. A study in vitro of the combined effects of soft drinks and tooth brushing with fluoride toothpaste on the wear of dentine. *Int J Dent Hyg* 2015;3:7–12.

Ramp MH, Suzuki S, Cox CF, et al. Evaluation of wear: enamel opposing three ceramic materials and a gold alloy. *J Prosthet Dent* 1997;77:523–530.

Robb ND, Cruwys E, Smith BG. Regurgitation erosion as a possible cause of tooth wear in ancient British populations. *Arch Oral Biol* 1991;36:595–602.

Robertson PB, DeRouen TA, Ernster V, et al. Smokeless tobacco use: how it affects the performance of major league baseball players. *J Am Dent Assoc* 1995;126:1115–1121.

Sakaguchi RL, Brust EW, Cross M, et al. Independent movement of cusps during occlusal loading. *Dent Mater* 1991;7:186–190.

Salas MMS, Nascimento GG, Vargas-Ferreira F, et al. Diet influenced tooth erosion prevalence in children and adolescents: results of a meta-analysis and meta-regression. *J Dent* 2015;43:865–875.

Schemoehorn BR, Moore MH, Putt MS. Abrasion, polishing and stain removal characteristics of various commercial dentifrices in vitro. *J Clin Dent* 2011;22:11–18.

Schlichting LH, Maia HP, Baratieri LN, Magne P. Novel-design ultra-thin CAD/CAM composite resin and ceramic occlusal veneers for the treatment of severe dental erosion. *J Prosthet Dent* 2001;105:217–226.

Schmidt U, Treasure J. Eating disorders and the dental practitioner. *Eur J Prosthodont Restor Dent* 1997;5:161–167.

Sehmi H, Colley RC. The effect of toothbrush abrasion force on dentine hypersensitivity in-vitro. *J Dent* 2015;43:1442–1447.

Seligman DA, Pullinger AG. The degree to which dental attrition in modern society is a function of age and of canine contact. *J Orofac Pain* 1995;9:266–275.

Seligman DA, Pullinger AG. A multiple stepwise logistic regression analysis of trauma history and 16 other history and dental cofactors in females with temporomandibular disorders. *J Orofac Pain* 1996;10:351–361.

Silness J, Berge M, Johannessen G. A 2-year follow-up study of incisal tooth wear in dental students. *Acta Odontol Scand* 1995;53:331–333.

Smith BG, Bartlett DW, Robb ND. The prevalence, etiology and management of tooth wear in the United Kingdom. *J Prosthet Dent* 1997;78:367–372.

Sognnaes RF, Wolcott RB, Xhonga FA. Dental erosion I. Erosion-like patterns occurring in association with other dental conditions. *J Am Dent Assoc* 1972;84:571–576.

Stewart B. Restoration of the severely worn dentition using a systematized approach for a predictable prognosis. *Int J Periodont Rest Dent* 1998;18:46–57.

Suzuki S, Cox CF, Leinfelder KF, et al. A new copolymerized composite resin system: a multiphased evaluation. *Int J Periodont Restor Dent* 1995;15:482–495.

Suzuki S, Suzuki SH, Cox CF. Evaluating the antagonistic wear of restorative materials when placed against human enamel. *J Am Dent Assoc* 1996;127:74–80.

Tay FR, Gwinnett AJ, Pang KM, Wei SH. Structural evidence of a sealed tissue interface with a total-etch wet-bonding technique in vivo. *J Dent Res* 1994;73:629–636.

Teo C, Young WG, Daley TJ, Sauer H. Prior fluoridation in childhood affects dental caries and tooth wear in a south east Queensland population. *Aust Dent J* 1997;42:92–102.

Tereza GPG, Oliveira GC, Machado MAAM, et al. Influence of removing excess of resin-based materials applied to eroded enamel on the resistance to erosive challenge. *J Dent* 2016;47:49–54.

Toole SO, Mistry M, Mutahar M, et al. Sequence of stannous and sodium fluoride solutions to prevent enamel erosion. *J Dent* 2015;43:1498–1503.

Tyas MJ. The Class V lesion—aetilogy and restoration. *Aust Dent J* 1995;40:167–170.

Ungar PS, Teaford MF. Preliminary examination of non-occlusal dental microwear in anthropoids: implications for the study of fossil primates. *Am J Phys Anthropol* 1996;100:101–113.

Ungar PS, Teaford MF, Glander KE, Pastor RF. Dust accumulation in the canopy: a potential cause of dental microwear in primates. *Am J Phys Anthropol* 1995;97:93–99.

Vandewalle KS, Vigil G. Guidelines for the restoration of Class V lesions. *Gen Dent* 1997;45:254–260.

Van Foreest A, Roeters J. Restorative dental treatment of abraded canine teeth in a Sumatran tiger *(Panthera tigris sumatrae)*. *J Vet Dent* 1997;14:131–136.

Villa G, Giacobini G. Dental microwear. Morphological, functional and phylogenetic correlations. *Ital J Anat Embryol* 1998;103:53–84.

West NX, Maxwell A, Hughes JA, et al. A method to measure clinical erosion: the effect of orange juice consumption on erosion of enamel. *J Dent* 1998;26:329–335.

Wiegand A, Burkhard JP, Eggmann F, Attin T. Brushing force of manual and sonic toothbrushes affects dental hard tissue abrasion. *Clin Oral Invest* 2013;17(3):815–822.

Wood I, Jawad Z, Paisley C, Brunton P. Non-carious cervical tooth surface loss: a literature review. *J Dent* 2008;36:759–766.

Yaacob HB, Park AW. Dental abrasion pattern in a selected group of Malaysians. *J Nihon Univ Sch Dent* 1990;32:175–180.

Yap AU, Neo JC. Non-carious cervical tooth loss: part 1. *Dent Update* 1995;22:315–318.

Yap AU, Neo JC. Non-carious cervical tooth loss. Part 2: management. *Dent Update* 1995;22:364–368.

Zero DT. Etiology of dental erosion—extrinsic factors. *Eur J Oral Sci* 1996;104(2 Pt 2):162–177.

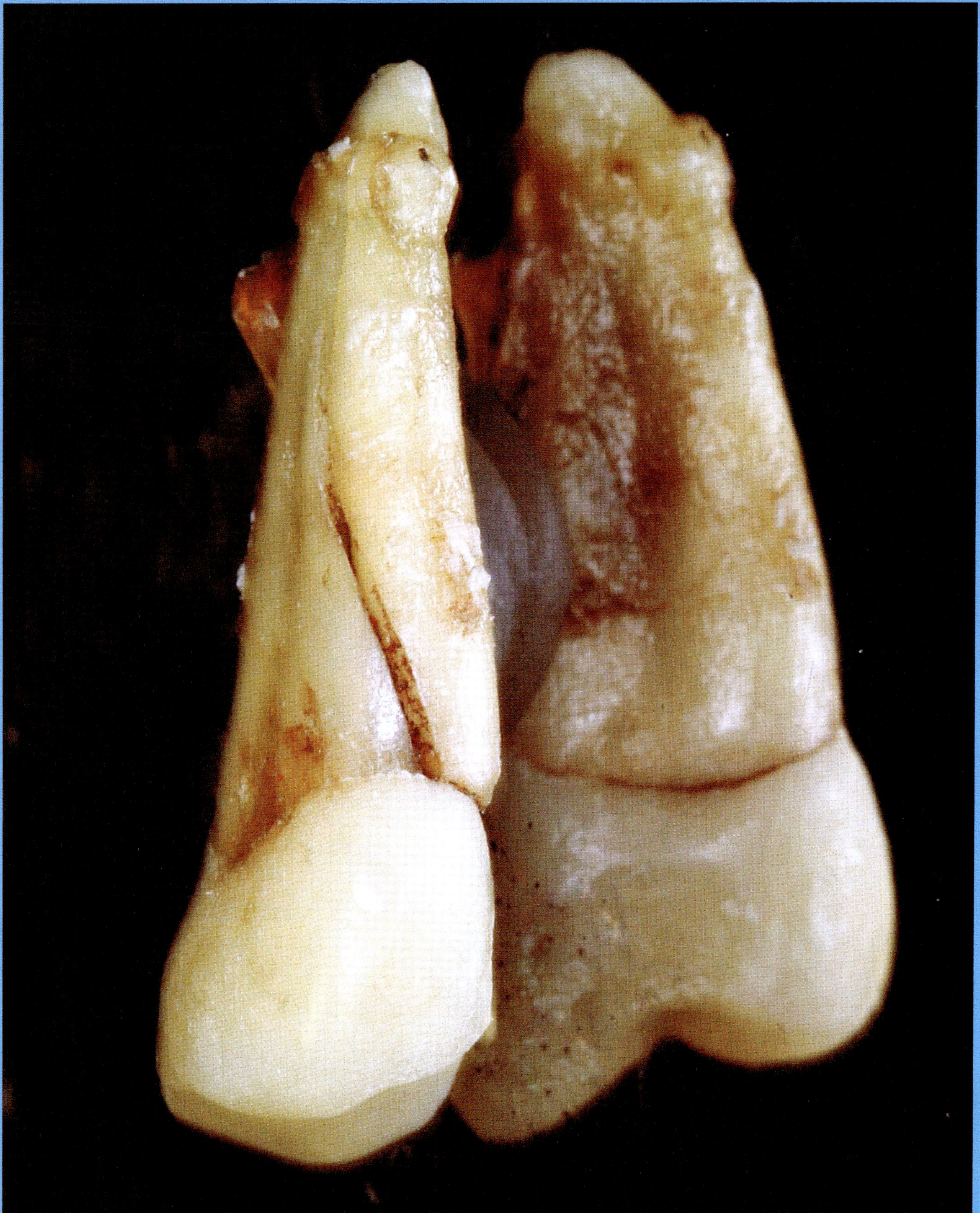

Chapter 23 Chipped, Fractured, or Endodontically Treated Teeth

Ronald E. Goldstein, DDS, Daniel C.N. Chan, DMD, MS, DDS, Michael L. Myers, DMD, and Gerald M. Barrack, DDS

Chapter Outline

Chips or fractures without pulpal involvement	724
Conservative bonding techniques for long-term results	724
Bonding original tooth fragment	726
Chips or fractures with pulpal involvement	727
Preservation of fractured maxillary central incisors through interdisciplinary therapy	728
Life expectancy with composite resins	730
Posterior restorations	731
Restoration of endodontically treated fractured teeth	732
Principles	732
Post design	734
Sequence of treatment for posterior teeth (molars and large premolars)	735
Sequence for anterior teeth	739
Post preparation	739
Sequence for premolars	743
Principles for crown preparation	743

New caries prevention and health measures and improved oral care will help more patients keep more of their teeth disease free for a lifetime. However, one thing in "dental life" is almost a certainty: teeth will continue to fracture. Although sports injuries can be greatly reduced with proper protective gear, our daily lives are conducive to all sorts of accidents causing patients to fracture their teeth. The frequency of permanent incisor fractures in children is reported to range from 5 to 20%.[1,2] The loss of tooth substance in these situations is likely to be more horizontal than vertical.

Most tooth fractures are minor and seldom involve pulp. This chapter discusses such simple fractures, as well as treatment of teeth with pulpal and endodontic intervention (Table 23.1). One example of a more serious fracture involving the pulp is also presented with an explanation of techniques for handling this problem. Difficult fracture cases are usually emergencies. With our population living longer and retaining most of their teeth, the incidence of cracks in teeth also seems to be increasing. A tabulated review of cracked tooth syndrome, treatment options, and other considerations is included for easy reference (Table 23.2).

Some important factors have to be considered in management of tooth fractures, including the extent of fracture, which can involve biological width violation, endodontic involvement, or alveolar bone fracture. Another factor is the pattern of fracture and restorability of the fractured tooth, which can be complicated with root fracture. Also, secondary trauma injuries, such as soft tissue status and presence/absence of fractured tooth fragment, have to be considered for the best treatment outcome.[3]

Conservative restorative dentistry is always the goal in treating esthetic problems, and the fractured tooth is no exception.

Table 23.1 Coronal Chips or Fractures

Diagnosis	Situation	Treatment Options	Considerations
No pulpal involvement	Small chip (enamel involvement only)	Recontour Composite repair	Occlusion
	Medium chip (dentin exposure)	Rebond fractured piece Composite repair	Shine-through effect; esthetics; occlusion
	Large chip (dentin exposure)	Rebond Repair Veneers (composite or porcelain)	Auxiliary retention; occlusion
Pulpal involvement	Direct pulp cap Endodontic treatment required: 1. conventional access with adequate tooth structure 2. extensive tooth loss; post and core required	Restore as for large chip Composite restoration Cast post and core Prefabricated post and core	Pulpotomy or partial pulpotomy Material choice: conventional glass ionomers, resin-modified glass ionomer, composite resin, and cast metal. Post materials: nickel-containing stainless steel, non-nickel-containing stainless steel, commercially pure titanium, titanium alloy, zirconia polycrystals, and carbon fibers

Table 23.2 Cracked Tooth Syndrome

Diagnosis	Situation	Treatment Options	Considerations
Intracoronal fractures	Affect enamel only Craze lines affecting enamel, dentin, and possibly the pulp	No treatment indicated	Long vertical craze line on anterior teeth
	Fractured cusp Supragingival	Remove the affected cusp; full crown/onlay coverage	Good prognosis
	Subgingival	Perisurgery, crown lengthening, orthodontic extrusion, full crown/onlay	Prognosis guarded
	Cracked tooth	Endodontics, full crown	Questionable prognosis
	Split tooth	Extraction; removal of mobile segment	Easily disclosed crack, movable segment; poor prognosis
	Vertical root fracture	Extraction or removal of fractured root	Difficult to diagnose; poor prognosis
Extracoronal fractures	Subgingival	Perisurgery, crown lengthening, orthodontic extrusion	Prognosis guarded
	Vertical root fracture	Extraction or removal of cracked root	Difficult to diagnose; poor prognosis

The most conservative treatment would obviously be cosmetic contouring, or the reshaping of the natural teeth, provided that it does not negatively alter the esthetics of the smile (Figure 23.1). Decades ago, the full crown restoration was the treatment of choice. Today, in addition to cosmetic contouring, the conservative solution is a choice between direct bonding with composite resin and laminating with porcelain.[4–6] Another option to consider when there is no or minimal violation of the biological width is the reattachment of the tooth fragment when it is available and has a good fit.[3,7] Tooth fragment reattachment offers a conservative, esthetic, and cost-effective restorative alternative.

The choice of restorative technique should be based on the following factors:

- **Amount of tooth destruction present.** Generally, small chips or fractures are easily restored with direct bonded composite resin (Figure 23.2). The esthetic result is excellent and provides the patient with an economic, one-appointment solution without any anesthesia.[8,9] However, if the patient continues to chip or fracture the bonding, then porcelain would be a better alternative (Figure 23.3). In the event that the enamel is severely compromised, requiring a more extensive restoration, the patient may ultimately be better off with a porcelain veneer. The fractured area is then replaced with the stronger and more durable porcelain. However, it may be a wise choice to select composite resin bonding as an interim restoration. This minimizes any further trauma to the tooth by additional preparation and allows observation time for any pulpal problem; moreover, the bonded solution can last for an indefinite period of time (Figure 23.4).[5] A more predictable long-term wear alternative to a composite resin restoration is reattachment of a tooth fragment with a dentin bonding agent or adhesive luting system.[7] Reattachment of a fragment to a fractured tooth is a great conservative solution to maintain the tooth's original form and

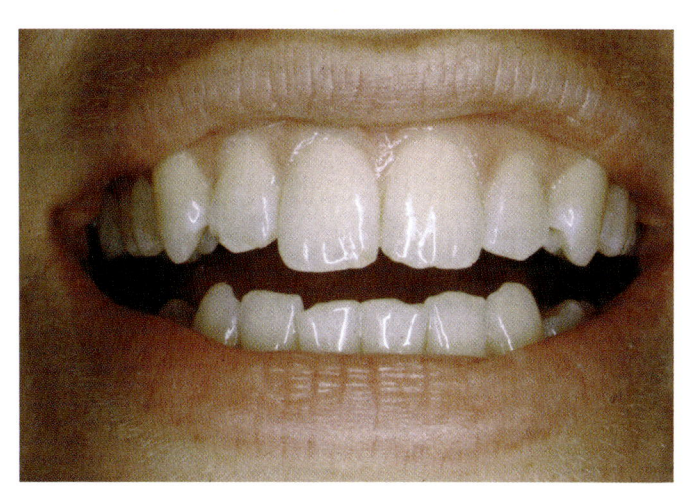

Chapter 23 Chipped, Fractured, or Endodontically Treated Teeth

Figure 23.1 **(A)** This 21-year-old girl had chipped her anterior incisors when she was a teenager.

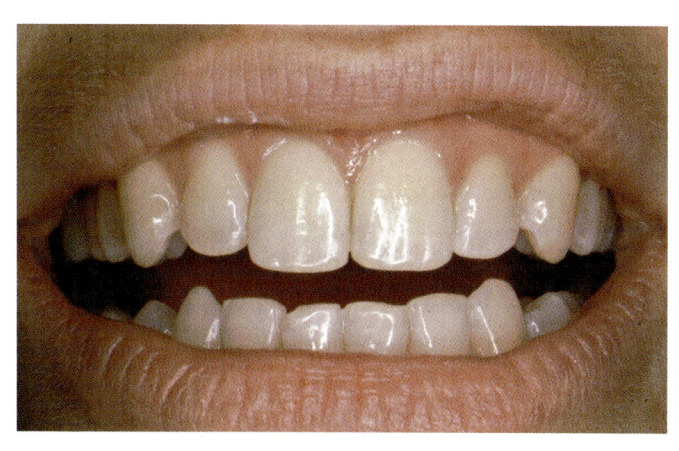

Figure 23.1 **(B)** Cosmetic contouring was the most conservative treatment available and was performed in a less than one-hour appointment.

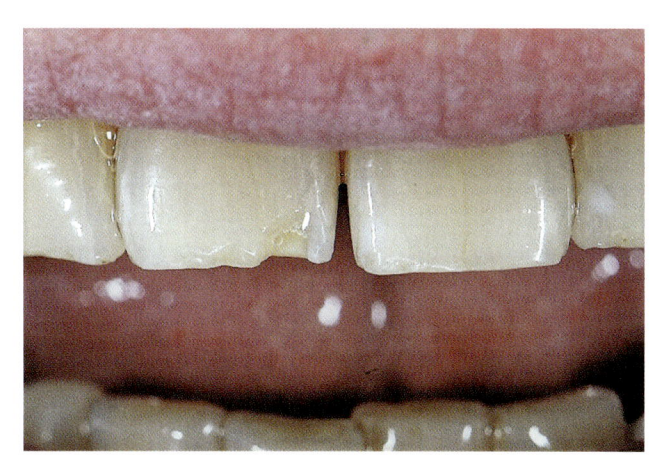

Figure 23.2 **(A)** This man chipped his maxillary right central incisor.

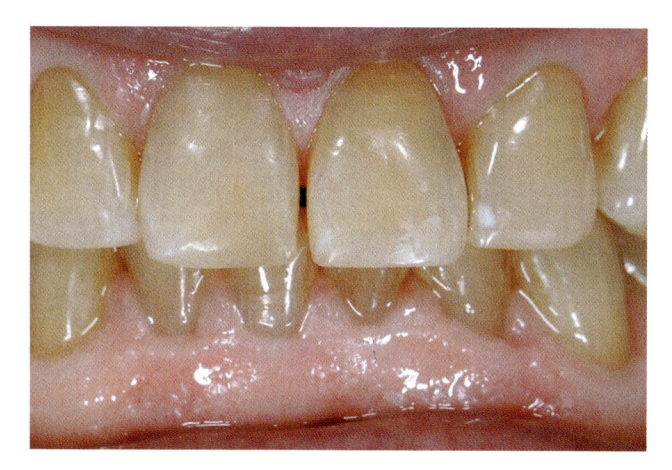

Figure 23.2 **(B)** The right central incisor was bonded with composite resin.

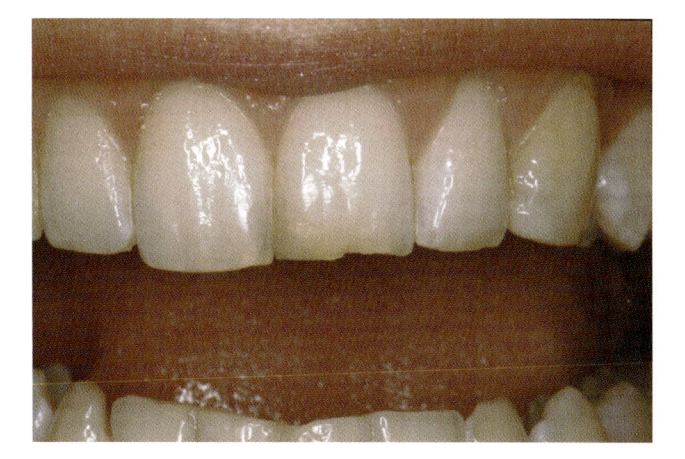

Figure 23.3 **(A)** This young lady fractured her maxillary anterior incisors. Despite numerous bonding repairs, she continued to refracture the teeth. Because she also objected to the incisal translucency, she was treatment planned for three porcelain veneers.

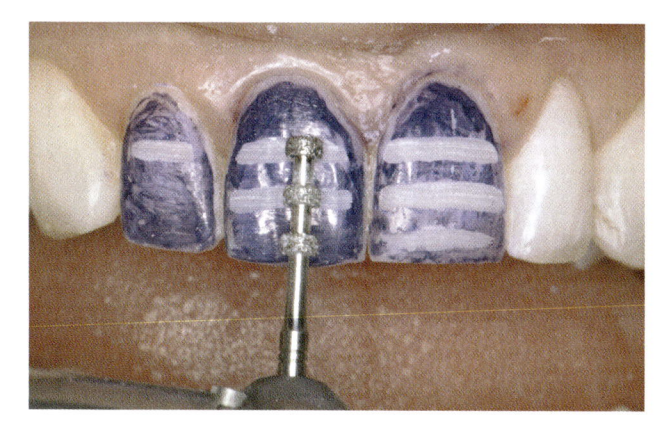

Figure 23.3 **(B)** The initial preparations for the three porcelain veneers were done with a 0.5 mm depth cutter (Brasseler LVS System, Brasseler USA).

texture and offers minimal compromise to the remaining tooth structure. Reattachment was shown to be successful in more complicated fracture cases when endodontic therapy had to be performed on the fractured tooth.[7]

- **Longevity required.** If the patient does not mind the added cost, increased longevity can be achieved with the porcelain veneer. However, the patient needs to be informed about the limited life expectancy of each restorative option. Patients must also be made aware of the

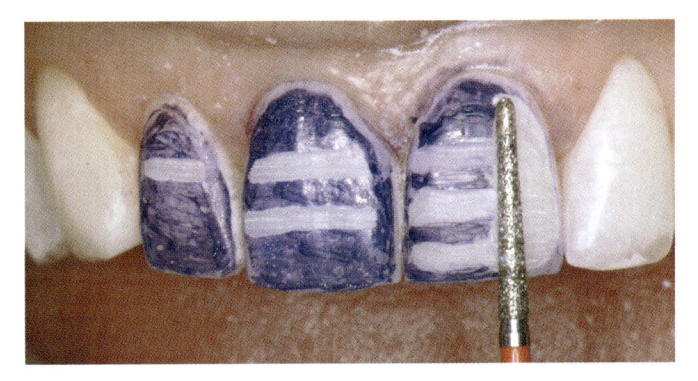

Figure 23.3 (C) The two-grit diamond is used to reduce the enamel to the predetermined depth cut.

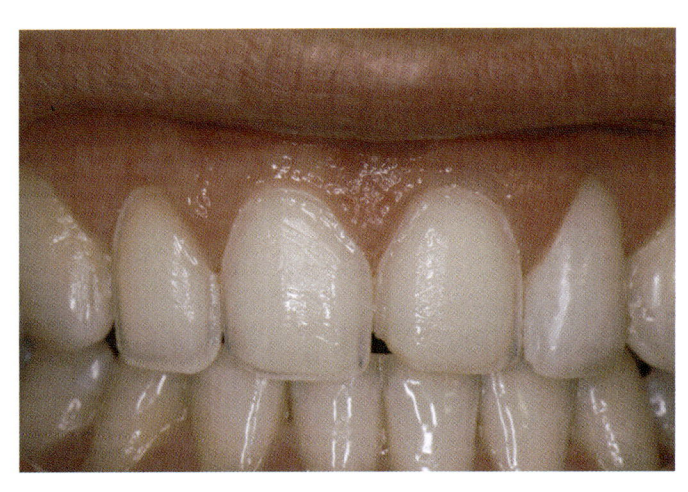

Figure 23.3 (D) The final preparations.

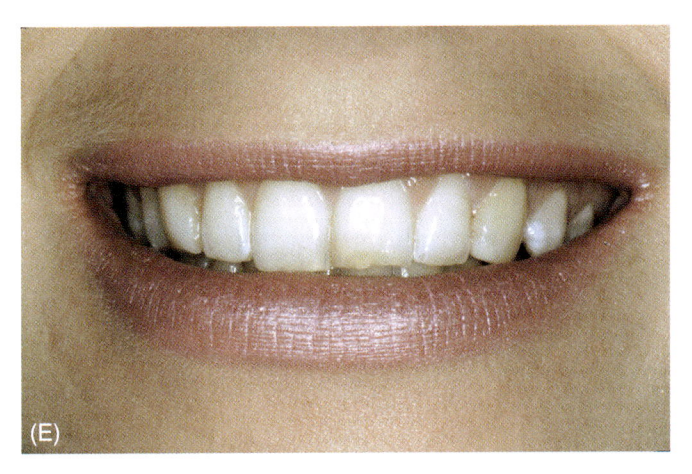

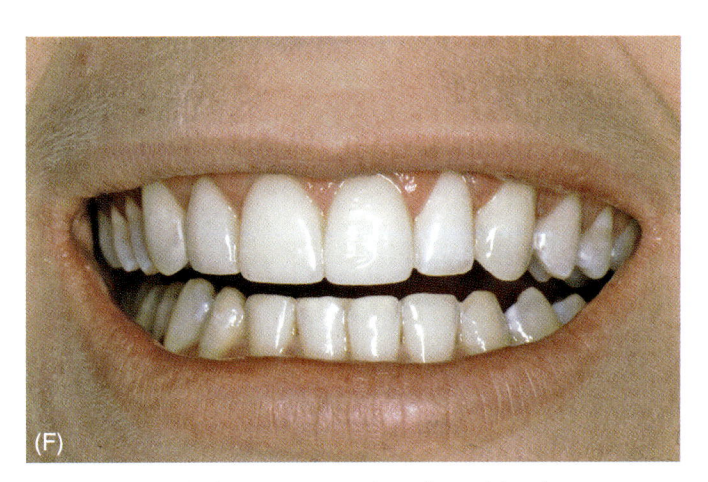

Figure 23.3 (E, F) Three porcelain veneers were placed on the central incisors and right lateral. The new veneers also achieved the objective to eliminate the incisal translucency.

periodic maintenance required, proper home care, and any dietary restrictions necessary to obtain the longest life possible.[6]

- **Economic considerations.** Although the cost savings of direct bonding might not be realized if numerous repairs are considered, it still may be easier for the patient to pay lesser amounts over the many years during which the direct bonded restoration can stay in place.
- **Occlusal factor.** If an end-to-end occlusal relationship or increased occlusal requirement exists, porcelain may again provide more durability, depending on the design of the veneer. It is essential to protect the incisal edge with sufficient porcelain to resist fracture. An example of this condition is seen in a patient who fractured his maxillary right central incisor (Figure 23.5A and B). During the clinical examination, this patient expressed his desire for a younger and brighter smile. The teeth were then prepared, and an impression was made for six porcelain veneers. To help protect the occlusion, porcelain was wrapped incisally to the lingual surface (Figure 23.5C). What began as an emergency visit to repair a fractured tooth resulted in enhancing this patient's entire smile (Figure 23.5D).

It is essential to use these opportunities to present each patient with alternatives that not only correct the immediate problem but also improve the entire smile.

In the final analysis, although direct bonding will generally be the method most often selected, there are definite situations for which porcelain veneers will be the technique of choice. The advantages and disadvantages of direct bonding, laminating, and crowns are outlined in Tables 23.3, 23.4, and 23.5 for comparison.[5]

Chips or fractures without pulpal involvement

Conservative bonding techniques for long-term results

Problem

A 27-year-old male presented with fractured maxillary central incisors involving the incisal edges (Figure 23.6A). Because the patient preferred not to reduce the tooth structure, a bonded composite resin was the material of choice to restore the fractured edges.

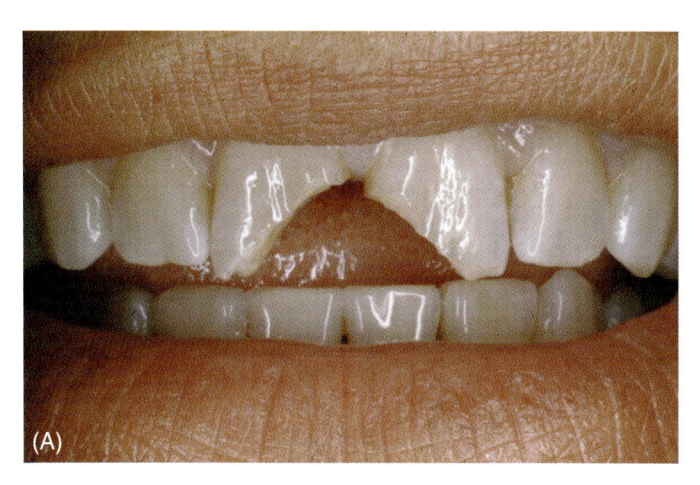

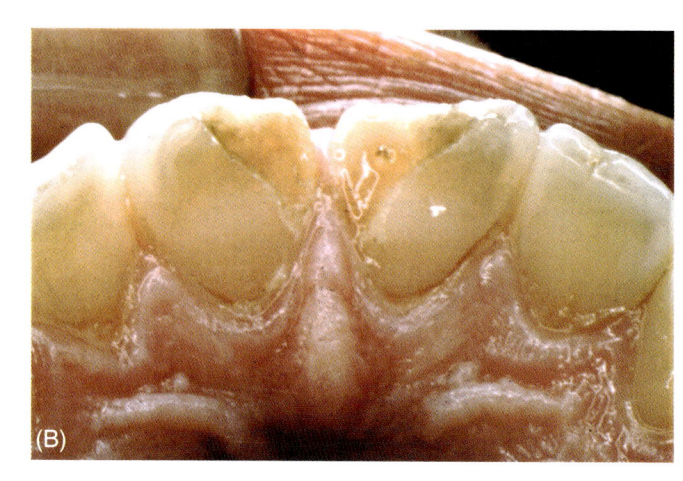

Chapter 23 Chipped, Fractured, or Endodontically Treated Teeth 725

Figure 23.4 **(A, B)** This 17-year-old student fractured her central incisors on the edge of a swimming pool.

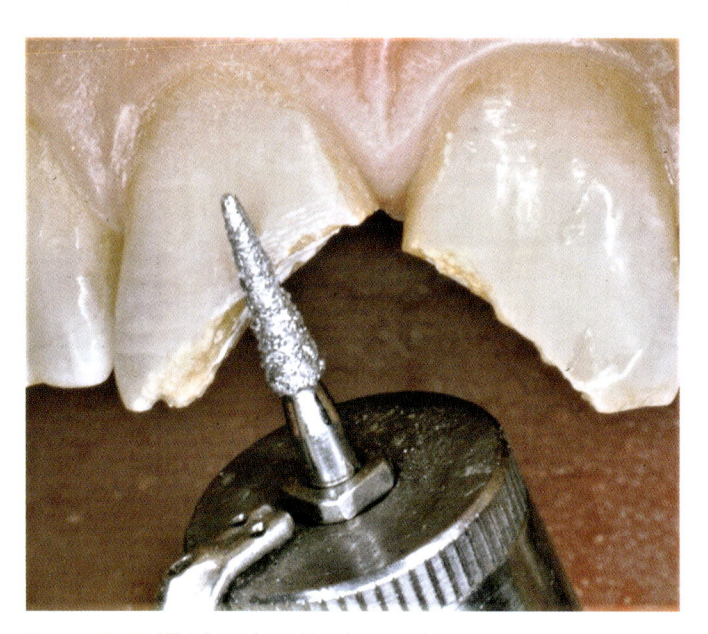

Figure 23.4 **(C)** A long bevel is placed using an extra-coarse diamond.

Treatment

Since the left central incisor overlapped the right one, the mesial surface of the left central was reshaped slightly to reduce the amount of overlapping in an attempt to create an illusion of straightness (Figure 23.6B). These fractures were old and not sensitive, so no protective base was required. In a new fracture or pulp exposure, the fracture site would have been protected first with glass ionomer or bioactive liner. A composite resin restoration was used for strength and to help blend in translucency. The restorations were finished with conventional composite resin finishing techniques (see Chapter 14).

Fourteen years later, the patient came in with a small fracture in the bonding material of the central incisor (Figure 23.6C). The teeth were reveneered with hybrid composite resin to improve his smile once more (Figure 23.6D). Although this patient may well be the exception to the rule of an average life expectancy of 5–8 years, his case does point out the fact that many patients would have preferred the restoration replaced long before the slight discoloration took place. However, careful maintenance, including good oral hygiene

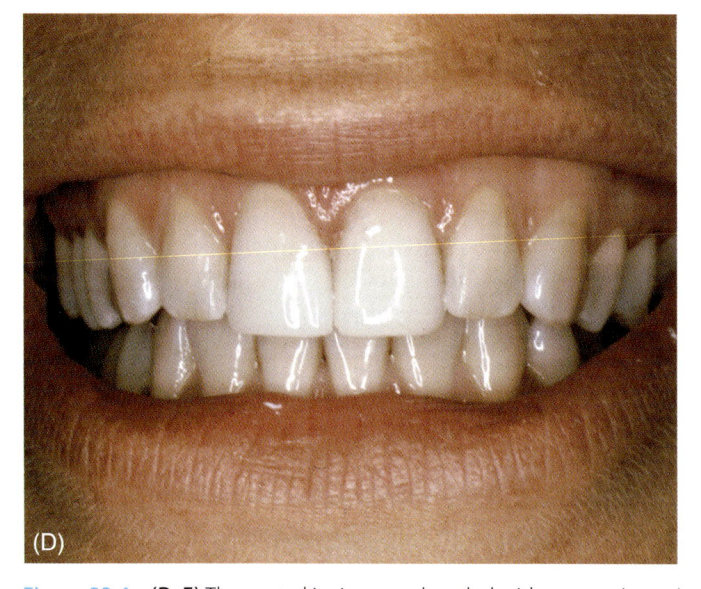

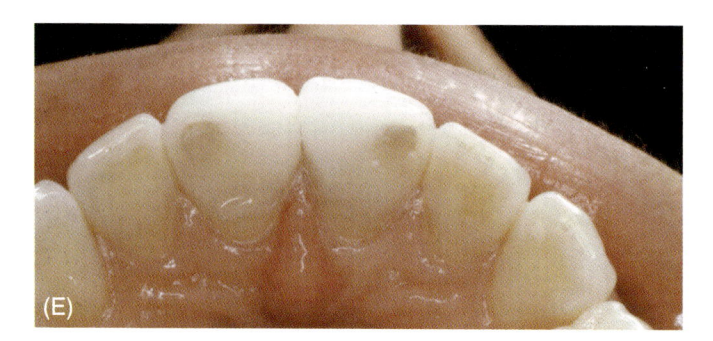

Figure 23.4 **(D, E)** The central incisors are bonded with composite resin.

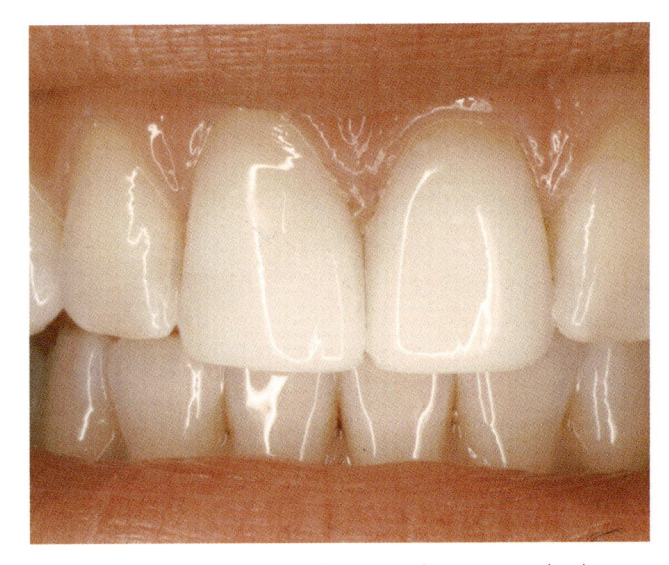

Figure 23.4 (F) Five years later, the patient has continued to be maintained with composite resin restorations.

and prudent dietary habits, helped account for the extended life of these restorations. The tooth can always be veneered or crowned if bonding does not work, but once the enamel is reduced for a full crown, it can never be bonded or veneered. In the future, better bonding and laminating materials will, no doubt, become available.

Bonding original tooth fragment

Simonsen first suggested that fractured original tooth segments could be bonded back together.[10] If the patient has a "clean" break and brings in the fractured piece of enamel, it is entirely possible and many times advisable to attempt reattachment by acid etching both the tooth itself and the fragment. Light-polymerized tooth-colored resin cement is applied to both pieces and the fracture piece is carefully fit and polymerized 1 min labially and 1 min lingually.

Additional modifications have taken place, and there are newer techniques that are variations on the original philosophy.[11] For instance, Croll advocated attaching the two segments

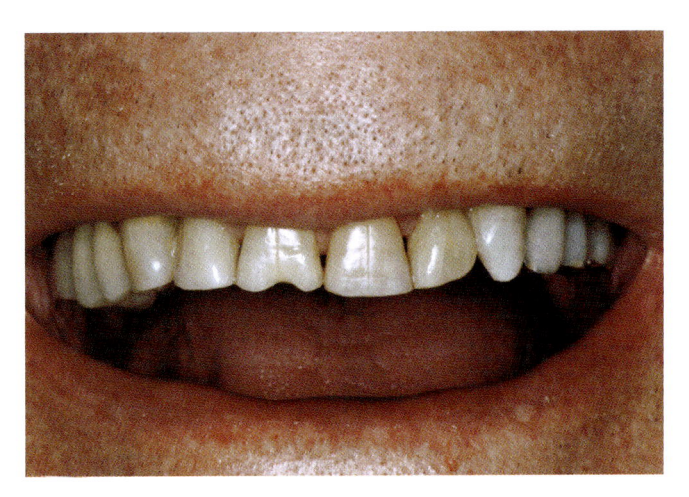

Figure 23.5 (A) This 65-year-old man had fractured his right central incisor. Because he desired a younger and brighter looking smile, six porcelain veneers were treatment planned.

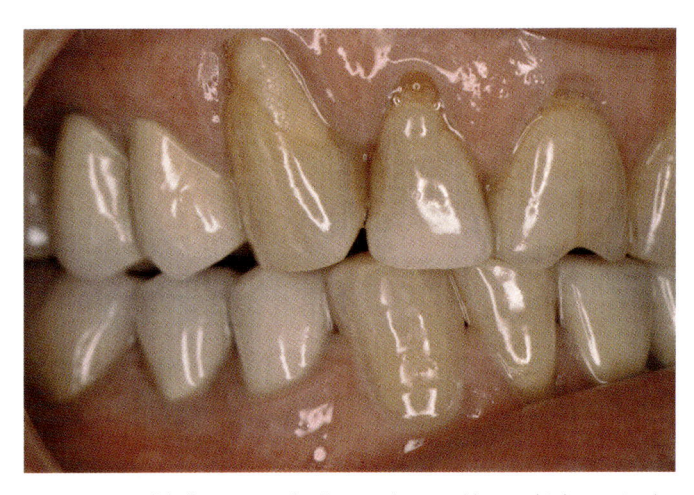

Figure 23.5 (B) This patient had an end-to-end bite, which required additional incisal edge reinforcement.

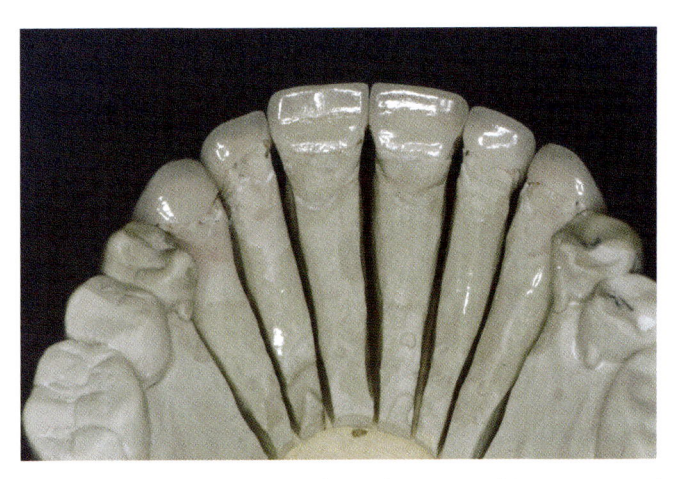

Figure 23.5 (C) To help protect the occlusion, porcelain was wrapped incisally to the lingual surface.

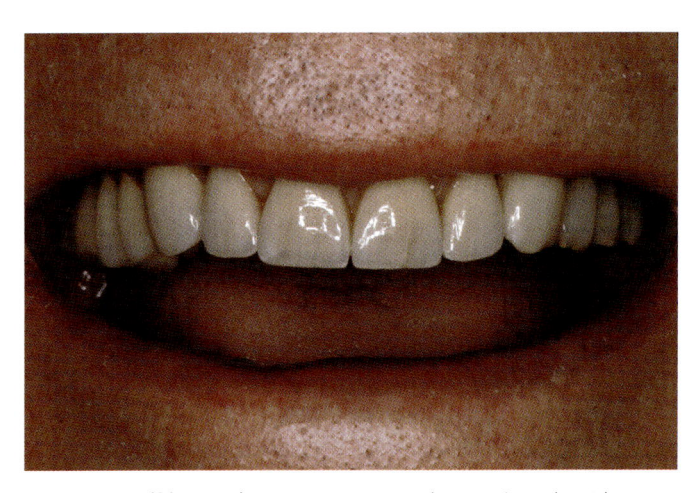

Figure 23.5 (D) Note the improvement in this man's smile with a lighter shade and teeth that are more proportionate to each other.

Table 23.3 Advantages and Disadvantages of Bonding

Advantages

Conserves tooth structure
Easier to match or blend in tooth shade
Less expensive than crowning
Immediate repair
Reduces possible trauma of a crown preparation for badly damaged teeth
No anesthesia required
Painless repair
Can improve shape and shade if necessary

Disadvantages

Can stain more easily than porcelain veneer or a crown
Needs periodic refinishing
Some maintenance required
Must have sufficient enamel left to be able to bond it
Must be repaired or replaced in approximately 5–8 years
Not appropriate for use in posterior teeth

Table 23.4 Advantages and Disadvantages of Porcelain Veneers

Advantages

Excellent esthetics
Improved edge strength
Better retention of surface finish
Fewer repairs required
Does not stain
Conserves tooth structure

Disadvantages

May require anesthesia
More costly than bonding
Usually requires two appointments
Some tooth preparation indicated
Cannot alter color once cemented

Table 23.5 Advantages and Disadvantages of Crowning

Advantages

Can ideally change color and shape of teeth
Longest lasting esthetic restoration
Lasts approximately 5–15 years
Less likely to require repairs

Disadvantages

Must reduce the enamel and dentin
Most expensive form of replacement
Possibility of pulp irritation
More chance for periodontal problems if margin is subgingival
Requires anesthesia
Difficult to repair

together, first with a glass ionomer light-polymerized liner (Vitrebond, 3M ESPE, St. Paul, MN) and then reinforcing labially and lingually with composite resin.[12] Many variations of such bonding are reported in the literature.[1,13–16]

Bonding the original tooth fragment is not limited to the anterior region. Posterior teeth fractures, especially in the case of premolars, can be successfully bonded together. The long-term survival of such repairs is reported to be in the region of 5 years.[1,17] However, in these cases, the bonded teeth are best viewed as a temporary restoration awaiting partial or full crown coverage. Liebenberg reported using resin-bonded partial-coverage ceramic restorations to treat incomplete fractures.[18,19]

Chips or fractures with pulpal involvement

In the event that the pulp is exposed, two choices exist:

- **Pulpotomy.** If the root apex is open, this is the preferred treatment according to several sources.[20,21] Ehrmann described the procedure beginning with coronal pulp removal, which will allow root maturation to proceed only with closure of the apex then taking place.[22] Following closure, a radicular pulpectomy is done and is usually followed by endodontic therapy plus construction of a post and core.

- **Partial pulpotomy.** Another view has been expressed by Cvek, who suggested a partial pulpotomy in permanent incisors with complex root fractures, regardless of whether the apex was open.[23] Basically, the technique consists of a 2mm depth removal of the coronal pulp with sterile saline being used to control bleeding. Next, a calcium hydroxide pulp liner (Dycal Caulk, DENTSPLY/Caulk, Milford, DE) is used and is covered with a composite resin. Ehrmann concluded that this latter technique seems to be the method of choice, citing fewer traumas and preserving most of the pulp as two advantages.[22] He reported that 33 of 35 cases were successful and retained their vitality, with the longest follow-up being 8 years.

The consideration for a chipped or fractured tooth is whether the pulp is damaged. If it has been exposed, the tooth should be protected with a pulp-capping material (calcium hydroxide, glass ionomer, or bioactive liner) and covered with a tooth-colored restorative material for at least 6 weeks. A recommended technique after pulp capping is bonding with a composite resin. Kanca reported the success of a case with a 5-year follow-up.[24]

The responsibility of the dentist is to preserve the natural dentition. In some circumstances, this is impossible, but it is the ideal for which to aim. To achieve this goal, it may be necessary to call on colleagues for assistance. Who is credited with the result is unimportant. What is important is for the patient to receive the best possible treatment and advice. This point is well illustrated by the actual treatment of a patient with fractures of the maxillary central incisors that extended lingually beneath the crest of the bone and exposed the pulps. The patient's dentist consulted an

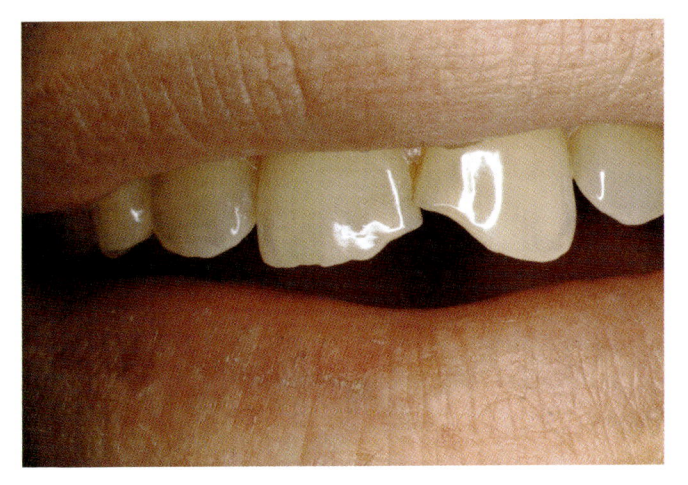

Figure 23.6 **(A)** This 27-year-old man fractured his maxillary central incisors.

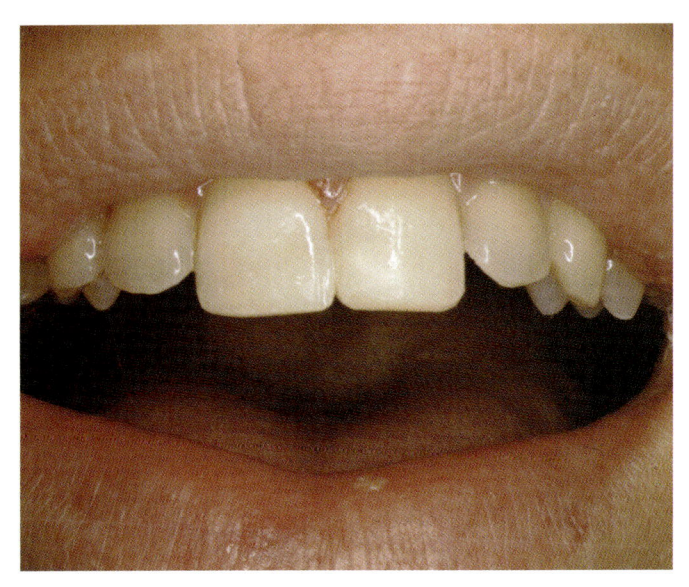

Figure 23.6 **(B)** After light cosmetic contouring to the left central incisor, both central incisors were bonded with composite resin.

oral surgeon who recommended endodontic treatment. Before final restorative therapy was chosen, consultations were held with an oral surgeon, a pediatric dentist, and two general practitioners. The case that follows involved consultation with other dental specialists and shows an esthetic result that was worth the effort.[25]

Preservation of fractured maxillary central incisors through interdisciplinary therapy

Problem

A general practitioner saw a 12-year-old girl who had been in an accident. He referred her to an oral surgeon for removal of both maxillary permanent central incisors, which had been fractured horizontally and vertically, exposing the pulps. The oral surgeon thought that the teeth might be saved and referred the patient to an endodontist. After endodontic therapy on both teeth (Figure 23.7A and B), the patient returned to the general practitioner, who consulted the pediatric dentist. The two agreed that someone skilled in cosmetic restorative procedures should be called on for the reconstruction.

Treatment

Because saving teeth was a step-by-step procedure involving endodontic treatment, periodontal surgery, and reconstructive techniques, the treatment plan could be changed if one of the suggested treatments failed. Endodontic therapy had already been completed on both central incisors. These following surgical procedures were then performed: removal of the tooth fragments that were fractured vertically; labial and lingual gingivectomy and gingivoplasty; palatal ostectomy; and labial frenectomy (Figure 23.7C). Approximately 5 mm of palatal plate was removed to expose new margins on the fractured teeth (Figure 23.7D). After the tissue healed, gold posts were constructed and cemented on the two maxillary incisors (Figure 23.7E–H). Final preparations were made, and

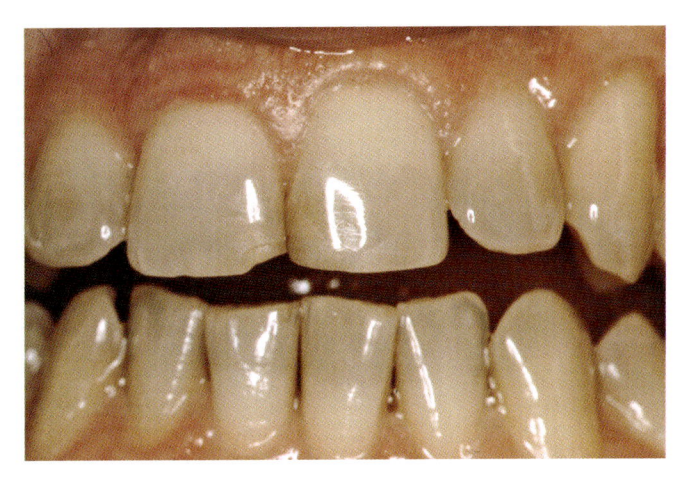

Figure 23.6 **(C)** Fourteen years later, this patient fractured the bonding on the right central incisor.

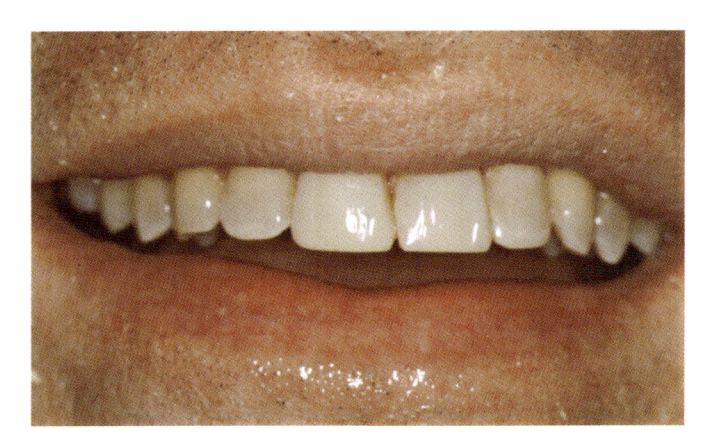

Figure 23.6 **(D)** The central incisors were reveneered and the left lateral was also bonded to achieve an even more attractive smile.

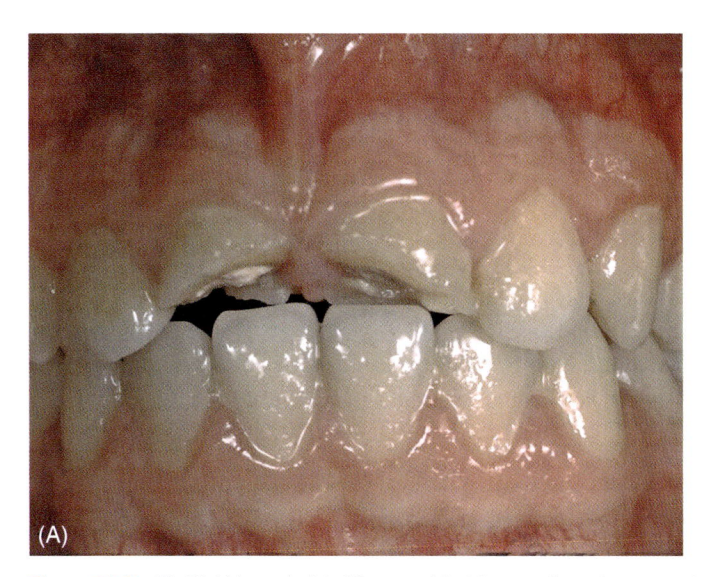

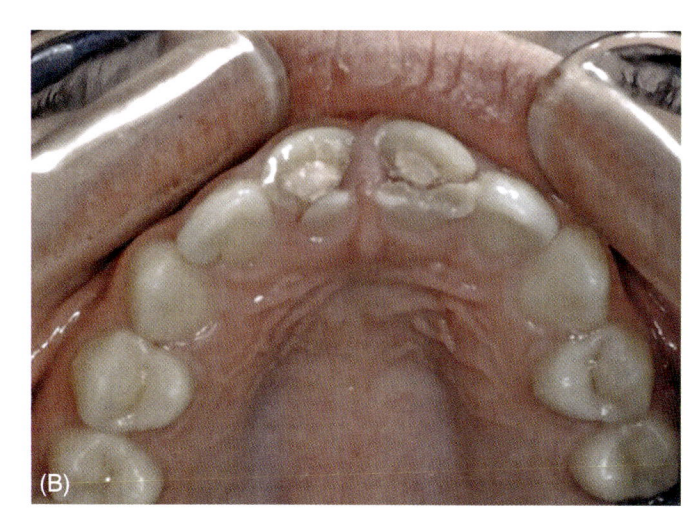

Figure 23.7 **(A, B)** Although this 12-year-old girl was referred to an oral surgeon for a postaccident extraction of both fractured central incisors, he wisely referred the patient to an endodontist in an attempt to save the teeth.

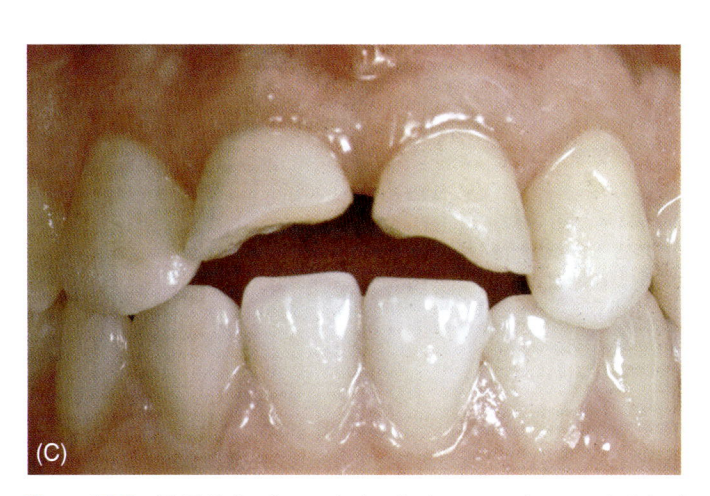

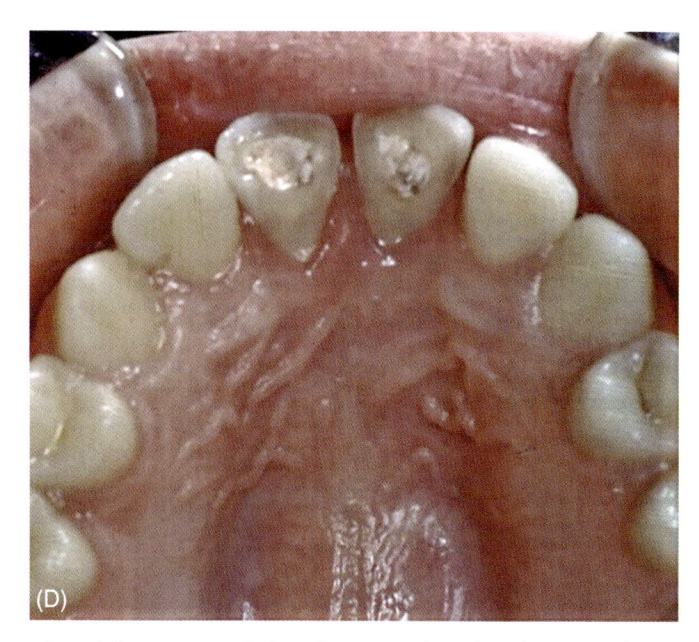

Figure 23.7 **(C, D)** Following endodontic therapy and removal of the fractured tooth fragments, periodontal surgery to lengthen the exposed crowns was performed.

impressions for all-ceramic crowns were made. The two crowns were seated (Figure 23.7I and J).

The parents were told that these crowns would probably have to be replaced when the patient is older because the margins may be exposed. However, they might last longer because of the higher marginal attachment. Because of the age of the child, the anticipated cost of the treatment, and the presumed lack of dental knowledge of the parents, the pediatric dentist and the general practitioner who were to do the treatment explained the reconstruction procedures at length. Although the endodontic therapy had been completed, the father informed the two dentists that he had decided to have "both teeth pulled and a plate put in." A subsequent conference convinced the parents that this would not be the wisest course to follow if restorative procedures could be performed. Their expression of thanks at the end of the treatment justified the time spent persuading the family to accept the outlined treatment plan (Figure 23.7 K and L).

Result

Dentists sometimes assume, incorrectly, that because a tooth is fractured beneath the periodontal ligament and into the bone, it cannot be saved. Proper surgical and reconstructive techniques can save these roots for many years, sometimes indefinitely.

Dentists may also assume, again incorrectly, that because of the expense or difficulty of treatment, a patient or their family would prefer to sacrifice a tooth. Not knowing what value the patient places on a tooth, the dentist should give the patient the opportunity to decide. It is almost always better to save a tooth. The patient can clean it more easily with floss, and the root support helps share occlusal load.

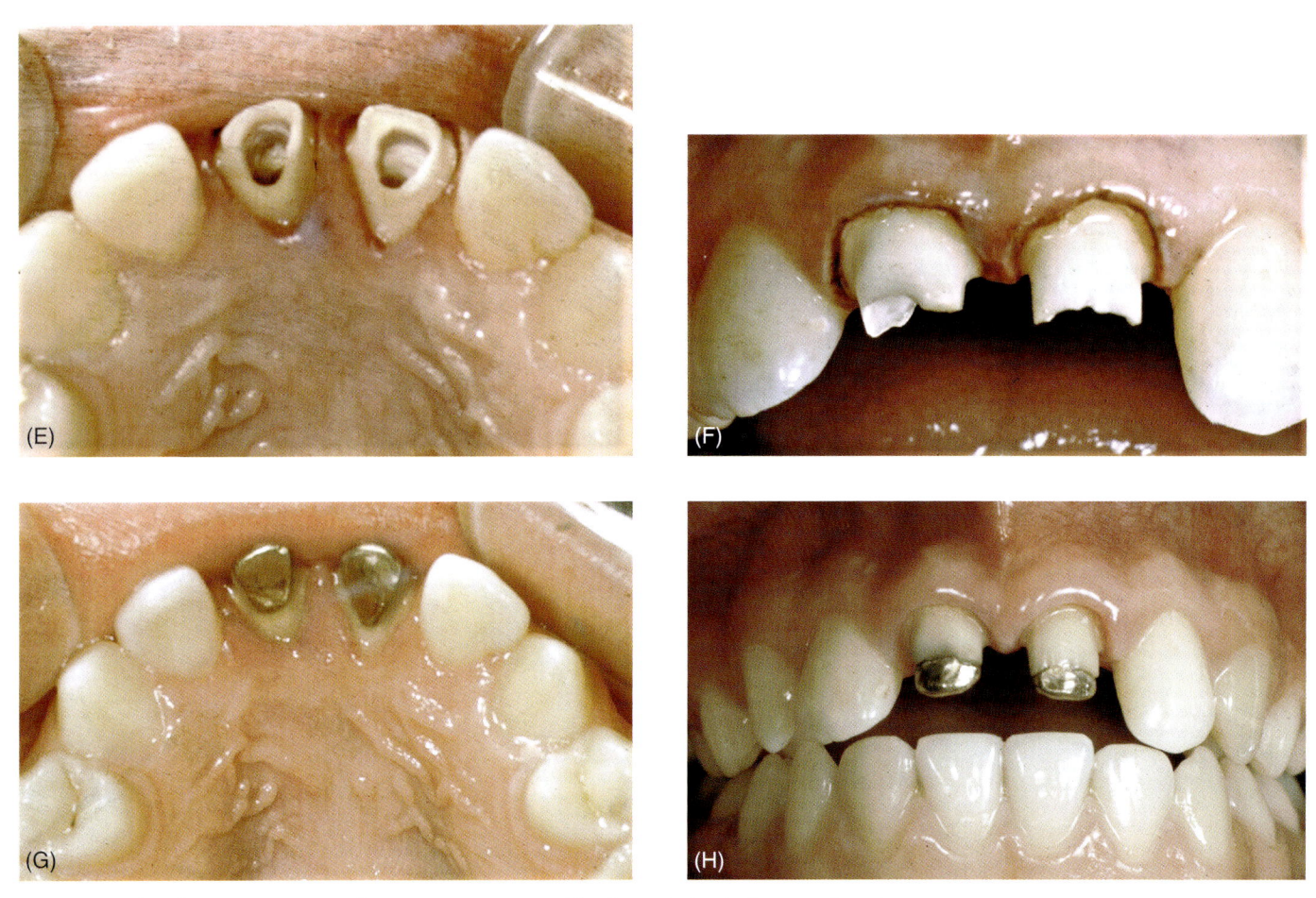

Figure 23.7 (E–H) Next, two posts and cores were constructed for the endodontically treated teeth.

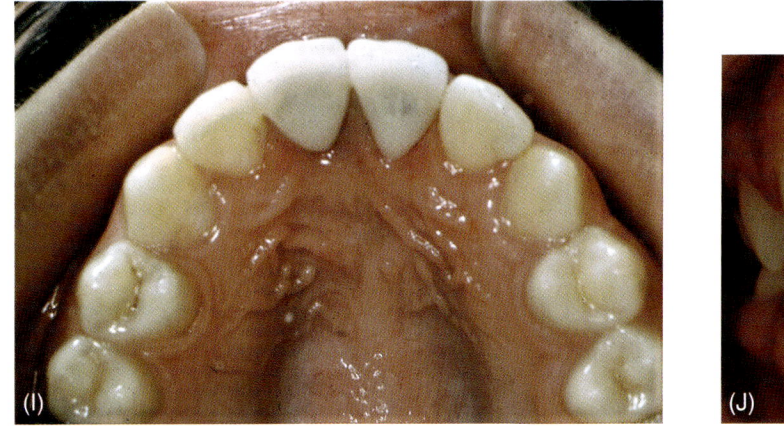

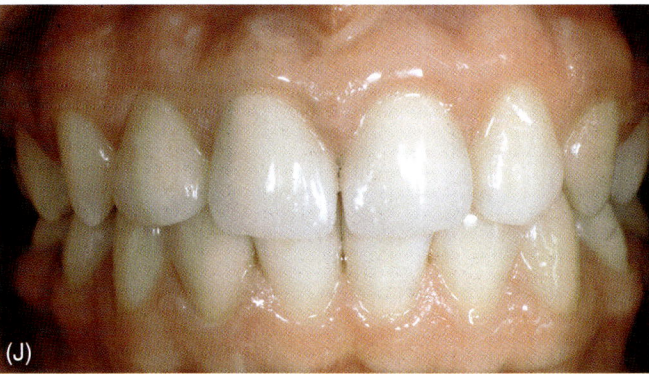

Figure 23.7 (I, J) Two aluminous porcelain crowns were constructed and inserted on the central incisors.

The purpose of this case is not to show the skill of the operator, but to call attention to the fact that, even though extraordinary measures are needed, it may be possible to preserve the natural dentition. To do so may involve multiple referrals and consultations, but the good result (Figure 23.7 J) and the knowledge that possibilities exist should be considered before a patient is allowed to lose a tooth. The function of dentistry is to maintain the integrity of the dental arch and to preserve the dentition. For this patient, at least, this goal was achieved.

Life expectancy with composite resins

Although the average life expectancy is 3–8 years, the fact is that some patients may experience a much longer and more useful restoration life (see Figure 23.8A–C).[6] These restorations are, for the most part, noninvasive, and the bonded restoration offers a good measure of protection to the tooth while odontoblastic activity is taking place at the damaged site. They can also continue to be reveneered rather than

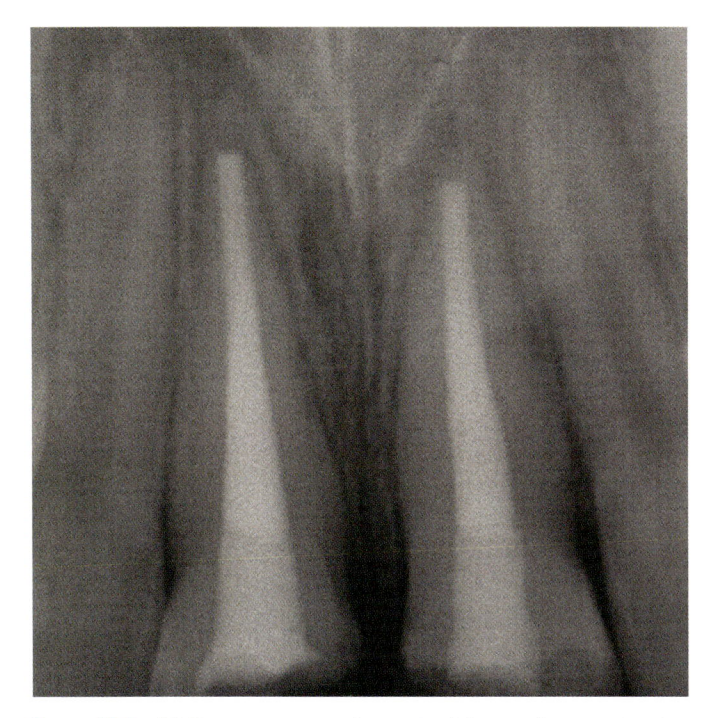

Figure 23.7 (K) Posttreatment radiograph of the two fractured and restored central incisors.

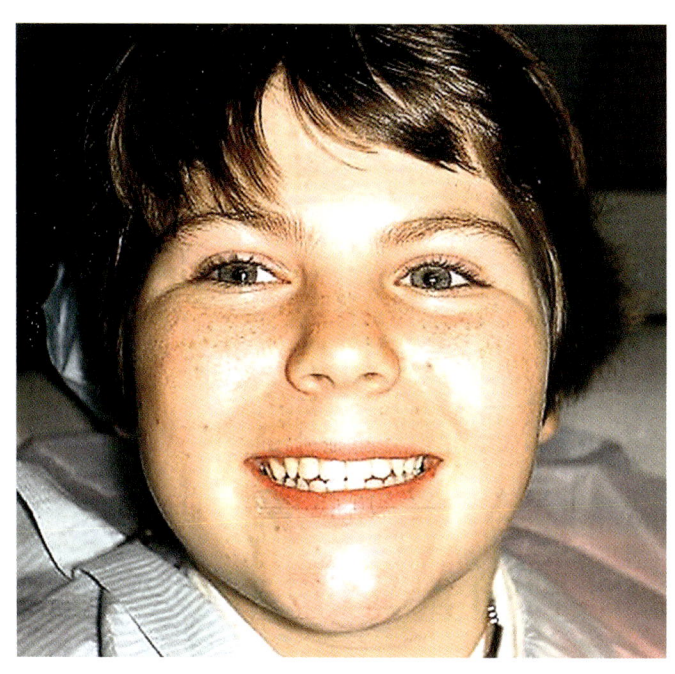

Figure 23.7 (L) A total team approach was necessary to save this young lady's maxillary incisors. Both she and her parents appreciated the benefits of interdisciplinary care.

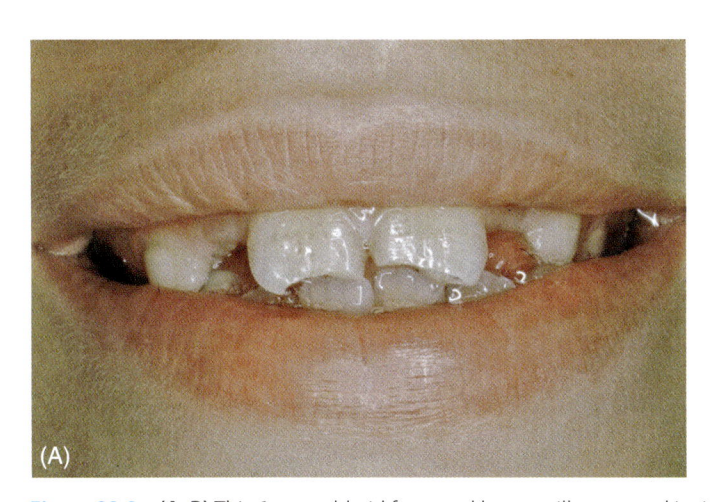

Figure 23.8 (A, B) This 6-year-old girl fractured her maxillary central incisors in an accident.

replaced for an indefinite period of time (Figure 23.8A–E). When replacement is necessary, if full crown coverage is the treatment of choice, it can be done with less chance of pulp involvement. The long-term success of this case is noteworthy because of the young age of the patient, high previous caries experience, deep cavities, and the saucer-shaped preparation technique predisposing to shorter longevity of resin-composite restorations. Literature reviews indicate that the annual failure rate of composite restorations is better than that of amalgam restorations. Principal reasons for composite restorations failure were secondary caries, fracture, marginal deficiencies, wear, and postoperative sensitivity.[26,27]

Posterior restorations

In these areas, it is even more important to place a protective base and use the etching technique on enamel walls and dentin. Marginal leaks can be minimized by this technique. In addition, patients must be advised of the possibility of replacing the restorations every 3–8 years.

Several methods of restoring the simple fracture have been shown in this chapter, although all seem to arrive at the same conclusion: the final measure of success is how these bonds respond to oral fluids. With further investigation, stronger materials and stronger bonds will be developed that may

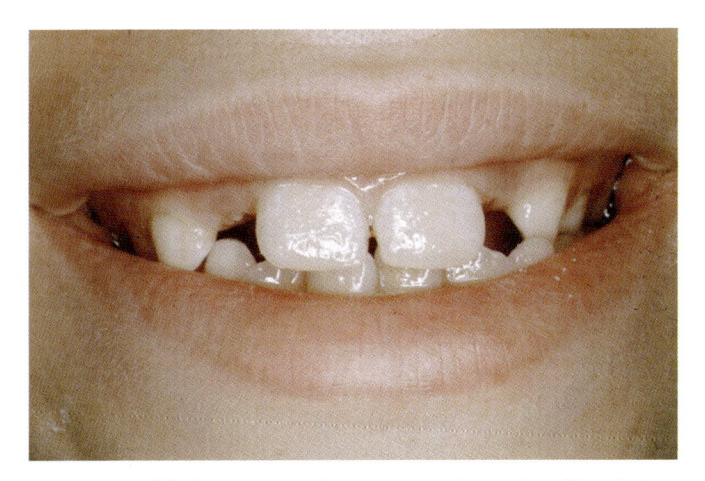

Figure 23.8 **(C)** The two central incisors were beveled and bonded with composite resin.

warrant reinserting restorations as improved materials become available. Thus, in certain cases, it may be to the patient's advantage not to destroy tooth structure for full-coverage procedures at present. However, when small pieces break off of posterior teeth, bonding can be used either as an interim or the final restoration if it is not in an occluding area where it may be under too much stress. If it is, then porcelain may be the best choice.

In the final analysis, the full crown remains a viable option, especially if esthetic changes are to be made that may not be possible with a more conservative treatment. Also, some patients prefer the long-lasting benefit that the full crown provides.[28]

Restoration of endodontically treated fractured teeth

Principles

The philosophy for the restoration of endodontically treated teeth has changed significantly in recent years. Traditional concepts were that nonvital teeth were so weakened by root canal therapy that they required a post to reinforce the root in the same manner that concrete is reinforced with steel rods. Further, it was believed that these teeth also needed to be crowned to protect the tooth from fracture.

Clinical experience and research studies have, in some cases, produced a dramatic shift in the way endodontically treated teeth are restored.[1,29-32] Endodontically treated teeth have certain characteristics that are well known by clinical dentists. They include changes in elasticity of dentin, resistance to fatigue, and changes in morphology.[33] Also, the loss of vitality results in a change in color over time. This can result in an unacceptable esthetic result. These teeth are structurally compromised due to the access opening required to accomplish root canal therapy. Additionally, these teeth often have extensive restorations or caries, further compromising their strength and structural integrity. Clinical experience has shown that these teeth seem to have an increased risk of fracture.

There is no large body of in vivo scientific literature to determine how to best restore endodontically treated teeth. However, there are several good retrospective studies that provide some guidance. From these studies, it is clear that anterior teeth have different characteristics and require a different clinical approach than posterior teeth. Another conclusion that can be made is that endodontically treated anterior teeth do not automatically require restoration with a crown. In fact, most endodontically treated

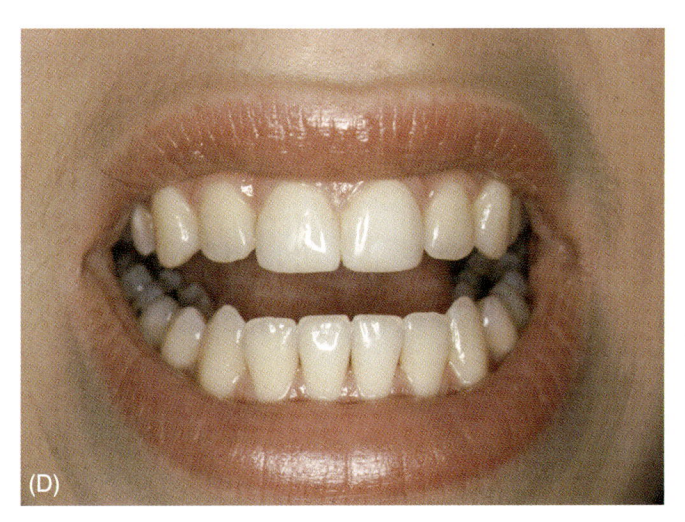

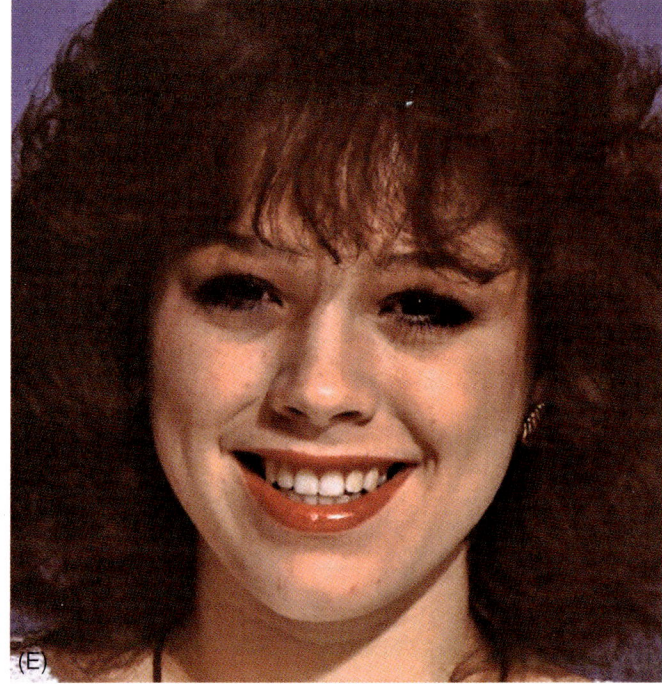

Figure 23.8 **(D, E)** Ten years later, the patient still retains her original bonding, although reveneering has been done to maintain appearance.

anterior teeth will have the same longevity whether or not they have been crowned. So, the clinical options for restoration of an anterior tooth are dictated by the condition and the functional and esthetic requirements of the tooth. If the tooth is relatively intact, it should simply be restored with a composite resin restoration. If it has changed color, then bleaching of the tooth would also be indicated. If the existing restorations or caries are moderate in size or include the incisal edge, then a porcelain veneer could be the appropriate choice for treatment. In many instances, bleaching of the endodontically treated tooth prior to restoration with composite resin or a porcelain veneer will provide a better esthetic result.

Three major reasons for using crowns are (1) if the tooth is badly broken down, (2) a significant change in tooth contour is desired, or (3) if the tooth is to be used as an abutment for a fixed or removable partial denture. Most anterior teeth in this condition have little sound remaining tooth structure and will require a post-and-core restoration to support and retain the crown. This concept is supported by most studies. Such a patient can be seen in Figure 23.9A–C. Post restorations used in anterior teeth fall into two broad types: (1) the prefabricated post with a core material to replace the missing coronal tooth structure and (2) the cast metal post and core that is custom made for the tooth (Figure 23.10A–J).

As previously mentioned, posterior teeth require a different treatment approach than is indicated for anterior teeth. Posterior teeth usually have a greater bulk of remaining tooth structure than anterior teeth. Also, the occlusal forces on posterior teeth are significantly greater than anterior teeth. Retrospective studies of posterior teeth that have had root canal therapy indicate that these teeth may be more likely to fracture if they are not crowned. The basic principle for posterior teeth is that the restoration should provide for cuspal coverage or protection. This can be accomplished with a crown (either full or partial coverage) or even an onlay. The logical exception to this rule might be for a molar or premolar that has a minimal endodontic access and at least one intact marginal ridge. In this instance, if the occlusion is favorable (i.e., canine disclusion), a small two-surface bonded composite could be considered.

Unlike anterior teeth, which many times require a post to retain the core, posterior teeth seldom need a post. The retention

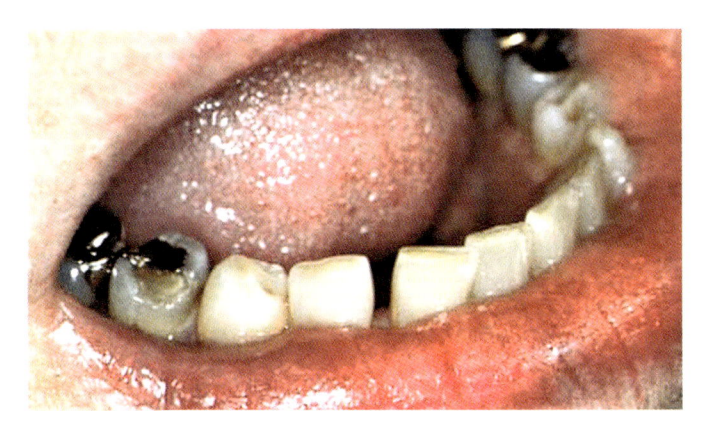

Figure 23.9 **(A)** This 60-year-old woman fractured the bucco-occlusal surface of her mandibular right second bicuspid. Because the fracture was in an occluding area and was previously repaired with composite resin bonding, plus aligned microcrack so the patient opted for the longer lasting protection of a full crown.

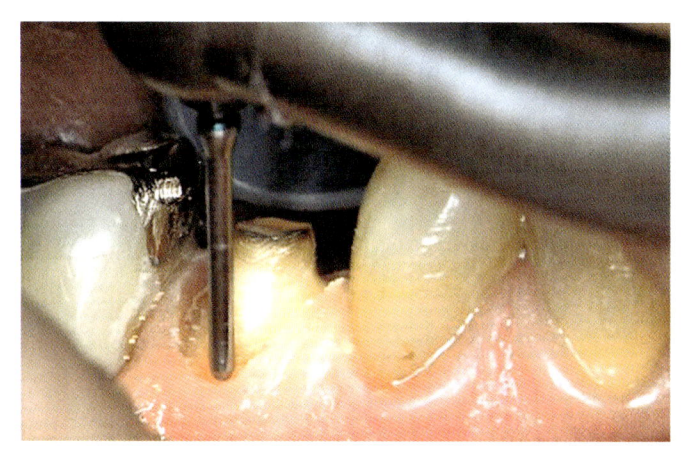

Figure 23.9 **(B)** Full shoulder margins are prepared with a TPE diamond (Shofu or AC11, Brasseler USA).

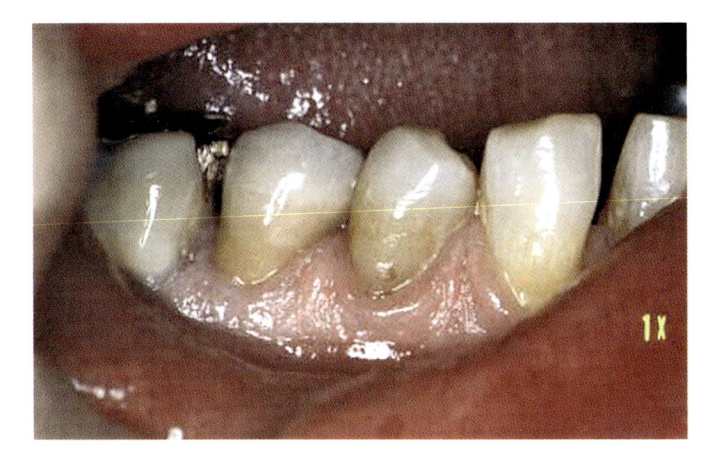

Figure 23.9 **(C)** The final crown shows how well ceramics can mimic the natural tooth and esthetically blend with the existing dentition.

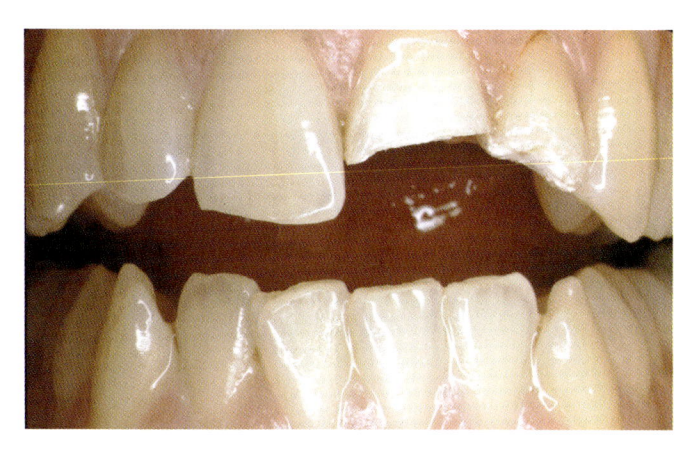

Figure 23.10 **(A)** This young lady fractured her left central and lateral incisors in an accident. Because the original teeth had protruded before fracturing, the patient requested that the restoration be accomplished with an improved appearance in the most permanent treatment available.

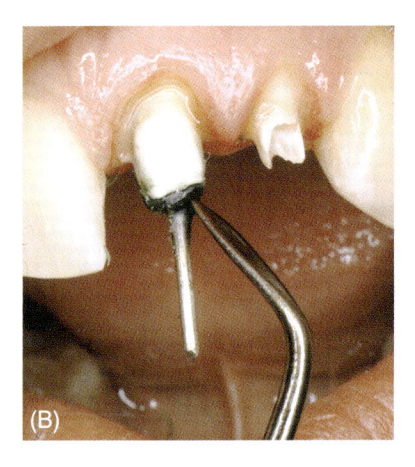

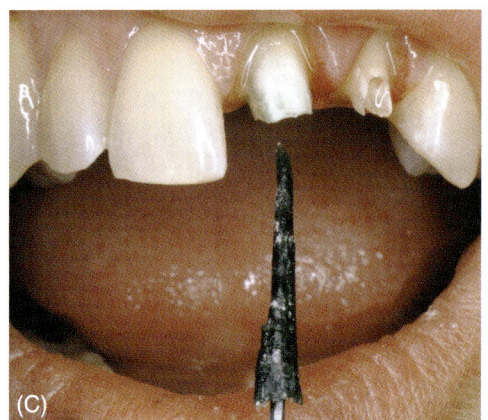

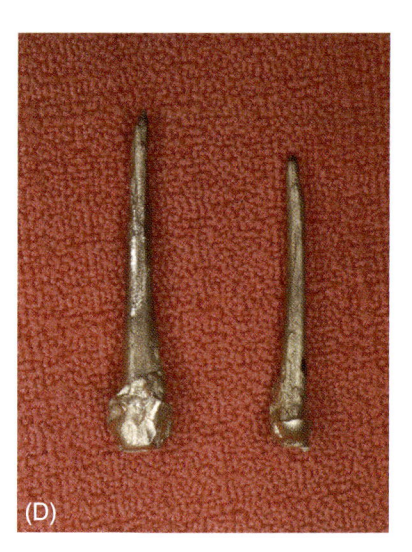

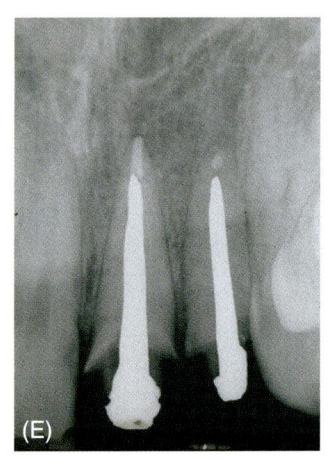

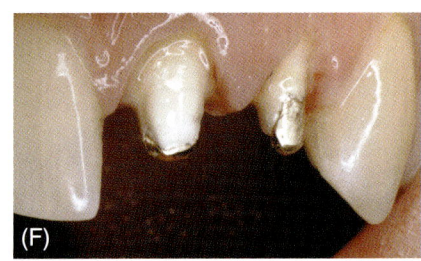

Figure 23.10 **(B–F)** Following endodontic therapy, two cast posts were constructed and cemented to place in the prepared incisors.

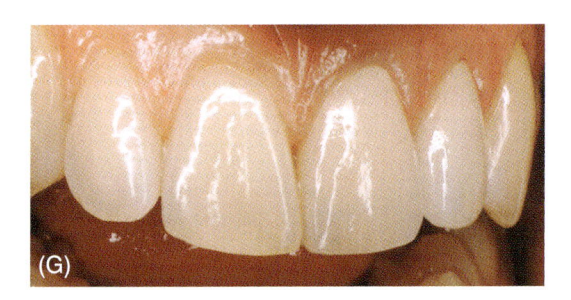

Figure 23.10 **(G)** The final all-ceramic crowns were bonded to place. Note how shade and texture help to blend in with the other teeth.

for the core or foundation can usually be obtained by taking advantage of the undercuts present in the pulp chamber, especially in molars. If a composite resin core material is used, it can be retained by both dentin bonding and the pulp chamber. If the tooth has hardly any coronal tooth structure (i.e., level with the gingival margin), a cemented, prefabricated post can be used to provide the required retention for the core restoration. Clinical research has supported the ability of posts to distribute stress in a favorable way that improves the fracture resistance of restored teeth.[34–36] Small premolars are more likely to need a post restoration because there may not be sufficient retention for the core.

In summary, endodontically treated anterior teeth do not always need to be crowned; when they are to be crowned, a post may or may not be required. Posterior teeth usually need a crown (i.e., cuspal coverage) but rarely require a post. The purpose of a post is to retain the core; it does not reinforce the root.[37,38]

Post design

Several principles must be considered in post selection and design. These principles apply for either prefabricated or cast posts. Design characteristics include length, diameter, shape, surface configuration or texture, method of attachment, and material. Many of these characteristics have been studied extensively by in vitro studies. In addition, several retrospective studies give guidance concerning optimum factors for post selection and design.

Retention of a post increases with increasing length. The post should at least be equal in length to the clinical crown or two-thirds of the root length, whichever is greater (Figure 23.10A and B). At least 4 mm of gutta-percha should be left in the apex of the root to maintain the apical seal. In contrast to post length, post diameter has little influence on retention. In fact, increasing post diameter requires removal of additional tooth structure and simply weakens the tooth, increasing the risk of a vertical root

(H) Prefabricated post and core	(I) Cast post and core	(J)

Figure 23.10 **(H)** The final all-ceramic crowns were bonded to place. Note the natural result of both the shade and texture of the crowned teeth. **(I)** Options for post-and-core restorations. **(J)** Optimum post length.

fracture. Therefore, the post should not be any larger in diameter than is absolutely necessary. The general guidelines are that the post should not be greater than one-third of the diameter of the root at the cement–enamel junction and that at least 1 mm of dentin thickness should be maintained at all levels of the root. Generally, it is best not to enlarge the post space any greater than the space created during root canal therapy. Too aggressive flaring of the canal during root canal therapy or enlargement of the canal space for a post will surely compromise the tooth. In the same vein, the shape of the post should be parallel rather than tapered. A tapered post design creates a wedging force within the root of the tooth. Conversely, parallel posts produce less stress and fewer vertical root fractures.

The surface configuration or texture has a significant influence on post retention. A smooth-surface or polished post is less retentive than a textured (e.g., sandblasted) post. Post designs that are serrated or crosshatched or have some other retentive design exhibit the best resistance to dislodgment.

One other design parameter is the mode of attachment. A post can have a passive fit in the tooth root and be retained by cement, or it can be actively retained (threaded like a screw) and retention gained by virtue of the threads (with or without the aid of cement). However, threaded posts create the potential for a significant wedging force within the tooth root and should be avoided. Parallel posts with proper length and a retentive surface design can obtain more than adequate retention. In situations when it is not possible to obtain the optimum length or shape, the required retention is much better and gained more safely by using a stronger cement (i.e., resin-modified glass ionomer or composite resin) than by using a threaded post.

There are several different materials that can be used for posts, including stainless steel, titanium, zirconium (tooth colored), ceramic, and polymers (Table 23.6). The material used for the post is much less important than the design and size of the post (i.e., preservation of tooth structure) unless esthetics becomes a consideration. If so, a tooth-colored post should be considered.

Sequence of treatment for posterior teeth (molars and large premolars)

The core buildup for a posterior tooth should be placed prior to crown preparation. A sufficient amount of time should have elapsed since completion of the root canal therapy to be confident that it has been successful. The tooth should be asymptomatic and not sensitive to percussion. Following root canal therapy, the typical molar will have a large existing restoration. All restorative materials and caries should be removed. The gutta-percha should be removed from the pulp chamber. The gutta-percha can be removed 1–2 mm into the canal orifices to increase retention (Figure 23.11). If there is at least one cusp remaining and the pulp chamber has walls of 2–3 mm in depth, a post is not required for retention of the core. The core should be composite resin (Table 23.7).

The advantage of composite resin is that it may be prepared immediately. Composite resin also offers the advantage of dentin bonding and a relatively simple technique for core placement. The main disadvantage of composite resin is that it is subject to water absorption and microleakage. It should only be used in posterior applications when it is possible to place the crown margins at least 2 mm beyond (i.e., apical to) the resin–tooth interface. A composite resin core material of contrasting color should be used to minimize the risk of inadvertently preparing the preparation margin on composite resin (Figure 23.12A–F).

For molars, if there is little remaining tooth structure or the pulp chamber is shallow, then a post should be used to provide retention for the core (Figure 23.13A). Usually, only one post is needed. A prefabricated post should be cemented into the largest

Table 23.6 Materials for Prefabricated Posts

	Material	Indications	Advantages	Disadvantages
Metallic stainless steel	Containing nickel (ASM 300)		Superior physical properties, radiopaque, excellent corrosion resistance	Nickel content (possible allergic response), metallic color
	No nickel (ASM 400)	General use; particularly suited for situations requiring high strength	Superior physical properties, radiopaque	Poor corrosion resistance, metallic color
Titanium	Commercially pure titanium (99%) Alloy Ti–Al–V		Moderate strength, biocompatibility / Superior physical properties, biocompatibility	Metallic color, not as radiopaque as stainless steel, difficult to cut
Nonmetallic Ceramic	Zirconia polycrystals	Situations requiring high esthetic demand; all-ceramic crowns	Tooth color, light transmission, high strength, white	Lack of long-term clinical results
Fiber–polymer composite	Carbon fibers		High strength, modulus of elasticity equal to dentin	No long-term clinical results, or white, fiber–polymer matrix interface may degrade

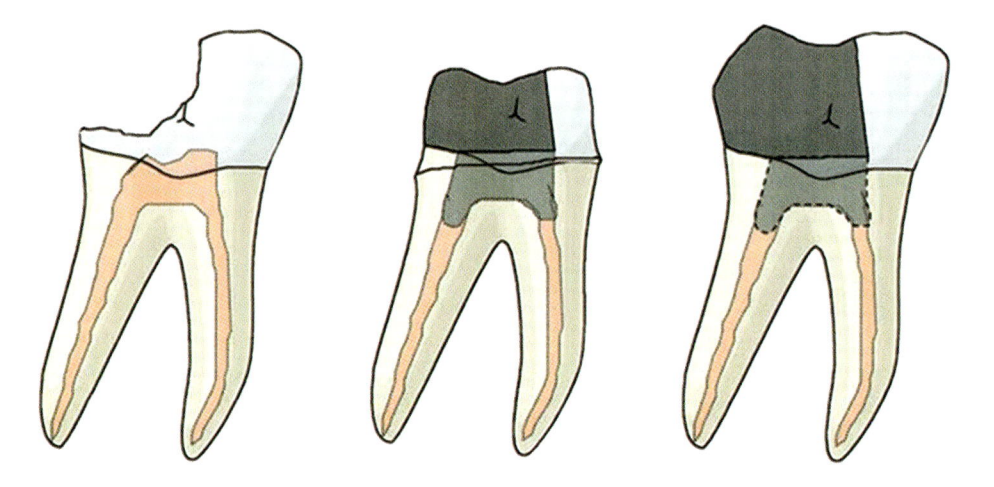

Figure 23.11 Composite resin core.

Table 23.7 Core Materials

	Indications	Advantages	Disadvantages
Conventional glass ionomers	Only for blockout of undercuts	Fluoride release	Low fracture toughness and strength, solubility
Resin-modified glass ionomer	Partial core buildup with adequate tooth structure present	Fluoride release, moderate strength, tooth color	
Composite resin	Core with prefabricated posts in anterior teeth	Tooth color, dentin bonding	Plastic deformation, absorbs moisture, dimensionally unstable
Cast metal	Cast post and core	Strength, core joined to post, biocompatibility	Cost, metallic color

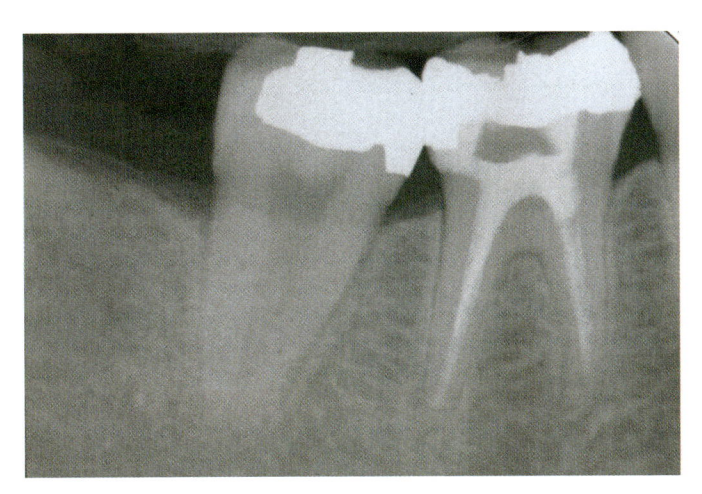

Chapter 23 Chipped, Fractured, or Endodontically Treated Teeth

Figure 23.12 **(A)** Periapical radiograph showing tooth #30 after successful root canal treatment.

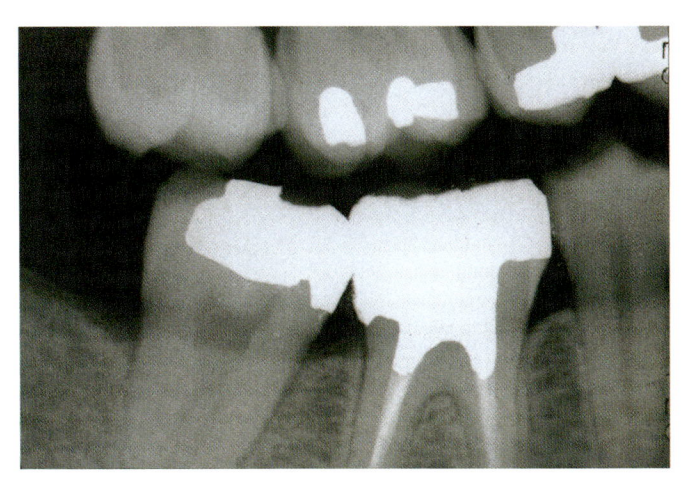

Figure 23.12 **(B)** Bitewing radiograph showing tooth #30 with amalgam core buildup completed. Note that the core material extends approximately 2 mm into the canal orifices for increased retention.

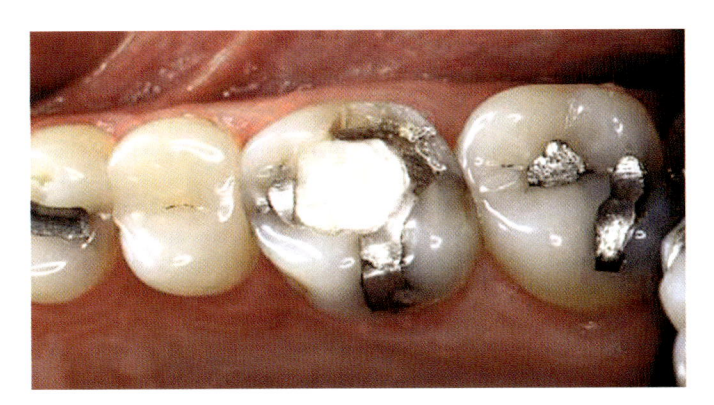

Figure 23.12 **(C)** Removal of temporary restorative material and remaining amalgam. Gutta-percha from the pulp chamber was removed for core retention.

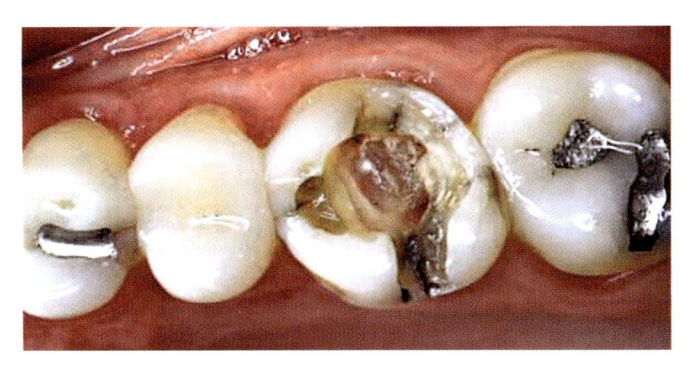

Figure 23.12 **(D)** Tooth #14 after successful root canal treatment. Note the crack on mesial and a photo should be made and a notation in the patient's chart since cracks may propagate.

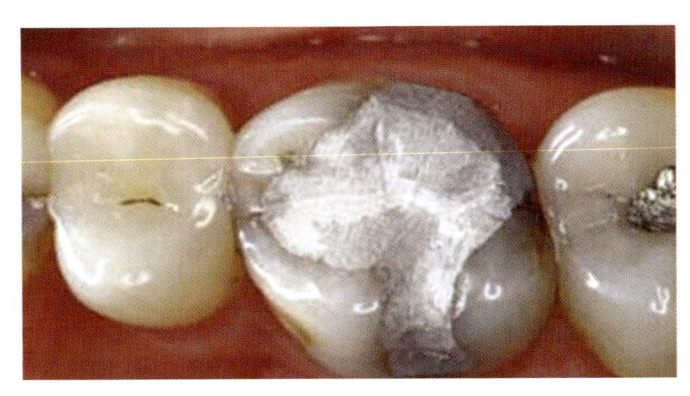

Figure 23.12 **(E)** Completed core buildup on tooth #14.

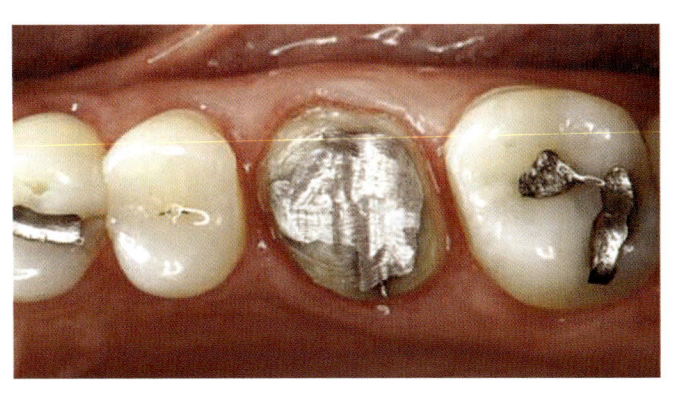

Figure 23.12 **(F)** Completed crown preparation on tooth #14.

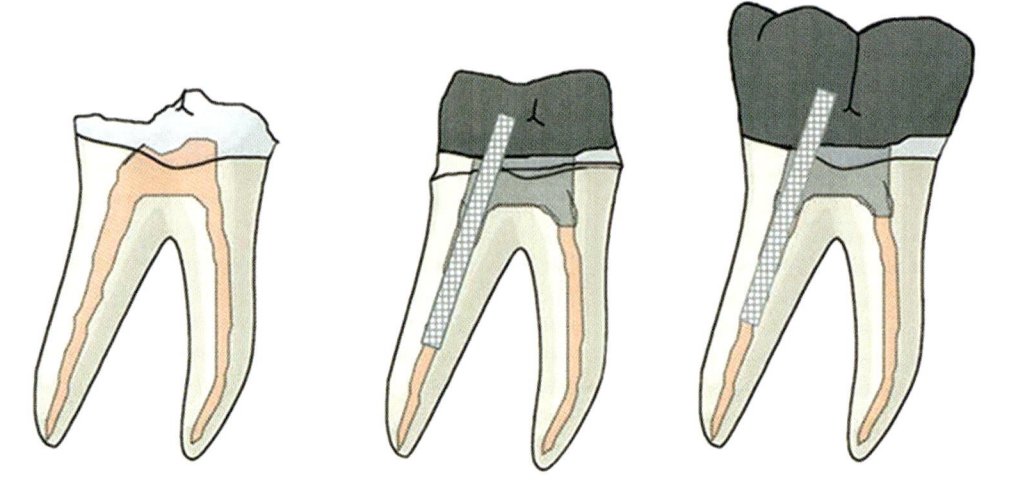

Figure 23.13 (A) Prefabricated post with core.

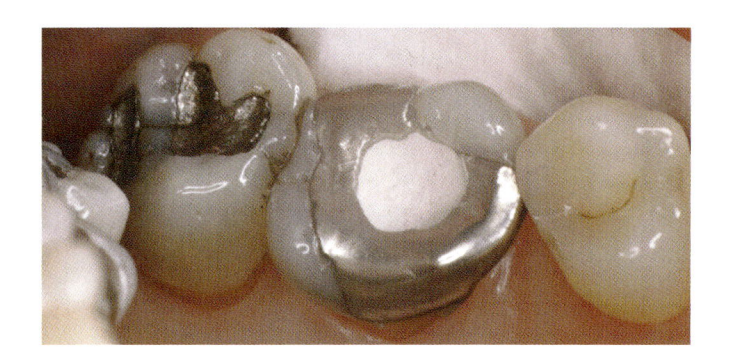

Figure 23.13 (B) Tooth #3 after successful root canal treatment.

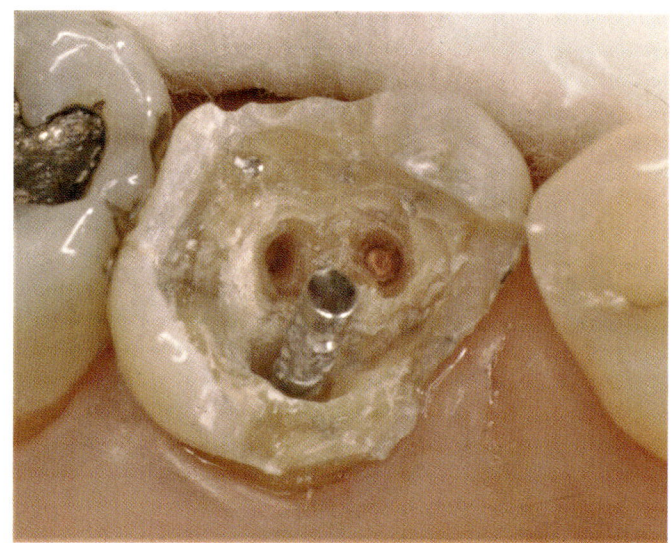

Figure 23.13 (C) Inadequate pulp chamber wall height and lack of remaining tooth structure evident after removal of previous restorative materials. Additional retention with prefabricated post is indicated.

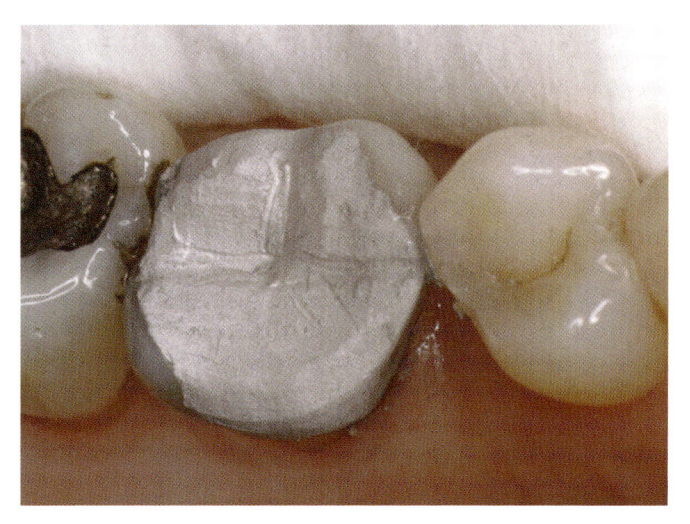

Figure 23.13 (D) Completed core buildup on tooth #3.

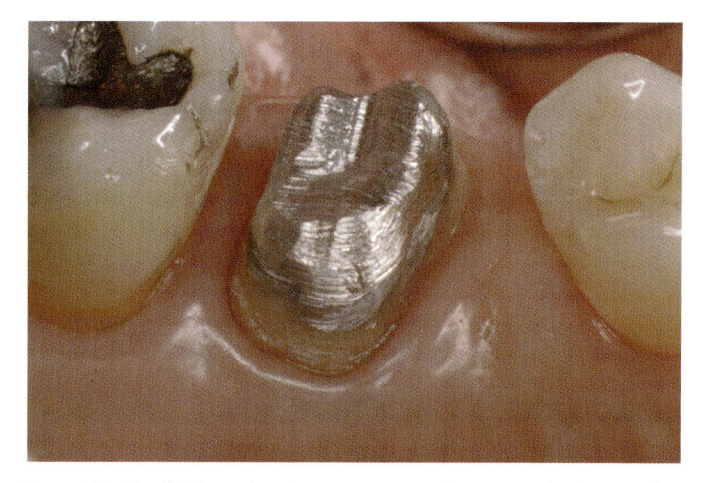

Figure 23.13 (E) Completed crown preparation on tooth #3. Note that the preparation margin extends apical to the core-tooth interface. (Although not esthetic, a metal 360 degree circumferential cord will improve long term retraction and fit of the final restoration.)

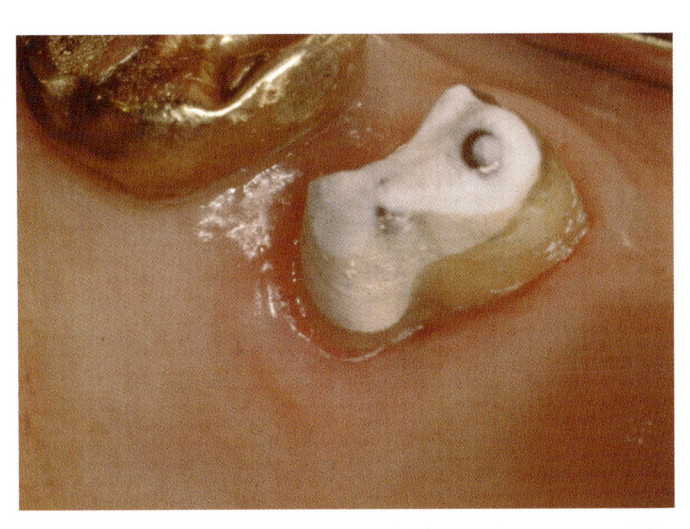

Figure 23.13 **(F)** Composite resin may also be used as core material, as is seen in another patient.

canal. In mandibular molars, this will typically be the distal canal. No attempt should be made to place a post in the mesial canal of a mandibular molar as the distal wall of the mesial root is thin and easily perforated. For maxillary molars, a single post in the lingual canal is adequate. Because the direction of the post is divergent from the pulp chamber, it creates excellent retention for the core (Figure 23.13B–F).

Sequence for anterior teeth

For anterior teeth, the decision to use a prefabricated post versus a cast post and core is best made after the crown preparation is completed (Table 23.8). The appropriate amount of incisal and axial reduction should be created. Then the amount of remaining sound tooth structure can be evaluated to make the decision about the post type. The prefabricated post and core is indicated when there is a moderate amount of remaining tooth structure or there are significant undercuts in the canal or pulp chamber that would require excessive removal of tooth structure. It should also allow the preparation of the crown margin to be at least 2 mm beyond the core to minimize the risk of water absorption. The advantage of this technique is that it conserves tooth structure, decreases the risk of root fracture, and is less expensive and time consuming. There are several disadvantages with the prefabricated post technique. The core of a prefabricated post and core is not as strong as a cast post and core. There is a risk of mechanical failure of the core since the composite resin core materials do not bond to cemented posts, unless a metal bonding agent is utilized, and, the resin core is susceptible to water absorption. It is also not indicated when the long axis of the root is significantly different from the long axis of the core.

The cast post and core is indicated when there is a minimal amount of remaining tooth structure or the core will be very close to the crown margin (less than 1 mm). It may also be needed when the core does not align with the root or there is a deep vertical overlap resulting in minimal occlusal clearance. The advantage of the cast post and core is that it is strong and will fit irregular or flared canals. The major disadvantages are that it is expensive, time consuming, and less conservative (requires more tooth reduction to eliminate undercuts or for canal enlargement).

Post preparation

After the decision has been made for either a cast post and core or a prefabricated post and core, the canal preparation should be initiated. The gutta-percha may be removed with either a hot instrument (plugger) or with a rotary instrument. The rotary instrument is more convenient, and there is no risk of burning the patient. A noncutting drill (Gates Glidden, Miltex, or Peeso reamer, Miltex) is the proper instrument for this step. The noncutting drill should be smaller in diameter than the existing canal space so that it only removes gutta-percha. A high-speed bur or an end-cutting drill from a prefabricated post kit should never be used to remove the gutta-percha because the risk of perforation is too great. The tooth is measured on a radiograph, a reference point is established on the tooth, and the gutta-percha is carefully removed to the desired depth, leaving a minimum of 4 mm for the apical seal. Ideally, a minimum of 10 mm of length should be obtained. The canal preparation should be the same at this point regardless of the type of post that is planned. No attempt should be made at this time to enlarge the canal; the goal of this step is to establish the proper post length.

Table 23.8 Post and Core Options for Anterior Teeth

	Indications	Advantages	Disadvantages
Prefabricated post and core	Moderate amount of remaining tooth structure Undercuts in canal or chamber Crown margin can be prepared ≥2 mm past core	Conserves tooth structure, decreased risk of root fracture, less expensive, simple technique, less time consuming	Not as strong as cast post and core, failure may occur at post–core interface
Cast post and core	Minimal amount of remaining tooth structure Core close to preparation margin Core does not align with root	Strong, fits irregular canals	Expensive, time consuming, less conservative

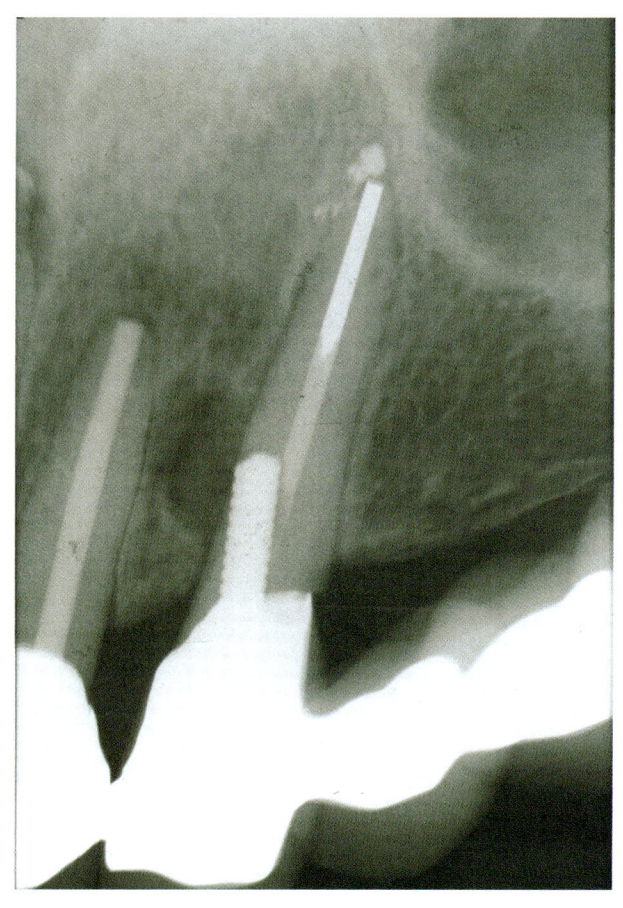

Figure 23.14 **(A)** Improper post and core technique leading to clinical failure.

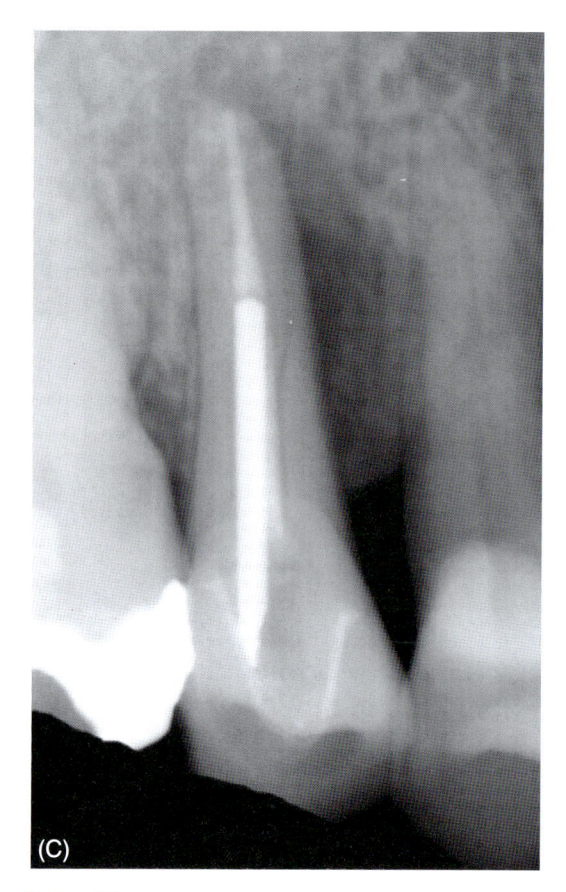

Figure 23.14 **(C)**

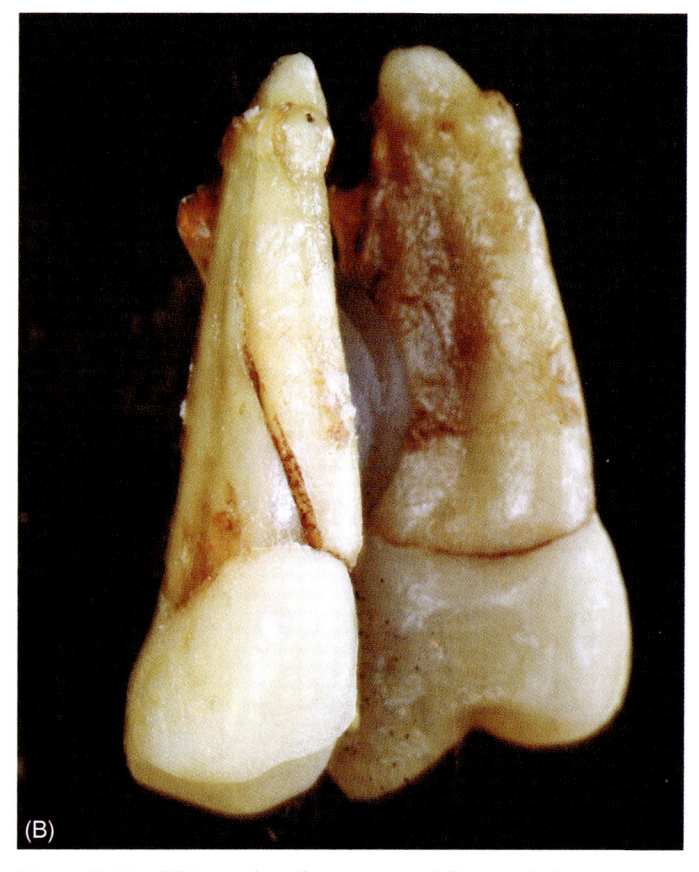

Figure 23.14 **(B)** Even when the proper guidelines are followed, endodontic-treated teeth can still lead to catastrophic fracture and end in extraction. Proper patient consent must be obtained before post placement in order to avoid future problems.

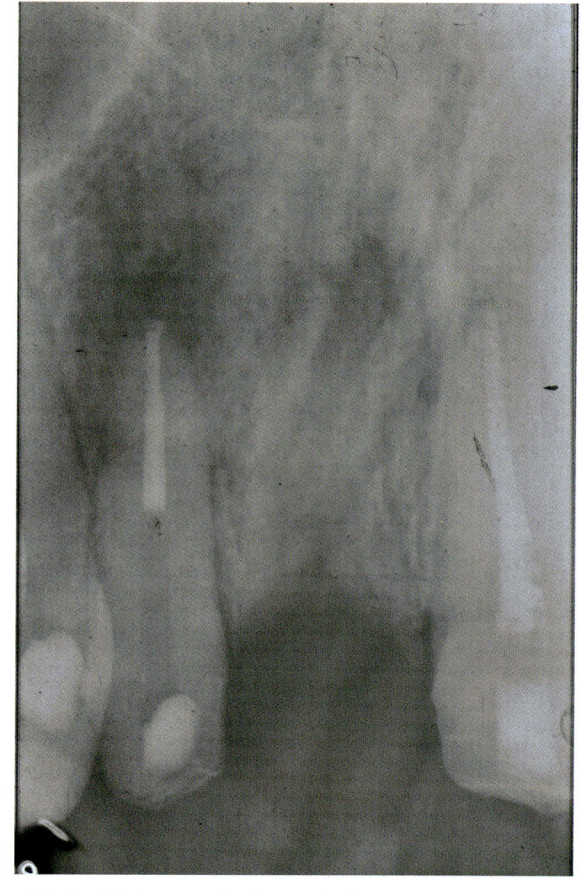

Figure 23.15 **(A)** Periapical radiograph showing tooth #7 after post space preparation.

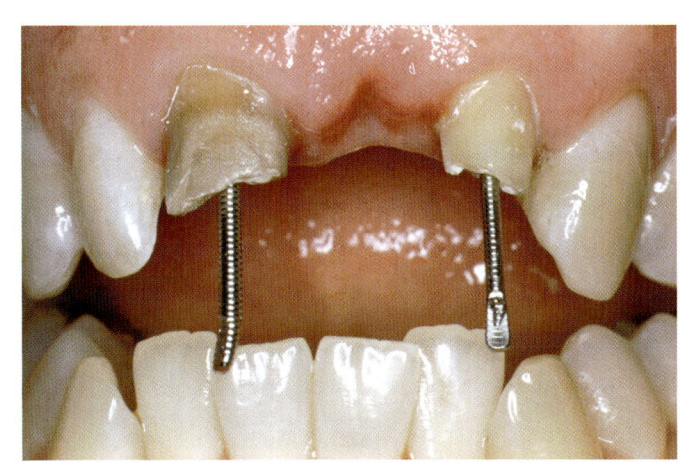

Figure 23.15 (B) Try-in of prefabricated posts. The post should be at least equal in length to the clinical crown or two-thirds of the root length.

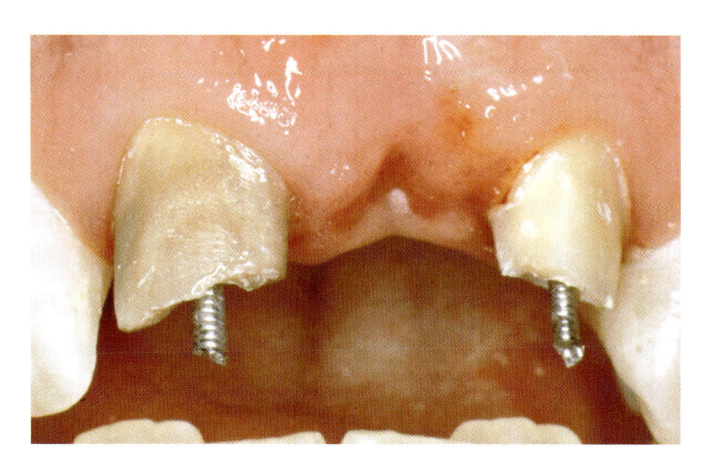

Figure 23.15 (C) Prefabricated post cut to length and cemented.

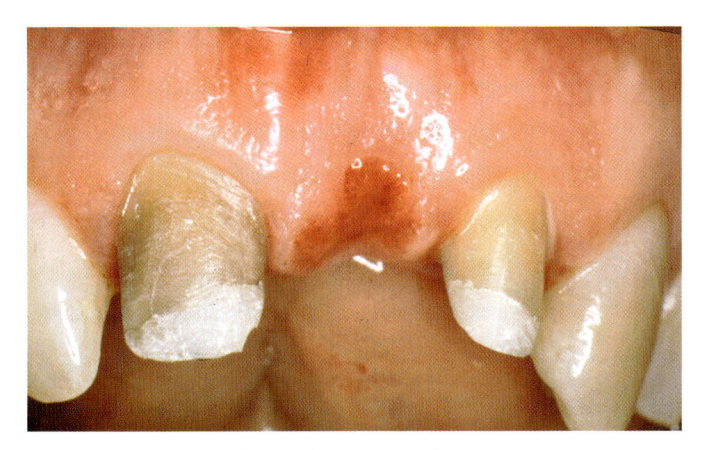

Figure 23.15 (D) Teeth #8 and #10 restored with composite core buildup material and prepared to receive porcelain-fused-to-metal crowns.

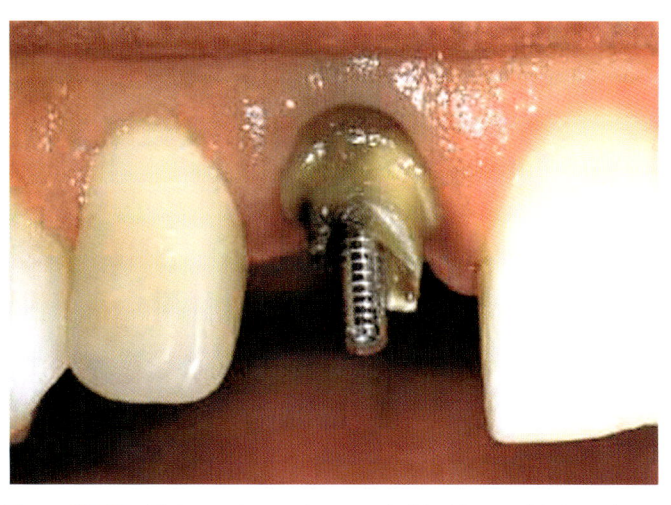

Figure 23.15 (E) In another patient, tooth #8 with a prefabricated post cut to length and cemented.

The post space length and preservation of gutta-percha in the apical portion of the root can be verified with a radiograph at this time. Digital radiographs are a distinct advantage as they save considerable time and require much less radiation, thus allowing the operator to take multiple views during the entire procedure. Combined with digital radiography, the use of an intraoral camera or surgical microscope can provide an excellent view of the canal and an inherent safety factor in preventing perforation. A tiny light source can also be a help in visualizing if you are still drilling in the center of the channel (Microlux, Addent). Next, the canal should be shaped with the drills provided with the post system. Enlargement of the canal should be kept to a minimum, remembering that the tooth becomes weaker as more tooth structure is removed. The canal should not be enlarged any greater than is necessary to accommodate the post (Figure 23.14A–C). The typical maxillary lateral incisor should not be enlarged to more than 0.040 inches (~1 mm) in diameter. Maxillary central incisors may be enlarged to a diameter of 0.050 inches (~1.3 mm). If the coronal portion of the canal is flared, the canal should not be enlarged to achieve

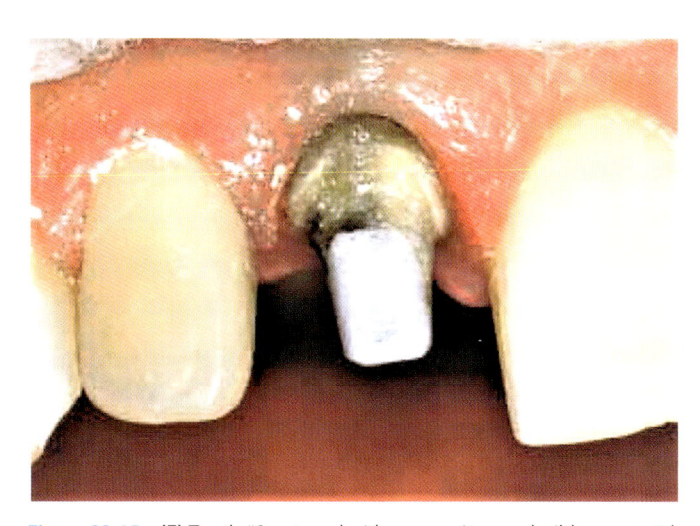

Figure 23.15 (F) Tooth #8 restored with composite core buildup material.

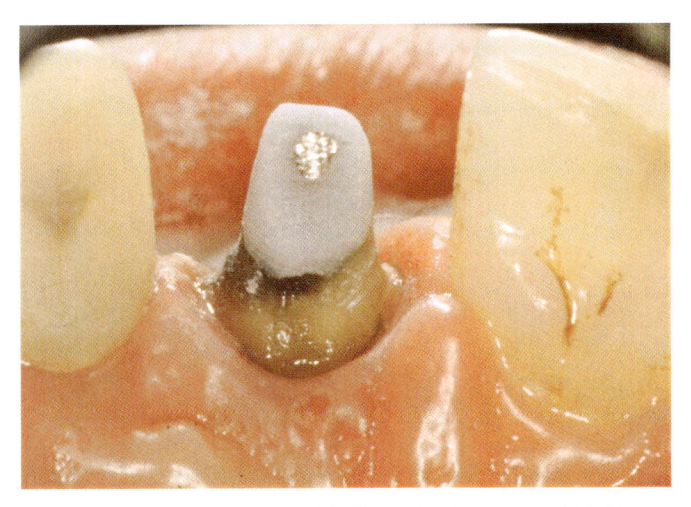

Figure 23.15 **(G)** Mirror view of the lingual surface of tooth #8. Note the ferrule design with 1–2 mm of vertical tooth structure beyond the restorative margin.

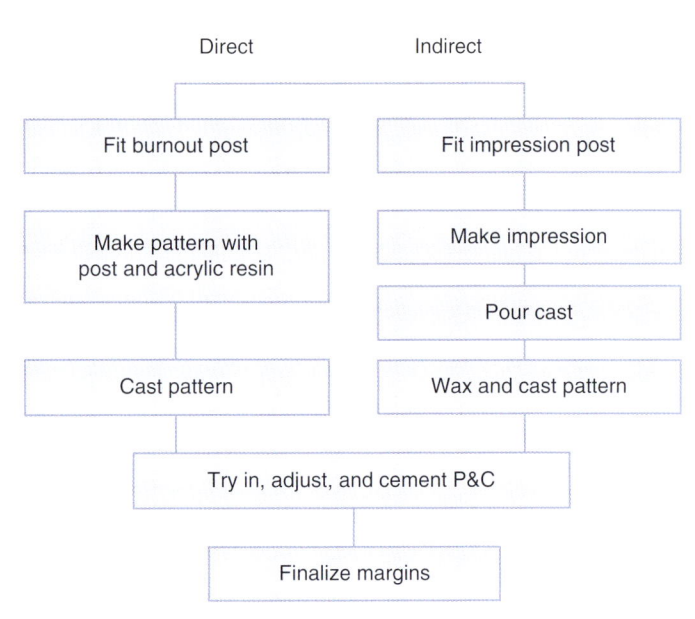

Figure 23.16 Direct and indirect techniques for cast post and core.

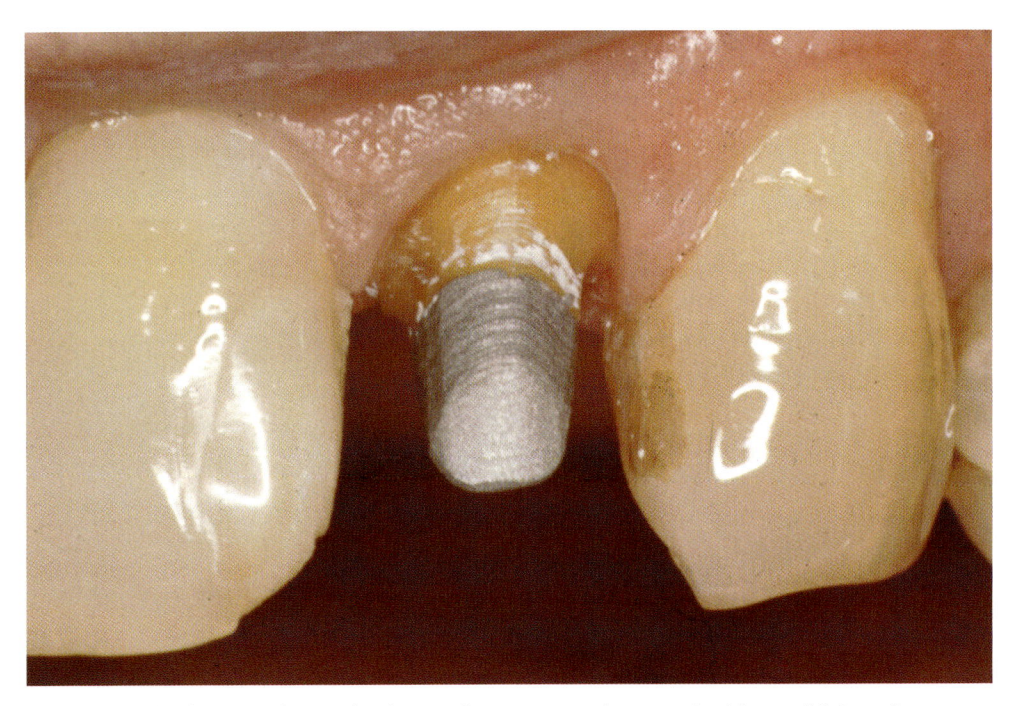

Figure 23.17 Similar case restored with post and core. The decision between restoring a tooth with a prefabricated post or cast post and core depends on how much intact tooth structure is remaining.

parallel walls as this will unnecessarily weaken the root. In this case, it may be better to use a tapered, prefabricated post design or a cast post and core in combination with a resin cement, but use a parallel drill below the tapered area.

The choice of material type is probably less significant than adhering to accepted design principles (i.e., adequate length, parallel shape). The most commonly used prefabricated post types are stainless steel, titanium, or titanium alloy. The prefabricated post can be cemented with any acceptable cement, including glass ionomer or resin cement. If the post is shorter than desired or the canal is tapered, a resin cement should be considered. For the core, composite resin has the necessary strength, provides dentin bonding, and is the material of choice to use with prefabricated posts in anterior teeth. Figure 23.15 shows two examples of the use of post and composite resin buildup.

Chapter 23 Chipped, Fractured, or Endodontically Treated Teeth

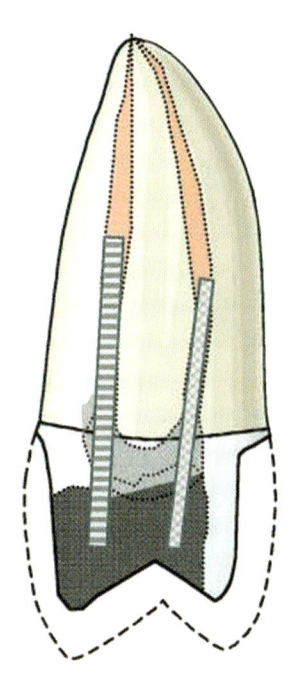

Figure 23.18 **(A)** Prefabricated post for additional core retention.

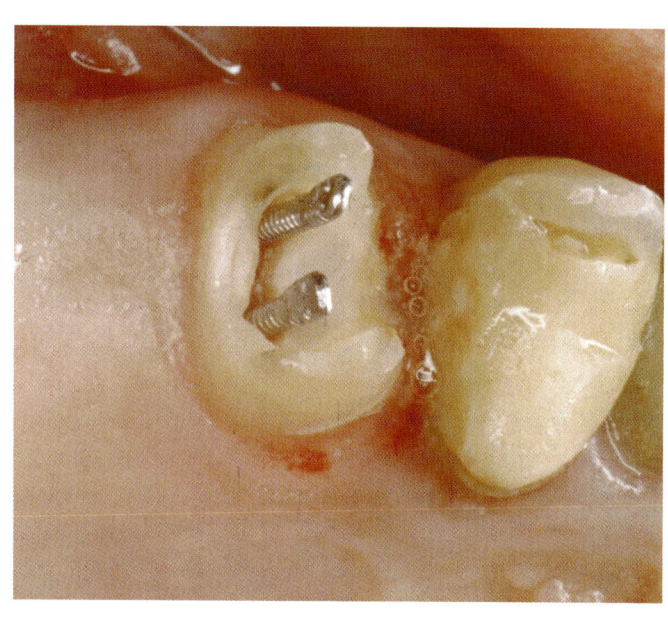

Figure 23.18 **(B)** Prefabricated posts in the two canals of a premolar prior to core placement. It is usually not possible to make these posts very long because of canal curvature. Because canals are usually not parallel to each other, the core is well retained by posts.

If a cast post and core is indicated, the pattern can be made by either a direct or an indirect technique (Figure 23.16). For the direct technique, undercuts in the canal or pulp chamber must be blocked out. Then a direct pattern can be made using the appropriate-size plastic post from the post system and making the core with autopolymerizing acrylic resin. With the indirect technique, an impression of the tooth is obtained using a plastic post to record the post space. The post can be cast in either a noble or non-noble metal (Figure 23.17). For smaller diameter posts, a type III gold alloy is inadvisable as it does not provide adequate strength. The use of a non-noble alloy (Ni–Cr–Be) provides the potential for resin bonding of the post to the dentin surface of the canal. This may be desirable for short posts or for tapered canals.

For cementation of the post, a groove or vent should be created along the length of the post to allow for excess cement to escape. If using resin or glass ionomer cements, a Lentulo spiral drill (DENTSPLY/Caulk) should be used to place the cement into the canal. This will result in the maximum retention for the post. After the cement has set, the excess is removed, and the core material is placed (prefabricated post) or the impression procedures are initiated (cast post and core).

For resin cement, the instructions for the bonding and cementation procedures for the cement should be followed. This may include placing cement on the post rather than into the canal to prevent overly rapid set of the cement. One advantage of using resin cement is that the core material can be placed immediately after the post is seated. Then the cement and core resin can set simultaneously and bond together. This technique works especially well when retrofitting a post to an existing crown (reverse post crown repair).

Sequence for premolars

The type of foundation restoration for a premolar is determined by the amount of available tooth structure. This requires making an estimation of the amount of tooth structure that will remain after the crown preparation. If there is a moderate amount of tooth structure, the tooth can be restored like a molar using composite resin as the core material. Similar to a molar, the retention for the core would be gained by either mechanical retention and/or dentin bonding. If there is minimal tooth structure, it is best to use the same treatment sequence as described for an anterior tooth. First, the tooth is prepared for the indicated crown. Then the amount of remaining tooth structure is evaluated. If the premolar has two roots, prefabricated posts can be cemented in the two canals (Figure 23.18A and B). It is usually not possible or even necessary to make these posts very long because of canal curvature. However, because the canals are usually not parallel, following placement of the core, the posts and core are virtually impossible to dislodge. For a small premolar, composite resin is an excellent material. If there is minimal or no coronal tooth structure, a cast post should be considered, especially for a single-rooted premolar.

Principles for crown preparation

The proper preparation of the tooth after completion of the post and core restoration is very important. Even with the ideal canal preparation and post restoration, the post has a tremendous potential to act as a wedge in the tooth root. This can result in initiation of a vertical root fracture and subsequent loss of the tooth. The best way to protect the tooth (i.e., the

Esthetic Problems of Individual Teeth

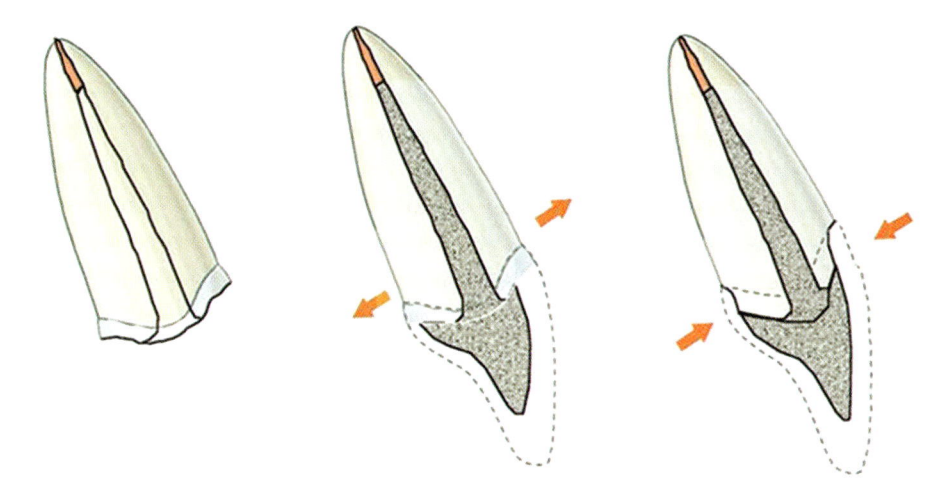

Figure 23.19 Ferrule design resists wedging force of post.

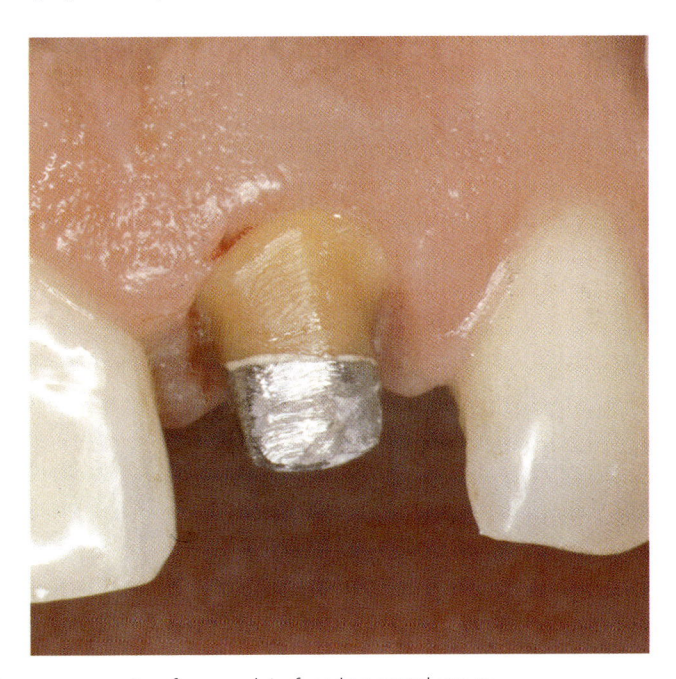

Figure 23.20 (A) Proper ferrule design on preparation for porcelain-fused-to-metal crown.

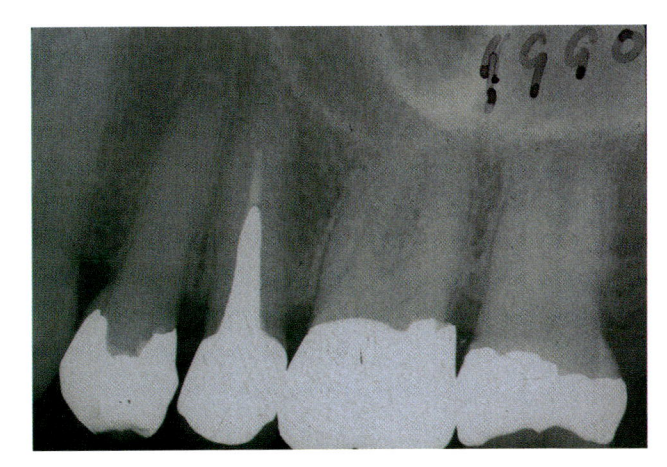

Figure 23.20 (B) Radiograph showing cast post and core after cementation. Note that the post is more than one-third of the diameter of the root at the cement–enamel junction and is tapered. Tooth preparation did not exhibit ferrule design.

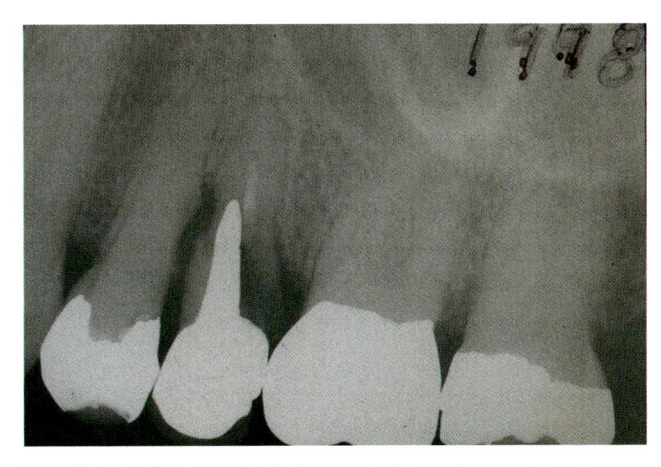

Figure 23.20 (C) Same clinical case as in Figure 23.20B after 8 years. Note the oblique root fracture. Such a fracture could be prevented by a more conservative post in combination with proper ferrule design in the crown preparation.

root) against this wedging force is by the creation of a ferrule design in the crown preparation on the tooth.[13,31,39–41] The ferrule design is the encirclement of 1–2 mm of vertical tooth structure by the crown. This encirclement, like metal bands on a barrel, helps protect the tooth from fracture. It resists the wedging forces that would be transmitted to the post from the occlusion. To create an adequate ferrule, the margin usually must be prepared further apically. Often, this requires a crown-lengthening procedure to gain sufficient tooth length to prepare the ferrule (Figure 23.19). This principle of creating a ferrule around the tooth is probably the single most important principle in the restoration of endodontically treated teeth (Figure 23.20). If an adequate ferrule is obtained, the type, material, and design of the post and core become much less important. Conversely, if a ferrule is not obtained, then the tooth is at risk of fracturing no matter what type of post or core is used. This is especially true for teeth that are expected to carry a heavy load, such as a removable partial denture or fixed partial denture abutment or in patients who exhibit excessive wear or bruxism.

References

1. Andreasen FM, Noren JG, Andreasen JO, et al. Long-term survival of fragment bonding in the treatment of fractured crowns: a multicenter clinical study. *Quintessence Int* 1995;26:669–681.
2. Hunter ML, Hunter B, Kingdon A, et al. Traumatic injuries to maxillary incisor teeth in a group of South Wales school children. *Endod Dent Traumatol* 1990;6:260–264.
3. Baratieri LN, Ritter AV, Junior SM, Filho JCM. Tooth fragment reattachment: an alternative for restoration of fractured anterior teeth. *Pract Periodont Aesthet Dent* 1998;10:115–127.
4. Goldstein RE. Chipped or fractured teeth. In: *Esthetics in Dentistry*. Philadelphia, PA: JB Lippincott; 1976:54–64.
5. Goldstein RE. Diagnostic dilemma: to bond, laminate, or crown. *Int J Periodont Restor Dent* 1987;7:5, 8–29.
6. Goldstein RE. Repairing fractured teeth. In: *Change Your Smile*, 3rd edn. Carol Stream, IL: Quintessence; 1997:89–106.
7. Macedo GV, Diaz PI, Fernandes CA, Ritter AV. Reattachment of anterior teeth fragments: a conservative approach. *J Esthet Restor Dent* 2008;20(1):5–18.
8. Fahl N Jr. Predictable aesthetic reconstruction of fractured anterior teeth with composite resins: a case report. *Pract Periodont Aesthet Dent* 1996;8(1):17–31.
9. Fahl N Jr. Optimizing the esthetics of Class IV restorations with composite resins. *J Can Dent Assoc* 1997;63:108–111, 114–115.
10. Simonsen RJ. Traumatic fracture restoration: an alternative use of the acid-etch technique. *Quintessence Int Dent Dig* 1979;10:15–22.
11. Simonsen RJ. Restoration of a fractured central incisor using original tooth fragment. *J Am Dent Assoc* 1982;105:646–648.
12. Croll TP. Rapid reattachment of fractured crown segment: an update. *J Esthet Dent* 1990;2:1–5.
13. Hyde TP. A reattachment technique for fractured incisor tooth fragments: a case history and discussion of alternative techniques. *Prim Dent Care* 1995;2(1):18, 20–22.
14. Strassler HE. Aesthetic management of traumatized anterior teeth. *Dent Clin North Am* 1995;39:181–202.
15. Vissichelli VP. Restoration of a fractured maxillary central incisor by using the original tooth fragment. *Gen Dent* 1996;44:238–240.
16. Walker M. Fractured-tooth fragment reattachment. *Gen Dent* 1996;44:434–436.
17. Munksgaard EC, Hojtved L, Jorgensen EH, et al. Enamel–dentin crown fractures bonded with various bonding agents. *Endod Dent Traumatol* 1991;7:73–77.
18. Liebenberg WH. Esthetics in the cracked tooth syndrome: steps to success using resin-bonded ceramic restorations. *J Esthet Dent* 1995;7:155–166.
19. Liebenberg WH. Use of resin-bonded partial coverage ceramic restorations to treat incomplete fractures in posterior teeth: a clinical report. *Quintessence Int* 1996;27:739–747.
20. Bader JD, Shugars DA, Robertson TM. Using crowns to prevent tooth fracture. *Community Dent Oral Epidemiol* 1996;24:47–51.
21. Cavalleri G, Zerman N. Traumatic crown fractures in permanent incisors with immature roots: a follow-up study. *Endodont Dent Traumatol* 1995;11:294–296.
22. Ehrmann EH. Restoration of a fractured incisor with exposed pulp using original tooth fragment: report of a case. *J Am Dent Assoc* 1989;118:183–185.
23. Cvek MA. A clinical report on partial pulpotomy and capping with calcium hydroxide in permanent incisors with complicated crown fracture. *J Endod* 1978;4:232–237.
24. Kanca J III. Replacement of a fractured incisor fragment over pulpal exposure: a long-term case report. *Quintessence Int* 1996;27:829–832.
25. Goldstein RE, Levitas TC. Preservation of fractured maxillary central incisors in an adolescent: report of a case. *J Am Dent Assoc* 1972;84:371–374.
26. Kopperud SE, Tveit AB, Gaarden T, et al. Longevity of posterior dental restorations and reasons for failure. *Eur J Oral Sci* 2012;120(6):539–548.
27. Goldstein GR. The longevity of direct and indirect posterior restorations is uncertain and may be affected by a number of dentist-, patient-, and material-related factors. *J Evid Based Dent Pract* 2010;10(1):30–31.
28. Goldstein RE. Esthetic principles for ceramo-metal restorations. *Dent Clin North Am* 1988;21:803–822.
29. Andreasen JO, Andreasen FM. *Essentials of Traumatic Injuries to the Teeth*. Copenhagen, NY: Munksgaard; 1990.
30. Isidor F, Brondum K, Ravnholt G. The influence of post length and crown ferrule length on the resistance to cyclic loading of bovine teeth with prefabricated titanium posts. *Int J Prosthodont* 1999;12:78–82.
31. Libman WJ, Nicholls JI. Load fatigue of teeth restored with cast posts and cores and complete crowns. *Int J Prosthodont* 1995;8:155–161.
32. Saupe WA, Gluskin AH, Radke RA Jr. A comparative study of fracture resistance between morphologic dowel and cores and a resin-reinforced dowel system in the intraradicular restoration of structurally compromised roots. *Quintessence Int* 1996;27:483–491.
33. Loquercio AD, Leski G, Sossmeier D, et al. Performance of techniques used for re-attachment of endodontically treated crown fractured teeth. *J Dent* 2008;36(4):249–255.
34. Salameh Z, Ounsi HF, Aboushelib MN. Fracture resistance and failure patterns of endodontically treated mandibular molars with and without glass fiber post in combination with a zirconia-ceramic crown. *J Dent* 2008;86:513–519.
35. Cagidiaco MC, Garcia-Godoy F, Vichi A, et al. Placement of fiber prefabricated or custom made posts affects the 3-year survival of endodontically treated premolars. *Am J Dent* 2008;21:179–184.

36. Ferrari M, Cagidiaco MC, Grandini S, et al. Post placement effects survival of endodontically treated premolars. *J Dent Res* 2007;86:729–734.
37. Sorensen JA, Martinoff JT. Intracoronal reinforcement and coronal coverage: a study of endodontically treated teeth. *J Prosthet Dent* 1984;51:780–784.
38. Sorensen JA, Martinoff JT. Clinical significant factors in dowel design. *J Prosthet Dent* 1984;52:28–35.
39. Assif D, Bitenski A, Pilo R, Oren E. Effects of post design on resistance to fracture of endodontically treated teeth with complete crowns. *J Prosthet Dent* 1993;69:36–40.
40. Hemmings KW, King PA, Setchell DJ. Resistance to torsional forces of various post and core designs. *J Prosthet Dent* 1991;66:325–329.
41. Sorensen JA, Engelman MJ. Ferrule design and fracture resistance of endodontically treated teeth. *J Prosthet Dent* 1990;63:529–536.

Additional resources

Bakland LK, Milledge T, Nation W. Treatment of crown fractures. *J Calif Dent Assoc* 1996;24(2):45–50.

Boscato N. Pereira-Cenci T. Moraes R. Swift, E. Self-adhesive resin cement for luting glass fiber posts. *J Esthet Rest Dent* 2014;26: 417–421.

Dietschi D, Duc O, Krejci I, Sadan A. Biomechanical considerations for the restoration of endodontically treated teeth: a systematic review of the literature—Part 1. Composition and micro- and macrostructure alterations. *Quintessence Int* 2007;38:733–743.

Dietschi D, Duc O, Krejci I, Sadan A. Biomechanical considerations for the restoration of endodontically treated teeth: a systematic review of the literature, Part II (Evaluation of fatigue behavior, interfaces, and in vivo studies). *Quintessence Int* 2008;39:117–129.

Gogna R, Jagadish S, Shashikala K, Keshava Prasad B. Restoration of badly broken, endodontically treated posterior teeth. *J Conserv Dent* 2009;12:123–128.

Goldstein RE. Current concepts in esthetic treatment. In: *Proceedings of the Second International Prosthodontic Congress; 1979; Los Angeles, CA*. Chicago, IL: Quintessence; 1979:310–312.

Goldstein RE. Esthetics in dentistry. *J Am Dent Assoc* 1982;104: 301–302.

Goldstein RE. Finishing of composites and laminates. *Dent Clin North Am* 1989;33:305–318.

Goldstein RE. *Change Your Smile*, 3rd edn. Carol Stream, IL: Quintessence; 1997.

Goldstein RE, Feinman RA, Garber DA. Esthetic considerations in the selection and use of restorative materials. *Dent Clin North Am* 1983;27:723–731.

Goldstein RE, Garber DA, Schwartz CG, Goldstein CE. Patient maintenance of esthetic restorations. *J Am Dent Assoc* 1992;123:61–66.

Goldstein RE, Garber DA, Goldstein CE, et al. The changing esthetic dental practice. *J Am Dent Assoc* 1994;125:1447–1457.

Loomba K, Loomba A, Bains R, Bains VK. A proposal for classification of tooth fractures based on treatment need. *J Oral Sci* 2010;52:517–529.

Meyenberg K. The ideal restoration of endodontically treated teeth-structural and esthetic considerations: a review of the literature and clinical guidelines for the restorative clinician. *Euro J Esthet Dent* 2013;8(2):238–268.

Patel DK, Burke FJ. Fractures of posterior teeth: a review and analysis of associated factors. *Dent Clin North Am* 1995;39:181–202.

Rauschenberger CR, Hovland EJ. Clinical management of crown fractures. *Dent Clin North Am* 1995;39:25–51.

Takatsu T, Sano H, Burrow MF. Treatment and prognosis of a vertically fractured maxillary molar with widely separated segments: a case report. *Quintessence Int* 1995;26:479–484.

Wahl MJ, Schmitt MM, Overton DA, Gordon MK. Prevalence of cusp fractures in teeth restored with amalgam and with resin-based composite. *J Am Dent Assoc* 2004;135:1127–1132

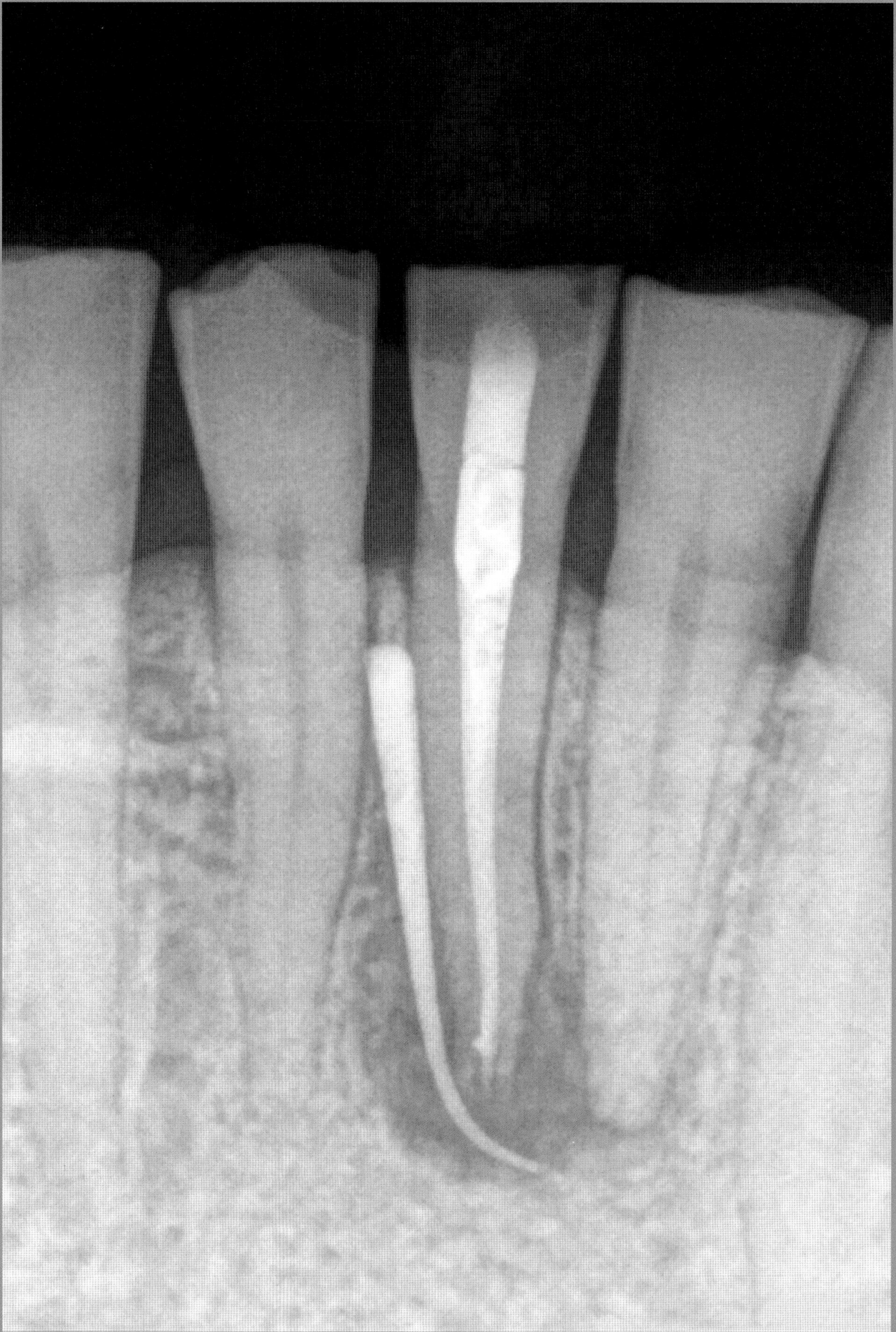

Chapter 24 Endodontics and Esthetic Dentistry

John West, DDS, MSD, Noah Chivian, DDS,
Donald E. Arens, DDS, MSD*, and Asgeir Sigurdsson, DDS, MS

Chapter Outline

Endodontics: an essential part of treatment planning	750	Ceramic restorations	776
Clinical evaluation	750	Aluminous porcelain	777
Dental history and building rapport	750	Porcelain-fused-to-metal crown	778
Communication: listen, learn, and record	751	Ceramic crowns: cast glass–all-ceramic crowns (aluminum oxide)–pressed ceramics (lithium disilicate)	778
Visual examination	751		
Periodontal probing	751		
Thermal pulp tests	754	Zirconia crowns	778
Electric pulp testing	756	Ceramic inlays and onlays	778
Cavity test	758	Etched cast restoration	779
Periradicular tests	759	Crown retention after endodontic treatment	779
Pretreatment radiographs	762	Removable partial denture abutments	780
Precementation radiographs	762	Instrumentation/debridement	780
Anesthetic test	763	Sealing the canal system	780
Diagnosis	764	Coronal seal background	781
Pulpal response to operative procedures	764	Restoration or removal of the endodontically diseased tooth	782
Pulpal repair	766		
Elective endodontics for pulpal reasons	767	Bleaching	783
Depth of preparation/remaining dentin	767	Walking bleach technique	784
Pulp capping	769	Trauma	790
Stressed pulp	770	Crown fractures	790
Elective endodontics for prosthetic reasons	770	Root fractures	790
Endodontic treatment protocols	771	Luxation and avulsion	793
Rubber dam is essential	771	Cracked tooth syndrome	794
Alternative methods of rubber dam for ceramic crowns	772	Increased prevalence	797
		Differential diagnosis	798
Access cavity preparation	774	Cracked tooth syndrome classes and treatment	798
Preparation and equipment	775	Endodontic surgery	804
Various types of restored teeth	776	Tissue discoloration (tattoo)	805
Gold crowns	776		

* Deceased

This chapter is dedicated to the memory of our colleague Donald E Arens, co-editor of the previous version of this chapter, whose passion for teaching was exceeded only by his humor and ability to see the finest qualities in his large circle of friends. May his memory be a blessing to all who were touched by him. Don was alive when we began this endodontic and esthetic chapter update, and his hand has had a profound positive influence and was his final contribution to dentistry, education, and the advancement of our profession.

Within the last three decades, dentists have witnessed a change in the number of patients who have shifted their priorities from prevention and repair to alignment and esthetics. In response, dental manufacturers have focused their attention on developing restorative materials that are color-fast and strong enough to resist maximum biting forces. As those materials became easier to manage and more reliable, dentists have designed and developed operative techniques that require minimal tooth reduction without losing their retentive and esthetic value.

The goal of esthetic dentistry is to create a smile that improves a patient's appearance and restores their self-image while also meeting biologic and structural considerations. However, reaching that goal goes beyond just reshaping a tooth or teeth and replacing the tooth's surface with a resin or ceramic. A comprehensive esthetic treatment plan must be all encompassing and take into consideration occlusive malpositioned teeth within the natural curvature of the arch, the health and welfare of the periodontal tissues, including pocket depth, and the loss of crestal soft tissue and bone. Of greatest importance is the diagnosis of pulp health before restorative procedures are scheduled. As such, the practitioner performing the endodontic procedures must either believe in their diagnosis and continue with the treatment plan or, when the prognosis is difficult, aggressively eliminate the potential for a latent endodontic problem by intentionally removing the pulp. This decision, as difficult as it is, is preferable to responding to pulpal disease after the esthetic restorations are in place.

Endodontics: an essential part of treatment planning

Endodontics should be incorporated into the interdisciplinary treatment process when the ultimate esthetic design is being determined. Treatment sequencing can be established and painful episodes and disruption of the restorative schedule avoided if the pulpal health and any previous endodontically treated teeth are evaluated early in the planning stages. The patient should be informed that the overall treatment plan is dynamic and may change as conditions arise. It is equally important to evaluate the patient's radiographs and, if deep existing amalgam or other restorations will be replaced as part of the treatment plan, the patient should be advised of future problems due to the depth and extent of those restorations. If, at a later time, there are complications such as an inflamed pulp or pain following final cementation, the patient has at least been informed and forewarned. The key here is to "pave your way with words." Irreversible pulpal inflammation and subsequent pulpal necrosis is often cumulative and multifactorial and can occur when the dentist least expects it, such as with a seemingly innocent and small facial restoration. However, a minor operative procedure may be the last pulpal insult needed to damage the pulp. After all, the pulp cannot benefit from the usual healing potentials in the body. It is incased in unyielding walls of dentin; it is a terminal circulation; it is a relatively large volume of tissue for a relatively small foraminal blood supply. This problem is sometimes complicated by difficulty not seeing or appreciating the depth of certain tooth-colored restorations. Magnification helps to overcome this obstacle.

The removal of existing restorations, excavation of decay, and the paralleling of multiple abutments may require periodic reassessment and endodontic reconsideration. Sensitive teeth that do not respond to palliative measures within a reasonable period of time may require endodontics. There is nothing more disheartening to a patient who has completed perhaps 18 months of combined orthodontic, periodontal, and restorative treatment than to experience a "toothache" shortly after final cementation. Although pulpal problems cannot always be predicted, a great majority can be avoided with insight, careful evaluation, and good interdisciplinary collaboration, sequencing, and judgment.

Clinical evaluation

The success of any reconstructive treatment plan begins with the question: is it predictable? Predictability begins with biology. Biology begins with health of periodontium (see Chapter 37), pulp, and surrounding attachment apparatus. The health of the pulp, the periradicular area, and the quality of the existing root canal treatment of the teeth to be restored need to be in the forethought and not an afterthought of treatment planning. That is why an endodontic chapter is included in this text about esthetics. Discussed in the following are standardized and time-tested procedures which help determine pulp and periradicular condition. Proper evaluation should include many, if not most of these.

- Communication that includes listening and recording
- Visual examination
- Periodontal probing
- Thermal tests
- Electric tests
- Cavity tests
- Periradicular tests: percussion and palpation
- Bite tests
- Radiographic evaluation
- Anesthetic test.

Dental history and building rapport

Besides knowing the medical condition of the patient, the diagnostician should ask the patient about previous dental experiences. Their desires and objectives should be clearly defined.

If neglect is evident, the reasons for the neglect should be determined and discussed. If phobia and anxieties exist, the extent of the case should be explained and relaxation techniques should be offered to assure a comfortable and pain-free treatment experience.

In addition, when a professional air of confidence, concern, and care are exhibited by the doctor and staff, the patient's trust, faith, and interest are earned and developed.

Once this rapport is established, the patient becomes far more receptive to accepting and entering a treatment plan regardless of its difficulty, fee, time, and patient apprehensions. The quality of treatment is inversely proportional to the level of stress experienced by the patient and the doctor during the dentistry. Again, informing your patient about the potential for existing restorations contributing to future endodontic treatment is essential for continued patient trust.

Communication: listen, learn, and record

As dentists, we are the professionals who must perform the tests, interpret the results, and design a treatment based on the information gathered. When the diagnosis is not evident, we must turn to the patient for that one pinpointing clue. Sir William Osler, the famous Canadian diagnostician, once said, "Listen, listen, listen, – for the patient is giving you the diagnosis." This statement is profound. The diagnostician must not only ask sufficient and leading questions to obtain as much information as possible but also listen carefully to interpret the verbal response and its expressed meaning. Patients should be quoted verbatim in the chart and their answers must become a permanent record for review.

Visual examination

Direct examination of each tooth with some method of magnification, loupes or a microscope, is essential to locate fracture lines, decay, or defective restorations. Transillumination through a fiber-optic light may be of great assistance in detecting color shifts in a crown (Figure 24.1A and B). A tooth with a pink or reddish hue could indicate internal hemorrhage from a recent injury (Figure 24.2), a dental procedure (Figure 24.3), or gingival tissue hyperplasia that has invaded a coronal cavity produced by caries or resorption (Figure 24.4A–D).

A gray, blue, or black color might indicate blood infiltrate hemostasis within the dentinal tubules and chamber, long-term necrotic tissue (Figure 24.5), or silver precipitants from certain root canal sealers and filling materials (Figure 24.6A–C). A yellow or brown (Figure 24.7A) unrestored crown often represents a physiologically calcified nonpathologic obliteration of the root canal chamber or root canal system (Figure 24.7B). Pharmacologically affected (i.e., tetracycline-stained) teeth may vary in color from yellow to black (Figure 24.8A–C) and their drug florescence and etiology may be verified by using an ultraviolet light or Woods black light. This situation is an infrequent finding now since the diminished use of tetracycline antibiotics in children. Many of these discolorations can be reduced or eliminated by oxidizing techniques and agents without requiring endodontic intervention (see Chapter 12).

Teeth with vertical fractures have a diagnostic constant. The transilluminated light does not pass through the fracture line, but the crown beyond the fracture (Figure 24.9A and B) or the opposite cusp(s) (Figure 24.10) appear darker. Periodontal probing, cold testing, and a bite test will possibly assist in confirming the diagnosis of cracked tooth syndrome (CTS).

Periodontal probing

Periodontal probing and evaluating the depth of the sulcus and individual pockets are of great importance to the treating dentist and the treatment plan. There are two main reasons for this:

1. If there is a combined periodontal–endodontal disease associated with a tooth, the true cause of the problem is not only difficult to diagnose but could be more difficult to manage during treatment.

Figure 24.1 **(A)** Transillumination of a maxillary left central incisor with a necrotic pulp.

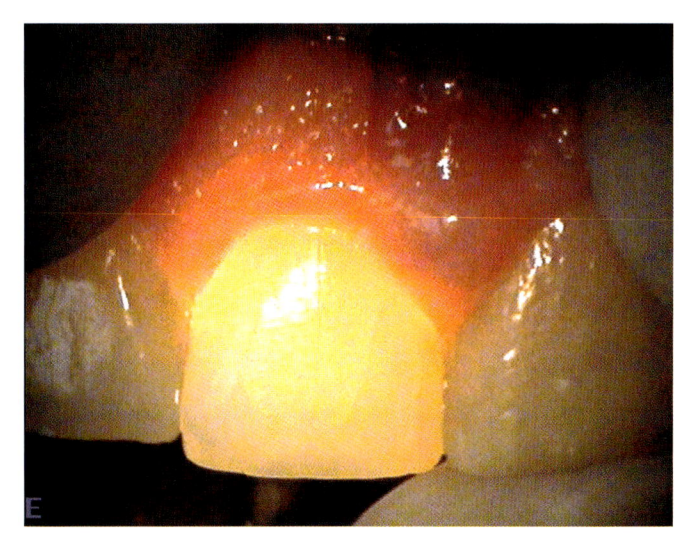

Figure 24.1 **(B)** Transillumination of the adjacent tooth with a vital pulp. Because there is an active blood flow through the live pulp tissue the tooth appears brighter to the fiber-optic light.

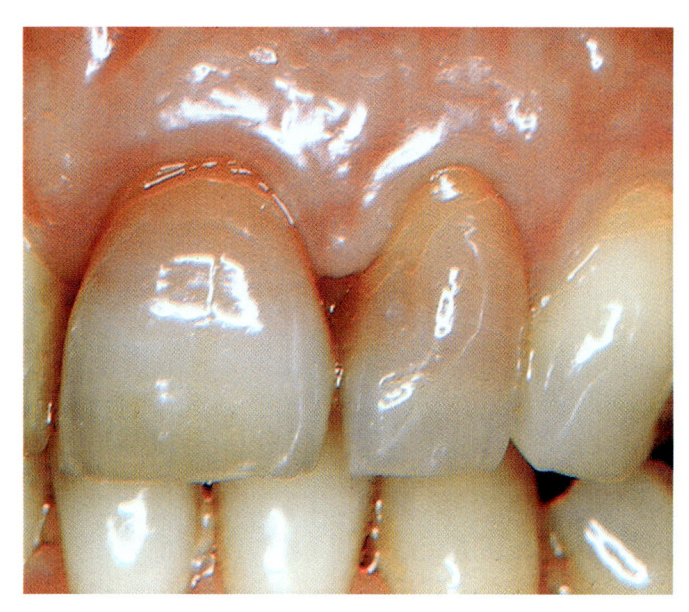

Figure 24.2 The maxillary central and lateral incisor teeth experienced a concussion injury and there was subsequent extravasation of blood causing the reddish hue.

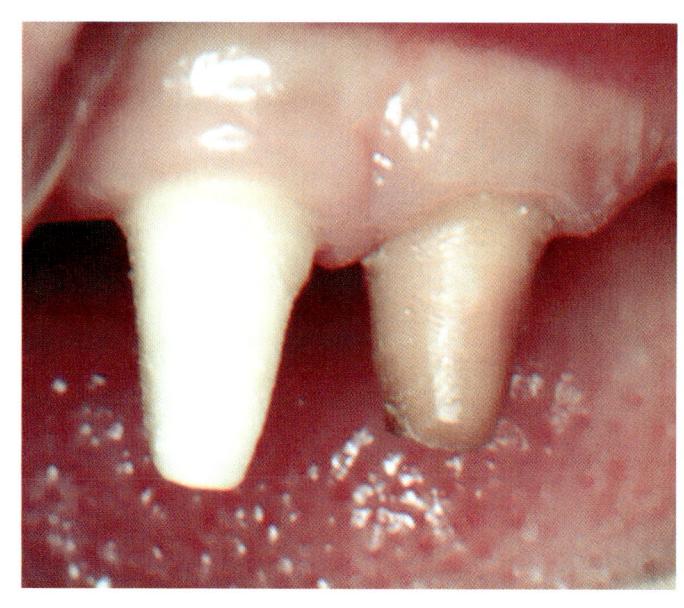

Figure 24.3 One week following crown preparation the tooth structure was red, signifying extravasations of blood and the need for pulp extirpation.

2. If there is an isolated, narrow but deep periodontal pocket somewhere around the tooth, a vertical root fracture must be ruled out before any further restorative treatment.

The pocket could simply be a draining sinus tract from a necrotic or infected pulp, especially if the pocket probing is precipitous and not conical as it would be in an independent lesion of periodontal origin. Accurate periodontal probing is essential to make the diagnosis of endodontic sinus tract versus periodontal pocket. Like a waterfall, the endodontic sinus tract may be narrow or wide. The key question is the probing conical suggesting a lesion of periodontal origin or is it precipitous suggesting a lesion of endodontic origin? If the sulcular sinus tract is part of a lesion of endodontic origin, endodontic treatment would then be indicated. The pocket should heal without any periodontal treatment within days after the initial root canal system cleaning visit. It is important to note that periodontal scaling or curettage

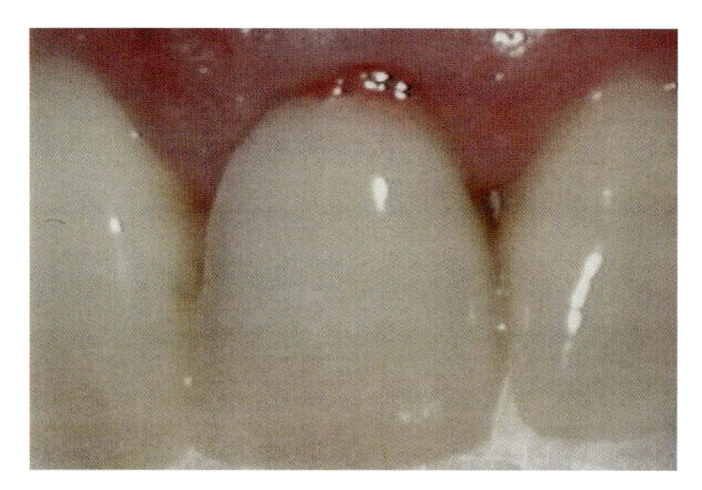

Figure 24.4 **(A)** Pink spot as a result of external resorption.

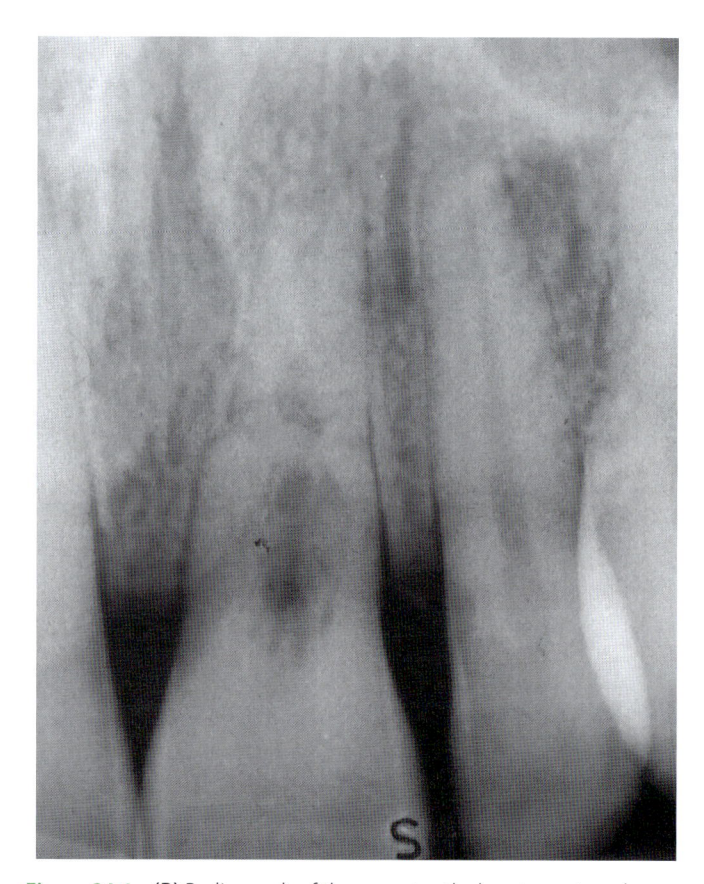

Figure 24.4 **(B)** Radiograph of the same tooth showing external resorption.

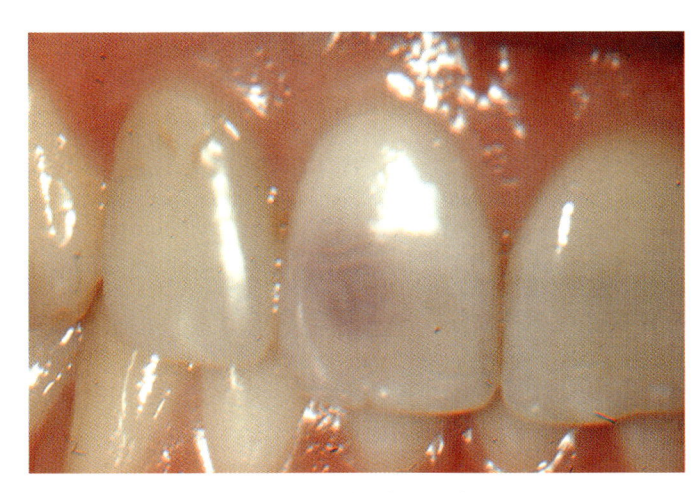

Chapter 24 Endodontics and Esthetic Dentistry

Figure 24.4 **(C)** Pink spot as a result of internal resorption.

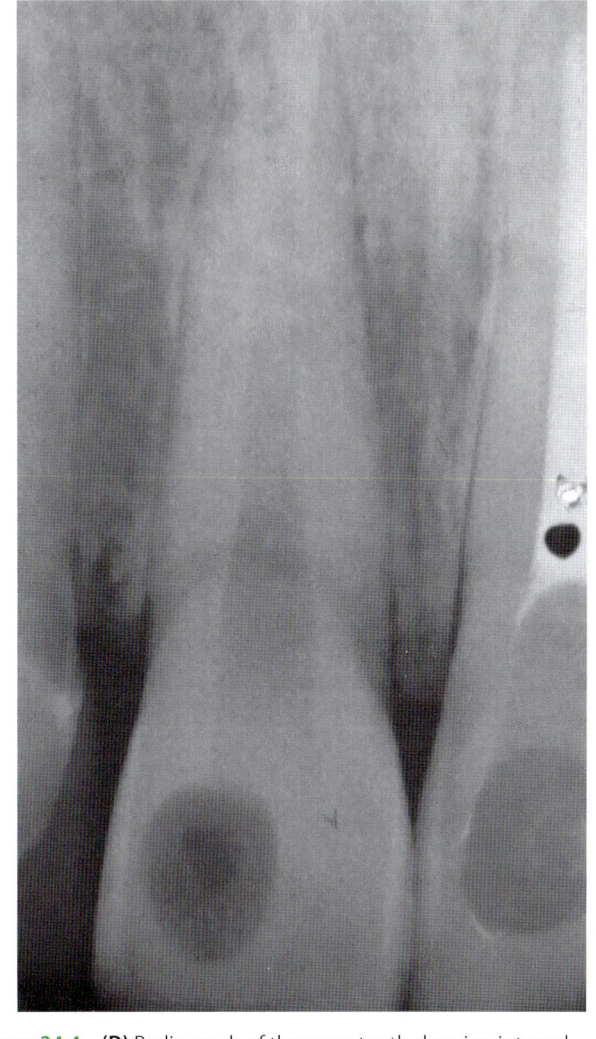

Figure 24.4 **(D)** Radiograph of the same tooth showing internal resorption.

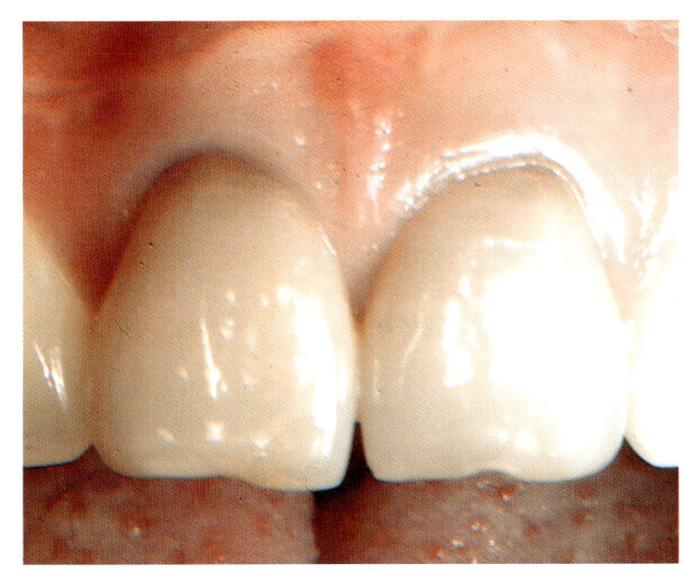

Figure 24.5 Maxillary central incisors with necrotic pulps.

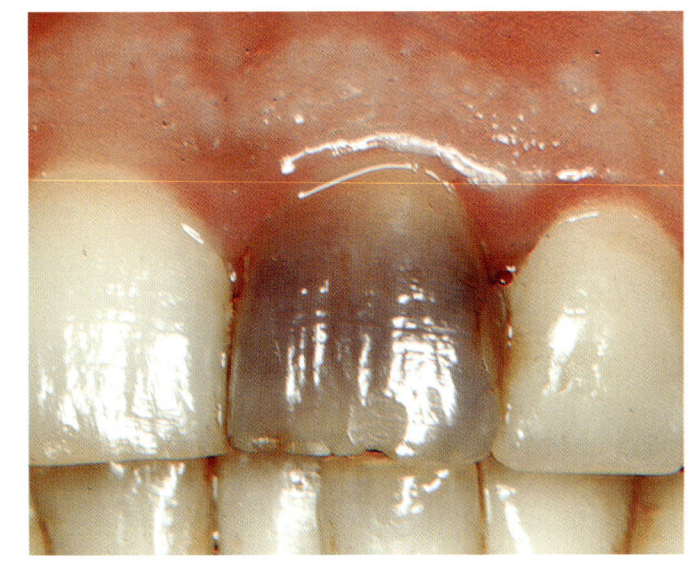

Figure 24.6 **(A)** Discoloration from silver containing root canal cement.

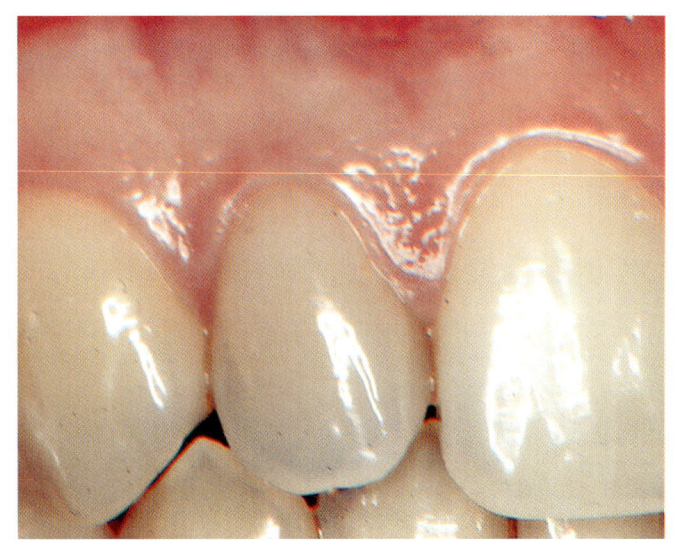

Figure 24.6 **(B)** Gray color of crown from a post.

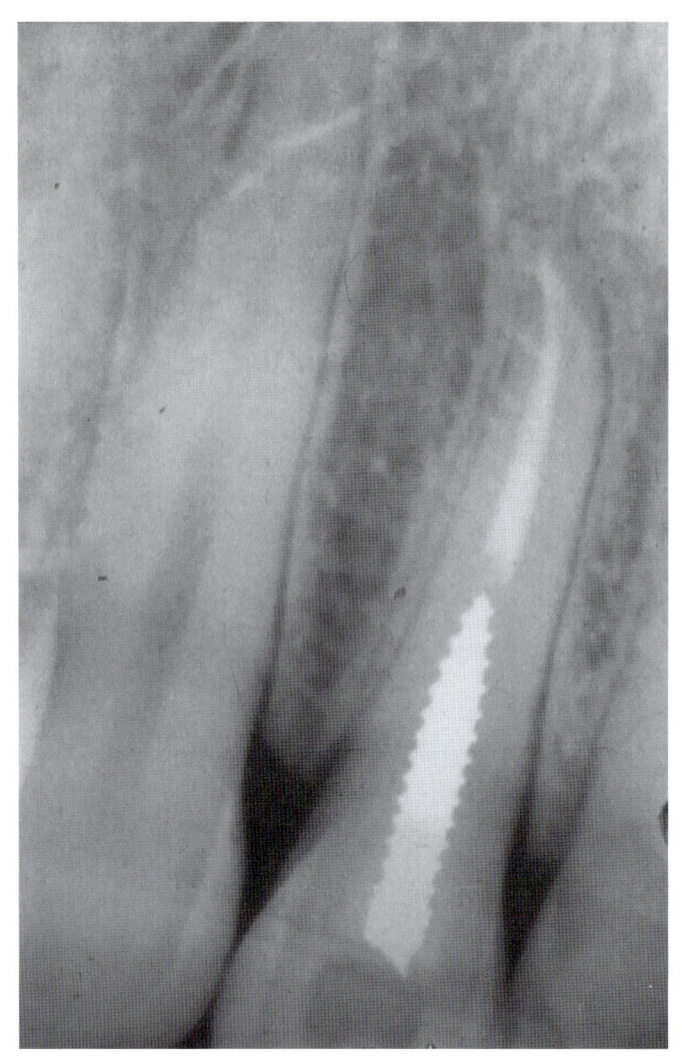

Figure 24.6 (C) An unnecessary post that caused the discoloration.

can be detrimental to healing of the pocket and, therefore, should postponed if the diagnosis is a lesion of endodontic origin. If the pocket has not healed after a few days of beginning endodontic treatment, the whole diagnosis needs to be reassessed and other possible diagnoses ruled out. The pocket could be associated with a vertical root fracture where the prognosis of the tooth is hopeless. Endodontic treatment would not resolve the pocket nor would periodontal treatment cure the condition. Removal and replacement of the tooth would be the only predictable treatment option.

Thermal pulp tests

Cold testing

In an effort to determine pulp vitality, cold testing is probably the most commonly advocated and the most accurate. In the past, an "ice pencil" (water frozen in sterilized anesthetic cartridge and removed) (Figure 24.11) or an ice cube was the only consistent way to chill a tooth. The problem with using frozen water is it may not be cold enough ($\geq 0\,°C$) to penetrate a porcelain crown. However, in a tooth with an acute pulpitis an "ice pencil" could be an effective diagnostic tool. Recently, 1,1,1,2-tetrafluoroethane spray (Endo-Ice®, Hygenic, Akron, OH) has become the cold testing method of choice (Figure 24.12A). The spray is cold enough ($-26\,°C$) to penetrate most crowns.

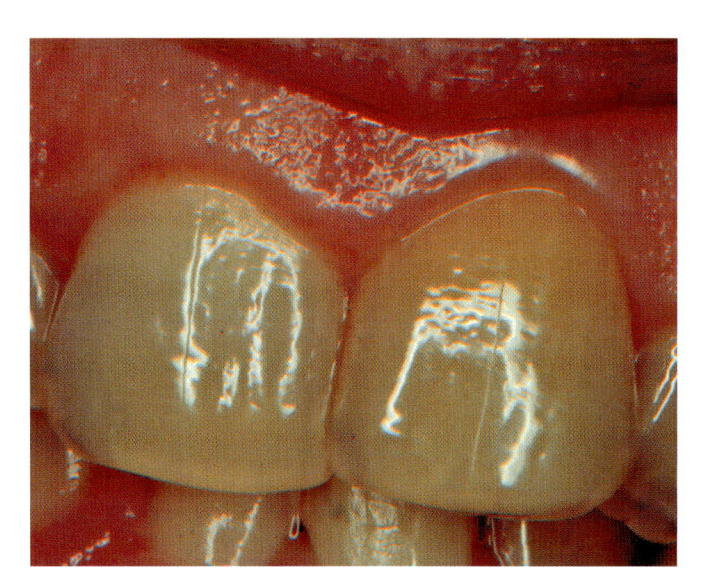

Figure 24.7 (A) The crown of this maxillary central incisor discolored gradually over a 3-year period following a concussion injury. The complete fill-in of the pulp chamber with dentin is the cause of the yellowish brown hue.

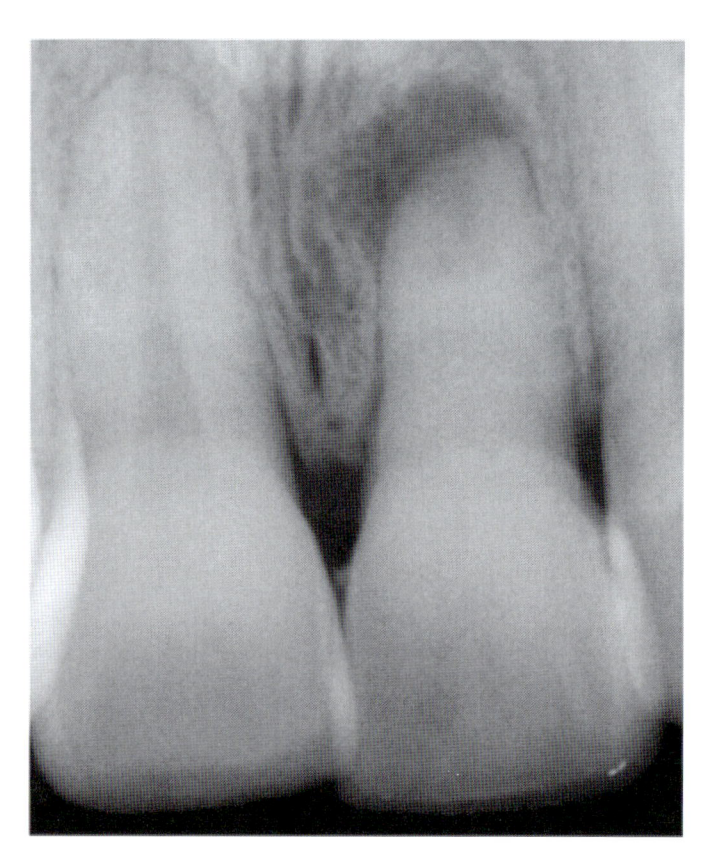

Figure 24.7 (B) Radiograph of a similar maxillary central incisor 10 years after a concussion injury. The pulp chamber is filled in with dentin producing the discoloration. In this case, there was pulp death after discoloration appeared. Because the pulp canal was obliterated, a surgical approach was used to seal the apex.

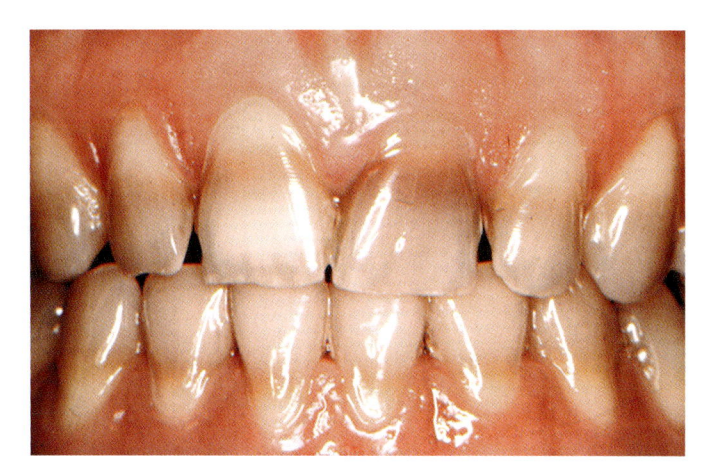

Chapter 24 Endodontics and Esthetic Dentistry

Figure 24.8 **(A)** Brown staining from Terramycin.

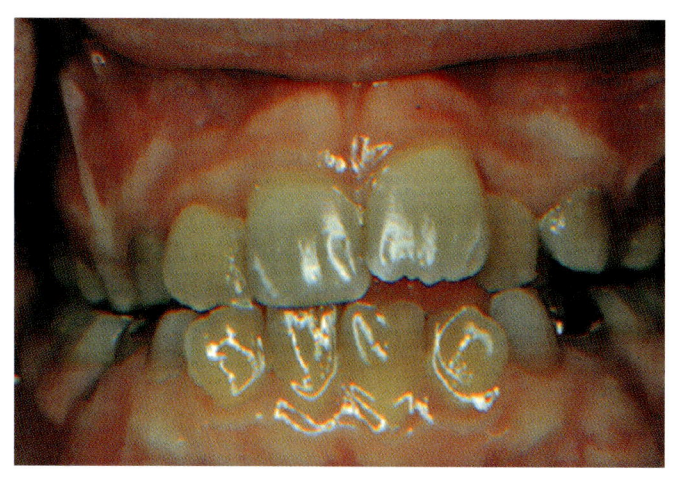

Figure 24.8 **(B)** Gray staining from Acromycin.

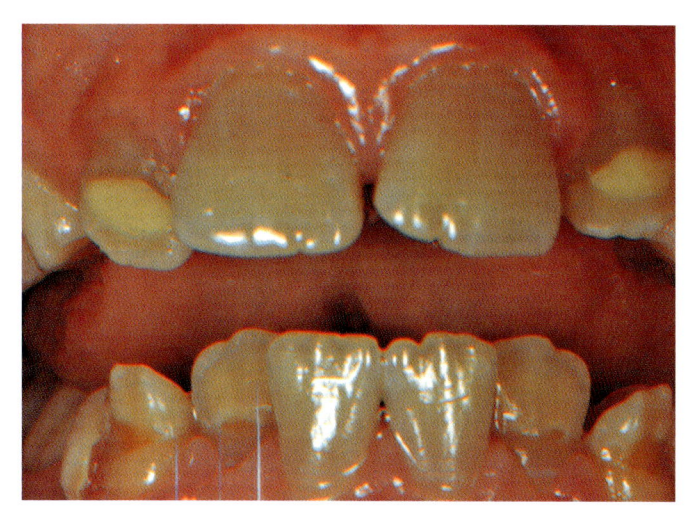

Figure 24.8 **(C)** Tan staining from Aureomycin.

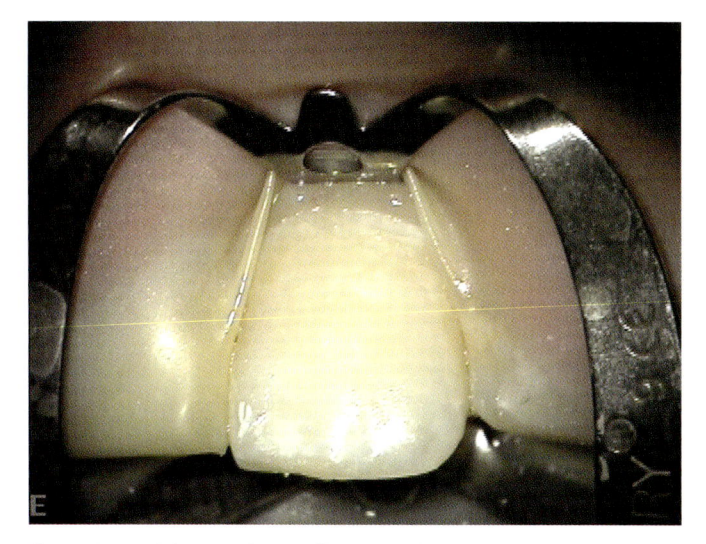

Figure 24.9 **(A)** View of a maxillary central incisor tooth with overhead lighting. No fracture is visible.

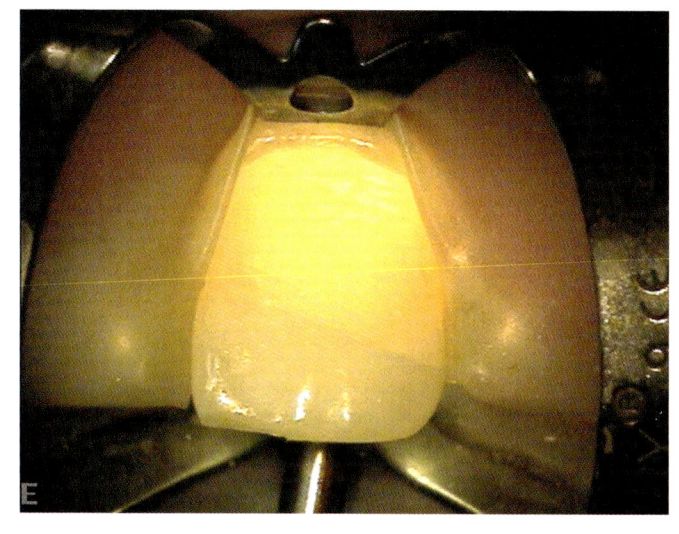

Figure 24.9 **(B)** Transilluminated view of the same tooth revealing the fracture line.

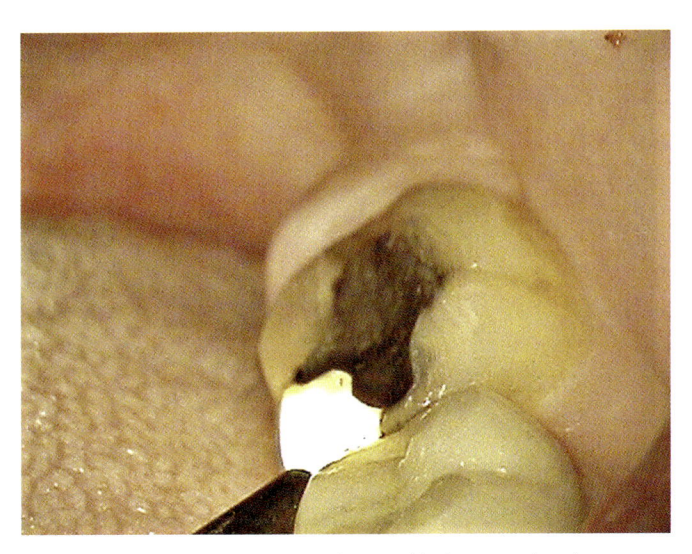

Figure 24.10 Transillumination of a mandibular second molar. The fracture lines at the mesial and lingual grooves do not allow the light to pass through.

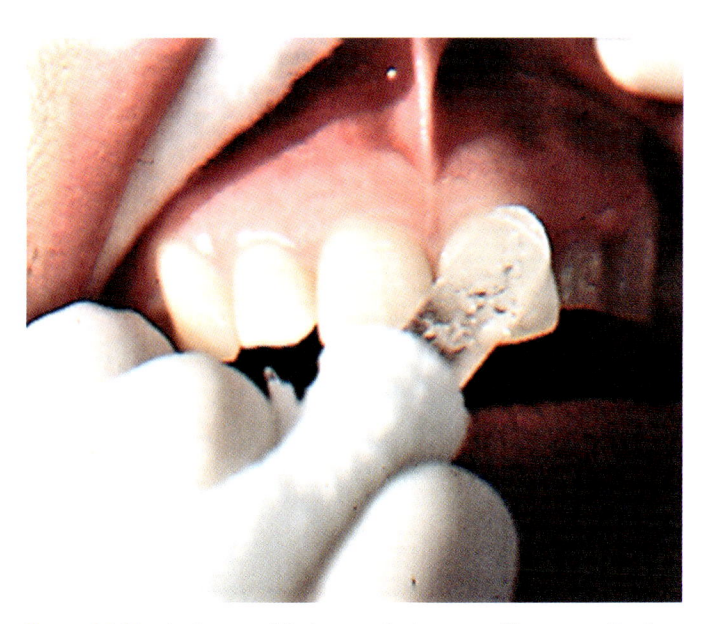

Figure 24.11 An ice pencil being applied to a maxillary central incisor tooth.

The procedure is easy to use, and it is safe for the pulp. The gas is sprayed on a cotton pellet (Figure 24.12B), and then the chilled cotton is placed on the buccal/facial of the tooth that is to be tested (Figure 24.12C). A baseline control should be established on an adjacent for comparison before testing the suspected tooth.

The response of a normal, healthy, vital pulp is sharp and quickly dissipates once the stimulus is removed. If the response is more intense and lingers after the pellet is removed, it usually indicates an irreversible pulpitis. When calcified pulp chambers or constricted canals exist, the response from an otherwise healthy tooth may be delayed or nonexistent. The reduced conductivity can mislead the operator. Therefore, other tests must be used to confirm negative responses.

When faced with teeth that are heavily restored, the final tests can be delayed until the caries has been excavated and the patient is in a provisional restoration. By thermal testing prior to anesthetizing but with the temporary crown removed, the true status of the pulp may be validated before final cementation and any changes that may have arisen during the fabrication interval can be appraised.

Heat testing

To duplicate patient heat symptom, heat can easily be applied to the buccal/facial of teeth using any warm gutta-percha heat source (Calamus, Tulsa Dental Products, Elements, Sybron Endo, Touch 'n Heat, Kerr). Special heat tips are made for heat testing. It is important to remember that heat is delayed and lasts, while cold in instant and fleeting. Heat pain will typically last from 8 to 36 h and then the pulp becomes necrotic.

Heat can be an informative of the pulp test; however, it is the most difficult test to apply. Heated water applied to an individual tooth after it has been carefully isolated by a rubber dam is the most reliable method. It is time consuming, and extreme care has to be taken so there is no leakage under the rubber dam. It is recommended to isolate and stimulate a tooth that is posterior to the one that is suspected to be heat sensitive first. Then move the rubber dam anteriorly and test tooth by tooth. Heated temporary stopping applied to the lateral surface of a natural tooth or a metal surface of a veneer casting has been recommended, but it is difficult to control the heat and the stopping has the tendency to stick on the tooth and may cause prolonged stimuli and thereby an inaccurate test. A rubber polishing wheel in a low-speed handpiece is another heat test alternative. Since it is difficult to control the heat generated, this method is not recommended. The antiquated method of touching a tooth with a red hot burnisher should be avoided because of the risk of overheating the tooth and creating a pulpal problem.

Electric pulp testing

Over the last 35 years, the Analytical Technology Vitality Scanner, more recently renamed Vitality Scanner (Sybron Endo) (Figure 24.13), has become the standard within the endodontic community. This battery-operated device is simple to use, accurate, and virtually trouble free. A small amount of an electrolytic gel (toothpaste, fluoride gels, or EKG paste) is applied to the end of the testing tip prior to its contact with the tooth. When the low-voltage electrical stimulation is transmitted to the teeth (Figure 24.14), the responses can be recorded from the patient's verbal identification of heat, tingling, or slight discomfort or pain. Credence should not be placed on the specific numbers displayed, nor should the differential between tests of individual teeth be used to determine stages of pulpal degeneration. The single purpose of electric pulp testing (EPT) is to test vital or nonvital and does not measure health versus inflammation. As previously stated, pulp testing heavily restored teeth can be inaccurate, and therefore unreliable. The Vitality Scanner "mini-tip" (Figure 24.15) is useful for full-coverage teeth to determine pulp vitality if root structure can be exposed with a plastic instrument or by first packing periodontal cord. The "mini-tip," when used

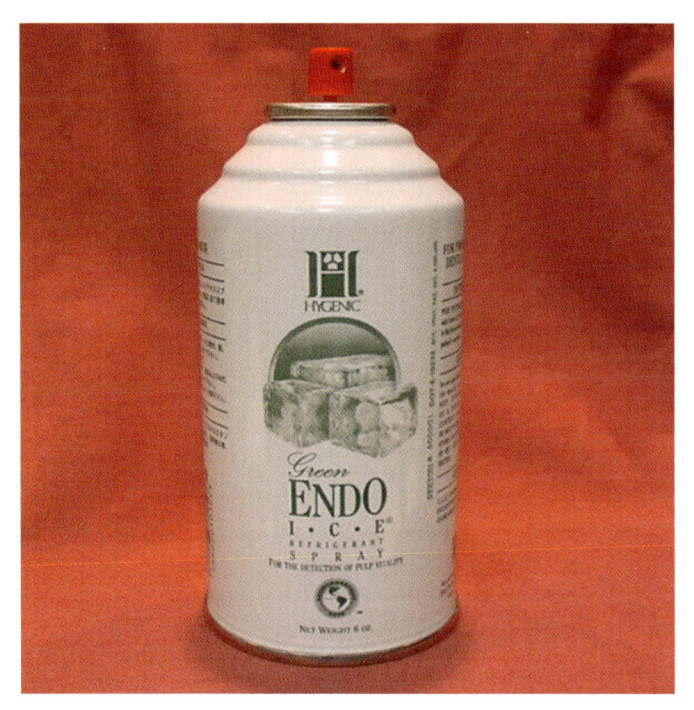

Figure 24.12 **(A)** Endo Ice (Hygienic).

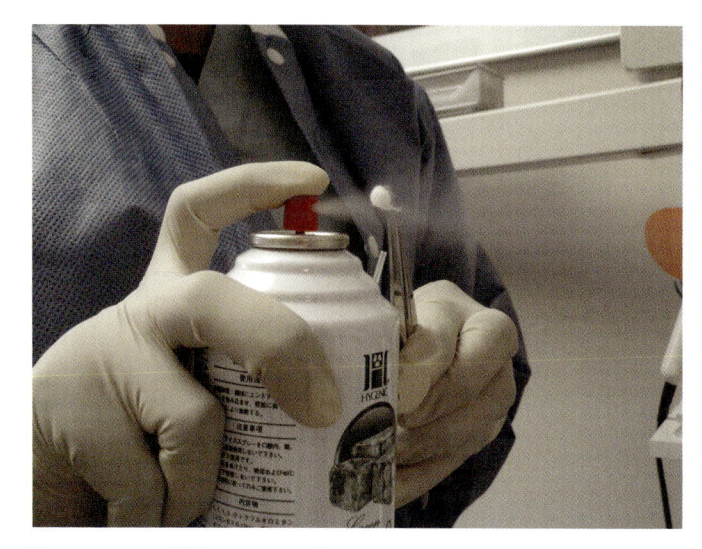

Figure 24.12 **(B)** Spraying Endo Ice on cotton pellet.

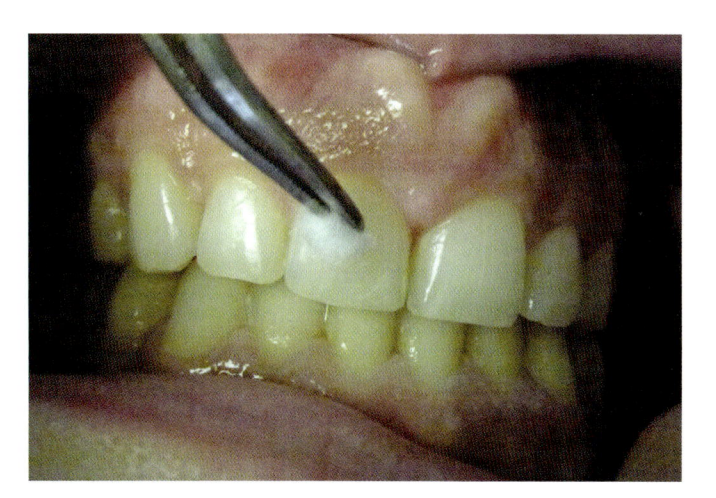

Figure 24.12 **(C)** Applying iced pellet to labial surface of tooth.

in conjunction with a prepared test cavity or a small opening in a cast crown (Figure 24.16A and B), on the other hand, is a very accurate pulp vitality test. The tip is then placed directly through the opening of the restoration or fabricated crown and onto the exposed dentin (see "Cavity test" section). Care should be taken to keep the electrolyte (tooth paste, fluoride gel, or EKG paste) from touching the metal of the casting.

If the dentist can determine that root canal treatment is indicated while the patient is still in the provisional restorations, the endodontic needs can be addressed without disturbing the crown margins. The patient should have been informed of such possibilities during the treatment plan discussion.

Ideally, no single test should be considered conclusive. Collaborative tests are, of course, more reliable and accurate. This is particularly true when dealing with apprehensive patients. Under stress, these patients will anticipate and respond even when no stimulus exists. The decision to treat these patients may be based on finesse, experience, intestinal fortitude of the dentist, and the intensity of the patient's pain. The option of when to treat what tooth should be communicated in detail. The records should indicate that the diagnosis and treatment plan is based on the patient symptoms, duplication of those symptoms and responses (or lack thereof), to vitality tests, as well as a thorough clinical, pulpal, periodontal, structural, functional, and esthetic evaluation. Your written informed consent document should be signed by you, the patient, and a witness, preferably the assistant who was in the treatment room during the discussion phase of the treatment. In the case of an emergency situation, the alternative should be offered to wait until the symptoms and signs localize. The patient decides whether to proceed or not.

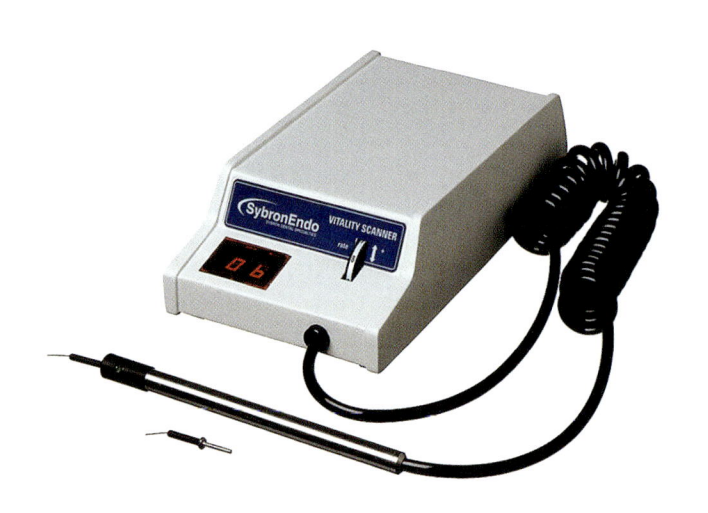

Figure 24.13 Vitality Scanner 2006 (Kerr Endodontics).

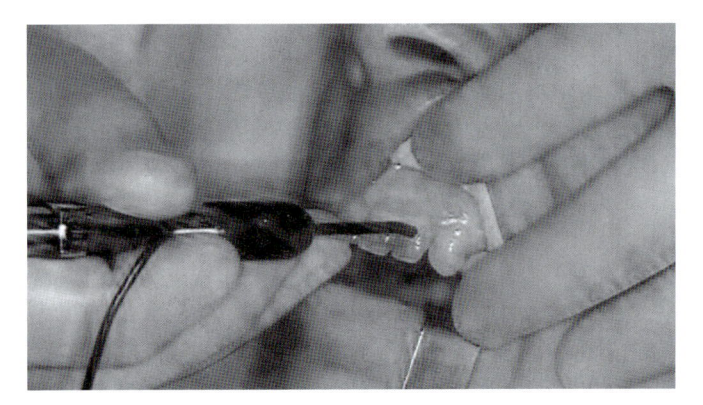

Figure 24.14 Vitality Scanner being applied to a dried tooth.

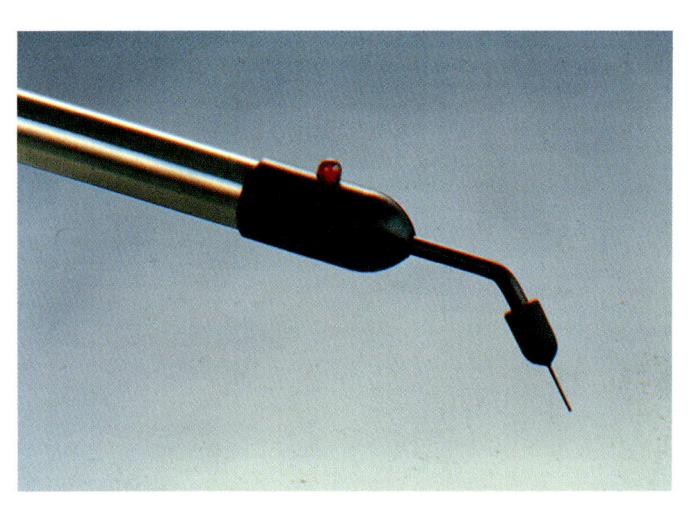

Figure 24.15 Mini-tip for the Vitality Scanner.

Cavity test

When tests are inconclusive with the less apprehensive patient, penetrating to the dentin with a new and small bur through the occlusal of a posterior crown or lingual of an anterior crown of an unanesthetized tooth is an excellent method of validating pulpal necrosis. This should only be done if the tooth has not responded to the electronic pulp testing and cold vitality tests. It should be carefully explained to the patient that, based on testing, it is likely that the pulp is already necrotic and therefore they should not feel any pain during the cavity test. If the patient reports pain/sensitivity when the cavity preparation has reached the dentin, this test indicates the EPT and ice tests were false positives and the cavity is restored and further diagnostic tests required. The cavity test to determine pulpal necrosis trumps the accuracy of both EPT and ice tests. If extensive caries is present, the patient should be anesthetized and the caries removed prior to restoring. This will allow visual evaluation of the cavity floor and the ability to estimate the strength of the abutment value of the tooth. If the patient does not report any pain or sensation, an endodontic access is

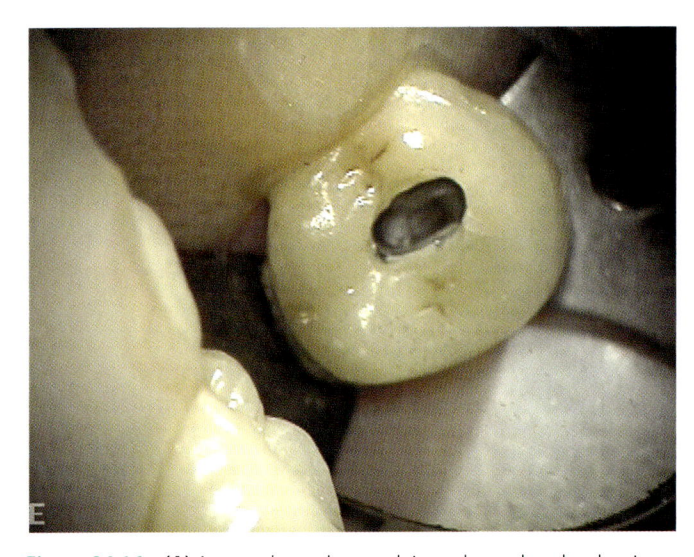

Figure 24.16 (A) Access through porcelain and metal to the dentin.

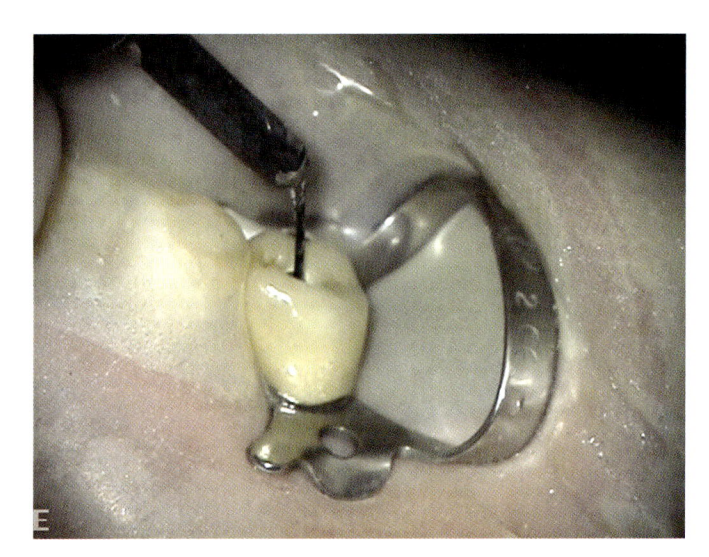

Figure 24.16 (B) Mini-tip placed on dentin through prepared cavity.

prepared and endodontic treatment is initiated after all decay excavation.

Electronic pulp testing with a "mini-tip" through a test cavity may be the key to making a diagnosis in a tooth with a radiolucency that cannot be differentiated as of either periodontal or endodontic origin. A necrotic pulp is diagnosed if the reading is negative. Endodontics would then be the treatment of choice (Figure 24.17A and B). If the reading is positive and there are no pulpal symptoms despite the radiographic appearance, periodontal therapy would be indicated if the tooth probed (Figure 24.17C–E). If the radiolucency is neither a lesion of endodontic nor periodontal origin, the patient should be referred to the oral surgeon for biopsy consideration. Finally, endodontic treatment may be required if the root apices are compromised during periodontal procedures (Figure 24.17 F and G).

Periradicular tests

Percussion

Gently tapping or pressing the forefinger on the incisal or occlusal surface of a tooth may elicit a painful response (Figure 24.18). In situations when the response generated is mild or absent, the test should be followed with gentle tap of a mirror handle (Figure 24.19). A painful response usually indicates inflammatory changes in the periodontal ligament caused by pulpal degeneration. When bacteria have entered the pulp, necrosis will follow. Endotoxins from the bacteria will eventually exit the canal and create an inflammatory reaction of the periodontal tissue surrounding the apex and/or lateral root portion of the tooth tested. The reaction is usually more intense when the inflammatory condition is endodontic rather than periodontal origin.

Occasionally, painful responses to percussion are elicited from teeth not undergoing pulpal degeneration. Acute sinusitis can cause the maxillary posterior teeth to be painful when percussed. Usually in this situation, more than one tooth responds painfully

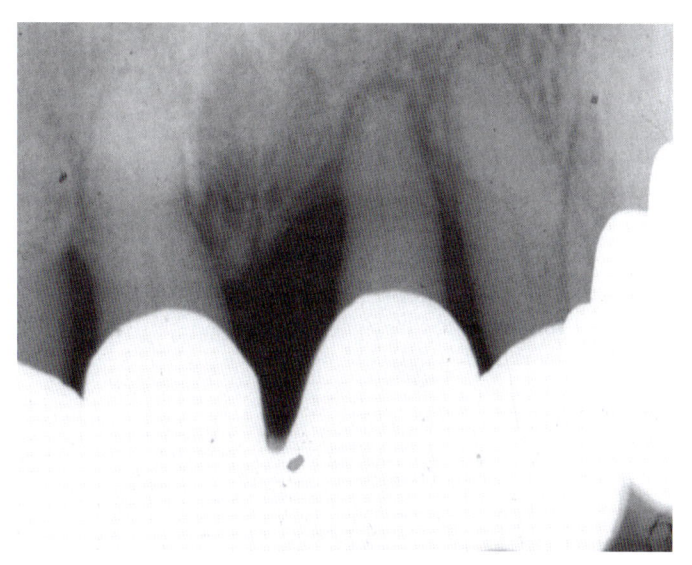

Figure 24.17 (A) Maxillary central incisor tooth with a vital pulp. Endodontic therapy was not indicated.

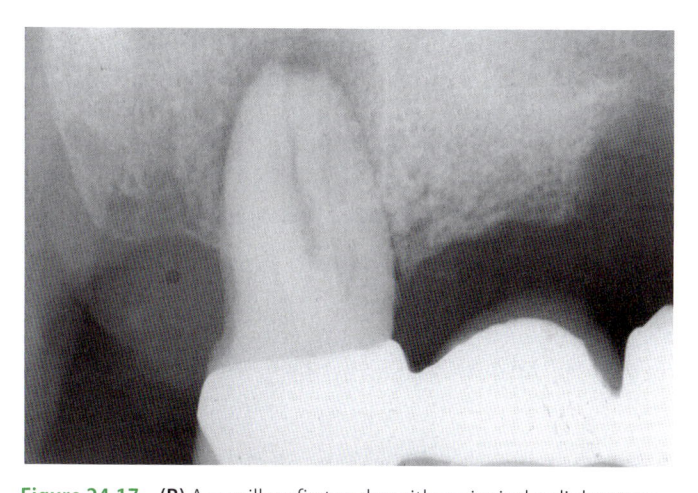

Figure 24.17 (B) A maxillary first molar with periapical radiolucency.

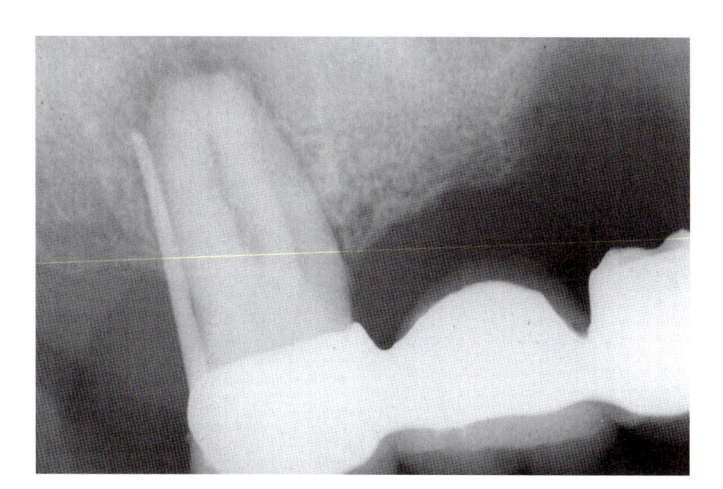

Figure 24.17 (C) A gutta-percha point placed in the distal periodontal pocket. Pulp testing through an occlusal opening revealed a vital pulp. The cause of the radiolucency was of periodontal origin, and therapy followed that course.

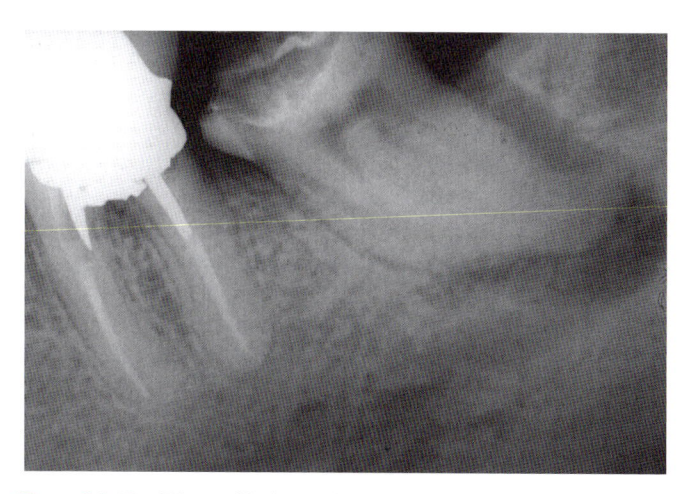

Figure 24.17 (D) Mandibular molar with a necrotic pulp. Root canal therapy was instituted.

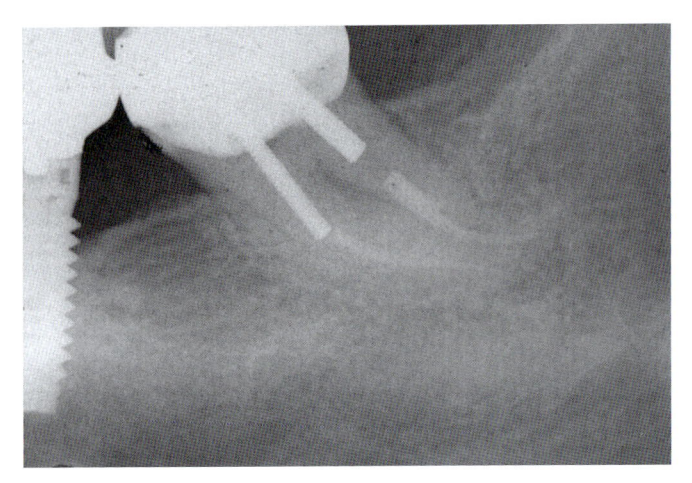

Figure 24.17 **(E)** Ten years after completion of root canal therapy, there is complete bone fill in. No periodontal treatments were performed on this tooth.

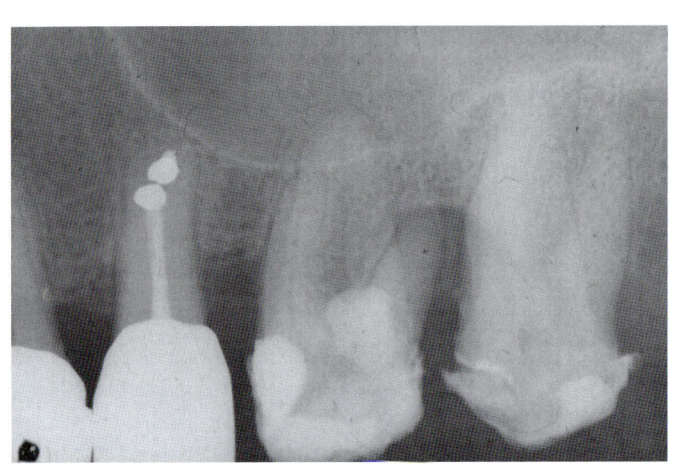

Figure 24.17 **(F)** Maxillary first molar with an uninflammed vital pulp. There was extensive bone loss surrounding the distobuccal root.

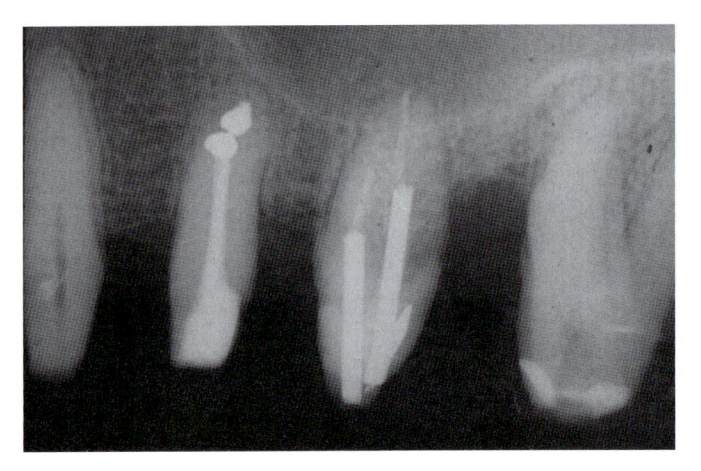

Figure 24.17 **(G)** Root canal therapy was performed to allow for the resection of the periodontally involved root.

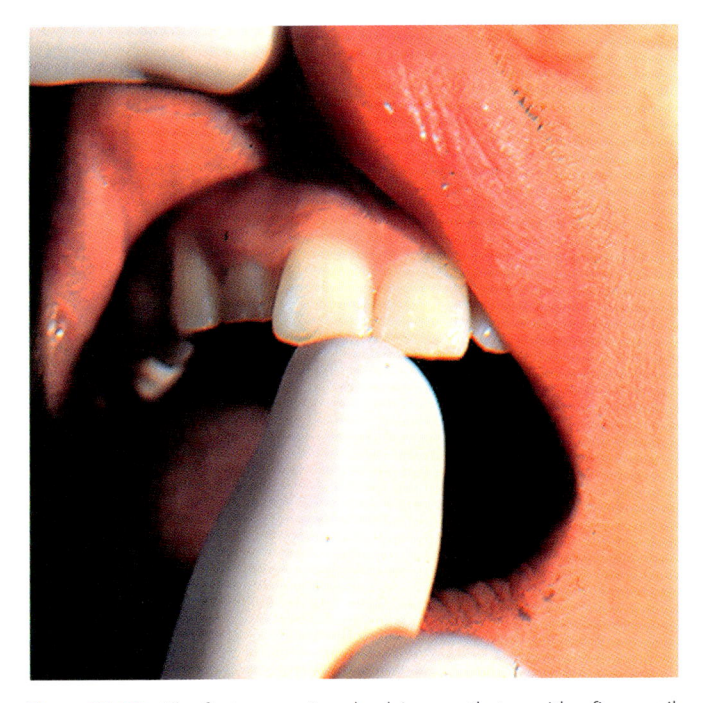

Figure 24.18 The first percussion check is a gentle tap with a fingernail.

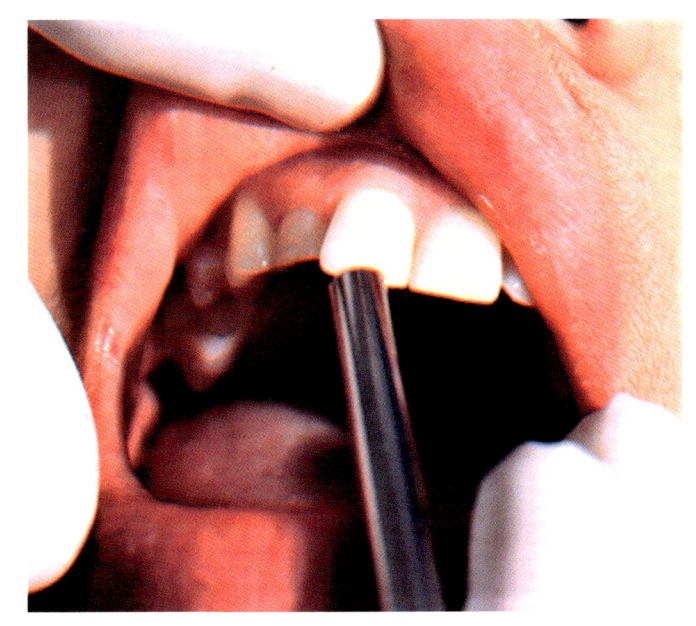

Figure 24.19 The second percussion check is a gentle tap with a mirror handle

to percussion. A careful history of the patient's respiratory experiences and allergies is essential in making the differential diagnosis, as well as history of pain in the affected area with sudden movements like bending over or running quickly up or down stairs. Teeth in traumatic occlusion are frequently sensitive to percussion but are also painful to cold. To exclude this possibility, a check for occlusal prematurity is indicated. A degenerative pulp does not usually respond to thermal pulp tests unless it is in the early stages of the process. If a tooth is painful to both percussion and sensitive or even hypersensitive to cold, the dentist should suspect a vertical fracture. Fractures are most frequently observed in mandibular second molars and maxillary bicuspids and occur irrespective of their restorative conditions. The use of the transilluminator or fiber-optic light is quite useful in diagnosing a fractured tooth (Figure 24.10).

Palpation

Pressure with a gloved forefinger over the root of a suspected tooth may reveal tissue distention and may also elicit a painful response (Figure 24.20). This indicates a radicular inflammatory response from the root canal system that must be validated with a negative pulp test (necrotic pulp) and a gingival crevice that probes within normal limits. A periapical radiograph may suggest the forming of a lesion of endodontic origin. The tender area may be so extensive that the teeth adjacent to the suspected tooth must also be tested. Once again a differential diagnosis of acute sinusitis should be considered when the maxillary posterior teeth are involved. The tissues painful to palpation with sinusitis usually spread away from the dentition and extend superiorly and facially. Although the area of pain is usually concentrated at the zygomatic process of the maxilla, the pain may extend around the orbit and incite headaches. Pulp testing and a careful history are essential in these situations.

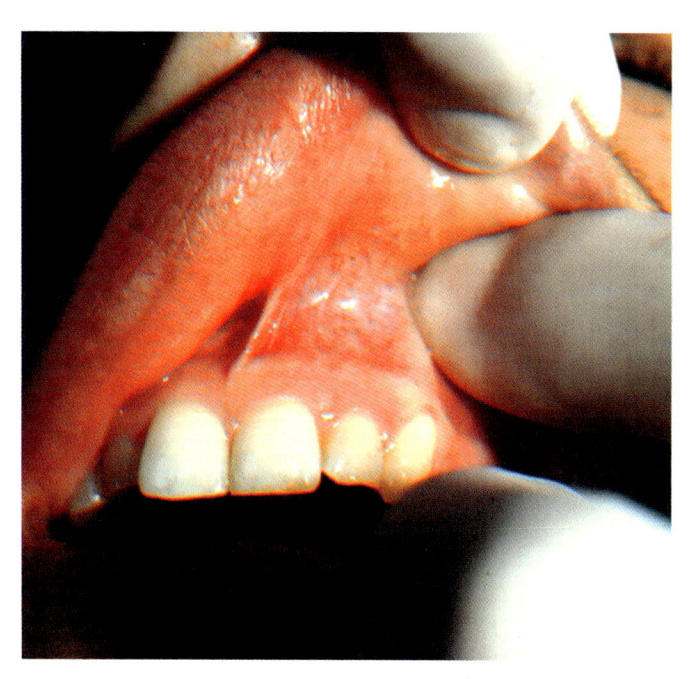

Figure 24.20 Palpation with forefinger in mucobuccal fold over suspected tooth.

Bite test

Every time that the patient's symptom is sensitivity to biting and/or chewing, it is important to investigate further which tooth and which part of the tooth is sensitive to biting pressure to distinguish between vertical crown/root fractures and periapical pathosis. A very helpful device for this investigation is Tooth Slooth® (Professional Results, Inc.; Figure 24.21). By design, this instrument has a slight depression in the biting surface so the patient will only bite on individual cusps (Figure 24.22A and B) without adjacent cusp interference during testing. If there is a

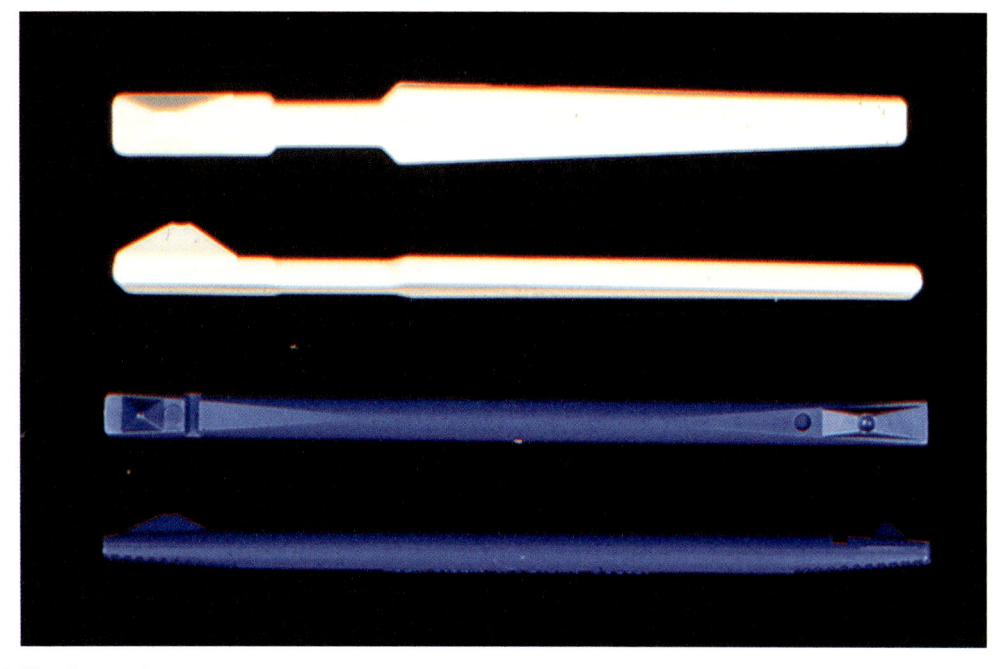

Figure 24.21 Tooth Slooth; two sizes.

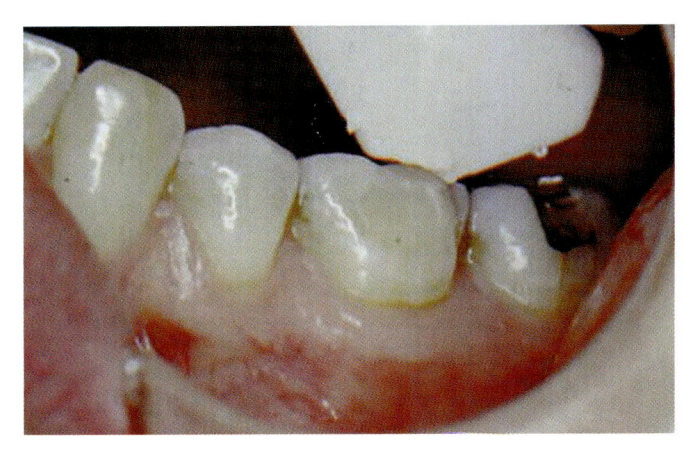

Figure 24.22 **(A)** Bite test with Tooth Slooth checking distobuccal cusp of mandibular molar.

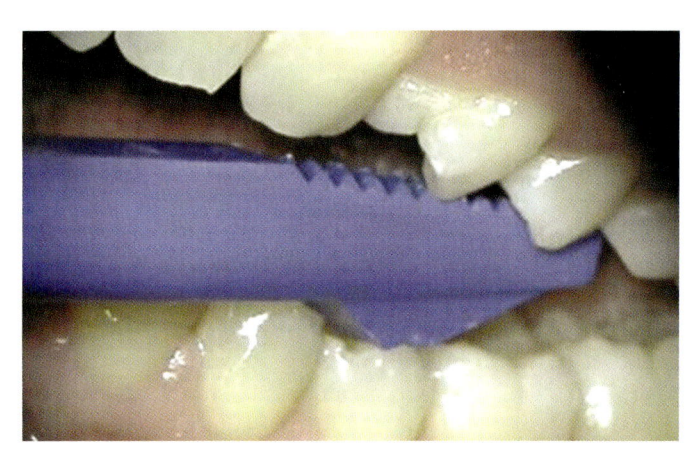

Figure 24.22 **(B)** Bite test with smaller-sized (blue) Tooth Slooth.

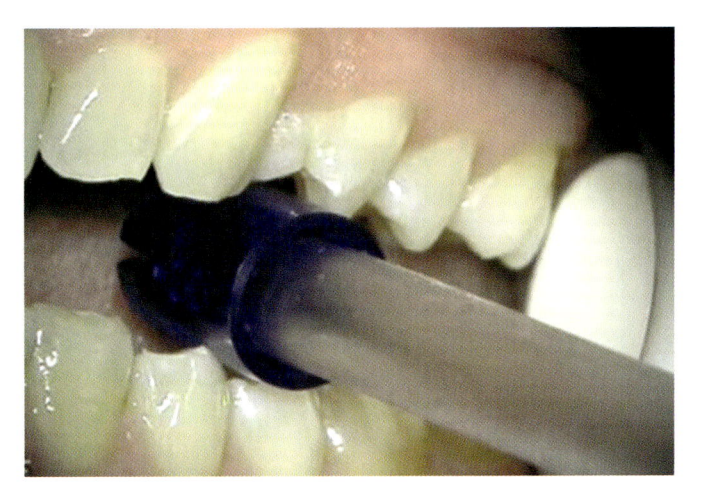

Figure 24.23 A plastic saliva ejector is useful in bite testing the entire tooth rather an individual cusp.

fracture in the crown, the patient is likely to report normal sensation to biting on all but the area/cusp that is fractured. It is advisable to start with having the patient bite on the Tooth Slooth on a tooth that is not suspected of being fractured to establish a normal baseline response. Then test from tooth to tooth around the mouth as the patient exerts pressure. The patient is asked to close slowly yet exert maximum pressure. Pain on bite release is indicative of an inflamed pulp/irreversible pulpitis requiring extirpation.

A plastic saliva ejector may be used as an alternative instrument for this test (Figure 24.23).

Pretreatment radiographs

Treatment planning requires a full set of well-angulated long cone exposed periapical films or digital images using film holders such as XCP (DENTSPLY RINN Corp.) or Kodak digital imaging that enables 90° angulation of the X-ray beam on the film or sensor. In addition to good angulations on the radiograph, these film holders will enable the operator to compare the images over time, which is essential when evaluating healing or failure. A bitewing and mesial, perpendicular, and distal periapicals images are diagnostically desirable.

When dealing with extensive situations, panoramic film is another diagnostic aid. If the patient requires endodontic treatment and is referred to the endodontist, then these films and a description of the goals and objectives of the referring dentist should be sent to the endodontist prior to the patient's first appointment. The endodontist may take additional films of the teeth to be treated to establish a complete record. In most cases, an endodontic procedure should not be initiated without evaluating at least two recent radiographs exposed at different horizontal angulations of the suspected tooth (Figure 24.24A and B). Examining varied views is essential in diagnosing the presence of additional roots, anatomical configurations, anomalies, and other unusual circumstances that may complicate the treatment.

Cone-beam computed tomography (CBCT), three-dimensional (3D) limited area scans, gives the clinician an additional instrument to help in diagnosis and treatment planning.[1] Endodontists often use the 3D scan as part of their regular preoperative regimen in teeth involved in periapical surgery, root resorption, retreatment (Figure 24.25A–F), dental alveolar trauma, periapical bone defects, unusual anatomy, root fractures, and so on. This noninvasive diagnostic radiographic procedure allows the clinicians to proceed with greater confidence and accuracy because of the additional information they have prior to treatment.

Precementation radiographs

Prior to cementation, Yamada (personal communication, June 2001) reradiographs the prepared teeth (Figure 24.26A and B). These images, unencumbered by the presence of the metal or ceramic castings, provide a chamber/canal road map record if the tooth requires endodontics in the future. Arens and Chivian[2] reported that over 40% of teeth requiring root canal therapy are crowned.

Prior knowledge of the size, location, and direction of the chamber and canal will reduce the possibility of the following:

- crown damage during access opening;
- lost time searching for the canal orifice;

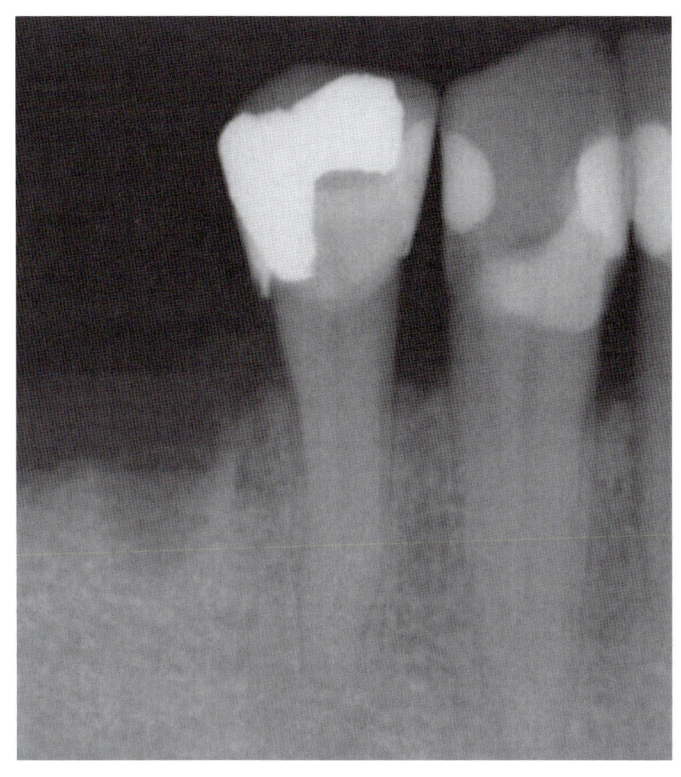

Figure 24.24 (A) Pretreatment radiograph of a mandibular premolar shows one canal.

- perforations of the chamber or the canal because of disorientation;
- crown dislodgement.

Each of these iatrogenic possibilities reduces the prognosis and jeopardizes the tooth's reliability as an abutment.

Anesthetic test

All the previously described tests are based on "duplicating" a patient's symptoms. Once the symptom is duplicated, the endodontic diagnosis can be made followed by appropriate treatment. Sometimes, however, a patient will present with "just pain" and the only test available to the dentist is the anesthetic test: administer anesthetic to the tooth or teeth where the patient "thinks" the pain is coming from and see if the pain vanishes. If the pain resolves, the anesthetic test indicates you have found the source but usually multiple teeth are anesthetized and a single source cannot be identified. The dentist should not guess which anesthetized tooth is the pain source. Instead, knowing that a pulpitis usually lasts from 8 to 36 h, administer a long-acting anesthetic such as Marcaine and have the patient return the next day or at end of the day if patient originally presents in the morning. If pain is still there when the patient returns, do anesthetic test again and see patient next day. Within a day or two, the pain will be gone (necrosis and gangrene) and the diagnosis is simple

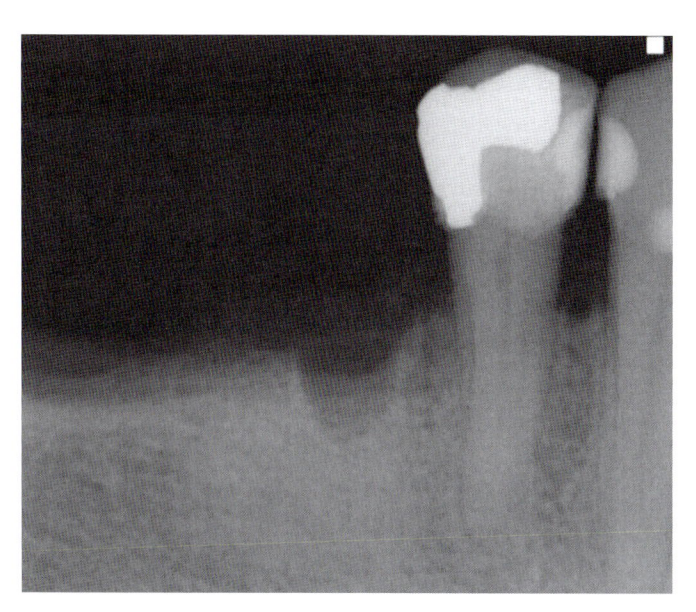

Figure 24.24 (B) A second radiograph taken from an angulation of 15° from the mesial discloses a second root.

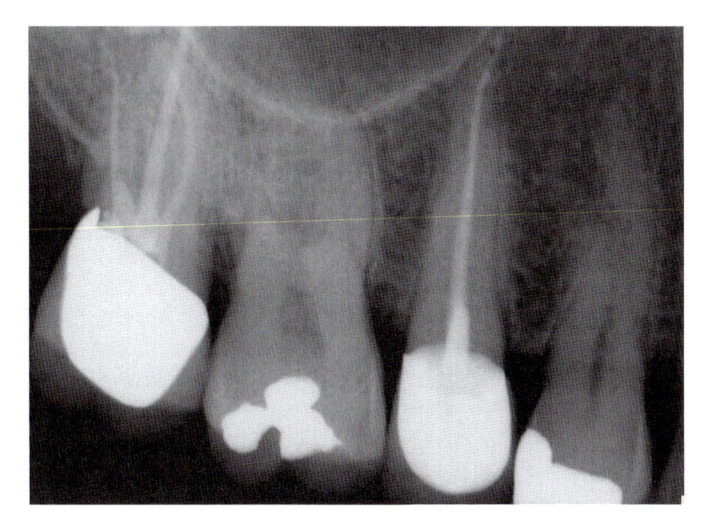

Figure 24.25 (A) Patient experienced pain 3 months after nonsurgical root canal treatment. Reproduced with permission of Dr J. Chikvashvili.

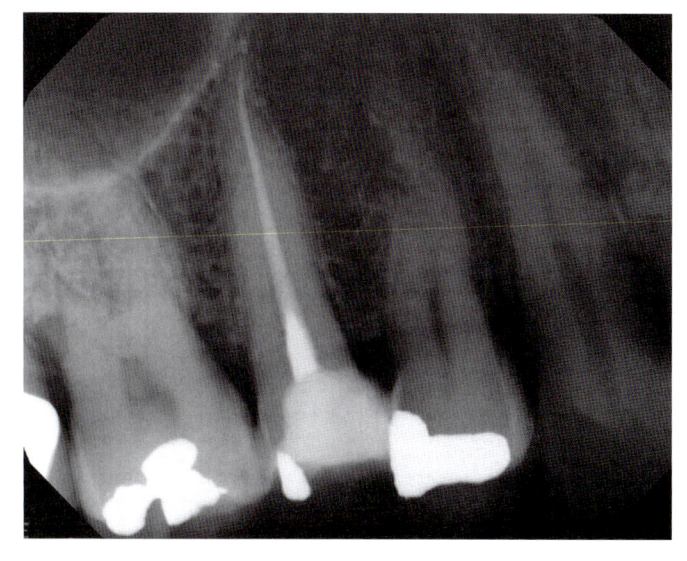

Figure 24.25 (B) Radiograph taken 15° from the mesial. Only one canal visible. Reproduced with permission of Dr J. Chikvashvili.

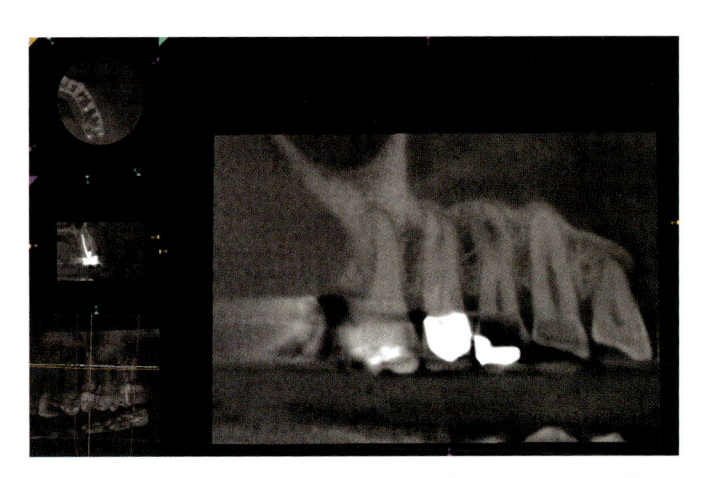

Figure 24.25 **(C)** CBCT sagittal plane image shows two untreated buccal canals. Reproduced with permission of Dr J. Chikvashvili.

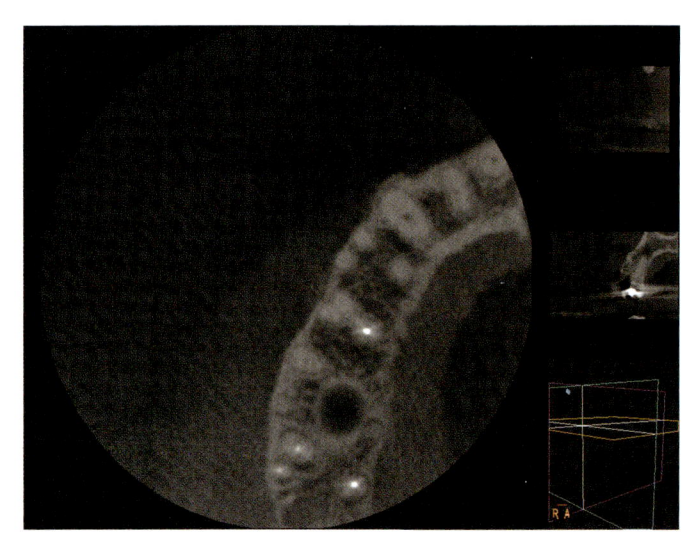

Figure 24.25 **(D)** CBCT axial plane image shows two untreated buccal canals. Reproduced with permission of Dr J. Chikvashvili.

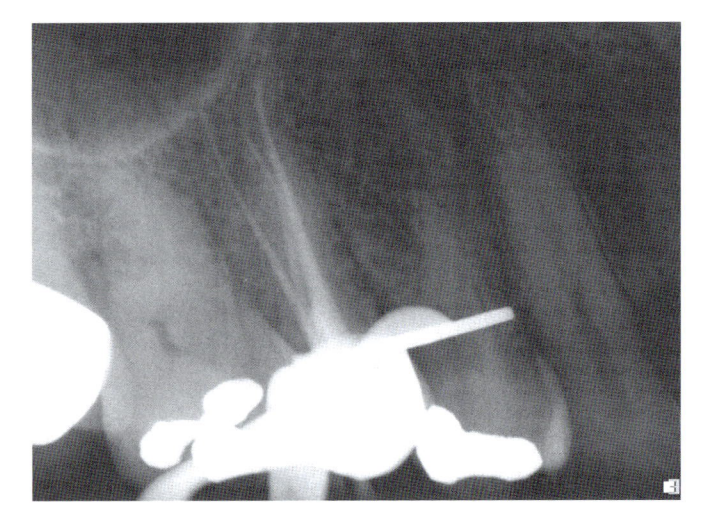

Figure 24.25 **(E)** Canals located and negotiated. Pain abated after canal debridement. Reproduced with permission of Dr J. Chikvashvili.

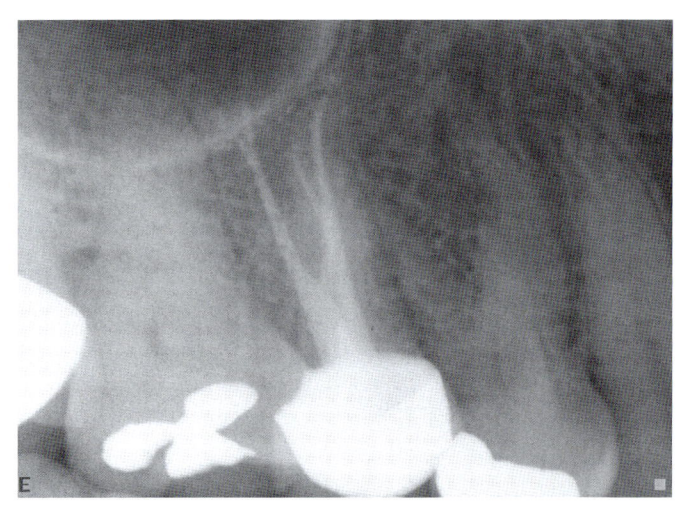

Figure 24.25 **(F)** Postoperative image showing three main and lateral canals obturated. Reproduced with permission of Dr J. Chikvashvili.

with pulp tests. Or in a day or two, the patient will be experience the beginning of an acute alveolar abscess. This tooth will be percussion sensitive and/or a periradicular radiolucency and/or cellulitis will be observable in its early stages. The pulp will test nonvital and the endodontic diagnosis is made. In summary, the anesthetic test buys time until patient symptoms can be duplicated or until nonodontogenic pain can be ruled out.

Diagnosis

By correlating all of the endodontic information, the dentist can, within reason, determine which tooth or teeth may or may not require root canal treatment prior to or during the reconstructive procedures. By far the most difficult pulpal tissue status to classify is found within the confines of a previously restored tooth. Therefore, it is important for the dentist and treatment team to understand endodontic biology and then to educate their patients how pulps react to dental procedures.

Pulpal response to operative procedures

Following caries, the single most influencing factor on pulp health (Figure 24.27) is the dentist correcting the ravages of caries and dental trauma. Simply modifying traumatic operative techniques could easily prevent adverse sequelae and reduce the eventual need for endodontics. A tooth with a healthy pulp, when operatively prepared, responds immediately to the dentinal injury. The dental tubules involved are vulnerable to the heat developed during the procedure, to the air during drying, and to any of the chemicals or materials used during the restorative procedures. Regardless of what the source, the odontoblasts will react. It is only a question of degree. With tooth reduction, the equation is simple: the higher the speed of the rotating instrument, the greater the heat generated and the greater the pulpal damage. Common sense would suggest that, in response to these predictable and undesirable insults, the surface of the

Figure 24.26 (A, B) Precementation radiographs provide a road map to the canals if endodontic therapy is necessary after cementation of the castings. *Source:* Courtesy of Dr Henry Yamada.

tooth should be reduced with well water-cooled high-speed dental handpieces and that the deepest excavation and final preparation should be achieved with low-speed handpieces. Adjunctively, a coolant spray should accompany all preparation cutting and every effort made to eliminate air blasts. Not only has Langeland[3] studies shown that 10 s of air is enough to displace odontoblastic nuclei (Figure 24.28) and present a definite hazard to the viability of the pulp, but Stanley's pulp studies[4] have also repeatedly demonstrated the pulp peril of cutting fast and dry.

In addition, unprotected dentinal tubules internal tooth bleaching, too rapid orthodontic tooth movement, impression taking, temporization, and cementation are other aggressive procedures within the normal dental regimen that demand attention and caution. The operator should also select materials and agents that have relatively neutral pH values, create little or no heat while curing, and control orthodontic forces within the physiologic tolerance of the periodontal ligament.

Despite using the utmost care during the course of restorative phase, there are situations that require the need for immediate root canal treatment:

- A tooth exhibiting exquisitely painful responses to cold liquids 10 weeks after deep decay excavation and pulp protection and sedation (Figure 24.29).
- The inability to exert full biting pressure on a crown 6–9 months after cementation even though the radiographs are negative (Figure 24.30).

Some postrestorative exacerbations are unavoidable, particularly when dealing with heavily restored teeth. Such episodes of acute or chronic pulpal inflammation more often stem from a preexisting pulpal condition that has been aroused before what appeared to be a simple operative procedure. Although the

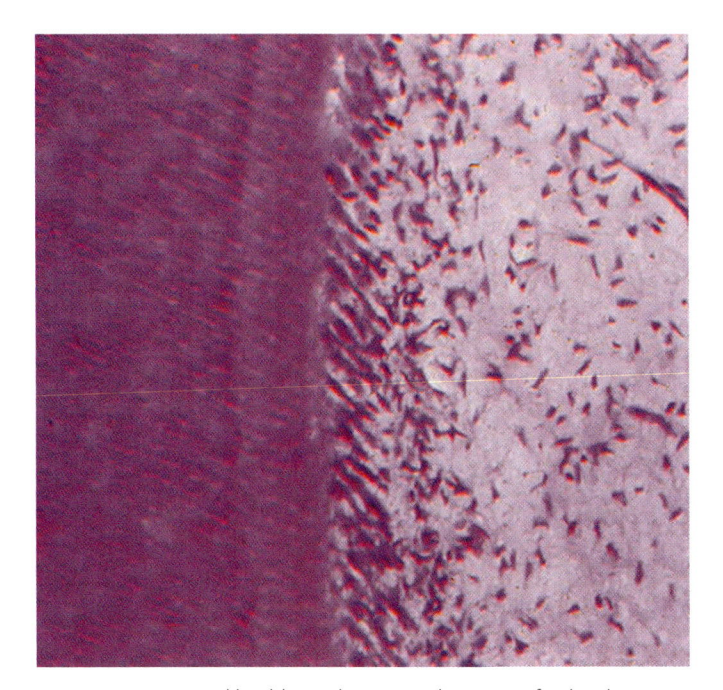

Figure 24.27 A vital healthy with its typical pattern of palisading odontoblasts. *Source:* Courtesy of Dr Harold R Stanley.

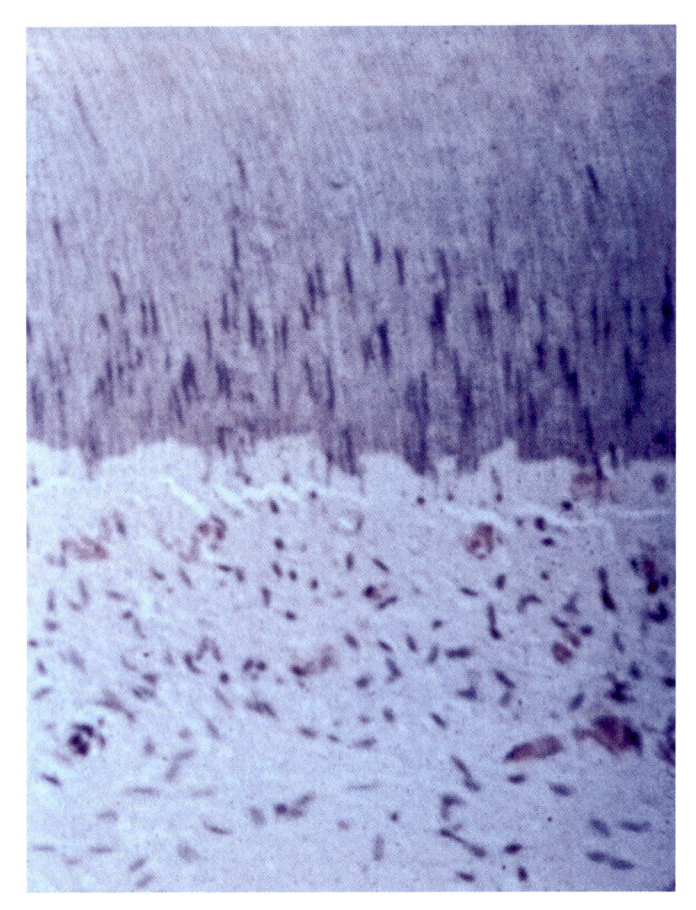

Figure 24.28 Displaced odontoblastic nuclei. *Source:* Courtesy of Dr Harold R Stanley.

healing potential of a healthy pulp following dental intervention has been well documented, the potential for complete repair has been known to decrease as the number of procedures is accumulated during a tooth's lifetime.

A healthy pulp's survival with resolution of acute inflammation will usually take place within 7–8 weeks after operative procedures provided there are no additional insults. Extending a patient's palliative treatment beyond that time frame is not only unjustified but also compromises the patient–doctor relationship. Rather, immediate endodontic treatment should be considered after this time, especially if diagnostic tests indicate pulpal distress.

Pulpal repair

Reparative dentin

Reparative or irregular dentin is deposited to form a protective barrier for the pulp tissue and is generally localized to the injury site. This abnormal dentin forms in response to intense and aggressive pulpal irritants that have reached the limit of pulp tolerance; for example, erosion, abrasion, caries, dentinal exposure by fracture, decay or mechanical tooth reduction, traumatic injury, caustic medicaments, and harmful restorative materials.

The histological appearance of reparative dentin (Figure 24.31) demonstrates dentinal tubules that are irregular, tortuous, or even absent. The increased thickness of the total dentin is likely

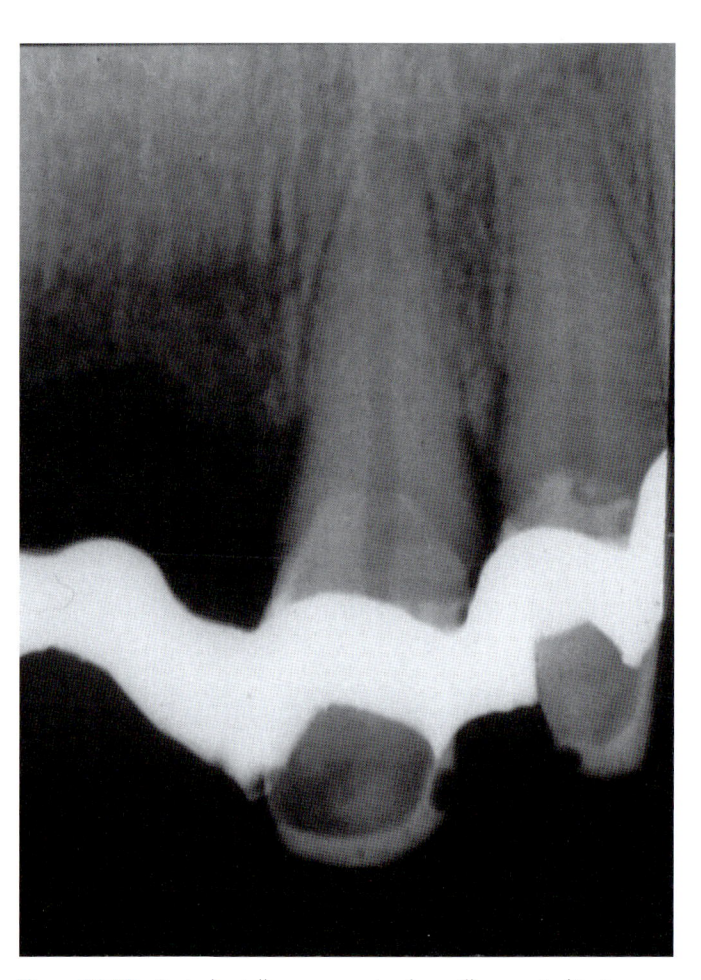

Figure 24.29 Periodontally compromised maxillary central incisor that is painful to minor temperature changes 10 weeks after deep caries excavation and crown preparation.

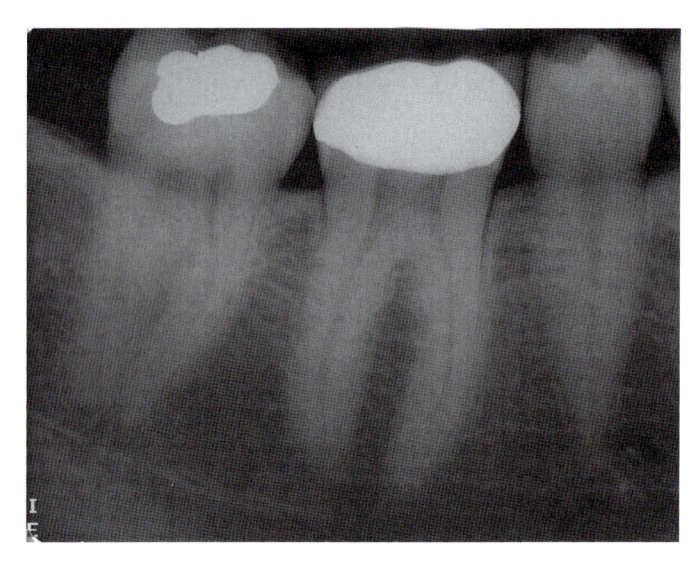

Figure 24.30 Mandibular molar with a normal radiographic appearance. However, the patient avoids using the tooth because of pain to chewing 9 months after cementation of the crown.

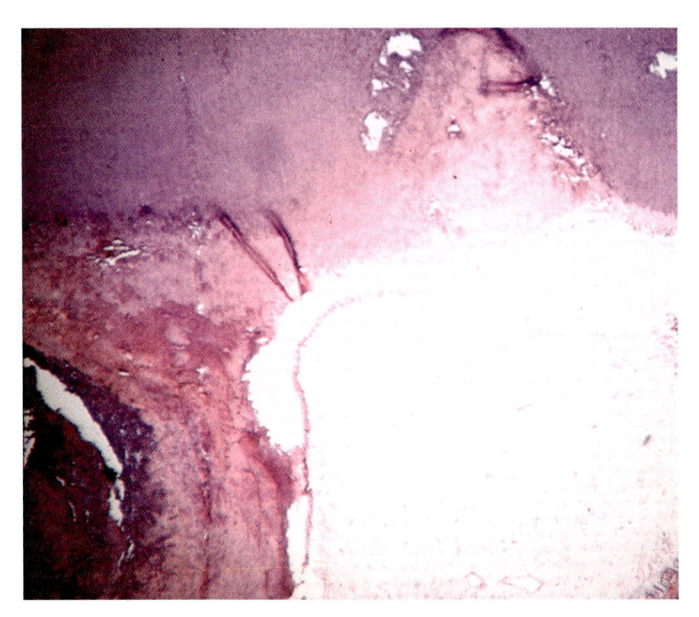

Figure 24.31 Reparative dentin. *Source:* Courtesy of Dr Harold R Stanley.

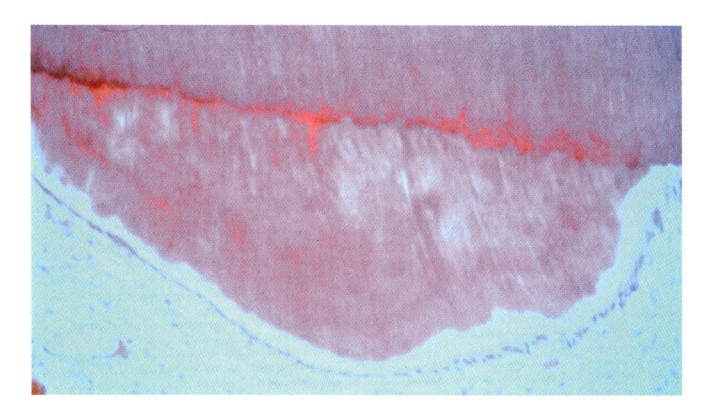

Figure 24.32 Secondary dentin. *Source:* Courtesy of Dr Harold R Stanley.

the reason patients have decreased responses to cold stimuli as time passes following a dental procedure. Quantitatively, it is noted the greater the degree of the "insult" caused by preparations and restorative materials, the greater the amount of reparative dentin that forms.

Although this calcified solid wall is considered beneficial and capable of resisting further episodes of irritation, the healing phenomenon decreases the ability of the tooth to respond to pulp testing at a later date.

Secondary dentin

Histologically and physiologically, there is a difference between reparative and secondary dentin. Secondary dentin begins forming soon after the tooth erupts into occlusion and continues to form throughout the pulp's life. This tooth structure is deposited over the primary dentin (Figure 24.32) throughout the entire chamber and the root canal system in response to stimuli within the limits of normal biological function, mastication, light thermal changes, chemical irritants, and slight trauma. The newly deposited dentinal tubules are smaller, exhibit more curves, and form a protective barrier for the pulp as the size of the pulp cavity is reduced. Reparative dentin, on the other hand, forms as a direct response to injury. Although secondary dentin deposition is not uniform in thickness, this dystrophic calcification may completely occlude the canal and complicate the eventual endodontic treatment. This diagnosis of calcific metamorphosis or calcific degeneration (CD) is a treatment decision-tree dilemma. Although historic dental literature has suggested nature has completed "her own root canal," many clinicians know differently. As the age of the human race rapidly increases, pulps will have to last longer and greater calcific metamorphosis or CD will occur, and as these pulps can eventually become necrotic, endodontic treatment will be increasingly technically difficult, sometimes resulting in access "accidents" such as loss of precious ferrule or even perforation. Calcific metamorphosis can be defined as a pulp calcifying that is out of sequence from other teeth or the tooth on the opposite side of the arch. Although this author (JDW) considers CD a pathology waiting to eventually become necrotic and symptomatic, most dentists would resist advising endodontics if the pulp were vital and patient asymptomatic. For those colleagues, you are obligated, however, to carefully monitor the CD condition for necrosis and eventual lesion of endodontic origin.

Elective endodontics for pulpal reasons

Depth of preparation/remaining dentin

According to Stanley, "The most important single factor in determining pulpal response to a given stimulus is the remaining dentin thickness between the floor of the cavity preparation or the surface of a crown preparation and the pulp chamber." Studies have shown that a 2 mm dentin thickness between the floor of the cavity preparation and the pulp (Figure 24.33) will provide an adequate insulation against the more traumatic thermogenic operative techniques in spite of intentional abuse and most restorative materials.[5]

Cavity or crown preparations cut with high-speed (200 000–300 000 rpm) air water spray and light touch produced minimal pathologic alteration to healthy pulps when the remaining dentin was 2 mm or more.

However Stanley[4] also states, "Although 2 mm of primary dentin between the floor of the cavity preparation and the pulp is usually a sufficient protective barrier against cutting techniques … the effluent of cements and self-curing resins can overcome this thickness of protection." To avoid such intrusions, calcium hydroxide lining materials capable of protecting the pulp tissue when appropriately used, should be placed in all deep-seated cavity preparations prior to building a secondary protective base of cement.

If the final restoration is a one-step procedure (i.e., amalgam or composite resin), then a dentin/pulpal floor protected with a calcium hydroxide dressing base can be permanently restored. The patient must be advised if there are pulpal risks involved. The records should reflect the risk condition and the discussion.

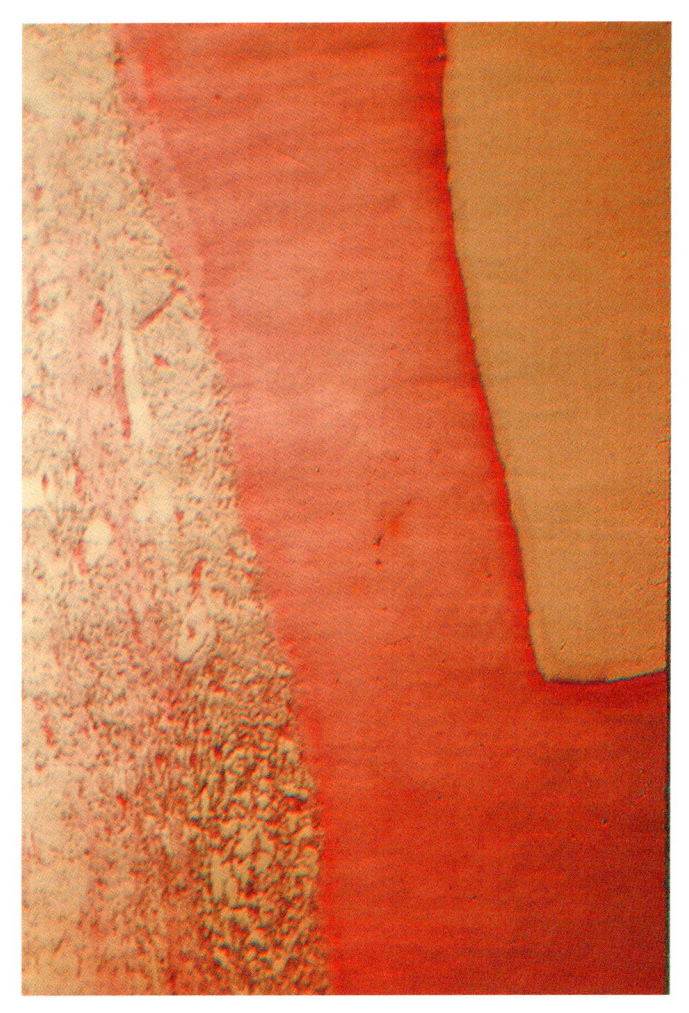

Figure 24.33 Cavity preparation with 2 mm of remaining dentin between its floor and the pulp tissue. *Source:* Courtesy of Dr Harold R Stanley.

The scenario differs with multiple-step restorations; that is, castings. If a tooth is compromised, the additional pulpal insults of preparation impression, try in, and cementation may exceed the pulp's ability to repair. If adverse symptoms persist, the pulp should be extirpated followed by endodontic treatment. Success rates justify this prophylactic approach.

If the requirements of the final restoration or the excavation of extensive caries results in less than 2 mm of remaining dentin, the expectation of a severe inflammatory reaction is greater. If a pink spot in the cavity or a blush on the tooth appears (Figure 24.34A and B) during or after preparation, it is possible that the 2 mm remaining dentin barrier has been violated. The probability of complete inflammatory reversibility and healing of a noticeably hemorrhagic pulp are minimal. Considering that additional procedures are required to finish the crown, endodontics should be performed before continuing. If at any time a patient elects to forego endodontic treatment following your recommendations, the records must indicate that the option to extirpate the pulp followed by endodontic treatment was strongly suggested and refused. However, an educated patient will always make the choice that is in their best interest. So the dentist's job is to pave your way with words and not only educate about esthetics, periodontics, structure, and function but also educate about endodontics. After a pulpitis occurs, it is often too late to inform your patient about pulpal risks that can occur during esthetic/restorative dentistry.

This presents a moral issue as to whether a patient should be allowed to dictate the final treatment when the risk of fracture is involved or other severe pulpal events are possible or likely. The dentist must realize they can always refuse to continue, provide palliative but temporary treatment to assure comfort, and suggest the patient see another dentist. If chosen, this decision, discussion, and referral must be recorded and witnessed. Irrespective of the remaining dentin thickness, the restoration has to be bacteria tight if the pulp is to have a chance to survive the insult. Care has to be taken to ensure the bacterial seal, because if there is leakage the bacteria will penetrate under the

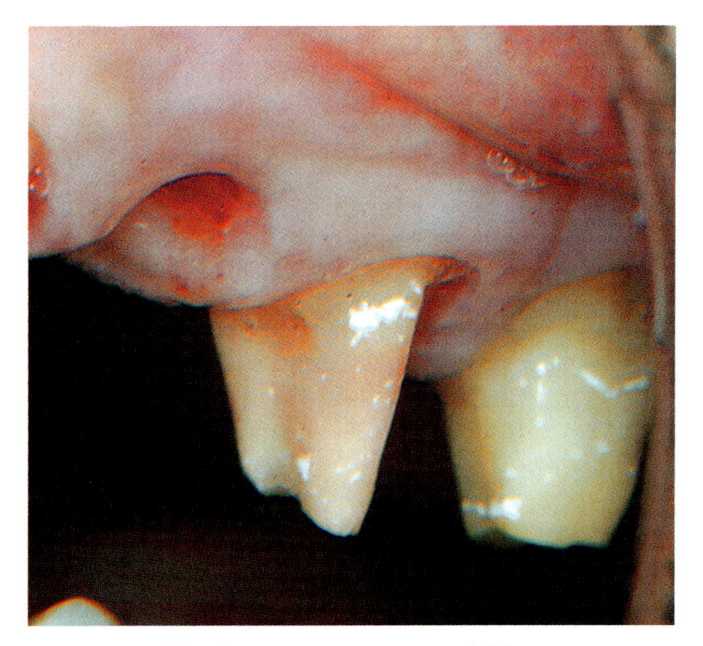

Figure 24.34 **(A)** Pink crown preparation 1 week following instrumentation. *Source:* Courtesy of Dr Harold R Stanley.

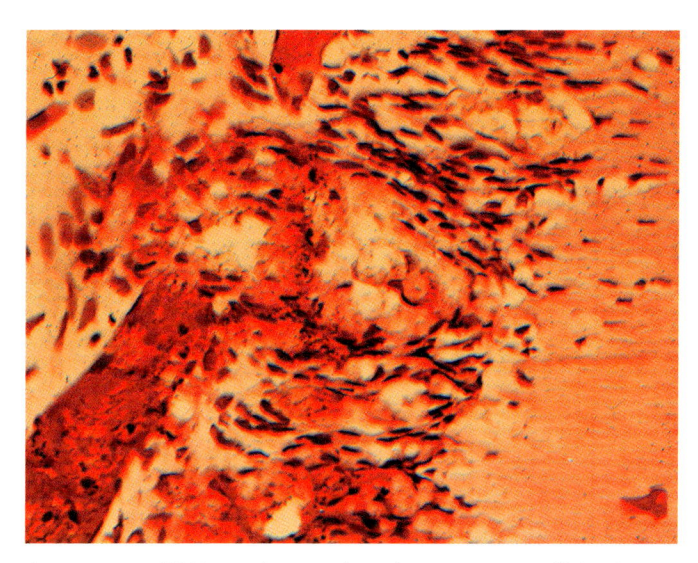

Figure 24.34 **(B)** Hemorrhagic pulp with extravasation of blood. *Source:* Courtesy of Dr Harold R Stanley.

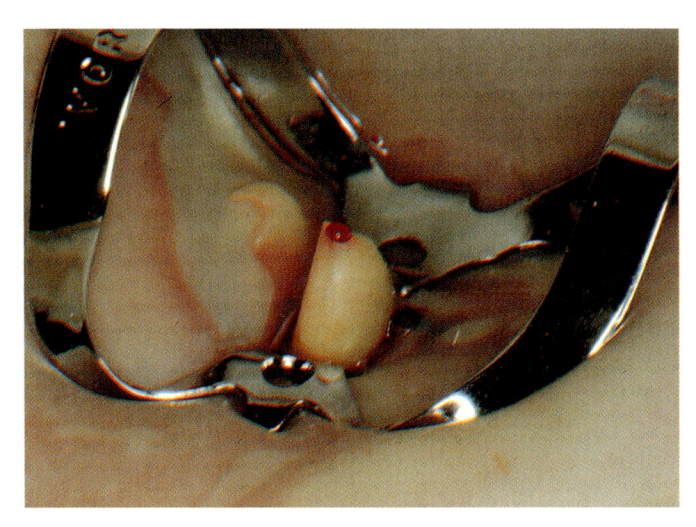

Figure 24.35 Pulp exposure during crown preparation. Extirpation is indicated.

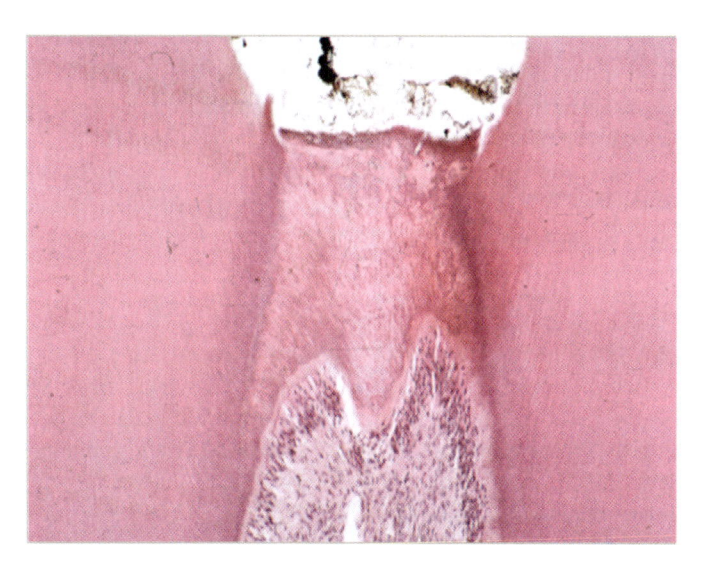

Figure 24.36 Dentin bridge following pulp capping with mineral trioxide aggregate (ProRoot MTA). Note thickness of bridge and absence of inflammation adjacent to the MTA. *Source:* Courtesy of Dr. Mahmoud Torabinejad.

restoration and through the dentinal tubules, initially cause pulpal irritation and eventually cause pulpal necrosis if the leakage is not stopped.

Pulp capping

Direct pulp capping in special situations has been shown to be safe, effective, and predictable. The ability of the pulp to repair when a mechanical exposure has been dressed with calcium hydroxide is well documented. The odontoblastic layer, once stimulated, forms a matrix that leads to the bridging of new dentin. This is because if the pulp were accidentally exposed by a dental bur (Figure 24.35) or by acute traumatic injury, then only the surface will show reversible inflammatory changes.[6] If the pulp exposure is under deep decay, there is good likelihood that the inflammation has affected a large portion of the pulpal tissue and even caused partial pulp necrosis. It is also important to remember that histologic pulpitis can be clinically asymptomatic, so the patient might not have any history of pain yet there can be a significant lesion in the pulpal chamber.[7]

Because of bacterial leakage risk into the pulp, direct pulp capping should only be considered with one-step restorations (i.e., amalgam or direct resin), and only when the patient is aware of the condition and the risk.

A thin calcium hydroxide mix of Dycal (acid resistant) is gently applied over the exposure. Care must be taken not to force the mix into the pulp because it could react adversely to an irritant like calcium hydroxide. However, healthy exposed tissue, unless insulted by pressure, contaminants, or leakage of the restoration, should respond favorably to the procedure. Successful pulp capping results have been reported by Torabinejad with mineral trioxide aggregate (Figure 24.36) (MTA pulp cap), ProRoot MTA (Tulsa/DENTSPLY).[8] Bogen et al. reported excellent results with MTA pulp capping in a two-visit procedure. The MTA was placed over an exposure, after caries removal, at the initial appointment.[9] At the following visit, the teeth were restored with a bonded composite. An analysis of the treated teeth after a 9-year observation period showed 97.76% favorable results based on radiographic appearance, cold testing, and subjective symptoms. However good the MTA may be for pulp capping, there is a downside to using it in a larger perforation as the material will probably need additional moisture in the form of moist cotton pellet placed on top of it to completely set. A larger perforation, therefore, will require an additional appointment to complete. More recently, Biodentine (Septodont), a calcium silicate-based capping material, has been suggested instead of MTA, because it completely sets in 15 min or less. It is important, though, to remember that most studies have not shown any significant difference in survival of the pulp when capped after accidental pulpal exposure with these three materials: calcium hydroxide, MTA, or Biodentine.

Pulp capping technique using direct acid etching and bonding has also been advocated. This concept is based on clinical observations but has little scientific data for support. Pameijer and Stanley studied the technique in a carefully controlled experiment on primates. Their results showed that pulp caps with acid etching and bonding agents produced 45% necrotic pulps and only 25% of the specimens developed dentin bridge formation,[10] whereas in the group pulp capped with calcium hydroxide only 7% of the pulps were necrotic and 82% of the teeth developed dentin bridge formation. Several more recent studies have all conclusively shown that, in human models, direct application of composite bonding or composite restorations on pulpal tissue is detrimental to its health.[11–13] Of note is that some animal studies have, at the same time, shown acceptable results. However, and because the animal evidence level is so low, these studies do not offer any treatment recommendation. It becomes obvious that if you elect to pulp cap, then calcium hydroxide, MTA,[14] or Biodentine are the materials of choice.

Even though there is a moderately good prognosis with pulp capping vital pulp exposures, the ease, predictability, and assurance of endodontic treatment certainly demands that the patient should be offered the option of root canal treatment when a definite exposure occurs; especially in teeth with fully formed apex. In teeth with pulp exposures and where multiple-step restorative procedures are contemplated (i.e., inlays, crowns, bridge abutments), nonsurgical root canal treatment is often the treatment modality of choice. Performing predictable endodontic outcomes prior to the prosthetic final cementation can obviate or avoid the aforementioned liabilities.

Stressed pulp

The dental literature is replete with methods and materials that demonstrate apparent success in preserving the integrity of the pulp, including the combination of sorghum molasses and English sparrow droppings.[15] But as time passes, subtle changes take place in the pulp, which create an unhealthy and unreliable tissue to depend upon as a sound foundation. This condition is often identified as stressed pulp. Abou-Rass considered the "stressed pulp" condition as an endodontic-restorative concept.[16] He believed it was of a clinical nature and not a histological entity. It should be considered a preexisting pulpal possibility in every restored tooth prior to subjecting the tooth to further restorative procedures. If the pulp is stressed, its ability to react favorably to the new insult will be diminished.

For example, a mandibular molar, although repeatedly restored, has remained without symptoms over a long period of time. A radiographic examination of the tooth demonstrates a deep occlusal amalgam and a large buccal composite restoration, recession of the pulp chamber, and narrowing of the root canals (Figure 24.37). Another example of stressed pulp is maxillary incisors that underwent concussion injuries and two previous crown preparations. Although there were no pulp exposures and there were minimal symptoms, intentional extirpations were performed because it was predicted the pulps would not survive another round of restorative procedures (Figure 24.38A–C). According to Abou-Rass's criteria, further insult to the affected (stressed) pulpal tissue would probably invite disaster. An intelligent decision would be elective endodontics, thereby intercepting potential problems.

Abou-Rass states that the pulp's ability to recover from "stressed" pulp is relative to:

- type of injury
- duration of injury
- physiologic age
- thickness of remaining dentin
- past trauma (impact injuries)
- repeated operative procedures.

When all of the aforementioned factors are examined and the patient's normal routine is changed because of vague symptoms, elective endodontic intervention should be considered. Another example of a stressed pulp is a patient with a maxillary anterior provisional restoration who required local anesthesia to remove the bridge 12 months after crown preparation and periodontal therapy because of pain from a maxillary central incisor tooth (Figure 24.39A). The combined dental procedure created additional stress and inflammation on the pulpal complex that was beyond its ability to repair. This scenario could have been avoided if elective endodontic intervention had been recommended to the patient.

Elective endodontics for prosthetic reasons

"No tooth or components of a tooth should be sacrificed if the prognosis of the remaining dentition can be improved by its retention."[17] Discussing elective endodontics vis-à-vis extensive restorations, Bohannan and Abrams felt that root canal therapy should be performed for[17]

- reorientation of occlusal planes;
- reduction of crown/root ratios;
- establishment of parallelism.

A clinician faces many such situations where the overall esthetic and restorative result could be enhanced if the pulp was extirpated and ideal root form was available. Unfortunately, the decision to perform the endodontics is often determined by issues other than what is beneficial to the patient; that is,

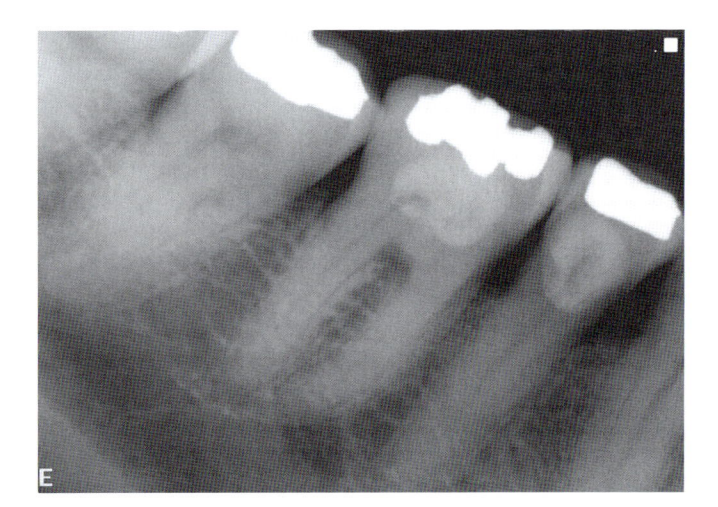

Figure 24.37 Mandibular molar with stressed pulp.

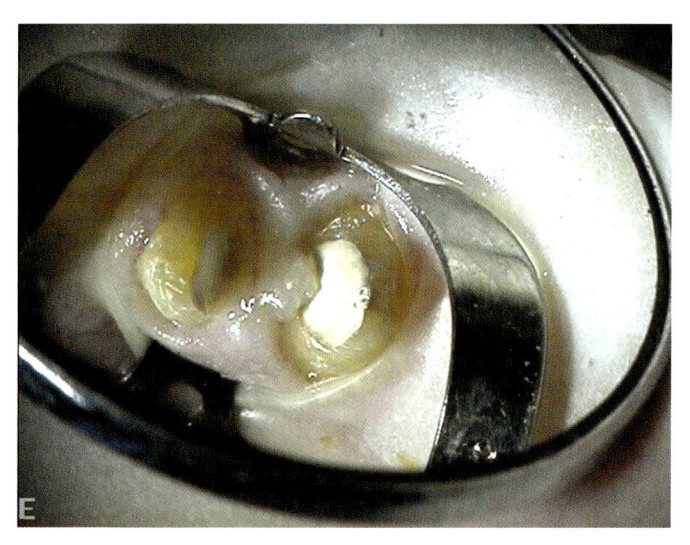

Figure 24.38 **(A)** Centrals incisor teeth after excavation of extensive caries. The pulps were not exposed.

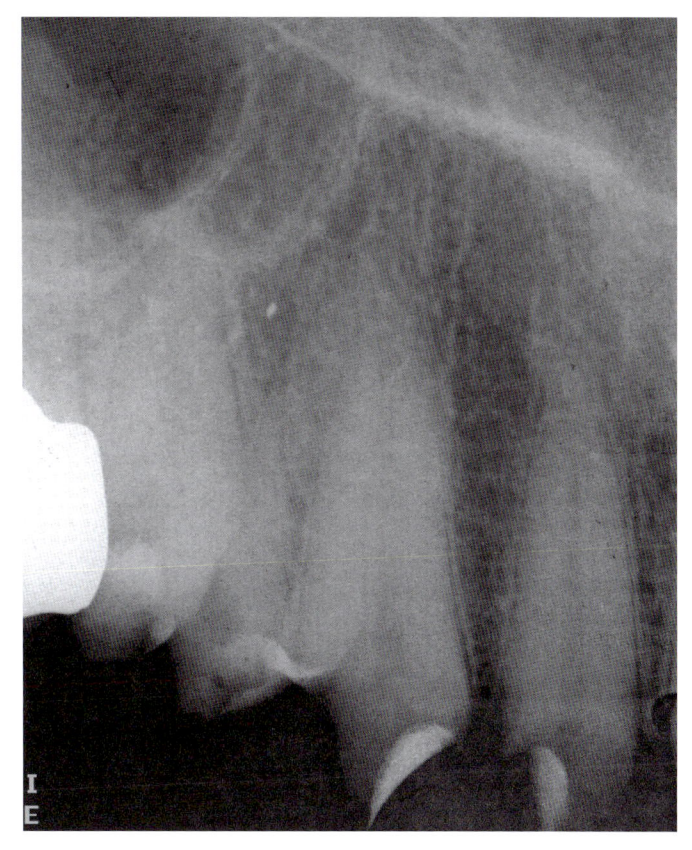

Figure 24.38 **(B)** Radiograph of same teeth. Note the minimal thickness of dentin adjacent to pulp chambers.

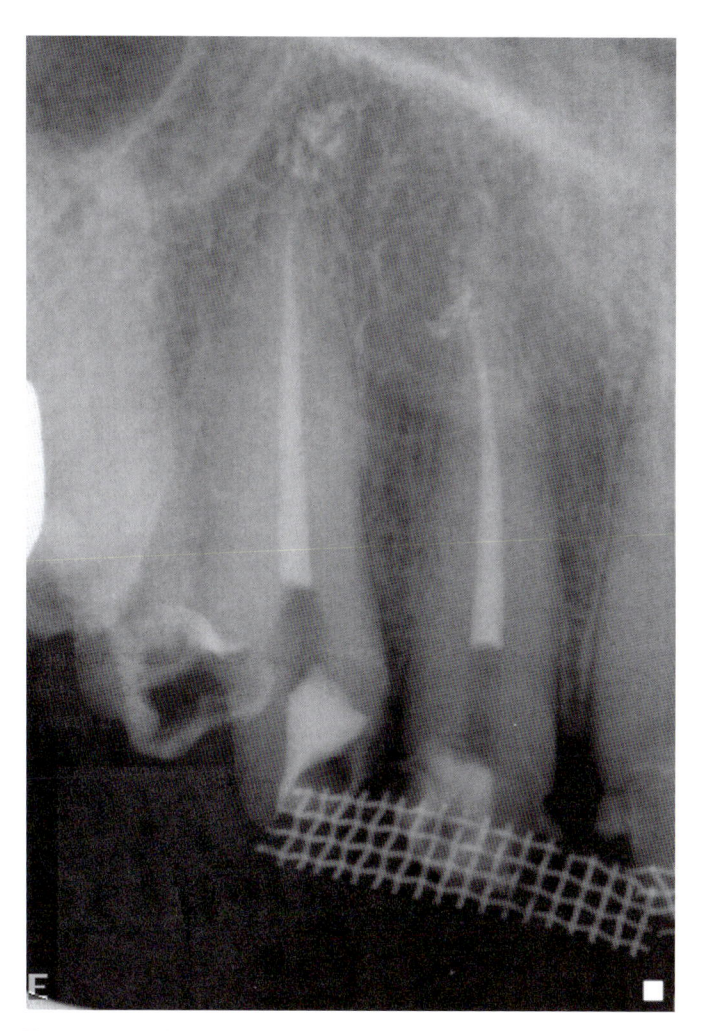

Figure 24.38 **(C)** Root canal treatment completed on the maxillary central incisors.

economics, time, lack of skill, or experience. Regardless, we must not lose sight that it is the duty of every dental diagnostician to evaluate and design each case with the goal of maximizing form, function, health, and esthetics. Therefore, when endodontic treatment enables the clinician to deliver the ideal restoration, why should the situation is compromised?

Endodontic treatment protocols

An understanding of basic endodontic principles and a clearly defined restorative plan are essential prior to beginning root canal treatment. The final esthetic result should not be compromised by an inadequate approach. Therefore, various phases of endodontic treatment will be examined to see how they may enhance or preserve esthetics rather than detract from it. Although this may seem repetitious, the risk of performing endodontic procedures for restored teeth must be explained and accepted by the patient, and all discussions should be documented and recorded before a procedure is attempted.

Rubber dam is essential

The use of the rubber dam in endodontics is mandatory for keeping risk of bacterial contamination to minimal and for patient safety.[18] Two studies have shown that 46% and 44% of general dentists do not routinely use a rubber dam when performing root canal treatment, although it is a deviation from standards of care.[19,20] It must be remembered that an untoward incident—that is, swallowing or aspirating a reamer or file when the rubber dam has not been used during therapy—leaves little doubt about legal liability. Other reports[20,21] showed that endodontists use a rubber dam 100% of the time. Crown lengthening may be required, prior to endodontic treatment, to expose sufficient tooth structure to accommodate the clamp. This is not a detriment since this procedure will be beneficial when establishing a finishing line for the restoration. "Even if the endodontically treated tooth is broken down and cannot be clamped, a rubber dam, regardless of the required modifications, should be used in all instances."[18]

The market offers over 100 different clamps, including wing, wingless, stainless, matte finish, and color coded, to cover a wide variety of clinical situations. One of the authors (NC) uses just three clamps in over 97% of his cases:

- #9 wing clamp—maxillary and mandibular anterior teeth and most crown preparations;
- #2 wing clamp—natural and restored premolar teeth;
- #4 wing clamp—natural and restored molar teeth.

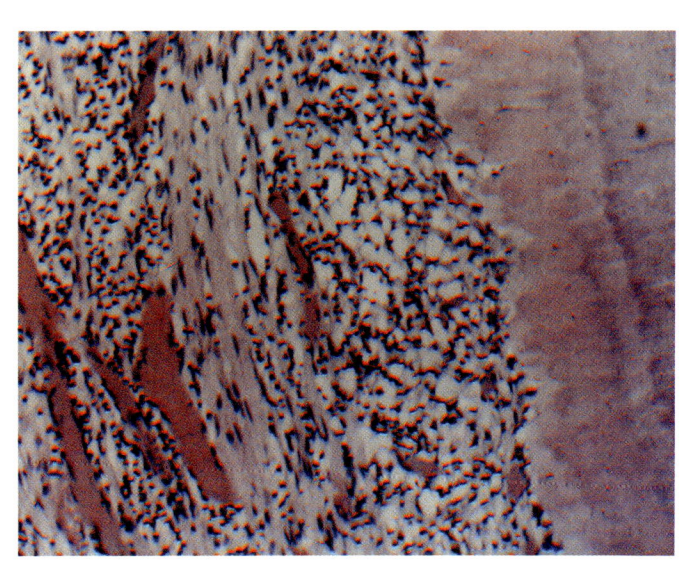

Figure 24.39 (B) A histological section of chronic inflammation, irreversible pulpitis, with round cell infiltration.

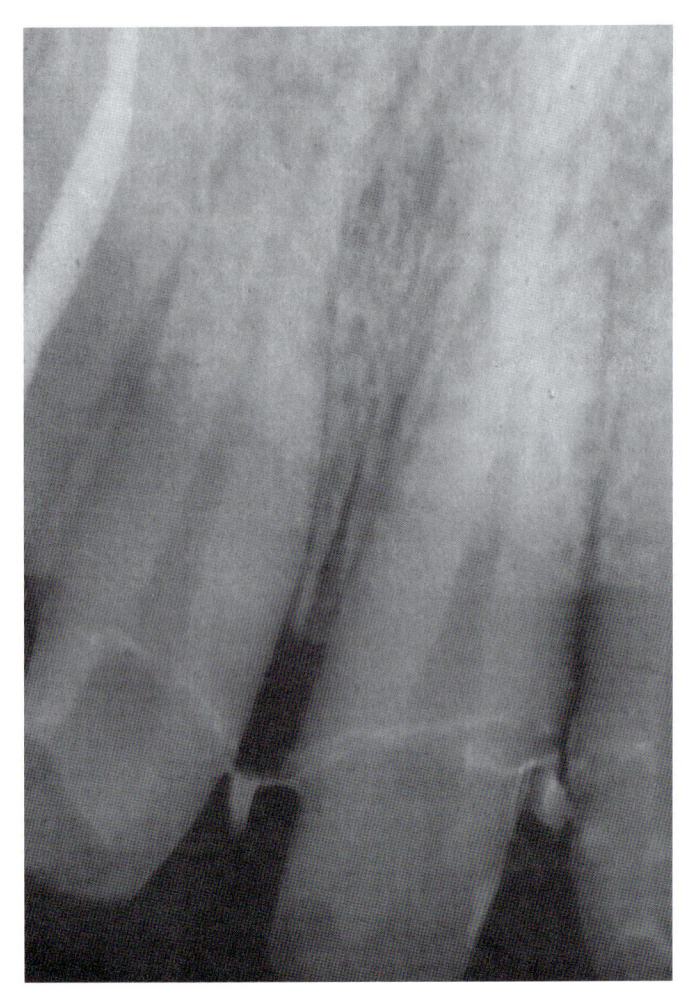

Figure 24.39 (A) Maxillary central incisor teeth with a chronic inflamed (stressed) pulp.

that, regardless of the crown margin design, all of the test samples displayed crazing of the porcelain in the area of the beaks of the clamp. Additional forces on the porcelain in clinical situations as the clamp is inadvertently moved during treatment would most certainly increase the probability of crazing. This problem could be eliminated when the teeth with questionable pulpal health are endodontically treated prior to cementation of the crown.

Since over 40% of root canal treatment is performed through existing restorations, the following alternative methods of rubber dam application are suggested for ceramic crowns to minimize potential problem.[2]

Alternative methods of rubber dam for ceramic crowns

- *Floss or Wedjets cord ligation.* Dental floss or rubber cord, Wedjets (Hygienic) (Figure 24.40A), can be used to retain a rubber dam when isolating a single tooth. Wedjets is a

Rubber dam clamps, when placed on ceramic restorations, have the potential to create problems.[22] In the study, porcelain-fused-to-metal (PFM) crowns, the clamps were placed on the crowns and left undisturbed for 1 h in the laboratory. They found

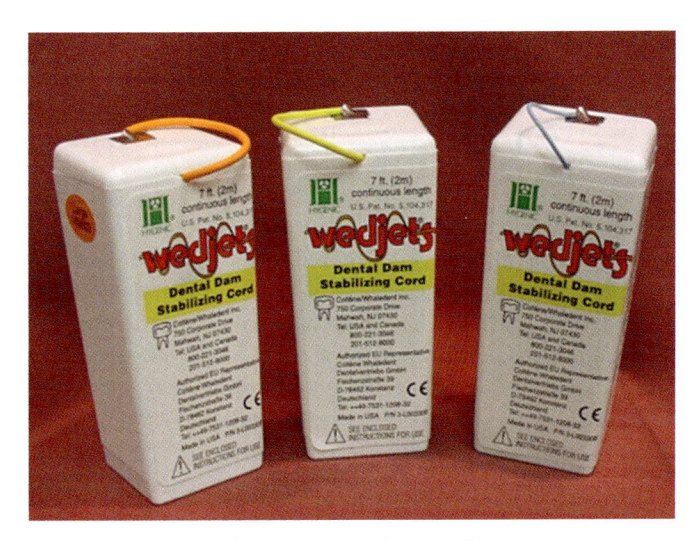

Figure 24.40 (A) Wedjets; three sizes (Hygienic).

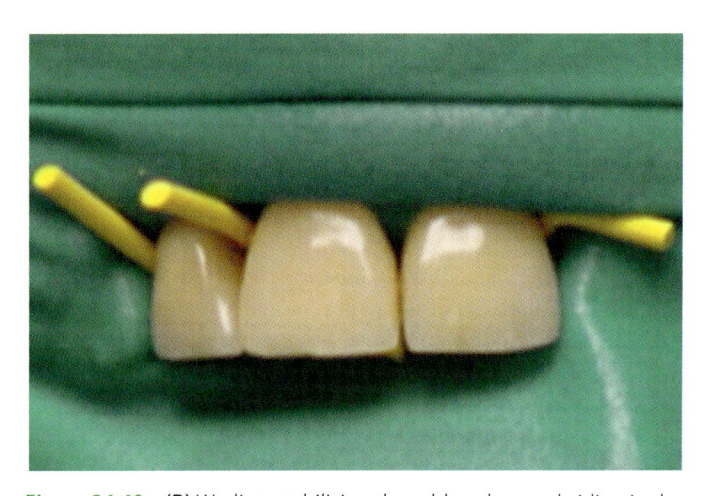

Figure 24.40 (B) Wedjets stabilizing the rubber dam and aiding in the isolation of a maxillary central incisor.

stretchable cord that is made from natural latex. The cord, available in three sizes, is placed like dental floss to hold the dam in place. Wedges can be used in conjunction with dental floss or Wedjets once the dam is in place. For convenience, it is recommended at least one tooth on either side of the treated tooth be included in the isolation (Figure 24.40B).

- *Cushee rubber dam clamp cushions (Practicon)* Cushees are soft silicone cushions that fit over the jaws of the standard steel clamps. The jaws of the clamp do not come in contact with the gingiva, tooth structure, or restoration. Patient comfort is increased and potential damage to ceramic restorations is decreased. They are available in two forms: yellow for anterior and bicuspid clamps (Figure 24.41A and B) and blue for molar clamps (Figure 24.41C).
- *Ingenuity/multiple teeth isolation* When dealing with splinted units, ingenuity is an important part of the problem-solving equation. This approach recommends the clamps be placed on unrestored adjacent teeth. Three or more contiguous holes are punched in the dam; the rubber is stretched over all the teeth to be isolated; and the most posterior tooth is clamped first. Then, the anterior tooth is addressed with the clamp placed in reverse with its bow facing anteriorly. The tooth to be treated remains unclamped and access is unrestricted (Figure 24.42). Once the dam is in place, Oraseal Putty (Ultradent) may be compacted around the gingival margin of the crown to block off any fluid leakage. When the entire arch is restored with ceramic restorations, you are faced with a difficult situation and must improvise to control esthetic damage. If there are individual crowns, avoid placing rubber dam clamps on any of the anterior or first premolar teeth. Surface damage to the porcelain when risked should be confined to the second premolar and molar teeth, which are less visible. Cushees or Wedjets should be used to protect the restorations.

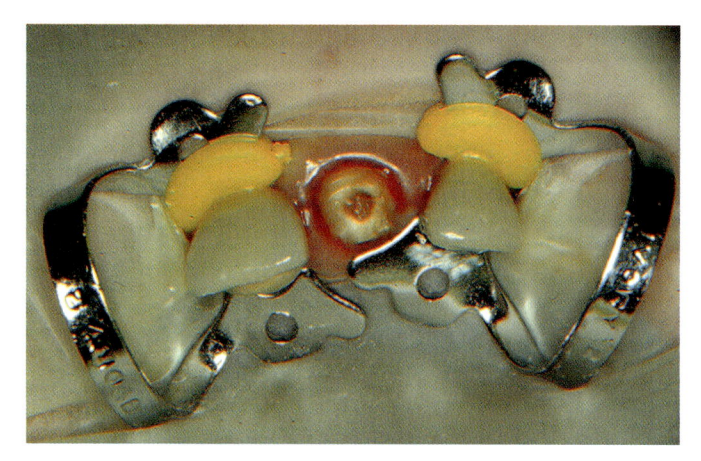

Figure 24.41 **(A)** Cushee rubber dam clamp cushions (Practicon) isolating multiple anterior teeth.

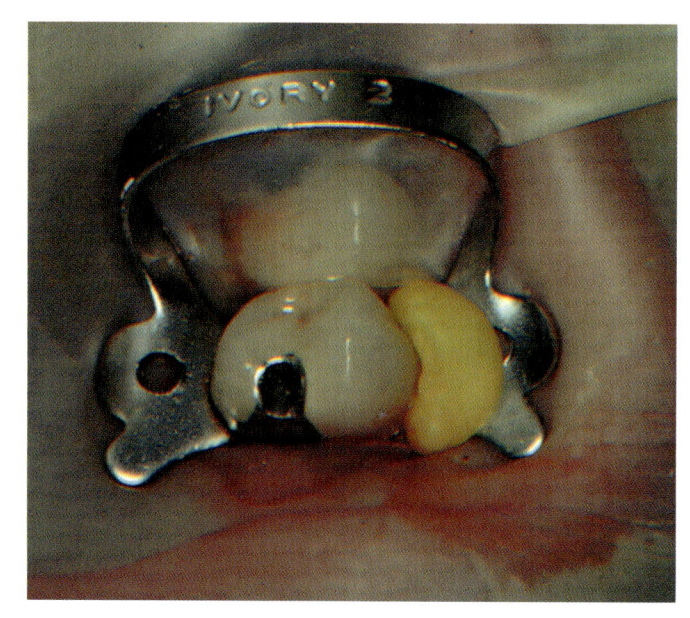

Figure 24.41 **(B)** Cushee rubber dam clamp cushions (Practicon) isolating maxillary premolar.

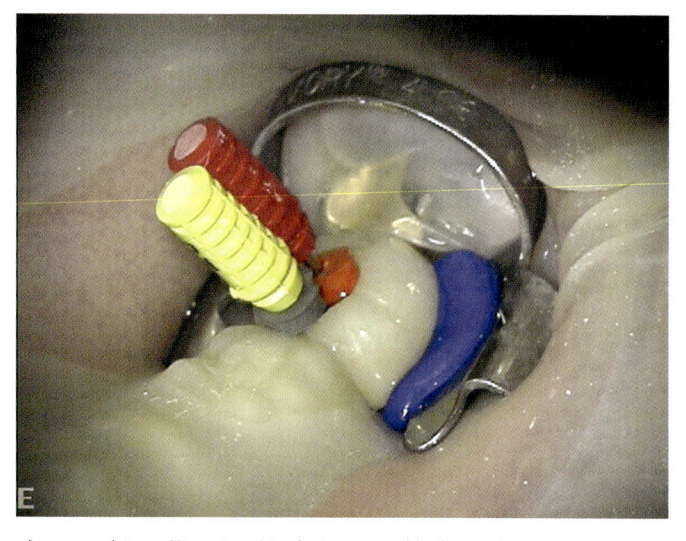

Figure 24.41 **(C)** Cushee rubber dam clamp cushions (Practicon) isolating mandibular molar.

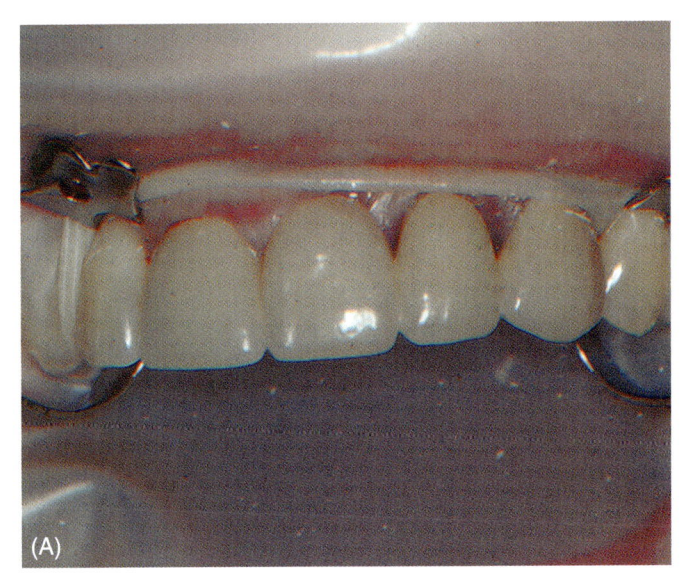

Figure 24.42 (A, B) Rubber dam isolation of multiple teeth.

Again for contamination and patient protection, as well as medicolegal reasons, endodontic treatment should never be attempted without rubber dam isolation. Nonlatex dam is available for those patients with known latex allergies. Apprehensive patients may be accommodated with use of Optra Dam Plus (Figure 24.43) (Ivoclar-Vivadent) or Insta-Dam Relaxed Fit (Zirc). It has a built-in frame and is smaller than the standard size of 5″ × 5″ rubber dam. It still affords similar protection and isolation.

Access cavity preparation

A carefully planned and well-executed access cavity preparation should maximize retained tooth structure, minimize weakening the tooth, provide for unobstructed visibility, and allow for straight-line entry into all of the root canal systems (Figure 24.44).

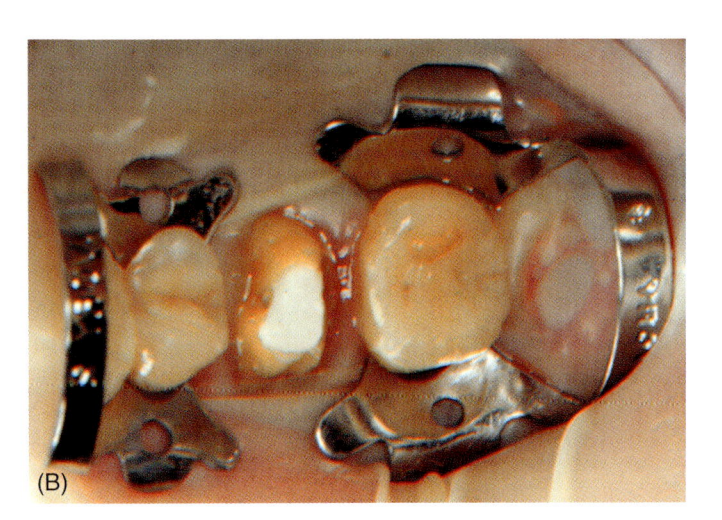

Entering the pulp chamber requires definitive knowledge of tooth morphology, the specific intricacies of the tooth to be treated, and proper instrumentation. As previously discussed, recent radiographs, taken with a paralleling device, ensuring minimal distortion, should be studied prior to picking up the handpiece. Two preoperative films exposed from different horizontal angles to give better information should be part of the pretreatment routine. Bitewing images are recommended for posterior teeth. The radiographs depict location of the chamber, presence or absence of calcification, number of roots and canals, and the relationship of the incisal or occlusal surfaces to the axial line of the root.

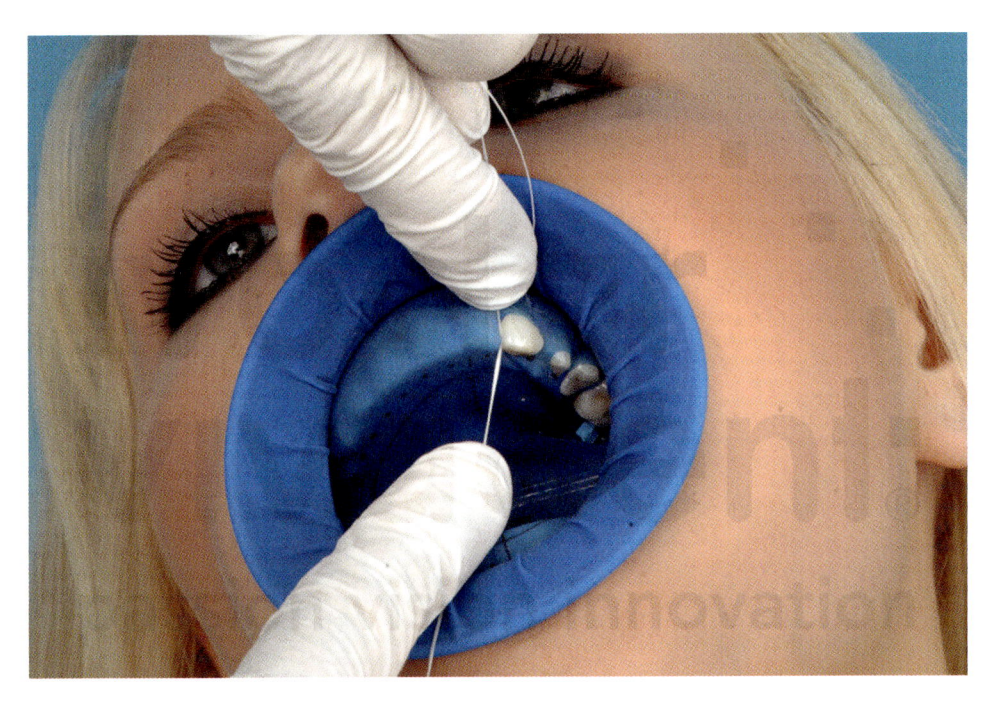

Figure 24.43 Optradam (Ivoclar).

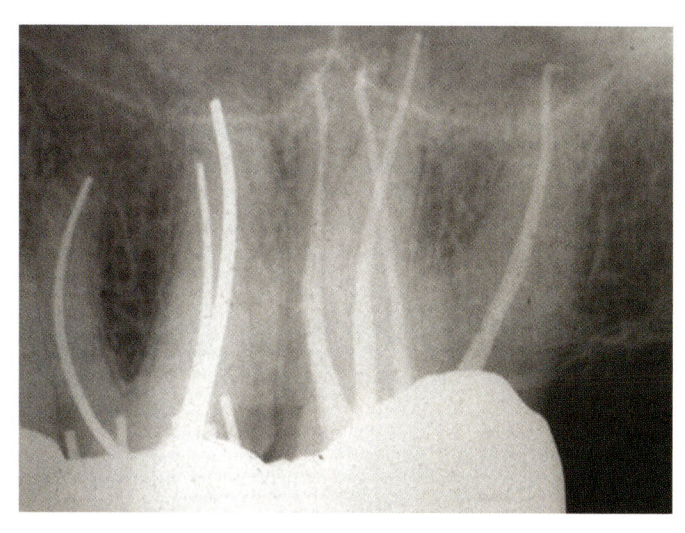

Figure 24.44 Straight-line access allowed for visualization of all four canals in the maxillary molar teeth. (First molar courtesy of Dr Hyman R Baer; second molar courtesy of Dr Stanley M Baer.)

Morphologically, the access cavity takes the shape of the underlying pulp chamber (Figure 24.45A–C). Variations in size and shape of the pulp chamber take place as the result of calcification resulting from caries, operative procedures, restorations, occlusal wear, abrasion, and so on. Therefore, by nature, the access cavity in a youngster's nonrestored tooth (Figure 24.46) would be larger than that of a similar tooth with multiple restorations in an older person (Figure 24.47).

Magnification is essential in searching for canals when calcification has obliterated the chamber. Magnification in conjunction with an auxiliary light source reduces the frustration of finding the canal orifices.

The access opening must be large enough to allow:

- visualization of the entire chamber;
- location of the root canal orifice(s);
- removal of all existing decay.

Preparation and equipment

The dentist should be aware that a tooth with a crown may be very different from the natural tooth it covers, both in regard to size and shape and to occlusal plane (Figure 24.48). A thorough examination of the preoperative radiograph(s) as well as careful periodontal probing of the tooth will provide important morphological information and should be part of the pretreatment process. It is customary to reduce the occlusal table if the final restoration will involve full coverage. This will provide flat surface for canal length measurement during the root canal treatment. It will also decrease the probably of postoperative discomfort since the tooth will not be in occlusion.

Natural tooth structure should be protected from heat during the access cavity preparation. Studies have shown deleterious crazing and cracking occurs in the enamel and dentin when access cavities are prepared dry. Regardless of the fact that the pulp will be extirpated, water should be used to cool both the bur and the tooth during this procedure.

Removal of existing occlusal and proximal restorations plus the decay should be completed prior to entering the pulp chamber. This will be the first step in establishing a bacteria-free environment. To facilitate canal orientation, some practitioners prepare the access and locate the orifices of the canals prior to placing the rubber dam. It is important, as always, to place the rubber dam before introducing an endodontic file into the tooth to eliminate the possibility of the aspiration or ingestion of the file.

Some manufacturers market endodontic access kits that include the instrumentation needed for this portion of the treatment:

- Endo Access Kit (Dentsply Tulsa Dental Specialties);
- CK Diamond Endodontic Access Kit (SS White);
- LAAXESS (SybronEndo).

Penetration and funneling are the two phases of an endodontic access cavity preparation, whether in natural tooth structure or teeth with full-coverage restorations. Penetration can be accomplished with high speed from various manufacturers: round burs #2 or #4 or round-ended fissure burs #1558.

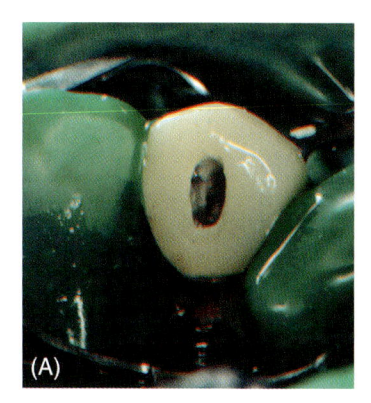

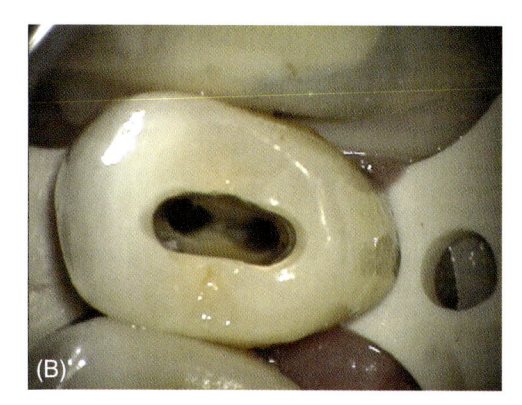

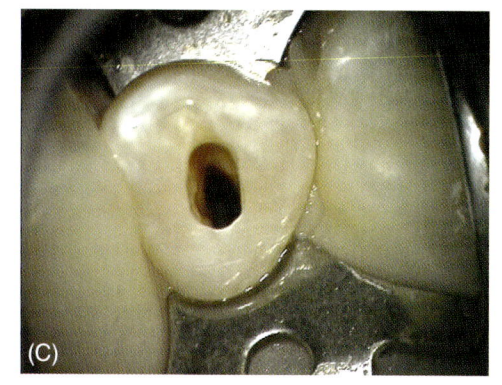

Figure 24.45 **(A)** Access cavity outlines reflect the shape of the pulp chamber: maxillary canine. **(B)** Access cavity outlines reflect the shape of the pulp chamber: maxillary premolar. **(C)** Access cavity outlines reflect the shape of the pulp chamber: mandibular premolar.

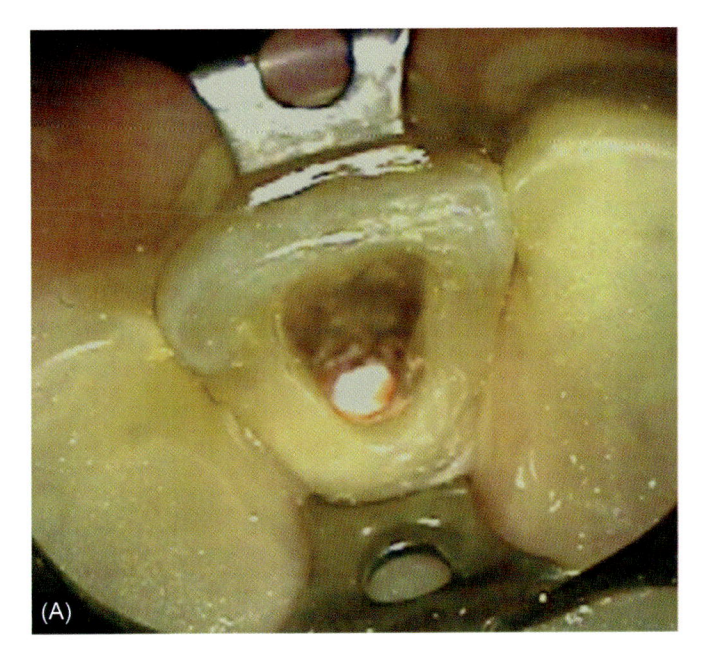

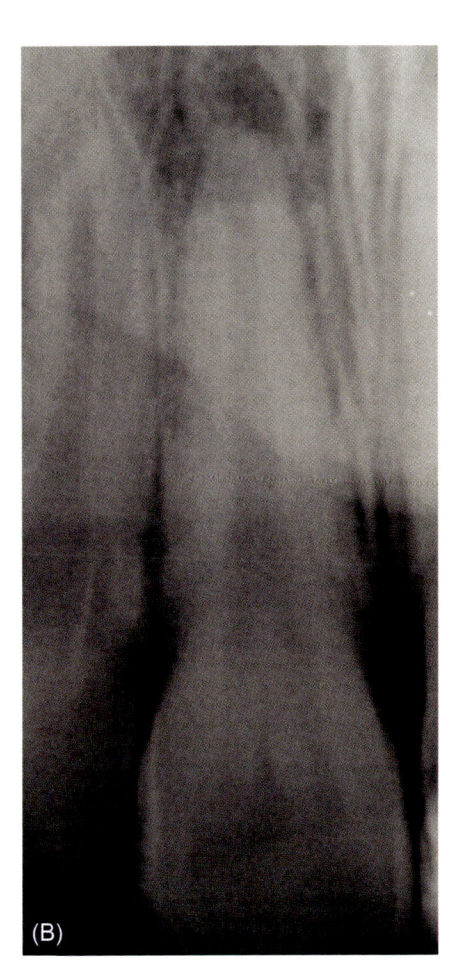

Figure 24.46 (A, B) Access cavity in a traumatized unrestored maxillary central incisor, 16-year-old person.

Round diamond burs are used for penetration in ceramic restoration. If decay is present in the chamber it can be removed with #2, #4, or #6 long-shank burs at low speed. A long-shank endodontic excavator #33 L is also very useful in the process.

Funneling is accomplished with tapered fissure diamonds or carbide fissure burs. A number of the diamonds have been specifically designed with noncutting tips to reduce the possibility of perforating the floor of the chamber while flaring the axial walls of the chamber:

- Endo-Z® bur (DENTSPLY Maillefer);
- LAAXXESS Diamond Bur (SybronEndo);
- Endo Safe End ESE018, ESE014 carbide, and CK Endo Access bur (SS White).

Tapered diamonds should be used for finishing access walls.

Various types of restored teeth

Teeth with partial or full-coverage restorations present additional obstacles in gaining entry into the pulp chamber. Gold, nonprecious metal, ceramo-metal, aluminum oxide cores with porcelain buildups, lithium disilicate and zirconium cores, and or all-zirconium crowns restorations require different types of instrumentation, burs, than natural tooth structure does.

Gold crowns

New transmetal burs, Transmetal Bur 19 mm (DENTSPLY Endodontics), are recommended for penetrating through gold. The sharpness of a new bur will maximize penetration and minimize the tendency to skip or skid. The bur is of similar shape to the #1558 used for access cavity preparation in natural tooth structure, but they are designed for efficient metal cutting. Electric-driven handpieces also facilitate minimal vibration during access preparations.

Ceramic restorations

Christensen found shallow microcracks in all samples tested after endodontic access cavities preparation. "... research results showed both a trend in glass ceramics (IPS Empress) and veneered ceramics (zirconia based) being more prone to cracks extending into body of restoration from endo access than monolithic ceramic materials (BruxZir, Lava Frame, Lava Ultimate, and IPS e.max CAD)."[23] One of his conclusions was, "Making access through a restoration thickness of less than 1 mm carries a greater risk of producing micro cracks

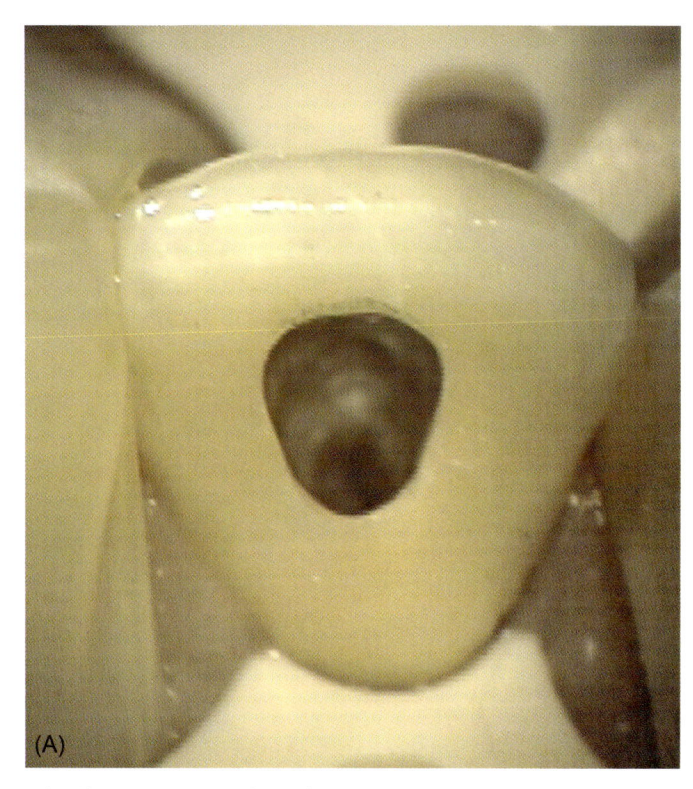

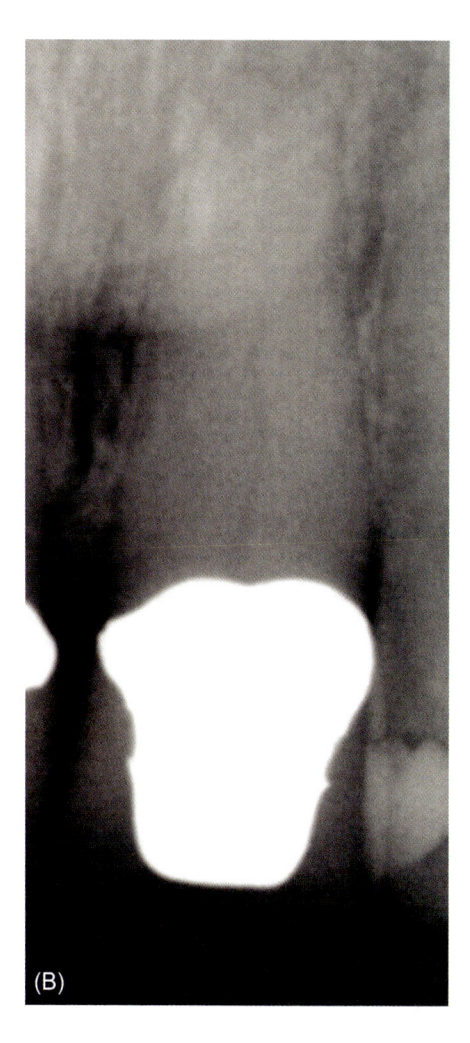

Figure 24.47 **(A, B)** Access cavities through PFM crowns in a middle-aged male.

which could propagate during service." To reduce this possibility, he suggested completing endodontic treatment before crown cementation. Since the need for treatment is not always predictable, Christensen recommends 1.5 mm or more of occlusal reduction when preparing the teeth for ceramic restorations. When endodontic treatment is needed after cementation, one-time-use diamonds, copious water spray, light pressure, and an electric handpiece are recommended to minimize cracking.[23]

Aluminous porcelain

Medium- or fine-cut diamonds accompanied by a water spray should be used to cut through porcelain. Carbide burs will generate incredible heat and the cutting action of the bur will significantly increase the possibility of porcelain failure.[24]

The dentist has the choice of the following round diamond stones:

- Brassier 801-016
- Premier 120 F
- Gnathos 801-016
- Premier 1116.8 round-end fissure diamond.

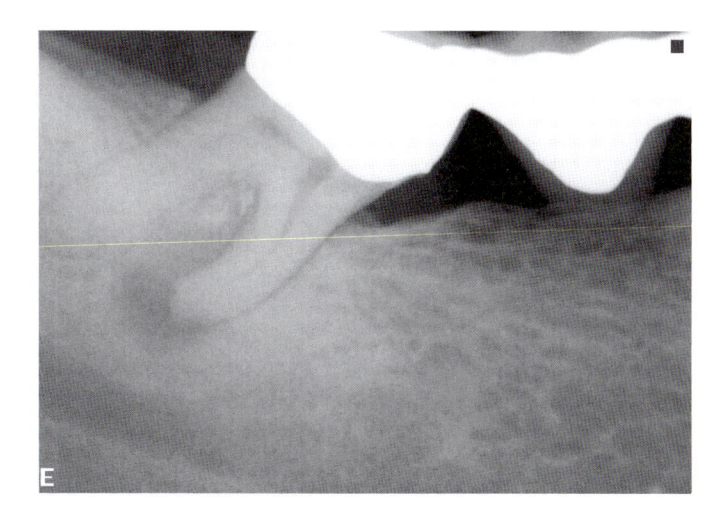

Figure 24.48 Mesially inclined mandibular second molar. Because of the tilt toward the mesial, the direction of the bur should be angled toward the distal to avoid perforation during access cavity preparation.

Disposable diamonds are efficient when cutting ceramic restorations. Being new, they tend to reduce crazing or cracking in the restoration and generate less heat.

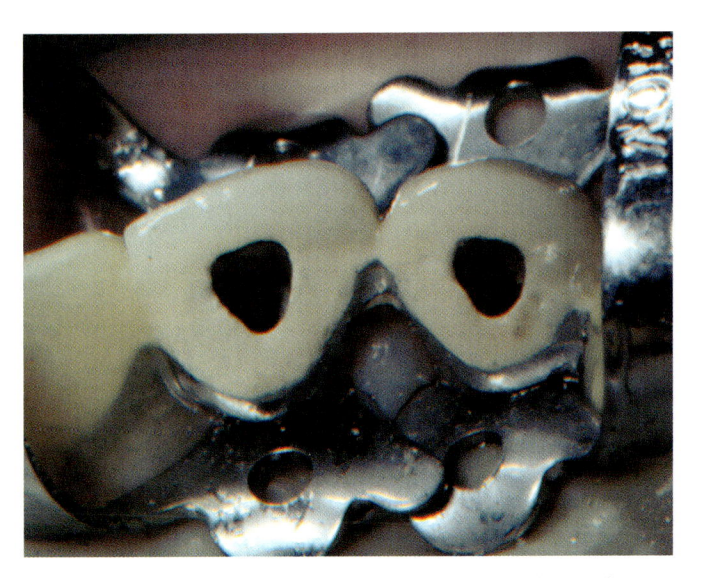

Figure 24.49 **(A)** Outline of access cavity traced through porcelain with a diamond stone.

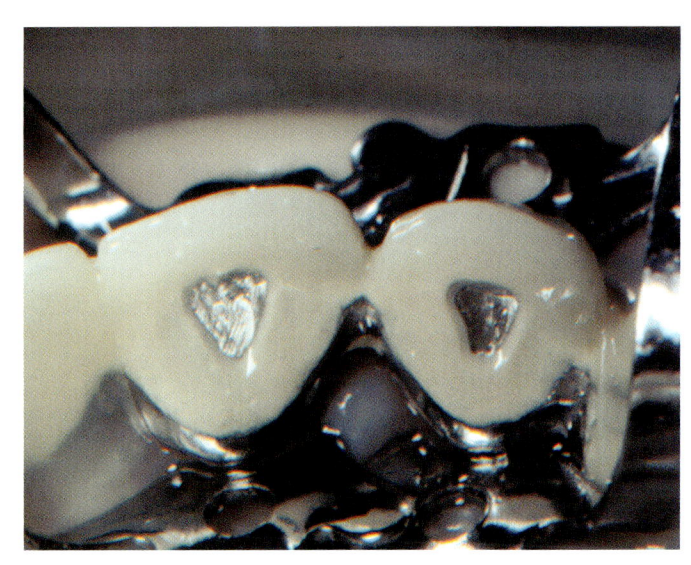

Figure 24.49 **(B)** Penetration and funneling of the access cavities.

Porcelain-fused-to-metal crown

A round diamond stone (Brasseler 801-016, Premier 120 F or Gnathos #801-016) accompanied by a copious water spray is best for the porcelain entry. Once the metal casting is met (Figure 24.49A), a classic access cavity is traced in the porcelain with the diamond stone. Penetration through the metal and dentin into the pulp chamber (Figure 24.49B) is accomplished with a new Transmetal Bur (DENTSPLY Maillefer). Carbide burs, cutting through metal, rapidly dull and should be discarded when they lose their efficiency. The funneling can be accomplished, as previously described, with flared fissure nonend cutting diamonds.

Ceramic crowns: cast glass–all-ceramic crowns (aluminum oxide)–pressed ceramics (lithium disilicate)

A laboratory study has shown that high-speed diamond instrumentation with water spray is efficient when cutting through Cerastore crowns.[25] The same study also indicated carbide burs used under similar conditions were inefficient. Years later, the ceramic technology has produced many new choices for use in patient care. However, the round diamond is still the choice for initiating the access cavity procedure.

Zirconia crowns

All-zirconia crowns or zirconia-core crowns have an unusual hardness and are difficult to cut through for removal or access cavity preparation. In preparing other ceramic crowns for endodontic access, the progress of cutting through the material can be observed in a matter of seconds. With zirconia, one questions the sharpness of the diamond stone or the rotation frequency of the handpiece when there is no progress in a reasonable period of time. It is not the diamond stones and handpieces that are the problem; it is the hardness of the zirconia that makes it difficult to cut. Research has shown zirconia is up to 10 times harder than other ceramic materials that we usually encounter. Therefore, a new classification of diamonds was developed by the dental manufacturing industry. The same preparation sequence is used for access with zirconia restorations: penetration, round diamond burs and funneling, and tapered fissure diamonds stones.

Zirconia cutting diamonds penetration funneling:

- Premier Dental round 125Z, tapered fissure 703.8 krz;
- Axis Dental round Z2801-18, tapered fissure Z856-18;
- Komet pear ZR 379 m, tapered fissure ZR379m.

If you inserted the zirconia crown and will be doing the endodontic treatment, you are ahead of the game and will be able to select the zirconia-appropriate diamond. If you are going to refer the patient to an endodontist, please let them know the crown is zirconia, so they will have the proper diamonds available. If you are doing the endodontic treatment for the patient and do not know what the type of ceramic material, try your usual and customary disposable diamond on the tooth. If there is no progress, in a reasonable period of time, assume the ceramic is zirconia and select a zirconia cutting diamond for the access cavity preparation.

Ceramic inlays and onlays

A twofold problem presents with these restorations vis-à-vis access preparation: fragility of the material and design of the restoration. Fracture and dislodgement are potential sequelae when cutting into these restorations. To avoid the problem, one must be certain of the pulpal health prior to selecting these restorations. If, however, faced with endodontic therapy through these restorations, the patient must be advised of the possible necessity of replacement. Once the risk is accepted, high-speed diamond instrumentation with copious water and minimal pressure will minimize the potential of rendering the restoration useless.

Etched cast restoration

Any tooth with a questionable pulp should be endodontically treated prior to placing an etched cast restoration. Frequently, this restoration is used to replace an anterior tooth that has been lost as a result of trauma. It is reasonable to assume the adjacent teeth may have sustained injury as well. Therefore, it is imperative that the pulp and periapical ligament status be ascertained before bonding the restoration in place. However, if faced with root canal therapy, the access cavity must be kept as small as possible. The likelihood of weakening the bond is great. In most cases, a new #2 or #1558 carbide bur and a copious water spray will minimize heat and reduce the vibration, which is the cause of debonding. Occasionally, it is more practical to prepare the access cavity through the labial surface, particularly when dealing with lower incisor teeth (Figure 24.50A–C). The distinct advantage of direct access without disturbing the casting is immeasurable. The opening can then be repaired with a light-cured composite resin (Figure 24.50D). Cosmetically, the lip and smile line should be considered before using this approach. Communicating the benefits of this approach and having the patient accept the technique before proceeding is essential.

Crown retention after endodontic treatment

In addition to esthetic compromises that occur as a result of access preparation, crown retention also becomes questionable. An in vitro study by McMullen et al. showed that the retentive value of a PFM crown was decreased 60.17% following access cavity preparation.[26] In a follow-up study, McMullen et al. showed that the retentive value of the crown could be increased 237% over its original value if the crown was recemented with poly carboxylate cement and the access cavity filled with amalgam.[27] However, it is rare that a crown or a bridge is removed after final cementation to allow for endodontic therapy.

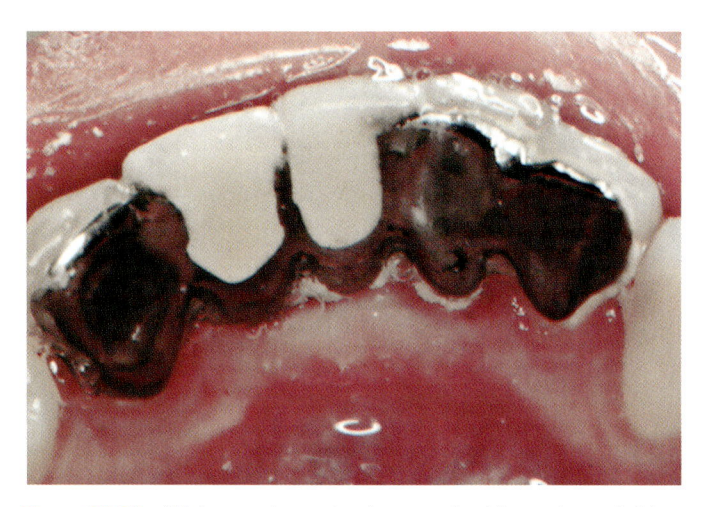

Figure 24.50 (A) Access alternative for an etched five unit cast bridge.

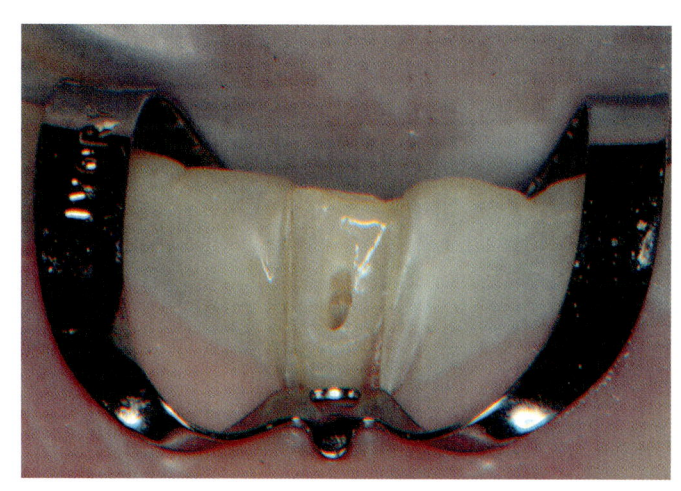

Figure 24.50 (B) Access cavity prepared on the labial surface.

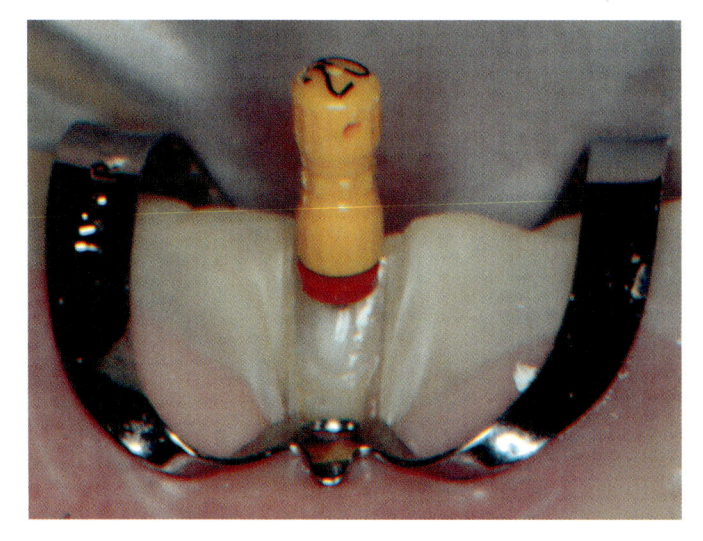

Figure 24.50 (C) Measurement file in place.

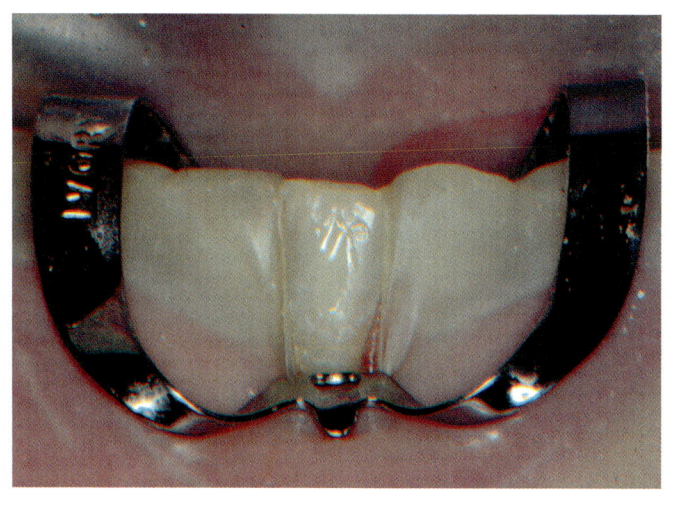

Figure 24.50 (D) Access opening repaired with composite resin.

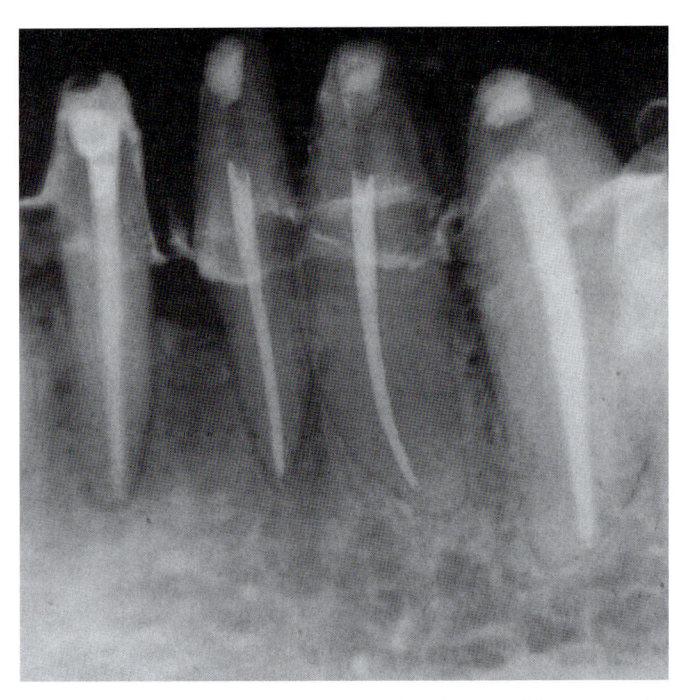

Figure 24.51 Endodontic therapy completed prior to fabrication of final castings on four mandibular anterior teeth with questionable pulpal health.

Unfortunately, retentive value following the restoration of the access cavities with amalgam alone has not been studied. With this in mind, repairing an access cavity with amalgam after endodontics may not restore it to an acceptable strength or esthetic level. This affirms the need to perform elective endodontics whenever a risk exists prior to the fabrication and cementation of a crown(s) (Figure 24.51).

Removable partial denture abutments

When faced with unusual situations—for example, occlusal rests and attachment receptacles in removable partial denture abutments—innovation enters the picture. To preserve their usefulness, attempts should be made to keep away from the attachment area. The final access preparation outline should be finished near the attachment but not encroach on it. The shape of the preparation may be decidedly atypical, but the preservation of the mechanical lock integrity will be retained.

Instrumentation/debridement

The goal of this phase of endodontic treatment is to eliminate all microorganisms from the canal system by completely removing organic, inorganic debris, biofilm, and smear layer. The objective is to accomplish cleaning and shaping the root canal system yet maintain the constriction of the canal apex and the funnel shape of the coronal aspect. This canal design will accommodate condensing instruments during the gutta-percha compaction yet confine the filling materials within the canal. Thorough debridement and hemorrhage control will not only insure endodontic success but also prevent discoloration of the crown. This is an extremely important esthetic consideration. Crown discoloration can stem from blood entering the dentinal tubules followed by latent red blood cell degeneration. Severe pulpal bleeding usually occurs when an acutely inflamed pulp is not entirely removed during extirpation. Once an accurate measurement is ascertained, further debridement of the canal and subsequent shaping coupled with copious irrigation with 2.5% sodium hypochlorite (NaOCl) will normally control hemorrhage. If, on occasion, the flow continues full strength, 6.25% NaOCl should be used as the irrigant. The solution should remain in the chamber for periods of 5–10 min.

Today's suggested medication in teeth with vital as well as necrotic pulps is calcium hydroxide, which does not cause tooth discoloration. However, clinicians still encounter discolored endodontically treated teeth when beechwood creosote, silver nitrate, azochloramid, or paraformaldehyde paste has been used as a treatment agent. Their removal as well as bleaching procedures may return the crown to its optimum color, but the duration of its esthetic improvement may be short. The patients should be advised of this fact.

Nickel titanium has enabled mechanical radicular shaping after a successful glide path is manually prepared. Mechanical rotary shaping has allowed dentists to consistently design endodontic preparations that can be predictably sealed using a variety of 3D obturation techniques.

Sealing the canal system

The final phase of treatment and the key to successful endodontics is the sealing of all portals of exit from the root canal system, including the access cavity. Here again, esthetic consideration revolves around discoloration of filling materials. A nonstaining root canal cement—that is, Roth #801 (Roth International, Inc., Chicago, IL), U/P Root Canal Sealer (Sultan Chemists Inc., Englewood, NJ), Thermaseal Plus (Tulsa/DENTSPLY), or RealSeal Sealer (SybronEndo, Anaheim, CA)—provides the necessary sealing capabilities when used in conjunction with gutta-percha. If silver precipitate is used in the cement, the chamber must be thoroughly cleaned before the esthetic access restoration is placed. The canal walls are coated with the cement and then gutta-percha or Resilon (RealSeal SybronEndo, Anaheim, CA) that is deformed by heat, pressure, or chemicals acts as a piston to drive the cement to the outer recesses of the prepared dentin walls. This results in the formation of a cement–dentin interface, which is necessary to produce successful results.

The canals should be filled completely and confirmed by radiographs. The excess gutta-percha and or Resilon and root canal cement should be removed 1–2 mm apical to the cervical line to prevent discoloration (Figure 24.52) in periodontally involved teeth where longer crowns are planned; the root filling materials should be removed to the bone level. Remnants of the cement may be removed with alcohol. A tooth-colored restorative material—that is, composite resin or glass ionomer cement—may be used to fill the rest of the canal and chamber when a post and core are not indicated.

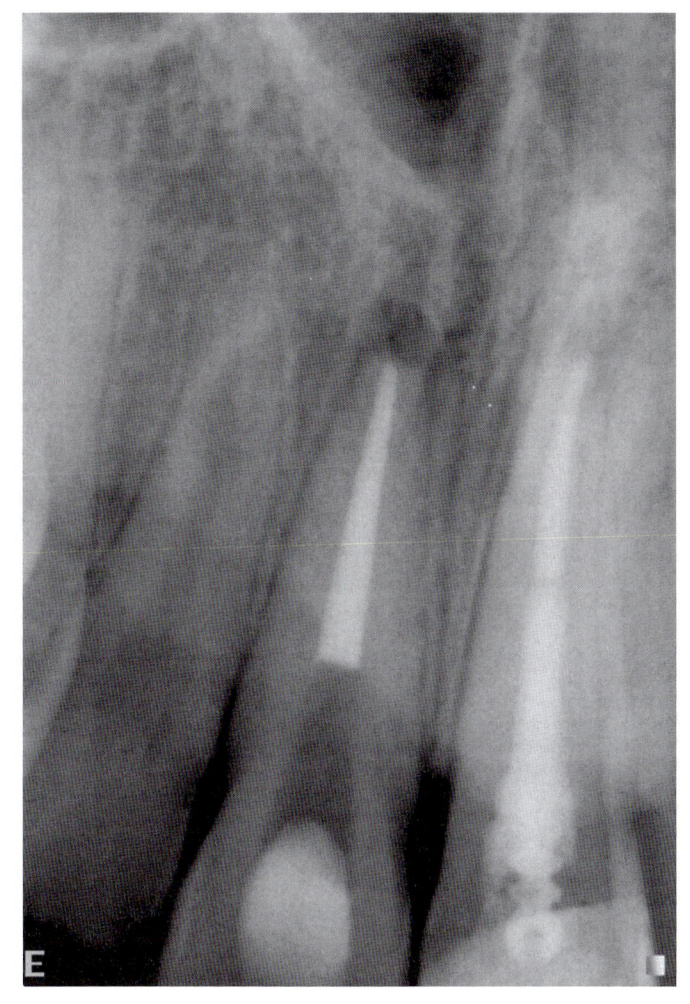

Figure 24.52 Gutta-percha root filling cut back 3 mm apical to the cervical line to prevent discoloration. This space will be restored with composite resin. The adjacent tooth will be restored with a crown.

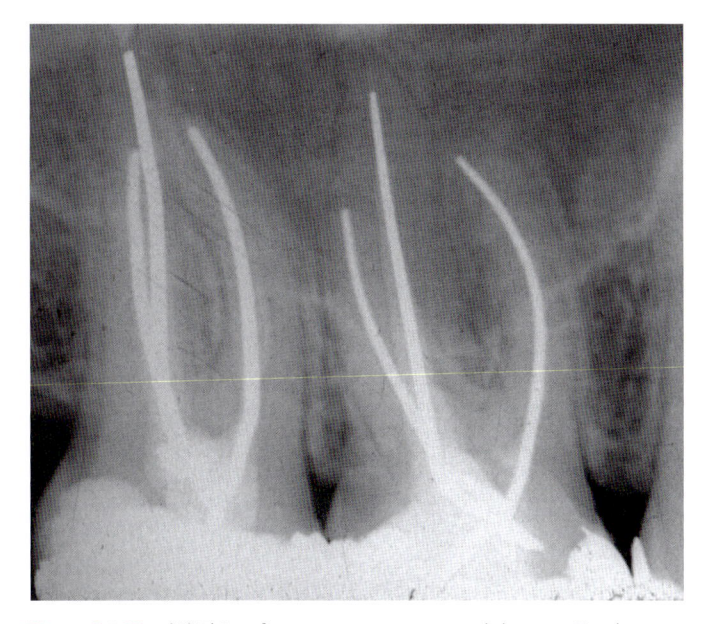

Figure 24.53 **(A)** Thirty-five years post root canal therapy. Teeth asymptomatic and no radiographic changes.

The coronal restoration should be placed as soon as possible after completion of the root canal treatment if it is not placed at the time when the canal(s) are filled. There is now building evidence that the coronal restoration is as important, if not more important, in microbiologically sealing the root canal system as the root canal obturation material (Figure 24.53A and B). Ray and Trope evaluated the radiologic quality of both coronal and canal obturations. They demonstrated that a tooth with good coronal and root seals had the best rate of absence of periapical lesions (91.4%).[28] Good restoration resulted in significantly less incidence of periapical lesions than good endodontic filling (80% versus 75.7%). Poor restoration resulted in significantly more periapical lesions than poor endodontic fillings (48.6% versus 30.2%). A few years later, a study by Tronstad et al. further confirmed that good endodontic filling with quality access restoration gave the highest success rate.[29]

A proper finish of both the temporary and the final filling material is essential so as not to irritate the patient's tongue or soft tissue. Thirty-bladed finishing instruments (ETUF, OS 1, and Brasseler) are perfectly suited to provide the smoothest margins for both the material and especially the marginal remnants of the existing restoration. Gold restorations are particularly susceptible to rough edges that need finishing with the 30-bladed instruments.

Coronal seal background

Three-dimensional obturation of the root canal system has long been the essential goal of successful endodontics. Obturation is, in fact, the third point of the time-tested endodontic triangle: (1) disinfection, (2) instrumentation, and (3) obturation.

Three-dimensional obturation refers to obturation of all foramina, which includes the endodontic access cavity, which is by far the largest bacterial entrance for root canal system recontamination. And yet a proper access endodontic seal is often neglected and is ultimately time sensitive and quality sensitive when measuring predictability (Figure 24.54). For

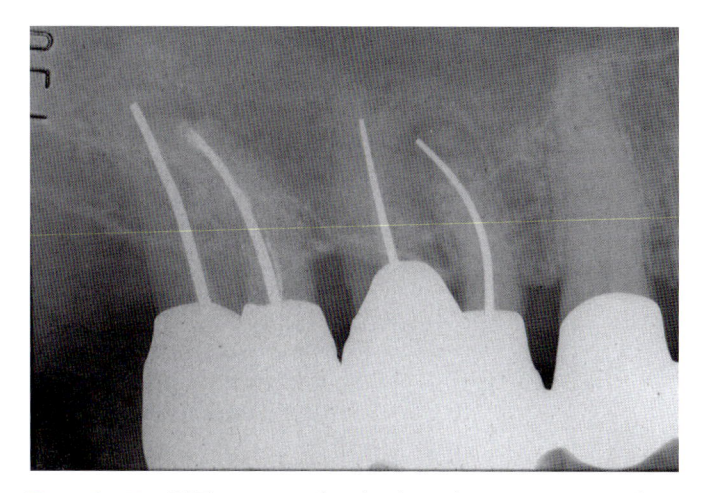

Figure 24.53 **(B)** Three years after distobuccal root resections and new castings. Periapical lesions developed around the mesiobuccal roots. During the extended treatment phase, the coronal ends of the silver points were periodically exposed to saliva.

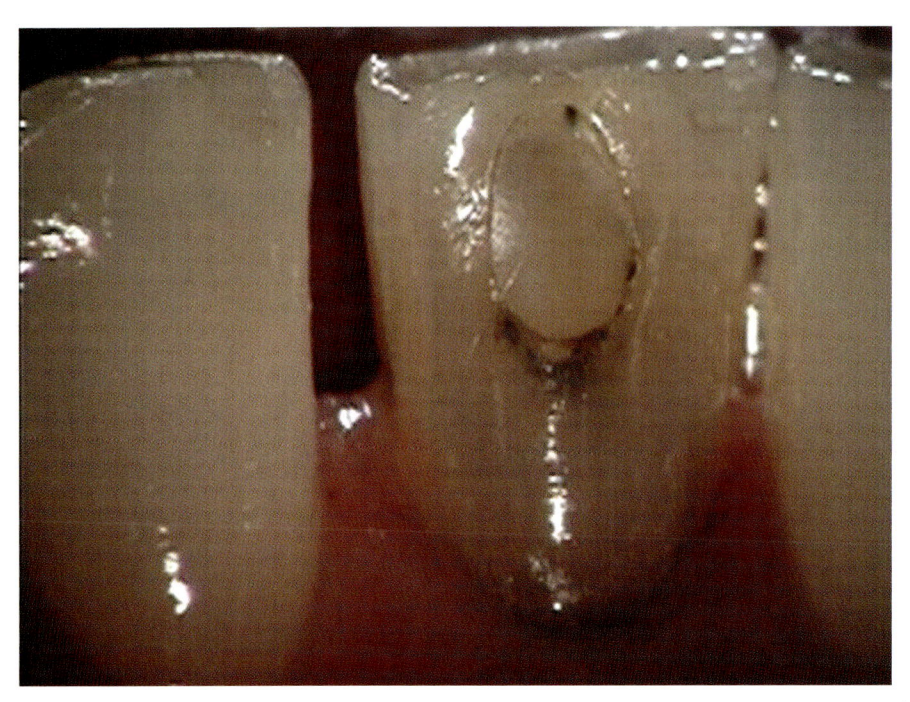

Figure 24.54 **(A)** Coronal access is the largest portal of exit needed to seal for predicable endodontic success. Lingual view of mandibular anterior tooth demonstrating microleakage at periphery of access cavity repair.

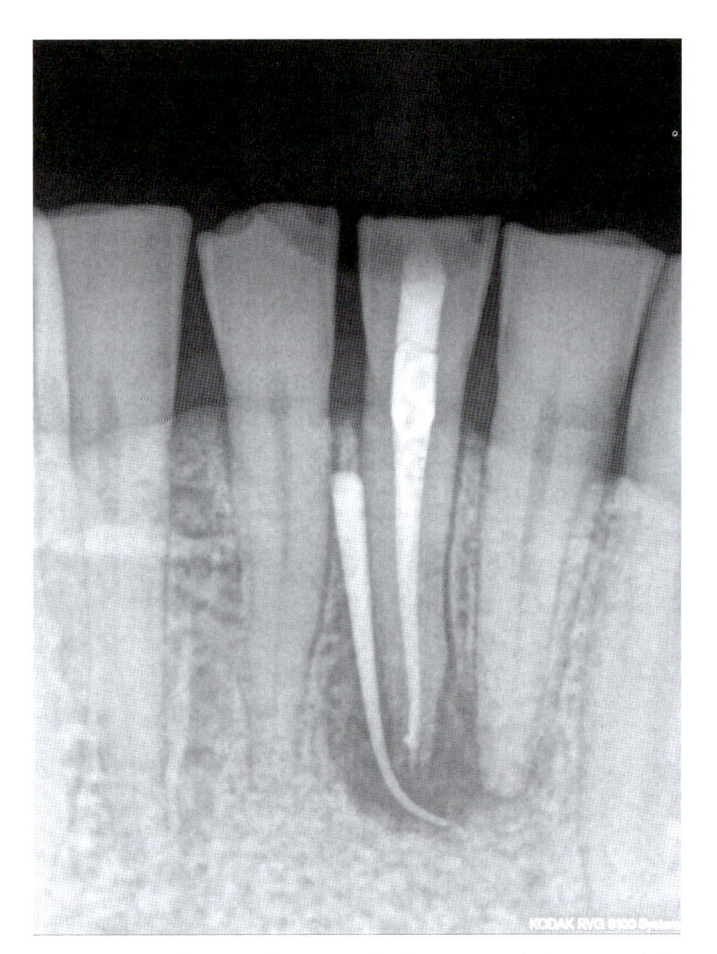

Figure 24.54 **(B)** Coronal access is the largest portal of exit needed to seal for predicable endodontic success. Periapical image of gutta-percha cone tracing sinus tract emanating from radiographic lesion of endodontic origin.

example, it is not appropriate to finish the endodontic treatment with cotton in the access and Cavit (3 M ESPE) or some other temporary access coverage. If the Cavit breaks down or salivary microleakage occurs prior to restorative, the endodontic seal is recontaminated, which prevents healing or creates a new lesion of endodontic origin.

West (clinical study, unpublished data, 2004) found approximately one-third (37%) of the consecutive 100 full-coverage molars with irreversible pulpitis or necrotic pulps with or without lesions of endodontic origin demonstrated marginal microleakage using caries indicator paste (Figure 24.55).[30] About two-thirds (67%) of consecutive 100 full-coverage molars with endodontic "failures" demonstrated marginal microleakage using caries indicator paste. The conclusion was "as much attention should be given to a quality access seal and repair as the 3D obturation of the entire root canal system which includes both radicular and coronal portals of exit." In addition to the quality of the coronal seal, focus should be made to make access cavity repair as "invisible" as possible by blocking out metal and choosing composites that mimic the surrounding porcelain.

Restoration or removal of the endodontically diseased tooth

The management of the endodontically diseased tooth in the esthetic zone has changed dramatically over the past two decades. Twenty years ago, most dentists had fewer endodontic technologies available to them and endodontists compared with what is available today.[30] In addition, implant technology was not yet a proven esthetic choice for replacing the diseased endodontic tooth. Endodontists would argue many teeth are experiencing wholesale, unnecessary, and inappropriate removal, particularly

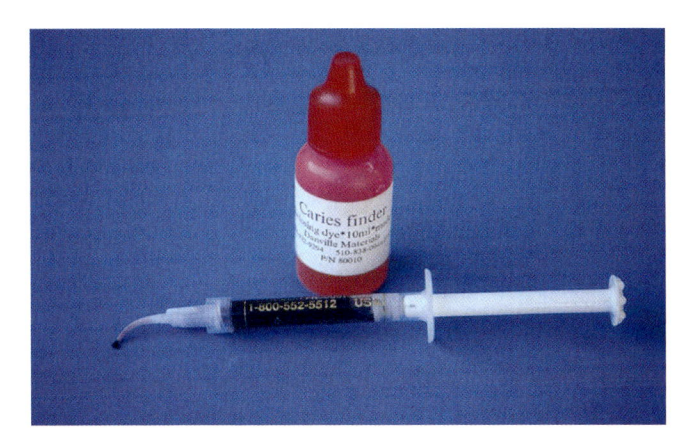

Figure 24.55 (A) Example of caries indicator paste, which is helpful in identifying mircroleakage and/or caries.

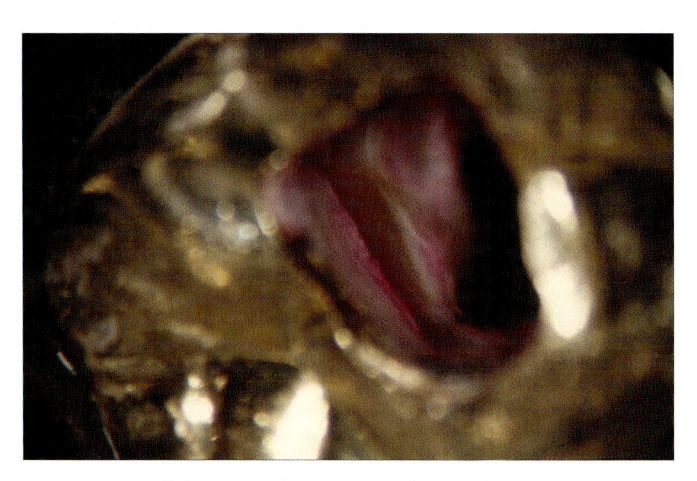

Figure 24.55 (B) Caries indicator paste observed in access cavity wall staining microleakage sites along junction of crown and crown preparation.

if the endodontically diseased tooth is not healing. Implant decisions are often based on the assumption that the tooth already has "two strikes" against it and that removal and implant placement is a biologic and cost-effective better choice. Which side of the argument is correct? What guidelines should be followed to present the patient with accurate options to make the decision that is in their best interest?

When making the decision to restore or remove a tooth, three important areas must be considered: biology, structure, and esthetics.

Two important questions must always be asked:

1. Is the tooth restorable?
2. Can the dentist create the endodontic seal?

Restorability guidelines

- 1.5–2.0 mm facial and lingual ferrule
- 1 mm ferrule wall thickness
- 2–2.5 mm biologic width
- crown/root ratio at least 1 : 1
- third, third, third

where the latter refers to desired diameter of radicular endodontic preparation. The mesial–distal width of the preparation should not exceed a third of the width of the root at the level of the cementoenamel junction (CEJ).

Endodontic seal guideline

The guideline for the endodontic seal is best summarized by the rationale for endodontics: Any endodontically diseased tooth can be predictably saved if the root canal system can be nonsurgically or surgically sealed and the periodontal condition is healthy or can be made healthy. In the case where a lesion of endodontic origin persists after treatment, the dentist must determine which approach, nonsurgical or surgical retreatment option, is best for the patient. Although many treatment plans are obvious, the dentist needs guidelines for teeth that may be in the gray area of a nonsurgical versus surgical endodontic seal.

The following five determinants will facilitate the thought process for dentist and patient (Figure 24.56A):

1. *Obturation.* If obturation is poor, nonsurgical retreatment offers the most predicable endodontic seal (Figure 24.56B).
2. *Lesion of endodontic (LEO) location.* If LEO is concentrated periapically, then a surgical seal may be the patient's best choice (Figure 24.56C).
3. *Structure.* If disassembly or previous endodontics, then surgical seal may be less invasive to the existing dentistry (Figure 24.56D).
4. *Coronal leakage.* Evidence of coronal leakage requires nonsurgical endodontic repair of undersealed root canal system and structural repair (Figure 24.56E).
5. *Esthetics.* If surgical seal is considered, dentist must take precautions to avoid a resulting gingival "black triangle" or scarring, particularly in a patient with a high smile line (Figure 24.56F).

Bleaching

Bleaching endodontically treated teeth has been a successful part of the endodontic treatment armamentarium. When indicated, the procedure should be instituted at the completion of the root fillings. The results are satisfying and the patient can readily see the change in tooth appearance.

Unfortunately, a liability associated with bleaching, external root resorption, has been noted by us, has appeared in the literature, and has been demonstrated in research studies.[31] External resorption is the result of an injury to and a subsequent reaction in the periodontal ligament. The use of 30% hydrogen peroxide (Superoxol) or heat has been demonstrated to increase the probability of resorption.[32] Microscopic opening in the dentinal wall in the cervical region, which is not covered by enamel or cementum, may allow for the penetration of the bleaching solution to the periodontal ligament. This morphologic abnormality

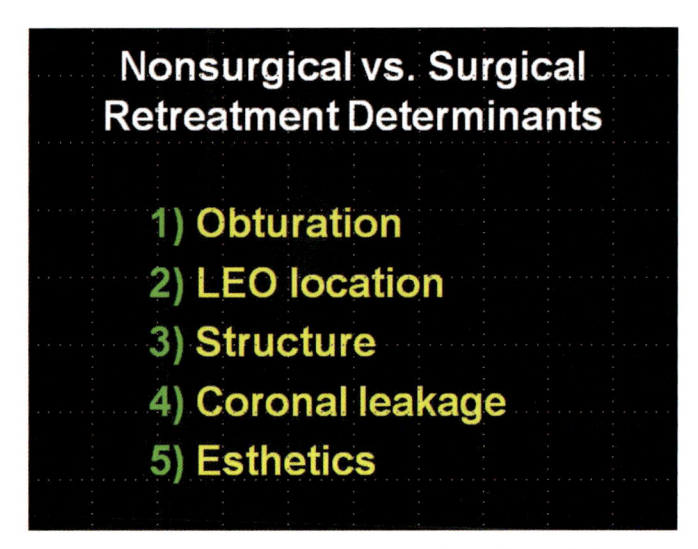

Figure 24.56 (A) Decision thought process for the five endodontic determinants that guide endodontic nonsurgical versus surgical retreatment.

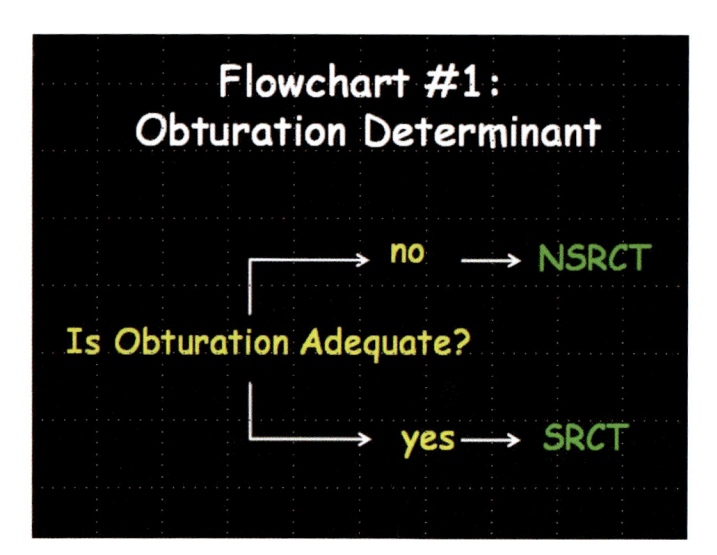

Figure 24.56 (B) *Obturation.* If obturation is poor, nonsurgical retreatment offers the most predictable endodontic seal. NSRCT: nonsurgical root canal treatment; SRCT: surgical root canal treatment.

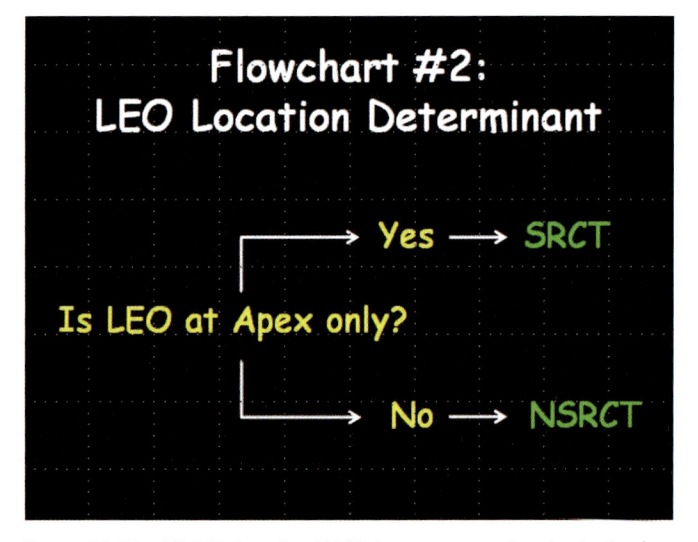

Figure 24.56 (C) *LEO location.* If LEO is concentrated periapically, then a surgical seal may be the patient's best and most efficient choice.

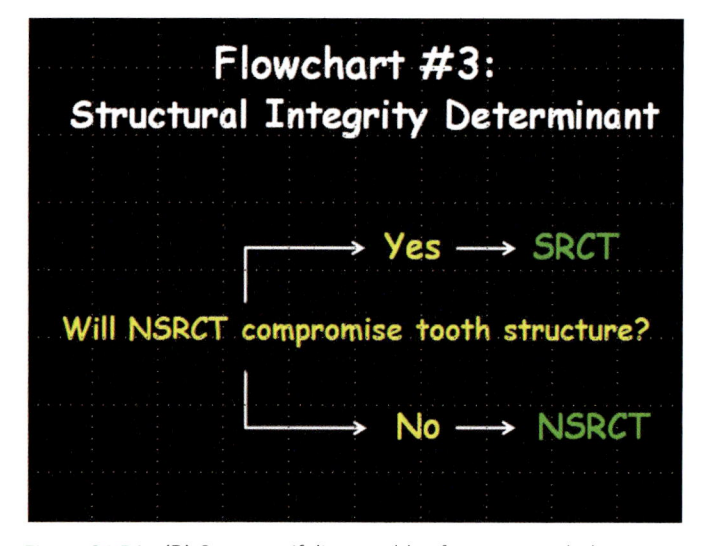

Figure 24.56 (D) *Structure.* If disassembly of previous endodontics presents a structural risk, then surgical endodontic seal may be less invasive to the existing dentistry.

occurred in 5–10% of the teeth examined.[33] Acid etching of the chamber has been advocated prior to bleaching to allow for deeper penetration of the Superoxol. Heat, Superoxol, and acid etching of the chamber increase the probability of resorption (Figure 24.57A and B) and should be avoided and a kinder, gentler technique should be used. However, the literature has never produced a report of a patient with cervical root resorption subsequent to internal nonvital bleaching, where "safe bleach" (described later) had been properly placed to protect the periodontal ligament.

Walking bleach technique

A solid, well-condensed gutta-percha root filling is a prerequisite to bleaching discolored endodontically treated teeth. This should be confirmed with a radiograph. If the root filling is inadequate, it should be redone. The bleach barrier must be placed 1 mm incisal to the undulating attachment apparatus to prevent possible migration of bleaching agents through unprotected dentinal tubules that exist in up to 6–8% of teeth. The "Bermuda Triangle" outline of endodontic resorption is identified by arrows (Figure 24.58). The incisally directed dentinal tubules serve as a direct bleach conduit that can ultimately initiate destructive resorption. Once it has been established that the gutta-percha obturation is adequate, it should be removed 2 mm apical to the cervical line and the reservoir that is created filled with zinc oxide eugenol temporary filling material, like IRM™ (DENTSPLY Caulk). All remnants of root and crown filling should be removed from the chamber. The chamber is washed with 70% alcohol. Sodium perborate powder mixed with water or 3% hydrogen peroxide to a resin-like consistency is packed into the chamber with a plastic instrument. Excess moisture is absorbed with a

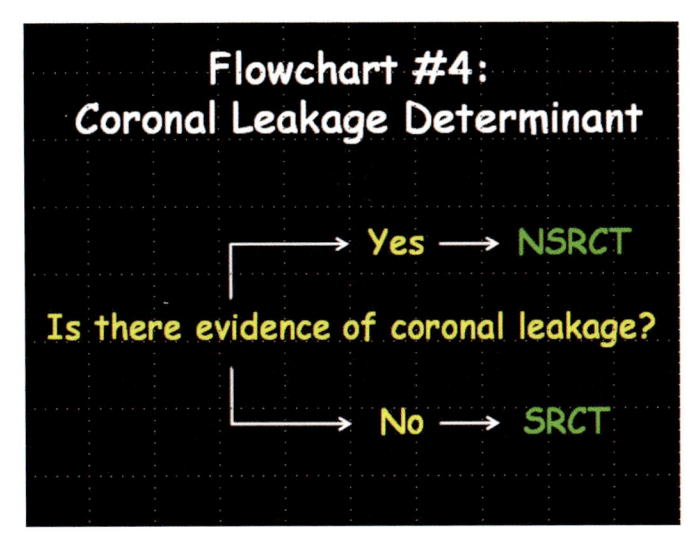

Figure 24.56 (E) *Coronal leakage.* Evidence of coronal leakage requires nonsurgical repair of undersealed root canal system.

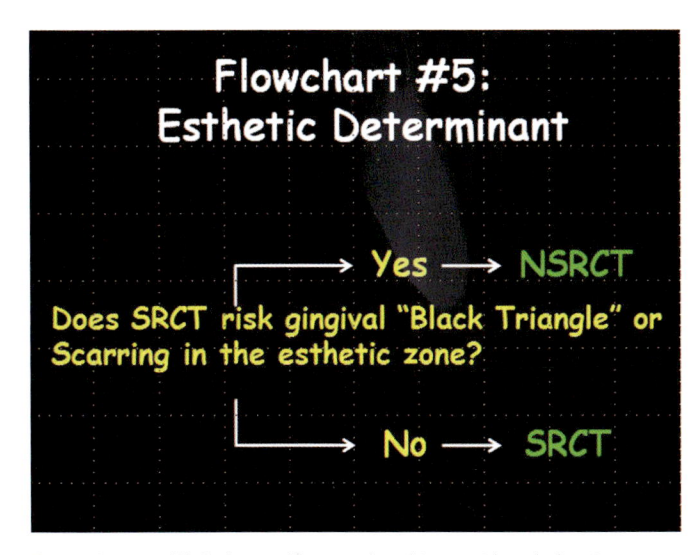

Figure 24.56 (F) *Esthetics.* If surgical seal is considered, dentist must take precautions to avoid a resulting gingival "black triangle" or surgical scarring, particularly in a patient with a high smile line.

cotton pellet. The access cavity is closed with good temporary filling material. An effort is made to ensure a total seal by removing the bleaching agent from the access walls. The maximum bleaching effect takes place within 48 h (Figure 24.59A and B).

The tooth is evaluated for improvement after that time. Application of the paste is repeated until an acceptable result is achieved (usually two to three applications). A case of severe discoloration could even take more applications.

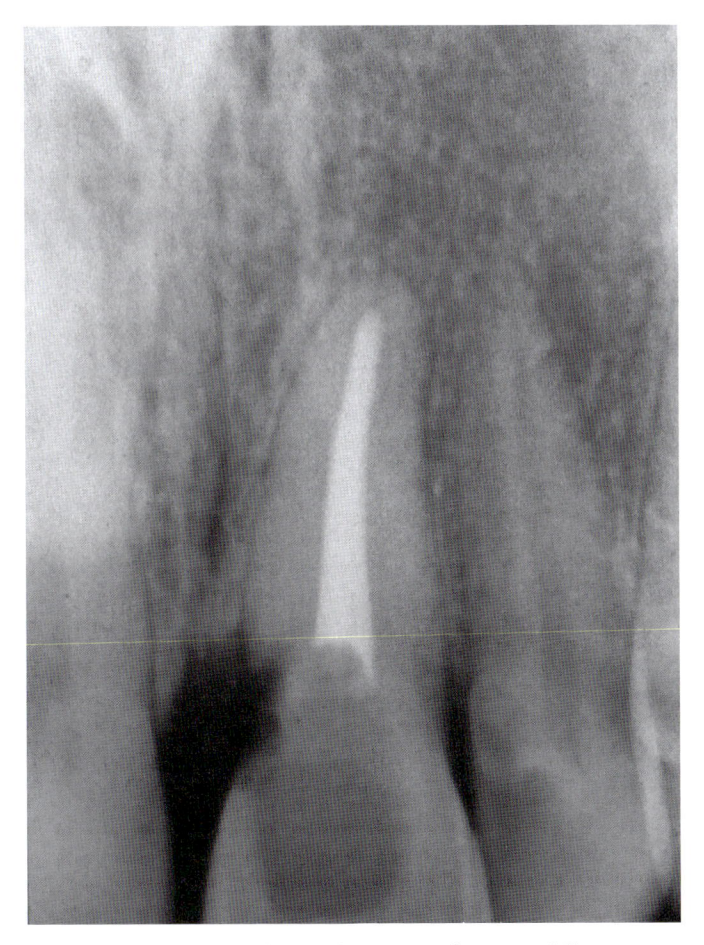

Figure 24.57 (A) External cervical resorption four years following bleaching with 30% Superoxol and heat.

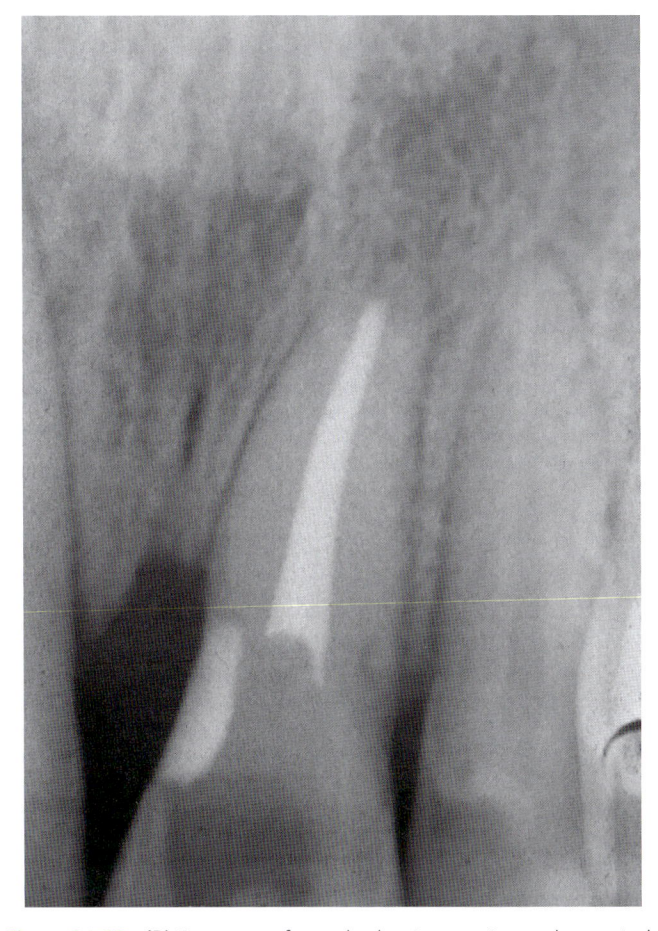

Figure 24.57 (B) Two years after orthodontic extrusion and a surgical approach to repair the resorptive defect.

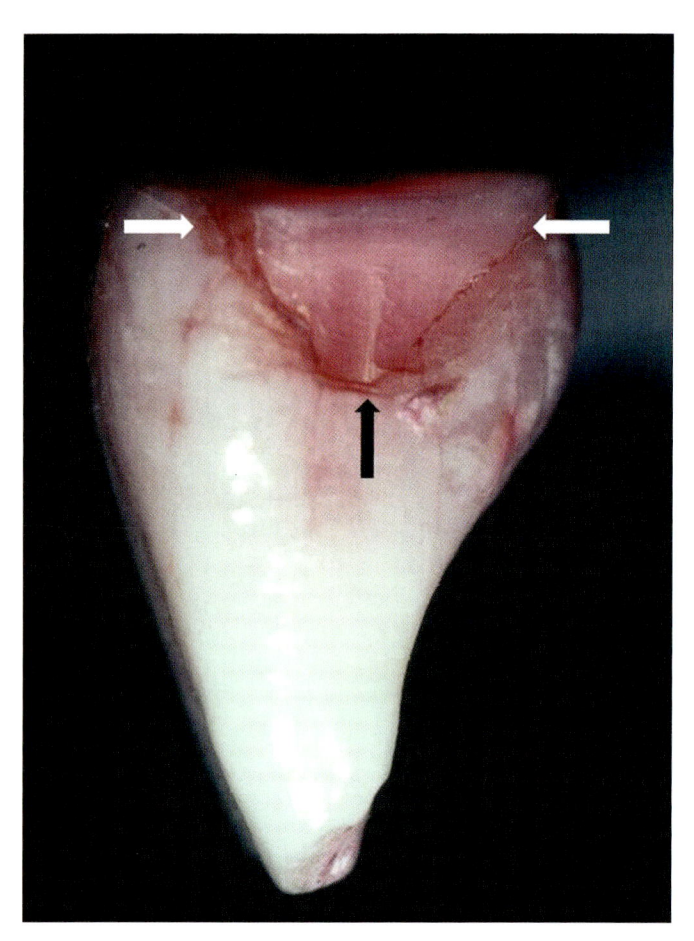

Figure 24.58 Three arrows identify the outer borders of the endodontic "Bermuda Triangle." The "safe" bleach barrier must be placed 1 mm incisal to the undulating attachment apparatus to prevent possible migration of bleaching agents through unprotected dentinal tubules that exist in up to 6–8% of teeth.

This "walking bleach" procedure was introduced by Spasser over 50 years ago.[34] The combination of sodium perborate and water apparently produces a sufficient oxygenating effect to bleach internal stains and is believed to be much gentler to the periodontal ligament.[3,35] In vivo and in vitro research studies have confirmed its efficacy. Its obvious advantage lies in its ability to produce the desired result without the liability of root resorption, which is associated with the use of Superoxol and heat.

Bleaching and endodontics

Bleaching pulpless teeth presents both a challenge and an opportunity. The challenge is to bleach the intact but discolored tooth while preventing cervical resorption. The esthetic treatment can be successful, safe, noninvasive, and cost effective.

Why discoloration?

Pulpal degeneration and subsequent endodontic access microleakage are the two main reasons for clinical crown discoloration, especially in the esthetic zone. Discoloration from an insufficient access seal is especially prominent where necrotic debris and endodontic sealer containing silver remains in the access cavity or its pulp horns. The initial discoloration after pulpal necrosis is due to extravasated red blood cells that undergo hemolysis and release of hemoglobin. Iron in the hemoglobin combines with hydrogen sulfide produced by bacteria to form dark-pigmented iron sulfide (Figure 24.60A). A pretreatment of maxillary left central incisor presents discolored and bleached. A clinical image after 6 weeks of walking bleach shows some improvement, but this is esthetically insufficient (Figure 24.60B). After 6 weeks the bleach was refreshed, and another 6 weeks later the color begins to match adjacent teeth (Figure 24.60C). Sometimes, color correction occurs in less the 24 h as well.

Preventing resorption

The literature suggests there are three key guidelines common to the "safe bleach."[36,37] In 10% of all teeth, a CEJ defect can be found between the cementum and enamel, where the dentin is nude of a cemented protective cover. In this region, dentinal tubules provide a direct conduit for internal bleaching agents to escape from the root canal system into the periodontal membrane. These tubules are particularly wide in younger patients and remain that

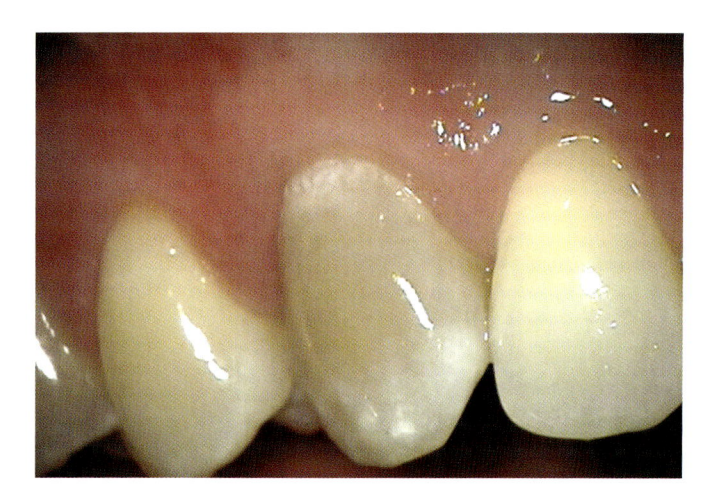

Figure 24.59 **(A)** Discolored maxillary canine with a necrotic pulp.

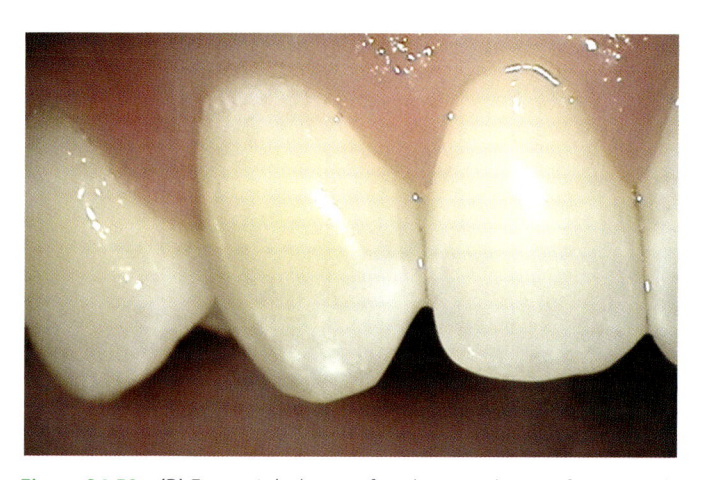

Figure 24.59 **(B)** Forty-eight hours after the completion of root canal therapy and walking bleach.

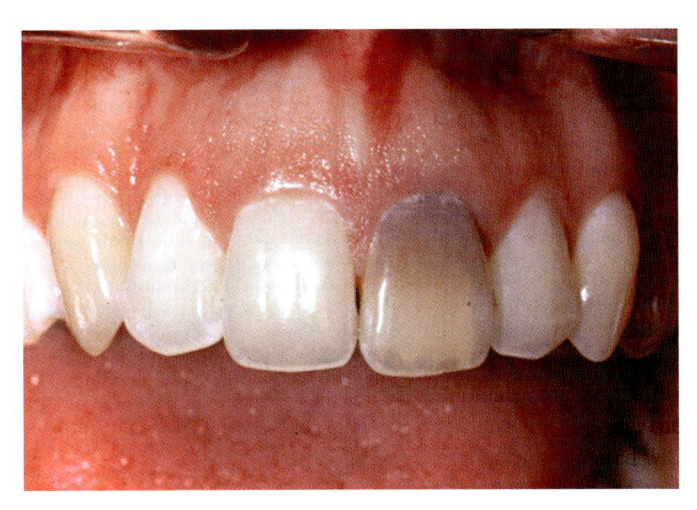

Figure 24.60 **(A)** Multiple walking bleaches are often necessary to achieve an appropriate esthetic result. Pretreatment of maxillary left central incisor.

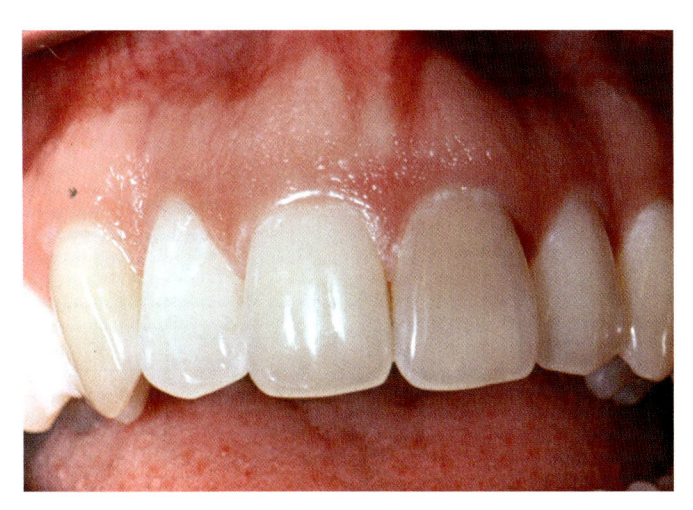

Figure 24.60 **(B)** Clinical image after 6 weeks of walking bleach.

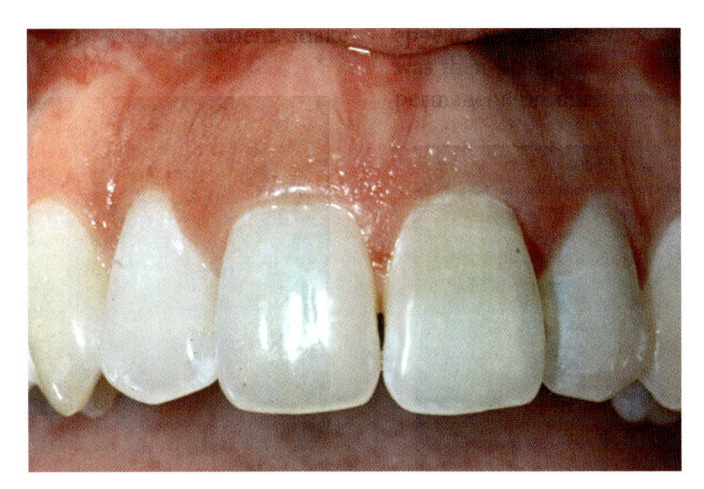

Figure 24.60 **(C)** After first 6 weeks, bleach was refreshed and another 6 weeks later the color begins to match adjacent teeth. Sometimes color correction occurs in less than 24 h as well.

way if pulpal necrosis occurs. Without sclerotic dentin closure, the periodontal ligament is vulnerable to being affected by bleaching agents. The combination of patent tubules, bare dentin, and bleaching agents running through the tubules represents a perfect storm for an inflammatory reaction that is the source of external root resorption at the cervical level.

Proximal dentinal

The CEJ runs up and down like a roll a coaster around the tooth where it curves incisally in the mesial and distal proximal areas. The potentially unprotected and also incisally directed trabecular must be protected by the location and protection of a bleach barrier. Figure 24.61A shows a discolored maxillary left lateral incisor. Figure 24.61B periapical reveals diagnosis of endodontically undersealed root canal system. In Figure 24.61C, endodontic retreatment was finished and safe bleach barrier appears similar to a "bobsled" cross-section protecting the incisal undulation of the epithelial attachment. Improved color occurs after a single day of walking bleach.

(Figure 24.61D). Posttreatment image of access repair and endodontic finish was successful enododontically and free of symptoms (Figure 24.61E). The patient was scheduled for 6-month follow-up to confirm nonsurgical retreatment healing and color preservation. Color relapse should not occur when proper and careful access cavities are restored.

Barrier transfer

This step is essential in preventing resorption. Three periodontal probings are made and recorded: mesial, facial, and distal. The probings measure the distance from the epithelial attachment to the incisal edge of the tooth. The internal level of the barrier is placed 1 mm incisal to the corresponding external probing of the epithelial attachment in order to block potential patent tubules from the root canal system to the epithelial attachment. The internal protective template shape and position are now identified and the shield can be placed using a variety of products, such as flowable composites, glass ionomers, and even Cavit.

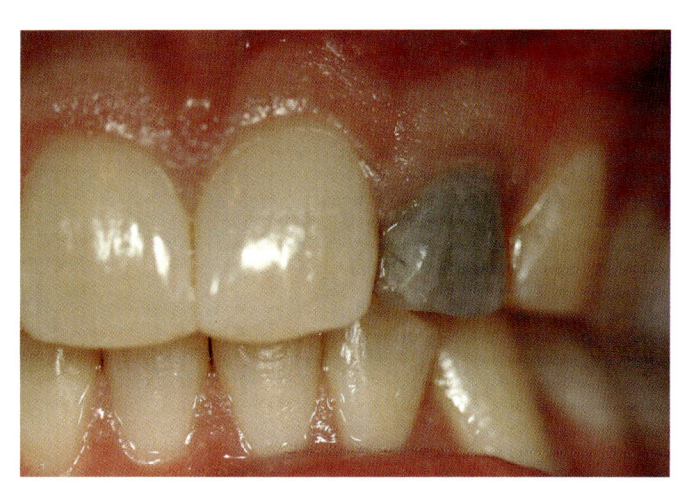

Figure 24.61 **(A)** Clinical example of nonsurgical endodontic retreatment, "safe" bleach barrier placement, and successful esthetic result. An overextended and undersealed endodontically treated discolored lateral incisor with persistent endodontic LEO.

Safest bleach barrier
- Tooth became pulpless in a patient older than 25 years.
- Properly positioned bleach barrier 1 mm incisal to epithelial attachment.
- Sodium perborate plus water.

Least safe bleach
- Tooth became pulpless in a patient younger than 25 years.
- No bleach barrier or incorrectly placed barrier.
- Superoxol plus heat.

Case selection for safe pulpless bleaching

There are two criteria for successful internal safe nonvital bleaching: (1) the root canal must be sealed in three dimensions to prevent endodontic failure, and (2) the tooth structure must be intact. Therefore, the ideal tooth for nonvital bleaching is a discolored unrestored crown. If minor restorations are needed, they should be placed before the bleaching but can be modified afterward if needed to match the color resulting from the nonvital bleaching. If larger restorations are present or are required, these teeth need to be treated with a veneer or full crown.

Technique

Once the safe bleach barrier is placed, place a thick mix of sodium perborate and Superoxol or sodium perborate and water. The mixture can usually be carried into the access cavity with a small amalgam carrier dedicated to carrying bleach paste, so that mercury amalgam remnants do not contaminate the paste color. The paste is compacted into place using an endodontic plugger. Excess bleach must be removed from the cavosurface to create a successful temporary seal; otherwise, the bleaching agents may leak out in between appointments. A 2 mm layer of Cavit is placed first around the rim, making a Cavit vortex, followed by a flat second layer. In this way, a Cavit positive seat is placed that prevents squeezing bleach out as well

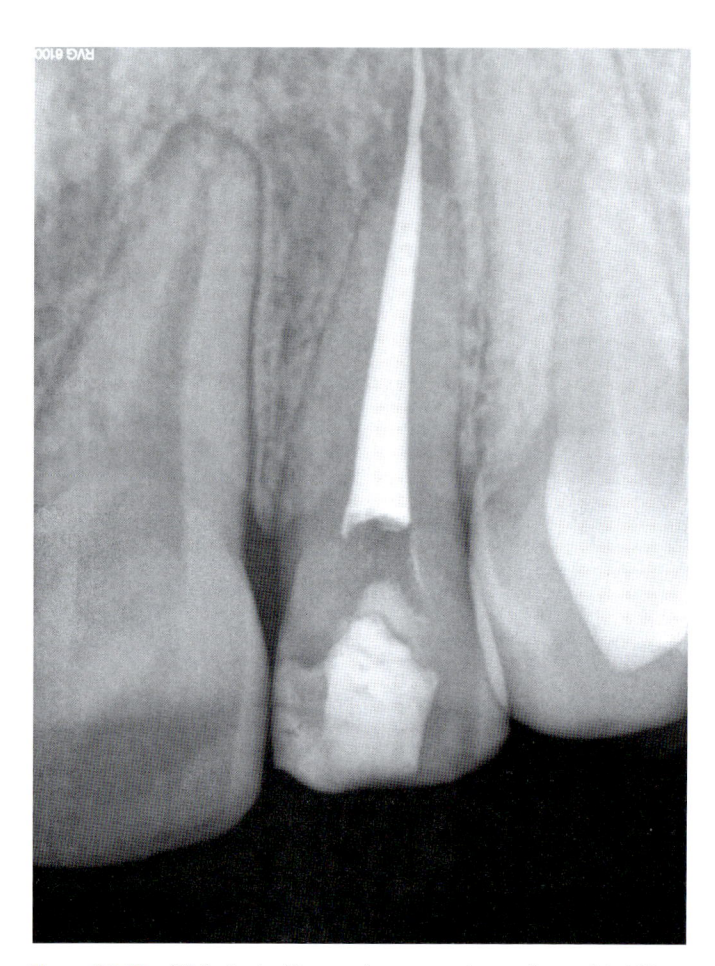

Figure 24.61 **(B)** Periapical image demonstrating radiographic LEO.

as creating a void when placing Cavit directly into the access cavity. The walking bleach is complete. One word of precaution is that, occasionally, a dramatic result happens overnight, and so it is wise to perform the first walking bleach on a day where you will be in your office the following day. Otherwise, these teeth may actually become too white after several days of inattention. This sequence may take two to four changes in stubborn discolorations. However, with the application of new walking bleach, there is usually improvement. When color is appropriate, place rubber dam, remove all traces of walking bleach and Cavit, etch, bond, and place layered light-activated composite resin. Light cure from the labial surface and then the lingual surface. A well-placed access material will prevent rediscoloration due to access microleakage.

Calcific metamorphosis and walking bleach

Trauma can cause an irreversible pulpitis, necrosis, resorption, or calcification. When a pulp chamber calcifies and pulp remains vital, the tooth can become discolored due to lack of light transmission through the calcified chamber. If the patient wants to correct the tooth discoloration and external bleaching is unsuccessful, a crown or veneer could correct the discoloration but is relatively invasive, especially if no caries or prior restorations are present. Endodontic treatment and bleaching of a tooth with a vital and healthy pulp is also invasive. However,

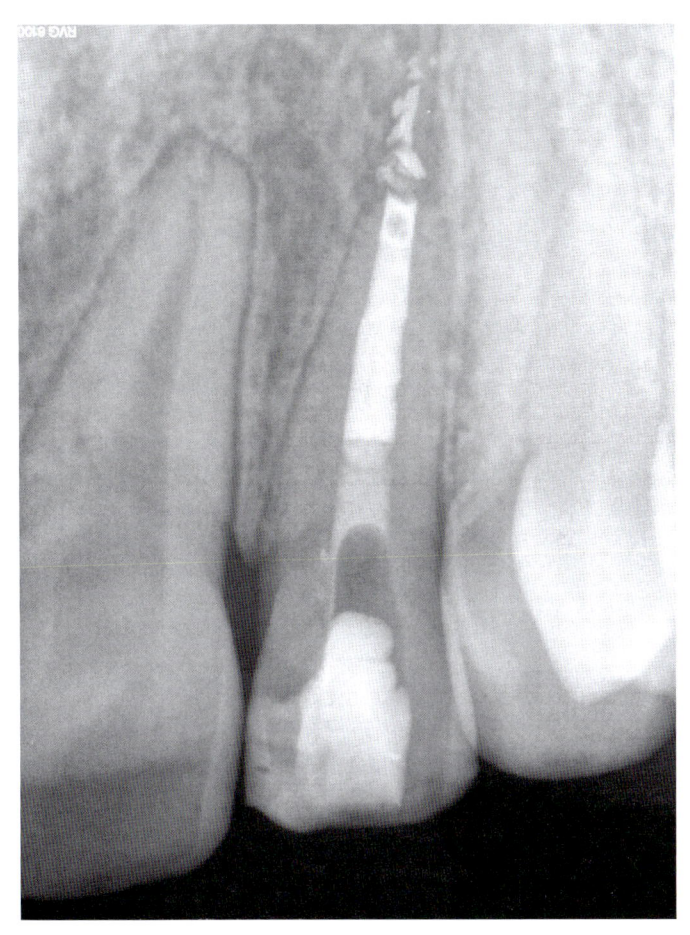

Figure 24.61 **(C)** Nonsurgical endodontic retreatment was finished, and "safe" bleach barrier resembles a "bobsled" cross-section protecting the incisal/apical undulation of the epithelial attachment.

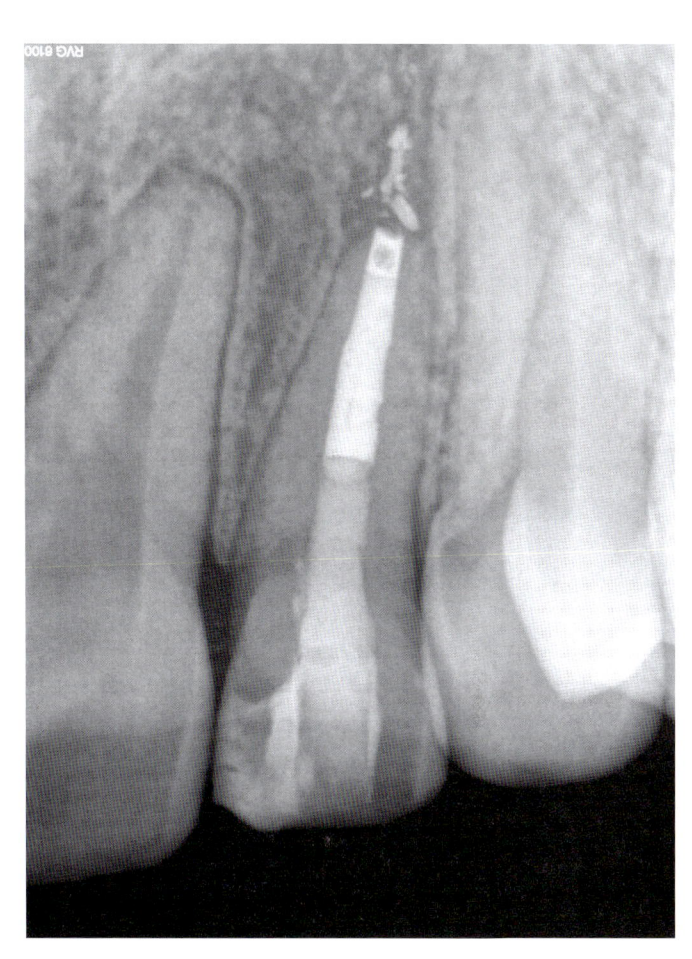

Figure 24.61 **(E)** Access repair finished and patient scheduled for 6-month posttreatment to confirm nonsurgical retreatment healing and color preservation. Color relapse should not occur when careful access cavities are restored properly.

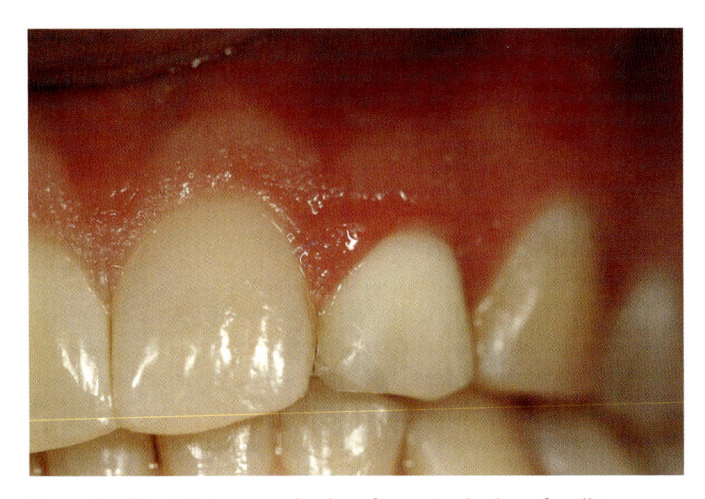

Figure 24.61 **(D)** Improved color after a single day of walking bleach.

a walking bleach can be performed without endodontics if the canal has receded far enough from the access cavity to allow space for a walking bleach without risking damaging the pulp. Figure 24.62A shows a pretreatment clinical of the maxillary left central incisor that reveals discoloration. A periapical radiograph demonstrates calcified chamber (Figure 24.62B). A follow-up periapical radiograph 9 years later shows that persistent chamber calcification has essentially remained unchanged while pulp remained vital to EPT and ice pulp tests (Figure 24.62C). Light could not naturally pass through the calcified chamber, giving the darker appearance to the tooth (Figure 24.62D). An external bleach tray was fabricated and used to improve color (Figure 24.62E). Although slight color improvement occurred with single-tooth external bleaching, it was unsatisfactory. High patient compliance is also required. A 3D CBCT image demonstrated complete calcification to #9 pulp chamber (Figure 24.62 F). A sagittal 3D section enables measurement from the incisal edge to the root canal system to be used for vertical access depth determination, which prevents pulp exposure during conservative access preparation (Figure 24.62G). Three-dimensional imaging also enables depth measurement from lingual, so safe access depth can be achieved (Figure 24.62H). A periapical image shows "bobsled" placement of safe bleach barrier and walking bleach sodium perborate paste and access seal (Figure 24.62I). A satisfactory esthetic result occurred during several weeks of walking bleach and prior to permanent restoration (Figure 24.62J). Pulp has remained vital and without symptoms.

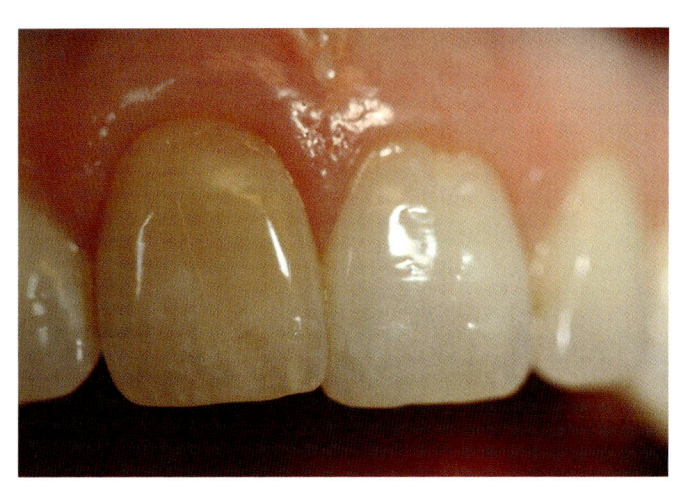

Figure 24.62 **(A)** Clinical example of walking bleach in tooth with calcified chamber and vital pulp. Clinical pretreatment of discolored maxillary right central incisor.

Trauma

The era of the new millennium has been one of participation in sports and speed. With it came the concurrent hazard of dental injury. Any blow to a tooth, regardless of its intensity, can cause pulpal damage or pulpal necrosis. The need for endodontic treatment is predicated on the physiologic response of the pulpal tissue and periodontal ligament.[30] The esthetic interest in traumatized teeth centers more around the hard tissue damage, even though the associated pulpal problems can greatly influence the treatment plan. Crown discolorations, fractured crowns, fractured roots, root displacements, and external resorption are the normal challenges. These problems and their endodontic implications will be discussed individually.

Crown fractures

In the fracture of a crown that does not involve the pulp or so-called uncomplicated crown fracture, the pulp most often survives without further compromise (Figure 24.63). Apparently, when the crown fractures, the force is dissipated and, therefore, is not transmitted to the root or periodontal ligament. For this reason, the internal tissues remain unharmed. When sufficient tooth structure exists to retain a crown or composite buildup, it is recommended to cover the exposed dentin with calcium hydroxide if there is less than 1 mm of dentin covering the pulp. If it is clear from the clinical appearance and/or radiographs that there is more than 1 mm of dentin then there does not seem to be any need to cover the exposed dentin; thus, etch and bond with composite resin until a deferred vitality analysis can be determined at 2, 6, and 12 weeks after the trauma. A true pulpal diagnosis may be determined at this time, and the final restoration may be safely considered.

If the remaining tooth structure is insufficient to adequately retain a restoration, endodontics should be considered. Although an argument may exist to support the use of pin-retained restorations, the degree of injury of pin placement and the risk of fracture predispose elective endodontics and a full

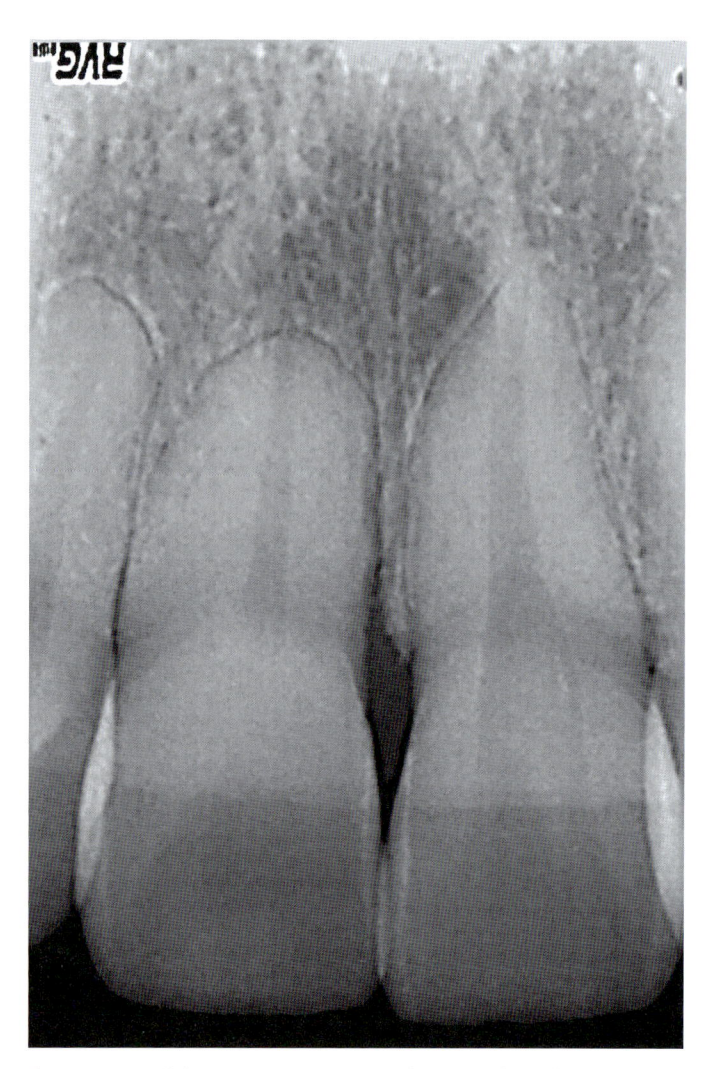

Figure 24.62 **(B)** Pretreatment periapical image of maxillary left central incisor with calcified pulp chamber.

crown. The only exception would be a tooth with incomplete root apex formation; then, every effort should be made to retain the vitality of the pulp; at least until the apex is fully formed. Once the root canal treatment is completed, a post and core can be fabricated to provide the ideal restorative condition. However, when the pulp is exposed, endodontic intervention is indicated (Figure 24.64). The root canal treatment is completed if the root is fully formed. or an apexification (root-end induction) procedure is advised for a tooth with an open apex.[38] Innovative solutions are required to provide for the esthetic needs of younger patients (Figure 24.65A–C).

Root fractures

Horizontal fractures of the root present unique problems, and the degree of difficulty is relative to the level of the break. It is very possible, and it occurs in a significant number of cases, that separation of the hard structure of a tooth can occur; yet, the elasticity of soft tissue thwarts pulpal separation. For this reason, no root canal treatment is indicated and should only be considered when signs or symptoms indicate that there is pulpal necrosis and infection in the canal space. Of note is that, most often, only the coronal segment becomes necrotic; the apical has almost always healthy pulpal tissue. Therefore, root canal treatment is only needed for the coronal segment; the apical root segment remains vital and care should be taken not to insert any instrument into that segment. When situations occur that warrant attention, the following alternatives are available.

For those fractures involving the apical third of the root, if the pulp necroses, endodontics is performed to the level of the break and the separated tip is monitored because most likely the pulpal tissue in it is healthy and does not need any treatment. In the case where a periradicular lesion develops, surgical extraction of the apical segment is the treatment of choice (Figure 24.66A and B). Considering restorative implications, there is usually sufficient root length that adequate post preparation can be accomplished without reaching the break level and jeopardizing the seal.

Mid root breaks create more challenging problems, the first of which is mobility. Owing to the crown/root ratio being reduced to less than 1 : 1, stability is impaired and a splint might has to be fabricated (Figure 24.67A–C). Recent studies indicate that there is minimal advantage of the splint for the longevity of the tooth. The advantage is mainly for patient comfort. These teeth must be monitored periodically to check pulp vitality and periodontal ligament damage. Many of these teeth maintain vital pulps and a healthy periodontium and need no endodontic intervention (Figure 24.68A and B). However, if the pulp becomes necrotic, extirpation of necrotic debris is required. Endodontic options

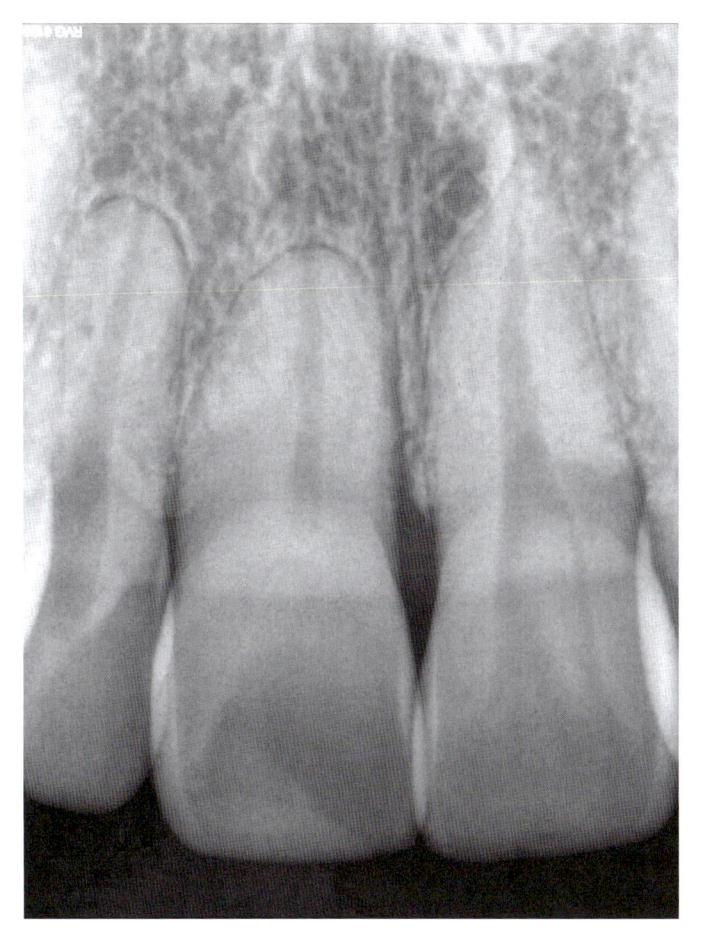

Figure 24.62 **(C)** Nine years later, a new periapical image shows the chamber size of maxillary right central incisor has remained essentially the same for more than 10 years and pulp still tests vital and healthy.

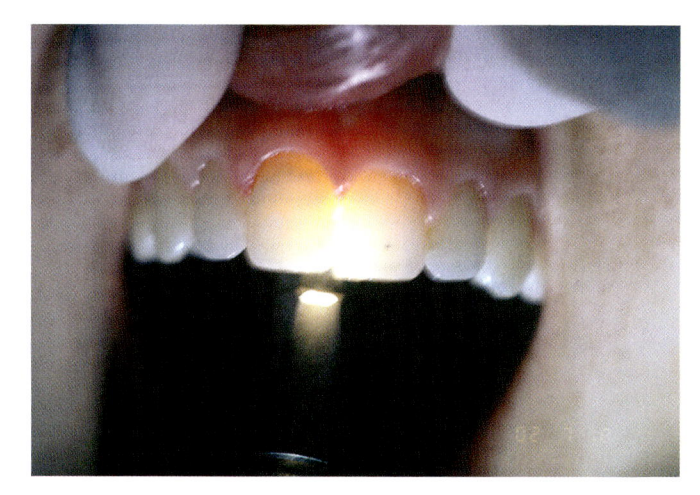

Figure 24.62 **(D)** Light does not transmit through the calcified maxillary right central incisor's chamber.

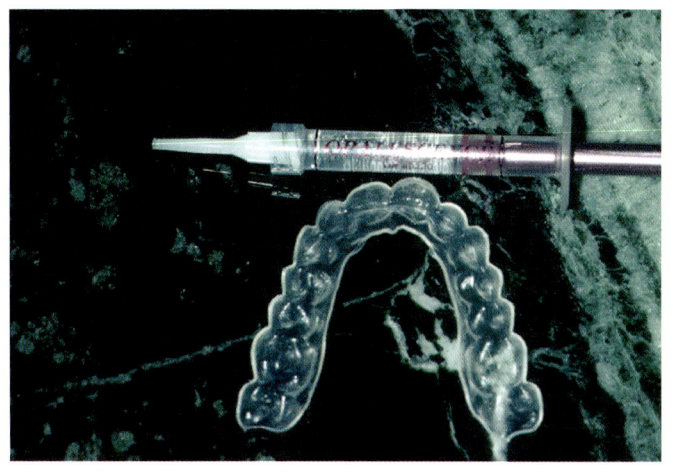

Figure 24.62 **(E)** A fabricated bleach tray was first used to improve color.

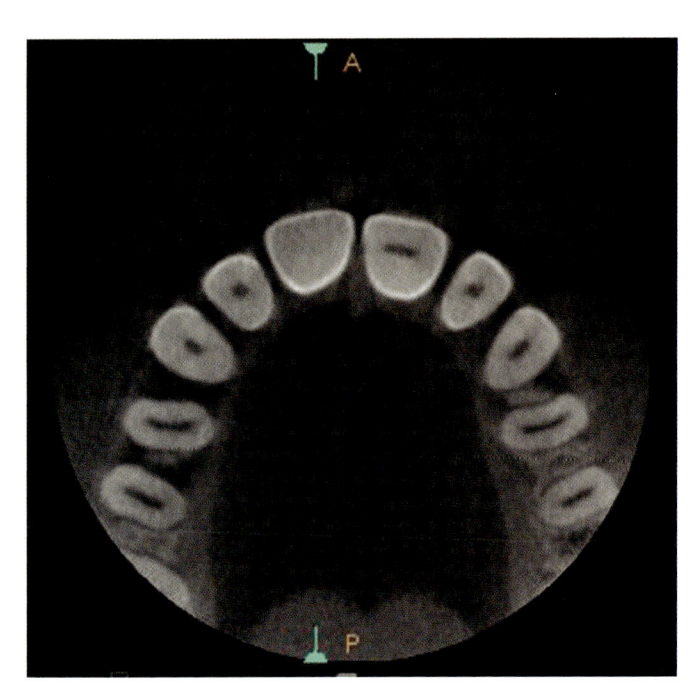

Figure 24.62 (F) The 3D CBCT image demonstrates complete calcification of #8 pulp chamber.

are: maintaining and filling the coronal segment to the break; instrumenting both segments and uniting the segments with either gutta-percha or the more solid vitallium pin; and removing the apical segment and inserting a vitallium pin through the coronal segment and extending it to the height of the vacant apical alveolus (Figure 24.69A–C). Such endosseous stabilizers are highly successful as long as there is no communication between the pin and the oral cavity by way of the crown or the periodontium. For this reason, the pin should be reduced to a coronal level within the canal to allow the chamber to be sealed

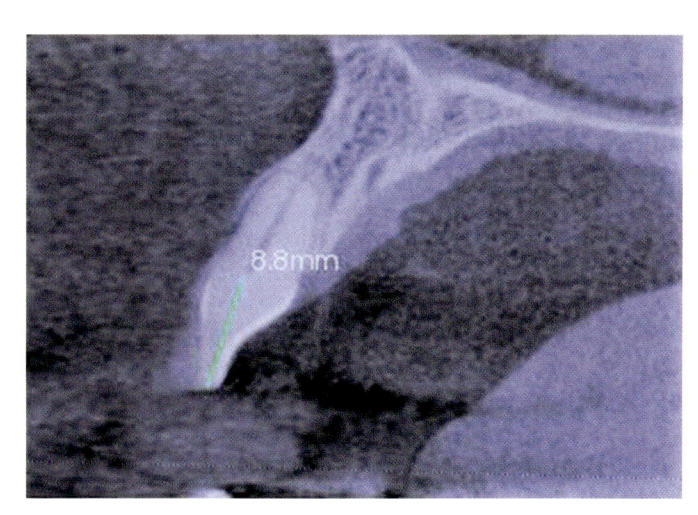

Figure 24.62 (G) The sagittal 3D CBCT section enables measurement from incisal edge to root canal system to be used for vertical access depth while at the same time preventing pulp exposure during conservative access preparation.

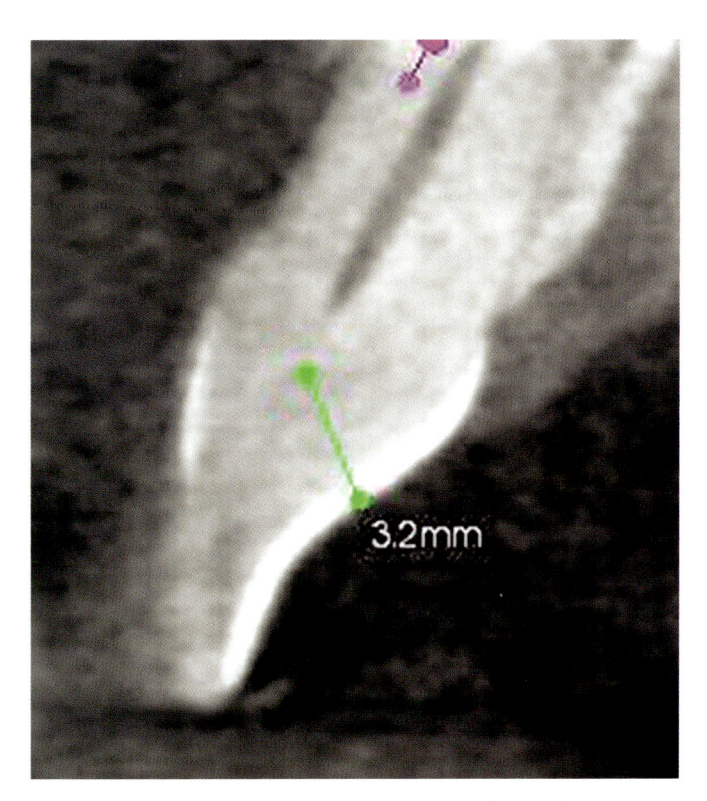

Figure 24.62 (H) The 3D CBCT imaging also enables depth measurement from lingual, so safe access depth can be achieved.

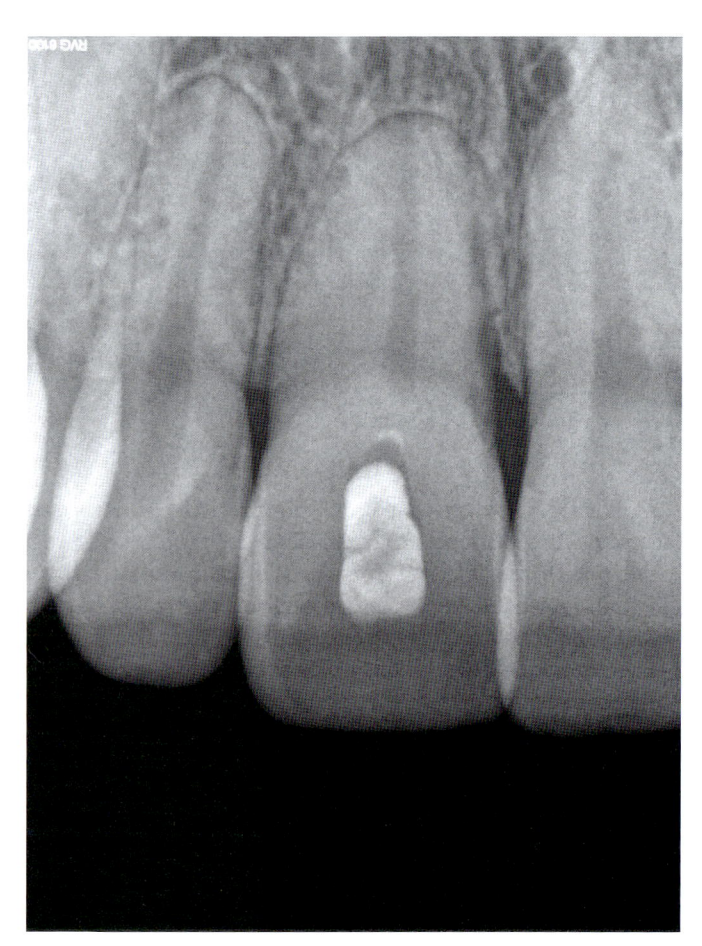

Figure 24.62 (I) Periapical image of walking bleach with small but accurately placed safe bleach barrier.

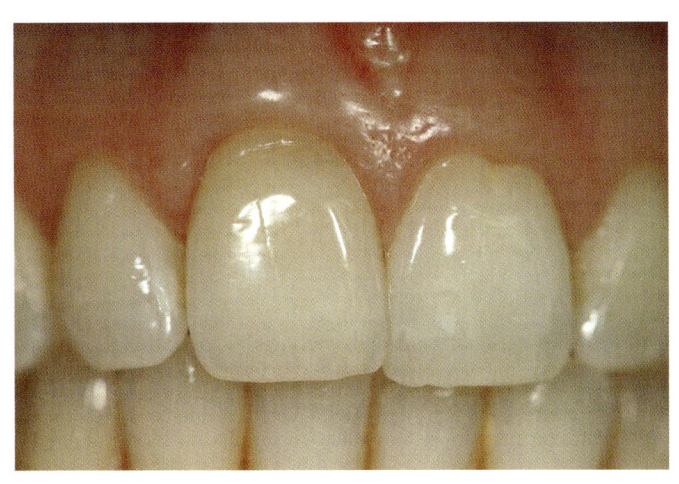

Figure 24.62 **(J)** Posttreatment clinical image of satisfactory esthetic result. Pulp has remained vital and without symptoms.

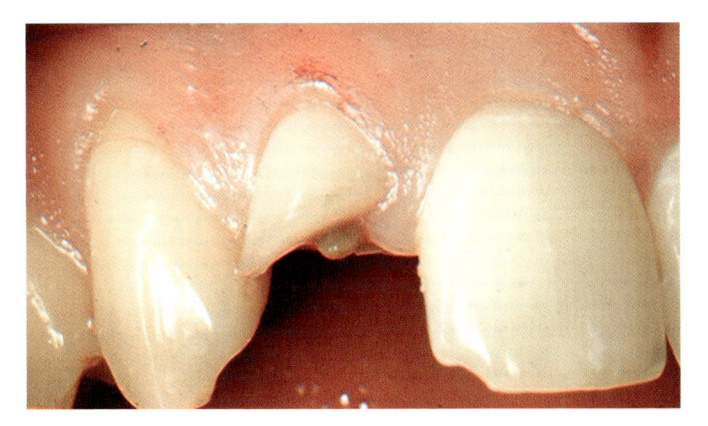

Figure 24.63 Crown fracture, no exposure, and the pulp remained vital.

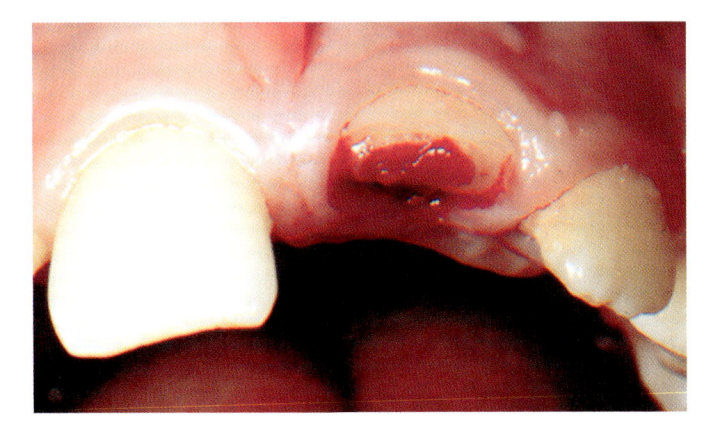

Figure 24.64 Crown fracture exposing the pulp. Root canal therapy was performed.

with a bonded resin filling. This obviously presents a problem when a post and core is needed to provide an adequate crown stump. Realizing post length will be curtailed; dentists must consider splinted units in the final treatment plan or extraction.

Root fractures that occur in the coronal third present by far the most difficult situations. The crown/root ratio is adverse, mobility is critical, and the prognosis is grave (Figure 24.70A and B). The coronal segment is too short to retain and the options for the root segment are extraction followed by a single tooth implant or bridge, vertical extrusion (Figure 24.71), or embedding of the apical segment. The loss of the root would ultimately lead to the loss of the alveolar integrity and the reduction of the alveolar height. Unless ridge augmentation is performed into the vacant alveolus an unesthetic bridge is inevitable. Endodontically treating the segment and further reducing the root coronally to a level at least 2 mm above/below the crestal height will enable bone to form across the coronal root surface. The embedded root will maintain the alveolar shape, form, and height. A fixed partial denture can then be fabricated without fear of alveolar shrinkage.

Perhaps the most favorable treatment would be extrusion of the root segment.[39] Endodontics is performed for the submerged root, and a post space is prepared to the normal depth. A stainless steel pin or post, pre-bent to form a hook that will extend approximately 4 mm into the oral cavity, occlusion permitting, is cemented in place. An arch wire is adapted to the labial surfaces of the two adjacent teeth on either side of the injured tooth. The wire is contoured to bend into the lingual space and create a 180° angle with the long axis of the root segment. The labial surfaces of the adjacent teeth are acid etched, and the wire is bonded in place. Ligature bands are wound around the wire and the hook. Owing to the perpendicular angle forces, the root will extrude into its predetermined position. Once the root segment is extruded to a level beyond the crest, it is prepared and an impression is made. The active force is eliminated, and the root is held in a passive position for a period of 6–10 weeks. This enables the resistant forces of the periodontal fibers to become stable and minimize the possibility of root regression. Occasionally, postextrusion periodontal probing will reveal the need for crown lengthening. Once confident of root stability, the final post and core and crown can be fabricated with certainty. However, extraction of the root and an implant may be part of the treatment planning decision. Displaced vertical root fractures offer very little hope unless the angle of the break terminates at a level that offers the options discussed for a horizontal coronal fracture.

Luxation and avulsion

Prognosis after severe luxation and avulsion injuries has dramatically improved in the last few years because of better understanding of how such injuries should be predictably treated. If a tooth is replaced into its original position within a few hours after the injury or, in the case of avulsion, replanted within 30–60 min after proper storage and then root canal therapy initiated 7–10 days later, the periodontal ligament will in most cases heal without any significant problems.[40] Luxated or avulsed teeth that were not properly treated or that suffered a massive injury to the periodontal ligament could present atypical problems created by subsequent ankylosis and root resorption.

Ankylosis without excessive resorption is not a serious problem unless the tooth fuses to bone in a location that creates an esthetic problem. Such is the possibility when the tooth is replanted in a child before the maxilla has had the opportunity to complete its growth. The maxilla continues to develop to adulthood, at which time the injured tooth is superior and labial to the adjacent uninjured incisors. When extracted, ridge augmentation and grafting are required to close the labial mucosa and reconstruct an esthetic alveolar ridge level. Currently, there is no treatment known to arrest ankylosis once it has started. Root canal treatment will not, in most cases, have any effect on the process because it is initially caused by massive damage to the periodontal ligament and then maintained with normal bone metabolisms of the body, which is impossible to reverse.

Inflammatory root resorption presents a somewhat different situation. It is characterized by rapid root resorption as well as lesions in the adjacent bone. The endodontic objectives are centered on the arrest of the inflammatory processes that were initiated by damage to the periodontal ligament, which are subsequently being maintained by irritation from an infected root canal system and dentinal tubules. Presently, treatment consists of periodic applications of calcium hydroxide dressings within the cleansed canals. If successfully arrested, the normal periodontal ligament will establish itself again over some period and the endodontic seal can be completed. When the damage is so extensive that it intrudes into the canal space from the root surface, additional repair is attempted by surgically exposing the defect, preparing a Class I cavity preparation and filling the defect with a nondiscoloring material. The choice of material depends on the location of the problem; however, Geristore (DenMat), a resin-modified glass ionomer cement, and MTA (ProRoot MTA Tulsa/Dentsply) are presently the materials of choice (Figure 24.72A–F). When the defect extends deep beneath the gingival crest, the crown shoulder may need to be prepared within the repair. This restorative solution, although not a desirable situation, may often be the only "best" alternative. However, Geristore resin ionomer is the material of choice when the preparation repair margin is coronal to the cervical line, since MTA is soluble in oral fluids.

Cracked tooth syndrome

CTS is a frequently misdiagnosed or undiagnosed dental pathology. It is not diagnosed with a periapical image since the pulp is vital without periradicular osseous change. Visual

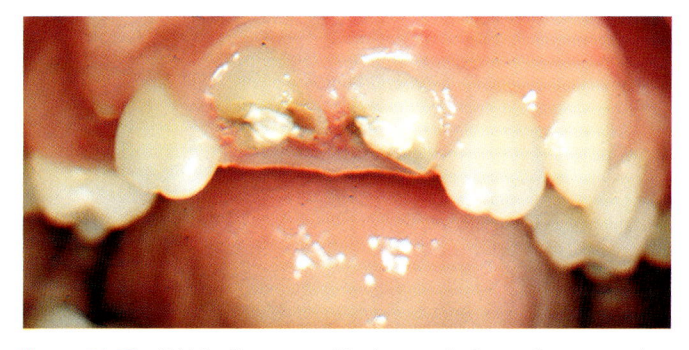

Figure 24.65 (A) Maxillary central incisor teeth. Crown fracture and pulp exposures requiring pulpectomies.

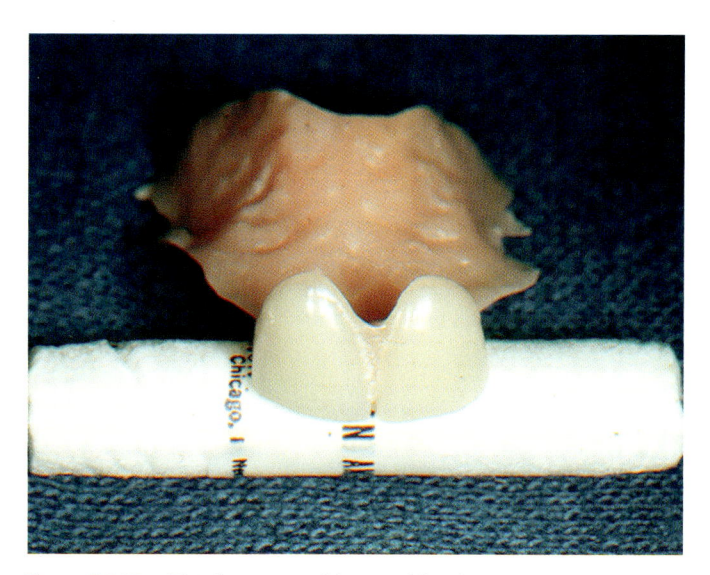

Figure 24.65 (B) A flipper was fabricated for this nine-year-old patient to satisfy the esthetic requirement.

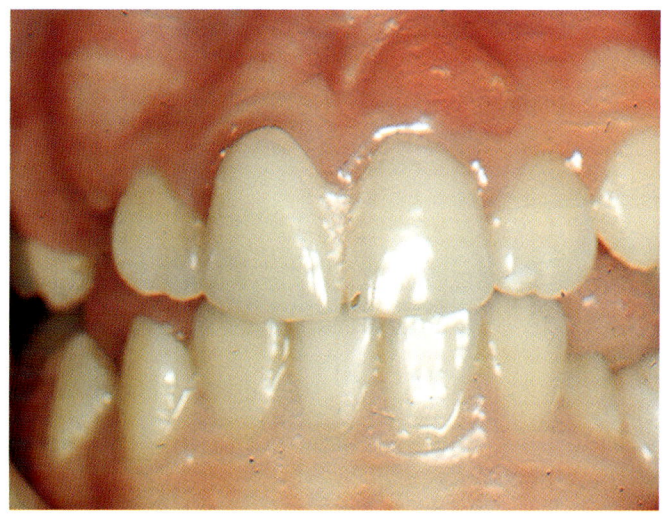

Figure 24.65 (C) The removable denture in place.

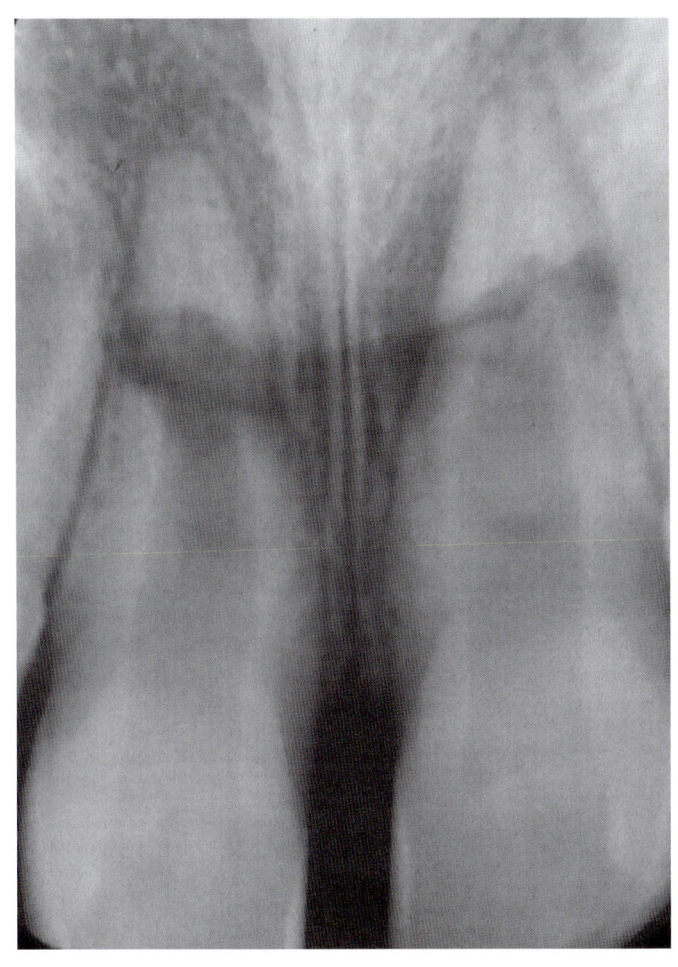

Figure 24.66 **(A)** Root fracture in the apical third. Maxillary central incisors, horizontal root fractures with pulp necrosis.

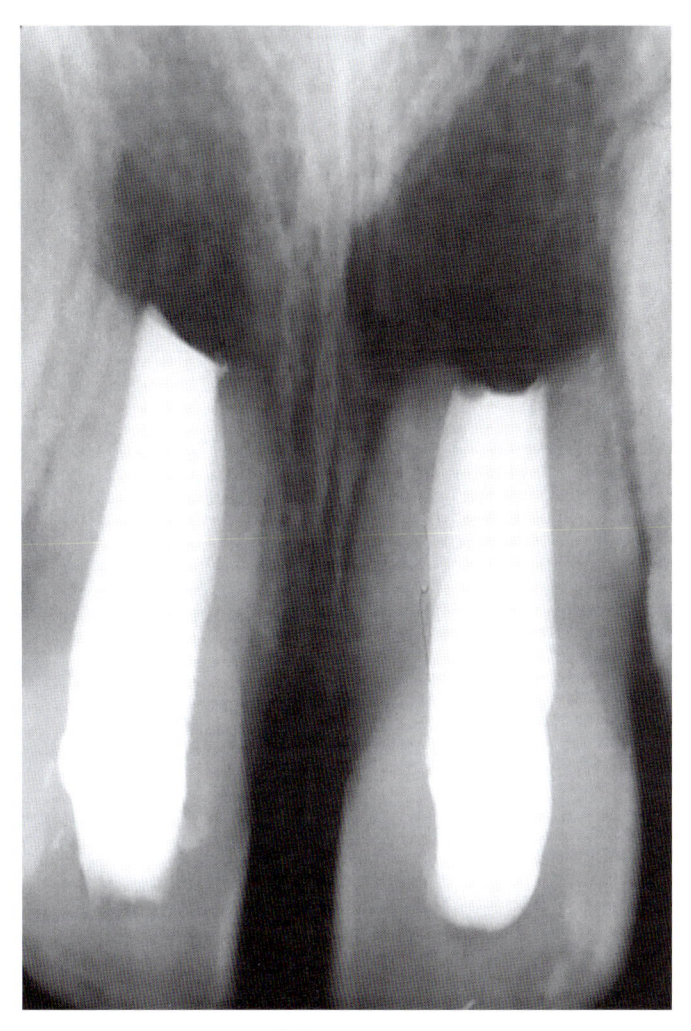

Figure 24.66 **(B)** Root canal therapy in the coronal segments the apical portions of the roots were surgically removed.

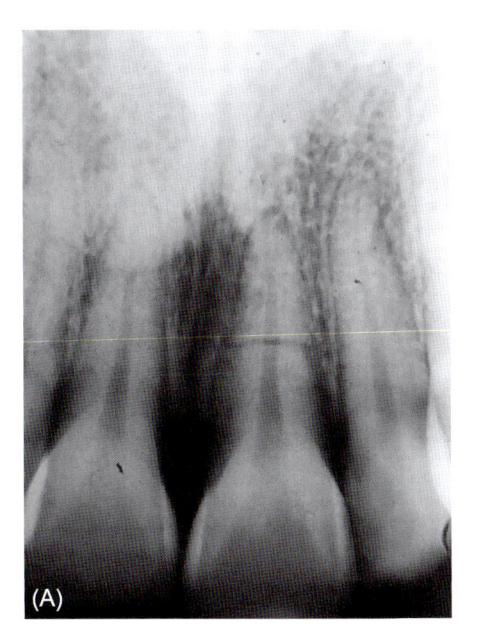

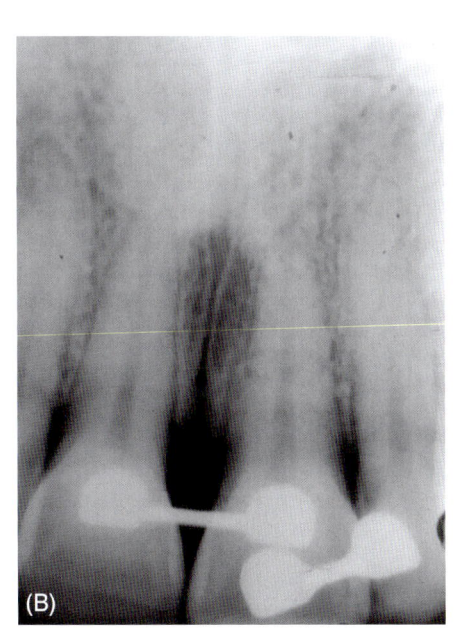

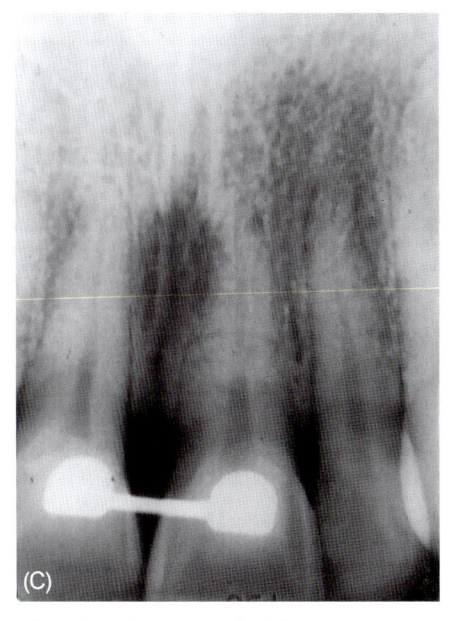

Figure 24.67 **(A)** Mid root fracture maxillary central incisor with minimal displacement. **(B)** Tooth splinted to adjacent teeth. **(C)** Six years postfracture: excellent root healing, and the pulp remained vital. The patient insisted on retaining the bonded bracket–arch bar splint.

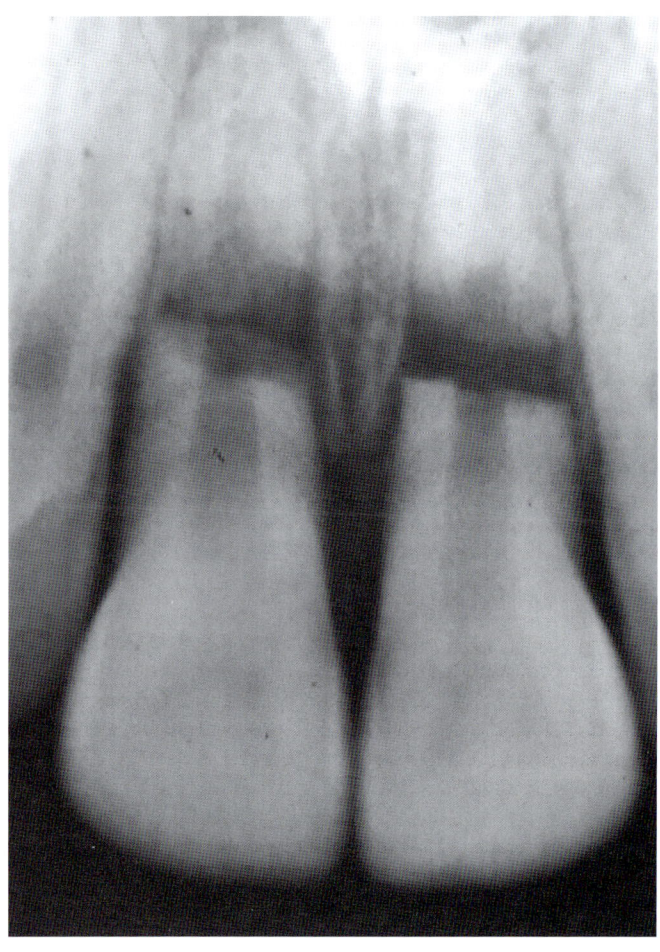

Figure 24.68 (A) Mid root fractures of maxillary central incisor teeth with severe displacement.

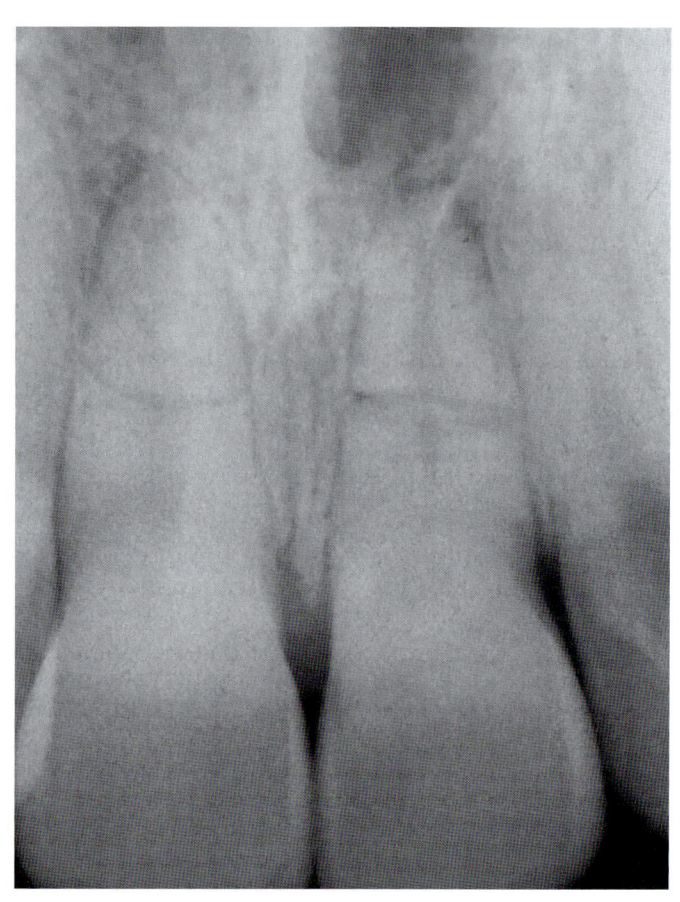

Figure 24.68 (B) Five year check radiograph. The treatment consisted of reducing the fracture and splinting with orthodontic brackets and an arch bar for 16 weeks. Vital pulps are present.

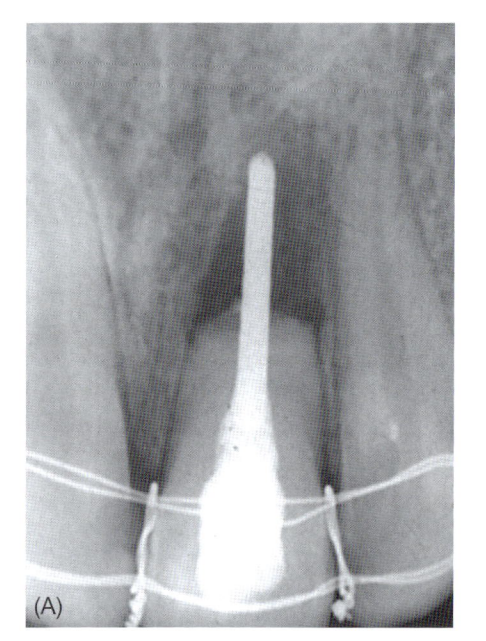

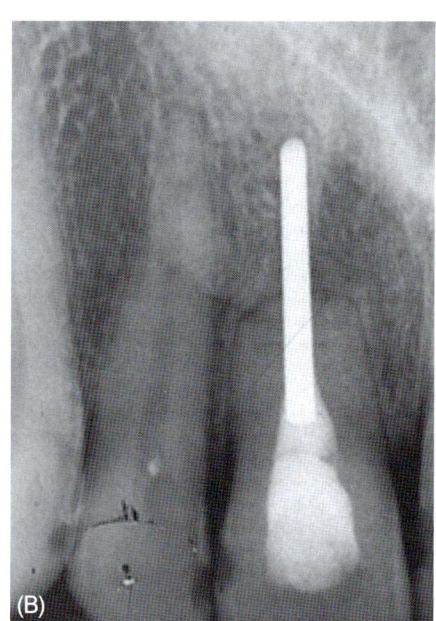

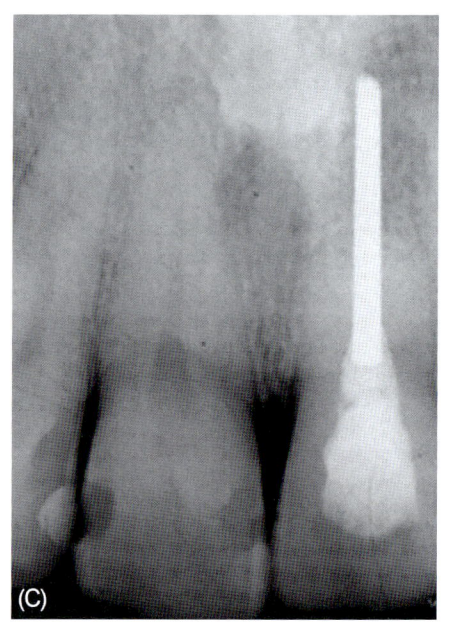

Figure 24.69 (A) Mid root fracture with pulp necrosis and apical periodontitis. Apical half of root extracted. Chrome cobalt endosseous implant (Austenal) cemented in remaining tooth structure. Tooth splinted. (B) Five years postsurgery. (C) Twenty-four years postsurgery. Tooth asymptomatic.

Figure 24.70 **(A)** Root fractures in coronal third requiring extraction. Maxillary lateral incisor

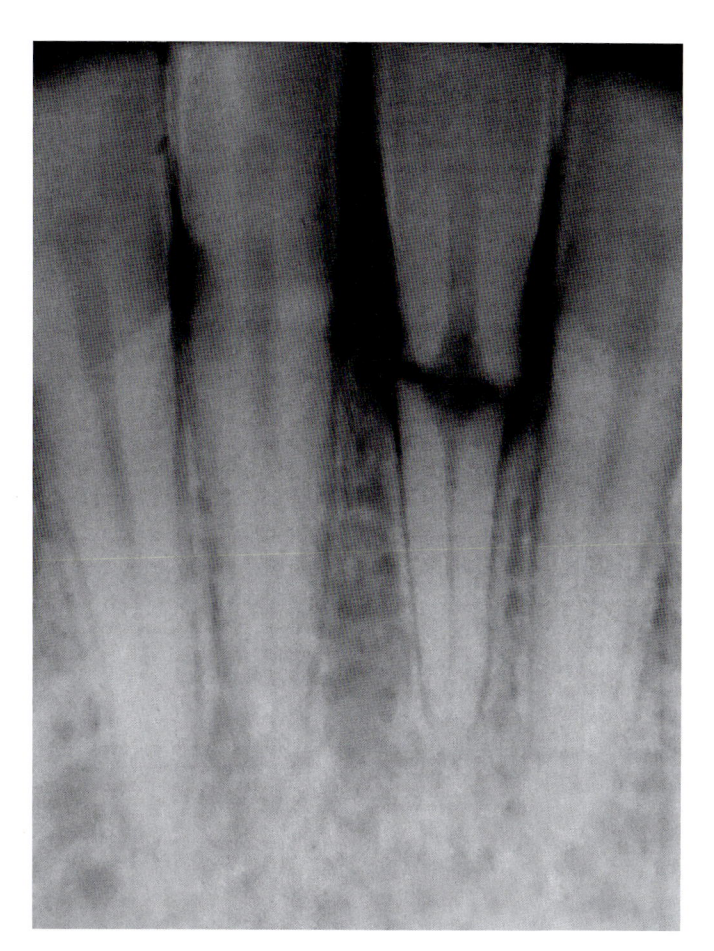

Figure 24.70 **(B)** Mandibular lateral incisor.

observation is unreliable since the extent of the hairline fracture cannot be fully observed. It must be diagnosed by properly clinically duplicating the symptoms for CTS. The seemingly elusive CTS is often a progressive condition that can result in an unrestorable fracture.[41]

Increased prevalence

A PubMed search reveals more than 11 500 articles have been published about CTS in the last 35 years. The condition of CTS was originally described by Cameron in 1964.[42] Because pretreatment diagnosis of the severity of the CTS is impossible, patients need to be advised about potential outcomes in diagnosis and how the diagnosis influences the CTS treatment plan and prognosis. Therefore, it is essential for the dentist to understand the guidelines for diagnosis and treatment of CTS.

It is important to note that CTS is one reason a patient may change dentists. The patient tells their dentist that they cannot chew on one side without discomfort. The dentist takes a periapical image of the area and there is no radiolucency. The pulps all test vital. The percussion test is negative. Without understanding the physiology of CTS, the dentist will not choose and interpret the right tests to actually make the diagnosis and recommend the proper treatment solution. The frequency of CTS is on the rise since humans are living longer, which means teeth need to last longer. More restorations are needed to retain teeth longer, and when teeth are more heavily restored they are more vulnerable to breakage.[43] In addition, grinding teeth, which may increase with increased daily stress, may exacerbate CTS. If left undiagnosed, CTS inevitably becomes worse, like a crack in glass. Sometimes the crack goes off to the side and the fragment of the tooth breaks off. The crack may also penetrate to the pulp or even a vertical root fracture. It is here where CTS can be diagnosed and usually successfully treated. Gibbs, who wrote one of the earliest reports on CTS, listed conditions that promote tooth fracture.[44] Cusps weakened by caries, by the shape and size of cavity preparations, and by improper restorations were generally considered the most important causes. He also described CTS as odontalgia secondary to cuspal fracture. His characteristic findings were (1) pain on mastication, (2) difficulty in locating pain, and (3) lack of other duplicable objective or subjective findings. Stanley suggested that considerations in cavity and crown preparations may reduce the incidence of CTS.[45] The restoration and remaining tooth structure must resist structural failure for restoration success. Cuspal protection is essential.

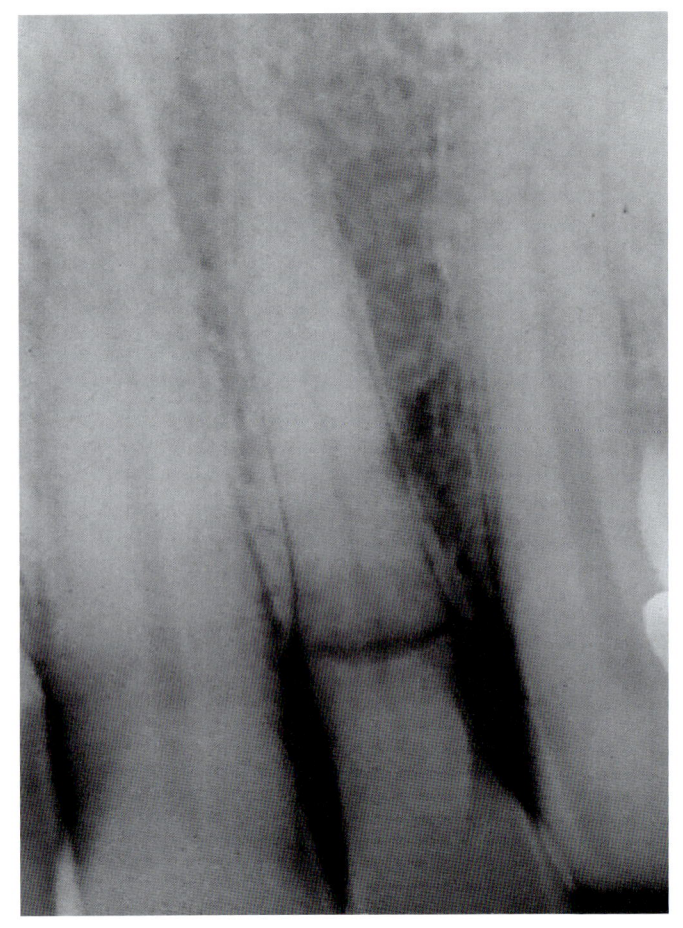

Figure 24.71 Maxillary lateral incisor with a root fracture in the coronal third. The root is long enough to consider a vertical extrusion.

Differential diagnosis

As part of the diagnostic process for CTS, the dentist must eliminate all other sources of pain when biting: endodontic acute alveolar abscess, periodontal abscess, pericoronitis, sinusitis, discomfort associated with orthodontic movement, hypersensitivity, poorly placed composite restoration, biologic width invasion, loose temporary or permanent restoration on tooth with vital dentin, open contact, a tooth ready to exfoliate, bruxism and clenching, or a parafunctional habit. Most of these conditions are easy to diagnose, but if the problem is none of these other possibilities the dentist must consider and test for a fractured tooth (CTS). What makes CTS such an elusive dental diagnosis?

Pulpal inflammation and necrosis occur in a coronal–apical direction because the cause of the insult cascade begins at the coronal end of the tooth: caries, restoration, cuspal fracture, new restorative and/or caries, and the insult cycle continues until the pulp cannot recover. Three anatomic conditions compromise the pulp's ultimate capacity for repair: (1) the pulp is surrounded by unyielding walls of dentin, preventing the recuperative swelling benefit of inflamed tissues elsewhere in the body; (2) the pulp is a relatively large volume of tissue for a relatively small blood supply through apical and lateral root canal system portals of exit; and (3) the pulp is an end-type circulation, such as the human appendix, which must be removed due to necrosis rather than repair when irreversibly inflamed. The single exception to the coronal–apical pulpal inflammatory direction would be, for example, the well-intended hygienist or dentist curetting an infrabony pocket and inadvertently severing a lateral blood supply, causing pulpal breakdown from a lateral direction. In this unlikely case, the pulp could test positive if the chamber tissue had not been affected or infected. This situation is more of a theoretical possibility than a clinical reality.

Unlike bone, pulps do not benefit from proprioception. Therefore, teeth with "toothaches," which are actually "pulp aches," cannot accurately identify themselves. The pain from stimuli such as sugar, cold, hot, and percussion must be duplicated by the dentist to diagnose the offending tooth/pulp. Not until the attachment apparatus is affected or infected from the root canal system can the patient reliably elicit pain and identify the pain offender through touching, moving, or biting on the source tooth.

Given the direction of most pulp death, teeth that have vital pulps do not have radiographic osseous lesions of endodontic origin, and teeth that have lesions of endodontic origin first have nonvital pulps and pulp testing must reveal negative electric, ice, and test cavity tests. Herein is the dilemma of CTS: How do you diagnose and treat to optimize the probability of success?

Cracked tooth syndrome classes and treatment

Class I: incomplete vertical fracture

In this class, there is incomplete vertical fracture through enamel and into dentin but not into the pulp (Figure 24.73A).

Symptoms

Class I fracture involves the dentinal tubules, and action potentials are produced when micromovement occurs due to the Class I crack. Although difficult to see without magnification and staining, the Class I fracture can be observed through the operating microscope and further revealed using transillumination. (Note: in the classification system described, Classes I–IV represent a progression of the Class I occlusal induced fracture.) If an early enough diagnosis is made and treated, the situation may not progress beyond a Class I fracture. If, on the other hand, the Class I diagnosis is missed and no treatment is provided, the crack may rapidly progress to Class III–V fractures, rendering the tooth unrestorable. Success depends on an accurate diagnosis, relief of occlusion, and proper cuspal coverage in a sequential and timely treatment plan.

The cleavage plane of a Class I fracture is usually in a mesiodistal direction. The patient with this problem often complains for months, years, or even decades that they experience a sharp pain when chewing. Again, radiographs are of no diagnostic value because there are no osseous changes and the fracture is perpendicular to the radiographic beam. Often, a patient will call one day to report that a portion of a tooth has broken off and the sharp pain has subsided.

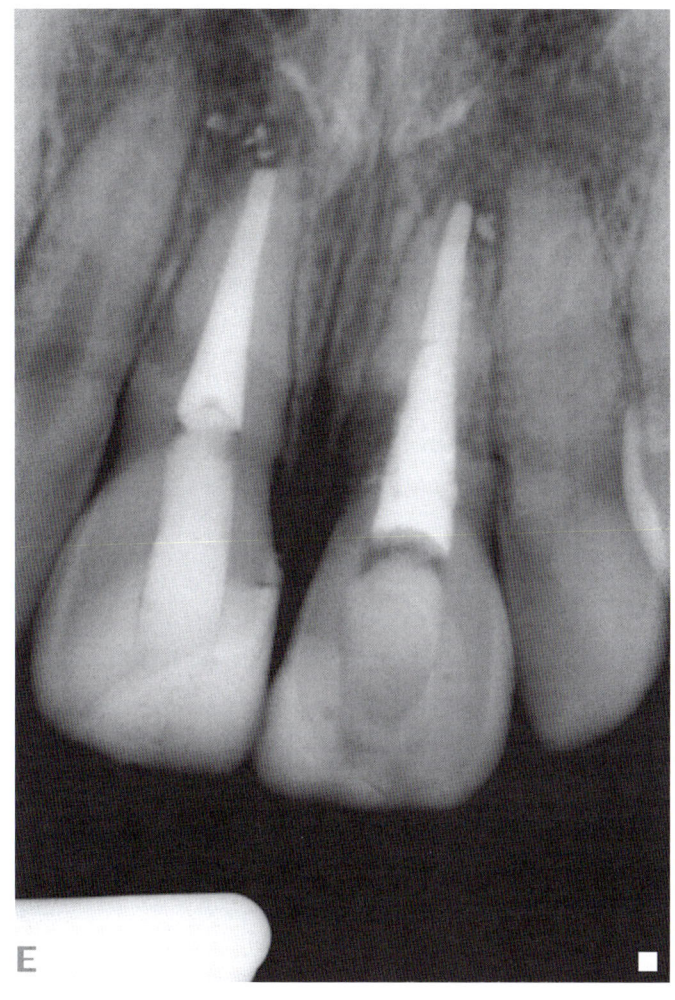

Figure 24.72 (A) Maxillary central incisor-surgical repair of resorptive defect 2 years following avulsion and replantation. Radiograph of a resorptive defect at cervical region following replantation, calcium hydroxide treatment, and root filling in a 10-year old patient.

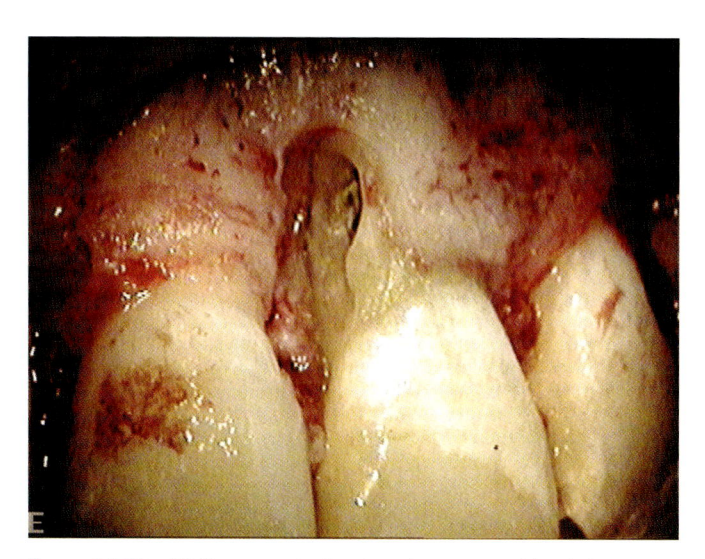

Figure 24.72 (B) Photograph showing the extent of the defect on the root.

Diagnosis

The key to the Class I CTS is to reproduce or duplicate ("dupe it") the symptoms of the patient's chief complaint or "felt need." The classic symptom is sharp pain when biting and yet the pulp is vital. The pain is often reported especially upon chewing release. A variety of diagnostic aids are available, such as an orange wood stick, "Tooth Sleuth," or wet cotton roll. The problem is the dentist directs the duplicating device and puts the onus on them. It is better to have the patient duplicate "their problem" using the "cotton wad" technique (Figure 24.73B). If they find it eating meals, they can find it now. The "cotton wad" is described as follows: place the patient in a sitting position and ask them to identify a substance that causes pain when chewing. If the answer is gum, for example, then wad and wet a sphere of cotton from a cotton roll that is the size of a piece of chewing gum. If the patient suggests another food, do the same thing and tell them to use their imagination. Have the patient chew with the cotton wad until they duplicate their biting pain. Give them time and some privacy to duplicate. Give them time to locate their own special occlusal position. The patient participates in the diagnosis versus the dentist doing something to them. It may take a few seconds or longer and you may need to change the cotton wad size a couple of times if the pain is not duplicated. The patient is instructed to keep their teeth together once they experience the pain. Then have the patient keep their teeth together and part their lips, so you can see where the cotton wad resides. If it is between two teeth such as the first and second molar, have the patient move the cotton wad to the forward tooth and test and repeat with the distal tooth until typically the patient's eyes squint and exclaims "that's it!" Literally, a wad of cotton is placed into the patient's mouth to simulate chewing and duplicate the symptom of pain when biting (Figure 24.73C). If bite pain duplication occurs, have the patient roll the cotton wad to the distal tooth, bite, and test. If not the second molar, have the patient move the cotton wad to the first molar. This is key to singularly isolating the CTS source. When your patient discovers the tooth by duplicating the symptom, a wince is often elicited (Figure 24.73D). You have diagnosed the bite source.

Treatment

Once the Class I CTS has been made, place a copper or stainless steel band with permanent cement. If the patient is asymptomatic to chewing after 1 week and has no thermal changes discomfort, then the tooth can be predictably restored with a full crown or onlay. In an unpublished clinical evaluation by the author (JDW), 133 cases of Class I CTS became asymptomatic after diagnosis and treatment performed from 1990 to 1993. One hundred patients were recalled in the year 2000, and 5% of the teeth required endodontic treatment, 2% were removed, and 93% were asymptomatic and did not require endodontic treatment.

Class II: pulpal involvement

In this class, the crown fracture is associated with irreversible pulpal inflammation of the pulp (Figure 24.73E).

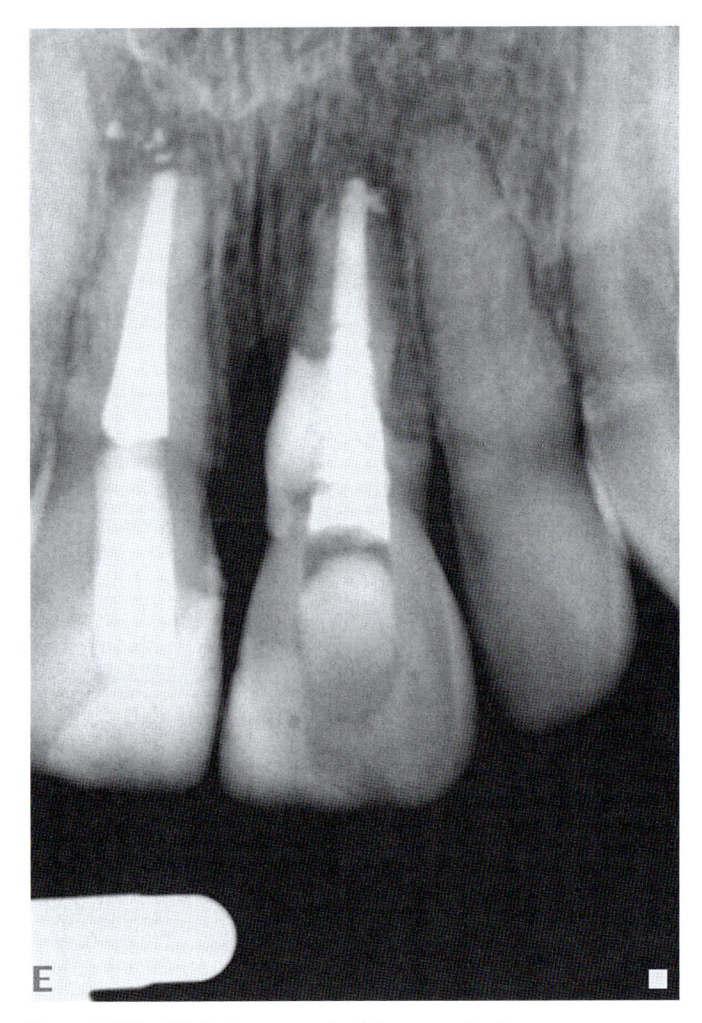

Figure 24.72 **(C)** Geristore repair of the resorptive lacunae.

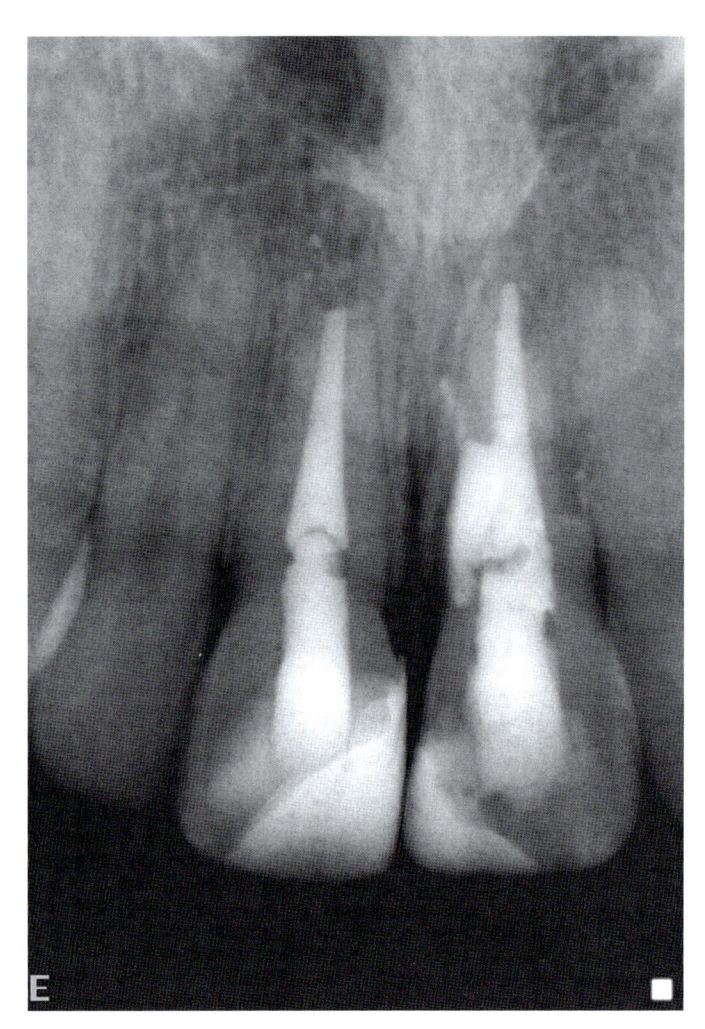

Figure 24.72 **(D)** Check-up after 4.5 years discloses a return to the normal periradicular bone pattern.

Symptoms

In addition to sharp biting pain, the patient will often experience discomfort with thermal changes and report a recent history of pain with thermal stimuli. The pulps may now have advanced to necrosis or the tooth may have advanced to an acute alveolar abscess. However, there will be a history of pain with thermal stimuli. The history is essential in identifying the class of the CTS. If the patient is questioned about when they had pain with biting—that is, was the pain first with biting or to thermal change—the patient will report that the pain occurred first with biting. This should lead to a diagnosis of a vertical fracture in the crown. If the fracture is not diagnosed, and the patient is treated just for pulpitis or acute alveolar access, failure will result. The reason for failure is that the tooth was not treated for the combined problem; that is, fracture and pulpal involvement.

Teeth in the Class II CTS category need to be treated with a copper or stainless steel band and cemented with permanent cement followed by initial endodontic treatment once the tooth has become asymptomatic. If the tooth is asymptomatic to chewing after the beginning of endodontic treatment, then endodontics should be finished and restored with a crown or at least cuspal coverage. It should be emphasized that the tooth must be completely asymptomatic to chewing or biting before preceding otherwise the symptom correction is unpredictable. Do not expect the tooth to be less symptomatic with the crown in place than it was with the cemented band.

Diagnosis

Duplicate symptoms of biting and pulpitis.

Treatment

Adjust the occlusion so that the tooth is not in occlusion. Band the crown immediately. Treat the pulpal pain appropriately. Check the mesial and distal surfaces for increased probing depth. If an isolated periodontal defect is observed, the fracture may involve the root surface in an apical direction and the prognosis is poor. If the tooth remains symptomatic to biting after the band is placed and endodontic treatment is complete, consider removal of the tooth. The reason the tooth remains symptomatic is that the fracture line has extended into the periodontal ligament and the patient experiences pain from the periodontal ligament and not the pulp. The symptoms will not improve when a crown is placed. If the tooth is asymptomatic with the band and following endodontic treatment, then continue with a cast crown. Within the next couple of years, some teeth in Class II

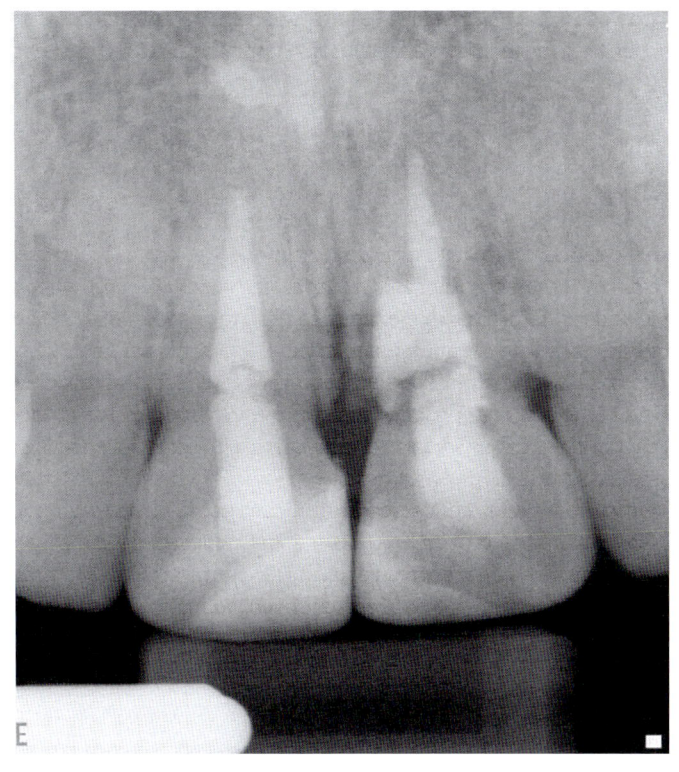

Figure 24.72 (E) Nine years postsurgery, 12 years posttrauma.

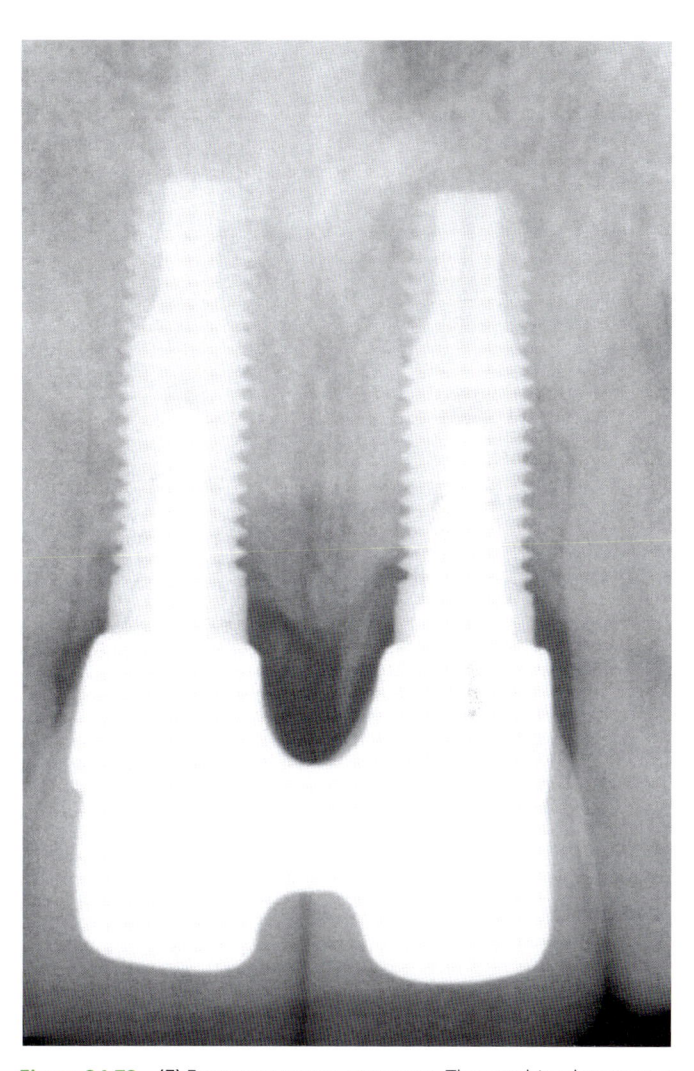

Figure 24.72 (F) Fourteen years post trauma. The combined treatment preserved the tooth as an esthetic "space maintainer" until there was sufficient jaw development to allow for implant placement in the now 22-year-old.

CTS will fail, but the majority will be as serviceable as any other endodontically treated tooth. Ultimately, it is difficult to measure the relationship of the depth of the fracture and pulpal involvement except measuring the patient symptoms after band placement. In summary, there are three possible outcomes after band placement (Figure 24.74A–D).

Class III: attachment involvement

The Class III CTS fracture is the most difficult to treat because the periodontal defect associated with the fracture is important to the prognosis. This dilemma was described by Hiatt;[46] he concluded that as the fracture proceeds deeper into structure of the tooth, bacteria invade the pulp or periodontal tissue and may result in pulpal lesions, periodontal lesions, or combined lesions. The attachment apparatus is often involved.

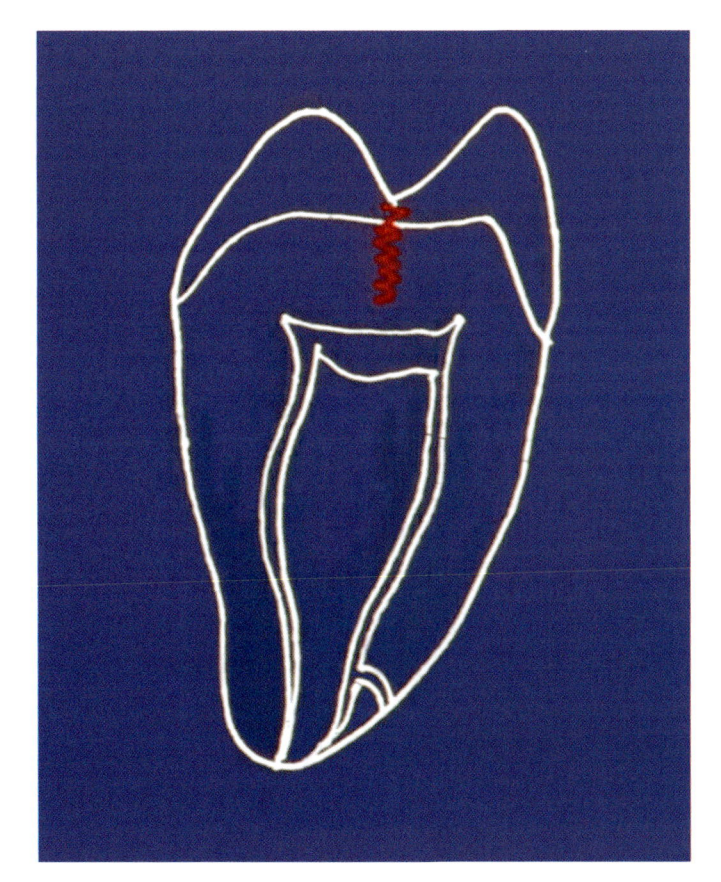

Figure 24.73 (A) CTS. Class I fracture occurs into dentin but does not involve pulp.

Symptoms
If the pulp is necrotic there are few symptoms.

Diagnosis

Often there is a history of Class I and Class II symptoms. Periradicular bone loss can often be seen radiographically.

Treatment

In most cases, the best treatment is extraction. However, certain procedures may be attempted if the tooth is particularly strategic either functionally or esthetically and an implant or bridge is not desired. The dentist can band the tooth, treat an acute symptom, and observe the result. Cleaning the root canal system will eliminate the endodontic component. If the tooth has shallow probing depths in the area of the fracture line and if the tooth becomes asymptomatic with biting following banding, then the dentist can consider proceeding with endodontic treatment and a crown. This should not be the treatment plan unless the patient fully understands the prognosis is uncertain.

Class IV: complete separation of tooth fragments

This type of fracture is through the crown, extends subgingivally, and one or more parts of the tooth are mobile. The mobile portion needs to be removed; if the remaining tooth structure is restorable, endodontics is performed and the tooth is restored. Usually, however, insufficient sound tooth remains after the fractured and loose portions are removed.

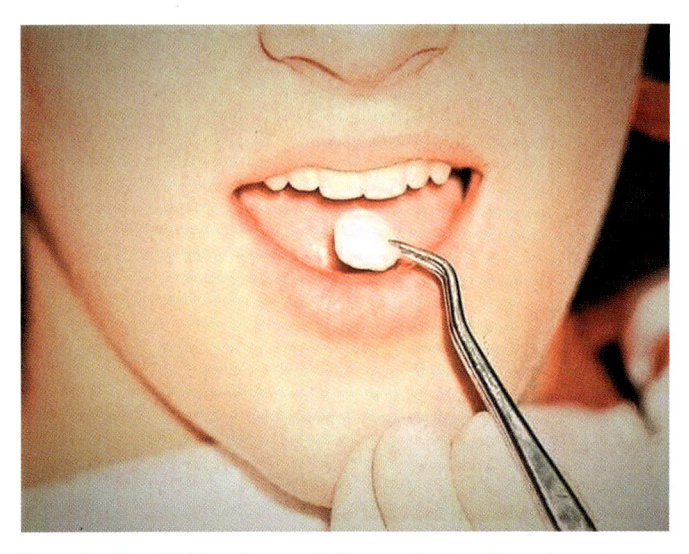

Figure 24.73 (B) Literally a wad of cotton is placed into the patient's mouth to simulate chewing and duplicate the symptom of pain when biting.

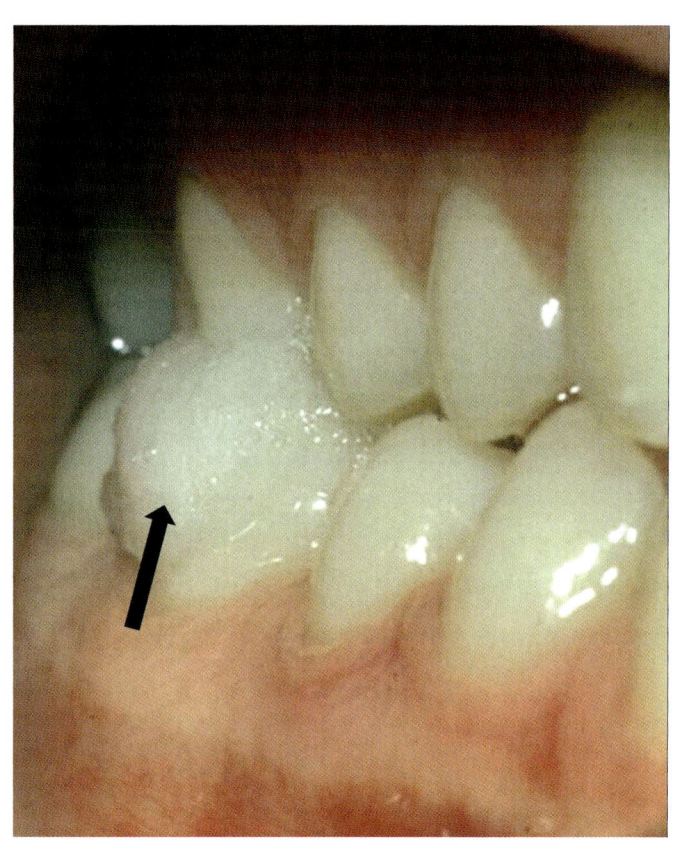

Figure 24.73 (C) Cotton wad is between first and second molar.

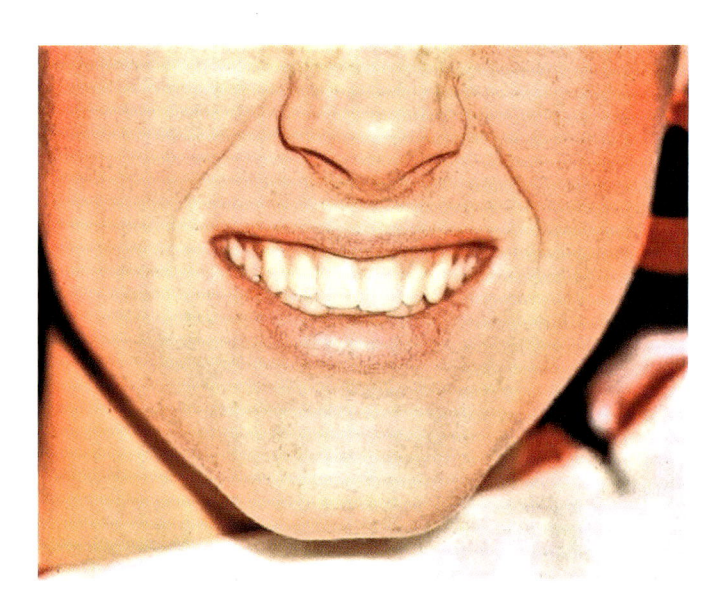

Figure 24.73 (D) When the patient discovers the tooth by duplicating the symptom, a wince is often elicited. You have diagnosed the bite source.

Symptoms
History of fracture symptoms, bite pain, and gingival inflammation and swelling.

Diagnosis
Deep and narrow periodontal defect usually in two locations around the circumference of the tooth.

Treatment
Extraction of all or a portion of the tooth if it were restorable.

Class V: retrograde root fracture

These fractures originate at the apex and travel coronally. They are iatrogenic in nature, resulting from overzealous root canal preparation and a resulting weakened root, forcible endodontic obturation, or from active post placement.

Symptoms
Tooth discomfort, but often vague.

Diagnosis
Radiographic, history, and observation during removal or endodontic microsurgery.

Treatment
Extraction or endodontic surgery.

Lastly, CTS occurs most frequently in the mandibular second molars followed by the maxillary first molars, mandibular first molars, and maxillary first premolars.[45]

Summary of cracked tooth syndrome guidelines

- Identify CTS tooth with patient chewing on cotton wad.

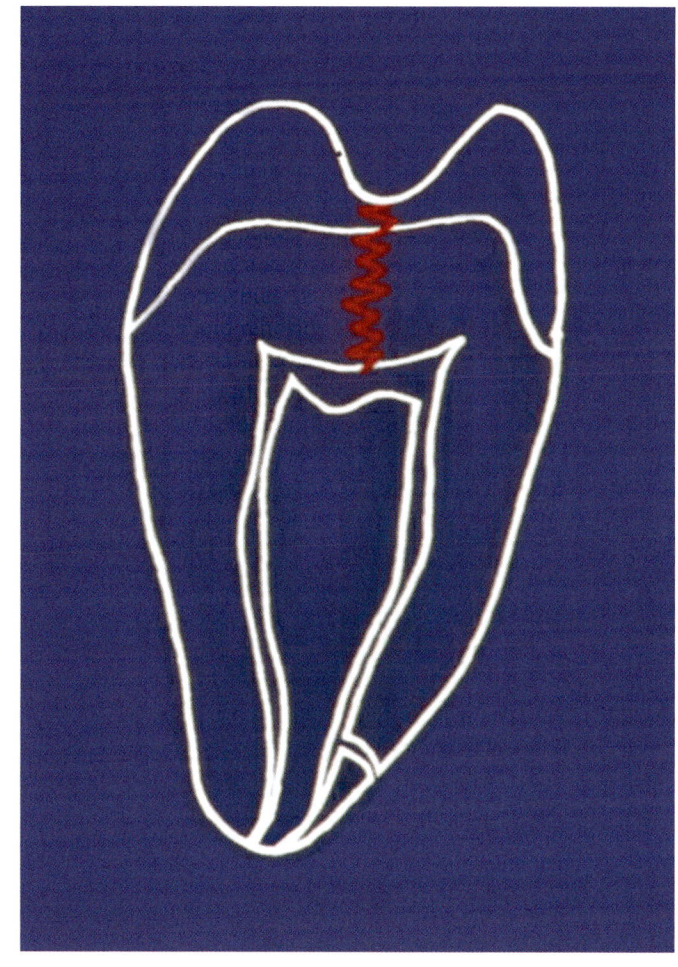

Figure 24.73 (E) Class II CTS involves the pulp.

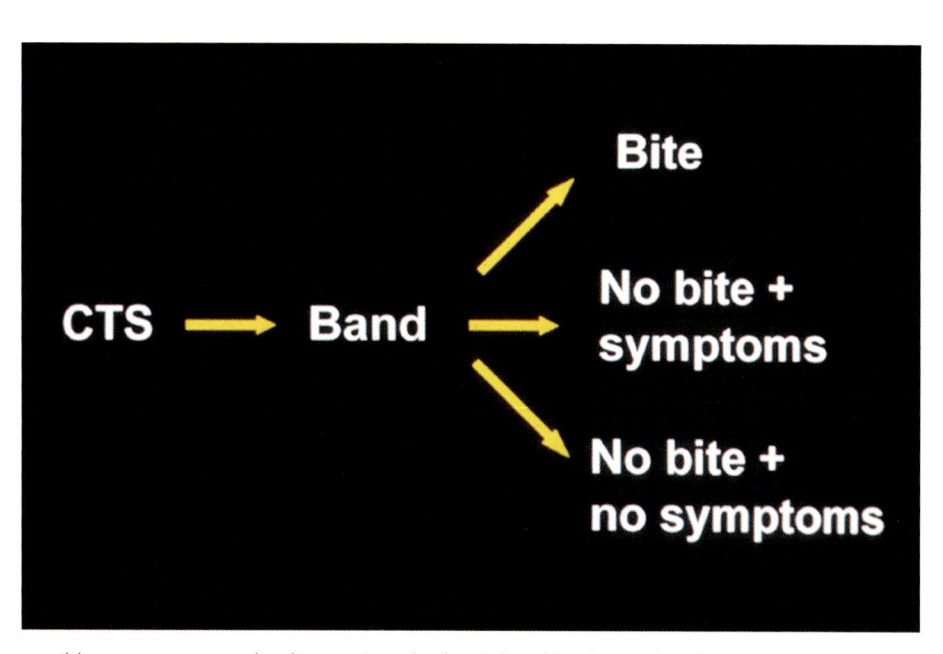

Figure 24.74 (A) Three possible outcomes once the diagnostic orthodontic band has been placed.

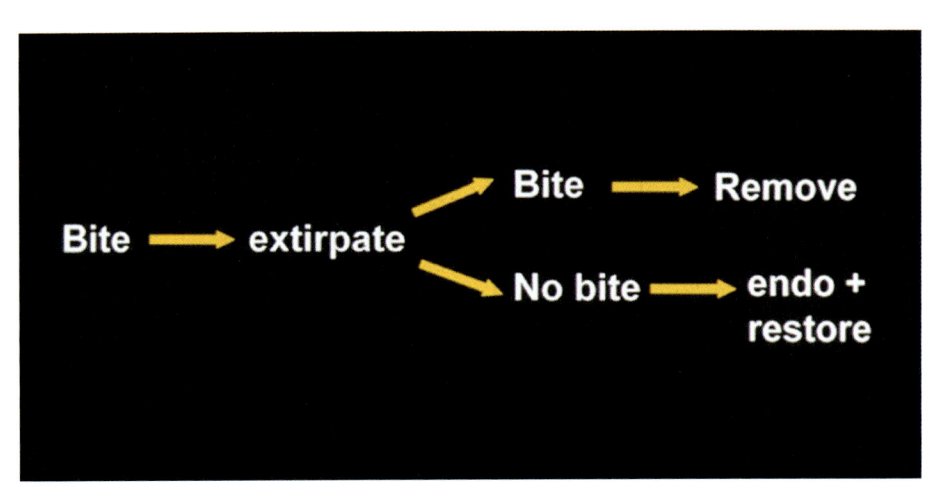

Figure 24.74 **(B)** Possible outcome #1.

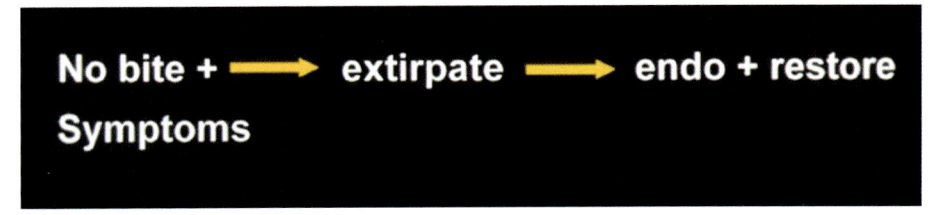

Figure 24.74 **(C)** Possible outcome #2.

Figure 24.74 **(D)** Possible outcome #3.

- Treat Class I CTS fractures with band and restore. Eliminate all centric and working contacts in noncentric holding cusps; that is, lingual cusps of mandibular posterior teeth and buccal cusps of maxillary posterior teeth.
- Treat Class II CTS fractures with band plus endodontic treatment and restore unless symptomatic (see flowchart).
- Treat Class III CTS fractures with band and perhaps endodontic treatment and restore, but extraction is likely.
- Treat Class IV CTS fractures by removal or root resection.
- Treat Class V CTS fractures by removal or endodontic surgical repair.

Conclusion

CTS presents both a diagnostic challenge for the dentist and an opportunity for the patient and the dentist. CTS is the reason many patients have a favorite side to chew on. In unpublished data, the author (JDW) has discovered approximately half of patients, when asked what their favorite side to chew on is, choose one side or the other. Approximately half of those patients, in other words, as many as a quarter of the patients in a dental practice, may have undiagnosed CTS that can and should be diagnosed and appropriately treated. But the dentist or hygienist must make this question part of every comprehensive dental examination or recall/cleaning appointment to diagnose this "silent" endodontic condition. In addition, CTS cases are increasing due to increased patient longevity, more wear, more restorations, and more stress.

Endodontic surgery

Although the technological advancements in endodontics have improved the rate of success, the demands of the populace to save teeth presents degrees of difficulty that test the best of endodontic mechanics. In an effort to satisfy these demands, dentists are often called on to overcome anatomic, iatrogenic, or traumatic complications by intervening surgically. Sealing portals of exit surgically, for example, post perforations (Figure 24.75A–D), root resorption lesions (Figure 24.72A–F), and inadequate root fillings, where nonsurgical treatment is not practical (Figure 24.76A–C). These modes of treatment constitute an extension of endodontic treatment and are an alternative to extraction.

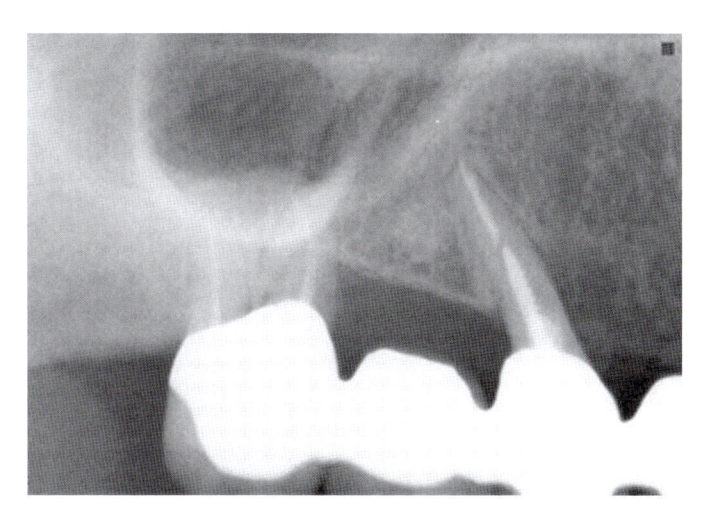

Figure 24.75 **(A)** Post perforation repair. Post perforation maxillary second premolar tooth.

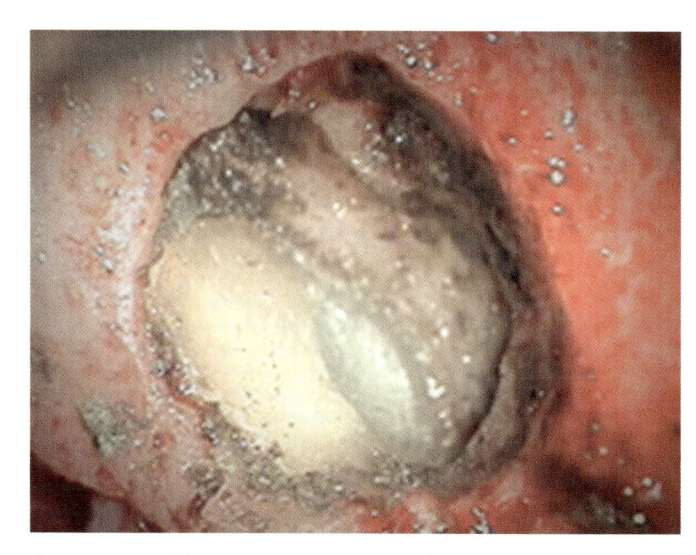

Figure 24.75 **(C)** Postoperative image perforation repaired with MTA repair.

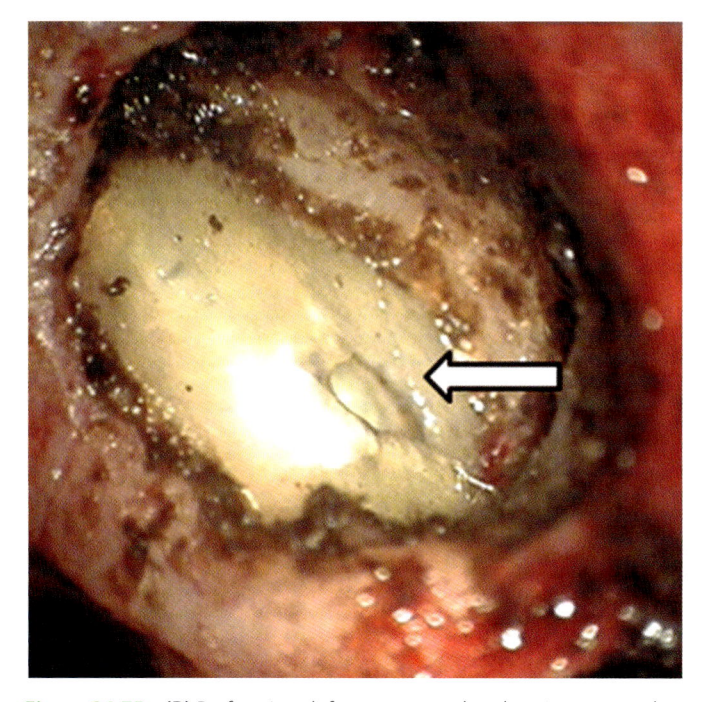

Figure 24.75 **(B)** Perforation defect uncovered and cavity prepared.

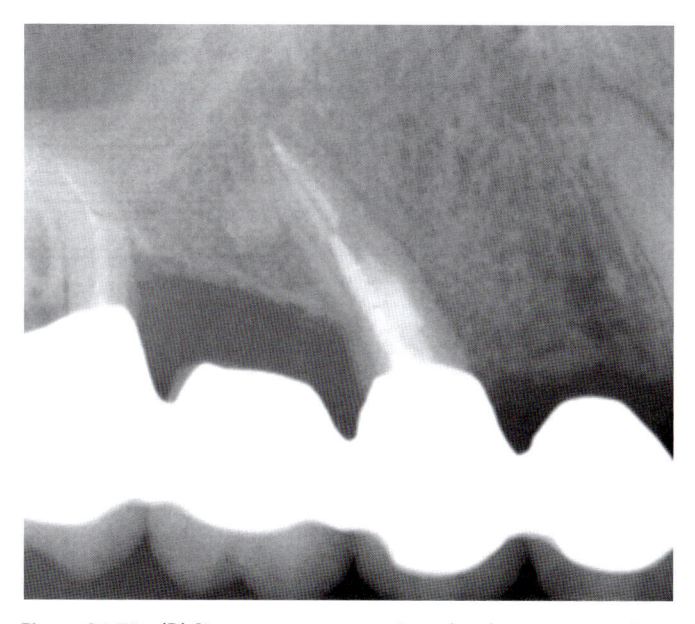

Figure 24.75 **(D)** Six years postsurgery. Complete bone regeneration, and tooth is asymptomatic.

Within the Endodontic community, there is an emphasis to retreat wherever possible and feasible rather than to choose endodontic surgery as the first treatment option. The advent of sophisticated techniques, equipment, and materials allows for the nonsurgical retreatment of teeth that were previous candidates for extraction (Figure 24.77A–C).

Since endodontic surgery requires incising and elevating the soft tissue from bone, the obvious esthetic consequences can be recession and scarring. For these reasons, the choice and location of the surgical flap must be carefully evaluated before a scalpel ever touches tissue.[47] There are several major flap designs that could be used, depending on existing restorations and anatomical factors.

Tissue discoloration (tattoo)

In the past, silver amalgam was the material of choice for retro filling, post perforation repairs, and sealing resorption defects. In a tissue environment, this material is notorious for its discoloring effect (Figure 24.78A and B). Once a black tattoo occurs, corrective treatment may require removal of the cause, excising the tattoo and grafting tissue across the defect. Such treatment can now be avoided by using Super EBA (Henry J Bosworth), Geristore (DenMat), or white MTA (ProRoot MTA Dentsply Tulsa Dental Specialties) Biodentine (Septodontics) because these products do not cause the staining/tattoo that is associated with the amalgam.

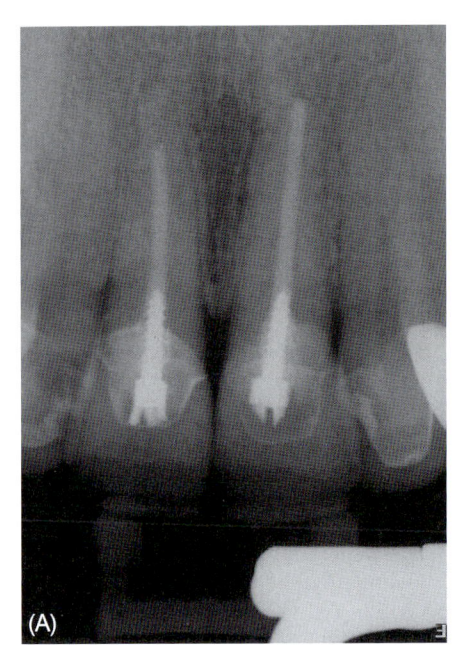

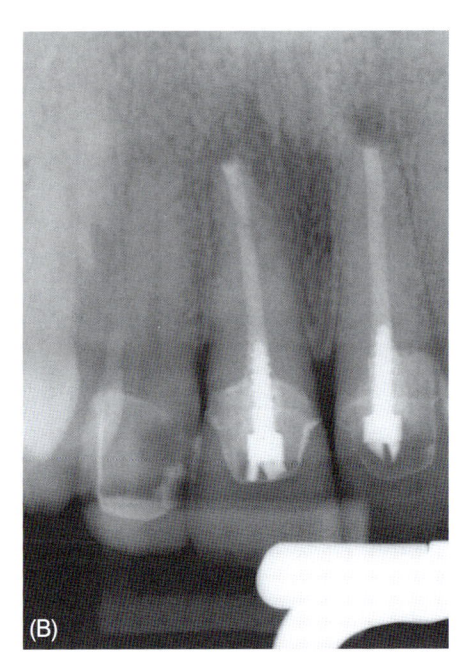

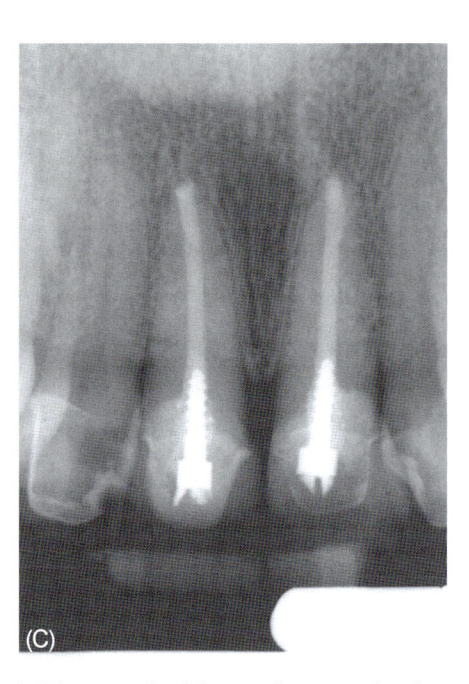

Figure 24.76 **(A)** Surgical retreatment of maxillary anterior periapical lesions. Preoperative radiograph. **(B)** MTA seals of the maxillary central and lateral incisors. **(C)** Ten-year checkup radiograph shows evidence of bone deposition.

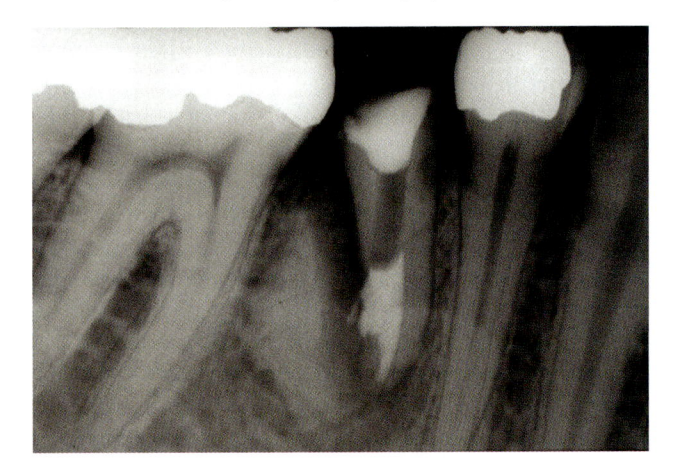

Figure 24.77 **(A)** Nonsurgical post perforation repair. Post perforation of a mandibular premolar tooth. The position of the strip perforation on the distal surface obviates the possibility of surgical repair.

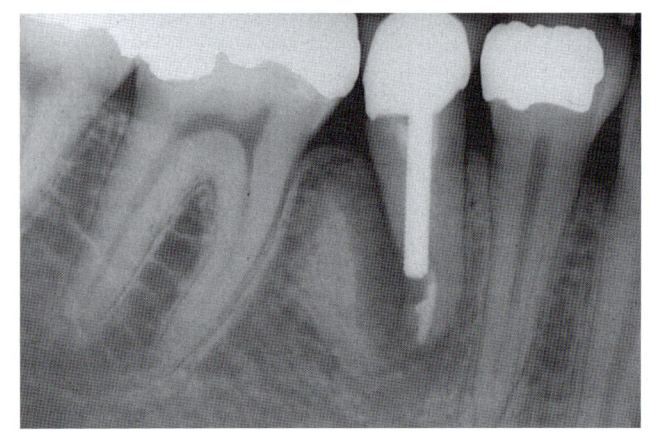

Figure 24.77 **(B)** The crown, core buildup, and the post were removed. The perforation was sealed with MTA. The tooth was restored with a cast post and a PFM crown.

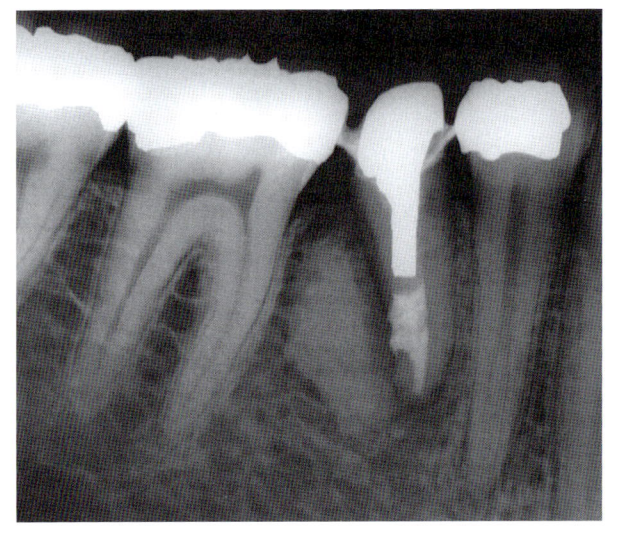

Figure 24.77 **(C)** Sixteen years after repair, the tooth is asymptomatic and there is complete regeneration of the bone in the defect site.

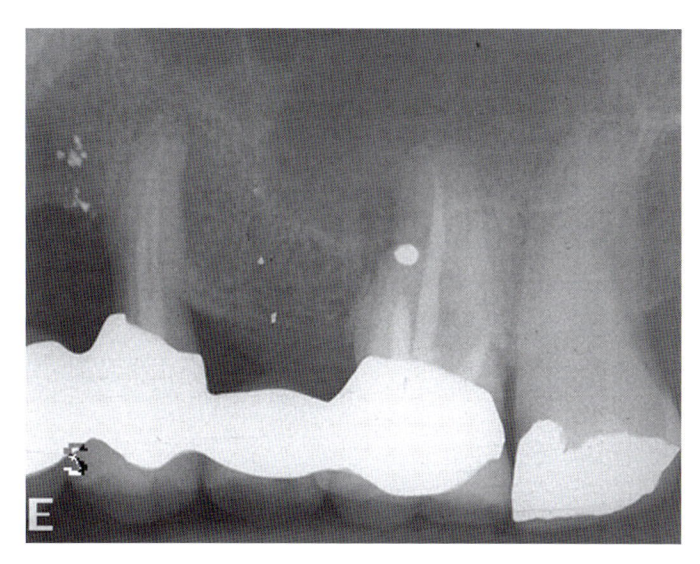

Figure 24.78 **(A)** Amalgam tattoo; 25 years after placement of an apical amalgam seal in the mesiobuccal root of a maxillary first molar and other apical amalgam repair procedures in the vicinity.

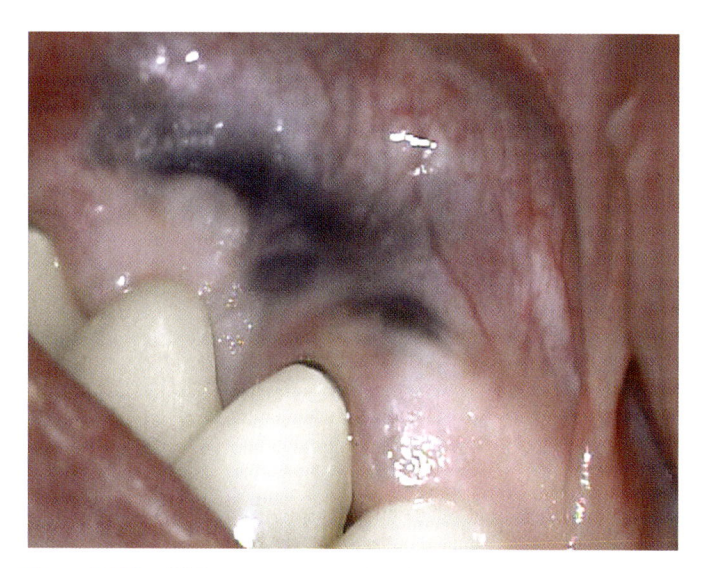

Figure 24.78 **(B)** Permanent tissue discoloration from the amalgam filling.

Summary

Endodontic treatment can be the key to long-term success of esthetic restorations. Since success and survival rates of endodontically treated teeth are equal to implants,[48–50] root canal treatment should be considered in the earliest phases of interdisciplinary treatment planning of endodontically diseased teeth. It is essential that your patient is aware that there are alternative methods to restoring the dentition to form, function, health, and esthetics. A well-informed patient will continue to be a trusting patient who values your services throughout their life and the life of the dental procedures.

References

1. Ball R, Barbizam JV, Cohenca N. Intraoperative endodontic applications of cone-beam computed tomography. *J Endod* 2013;39:548–557.
2. Arens DE, Chivian N. Endodontic contributions to esthetic dentistry. In: Annual Meeting of the American Academy of Esthetic Dentistry, Los Angeles, CA; 1993.
3. Langeland K. Prevention of pulpal damage. *Dent Clin North Am* 1972;16:709–732.
4. Stanley HR. *Human Pulp Response to Restorative Dental Procedures*. Gainesville, FL: University of Florida College of Dentistry; 1981.
5. Stanley HR, Swerdlow H. Reaction of the human pulp to cavity preparation: results produced by eight different operative techniques. *J Am Dent Assoc* 1959;58:49–59.
6. Robertson A, Andreasen FM, Bergenholtz G, et al. Pulp reactions to restoration of experimentally induced crown fractures. *J Dent* 1998;26:409–416.
7. Michaelson PL, Holland GR. Is pulpitis painful? *Int Endod J* 2002;35:829–832.
8. Torabinejad M, Chivian N. Clinical applications of mineral trioxide aggregate. *J Endod* 1999;25:197–205.
9. Bogen G, Lee SJ, Bakland LK. Direct pulp capping with mineral trioxide aggregate: an observational study. *J Am Dent Assoc* 2008;139:305–315.
10. Pameijer CH, Stanley HR. The disastrous effects of the "Total Etch" technique in vital pulp capping in primates. *Am J Dent* 1998;11:S45–S54.
11. About I, Murray PE, Franquin JC, et al. The effect of cavity restoration variables on odontoblast cell numbers and dental repair. *J Dent* 2001;29:109–117.
12. Subay RK, Demirci M. Pulp tissue reactions to a dentin bonding agent as a direct capping agent. *J Endod* 2005;31:201–204.
13. Silva GA, Gava E, Estrella AC, Alves JB. Subclinical failures of direct pulp capping of human teeth by using a dentin bonding system. *J Endod* 2013;39:182–189.
14. Cho S-Y, Seo D-G, Lee S-J, et al. Prognostic factors for clinical outcomes according to time after direct pulp capping. *J. Endod* 2013;39:327–331.
15. Hunter FA. Saving pulps. A queer process. *Dent Item Int* 1883;5:352.
16. Abou-Rass M. The stressed pulp condition: an endodontic-restorative diagnostic concept. *J Prosthet Dent* 1982;48:264–267.
17. Bohannan H, Abrams L. Intentional vital extirpation in periodontal prosthesis. *J Prosthet Dent* 1961;11:781–789.
18. Zinman EJ. Endodontic records and legal responsibilities. In: Cohen S, Burns RC eds. *Pathways of the Pulp*, 7th edn. St. Louis, MO: Mosby; 2002:379.
19. Survey of general dentists rubber dam usage during root canal treatment. *Dental Products Report*, November 2004.
20. Anabtawi MF, Gilbert GH, Bauer MR, et al. Rubber dam use during root canal treatment: findings from the dental practice-based research network. *J Am Dent Assoc* 2013;144:179–186.
21. Survey of endodontists rubber dam usage during root canal treatment. *Dental Products Report*, December 2002.
22. Madison S, Jordan RD, Krell KV. The effects of rubber dam retainers on porcelain fused-to-metal restorations. *J Endod* 1986;12:183–186.
23. Christensen GJ. The all-ceramic restoration dilemma: where are we? *J Am Dent Assoc* 2011;142:668–671.

24. Michanowicz AE, Michanowicz JP. Endodontic access to the pulp chamber via porcelain jacket crowns. *Oral Surg* 1962;15(Suppl 2):1483–1488.
25. Teplitsky PE, Sutherland JK. Endodontic access of Cerestore crowns. *J Endod* 1985;11:555–558.
26. McMullen AF III, Himmel VT, Sarkar NK. An in vitro study of the effect endodontic access preparation has upon the retention of porcelain fused to metal crowns of maxillary central incisors. *J Endod* 1989;15(4):154–156.
27. McMullen AF III, Himmel VT, Sarkar NK. An in vitro study of the effect endodontic preparation and amalgam restoration have upon incisor crown retention. *J Endod* 1990;16(6):269–272.
28. Ray HA, Trope M. Periapical status of endodontically treated teeth in relation to the technical quality of the root filling and the coronal restoration. *Int Endo J* 1995;28:12–18.
29. Tronstad L, Asbjørnsen K, Døving L, et al. Influence of coronal restorations on the periapical health of endodontically treated teeth. *Endod Dent Traumatol* 2000;16:218–221.
30. West JD. Endodontic predictability—"Restore or remove: how do I choose?" In: Cohen M, ed. *Interdisciplinary Treatment Planning: Principles, Design, Implementation*. Chicago, IL: Quintessence; 2008:123–164.
31. Trope M, Chivian N, Sigurdsson A. Trauma injuries. In: Cohen S, Burns RC (eds), *Pathways of the Pulp*, 7th edn. St. Louis, MO: Mosby; 1998.
32. Madison S, Walton R. Cervical root resorption following bleaching of endodontically treated teeth. *J Endod* 1990;16:570–574.
33. Lado EA, Stanley HR, Weissman MI. Cervical resorption in bleached teeth. *Oral Surg* 1983;55:78–80.
34. Spasser HF. A simple bleaching technique using sodium perborate. *N Y State Dent J* 1961;27:332–334.
35. Jimenez-Rubio A, Segura JJ. The effect of the bleaching agent sodium perborate on macrophage adhesion in vitro: implications in external cervical root resorption. *J Endod* 1998;24:229–232.
36. Steiner DR, West JD. A method to determine the location and shape of an intracoronal bleach barrier. *J Endod* 1994;20:304–306.
37. Plotino G, Buono L, Grande NM, et al. Nonvital tooth bleaching: a review of the literature and clinical procedures. *J Endod* 2008;34:394–407.
38. Andreasen JO, Andreasen FM. *Essentials of Traumatic Injuries to Teeth*. Copenhagen: Munksgaard; 1990.
39. Heithersay GS. Combined endodontic–orthodontic treatment of transverse root fractures in the region of the alveolar crest. *Oral Surg* 1973;3:404–415.
40. Andreasen JO, Borum MK, Jacobsen HL, Andreasen FM. Replantation of 400 avulsed permanent incisors. 4. Factors related to periodontal ligament healing. *Endod Dent Traumatol* 1995;11:76–89.
41. Rivera EM, Williamson A. Diagnosis and treatment planning: cracked tooth. *Tex Dent J* 2003;120:278–283.
42. Cameron CE. Cracked-tooth syndrome. *J Am Dent Assoc* 1964;68:405–411.
43. Seo DG, Yi YA, Shin SJ, Park JW. Analysis of factors associated with cracked teeth. *J Endod* 2012;38:288–292.
44. Gibbs JW. Cuspal fracture odontalgia. *Dent Dig* 1954;60:158–160.
45. Stanley HR. The cracked tooth syndrome. *J Am Acad Gold Foil Oper* 1968:11:36–47.
46. Hiatt WH. Incomplete crown–root fracture in pulpal–periodontal disease. *J Periodontol* 1973;44:369–379.
47. Arens DE, Torabinejad M, Chivian N, Rubinstein R. *Practical Lessons in Endodontic Surgery*. Carol Stream, IL: Quintessence Publishing Co.; 1998.
48. Salehrabi R, Rotstein I. Endodontic treatment outcomes in a large patient population in the USA: an epidemiological study. *J Endod* 2004;30:846–850.
49. Doyle S, Hodges JS, Pesun IJ, et al. Factors affecting outcomes for single-tooth implants and endodontic restorations. *J Endod* 2007;33:399–402.
50. Iqbal M, Kim S. For teeth requiring endodontic treatment, what are the differences in outcomes of restored endodontically treated teeth compared to implant-supported restorations? *Int J Oral Maxillofac Implants* 2007;22(Suppl):96–116.

PART 5
ESTHETIC CHALLENGES OF MALOCCLUSION

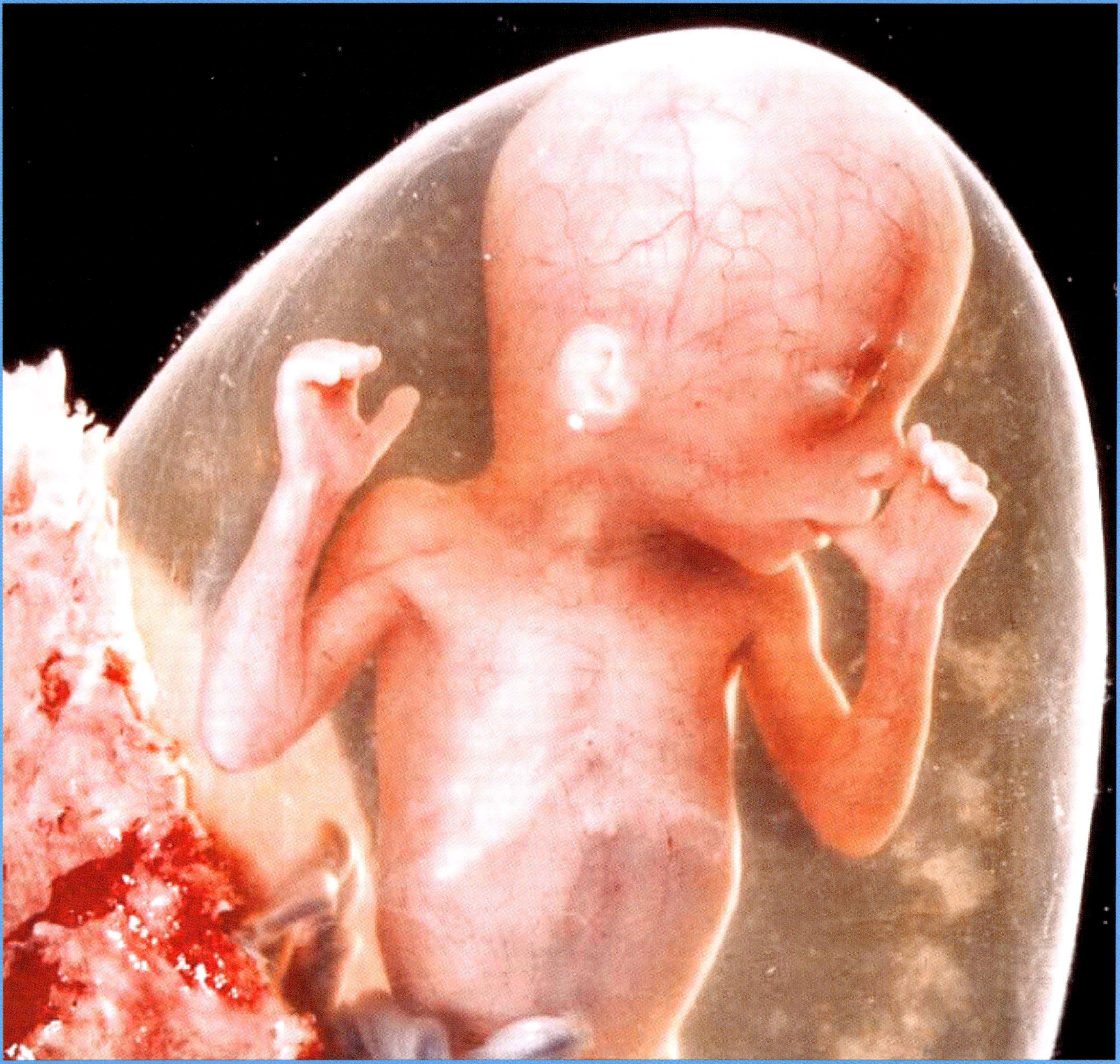

Chapter 25 Oral Habits

Ronald E. Goldstein, DDS, James W. Curtis Jr, DMD,
Beverly A. Farley, DMD*, and Daria Molodtsova, MS

Chapter Outline

Digit sucking	811	Fingernails	825
Negative adult oral habits	813	Pins placed between the teeth	825
Signs of destructive oral habits	813	Thread biting	826
Bruxism	814	Oral piercing and metal mouth jewelry	826
Bruxism with temporomandibular joint pain	815	Stim-u-dents or toothpicks used as wedges	826
Chewing habits	816	Incorrect use of dental floss and toothbrush	827
Tongue habits	816	Pen or pencil chewing	827
Lip or cheek biting	819	Pipe smoking	831
Mouth breathing	821	Eyeglasses or other objects held between the teeth	831
Eating disorders and poor dietary habits	822	Ice chewing	831
Alcohol and drug abuse	825	Cracking nuts with the teeth	833
Foreign objects in the mouth	825	Diagnosis and treatment of damaging oral habits	833

Oral habits can, and all too frequently do, cause esthetic and/or functional problems in the mouth. For this reason, destructive habits need to be diagnosed and corrected as early as possible. Most patients are unaware that their oral habits are causing permanent damage to their teeth, such as bruxism, holding their eyeglasses between their teeth, or chewing on ice. Adequate diagnosis of damaging habits requires a thorough evaluation of each patient's stomatognathic state. This must include examination of the form and function of the teeth and the status of the temporomandibular joints and related musculature.

Oral habits should be foremost in the examination and diagnosis of pediatric patients. Later in life, the permanent teeth and mouth should be carefully examined for changes related to oral habits that often occur in response to stress. Hygienists can play a key role in initially detecting wear patterns in teeth that could be arrested. Most people are surprised, but pleased, that their destructive habits can be stopped or the damage from them can be controlled. Dental procedures and corrective behavioral techniques may be helpful in breaking such oral habits. However, unless these habits are totally discontinued, treatment will inevitably serve as only a temporary measure.

Digit sucking

Digit sucking is a habit that usually begins and ends in childhood (Figure 25.1). Failure to stop this behavior can result in adult arch deformities that make correction more difficult (Figure 25.2A–C).

* Deceased

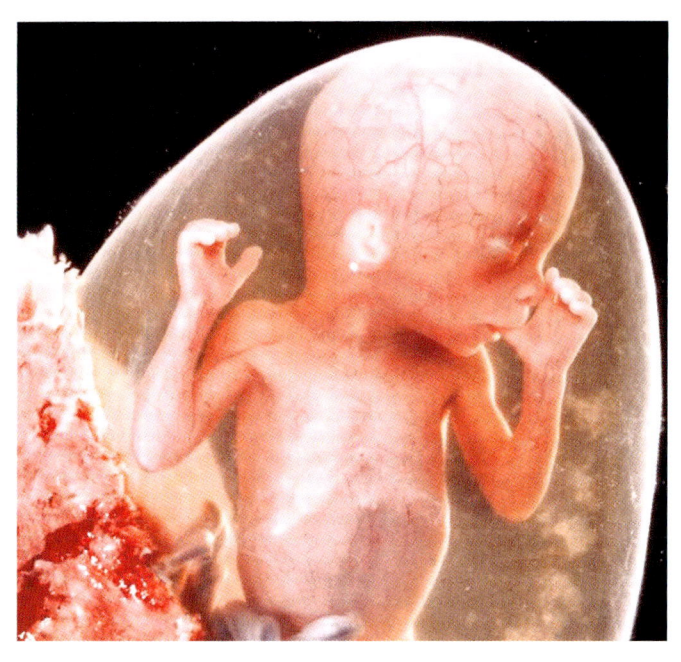

Figure 25.1 This unusual photograph demonstrates the early age (18-week-old fetus) at which thumb sucking may be manifested. Whereas many habits may be acquired, some seem to be genetically inbred, as evidenced in this magnificent photograph. Reproduced with permission from Nilsson.[1]

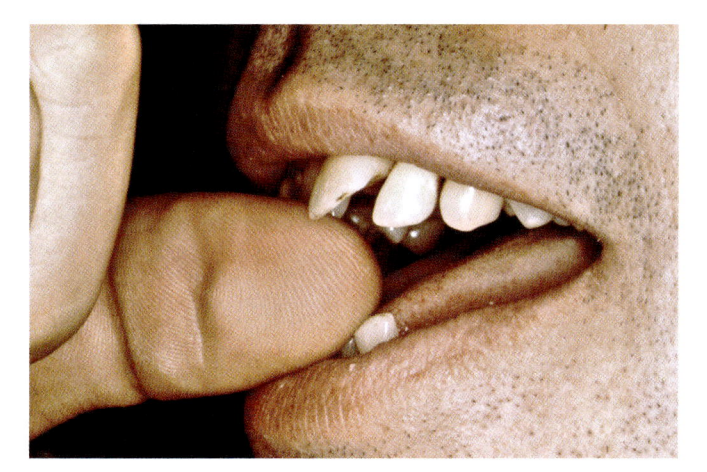

Figure 25.2 **(A)** This 33-year-old education director told of sucking his thumb as a child, which graduated into a finger-biting habit. Note the position of the thumb during the biting habit.

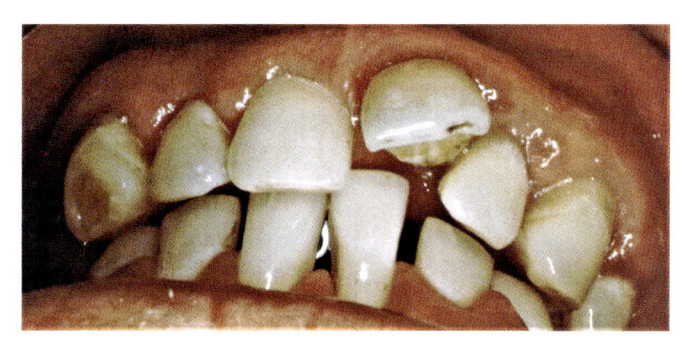

Figure 25.2 **(B)** Both maxillary and mandibular left central incisors are in labioversion as a result of the finger-biting habit.

It is estimated that roughly 4 of 10 children between the ages of birth and 16 years of age engage in digit sucking at some time during their lives. This habit may also involve several digits or fist sucking as well. Chandler, in 1878, was among the first dentists to correlate thumb- and finger-sucking habits with specific facial deformities.[2] He felt that displacement of teeth, as well as frequent elongation and narrowing of the bones of the nose, resulted from this habit. Much attention has been given to this widespread habit and the adverse dental effects that prolonged frequent digit sucking can produce. Digit sucking may damage the primary dentition and contribute to an atypical resorption pattern of maxillary primary central incisors.[3,4] Detailed reviews of the effects of prolonged thumb and finger sucking on the dental, soft-tissue, and skeletal structures have been written by numerous authors.[5–11] These orofacial malformations are usually unesthetic and may cause malocclusion and speech dysfunction. What is striking about the anomalies described in such abundance in the pediatric dentistry and orthodontic literature is the frequency with which some self-correction occurs if the behavior can be stopped.

For example, Larsson has presented the results of longitudinal studies of children using lateral cephalometric radiographs and observation of the occlusion.[6–8] In the younger children, thumb sucking increased the incidence of open bite with proclined and protruded maxillary incisors, a lengthened maxillary dental arch, and anteriorly displaced maxillary base. He found that finger sucking frequently caused a unilateral abnormal molar relationship on the sucking side of the mouth when the child consistently sucked a thumb. Finger sucking was also an important etiologic factor in the development of a posterior cross-bite in the primary dentition. However, if the children stopped thumb sucking, these malocclusions were somewhat corrected by increased growth of the alveolar process and the eruption of the incisors. Similarly, others have found a tendency to an open bite and an elongated maxillary arch length among children with

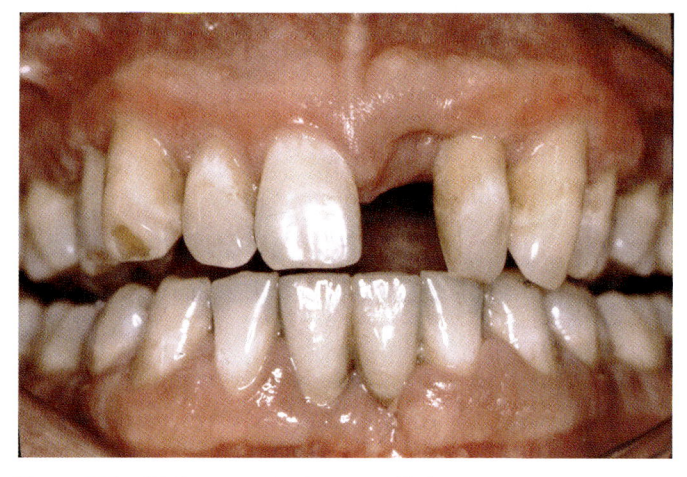

Figure 25.2 **(C)** Treatment in this type of habit sometimes consists of orthodontics and/or prosthodontics, depending on whether bone loss is present. Since there was considerable bone loss in this patient, treatment consisted of extraction of maxillary and mandibular left central incisors, plus additional periodontal therapy. Maxillary and mandibular resin bonded fixed partial dentures followed.

strong sucking habits between ages 7 and 16 years.[11-13] The dental effects of the thumb sucking were primarily in the anterior region of the mouth, with 80% of the children shoving the tongue over the lower incisors during swallowing. Eliminating the sucking habit tended to produce spontaneous closure of the open bite and cessation of the tongue thrust.

Bowden found yet other disturbances in persistent thumb suckers: significant increases in the proportion of the protrusive maxillary dental base relationships, tongue thrust activities, tongue-to-lip resting positions, and open bite tendencies.[14] Haryett et al. noted crowding of the mandibular incisors and facial asymmetries resulting from tooth interferences in the molar area because of maxillary contraction from sucking.[15] Infante's study of preschool children found posterior lingual cross-bite and protrusive position of the maxillary molars relative to the mandibular molars to be more prevalent and pronounced among those children who were thumb suckers.[16] Popovich and Thompson concluded that, as the habit persisted, the probability increased that a child would develop a Class II malocclusion.[17] In each of these studies, the problems appeared to diminish in prevalence and severity as digit sucking declined, usually occurring naturally as the child grew older.

Massler believes that some of these displacements can be self-corrected by the molding action of normal labial and lingual musculature once thumb sucking is discontinued. For example, the continued and forceful placement of the thumb against the long axis of the erupting tooth may temporarily displace the erupting anterior teeth.[18] Massler suggested that more marked protrusions probably have a genetic basis. Although this protrusive tendency can be maximized by thumb-sucking behaviors, it can also manifest itself in children who have never been habitual digit suckers.

In addition to the orofacial effects caused by digit sucking, other injuries may arise as a result of this habit. Rayan and Turner described hand complications that may develop from prolonged digit sucking.[19]

Because thumb sucking is such an obvious oral habit, and perhaps because it occurs at a time when parental attention is most focused on the child, the general public has taken part in a sometimes acrimonious open debate over the possible permanent effect of the habit. The debate extends to when, or even if, the parent and/or dentist should intervene. In the 1930s and 1940s, pediatricians, pediatric dentists, and parents were frequently united in their battle against thumb sucking to prevent malocclusion. Infants were sometimes wrapped in elbow cuffs or had the sleeves of their nightgowns tied to prevent fingers from reaching their mouth. However, as Massler described, the result was "that we now are treating a generation of tongue suckers with anterior open bites and lip suckers with the so-called mentalis habit."[18] These habits, he pointed out, persist much longer than thumb sucking and are considerably more difficult to discontinue.

The accepted wisdom of our own age is that most children give up sucking by the age of 3–7 years. Until a child passes this age, it is just as well, and much simpler, to avoid intervention. There is much agreement that digit-sucking habits are unlikely to produce permanent damage to the orofacial structures if the habits are abandoned by 4–5 years of age. Beyond this period, the likelihood of harmful effects is increased. At that time, the help of a behavioral therapist or psychiatrist may be warranted. Techniques available for eliminating the habit include (1) prevention of the habit, (2) positive reinforcement, and (3) aversive conditioning methods.

Management of the habit should involve enlisting the parent and child in a cooperative effort to stop the digit sucking.[20-22] Treatment may require the insertion of a fixed intraoral appliance to stop the sucking activity. For example, a palatal crib appliance blocks the habitual placement of the thumb, alleviates the suction stimuli, and works to restrain the tongue from thrusting against the incisors.

Negative adult oral habits

None of us outgrows the need for oral gratification. Few adults lack some type of learned oral habit to meet these needs. Levitas explains that an action repeated constantly becomes a habit.[23] Usually, the original stimulus or cause quickly becomes lost in the unconscious. Because the need for oral gratification never quite disappears, even as adults, the most common of the unconscious habits center in and around the mouth.

It is the dentist's responsibility to detect habits that are destructive. Unlike children, adult patients seldom make your task easier by displaying the action. Most often, you cannot look for the habit itself but rather only the byproducts of the habit. Unfortunately, by the time the problems are visible, the habit has been present for a long time and is fairly ingrained. This is even more reason for vigilance in detection. Evaluate the patient's stomatognathic state, including examination of the teeth in form and function and the temporomandibular joints and related musculature.

Signs of destructive oral habits

The following are signs that reveal destructive occlusal habit patterns:

- Loss of enamel contour, especially on the incisal edges of the anterior teeth.
- A change in the smile line over the years. This can be observed by asking the patient for earlier photographs beginning at age 13 or 14 years and studying the progressive facial changes. An 8× loop should magnify photographs enough to see these changes.
- Changes in vertical dimension showing facial collapse.
- Wear facets that are destroying the natural esthetic contour of the teeth. In particular, any change in the canine's silhouette form should be noted.
- Newly apparent spaces in the mouth or the enlargement of previously existing spaces.
- Newly flared, erupted, or submerged teeth.
- Ridges, lumps, or masses in the tissue of the tongue, lips, or inside the mouth.

Bruxism

The most damaging, most frequently seen, and most frequently missed of all of the destructive oral habits is bruxism, which can destroy the form and integrity of the incisal edges of the anterior teeth (Figure 25.3A).

Esthetic treatment of the ravages of bruxism first involves habit correction control and or treatment. Second, if possible, restore the lost tooth form with bonding, veneering, or crowning combined with cosmetic contouring (Figure 25.3B) of the opposing teeth.[24-27] This usually consists of beveling the opposing teeth and replacement of the worn tooth structure. Sinuocclusal pathways must remain the same; try not to contour areas that are involved in excursive movement. If it is not possible to restore missing tooth structure, it may be possible to restore esthetics through cosmetic contouring. Also, if the anterior teeth have worn evenly, reshape the laterals to create more interincisal distance. This technique can be effective in achieving an illusion of greater incisal length, thus providing enhanced esthetics.

Bruxism may be a learned behavior that is a reaction to stress associated with various dental or medical conditions, such as malocclusions, missing or rough teeth, infections, malnutrition, and allergies.[28-33] These conditions may contribute to the extent to which bruxism is manifested (Figure 25.4A and B). Studies by Hicks and colleagues showing an increase in bruxism among college students implicated stress as a major etiologic factor.[31,34]

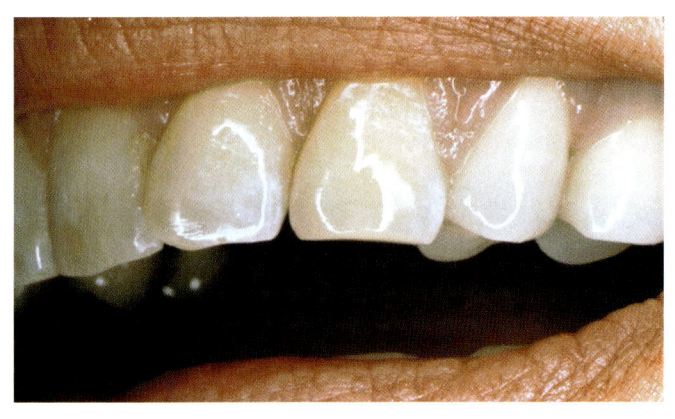

Figure 25.3 **(A)** This 30-year-old teacher had worn her left canine flat due to bruxism.

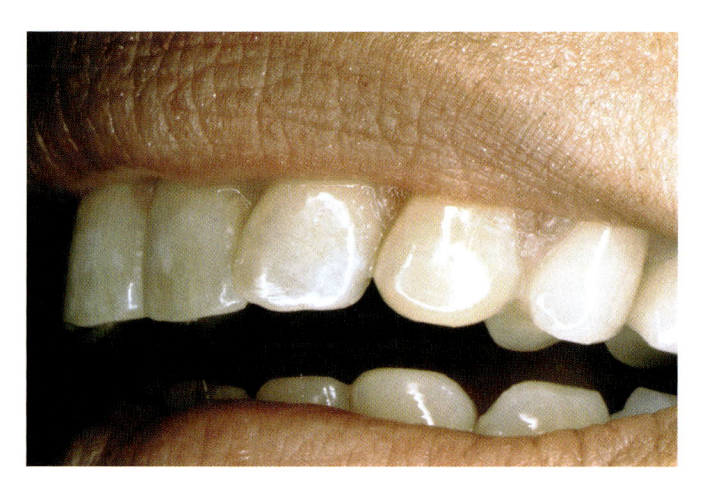

Figure 25.3 **(B)** After treatment for the condition, which consisted of appliance therapy, the anteriors were cosmetically contoured rather than adding to the tooth surface. In cases like this, it is important for the patient to wear an appliance afterward to make certain that additional bruxism will no longer destroy enamel.

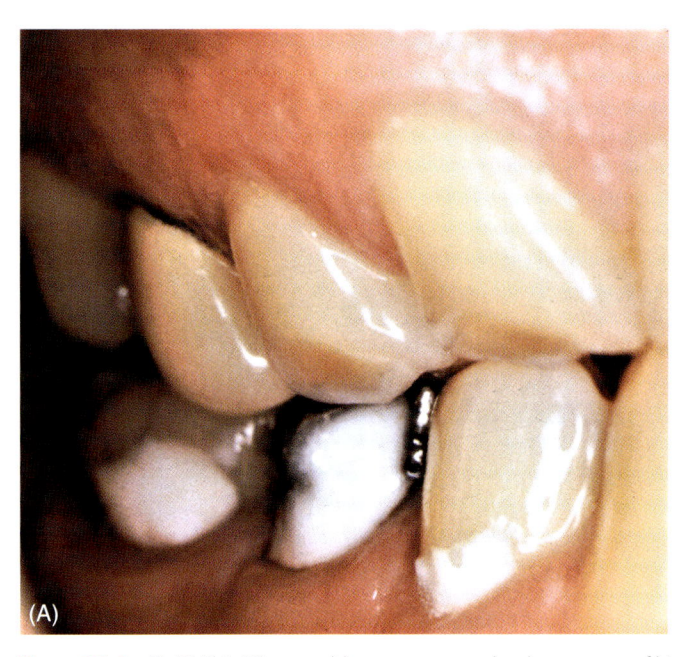

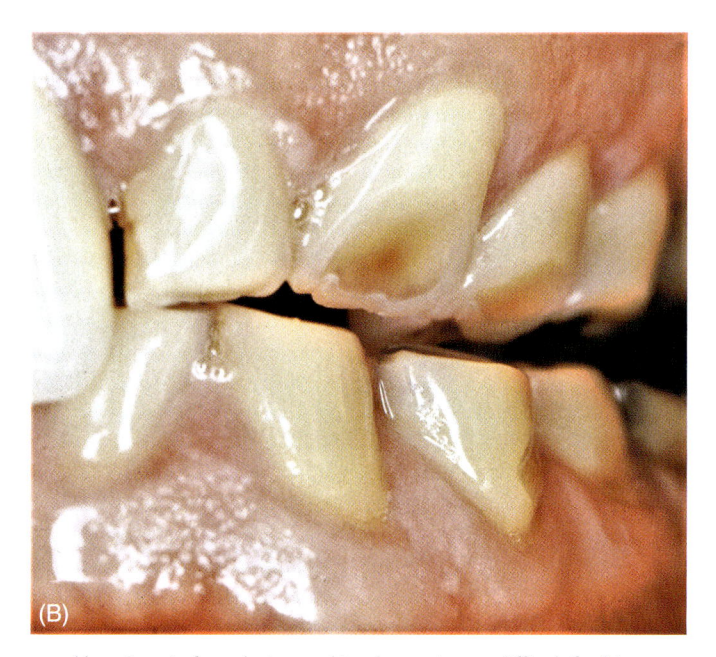

Figure 25.4 **(A, B)** This 50-year-old man was completely unaware of his nocturnal bruxism. In fact, during waking hours, it was difficult for him to get his teeth to fit together in the eccentric position.

Cigarette smoking has been shown to exacerbate nocturnal bruxism.[9,35] Numerous reports have shown bruxism to be related to sleep disorders and sleep apnea.[36–39]

Bruxism can sometimes begin after orthodontic treatment for crowded teeth. After incisors are realigned, the patient can develop a habit of clinching and grinding in the anterior region that can eventually destroy incisal anatomy.

Bruxism with temporomandibular joint pain

Esthetic destruction of the patient's teeth can be sufficient to enable us to recognize the disease process of temporomandibular joint pain long before the patient actually begins treatment.[40–48]

The following case illustrates this position. A young woman had been treated without success by several physicians for headaches, dizzy spells, and neck, back, and shoulder pain (Figure 25.5A–E). Her problems with pain, as well as with the destruction of her teeth, appeared to be related to her bruxism. When asked to open her mouth, she deviated sharply to one side. The intraoral muscles (pterygoid and masseter) and ligaments were in acute spasm and tender to palpitation. Treatment began with insertion of a maxillary bruxing appliance. (With bruxism patients, it is important to obtain study casts to determine if there are wear facets, where they are located, and why they occurred.) The bruxing appliance was constructed to help stop the incisal wear. The patient's teeth were then reshaped to improve the smile line. Most pain and headaches stopped within a period of 3–6 weeks after the insertion of this appliance, together with muscle therapy to the affected areas.

The patient must realize the importance of continuing to wear the bruxing appliance to maintain the esthetic correction and to avoid reintroducing temporomandibular joint pain and dysfunction.[49]

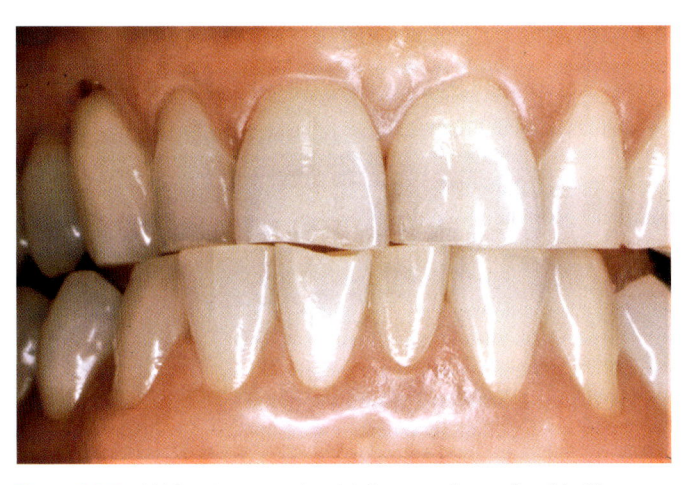

Figure 25.5 **(A)** Bruxism was the chief cause of wear for this 31-year-old woman.

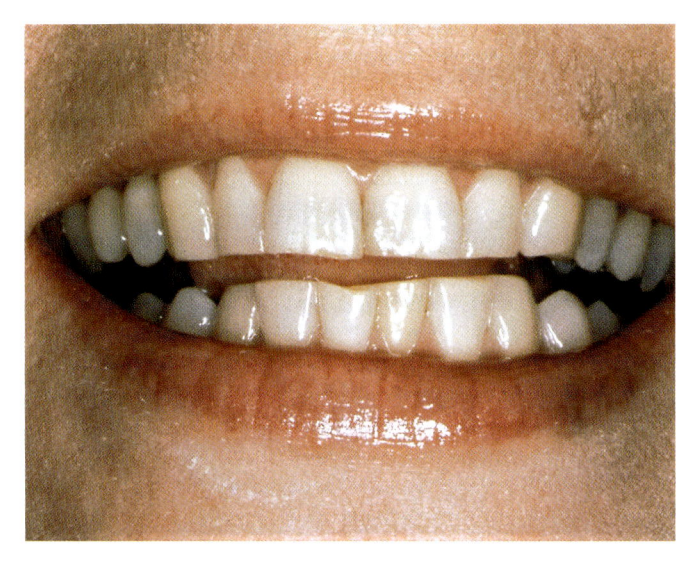

Figure 25.5 **(B)** Note how she would unconsciously put the tongue behind the front teeth to hide the space that shows a jagged outline. In addition to poor esthetics, the patient also suffered constant headaches and neck and back discomfort because of further temporomandibular joint dysfunction.

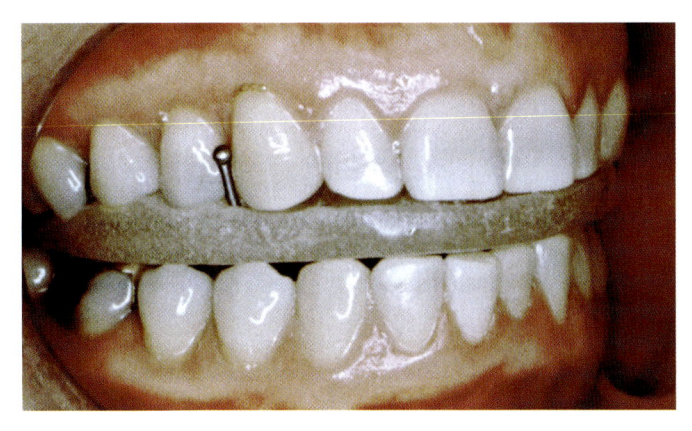

Figure 25.5 **(C)** A removable appliance was made to correct the temporomandibular joint dysfunction and prevent teeth from further wearing away. Following 3 months of temporomandibular joint treatment to cure the symptoms and relax the muscles, the patient wore the appliance only at night.

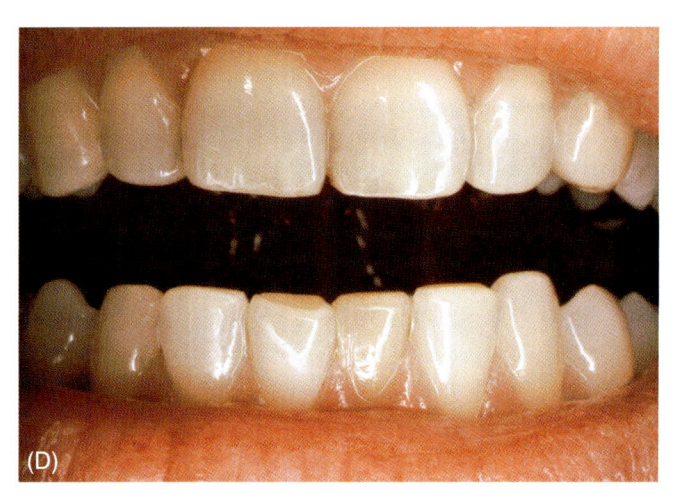

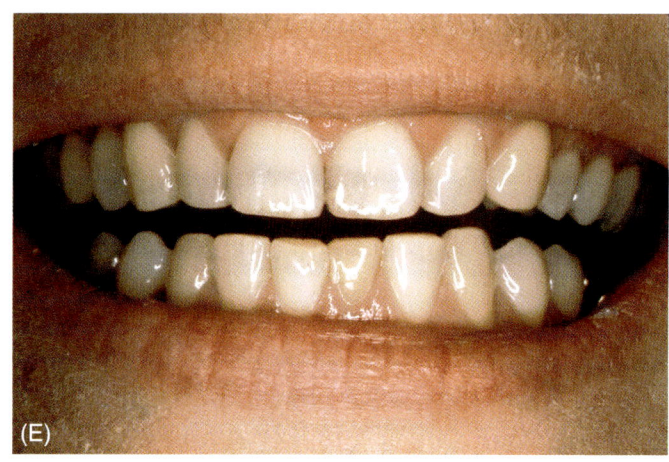

Figure 25.5 (D, E) After several months of appliance therapy, the square, masculine-looking upper and lower teeth were cosmetically contoured to produce a more feminine and attractive smile.

Chewing habits

The use of smokeless tobacco is another habit that causes excessive wear on the dentition, in addition to the potential of causing oral cancer.[50–52] The lingual cusps of maxillary teeth and buccal cusps of mandibular teeth are the most affected, often worn to the gingival margin. Staining of exposed dentin is also readily apparent.

Dark brown/black stains on the teeth, marked abrasion of anterior teeth, and pathologic changes of the oral mucosa are seen in many eastern countries, such as India, Malaysia, and Thailand, in those who chew betel nuts for medicinal and/or psychological purposes[53–55] (Figure 25.6). Patients who refuse or cannot stop the habit should be on monthly "cosmetic" cleanings. This type of prophylaxis is most readily accomplished using a high-powered, mildly abrasive spray. These patients should be warned that the sharp edges of the betel nut may cut the gingiva, leading to ulceration. In addition, the betel nut contains carcinogens that can lead to the development of oral cancer in habitual users. Coca leaf chewing was shown to cause similar effects on the dentition in ancient cultures.[56]

Tongue habits

The tongue is one of the strongest muscles in the human body. The most frequent signs of tongue thrust are protrusion of the tongue against or between the anterior teeth and excessive circumoral muscle activity during swallowing. Although pushing the tongue against teeth, particularly between spaces in the teeth, does not invariably cause harm, it is certainly a potential cause of damage. Either maxillary or mandibular teeth can become involved (Figure 25.7). Indentations in the tongue have been reported to provide an indication of clenching.[57] Gellin, however, feels that anterior tongue positioning does improve with time, and the continual growth and development of the lower face allow for diminishing anterior tongue positioning.[20] Various studies showed the relationship between tongue thrust and malocclusion.[58–60]

There are clinicians who have observed a large number of patients with malocclusions who demonstrate a protrusive tongue tip pattern against or between the anterior teeth while speaking or swallowing. This group suggests that tongue thrusting is one of the primary etiologic factors in open bite and incisor protrusion. There is also much controversy concerning the use of removable appliances in the treatment of tongue twisting.

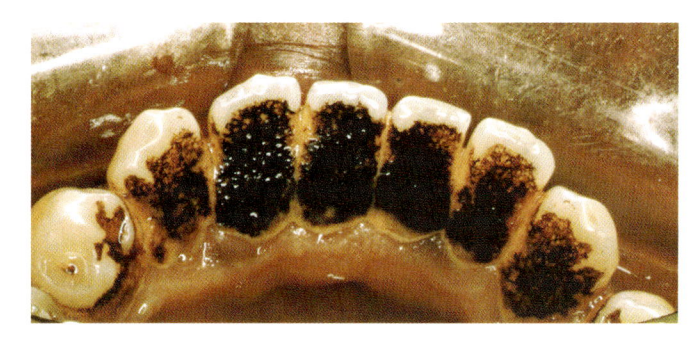

Figure 25.6 This 35-year-old male had the habit of placing betel nuts under his tongue, which helped to produce the black stain shown.

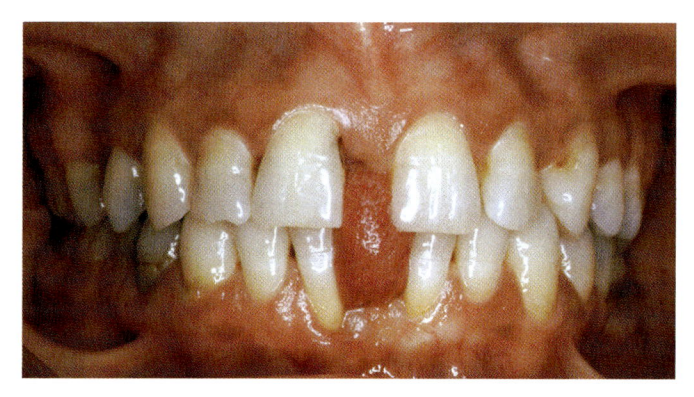

Figure 25.7 This 47-year-old teacher developed a habit of forcing her tongue between her maxillary and mandibular incisors. Note the large space created as a result of years of tongue pressure.

The young woman in Figure 25.8A and B would like to advance her modeling career, but a space between her teeth appears as a black hole in photographs. Consequently, she poses with her tongue pressed behind the space in her teeth in an attempt to hide the darkness. This trick helps with the photographic illusion, but if she presses her tongue too much in a labial direction, the space can increase over the years. The habit of putting the tongue between the teeth to disguise a space will almost certainly cause the space to increase with time (Figure 25.8C). Treatment of spaces between the teeth is usually best handled through orthodontic care and possibly myofunctional therapy to promote a more positive resting and swallowing tongue position. However, some patients may not mind, and may even prefer their teeth with a space. Although no space should be corrected without approval from the patient, even these patients need to be referred to an orthodontist for monitoring and control of any further widening that might have functional implications.

For those patients who desire closure of the diastema, referral to an orthodontist can determine if repositioning of the teeth is appropriate. In discussing the referral with the patient, make certain that it is understood that orthodontics does not need to be a matter of metal brackets. One of the most common solutions to gaps is the construction of a retainer that the patient wears at night. After the teeth have stabilized, the retainer can be worn a few nights each week to maintain tooth position and prevent reopening the space.

An alternative or compromise treatment consists of bonding composite resin to close the spaces. Crowns and porcelain veneers can also serve this function, but bonding has the advantage of reversibility. The patient could later elect to have orthodontic treatment, especially if the spaces continue to widen.

Sometimes, orthodontics may not be the patient's choice, and the following case illustrates an alternative, restorative means of treatment. The young man shown in Figure 25.9A–H was extremely self-conscious about a space between his central incisors caused by a tongue thrust. He was referred for orthodontics, both to correct the space and to correct his destructive habit. However, the appliance needed to correct the spacing between this young man's teeth gave him what he considered a freakish appearance, and he asked for an alternative treatment. Treatment was then planned using composite resins, which, although not permanent, produce immediate results.

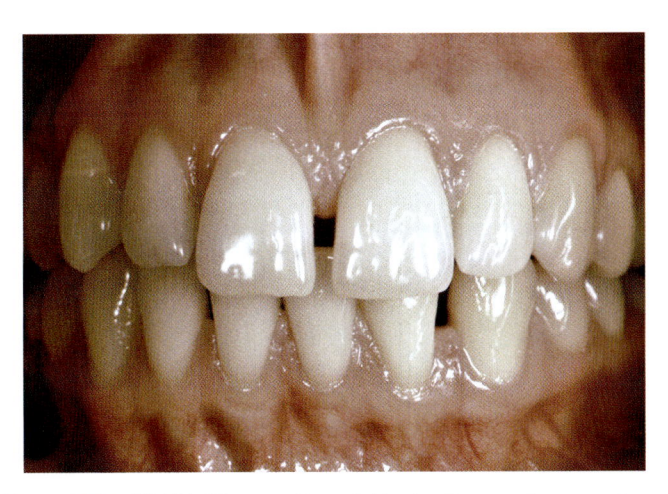

Figure 25.8 **(A)** This 23-year-old model had a diastema between the maxillary central incisors.

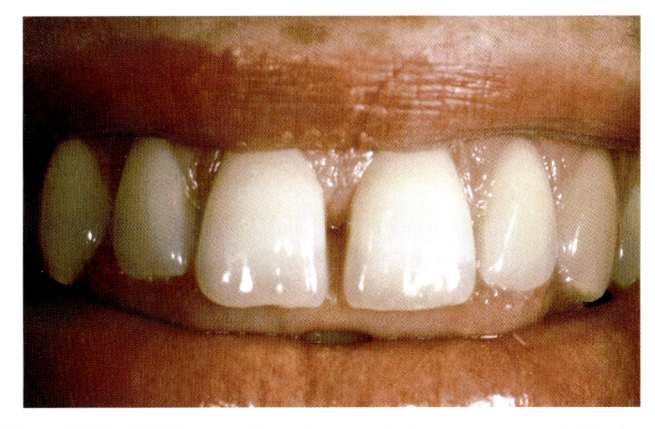

Figure 25.8 **(B)** When smiling, she would place her tongue behind the two front teeth to hide the space, which would otherwise show up dark. Note how the tongue creates a pink filler similar to gingival tissue. Many models unconsciously develop similar habits, which can create additional space because of the tongue pressure if done over a long period of time. It is much wiser to either close these spaces orthodontically or compromise with restorative means.

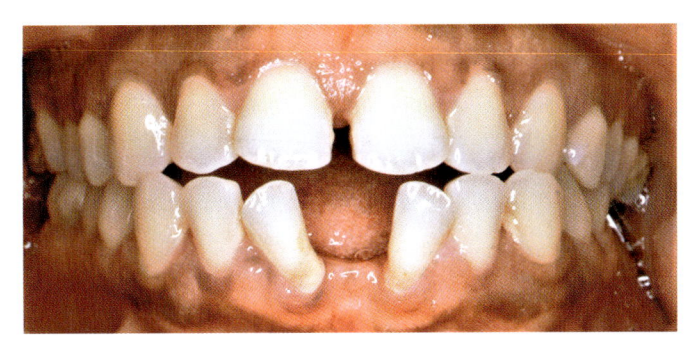

Figure 25.8 **(C)** The habit of placing the tongue between the teeth to disguise a space will almost certainly cause the space to increase with time.

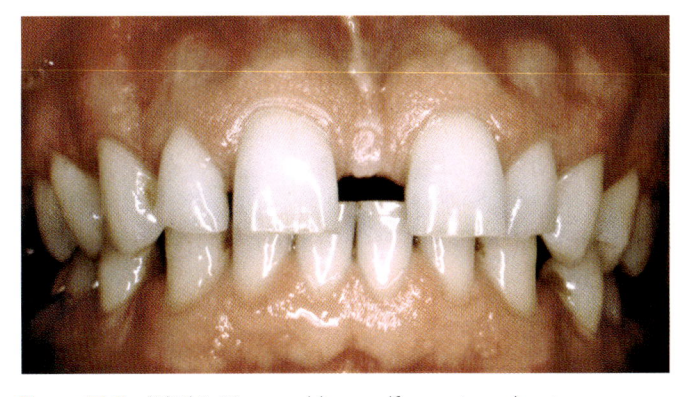

Figure 25.9 **(A)** This 32-year-old was self-conscious about a space between his front teeth that was originally caused by tongue thrusting.

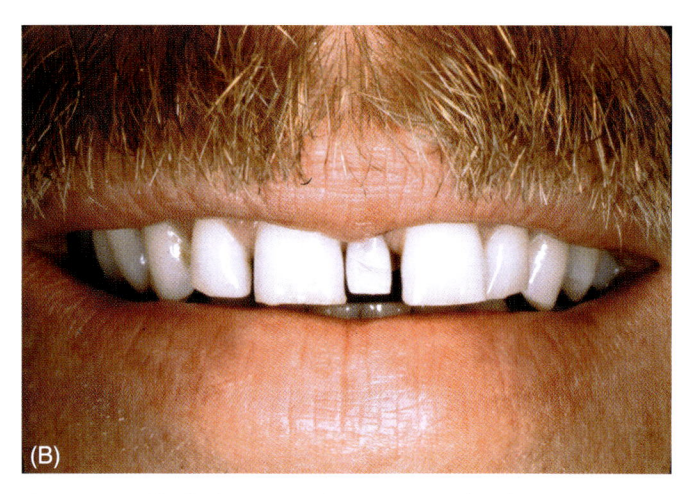

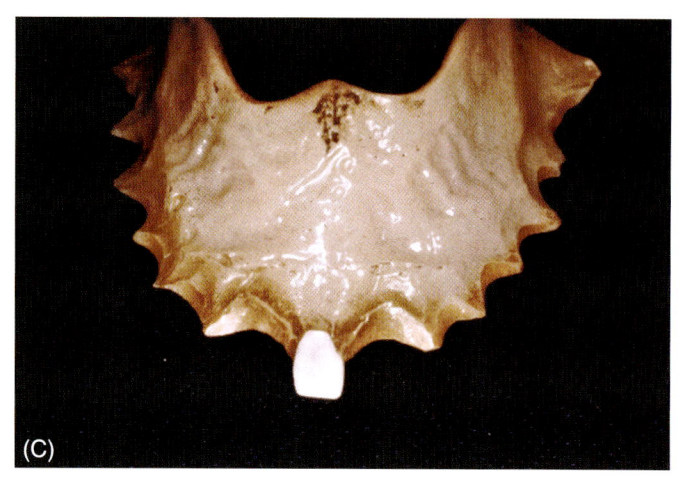

Figure 25.9 **(B, C)** The patient shown in 25.9A felt that people were noticing his smile, and since he did public speaking, he wanted to improve his appearance. This replacement had been in the mouth for 16 years.

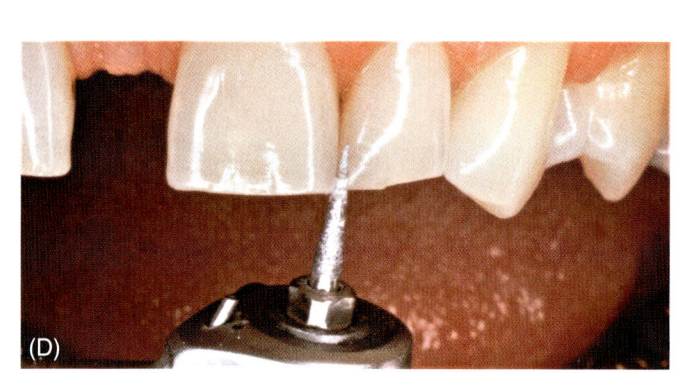

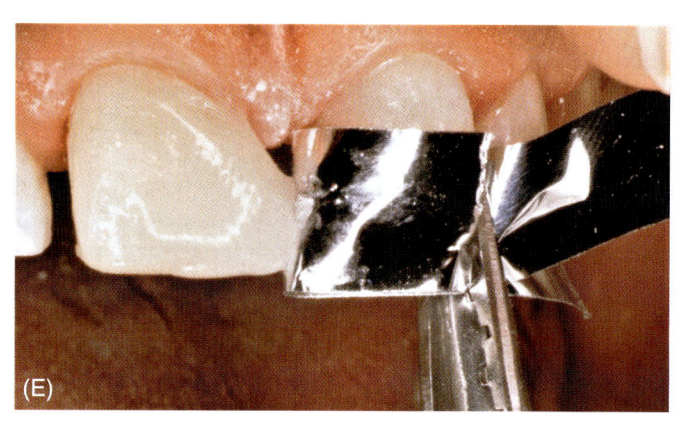

Figure 25.9 **(D, E)** The patient was referred for orthodontic consultation but elected to have composite resin bonding as a compromise treatment.

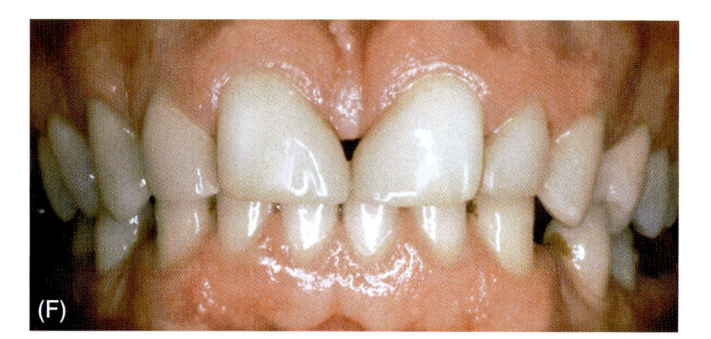

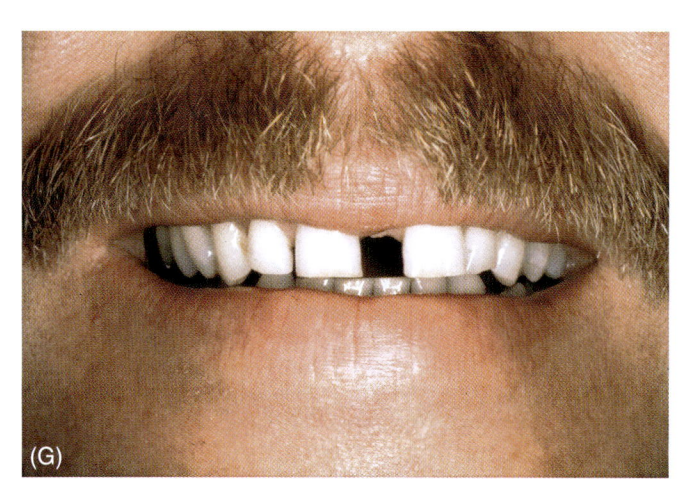

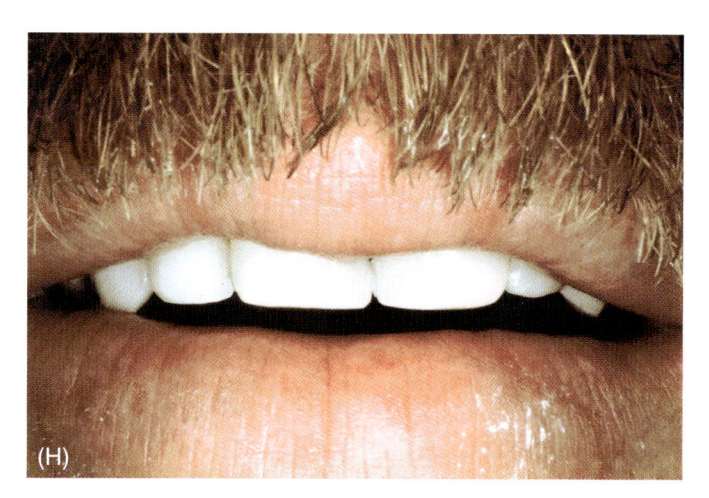

Figure 25.9 **(F–H)** Although closing the space created a disproportionate overbuilding of the two central incisors, through judicious carving of the finished bonded restorations, a more proportionate and not unattractive arrangement can be achieved. This consisted of opening the incisal embrasures, as well as creating a greater interincisal distance.

Lip or cheek biting

The signs of lip or cheek biting are usually telltale marks from the teeth (Figure 25.10A and B). Glass and Maize have described the appearance of oral tissues that have been chewed or bitten over a period of time.[61] This results in the appearance of hard fibrous knots or masses known as morsicatio buccarum et labiorum. Sometimes, the patient uses the teeth to suck or knead the altered tissue. If the habit continues over an extended period of time, it can also cause tooth abnormalities by enlarging any small diastema or interdental space. The more a patient chews or sucks, the more pressure is created between the teeth and the wider the space.

Other lip habits, such as lip wetting or lip sucking, and a swallowing pattern that includes a hyperactive mentalis muscle can cause damage to developing orofacial structures in children. Lip wetting is frequently unnoticed by the average dental practitioner. Clinically, the entire lip looks soft and moist and does not have a sharply demarcated vermilion border.

Cheek biting is one of the most frequently seen destructive oral habits and can reflect a circular pattern (Figure 25.10C). Sometimes, loss of part of a tooth or an entire tooth can initiate cheek biting. The presence of resulting fibrous tissue may cause the patient to pull the knot of tissue between the teeth and begin to suck. Diagnosis of cheek biting can be made by examining the inside border of the cheek for a flickered, sometimes white fibrous ridge midway between the arches.

Treatment of lip biters and cheek biters consists of several steps. The first usually involves reshaping the teeth to round, smooth, and polish any sharp edges. It is also important in working with such patients to find out if there has been any recent crowning, lengthening, or shortening of the teeth or other changes that might have induced this habit. If so, they may need to be modified.

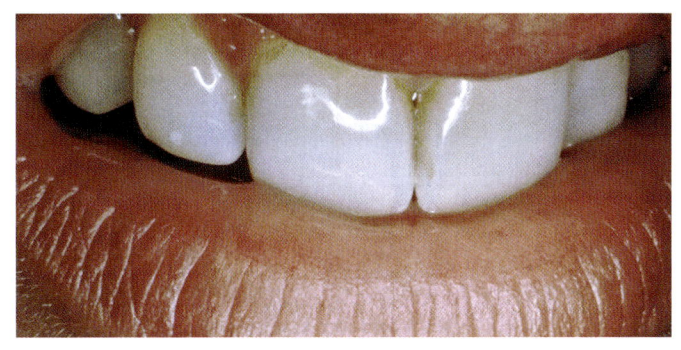

Figure 25.10 **(A)** This 29-year-old woman felt that her upper teeth were "growing down more" and irritating her lower lip. She was told to let us know exactly when she closed her lip and felt that it was fitting tightly into the teeth.

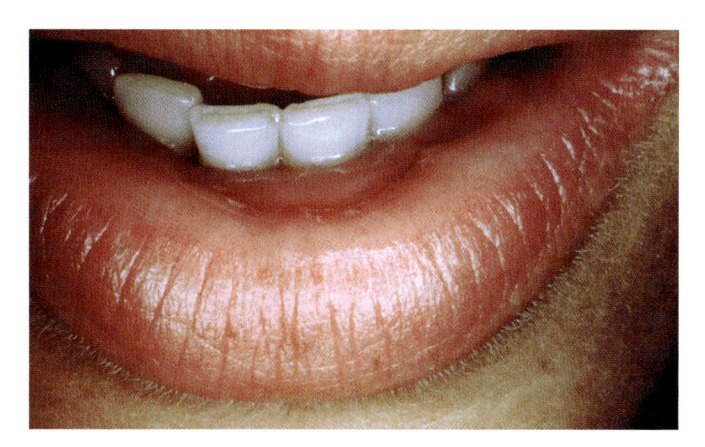

Figure 25.10 **(B)** During her next appointment, she stated that she realized that she is both sucking and biting down on her lip at the same time.

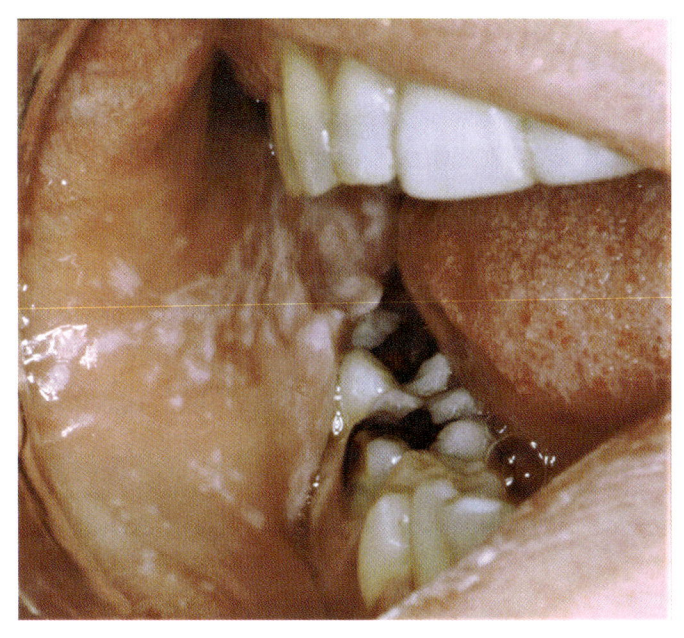

Figure 25.10 **(C)** This 50-year-old woman had a habit of biting her cheek. Note the pattern of white fibrous tissue.

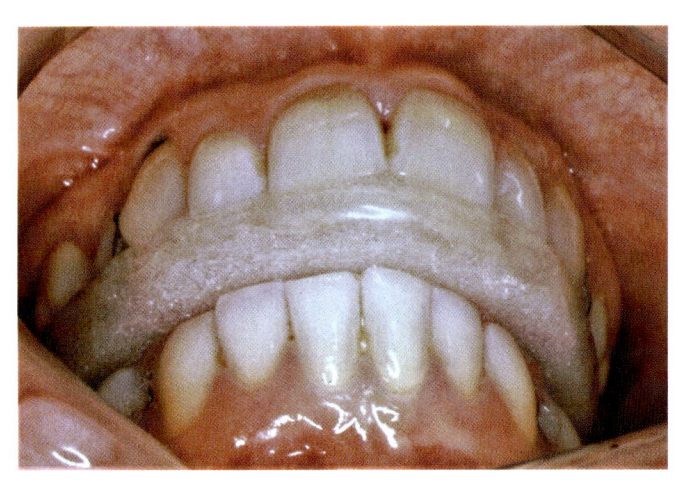

Figure 25.10 **(D)** Since her external pterygoid muscles were in spasm, it was also felt that she could be grinding her teeth, so an upper temporomandibular joint appliance was constructed, rounding the labial incisal angle in particular.

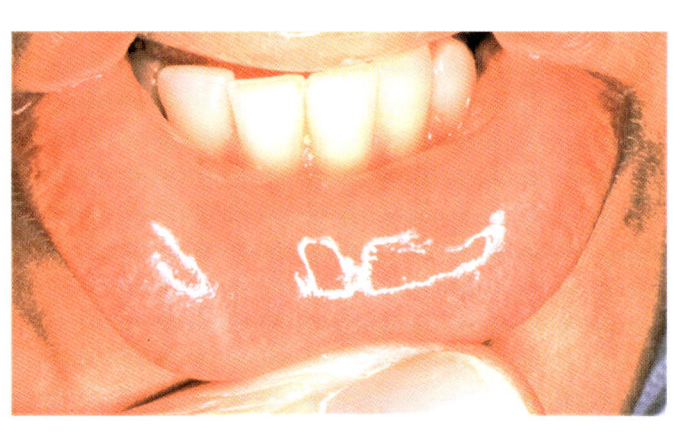

Figure 25.10 **(E)** After 5 months of wearing the appliance, at first all of the time and then at night only, the patient's tissue returned to normal. In addition, her muscle spasms disappeared, and all other symptoms subsided.

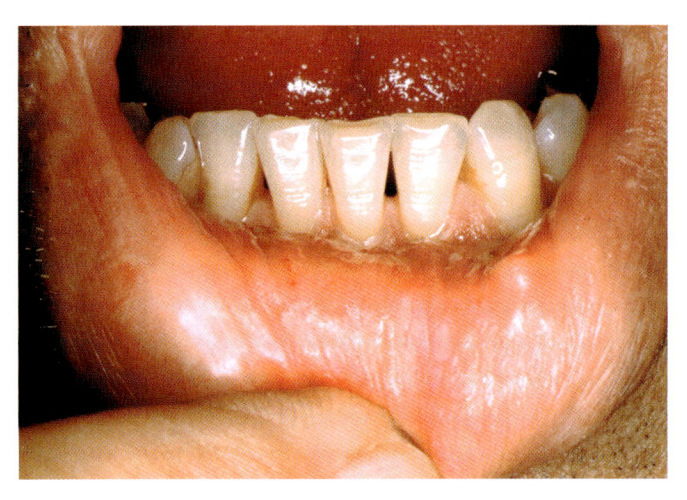

Figure 25.11 **(A)** This 50-year-old man had been sucking the lower left lip into an open interdental space between the mandibular left central and lateral. Note the lesion created on the lower left inner border of the lip due to the patient's sucking habit.

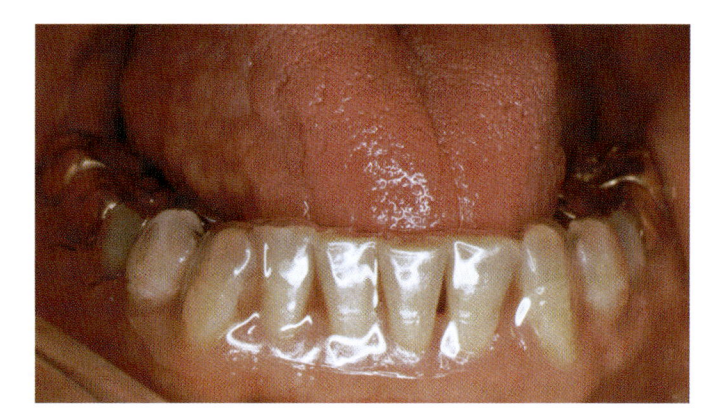

Figure 25.11 **(B)** A vacuform matrix was made to close up this area to see if the patient could break the sucking habit. Unfortunately, the only time the patient could eliminate the habit of sucking was when the appliance was being worn.

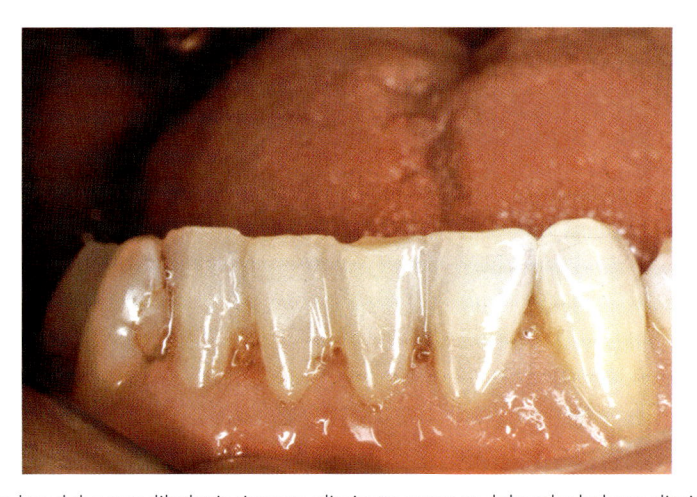

Figure 25.11 **(C)** It was decided to bond the mandibular incisors to eliminate space and thereby help to eliminate his sucking habit. Had the patient been able to alleviate the habit with the matrix, it would have been possible to eliminate the need for closure of this space.

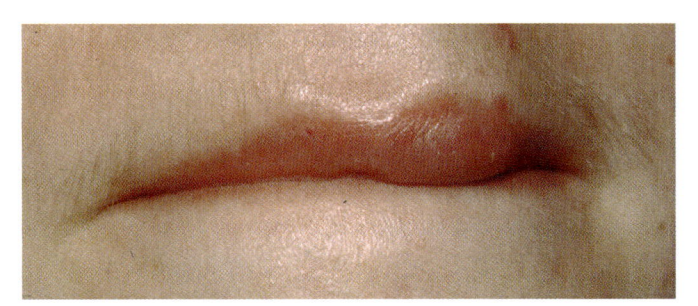

Figure 25.12 **(A)** This young lady developed a habit of sucking her upper lip.

The second part of treatment usually involves creating an appliance to prevent the patient from biting the lip or cheek (Figure 25.10D and E).[62] This should be as thick as feasible and rounded on the labial surface. As a temporary measure, a removable acrylic interdental spacer or a vacuform matrix can be used to prevent the patient from biting or sucking (Figure 25.11A–C).

One of the added advantages of such devices, which are worn around the clock during the early phases of treatment, is that they make the patient more aware of the intensity and frequency of such habits and the circumstances under which they most often manifest themselves. Many patients are not aware that they bite or suck their lips or cheeks, especially in relation to stress. Once the patient stops biting the lip, the use of the appliance can be reduced to evenings only. Most patients will require between 3 and 6 months to correct the problem (Figure 25.12A–D).

Finally, any space between the teeth can be corrected via orthodontics or the application of composite resin bonding or porcelain veneers to close the diastema (see Figure 25.11C). The use of full crowns would be a third choice to close the space.

Mouth breathing

Common in childhood, mouth breathing is the habit of using the mouth instead of the nose for respiration regardless of whether the nose is obstructed. However, there are often specific reasons

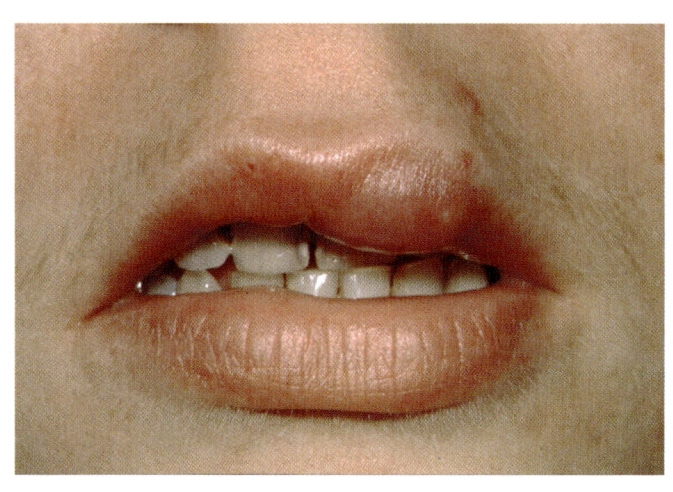

Figure 25.12 **(B)** A bulbous lesion was the result of the constant suction action that prompted the patient to seek treatment only for the lip but not the obvious caries. *Source:* Reproduced with permission from Goldstein.[63]

for mouth breathing, such as allergies, enlarged nasopharyngeal lymphoid tissues, and asthma.[64–67] The prevailing hypothesis is that prolonged mouth breathing during certain critical growth periods in childhood causes a sequence of events that results in dental and skeletal changes. Excessive eruption of the molars is almost always a constant feature of chronic mouth breathing. This molar eruption causes clockwise rotation of the mandible during growth, with a resultant increase in lower facial height. The increased lower facial height is often associated with retrognathia and anterior open bites. Low tongue posture is seen with mouth breathing and impedes the lateral expansion and anterior development of the maxilla.[68–79] The dentofacial effects that develop in children persist into adulthood, and the mouth-breathing and tongue-thrusting behavior may continue. Barber has found that mouth breathing can lead to dryness and

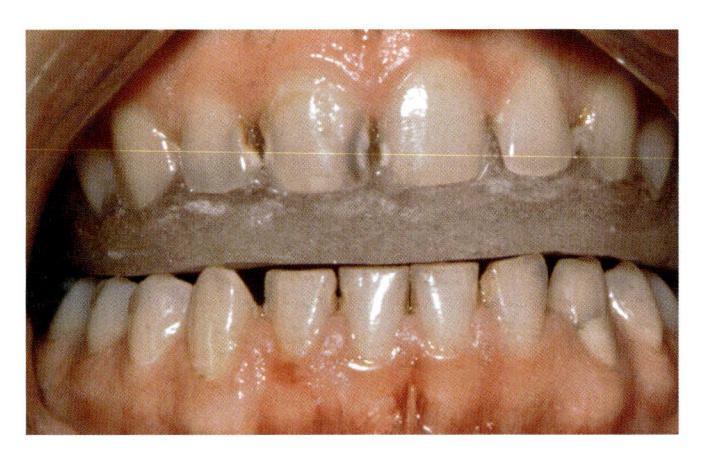

Figure 25.12 **(C)** A removable maxillary appliance was made for the patient to wear full time until she completely broke the habit. Note also advanced caries, which needed to be treated.

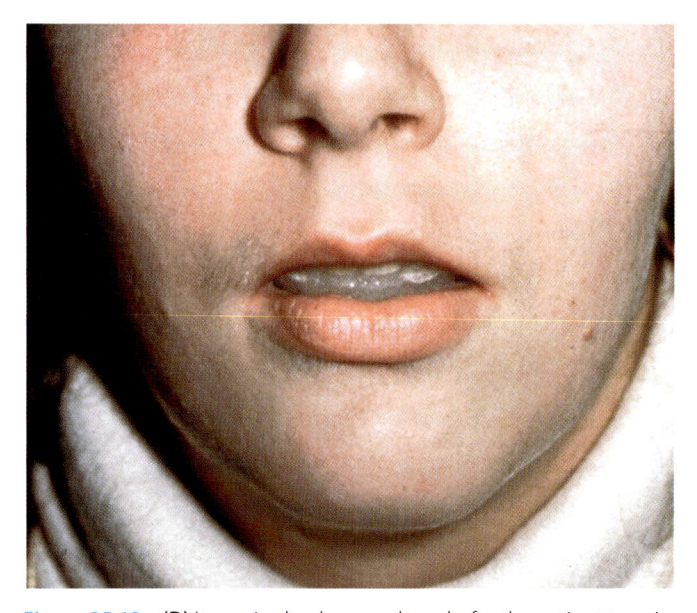

Figure 25.12 **(D)** It required only several weeks for the patient to gain back her normal-appearing lip. Then the patient could focus her attention on her other dental treatment.

irritation of the throat, mouth, and lips, as well as chronic marginal gingivitis.[80] Also, it is strongly associated with both lip-biting and lip-wetting habits. It may be necessary to treat the mouth-breathing habit prior to or in conjunction with the treatment of the lip habit.

Eating disorders and poor dietary habits

Anorexia nervosa and bulimia are psychosomatic eating disorders that have associated oral symptoms. The exact prevalence of these eating disorders is unknown. However, they are most frequently seen in young women, ranging from adolescence into early adulthood. In some studies,[81–84] it has been estimated that eating disorders affect up to 20% of the women on college campuses. As our culture continues to emphasize outward appearance, it is likely that this problem will not resolve soon. Dentists are often the first health-care professionals to recognize the signs of eating disorders, particularly bulimia. It may well be that the obsession to improve outward appearances that drives some individuals to develop eating disorders may also fuel their desire for esthetic dental services. Thus, practices that have a strong emphasis on esthetic care should be diligent in assessing their patients, especially young women, for signs of eating disorders.

The bulimic patient ingests large amounts of food, followed by voluntary or involuntary purging. The purging may occur with the use of high doses of laxatives or induced vomiting. In those bulimics who purge by vomiting, the pH of the gastric acid is low enough to initiate dissolution of the enamel. Further compounding the problem is the frequent vigorous tooth brushing that is used to rid the mouth of the taste and telltale odor of the vomitus. Brushing the teeth immediately after they have been exposed to gastric acids will accelerate the loss of enamel. Numerous studies show that a high percentage of patients seen with bulimia exhibit lingual erosion of the maxillary anterior teeth caused by regurgitation of gastric acids (Figure 25.13A–D).[85–89] If the disorder persists, the erosion will eventually affect the occlusal surfaces of the molars and premolars. If the bulimia is not controlled, the entire dentition may be destroyed, necessitating complete dental rehabilitation with full-coverage restorations.

Unfortunately, if the habit persists after the rehabilitation, these patients are likely to develop recurrent caries around the margins of the crowns.

Patients with anorexia nervosa pose an entirely different set of problems. Although bulimia and anorexia are disorders that involve a severely altered self-perception, individuals with anorexia may tend to fully lose self-esteem and fall into a state of total oral neglect. In its severest form, patients with anorexia may present with rampant caries and notably dry mucosa (Figure 25.14A–C). They are very prone to the effects of metabolic imbalance and should be treated cautiously in the dental office.

In addition to the intraoral ravages of bulimia and anorexia, outwardly visible signs of these disorders can be seen. Figure 25.15 shows a 35-year-old female who suffered from both bulimia and anorexia. Notice the swelling of the parotid gland, clearly seen at the angle of the mandible. This hypertrophy of the gland is commonly seen in bulimics. It is caused by repeated vomiting and is present bilaterally. Also, on close examination of the photograph, a fine, downy facial hair can be detected. This facial hair is called lanugo and may be found in anorexics.

The dental manifestations of eating disorders can be treated immediately, but treatment must be limited to emergency, preventive, and/or temporary measures until the disorder is brought under control. Preventive measures to reduce the damaging effects of gastric acids can be immediately employed. The first measure is to have the individual refrain from brushing the teeth after vomiting. Second, oral rinses to reduce the pH in the mouth can be extremely helpful. Water can be used to rid the mouth of the acids that are present. If available, sodium bicarbonate (baking soda) rinses can neutralize the acidity in the mouth following an episode of vomiting. Various topical fluoride preparations will aid in minimizing the acidic destruction of the enamel and dentin. Because of the psychosomatic nature of anorexia and bulimia, it is imperative for the dentist to approach these patients in a factual, nonconfrontational, concerned manner that will encourage them to seek proper medical attention.

People who habitually eat or suck on lemons or drink large amounts of lemon-flavored water may exhibit acid erosion (Figure 25.16A and B). This erosion is seen on the labial surfaces

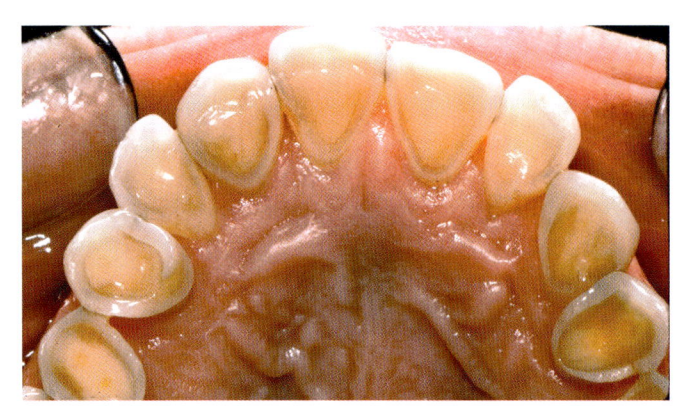

Figure 25.13 **(A)** Preoperative upper anterior palatal view of a bulimic patient shows extreme erosion of the lingual and occlusal surfaces. *Source:* Figure courtesy of Dr Vincent Celenza.

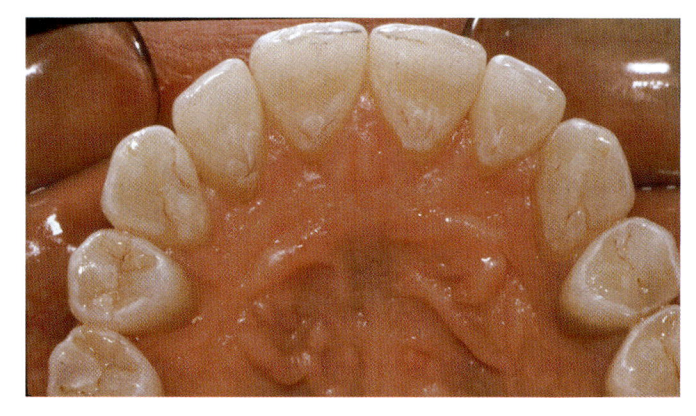

Figure 25.13 **(B)** Final restorations in place. *Source:* Figure courtesy of Dr Vincent Celenza.

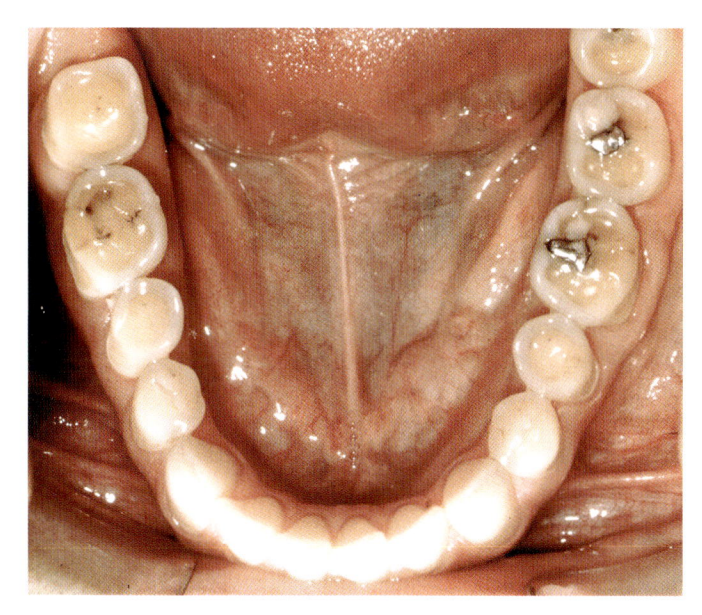

Figure 25.13 **(C)** Preoperative occlusal view of the lower arch showing extreme occlusal acid erosion. *Source:* Figure courtesy of Dr Vincent Celenza.

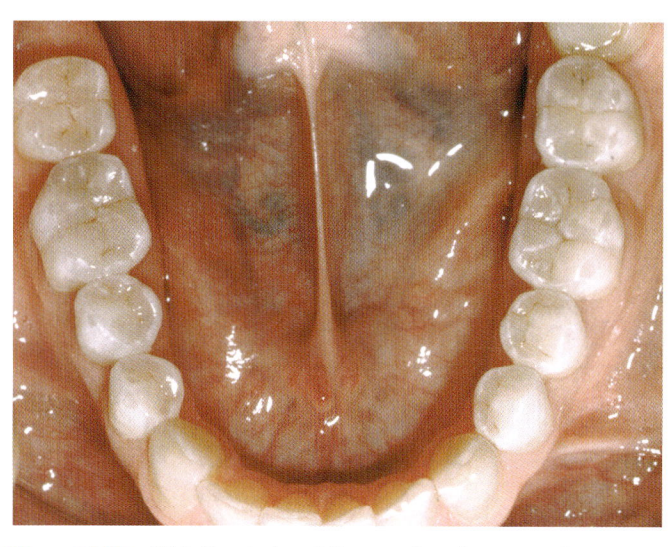

Figure 25.13 **(D)** Full arch view, 2.5 years after placement. *Source:* Figure courtesy of Dr Vincent Celenza.

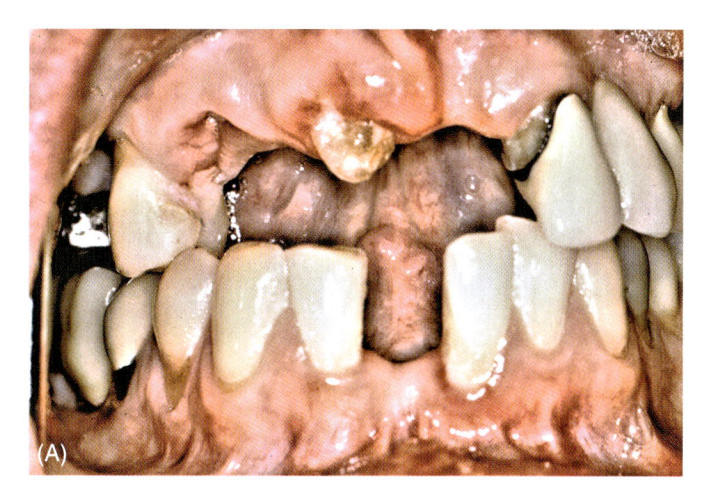

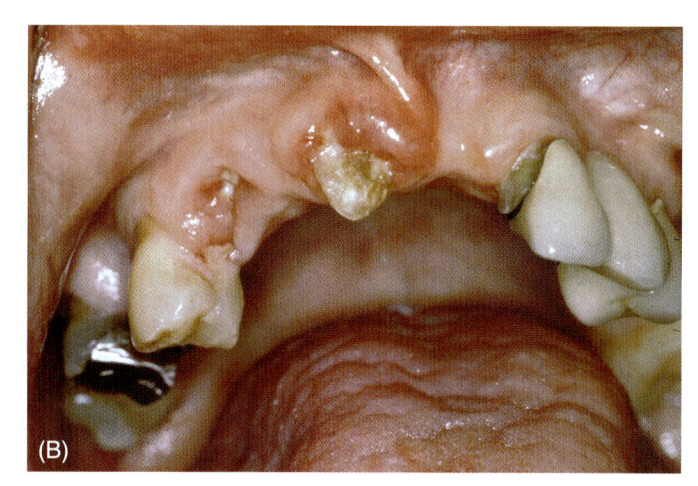

Figure 25.14 **(A, B)** This 28-year-old female had been anorexic since age 17. She had unsuccessfully participated in numerous counseling programs, and her self-image continued to be extremely poor. Although she weighed only 92 lb, she perceived herself to be grossly overweight. She was so focused on her body's appearance that she totally neglected her oral health. Note the loss of teeth and decay.

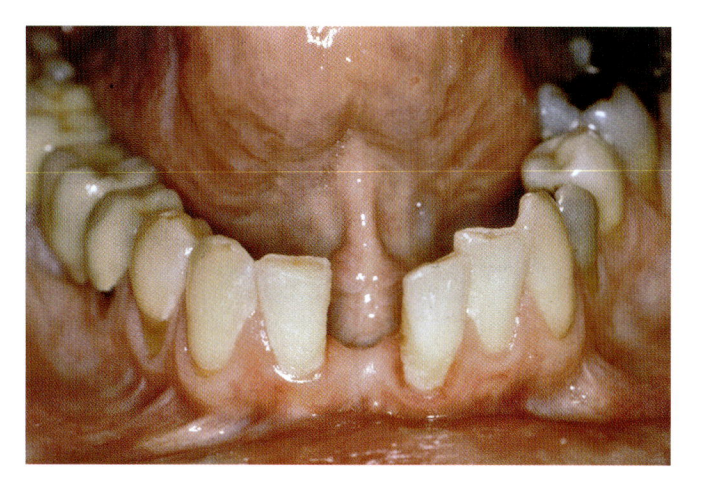

Figure 25.14 **(C)** Although not completely visible, this photograph illustrates drying and atrophy of the oral mucosa as seen on the lateral and ventral surfaces of the tongue.

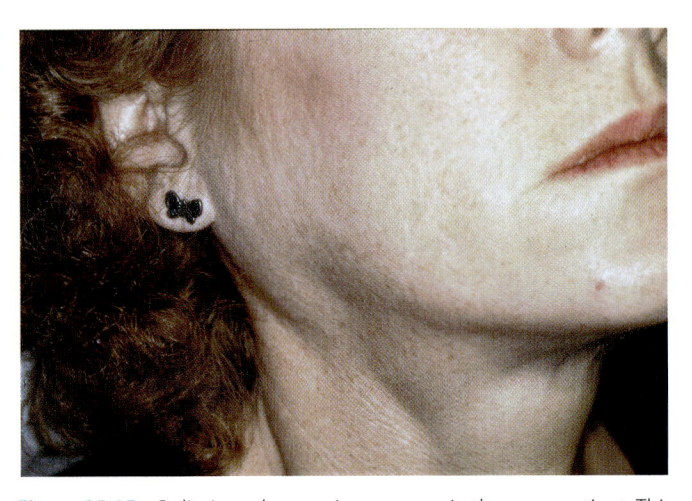

Figure 25.15 Bulimia and anorexia can occur in the same patient. This 35-year-old female initially manifested her eating disorder as bulimia when she was about 15 years old. Over the years, she has continued her purging, and while in college she began to exhibit behavior characteristic of anorexia. She is now firmly entrenched in both bulimia and anorexia. Her parotid hypertrophy is a manifestation of her bulimia. The lanugo (fine facial hair) is a sign sometimes seen in anorexics.

of the anterior teeth if they suck the fruit or the lingual surfaces if they chew it. Those who actually eat lemons may present with lingual erosion that mimics that of bulimia. Excessive consumption of fruits and drinks with high acid such as kombucha content can cause decalcification of enamel and dissolution of dental tissues (refer to Chapter 22).

In cases of dental erosion, the teeth first exhibit a diminished luster. As continual erosion leads to smoothing of enamel pits, the eroded areas eventually appear smooth and polished. Advancing erosion results in exposed dentin that wears down rapidly and often exhibits extensive sensitivity.

Early detection of erosive lesions and identification of patients at high risk for developing erosion are most important. If you detect erosion, it is essential to ask if the patient has changed their eating habits or diet recently.

Caries is frequently seen in patients who have a habit of sucking hard citrus-flavored candies with high sugar content (Figure 25.16C). Thus, rebuilding the lost tooth structure offers only palliative therapy. Dietary changes must be made in these patients who insist on continuing with this habit pattern. Dental management of patients with these disorders should be

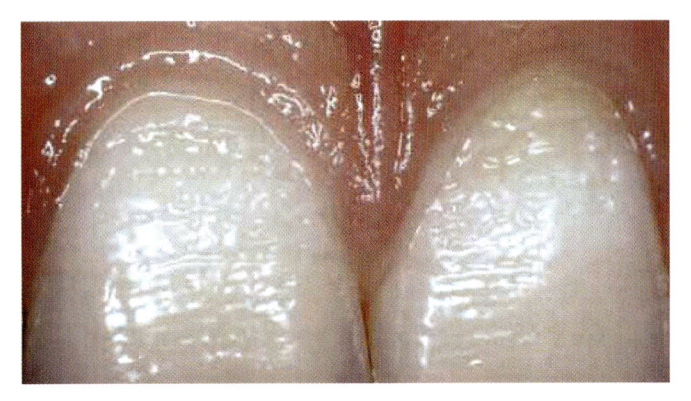

Figure 25.16 **(A)** People who have a habit of sucking lemons seldom are aware of the potential for damage to their enamel. This patient was diagnosed early in her habit, so a minimum of damage was done.

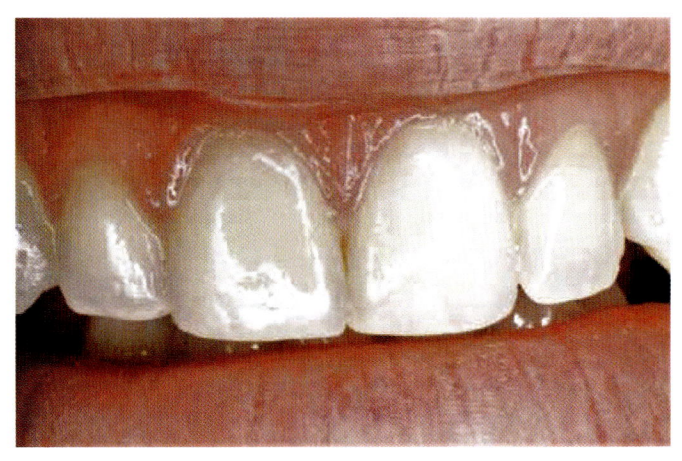

Figure 25.16 **(B)** Composite resin bonding was the treatment of choice.

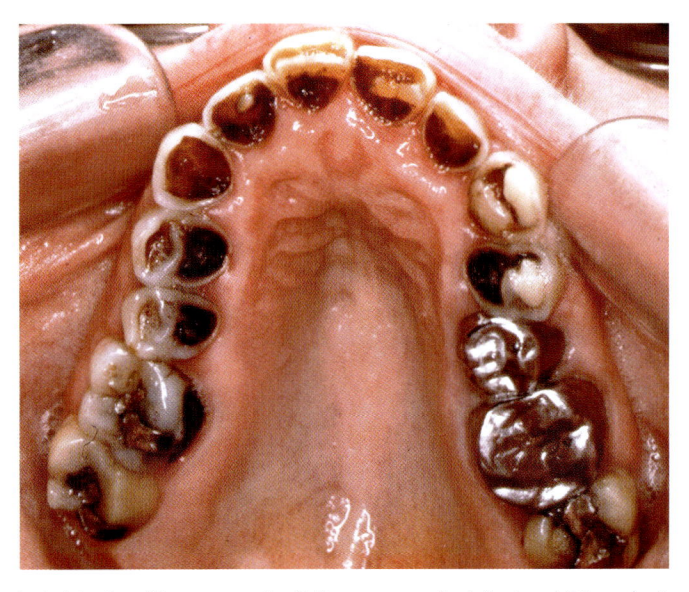

Figure 25.16 **(C)** This 63-year-old had a habit of sucking one pack of Lifesavers candy daily. In addition, she ingested two tablespoons of vinegar and 500 mg of vitamin C. Her maxillary teeth showed considerable damage due to caries and erosion. Treatment included full-mouth restoration with full crowns on the maxillary teeth.

conservative. Bonded composite resin or glass ionomer materials may reduce sensitivity and prevent the erosion from progressing. Any extensive dental treatment, such as crown and bridge, should be postponed until the disorder/habit itself is controlled or stabilized. Otherwise, dental treatment may not be effective.

Alcohol and drug abuse

Chronic alcoholism is another disorder that has oral implications (Figure 25.17). Case studies describe patients with a history of chronic alcoholism that have extensive wear of the teeth.[90–92] All had loss of lingual and incisal surfaces of the maxillary anterior teeth consistent with regurgitation erosion. This regurgitation results from a gastritis that is produced by ingestion of excessive amounts of alcohol.

Abuse of specific drugs has been shown to have adverse effects on the dentition. Individuals who regularly use methylenedioxymethamphetamine ("ecstasy") may have excessive wear of the teeth.[93,94] This occurs through a dual mechanism of decreased salivation and hyperactivity of the muscles of mastication. In essence, this drug evokes a form of bruxism that occurs in a dry mouth. Although not reported, other amphetamines may cause similar conditions. Cocaine has been reported to cause dental erosions because of its acidic nature.[95] Some abusers obtain their high by wetting the tip of their finger, dipping it into the cocaine, and wiping the drug into the buccal vestibule or onto the gingival tissues. When the acidic drug comes in contact with the tooth surface, erosive lesions can develop.

Other substances such as anabolic steroids can also be detrimental to oral health. It was found that the use of anabolic steroids by athletes caused gingival overgrowth.[96] Gingival overgrowth is a condition in which the gingival tissues become swollen and grow over the teeth. Overgrown gums make it easier for bacteria found in plaque to accumulate and attack supporting structures of the teeth, potentially leading to severe periodontal infection.

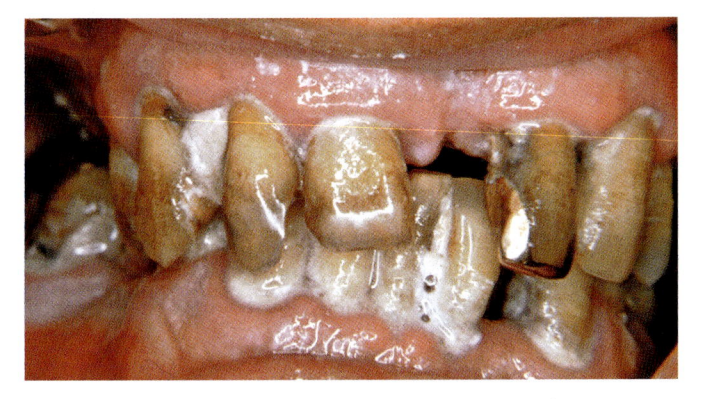

Figure 25.17 Chronic alcoholism is a habit that can produce various intraoral problems. This retired gentleman is a good example of how loss of self-respect can lead to greater oral disease. He quit caring about his appearance and completely gave up oral hygiene, as evidenced in this image.

Furthermore, cigarette smoking is one of the most addictive habits in contemporary life. People who smoke are more likely to accumulate calculus and plaque due to reduced salivary flow. Tobacco also limits blood flow to gum tissues, restricting the necessary nutrients to the bone and periodontal support of the teeth, thus leading to gum recession and bone loss. Cigarette smoking has also been shown to exacerbate nocturnal bruxism, which induces loss of tooth structure.[9,35] In addition, tobacco smoke contains a number of carcinogens, and leads to the development of oral and/or lung cancer.

Foreign objects in the mouth

Another habit that can produce permanent damage to the dentition relates to placing foreign objects in the mouth. The resultant damage is caused by abrasion, which is a term used to describe wear or defects in tooth tissues resulting from contact with a foreign object. The following are some of the more common types of habits that can cause this damage.

Fingernails

Since the fingernail is an extension of the finger, one may wonder if the common practice of placing the fingernails between the teeth is a continuation of a previous thumb- or finger-sucking habit. It may also begin suddenly, well into adult life, because of a chipped or spaced tooth or some roughness in the mouth that acts like a magnet for some people, perhaps in an effort to smooth out the roughness.

The most destructive of the fingernail habits involves the patient's wedging the fingernail in an interdental area that eventually becomes a space (Figure 25.18A–D). Treatment involves closure of the space. It is important that the patient be aware that continuation of this habit can quickly reopen the space. In some cases, it may be necessary to restrain the individual by constructing a vacuform matrix to cover the entire arch or an orthodontic retaining appliance (see Figure 25.18C and D). The patient should wear this appliance full time for 6 weeks. Closure of the space during this period, together with a 3-month retaining period, should be sufficient to break the habit. You can help ensure that the habit does not recur by cosmetically contouring the teeth to remove any rough or sharp edges.

Nail biting is also a learned habit that may provide a physical mechanism for stress relief. Encourage your patients to have short, well-manicured nails. Rough edges in the nail may cause the patient to smooth the nail unconsciously by rubbing it in the incisal embrasure. Also, advise the nail biter to carry a fingernail clipper at all times so that "nervous energy" can be converted into self-manicuring the nails when a possible urge to bite the nails exists. Behavioral techniques to reduce stress levels will aid in eliminating this type of habit.

Pins placed between the teeth

Placing various types of pins, needles, or even bobby pins in one's mouth is not an uncommon habit, particularly among people

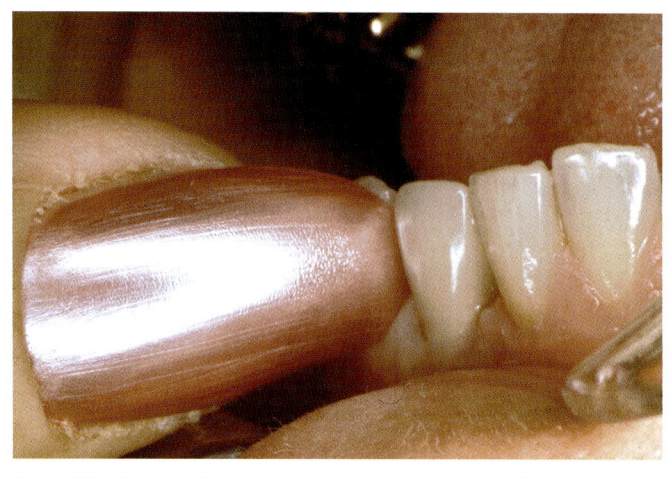

Figure 25.18 **(A)** This 30-year-old developed a habit of putting her nail between her lower incisors.

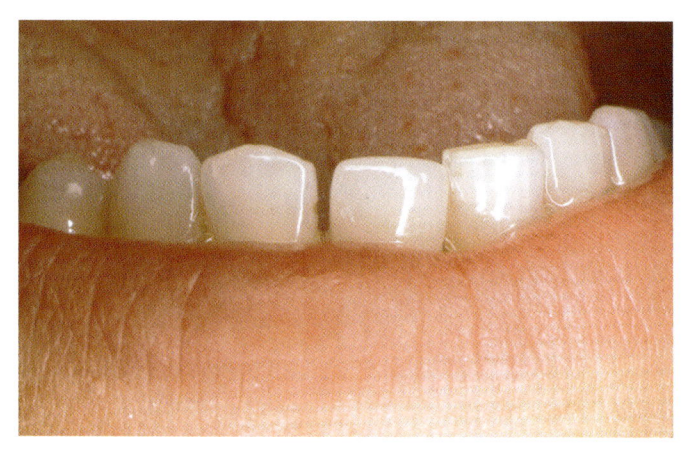

Figure 25.18 **(B)** Note the space created between the lateral and central incisors on the lower right side due to fingernail pressure.

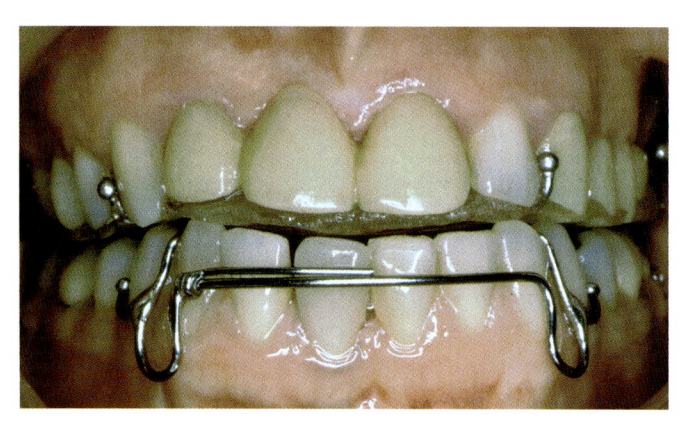

Figure 25.18 **(C)** A removable Hawley-type orthodontic appliance was constructed to reposition the lower anteriors. Because of the nature of this appliance, it also helped the patient to break the habit, since she could not put the fingernail into the same space.

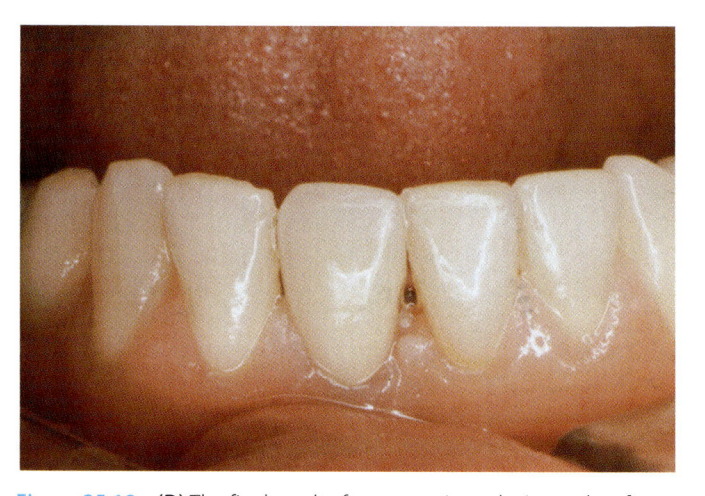

Figure 25.18 **(D)** The final result after approximately 6 months of treatment.

who knit and sew. People suffering tooth deformity from this habit usually hold the pin or needle between their anterior teeth (Figure 25.19A–D). Diagnosis can often be made by checking the patient's protrusive end-to-end relationship to see if a perfect matching groove is present. It is helpful to ask patients about their work and hobbies. Taking a thorough habit history, such as the one in Figure 25.20, is helpful. Treatment follows the pattern of other habits described in this section; that is, appearance is restored and whatever appliances and means necessary to discourage continuance of the habit are used. With this problem, it is also useful to tell the patient to at least vary the location where the pins are held.

Thread biting

Thread biting may produce notches in the incisal edges of anterior teeth. This is an occupational habit. Patients who are seamstresses should be warned against this behavior. Sharp edges of enamel that produce irritation should be eliminated by careful rounding or restorative treatment (Figure 25.21A and B).

Oral piercing and metal mouth jewelry

Metal mouth jewelry is often the culprit in cracked or broken teeth. Plastic jewelry reduces this risk, though cannot eliminate it entirely. For piercings of the lips, the "backside" of the jewelry, attached inside the mouth, can be a source of irritation to the opposing tissue. As the metal or plastic rests on the gum tissue, it can abrade and literally wear it away as it moves back and forth. For this reason, it is especially important to check the tissue around and touching any metal or plastic in the mouth regularly to ensure the continued health of these tissues. If the jewelry is causing damage or infection, it is essential to discover this early in the process (Figure 25.21C–F).

Stim-u-dents or toothpicks used as wedges

Toothpicks or Stim-u-dents can provide an effective means of cleaning tooth surfaces. If the object is forced between the teeth, however, it can create unwanted spaces. Patients should be told to use the toothpick or Stim-u-dent like a soft brush to clean plaque or debris from the smooth surface of the tooth (Figure 25.22A and B).

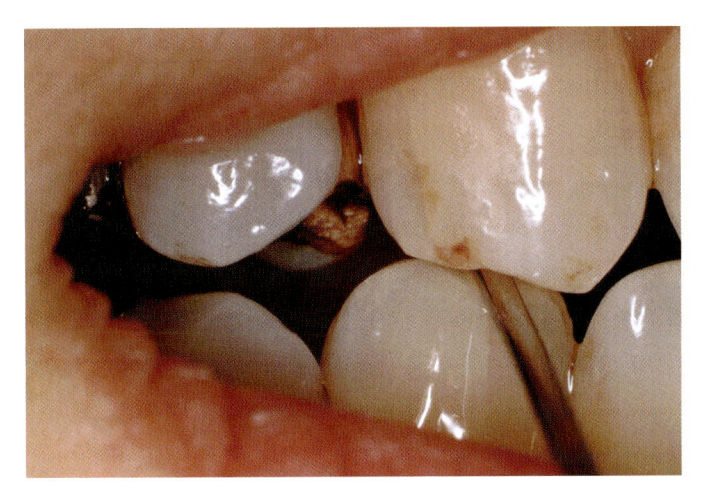

Figure 25.19 (A) This 39-year-old interior designer had a habit of holding sewing needles and pins between her cuspids.

Incorrect use of dental floss and toothbrush

Abnormal tooth wear may result from improper oral hygiene procedures. Misuse of dental floss may cause abnormal tooth wear. Excessive and strenuous use of dental floss apical to the cementoenamel junction may result in notching of the root surfaces. In addition, tooth abrasion may occur from incorrect use of a toothbrush. Toothbrush abrasion can be extreme, particularly if related to obsessive or compulsive behavior (Figure 25.23A–C).

Finally, incorrect use of dental floss can lead to abnormal loss of interdental space. Figure 25.24A–D shows a patient who has had bonding of her anterior teeth and unfortunately developed an incorrect method of flossing.

Pen or pencil chewing

This habit became considerably more destructive when pencils changed from wood to the newer plastic types (Figure 25.25A–E). It is not uncommon to see this habit in business people who spend a great deal of time at their desks working figures. Treatment involves wearing an appliance that prevents the patient from placing the pen or pencil between the teeth.

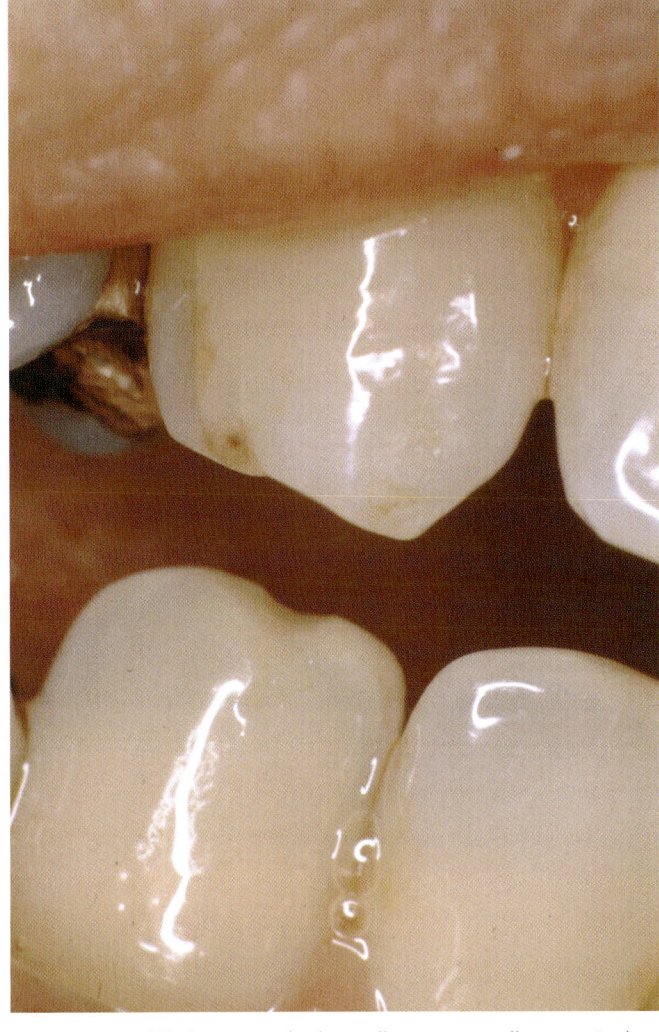

Figure 25.19 (B) The patient had actually worn a small groove in the biting edge of the teeth that exactly fit the sewing needle she used. In addition to cosmetic contouring or composite resin bonding to add to the worn spot, be sure to have the patient avoid consistently placing any foreign objects between the teeth.

(C)

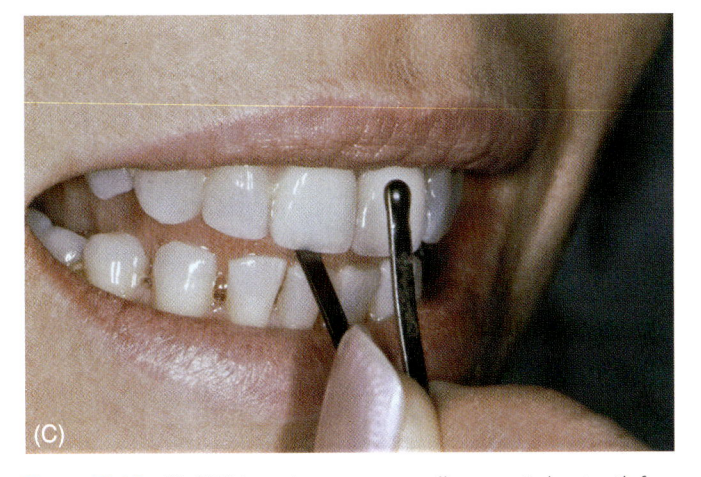

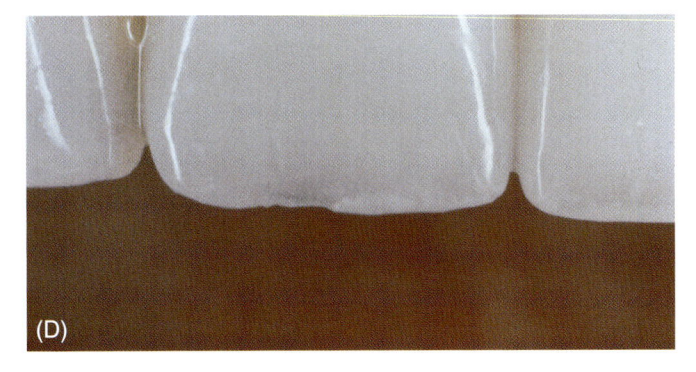

(D)

Figure 25.19 (C, D) This patient wore a small groove in her tooth from constant use of bobby pins.

Habit Questionnaire
Does Your Habit Affect Your Smile?

(Please check the appropriate space)
Do you now or did you ever

	Yes	No
1. Chew your lips or cheeks?	___	___
2. Suck your fingers, thumbs, or lemons?	___	___
3. Chew ice?	___	___
4. Bite your fingernails?	___	___
5. Hold pins or needles in your mouth?	___	___
6. Chew pencils or plastic pens?	___	___
7. Chew or hold your glasses in your mouth?	___	___
8. Crack nuts or ice with your teeth?	___	___
9. Play a musical instrument that requires you to hold the instrument with your teeth?	___	___
10. Smoke a pipe, cigar, or cigarettes?	___	___
11. Bite or suck your lips?	___	___
12. Use Stimudents or toothpicks?	___	___
13. Keep your tongue pressed against the upper teeth?	___	___
14. Place your tongue in a space between your teeth?	___	___
15. Grind or clench your teeth?	___	___

If you answer "yes" to two or more of the above questions, you may have a habit problem. Ask your dentist to see if your habit or habits are causing potential damage to your teeth.

Figure 25.20 The first step in either preventing or stopping a destructive oral habit is to help patients to discover their habits. *Source:* Reproduced with permission from Goldstein.[63]

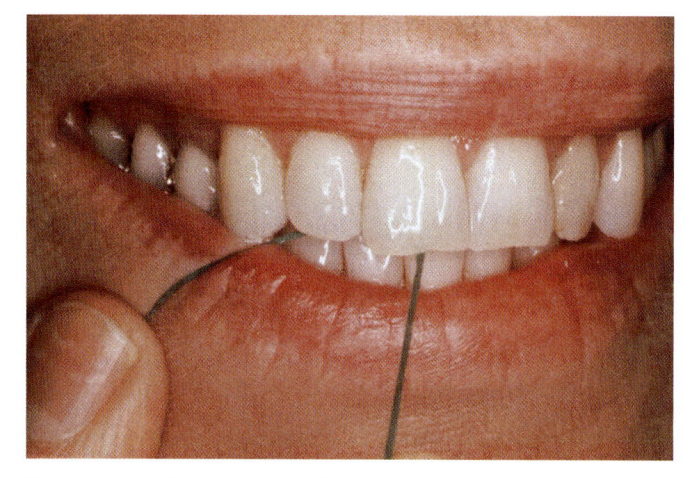

Figure 25.21 **(A)** This 55-year-old woman developed a habit of cutting sewing thread with her incisors.

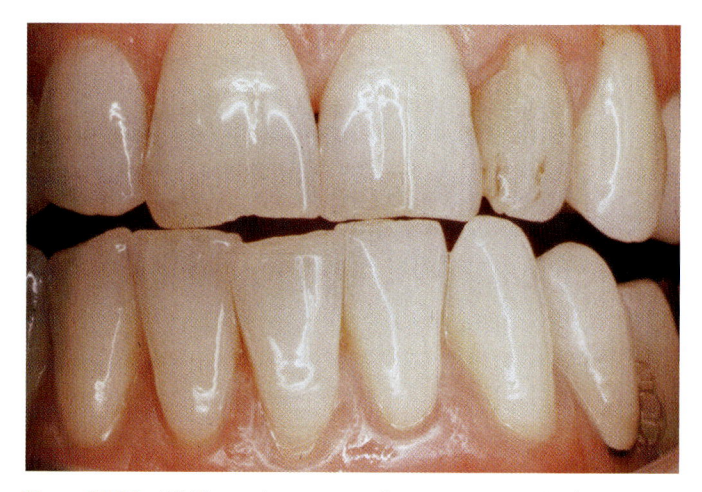

Figure 25.21 **(B)** The patient eventually wore a groove in the maxillary right central incisor.

Chapter 25 Oral Habits

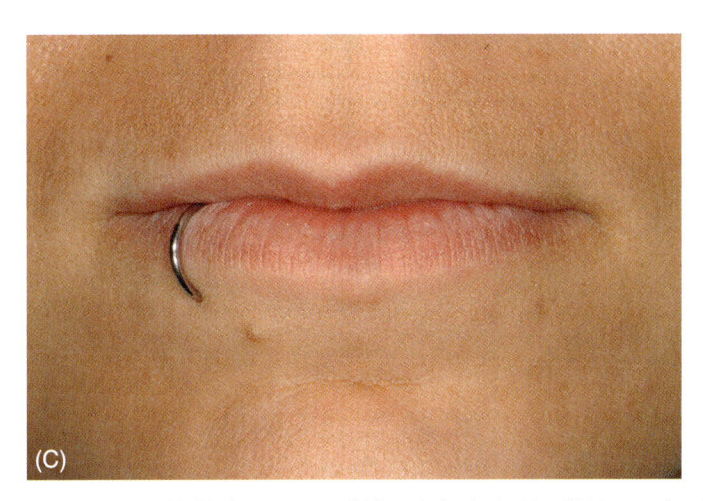

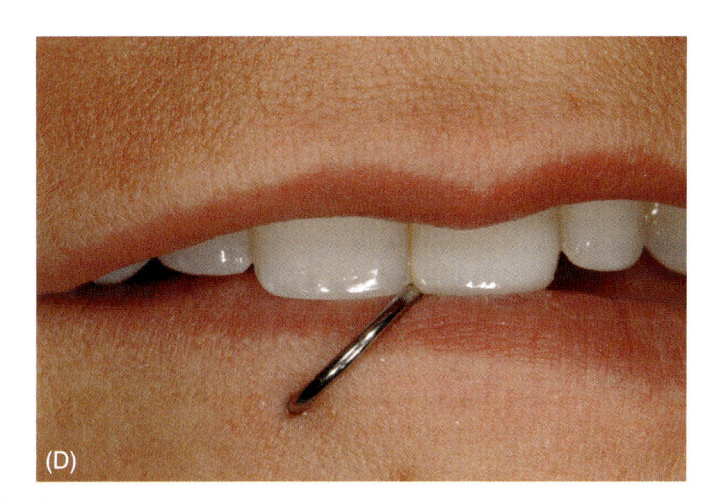

Figure 25.21 (C, D) This 25-year-old female had a habit of biting on her lip piercing.

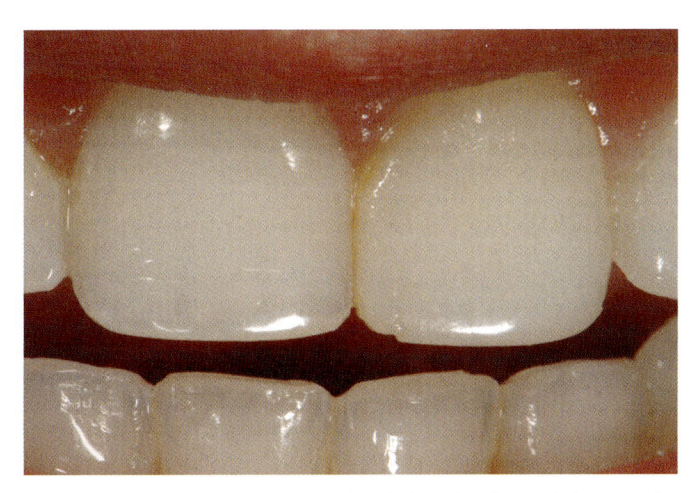

Figure 25.21 (E) As a result of her bad habit, she chipped the mesial of her left central incisor.

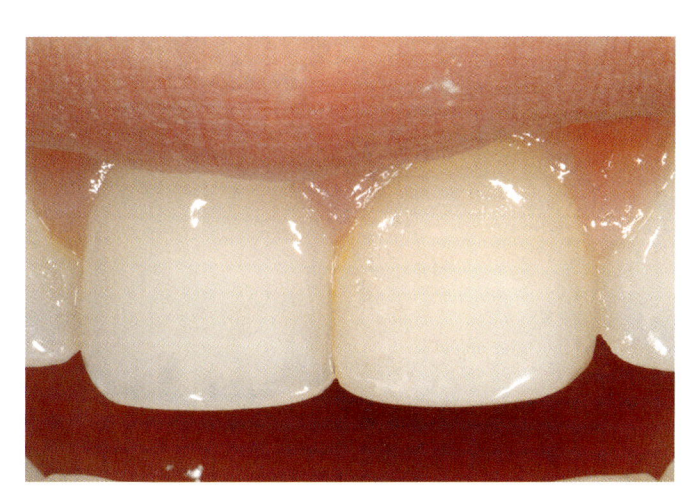

Figure 25.21 (F) Composite resin bonding was used to restore the chip in her tooth. In addition, the patient was advised to quit the habit or remove the lip piercing.

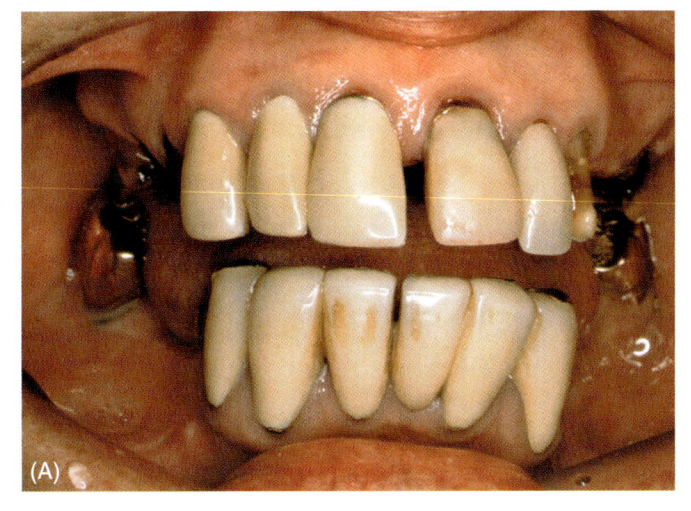

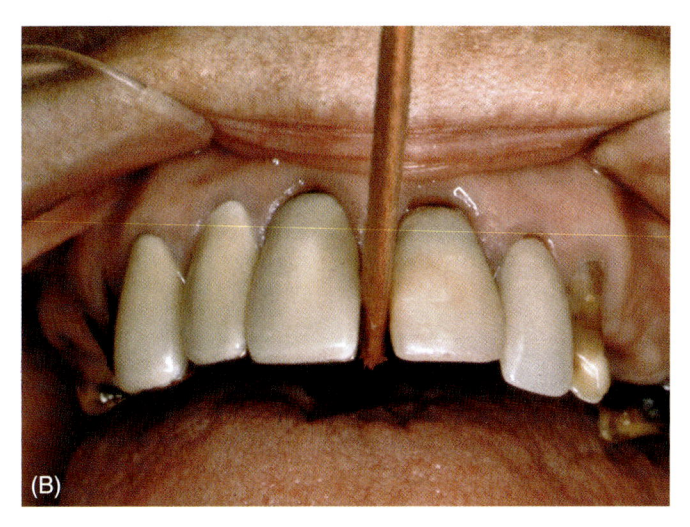

Figure 25.22 (A, B) These photographs show a patient who constantly placed Stim-u-dents between her front teeth. Although these teeth were originally together with no spaces, the patient quickly separated the teeth to create a space. Her goal was to expand her arch to give more fullness to her face. She had previously been referred for orthodontic treatment but rejected this treatment plan.

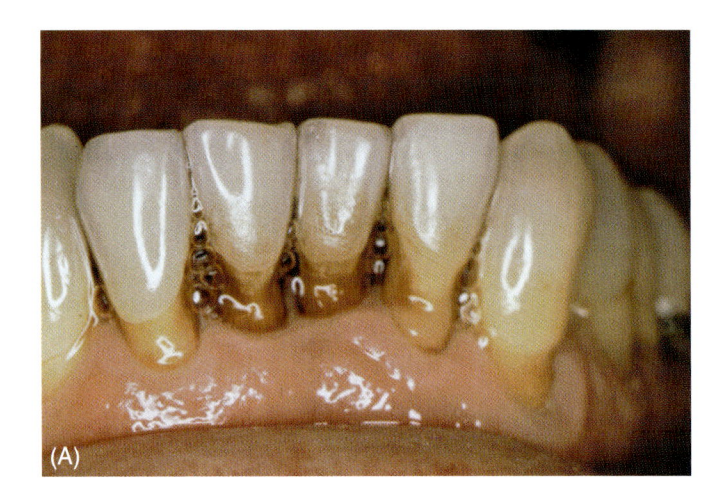

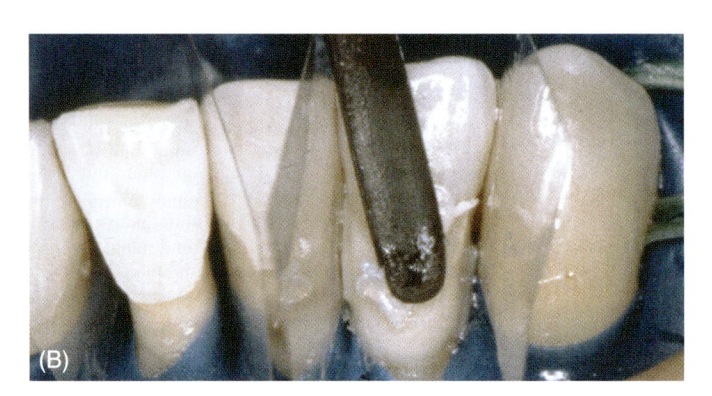

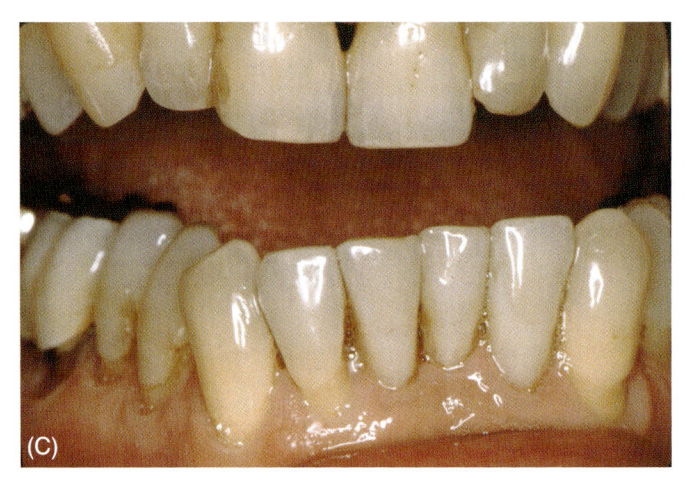

Figure 25.23 **(A–C)** This is severe toothbrush abrasion and gingival recession seen in a 37-year-old male with a known obsessive–compulsive disorder. The aggressive brushing of his teeth was one of his extreme habits (see also Chapter 22, Figure 22.10B and C). Composite resin bonding was done to restore the cervical deformities.

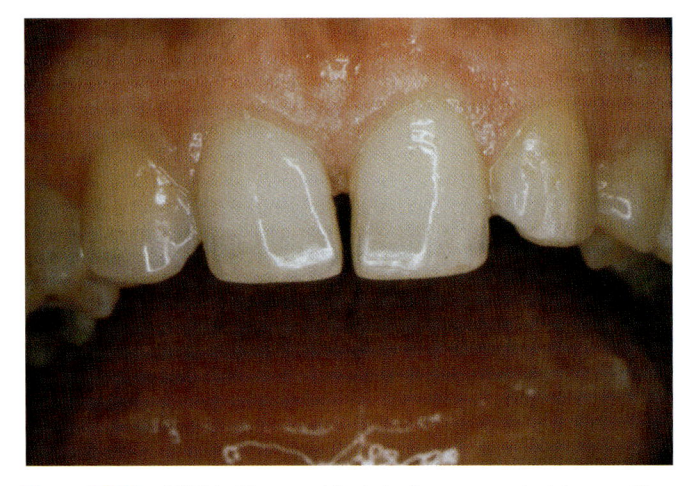

Figure 25.24 **(A)** This 25-year-old originally presented with a maxillary diastema.

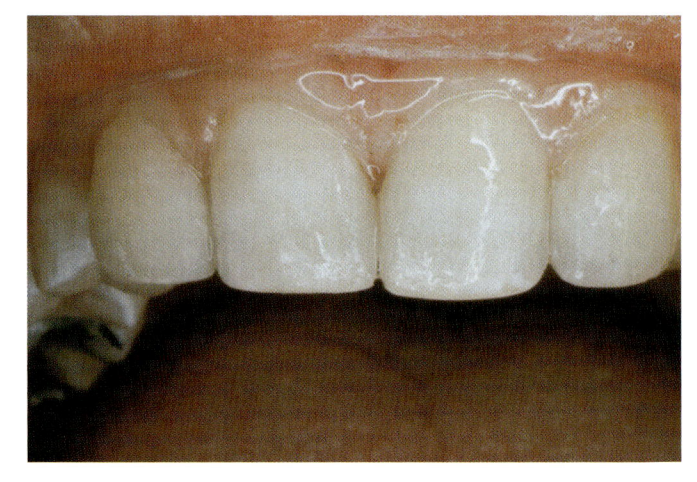

Figure 25.24 **(B)** Composite resin bonding was chosen to close the space between the central incisors and convert her canines into laterals. Note that the interdental space looks good between the central incisors.

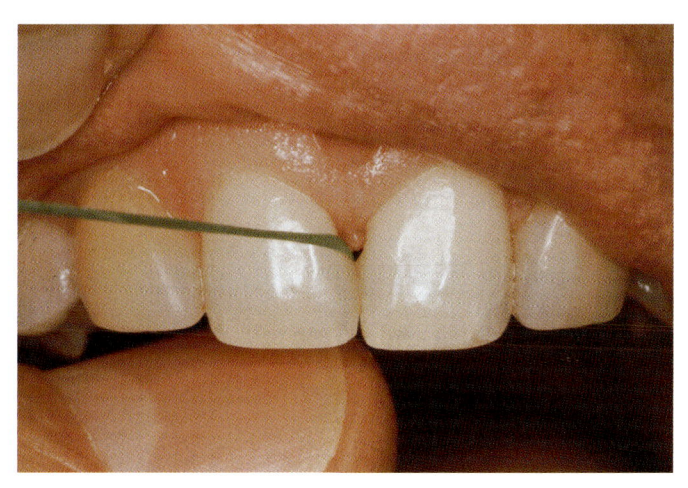

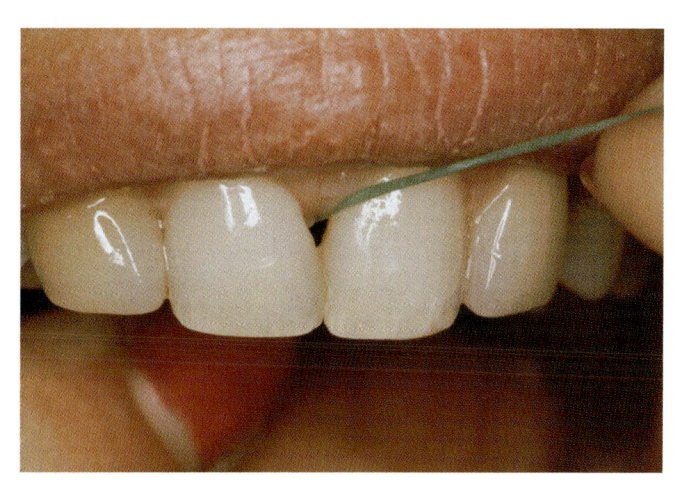

Figure 25.24 (C–D) At a two week post-operative visit, we noticed her interdental tissue had receded. After questioning the patient about habits, she was requested to demonstrate exactly how she flossed her teeth. What she was doing was pushing the floss into the teeth on one side and then going straight across to the other side without coming back into the contact area; thus, she was "guillotining" her interdental papilla away. Treatment involved new oral care instructions to prevent further tissue loss and provide an opportunity for the gingiva to regenerate and fill in the interdental space.

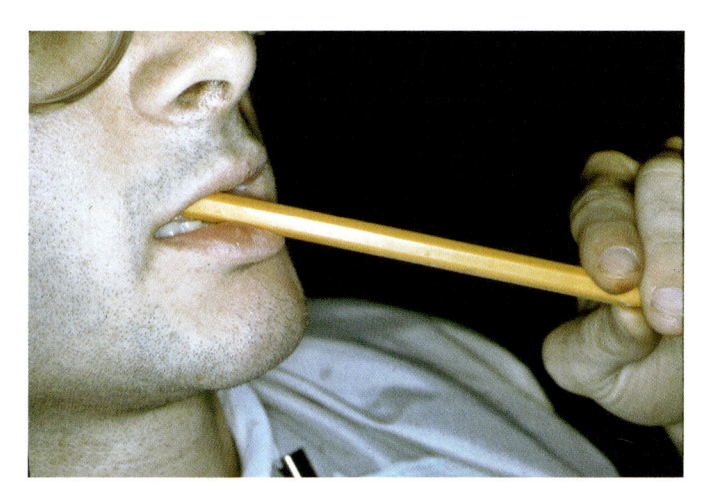

Figure 25.25 (A) This 21-year-old developed a habit of chewing pencils.

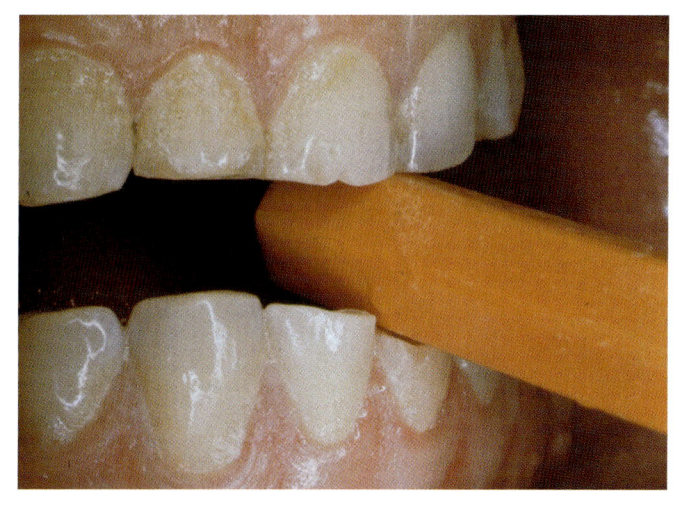

Figure 25.25 (B) Eventually, wooden pencils were replaced with plastic ones, which he began to turn with his fingers, causing incisal wear.

Pipe smoking

Any kind of smoking creates its own unesthetic results, staining the teeth and affecting the health of the oral soft tissues. Pipe smoking has the most potential for changing tooth relationships. Continually holding a pipe in one location may cause large notches in several teeth. The problem is that the patient usually places the pipe stem in the same position, most often the premolar area. These teeth then become worn or submerged (Figure 25.26A and B).

Treatment involves correcting the deformity and helping the patient break the habit. In this case, it may be easier to teach the patient to change the pattern of holding the pipe rather than give up the habit altogether. At the very least, this would make certain that the occlusal forces are distributed among many teeth. Although the submerged teeth can usually be orthodontically repositioned, restorative means may provide an easier solution.

However, some tooth structure would probably have to be removed so that the bonded restoration could be attached using the etched occlusal surface enamel.

Eyeglasses or other objects held between the teeth

Most persons who consistently place eyeglasses, plastic swizzle sticks, or other objects in their mouths are not aware of the habit, much less the resulting functional and esthetic deformity (Figure 25.27A and B). Treatment is the same as noted earlier.

Ice chewing

Patients seldom realize the damage that chewing ice, a seemingly innocuous habit, can cause. Chewing ice can fracture the teeth and can also produce microcracks in the enamel.

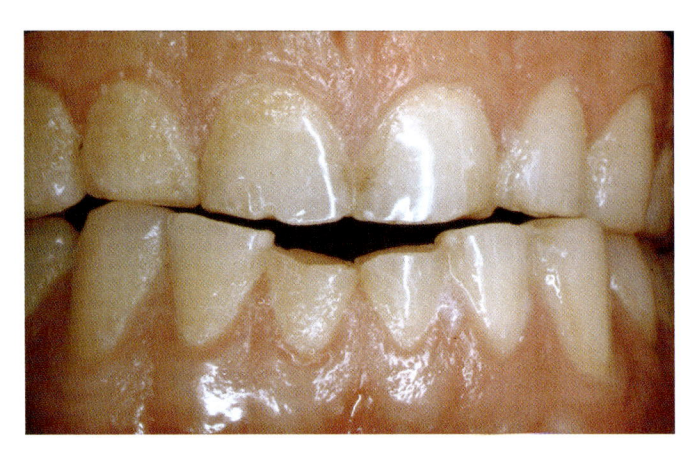

Figure 25.25 **(C)** Note the amount of damage caused by the pencil chewing. Composite resin bonding was used as an economic and immediate esthetic replacement for the missing tooth structure. The patient was also given a plastic bite appliance for the maxillary arch that he would wear anytime he felt the need to put a pencil in his mouth.

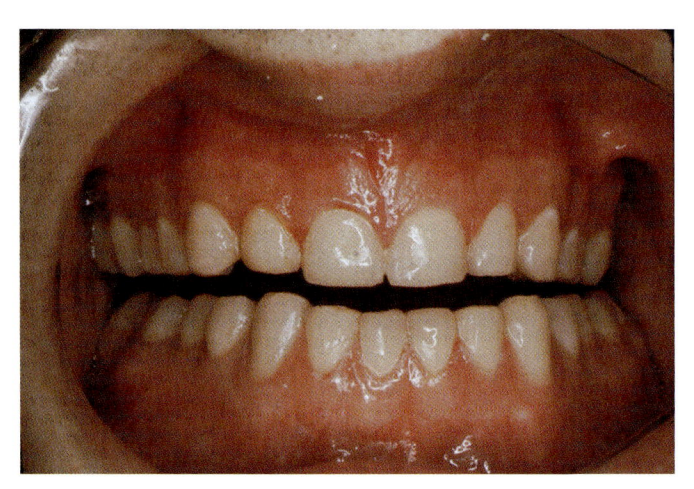

Figure 25.25 **(D)** He successfully broke the habit, and the bonding held up for approximately 12 years, when, unfortunately, the patient restarted his previous habit.

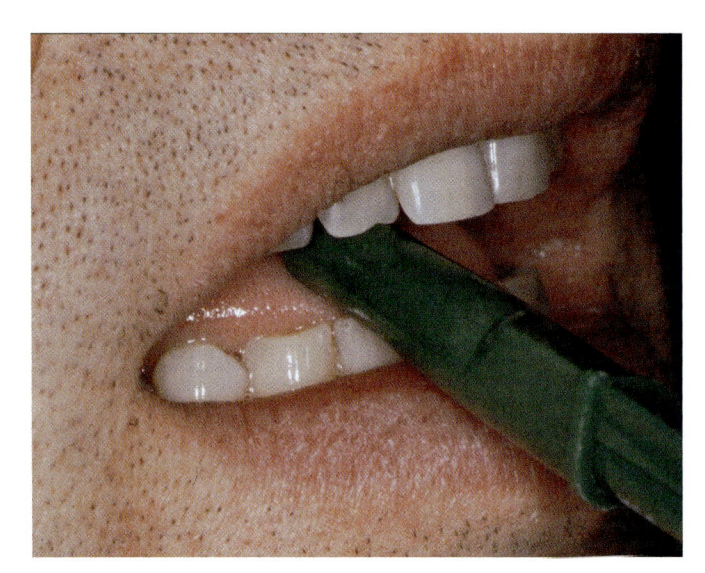

Figure 25.25 **(E)** This 46-year-old man had an unconscious habit of not only placing plastic pens in his mouth but also sliding the pen in and out. This wore a groove in the center of the incisal edge.

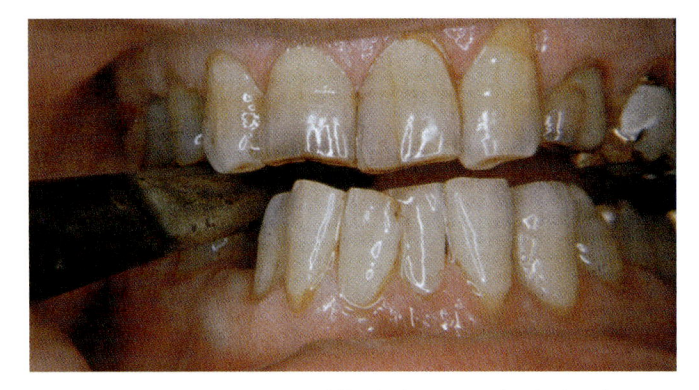

Figure 25.26 **(A)** This 56-year-old had a long-standing habit of pipe smoking.

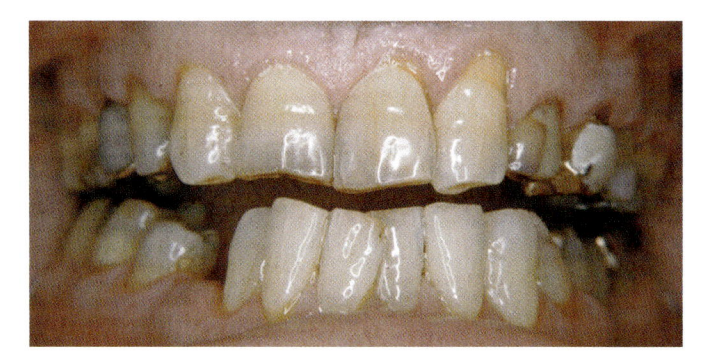

Figure 25.26 **(B)** After the pipe was removed, and the patient bit down, the amount of damage caused by the pipe being held in the premolar positions was evident. Particularly note how he favored the right side, which showed a greater amount of abnormal space.

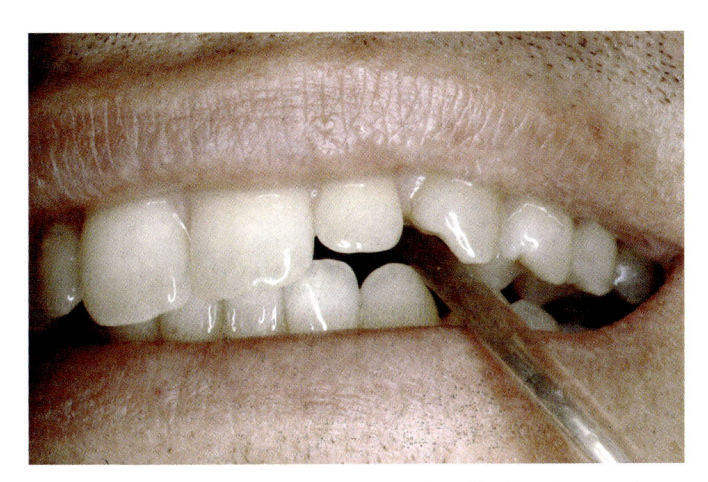

Figure 25.27 **(A)** This 31-year-old had a habit of holding his eyeglasses with his teeth.

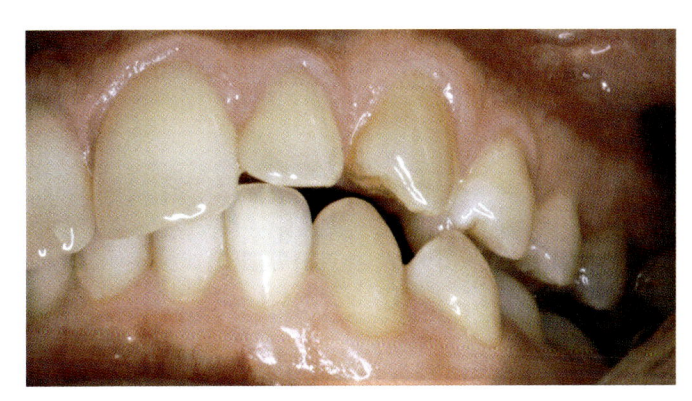

Figure 25.27 **(B)** He always held them in the same position, causing the left canine to flare out, thus creating an unattractive and unnecessary space between his front teeth. Patients should always be advised never to hold anything but food between their teeth.

The microcracks themselves are usually not visible to the eye, but they stain much more readily than normal, especially with coffee, tea, and soy sauce. If the person chewing ice has defective restorations, a sliver of ice can also act as a wedge that can split the tooth.

Cracking nuts with the teeth

Using teeth to open the shell of a nut may be the handiest way to reach the nutmeat, but it may also be the quickest way to break a tooth. A common offender is the pistachio nut. The harder the nut is, the more chance there is of a fractured tooth. The only preventive measure you can take is to warn patients of the potential damage, particularly if any incisal edge has been bonded with composite resin.

Diagnosis and treatment of damaging oral habits

There are many more examples of damaging oral habits, but the principles of diagnosis and treatment are similar for all of them. There are two most important principles to remember:

1. Early diagnosis means prevention.
2. Treating the symptoms is only a temporary solution—the patient must break the habit.

Keys to helping patients break damaging oral habits include the following:

- Precise diagnosis of the exact nature of the habit.
- Help the patient recognize the habit and tactfully suggest counseling or other methods to deal with stress and tension.
- Correct the damage caused by the habit so that rough edges, open gaps, or tissue changes do not contribute to resumption of the habit. Preventive appliances are also useful in helping to make patients more aware of these behaviors and break the cycle of "habit–sign–habit."

The treatment of children's oral habits, particularly digit sucking, is somewhat easier because there is usually an adoring adult to reinforce changed behavior. The therapists who participated in a convention of speech pathologists concerned with such behavior almost uniformly suggested methods that require commitment on the part of the patient, removal of guilt about the habit, and a willingness of the parent to give the child some extra attention as the habit is relinquished. Charts with checkmarks or gold stars are often used as reinforcement, as are kisses and praises.[21]

Tips for adult patients to modify their negative oral habits are as follows:

- An extremely precise diagnosis of the problem is an essential first step since many adults may not realize that they have a destructive habit.
- Once the patient has become aware of the habit, they can monitor the behavior, writing down when, how intensely, and under what circumstances it occurs. This will reinforce the patient's awareness of the habit, provide some clues as to what evokes it (such as cheek biting occurring most often in stressful situations or when tired), and provide many occasions in which not using the habit can be reinforced. Suggest to your patient that they enlist the assistance of someone else to help identify various aspects of the habit. A colleague would be a good source if the habit occurs primarily during working hours. Spouses, relatives, or friends may provide assistance if the habit takes place during nonworking hours.
- Some behavioral scientists believe that one habit replaces another. Certainly, it is easier to create a habit than to break one, so it could be suggested to patients that they attempt to temporarily replace the destructive oral habit with a less destructive one, such as chewing sugarless gum.
- Finally, the use of orthodontic devices such as those described in this chapter will help the patient recognize and break this habit.

An important part of treatment, as well as the record of each new patient, should be a completed thorough habit questionnaire, such as the one in Figure 25.20. The patient can fill this out unless they are so young that a parent or guardian would be a more appropriate source of information. This questionnaire should be updated as regularly as a patient's medical history. Destructive habits can start anytime, and it is the dentist's responsibility—and opportunity as a professional with diagnostic ability and an inquisitive nature—to identify these habits and stop them before more damage is done.

References

1. Nilsson L. *A Child is Born*. Stockholm: Albert Bonniers; 1976:125.
2. Chandler TH. Thumbsucking in childhood as a cause of subsequent irregularity of the teeth. *Boston Med Surg J* 1878;99:204–208.
3. Fukuta O, Braham RL, Yokoi K, Kurosu K. Damage to the primary dentition resulting from thumb and finger (digit) sucking. *ASDC J Dent Child* 1996;63:403–407.
4. Taylor MH, Peterson DS. Effect of digit-sucking habits on root morphology in primary incisors. *Pediatr Dent* 1983;5:61–63.
5. Johnson ED, Larson BE. Thumb-sucking: literature review. *ASDC J Dent Child* 1993;60:385–391.
6. Larsson E. Dummy- and finger-sucking habits with special attention to their significance for facial growth and occlusion. *Swed Dent J* 1978;2:23–33.
7. Larsson E. The effect of finger-sucking on the occlusion: a review. *Eur J Orthod* 1987;9:279–282.
8. Larsson E. Artificial sucking habits: etiology, prevalence and effect on occlusion. *Int J Orofac Myol* 1994;20:10–21.
9. Lavigne GL, Lobbezoo F, Rompe PH, et al. Cigarette smoking as a risk factor or an exacerbating factor for restless legs syndrome and sleep bruxism. *Sleep* 1997;20:290–293.
10. Luke LS, Howard L. The effects of thumb sucking on orofacial structures and speech: a review. *Compend Cont Educ Dent* 1983;4:575–579.
11. Van Norman RA. Digit-sucking: a review of the literature, clinical observations and treatment recommendations. *Int J Orofac Myol* 1997;23:14–34.
12. Ngan P, Fields HW. Open bite: a review of etiology and management. *Pediatr Dent* 1997;19:91–98.
13. Subtelny JD, Subtelny J. Oral habits—studies in form, function and therapy. *Angle Orthod* 1973;43:349–383.
14. Bowden BD. A longitudinal study of the effects of digit- and dummy-sucking. *Am J Orthod* 1966;52: 887–901.
15. Haryett RD, Hansen FC, Davidson PO, Sandilands ML. Chronic thumb sucking: the psychologic effects and the relative effectiveness of various methods of treatment. *Am J Orthod* 1967;53:569–585.
16. Infante PF. An epidemiological study of finger habits in preschool children as related to malocclusion, socioeconomic status, race, sex, and size of community. *J Dent Child* 1976;43:33–38.
17. Popovich F, Thompson GW. Thumb and finger-sucking—its relation to malocclusion. *Am J Orthod* 1973;63:148–155.
18. Massler M. Oral habits: development and management. *J Pedod* 1983;7:109–119.
19. Rayan GM, Turner WT. Hand complications in children from digit sucking. *J Hand Surg* 1989;14:933–936.
20. Gellin ME. Digit sucking and tongue thrusting in children. *Dent Clin North A* 1978;22:603–618.
21. Greenly L. Suggestions for combating digit sucking as offered by members at the 1982 I.A.O.M. Convention. *Int J Orofac Myol* 1982;8:22–23.
22. McSherry PF. Aetiology and treatment of anterior open bite. *J Irish Dent Assoc* 1996;42:20–26.
23. Levitas TC. Examine the habit—evaluate the treatment. *ASDC J Dent Child* 1970;37:122–123.
24. Bartlett DW, Ricketts DN, Fisher NL. Management of the short clinical crown by indirect restorations. *Dent Update* 1997;24:431–436.
25. Becker W, Ochsenbein C, Becker BE. Crown lengthening: the periodontal-restorative connection. *Compend Cont Educ Dent* 1998;19:239–240, 242,244–246.
26. Bishop K, Bell M, Briggs P, Kelleher M. Restoration of a worn dentition using a double-veneer technique. *Br Dent J* 1996;180:26–29.
27. Quinn JH. Mandibular exercises to control bruxism and deviation. *Cranio* 1995;13:30–34.
28. Da Silva AM, Oakley DA, Hemmings KW, et al. Psychosocial factors and tooth wear with a significant component of attrition. *Eur J Prosthodont Restor Dent* 1997;5:51–55.
29. Faulkner KD. Bruxism: a review of the literature. Part I. *Aust Dent J* 1991;35:266–276.
30. Faulkner KD. Bruxism: a review of the literature. Part II. *Aust Dent J* 1991;36:355–361.
31. Hicks RA, Conti PA, Bragg HR. Increases in nocturnal bruxism among college students implicate stress. *Med Hypotheses* 1990;33:239–240.
32. Hublin C, Kaprio J, Partinen M, Koskenvuo M. Sleep bruxism based on self-report in a nationwide twin cohort. *J Sleep Res* 1998;7:61–67.
33. Kampe T, Edman G, Bader G, et al. Personality traits in a group of subjects with long-standing bruxing behaviour. *J Oral Rehabil* 1997;24:588–593.
34. Hicks RA, Conti PA. Changes in the incidence of nocturnal bruxism in college students: 1966–1989. *Percept Mot Skills* 1989;69:481–482.
35. Madrid G, Madrid S, Vranesh JG, Hicks RA. Cigarette smoking and bruxism. *Percept Mot Skills* 1998;87:898.
36. Bailey DR. Tension headache and bruxism in the sleep disordered patient. *Cranio* 1990;8:174–182.
37. Macaluso GM, Guerra P, Di Giovanni G, et al. Sleep bruxism is a disorder related to periodic arousals during sleep. *J Dent Res* 1998;77:565–572.
38. Okeson JP, Phillips BA, Berry DT, et al. Nocturnal bruxing events in subjects with sleep-disordered breathing and control subjects. *J Craniomandib Disord* 1991;5:258–264.
39. Weideman CL, Bush DL, Yan-Go FL, et al. The incidence of parasomnias in child bruxers versus non-bruxers. *Pediatr Dent* 1996;18:456–460.
40. Allen JD, Rivera-Morales WC, Zwemer JD. Occurrence of temporomandibular disorder symptoms in healthy young adults with and without evidence of bruxism. *Cranio* 1990;8:312–318.
41. Kieser JA, Groeneveld HT. Relationship between juvenile bruxing and craniomandibular dysfunction. *J Oral Rehabil* 1998;25:662–665.
42. Lobbezoo F, Lavigne GJ. Do bruxism and temporomandibular disorders have a cause-and-effect relationship? *J Orofac Pain* 1997;11:15–23.
43. Molina OF, dos Santos J Jr, Nelson SJ, Grossman E. Prevalence of modalities of headaches and bruxism among patients with craniomandibular disorders. *Cranio* 1997;15:14–25.

44. Rugh JD, Harlan J. Nocturnal bruxism and temporomandibular disorders. *Adv Neurol* 1988;49:329–341.
45. Seligman DA, Pullinger AG. A multiple stepwise logistic regression analysis of trauma history and 16 other history and dental cofactors in females with temporomandibular disorders. *J Orofac Pain* 1996;10:351–361.
46. Tsolka P, Walter JD, Wilson RF, Preiskel HW. Occlusal variable, bruxism and temporomandibular disorders: a clinical and kinesiographic assessment. *J Oral Rehabil* 1995;22:849–856.
47. Vanderas AP. Relationship between craniomandibular dysfunction and oral parafunctions in Caucasian children with and without unpleasant life events. *J Oral Rehabil* 1995;22:289–294.
48. Vanderas AP, Manetas KJ. Relationship between malocclusion and bruxism in children and adolescents: a review. *Pediatr Dent* 1995;17:7–12.
49. Yustin D, Neff P, Rieger MR, Hurst T. Characterization of 86 bruxing patients with long-term study of their management with occlusal devices and other forms of therapy. *J Orofac Pain* 1993;7:54–60.
50. Bowles WH, Wilkinson MR, Wagner MJ, Woody RD. Abrasive particles in tobacco products: a possible factor in dental attrition. *J Am Dent Assoc* 1995;126:327–331.
51. Magnusson T. Is snuff a potential risk factor in occlusal wear? *Swed Dent J* 1991;15:125–132.
52. Robertson PB, DeRouen TA, Ernster V, et al. Smokeless tobacco use: how it affects the performance of major league baseball players. *J Am Dent Assoc* 1995;126:1115–1121.
53. Reichart PA, Phillipsen HP. Betel chewer's mucosa—a review. *J Oral Pathol Med* 1998;27:239–242.
54. Zain RB, Gupta PC, Warnakulasuriya S, et al. Oral lesions associated with betel quid and tobacco chewing habits. *Oral Dis* 1997;3:204–205.
55. Zain RB, Ikeda N, Gupta PC, et al. Oral mucosal lesions associated with betel quid, areca nut and tobacco chewing habits: consensus from a workshop held in Kuala Lumpur, Malaysia, November 25–27, 1996. *J Oral Pathol Med* 1999;28:1–4.
56. Langsjoen OM. Dental effects of diet and coca-leaf chewing on two prehistoric cultures of northern Chile. *Am J Phys Anthropol* 1996;101:475–489.
57. Sapiro SM. Tongue indentations as an indicator of clenching. *Clin Prev Dent* 1992;14:21–24.
58. Andrianopoulos MV, Hanson ML. Tongue-thrust and the stability of overjet correction. *Angle Orthod* 1987;57:121–135.
59. Melsen B, Attina L, Santuari M, Attina A. Relationships between swallowing pattern, mode of respiration, and development of malocclusion. *Angle Orthod* 1987;57:113–210.
60. Mikell B. Recognizing tongue related malocclusion. *Int J Orthod* 1985;23:4–7.
61. Glass LF, Maize JC. Morsicatio buccarum et labiorum (excessive cheek and lip biting). *Am J Dermatopathol* 1991;13:271–274.
62. Walker RS, Rogers WA. Modified maxillary occlusal splint for prevention of cheek biting: a clinical report. *J Prosthet Dent* 1992;67:581–582.
63. Goldstein RE. *Change Your Smile*, 3rd edn. Carol Stream, IL: Quintessence; 1997.
64. Bayardo RE, Mejia JJ, Orozco S, Montoya K. Etiology of oral habits. *ASDC J Dent Child* 1996;63:350–353.
65. Coccaro PJ, Coccaro PJ Jr. Dental development and the pharyngeal lymphoid tissue. *Otolaryngol Clin North Am* 1987;20:241–257.
66. Linder-Aronson S, Woodside DG, Lundstrom A. Mandibular growth direction following adenoidectomy. *Am J Orthod* 1986;89:272–284.
67. Venetikidou A. Incidence of malocclusion in asthmatic children. *J Clin Pediatr Dent* 1993;17:89–94.
68. Cooper BC. Nasorespiratory function and orofacial development. *Otolaryngol Clin North Am* 1989;22:413–441.
69. Ellingsen R, Vandevanter C, Shapiro P, Shapiro G. Temporal variation in nasal and oral breathing in children. *Am J Orthod Dentofac Orthop* 1995;107:411–417.
70. Gross AM, Kellum GD, Franz D, et al. A longitudinal evaluation of open mouth posture and maxillary arch width in children. *Angle Orthod* 1994;64:419–424.
71. Gross AM, Kellum GD, Michas K, et al. Open-mouth posture and maxillary arch width in young children: a three-year evaluation. *Am J Orthod Dentofac Orthop* 1994;106:635–640.
72. Gross AM, Kellum GD, Morris T, et al. Rhinometry and open-mouth posture in young children. *Am J Orthod Dentofac Orthop* 1993;103:526–529.
73. Hartgerink DV, Vig PS. Lower anterior face height and lip incompetence do not predict nasal airway obstruction. *Angle Orthod* 1989;59:17–23.
74. Kellum GD, Gross AM, Walker M, et al. Open mouth posture and cross-sectional nasal area in young children. *Int J Orofac Myol* 1993;19:25–28.
75. Kerr WJ, McWilliam JS, Linder-Aronson S. Mandibular form and position related to changed mode of breathing—a five-year longitudinal study. *Angle Orthod* 1989;59:91–96.
76. Klein JC. Nasal respiratory function and craniofacial growth. *Arch Otolaryngol Head Neck Surg* 1986;112:843–849.
77. Shapiro PA. Effects of nasal obstruction on facial development. *J Allergy Clin Immunol* 1988;81:967–971.
78. Stokes N, Della Mattia D. A student research review of the mouthbreathing habit: discussing measurement methods, manifestations and treatment of the mouthbreathing habit. *Probe* 1996;30:212–214.
79. Vickers PD. Respiratory obstruction and its role in long face syndrome. *Northwest Dent* 1998;77:19–22.
80. Barber TK. Lip habits in preventive orthodontics. *J Prev Dent* 1978;5:30–36.
81. Fombonne E. Increased rates of psychosocial disorders in youth. *Eur Arch Psychiatry Clin Neurosci* 1998;248:14–21.
82. Keel PK, Mitchell JE. Outcome in bulimia nervosa. *Am J Psychiatry* 1997;154:313–321.
83. Ressler A. "A body to die for": eating disorders and body-image distortion in women. *Int J Fertil Womens Med* 1998;43:133–138.
84. Schwitzer AM, Bergholtz K, Dore T, Salimi L. Eating disorders among college women: prevention, education, and treatment responses. *J Am Coll Health* 1998;46:199–207.
85. Bouquot JE, Seime RJ. Bulimia nervosa: dental perspectives. *Pract Periodont Aesthet Dent* 1997;9:655–663.
86. Brown S, Bonifazi DZ. An overview of anorexia and bulimia nervosa, and the impact of eating disorders on the oral cavity. *Compend Cont Educ Dent* 1993;14:1594, 1596–1602, 1604–1608.
87. Roberts MW, Li SH. Oral findings in anorexia nervosa and bulimia nervosa: a study of 47 cases. *J Am Dent Assoc* 1987;115:407–410.
88. Ruffs JC, Koch MO, Perkins S. Bulimia: dentomedical complications. *Gen Dent* 1992;40:22–25.
89. Rytomaa I, Jarvinen V, Kanerva R, Heinonen OP. Bulimia and tooth erosion. *Acta Odontol Scand* 1998;56:36–40.
90. Harris CK, Warnakulasuriya KA, Johnson NW, et al. Oral health in alcohol misusers. *Community Dent Health* 1996;13:199–203.
91. Robb ND, Smith BG. Prevalence of pathological tooth wear in patients with chronic alcoholism. *Br Dent J* 1990;169:367–369.

92. Smith BGN, Robb ND. Dental erosion in patients with chronic alcoholism. *J Dent* 1989;17:219–221.
93. Duxbury AJ. Ecstasy—dental implications. *Br Dent J* 1993;175:38.
94. Redfearn PJ, Agrawal N, Mair LH. An association between the regular use of 3,4 methylenedioxy-methamphetamine (ecstasy) and excessive wear of the teeth. *Addiction* 1998;93:745–748.
95. Krutchkoff DJ, Eisenberg E, O'Brien JE, Ponzillo JJ. Cocaine-induced dental erosions. *N Engl J Med* 1990;322:408.
96. Ozcelik O, Haytac MC, Seydaoglu G. The effects of anabolic androgenic steroid abuse on gingival tissues. *J Periodontol* 2006;77(7):1104–1109.

Additional resources

Aanestad S, Poulsen S. Oral conditions related to use of the lip plug (ndonya) among the Makonde tribe in Tanzania. *Acta Odontol Scand* 1996;54:362–364.

Abreu Tabarini HS. Dental attrition of Mayan Tzutujil children—a study based on longitudinal materials. *Bull Tokyo Med Dent Univ* 1995;42:31–50.

Al-Hiyasat AS, Saunders WP, Sharkey SW, et al. The abrasive effect of glazed, unglazed, and polished porcelain on the wear of human enamel, and the influence of carbonated soft drinks on the rate of wear. *Int J Prosthodont* 1997;10:269–282.

Al-Hiyasat AS, Saunders WP, Sharkey SW, et al. Investigation of human enamel wear against four dental ceramics and gold. *J Dent* 1998;26:487–495.

Al-Hiyasat AS, Saunders WP, Sharkey SW, Smith GM. The effect of a carbonated beverage on the wear of human enamel and dental ceramics. *J Prosthodont* 1998;7:2–12.

Altshuler BD. Eating disorder patients. *Recognition and intervention.* J Dent Hyg 1990;64:119–125.

Attanasio R. Nocturnal bruxism and its clinical management. *Dent Clin North Am* 1991;35:245–252.

Attin T, Zirkel C, Hellwig E. Brushing abrasion of eroded dentin after application of sodium fluoride solutions. *Caries Res* 1998;32:344–350.

Bader GG, Kampe T, Tagdae T, et al. Descriptive physiological data on a sleep bruxism population. *Sleep* 1997;20:982–990.

Bader JD, McClure F, Scurria MS, et al. Case–control study of non-carious cervical lesions. *Community Dent Oral Epidemiol* 1996;24:286–291.

Bartlett DW. The causes of dental erosion. *Oral Dis* 1997;3:209–211.

Bartlett DW, Coward PY, Nikkah C, Wilson RF. The prevalence of tooth wear in a cluster sample of adolescent schoolchildren and its relationship with potential explanatory factors. *Br Dent J* 1998;184:125–129.

Bartlett DW, Evans DF, Smith BG. The relationship between gastro-oesophageal reflux disease and dental erosion. *J Oral Rehabil* 1996;23:289–297.

Bartlett DW, Smith BG. Clinical investigations of gastro-oesophageal reflux: part 1. *Dent Update* 1996;23:205–208.

Bartlett DW, Smith BG. The dental impact of eating disorders. *Dent Update* 1994;21:404–407.

Bauer W, van den Hoven F, Diedrich P. Wear in the upper and lower incisors in relation to incisal and condylar guidance. *J Orofac Orthop* 1997;58:306–319.

Beckett H. Dental abrasion caused by a cobalt-chromium denture base. *Eur J Prosthodont Restor Dent* 1995;3:209–210.

Beckett H, Buxey-Softley G, Gilmour AG, Smith N. Occupational tooth abrasion in a dental technician: loss of tooth surface resulting from exposure to porcelain powder—a case report. *Quintessence Int* 1995;26:217–220.

Behlfelt K. Enlarged tonsils and the effect of tonsillectomy. Characteristics of the dentition and facial skeleton. Posture of the head, hyoid bone and tongue. Mode of breathing. *Swed Dent J Suppl* 1990;72:1–35.

Berge M, Johannessen G, Silness J. Relationship between alignment conditions of teeth in anterior segments and incisal wear. *J Oral Rehabil* 1996;23:717–721.

Bigenzahn W, Fischman L, Mayrhofer-Krammel U. Myofunctional therapy in patients with orofacial dysfunctions affecting speech. *Folia Phoniatr* 1992;44:238–244.

Bishop K, Kelleher M, Briggs P, Joshi R. Wear now? An update on the etiology of tooth wear. *Quintessence Int* 1997;28:305–313.

Blair FM, Thomason JM, Smith DG. The traumatic anterior overbite. *Dent Update* 1997;24:144–512.

Bohmer CJ, Klinkenberg-Knol EC, Niezen-de Boer MC, et al. Dental erosions and gastro-oesophageal reflux disease in institutionalized intellectually disabled individuals. *Oral Dis* 1997;3:272–275.

Brenchley ML. Is digit sucking of significance? *Br Dent J* 1992;171:357–362.

Burke FJ, Whitehead SA, McCaughey AD. Contemporary concepts in the pathogenesis of the Class V non-carious lesion. *Dent Update* 1995;22:28–32.

Carlson-Mann LD. Recognition and management of occlusal disease from a hygienist's perspective. *Probe* 1996;30:196–197.

Cash RC. Bruxism in children: a review of the literature. *J Pedodont* 1988;12:107–112.

Champagne M. Upper airway compromise (UAC) and the long face syndrome. *J Gen Orthod* 1991;2:18–25.

Cook DA. Using crayons to educate patients about front-tooth wear patterns. *J Am Dent Assoc* 1998;129:1149–1150.

De Cuegas JO. Nonsurgical treatment of a skeletal vertical discrepancy with a significant open bite. *Am J Orthod Dentofac Orthop* 1997;112:124–131.

Delcanho R. Screening for temporomandibular disorders in dental practice. *Aust Dent* 1994;39:222–227.

Djemal S, Darbar UR, Hemmings KW. Case report: tooth wear associated with an unusual habit. *Eur J Prosthodont Restor Dent* 1998;6:29–32.

Dodds AP, King D. Gastroesophageal reflux and dental erosion: case report. *Pediatr Dent* 1997;19:409–412.

Donachie MA, Walls AW. Assessment of tooth wear in an ageing population. *J Dent* 1995;23:157–164.

Douglas WH. Form, function and strength in the restored dentition. *Ann R Austr Coll Dent Surg* 1996;13:35–46.

Edwards M, Ashwood RA, Littlewood SJ, et al. A video-fluoroscopic comparison of straw and cup drinking: the potential influence on dental erosion. *Br Dent J* 1998;185:244–249.

Ehrlich J, Hochman N, Yaffe A. Contribution of oral habits to dental disorders. *Cranio* 1992;10:144–147.

Evans RD. Orthodontics and the creation of localised inter-occlusal space in cases of anterior tooth wear. *Eur J Prosthodont Restor Dent* 1997;5:69–73.

Evans RD, Briggs PF. Tooth-surface loss related to pregnancy-induced vomiting. *Prim Dent Care* 1994;1:24–26.

Formicola V. Interproximal grooving: different appearances, different etiologies. *Am J Phys Anthropol* 1991;86:85–87.

Frayer DW. On the etiology of interproximal grooves. *Am J Phys Anthropol* 1991;85:299–304.

Friman PC, Schmitt BD. Thumb sucking: pediatrician's guidelines. *Clin Pediatr* 1989;28:438–440.

Gilmour AG, Beckett HA. The voluntary reflux phenomenon. *Br Dent J* 1993;175:368–372.

Goldstein RE. Diagnostic dilemma: to bond, laminate, or crown? *Int J Periodont Restor Dent* 1987;87(5):9–30.

Goldstein RE. The difficult patient stress syndrome: Part 1. *J Esthet Dent* 1993;5:86–87.

Goldstein RE. Esthetics in dentistry. *J Am Dent Assoc* 1982;104:301–302.

Goldstein RE, Garber DA, Schwartz CG, Goldstein CE. Patient maintenance of esthetic restorations. *J Am Dent Assoc* 1992;123:61–66.

Goldstein RE, Parkins F. Air-abrasive technology: its new role in restorative dentistry. *J Am Dent Assoc* 1994;125:551–557.

Gregory-Head B, Curtis DA. Erosion caused by gastroesophageal reflux: diagnostic considerations. *J Prosthodont* 1997;6:278–285.

Grippo JO. Abfractions: a new classification of hard tissue lesions of teeth. *J Esthet Dent* 1991;3:14–19.

Grippo JO. Noncarious cervical lesions: the decision to ignore or restore. *J Esthet Dent* 1992;4(Suppl):55–64.

Hacker CH, Wagner WC, Razzoog ME. An in vitro investigation of the wear of enamel on porcelain and gold in saliva. *J Prosthet Dent* 1996;75:14–17.

Harris EF, Butler ML. Patterns of incisor root resorption before and after orthodontic correction in cases with anterior open bites. *Am J Orthod Dentofac Orthop* 1992;101:112–119.

Hazelton LR, Faine MP. Diagnosis and dental management of eating disorder patients. *Int J Prosthodont* 1996;9:65–73.

Hertzberg J, Nakisbendi L, Needleman HL, Pober B. Williams syndrome—oral presentation of 45 cases. *Pediatr Dent* 1994;16:262–267.

Heymann HO, Sturdevant JR, Bayne S, et al. Examining tooth flexure effects on cervical restorations: a two year clinical study. *J Am Dent Assoc* 1991;122:41–47.

Hicks RA, Conti P. Nocturnal bruxism and self reports of stress-related symptoms. *Percept Mot Skills* 1991;72:1182.

Hicks RA, Lucero-Gorman K, Bautista J, Hicks GJ. Ethnicity and bruxism. *Percept Mot Skills* 1999;88:240–241.

Horsted-Bindslev P, Knudsen J, Baelum V. 3-year clinical evaluation of modified Gluma adhesive systems in cervical abrasion/erosion lesions. *Am J Dent* 1996;9:22–26.

Hsu LK. Epidemiology of the eating disorders. *Psychiatr Clin North Am* 1996;19:681–700.

Hudson JD, Goldstein GR, Georgescu M. Enamel wear caused by three different restorative materials. *J Prosthet Dent* 1995;74:647–654.

Hugoson A, Ekfeldt A, Koch G, Hallonsten AL. Incisal and occlusal tooth wear in children and adolescents in a Swedish population. *Acta Odontol Scand* 1996;54:263–270.

Ikeda T, Nishigawa K, Kondo K, et al. Criteria for the detection of sleep-associated bruxism in humans. *J Orofac Pain* 1996;10:270–282.

Imfeld T. Dental erosion. Definition, classification and links. *Eur J Oral Sci* 1996;104:151–154.

Imfeld T. Prevention of progression of dental erosion by professional and individual prophylactic measures. *Eur J Oral Sci* 1996;104:215–220.

Ingleby J, Mackie IC. Case report: an unusual cause of toothwear. *Dent Update* 1995;22:434–435.

Jagger DC, Harrison A. An in vitro investigation into the wear effects of selected restorative materials on enamel. *J Oral Rehabil* 1995;22:275–281.

Jagger DC, Harrison A. An in vitro investigation into the wear effects of selected restorative materials on dentine. *J Oral Rehabil* 1995;22:349–354.

Jarvinen VK, Rytomaa II, Heinonen OP. Risk factors in dental erosion. *J Dent Res* 1991;70:942–947.

Johansson A. A cross-cultural study of occlusal tooth wear. *Swed Dent J Suppl* 1992;86:1–59.

Josell SD. Habits affecting dental and maxillofacial growth and development. *Dent Clin North Am* 1995;39:851–860.

Josephson CA. Restoration of mandibular incisors with advanced wear. *J Dent Assoc S Afr* 1992;47:419–420.

Kaidonis JA, Richards LC, Townsend GC, Tansley GD. Wear of human enamel: a quantitative in vitro assessment. *J Dent Res* 1998;77:1983–1990.

Kampe T, Hannerz H, Strom P. Ten-year follow-up study of signs and symptoms of craniomandibular disorders in adults with intact and restored dentitions. *J Oral Rehabil* 1996;23:416–423.

Kelleher M, Bishop K. The aetiology and clinical appearance of tooth wear. *Eur J Prosthodont Restor Dent* 1997;5:157–160.

Khan F, Young WG, Daley TJ. Dental erosion and bruxism. A tooth wear analysis from south east Queensland. *Aust Dent J* 1998;43:117–127.

Kidd EA, Smith BG. Toothwear histories: a sensitive issue. *Dent Update* 1993;20:174–178.

Kiliaridis S, Johansson A, Haraldson T, et al. Craniofacial morphology, occlusal traits, and bite force in persons with advanced occlusal tooth wear. *Am J Orthodont Dentofac Orthop* 1995;107:286–292.

Kleinberg I. Bruxism: aetiology, clinical signs and symptoms. *Aust Prosthodont J* 1994;8:9–17.

Knight DJ, Leroux BG, Zhu C, et al. A longitudinal study of tooth wear in orthodontically treated patients. *Am J Orthod Dentofacial Orthop* 1997;112:194–202.

Kokich VG. Esthetics and vertical tooth position: orthodontic possibilities. *Compend Cont Educ Dent* 1997;18:1225–1231.

Lambrechts P, van Meerbeek B, Perdigao J, et al. Restorative therapy for erosive lesions. *Eur J Oral Sci* 1996;104:229–240.

Lavigne GL, Rompre PH, Montplaisir JY. Sleep bruxism: validity of clinical research diagnostic criteria in a controlled polysomnographic study. *J Dent Res* 1996;75:546–552.

Lee CL, Eakle WS. Possible role of tensile stress in the etiology of cervical erosive lesions of teeth. *J Prosthet Dent* 1984;52:374–380.

Lee CL, Eakle WS. Stress-induced cervical lesions: review of advances in the past 10 years. *J Prosthet Dent* 1996;75:487–494.

Leinfelder KF, Yarnell G. Occlusion and restorative materials. *Dent Clin North Am* 1995;39:355–361.

Leung AK, Robson WL. Thumb sucking. *Am Fam Physician* 1991;44:1724–1728.

Levine RS. Briefing paper: oral aspects of dummy and digit sucking. *Br Dent J* 1999;186:108.

Lussi A. Dental erosion clinical diagnosis and case history taking. *Eur J Oral Sci* 1996;104:191–198.

Lussi A, Portmann P, Burhop B. Erosion on abraded dental hard tissues by acid lozenges: an in situ study. *Clin Oral Investig* 1997;1:191–194.

Mair LH, Stolarski TA, Vowles RW, Lloyd CH. Wear: mechanisms, manifestations and measurement. Report of a workshop. *J Dent* 1996;24:141–148.

Marchesan IQ, Krakauer LR. The importance of respiratory activity in myofunctional therapy. *Int J Orofac Myol* 1996;22:23–27.

Maron FS. Enamel erosion resulting from hydrochloride acid tablets. *J Am Dent Assoc* 1996;127:781–784.

Matis BA, Cochran M, Carlson T. Longevity of glass-ionomer restorative materials: results of a 10-year evaluation. *Quintessence Int* 1996;27:373–382.

McCoy G. The etiology of gingival erosion. *J Oral Implantol* 1982;10:361–362.

McCoy G. On the longevity of teeth. *J Oral Implantol* 1983;11:248–267.

McIntyre JM. Erosion. *Aust Prosthodont J* 1992;6:17–25.

Mehler PS, Gray MC, Schulte M. Medical complications of anorexia nervosa. *J Womens Health* 1997;6:533–541.

Menapace SE, Rinchuse DJ, Zullo T, et al. The dentofacial morphology of bruxers versus non-bruxers. *Angle Orthod* 1994;64:43–52.

Mercado MD. The prevalence and aetiology of craniomandibular disorders among completely edentulous patients. *Aust Prosthodont J* 1993;7:27–29.

Mercado MD, Faulkner KD. The prevalence of craniomandibular disorders in completely edentulous denture-wearing subjects. *J Oral Rehabil* 1991;18:231–242.

Metaxas A. Oral habits and malocclusion. A case report. *Ont Dent* 1996;73:27–33.

Millward A, Shaw L, Smith AJ. Dental erosion in four-year-old children from differing socioeconomic backgrounds. *ASDC J Dent Child* 1994;61:263–366.

Millward A, Shaw L, Smith AJ, et al. The distribution and severity of tooth wear and the relationship between erosion and dietary constituents in a group of children. *Int J Paediatr Dent* 1994;4:151–157.

Milosevic A. Tooth wear: an aetiological and diagnostic problem. *Eur J Prosthodont Restor Dent* 1993;1:173–178.

Milosevic A, Brodie DA, Slade PD. Dental erosion, oral hygiene, and nutrition in eating disorders. *Int J Eat Disord* 1997;21:195–199.

Milosevic A, Dawson LJ. Salivary factors in vomiting bulimics with and without pathological tooth wear. *Caries Res* 1996;30:361–366.

Milosevic A, Lennon MA, Fear SC. Risk factors associated with tooth wear in teenagers: a case control study. *Community Dent Health* 1997;14:143–147.

Morley J. The esthetics of anterior tooth aging. *Curr Opin Cosmet Dent* 1997;4:35–39.

Moses AJ. Thumb sucking or thumb propping? *CDS Rev* 1987;80:40–42.

Moss RA, Lombardo TW, Villarosa GA, et al. Oral habits and TMJ dysfunction in facial pain and non-pain subjects. *J Oral Rehabil* 1995;22:79–81.

Murray CG, Sanson GD. Thegosis—a critical review. *Aust Dent J* 1998;43:192–198.

Nel JC, Bester SP, Snyman WD. Bruxism threshold: an explanation for successful treatment of multifactorial aetiology of bruxism. *Aust Prosthodont J* 1995;9:33–37.

Nel JC, Marais JT, van Vuuren PA. Various methods of achieving restoration of tooth structure loss due to bruxism. *J Esthet Dent* 1996;8:183–188.

Nemcovsky CE, Artzi Z. Erosion-abrasion lesions revisited. *Compend Cont Educ Dent* 1996;17:416–418.

Neo J, Chew CL. Direct tooth-colored materials for noncarious lesions: a 3-year clinical report. *Quintessence Int* 1995;27:183–188.

Neo J, Chew CL, Yap A, Sidhu S. Clinical evaluation of tooth-colored materials in cervical lesions. *Am J Dent* 1996;9:15–18.

Nunn JH. Prevalence of dental erosion and the implications for oral health. *Eur J Oral Sci* 1996;104:156–161.

Nunn J, Shaw L, Smith A. Tooth wear—dental erosion. *Br Dent J* 1996;180:349–352.

Nystrom M, Kononen M, Alaluusua S, et al. Development of horizontal tooth wear in maxillary anterior teeth from five to 18 years of age. *J Dent Res* 1990;69:1765–1770.

Okeson JP. Occlusion and functional disorders of the masticatory system. *Dent Clin North Am* 1995;39:285–300.

Osborne-Smith KL, Burke FJ, FarlaneTM, Wilson NH. Effect of restored and unrestored non-carious cervical lesions on the fracture resistance of previously restored maxillary premolar teeth. *J Dent* 1998;26:427–433.

O'Sullivan EA, Curzon ME, Roberts GJ, et al. Gastroesophageal reflux in children and its relationship to erosion of primary and permanent teeth. *Eur J Oral Sci* 1998;106:765–769.

Owens BM, Gallien GS. Noncarious dental "abfraction" lesions in an aging population. *Compend Cont Educ Dent* 1995;16:552–562.

Paterson AJ, Watson IB. Case report: prolonged match chewing: an unusual case of tooth wear. *Eur J Prosthodont Restor Dent* 1995;3:131–134.

Pavone BW. Bruxism and its effect on the natural teeth. *J Prosthet Dent* 1985;53:692–696.

Pierce CJ, Chrisman K, Bennett ME, Close JM. Stress, anticipatory stress, and psychologic measures related to sleep bruxism. *J Orofac Pain* 1995;9:51–56.

Pintado MR, Anderson GC, DeLong R, Douglas WH. Variation in tooth wear in young adults over a two-year period. *J Prosthet Dent* 1997;77:313–320.

Powell LV, Johnson GH, Gordon GE. Factors associated with clinical success of cervical abrasion/erosion restorations. *Oper Dent* 1995;20:7–13.

Principato JJ. Upper airway obstruction and craniomandibular morphology. *Otolaryngol Head Neck Surg* 1991;104:881–890.

Ramp MH, Suzuki S, Cox CF, et al. Evaluation of wear: enamel opposing three ceramic materials and a gold alloy. *J Prosthet Dent* 1997;77:523–530.

Ribeiro RA, Romano AR, Birman EG, Mayer MP. Oral manifestations of Rett syndrome: a study of 17 cases. *Pediatr Dent* 1997;19:349–352.

Ritchard A, Welsh AH, Donnelly C. The association between occlusion and attrition. *Aust Orthod J* 1992;12:138–142.

Rivera-Morales WC, McCall WD Jr. Reliability of a portable electromyographic unit to measure bruxism. *J Prosthet Dent* 1995;73:184–189.

Robb ND, Cruwys E, Smith BG. Regurgitation erosion as a possible cause of tooth wear in ancient British populations. *Arch Oral Biol* 1991;36:595–602.

Rogers GM, Poore MH, Ferko BL, et al. In vitro effects of an acidic by-product feed on bovine teeth. *Am J Vet Res* 1997;58:498–503.

Schmidt U, Treasure J. Eating disorders and the dental practitioner. *Eur J Prosthodont Restor Dent* 1997;5:161–167.

Schneider PE. Oral habits—harmful and helpful. *Update Pediatr Dent* 1991;4:1–4, 6–8.

Schwartz JH, Brauer J, Gordon-Larsen P. Brief communication: Tigaran (Point Hope, Alaska) tooth drilling. *Am J Phys Anthropol* 1995;97:77–82.

Seligman DA, Pullinger AG. The degree to which dental attrition in modern society is a function of age and of canine contact. *J Orofac Pain* 1995;9:266–275.

Seow WK. Clinical diagnosis of enamel defects: pitfalls and practical guidelines. *Int Dent J* 1997;47:173–182.

Sherfudin H, Abdullah A, Shaik H, Johansson A. Some aspects of dental health in young adult Indian vegetarians. A pilot study. *Acta Odontol Scand* 1996;54:44–48.

Silness J, Berge M, Johannessen G. A 2-year follow-up study of incisal tooth wear in dental students. *Acta Odontol Scand* 1995;53:331–333.

Silness J, Berge M, Johannessen G. Longitudinal study of incisal tooth wear in children and adolescents. *Eur J Oral Sci* 1995;103:90–94.

Silness J, Berge M, Johannessen G. Re-examination of incisal tooth wear in children and adolescents. *J Oral Rehabil* 1997;24:405–409.

Smith BG, Bartlett DW, Robb ND. The prevalence, etiology and management of tooth wear in the United Kingdom. *J Prosthet Dent* 1997;78:367–372.

Smith BG, Robb ND. The prevalence of toothwear in 1007 dental patients. *J Oral Rehabil* 1996;23:232–239.

Sognnaes RF, Wolcott RB, Xhonga FA. Dental erosion I. Erosion-like patterns occurring in association with other dental conditions. *J Am Dent Assoc* 1972;84:571–576.

Speer JA. Bulimia: full stomach, empty lives. *Dent Assist* 1991;60:28–30.

Spranger H. Investigation into the genesis of angular lesions at the cervical region of teeth. *Quintessence Int* 1995;26:183–188.

Steiner H, Lock J. Anorexia nervosa and bulimia nervosa in children and adolescents: a review of the past 10 years. *J Am Acad Child Adolesc Psychiatry* 1998;37:352–359.

Stewart B. Restoration of the severely worn dentition using a systematized approach for a predictable prognosis. *Int J Periodont Restor Dent* 1998;18:46–57.

Suzuki S, Suzuki SH, Cox CF. Evaluating the antagonistic wear of restorative materials when placed against human enamel. *J Am Dent Assoc* 1996;127:74–80.

Taylor G, Taylor S, Abrams R, Mueller W. Dental erosion associated with asymptomatic gastroesophageal reflux. *ASDC J Dent Child* 1992;59:182–185.

Teaford MF, Lytle JD. Brief communication: diet-induced changes in the rates of human tooth microwear: a case study involving stone-ground maize. *Am J Phys Anthropol* 1996;100:143–147.

Teo C, Young WG, Daley TJ, Sauer H. Prior fluoridation in childhood affects dental caries and tooth wear in a south east Queensland population. *Aust Dent J* 1997;42:92–102.

Thompson BA, Blount BW, Krumholz TS. Treatment approaches to bruxism. *Am Fam Physician* 1994;49:1617–1622.

Timms DJ, Trenouth MJ. A quantified comparison of craniofacial form with nasal respiratory function. *Am J Orthod Dentofac Orthop.*1988;94:216–221.

Touyz LZ. The acidity (pH) and buffering capacity of Canadian fruit juice and dental implications. *J Can Dent Assoc* 1994;60:448–454.

Turp JC, Gobetti JP. The cracked tooth syndrome: an elusive diagnosis. *J Am Dent Assoc* 1996;127:1502–1507.

Tyas MJ. The Class V lesion—aetilogy and restoration. *Aust Dent J* 1995;40:167–170.

Ung N, Koenig J, Shapiro PA, et al. A quantitative assessment of respiratory patterns and their effects on dentofacial development. *Am J Orthod Dentofac Orthop* 1990;98:523–532.

Villa G, Giacobini G. Subvertical grooves of interproximal facets in Neandertal posterior teeth. *Am J Phys Anthropol* 1995;96:51–62.

Waterman ET, Koltai PJ, Downey JC, Cacace AT. Swallowing disorders in a population of children with cerebral palsy. *Int J Pediatr Otorhinolaryngol* 1992;24:63–71.

West NX, Maxwell A, Hughes JA, et al. A method to measure clinical erosion: the effect of orange juice consumption on erosion of enamel. *J Dent* 1998;26:329–335.

Westergaard J, Moe D, Pallesen U, Holmen L. Exaggerated abrasion/erosion of human dental enamel surfaces: a case report. *Scand J Dent Res* 1993;101:265–269.

Woodside DG, Linder-Aronson S, Lundstrom A, McWilliam J. Mandibular and maxillary growth after changed mode of breathing. *Am J Orthod Dentofac Orthop* 1991;100:1–18.

Yaacob HB, Park AW. Dental abrasion pattern in a selected group of Malaysians. *J Nihon Univ Sch Dent* 1990;32:175–180.

Yamaguchi H, Tanaka Y, Sueishi K, et al. Changes in oral functions and muscular behavior due to surgical orthodontic treatment. *Bull Tokyo Dent Coll* 1994;35:41–49.

Young DV, Rinchuse DJ, Pierce CJ, Zullo T. The craniofacial morphology of bruxers versus nonbruxers. *Angle Orthod* 1999;69:14–18.

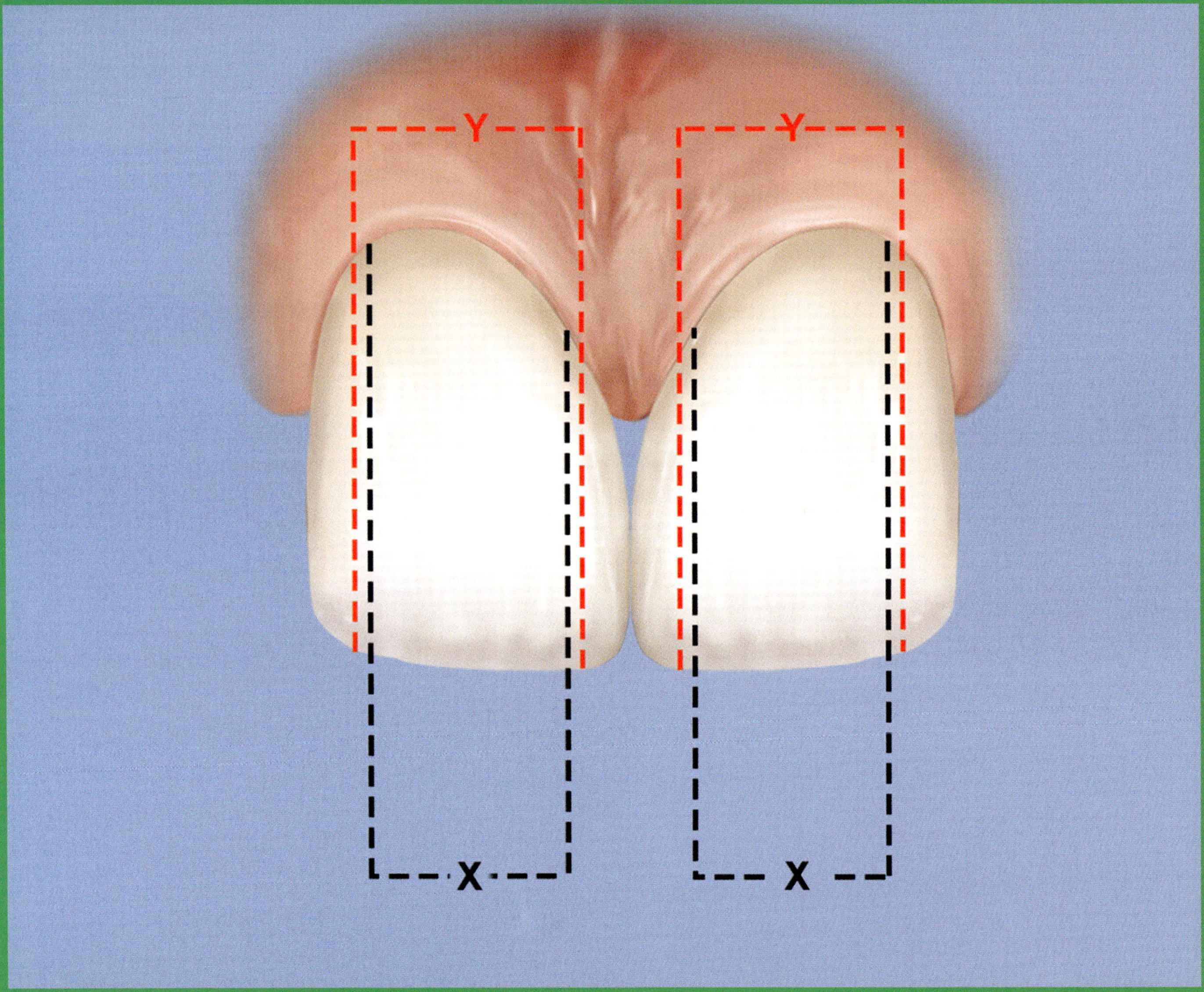
Y
Y
X
X

Chapter 26 Restorative Treatment of Diastema

Barry D. Hammond, DMD, Kevin B. Frazier, DMD, EDS,
Anabella Oquendo, DDS, and Ronald E. Goldstein, DDS

Chapter Outline

Etiology of diastema	842	Functional considerations in restoring diastemata	848
Diagnosis and treatment planning	843	Restorative treatment options	849
Treatment options for correction of diastemata	844	Direct bonding with composite resin	849
Esthetic considerations in restoring diastemata	844	Porcelain veneers	864
Incisal edge position	846	Closing single midline diastema with porcelain	866
Tooth proportion	846	Closing multiple diastemata with porcelain veneers	867
Gingival esthetics	847	Combination crowns/veneers	869
Esthetic illusions	847		

One of the most challenging tasks of modern restorative dentistry is resolving the dilemma of spaces between the anterior teeth. The presence of a diastema is desirable in some cultures; however, it is always a matter of personal choice for those who believe closing it will improve the appearance of their smile.[1] Self-consciousness, low self-esteem, and awkward attempts to conceal a perceived anatomical defect are frequent consequences of smiles that are perceived as esthetically compromised.[2] A diastema usually distorts a pleasing smile by concentrating the observer's attention not on the overall dental composition but instead on the interdental space.[3]

The general public has been shown to have definite preferences for anterior tooth variations. Rosentiel and Rashid observed that 90% of the interviewed adults preferred an image without a diastema against one with even a minimal diastema as small as 0.5 mm.[4] Those who dislike the appearance of a diastema often attempt to hide it with intentional habits, such as lip or tongue posturing.[5] Some patients have even resorted to daily applications of wax or cotton to disguise the spaces (Figure 26.1A and B). The use of removable veneers has increased in popularity and they can be worn in public to disguise a myriad of dental deficiencies (including diastemata) or to preview proposed esthetic changes (Figure 26.2A and B). However, the personal values and preferences of the patient are the principles that are most important. Consideration of the patient's needs and expectations is paramount. Satisfaction with the final treatment outcome is ensured by careful questioning about their preferences.[6]

Treatment planning to correct a diastema may include orthodontics, restorative dentistry (by direct or indirect methods), surgery, or a combination of several therapies. Like most esthetic problems, diastema treatment requires careful analysis and often involves an interdisciplinary approach for more complex

Ronald E. Goldstein's Esthetics in Dentistry, Third Edition. Edited by Ronald E. Goldstein, Stephen J. Chu, Ernesto A. Lee, and Christian F.J. Stappert.
© 2018 John Wiley & Sons, Inc. Published 2018 by John Wiley & Sons, Inc.

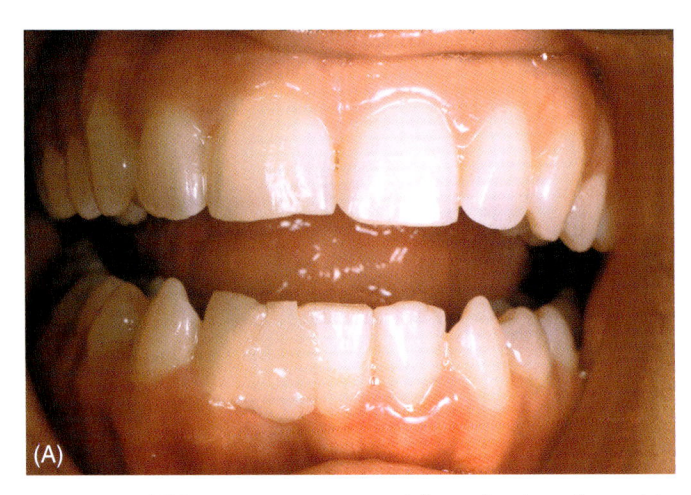

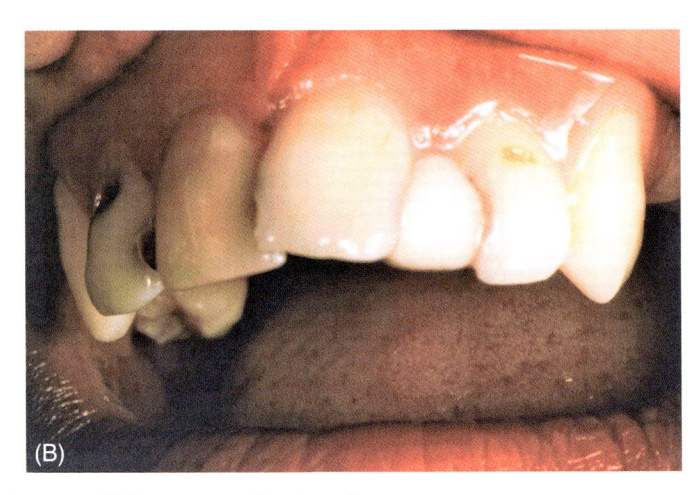

Figure 26.1 **(A)** Some patients resort to daily applications of materials such as wax **(B)** Or cotton to disguise a diastema.

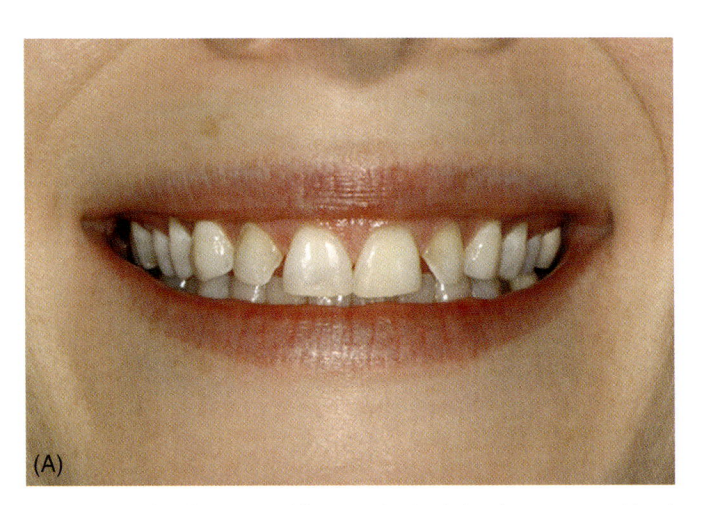

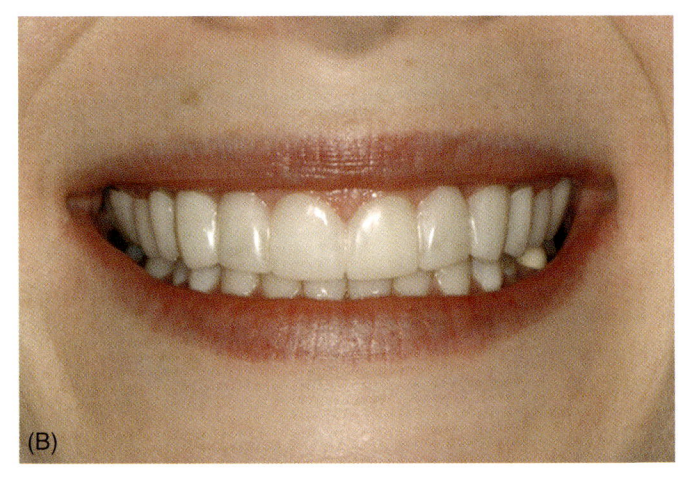

Figure 26.2 **(A, B)** A removable Snap-On Smile has been inserted by the patient to close the spaces and improve her smile as desired for social occasions. *Source:* Reproduced with permission of Denmat© Corporation.

scenarios. While closure of these spaces in many cases can be relatively straightforward, obtaining a result that is esthetically pleasing and stable requires careful analysis of tooth positions as they relate to facial esthetics, tooth proportions and shape, soft tissue architecture, periodontal health, and occlusion. Besides the clinical exam, access to diagnostic casts, radiographs, photographs, and digital imaging may be necessary to thoroughly evaluate a diastema and develop a suitable treatment plan. Before providing treatment to close an anterior diastema, one should attempt to identify and treat the underlying cause(s) if possible and applicable. All appropriate options, along with advantages and disadvantages of each, should be presented to allow the patient to be fully informed, and thus able to make the most appropriate choice in terms of treatment modality and preference of materials.

Etiology of diastema

The etiology of diastemata (multiple diastemas) may be attributed to hereditary and/or developmental factors (Table 26.1).[7,8] Since hereditary determinants play a major role in causing diastemata, there is nothing that can be done to prevent most of them; however, many of the developmental causes of diastema formation are preventable or manageable. It is important to distinguish the origin of such spaces to determine whether they are hereditary or developmental, since the latter category often indicates instability within the oral cavity as a result of tooth loss, reduced periodontal support, and/or occlusal trauma.[9] Although racial and gender differences for diastemata prevalence have been found to exist, approximately 50% of all children between 6 and 8 years old exhibit maxillary midline spaces that typically decrease in size with age,[7] except for approximately 6% that persist into adulthood.[10]

Table 26.1 Factors Contributing To Diastemata

Hereditary Factors	Developmental Factors
Congenitally missing teeth	Habits
Tooth/jaw size discrepancy	Periodontal disease
Supernumerary teeth	Tooth loss
Frenal attachments	Posterior bite collapse
Tooth shape	Occlusal trauma

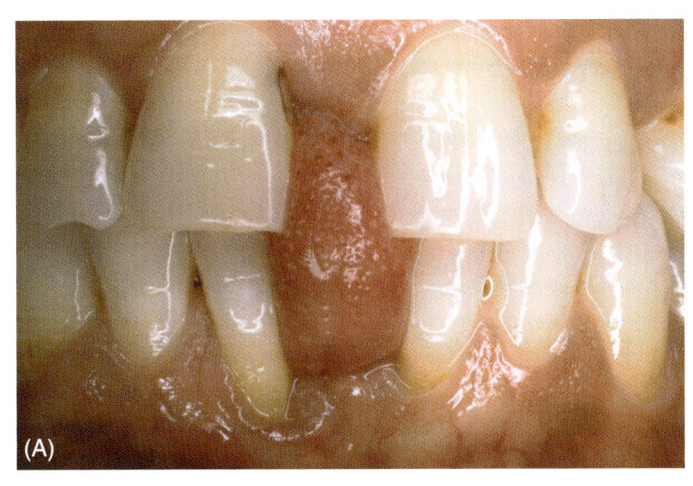

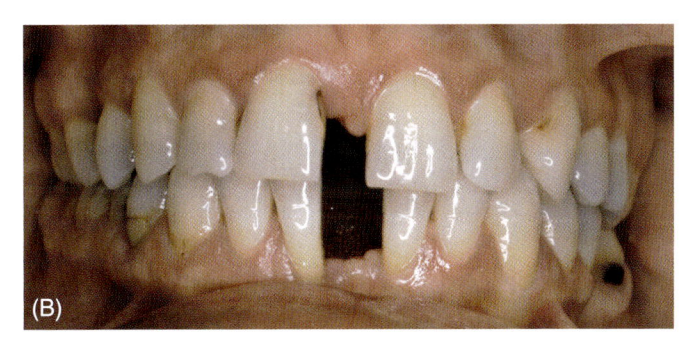

Figure 26.3 **(A, B)** This patient had a habit of forcing her tongue between both maxillary and mandibular anterior teeth, which caused her diastema to continue to enlarge.

With the exception of third molars; maxillary lateral incisors and mandibular second premolars are the most commonly congenitally missing permanent teeth.[10] A missing tooth creates an obvious space problem in the immediate area and may lead to undesirable spacing in adjacent regions as the position of several teeth in a quadrant (or the opposing quadrant) can be affected by the absence of a single tooth. Small teeth and large jaws (tooth size/jaw size discrepancy) can lead to generalized spacing, whereas unerupted supernumerary teeth can create a diastema by their position between the roots of other teeth.[11] Microdontia, a condition seen in conjunction with other hereditary conditions (e.g., exhibited in higher incidence in patients with dental agenesis),[12] often leads to diastemata as well. Anatomic factors such as those seen in atypical frenum positions may also contribute to diastema formation[13] and may require a combined surgical/restorative and/or orthodontic approach for long-term stability.

Among the most common developmental causes of diastemata are habits, one of which is tongue thrusting. Large tongues (macroglossia) or abnormal swallowing patterns can cause tooth separation by the habitual forcing of the tongue into the lingual embrasures of teeth (Figure 26.3A and B) creating pressure that can eventually wedge them apart. Pernicious habits such as chronic lip biting may also contribute to tooth movement and diastema formation, in a similar manner as tongue thrusting, through chronic labially directed pressure.[7] Periodontal trauma with resultant spacing between the incisors can be caused by habits such as wedging a fingernail, toothpick, or other foreign object between the teeth (see Chapter 25). Other developmental causes of diastemata are obvious, such as the loss of a permanent tooth, or more subtle, such as chronic periodontal disease.[14] Tooth loss in the posterior region has been associated with anterior diastema formation as a result of posterior bite collapse or from mesial–distal drift or tipping of posterior teeth.[15] In this case, the loss of posterior occlusal contacts alters the pattern of occlusal function, often leading to tooth migration and the potential for decreased vertical dimension. The indirect result of this condition can be a labial flaring of the maxillary incisors (pathologic tooth migration) with resultant space formation. Prevention of tooth loss, preventive or corrective occlusal therapy to maintain vertical dimension or minimize occlusal trauma, and maintenance of periodontal health can reduce the likelihood of diastema formation that results from deterioration of the normal structure and function of the oral cavity. Although it was shown by Martinez-Canut et al. that bone loss is the factor most often related to pathologic tooth migration, it was also concluded that pathologic tooth migration was rarely the result of any one single factor.[15]

The presence of fibrous frenal attachments (often found in the maxillary midline) can result in a persistent midline diastema that often requires surgical intervention to enable space closure or prevent relapse. In these cases, consultation between the restoring dentist, the orthodontist, and the periodontist is highly recommended to determine the appropriate timing for frenal resection as a part of the overall treatment.

The etiology of diastema and the prognosis for successful closure following treatment, along with patient's desires, must all be factored into the decision as to whether or not to treat, and, if indicated, the appropriate mode of treatment chosen. Understanding the reason(s) for the spacing and attempting to correct or minimize the causative factors can improve the odds for success of corrective therapy.

Diagnosis and treatment planning

Although the presence of a diastema and an initial opinion regarding its treatment may seem obvious, careful evaluation and thorough planning is essential prior to rendering treatment to obtain a successful, esthetic, and stable result. As previously discussed, the etiology of diastema may be attributed to hereditary and developmental factors. Upon identifying these factors, the dentist should include the patient in the treatment planning process by presenting appropriate treatment alternatives, prognoses, and fees.

Identifying the cause(s) of a diastema will often indicate the most appropriate corrective treatment plan.[16] For example, diastemata due to periodontal problems cannot be corrected predictably with restorations alone if alveolar bone has been lost and the teeth are mobile. When periodontal disease is causing the teeth to drift and separate, any active pathology (acute or chronic) must first be resolved. Referral for a periodontal consultation is often warranted as the disease process itself may be advanced and carry a poor or guarded prognosis. Once the periodontal condition has been treated and stabilized, other therapies can be instituted, such as orthodontics and/or restorative dentistry. Either option may also include splinting to compensate for lost periodontal support. Properly sequenced treatment in these cases enables the clinician to achieve a final esthetic result that may be performed with better confidence for a more stable and predictable result.[17]

Although restorations are usually indicated to close multiple diastemata due to small teeth, other coordinated therapies may be needed to achieve an optimal esthetic result. Tooth repositioning may be necessary to create uniform or more manageable spaces prior to restoration placement. However, if one is considering orthodontics to close spaces but the associated teeth need restorations to restore lost form or function, then restorative therapy alone may be an acceptable option depending on the size of the spaces and proportions of the teeth. Short teeth diastemata cases may require periodontal surgery to provide additional clinical crown height to balance the increase in tooth width (i.e., create more pleasing tooth proportions; specifically, width-to-length ratios) from planned restorations intended to close spaces. Part of the diagnostic phase should include evaluation of tooth and gingival exposure, in the full and exaggerated smile, to assess whether additional treatment (e.g., crown lengthening) purely for esthetics is even warranted. Short or hypermobile upper lips, supra-eruption of teeth, and vertical maxillary excess can contribute to excessive tooth/tissue display that may require consideration for additional therapy, beyond that of diastema closure, to achieve the most ideal esthetic result. However, if only a small part of the vertical height of the teeth is seen (even in the exaggerated smile), then the additional cost, time, and discomfort of elective periodontal treatment may not be worth it to the patient. Additional teeth not directly affected by a diastema may also need to be included in the restorative treatment plan to provide a proportional smile. Anytime a patient is considering extensive restorative treatment, they should first be given the opportunity to change their existing tooth color. Prerestorative bleaching can improve the esthetic result of any type of restorative therapy and should always be considered when extensive dental treatment is planned. Tooth-whitening procedures allow thinner or more translucent restorations to be used (e.g., porcelain veneers, all-ceramic crowns with reduced core opacity, or direct composite resin bonding) when dark/stained tooth structure does not have to be masked.[18,19] The preceding factors illustrate the importance of thorough diagnosis and comprehensive treatment planning for all types of diastema cases.

As patient acceptance of ideal treatment is the ultimate objective for the dentist in this phase, it is often necessary to allow the patient to visualize and approve the anticipated result.[5] For simple diastema closures involving restorations, the chairside application of tooth-colored wax or unbonded composite resin (for an esthetic preview or "mockup") to the patient's proximal tooth surfaces should provide a good preview of the proposed result. For complex cases that involve several teeth or combination therapies (orthodontics and restorations), a diagnostic wax-up and/or computer imaging may be required to enable the patient to fully appreciate the anticipated result of extensive treatment (see Chapter 3).[20] Alternatively, and when applicable, a more detailed esthetic preview can be utilized to confirm the proposed changes or need for additional refinement. The use of laboratory-fabricated templates or removable veneers (i.e., Snap-On Smile®) (see Figure 26.2A and B) or bis-acryl-type provisional materials added to the teeth via a matrix (fabricated from a diagnostic wax-up) (see Figure 26.4A–C) can be a valuable adjunct for the patient to enable them to preview their new smile directly in their own mouth and provide valuable diagnostic information to the clinician. When multiple disciplines are involved, such as orthodontics, surgery, and restorative dentistry, a case presentation conference (or teleconference) with all involved clinicians and the patient may facilitate acceptance of complex treatment plans.

Pre- and postoperative photographs or digital images can provide many benefits. Photographs of the results of treatment completed for other patients with similar conditions can be used to help current patients envision the possibilities associated with their own treatment and inspire confidence in the dentist's abilities to treat these types of cases. If computer imaging is utilized to enable patients to visualize anticipated treatment results, it would be advisable to provide both close-up and full-face before and after images for best patient and doctor visualization of the possible outcome. However, care must be exercised to present the proposed treatment in a way that does not imply a "guarantee" of results. One must always remember that due diligence is required in the diagnostic phase to give the best chance for a successful outcome based on achieving realistic patient expectations. Photographs used to document the procedure can also be used to improve the chances for reimbursement from third-party payers in certain cases. A duplicate set of pre- and posttreatment images given to patients following treatment helps to prevent "buyer's remorse" by reminding them of their presenting condition, and allows them to serve as marketing advocates for the office when dramatic, successful before and after photographs are displayed to family and friends.

Treatment options for correction of diastemata

Esthetic considerations in restoring diastemata

When restorations are indicated for diastema closure, several esthetic factors must be considered. First and most obvious is how the teeth fit within the frame of the face and the smile, the so-called macroesthetics.[21] Second are the considerations associated with the esthetic appearance of the individual teeth, the microesthetic component. Regarding the macroesthetic factors, it is necessary to evaluate the elements that make up facial composition before focusing on the teeth. Considering the teeth first will reduce the scope of the investigation. Frontal and lateral examinations of the subject, including analysis of the position of the eyes, nose, chin, and lips, allows identification of the reference points and lines that are indispensable to the diastema closure. The facial features have an important influence on the perception of an individual's personality. The somatic traits are in fact often correlated with precise psychological characteristics, and some features are associated with specific individual aspects. Analysis of these features is made using horizontal and vertical reference lines which allow correlation of the patient's face and dentition.[22]

A variety of factors should be considered when determining the most appropriate treatment for closing anterior spaces. Clinical evaluation of the lateral facial (profile) view should be one consideration. Anterior tooth position can affect lip support, lip fullness, vermillion exposure, and the nasolabial angle. When space closure includes incisor retraction, its effect on the lips must be considered.

Both restorative and/or orthodontic treatment can produce changes in lip support, and thus if not well planned may compromise the final treatment outcome. Taking into account perioral tissue contours will minimize the potential of producing an orthodontically induced unesthetic facial profile. The patient with thin lips or minimal muscular tone is most at risk of losing lip support when incisors are retracted to close anterior spaces.

Changes to the position and outline of the maxillary central incisors can significantly impact the treatment result. These changes should not interfere with the tooth's position of equilibrium, between the tongue lingually, the lips labially, and the cheeks laterally. Alterations of this type could alter the positional equilibrium of the teeth, thereby increasing the chance of tooth movement in the form or crowding or spacing, as well as negatively affecting the patient's unique facial form in an undesirable fashion.[22]

Conventional wisdom would dictate that alignment of the facial and dental midlines is desirable. In nature, this occurrence is rare. Kokich et al. have found that discrepancies between the facial and dental midlines that are 4 mm or less are not readily noticeable to either patients or general dental practitioners.[23] Therefore, as a rule, limited midline discrepancies need not affect treatment considerations unless requested by the patient.[22]

During speech and facial expression, a different amount of tooth exposure may be seen. The face and lips together create a dynamic, constantly changing frame. The fluid nature of the relationship between soft and hard tissues must be considered in the treatment plan for diastema closure. The dentolabial analysis is essential for evaluating the correct ratio between the teeth and lips during the various phases of speaking and smiling. When the mandible is in the rest position, the teeth do not come into contact, the lips are slightly apart, and a portion of the incisal third of the maxillary incisors should be visible. This "incisal display" varies from 1 to 5 mm, depending on the length of the upper lip and the patient's age and sex.[22,24]

Patients who require prosthetic treatment frequently request a younger looking smile. Tooth wear and loss of perioral muscle tone, common to the aging process, diminish the amount of maxillary incisor visibility. Consequently, there is a greater exposure of the mandibular incisors as part of the aging process.

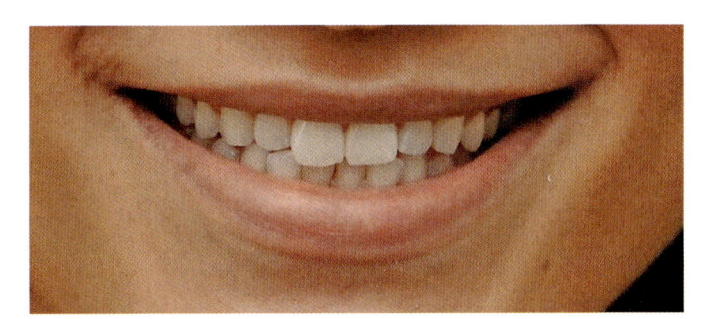

Figure 26.4 (**A**) Patient is unhappy with the unevenness of her teeth and wants a straighter, more uniform smile.

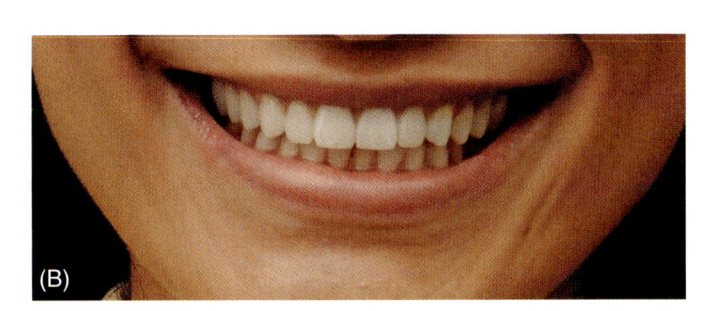

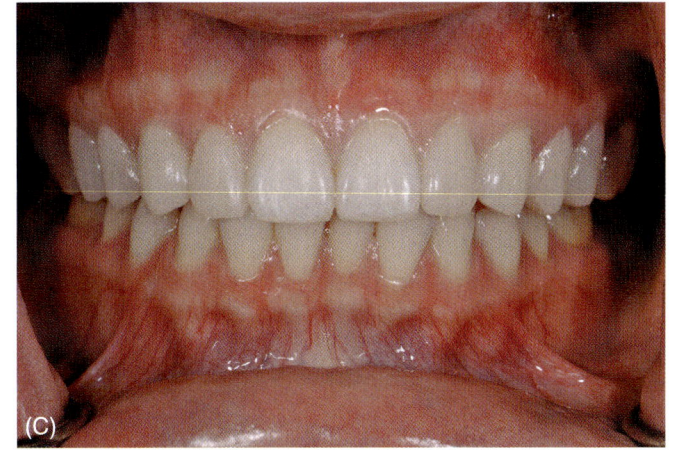

Figure 26.4 (**B, C**) Patient is able to preview the proposed changes for her smile from the bis-acryl template applied to her teeth chairside. Diagnostic wax-up compliments of Viet Tran (Master Ceramist, The Dental College of Georgia at Augusta University) and intraoral diagnostic mockup performed by Dr. Eduardo Britton (Dental College of Georgia Prosthodontic Graduate Resident). *Source:* Reproduced with permission of Gerard Chiche.

Maxillary incisor tooth display, with the lips at rest, is a major determining parameter in justifying incisal edge lengthening.[22] Incisal edge lengthening can work in the patient's favor during diastema closure. In a best case scenario, to maintain the correct tooth proportion, the teeth widened during the diastema closure must also be lengthened. When esthetically and functionally appropriate, this approach will result in an incisal edge display, which is usually consistent with the patient's desires.

Incisal edge position

Appropriate vertical tooth position (incisal edge position) and vertical gingival margin control are as important as correcting horizontal deficiencies in achieving an ideal result when closing diastemata.[25] Identification of the position of the incisal edge, in both the apicocoronal (incisal curve) and anterior–posterior (incisal profile) directions, represents a fundamental aspect of the esthetic diagnosis for diastema closure. Many of the procedural choices that the clinician and dental technician will make, to provide suitable prosthetic restorations, are significantly affected by the correct incisal edge position.[22] An esthetically pleasing and functionally stable final result must begin with correct determination of the incisal edge position of the maxillary anterior teeth. It is this incisal edge position that plays a major role in determining the proper width-to-length ratio of the clinical crowns.[25] Providing the appropriate amount of maxillary incisor display with the lips at rest is a key factor in the development of a more "youthful" smile.

The incisal plane, as a rule, when observed from the front, has a convex curve that follows the natural curve of the lower lip. Maintaining or reestablishing an incisal curvature in harmony with the lower lip is integral to ideal diastema closure treatment. In closing diastemata, esthetically pleasing tooth shape and proportion are enhanced by ensuring parallelism with the lower lip.[22] Even in patients with a relatively flat lower lip contour, it is still desirable to provide at least some degree of curvature to the upper incisal smile line.

The incisal profile is the position of the incisal edge in the anterio-posterior direction and, as a rule, is contained within the inner border of the lower lip. Properly positioned incisal edges allow for adequate closure of the lips without interference. The incisal plane is the anterior portion or continuation of the posterior occlusal plane. When viewed from the front, it should be parallel to the horizontal reference lines, such as the interpupillary line and the labial commissural line (assuming they are horizontally level), to maintain natural facial harmony.[22] If the teeth are too far forward and if proportions allow, the use of orthodontics to close the spaces should be considered. Prosthetic or direct restorative rehabilitation in such cases should involve modifying the incisal profile as needed to correct for any deficiency in this horizontal plane and allow for proper lip closure and speech.

Tooth proportion

The optimal mesiodistal width to incisogingival length (width-to-length ratio) proportion for Caucasian patients as described by Magne, Sterrett, Duarte, and Chu for naturally appearing, esthetic maxillary central incisors ranges from 72% to 81%.[26] When these proportions are violated, as often happens when large diastemas are closed solely with restorations, the restored teeth look "wrong" because they are out of proportion (see Chapter 9). Methods available to compensate for the extra tooth width include lengthening the anatomic crown with a restoration, increasing the clinical crown length with periodontal surgery, or using restorative "optical illusions" to make a wide tooth appear narrower (see Chapter 8). Lengthening a tooth by extending the incisal edge is the simplest method of maintaining proportionality of the individual tooth when additional width is required to close spaces. However, the patient's occlusal scheme may not allow for the additional incisal length needed to compensate for the added width. Potential complications include a steepened bite with the possibility for increased muscle force and interference with speech or lip closure. A complete examination and thorough analysis of the patient's occlusion should reveal this potential complication prior to starting the treatment phase along with trial lengthening by addition of composite resin to confirm or refute these concerns. Lengthening the clinical crown by gingivectomy or an apically repositioned flap with osseous recontouring may provide the needed length to offset the additional width without creating potential occlusal interferences. However, a careful periodontal evaluation must be rendered to ensure an adequate crown-to-root ratio remains following osseous surgery and that sufficient interdental soft tissue will remain to reduce the risk of open gingival embrasures (i.e., "black triangles") following placement of restorations.[27] Either of these tooth lengthening options can allow for diastema closure with natural-looking, proportional restorations, although the esthetic harmony of all of the anterior teeth should also be considered as a whole.

The concept of the "golden proportion" or "divine proportion" as applied to a smile and described by Lombardi, Levin, and others[28–30] was based on a ratio (1 : 1.618) of the apparent width of each anterior tooth (as viewed from a direct facial perspective) compared with the tooth immediately anterior and posterior to it. This concept was utilized for many years as the most harmonious or appealing tooth-to-tooth ratio for an esthetic smile. In more recent years, however, it has been shown that the majority of beautiful smiles do not have proportions coinciding with the golden proportion formula[31] and that this proportion does not occur naturally in the average natural dentition, although it can still provide an esthetically pleasing result.[32–34] Although the golden proportion can be a valuable aid as a starting point for esthetic evaluation and diagnostic modeling, the reality is that any interdental width ratio from 65% to 85% can be esthetically acceptable, and thus the golden proportion ratio should be used as a tool, not as a rule.

More recently, an alternative option for determining tooth-to-tooth relationships was introduced, the "recurring esthetic dental" (RED) proportion.[33,35] Using this method, the clinician may choose any proportion that looks appropriate, as long as it remains consistent as it proceeds from the midline distally in the arch. Seventy-five percent of North American dentists preferred using the RED proportion when designing smiles with normal length teeth over using the golden proportion.[36] The 70% RED proportion has been recommended for normal length teeth (with a 78% width : length ratio of the maxillary central incisors). Using this concept and the 70% ratio, the width of the maxillary lateral incisor is 70% of frontal view width of the maxillary central incisor, and the canine is 70% of the width of the resulting lateral incisor width. RED ratios of 62–80% are recommended, dependent on the teeth length (larger ratio for shorter teeth and smaller ratio for longer teeth). The mean maxillary tooth widths for the anterior teeth as shown by Chu were 8.5 mm for the central incisor, 6.5 mm for the lateral incisor, and 7.5 mm for the canines and that 82% of patients fell within ±0.5 mm of the mean values.[26] Other ratios that can be used with esthetic success include restoring the optical width of the maxillary lateral incisor at about 65% of the central incisor and the canine at approximately 75–80% of the optical width of the lateral incisor.[37] Studies by Magne et al. showed ranges of unworn maxillary central incisor widths from 8.46 to 11.07 mm, lateral incisors from 5.51 to 8.22 mm, and canines from 6.8 to 9.02 mm with average width-to-length ratios of 78% for unworn centrals, 73% for laterals, and 73% for canines.[38] Regardless of the ratio used, when treatment planning esthetics for the anterior part of the mouth, the central incisors should "dominate" the smile in terms of both position and size.[30,39] However, as stated by Magne and Belser, dominance must be measured according to personality (see Chapter 9).[40]

Gingival esthetics

There are esthetic considerations for periodontal surgery that, in many cases, are as important as those for teeth. The appearance of the teeth and gingival tissues must act in concert to provide a balanced and harmonious smile. A defect in the surrounding pink tissue may not be adequately compensated for by the quality of the dental restoration and vice versa.[41] In the past decade there has been a remarkable upswing in interdisciplinary collaboration between dentist, orthodontist, and periodontist in smile enhancement. In fact, the pseudo-specialty of "cosmetic periodontics" has evolved in conjunction with the pseudo-specialty of cosmetic dentistry.[42]

In creating an esthetically pleasing and natural smile, the perfect balance between white architecture (teeth) and pink architecture (gingiva) is often difficult to achieve.[43] Evaluation of the smile line also reveals the amount of exposure of the anterior teeth (including the cervical portion of the teeth) and soft tissue when smiling. Based on the amount of dental and gingival display of the anterior maxillary arch, Tjan and Miller identified three types of smile lines: low, average, and high. A pleasant smile can be defined as one that exposes the maxillary teeth completely, along with approximately 1 mm of gingival tissue. Gingival exposure that does not exceed 2–3 mm is nevertheless considered esthetically pleasant, while an excessive display (>3 mm) is generally considered unattractive.[44]

When closing diastemata in patients with a high smile line, recommended treatment will often include increasing tooth length apically to offset the increase in tooth width. Periodontal plastic surgical procedures are often needed and utilized to correct tooth–soft tissue relationships or to improve tooth proportions. Resective surgeries (e.g., gingivectomy, osseous crown lengthening) or additive surgeries (e.g., gingival grafting, coronal soft tissue repositioning) are recommended when discrepancies in the soft tissue interfere with the proposed tooth proportion.[25] Ideally, the position of the midfacial portion of the free gingival margin of the maxillary central incisors and the canines should be at the same height, with the free gingival margin of the lateral incisors being slightly more coronal to a line drawn between the central incisors and canines.[45-47] Symmetry of tissue height and contour between the maxillary central incisors is, however, the more critical factor over bilateral symmetry between the central and lateral incisors and canines.[45] Crown lengthening one tooth to achieve width-to-length proportionality may result in a decreased esthetic result because of the asymmetry of the gingival margins. Gingivectomy or apically positioned flap procedures should usually be carried out over as many teeth as needed to maintain esthetic harmony of the gingival contours. Occasionally, a single tooth may exhibit an improper gingival contour due to supra-eruption or malposition within the arch (e.g., a palatally inclined maxillary incisor will likely have a more coronally placed free gingival margin), and in this case a periodontal procedure for the individual tooth may be appropriate.

Altering soft tissue levels can also be accomplished successfully in many cases through orthodontic intrusion or extrusion. Among the benefits of the nonsurgical orthodontic approach are the preservation of supporting tissues and maintenance of the crown-to-root ratio. From an esthetic perspective, a major advantage for considering orthodontic correction is the ability to restore ideal cervical gingival morphology and emergence profile. In addition, the possibility of inadvertently surgically exposing the root portion of the tooth, with its inherent negative consequences is eliminated.[25]

Esthetic illusions

A wide tooth can be made to appear smaller (narrower) than it is in reality by altering its contours and using different color values in various parts of the tooth or by selecting a darker shade. The apparent face of the tooth (X) is that portion of the facial surface that is isolated by the facial/interproximal line angle (Figure 26.5A and B). The mesiofacial and distofacial line angles will influence what the eye perceives as the apparent width of the facial surface of a tooth. A wide tooth can be made to look narrower by moving the mesiofacial and distofacial line angles closer together and rounding slightly the tooth surfaces lateral to these line angles (S), opening the incisal embrasures (IE) and rounding the incisal line angles (Figure 26.5C and D). Thus, two adjacent teeth with different actual mesiodistal widths can be made to appear similar in width if the distance between the facial line angles is the same (maintaining the same "apparent face width") along with the use of other artistic illusions. Proximal contours, facial surface features, and color values can

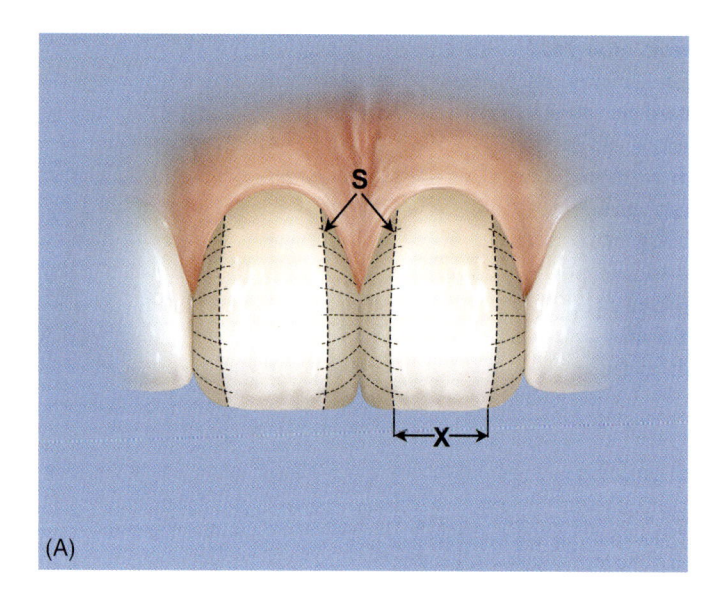

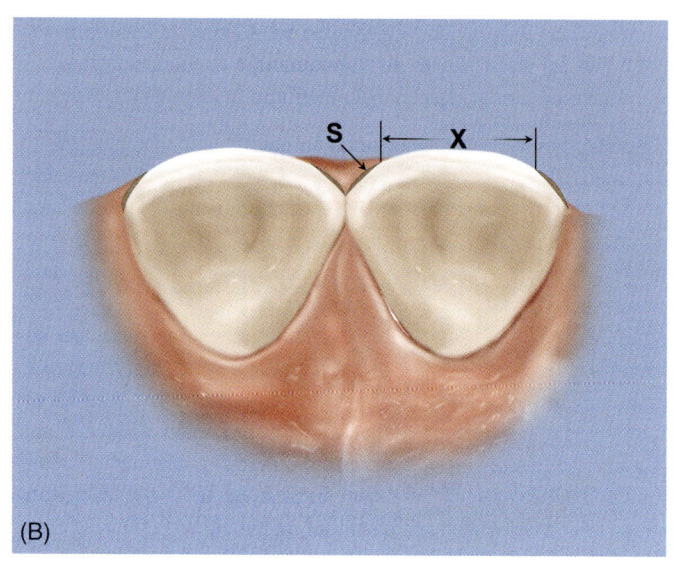

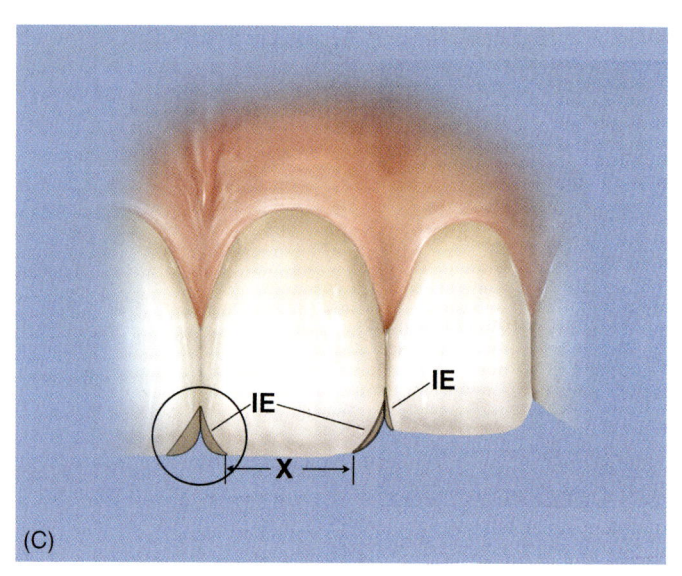

Figure 26.5 (A–C) Principles for closing a diastema. The apparent width of a tooth ("X") can be altered to appear wider or narrower by moving the facial interproximal line angles mesially or distally, rounding the tooth surfaces lateral to these line angles ("S") along with the line angles themselves, opening the incisal embrasures ("IE"), and rounding the incisal line angles (see text for more details). (S = Shaping, IE = Incisal Embrasures). *Source:* illustrations by Zach Turner.

further enhance the illusion provided by line angles. Wide and deep facial embrasures with lingually positioned contact areas give the illusion of narrow teeth, whereas constricted and shallow facial embrasures make teeth look wider. Horizontal or vertical "lines" (e.g., developmental depressions or other secondary anatomical features) added to the facial surfaces of teeth can make the tooth look artificially wider or longer as needed. Lighter color values on the facial surface of a tooth and darker values on the proximal surfaces will further contribute to the deception of tooth size. These illusions enable the dentist to make several teeth of different actual sizes look proportional in their widths by manipulating line angle location, proximal contours, surface texture, and color value. They can be valuable adjuncts to treatment when compromises have to be made and ideal conditions are not available for closing diastemata and maintaining tooth proportionality and harmony within the overall smile.

Functional considerations in restoring diastemata

The requirement that the occlusion be stable following diastema closure holds true regardless of the esthetics achieved, and whether the result was achieved by means of orthodontics, restorative space management, or a combination of both. Careful attention must be given to avoid converting a stable occlusion into an unstable occlusal scheme in the process of diastema correction. The signs of a stable occlusion are asymptomatic, normally functioning temporomandibular joints, firm teeth with no signs of excessive wear, teeth that do not migrate from their position, and supportive structures that can be maintained in a healthy condition.[48] A dentition composed of spaces can present with varying occlusal patterns, including an increased or decreased overjet or overbite. The treatment of the malocclusion can be a challenge because of these spatial discrepancies.

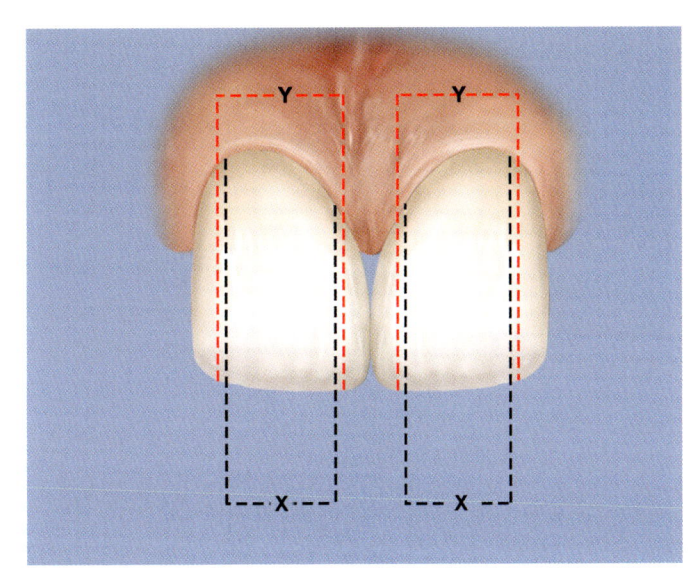

Figure 26.5 **(D)** When teeth are too wide, they should be contoured so that the labial surface does not appear as wide. Thus, the line angles should be more to the center of the tooth or closer together (*X* instead of *Y*). Source: illustration by Zach Turner.

Therefore, an occlusal analysis should be included in the treatment planning process, and the best option for incorporating orthodontics, restorative, or a combination of both must be clearly identified to achieve the most predictable esthetic and functional result.[25] The envelope of function must also be considered when planning to close spaces that exist in the esthetic zone. Any preexisting, nonpathogenic neurologically programmed tooth closure pattern may be interrupted when the diastema is closed, especially if tooth position is altered. The mandible has a favored pathway of motion. Occlusal instability may occur as a result of teeth or restorations that interfere with this jaw closure pathway. Signs of instability may include fremitus, excessive wear, tooth movement, and fracture of restorations[49] or any combination of these.

Orthodontics, operative (direct restorative) dentistry, prosthodontics, or combinations of these therapies are the most suitable of suggested options for the closing of diastemata. Orthodontics requires the use of appliances, which means a more complex, longer, and often more expensive treatment. Prosthodontics requires indirect and more invasive procedures with laboratory involvement at an increased cost to the patient. Factors such as the number and size of the diastemata influence the choice of restorations or other treatment options. Direct adhesive composite resin restorations and indirect porcelain veneer restorations present excellent treatment alternatives to reestablish the esthetics, function, and biologic characteristics of oral tissues when closing diastemata.[43] The advantage of modern materials and techniques often allows for preservation of tooth structure by means of conservative, less-invasive procedures.

The specific goals of treating diastemata remain unchanged regardless of the technique used: (1) create a tooth form in harmony with adjacent teeth, arch, and facial form; (2) maintain an environment for excellent gingival health; and (3) attainment as well as maintenance of a stable, functional occlusion. The final result should be one that is harmonious and pleasing to the patient. These goals, and consequent clinical success, can be met and achieved by applying contemporary principles of smile design and following an appropriate sequence of treatment.[25]

Restorative treatment options

Direct bonding with composite resin

Simple diastema

Use of directly bonded composite resin is considered by many to be the first line of treatment for a single diastema or when ultraconservative restorations are indicated (e.g., young patient, unrestored teeth, need for reversible procedure). In the hands of a skillful clinician, the use of composite resin can yield very acceptable results that, when maintained properly, can last for years. Other advantages of using composite resin include: accurate mock-ups for color verification and approval; relative ease of repair; maximum conservation of tooth structure, since mechanical tooth preparation is often unnecessary;[50] the ability to complete the procedure often in one visit, allowing for immediate results; and lower cost (compared with indirect restorations).[51] Thus, the ability to save time, money, and tooth structure makes composite resin a popular choice with many dentists and patients. By choosing a conservative restorative option, such as direct composite resin bonding, both the patient and the clinician have the full range of treatment options available (since most of the pretreatment tooth structure remains) for whatever subsequent treatment is available or recommended in the future. As mentioned previously, patients should always be given the chance to alter their tooth color through bleaching prior to restorative treatment. If tooth bleaching is accepted as a part of therapy, it should always be performed prior to adhesive dentistry with bonding being delayed for 10–14 days following completion of bleaching to allow for tooth color stabilization and tooth–resin bond strength levels to return to normal values.[52–54]

One key element to closing diastemata with composite resin is developing a natural interproximal emergence profile that will eliminate or at least minimize unesthetic gingival embrasures and allow for proper oral hygiene. Figure 26.6A and B shows how facial, mesial, and lingual surfaces are contoured to close the interdental space (gingival embrasure). Improper emergence contours can lead to food entrapment and greater difficulty in cleaning with dental floss. Figure 26.6C and D depicts correct versus incorrect gingival embrasure contours and is applicable whether restoring with direct composite resin or by indirect means (i.e., crowns or veneers). With wider diastemas or gingival embrasures, it may be necessary to reshape (using electrosurgery or soft tissue laser) or displace (with retraction cord or semi-rigid metal matrix) the interdental papilla in order to develop better interproximal emergence contours. In most cases involving a wide diastema, however, the patient must be accepting of a less than ideal interdental papilla or resort to restorative options such as the use of pink porcelain (or

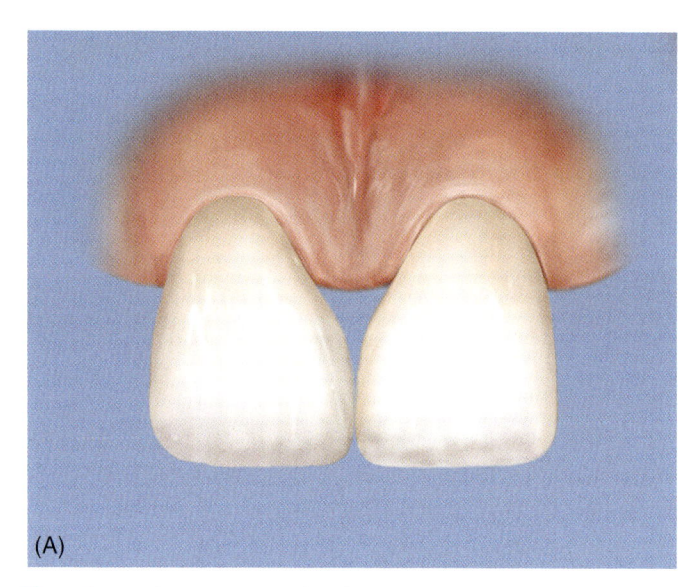

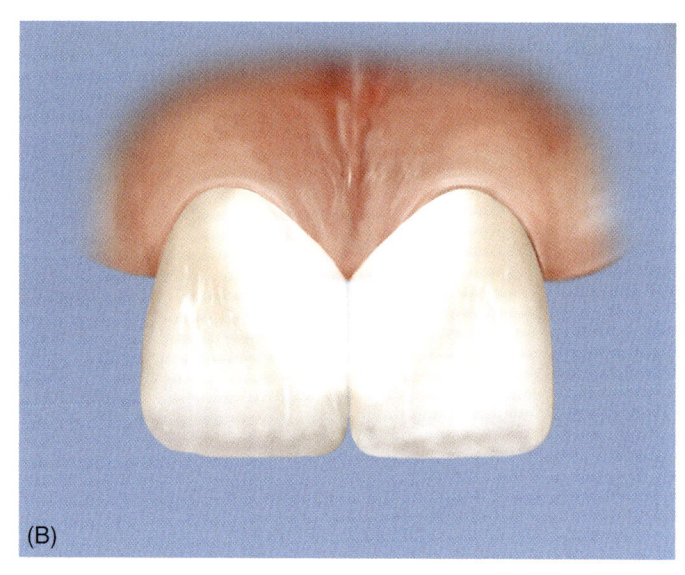

Figure 26.6 Composite resin bonding is the most conservative method to close a cervical interdental space ("black triangle"). **(A)** Before the restoration. **(B)** After the restoration, outlining the surfaces involved with the restoration. *Source:* illustrations by Zach Turner.

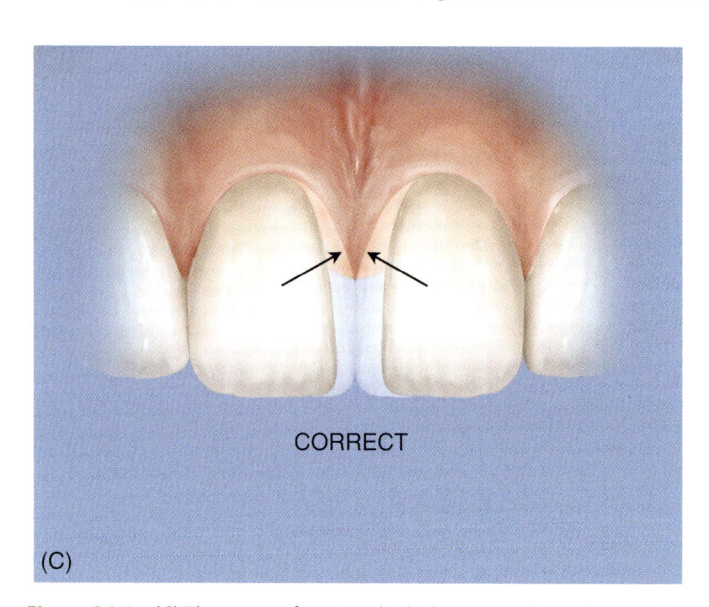

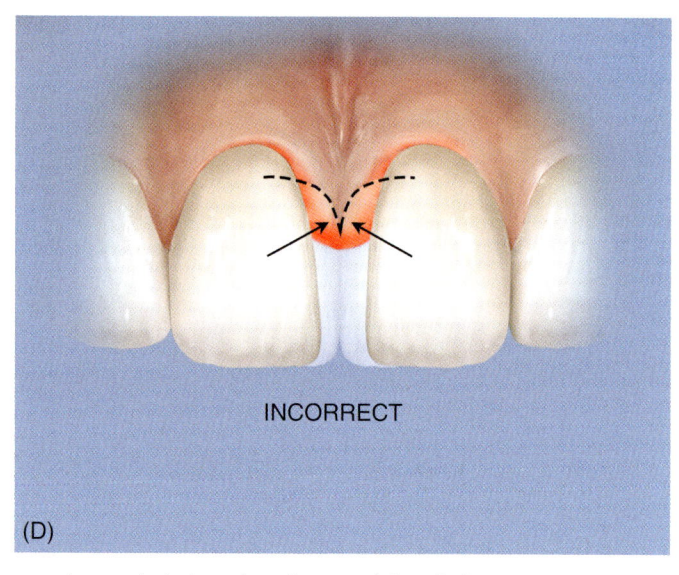

Figure 26.6 **(C)** The proper form in which the composite resin must be contoured to mask the interdental space while still allowing easy cleaning with dental floss. **(D)** The improper form. *Source:* illustrations by Zach Turner.

composite resin) or longer interproximal tooth contacts to lessen the visual effect of missing soft tissue. The reshaping of the papilla is most commonly performed by electrosurgery or laser treatment, which will subsequently allow for bonding at the same appointment. In cases of smaller diastemata, contouring the restorations at the cervical interproximal aspect to apply lateral pressure to the papilla will typically result in coronal migration of the interproximal soft tissue.

Figure 26.7A–F depicts closure of a midline diastema by direct composite resin. There are at least three pretreatment measurements needed before closing even the most straightforward or uncomplicated single diastema: the width of each tooth adjacent to the space, the width of the space, and the width-to-length ratio of these teeth. If the teeth are equally wide and their length can proportionally accommodate the additional width necessary to close the space, it is a simple matter of equally dividing the space closure requirement between the two teeth regarding how much composite resin to add. Unevenly wide teeth, unbalanced post-treatment ratios, or asymmetry within the smile require broader considerations and planning beyond a simple local space closure. Assuming that the incisors are the same width (preoperatively), an equal amount of composite resin should be added to each tooth (one tooth at a time) and the width measured again with calipers to ensure that following reshaping and polishing that 50% of the space has been successfully closed with the first addition of resin. Some clinicians, however, may choose to add composite resin to the adjacent teeth at the same time. This option can be acceptable as long as composite resin is added and contoured equally between the adjacent teeth and corrected as needed prior to polymerization. Note how in Figure 26.8A–C that the addition of composite resin to only one tooth or unequal application to both teeth will typically lead to a less than ideal

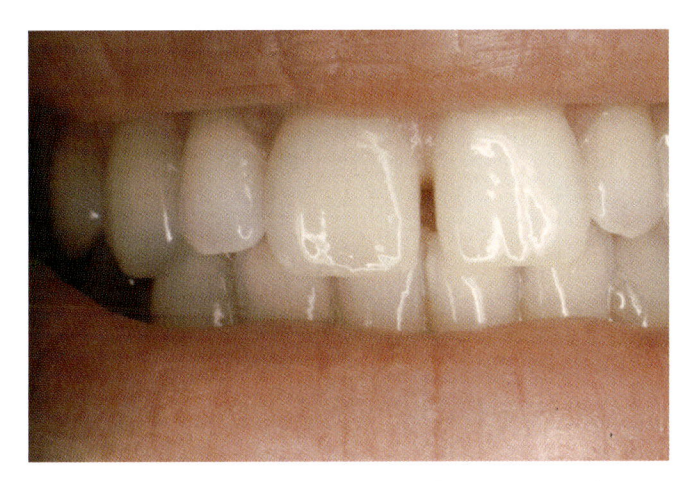

Figure 26.7 (A) The most practical method for closing a simple diastema is with composite resin bonding.

result. However, adding resin to only one tooth can be an acceptable strategy if it is narrower than the contralateral tooth preoperatively.

For cases involving multiple diastemata, it can be a bit more challenging and time consuming to restore with direct composite resin, and thus many clinicians resort to indirect methods. However, the guidelines and restorative protocol remain the same as with a single diastema, but the treatment requires more time and patience. Among common decision factors to be considered in restoring multiple diastemata distal to the midline involves whether to add only to the proximal surface of one tooth or include the proximal surface of the adjacent tooth as well. Obviously the interproximal contour and size of the teeth in question as well as size of the space to be closed must be taken into account. It is important, however, to keep in mind that the maxillary central incisors should be nearly mirror images of each other in terms of size, contour, and color and should "dominate" the smile. A slight variance in size, contour, and position of lateral incisors is, however, acceptable in many cases and can even result in a more natural appearance. Figure 26.9A–C demonstrates how composite resin can be utilized to restore multiple diastemata following orthodontic care and restore the smile to a very pleasing and esthetic appearance. Composite resin was chosen as the restorative material based on the patient's age, desire for conservative treatment, and finances.

Cases where a diastema exists but the teeth currently have a pleasing proportion, or such that the application of composite

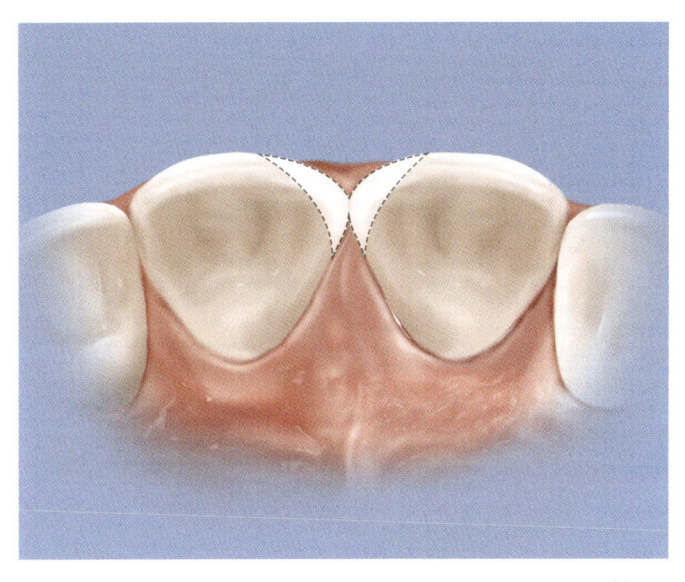

Figure 26.7 (C) This drawing illustrates that composite resin will be bonded to the labial, mesial, and palatal surfaces. *Source:* illustration by Zach Turner.

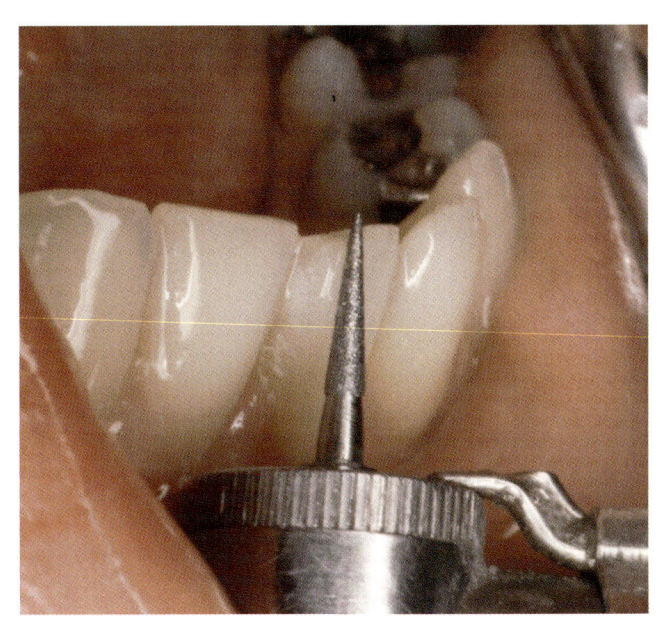

Figure 26.7 (B) Many times, it will be necessary to adjust the occlusion on the opposing arch to lessen the stress on the bonded incisors. Care should be exercised however to maintain a definitive lower incisal edge.

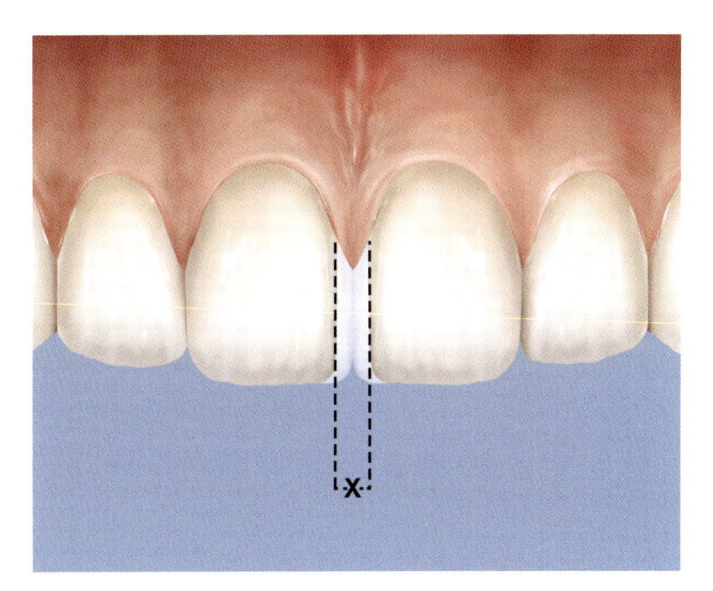

Figure 26.7 (D) The midline diastema is closed by measuring the size of the interdental space (*X*) and adding composite in equal amounts (*X*/2) to each tooth (assuming teeth are of equal width preoperatively). *Source:* illustration by Zach Turner.

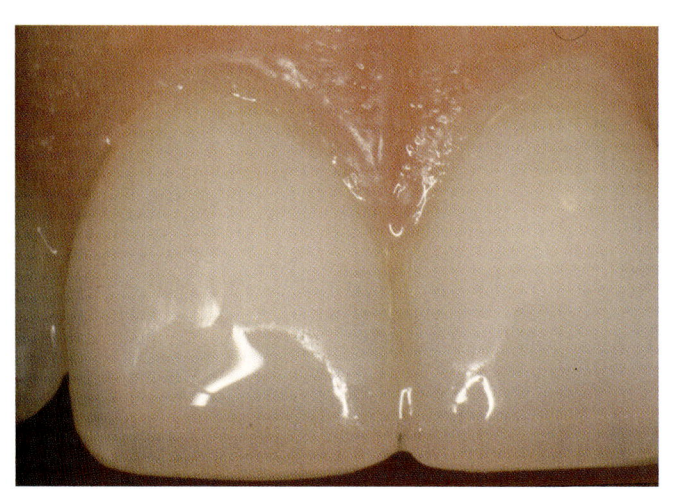

Figure 26.7 **(E)** The space is now closed. Note how invisible a properly contoured and well-blended restoration can be.

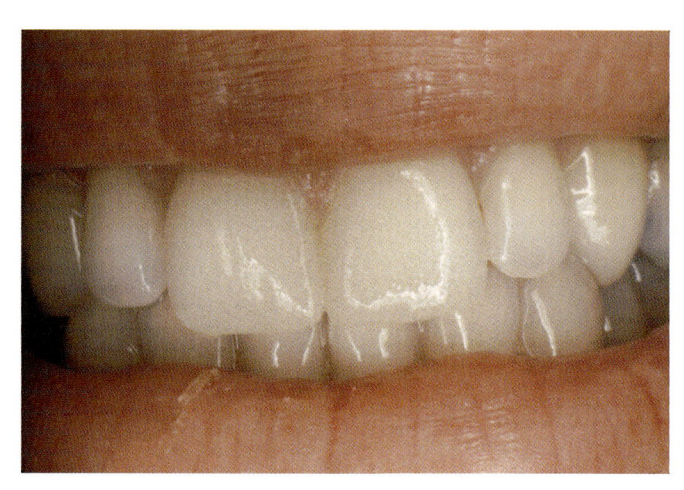

Figure 26.7 **(F)** The post-treatment view confirms what the patient said, "that even a small diastema can distract from one's smile."

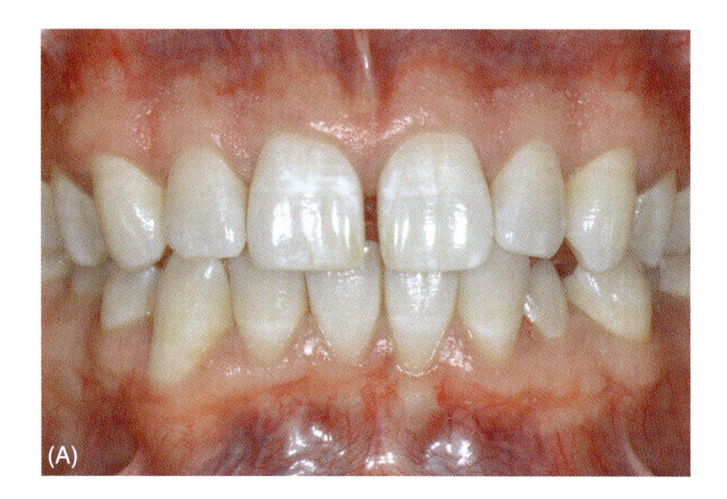

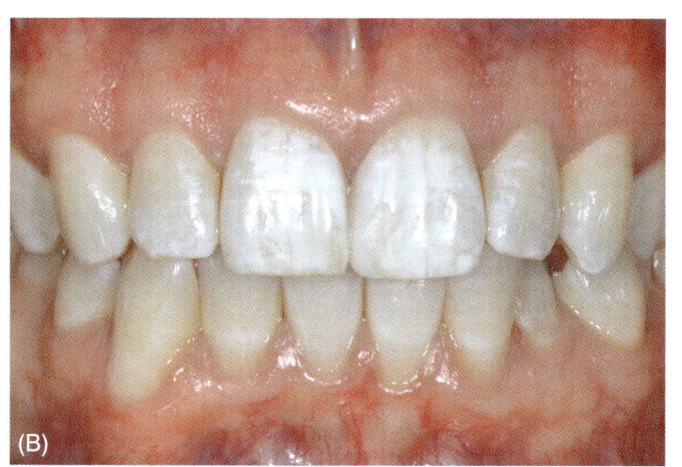

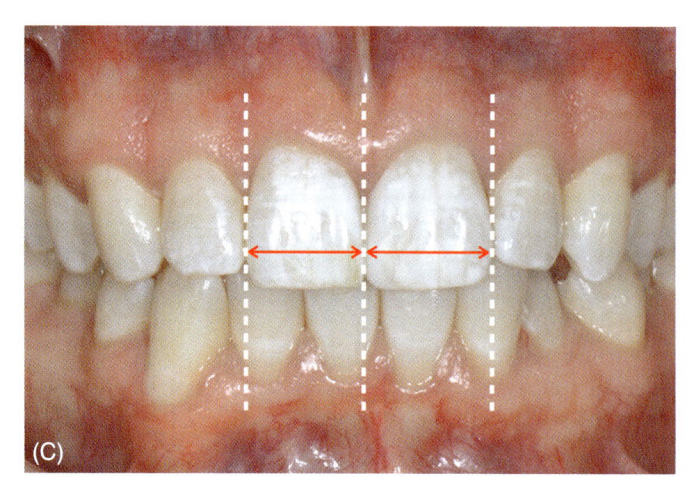

Figure 26.8 (A–C) Notice how the addition of composite resin to one central incisor (#9), in an attempt to close a midline diastema, results in uneven widths of the incisors and a less than desirable esthetic result.

resin to close the space would result in teeth that appear excessively wide, present more of a diagnostic challenge. An alternative to bonding to the central incisors, for example, may be to orthodontically approximate the teeth, followed by application of composite resin to the adjacent teeth as long as it does not make the lateral incisors appear too wide and cause them to compete for dominance with the central incisors. Clinical case 26.1 illustrates this technique.

An often misdiagnosed etiology of diastemata is related to tooth shape. Narrow teeth can present challenges to achieving the ideal 75–80% width-to-length ratio and may exhibit long interproximal contacts (accompanied by a lack of ideal interproximal soft tissue contours) that are not esthetically pleasing. Understanding not only how tooth size but also tooth shape plays a role in the development of pleasing esthetics is important to the overall outcome in diastema closure. Clinical case 26.3 describes how composite resin bonding was utilized to close residual post-orthodontic spaces due to tooth shape inadequacies and create an overall esthetically pleasing and hygienic result. Although this case may not be considered to be an example of simple diastema closure treatment, it does demonstrate how appropriate diagnosis, including a pretreatment diagnostic wax-up, when needed, and subsequent well-planned orthodontic treatment allow similar cases to be finished in an expedient and pleasing manner. These types of interdisciplinary care must involve frequent and clear communication between the restorative dentist and specialist.

Localized spacing due to missing teeth may require a combination of orthodontic and restorative treatment. Minor tooth movement to correct uneven mesial or distal drifting of spaced teeth can improve the esthetic result of corrective restorations by creating symmetric interdental spaces for individual restorations, or through the formation of normal-sized edentulous spaces for prosthetic restorations. Although orthodontic repositioning may offer the most noninvasive or conservative method for diastema correction, this approach may be impractical, unaffordable, or unacceptable to some patients and may not even result in permanent closure of the diastemata. In these situations, restorations are used as a means of closing a diastema rather than orthodontics, or to splint teeth following tooth repositioning[55] to minimize any potential for relapse. The size and number of the diastemata, functional and esthetic requirements of the patient, and pretreatment condition of the affected teeth influence the choice of restoration and restorative material. Composite resin bonding can often be used to complete the final esthetic correction of remaining interdental spaces or serve as interim restorations until more definitive care can be rendered. It is important to remember that the end result of diastema closure should conform to the esthetic ideals of smile design.[21,56] Esthetic parameters for pleasing tooth proportions in terms of width-to-length ratios and tooth-to-tooth relationships should be followed wherever possible for the most esthetically pleasing result.

Closing multiple diastemas

As mentioned previously, treating a case of multiple diastemas (diastemata) presents a greater challenge. Often a "mock-up" or "esthetic preview" using a bis-acryl-type material in a polyvinyl siloxane matrix (made from a diagnostic wax-up) can be very helpful in evaluating the anticipated results prior to definitive treatment. Pretreatment clinical assessments including incisal edge position, tooth shape and width-to-length ratios, periodontal–esthetic relationships, restoration influence on speech, etc. can be evaluated prior to initiating treatment and alterations made as needed. Clinical case 26.4 depicts the closure of multiple interdental spaces using direct composite resin.

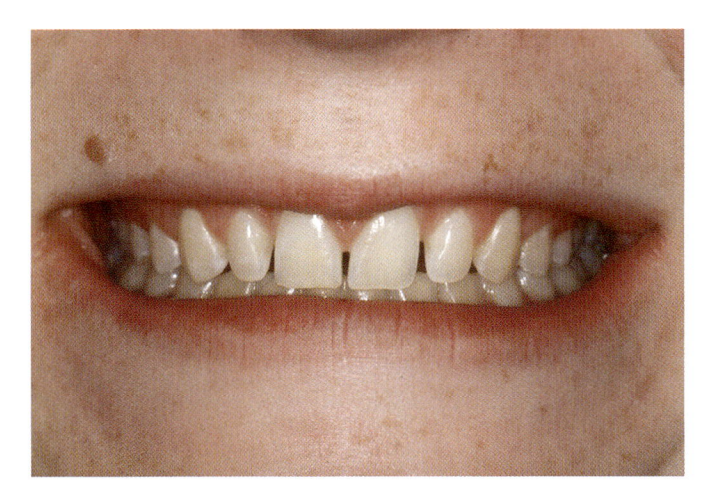

Figure 26.9 **(A)** This patient was unhappy with the appearance of her smile due to the spaces and small size of her teeth. These residual spaces were intentionally left by the orthodontist to allow for future bonding. *Source:* Reproduced with permission of Jim Peyton.

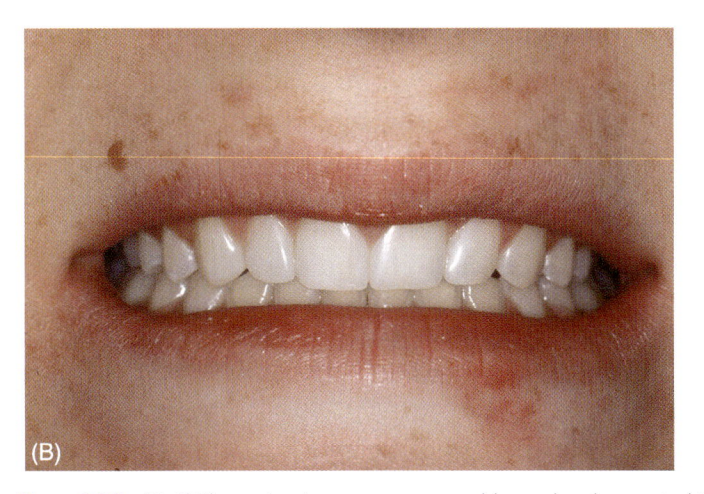

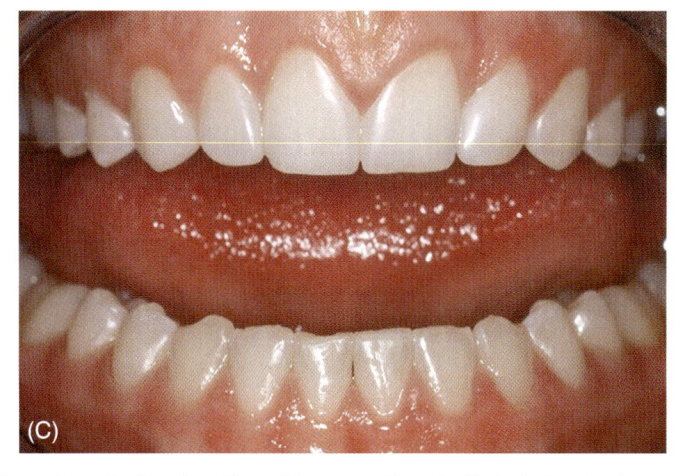

Figure 26.9 **(B, C)** The patient's concerns were addressed and corrected through meticulous bonding with composite resin. Note that not only were the spaces closed but also the teeth are now more appropriately proportioned. *Source:* Reproduced with permission of Jim Peyton.

Clinical case 26.1

Problem

This 23-year-old man stated as his chief complaint that the space between his two front teeth had returned after having been restored several years before with full porcelain crowns to correct the diastema (Figure 26.10A). It was believed that the teeth had drifted apart because of an existing periodontal condition that was further complicated by an occlusal problem.

Treatment

The mandibular incisors were adjusted to eliminate anterior interference and traumatic occlusion, followed by initiation of periodontal therapy. Upon completion of conservative periodontal therapy, an elastic ligature was placed around the maxillary central incisors to close the diastema. After wearing the elastic for several days, the patient returned with the space closed (Figure 26.10B). To prevent future drifting of the central incisors and reformation of the diastema, the newly created space between the central and lateral incisors must be treated. Artus's shim-type articulating ribbon (Artus Corp.) was used to protect the adjacent centrals from acid etching and bonding to the lateral incisors. This extremely thin material (5/10 000th of an inch) is preferred over the much thicker Mylar or other materials to achieve the tightest contact possible. Figure 26.10C shows the shim stock in place with the lateral incisor etched and ready for application of composite resin bonding agent, followed by light curing (see Figure 26.10D). Alternatively, Teflon tape (also known as "plumber's tape") can be used for protection of adjacent teeth from acid etching (see Figure 26.10E). The addition of composite resin is next adapted to the lateral incisor to close the diastema (Figure 26.10E). This material is then polymerized from the labial and palatal surfaces. Some clinicians choose not to use any matrix during the placement of the composite resin itself (matrix removed after etch and

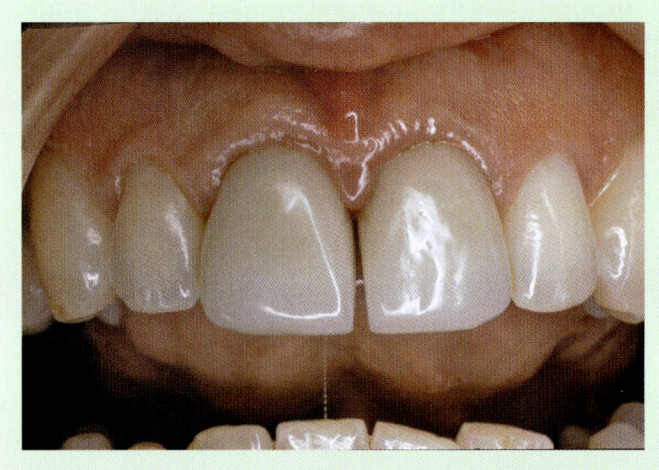

Figure 26.10 **(A)** This 23-year-old man presented with a new diastema formation between his previously crowned central incisors. The space had opened because of a periodontal condition complicated by traumatic occlusion.

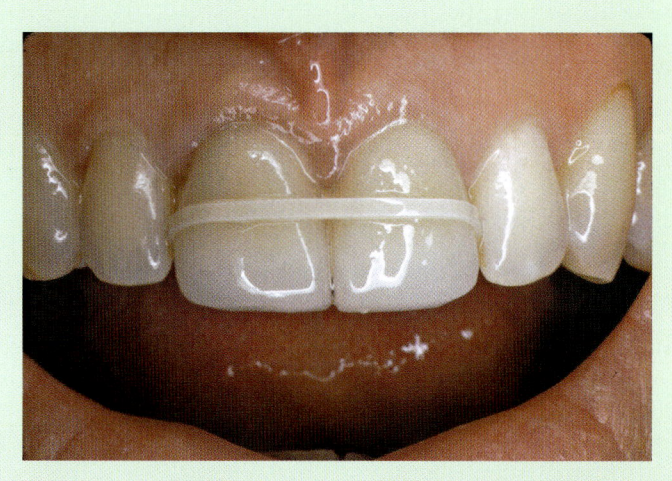

Figure 26.10 **(B)** After conservative periodontal therapy and occlusal equilibration, a rubber elastic was placed on the central incisors to reapproximate the teeth.

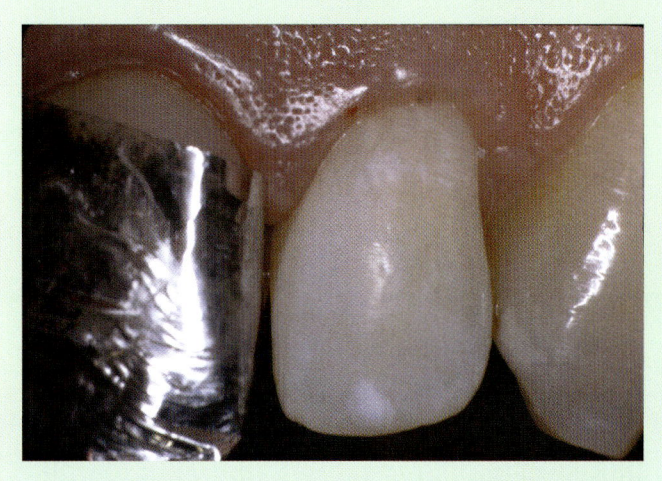

Figure 26.10 **(C)** The adjacent lateral incisors were tightly bonded using Artus shim stock (5/10 000th of an inch thick) to achieve the tightest closure possible.

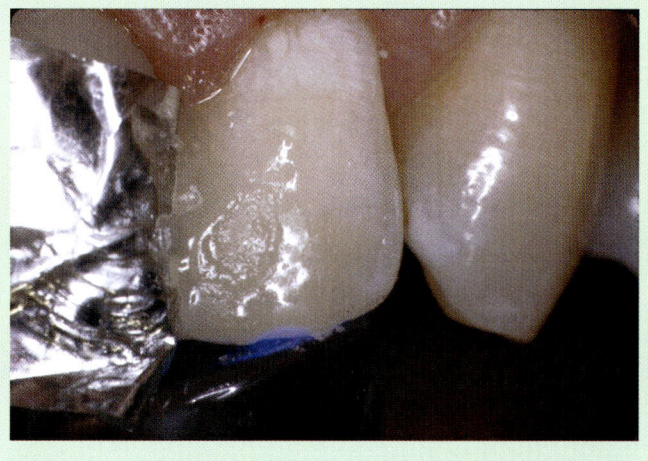

Figure 26.10 **(D)** As Figure 26.10C, but with the addition of composite resin to close the diastema.

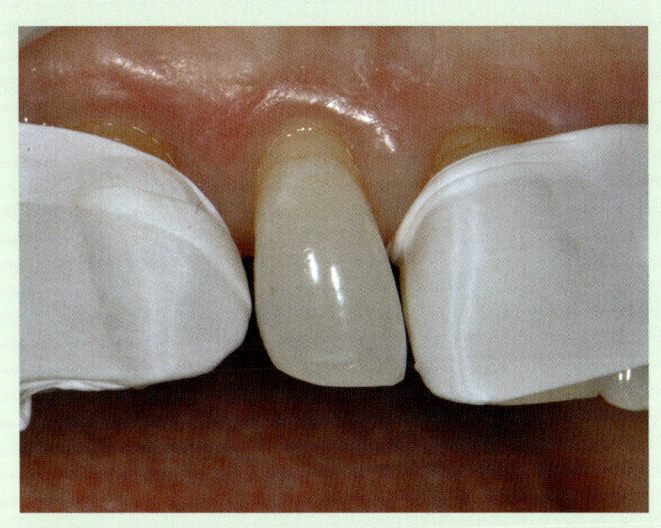

Figure 26.10 (E) Use of Teflon tape wrapped around the adjacent teeth to prevent contact with acid etchant to follow. The tape can be removed following rinsing of the etchant to allow composite resin to be built up directly against the adjacent teeth to achieve a tight contact.

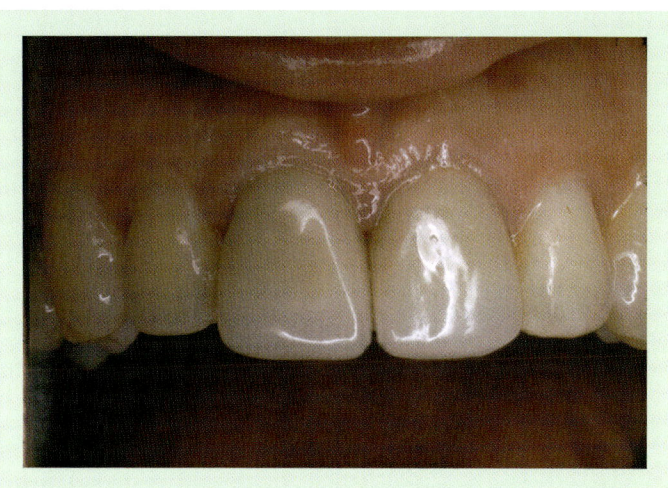

Figure 26.10 (F) After 24 months, the teeth continue to be held in position by the tightly bonded lateral incisors and a stabilized occlusion.

application of adhesive layer) and prefer to build the composite resin layer(s) directly against the adjacent tooth or adjacent composite resin restoration as long as it is smooth and highly polished. This approach provides exceptional interproximal contacts without the use of wedges that can cause gingival "black" triangles. Once completed, the teeth can be separated by the use of a small instrument inserted between the teeth below the contact using a gentle twist. The occlusion should be checked carefully, with the patient reclined and in a fully upright position, to ensure that excessive centric or excursive contacts are eliminated to avoid mobility and possible tooth movement which could lead to the recurrence of a diastema.

Result

Figure 26.10F shows the closed diastema, sufficiently stabilized by the lateral incisors. Regardless of whether the lateral incisors were crowned, laminated, or bonded, it is essential that the contact area be broad, so that the central incisors are held securely in place. During closure, it is recommended to stabilize the central incisors by temporarily holding them together on the lingual with composite resin (with minimal use of etchant and adhesive) until the lateral incisors can be bonded. Following completion of the final bonding process, the composite resin on the lingual of the central incisors can be easily removed.

Clinical case 26.2

Figure 26.11A shows a similar case where the patient had a midline diastema but was happy with the shape and size of her maxillary central incisors and elected orthodontic treatment to close the space between teeth #8 and #9. Diastemata remained bilaterally (due to the small lateral incisors) following completion of orthodontic care; see Figure 26.11B. The patient was pre-advised of this likelihood prior to initiating orthodontic treatment as part of informed consent. Teflon tape was used to protect the adjacent teeth from acid etchant (as in Figure 26.10D). Following etching and application of adhesive (no primer was needed as only bonding to enamel), composite resin was added to the mesial and distal of both lateral incisors. The composite resin additions were built directly in contact with the adjacent teeth without the use of any separating matrix. The final result can be seen in Figure 26.11C with a well-proportioned lateral incisor. One can also see the results of gingival grafting over the root of tooth #11 (#6 was also treated simultaneously) that was completed prior to orthodontic therapy. The patient was very pleased with the overall interdisciplinary combination of periodontal, orthodontic, and restorative care.

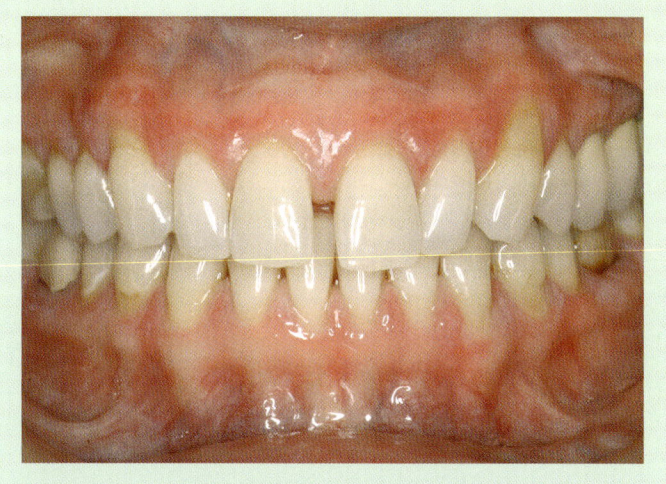

Figure 26.11 (A) This patient was unhappy with her midline diastema and tissue recession over her maxillary canines. The patient was given options for treatment and elected an interdisciplinary approach to achieve her desired result.

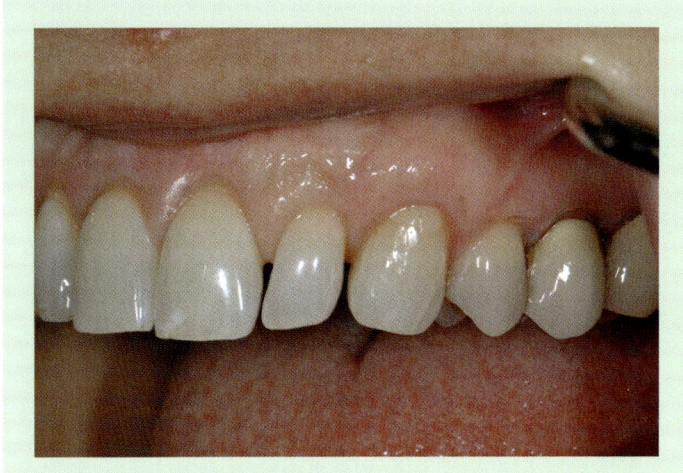

Figure 26.11 (B) Postorthodontic spaces remain mesial and distal to her lateral incisor (right side is identical) due to the small size of these teeth.

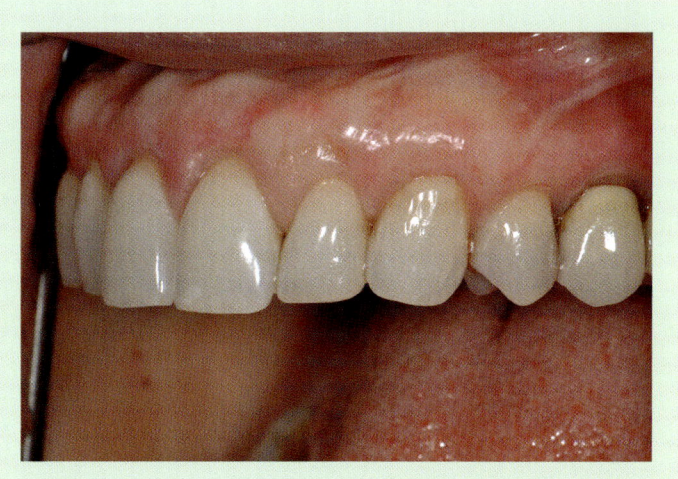

Figure 26.11 (C) Spaces closed by use of composite resin. Note the more appropriately sized lateral incisor following direct bonding and the nice result of root coverage following gingival grafting over the canine tooth. (The patient's right side was similarly treated.)

Large diastemata

Certain esthetic dilemmas are inherent with large diastemata that create more difficult challenges in trying to produce esthetically acceptable results. In many cases, without orthodontic intervention, some compromise in esthetics is likely. The first challenge is obviously attempting to create esthetically pleasing tooth width-to-length ratios. Along with this challenge is the need for more aggressive tooth preparations and the likely involvement of more teeth to attempt to compensate for and prevent excessively wide teeth. The second challenge is with soft tissue contours (i.e., gingival papillae). Large diastemata are usually associated with broad, flat interdental papillae. Without

Clinical case 26.3

Problem

A teenage male underwent orthodontic therapy for a Class II, Division II dental malocclusion (Figure 26.12A) requiring preliminary skeletal growth modifications and Class II correction. Pretreatment evaluation revealed that the shape of the teeth would in all likelihood require restorative therapy to improve their contours following tooth movement, and this finding was discussed with the patient and his parents (as part of informed consent) prior to orthodontic treatment. Following completion of his orthodontic therapy, residual maxillary anterior diastemas were apparent (maintained intentionally in preparation for future bonding, see Figure 26.12B) as a result of this tooth shape deficiency. Following debanding, the patient was unwilling to return to school until the spaces were closed, and thus the direct restorative procedure was carried out within 24 h of orthodontic appliance removal.

Treatment/result

The patient underwent 2 years of orthodontic therapy to correct his malocclusion and gingival levels. Following removal of appliances, the patient was instructed to return to his restorative dentist for composite resin bonding of the interproximal surfaces of the maxillary lateral and central incisors. Composite resin was added to close the diastemata, resulting in esthetically and periodontally ideal tooth contours (Figure 26.12C).

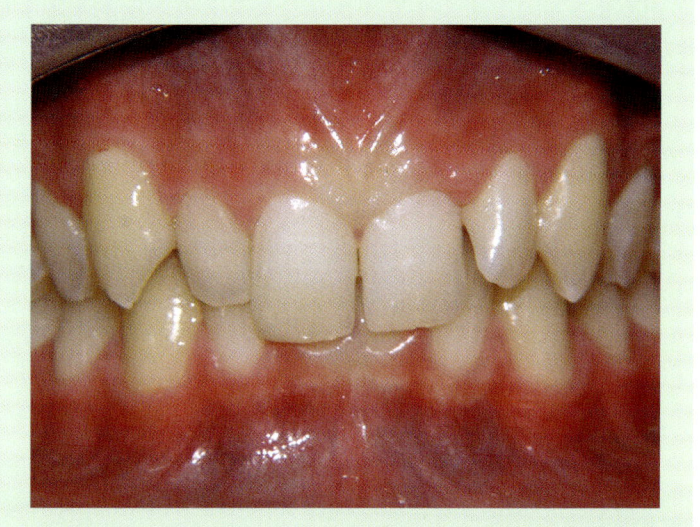

Figure 26.12 (A) Pretreatment orthodontic consultation for this male teen included the likelihood of posttreatment restorative care to improve tooth proportions as a result of tooth shape (slender teeth). *Source:* Reproduced with permission of Amara Abreu.

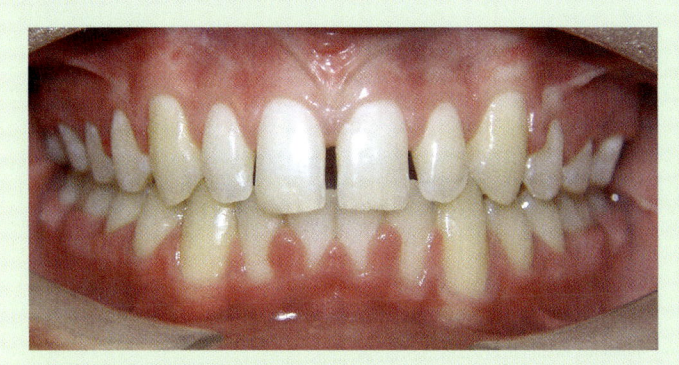

Figure 26.12 **(B)** The patient's smile and orthodontic results immediately following debanding. Note the significant enhancement in tooth alignment in both the horizontal and vertical planes. The health and appearance of the edematous lower gingival tissues were greatly improved following subsequent dental hygiene visits and improved home care. *Source:* Reproduced with permission of Amara Abreu.

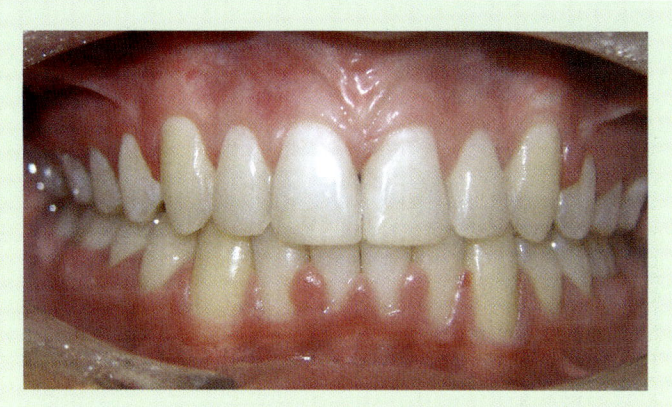

Figure 26.12 **(C)** An improvement in tooth size and shape is shown following closure of the diastemata with composite resin the day after orthodontic appliances removal. *Source:* Reproduced with permission of Amara Abreu.

Clinical case 26.4

Problem

A 26-year-old female presented with desire to close the spaces between her front teeth (see Figure 26.13A–C) as well as replace the missing maxillary premolar teeth. Her dental history included previous orthodontics with extractions, and she subsequently had an acid-etch retained bridge ("Maryland bridge") placed from tooth #3 to #6 to replace the missing premolar (space was limited to a single pontic). This Maryland bridge eventually fractured and tooth #3 exhibited significant decay.

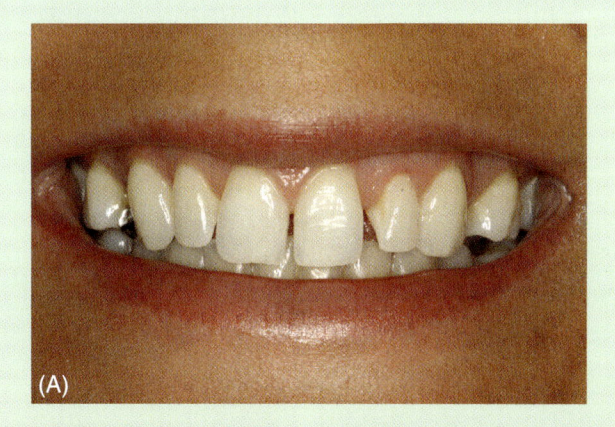

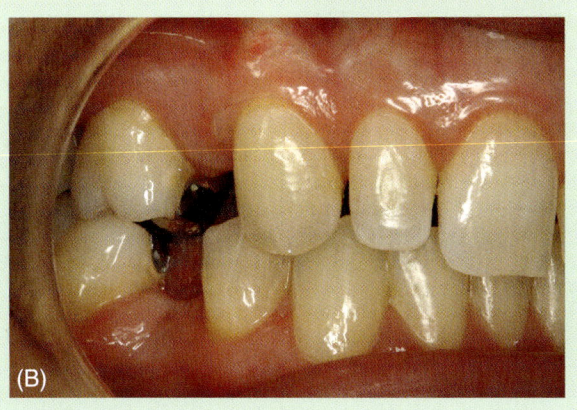

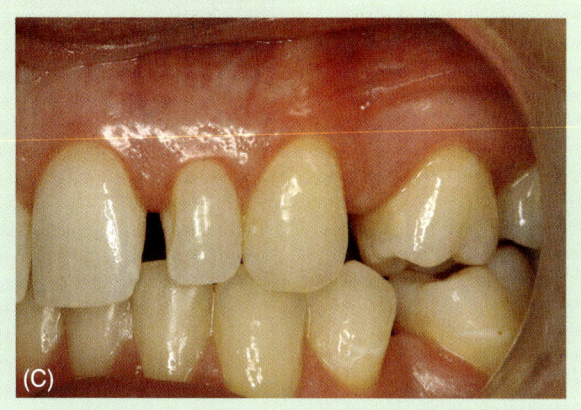

Figure 26.13 **(A–C)** A 26-year-old female presents wanting to close the spaces between her teeth. *Source:* Reproduced with permission of Robert C. Margeas.

Treatment

Esthetic analysis revealed narrow central incisors for which composite resin addition would not only close the interdental space but also improve the width-to-length ratios. The patient had been presented with the option of porcelain veneers by other dentists, but her desire was for a more conservative approach and instead chose composite resin bonding as both an economic and immediate solution.

Prior to acid etching, shade selection was accomplished by trial addition of composite resin to simulate the desired result. A polyvinyl siloxane putty matrix (Template, Clinician's Choice Dental Products, Inc., New Milford, CT) was fabricated on the cast of the diagnostic wax-up and used as a template intraorally to establish incisal length and midline position (Figure 26.13D). Use of such a matrix removes the guesswork as the proportions have been predetermined via the diagnostic wax-up. The bonding process was carried out starting first with the central incisors in order to ensure tooth width symmetry (Figure 26.13E). Teflon tape was utilized to protect adjacent teeth from etchant and adhesive. Following completion of the central incisors, the lateral incisors were similarly treated. The putty matrix was again utilized as support for the lingual (palatal) increment or "shelf" of composite resin (Figure 26.13F). The remaining facial increments of composite resin were freehand sculpted to complete the buildup. A clear Mylar strip was inserted between the central and lateral incisors and a "pull through" technique was used to draw the composite resin into the interproximal space as the Mylar strip was slowly pulled from a facial to palatal direction. This technique can be used to develop interproximal contacts directly against the adjacent teeth without the use of wedges, which can cause bleeding, undercontoured axial surfaces, and often result in unsightly "black triangles."

The restorations were then shaped and polished using Sof-Lex discs (3M ESPE, St. Paul, MN) and ET diamonds (Brasseler USA, Savannah, GA) followed by rubber FlexiCups and FlexiPoints (Cosmedent, Chicago, IL), Jiffy composite polishing brushes (Ultradent Products, Inc., South Jordan, UT), and finally polished with Enamelize Polishing Paste on a FlexiBuff felt-coated disc (Cosmedent) (Figure 26.13G–I). Interproximal polishing was accomplished by use of very thin polishing Epitex strips (GC America, Alsip, IL) (Figure 26.13J). Tooth #3 was then prepared to receive a monolithic zirconia crown and cantilever pontic #4. Tooth #13 was replaced by the direct bonding of a composite resin pontic to the mesial of #14 (see "Immediate closure of posterior diastema" section).

Result

The end result shows a beautiful, well-proportioned smile that met the patient's objectives of using a conservative technique to close the anterior diastemata (Figure 26.13K–N). The conservative nature of the treatment performed allows the patient the opportunity to have porcelain veneers placed at a later date should she so choose.

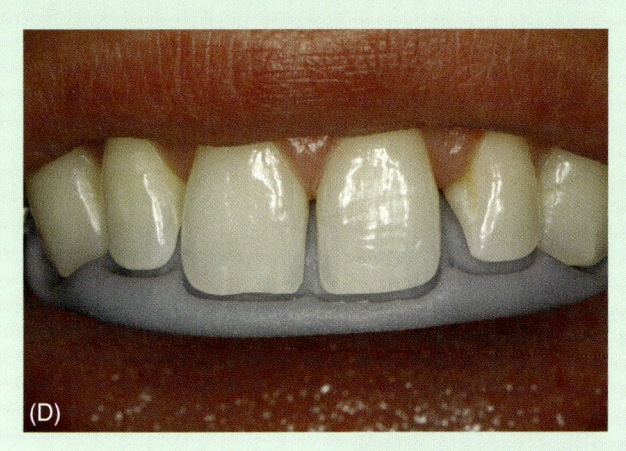

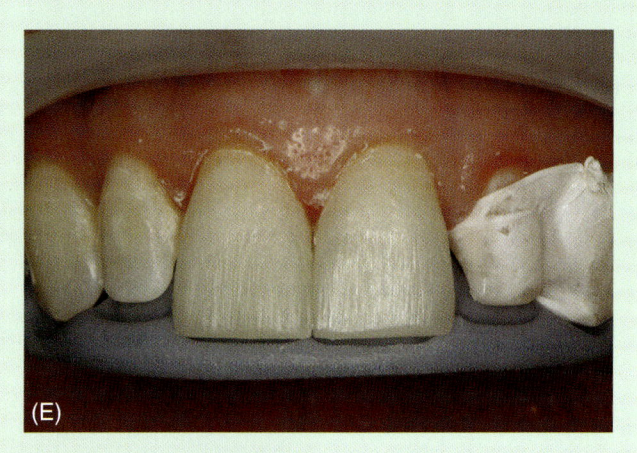

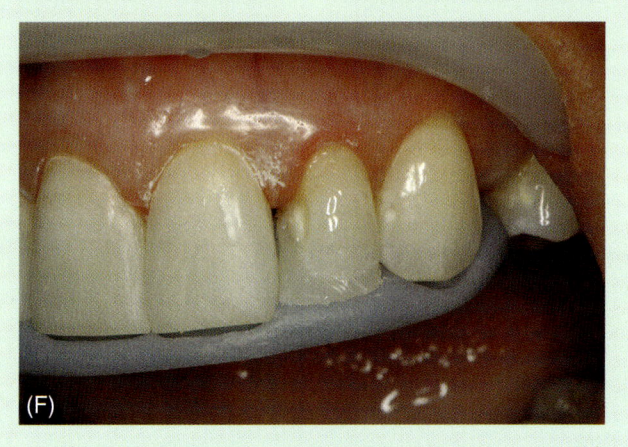

Figure 26.13 **(D–F)** Illustration of the use of a polyvinyl siloxane putty matrix to aid in composite addition to close the interdental spaces as predetermined from the diagnostic wax-up. *Source:* Reproduced with permission of Robert C. Margeas.

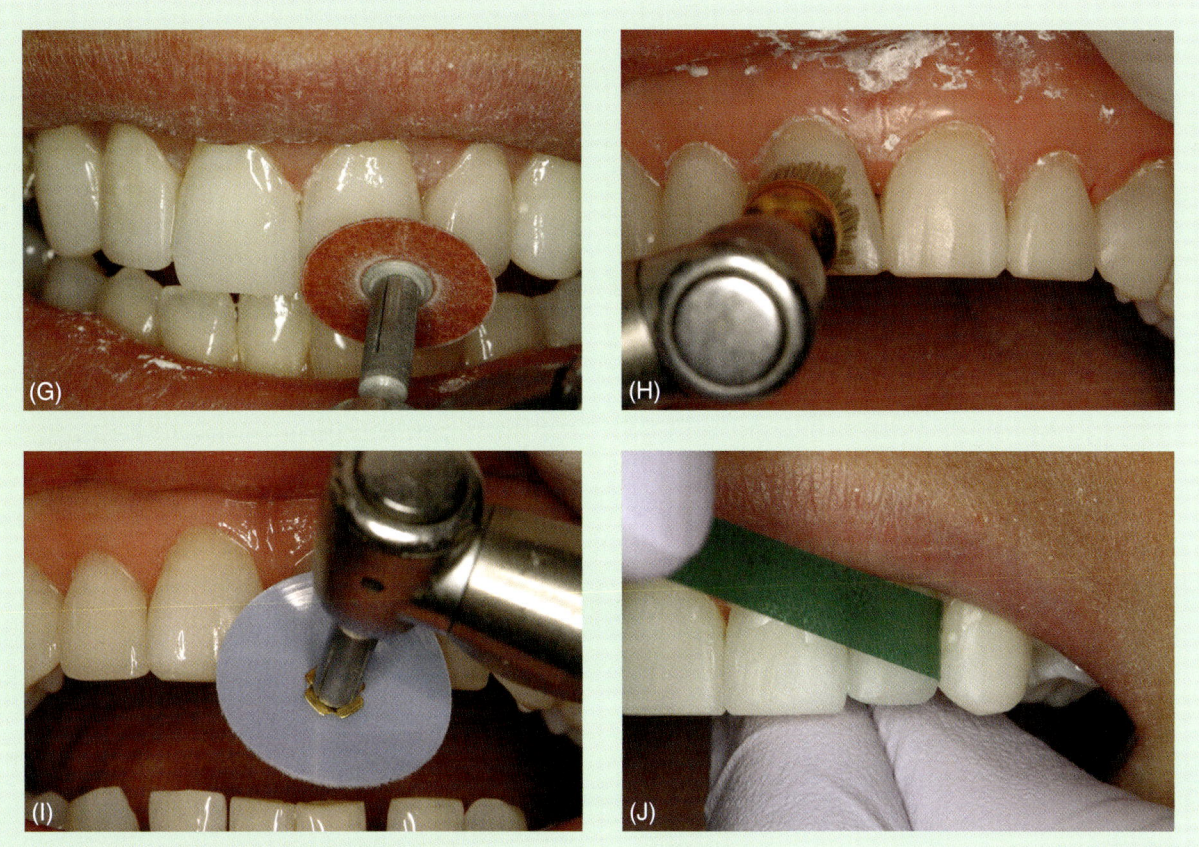

Figure 26.13 **(G to J)** Multiple steps are used to contour, finish, and polish the restorations to achieve the esthetic result desired. *Source:* Reproduced with permission of Robert C. Margeas.

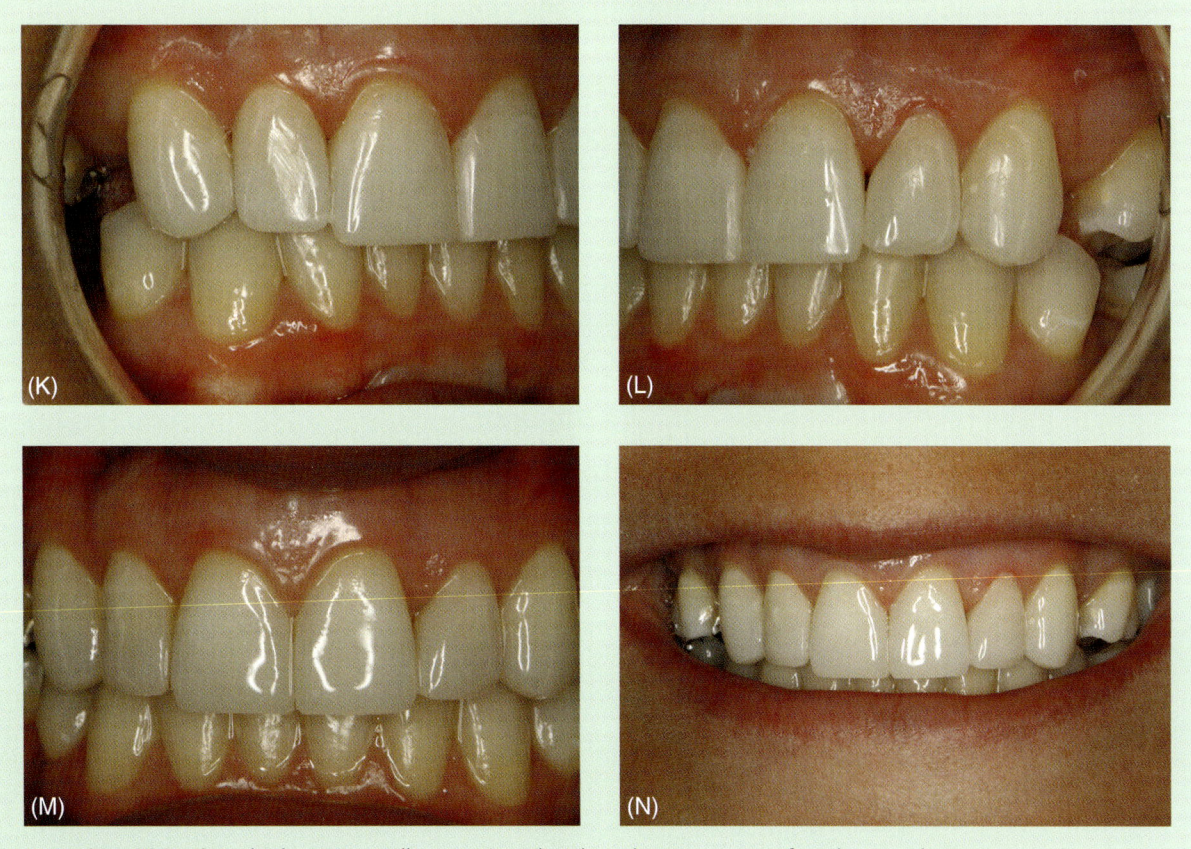

Figure 26.13 **(K to N)** Final result, showing a well-proportioned smile and improvement of tooth-to-tooth proportions. *Source:* Reproduced with permission of Robert C. Margeas.

Clinical case 26.5

Problem
A 60-year-old airline travel agent presented with a large diastema between the maxillary central incisors (see Figure 26.14A–E). Advanced cervical erosion was also evident on her maxillary anterior teeth, especially on her right side.

Treatment
The teeth were slightly reproportioned by stripping and disking the distal surfaces of the central incisors (Figure 26.14B). The key to successful restorative diastema closure is creating the illusion of a believable "natural" tooth width in the central and lateral incisors. Figure 26.14C shows a narrower width of the central incisors after the distal surfaces have been sufficiently reduced and prepared for full-veneer bonding to close the central incisor diastema and restore the cervical defects. The definitive bonded composite resin restorations can be seen in Figure 26.14D.

Result
Figure 26.14 F shows an entirely new smile with better proportioned teeth rather than two oversized teeth. Note that the cervical erosion on the maxillary right side has been simultaneously restored with composite resin bonding (occlusion should be meticulously checked and adjusted to minimize any occlusal etiology to these types of noncarious cervical lesions). The mandibular anterior incisors were also cosmetically contoured to give them a level plane of occlusion. Comparing the before and after smiles (see Figure 26.14E and F) specifically illustrates how the patient's mid-upper lip naturally drops rather low, forming a classic "cupid's bow" contour. This lowered lip line tends to mask the extra width of the central incisors, which also contributes to the illusion.

A schematic drawing of how this case was restored can be seen in Figure 26.15A and B. X denotes the distal surface of the central and lateral incisors, which were reduced to compensate for the

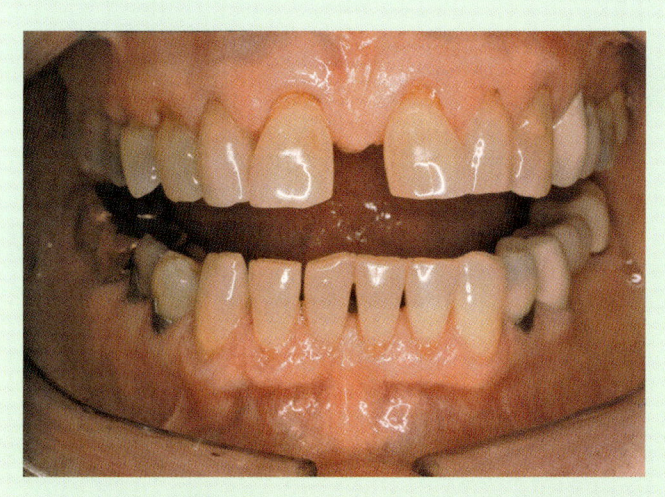

Figure 26.14 (A) This 60-year-old woman presented with a large diastema between her central incisors and cervical erosion on her maxillary anterior teeth.

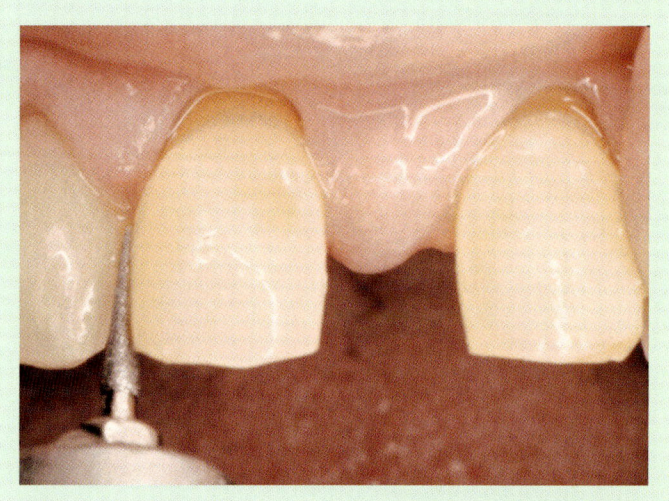

Figure 26.14 (B) Stripping and disking of the distal surfaces of the central incisors were done to slightly reproportion the teeth.

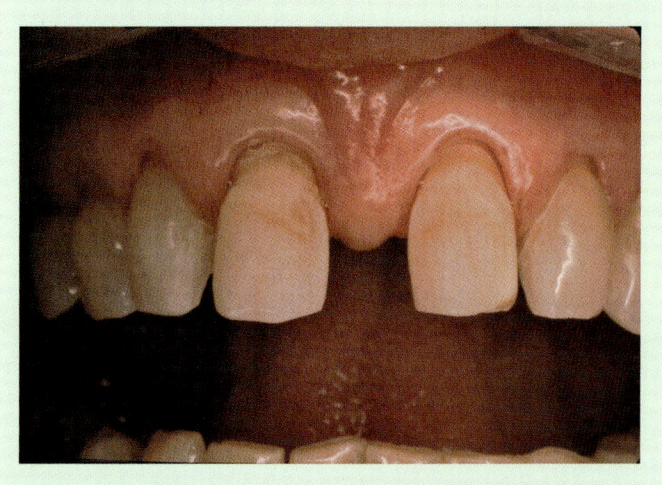

Figure 26.14 (C) The narrowed width of the central incisors (from disking of the distal surfaces) will allow for addition of composite to the mesial surfaces to close the diastema while attempting to avoid excessively wide teeth.

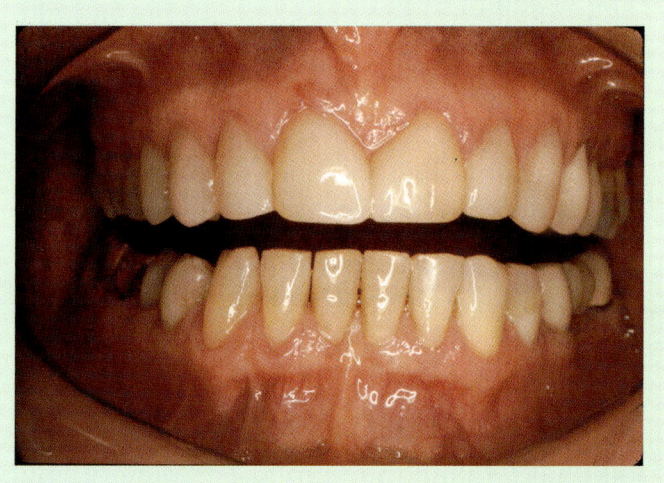

Figure 26.14 (D) The final full-veneer bonding closed the diastema and restored the cervical defects.

addition of composite resin to the mesial surface of the teeth. This reduction of the distal surface helps to keep the mesially bonded aspects (Y) of the central incisors in proper proportion. Residual spacing between the canines and lateral incisors can then be subsequently closed as well by the addition of composite resin. Any subgingival bonded areas must be meticulously contoured and finished so that the patient can maintain good dental hygiene and tissue health with the use of dental floss (Figure 26.15C).

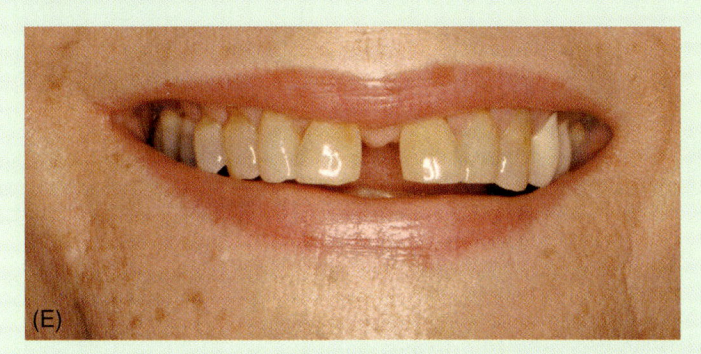

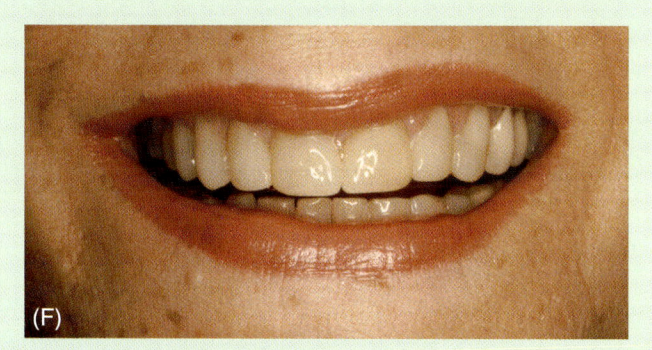

Figure 26.14 (E, F) Comparison of the before and after smiles shows an entirely new smile that is better proportioned by treating four anterior teeth. If only the central incisors had been bonded, two oversized central incisors would have resulted.

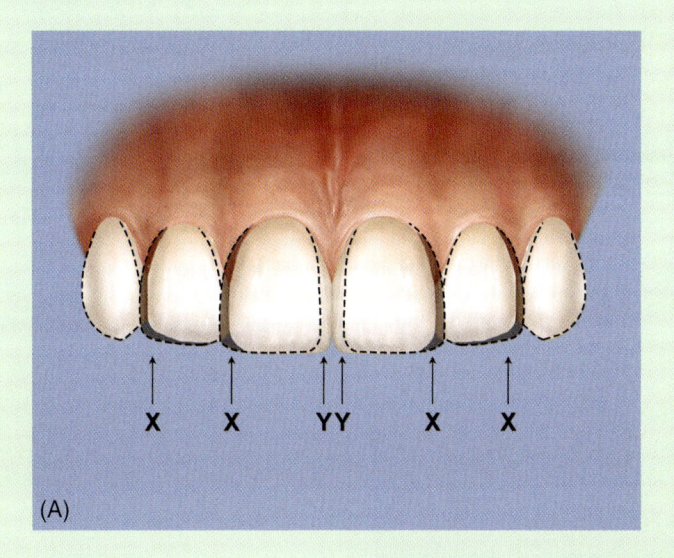

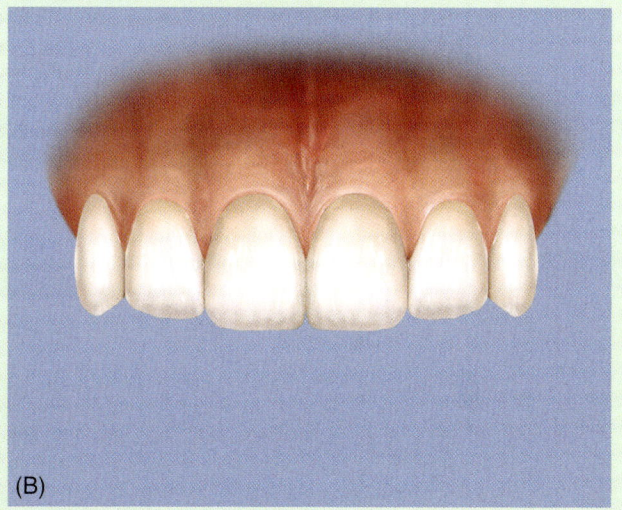

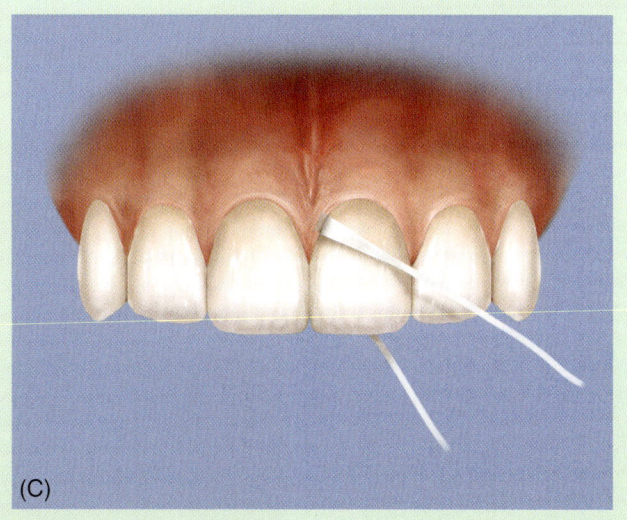

Figure 26.15 (A, B) These drawings illustrate how the teeth of the patient in Figure 26.14 were restored. Additional tooth reduction was performed on the distal surfaces of the central and lateral incisors ("X") to allow for the addition of composite resin to the mesial surfaces ("Y") (Note: composite resin was added to the mesial surfaces of central and lateral incisors and canines), resulting in more ideal width to length ratios and a better proportioned smile as can be seen in Figure B (see text for more details). (C) The shape of the bonding should be conducive to easy flossing to maintain periodontal health. *Source:* illustrations by Zach Turner.

orthodontic treatment to approximate the tooth roots closer together, restorative treatment of the teeth in the cervical interproximal areas can only minimally alter this type of soft tissue contour. In the ideal situation, the interdental tissue should occupy approximately 40% of the incisogingival length of the incisors. Papillae heights, as shown by Chu et al., were determined on average to be 40% of the clinical crown length as measured from gingival zenith to incisal edge.[57]

Two design options are possible with composite resin to close a diastema: full labial veneer versus proximal addition with labiolingual overlap. The following are factors that influence the choice:

- Full labial veneering offers the advantages of concealing the restoration margins by moving them further into the interproximal zone and covering any other imperfections of the facial surface. Hidden restoration margins are useful for disguising slight shade mismatches with tooth structure and to minimize the visibility of stain accumulation that may eventually occur at the margins.
- A full veneer restoration offers the advantage of increased retention, which is essential when tooth lengthening is desired in addition to interproximal space closure. Tooth lengthening is often needed to maintain an esthetic proportion of width to length for teeth when proximal additions are made to close spaces.
- If only one diastema is to be closed, composite resin is typically added to the proximal surface of one or both adjacent teeth (dependent on the size of the diastema and current width of approximating teeth) extending to the facial and lingual proximal line angles unless previous existing restorations dictate otherwise. Thus, when only the proximal surfaces require addition of composite resin, there is less indication for a complete labial veneer. This amount of coverage generally provides adequate retention and allows a sufficient amount of material to be removed by polishing if future staining occurs. Thoroughly polishing the tooth surfaces to be bonded to remove accumulated plaque and acquired pellicle prior to acid etching will help reduce future staining at the tooth resin interface. If composite resin bonding is required on both proximal surfaces of the same tooth, and especially if it extends significantly beyond the facial proximal line angles or if the incisal length needs to be increased, then full composite resin veneer coverage may be better suited for enhanced retention and esthetics. Proximal composite resin restorations that extend significantly past the facial line angles place the tooth resin interfaces more in the zone of direct vision of observers. Subsequently, staining that may occur at this interface would be more readily visible and require more frequent maintenance to polish and "renew" the restoration.
- Extremely translucent incisal edges on the teeth to be bonded may be a contraindication to using a complete labial veneer of composite resin. In this situation, confining the bonding material to the proximal surfaces will maintain the translucency of the incisal edges. When the incisal edge must be

included as part of the restoration, composite resin with varying degrees of translucency or opacity can be selected to match the optical qualities of the existing incisal edge.

Historically, the choice of composite resin was influenced by the size of the space being closed in addition to the functional and esthetic requirements of the restoration.[58] If the space was small (≤1.5 mm), a microfilled composite resin material was used alone to close the diastema. However, it should be noted that deep overbites or heavy functional contacts may contribute to excessive wear or fracture of microfilled composite resins. Currently, for these situations or in the case of a larger diastema (>1.5 mm), modern, microhybrids or nanofilled resins can be used, which offer the combination of improved strength with greater fracture resistance (compared with microfills) and good polishability.[59,60] If so desired, however, a microfilled material can be veneered over the labial surface to provide the highest degree of luster and esthetics (Figure 26.16A–C).

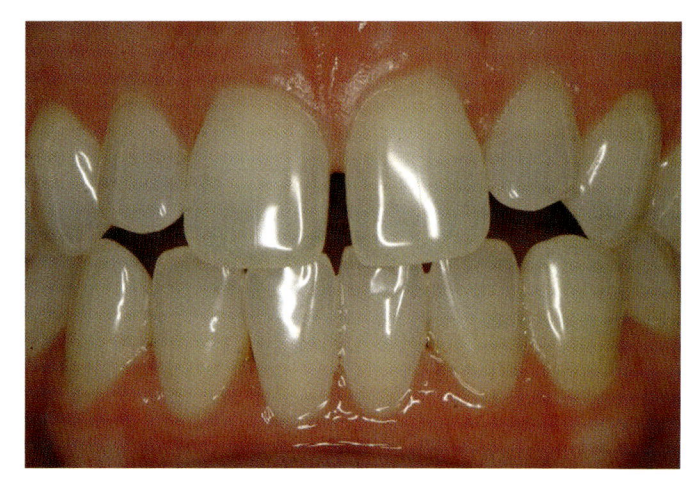

Figure 26.16 **(A)** When a diastema of this size or larger is to be closed using composite resin bonding, a micro- or nanohybrid material should be applied to the lingual surface for strength. *Source:* Reproduced with permission of Robert C. Margeas.

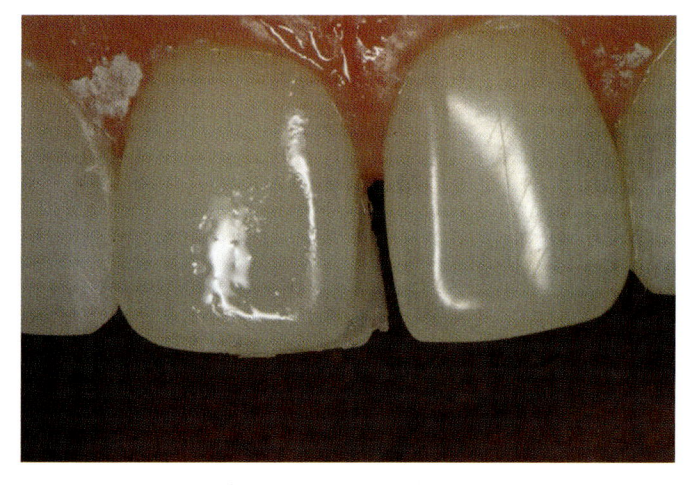

Figure 25.16 **(B)** To obtain a maximum "glaze" or polish to match existing enamel, a microfilled composite resin can be used on the labial surface. *Source:* Reproduced with permission of Robert C. Margeas.

Chapter 26 Restorative Treatment of Diastema

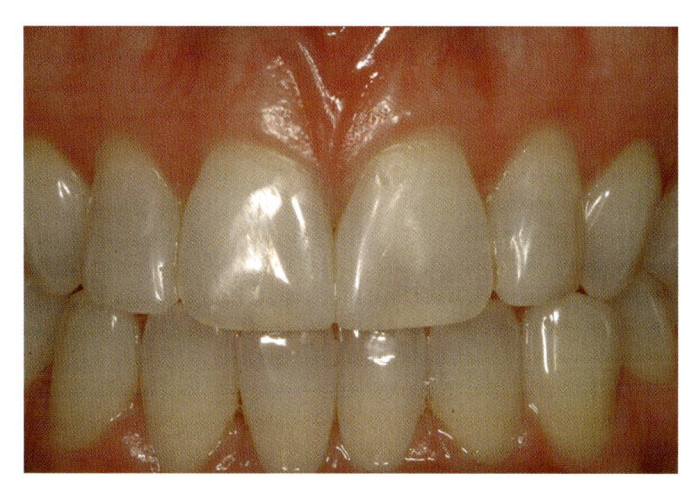

Figure 26.16 **(C)** Note the glazed appearance of the microfilled, highly polished labial enamel composite resin layer. *Source:* Reproduced with permission of Robert C. Margeas.

Immediate closure of posterior diastema

For a small posterior interdental space, a direct resin-bonded pontic could be considered as an option to improve the esthetic continuity from anterior to posterior. The patient, as described in Figure 26.13, was unhappy with the remaining space following orthodontic treatment (and accompanying extractions). As described previously, the space on the upper right was restored with a full-coverage ceramic crown and cantilevered pontic. However, the remaining space on the upper left quadrant was not of sufficient size to consider a dental implant and the adjacent teeth did not need any type of full- or partial-coverage restoration. Placing a full-coverage restoration on the first molar was discussed as an option but the patient was not willing to have an elective restoration placed in order to retain the pontic. Thus, the decision was made to close the space with a small, composite resin pontic directly bonded to the adjacent molar (tooth #14). The only preparation to the molar was to lightly roughen the mesial surface with a fine diamond bur to remove the fluoride-rich, aprismatic enamel for better etching. The connector size was kept as large as possible to decrease risk of fracture of the pontic from the adjacent molar (Figure 26.17E). Again, occlusion was carefully checked and adjusted to minimize excessive occlusal forces on the pontic or any lateral interferences in excursive movements. The final result can be seen in Figure 26.17F and G. The patient was very happy with the overall outcome of resin bonding to solve her esthetic dilemma, both anteriorly and posteriorly.

Fortunately, posterior diastemata are not typically considered as much of an esthetic concern as those in the anterior region, and more often than not they are just a nuisance as a result of food entrapment. For larger diastemata, and especially in patients who demonstrate destructive habits such as clenching or bruxing, the prognosis of using direct resin materials should be considered guarded. As mentioned previously, use of resins with improved strength would be preferred over a microfilled

Clinical case 26.6

Problem

A 26-year-old female had undergone orthognathic surgery for her Class III protrusive malocclusion, which left a small diastema between the mandibular right cuspid and first bicuspid. The patient was very self-conscious of this space and adamantly declined other needed dental treatment until the space was closed (Figure 26.17A and B).

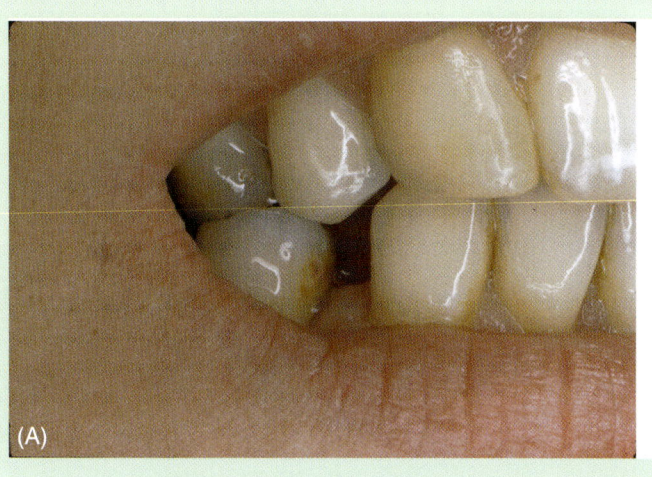

Treatment

Because a lack of sufficient space prevented the construction of a two- or three-unit fixed partial denture that would look symmetrical and attractive, an alternative treatment approach was needed. The option of a second orthodontic treatment was deemed impractical as surgical orthodontics had already been employed as long-term treatment. A direct placement

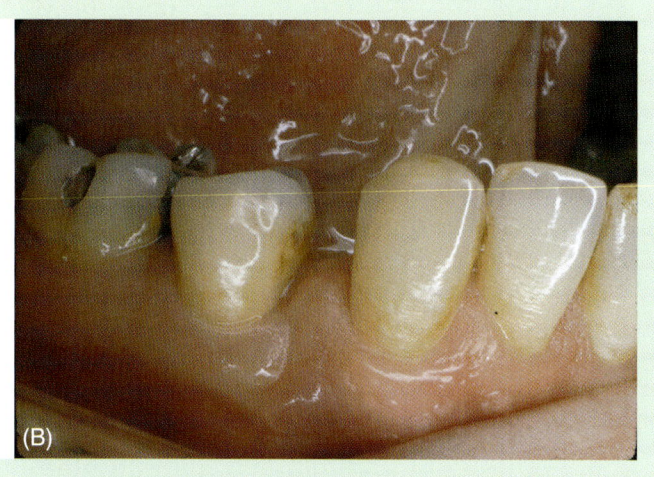

Figure 26.17 **(A, B)** This 26-year-old female was unhappy with the large diastema between the mandibular right cuspid and bicuspid following orthognathic surgery.

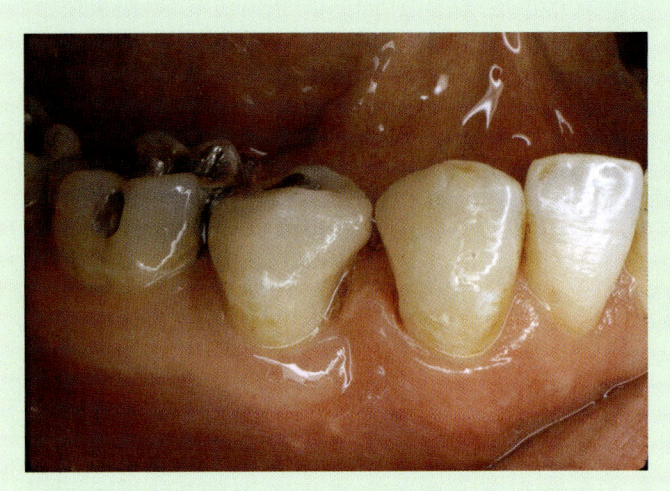

Figure 26.17 (C) Composite resin was added to the adjacent proximal surfaces.

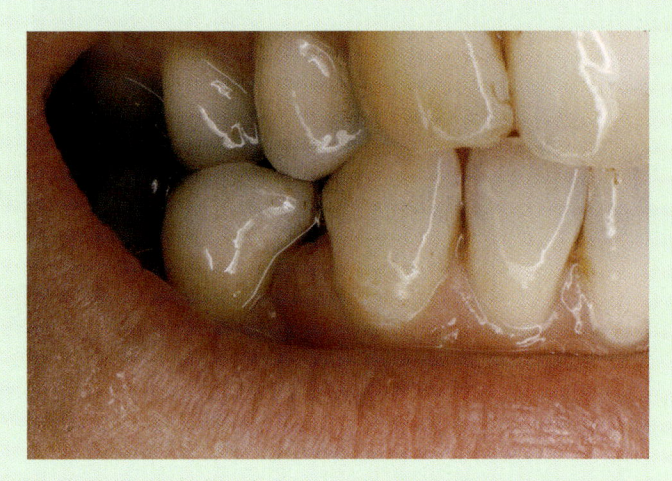

Figure 26.17 (D) The teeth remained acceptably closed after 5 years.

composite resin technique was chosen as both an immediate and economical solution. In the case of a larger diastema, it will usually be necessary to add restorative material to both teeth to maintain better proportionality and minimize the overcontouring of any one tooth. In this case, the distal surface of the cuspid and the mesial surface of the first bicuspid were etched and restored with composite resin to close the diastema (Figure 26.17C). Because esthetics was the patient's chief concern, it was not imperative to completely close the space or obtain tight contact between these teeth. As each tooth was minimally bonded, neither appeared from a distance to be overly contoured or too large.

Result

The 5-year follow-up result can be seen in Figure 26.17D. It is important to inform the patient that no dental restoration is truly "permanent" and that composite resin closure of a diastema may require refinishing, repair, or replacement every few years as discoloration, wear, and fractures may occur. Appropriate case selection, delivery of care, and pre- and posttreatment preventive measures (such as occlusal evaluation and adjustment as needed, elimination of noxious habits, occlusal guard, etc.) can improve the odds for long-term success.

composite resin due to added strength, and thus a reduced risk for fracture. Attempting to establish broad contacts occlusogingivally would be advantageous to improve the strength of the marginal ridge and reduce the size of the gingival embrasure as a food trap. Occlusion must be carefully checked and adjusted, perhaps even to the opposing cusp as well, and especially in cases where a plunger cusp exists, to minimize risk of excessive wear or fracture of the restoration. An occlusal guard should be considered for those patients with parafunctional activity.

Porcelain veneers

The choice of porcelain veneers for diastema closure offers superb esthetics as the major indication for their use. Ceramics have the capacity to replicate the esthetically pleasing characteristics and vitality of natural teeth.[61] In addition, indirectly fabricated restorations are considered easier for many dentists as most of the contouring, shading, and anatomy is created by the laboratory technician. Other advantages of incorporating all-ceramic restorations, especially for anterior teeth, include improved strength, durability, marginal integrity, color match, and wear resistance.[62] Owing to its crystalline matrix, ceramics are more resistant to attritional wear than composite resin.[63] However, owing to the brittle nature of porcelain,[63] the failures with porcelain tend to be more catastrophic in nature, especially under tensile and torsional stresses[61,64,65] and, therefore, more likely to require a remake of the restoration. Although composite resin restorations often require no or minimal mechanical tooth preparation, porcelain veneers almost always require some enamel preparation for the best results and, therefore, should not be considered to be a reversible procedure. It is possible in select

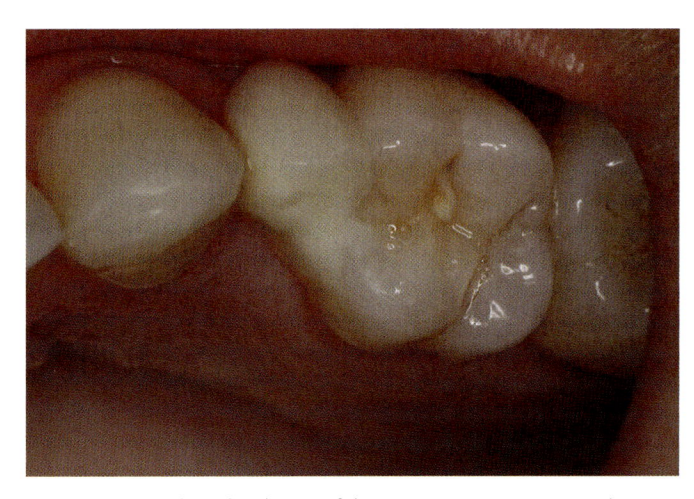

Figure 26.17 (E) Occlusal view of the composite resin pontic showing the large connector size (patient from Clinical case 26.4 (Figure 26.13)).
Source: Reproduced with permission of Robert C. Margeas.

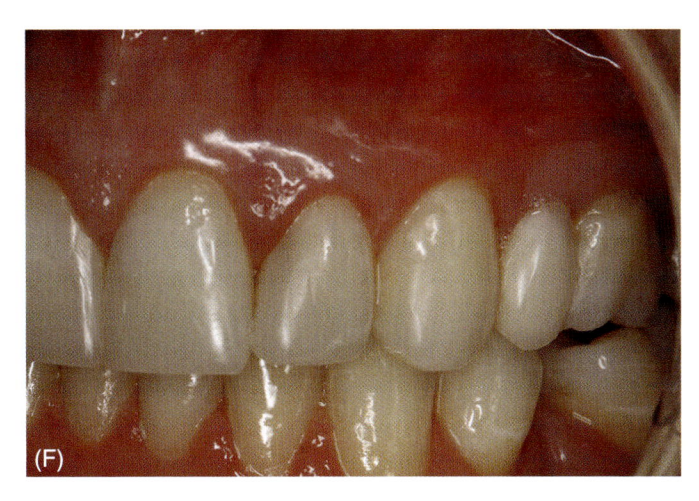

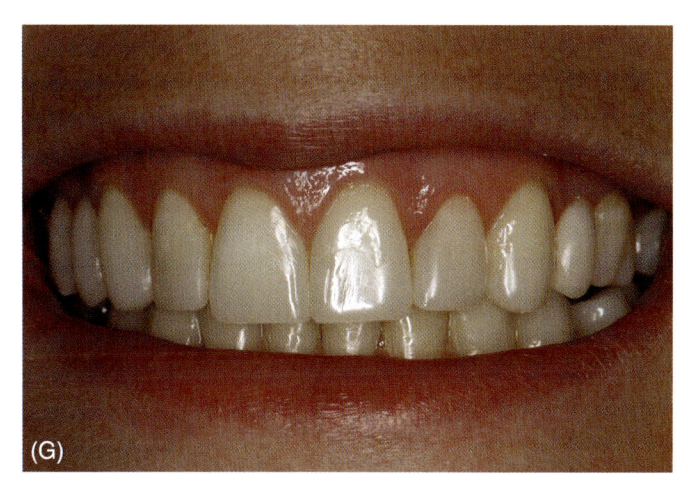

Figure 26.17 (F, G) The final result of closing the posterior space via a resin-bonded composite pontic was very pleasing esthetically to the patient. *Source:* Reproduced with permission of Robert C. Margeas.

cases, however, to use minimal preparation veneers that can be fabricated as thin as 0.3 mm[66–68] and provide excellent esthetics with minimal tooth preparation as seen in Clinical case 26.7.

As mentioned previously, it is important to keep in mind that most cases of porcelain veneers do require some degree of tooth preparation to sufficiently align and contour the restored teeth, reduce sharp edges (to minimize risk of internal crack propagation of the overlying ceramic material), and to allow for proper gingival health. The amount of preparation is case dependent, and the practitioner should advise the patient that conservative preparation does not always mean insignificant tooth reduction, but rather reduction of the least amount of tooth structure possible to achieve the goals of the case. The final desired position, color, and shape of the restoration(s) should be the main determinants for the amount of tooth preparation. Just as the amount of reduction is specific to each case, the design of veneer preparations must also be case specific and not be generalized as a single protocol for use in every situation.[68]

Clinical case 26.7

Problem

This patient was unhappy with the appearance of his smile (Figure 26.18A and B) and was getting married in 8 weeks; thus, orthodontic treatment was not an option. The patient's goals included closing the spaces, straightening his teeth to make them show more evenly in his smile, and brightening them.

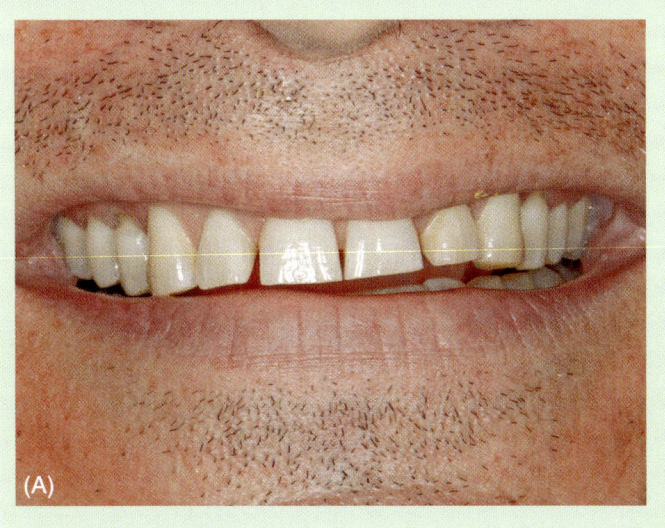

Treatment

The teeth were minimally prepared to round and soften sharp corners, remove any undercuts to the path of insertion, and to develop a very slight chamfer finish line (for gingival health) and to minimize staining at restoration–resin cement–tooth interface (Figure 26.18C). Lithium disilicate veneers were

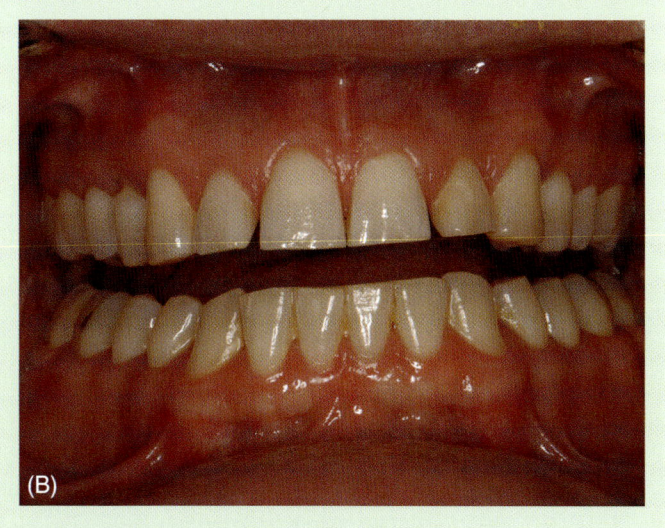

Figure 26.18 (A, B) This adult male patient desired to improve the evenness and color of his smile and close the spaces. Owing to time restrictions, orthodontic care was not an option. *Source:* Reproduced with permission of James Fondriest.

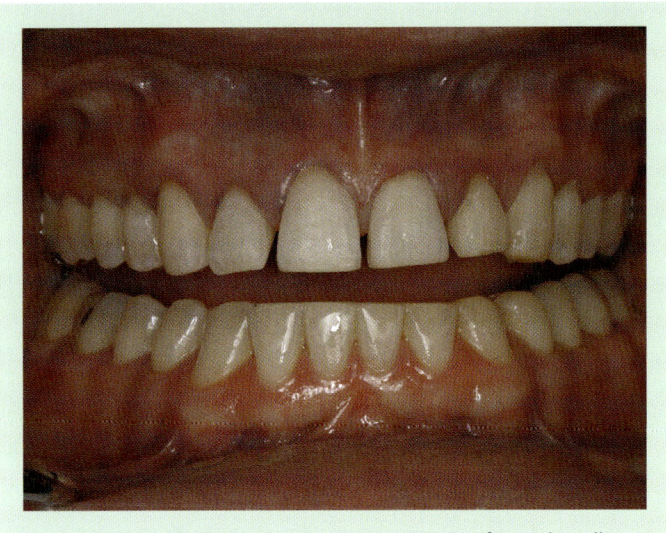

Figure 26.18 (C) Minimal preparations were performed to allow for porcelain veneers that would fulfill the patient's desires. *Source:* Reproduced with permission of James Fondriest.

chosen because of their strength at minimal thicknesses. A shade was chosen that would brighten his smile and give him the look he was seeking.

Result

The patient's goals for treatment were successfully met without significant sacrifice of healthy tooth structure. In addition, occlusal function was improved and anterior guidance was restored. The before and after final results can be seen in Figure 26.18D and E. The patient was very happy with the results obtained and advised of necessary home care techniques and need for follow-up recall visits.

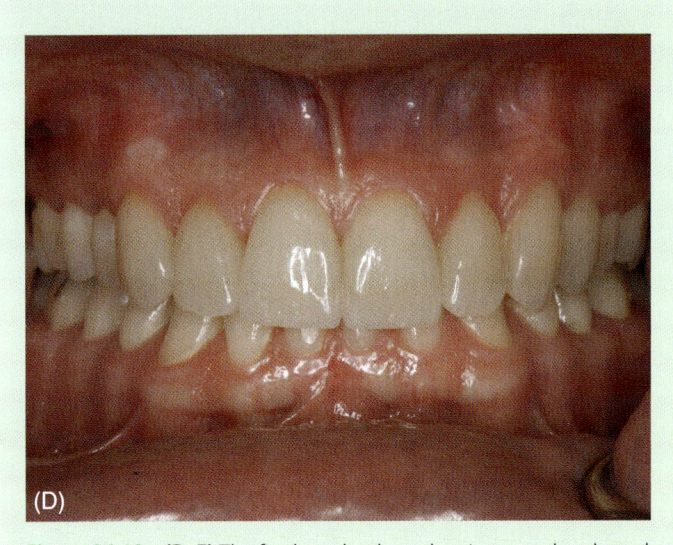

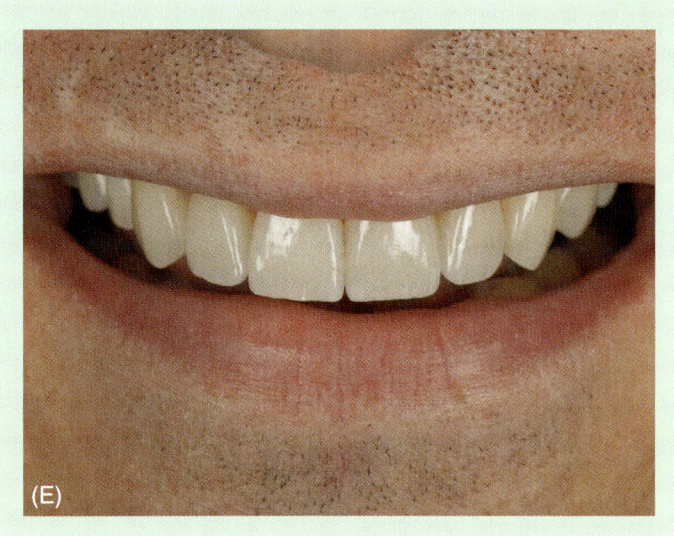

Figure 26.18 (D, E) The final results show that, in properly selected cases, minimal prep veneers can be very esthetic, preserve tooth structure for improved bond strength, and provide for acceptable cervical contours to maintain periodontal health. *Source:* Reproduced with permission of James Fondriest.

The normal proximal finish line employed for a traditional porcelain veneer preparation is typically a chamfer prepared labial to the interproximal contact when there are no interdental spaces present. However, when attempting to close diastemata or modify interproximal tooth contours, the lingual margin in most cases should be carried through the embrasure to the linguoproximal line angle, but without extending onto the lingual surface, thereby creating a potential path-of-draw issue (Figure 26.19A and B). The finish line for a porcelain veneer that is being used to close a diastema may approach a featheredge at the linguoproximal line angle, although a chamfer provides more edge strength.[69] A lingually positioned proximal finish line on the diastema side of the tooth avoids preparation undercuts with the linguoincisal extension and also allows for a thicker interproximal increment of porcelain to reduce translucency. In addition, it allows the laboratory technician to begin the interproximal emergence profile from the linguoproximal line angle, creating broader and more gradual contours for enhanced esthetics and patient hygiene.

Consultation with one's ceramist is important in treating diastema patients with indirect restorations. Additionally, the radiographic location of the osseous crest and periodontal pocket depths should be evaluated as interproximal subgingival margins are often needed to achieve a natural-looking diastema closure.

Closing single midline diastema with porcelain

In most cases of a single midline diastema where the teeth have normal proportion and the size of the diastema is not too large, the clinician will likely choose to close it with composite resin (given the advantages discussed previously). The results are

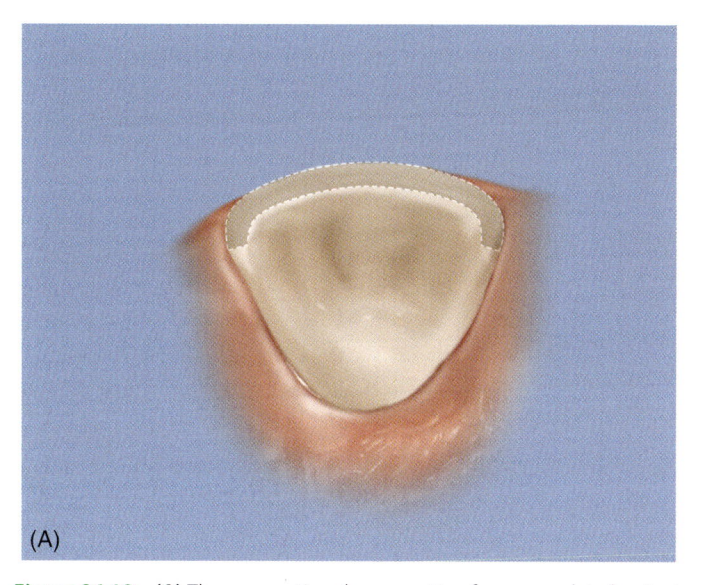

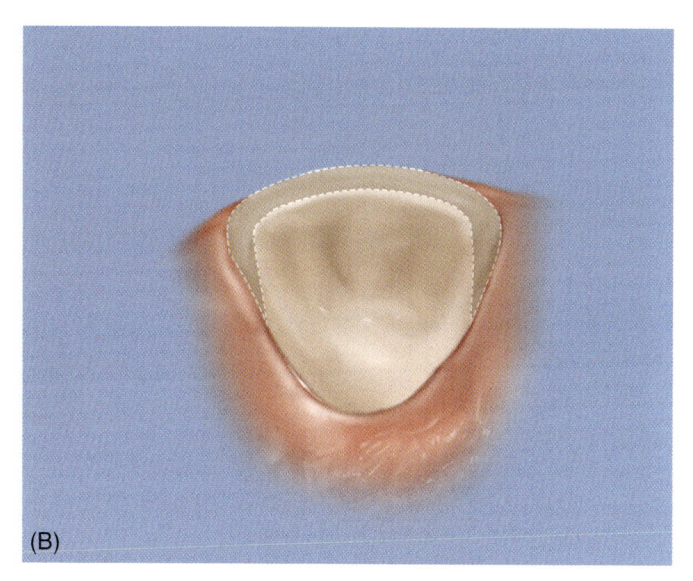

Figure 26.19 **(A)** The conventional preparation for a porcelain laminate, when there is no space to close, usually extends one-third to midway into the proximal surface. **(B)** This revised preparation extending to the linguoproximal line angle is indicated when closing interdental spaces. *Source:* illustrations by Zach Turner.

immediate and can be long lasting with proper maintenance. For those occasions when the dentist and patient prefer to close a diastema using porcelain (e.g., enhanced esthetics, larger diastema, personal preference) and the facial surfaces of the abutment teeth are unrestored and esthetic, an alternative approach may include the use of porcelain sectional veneers, or so-called "porcelain pieces." Sectional veneers enable the diastema to be closed with minimal or no tooth preparation other than creating a path of draw and rounding any sharp line angles. The disadvantages of this option are that it involves an additional appointment, the porcelain pieces can be more difficult to handle (i.e., fragile) and stabilize during the bonding procedure, and it requires exceptional laboratory support, and thus an accompanying laboratory fee. However, with good laboratory support and proper case selection, the results can be exceptional, as shown in Clinical case 26.8.

Closing multiple diastemata with porcelain veneers

When several restorations will be required (multiple diastemata), laboratory-fabricated restorations can allow the dentist to achieve more ideal results in terms of proportioning multiple teeth (assuming the teeth are relatively evenly spaced) and provide for better symmetry. Clinical case 26.9 describes use of porcelain veneers to accomplish this objective.

For the more discriminating patient who seeks results over tooth preservation, in most instances additional preparation will be required. In any case, however, it should always be the goal of the practitioner to preserve as much tooth structure, and specifically enamel, as possible to improve the bond strength and maintain the overall flexural strength of the

Clinical case 26.8

Problem

A female patient was unhappy with the space between her front teeth and the chipped edge of the right incisor and wanted to know the options for treatment, but was otherwise satisfied with the appearance of her smile (see Figure 26.20A and B). She was not interested in orthodontics to close the space, and she wanted to preserve her natural tooth structure and have the most esthetic, longest lasting result possible.

Treatment

The patient elected to have the diastema closed and incisal edge of tooth #8 repaired with ceramic. The interproximal surfaces were disked to ensure smoothly contoured surfaces, but no other preparation was made. Porcelain pieces were fabricated from feldspathic porcelain with clear porcelain added to the facial margins to create a "contact lens effect"

(Figure 26.20C) and bonded using the etch-and-rinse technique and clear light-cured composite resin cement. Prior to the adhesive bonding step, the sectional veneers were carefully inserted in order to evaluate the fit, esthetics, and ultimate path of insertion needed (Figure 26.20D). After bonding to place, the excess porcelain was carefully reduced with a fine diamond bur followed by final contouring and polishing of the teeth and ceramic.

Result

The final result was very esthetic, with the patient being extremely satisfied with the outcome (see Figure 26.20E and F). The exquisite detail to emergence profile and hygienic contours, and the artistic ability of the master ceramist were paramount to the ultimate success of this case.

868 — Esthetic Challenges of Malocclusion

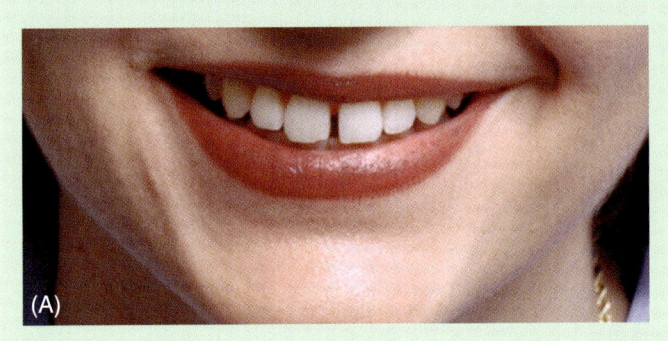

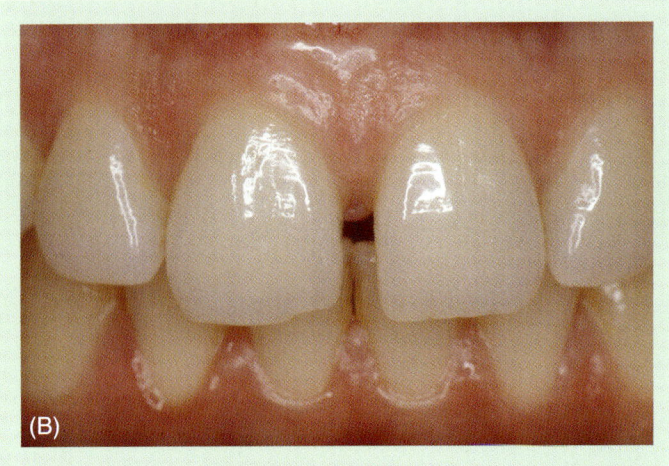

Figure 26.20 **(A, B)** This female patient was unhappy with the space between her front teeth and wanted the most esthetic option available for closing it while remaining as conservative as possible. *Source:* Figure B from Chiche et al.[45(p53)] Reproduced with permission of Quintessence Publishing.

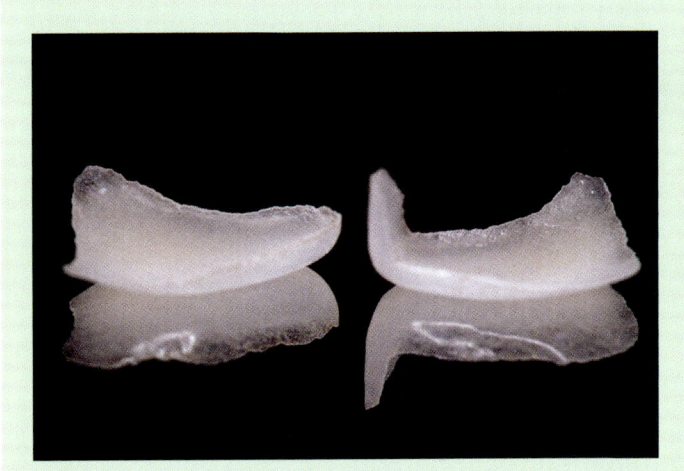

Figure 26.20 **(C)** Feldspathic sectional veneers (porcelain pieces) were fabricated that would be bonded with resin cement. *Source:* Chiche et al.[45(p45)] Reproduced with permission of Quintessence Publishing.

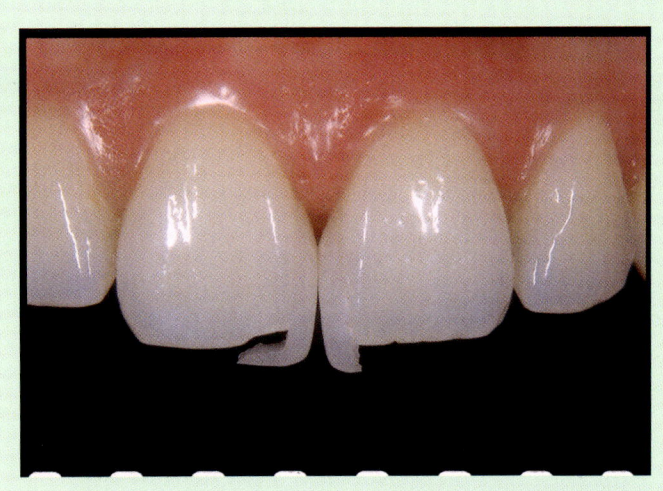

Figure 26.20 **(D)** Sectional veneers are shown being inserted during the try-in phase in order to evaluate fit and path of placement required for the final bonding process.

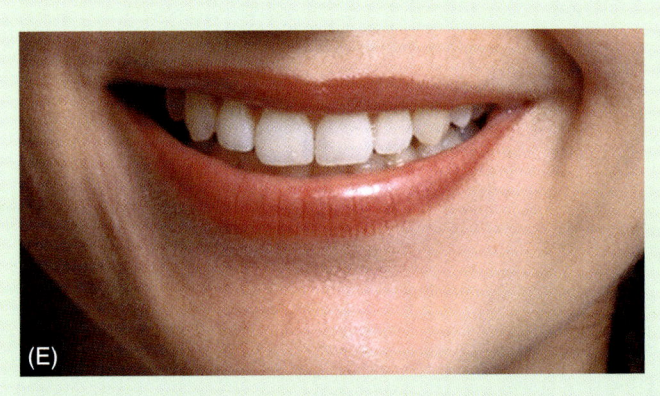

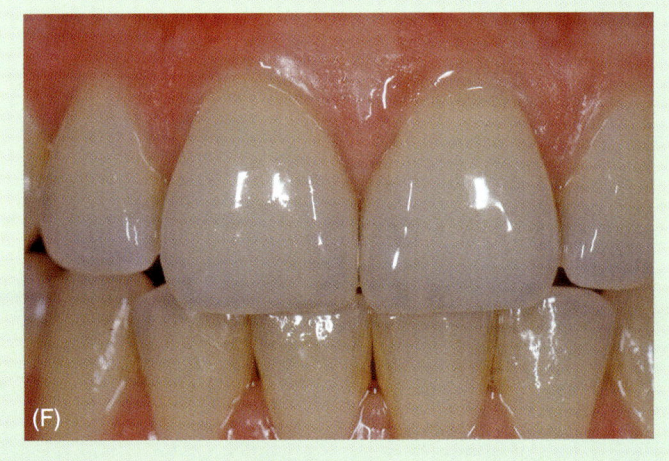

Figure 26.20 **(E, F)** The final result shows the conservative nature of this diastema closure and the extreme attention to detail in the laboratory phase and bonding technique (to ensure correct alignment of these porcelain sectional veneers). *Source:* Figure E from Chiche et al.[45(p53)] Reproduced with permission of Quintessence Publishing.

tooth as it has been shown that bonding ceramic to the tooth recovers strength that is lost as an inherent part of tooth preparation for restorative procedures.[70] In fact, bonded ceramic veneers are capable of restoring the fracture strength of teeth to values of intact teeth.[40,71,72] Clinical case 26.10 depicts a more typical porcelain veneer preparation utilized to close multiple diastemata.

Combination crowns/veneers

One of dentistry's goals is to be as conservative as possible while accomplishing the best functional and esthetic result. However, at times it becomes necessary to combine full-coverage restorations with veneers in closing diastemata. Figure 26.23A illustrates the principle of space reallocation, through specific preparation

Clinical case 26.9

Problem

Figure 26.21 shows a 21-year-old male model who hesitated to smile because of his diastemata (see Figure 26.21A, D, and F). The patient was also concerned about the appearance of his inflamed gingiva adjacent to the left central incisor, and subsequent examination showed an overextension of existing composite resin bonding. A main requirement of this patient was immediate esthetic treatment since he was leaving the country the following week. A second requirement was that no additional tooth be reduced, including the opposing teeth.

Treatment

In order to maximize longevity and esthetics, porcelain laminates were chosen as the most conservative treatment. Figure 26.21B shows the occlusal view, indicating just how much the left central incisor protruded before restoration. Four porcelain laminates were used to create a symmetric arch with proper spacing (see Figure 26.21C). The improvement by the final result can be seen by comparing the before and after smiles (see Figure 26.21D–G). Note how the increased tooth size is well proportioned to the face. As mentioned previously, altering tooth size and controlling interproximal contours for diastema cases requires extending the lingual finish line of the veneer preparations close to the lingual–proximal line angles. By extending the finish line to the lingual, it enables the laboratory technician more flexibility in controlling the final esthetics of the case.

Result

Frequently, orthodontic treatment is required to reposition teeth together to avoid the overly contoured appearance of restored teeth. Although this treatment could have been employed and allowed for more ideal tooth proportions, the patient chose immediate esthetic correction over lengthy orthodontic treatment and was accepting of slight compromises to ideal esthetics for the sake of tooth conservation and expedience.

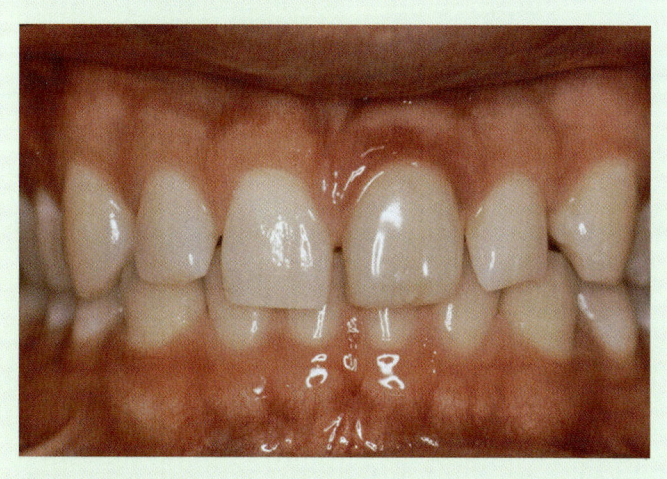

Figure 26.21 (A) This 21-year-old male model performed both runway and photography modeling without smiling because he disliked the spaces between his teeth.

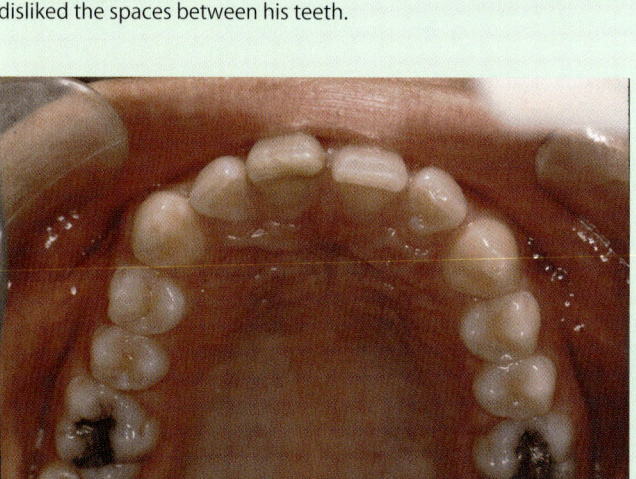

Figure 26.21 (B) This before occlusal view shows how much the left central incisor protruded prior to treatment. (Note: image is reversed).

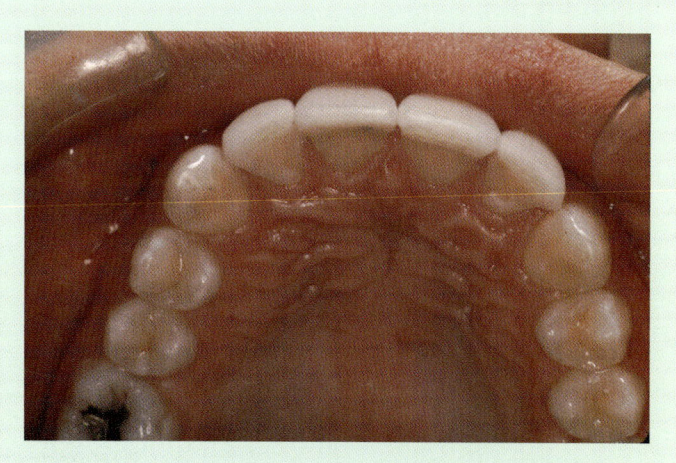

Figure 26.21 (C) Only four porcelain laminate veneers were necessary to eliminate the dark spaces between his teeth. Also note that tooth #9 was brought back into arch alignment.

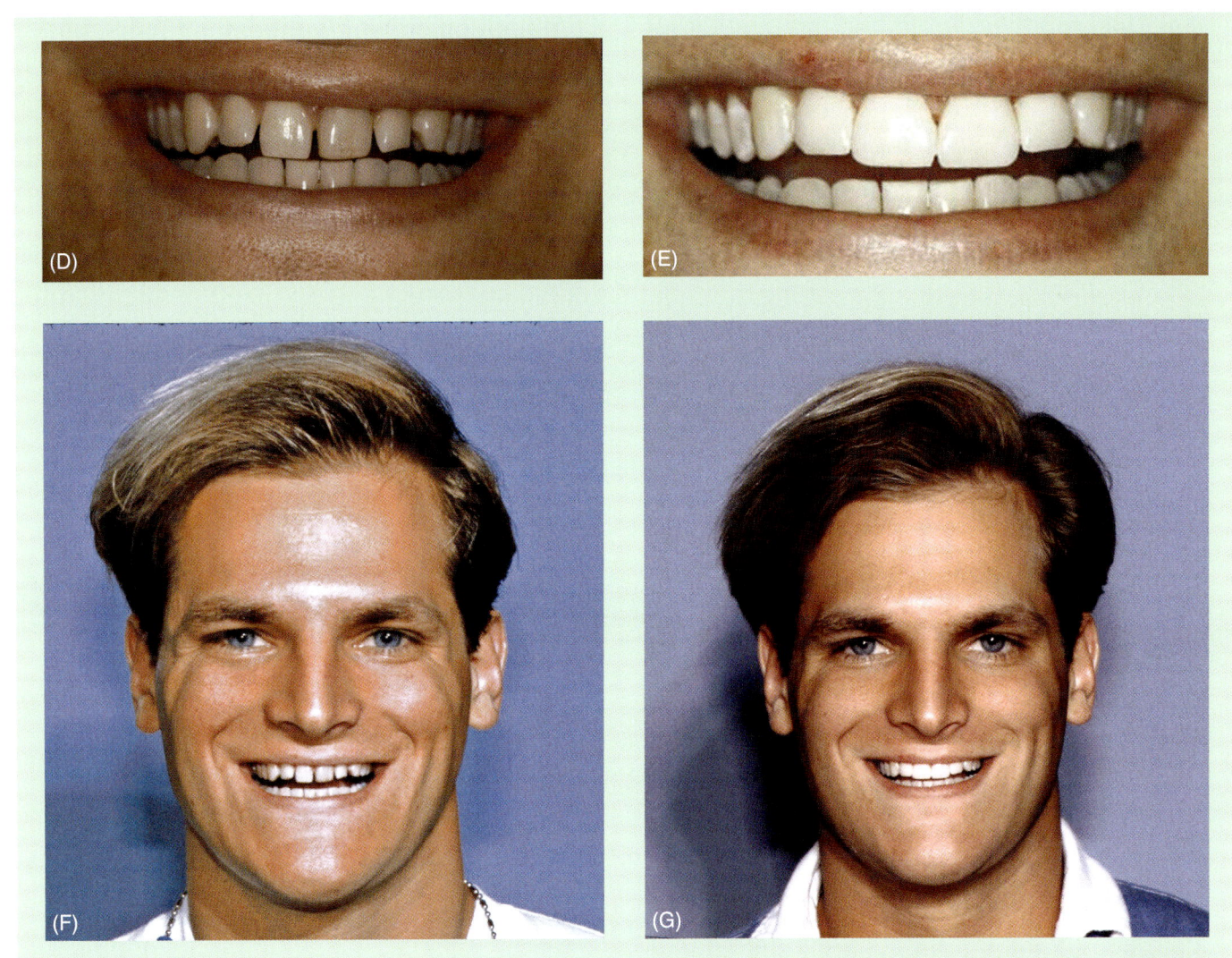

Figure 26.21 **(D–G)** These before and after pictures show how much better proportioned the larger teeth appear in the full face view.

guidelines, to allow for better proportioned teeth as if often required when closing diastemata. Tooth preparation needs to be carefully planned and carried out by means of tooth reduction guides (fabricated from accurate diagnostic wax-ups), keeping in mind that lateral incisors should not be made too wide, thereby competing for central incisor dominance. Adequate tooth reduction is paramount in providing the ceramist with appropriate space in which to create a beautiful and well-proportioned smile (Figure 26.23B–F).

Summary

The esthetic significance of a diastema and the decision to close it is predominantly the choice of the patient. The dentist must possess a full appreciation of the factors contributing to diastemata and the various options available to treat them. Once the etiology of a diastema is identified, the patient should be informed of treatment alternatives, therapeutic time commitments, prognoses, and costs. Consideration of etiologic factors, appropriate treatment planning of the dental patient as an individual, and mutually agreed-upon expectations for outcomes of treatment are essential in the successful management of anterior diastemata and other modalities of esthetic care.

Selecting the proper treatment involves the usual challenges of addressing the needs and expectations of the patient and determining what degree of accommodation is necessary to achieve the desired result. An integrated orthodontic restorative or totally restorative approach may enhance the esthetic result only when a pure orthodontic therapy solution is not feasible or

Clinical case 26.10

Problem
This patient desired to close the spaces between her teeth but did not wish to undergo orthodontic treatment. The teeth were determined to need additional width to improve the proportions, and thus it was decided to treat her case restoratively. In addition, she wanted to have brighter teeth while maintaining a natural appearance. The pretreatment photo can be seen in Figure 26.22A.

Treatment
Following diagnostic wax-up and surgical guide fabrication, the gingival margins of teeth #7 and #8 were altered via osseous reduction for tooth #7 and very slight soft tissue modification over #8 to match the height and gingival zenith position with that of #9. Following adequate healing, teeth #6–#11 were prepared as conservatively as possible for ceramic veneers (see Figure 26.22B). The canines were included for better proportion of her smile, especially with respect to achieving pleasing widths and proportions of the incisors while maintaining central incisor dominance. Tooth preparations involved the proximal surfaces and were extended slightly subgingivally to allow the laboratory technician to have better control of the emergence profile and interproximal contours. Feldspathic veneers were fabricated following the guidelines of the diagnostic wax-up and approved provisional restorations.

Result
As seen in Figure 26.22C and D, the patient's goals of space closure and additional brightness were accomplished very successfully. The teeth are well proportioned, and the gingival architecture developed through minor periodontal surgery balanced out the soft tissue profile to give a very pleasing and esthetic result.

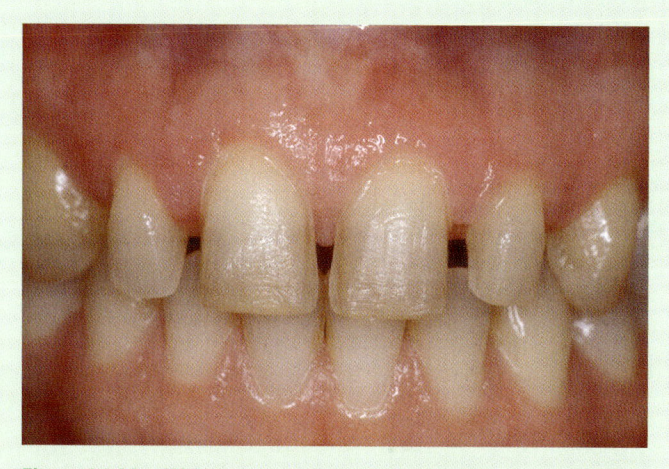

Figure 26.22 **(B)** The six maxillary anterior teeth were prepared for feldspathic porcelain veneers. The canines were included to prevent excessively wide lateral incisors. *Source:* Chiche et al.[45(p53)] Reproduced with permission of Quintessence Publishing.

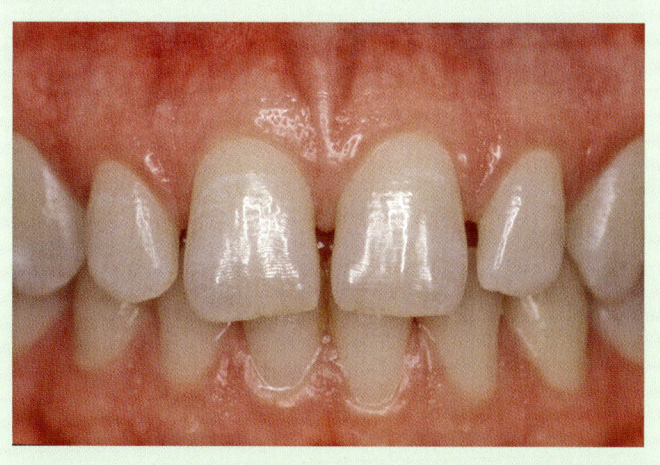

Figure 26.22 **(A)** This patient desired to improve her smile nonorthodontically as well as brighten her teeth. *Source:* Chiche et al.[45(p53)] Reproduced with permission of Quintessence Publishing.

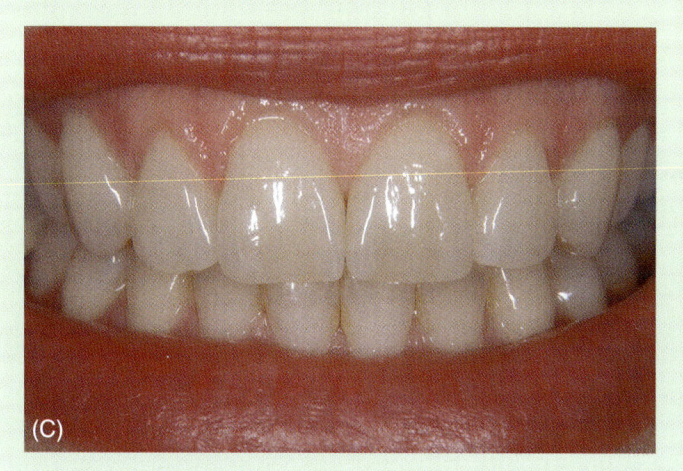

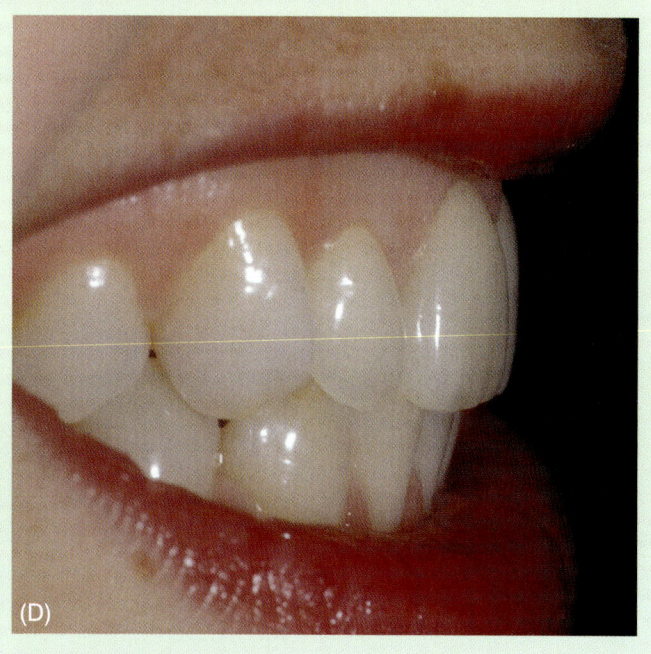

Figure 26.22 **(C, D)** The final result shows a very pleasing and natural smile that met the patient's goals. *Source:* Figure C from Chiche et al.[45(p53)] Reproduced with permission of Quintessence Publishing.

practical. For larger diastemata where teeth will appear excessively wide when restored, periodontal therapy should be considered to improve tooth proportionality and bring better balance to the overall smile.

Regardless of the choice of treatment, the objective is to improve esthetics while preserving as much healthy tooth structure as possible. For the highly esthetic-driven patient, however, the ultimate esthetic result may come at the price of greater tooth reduction, and the patient must be made aware of this trade-off and its inherent risks. Good occlusion and maintenance of the supporting tissues are equally important to prevent diastema reformation and failure of corrective therapies. The ability of the dentist to successfully manage diastemata is the mark of a clinician who practices esthetic dentistry according to sound, interdisciplinary, evidence-based principles.

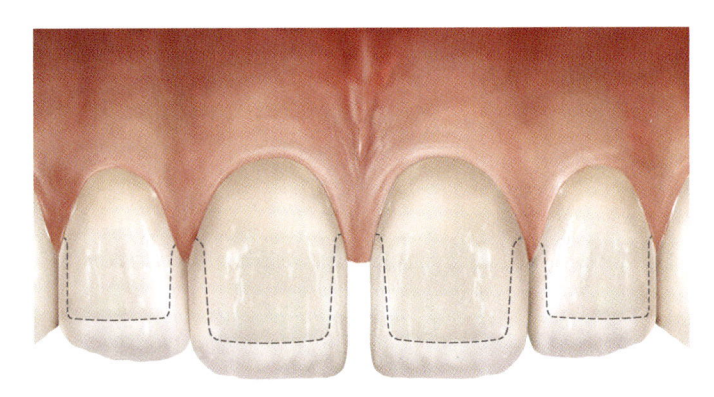

Figure 26.23 **(A)** This drawing illustrates the principle of additional reduction on the distal surfaces of the central incisors to prevent excessively wide centrals when closing a midline diastema in cases where the teeth are currently correctly proportioned. Additional porcelain or composite resin will be subsequently added to the mesial of the lateral incisors to close the space created by this preparation design. *Source:* Illustrations by Zach Turner

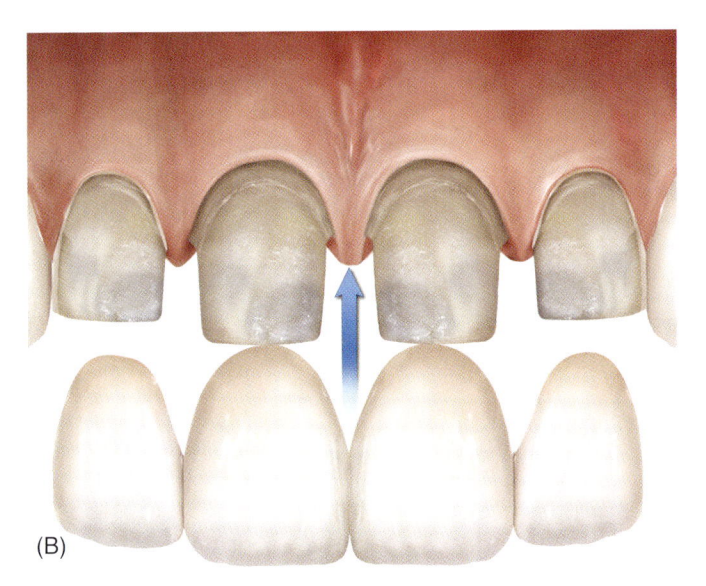

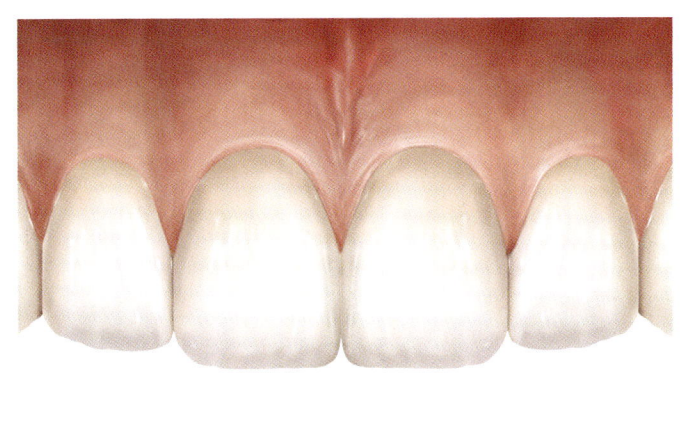

Figure 26.23 **(B, C)** These illustrations show the preparation design as drawn in Figure 26.23A and the definitive restorations (full-coverage crowns on central incisors and porcelain veneers on lateral incisors) created to close the midline diastema and maintain proportionality between the central and lateral incisors.

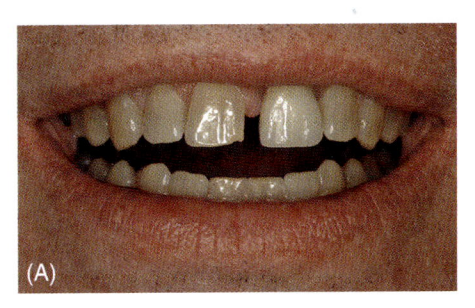

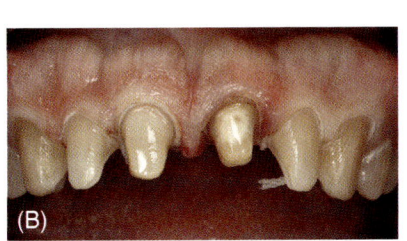

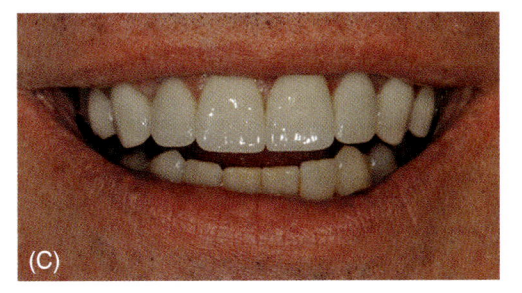

Figure 26.23 **(D)** This patient wanted to close his maxillary diastema plus improve his smile with brighter and better looking teeth. **(E)** The left central crown was removed and the right central was prepared for full crown, and the canines and lateral incisors prepared for porcelain veneers. **(F)** The final result corrects the patient's previous reverse smile line and illustrates using both porcelain veneers and crowns to provide a more attractive smile.

References

1. Chalfifoux PR. Perception esthetics: factors that affect smile design. *J Esthet Rest Dent* 2007;8:189–192.
2. Lowe E. Simplifying diastema closure in the anterior region. *Dent Today* 2003;22(12):50–55.
3. Gurel G. PLVs for diastema closure. In: *The Science and Art of Porcelain Laminate Veneers*. New Malden: Quintessence; 2003:369–392.
4. Rosentiel SF, Rashid RG. Public preferences for anterior tooth variations: a web-based study. *J Estht Rest Dent* 2002;14(2):97–106.
5. Goldstein RE. *Change your Smile*, 3rd edn. Chicago: Quintessence; 1997.
6. Furuse AY, Herkrath FJ, Franco EJ, et al. Multidisciplinary management of anterior diastemata: clinical procedures. *Pract Proced Aesthet Dent* 2007;19(3):185–191.
7. Huang WJ, Creath CJ. The midline diastema: a review of its etiology and treatment. *J Ped Dent* 1995;17(3):171–179.
8. Oesterle LJ, Shellhart WE. Maxillary diastemas: a look at the causes. *J Am Dent Assoc* 1999;130:85–94.
9. Fradeani M, Barducci G. Tooth analysis. In: Fradeani M, ed. *Esthetic Rehabilitation in Fixed Prosthodontics. Volume 1, Esthetic Analysis: A Systematic Approach to Prosthetic Treatment*. Chicago, IL: Quintessence; 2004:137–242.
10. Profitt W, Fields H, Sarver D. *Contemporary Orthodontics*, 4th edn. St. Louis, MO: Mosby; 2007.
11. Yamaoka M, Furusawa K, Yasuda K. Effects of maxillary anterior supenumerary impacted teeth on diastema. *Oral Surg Oral Med Oral Pathol Oral Radiol Endod* 1995;80:252.
12. Garib D, Alencar B, Lauris J, Baccetti T. Agenesis of maxillary incisors and associated dental anomalies. *Am J Orthod Dentofacial Orthop* 2010;137:732.e1–732.e6.
13. Leonard MS. The maxillary frenum and surgical treatment. *Gen Dent* 1998;46:614–617.
14. Towfighi PP, Brunsvold MA, Storey AT, et al. Pathologic migration of anterior teeth in patients with moderate to severe periodontitis. *J Periodont* 1997;68:967–972.
15. Martinez-Canut P, Carrasquer A, Magan R, Lorca A. A study on factors associated with pathologic tooth migration. *J Clin Periodont* 1997;24(7):492–497.
16. Popovich F, Thompson GW. Maxillary diastemas: a look at the causes. *J Am Dent Assoc* 1999;130:85–94.
17. Attia Y. Midline diastemas: closure and stability. *Angle Orthod* 1993;63:209–212.
18. Haywood VB, Parker H. Niteguard vital bleaching beneath existing porcelain veneer: a case report. *Quintessence Int* 1999;30(11):743–774.
19. Haywood VB, Pahjola R. Bleaching and esthetic bonding of tetracycline-stained teeth. *Contemp Esthet Restor Pract* 2004;8(10):16–23.
20. Newitter DA. Predictable diastema reduction with filled resin: diagnostic wax-up. *J Prosthet Dent* 1986;55:293–296.
21. Morley J, Eubank J. Macoesthetic elements of smile design. *J Am Dent Assoc* 2001;132(1):39–45.
22. Fradeani M, Corrado M. Facial analysis. In: Fradeani M, ed. *Esthetic Rehabilitation in Fixed Prosthodontics. Volume 1, Esthetic Analysis: A Systematic Approach to Prosthetic Treatment*. Chicago, IL: Quintessence Publishing; 2004:28.
23. Kokich VO, Kiyak HA, Shapiro PA. Comparing the perception of dentist and lay people to altered dental esthetics. *J Estht Dent* 1999;11:311–324.
24. Vig RG, Brundo GC. The kinetics of anterior tooth display. *J Prosthet Dent* 1978;39(5):502–504.
25. Oquendo A, Brea L, David S. Diastema: correction of excessive spaces in the esthetic zone. *Dent Clin North Am* 2011;55(2):265–281.
26. Chu SJ. Range and mean distribution frequency of individual tooth width of the maxillary anterior dentition. *Pract Proced Aesthet Dent* 2007;19(4):209–215.
27. Tarnow DP, Magner AW, Fletcher P. The effect of the distance from the contact point to the crest of bone on the presence or absence of the interproximal dental papilla. *J Periodontol* 1992;63:995–996.
28. Levin EI. Dental esthetics and the golden proportion. *J Prosthet Dent* 1978;40:244–252.
29. Ricketts RM. The biologic significance of the divine proportion and Fibonacci series. *Am J Orthod* 1982;81:351–370.
30. Lombardi RE. The principles of visual perception and their clinical application to denture esthetics. *J Prosthet Dent* 1973;29:358–382.
31. Mahshid M, Khoshvaghti A, Varshosaz M, Vallaei N. Evaluation of "golden proportion" in individuals with esthetic smile. *J Esthet Restor Dent* 2004;16:185–192.
32. Preston JD. The golden proportion revisited. *J Esthet Dent* 1993;5:247–251.
33. Rosenthiel SF, Ward DH, Rashid RG. Dentists' preferences of anterior tooth proportion—a web based study. *J Prosthodont* 2000;9:123–136.
34. Hasanreisoglu U, Berksun S, Aras K, Arslan I. An analysis of maxillary anterior teeth: facial and dental proportions. *J Prosthet Dent* 2005;94:530–538.
35. Ward DH. Proportional smile design using the recurrent esthetic dental (RED) proportion. *Dent Clin North Am* 2001;45:143–154.
36. Ward DH. A study of dentists' preferred maxillary anterior tooth width proportions: comparing the recurring esthetic dental proportions to other mathematical and naturally occurring proportions. *J Esthet Restor Dent* 2007;19:324–339.
37. McLaren EA, Phong TC. Smile analysis and esthetic design: "in the zone". *Inside Dent* 2009;5(7):44–48.
38. Magne P, Gallucci G, Belser U. Anatomic crown width/length ratios of unworn and worn maxillary teeth in white subjects. *J Prosth Dent* 2003;89:453–461.
39. Frush JP, Fisher RD. The dynesthetic interpretation of the dentogenic concept. *J Prosthet Dent* 1958;8:558–580.
40. Magne P, Belser U. *Bonded Porcelain Restorations in the Anterior Dentition: A Biomimetic Approach*. Berlin: Quintessence; 2002.
41. Chu S, Tarnow D, Bloom M. Diagnosis, etiology. In: Tarnow D, Chu S, Kim J, eds. *Aesthetic Restorative Dentistry Principles and Practice*. Mahwah, NJ: Montage Media; 2008:1–25.
42. Sarver DM. Principles of cosmetic dentistry in orthodontics: Part 1. Shape and proportionality of anterior teeth. *Am J Orthod Dentofacial Orthop* 2004;126(6):749–753.
43. De Araujo EM Jr, Fortkamp S, Baratieri LN. Closure of diastema and gingival recontouring using direct adhesive restorations: a case report. *J Esthet Restor Dent* 2009;21(4):229–240.
44. Tjan A, Miller G. Some esthetic factors in a smile. *J Prosthet Dent* 1984;51(1):24–28.
45. Chiche GJ, Kokich VG, Caudill R. Diagnosis and treatment planning of esthetic problems. In: *Esthetics of Anterior Fixed Prosthodontics*. Chicago, IL: Quintessence; 1994:33–52.
46. Rufenacht CR. Structural esthetic rules. In: *Fundamentals of Esthetics*. Chicago, IL: Quintessence; 1990:67–134.

47. Chu SJ, Tan JP, Stappert CFJ, Tarnow DP. Gingival zenith positions and levels of the maxillary anterior dentition. *J Esthet Restor Dent* 2009;21:113–120.
48. Dawson P. Requirements for occlusal stability. In: Dawson P, ed. *Functional Occlusion from TMJ to Smile Design*. St Louis, MO: Mosby; 2007:345–348.
49. Gurel G. Porcelain—bonded restorations and function. In: Galip G, ed. *The Science and Art of Porcelain Laminate Veneers*. New Malden: Quintessence; 2003:135–155.
50. Lacy AM. Application of composite resin for single-appointment anterior and posterior diastema closure. *Pract Periodont Aesthet Dent* 1998;10:279–286.
51. Clark D, Sarrett D, Antonson D. Preliminary report of the use of acid etch composite build-ups to treat diastemas. *Quintessence Int* 1982;13(2):147–152.
52. Haywood VB. *Tooth Whitening: Indications and Outcomes of Nightguard Vital Bleaching*. Hanover Park, IL: Quintessence; 2007.
53. Nour El-Din AK, Miller BH, Griggs JA, Wakefield C. Immediate bonding to bleached enamel. *Oper Dent* 2006;31(1):106–114.
54. Dishman MV, Covey DA, Baughan LW. The effects of peroxide bleaching on composite to enamel bond strength. *Dent Mater* 1994;10(1):33–36.
55. Gribble AR. Multiple diastema management: an interdisciplinary approach. *J Esthet Dent* 1994;6:97–102.
56. Davis NC. Smile design. *Dent Clin North Am* 2007;51(2):299–318.
57. Chu SJ, Tarnow DP, Tan JP, Stappert CFJ. Papilla proportions in the maxillary anterior dentition. *Int J Periodontics Restorative Dent* 2009;29:385–393.
58. Radz GM. Anterior esthetic bonded restorations using an improved hybrid composite. *Compend Cont Educ Dent* 1995;16:1204–1210.
59. Beun S, Glorieux T, Devaux J, et al. Characterization of nanofilled compared to universal and microfilled composites. *Dent Mater* 2007;23:51–59.
60. Mitra SB, Wu D, Holmes BN. An application of nanotechnology in advanced dental materials. *J Am Dent Assoc* 2003;134:1382–1390.
61. Webber B, McDonald A, Knowles J. An in vitro study of the compressive load at fracture of Procera AllCeram crowns with varying thickness of veneer porcelain. *J Prosthet Dent* 2003;89:154–160.
62. Fradeani M. The application of all-ceramic restorations in the anterior and posterior regions. *Pract Proced Aesthet Dent* 2003;(Suppl):13–17.
63. Heintze SD, Zappini G, Rousson V. Wear of ten dental restorative materials in five wear simulators—results of a round robin test. *Dent Mater* 2005;21:304–317.
64. Denry IL. Ceramics. In: Craig RG, Powers JM, eds. *Restorative Dental Materials*, 11th edn. St. Louis, MO: Mosby; 2002:551–574.
65. Craig RG. Ceramic–metal systems. In: Craig RG, Powers JM, eds. *Restorative Dental Materials*, 11th edn. St. Louis, MO: Mosby; 2002:575–592.
66. Ritter RG, Rego NA. Material considerations for using lithium disilicate as a thin veneer option. *J Cosmetic Dent* 2009;25:111–117.
67. Strassler HE. Minimally invasive porcelain veneers: indications for a conservative esthetic dentistry treatment modality. *Gen Dent* 2007;55(7):686–694.
68. Javaheri D. Considerations for planning esthetic treatment with veneers involving no or minimal preparation. *J Am Dent Assoc* 2007;138:331–337.
69. Rouse JS. Full veneer versus traditional veneer preparation: a discussion of interproximal extensions. *J Prosthet Dent* 1997;78:545–549.
70. Magne P, Douglas WH. Cumulative effects of successive restorative procedures on anterior crown flexure: intact versus veneered incisors. *Quintessence Int* 2000;31:5–18.
71. Magne P, Douglas WH. Design optimization and evolution of bonded ceramics for the anterior dentition: a finite-element analysis. *Quintessence Int* 1999;30:661–672.
72. Stappert CF, Ozden U, Gerds T, Strub JR. Longevity and failure load of ceramic veneers with different preparation designs after exposure to masticatory stimulation. *J Prosthet Dent* 2005;94:132–139.

Additional resources

De Araujo EM Jr, Fortkamp S, Baratieri LN. Closure of diastema and gingival recontouring using direct adhesive restorations: a case report. *J Esthet Resor Dent* 2009; 21:229–240.

Dietschi D. Optimizing smile composition and esthetics with resin composites and other conservative esthetic procedures. *Eur J Esthet Dent* 2008;3:14–74.

Fahl N Jr. A polychromatic composite layering approach for solving a complex Class IV/direct veneer-diastema combination: part I. *Pract Proced Aesthet Dent* 2006;18:641–645.

Fahl N Jr. A polychromatic composite layering approach for solving a complex Class IV/direct veneer-diastema combination: part II. *Pract Proced Aesthet Dent* 2007;19:17–22.

Frese C, Schiller P, Staehle HJ, Wolff D. Recontouring teeth and closing diastemas with direct composite buildups: a 5-year follow up. *J Dent* 2013;41:979–985.

Gurrea J. Bruguera A. Wax-up and mock-up. A guide for anterior periodontal and restorative treatments. *Int J Esthet Dent* 2014;9:146–160.

Rosales AB, Carvacho DDN, Cacciutolo RS, et al. Conservative approach for the esthetic management of multiple interdental spaces; a systemic approach. *J Esthet Restor Dent* 2015;27(6):344–354.

Wolff D, Kraus T, Schach C, et al. Recontouring teeth and closing diastemas with direct composite buildups: a clinical evaluation of survival and quality parameters. *J Dent* 2010;38:1001–1009.

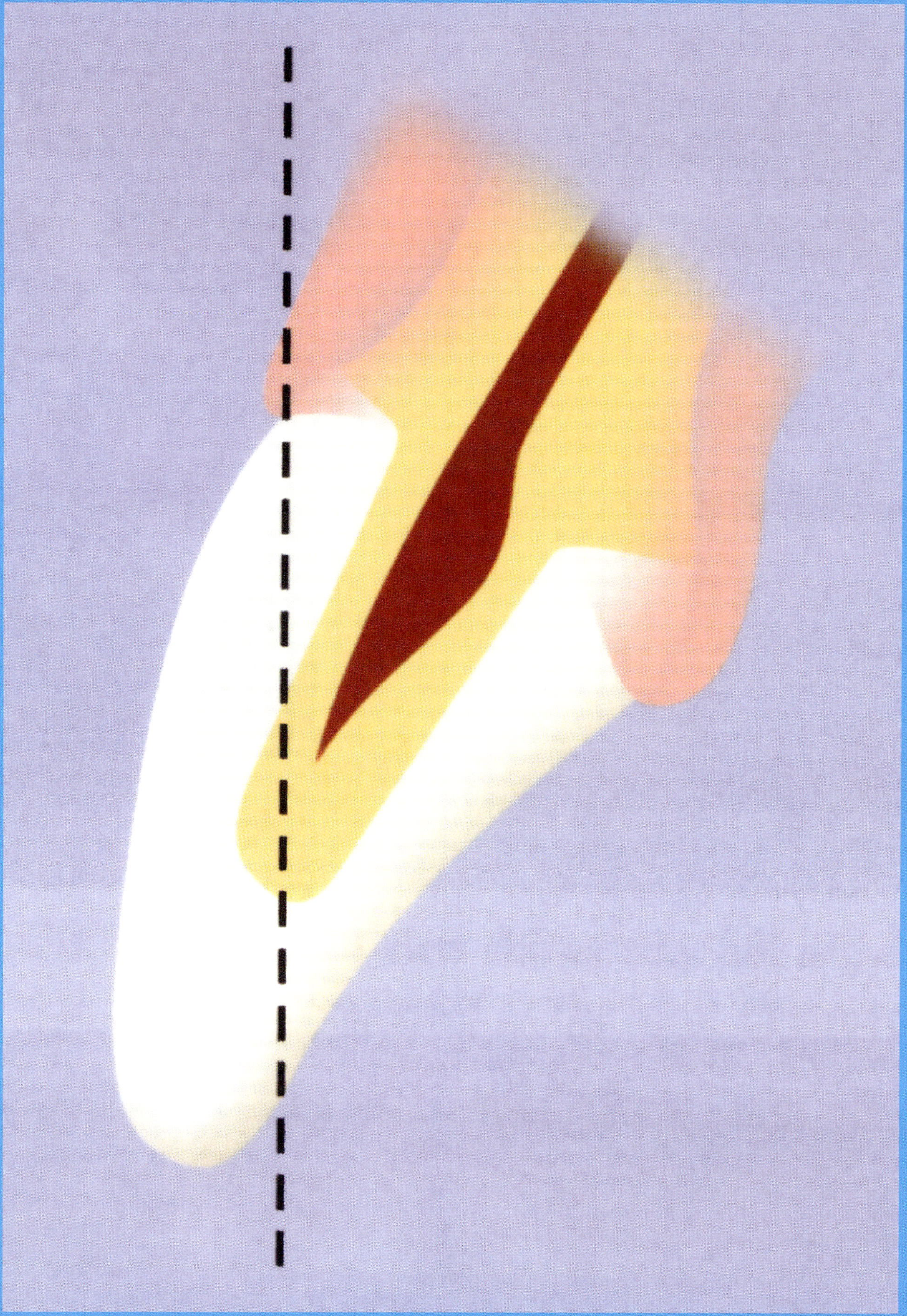

Chapter 27 Restorative Treatment of Crowded Teeth

Ronald E. Goldstein, DDS, Geoffrey W. Sheen, DDS, MS, and Steven T. Hackman, DDS

Chapter Outline

Treatment considerations	877
Arch space	878
Gingival architecture	878
Influence of root proximity	881
Smile line	881
Emergence profile and oral hygiene	881
Treatment strategy	881
Identifying the degree of esthetic correction required	881
Identifying the type of restoration required	882
Treatment options	883
Cosmetic contouring	883
Correction by disking	883
Correction by bonding	883
Correction by porcelain veneers	884
Cosmetic contouring and porcelain veneers to eliminate crowding	886
Correction by crowning	887
Crowning to eliminate crowding	888
Crowning and repositioning of mandibular anteriors	890
Unusual or rare clinical presentations	890
Malposed and misaligned teeth	890
The protruding tooth	891
The retruded tooth	891
The lingually locked tooth	891
To bond, veneer, or crown?	893

Orthodontics should be the first consideration when the patient presents with crowded teeth.[1-4] If a patient is unable to accept orthodontic solutions, the general practitioner must determine whether the patient can be treated with minor tooth movement, restorations, or extraction, or a combination of these procedures.

To analyze the treatment of crowded teeth, this chapter has been organized into the following sections: treatment considerations, treatment strategy, treatment options, and unusual or rare clinical presentations.

Treatment considerations

Many patients have slightly crowded or overlapping anterior teeth that are not an esthetic problem. However, when an individual feels their crowded teeth are unesthetic and seeks treatment, it may present a challenge for the dentist. Choosing the correct approach is the most important aspect of the treatment.[5]

Before properly developing a plan of treatment, consider a number of preoperative conditions. A thorough evaluation of the patient will establish the basis for potential treatment options.[6] The areas to be evaluated include arch space, gingival architecture, influence of root proximity, smile line, emergence profile, occlusion, and oral hygiene.

Arch space

The most significant factor in the treatment of crowded teeth is the available arch space, and how that space is occupied by the dentition. Locating space deficiencies and their degree will determine which teeth will require modification (Figure 27.1A–D).

Berliner presented a classic formulation and clinical rule in his text that helps to make treatment of crowding more predictable. He stated:[7]

> When the sum of the mesiodistal widths (at contact-point level from distal of right lateral to distal of left lateral) in any given segment measures more than the available arch space, when measured between the two points (obtained by dropping perpendicular lines from the mesial contact-point levels of the right and the left cuspids to the gingival line), the central and the lateral teeth will be buckled (displaced labially or lingually) or overlapped; conversely, when the sum of the combined mesiodistal widths of the central and the lateral teeth measure less than the available arch space (as indicated above), the involved teeth present diastemas.

This formula can aid in the correction of crowded or spaced teeth by measuring the amount to be added or subtracted for the desired objective (Figure 27.2A–C).

Gingival architecture

An often overlooked component of an esthetic smile is the gingival architecture. When there is crowding in the anterior region, certain teeth will be forced facially or lingually. In a Class II, Division 2 occlusion, for example, the maxillary lateral incisors may be positioned labially, and the gingival tissue will be forced more apically. This creates a discontinuity in the overall smile of

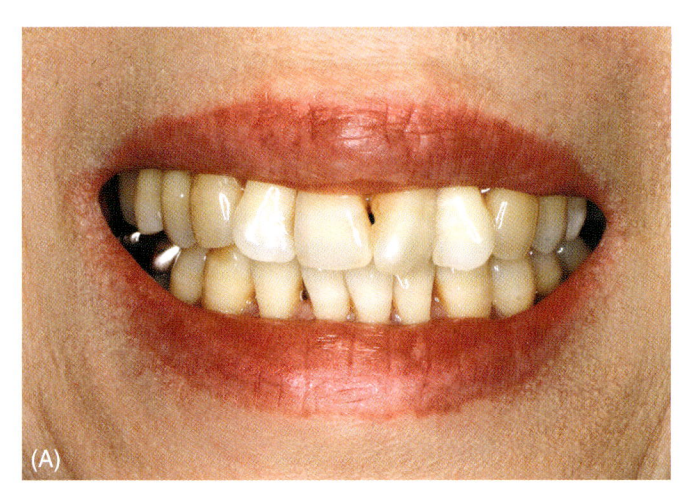

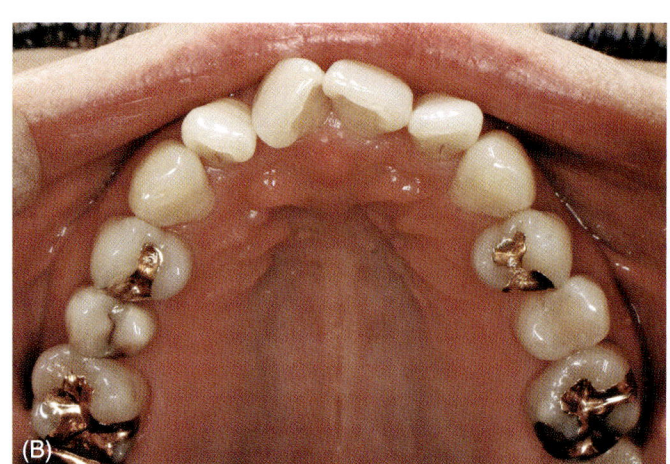

Figure 27.1 **(A, B)** This dental assistant wanted to change her smile without orthodontics or crowning. After measuring her arch space, reviewing her radiographs, plus doing mock contouring and bonding on the diagnostic casts, it was decided that direct bonding with composite resin could be a compromise solution.

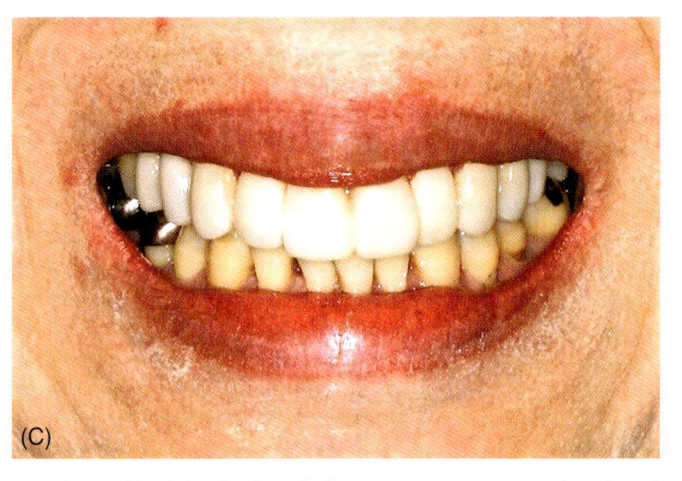

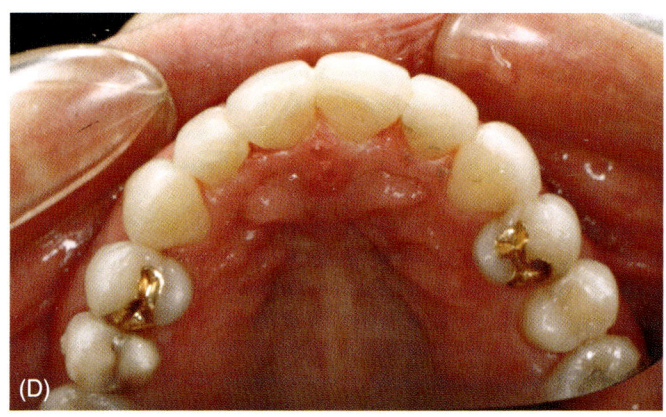

Figure 27.1 **(C, D)** The final result shows proportionate-sized teeth and a much improved smile were accomplished in a 1-day appointment. (The step-by-step procedures for this patient can be seen at http://www.dentalxp.com/video/contouring-mock-bonding-using-diagnostic-99131.aspx?locale.)

Chapter 27 Restorative Treatment of Crowded Teeth

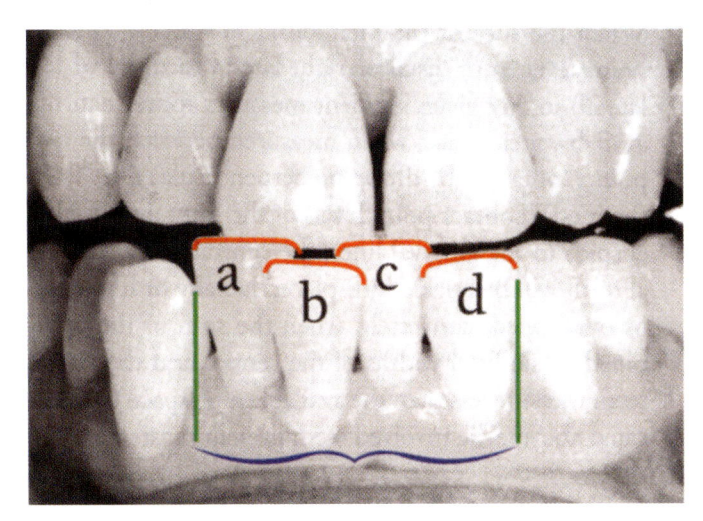

Figure 27.2 **(A)** Preoperative view: note the relationship of the combined widths of the lower central and lateral teeth (a, b, c, d) to the extent of available arch space. Sum of combined tooth widths is greater than available arch space, resulting in buckling.

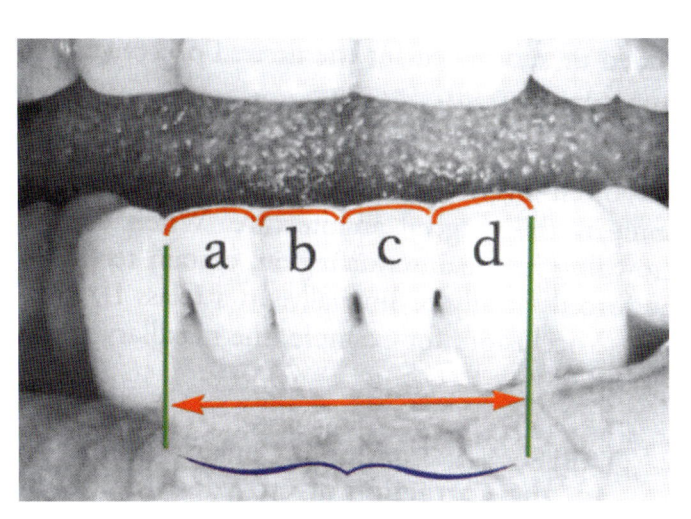

Figure 27.2 **(B)** Postoperative measurement, after remodeling of the lower central and lateral incisor teeth: the combined tooth widths equal the available arch space, and repositioning of the teeth became a feasible clinical procedure.

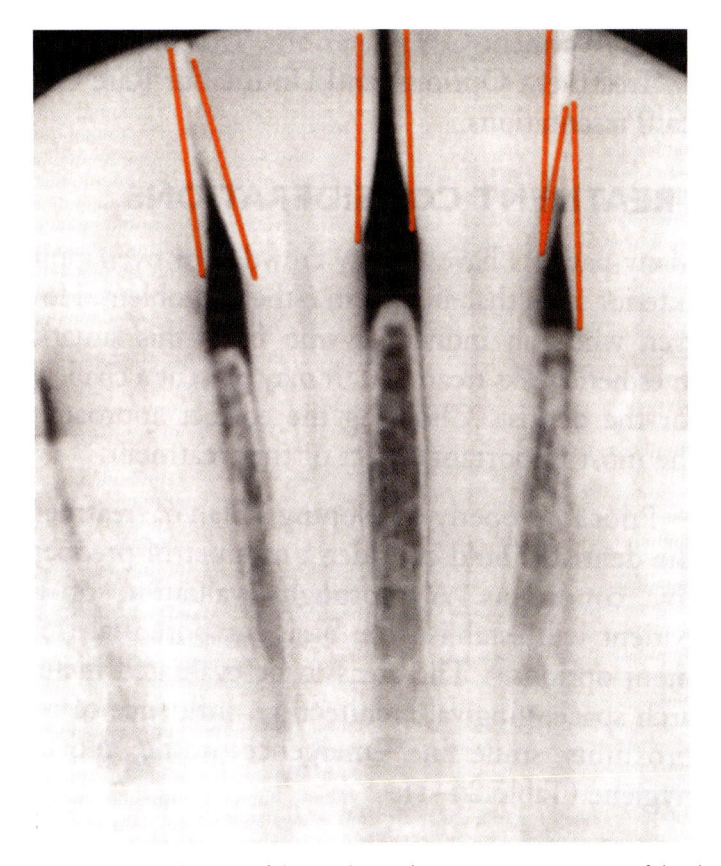

Figure 27.2 **(C)** The proximal thickness of the enamel "caps" of the teeth on a lower anterior segment of the dental arch is indicated in outline. *Source:* Reproduced with permission from Berliner.[7(p65)]

the patient. Treatment considerations in this situation may require slight modification to the gingival architecture around the central incisors to create a more harmonious smile. If the patient's lip line hides the gingival discrepancy, then surgical intervention may not be necessary (Figure 27.3A–F).

Likewise, crowding in the mandibular anterior incisors often results in the rotation or lingualization of the central or lateral incisors. Therefore, the gingival tissue will be positioned more incisally. It may be necessary to perform a crown-lengthening procedure prior to esthetic restoration of these teeth.[8,9]

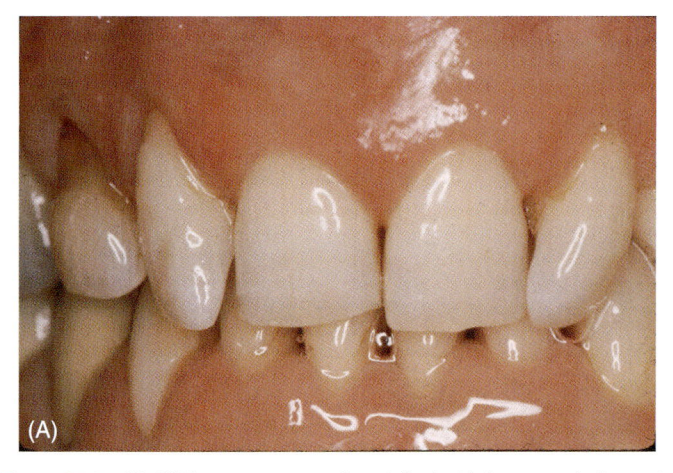

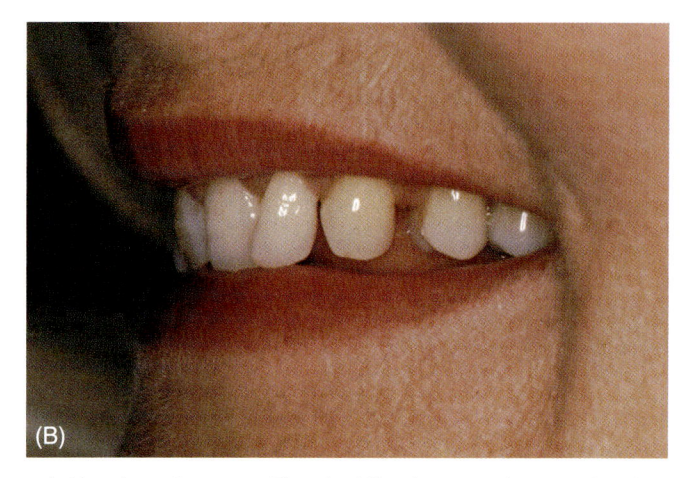

Figure 27.3 **(A, B)** This patient was dissatisfied with her crowded anterior teeth. Note how the gingival height differs between the central and lateral incisors and the maxillary right cuspid was a retained deciduous tooth.

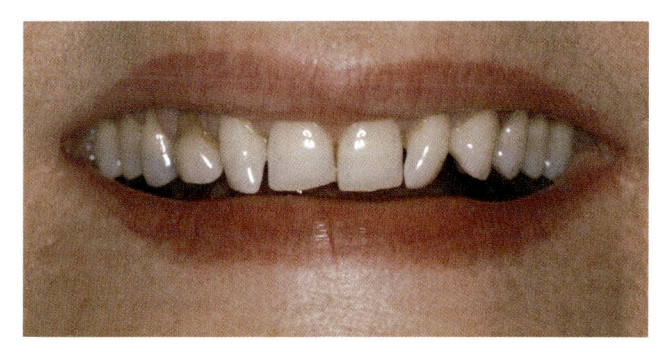

Figure 27.3 **(C)** The dissimilar gingival heights did not bother the patient because her natural smile line concealed these irregularities.

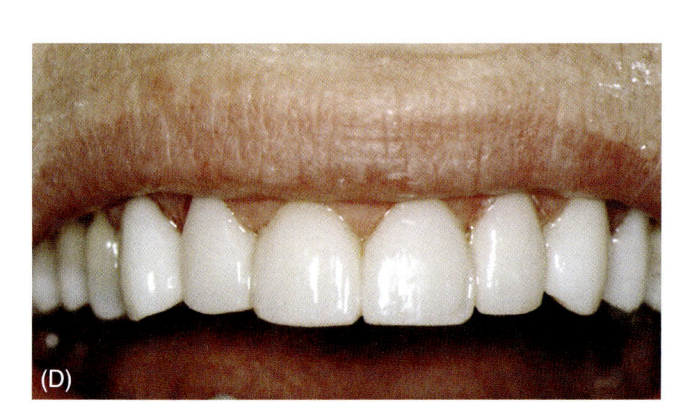

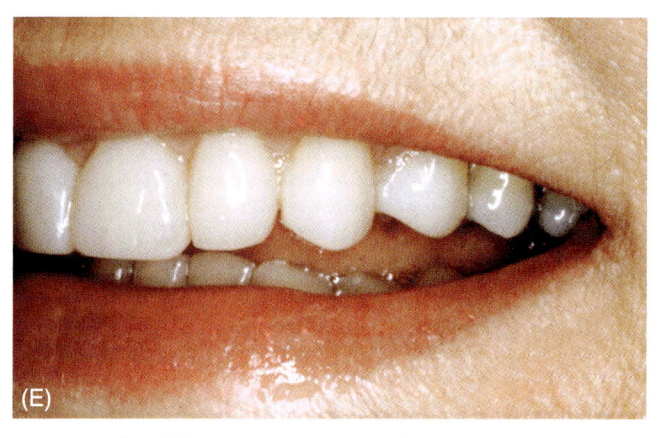

Figure 27.3 **(D, E)** After cosmetic contouring of the six anterior teeth, direct composite bonding was completed. The final result shows improved proportion in tooth size and form.

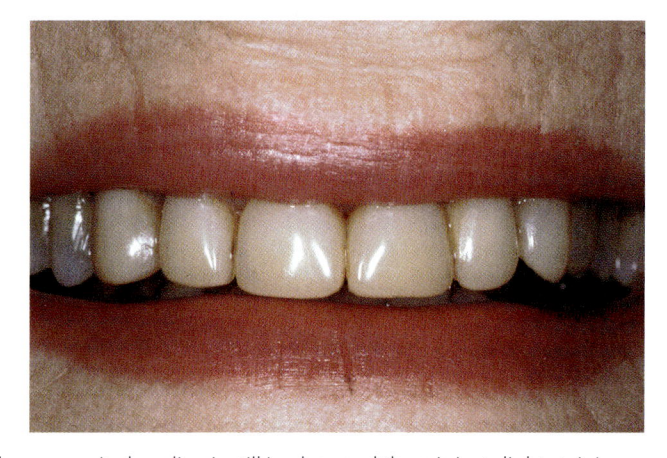

Figure 27.3 **(F)** Sixteen years later, the composite bonding is still in place and there is just slight staining.

Influence of root proximity

Root proximity may complicate the restoration of crowded mandibular anterior teeth. Root structures may be so close to one another that a separation is not possible. This creates gingival impingement that can be almost impossible to treat.

It may be necessary to extract one of the crowded teeth, leaving three incisors in place of four.[10] The decision should be based on radiographs and a study of the periodontium to determine the amount of bone present. If bone loss exists due to crowding, then extraction and repositioning are generally the treatment of choice. This can be successful when the teeth are properly proportioned. It is seldom noticeable to the patient. The tooth is extracted, and the remaining anterior teeth are repositioned, providing additional bone support. When small diastemas remain, the teeth can be bonded with composite resin or splinted to prevent further tooth movement.

In almost every case, some form of retainer is necessary. The patient should be informed that they can reduce the wearing time of the retainer only if it does not fit too tightly each time it is placed. A tight fit might indicate some relapse, and the retainer should continue to be worn each night. The patient can also return for possible further treatment either to surgically relax retentive gingival fibers or to adjust the occlusion to help equilibrate the stressful occlusal forces. But failure to wear the retainer can result in relapse.

Smile line

It is important to study the patient's smile line. The extent to which incisogingival tooth structure will show in the widest smile and in other expressions should be noted. If the patients cervical margins show during the widest smiles, the treatment of choice should be an all-ceramic crown with shoulder or deep chamfer margins. If there are occlusal demands for the strongest restoration possible, choose a zirconia crown. If occlusion is not a problem, a lesser strength all-ceramic crown or other esthetic restoration, such as bonding or porcelain veneer, should be considered.[11]

Emergence profile and oral hygiene

Many of the nonorthodontic treatment options discussed in this chapter are meant to "camouflage" malposed or malaligned teeth. Consideration must be given to the contours that will be created by the restorative process.[12–14] Often, these contours are unnatural and create areas around the teeth that the patient will find difficult to maintain with good oral hygiene. If these esthetic restorations are to survive, consider the final contours being created, and the patient must be given the necessary instructions to maintain them.

Treatment strategy

Development of an appropriate treatment plan for the correction of crowded teeth should follow a strategy. First, it is necessary to identify what type of correction and how much correction of tooth contours are required to achieve the desired esthetic results.[4,15] Then, it becomes necessary to evaluate the dentition, identify clinical limitations to treatment, and select appropriate restorative options that will accomplish the desired esthetic outcome.

Identifying the degree of esthetic correction required

Following a process of evaluation and development of a problem list, utilize this information to determine the degree of corrections required. Esthetic computer imaging can assist both you and the patient to visualize the proposed treatment.[16,17] The development of a diagnostic wax-up is a necessary procedure and may be used to confirm the viability of the proposed treatment developed by computer imaging. It will also enable you to perform a trial smile so the patient can see your proposed treatment plan.

Two sets of diagnostic casts should be made. One set will serve as a historical record of the patient's preoperative condition and should never be modified. The second set of casts should be used for the diagnostic wax-up.

Developing a diagnostic wax-up involves both the addition of wax to deficient areas of the dentition and the removal of stone as necessary to achieve the desired esthetic results. The diagnostic wax-up should be accomplished with attention to detail. Line angles, embrasure spaces, incisal lengths, and gingival contours must represent the desired results if this effort is to be an effective tool in the esthetic treatment plan.[18] Through this process, arch space deficiencies can be worked out, and specific modifications to each tooth involved can be identified.

Once completed, the diagnostic wax-up is used to develop additional clinical aids for the accurate and successful completion of the esthetic treatment plan. Polyvinyl siloxane material is applied to the palate, lingual surface, and incisal edge of the wax-up to form a simple reduction guide. After the material has set, the matrix is carefully trimmed just to the facioincisal line angle. During preparation, the matrix is placed against the lingual surfaces of the teeth (the palatal coverage stabilizes the matrix). The desired incisal length and position of the facial surface (as developed in the diagnostic wax-up) can be identified, and adequate tooth reduction can be determined.

A provisional matrix can also be fabricated by using the same materials and technique. In addition to the palate, lingual surfaces, and incisal edges, the interocclusal record material also covers the facial surfaces and extends several millimeters onto the gingival tissue. The matrix formed will accurately duplicate the subtleties of the diagnostic wax-up. With proper embrasure form and gingival contours accurately duplicated in the provisional restorations, chairside adjustment will be significantly reduced.

A well-planned and executed diagnostic wax-up is an essential communication tool for both the patient and the laboratory.[19–21] Dental esthetics is truly in the eyes of the beholder. Everyone has a certain concept of how the teeth should look. Since provisional restorations are closely fabricated to the contours of the diagnostic wax-up,[22] the patient will have a chance to observe and identify any changes in contour and function they may desire. If necessary, changes can be made in the provisional restorations, and an impression of these newly contoured restorations can be made. The new cast will serve as a clinically evaluated diagnostic tool used to communicate this vital information to the laboratory.

In summary, a diagnostic wax-up will identify to what degree corrective contours must be made to idealize a crowded dentition. With knowledge of the specific modifications required for each tooth, you can begin to select the proper treatment options.[23] This process should be undertaken whether the treatment is minor cosmetic contouring or as comprehensive as a complete restoration of the anterior region with full-coverage crowns.

Identifying the type of restoration required

There are many treatment options available for correcting crowded teeth,[24–27] including cosmetic contouring, bonding, porcelain veneers, and crowns (Table 27.1). The condition of the existing dentition is a factor in determining which restorative option is ideal.

Teeth without any restorations or caries should be treated as conservatively as possible. If only minor modifications to tooth contours are required to achieve the desired esthetic result, cosmetic contouring and bonding provide the least invasive treatment options. Small existing restorations are easily incorporated into other restorative treatments.

If caries in the teeth to be treated are too large for composite resin, then more extensive restorations, such as porcelain veneers or crowns, need to be considered. The size and location of the caries may dictate the design of these restorations.

The presence of an endodontically treated tooth,[28] with or without a post and core, may or may not require a crown. In the crowded tooth scenario, a full crown may be beneficial to create a more esthetic arrangement in the anterior region. Care must be taken, however, not to overextend or overcontour the final restoration, which would result in possible gingival irritation.

In summary, conservative treatments such as esthetic contouring,[29] disking combined with minor tooth movement, and bonding are available for minor corrections of crowded teeth.

Table 27.1 Treatment Options and Indications for the Correction of Crowded Teeth

Procedure	Indications	Contraindications	Sequence	Criteria
Disking and orthodontics	Usually the first and best option for redistribution of significantly crowded teeth in the anterior region Disking used to slightly modify the width of specific teeth to reposition them into the dental arch	Inadequate supporting structures–bone, tooth roots, or gingival tissue When immediate solutions are demanded by the patient	Study model analysis of available arch space and tooth size Orthodontic consult to reposition teeth into desired final position	
Cosmetic contouring	Modification of line angles, incisal edges, or defects to create illusions of proper tooth size, shape, or position Minimal alteration of tooth position	If contouring would expose dentin If contouring would eliminate desirable occlusal or functional contacts	Following determination of the desired results by diagnostic wax-up	<0.5 mm of facial reduction <1.0 mm of incisal reduction
Bonding	Addition of composite resin to modify apparent height and width of natural tooth by alteration of the shape and location of line angles Diastema closure Incisal edge modification of sound tooth structure	Inadequate enamel or supporting tooth structure Severe occlusal loads placed on composite restoration Severe tooth discoloration	Following color modification (bleaching, etc.) of natural tooth structure Following diagnostic wax-up to determine need for preoperative cosmetic contouring	<1.0 mm addition of composite resin
Porcelain veneers	Indicated for esthetic rehabilitation of entire anterior segments Individual teeth must be structurally sound Changes can be additive, subtractive, or both Shape/size, alignment, and color of the teeth may be modified	Weak supporting tooth structure Multiple, large existing restorations Minimal bondable tooth structure Bruxism	Following diagnostic wax-up to determine need for preoperative esthetic contouring	0.5 mm of reduction possible within enamel <25% exposed dentin 2 mm maximum thickness of porcelain
All-ceramic crowns	Indicated for structurally weak teeth with large multiple restorations or when a more conservative restoration is contraindicated A favorable occlusal scheme should exist (canine guidance) Compatible opposing dentition or restorations	Unfavorable occlusal scheme Significant vertical overlap with minimal occlusal clearance When a more conservative restoration is indicated to achieve desired esthetic results	Following diagnostic wax-up to clearly define esthetic and functional objectives Following proper buildup procedures	1.0 mm marginal reduction Uniform, circumferential 90° shoulder margin 2 mm incisal reduction

When corrections that are more substantial are required, porcelain veneers and crowns become the treatment of choice.[12]

Treatment options

Cosmetic contouring

Certainly, the most economic and simplest of treatments to improve crowded teeth is through cosmetic contouring. This one appointment procedure can make a dramatic difference to the smile in most patients who may not have the funds for either the more time consuming procedure such as orthodontic treatment or either bonding or porcelain veneers (see Chapter 11).

Although cosmetic contouring by itself can make a major difference (Figure 27.4A and B), it can also help make the difference between ordinary and extraordinary results when other restorative procedures are included. Thus, this chapter will include results featuring bonding, veneering, and crowning with help from cosmetic contouring techniques.

Correction by disking

If the evaluation of arch space, as previously described by Berliner,[7] shows that the combined addition of a, b, c, and d in the lower arch equals 21 mm (see Figure 27.2A) but the available space is 20 mm, the amount of crowding is 1 mm. Therefore, if minor movement or repositioning is attempted to realign the teeth, 1 mm of combined mesiodistal width can be sacrificed through disking. However, not all of the tooth surface will have to be lost from the central and lateral incisors. The mesial surfaces of the cuspids are also available and, under certain rare conditions, the distal surfaces of cuspids as well.

One limitation on reducing tooth structure through disking is the thickness of enamel on the teeth. Radiographs must be accurate enough to measure the available enamel. A measurement can be made of the proximal surfaces on each of the anterior teeth to predict the maximum reduction possible without perforating the dentin.

For example, if 0.25 mm is found to be the amount that can be reduced per proximal surface, then 0.5 mm can be reduced per tooth. Therefore, 3.0 mm could theoretically be reduced from the six anterior teeth by disking to increase the available arch space. In applying this to the earlier example of 1 mm crowding, there should be no repositioning problem.

The procedure for applying the aforementioned principle is as follows:

1. Measure the mesiodistal width of the individual teeth and the available arch space with a dental dial caliper (Erskine).
2. Measure the enamel thickness by studying the radiographs of the involved anterior teeth (see Figure 27.2C). Peck and Peck caution that accessing enamel thickness from radiographs alone is subject to possible distortion.[30] Instead, they offer an arbitrary, but safe, guideline of 50% of the mesiodistal enamel thickness as the maximum limit of reproximation.
3. After determining that the amount of space necessary to realign the teeth is attainable without perforating dentin, disk the teeth accordingly. This can be done at one time, if the space is minimal, or over a period of time, depending on the conditions present. The patient can be instructed to return weekly or biweekly for stripping. Diamond separating strips should be used. If the teeth are extremely tight, use a diamond separator disk or mini strip first for ease in initial disking. If considerable space is necessary, consider using coarser strips which have a diamond abrasive on each side or an ET3, ET4, or 30 μm diamond bur (Brasseler, USA).
4. Repositioning can now be accomplished by any of several different methods shown in Chapter 28.

Correction by bonding

The success of composite resin bonding has made immediate restorative correction of crowded teeth possible.[31,32] In most cases, it will be necessary to combine the treatments of composite resin bonding with esthetic contouring (see Chapter 11) to

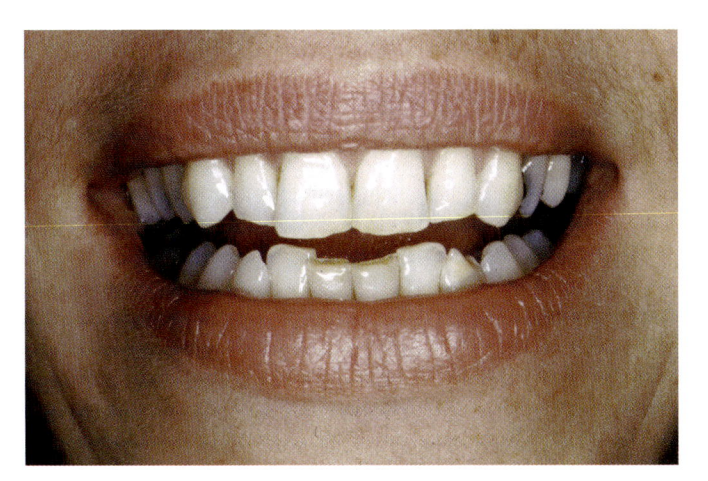

Figure 27.4 **(A)** This patient wanted to improve her smile as economically as possible, so cosmetic contouring was selected as the treatment of choice.

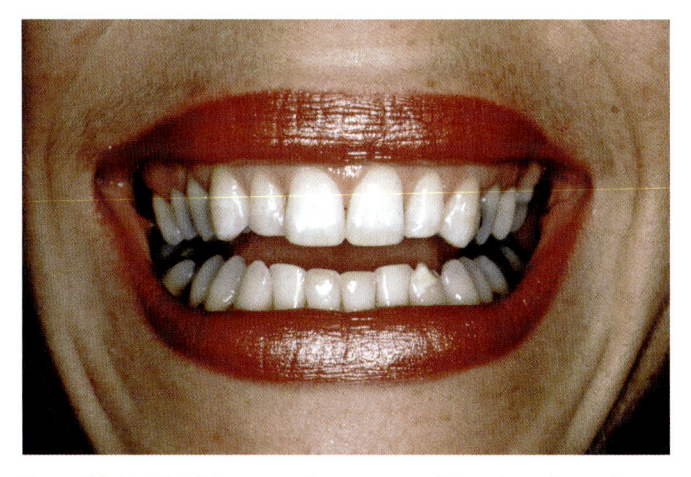

Figure 27.4 **(B)** A 1 hour appointment was all it took to please the patient with her new improved smile.

produce the greatest effect. As with all bonding techniques, the patient must be apprised of not only the esthetic life expectancy and limitations of the bonded restoration, but also an estimate of how much maintenance may be required.

In cases of severe crowding, it is always best to take diagnostic models and actually perform the proposed procedure before telling the patient you think you can do it. This way you can also show the patient what the "after" will look like.

The combination of cosmetic contouring and composite resin bonding is one of the most economical treatments to transform the smile in a single appointment (Figure 27.5A–G). However, when space is a problem, you do need to let your patient see how much narrower each tooth will be and how it may change their perception of what is envisioned. One major advantage of first doing direct bonding is that the patient can see a dramatic change. Later, the patient can always opt for a ceramic alternative.

Correction by porcelain veneers

The advantage in selecting porcelain veneers to correct crowded teeth is the ability for the laboratory to properly proportion the new restorations. This permits a conservative solution to be used that will need less maintenance.[12,33]

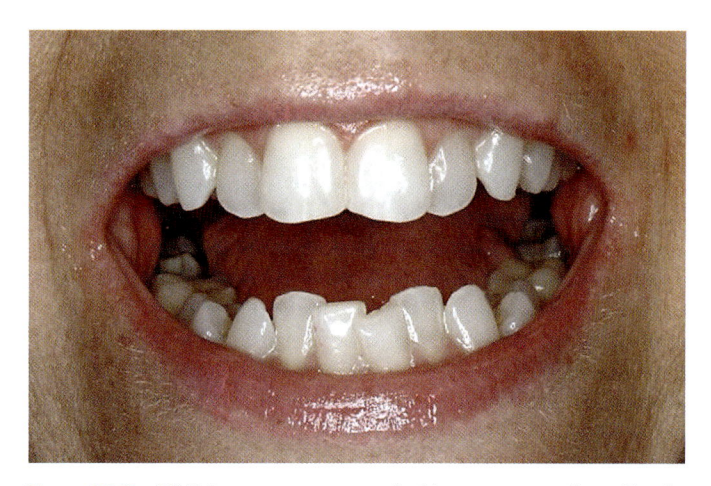

Figure 27.5 **(A)** This woman presented with severe crowding of both maxillary and mandibular arches, but refused orthodontic treatment, even with Invisalign. Diagnostic casts were made and the proposed treatment was performed on the models to see if the patient could be pleased with the result.

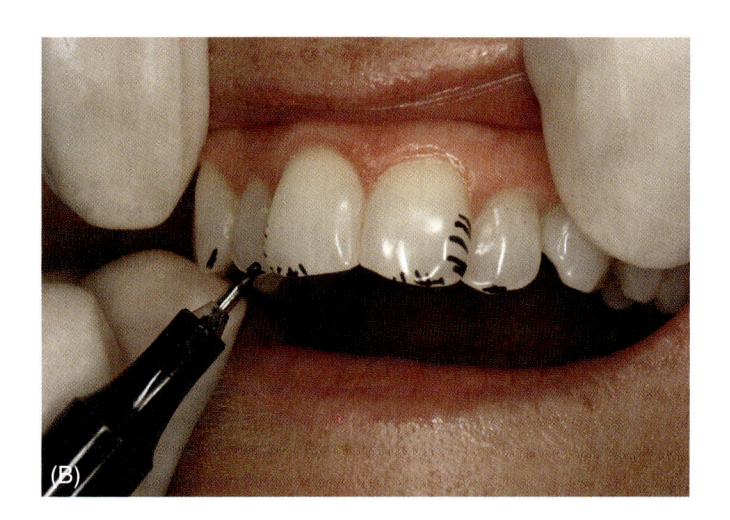

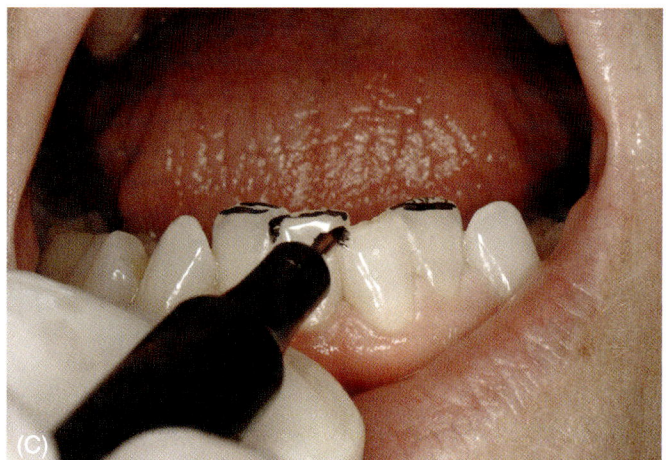

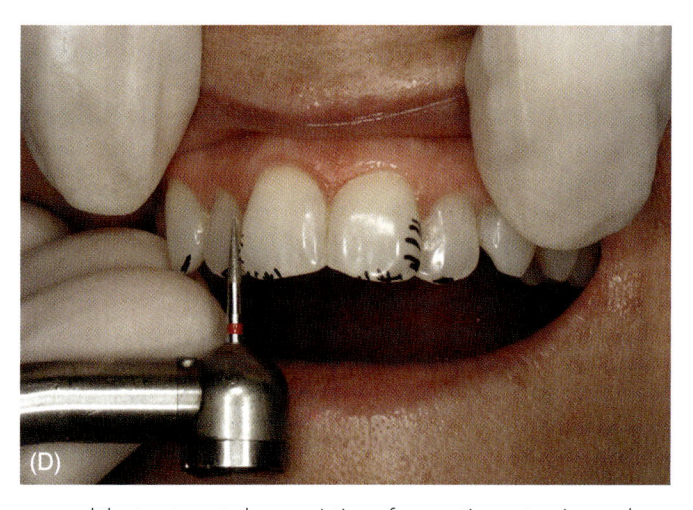

Figure 27.5 **(B–D)** After the patient approved the treatment plan consisting of cosmetic contouring and composite resin bonding, the teeth were marked with an alcohol marker and contoured using a 30 μm diamond (ET6, Brasseler USA).

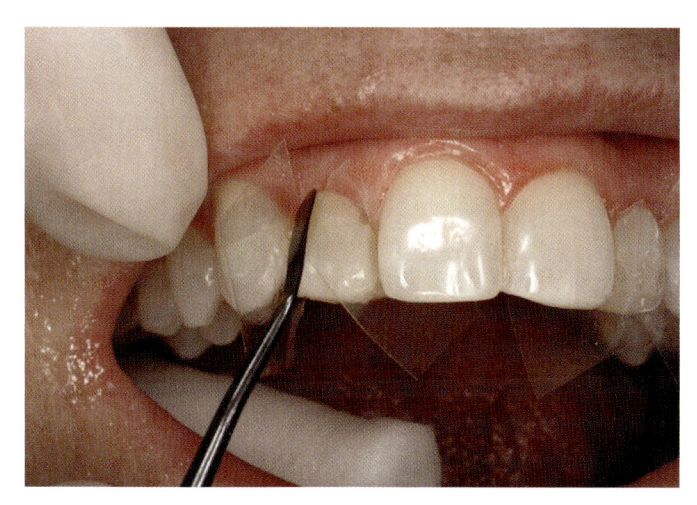

Figure 27.5 **(E)** Next, the left and right maxillary lateral incisors and lower central and laterals were bonded with a microfill composite resin using an extra-thin nonstick bonding instrument (TNCIGFT3, Hu-Friedy).

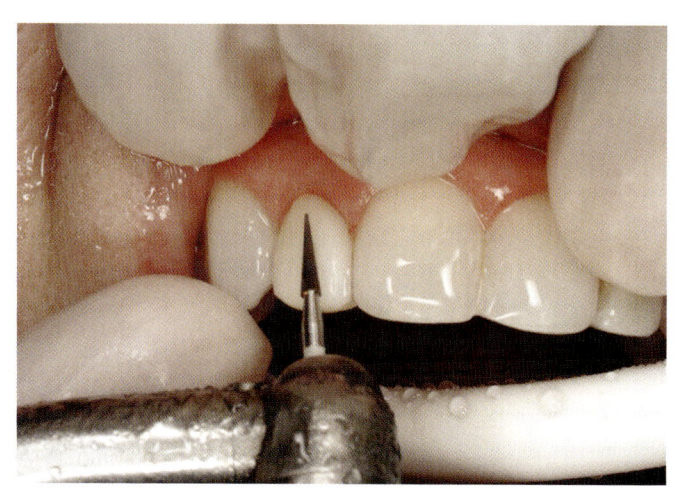

Figure 27.5 **(F)** Next, the final contour was done using a 30 blade carbide (ET6UF, Brasseler USA).

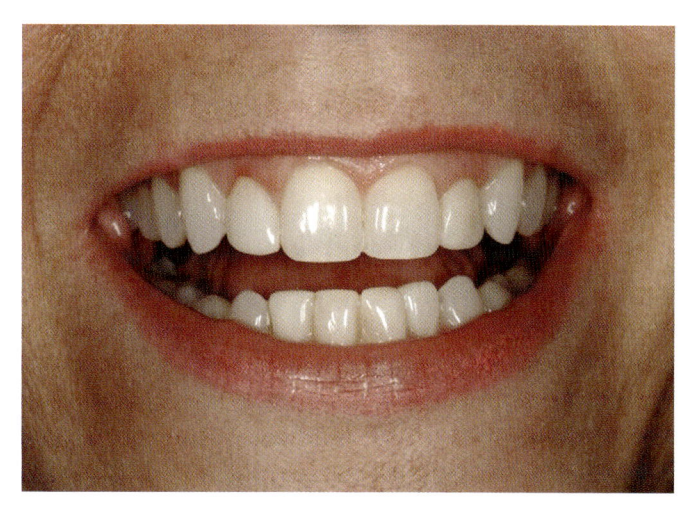

Figure 27.5 **(G)** The patient was happy with a much improved smile.

When selecting porcelain veneers, determine arch space deficiencies on each side. Both lateral incisors may be rotated in a similar fashion, resulting in an equal amount of space on both sides of the arch. However, if one lateral is overlapped more than the other, the available space may be asymmetric. Correction may require shifting of line angles in the final restorations to create an illusion of equal dimension in the final restorations.

After reproportioning the anterior space, if the total space will result in teeth that would look much too narrow, building out the teeth in a slight labioversion should be considered. The more the buccal surface is positioned anteriorly, the wider the teeth will become. The added thickness will go unnoticed if it occurs throughout the restored teeth and results in an entire arc that is positioned labially from bicuspid to bicuspid. A curve that will look good from an occlusal and a labial view should be selected. It is usually possible to compromise by building out the other teeth slightly and lingualizing the most labially positioned teeth. How much and where the existing teeth will need reducing during the preparation of the teeth should be determined. This is easily accomplished by using a reduction matrix fabricated from a diagnostic wax-up.

Usually, the most severe reduction would resemble a similar amount of dentin loss as in a full crown. Even if a tooth will have to be severely prepared for a veneer, the total tooth structure removed would be much less with a veneer preparation than for a crown preparation. The worst scenario would be to require endodontic therapy by doing a vital extirpation of the pulp. If you are considering building out the teeth you must consider any possible effect this action will have on the smile line. Will this result make the patient too "toothy"? Also consider any possible change in tooth shade the patient may want. A lighter tooth tends to make the teeth appear to stand out even more. Of major importance is to always let the patient see and understand how their tooth sizes will change with your treatment plan.

The following sections give examples of the use of porcelain veneers to correct crowding in the anterior region.

Cosmetic contouring and porcelain veneers to eliminate crowding

Case study 27.1

Problem

Figure shows a 58-year-old housewife with concerns about her eroded, crowded, and stained front teeth. Measurement with a dental dial caliper (Erskine) helped to accurately determine available space for reproportioning tooth size. Although orthodontics was mentioned as a first step to an ideal solution, the patient preferred to accept a compromise treatment of porcelain veneers and cosmetic contouring. Although crowding was less of a concern to the patient, she nevertheless decided to have straighter-looking teeth through a compromise treatment of porcelain veneers that would also esthetically correct the erosion and discoloration.

Treatment

Figure 27.6D shows the areas that will be esthetically contoured. Following contouring to reproportion spaces, Figure 27.6E demonstrates the gingival chamfer margin being placed with a two-grit LVS diamond bur (Brasseler USA). The occlusal view (Figure 27.6C) reveals just how much overlapping existed. Figure 27.6F shows the teeth after esthetic contouring and tooth preparation have occurred, and also how defective amalgam restorations were removed and glass ionomer bases were placed. Figure 27.6G shows finished veneers in place. Note the newly proportioned, straighter, and lighter-looking teeth. The final occlusal view also shows a new arch created by the veneers, building out teeth #9 and #10 and the new posterior veneer onlays on the upper right side.

Result

Before and after smiles can be seen by comparing Figure 27.6A and H. Cosmetic contouring has also improved the alignment of the lower anteriors. Constructing the porcelain veneers indirectly allows the laboratory to better proportion the tooth size.

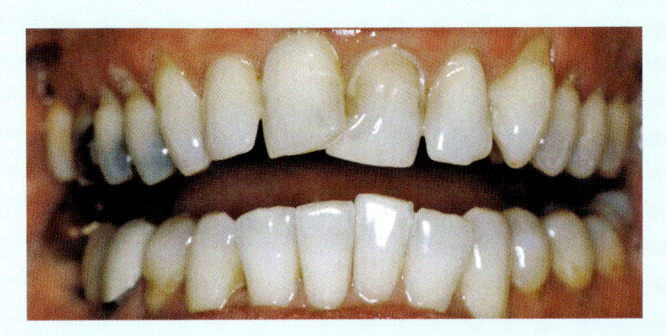

Figure 27.6 (A) This 58-year-old woman was dissatisfied with her crowded, eroded, and discolored teeth.

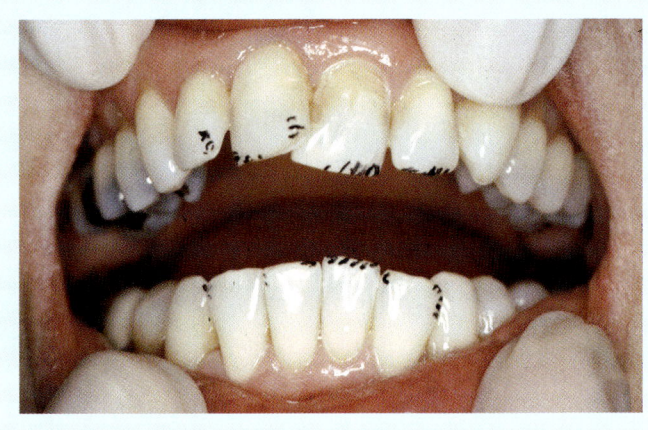

Figure 27.6 (B) The teeth are first esthetically contoured to begin creating the illusion of straighter teeth.

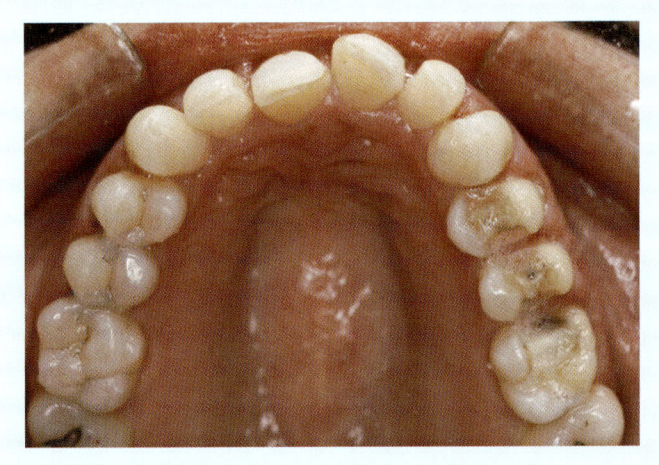

Figure 27.6 (C) This occlusal view shows the final tooth contouring. Note the patient's right posterior quadrant. The teeth were prepared for combination laminate/onlays.

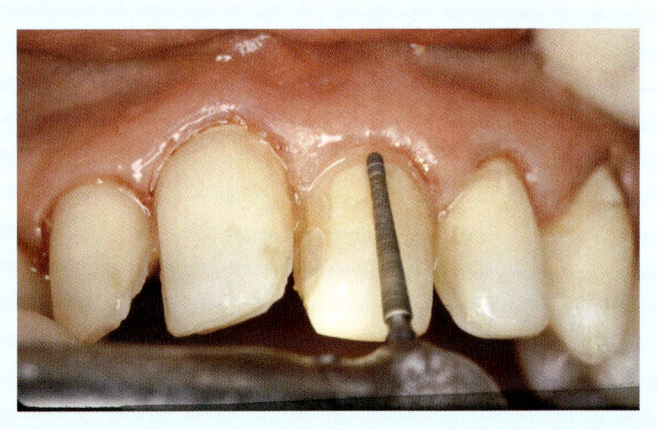

Figure 27.6 (D) Next, the anterior teeth are prepared for porcelain veneers. A special two-grit diamond bur (LVS2, Brasseler USA) helps prepare both the body and margin of the tooth.

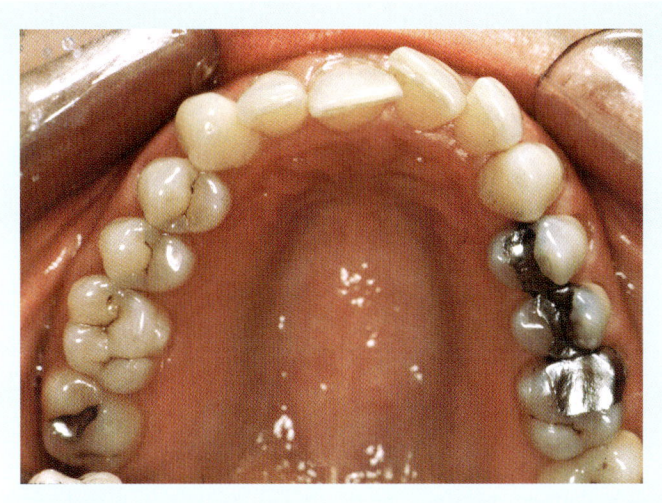

Figure 27.6 **(E)** The occlusal view shows the extent of overlapping in the central incisors.

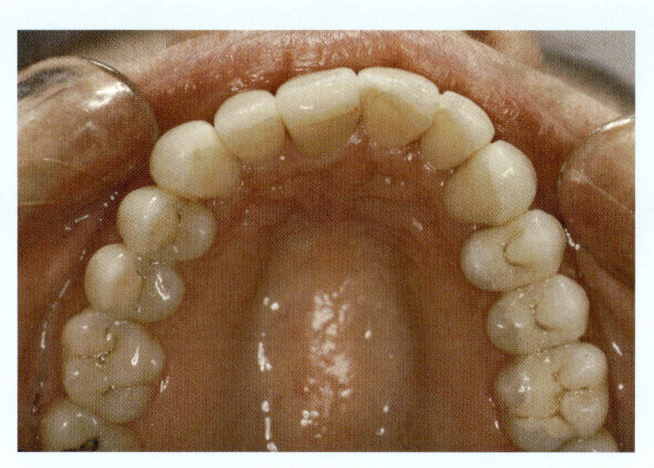

Figure 27.6 **(F)** Porcelain veneers were cemented from the right cuspid to the left second bicuspid; the laminate onlays were inserted on the maxillary right bicuspids and first molar.

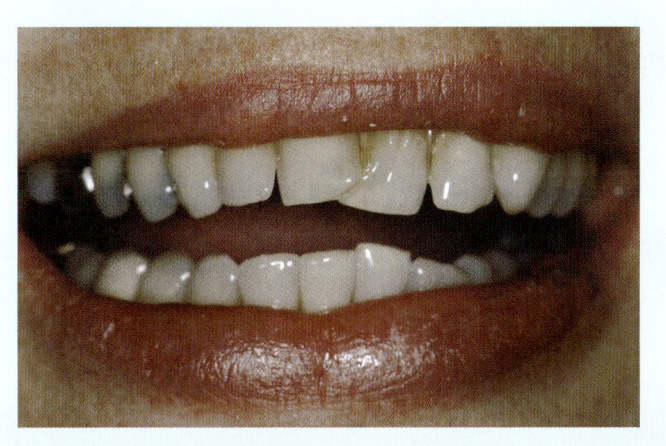

Figure 27.6 **(G)** Preoperative smile view.

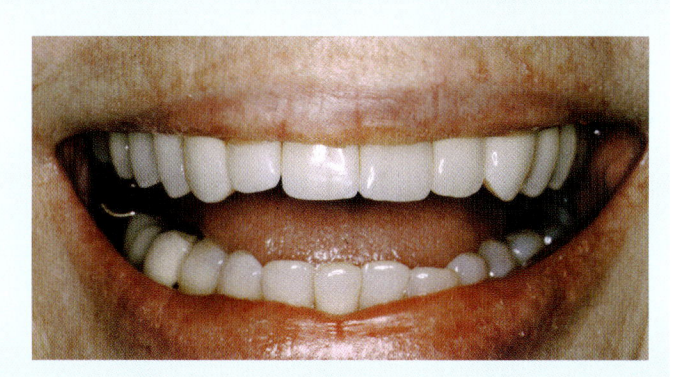

Figure 27.6 **(H)** Postoperative view of improved smile created by use of porcelain veneers and cosmetic contouring.

Correction by crowning

As in bonding, the first problem in restoring crowded teeth by crowning is tooth size. Each tooth needs to be or appear to be proportional. The more teeth that are crowned, the less distortion there is.[34–36] This means that if only one or two teeth are crowned, there may be a noticeable difference between the crowned teeth (which would be smaller) and the natural ones, depending on the space involved. However, it is possible to accomplish this by carefully shaping both the tooth to be crowned and the adjacent teeth to appear harmonious in size.

An alternative solution is to reshape the existing teeth.[37] For example, in a maxillary anterior crowded condition, instead of merely crowning two central incisors, the lateral incisors can be reshaped by reducing the mesial surface slightly, so that the adjacent central incisors can be enlarged. This same principle can be applied to other areas of the mouth. The teeth adjacent to crowns are always reduced to recover some of the space lost because of crowding. The more the adjacent teeth are reduced, the less noticeable is the distortion. An example of crowning six incisors to eliminate the crowding of anteriors follows.

Crowning to eliminate crowding

Case study 27.2

Problem

Figure 27.7A and B shows a 38-year-old store owner who presented with crowded and discolored maxillary and mandibular teeth. Although orthodontic treatment was suggested as ideal treatment, he elected a compromise that consisted of bonding the mandibular and crowning the maxillary teeth.

Treatment

When teeth are as crowded as this, it is sometimes necessary to do a vital pulp extirpation to prepare the teeth for adequate porcelain thickness. Thus, tooth preparation and diagnostic wax-up were first completed on the study casts (Figure 27.7C and D). The patient was fully informed of the possibility of endodontic therapy. The actual tooth preparation can be seen in Figure 27.7E and F. Fortunately, the pulp had receded, so extirpation was not necessary. Electrosurgery was completed prior to impressions to improve access to the preparation margins. Six full porcelain crowns restored the esthetics of the maxillary arch (Figure 27.7G), whereas composite resin bonding helped restore mandibular esthetics. A maxillary occlusal night appliance was constructed for the patient to wear since the patient had a history of clenching while sleeping.

Result

The resulting smile with straighter and lighter teeth (Figure 24.7H and I) was most appreciated by the patient. In fact, at the next postoperative appointment I noticed he had shaved off his facial hair. When I asked why, he told me he felt he did not have to hide his "crooked tooth smile" any longer.

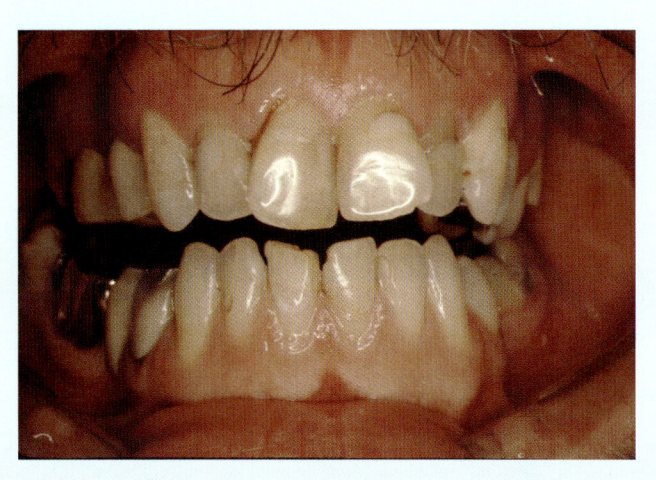

Figure 27.7 (A) This 38-year-old man wanted to improve his crowded maxillary and mandibular teeth.

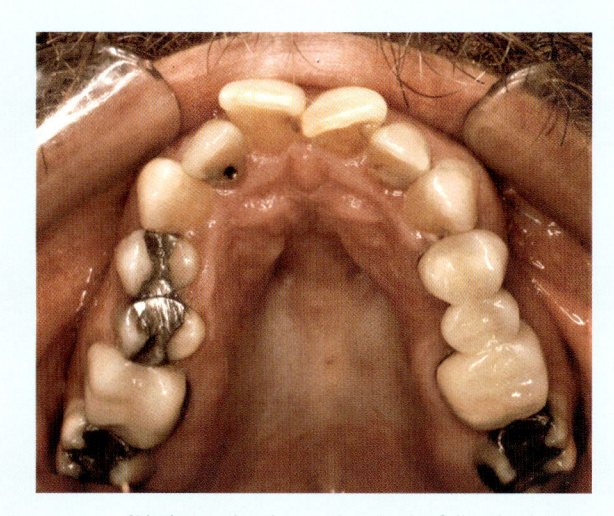

Figure 27.7 (B) This occlusal view shows why full orthodontic treatment was originally presented as the ideal treatment. The patient insisted on a "quick fix" solution.

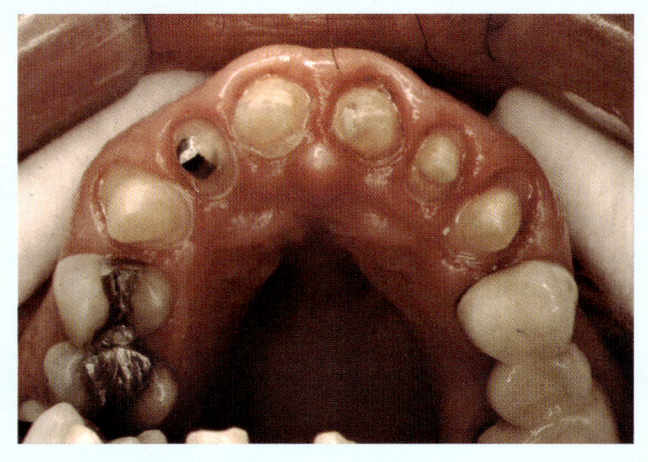

Figure 27.7 (C) The occlusal view shows the patient ready for impressions after electrosurgery for effective tissue displacement.

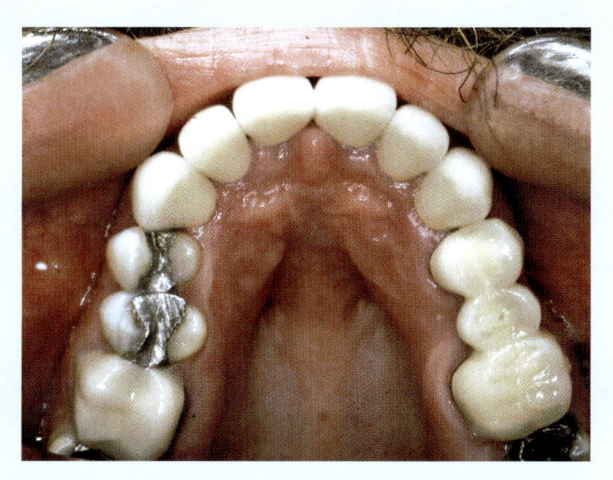

Figure 27.7 (D) The final six crowns show improved proportion and symmetry in the arch.

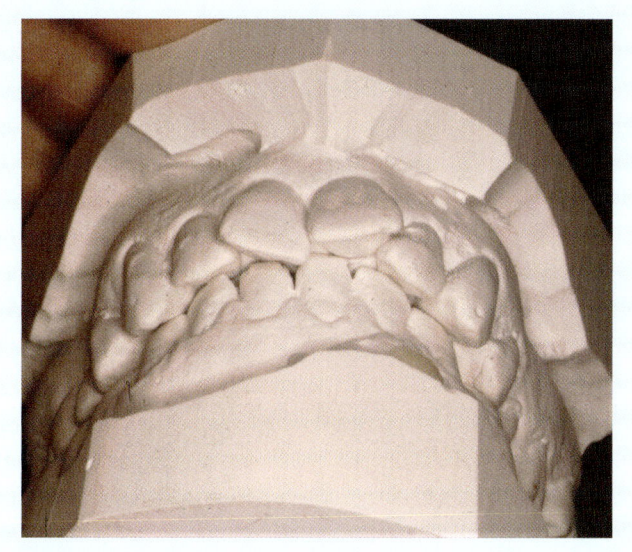

Chapter 27 Restorative Treatment of Crowded Teeth

Figure 27.7 **(E)** Diagnostic casts show the extent of crowding in the maxillary anterior teeth.

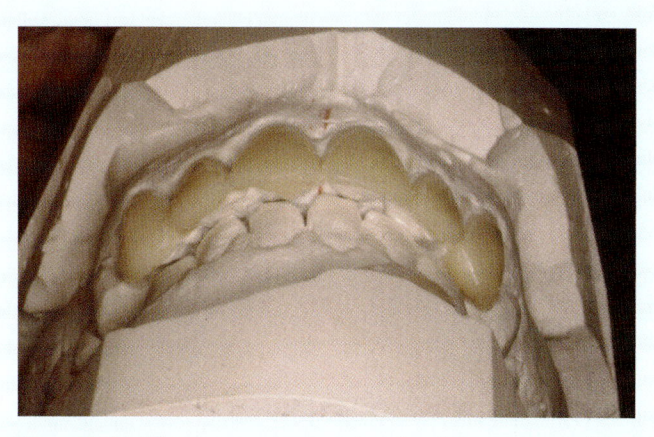

Figure 27.7 **(F)** A wax-up was completed to demonstrate to the patient and dental team how crowns could be used to accomplish the esthetic goal.

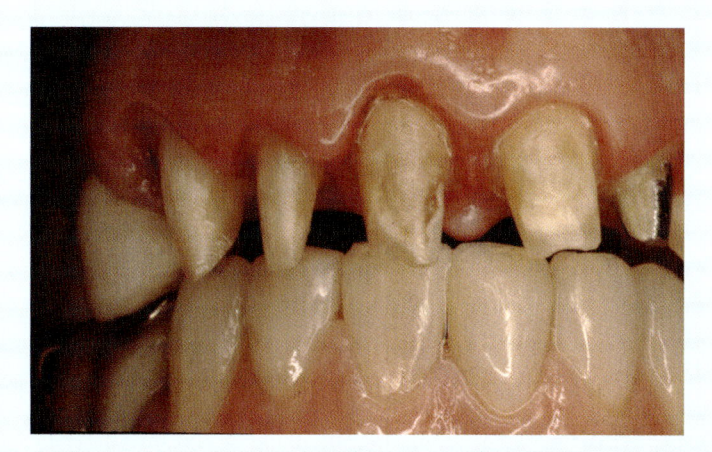

Figure 27.7 **(G)** Although the patient was warned that endodontic therapy might be necessary on the maxillary incisors, the teeth were prepared without pulpal exposures.

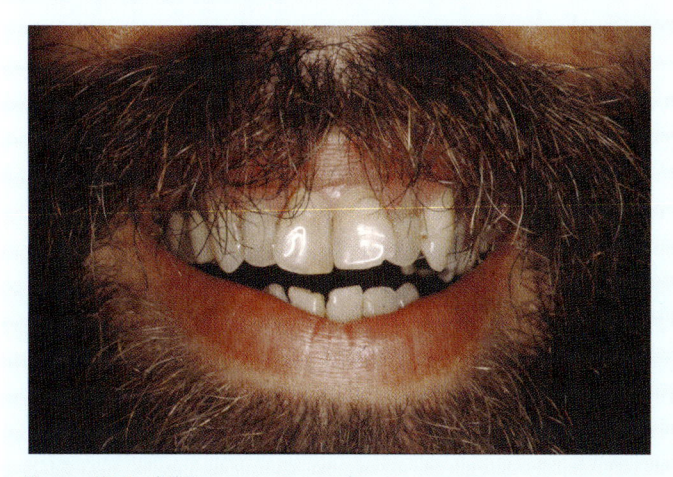

Figure 27.7 **(H)** Pretreatment smile.

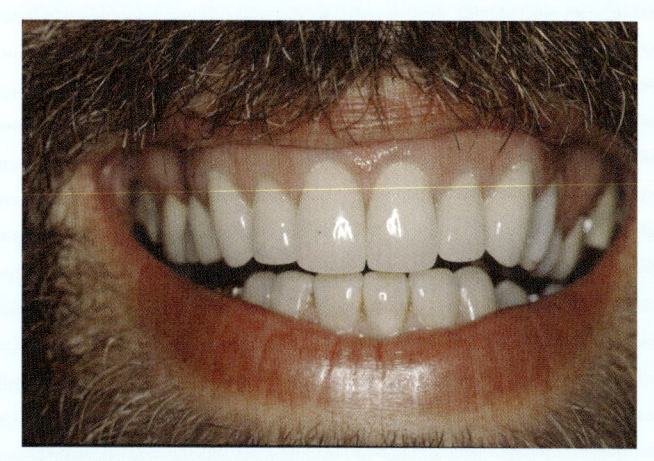

Figure 27.7 **(I)** Posttreatment smile with six maxillary full porcelain crowns and four mandibular incisors with bonded composite resins.

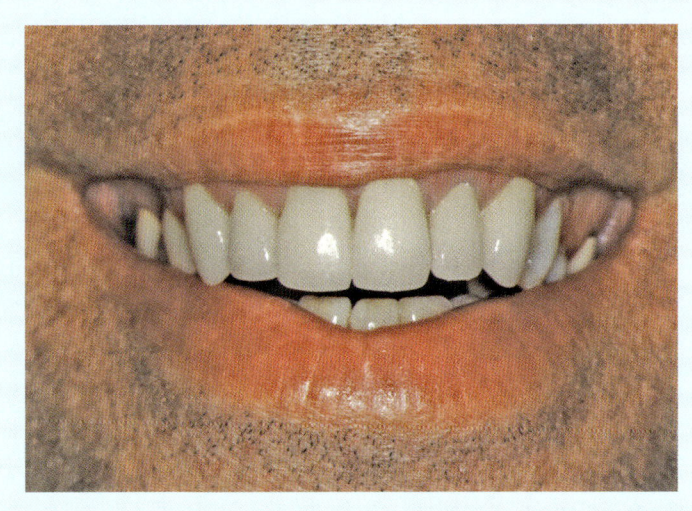

Figure 27.7 **(J)** At the next postoperative appointment I noticed the patient had shaved off his facial hair because he felt he did not need to hide his "crooked tooth smile" now.

If crowded teeth are to be corrected with bonding, veneering, or full crowns, the central incisors must be proportioned correctly. This can be accomplished by either disking the mesial surfaces of adjacent uninvolved teeth or reducing the size of adjacent crowned teeth. For final esthetics, contouring of adjacent teeth should be considered.

The decision whether to veneer or crown should be made primarily on the position of the overlapping (protruding) teeth. To restore the arch on or near the labial-most position of the teeth, porcelain veneers can be used. However, if the choice is to use maximum position (including vital pulp extirpation), then crowns will probably be the best choice.

Crowning and repositioning of mandibular anteriors

Although crowding can occur in both arches, it is more common in the mandibular anterior teeth. Treatment for these teeth is usually repositioning. There may be occasions when the orthodontist will choose not to reposition, and the patient may want these teeth bonded, veneered, or crowned. For teeth that are badly broken down or have significant gingival recession that has made them unattractive, bonding, veneering, or crowning can accomplish two things: it can restore and straighten each tooth to its proper form. How much correction can be achieved by repositioning is governed partially by root structure and crown inclination. If the axial alignments of the teeth are divergent, there is a limit to how much they can be straightened. If one of the teeth is in extreme labioversion, it is difficult to do much straightening without building the adjacent tooth somewhat thicker. This may create a gingival impingement on the tooth that is being overcontoured. Excessive labial reduction could cause pulp damage, so some compromise has to be reached. For this reason, repositioning is generally the better solution. Sometimes, a combination approach is the best solution. If the teeth are broken down and discolored, and have unattractive, large restorations, partial repositioning can be attempted, and crowning may take care of the remainder of the problem. This way, the patient might not mind wearing an appliance for a short while. One of the main objections that patients have to orthodontic treatment is the length of time the appliances have to be worn. However, if Invisalign or lingual brackets can be utilized, then patients have much less objection to orthodontic therapy.

Unusual or rare clinical presentations

Occasionally, you are presented with unusual dental problems associated with crowded dentitions, such as severely malposed and misaligned teeth, a protruding tooth, a retruded tooth, or the "lingually locked" tooth.[38–43]

Malposed and misaligned teeth

The method of choice for correcting malposition or misalignment of a tooth or teeth is orthodontics. For adults, consideration should be given to the easiest and less noticeable method if the patient has any fear of others knowing the treatment is taking place. We have had tremendous success with suggesting Invisalign whenever it is possible to obtain the desired result. If the patient is not concerned with appearance, then removable appliances, ceramic brackets, or even lingual braces are options.

An effective technique for repositioning crowded lower incisors is the use of the provisional splint with small hooks. A composite resin stop that is mechanically bonded to the teeth helps keep the elastic from slipping. Some disking in the interproximal surfaces of the anterior teeth is necessary to create space for the incisors to move lingually. Finally, it is vital to plan some sort of retention—if the typical removable retainer is not acceptable to the patient, then either an A-splint or direct bonding with a composite resin splint can be used. Auxiliary products such as tooth-colored reinforced fibers, such as Ribbond and Dentapreg, have been quite useful. Adult patients may think that they are too old for orthodontic therapy. You will have to judge the importance of immediate facial esthetics to the patient. If repositioning is the best solution to the esthetic problem, then the patient should be motivated to accept this therapy. Obviously if you have staff or other patients who do not mind showing your patient how pleased they are with the treatment in their own mouths this can be quite effective in motivating the patient to accept treatment. Generally, fear of the unknown can be cured by personal contact with those who may have had the same fear but are so happy with their ongoing treatment.

If the patient will accept only those procedures that offer an immediate solution, then bonding, veneering, or crowning may be the only feasible compromises. Cosmetic contouring should also be considered. Rather than no treatment, cosmetic contouring may provide some compromise benefit.

The protruding tooth

In restoring a crowded labially positioned incisor, careful preparation can make the protruding tooth appear to be in a more lingual position. Care must be taken to avoid a short preparation. The labial surface is reduced as far as possible without damaging the pulp; very little tooth structure is removed from the linguoincisal surface (Figure 27.8A and B). It is extremely important not to reduce the incisogingival height until the preparation is essentially complete. This will help avoid a short preparation. If the labial protrusion is so extreme that the pulp may become involved, explain to the patient that vital pulp extirpation may be necessary.[7] Such aggressive procedures should be undertaken only when appearance is extremely important and the patient is completely aware of the possible consequences and has signed an informed consent for treatment.

The retruded tooth

This esthetic problem is similar to that of the protruded tooth. However, realignment of the tooth in linguoversion frequently necessitates reduction and recontouring of the opposing teeth to allow for clearance of the newly crowned, bonded, or veneered tooth. To achieve the desired result, a large amount of the tooth structure may have to be removed from the linguoincisal surface of the opposing tooth. Esthetic results can then be achieved by crowning or veneering. If a full crown is desired, then the lingual side can be covered with a thin layer of porcelain and perhaps an all-zirconia crown could be utilized. The labial porcelain may be built out to correct alignment. Veneering can be especially useful since virtually no enamel needs to be reduced on the labial surface, with only linguoincisal enamel being reshaped to mask the amount of retrusion present. One potential problem may be the amount of impingement on the labial gingival tissue, so consultation with a periodontist could be beneficial.

The lingually locked tooth

If a lingually locked tooth is fully erupted, it can be restored to correct position by pulp extirpation and placement of an off-center endodontic post and porcelain crown. However, if the tooth is too short and in moderate linguoversion, this treatment may be impractical. A porcelain shoulder is prepared on the labial, and the porcelain is built up butted against the labial gingiva. The patient must be warned that oral hygiene must be scrupulous. It is far better to try to convince the patient of the

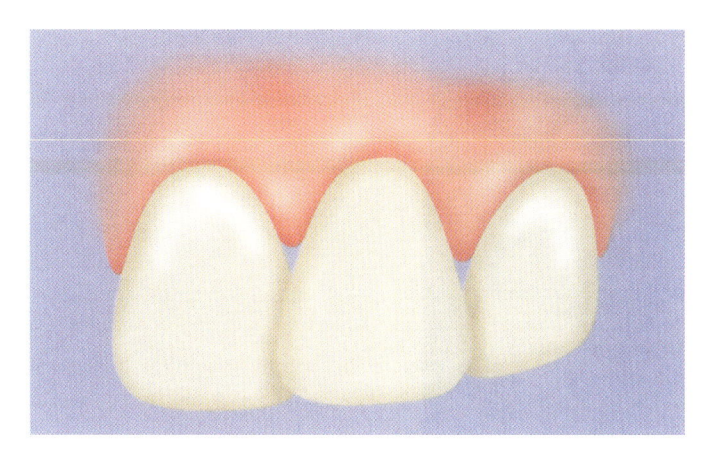

Figure 27.8 **(A)** The crowded labially positioned incisor requires a careful preparation to make it appear to be in a more lingual position.

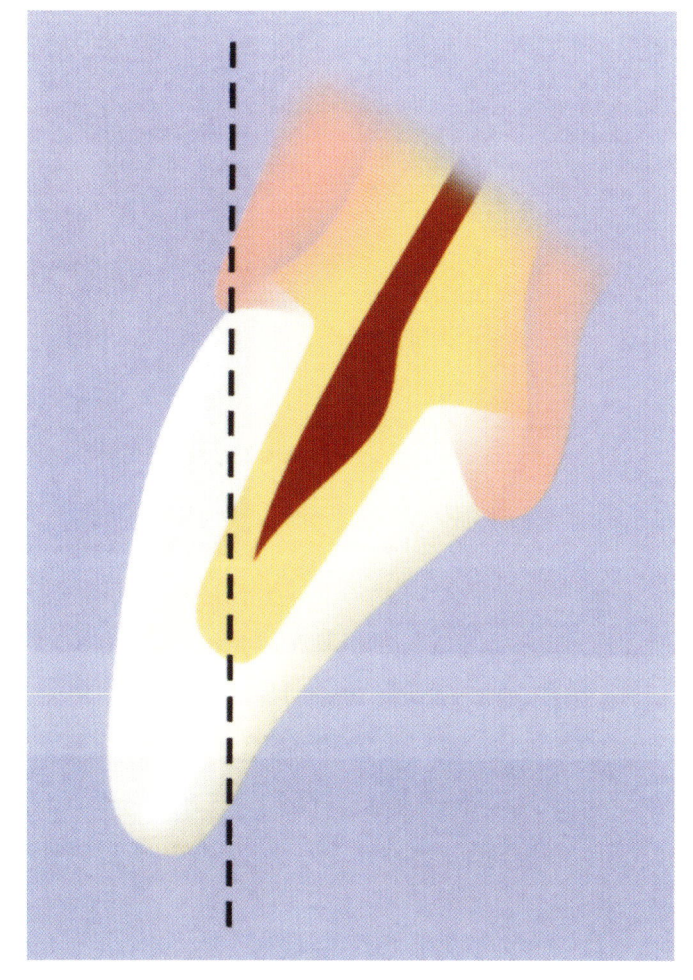

Figure 27.8 **(B)** The labial surface is reduced as far as possible without damaging the pulp. It is extremely important not to reduce the incisogingival height until the preparation is essentially complete.

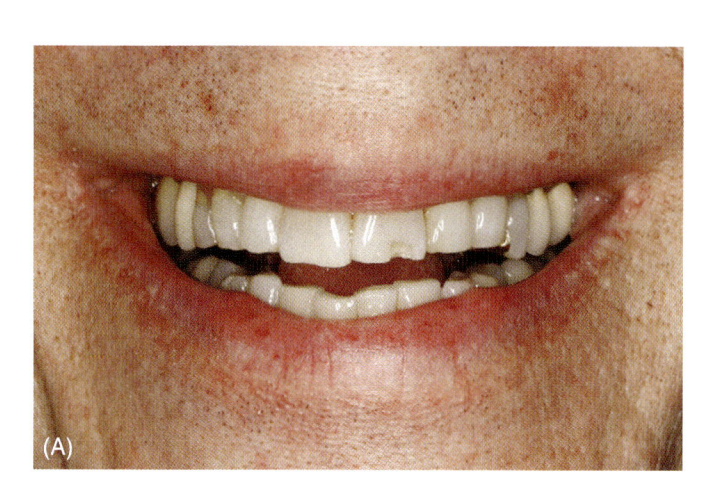

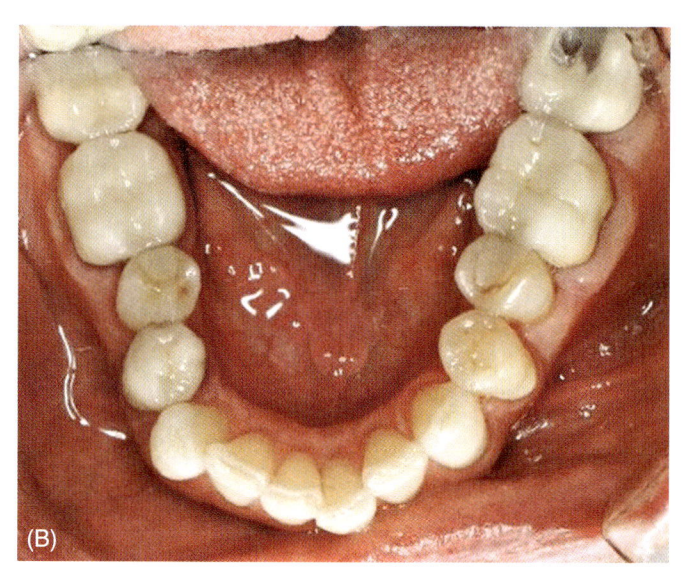

Figure 27.9 **(A, B)** This man wanted to improve his smile both esthetically and functionally.

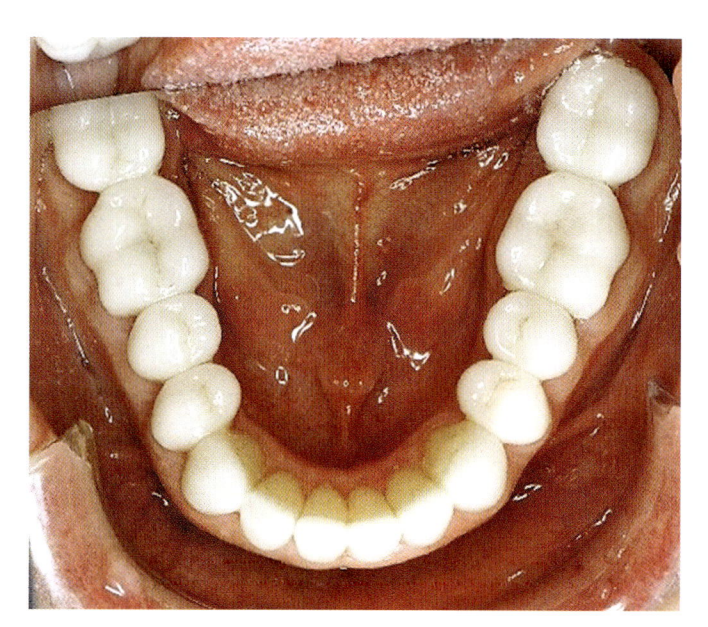

Figure 27.9 **(C)** The patient was accepting of conventional orthodontics for a short period that would improve the crowding on the lower arch for a better eventual result.

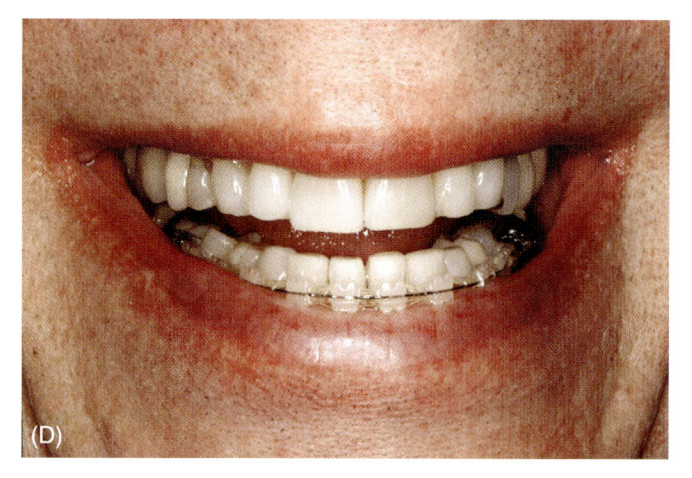

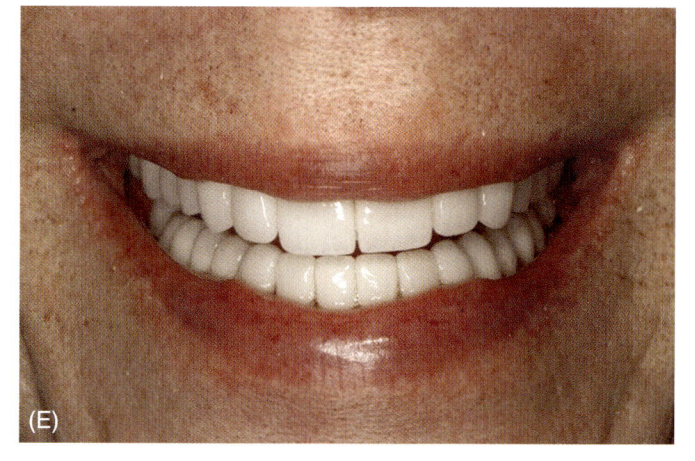

Figure 27.9 **(D, E)** The final result is a combination of orthodontics, all-ceramic crowns, and porcelain veneers, which pleased the patient.

advantages of repositioning the lingually locked tooth than to try to restore it in place. In severe situations, a third choice involving extraction and moving the remaining teeth together with bonded brackets may be indicated.

To bond, veneer, or crown?

The following questions should be considered:

- What is the size of the crowded tooth? Will bonding make the tooth too bulky? Bonded lower anteriors are more susceptible to this problem.
- How much enamel is left for bonding? Are there very large existing restorations that, once removed, will lessen the retention for a new bonded restoration? Also, if the patient normally has a tendency to build plaque and calculus on the lingual surfaces of lower anteriors, bonding may not be the best choice.
- What is the appearance of the enamel? Is it badly stained or discolored so that a large amount of opaquer plus several layers of composite resin will be required to mask the defects? If so, then veneering or crowning is the better choice.
- Does the patient have a bad habit that may stain a bonded restoration? Heavy smokers or coffee/tea drinkers may choose veneering or crowning to lessen the amount of postoperative discoloration.
- Is there an economic problem? Frequently, patients may wish to have their teeth veneered or crowned, but finances enter into the decision since bonding with composite resin is less expensive than either crowning or veneering with porcelain.
- How long does the patient expect the restoration to last? Chances are that both veneering and crowning can provide much longer life than direct bonding with composite resin.

In the final analysis, most patients could benefit from a combination of orthodontics and restorative dentistry (Figure 27.9A–E). Those patients who select a more conservative option should also be informed whether later on it will be possible to proceed with a more ideal or optimal treatment plan. In this regard, so many of my earlier bonding patients have opted to change from composite resin to porcelain veneers or even all-ceramic crowns. Others even decided to undergo some orthodontic therapy before their final restoration option. Thus, it is always appropriate to present both an ideal and compromised treatment plan as well as a long-term option. Patients who may need a quick smile transformation but are restricted by financial considerations may be in a much better financial situation in later years.

References

1. Burstone CJ, Marcotte MR. *Problem Solving in Orthodontics: Goal-Oriented Treatment Strategies*. Chicago, IL: Quintessence; 2000.
2. Foster TD. *A Textbook of Orthodontics*, 2nd edn. Oxford: Blackwell Scientific; 1982.
3. Graber TM, Vanarsdall RL. *Orthodontics: Current Principles and Techniques*. St. Louis, MO: Mosby; 2000.
4. Proffit W, Fields HW. *Contemporary Orthodontics*, 3rd edn. St. Louis, MO: Mosby; 2000.
5. Roblee RD. *Interdisciplinary Dentofacial Therapy*. Chicago, IL: Quintessence; 1994.
6. Rufenacht CR. *Principles of Esthetic Integration*. Chicago, IL: Quintessence; 2000.
7. Berliner A. *Ligatures, Splints, Bite Planes, and Pyramids*. Philadelphia, PA: JB Lippincott; 1964.
8. Oringer RJ, Iacono VJ. Periodontal cosmetic surgery. *J Int Acad Periodontol* 1999;1:83–90.
9. Wilson TG, Korman KS. *Esthetic Periodontics (Periodontal Plastic Surgery)*. Chicago, IL: Quintessence, 1996.
10. Lieberman MA, Gazit E. Lower incisor extraction—a method of orthodontic treatment in selected cases in the adult dentition. *Isr J Dent Med* 1973;22:80–83.
11. Bello A, Jarvis RH. A review of esthetic alternatives for the restoration of anterior teeth. *J Prosthet Dent* 1997;78:437–440.
12. Goldstein RE. *Esthetics in Dentistry*, Vol. 1, 2nd edn. Hamilton, ON: BC Decker; 1998.
13. Kokich VG. Esthetics: the orthodontic–periodontic restorative connection. *Semin Orthodont* 1996;2(1):21–30.
14. Studer S, Zellweger V, Scharer P. The aesthetic guidelines of the mucogingival complex for fixed prosthodontics. *Pract Periodont Aesthet Dent* 1996;8:333–341.
15. Levine JB. Esthetic diagnosis. *Curr Opin Cosmet Dent* 1995;3:9–17.
16. Crispin B. *Contemporary Esthetic Dentistry: Practice Fundamentals*. Chicago, IL: Quintessence; 1994.
17. Goldstein CE, Goldstein RE, Garber DA. *Imaging in Esthetic Dentistry*. Chicago, IL: Quintessence; 1998.
18. Magne P, Magne M, Belsor V. The diagnostic template: a key element to the comprehensive esthetic treatment concept. *Int J Periodont Restor Dent* 1996;16:560–569.
19. Derbabian K, Marzola R, Arcidiacono A. The science of communicating the art of dentistry. *J Calif Dent Assoc* 1998;26:101–106.
20. Jun S. Communication is vital to produce natural looking metal ceramic crowns. *J Dent Technol* 1997;14(8):15–20.
21. Small BW. Laboratory communications for esthetic success. *Gen Dent* 1998;46:566–568, 572–574.
22. Donovan TE, Cho C. Diagnostic provisional restorations in restorative dentistry: the blueprint for success. *J Can Dent Assoc* 1999;65:272–275.
23. Rada RE. Interdisciplinary management of a common esthetic complaint. *Gen Dent* 1999;47:387–389.
24. Heyman HO. Conservative concepts to achieving anterior esthetics. *J Calif Dent Assoc* 1997;25:437–443.
25. Margolis MJ. Esthetic considerations in orthodontic treatment of adults. *Dent Clin North Am* 1997;41:29–48.
26. Okuda WH. Creating facial harmony with cosmetic dentistry. *Curr Opin Cosmet Dent* 1997;4:69–75.
27. Portalier L. Composite smile designs: the key to dental artistry. *Curr Opin Cosmet Dent* 1997;4:81–85.
28. Fradeani M, Aquilino A, Barducci G. Aesthetic restoration of endodontically treated teeth. *Pract Periodont Aesthet Dent* 1999;11:761–768.
29. Epstein MB, Mantzikos T, Shamus IL. Esthetic recontouring: a team approach. *N Y State Dent J* 1997;63(10):35–40.
30. Peck H, Peck S. Reproximation (enamel stripping) as an essential orthodontic treatment ingredient. In: *Transactions of the Third International Orthodontics Congress*. London: Crosby Lockwood Staples; 1975.

31. Dietschi D. Free-hand composite resin restorations: a key to anterior esthetics. *Pract Periodont Aesthet Dent* 1995;7(7):15–25.
32. Fahl N Jr, Denehy GE, Jackson RD. Protocol for predictable restoration of anterior teeth with composite resins. *Pract Periodont Aesthet Dent* 1995;7(8):13–21.
33. Garber DA, Goldstein RE, Feinman RA. *Porcelain Laminate Veneers*. Chicago, IL: Quintessence; 1988.
34. Chiche GJ, Pinault A. *Esthetics of Anterior Fixed Prosthodontics*. Chicago, IL: Quintessence; 1993.
35. Narcisi EM, Culp L. Diagnosis and treatment planning for ceramic restorations. *Dent Clin North Am* 2001;45:117–142.
36. Paul SJ, Pietrobon N. Aesthetic evolution of anterior maxillary crowns: a literature review. *Pract Periodont Aesthet Dent* 1998;10(1):87–94.
37. Singer BA. *Esthetic Dentistry: A Clinical Approach to Techniques and Materials*. Philadelphia, PA: Lea & Febiger; 1993.
38. Curry FT. Restorative alternative to orthodontic treatment: a clinical report. *J Prosthet Dent* 1999;82:127–129.
39. Cutbirth ST. Treatment planning for porcelain veneer restoration of crowded teeth by modifying stone models. *J Esthet Restor Dent* 2001;13:29–39.
40. Gleghorn TA. Use of bonded porcelain restorations for nonorthodontic realignment of the anterior maxilla. *Pract Periodont Aesthet Dent* 1998;10:563–565.
41. Narcisi EM, DiPerna JA. Multidisciplinary full-mouth restoration with porcelain veneers and laboratory-fabricated resin inlays. *Pract Periodont Aesthet Dent* 1999;11:721–728.
42. Salama M. Orthodontics vs. restorative materials in treatment plans. *Contemp Esthet Restor Pract* 2001;5:20–30.
43. Shannon A. Reconstruction of the maxillary dentition utilizing a nonorthodontic technique. *Pract Periodont Aesthet Dent* 1999;11:973–978.

Additional resources

Gkantidis N, Sanoudos M. Lower anterior crowding correction by a convenient lingual method. *J Esthet Restor Dent* 2013;25(2):96–100.

Viswanath D, Shetty S, Mascarenhas R, Husain A. Treatment of mandibular anterior crowding with incisor extraction using lingual orthodontics: a case report. *World J Orthod* 2010;11:e99–e103.

Zachrisson BU. Long-term experience with direct-bonded retainers: update and clinical advice. *J Clin Orthod* 2007;41:728–737.

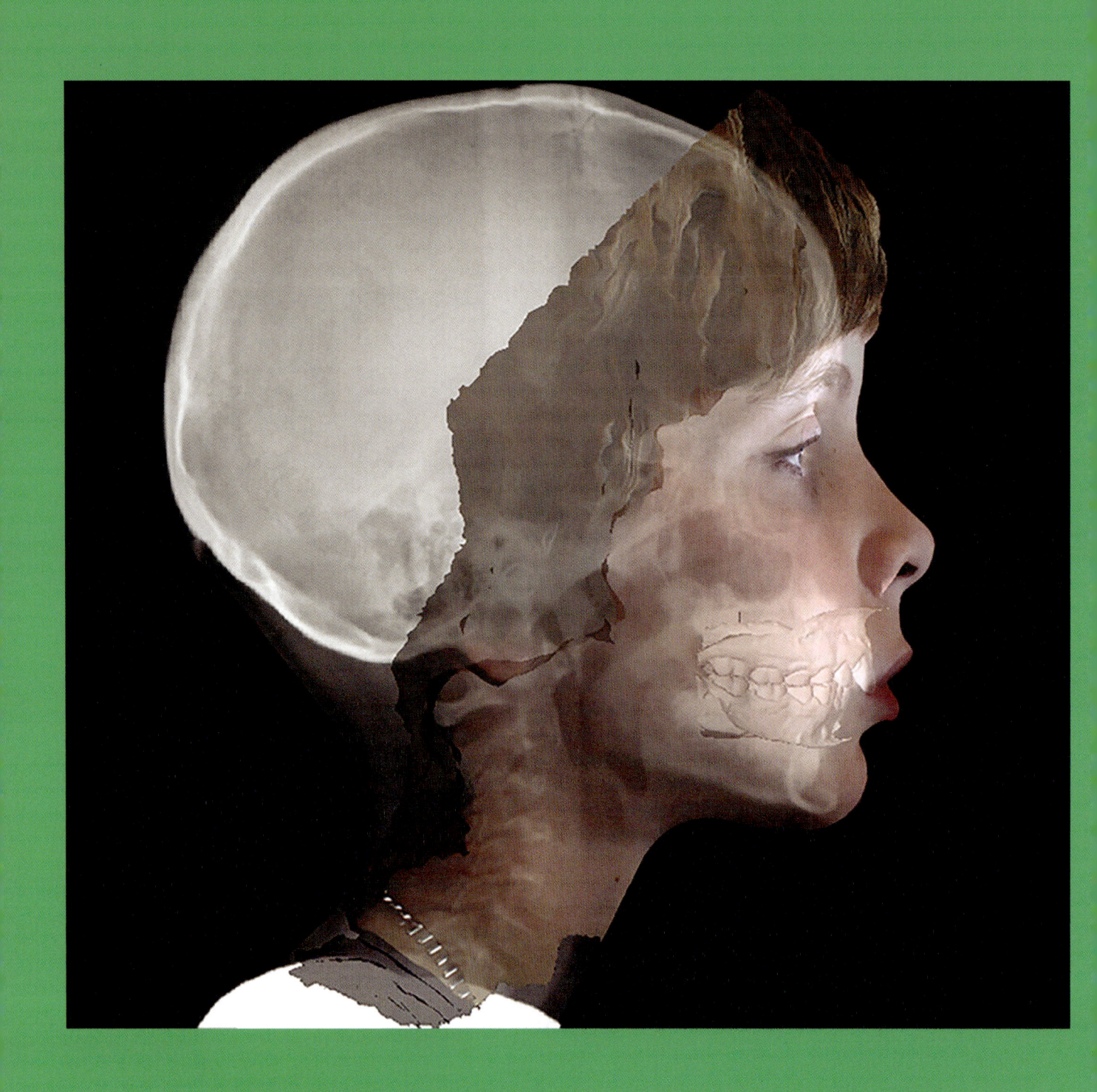

Chapter 28 Esthetics in Adult Orthodontics

Eladio DeLeon Jr, DMD, MS

Chapter Outline

Impact of orthodontic treatment on facial esthetics	898	What is the ideal functional occlusal scheme?	915
Integrating orthodontics into the interdisciplinary treatment plan	905	Achieving a "realistically ideal" occlusion in adult orthodontic patients	916
Technological advances in orthodontics	909	Tooth size–arch length discrepancies in the adult patient	919
Periodontal considerations with adult orthodontic treatment	909	Arch length/perimeter	920
Occlusal considerations for the adult orthodontic patient	915	Curve of Spee	921
Ideal static occlusion: an historical and contemporary perspective	915	Incisor protrusion	922
		Tooth size discrepancies	923

In honor and memory of Dr Marvin C. Goldstein.

Over the past few decades, the focus of dentistry has undergone a significant paradigm shift. The increasing esthetic awareness of the adult patient has expanded the therapeutic realm of dental practitioners from solely controlling dental disease to optimizing smile esthetics.

Although orthodontic treatment is primarily perceived as based on achieving "straight teeth" and ideal occlusal relationships, greater attention is increasingly directed toward enhancing the smile, the face, and the ability to masticate. The scope of "adult orthodontics" simply includes the alignment of teeth and jaws of those persons who are beyond the normal growth phase. These are typically individuals over the age of 16. Given the expanded and often prolonged dental history of this patient population, an interdisciplinary approach is often required to maximize the esthetic result.

There are positive and negative aspects of treating adult patients. The advantages are threefold: enhanced motivation, increased pain tolerance, and autonomous fiscal responsibility. The adult patient is obviously reluctant to be seen wearing the "braces" that are usually associated with adolescent and preadolescent therapy. The advent of esthetic removable and fixed appliances, coupled with the prospects of improved esthetics and function, is generally sufficient to overcome this hesitation. The limited ability of the orthodontist to channel the facial growth of the child to improve facial esthetics is a luxury that is unavailable to the adult orthodontic patient. In those adults who require skeletal movement to enhance esthetics, surgical intervention may be required.

There are two basic reasons that adults seek orthodontic treatment: to improve appearance and/or to improve chewing or speaking function. Obviously, the former comprises the majority of the motivation in the adult seeking treatment. It is therefore valuable to distinguish between esthetic and cosmetic services. Esthetic treatment involves an effort to improve appearance by providing permanent structural changes. Cosmetic treatment generally involves obscuring or covering unsightly imperfections.

The intent is to enhance certain facial features with temporary applications. However, the field of cosmetics has expanded to mildly invasive procedures such as injections of botulinum toxin type A (Botox) and/or injectable fillers to eliminate age-related facial wrinkles and furrows. Treatment with Botox now includes the treatment of wrinkles lateral to the eyes ("crow's feet") and to treat the gummy smile. Other cosmetic procedures include soft tissue revisions, such as blepharoplasties and rhinoplasties, and extensive dental prosthetic procedures, which are extensively explored in other chapters of this volume.

Cosmetic dentistry likewise seeks to merely camouflage the underlying defects (Figure 28.1). In contrast, esthetic dentistry seeks to correct the underlying problems, such as improper dental, skeletal, and functional relationships, and those involved in arch coordination and symmetry. Only when these goals have been achieved, can subsequent esthetic restorative procedures create a truly esthetic smile. Faced with this growing demand, the responsibility of the dental practitioner is to first and foremost educate the patient that the foundation of an esthetic smile lies in controlling disease as well as the achievement of proper orthodontic form and function. When educating the patient about treatment options, it is essential to differentiate between cosmetic dentistry and esthetic dentistry. Attempting to achieve esthetic results without the realization of these goals can only lead to a compromised treatment outcome. Thorough patient education of the discriminating, self-motivated adult patient is essential to generate an informed treatment decision tailored to the patient's goals and economic resources.

This chapter will illustrate tooth movement to relieve tooth crowding, spacing, and to provide simple alignment. Chapter 29 will avail the reader of a comprehensive review of the diagnosis, treatment planning, and appliance selection with treatment of complex orthodontic and facial abnormalities that negatively impact facial and dental esthetics.

Although the contemporary identity of the profession is orthodontics and dentofacial orthopedics, the expanded domain requires a team approach involving oral and maxillofacial surgeons, periodontists, and restorative dentists, all collaborating to enhance the smiles of patients of all ages.

Impact of orthodontic treatment on facial esthetics

Facial esthetics is a blend of the health, symmetry, and proportionality of facial and dental hard and soft tissues and, accordingly, a comprehensive evaluation of all factors must be evaluated in order determine the most effective and efficient treatment plan for the adult orthodontics patient. The following factors all play a role in treatment planning orthodontics in the adult patient and ultimately determine whether or not the treatment was successful: preexisting dental conditions, preexisting

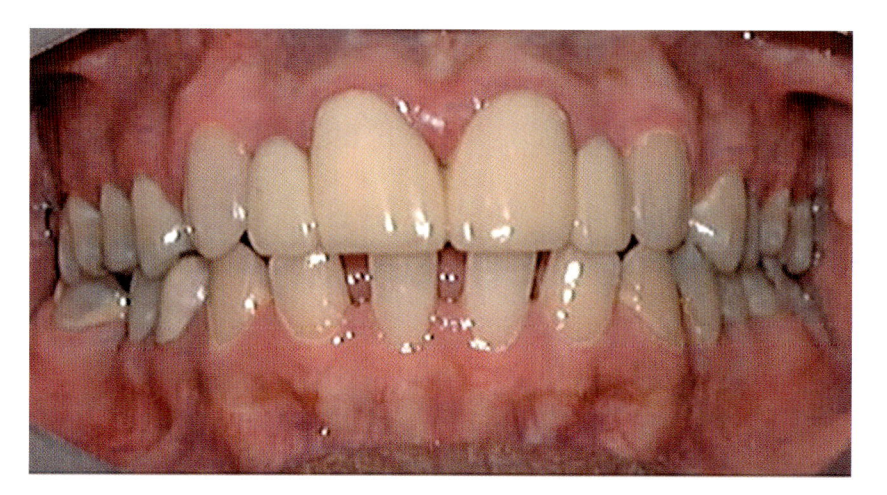

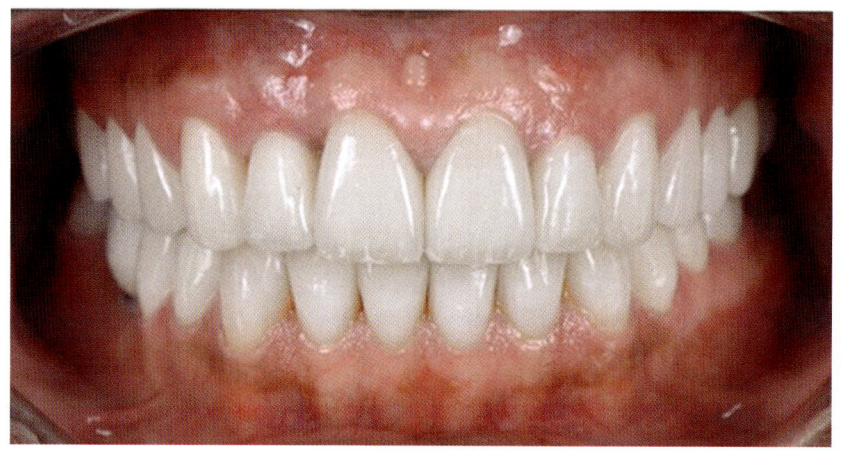

Figure 28.1 Camouflaging defects: orthodontics, implants to replace congenitally missing maxillary laterals.

facial features, and preexisting temporomandibular conditions, based upon comprehensive facial, dental skeletal analyses, patient finances, and patient intangibles.

Historically, some adults have sought orthodontic care for their children before seeking it themselves, but recently that paradigm has begun to shift. According to the American Association of Orthodontists (AAO), adults now make up 20%[1] of all orthodontic patients seen by AAO members. Traditionally, orthodontists have treated almost exclusively patients under the age of 18, with the majority of them having healthy, intact dentitions. Adults can pose added complexity to treating their facial, skeletal, and dental problems successfully, as Dr Vincent Kokich[2] points out: "Adults may have old and failing restorations, edentulous spaces, abraded teeth, periodontal bone defects, gingival level discrepancies, and teeth beyond any sustained useful purpose...that could compromise the orthodontic result."

To fully understand the needs of adult patients, a lengthy medical and dental history is needed and extensive clinical records to include extra-/intraoral exams and photographs, lateral cephalogram, panoramic radiograph, full periodontal charting, and a recent full mouth series of radiographs. In the present stage of digital images, there is simply no excuse for poor quality of images, and staff should be trained properly and be expected to deliver the best diagnostic records that current technology has to offer (Figures 28.2, 28.3, and 28.4).

One of the first analyses that should be conducted, both in person and with the aid of high-quality digital images, is a smile analysis. According to Dr David Sarver,[3] "smile and facial animation…should be of great interest to orthodontist." As Sarver writes, orthodontists typically evaluate the "posed smile" even with the knowledge that there are two different types of smiles: the posed and the spontaneous smile. The posed smile is evaluated due to its reproducibility and predictability with two major characteristics being scrutinized: the amount of incisor and gingival display and the transverse dimension of the smile. The posed smile and the spontaneous smile must be acceptable to the patient to prevent a self-conscious or affected smile (Figure 28.5).

The amount of incisor and gingival display for the maximum esthetic result has been found to not always be congruent, according to orthodontists and laypeople alike. Truly, beauty is in the eye of the beholder and is supported by the following studies. In 2008, Gul-e-Erum and Fida[4] asked 12 laypeople who were orthodontic patients to evaluate 46 frontal full-face pictures of a man and woman with digitally altered characteristics of buccal corridors, incisal show/lip line, and smile arc, among others. Results showed that "zero gingival display with zero incisal coverage was preferred in the photograph of the man, incisal display with 2 mm gingival display preferred in the photograph of the woman." In similar studies by Hulsey,[5] Hunt et al.,[6] and Kokich et al.,[7] upper lip height at the gingival margin of the upper incisor, tolerance of −2 to +2 mm from gingival margin, and gingival display threshold of 3.0 mm were the preferences of their respective studies.

This deviation in study results holds true for preferences on buccal corridors, gingival zeniths, smile arcs, and midline deviations.[8] Although there seems to be agreement as to what is

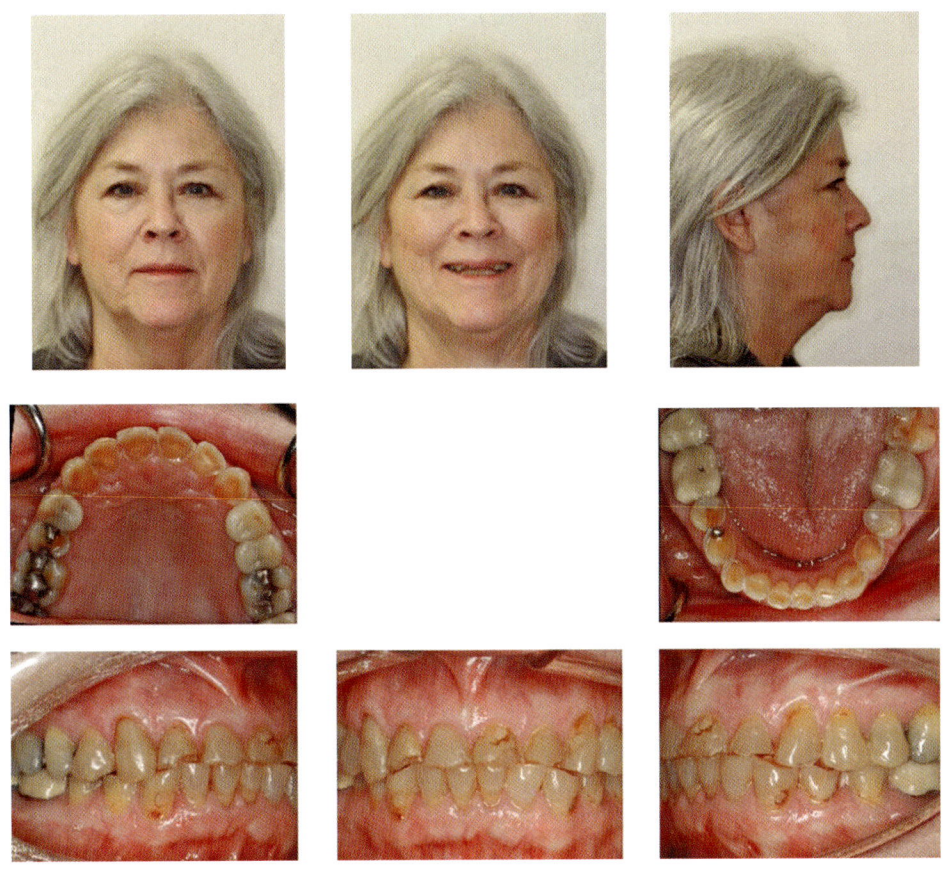

Figure 28.2 Photographic montage, close-up smile, periodontal charting.

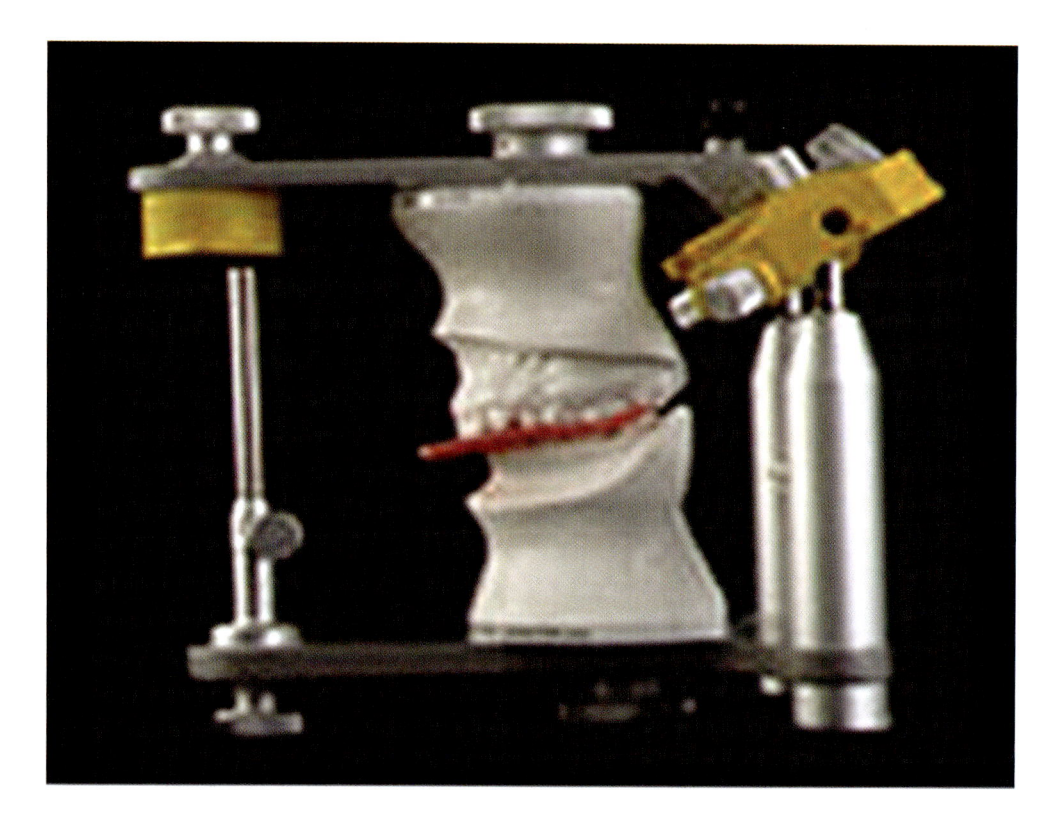

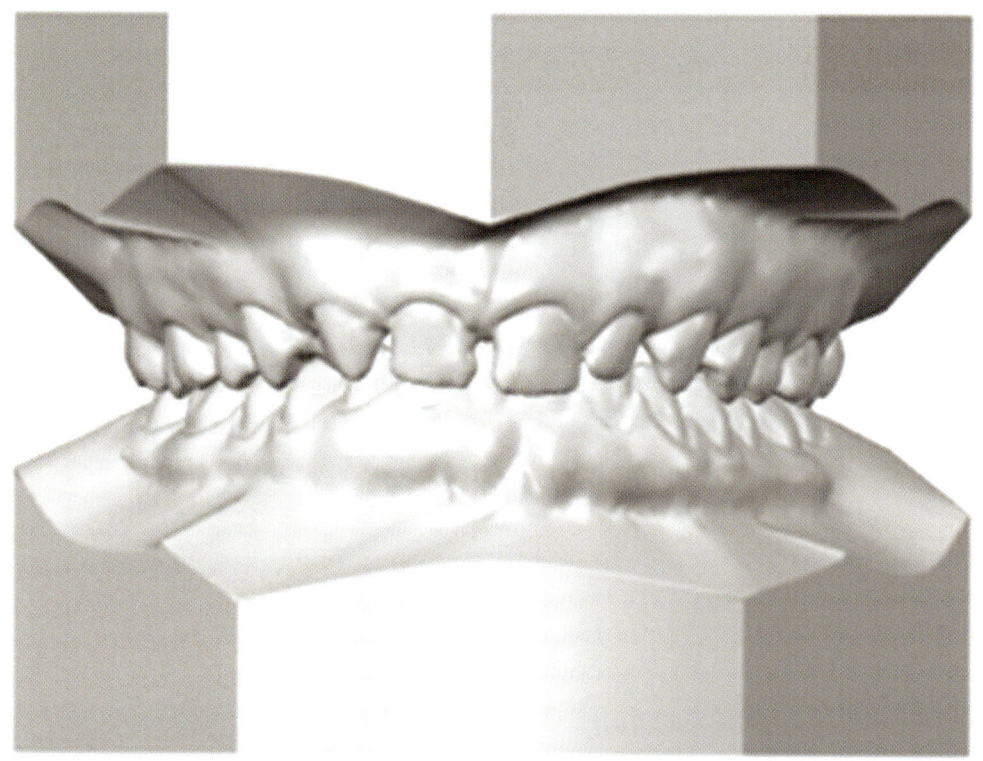

Figure 28.3 Mounted models and American Board of Orthodontists (ABO) dental models.

"not esthetic," there is a slight variation among dental professionals and laypeople as to what consists of maximum esthetics (Figures 28.6, 28.7, and 28.8).

As a part of smile and facial analysis, the orthodontist must also evaluate for proper dental and facial proportions, and also display and length of teeth. With the incorporation of high-quality digital images into the treatment planning of orthodontics, it is very important to scrutinize facial symmetry in all three planes of space: height, width, and depth. According to Sarver,[9] when determining proportionality in the horizontal plane, the face is divided into three equal planes, with the distances measured between the chin to the bottom of the nose,

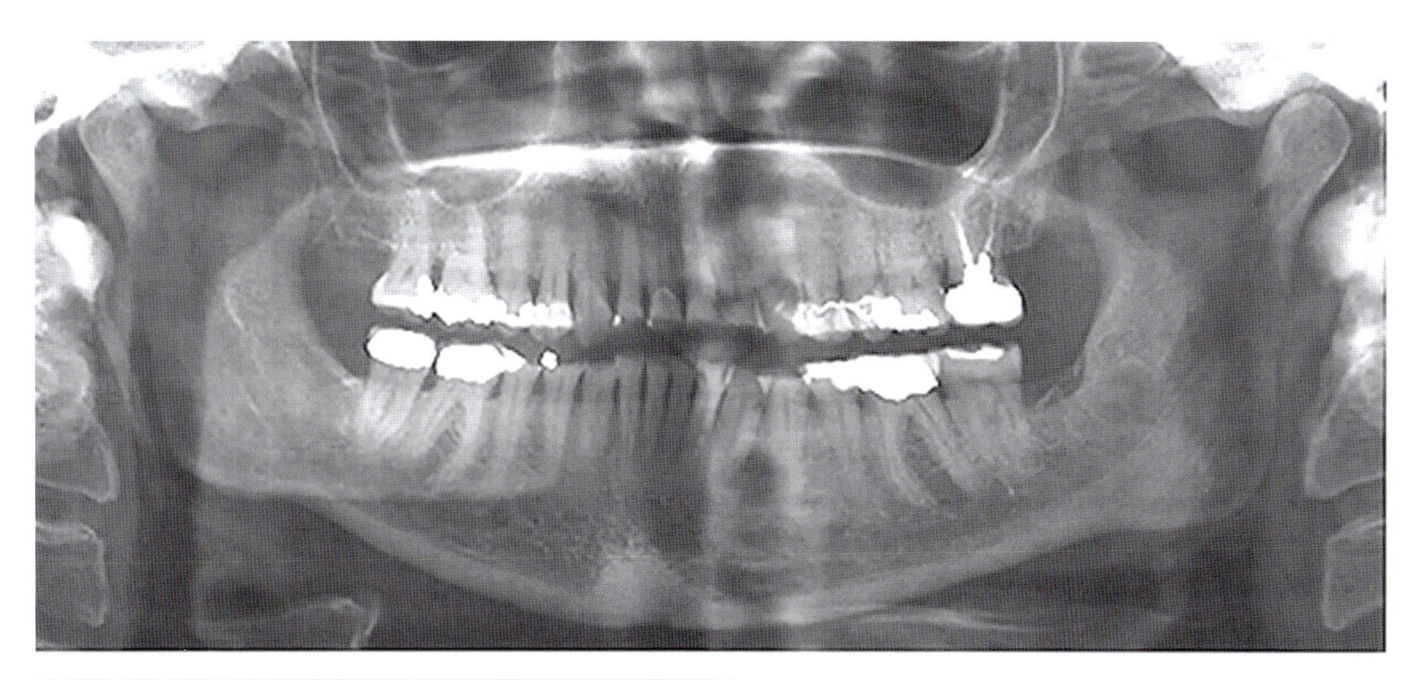

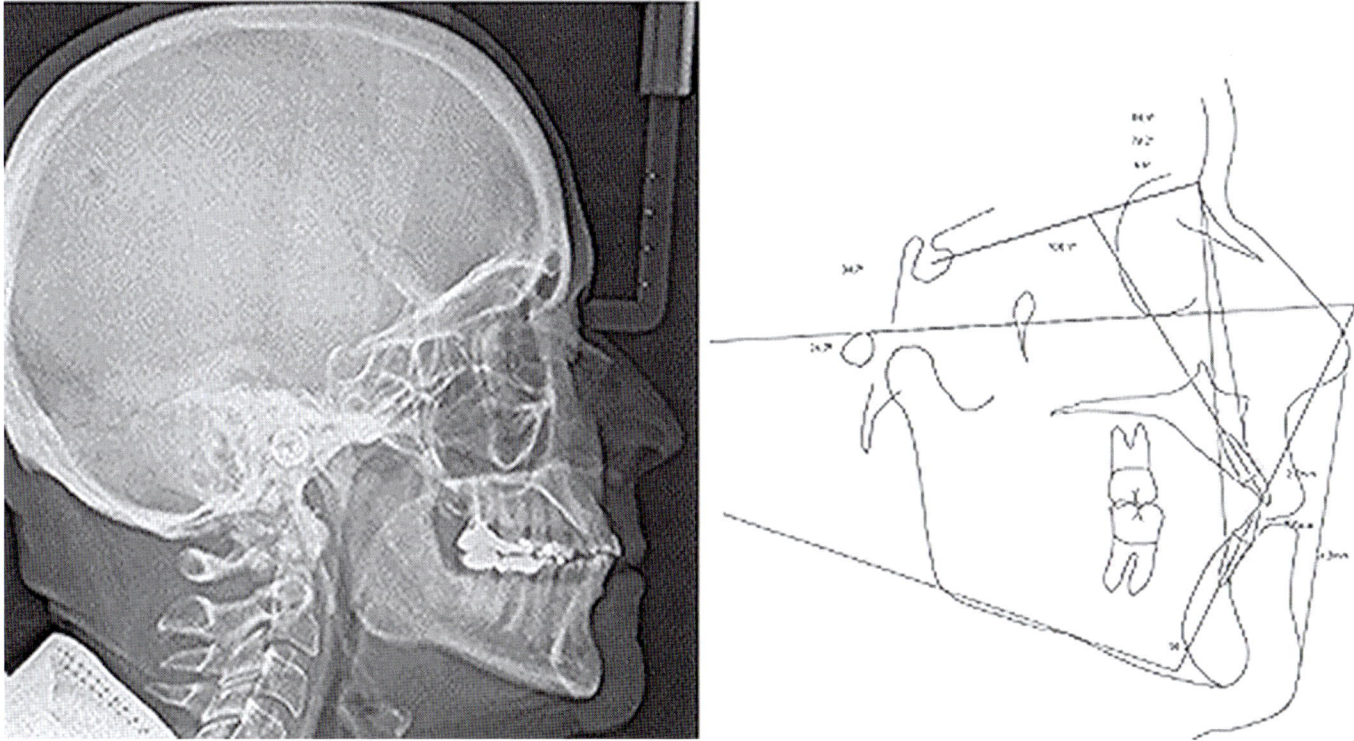

Figure 28.4 Panoramic and cephalometric radiographs and cephalometric analysis.

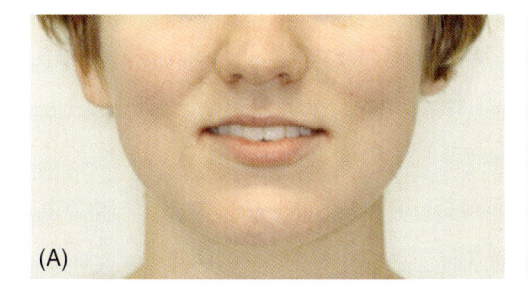

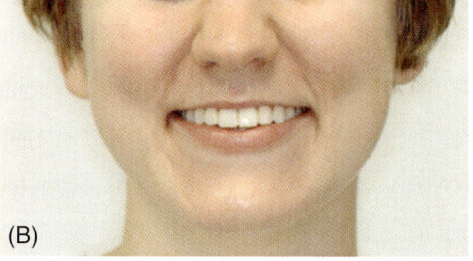

(A)   (B)

Figure 28.5 (A) Posed smile. (B) Spontaneous smile.

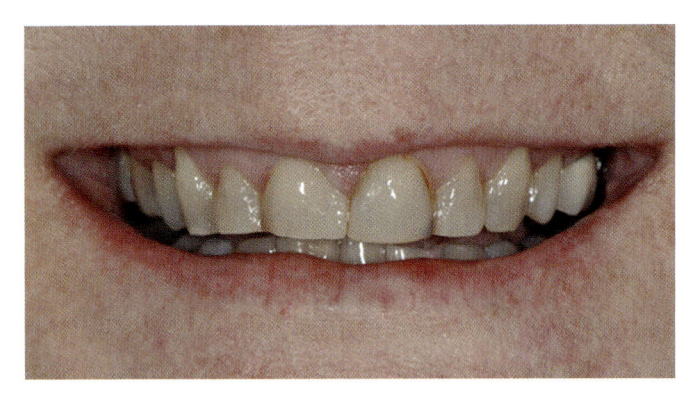

Figure 28.6 Excessive buccal corridors.

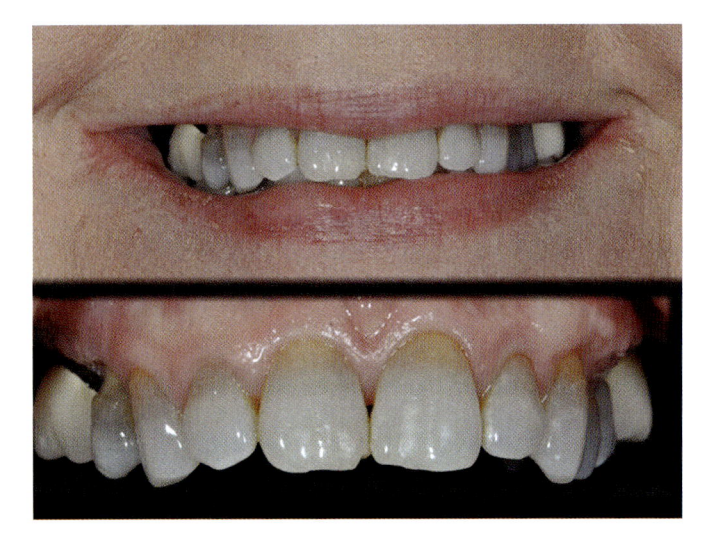

Figure 28.7 Reverse smile line.

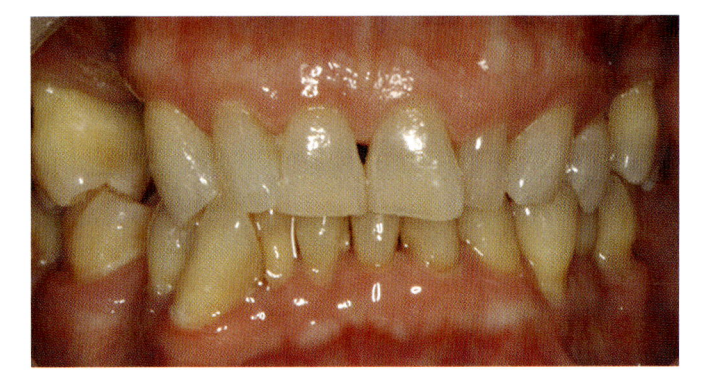

Figure 28.8 Midline deviation, black triangle, and gingival recession with significant crowding

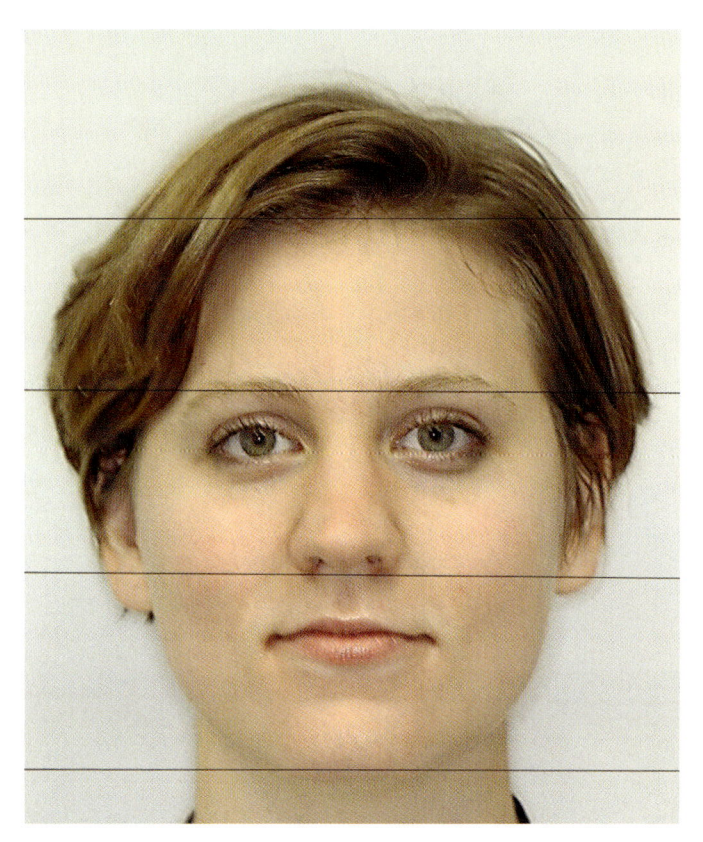

Figure 28.9 The rule of thirds.

from the bottom of the nose to the brow, and from the brow to the hairline being of equal value (the rule of thirds). Of distinct importance to orthodontists are the proportions of the lower face, because that is where the orthodontic impact is the greatest. The upper lip to the nose should represent a third, while the lower lip to chin should equal two-thirds. If these proportions are not correct prior to treatment, they should be noted in the findings section and can figure into the objectives of treatment if the orthodontist so chooses. Vertically, the face should follow the rule of fifths, with one-fifth equaling the width of an individual's eye. The boundaries in which there should be equal fifths are from the lateral portion of the ear to the lateral portion of the eye to medial aspect of the eye, with the distances being congruent and symmetric on the right and left sides of a person's face (Figures 28.9 and 28.10).

Symmetric and proportional facial components are an absolute for maximum orthodontic esthetics, but orthodontists face an uphill battle without proper dental proportions that include display of teeth. When treating adults, those who venture into esthetic and functional reconstruction should be fully aware of the potential compromising factors so clearly outlined by Dr Kokich. He listed and expanded on key compromising factors of adult treatment: attrition of teeth, iatrogenic width/height changes with permanent dental restorations, and periodontal considerations. Simplified, the greater the attrition of teeth, the greater the width compared with the height. Dentists also restore teeth to the best of their abilities, but often times change the anatomic width/height ratios with restorative treatment.

Periodontal disease affects the proportionality of teeth because the receding gums reveal greater amounts of tooth structure, which alters the natural width/height ratios. In addition to single tooth width/height ratios, one of the longest standing ratios was proposed to relate to dentistry: the golden proportion. When used in dentistry, the golden proportion of 1.618 to 1 has been shown to relate to the perceived width of the maxillary teeth starting at the midline and working distally, but only when the onlooker is positioned directly in front of the subject being examined. Using the lateral incisor as the value "1," the most esthetic width of the central would be 1.618 and the width of the canine would be 0.618.[10,11] However, according to references on

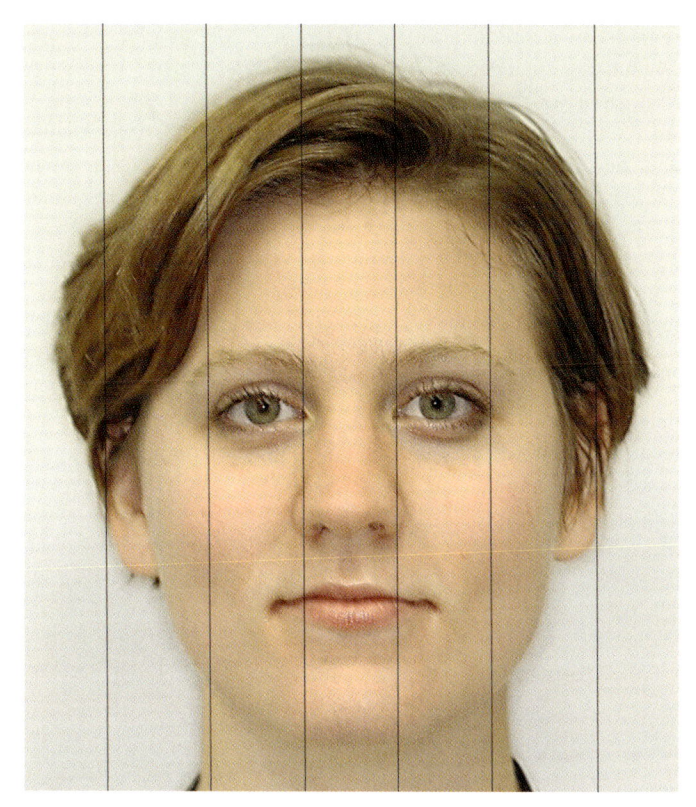

Figure 28.10 The rule of fifths.

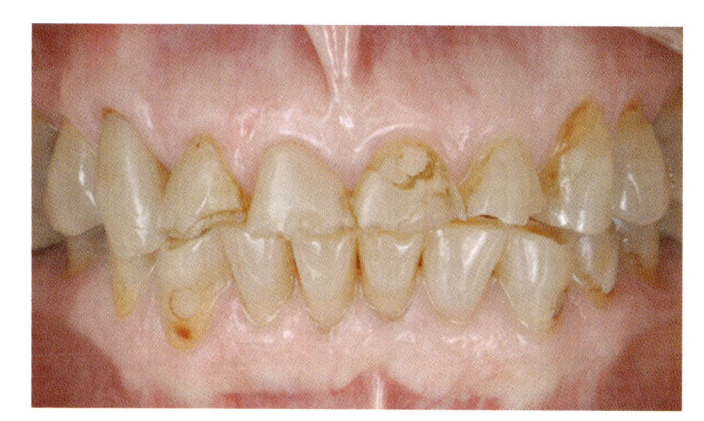

Figure 28.11 Severe attrition.

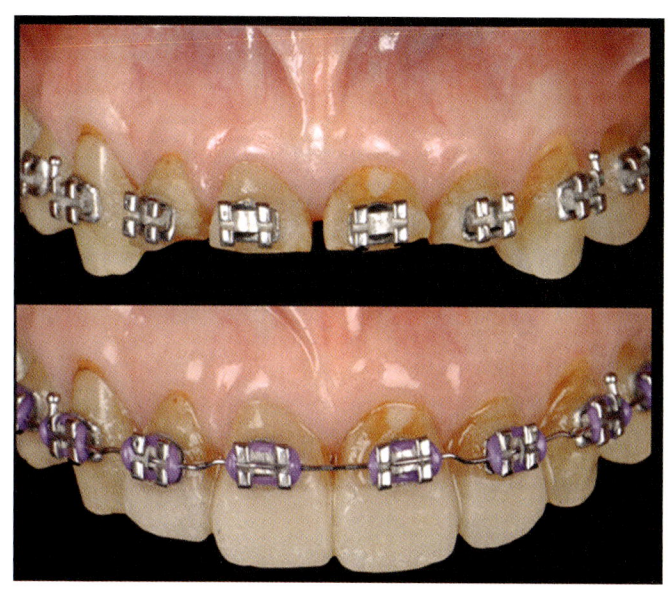

Figure 28.12 Orthodontic–restorative preparation in establishing the proper ratio and symmetry.

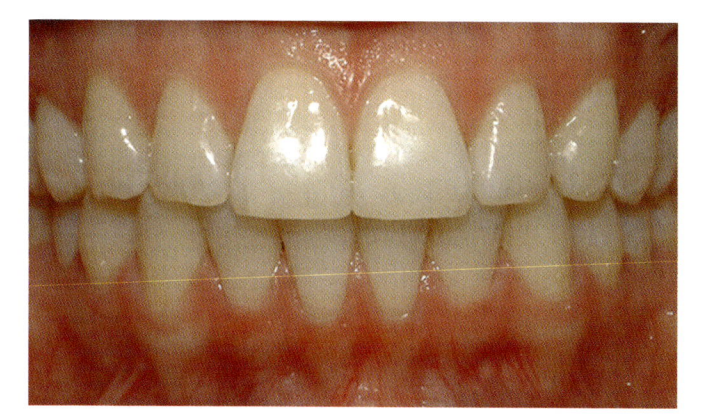

Figure 28.13 Ideal tooth size proportions.

tooth size, there is no correlation of the golden proportion with the actual dimensions of incisors.[12]

The actual width of maxillary lateral incisor to maxillary central incisor proportionally is better estimated at 77.5%, with a range of 71–82%. As a result, the use of the golden proportion to determine tooth size or space appropriation for replacement or restoration of missing or anomalous crown would not be appropriate.[13]

To determine proper width-to-height ratio, we again rely upon the research of Dr Sarver,[14] who states that although there is some variability in the data of width-to-height ratios of maxillary central incisors, which varies between 66% and 80%, he and Dr G. Gurel,[15] in a published study on the art of laminate veneers, believe the most esthetic width-to-height ratio is 0.8. While well stated, this is a guideline and not an absolute rule, since natural teeth undergo attrition during their lifetime and it may be difficult to determine what the preattrition ratio was. In all of esthetics, proper ratio amounts and symmetry appear to be the most important factors (Figures 28.11, 28.12, and 28.13).

Beyond the world of diagnosing and treatment planning in three dimensions, orthodontists continue to rely upon two-dimensional radiography, especially panoramic and cephalometric radiographs. Prior to cone beam computed tomography (CBCT) being available on the market for reasonable prices, these two radiographs were two of the most important pieces of the treatment planning puzzle (Figure 28.4). Today, cephalograms and panoramic radiographs are used adjunctively with three-dimensional radiographs. It has always been imperative that orthodontists do not take normal values created with population statistics from cephalograms as absolute treatment values for their patients in hopes of achieving "normal values." With that said, normal values are extremely helpful in understanding where an individual deviates and possibly needs correction. In 1988, McNamara and Ellis[16] established normal cephalometric values based on their sample size of 125 untreated individuals with "ideal" occlusal and facial relationships. It was stressed in this particular study that infinite combinations of dentoskeletal relationships could lead to normal values; again, these cephalometric "norms" were not numbers to treat to, but rather "guides for the clinical assessment of the patient. The final diagnosis and treatment plan will rely on a number of other factors that cannot be obtained from a radiograph." Taking into account that different researchers and clinicians have established their own cephalometric analyses, the McNamara and Ellis study aimed to evaluate the parameters from some of the more popular analyses, including Steiner, Downs, and McNamara. The results of this study continue to substantiate the norms established by the creators of the different cephalometric analyses and further prove that there is large variation as to how an individual may reach a point of ideal facial and dental esthetics when evaluating the dentoskeletal relationships (Figures 28.14 and 28.15).

When treating adults, orthodontically, the practitioner must be keenly aware that faces change with age and that there are several very predictable facial features we should consider when doing treatment planning. In 2009, Desai et al.[17] concluded that, after looking at 221 subjects placed into five age groups, "a significant decrease of 1.5–2 mm in maxillary display at smile was found with increasing age. Similarly, upper lip thickness also decreases by 1.5 mm at rest and at smile." In addition, "no subject in the 50 and over age group had a high smile and no subject 15–19 year group had a low smile. Most subjects (78%) had average smile height." Their conclusions were that the smile gets narrower vertically and wider transversely, and this is due to the decreasing ability of a subject's facial muscles to frame a smile with increasing age. For orthodontists, this is critical evidence in determining what harmony must exist between the hard and soft tissues of the lower face. For instance, gingival height discrepancies are of less importance in an adult that shows no gingiva on full smile compared with a teenage patient who shows full incisors plus a small amount of soft tissue. Although we strive for perfection in all of our patients, the amount of reveal of the

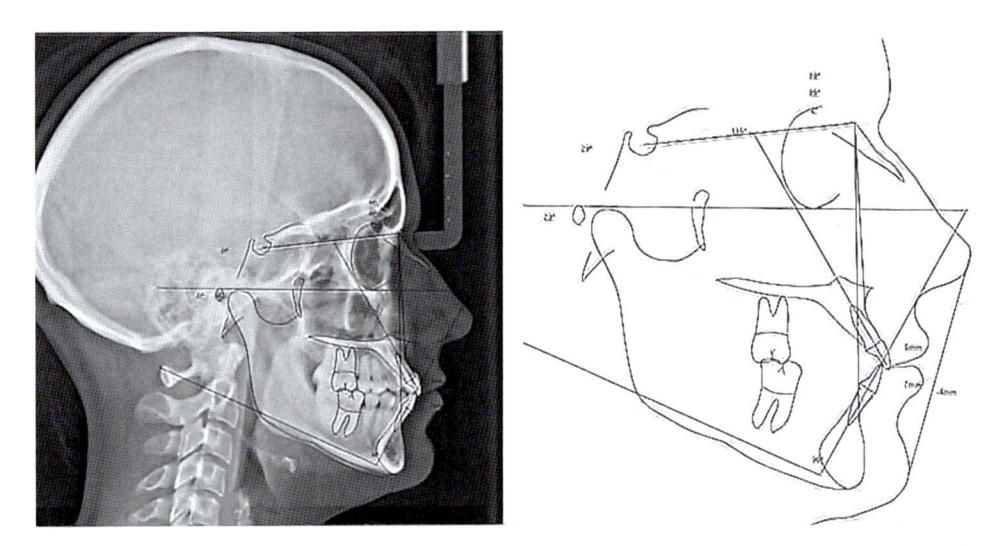

Figure 28.14 Cephalometric analyses are used to evaluate the formation of the facial skeleton, jaw relationships, axial inclination of the incisors, soft-tissue morphology, and growth patterns. Cephalometric norms for various ethnic and racial groups are available and should be used in the analysis.

Measurement Name	Norm (American white)
SNA	82°
SNB	80°
ANB	2°
1̲-NA	4 mm
1̄-NB	4 mm
1̲ to 1̄	131°
GoGn - SN	32°
1̄-MnPl	93°
1̲-|FH	62°
Y axis	61°

Figure 28.15 Steiner cephalometric norm measurements: sample population, white North American children and young adults.

anterior teeth in the adult smile can be a compromise in the adult patient (Figures 28.16, 28.17, and 28.18).

Within the past decade, one treatment modality that has been highly sought after in the world of plastic surgery has crept into the world of dentistry: the use of Botox. Botox has historically been used to help alleviate some of the effects of aging, namely wrinkles and frown lines. However, within the past decade, dentists have found a novel use for it in treating one of the most difficult problems in facial esthetics, the "gummy smile." The gummy smile can be attributed to being caused by several different etiologies: delayed passive eruption, vertical maxillary excess, and a hyperfunctional upper lip musculature. Traditional methods of treating these etiologies have consisted of periodontal osseous recontouring, orthognathic surgery impacting the maxilla, or simply patient restriction of their full smile. A gummy smile has been reported to truly affect one's self-esteem, making them incredibly self-conscious about smiling and embarrassed in social settings. As such, Dr Mario Polo[18] published a study in 2008 relating to the use of Botox in the correction of excessive gingival display during smiling that was of neuromuscular origin, meaning a hyperfunctioning lip. His sample of 30 patients was injected with 2.5 units of Botox on the right and left sides of their faces in several places to hopefully attenuate the activity of the upper lip. Results showed that the average lip drop 2 weeks postinjection was 5.1 mm for the 30 patients. Secondarily, what Dr Polo also found was that the Botox began to be less effective over time, but even at 24 weeks postinjection the gingival display was still less than the baseline. His prediction, based on third-order polynomial equations, was the Botox would not become 100% ineffective until 30–32 weeks postinjection. With this study and results, it is only a matter of time before dental professionals begin to prescribe this possible short-term treatment modality for their patients.

Integrating orthodontics into the interdisciplinary treatment plan

Orthodontics alone can solve many esthetic problems of the face, jaws, and teeth, but many others require an interdisciplinary approach.[19] Such an interdisciplinary approach requires teamwork and constant communication between the restorative dentist and each specialist involved.[20] Failure of effective communication between the practitioners involved results in disjointed and uncoordinated multidisciplinary treatment of the patient rather than a stepwise integrated interdisciplinary treatment, and this lack of communication and consensus can compromise the final esthetic result.

Orthodontics can serve as an adjunct to esthetic restorative treatments in several different ways. One of the most common orthodontic–restorative treatments involves the restoration of peg laterals (Figures 28.19, 28.20, 28.21, and 28.22). Orthodontics can also facilitate restorative treatment in the esthetic zone by extruding teeth (planned for future extraction or as a result of a traumatic injury) to avoid the need for bone grafting prior to placement of an implant to replace that hopeless tooth,[21] aligning incisors to maximize restorative effect, and adjusting vertical

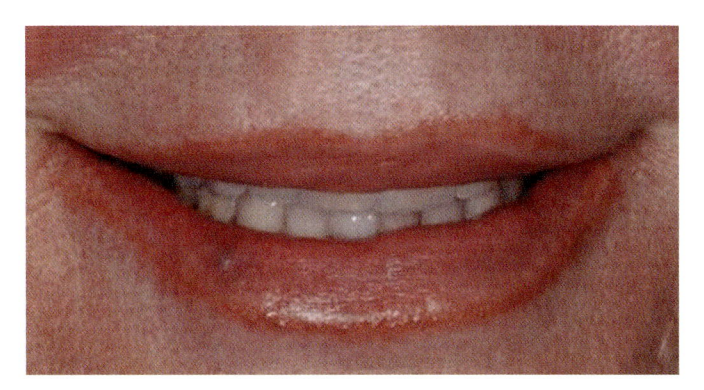

Figure 28.16 Low smile line.

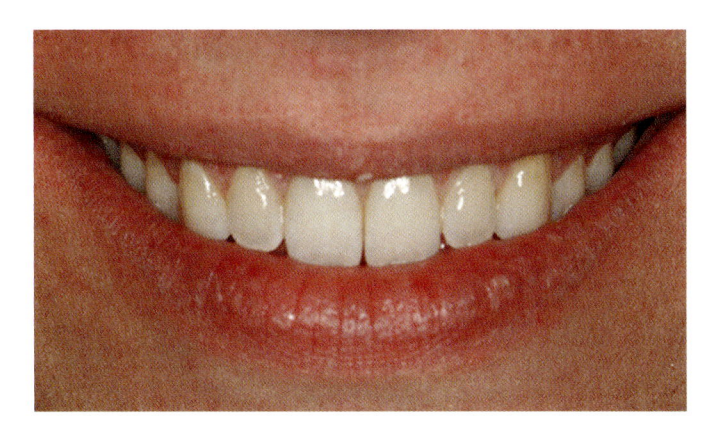

Figure 28.17 Medium smile line.

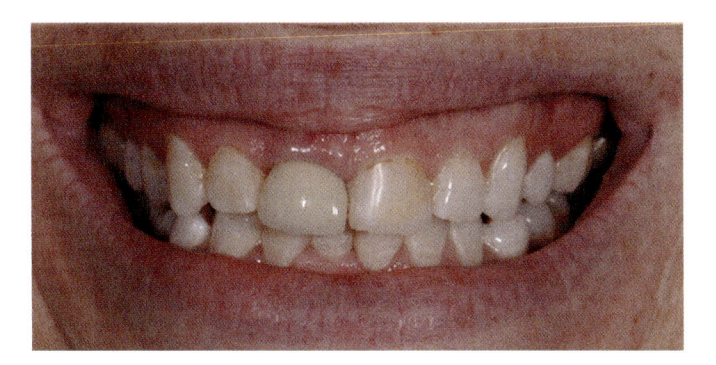

Figure 28.18 High smile line.

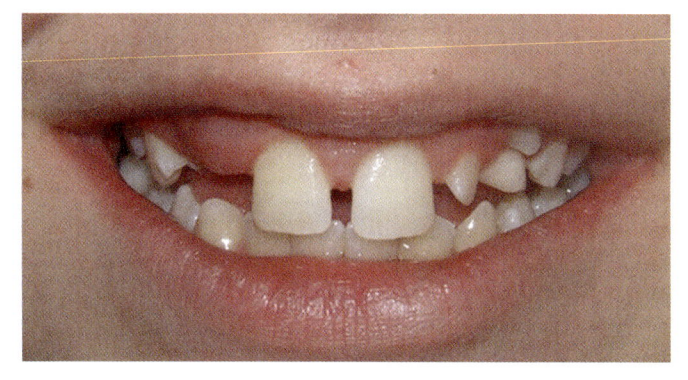

Figure 28.19 Close-up smile of congenitally missing right lateral and pegged left lateral.

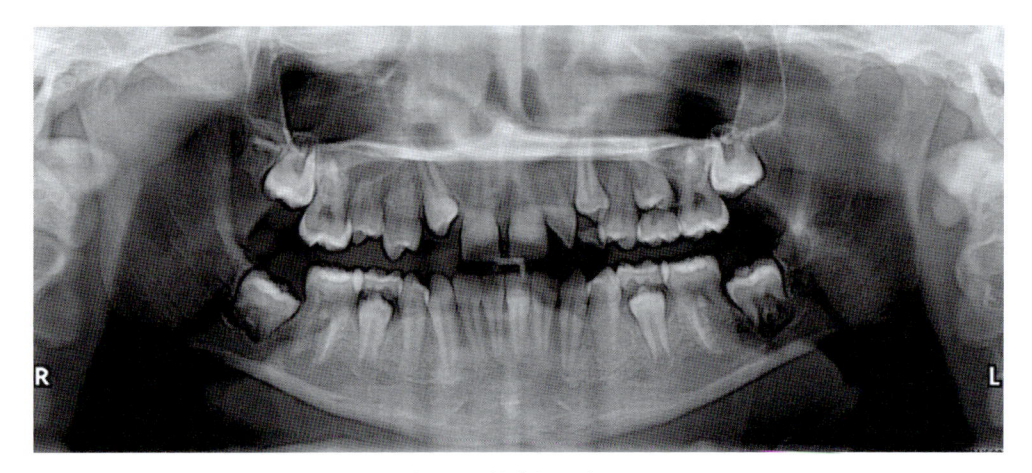

Figure 28.20 Panorex of congenitally missing right lateral and pegged left lateral.

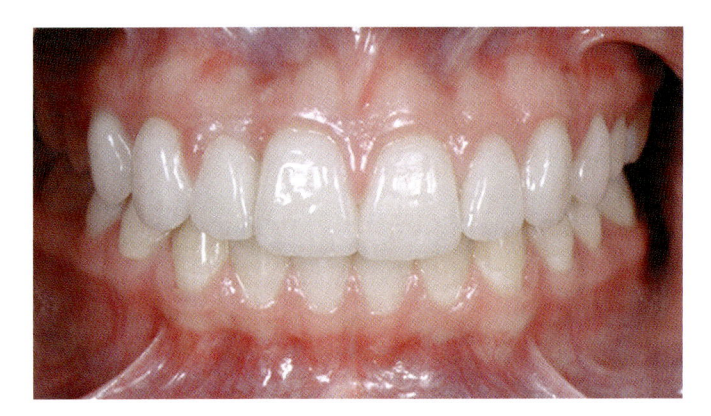

Figure 28.21 Orthodontic–restorative treatment of congenitally missing right lateral and pegged left lateral restored with an acid etch bonded bridge for the maxillary right lateral and veneer maxillary left lateral.

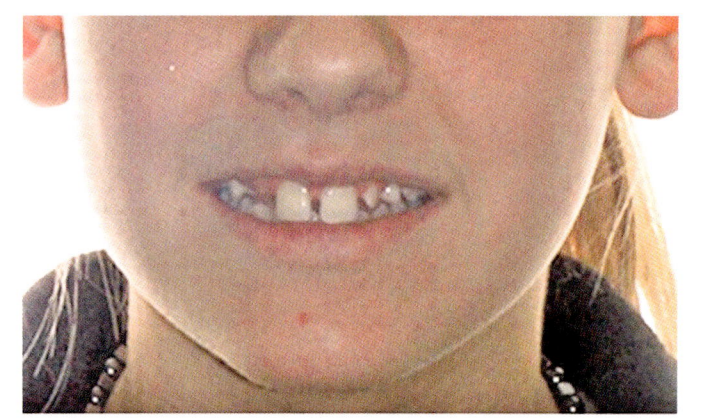

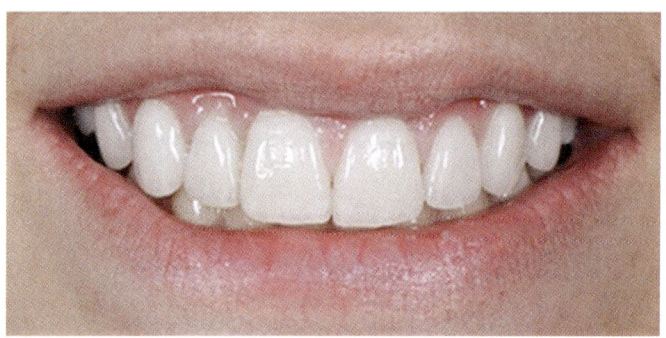

Figure 28.22 Initial and final photographs of the orthodontic–restorative treatment of congenitally missing right lateral and pegged left lateral.

position of teeth to restore symmetry of gingival heights (Figures 28.23, 28.24, 28.25, and 28.26). Kokich and Spear define a series of eight guidelines that, if followed, can help the dental team to integrate orthodontics into the restorative treatment:

1. Establishing realistic treatment objectives.
2. Creating a vision of the treatment outcome.
3. Determining the treatment sequence.
4. Building up small or malformed teeth (i.e., peg laterals).
5. Positioning the teeth in a way that facilitates the planned restorative treatments.
6. Evaluating the gingival esthetics during the orthodontic finishing.
7. Taking radiographs during the orthodontic finishing.
8. Interaction between the orthodontist and the restorative dentist.

When establishing treatment objectives for the orthodontic–restorative patient, "It is important to establish achievable/realistic, not idealistic treatment objectives."[20] Such treatment objectives must be financially realistic, occlusally realistic, and realistic for the restorative dentist. If the team does not establish financially realistic treatment objectives, the patient might be unable to continue with the restorative work following the orthodontic treatment. Because the orthodontist may be unaware of the restorative requirements, and the restorative dentist may have difficulty visualizing the possibilities of orthodontic treatment, the team should use a diagnostic wax setup to illustrate the possibilities and requirements of each stage of treatment[20] (Figures 28.27, 28.28, and 28.29).

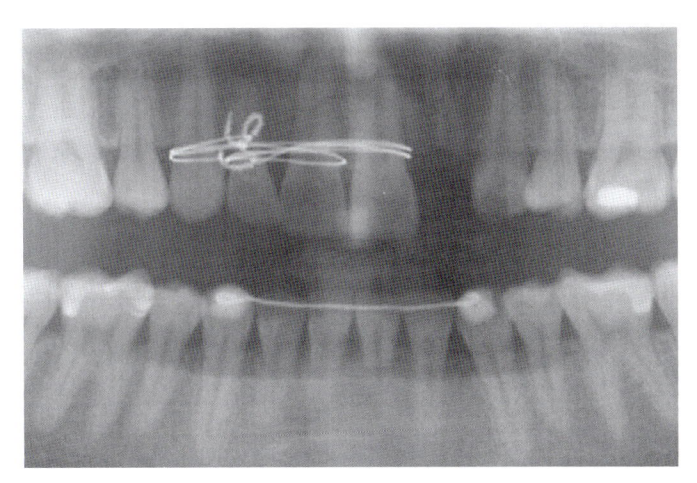

Figure 28.23 Traumatic injury of maxillary lateral. Treatment plan was to promote alveolar bone development by extruding maxillary lateral root, thus avoiding the need for bone grafting prior to implant placement.

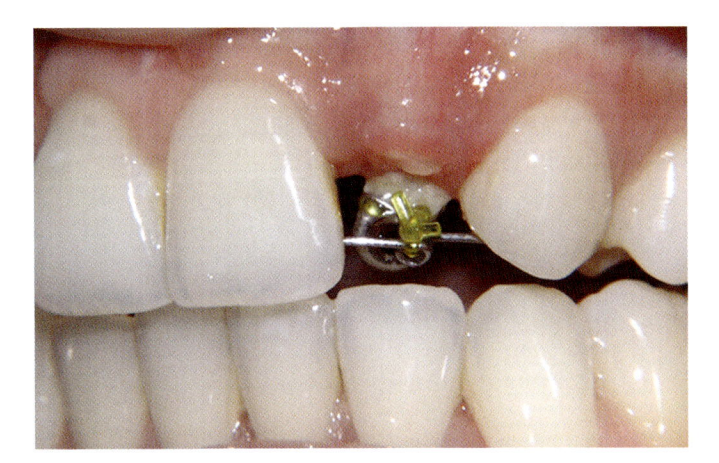

Figure 28.24 Orthodontic lingual appliance to extrude maxillary lateral root.

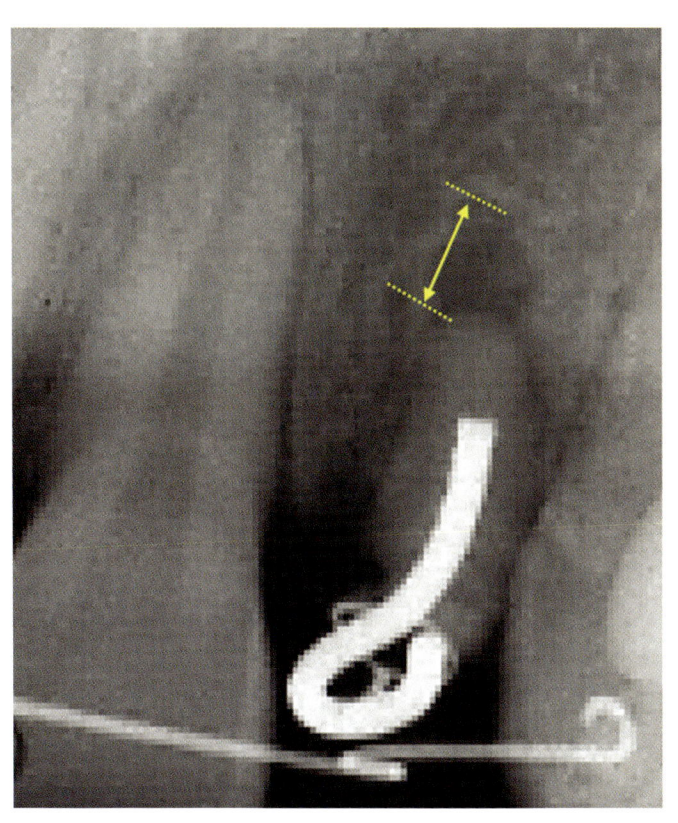

Figure 28.25 Periapical radiograph revealing extrusive movement of maxillary lateral root.

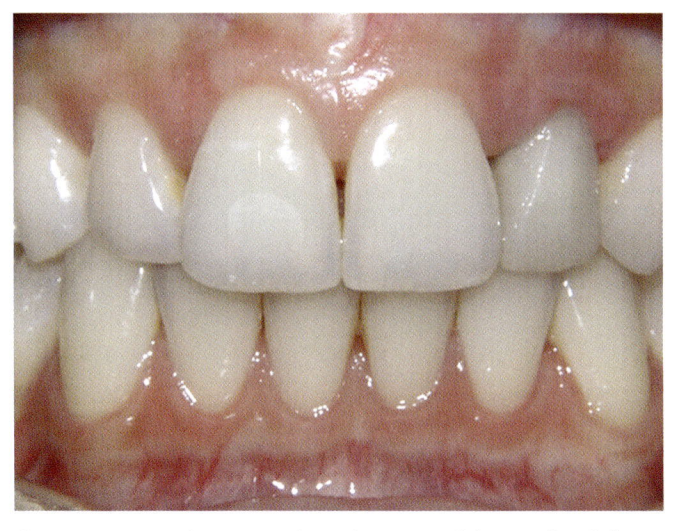

Figure 28.26 Implant/crown for replacement of the maxillary left lateral after orthodontic extrusion as an alternative to bone grafting prior to implant placement.

After setting treatment objectives, creating a vision for treatment, and discussing the treatment plan with the patient, the team must establish a sequence for the treatment. Many orthodontic–restorative patients also require treatment from a periodontist, endodontist, and an oral surgeon. The greater the number of specialists involved, the more complex the treatment becomes. Often, the patient must undergo treatment from each specialist at multiple times during the entirety of the treatment. This necessitates that an accurate sequence of treatment be established to avoid each practitioner from operating in a vacuum and carrying out *multi*disciplinary treatment rather than *inter*disciplinary treatment. Each of the participating practitioners should have a copy of the sequence of treatment.[20]

If the patient has small or malformed teeth, such as peg lateral incisors, that are involved in the treatment plan, the issue of when to build these teeth up must be addressed in the treatment sequence. In many instances, the orthodontist will need to create space around these teeth for a proper buildup to be completed by the restoring dentist. This issue is most common in two situations: peg-shaped lateral incisors and retained primary teeth. In the instance of peg lateral incisors, sufficient space may exist prior to initiating orthodontic therapy, and a composite buildup may be completed prior to the orthodontist bonding brackets. More commonly, however, insufficient space exists adjacent to the peg lateral, and the orthodontist must open space for a proper composite buildup. Kokich and Spear raise four key issues that the orthodontist and restorative dentist must discuss related to the positioning of pegged lateral incisors:

1. *How much space is needed for an adequate build-up?* Once this has been determined, the restorative dentist may find it helpful for the orthodontist to open slightly more space than is deemed necessary. This allows easier contouring and polishing of the interproximal surfaces of the buildup. The orthodontist can then close the space during finishing of the case.[20]

2. *Where should the peg lateral incisor be positioned mesiodistally relative to the central incisor and canine?* With the lateral too close to the canine, the restorative dentist must overcontour the mesial surface of the lateral. Because natural lateral incisors have a relatively flat emergence profile on their mesial surfaces and a more convex emergence profile on their distal surfaces, the peg lateral should be positioned closer to the central incisor than to the canine.[20]

3. *Where should the lateral incisor be positioned buccolingually?* The buccolingual position of the lateral depends largely on the type of planned restoration for the peg lateral incisor. If the definitive restoration will be a porcelain crown, the lateral should be positioned in the center of the ridge, with 0.50–0.75 mm of overjet. This helps to minimize unnecessary preparation of the tooth. If the definitive restoration will be a porcelain veneer, the orthodontist should position the lateral lingually so that it contacts the mandibular incisor.[20]

4. *Where should the peg lateral incisor be positioned incisogingivally?* This decision is based on the relationship of the gingival margins. The gingival margin of the peg lateral should be aligned with the contralateral lateral incisor, slightly apical to the gingival margin of the central incisors.[20]

In a patient with a retained primary tooth, the primary tooth may be replaced in the future with an implant. If this is the case, the primary tooth will need to be retained for as long as possible to maintain as much alveolar bone as possible for placement of the implant in the future. The orthodontist should open space mesial and distal to the primary tooth so that the restorative dentist can build up the primary tooth temporarily during the orthodontic treatment. A diagnostic wax-up may be necessary to determine the correct width of the composite restoration.[20]

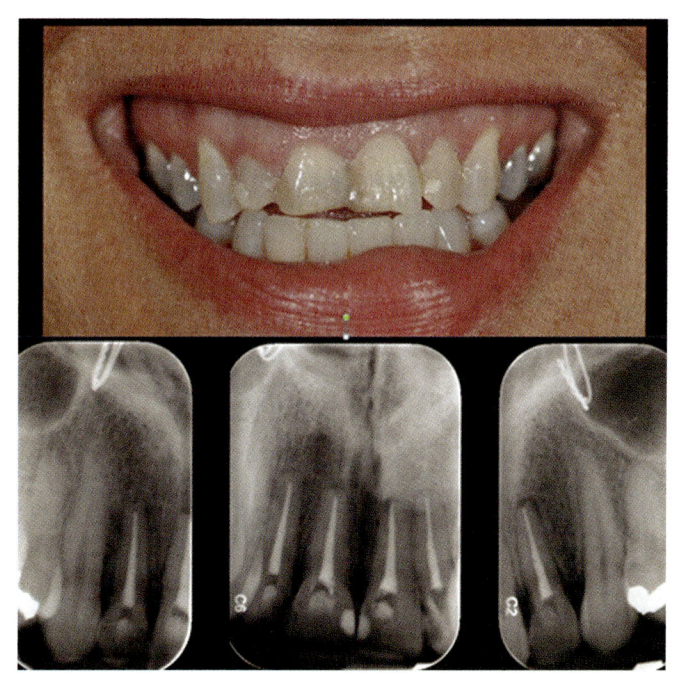

Figure 28.27 Traumatic injury to maxillary anteriors resulting in the need to visualize the treatment possibilities.

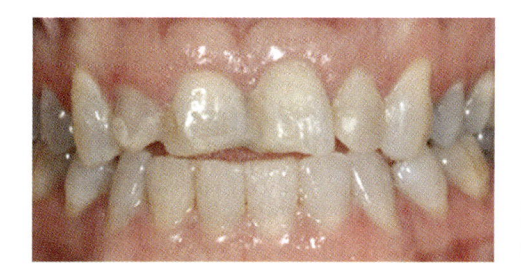

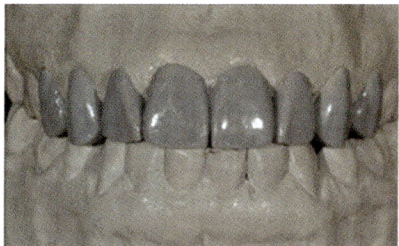

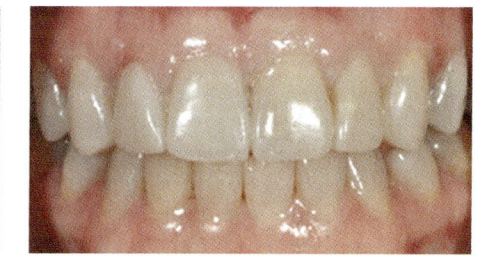

Figure 28.28 Diagnostic setup.

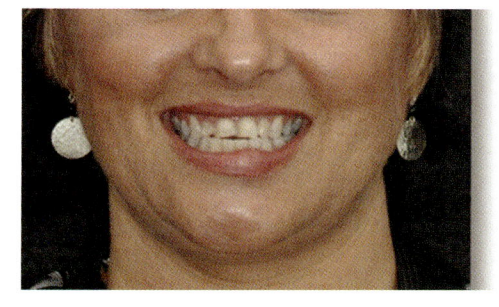

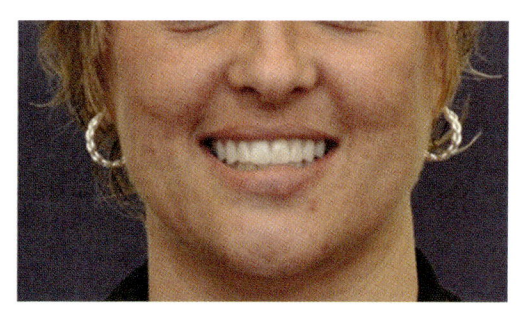

Figure 28.29 Comparison of the pretreatment and final close-up smile after completing an interdisciplinary orthodontic and restorative treatment.

The orthodontist should consider the planned restorative treatment when determining the final position of teeth in the orthodontic–restorative patient. If a resin-bonded bridge is planned, it is important to position the abutment teeth with sufficient overjet and appropriate overbite. With the overbite minimized, more of the lingual surface of the abutment teeth can be covered with the bonded metal framework, increasing the retention of the resin-bonded bridge. Owing to the greater shear strength of the resin-bonded bridge, incisors should be oriented more upright to direct forces on the bridge more vertically. If a conventional anterior fixed partial denture is planned, the orthodontist should create 0.50–0.75 mm of excess overjet. This will allow for material thickness when restoring the missing tooth. In most patients with an abraded anterior dentition, the teeth have supraerupted to accommodate for the attrition, and the incisors are shorter in height than unworn teeth. In such a patient, the orthodontist should intrude the abraded teeth and reestablish the appropriate gingival heights. As the orthodontist is intruding the incisors, the restorative dentist may restore the incisal edges of these teeth.[20]

The orthodontist, restorative dentist, and a periodontist should evaluate the gingival esthetics. Kokich and Spear recommend four criteria for the orthodontist to evaluate (Figure 28.12) as follows:

1. Gingival levels of two central incisors should be at same height.
2. Gingival margin over lateral incisor should be about 0.50 mm incisal to central incisor gingival margin, and the gingival margin of the canines should be at the same height as the central incisor.
3. The labial gingival contour of each tooth should follow the contour of the cementoenamel junction.
4. The interproximal papilla should fill the space gingival to the proximal contact.

While finishing the case, the orthodontist should take radiographs to evaluate root position. While proper root position is important in all orthodontic patients, it becomes even more critical in the orthodontic–restorative patient in whom implants are planned. The orthodontist should be careful to create adequate space between the roots for proper placement of the planned implant. The orthodontists should maintain close contact with the restorative dentist during finishing in the orthodontic–restorative patient so that the restorative dentist has input on the final tooth position prior to restorations.[20]

Technological advances in orthodontics

There have been many technological advances in orthodontics that have enhanced the orthodontic treatment of patients seeking esthetic enhancement. These advances have come in ceramic brackets, self-ligating brackets, clear aligners, CBCT, digital photography, digital models, and three-dimensional photography. The advances in ceramic brackets to reduce the friction, enhance debonding protocols, and decrease the bulk of brackets have made them a more viable option for the patient concerned with the appearance of traditional braces.[22] Newer, self-ligating ceramic brackets have even been shown to have less friction than traditionally ligated metal brackets.[22] Many have claimed that the lower level of friction associated with self-ligating brackets results in faster initial alignment, shorter overall treatment time, and fewer patient visits to the orthodontist; however, more research is needed to substantiate such claims.[23,24] Along with tooth-colored brackets, tooth-colored wires have become a more viable option for use in the esthetic-minded patient. While some of these esthetic archwires have been fabricated from various silica polymers, newer esthetic archwires are metallic archwires coated with polymers such as Teflon and epoxy resin. These esthetic archwires have been shown to be rougher than their metallic counterparts, and the coatings may affect their three-point bending properties.[25]

Other, less visible orthodontic appliances have also made substantial advances. Customized lingual brackets and wires can be fabricated using computer-aided design/manufacturing technology and have been shown to be an accurate means of positioning teeth.[26] These appliances have the esthetic benefit of being virtually invisible to the patient and third parties, but have the disadvantage of being extremely expensive and sometimes difficult to manipulate. Another esthetic treatment option is a clear aligner system, commonly referred to as clear aligner therapy. While anecdotal evidence and advertising claims are strongly in favor of the treatment effects of such systems, neither the treatment indications nor the limitations of clear aligner therapy have been defined or supported with scientific evidence.[27] This leaves clinicians to rely on the experience of respected colleagues, personal clinical experience, and advertising claims when using clear aligner therapy.

Other technologies have enhanced the communication and treatment planning capabilities between specialists and the restorative dentist. CBCT three-dimensional radiographs have enhanced the ability of orthodontists and oral surgeons to locate impacted teeth[28] (Figure 28.30). Three-dimensional imaging enhances the treatment planning for patients with impacted maxillary canines, and helps the orthodontist and restorative dentist decide whether to bring an impacted canine into the arch or have it extracted and replaced with a prosthesis. Digital photographs and radiographs have made communication easier between orthodontist and the restorative dentist, with the two being able to send images to each other easily and inexpensively.[29,30] As digital models have become more widely available and affordable, accurate measurements are able to be made by multiple practitioners on a single set of models[31] (Figure 28.31). With CBCT, digital models, and three-dimensional photography[32] (Figure 28.32), a virtual patient that practitioners could use to make treatment decisions is on the horizon.

Periodontal considerations with adult orthodontic treatment

With an increasing number or adults seeking orthodontic treatment, periodontal concerns have become a major consideration for treating adult patients. In 1985–1986, a national survey of adults showed 8% of employed adults aged greater than

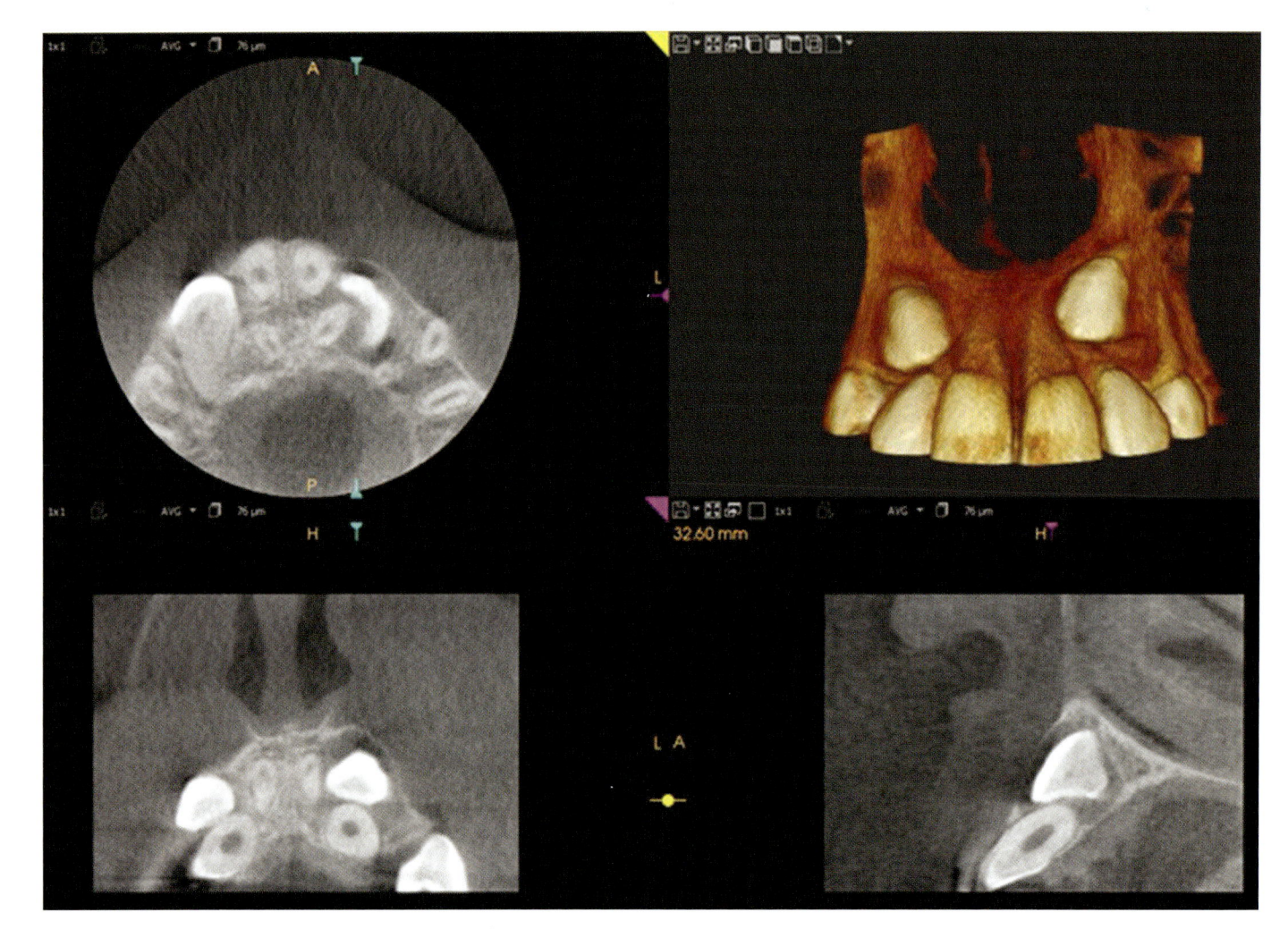

Figure 28.30 CBCT, CS 3D imaging Carestream Dental.

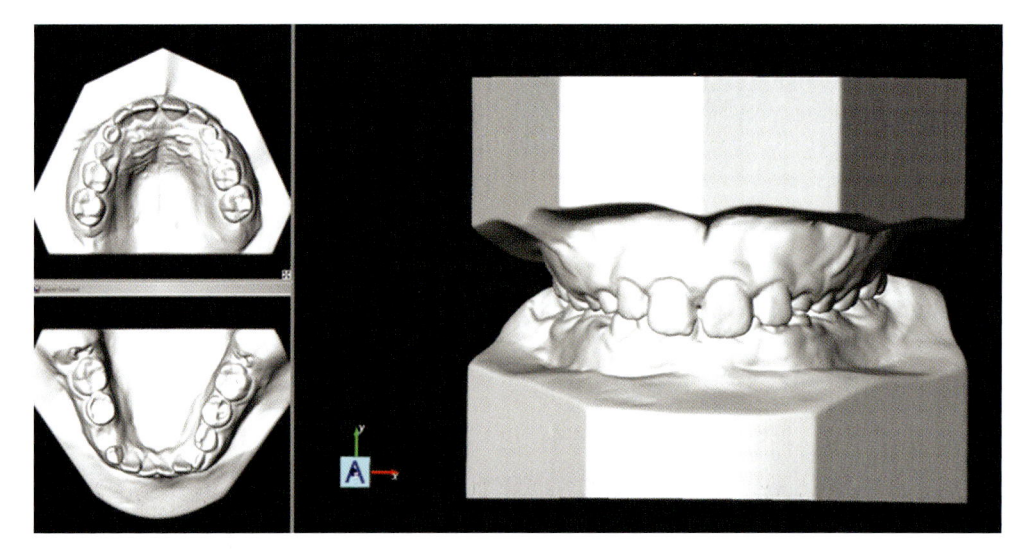

Figure 28.31 Digital models by Ortho Insight 3D™ by Motion View Software, LLC.

or equal to 18 years and 34% of retired adults aged greater than or equal to 65 years had at least one periodontal site with greater than or equal to 6mm loss of attachment.[33] When an adult patient presents for orthodontic treatment, a clinician must first determine which patients are at risk for developing periodontal disease or have a history of periodontal disease. Despite the high prevalence of periodontal problems in adult patients, orthodontic treatment is not contraindicated as long as the disease process is under control. On the contrary, orthodontics has been shown to improve some periodontal defects and the ability to restore a

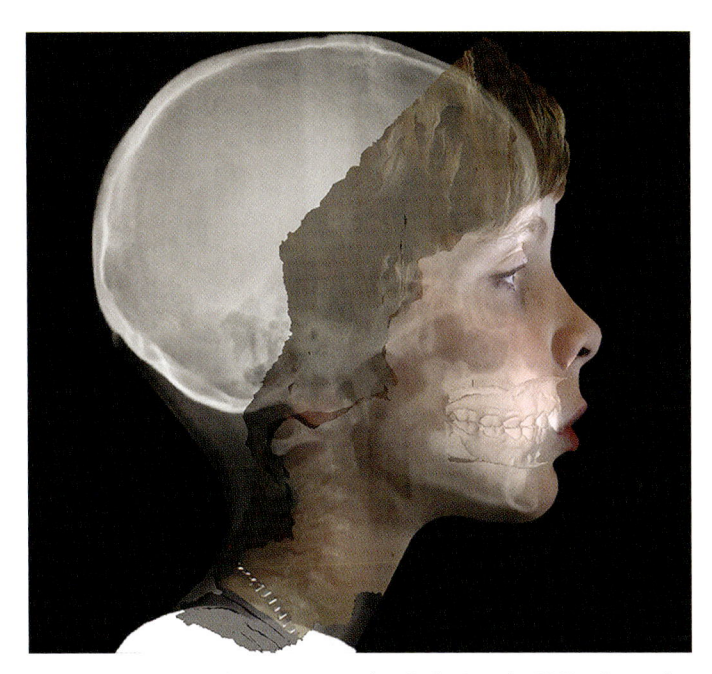

Figure 28.32 Virtual patient created in Ortho Insight 3D™ software by Motion View Software, LLC.

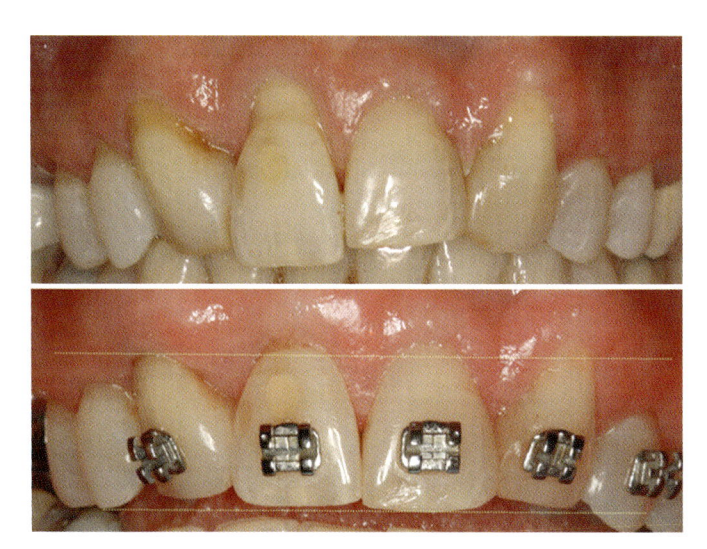

Figure 28.33 Orthodontics and periodontics to improve a compromised dentition.

compromised dentition[34–36] (Figure 28.33). However, considerations such as treatment schedules, tooth movement, tissue response, esthetics, and retention must all be taken into consideration during the treatment planning of adult orthodontic treatment.

Evaluating adult orthodontic patients for risk of periodontal disease during treatment is of utmost importance. Aside from pretreatment records and close communication with the patient's general dentist and periodontist, several recommendations have been made concerning adult orthodontic patients. The first involves a thorough medical and dental history. Important questions that should be answered on the patient's history include the interval at which the patient receives regular dental care, use of tobacco products, history of diabetes and other metabolic diseases, a list of their medications, and a history of past periodontal treatment. Intraoral radiographs are another important screening tool to help assess risk and disease. These radiographs should include anterior periapical radiographs and posterior bitewing radiographs. Radiographs not only allow a clinician to assess the periodontal condition of the patient, but also establish a baseline at the start of treatment. Clinical exam, including full-mouth periodontal probing, is also recommended to help assess periodontal risks and disease (Figure 28.34). Appropriate measures should be taken if a patient demonstrates periodontal disease or be at risk of developing periodontal disease.

Treatment planning patients with a history of periodontal disease must receive major attention prior to initiating orthodontic treatment. It is recommended to allow at least 2–6 months after the last periodontal therapy to ensure proper periodontal tissue remodeling.[37] Regenerative periodontal techniques are usually implemented prior to orthodontic treatment, but some studies indicate that it may be performed after treatment.[38–41]

In patients with thin attached gingiva, it is often recommended to improve the tissue width before labial orthodontic movement in an attempt to prevent the development of bony dehiscences.[42–44] Timing of preventative surgical measures ranges from several weeks to 6 months and needs to be further investigated to establish guidelines.[45] Whatever the recommended treatment prior to orthodontics, it is critical for the patient to exhibit sound oral hygiene to minimize risks and optimize treatment results.

During orthodontic treatment of adults with a history of periodontal problems, it is recommended that the patient continues regular periodontal maintenance.[37] The maintenance intervals should be determined based on the patient's risks and the planned tooth movements. If a patient fails to maintain good oral hygiene practices, treatment may be discontinued at the clinician's discretion. Procedures that are considered elective (i.e., frenectomy, esthetic recontouring, etc.) should be completed at the end of orthodontic treatment when the final positions of hard and soft tissues can be determined.[46–48] Despite proper planning and preventative periodontal treatments to help reduce anticipated problems in patients with a history of periodontal disease, the adult periodontium can respond unpredictably to forces placed on teeth.

As a result of the current ability to control orthodontic forces on teeth, force systems can be adjusted for the needs of adult patients. Adult patients may have experienced alveolar bone loss and a reduced periodontium over time, thus positioning the center of resistance more apically. As a result of a more apical center of resistance, it is more likely for a tooth to be tipped and extruded rather than bodily moved.[49,50] Therefore, it is recommended to use light forces of between 30 and 60 gf per tooth, often using segmental arch mechanics (Figures 28.35 and 28.36).[51,52] Treatment time is often prolonged due to the complexity of treatment mechanics and the age of the patient.[53]

In adult patients, tooth movement may become slower due to the lack of collagen conversion and cell mobilization.[53] Adults also form hyalinized zones more easily on the pressure side of

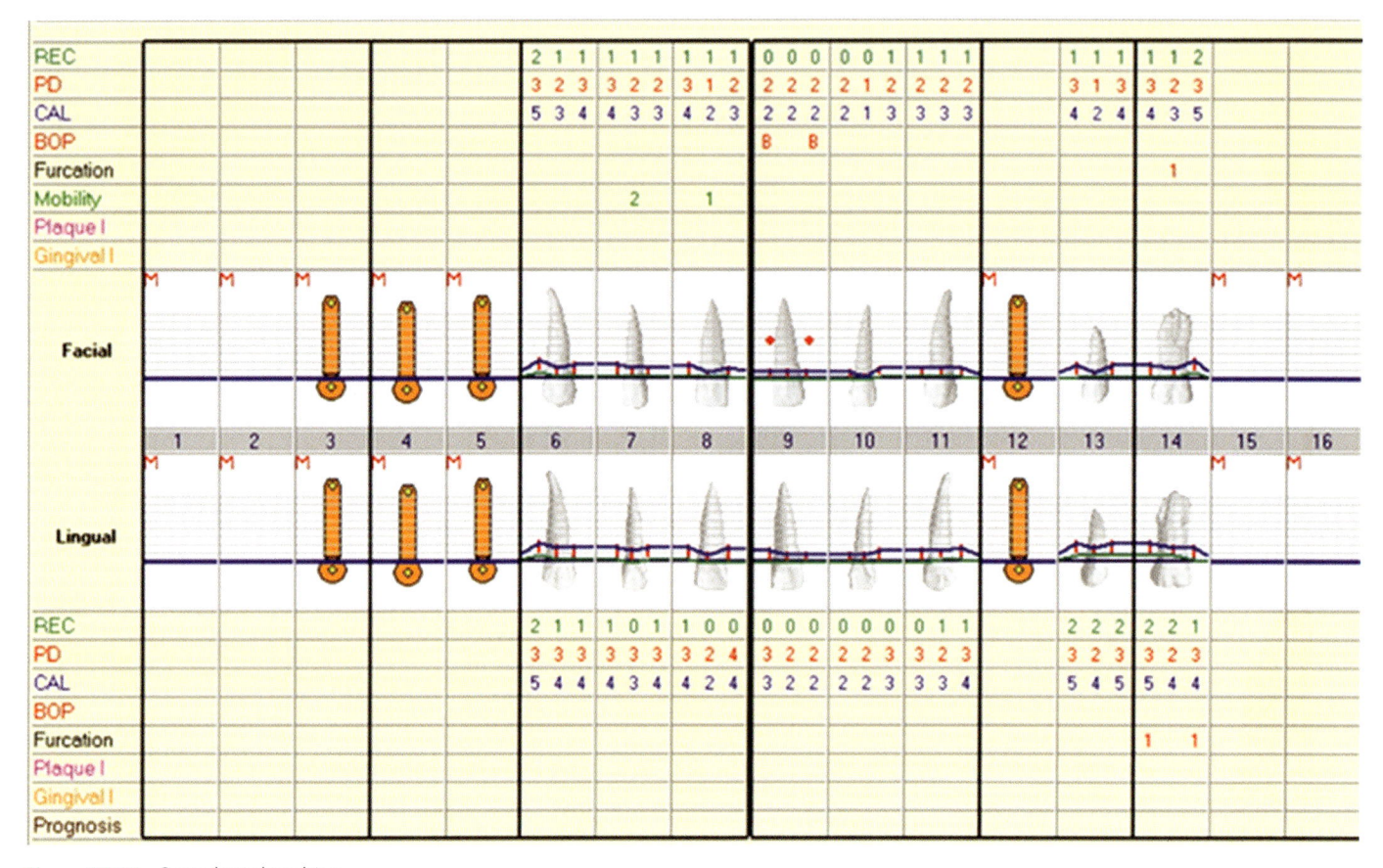

Figure 28.34 Periodontal probing.

Types of Tooth Movement	Force (grams)
Tipping	30–60
Rotation	30–60
Root Uprighting	50–100
Translation	70–120
Extrusion	30–60
Intrusion	5–20

Force requirements will vary based on the available root area (single versus multirooted). Reduced periodontal support will alter the center of resistance of a tooth. As the center of resistance moves apically, the magnitude of the tipping moment produced is equal to the force times the distance from the point of force application to the center of resistance. As the distance of force application to center of resistance increases, force levels should be lighter.

Figure 28.35 Forces systems. Reproduced with permission of Elsevier.

tooth movement, thus initially preventing the tooth from being moved to the intended position.[54] Once the hyalinized zone (acellular) is eliminated by periodontal ligament regeneration, tooth movement may continue.[55] Throughout the history of orthodontics, there have been attempts to overcome the factors that contribute to delayed tooth movement. In recent times, periodontally accelerated osteogenic orthodontics (PAOO), also known as Wilckodontics, has gained attention in the field of orthodontics.

PAOO is a treatment technique that uses full-flap periodontal surgery to improve osseous contours and mechanical injury to bone surrounding teeth to induce cell mobilization needed for tooth movement (Figures 28.37 and 28.38). To date, numerous case presentations have shown decreased treatment times in adult patients, but long-term controlled data are lacking.

Improving dental and facial esthetics has been shown to be the primary motivating factor for adult patients seeking orthodontic

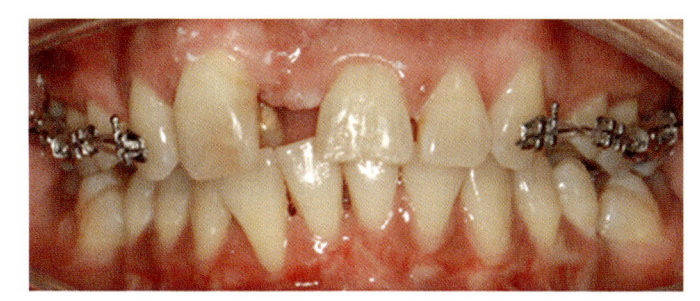

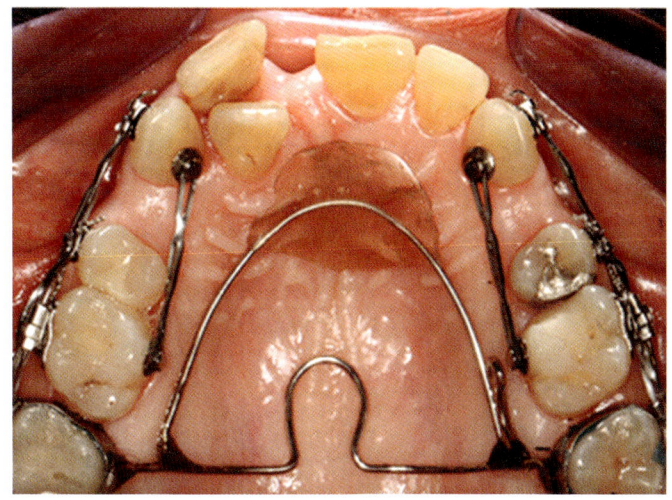

Figure 28.36 Segmental mechanics.

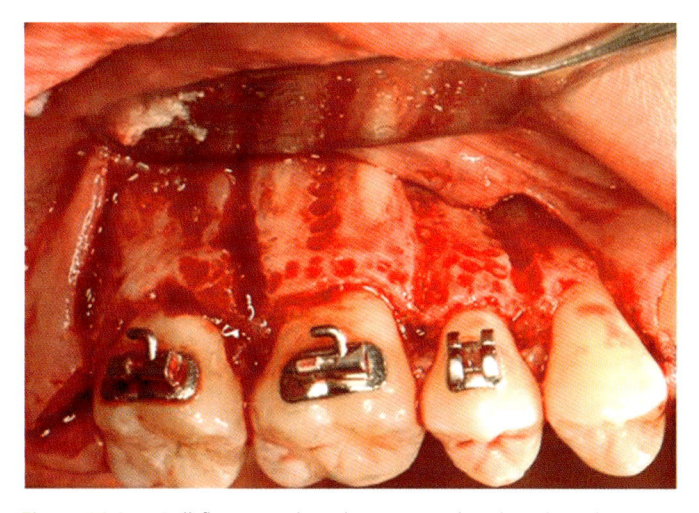

Figure 28.37 Full-flap periodontal surgery with induced mechanical injury to induce cell mobilization needed for tooth movement.

treatment.[56] Gingival tissues play an integral part in dental esthetics and should be considered during orthodontic treatment planning in adult patients. Two problems that may develop during orthodontic treatment concerning gingival tissues include gingival margin discrepancies and lack of interdental papilla, also known as "black triangles."[57]

The gingival margins are the negative space that frames the clinical crown. For optimal esthetics, it has been noted that the central incisors and canines should share the same gingival margin height. The lateral incisors should be placed slightly coronal to the gingival margins of the central incisors and canines (see

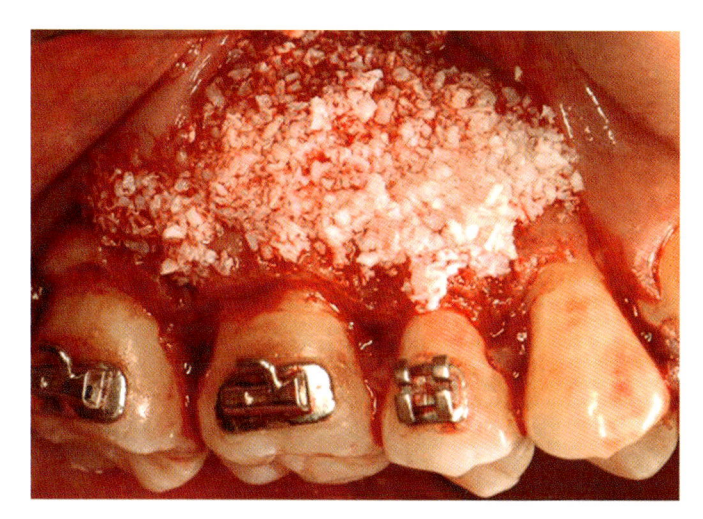

Figure 28.38 PAOO: a surgical procedure that combines selective alveolar corticotomy, particulate bone grafting, and the application of orthodontic forces.

Figure 28.51).[57] The labial margins should also mimic the contours of the cementoenamel junction. When gingival margins are less than ideal, the clinician must make one of two decisions: orthodontically attempt to reposition the gingival margin, or surgical reposition the gingival margin. It must be noted that if the gingival margins are hidden by the upper lip upon smiling, there is no need to reposition the gingival margins to an ideal position. If the gingival margins are displayed upon smiling, the next step is to determine the labial sulcus depth of the central incisors. If the shorter of the teeth has a deeper sulcus depth, gingival surgery may be indicated to lengthen the shorter tooth. If they have the same sulcular depth, gingival surgery will not correct the problem. It is also important to compare the shortest central incisor with the lateral incisors. If the shortest central incisor is longer than the lateral incisors, it may be possible to extrude the longer incisor and equilibrate the incisal edge. On the contrary, if the shortest central incisor is the same size or smaller than the lateral incisor, extruding and equilibrating the longer incisor will produce suboptimal esthetics. The next step is to determine whether the incisal edges have been abraded. If the edges are thicker than the adjacent teeth due to attrition, it may be indicated to intrude the teeth to allow for proper restoration.[57] The gingival margin is also formed by the papilla, or lack thereof.

For optimal esthetics, there should be papilla between each tooth and the tip should extend halfway between the incisal edge and labial gingival height of contour over the center of each anterior tooth. In some adult patients, the papilla may be absent, creating the appearance of "black triangles" (Figure 28.39). The lack of papilla may be due to several problems. The first problem involves divergent roots. If the roots are divergent, the brackets may be placed parallel to the long axis of the tooth or a bend may be placed in the tooth to help produce more parallel roots. Another cause may involve abnormal tooth shape. If this is the case, the tooth may be recontoured interproximally to help eliminate the space. In patients with lack of papilla due to the destruction of crestal bone, the mesial contours of the central incisors may be flattened to move the contact more distally, creating a larger contact point. Although this may not completely eliminate the negative space from the lack of papilla, it will most likely improve the esthetics significantly (Figure 28.40).[45,57] After optimal esthetics is achieved, it is important to create and maintain a stable periodontium to prevent relapse (Figure 28.41).

Gingival tissues are compressed in the direction of tooth movement, creating an increase in elasticity that is often associated with orthodontic relapse.[58] Periodontal fibers have been shown to undergo rearrangement even after a retention period of 4–6 months.[59,60]

It is recommended to allow at least 12 months of retention to provide appropriate time for remodeling of periodontal fibers.[61] Stability of periodontal tissues has shown to have been accomplished by long-term fixed retention, adjunctive periodontal surgery, orthodontic overcorrection, or a combination of the latter two (Figure 28.41).[62,63]

Orthodontically treated patients with significantly reduced periodontal support are in need of definitive retention.[64] Fixed retention as a means of permanent splinting is often preferred to removable retention due to unwanted forces exerted by insertion and removal of the removal retainer.[49] Retention may also involve prosthetic reconstruction in patients with loss of teeth, occlusal trauma, progressive mobility, or pain in function.[45,65]

Adjunctive periodontal procedures may also be advised to help improve stability in orthodontically treated patients.

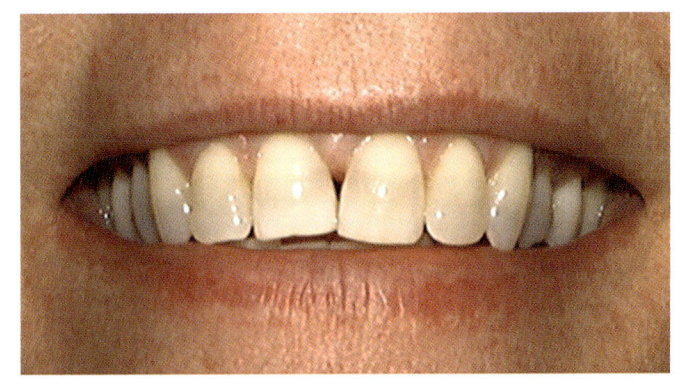

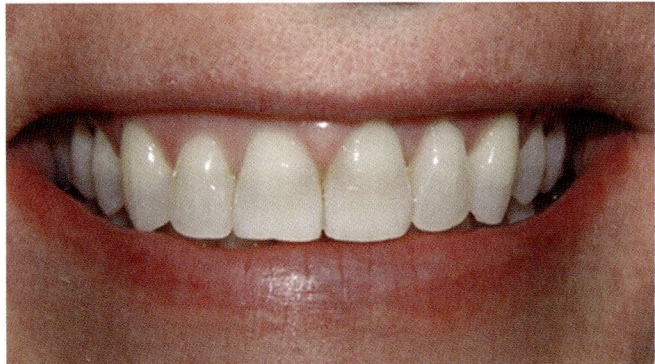

Figure 28.39 Absence of papilla, resulting in "black triangle."

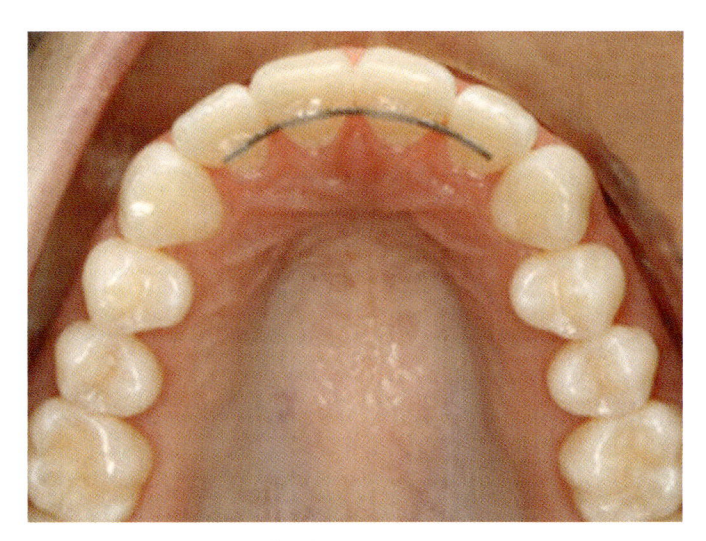

Figure 28.41 Long-term fixed retainer.

Base of proximal contact to Bone Crest	Presence of interdental papilla
5 mm	98%
6 mm	56%
7 mm	27%

Figure 28.40 Presence of interdental papilla. Reproduced with permission of John Wiley and Sons.

Periodontal surgery may help provide stability to an orthodontically treated dentition. The cause–effect relationship between a thick frenum with a high insertion and maxillary midline diastema is well documented.[66] Therefore, it is often advisable to perform a frenectomy after closure of a midline diastema caused by prominent frenum.[45] Other periodontal procedures, such as circumferential fiberotomy of supracrestal gingival fibers (CSF), have been effective preventing relapse of teeth that were severely rotated prior to treatment.[67,68] CSF should be done toward the finishing stages of orthodontic treatment, since studies have shown that relapse can occur as soon as 5 h after removal of orthodontic appliances.[59,69] Long-term studies have shown CSF to be more effective in alleviating pure rotational relapse than in labiolingual relapse and more effective in the maxillary anterior segment than in the mandibular anterior segment.[68]

Occlusal considerations for the adult orthodontic patient

Although a consensus exists among restorative dentists, periodontists, and orthodontists on the parameters of an "ideal" occlusion, when evaluating the occlusion of an adult orthodontic patient the occlusal goals must be determined on a patient-by-patient basis. Many adults present for orthodontic treatment with a myriad of preexisting conditions that can make achieving an "ideal" occlusion challenging and even detrimental to either the esthetics or functional integrity of the patient's occlusal health. For these adult patients, the goal should be to achieve a "compromised and sustainable" occlusion.

Such a compromised goal should be clearly understood by all parties involved that includes a signed understanding by the patient of the intended outcome.

Ideal static occlusion: an historical and contemporary perspective

One of the classic papers on evaluating static occlusion is by Lawrence F. Andrews, wherein he outlines six characteristics that were noted in a study of 120 casts of nonorthodontic patients with normal occlusion.[70]

Normal occlusion was determined by teeth which, "(1) had never had orthodontic treatment, (2) were straight and pleasing in appearance, (3) had a bite which looked generally correct, and (4) in my [Andrews'] judgment would not benefit from orthodontic treatment."[70] The six keys were also validated by studying 1150 treated orthodontic cases that were presented at national orthodontic meetings, and it was found that the lack of one of the six keys of occlusion was an error that was predictive of an incomplete end result in the treated cases.[70] Andrews' six keys of occlusion are as follows:

1. Angle Class I molar relationship and the distal surface of the distobuccal cusp of the upper first molar occluded with the mesial surface of the mesiobuccal cusp of the lower second molar.
2. Mesial inclination of the incisal aspect of the crown (toward the midline).
3. Ideal crown inclination (labiolingual or buccolingual) of maxillary and mandibular anterior teeth and lingual inclination of the crowns of maxillary and mandibular posterior teeth.
4. Teeth should be free of undesirable rotations.
5. No spacing present, with tight contact points.
6. Flat to slight curve of Spee.[70]

The current reference that many orthodontists use to evaluate whether they have achieved an ideal static occlusion is the standards set forth by the ABO.[71] The criteria that the ABO use to evaluate posttreatment results of orthodontic treatment are as follows:

1. Alignment. The incisal edges of the maxillary and mandibular anteriors are evaluated as the lingual surfaces of the maxillary anteriors and the labial–incisal surfaces of the mandibular anteriors.[71] In the maxillary posterior segments, the central groove is evaluated, whereas in the mandibular posterior segments the buccal cusps are used for evaluation.[71]
2. Marginal ridges must be leveled.
3. Buccolingual inclination. There should not be significant differences between the heights of the buccal and lingual cusps of the maxillary and mandibular molars and premolars.
4. Occlusal relationship. The mesiobuccal cusp on the maxillary first molar must align within 1 mm of the buccal groove of the mandibular first molar, and the buccal cusps of the maxillary molars, premolars, and canines must align within 1 mm of the interproximal embrasures of the mandibular posterior teeth.
5. Occlusal contact between the lingual cusps of maxillary dentition and occlusal contact of the buccal cusps of the mandibular dentition with their complementary arches' marginal ridges/fossae.
6. Proper buccal overjet in the posterior segments and proper mandibular incisal edge contact with the lingual surfaces of the maxillary anterior teeth.
7. Interproximal contact between adjacent teeth.
8. Proper angulation of the roots of teeth such that they closely parallel each other and are perpendicular to the occlusal plane, allowing sufficient interradicular bone between adjacent teeth.[71]

What is the ideal functional occlusal scheme?

Dentists and orthodontists alike both seek to find the ideal functional occlusal scheme for their patients that will provide them with the best opportunity to function in the short and long term in an efficient, sustainable, symptom-free manner. This search has led to many different viewpoints as to which functional occlusal scheme truly is "ideal." Popular functional occlusal schemes include the following:

1. Canine protected occlusion (CPO). Only the canines contact on the working side during eccentric lateral mandibular movements with no nonworking contacts.

2. Group function. Multiple posterior teeth contact on the working side during eccentric lateral mandibular movements with no nonworking contacts.
3. Balanced occlusion. Multiple posterior teeth contact on the working and nonworking sides during eccentric lateral mandibular movements. CPO and group function are the two theories that predominate current thinking, with certain individuals believing that one occlusal scheme is superior to the other.

In order to determine which, if any, functional occlusal scheme is superior, we must look at the relevant literature to practice evidence-based decision making, which is the standard of care. Rinchuse et al. performed an exhaustive and comprehensive review of the literature (172 different books/articles) concerning functional occlusion and found the following:[72]

1. A single type of functional occlusion has not been demonstrated to predominate in nature.
2. CPO as the optimal type of functional occlusion to establish in orthodontic patients is equivocal and unsupported by the evidence-based literature.
3. CPO might be merely one of several possible optimal functional occlusion types toward which to direct orthodontic patients' treatments.
4. Group function occlusion and balanced occlusion (with no interferences) appear to be acceptable functional occlusion schemes, depending on the patient's characteristics.
5. The stability and longevity of CPO is questionable (i.e., as the cusp tip of the canine wears over a patient's life, CPO can change to group function).

Achieving a "realistically ideal" occlusion in adult orthodontic patients

Certain conditions prevalent in some adults may prevent practitioners from achieving the aforementioned criteria that are used to define an ideal static and functional occlusion. These conditions can include skeletal discrepancies, missing/extracted teeth, existing prosthetic appliances (such as dental implants), an altered vertical dimension of occlusion (VDO), and previous or existing periodontal disease.[73] These conditions, along with the patient's level of motivation for treatment, must be taken into account when the pretreatment occlusal goals are set. Thus, determining the occlusal scheme that is "realistically ideal" for each individual patient, based upon their pretreatment condition and motivation for treatment, is vital to developing a treatment plan that can be successfully achieved (Figures 28.42, 28.43, 28.44, 28.45, and 28.46).[73]

In adult patients with significant skeletal discrepancies, growth modification to help correct these discrepancies is not a treatment option. Therefore, the practitioner and the patient are left with two options to help correct the discrepancy: orthognathic surgery or dental compensation. The patient needs to be informed in cases in which the dental camouflage that must be made to compensate for the skeletal discrepancy will result in

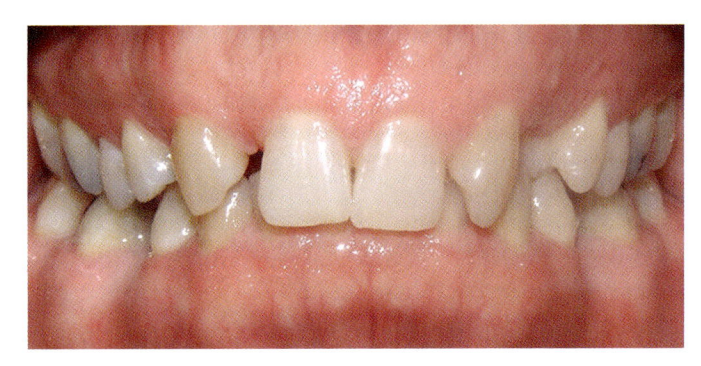

Figure 28.42 Malocclusion requiring realistic treatment plan and occlusal scheme.

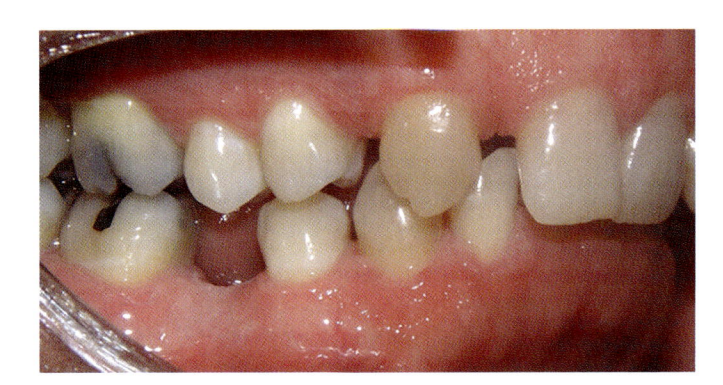

Figure 28.43 Malocclusion/occlusal scheme right.

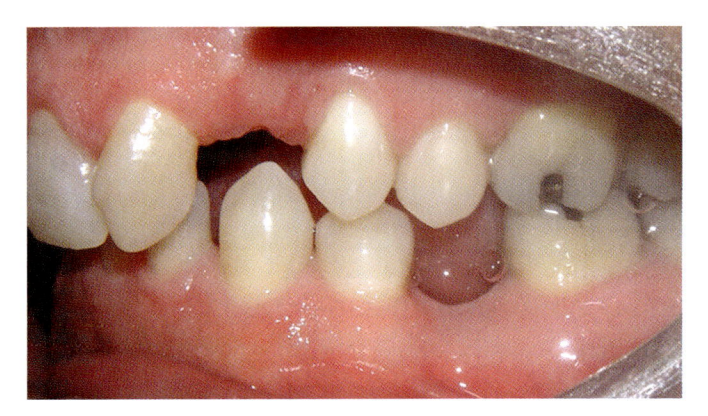

Figure 28.44 Malocclusion/occlusal scheme left.

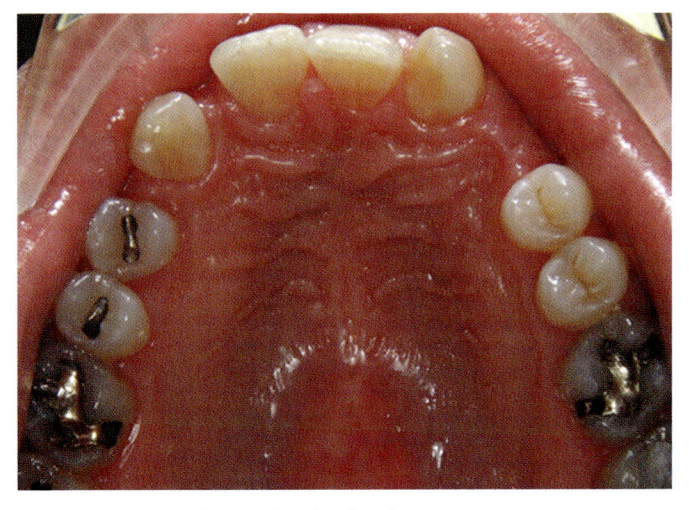

Figure 28.45 Maxillary occlusal malocclusion.

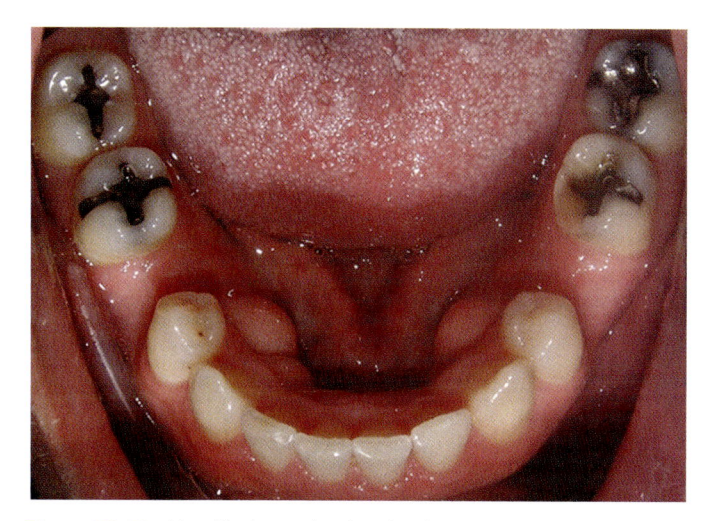

Figure 28.46 Mandibular occlusal malocclusion.

the patient having a less than ideal outcome esthetically and/or functionally so that they can make an educated decision as to which treatment option to pursue (Figure 28.47).

Some adult patients present for orthodontic treatment with multiple missing teeth. There are a very large number of scenarios and treatment options that can present themselves in these situations. The decision on whether to replace or not replace missing teeth will have an effect on the occlusal scheme that the patient will have at the end of treatment, and this must be taken into account during diagnosis and treatment planning to ensure a favorable posttreatment outcome.[20] If missing teeth are to be replaced prosthetically, it is vitally important that the orthodontist is allowed to treat the patient before the placement of the prosthesis to ensure that the prosthesis functions with the patient's postorthodontic occlusion correctly.[20] It is also important for the orthodontist to know the restorative dentist's prosthetic plan so that the most ideal occlusal relationship can be created.[20]

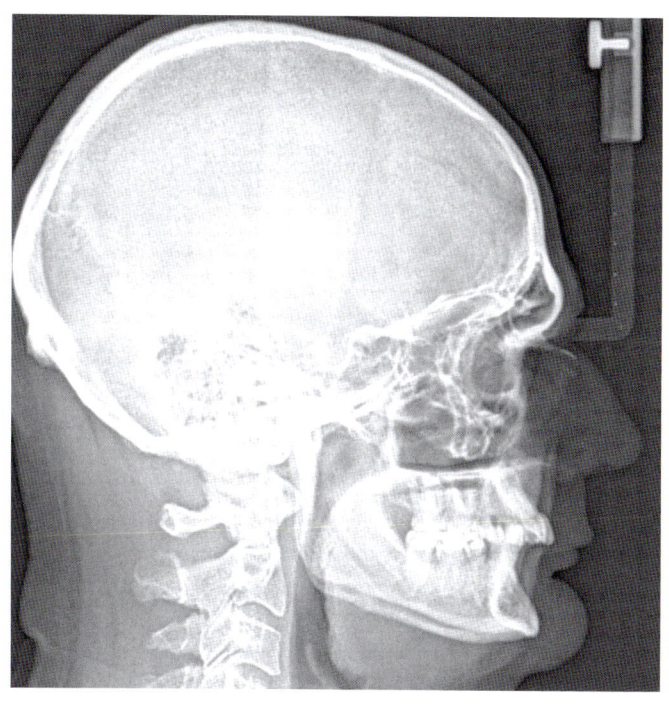

Figure 28.47 Adult Class II skeletal malocclusion. Treatment options: orthognathic surgery or dental compensation.

Many types of dental restorations are more prone to failure during excursive, nonaxial loading. This should be taken into account when the ideal functional occlusal scheme is chosen for the patient (Figures 28.48, 28.49, 28.50, 28.51, and 28.52).

Many adult patients are presented for orthodontic treatment with preexisting prosthetic restorations, such as fixed partial dentures, dental implants, fixed prosthetic crowns, removable partial dentures, full dentures, and so forth. These preexisting restorations/prostheses may necessitate removal and/or replacement to achieve a more ideal occlusal result. However, the

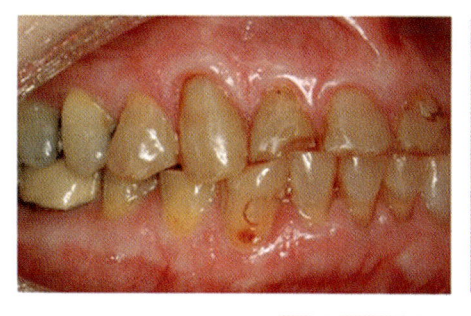

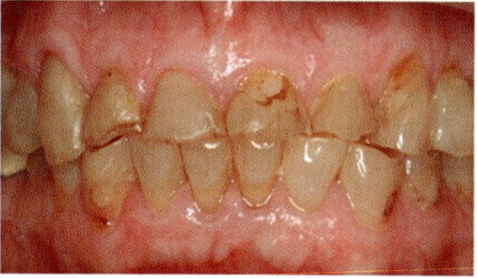

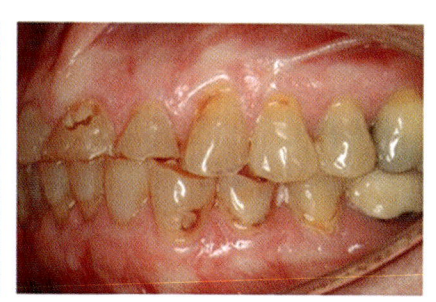

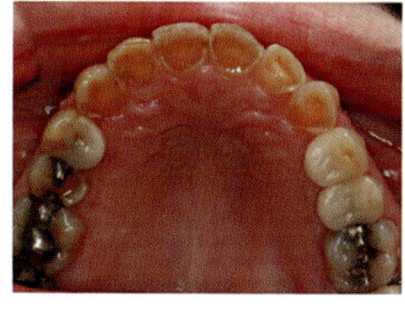

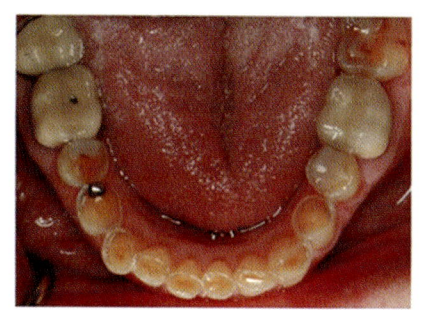

Figure 28.48 Initial intraoral photographs.

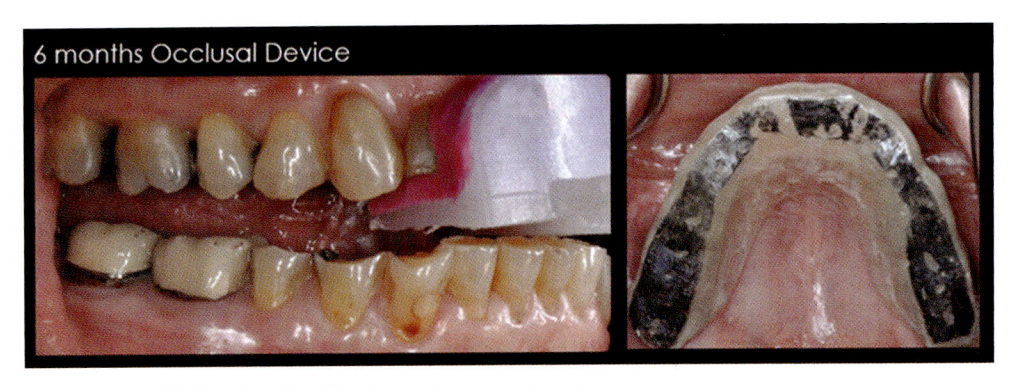

Figure 28.49 Occlusal splint to establish occlusal positioning and treatment goals.

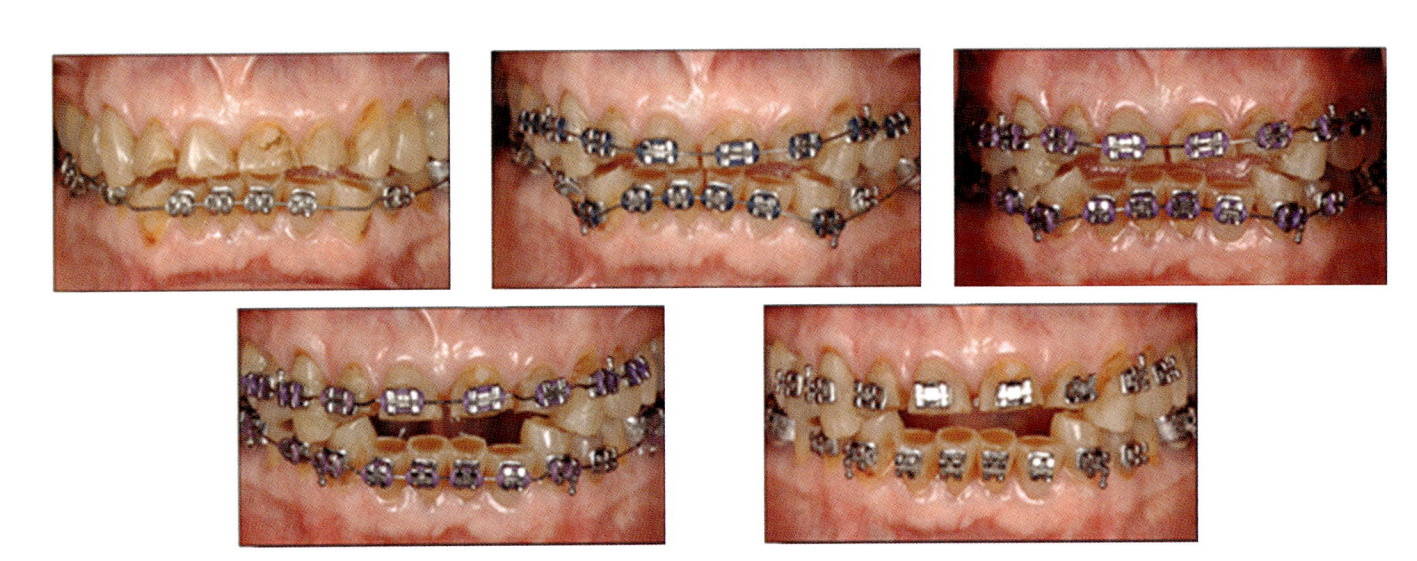

Figure 28.50 Orthodontic treatment progress.

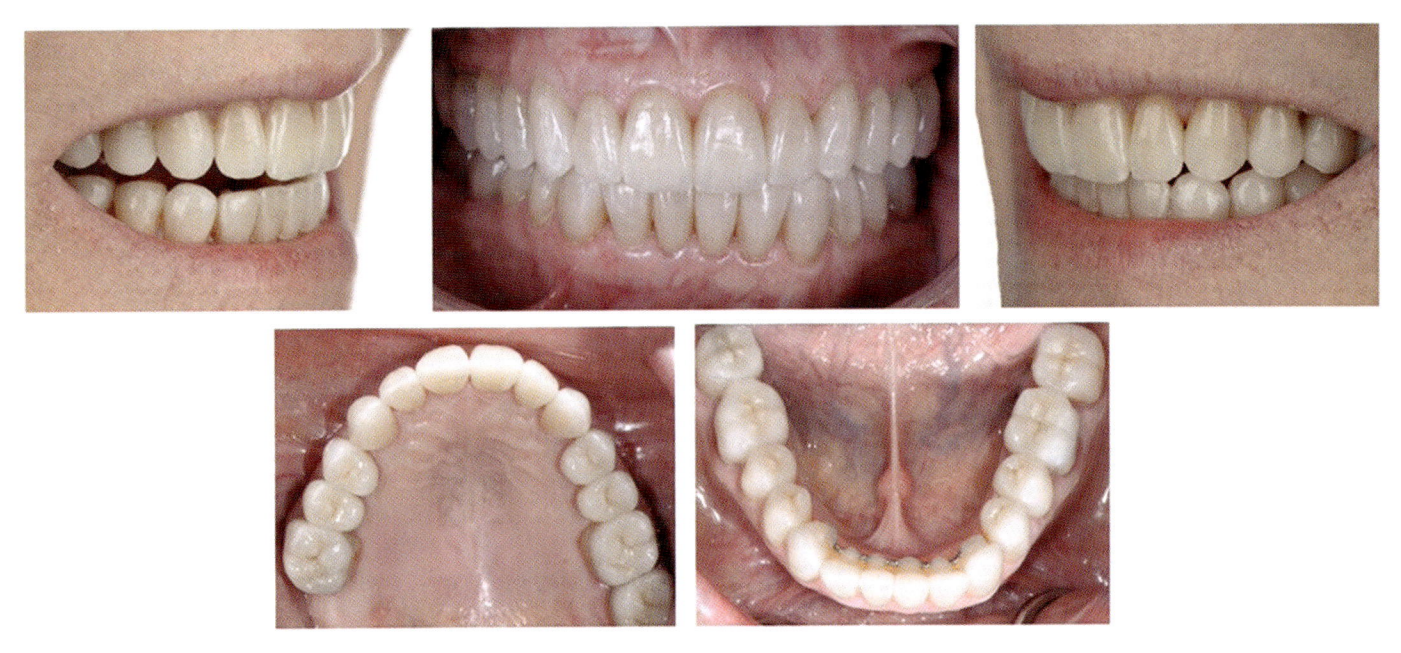

Figure 28.51 Final extra- and intraoral images.

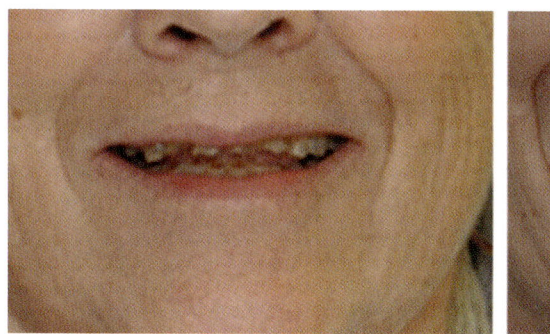

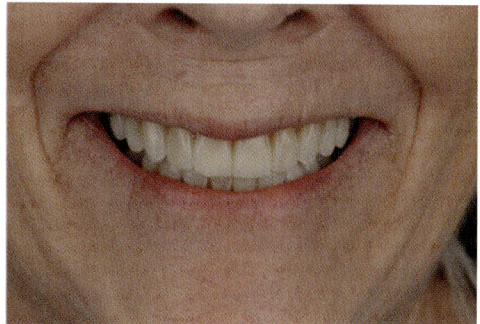

Figure 28.52 Initial and final close-up smile.

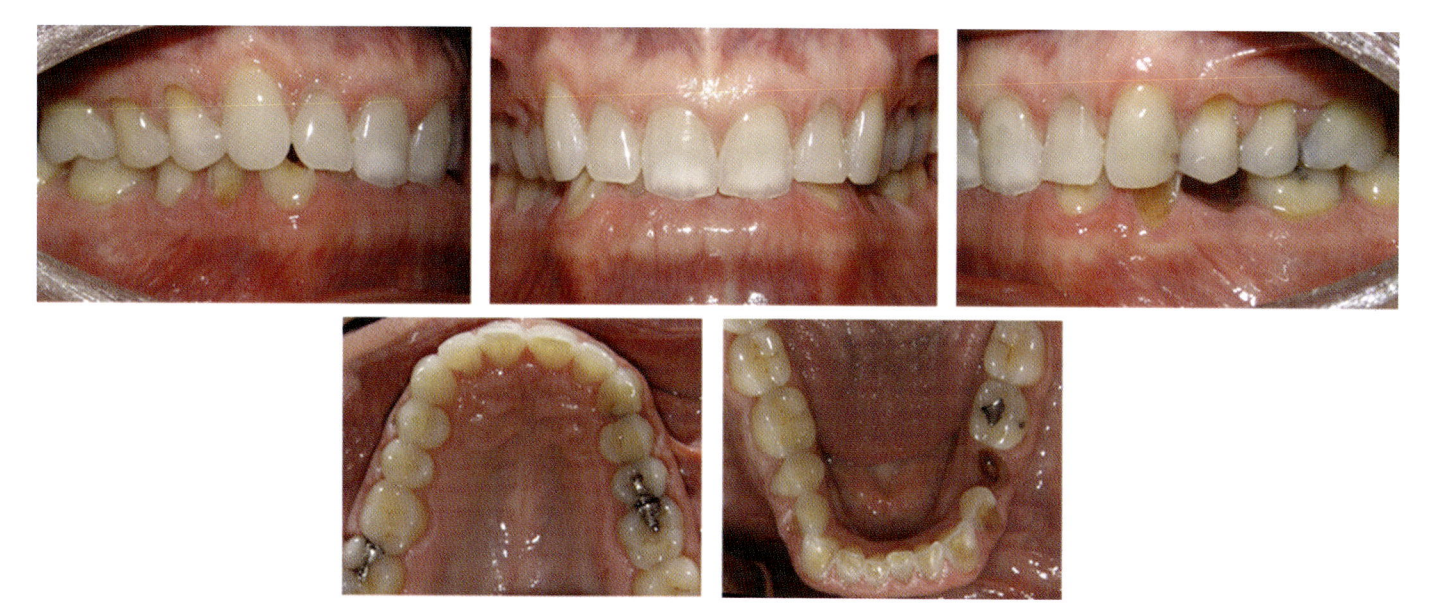

Figure 28.53 Adult with altered VDO, severe attrition, and 100% overbite.

benefits of achieving this result must be weighed against the cost that the patient must go through to have these restorations removed and/or replaced. It is our duty as orthodontic practitioners to educate our patients on these issues so that the patient can make an informed decision about which treatment option they would like to pursue.

Adult patients may also present with an increased or decreased VDO. An altered VDO is typically seen due to multiple missing teeth, severe attrition, or an existing dental prosthesis made at an incorrect VDO. In patients that appear to have an altered vertical dimension, a thorough clinic examination with documentation and mounted models is needed. Establishing a patient at the correct vertical dimension or maintaining the vertical dimension if it is correct is of the utmost importance in establishing an ideal occlusal scheme (Figures 28.53 and 28.54).

Periodontal status also must be taken into account when developing the occlusal scheme for adult orthodontic patients.[74] For example, lack of periodontal support around the maxillary and mandibular canines may be an indication to make the patient's functional occlusal scheme group function instead of CPO. Another example would be avoiding a deep overbite with heavy anterior guidance on a patient with significantly compromised periodontal support in the maxillary and mandibular incisors.[74] Also, in adult patients that have had a combination of bone loss and uneven attrition of the posterior dentition, leveling the marginal ridges to meet ABO standards should not take precedence over achieving interproximal bone levels free of vertical defects.[74,75] Therefore, the occlusal relationship that may be achieved postorthodontically may be less than "ideal" when evaluated by board standards to achieve a more favorable periodontal situation.[74,75] For all these reasons, a comprehensive periodontal evaluation complete with vertical bite wings should be performed before establishing the occlusal goals for an orthodontic patient.[75,76]

Tooth size–arch length discrepancies in the adult patient

As one ages, there are notable changes that occur to both the craniofacial complex and the dental arches. Cephalometric studies by Behrents demonstrate that craniofacial growth continues

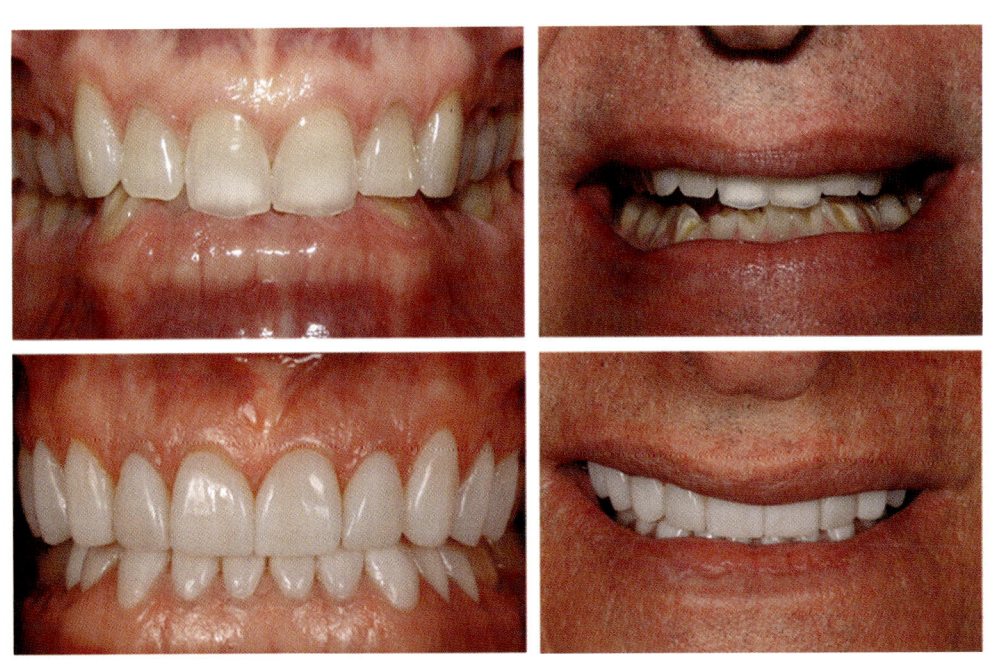

Figure 28.54 Altered VDO, severe attrition, and 100% overbite treated with an interdisciplinary treatment approach combining orthodontics and restorative.

into adulthood.[77,78] Although the curve of Spee, overjet, and overbite may appear to remain stable throughout adulthood, studies[79–83][84] have found statistically significant decreases in arch width, depth, and perimeter over the course of one's life. Carter and McNamara's results found that these decreases were no more than 3 mm in any one dimension.[79] The etiology for these decrements is unclear; however, the changes appear not to occur independently of each other and are not statistically associated with any one factor.[82] Dr Begg's study of Stone Age human dentition demonstrates excessive occlusal and interproximal wear that contributed to the reduction in arch perimeter.[85] He attributed the excessive wear to the primitive diet of early humans. One may speculate that that a light consistent force from one's musculature or function may cause these arch changes, but Proffit[86] notes that tongue pressure is greater than lip pressure during swallowing and at rest. If tooth position was determined solely by muscular forces from the tongue and lip alone, one would expect an increase in arch dimensions rather than a decrease.

Decreases in arch width, depth, and perimeter all contribute to potential arch length discrepancies that result in crowding, especially in the mandibular anterior region. There are several other hypotheses that attempt to explain the reason behind late mandibular crowding. Some studies have attributed third molars to anterior malalignment, claiming that they exert forces that direct the dentition mesially.[84,87–89] However, later studies showed no correlation between the two.[90–93] Other researchers have suggested that skeletal growth changes can lead to lower crowding,[94–96] but a study by Levin found no significant association between jaw growth and late mandibular incisor malalignment.[97] Tooth morphology and tooth size are other variables that have been studied. Fastlicht[91] concluded that the larger the mesiodistal width of the mandibular incisors, the greater the crowding, but others have shown that the size and the shape of mandibular incisors do not significantly contribute to their alignment.[97,98]

Regardless of etiology, lower, and to a lesser extent upper, malalignment increases with age. The Third National Health and Nutrition Examination Survey (NHANESIII) study used the irregularity index to quantify incisor crowding among subjects. The irregularity index is the sum of the distance (in millimeters) from the intended contact point of one incisor to the adjacent contact point of the neighboring incisor. Data taken from NHANESIII show that 55% of children from age 8 to 11 have well-aligned incisors, while this percentage decreases during adolescence (44%) and further decreases in adults. Only 34% of adults have well-aligned incisors. As one ages, there appears to be about a 50% chance of increased crowding in the maxillary arch, and an 85% chance of increased crowding in the mandibular arch.[86] Furthermore, McNamara and Carter found that males displayed more incisor irregularity than females. However, the change in irregularity throughout adulthood was the same in both sexes.[79]

When evaluating an adult for orthodontic treatment, one must consider four factors involving the total tooth size–arch length discrepancy: (1) arch length/perimeter; (2) curve of Spee; (3) incisor protrusion; and (4) tooth size discrepancies.

Arch length/perimeter

Arch perimeter is defined as the distance between the mesial of the first molars, measuring with the line traveling over the contact points of the posterior teeth and the incisal edges of the anterior teeth. Carter and McNamara found a statistically

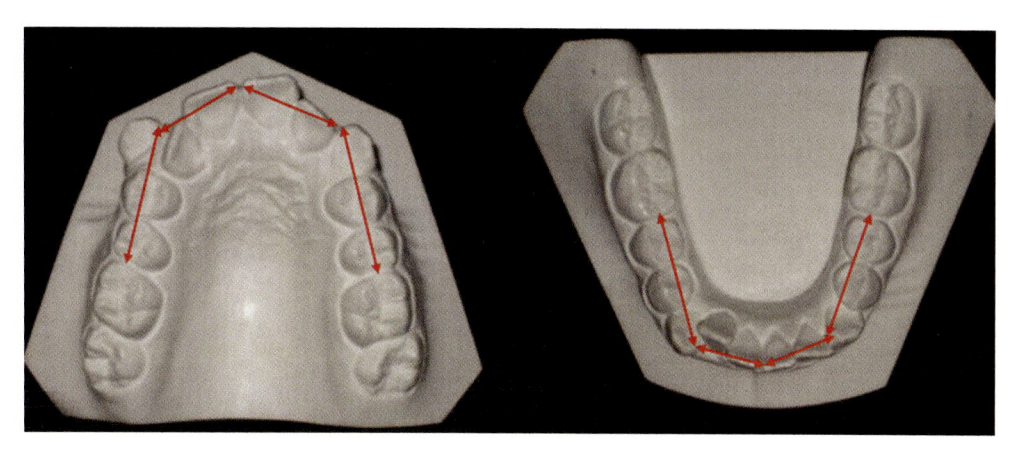

Figure 28.55 Calculating arch perimeter.

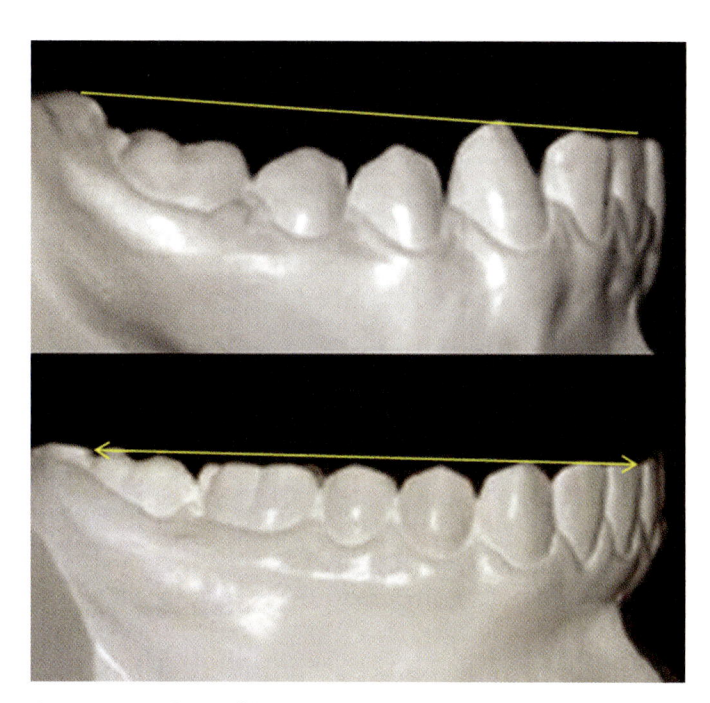

Figure 28.56 Curve of Spee.

significant decrease in maxillary perimeter is similar over time for males (1.8 ± 1.2 mm) and females (2.0 ± 1.2 mm); however, mandibular arch perimeter in males decreased significantly more from 17 to 48 years of age (2.4 ± 1.2 mm) than the same perimeter in females (1.7 ± 1.3 mm).[79] Arch perimeter can be estimated by analyzing a patient's dental casts. This is done by dividing the casts into four straight-line segments: the posterior segments are measured from the mesial of the first molars to the mesial of the canines, and the anterior segments are measured from the mesial of the canines to the mesial of central incisors (Figure 28.55). The sum of these four segments is considered as the space available. To calculate the space required, sharpened calipers are used to measure mesiodistal of each tooth mesial of the first molars. Subtracting space available from space required will estimate the amount of crowding or spacing that is present. It is important to realize that this measurement is only one of four factors that helps predict a tooth size–arch length discrepancy. This measurement would only be accurate if the arches had ideal protrusion, minimal curve of Spee, and no apparent tooth size discrepancy, which is seldom the case. Molar distalization is one way to provide space for maxillary crowding.

With the use of miniplates as anchorage, it has been demonstrated that an entire arch can be distalized.[99] Miniplates allow the roots of teeth to be moved more predictably through the alveolar bone without interference of screws. If a greater amount is necessary, extractions of second molars can allow more space for posterior segment distalization, or extraction of premolars so that only the anterior segment has to be moved.

Curve of Spee

The curve of Spee was described by F. Graf von Spee in 1890. He used skulls with abraded teeth to define the line of occlusion as the line on a cylinder tangent to the anterior border of the condyle, the occlusal surface of the second molar, and the incisal edges of the mandibular incisors. Studies show that, as one ages, the curve of Spee remains relatively stable.[79]

A significant curve of Spee is often evident in malocclusions with deep overbites. This curve is frequently leveled as part of overbite reduction and represents a routine procedure in orthodontic practice (Figure 28.56). Clinicians have been concerned for some time with the degree of reduction in arch circumference that accompanies leveling of the curve of Spee because they believe that this leads to incisor protrusion.[100]

One popular rule of thumb for estimating the resulting loss of arch circumference is that 1 mm of arch circumference is needed for each millimeter of curve of Spee depth present.[101] Baldridge[100] and Garcia[101] found the ratio to be more accurately expressed by the formulas $Y = 0.488X - 0.51$ and $Y = 0.657X + 1.34$ respectively, where Y is the arch length differential in millimeters and X is the sum of right and left side maximum depths of the curve of Spee in millimeters. In a mathematical model, Germane et al.[102] determined the relationship to be nonlinear and the arch circumference differential less than a one-to-one ratio for curves of Spee having a depth of 9 mm or less. Woods[103] showed that incisor flaring may be primarily related to the mechanics of leveling the curve of Spee, not necessarily due to the differential in arch circumference. He stated that the reduction of the curve may be achieved through anterior teeth intrusion and/or tip-back mechanics without flaring the incisors.

Incisor protrusion

When incisors protrude they align on a large arc with a greater circumference, creating space to minimize crowding. On the other hand, retroclined incisors, a much rarer occurrence,

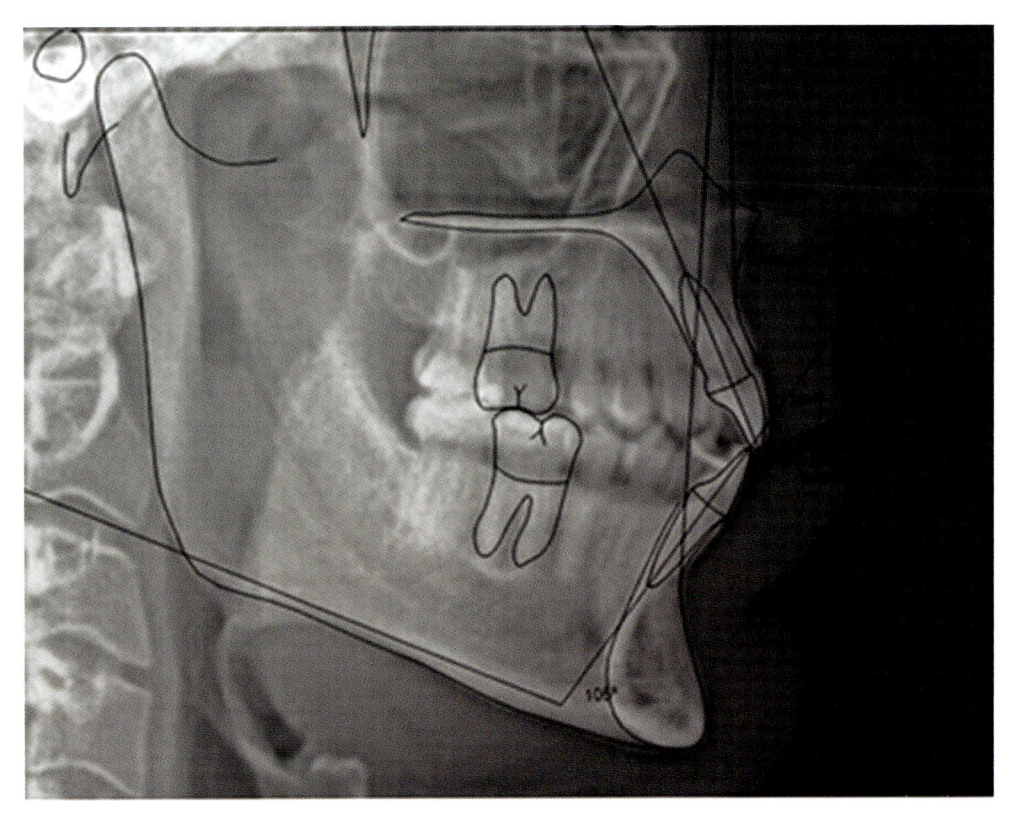

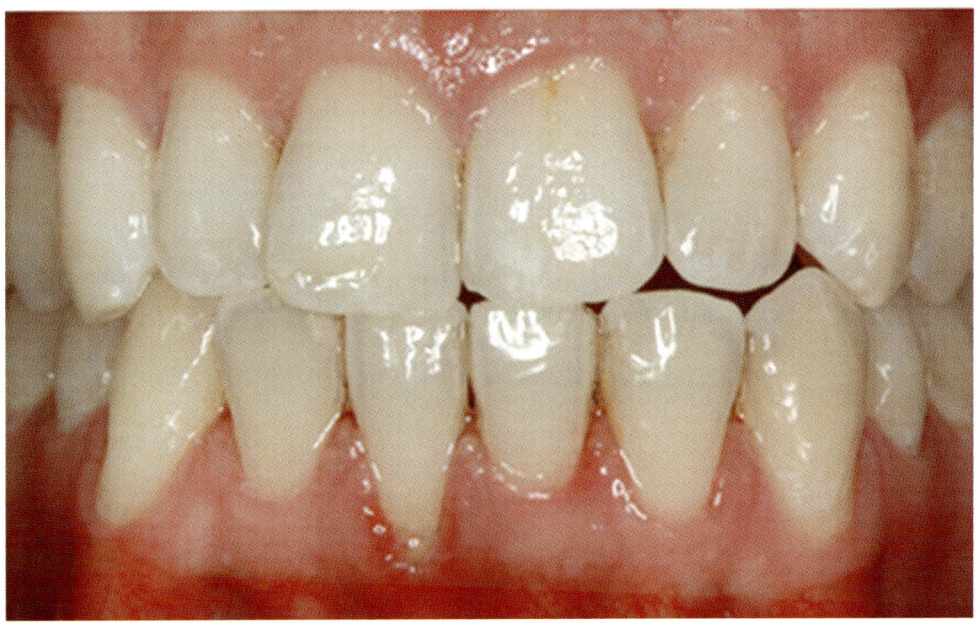

Figure 28.57 Excessive incisor proclination.

decrease arch circumference and increase the likeliness of crowding. Proffit et al.[62] state that "protrusion and crowding are really different aspects of the same phenomenon. If there is not adequate space to align teeth, the result can be crowding, protrusion, or most likely a combination of the two." Therefore, one must be aware of the amount of incisor protrusion to appreciate the results from a space analysis. The amount of incisor protrusion can be determined by cephalometric or facial from analysis. When a clinician decides to procline incisors to create more space within the arch, they must be careful not to do so excessively, which would position the teeth off the underlying alveolar bone. Excessive proclination not only makes proper overjet difficult to achieve, but also increases the likelihood of relapse, and serious periodontal complications (i.e., recession and attachment loss) on the facial aspect of incisors (Figure 28.57).

Tooth size discrepancies

In addition to interarch tooth size discrepancies due to morphology (Figure 28.58) or restorative procedures (Figure 28.59), a patient can also present with interarch tooth size discrepancies. For one to have appropriate interdigitation, overbite and overjet, maxillary and mandibular teeth must be dimensionally proportional to each other. Interarch discrepancies can be found anywhere in the arch; however, Smith et al. found that the mandibular second premolars explained most of the observed differences in the interarch discrepancy, followed by the maxillary lateral incisors, maxillary second premolars, and lower central incisors. Discrepancies in the sizes of these four teeth accounted for approximately 50% of the observed interarch discrepancies.[104]

If interarch discrepancies are not identified before treatment and are not addressed during treatment, compromised results will follow. The most common method used to identify interarch discrepancies is Bolton's analysis. It is performed by measuring the mesiodistal width of each permanent tooth from one first molar to the other. Two standard tables (developed by Bolton, based on his studies) are used to compare the summed widths of the maxillary teeth to the mandibular teeth: one table for the anterior teeth, and another table for the full arch, excluding second and third molars (Figure 28.60). Using both tables together can help identify where the majority of the interarch tooth discrepancy exists, either in the anterior or posterior segments. However, it is important to note that Smith et al. found significant differences in the overall, anterior, and posterior interarch ratios between gender and different ethnicities (whites, blacks, and Hispanics).[104] They found that Bolton's analysis is the most accurate for white females, but suggests that population-specific and male standards are necessary for clinical assessments.[104] Furthermore, they found that the larger the maxillary arch segment length, the greater the discrepancy between Bolton's ratios and the actual ratios. Other methods used to identify interarch tooth discrepancies, which are rarely used, include Kesling's diagnostic setup, Howes' ratio of canine fossa width to total maxillary tooth width, and Neff's anterior coefficient.[105–108]

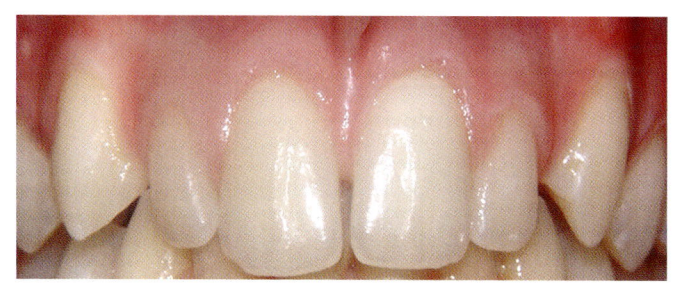

Figure 28.58 Interarch tooth size discrepancy due to amorphous morphology of the maxillary incisors.

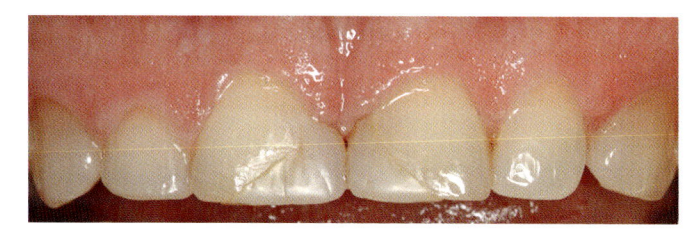

Figure 28.59 Interarch tooth size discrepancy due to restorative procedures.

Tooth deficiencies are corrected restoratively with direct composite, veneers, or full-coverage crowns, while tooth excess is corrected by judicious interproximal stripping. When treating adult patients, the clinician must be aware of the patient's previous restorative procedures (i.e., overcontoured crowns/restorations) that may create Bolton's ratios that appear to be out of balance. When a patient presents with missing teeth, their contralateral equivalents, assuming they are not extensively restored, may be measured and used for Bolton's analysis. However, this is clearly an assumption and should not be solely relied upon for treatment decisions. The more restorations present, the more difficult it is to accurately assess interarch discrepancies accurately.

In summary, the increased awareness of the benefits of a healthy dentition and appealing smile has motivated adult patients to seek a comprehensive approach to their dental treatment. At the same time, the restorative dentist has also come to appreciate the value of integrating orthodontics into a comprehensive rehabilitative treatment plan. Eliminating unfavorable occlusal relationships, positioning teeth to enhance esthetics and periodontal health, can greatly enhance the overall treatment outcome. The goal of achieving an excellent functional and esthetic outcome can be best achieved with an interdisciplinary treatment approach. This comprehensive/interdisciplinary approach brings together various specialty areas of dentistry and their respective recent advances, which greatly benefits the patient and the interdisciplinary team.

Acknowledgements

This chapter represents the primary work of Dr Marvin C. Goldstein, deceased uncle of the primary author of this work. Dr Marvin C. Goldstein was a major benefactor of the Department

Bolton's Tooth-size Relationships			
Maxillary anterior sum of 3–3	Mandibular anterior sum of 3–3	Maxillary total sum of 6–6	Mandibular total sum of 6–6
40	30.9	86	78.5
41	31.7	88	80.3
42	32.4	90	82.1
43	33.2	92	84.0
44	34.0	94	85.8
45	34.7	96	87.6
46	35.5	98	89.5
47	36.3	100	91.3
48	37.1	102	93.1
49	37.8	104	95.0
50	38.6	106	96.3
51	39.4	108	98.6
52	40.1	110	100.4
53	40.9		
54	41.7		
55	42.5		

Figure 28.60 Bolton's analysis.

of Orthodontics, The Dental College of Georgia, Augusta University, Augusta, Georgia.

I thank The Dental College of Georgia (DCG) orthodontic residents, the DCG esthetic team, and Dr Thomas J. Zwemer for their support and contributions to this chapter.

References

1. American Association of Orthodontics. Orthodontic treatment contributes to good dental health for adults. https://www.aaoinfo.org/adult-orthodontics (accessed November 29, 2017).
2. Kokich VG. *Adult Orthodontics in the 21st Century: Guidelines for Achieving Successful Results.* http://www.dentalxp.com/articles/Kokich-Adult%20Ortho%20in%20the%2021st%20Century.pdf (accessed October 31, 2017).
3. Sarver DM. The importance of incisor positioning in the esthetic smile: the smile arc. *Am J Orthod Dentofacial Orthop* 2001;120(2):98–111.
4. Gul-e-Erum, Fida M. Changes in smile parameters as perceived by orthodontists, dentists, artists, and laypeople. *World J Orthod* 2008;9(2):132–140.
5. Hulsey CM. An esthetic evaluation of lip-teeth relationships present in the smile. *Am J Orthod* 1970;57:132–144.
6. Hunt O, Johnston C, Hepper P, et al. The influence of maxillary gingival exposure on dental attractiveness ratings. *Eur J Orthod* 2002;24(2):199–204.
7. Kokich VO, Kokich VG, Kiyak HA. Perceptions of dental professionals and laypersons to altered dental esthetics: asymmetric and symmetric situations. *Am J Orthod Dentofacial Orthop* 2006;130(2):141–151.

8. Witt M, Flores-Mir C. Laypeople's preferences regarding dentofacial esthetics. *J Am Dent Assoc* 2011;142(8):925–937.
9. Sarver DM. *The Face as the Determinant of Treatment Choice*. http://sarvercourses.com/Portals/0/pdfs/facedetrmtx.pdf (accessed October 31, 2017).
10. Levin EI. The golden proportion. 2015. http://www.goldenmeangauge.co.uk/ (accessed October 31, 2017).
11. Levin EI. Dental esthetics and the golden proportion. *J Prosthet Dent* 1978;40:244–252.
12. Preston JD. The golden proportion revisited. *J Esthet Dent* 1993;5:247–251.
13. Magne P, Gallucci GO, Belser UC. Anatomic crown width/length ratios of unworn and worn maxillary teeth in white subjects. *J Prosthet Dent* 2003;89:453–461.
14. Sarver DM. Principles of cosmetic dentistry in orthodontics: part 1. Shape and proportionality of anterior teeth. *Am J Orthod Dentofacial Orthop* 2004;126(6):749–753.
15. Gurel G. *The Science and Art of Porcelain Laminate Veneers*. New Malden, UK: Quintessence; 2003.
16. McNamara JA Jr, Ellis E III. Cephalometric analysis of untreated adults with ideal facial and occlusal relationships. *Int J Adult Orthodon Orthognath Surg* 1988;3(4):221–231.
17. Desai S, Madhur U, Nanda R. Dynamic smile analysis: changes with age. *Am J Orthod Dentofacial Orthop* 2009;136(3):310.e1–310.e10.
18. Polo M. Botulinum toxin type A (Botox) for the neuromuscular correction of excessive gingival display on smiling (gummy smile). *Am J Orthod Dentofacial Orthop* 2008;133(2):195–203.
19. Goldstein RE, Goldstein CE. Is your case really finished? *J Clin Orthod* 1988;22:702–713.
20. Kokich VG, Spear VM. Guidelines for managing the orthodontic–restorative patient. *Semin Orthod* 1997;3:3–20.
21. Korayem M, Flores-Mir C, Nassar U, Olfert K. Implant site development by orthodontic extrusion: a systematic review. *Angle Orthod* 2008;78(4):752–760.
22. Voudouris JC, Schismenos C, Lackovic K, Kuftinec MM. Self-ligation esthetic brackets with low frictional resistance. *Angle Orthod* 2010;80:188–194.
23. Fleming PS, Johal A. Self-ligating brackets in orthodontics: a systematic review. *Angle Orthod* 2010;80:575–584.
24. Chen SS-H, Greenlee GM, Kim JE, et al. Systematic review of self-ligating brackets. *Am J Orthod Dentofacial Orthop* 2010;137:726.e1–726.e18.
25. Iijima M, Muguruma T, Brantley W, et al. Effect of coating on properties of esthetic orthodontic nickel–titanium wires. *Angle Orthod* 2012;82(2):319–325.
26. Grauer D, Proffit WR. Accuracy in tooth positioning with a fully customized lingual orthodontic appliance. *Am J Orthod Dentofacial Orthop* 2011;140:433–443.
27. Lagravere MO, Flores-Mir C. The treatment effects of Invisalign orthodontic aligners: a systematic review. *J Am Dent Assoc* 2005;136:1724–1729.
28. DeVos W, Casselman J, Swennen RJ. Cone-beam computerized tomography (CBCT) imaging of the oral and maxillofacial region: a systematic review of the literature. *Int J Oral Maxillofac Surg* 2009;38:609–625.
29. Paredes V, Gandia JL, Cibrián R. Digital diagnosis records in orthodontics: an overview. *Med Oral Patol Oral Cir Bucal* 2006;11:E88–E93.
30. Wenzel A, Gotfredsen E. Digital radiography for the orthodontist. *Am J Orthod Dentofacial Orthop* 2002;121:231–235.
31. Fleming PS, Marinho V, Johal A. Orthodontic measurements on digital study models compared with plaster models: a systematic review. *Orthod Craniofac Res* 2011;14:1–16.
32. Kau CH, Richmond S, Zhurov A, et al. Use of 3-dimensional surface acquisition to study facial morphology in 5 populations. *Am J Orthod Dentofacial Orthop* 2010;137:S56.e1–S56.e9.
33. U.S. Public Health Service, National Institute of Dental Research. *Oral Health of United States Adults; National Findings*. NIH publication number 87-2868. Bethesda, MD: National Institute of Dental Research; 1987.
34. Corrente G, Abundo R, Re S, et al. Orthodontic movement into infrabony defects in patients with advanced periodontal disease: a clinical and radiological study. *J Periodontol* 2003;74:1104–1109.
35. Nemcovsky CE, Beny L, Shanberger S, et al. Bone apposition in surgical bony defects following orthodontic movement: a comparative histomorphometric study between root- and periodontal ligament-damaged and periodontally intact rat molars. *J Periodontol* 2004;75:1013–1019.
36. Nemcovsky CE, Sasson M, Beny L, et al. Periodontal healing following orthodontic movement of rat molars with intact versus damaged periodontia towards a bony defect. *Eur J Orthod* 2007;29:338–344.
37. Sanders NL. Evidence-based care in orthodontics and periodontics: a review of the literature. *J Am Dent Assoc* 1999;130:521–527.
38. Diedrich P. Guided tissue regeneration associated with orthodontic therapy. *Semin Orthod* 1996;2:39–45.
39. Re S, Corrente G, Abundo R, Cardaropoli D. Orthodontic movement into bone defects augmented with bovine bone mineral and fibrin sealer: a reentry case report. *Int J Periodontics Restorative Dent* 2002;22:138–145.
40. Rabie ABM, Gildenhuys R, Boisson M. Management of patients with severe bone loss: bone induction and orthodontics. *World J Orthod* 2001;2:142–153.
41. Passanezi E, Janson M, Janson G, et al. Interdisciplinary treatment of localized juvenile periodontitis: a new perspective to an old problem. *Am J Orthod Dentofacial Orthop* 2007;131:268–276.
42. Melsen B, Allais D. Factors of importance for the development of dehiscences during labial movement of mandibular incisors: a retrospective study of adult orthodontic patients. *Am J Orthod Dentofacial Orthop* 2005;127:552–561.
43. Wennström JL. Mucogingival considerations in orthodontic treatment. *Semin Orthod* 1996;2:46–54.
44. Holmes HD, Tennant M, Goonewardene MS. Augmentation of faciolingual gingival dimensions with free connective tissue grafts before labial orthodontic tooth movement: an experimental study with a canine model. *Am J Orthod Dentofacial Orthop* 2005;127:562–572.
45. Gkantidis K, Christou P, Topouzelis N. The orthodontic–periodontic interrelationship in integrated treatment challenges: a systematic review. *J Oral Rehabil* 2010;37:377–390.
46. Spear FM, Kokich VG, Mathews DP. Interdisciplinary management of anterior dental esthetics. *J Am Dent Assoc* 2006;137:160–169.
47. Konikoff BM, Johnson DC, Schenkein HA, et al. Clinical crown length of the maxillary anterior teeth preorthodontics and postorthodontics. *J Periodontol* 2007;78:645–653.
48. Theytaz GA, Kiliaridis S. Gingival and dentofacial changes in adolescents and adults 2 to 10 years after orthodontic treatment. *J Clin Periodontol* 2008;35:825–830.
49. Williams S, Melsen B, Agerbaek N, Asboe V. The orthdontic treatment of malocclusion in patients with previous periodontal disease. *Br J Orthod* 1982;9:178–184.
50. Melsen B. Limitations in adult orthodontics. In: Melsen B, ed. *Current Controversies in Orthodontics*. Chicago, IL: Quintessence; 1991:147–180.
51. Burstone CJ. Deep overbite correction by intrusion. *Am J Orthod* 1977;72:1–22.

52. Melsen B, Agerbaek N, Markenstam G. Intrusion of incisors in adult patients with marginal bone loss. *Am J Orthod Dentofacial Orthop* 1989;96:232–241.
53. Reitan K. Biomechanical principles and reactions. In: Graber TM, Swain BF, eds. *Current Orthodontic Concepts and Techniques.* St Louis, MO: Mosby; 1985:101–192.
54. Reitan K. Effects of force, magnitude and direction of tooth movement on different alveolar bone types. *Angle Orthod* 1964;34:244–255.
55. Ericsson I, Thilander B, Lindhe J, Okamoto H. The effect of orthodontic tilting movements on the periodontal tissues of infected and non-infected dentitions in dogs. *J Clin Periodontol* 1977;4:278–293.
56. McKiernan EX, McKiernan F, Jones ML. Psychological profiles and motives of adults seeking orthodontic treatment. *Int J Adult Orthod Orthognath Surg* 1992;7:187–198.
57. Kokich VG. Esthetics: the ortho-perio-restorative connection. *Semin Orthod* 1996;2(1):21–30.
58. Redlich M, Shoshan S, Palmon A. Gingival response to orthodontic force. *Am J Orthod Dentofacial Orthop* 1999;116:152–158.
59. Reitan K. Tissue rearrangement during retention of orthodontically rotated teeth. *Angle Orthod* 1959;29:105–113.
60. Reitan K. Principles of retention and avoidance of post-treatment relapse. *Am J Orthod* 1969;55:776–790.
61. Destang DL, Kerr WJS. Maxillary retention: is longer better? *Eur J Orthod* 2003;25:65–69.
62. Proffit WR, Fields HM, Sarver DM. *Contemporary Orthodontics*, 4th edn. St. Louis, MO: Mosby; 2007.
63. Türkkahraman H, Sayin MO, Bozkurt FY, et al. Archwire ligation techniques, microbial colonization, and periodontal status in orthodontically treated patients. *Angle Orthod* 2005;75:231–236.
64. Artun J, Urbye KS. The effect of orthodontic treatment on periodontal bone support in patients with advanced loss of marginal periodontium. *Am J Orthod Dentofacial Orthop* 1988;93:143–148.
65. Corrente G, Vergano L, Re S, et al. Resin-bonded fixed partial dentures and splints in periodontally compromised patients: a 10-year follow-up. *Int J Periodontics Restorative Dent* 2000;20:628–636.
66. Gkantidis N, Kolokitha OE, Topouzelis N. Management of maxillary midline diastema with emphasis on etiology. *J Clin Pediatr Dent* 2008;32:265–272.
67. Boese LR. Fiberotomy and reproximation without lower retention 9 years in retrospect: part II. *Angle Orthod* 1980;50:169–178.
68. Edwards JG. A long-term prospective evaluation of the circumferential supracrestal fiberotomy in alleviating orthodontic relapse. *Am J Orthod Dentofacial Orthop* 1988;93:380–387.
69. Ong, MA, Wang HL. Periodontic and orthodontic treatment in adults. *Am J Orthod Dentofacial Orthop* 2002;122:420–428.
70. Andrews LF. The six keys to normal occlusion. *Am J Orthod* 1972;62(3):296–309.
71. Casko J, Vaden J, Kokich V, et al. Objective grading system for dental casts and panoramic radiographs. *Am J Orthod Dentofacial Orthop* 1998;114(5):589–599.
72. Rinchuse D, Kandasamy S, Sciote J. A contemporary and evidence-based view of canine protected occlusion. *Am J Orthod Dentofacial Orthop* 2007;132(1):90–102.
73. Kokich VG. Create realistic objectives. *Am J Orthod Dentofacial Orthop* 2011;139(6):713.
74. Geiger A. Malocclusion as an etiologic factor in periodontal disease: a retrospective essay. *Am J Orthod Dentofacial Orthop* 2001;120(2):112–115.
75. Mathews D, Kokich V. Managing treatment for the orthodontic patient with periodontal problems. *Semin Orthod* 1997;3(1):21–38.
76. Grubb J. Radiographic and periodontal requirements of the American Board of Orthodontics: a modification in the case display requirements for adult and periodontally involved adolescent and preadolescent patients. *Am J Orthod Dentofacial Orthop* 2008;134(1):3–4.
77. Behrents RG. *Growth in the Aging Craniofacial Skeleton*. Monograph No. 17, Craniofacial Growth Series. Ann Arbor, MI: Center for Human Growth and Development, The University of Michigan; 1985.
78. Behrents RG. *An Atlas of Growth in the Aging Craniofacial Skeleton*. Monograph No. 18, Craniofacial Growth Series. Ann Arbor, MI: Center for Human Growth and Development, The University of Michigan; 1985.
79. Carter GA, McNamara JA Jr. Longitudinal dental arch changes in adults. *Am J Orthod Dentofacial Orthop* 1998;114(1):88–99.
80. Moyers RE, van der Linden FPGM, Riolo ML, McNamara JA Jr. Standards of human occlusal development. Monograph 5, Craniofacial Growth Series. Ann Arbor, MI:Center for Human Growth and Development, The University of Michigan; 1976.
81. Sillman JH. Dimensional changes of the dental arches: longitudinal study from birth to 25 years. *Am J Orthod* 1964;50:824–841.
82. Brown VP, Daugaard-Jensen I. Changes in the dentition from the early teens to the early twenties. *Acta Odontol Scand* 1951;9:177–192.
83. Lundström A. Changes in crowding and spacing of the teeth with age. *Dent Pract* 1969;19:218–224.
84. Bishara S, Treder JE, Jakobsen JR. Facial and dental changes in adulthood. *Am J Orthod Dentofacial Orthop* 1994;106(2):175–186.
85. Begg, PR. Stone age man's dentition. *Am J Orthod* 1954;40:298–312.
86. Proffit WR. Equilibrium theory revisited: factors influencing positions of the teeth. *Angle Orthod* 1978;48:175–186.
87. Bergstrom K, Jensen R. Responsibility of the third molar for secondary crowding. *Dent Abstr* 1961;6:544.
88. Vego L. A longitudinal study of mandibular arch perimeter. *Angle Orthod* 1962;32:187–192.
89. Richardson ME. Late lower arch crowding: facial growth or forward drift? *Eur J Orthod* 1979;1:219–225.
90. Richardson ME. The role of the third molar in the cause of later lower arch crowding: a review. *Am J Orthod Dentofacial Orthop* 1989;95:79–83.
91. Fastlicht J. Crowding of mandibular incisors. *Am J Orthod* 1970;58:156–163.
92. Solomon AG. *The Role of Mandibular Third Molars in the Aetiology of Mandibular Incisor Crowding and Changing Growth Patterns in the Dentofacial Complex* [thesis]. University of Toronto; 1973.
93. Kaplan RG. Mandibular third molars and postretention crowding. *Am J Orthod* 1974;66:411–430.
94. Southard TE, Southard KA, Weeda LW. Mesial force from unerupted third molars. *Am J Orthod Dentofacial Orthop* 1991;99:220–225.
95. Moore AW, Hopkins SC. Inadequacy of mandibular anchorage. *Am J Orthod* 1960;46:440–451.
96. Björk A. Prediction of mandibular growth rotation. *Am J Orthod* 1969;55:585–599.
97. Levin PC. *The Role of Differential Horizontal Jaw Growth in the Etiology of Mandibular Incisor Crowding* [thesis]. University of Toronto; 1975.
98. Puneky PJ, Sadowsky C, BeGole EA. Tooth morphology and lower incisor alignment many years after orthodontic therapy. *Am J Orthod* 1984;86:299–305.

99. Hsiang-Hua Lai E, Yao CC, Chang JZ, et al., Three-dimensional dental model analysis of treatment outcomes for protrusive maxillary dentition: comparison of headgear, miniscrew, and miniplate skeletal anchorage. *Am J Orthod Dentofac Orthop* 2008;134(5):636–645.
100. Baldridge DW. Leveling the curve of Spee: its effect on mandibular arch lengths. *J Pract Orthod* 1969;3:26–41.
101. Garcia R. Leveling the curve of Spee: a new prediction formula. *J Tweed Found* 1985;13:65–72.
102. Germane N, Staggers JA, Rubinstein L, Revere JT. Arch length considerations due to the curve of Spee: a mathematical model. *Am J Orthod Dentofac Orthop* 1992;102:251–255.
103. Woods M. A reassessment of space requirements for lower arch leveling. *J Clin Orthod* 1986;20:770–778.
104. Smith SS, Buschang PH, Watanabe E. Interach tooth size relationships in three different populations: does Bolton's analysis apply? *Am J Orthod Dentofacial Orthop* 2000;117:169–174.
105. Kesling HD. The philosophy of the tooth positioning appliance. *Am J Orthod* 1945;31:297–340.
106. Howes AE. Case analysis and treatment planning based upon the relationship of the tooth material to its supporting bone. *Am J Orthod* 1947;33:499–533.
107. Neff CW. Tailored occlusion with anterior coefficient. *Am J Orthod* 1949;35:309–313.
108. Neff CW. The size relationship between the maxillary and mandibular anterior segments of the dental arch. *Angle Orthod* 1957;27:138–147.

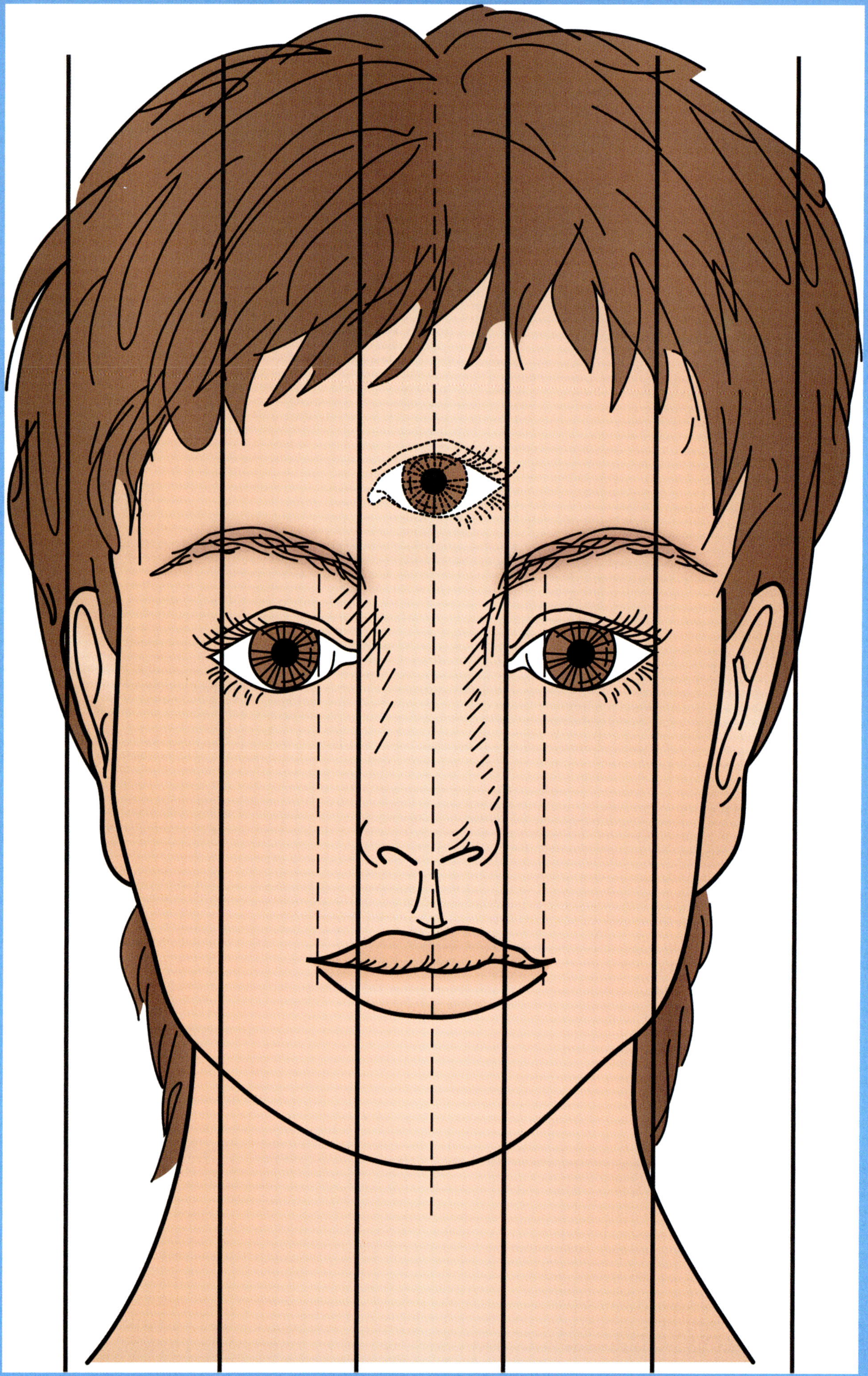

Chapter 29 Surgical Orthodontic Correction of Dentofacial Deformity

John N. Kent, DDS, John P. Neary, MD, DDS,
John Oubre, DDS, and David A. Bulot, DDS, MD

Chapter Outline

Facial esthetics	930	Injury to teeth	939
Age	930	Blood loss	939
Body type	930	Stabilization of operated segments	940
Racial characteristics	930	Postoperative discomfort and symptoms	940
Symmetry and proportion	930	Diagnosis and treatment	940
Who are the candidates?	933	Mandibular excess	940
Patient expectations	933	Mandibular deficiency	942
Pediatric patients	933	Maxillary excess	948
Severe skeletal disharmony	933	Maxillary deficiency	948
First visit	933	Facial asymmetry	951
Diagnostic records	934	Distraction osteogenesis	955
Case presentation visit	935	Surgically assisted orthodontics	956
Presurgical visit	937	Adjunctive hard- and soft-tissue procedures	959
Postsurgical treatment	937	Role of orthognathic surgery in treating obstructive	
Surgical complications and risks	939	sleep apnea	959

Dentistry has become more aware of the relationship between the dentition and the facial bones, and its impact on facial appearance. The precise, artistic work of the esthetic restorative dentist can be enhanced by orthodontic and surgical optimization and rejuvenation of the facial hard- and soft-tissue framework for the dentition. Such things as abnormal muscle function, lip incompetence, a variety of occlusal problems, and disturbances in facial bone growth contribute to facial disharmony. Today, the recognition and demand for correction of malocclusion and abnormal facial contour in adults are a significant topic in the practice of dentistry and in the specialties of orthodontics and oral and maxillofacial surgery. It is essential that all practitioners continually update their knowledge of the expanding treatment options provided by general dentists and specialists alike.

From the turn of the 20th century through the 1950s, the treatment of dentofacial abnormalities was limited largely to correction of mandibular prognathism by osteotomies of the ramus or body of the mandible. During the following decade, owing to the pioneering efforts of Hugo Obwegesser and other European surgeons, surgical procedures were developed to correct mandibular retrognathism, chin deformities, and excessive maxillary growth. Since that time, numerous procedures to treat the entire spectrum of dental, skeletal, and soft-tissue abnormalities have been developed. Optimal esthetic and functional results are now obtainable for all patients with a variety of occlusal and facial defects, as seen in various textbooks today (and in books no longer in print, such as those by Hinds and Kent; Satorianos and Sassouni; Bell, Proffit, and White; Epker and Wolford; and Epker and Fish). Significant clinical and basic science research articles in the oral and maxillofacial surgery and orthodontic literature continue to provide outcome analyses of traditional orthodontic and orthognathic procedures and innovative progress in areas such as adjunctive soft-tissue procedures and evaluation of emerging biomaterials. The introduction of rigid fixation principles with bone plates and screws in the 1980s has eliminated intermaxillary fixation (jaws wired shut) in the large majority of patients. Applications in the 1990s of distraction osteogenesis and continued advancement of these devices offer innovative solutions to difficult deformities. Applications include single jaw distraction, combined maxillomandibular distraction, and mandibular widening.

Unquestionably, some dental malocclusions do not need concomitant orthodontic and surgical procedures and will respond nicely to either modality alone. However, most skeletal malocclusions are too severe to be treated by either specialty alone. A successful outcome that remains stable for the long term often requires a multidisciplinary approach. Following an appropriate diagnosis, the restorative dentist, orthodontist, and surgeon must evaluate the patient and then together formulate a comprehensive treatment plan, clearly communicating the proper sequence for the satisfactory completion of all dental, orthodontic, and surgical procedures. Communication among all parties involved must continue throughout treatment and long-term follow-up. This chapter presents the sequence of events the patient will encounter, including the examination, case presentation, orthodontic treatment, surgical procedures, and follow-up management. Finally, a detailed description of common dentofacial abnormalities is presented in a problem-oriented fashion with illustration of treatment results.

Facial esthetics

The planning of corrective surgery for dentofacial deformities is surely one of the best examples of the interaction of art and science in the field of dentistry. Although it has been often said that beauty is skin deep, understanding facial esthetics requires an in-depth knowledge of how subcutaneous fat, muscle tone, and particularly the underlying supporting skeleton combine and interact to produce the facial appearance.

Modern concepts of facial esthetics, especially in America, are influenced by classical ideals. As professionals, we must strive to be objective in our analysis and planning but must also be aware of cultural biases, physical and racial characteristics, and, most importantly, the patient's desires. The evaluation of the face must be critical of form as it relates to function. Treatment should never alter one to the detriment of the other. In an attempt to evaluate facial form, there are five significant factors that should be considered objectively: age, body type, race, symmetry, and proportion.

Age

The age of a patient is an important determinant of facial form. Underlying skeletal structures are not fully expressed until late adolescence. In adults, there is relative stability of the facial skeletal structure; however, during the aging process, generalized demineralization of bone occurs, which can have subtle effects on form. The distribution of subcutaneous tissue shifts with age, particularly with changes in fat deposits that may result in ocular, temporal, and buccal fat loss and accentuation of the underlying skeletal structures. The skin loses elasticity and begins to wrinkle and sag. Hair may recede, thin, and gray. Dimensional changes can also occur with the loss of teeth and associated alveolar bone.

Body type

Body type relates to age and sex and is generally reflected in facial form. Basic body types include ectomorph (asthenic) types who are thin and angular, mesomorph (sthenic) types who are well proportioned and square, and endomorph (pyknic) types who are heavy set and rounded. Proper relation of facial form to body type is essential for desirable balance.

Racial characteristics

Racial characteristics are increasingly important in today's society. These qualities should be appreciated and should not limit the achievement of esthetic improvement in facial reconstructions. Asians will tend to have rounded faces, and their profile will be straight or slightly concave without defined anterior projection of the zygomas, nasal dorsum, or chin. Those of African origin will tend toward a convex profile with a flat forehead and nasal dorsum juxtaposed with bimaxillary dental alveolar protrusion, prominent lips, and a less-defined chin. Northern Europeans, after whom most cephalometric norms were developed, tend to exhibit a straight or slightly convex profile with a defined anterior projection of the nose, zygomas, and chin.

Symmetry and proportion

The last two factors, symmetry and proportion, are most easily discussed together; also more readily lending themselves to quantification than all five factors listed. Soft- and hard-tissue measurements are recorded in the frontal and profile views, and the treatment can be designed to maximize the esthetic end result.

On frontal view, the face can be divided vertically into thirds (Figure 29.1): the upper third is from the upper hairline to the glabella, the middle third is from the glabella to the subnasale, and the lower third is from the subnasale to the menton. A one-to-one ratio indicates ideal esthetic proportions. The lower third can further be divided in half, with the division at the vermilion

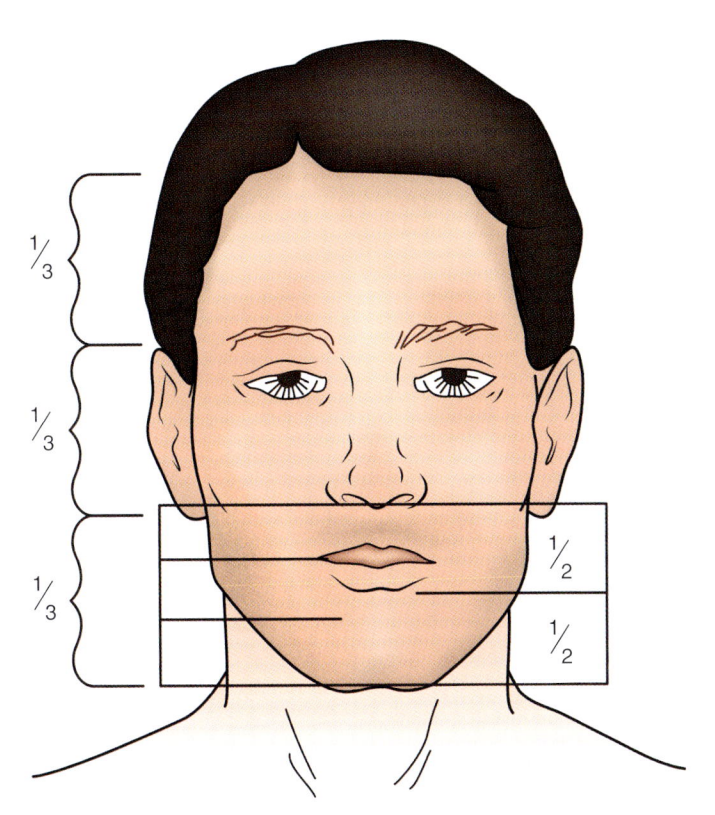

Figure 29.1 Frontal view of the face. Upper, middle, and lower thirds are delineated. Lower third is further divided into halves and thirds.

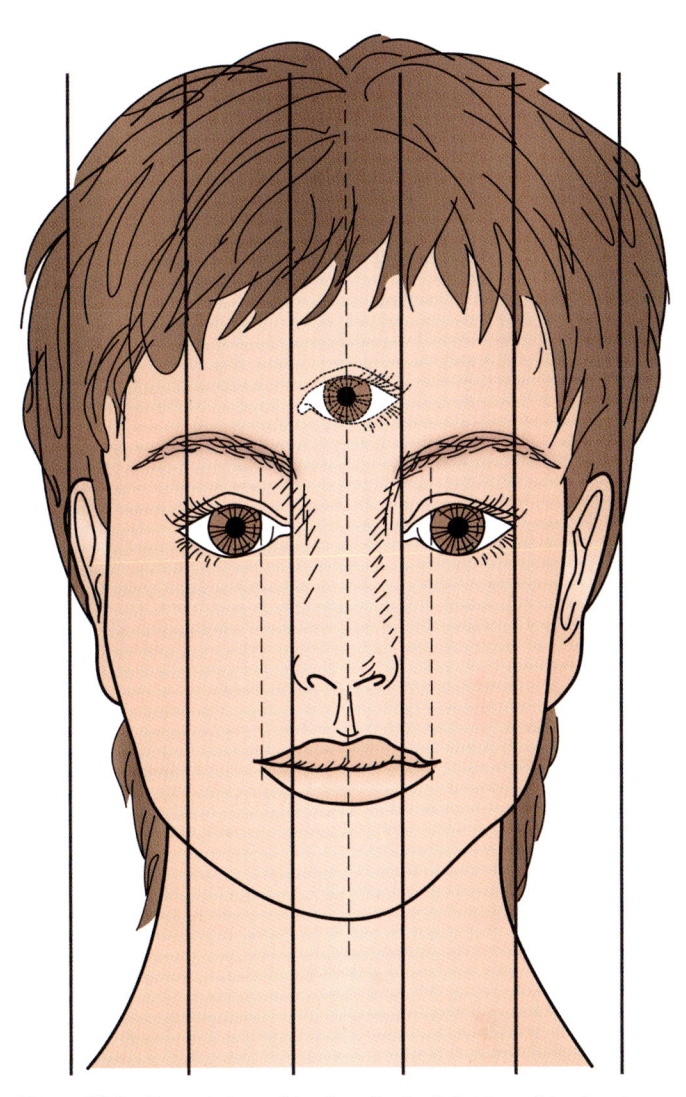

Figure 29.2 Frontal view of the face. Sagittal division of the face into fifths with each fifth equal to one eye width.

border of the lower lip, or in thirds, with the upper third ending at the oral commissure (see Figure 29.1).

The smile line is also evaluated on the frontal view. The patient is first evaluated with lips in a relaxed position (or repose); 2–4 mm of the central incisors should be visualized in this relaxed lip position. As the patient is asked to smile, generally 10–12 mm of incisor display is seen. There are minor differences for male and females. Generally, females will tend to show more tooth display both at repose and animation. Note excessive display of incisors and gingiva and corrected normal display in Figure 29.13A and B.

Symmetry and proportion can be judged on frontal examination by dividing the face into fifths, with each fifth being equal to the eye width (Figure 29.2). Midline points should lie on an axis, dividing the face in half, and all paired facial structures should be nearly equidistant from this axis. The intercanthal distance should be one eye width and should correspond to the width of the alar cartilages. The oral commissures should lie on vertical axes tangent to the medial limbus of each eye, and the distance between each axis should be 1.5 times the width of the eye (see Figure 29.2).

Additional proportion evaluations are evident on profile examination. Nasal projection can be judged by the nasofrontal angle (115–130°), the nasofacial angle (30–40°), and a nasomental angle (120–132°). Using a vertical line from the glabella to the menton, a perpendicular line drawn to the nasal tip should be 55–60% of the distance from the point of intersection to the nasion. The distance from the nasal tip to the subnasale should equal the distance from the subnasale to the vermilion border of the upper lip Figure 29.3). Also, on profile examination, the interplay among the lip, chin, and neck can be evaluated (Figure 29.4). The mentocervical angle should be 80–95°. The depth of the labiomental sulcus, measured using a line from the lower lip to the soft-tissue pogonion, should be approximately 4 mm.

The "ideals" described earlier should not be used to establish definitive treatment objectives in all patients. These are only guidelines by which facial harmony may be defined and from which ideas regarding treatment planning may be derived. There are numerous other measures, angles, and analyses that may be used to aid in the diagnosis of a dentofacial deformity. Regardless of what data are collected and which analysis is used, final treatment decisions must be tailored to the individual patient. It is probable that the most important treatment planning information obtained will come from listening to the patient's own treatment goals.

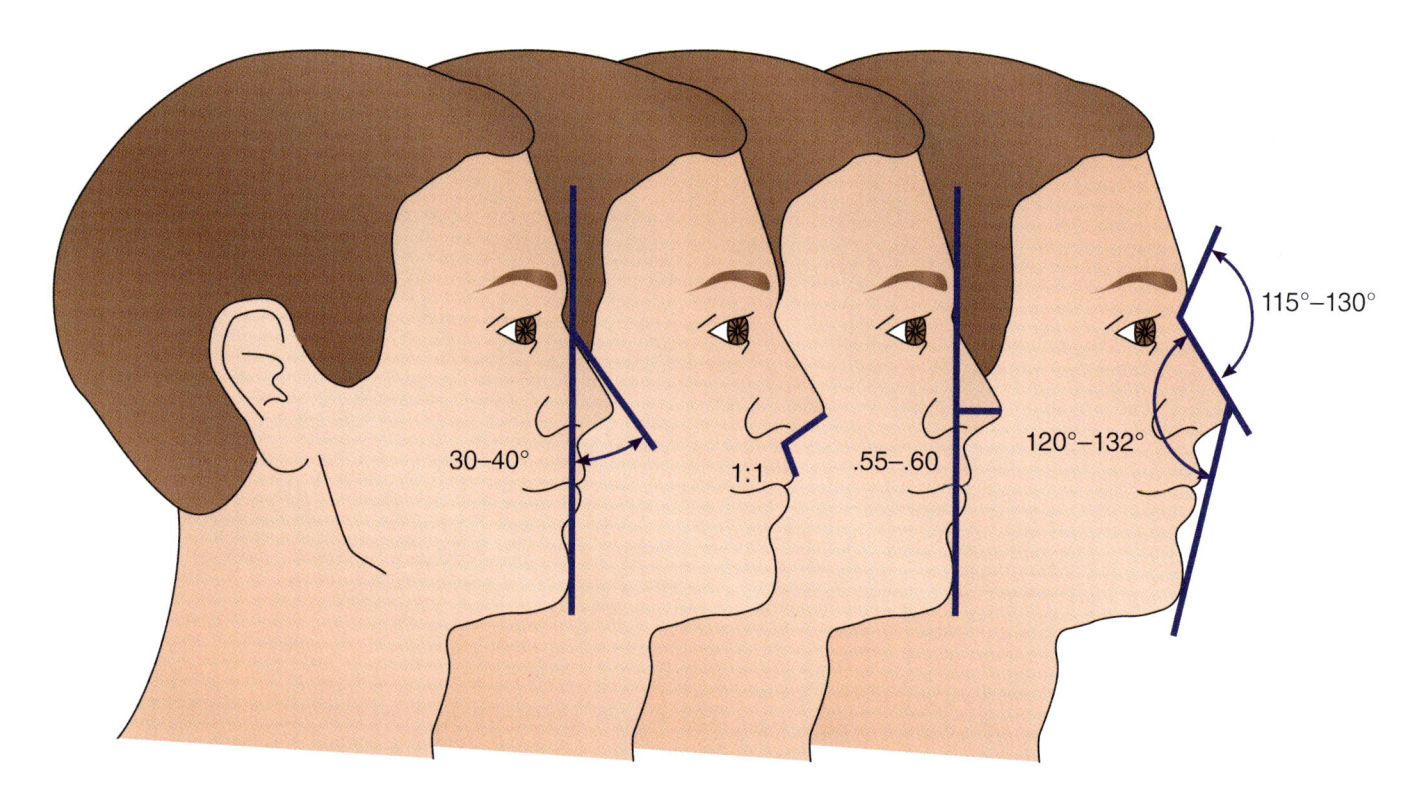

Figure 29.3 Profile views of the face relating the nose to the forehead, lips, and chin. Nasofrontal, nasofacial, and nasomental angles are described, as well as linear measurements of nasal tip projection.

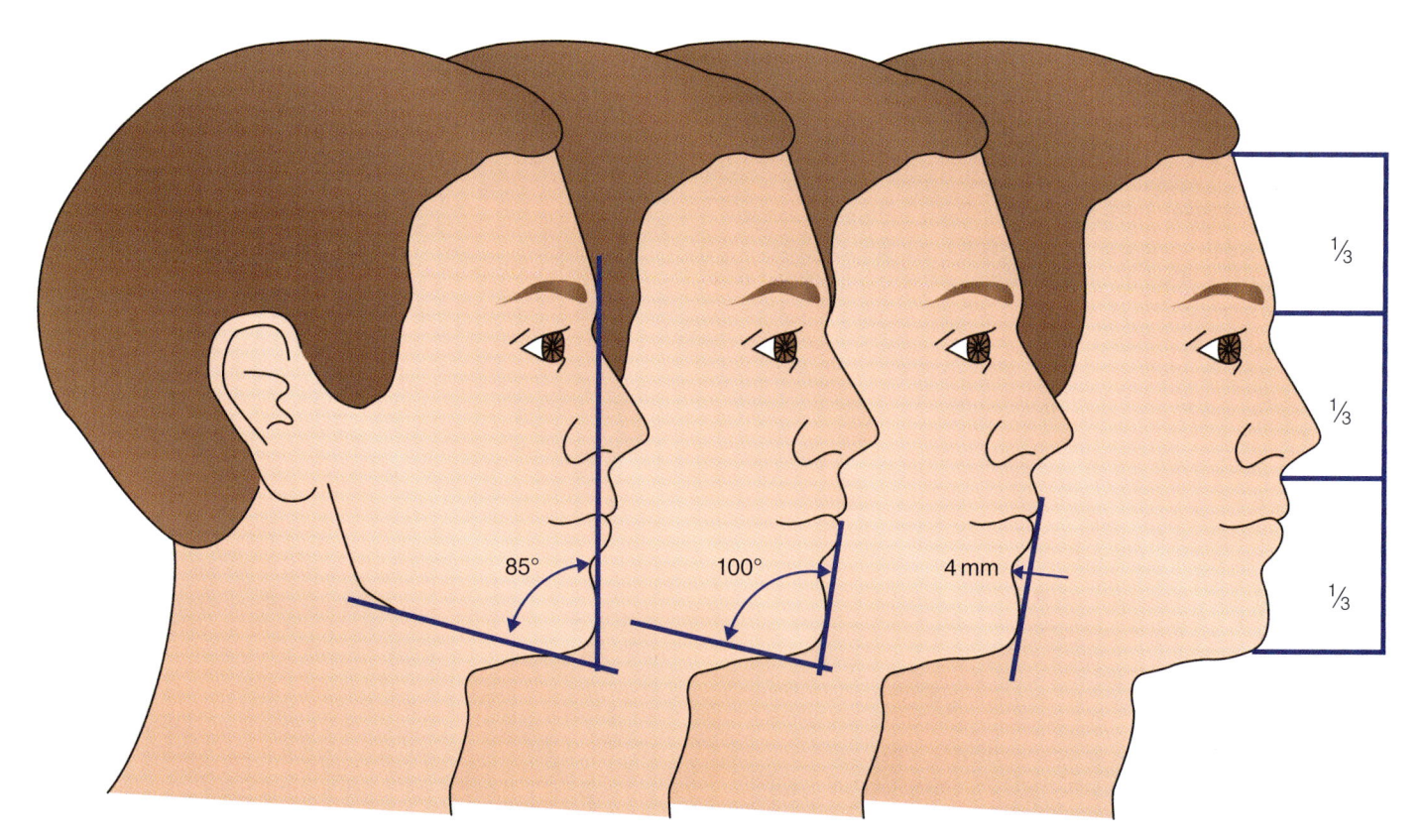

Figure 29.4 Profile views of the face relating the chin to the lips and neck and the labial mental sulcus to the lower lip and chin. The mental cervical angle is described.

Who are the candidates?

Patient expectations

Combined surgical–orthodontic management is a complex process, which requires coordinated efforts among all three dental professionals. Surgical treatment of these dentofacial deformities does not come without risks, costs, and inconvenience. The prospective patient must understand what is involved without "glossing over" the facts. It is especially important to listen to the patient's perception of the problem and then determine what they want to achieve as a result of treatment. If their expectations are inconsistent with their overall behavior, mode of dress, and level of health awareness, questions about their motives should be forthright. If they have a significant deformity and want to be "perfectly normal" or are suffering psychologically, they may be desperately hoping that treatment will enhance their image and success in life. The best possible result of treatment may not satisfy them.

Pediatric patients

In growing individuals, combined surgical–orthodontic treatment is generally avoided. Although most juvenile deformities can be rectified by influencing the growth process, psychological embarrassment or significant impairment of speech and masticatory function may warrant surgical procedures before facial growth is complete. In such cases, it is clearly explained to the patient and parents that further treatment may be necessary. Typically, the surgical phase of treatment is deferred until late adolescence, when growth is complete. Serial hand radiographs are compared to ensure maturation of epiphyseal plates.

The exception to this is the syndromic patient with significant facial deformity. Distraction osteogenesis is increasingly being used to correct deformities in this patient population. Typically, these patients will undergo several orthognathic procedures. The initial procedures such as distraction are aimed at increasing the native airway to eliminate the need for tracheotomies to establish a stable airway. Exciting research in this area is progressing rapidly as innovative applications of distraction are being applied not only to growing patients but also to adults.

Severe skeletal disharmony

There are many adults with malocclusions who exhibit little or no facial disharmony and who can be properly treated with orthodontics alone. However, if a true skeletal imbalance exists, orthodontic treatment cannot achieve proper gnathologic relationships, esthetics, and tooth position over basal bone simultaneously. In cases of severe skeletal disharmony, orthodontic treatment alone usually will not satisfactorily improve the facial profile. In fact, the occlusion may be improved at the expense of the esthetic relationships. The orthodontist should determine prior to initiating treatment whether and to what degree there is a skeletal component to the deformity. In the case of a significant skeletal deformity, the oral and maxillofacial surgeon should be consulted to discuss surgical options.

Adult Class II malocclusions corrected orthodontically are classically treated by extractions in the upper arch only and maximum retraction of the upper anterior segment. With the advent of temporary anchorage devices (TADs), bodily retraction of the maxillary incisors is possible without maxillary posterior teeth moving forward. However, overretraction and flattening of the upper lip need to be considered and are often an esthetic compromise.

Orthodontic treatment of Class III malocclusions can result in severe lingual inclination of the lower incisors and does not correct excess chin prominence. There is little opportunity to bodily retract the lower incisors owing to the very narrow alveolus. In cases where the lower incisors are protruded, extraction of mandibular first premolars along with use of TADs allow for retraction of the lower anterior teeth to establish incisor coupling. Usually, occlusal equilibration is needed to make the Class III molar relationship function well. One of the most difficult factors to overcome is the bilateral posterior crossbites often found with this type. If the midpalatal raphe is patent, it is possible to orthopedically expand the maxilla using "jackscrew"-type devices. Since this raphe will be fused in the late teens or early twenties, many adults cannot be treated with palatal expansion. Compromises will need to be accepted if orthodontics alone is the only alternative.

Since extraction therapy will average a minimum of 18–24 months, many adults will not accept treatment because of the time factor. Some will balk at using headgear, TADs, or rubber bands. Others will insist on wearing ceramic or lingual brackets, making incisor retraction even more difficult.

First visit

The first and most important step for the patient is the recognition that a dentofacial abnormality exists. The patient may have abnormalities in both the maxillary and mandibular regions requiring eventual orthodontic and surgical treatment of both jaws. At this point, the patient should be instructed that additional examination and tests are necessary to accurately locate the deformity and describe treatment possibilities. Each member of the team (general dentist, orthodontist, and oral and maxillofacial surgeon) examines the patient, formulates a diagnosis, and prepares a treatment sequence. The length of orthodontic treatment, types of surgical procedures, cost, and complications cannot be discussed until the diagnostic records are taken and a treatment plan is formulated.

In these days of increased consumer awareness, the orthodontist and surgeon must be scrupulously truthful about all details and risks of proposed treatments even if they cause the patient to decline treatment. When the patient needs and receives guarantees and when the team members are overly enthusiastic, the situation is ripe for mishap. It is common practice to write out in detail a complete diagnostic report citing the treatment modalities and risks and mail signed copies to the patient and other team members. A report such as this, when accompanied by a signed-consent form and signed-prediction tracings, will substantiate a claim that the patient was fully informed and consented to the treatment.

Diagnostic records

To identify the dentofacial deformity and formulate treatment recommendations, diagnostic records usually include a panoramic radiograph, a lateral cephalogram, study casts, and facial, profile, and intraoral photographs. The panoramic radiograph is preferred by the orthodontist and surgeon for assessment of bone size, shape, pathology, and determination of osteotomy sites. The standardized lateral cephalogram is used for performing cephalometric analyses and subsequently making cephalometric prediction tracings. Additional records, such as temporomandibular joint (TMJ) films, frontal cephalograms, and mounted casts, are also used in selected cases. Cone beam computed tomography has become more popular, especially in evaluating asymmetries.

Cephalometric analysis

There are over 300 cephalometric measurements or analyses described in the literature for facial soft-tissue and bony architecture. Even though they provide language by which we communicate, they have limitations. Unavoidable error exists in taking and analyzing the cephalogram, partly because it is susceptible to geometric distortions. The "normal" data to which comparisons are made are derived from "ideal" individuals, and comparisons become less reliable as extremes in skeletal deformity are approached. Neither the cephalogram nor the particular analysis to which the derived data are compared is most important from the diagnostic standpoint—rather, it is how these data correlate with the overall examination and treatment goals. Cephalometrics is more useful for documenting progress and change as the treatment unfolds than for the actual diagnostic process itself. The cephalometric tracing is created utilizing imaging software programs, or acetate paper overlaid on the cephalogram (Figure 29.5A). Changes over time can be compared by superimposing tracings on each other.

Cephalometric prediction tracings

The cephalometric prediction tracing predicts the changes that should occur as a result of orthodontic or surgical treatment. For example, the work-up of a patient with a Class II malocclusion with vertical maxillary excess (VME), mandibular retrognathism, and chin deficiency requires several tracings. Tracing 1 is the patient's existing dentofacial deformity (see Figure 29.5A). An overlay of tracing 2 (Figure 29.5B) on tracing 1 demonstrates maxillary orthodontic tooth movement, superior repositioning of the maxilla by Le Fort I osteotomy, and autorotation of the mandible. Tracing 3 demonstrates the advancement of the mandible by sagittal split osteotomy performed simultaneously with the maxillary surgery (Figure 29.5C). If necessary, a horizontal osteotomy of the chin or a chin implant is placed for augmentation, as shown in tracing 4 (Figure 29.5D). Tracing 5 demonstrates a superimposition of all predicted hard- and soft-tissue changes on tracing 1 (Figure 29.5E). It is important to use the tracings without cephalometric lines, angles, and measurements, which are necessary for diagnostic purposes, as they may be confusing to the patient.

Most orthodontic–orthognathic work-ups today are done with any one of several sophisticated computerized software programs. Digital cephalograms are superimposed on digital lateral facial photographs and captured into the prediction software application. Proposed orthodontic and orthognathic movements are made with the mouse, and the predicted facial form is displayed. Although these visual representations have great value in showing patients what changes can be made, it must be made clear that these are ideal treatment goals. One cannot guarantee that the end result will always be as predicted ideally.

When there are multiple treatment options, it is beneficial to show the patient computer treatment simulations, so that their input can be considered in finalizing the treatment plan.

Figure 29.6A–D shows a patient presenting with a Class III malocclusion. The treatment options are not always clear, and the benefit of diagnostic computer software is that it is relatively easy to do different treatment simulations. When laypeople can compare morphed images of different treatment options, it is easier for them to understand and make informed choices.

Since this patient had a Class III malocclusion that could be treated effectively with different procedures, visual treatment objectives (mandibular set back versus Le Fort I maxillary advancement) helped the patient decide on the best approach to satisfy her individual desires. She liked the fuller midface achieved with the Le Fort I simulation, and that is the treatment approach that was used (Figure 29.6E).

The dental arches were decompensated with a nonextraction treatment plan. Her maxilla was advanced to a Class I dental relationship. The facial changes achieved were more congruent with the patient's needs (Figure 29.6 F–L).

Facial and intraoral photographs

All facial portraits should be of the head in an erect, natural, unstrained posture against a neutral-colored background. Teeth should be in occlusion, with the lips relaxed. For patients with lip incompetence, a second portrait should be taken with the lips closed to depict the amount of lip strain present. Frontal and profile portraits are taken. In Class II deformities, it is helpful for diagnostic purposes to take a second profile view with the mandible postured forward. In Class III deformities secondary to horizontal maxillary deficiency, it is demonstrative to take an additional profile portrait with a layer of gauze under the upper lip. In patients that exhibit a pseudo Class III deformity, a second photograph with the mouth slightly open will help show a more pleasing profile as the mandible rotates downward (clockwise). Facial photographs also include smiling and maximum opening views if hypomobility exists. Finally, photographs of the patient's anterior and posterior occlusion in centric relationship and centric occlusion are taken, as well as occlusal views of the maxilla and mandible denoting arch form.

Study casts

Full-arch casts should be trimmed in centric relation according to the methods described in undergraduate orthodontic textbooks. This trimming is necessary since many of the deformities are "nonocclusions," which cannot be accurately articulated

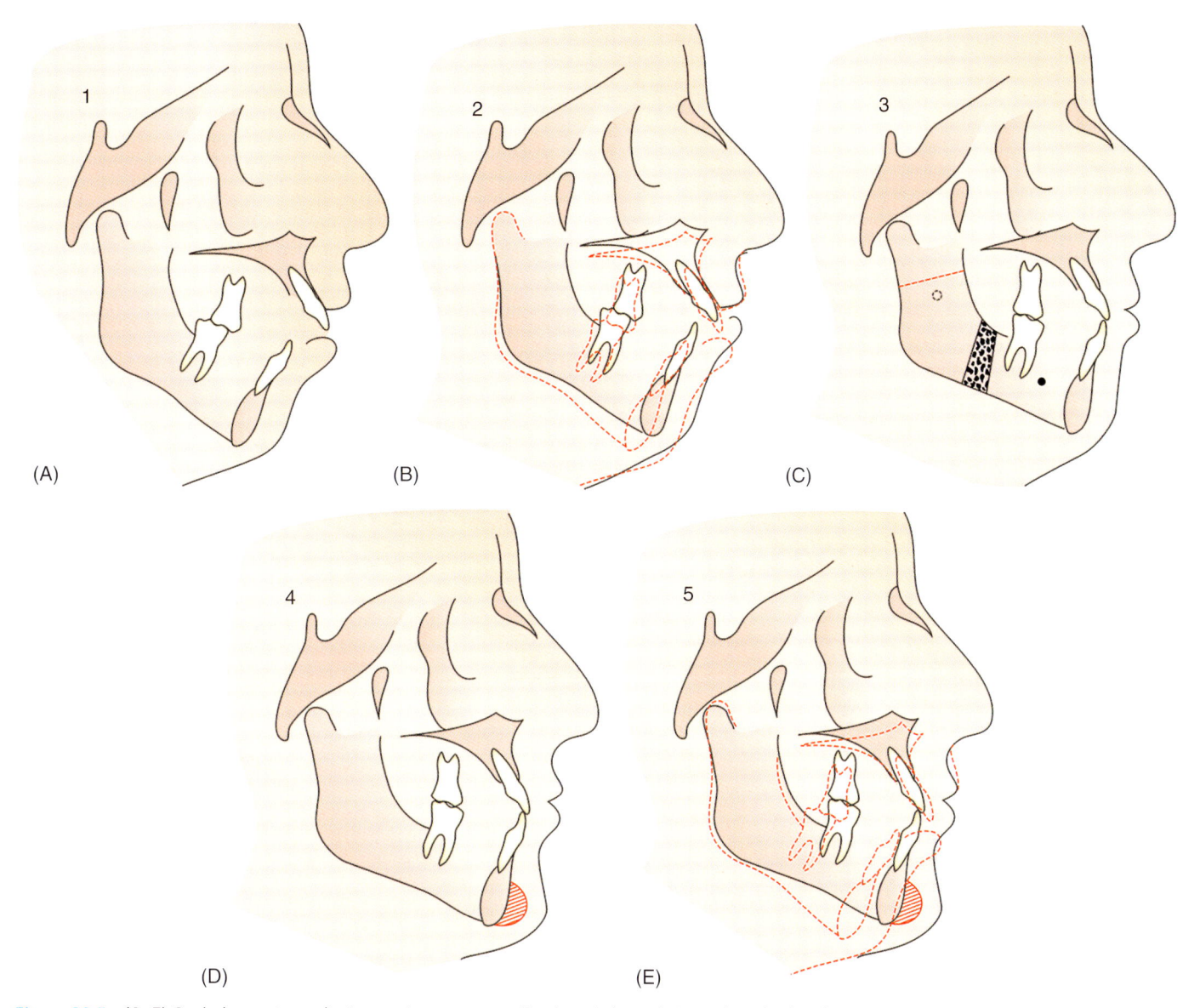

Figure 29.5 **(A–E)** Cephalometric prediction tracing sequence. Tracings 1 through 5 are described in the text.

when the models are held by hand. In severe cases, as well as cases that will undergo significant vertical changes as a result of treatment, mounting of the casts on an articulator with hinge-axis records will be necessary. The decision of precision hinge-axis versus the arbitrary hinge-axis determination is dictated by individual circumstances, such as TMJ deterioration or dysfunction, degree of mandibular autorotation, and obvious asymmetry, among others.

Case presentation visit

Once the diagnosis and general treatment plans have been formulated, the team, consisting of the patient's dentist, orthodontist, and oral and maxillofacial surgeon, renders a final integrated treatment plan. The most effective manner in which to coordinate and present all of this information would be a joint conference among all of the parties involved.

The role of the primary dentist is to coordinate the efforts of the specialists through the diagnostic process and treatment period, since maintenance of the final result will be relegated to them. The general dentist should restore the dentition only to prevent dental emergencies during the surgical and orthodontic treatment. Defective restorations, caries, infection, and periodontal disease must be controlled, and oral hygiene must be monitored. Since the periodontal structures will be challenged during orthodontic and surgical treatment, optimal control and management of periodontal disease should be corrected immediately and monitored throughout the treatment.

It is beneficial to decide at the outset whether conventional orthodontics or a combined surgical–orthodontic treatment plan will be followed. Because of existing skeletal imbalance and facial disharmony, the axial relationships of the teeth are often compromised. For example, lingually inclined lower incisors in mandibular prognathism or labially inclined lower incisors in mandibular retrognathism are naturally occurring dental

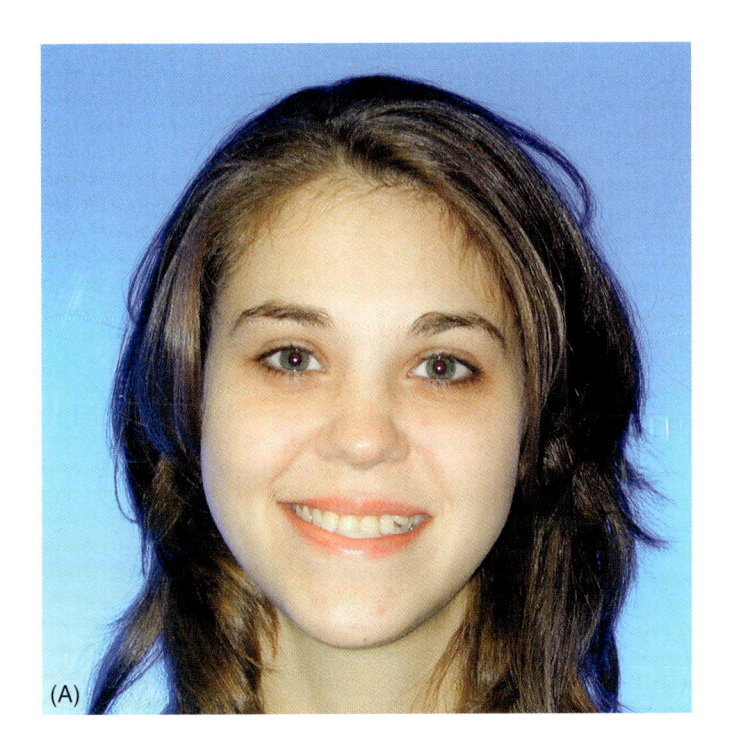

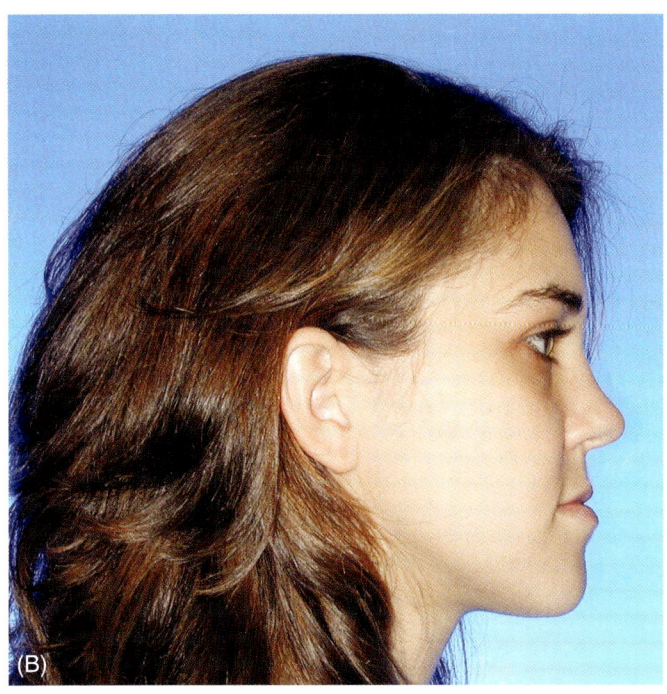

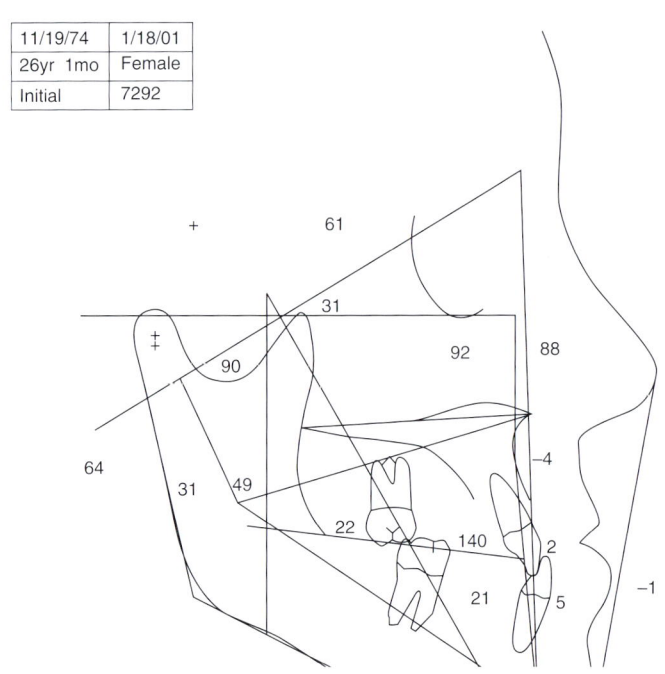

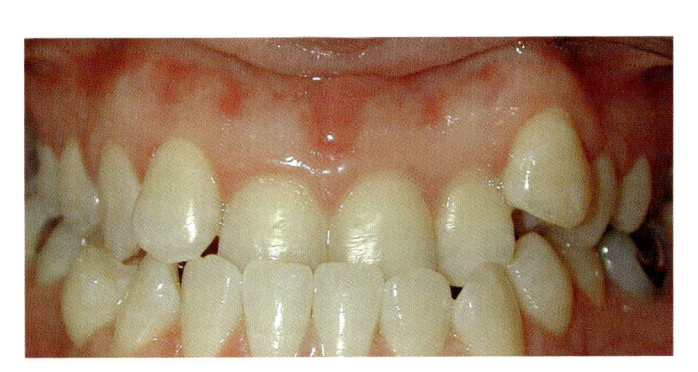

Figure 29.6 (A–D) Initial records of an adult with a Class III malocclusion.

"compensations" that must be corrected before any surgery is performed. This idealization of the tooth-to-bone relationship will not only enhance the final skeletal–dental balance but will also provide the surgeon with a greater opportunity to reorient the skeletal framework sufficiently to render a substantial improvement in the facial appearance.

Therefore, it is essential that the orthodontist explains to the patient that the presurgical "decompensation" of the dentition accentuates the deformity and can make the malocclusion, facial profile, and speech temporarily worse (Figure 29.7A–F). The patient must understand that this ultimately improves the bony support for the teeth and maximizes the esthetic changes resulting from upcoming surgical procedures.

In most instances, considerable effort is extended in the presurgical phase to arrange the dental arches so that a nearly ideal occlusion is achieved by the surgical procedure. This will leave

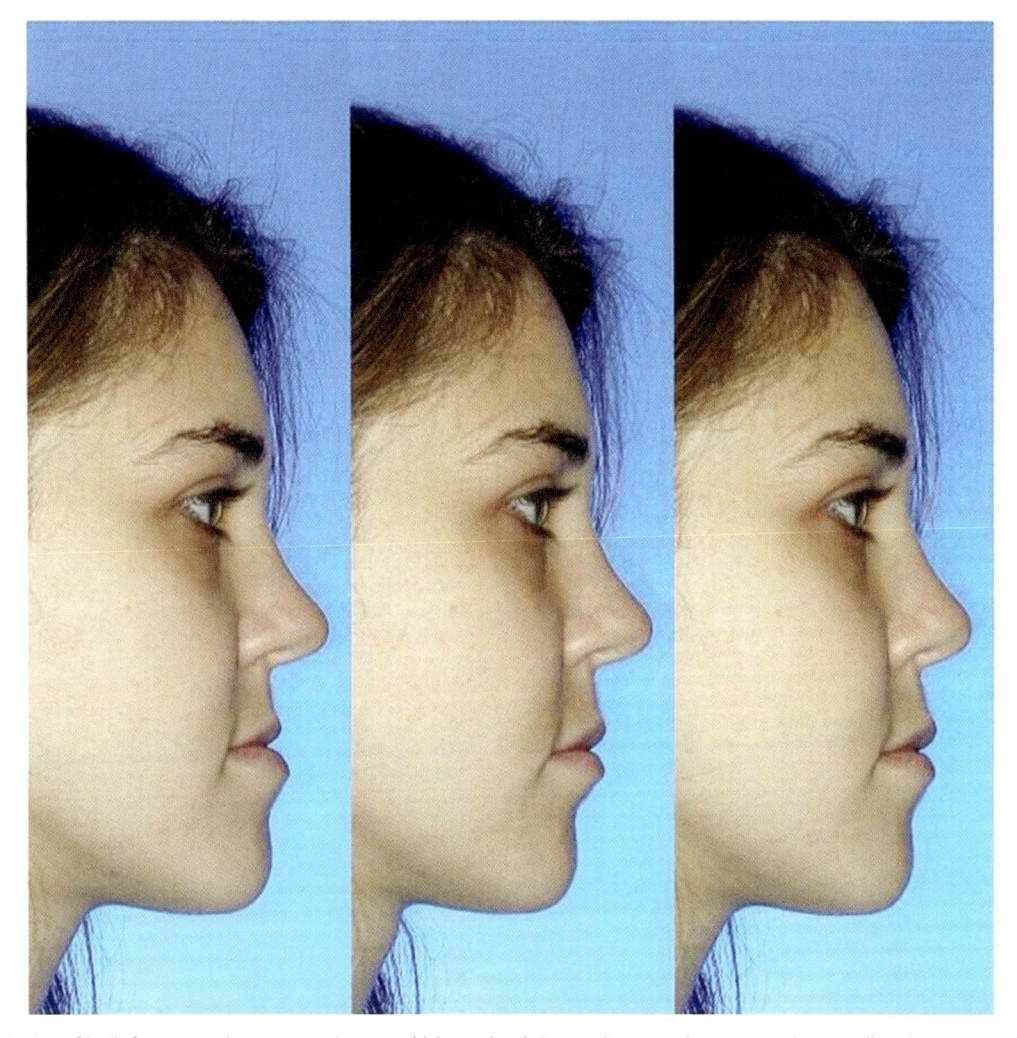

Figure 29.6 (E) Initial profile (left); surgical treatment by mandible set back (center); surgical treatment by maxilla advancement (right).

only short-term orthodontic detailing and refinement of the final occlusal scheme postsurgically. This approach offers several important advantages. Once surgery is completed, the patient is usually anxious to be finished. Second, and most importantly, if the immediate postoperative occlusion is stable, then the occlusion is more likely to remain stable for the long term.

Presurgical visit

When it is felt that the presurgical goals of arch alignment have been achieved, a set of progress records consisting of models, a cephalogram, and a panoramic radiograph will be obtained to verify that the patient is ready for surgery. Additional orthodontic treatment may be necessary to satisfy surgical goals.

A week or two before surgery, the patient should visit their general dentist for a thorough prophylaxis and fluoride treatment. The orthodontist will crimp or solder hooks to full-sized passive rectangular arch wires. This gives the surgeon options for intermaxillary fixation or elastics at the time of surgery. Even though the surgeon will be primarily responsible for the care of the patient during the postsurgical healing phase, the general dentist and orthodontist should be available.

Postsurgical treatment

At the conclusion of a 6- to 8-week period, whether intermaxillary fixation (IMF; jaws wired) is used or not, the surgeon will notify the orthodontist that they may begin definitive orthodontic treatment if clinical and radiographic examination indicates satisfactory healing. If bone segments begin to relapse, the orthodontist, working in concert with the surgeon, can nonsurgically reestablish the correct maxillomandibular relationship with elastics.

When occlusal splints are removed, the surgeon instructs the patient in the use of "training" elastics to preserve the skeletal alignment. Orthodontic follow-up as soon as possible is recommended. The orthodontist will inspect the mouth for loose or damaged brackets, wires, and so on. Patients will typically continue the training elastics on a tapering basis for 1–2 months. The surgery wires are removed as soon as the patient is opening comfortably and are replaced with light passive rectangular wires. The objective during and immediately after the surgery is to not produce orthodontic movement and possible surgical relapse. The patient should also be instructed in mobilization exercises to regain the full range of condylar motion. Occasionally, a physical therapy referral will be indicated.

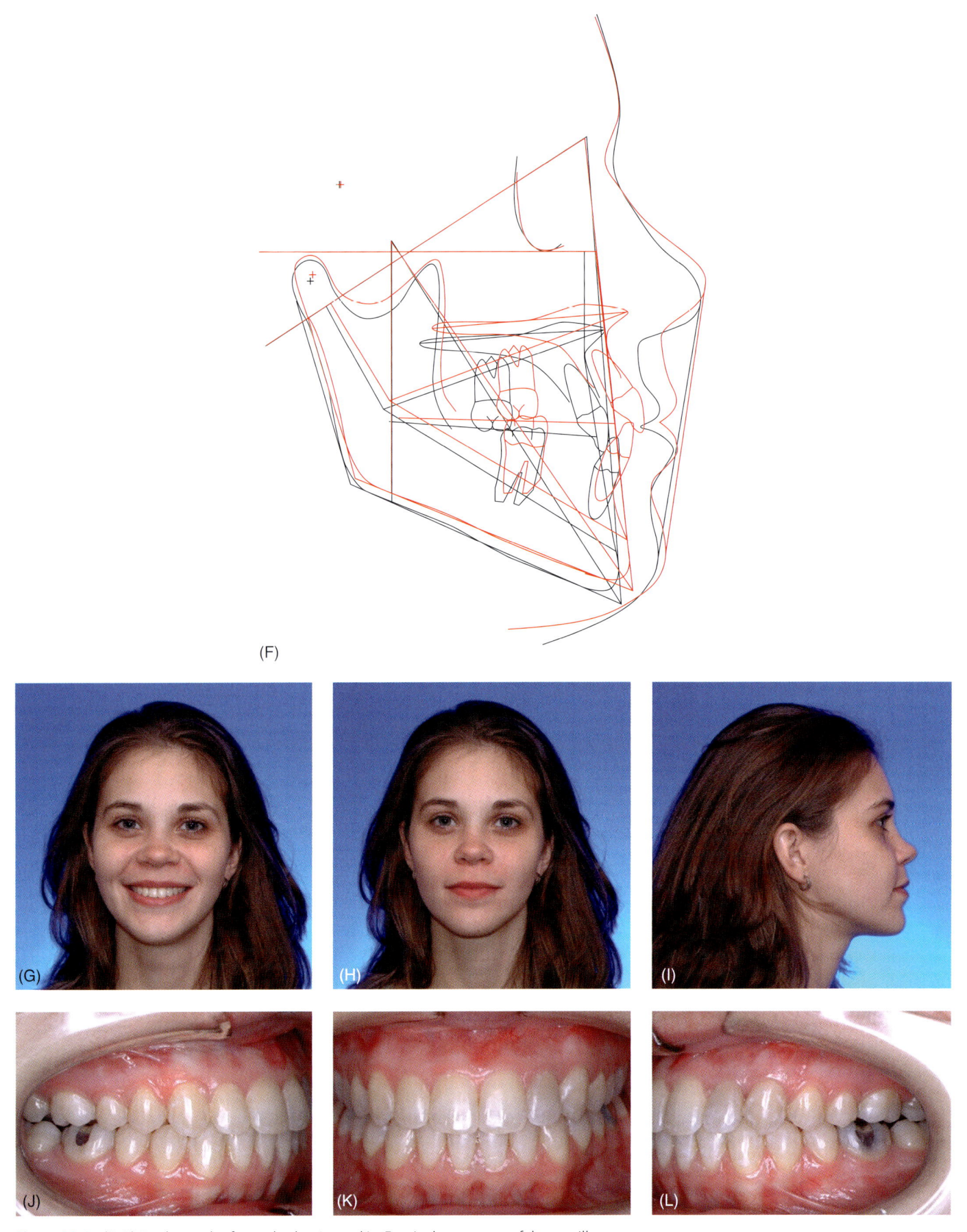

Figure 29.6 (F–L) Final records after orthodontics and Le Fort I advancement of the maxilla.

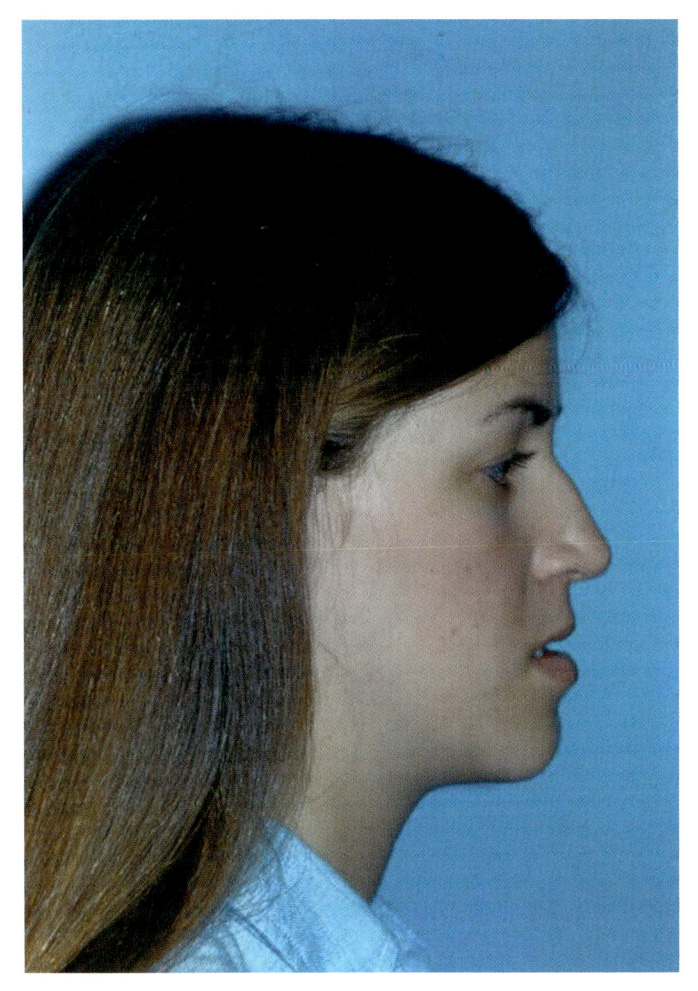

Figure 29.7 **(A)** Correction of mandibular prognathism and Class III malocclusion. Preorthodontic profile of a patient with mandibular prognathism and flat cheekbones.

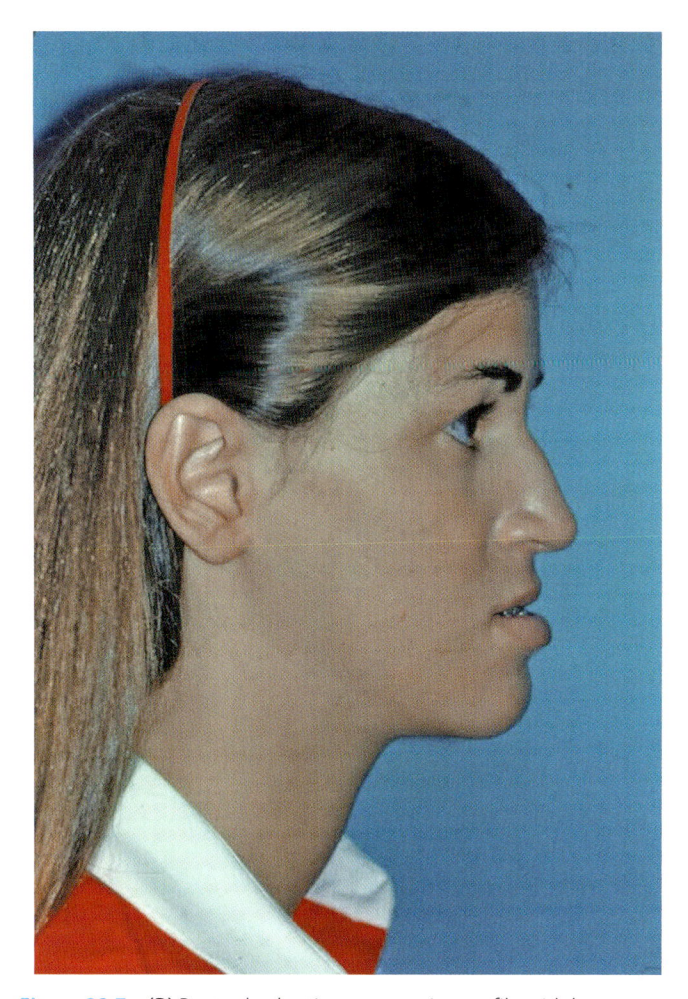

Figure 29.7 **(B)** Postorthodontic, preoperative profile with lower incisors flared to remove dental compensations. Patient intentionally looks worse from orthodontic treatment.

Ideally, the final phase of orthodontic treatment should be straightforward, with most patients completing treatment 4–8 months after surgery. Tooth positioners may be used for a short period after the braces are removed. In open bite cases, a true hinge-axis positioner is desirable. They are usually followed by more traditional retentive devices such as Hawley appliances and bonded lingual wires. Occasionally, a chin-cup is worn at night if relapse or additional growth is anticipated.

Surgical complications and risks

Fortunately, severe complications are rare. Certain surgical procedures carry a higher risk and are discussed in their respective sections. Patients must be adequately informed of these risks, particularly if there is no alternative in the selection of a surgical procedure. Complications, particularly infections, from orthognathic surgery were not uncommon in the past. Today, however, proper selection of surgical procedures, refinement of surgical techniques, improved methods of postoperative fixation with bone plates, control of edema, use of antibiotics, and increased knowledge of the treatment of postoperative infections have resulted in a low incidence of complications.

Injury to teeth

Most common surgical procedures last 2–5 h. The intraoral approach is most common and provides wide exposure of the maxilla and mandible while minimizing facial scars. An exceptional case may require an extraoral approach, particularly when mandibular bone grafts are used. Injuries to the teeth can occur with segmental alveolar osteotomies. With preoperative widening of the interdental space by orthodontics and careful technique, the injury to teeth can be avoided.

Blood loss

Blood loss can be significant during these procedures but is reduced with the increased use of hypotensive anesthesia. Transfusions of blood may be necessary in "double jaw" or more lengthy cases. The technique of autologous transfusion, in which the patient donates blood 2–3 weeks preoperatively, has significantly decreased the incidence of complications associated with transfusions.

Stabilization of operated segments

Stabilization of the operated segments is tantamount to proper healing, prevention of infection, and predictability of long-term stability. Bone segments are stabilized with bone plates and screws. Intermaxillary fixation, routinely required in the past, is now used primarily for cases involving significant mandibular setbacks or if bone plates and screws fail to immobilize jaw segments or are not possible. Early mobilization promotes faster functional bone healing, more rapid return of masticatory function, and facilitation of nutritional maintenance during the early postoperative period.

Postoperative discomfort and symptoms

Postoperative discomfort is generally mild and can be handled with the conservative use of analgesics. Most patients are given a pain regimen not much more significant than third molar surgery. Since there is a potential for significant postoperative edema, it is imperative to have informed the family that the patient may look much worse than they feel. Intraoperative as well as postoperative steriods tend to help manage the postoperative edema. Surgical dietary counseling and the availability of commercially prepared high-calorie, high-protein supplements can minimize weight loss postoperatively and maintain the nutritional balance required for normal wound healing.

Diagnosis and treatment

Common dentofacial deformities are described in terms of their facial, skeletal, and dental characteristics. Treatment sequencing, orthodontic principles, and surgical procedures are now presented as a guide to the most frequently occurring deformities.

Mandibular excess

The facial soft-tissue characteristics of classic mandibular skeletal prognathism or excess are primarily manifested in the profile view (see Figure 29.7A). There is a prominence of the lower lip and chin, a flat mentolabial fold, a normal to slight increase in the lower anterior facial height, a normal to obtuse gonial angle, and an appearance of sallow or deficient zygomas. From the frontal view, an increase in the lower anterior facial height and a flatness or lack of contour in the area of the zygomas and chin is usually evident. Cephalometrically, the point A–nasion–point B (ANB) angle is decreased, whereas the facial angle, sella–nasion–point B (SNB) angle, and the lower anterior facial height are increased. The maxillary incisors are flared, and the lower incisors are lingually inclined. A negative overjet, Class III cuspid and molar relationships, and bilateral crossbites are common. In addition, these cases are generally characterized by severe arch length discrepancies in both arches.

Orthodontically, upper first bicuspids may be removed to correct crowding and flaring of the upper incisors. The lower arch is often treated without extractions, since arch length is gained by tipping the incisal edges forward. This produces proper axial inclination of the incisors and fullness in the lower lip (see Figure 29.7B). The resulting worsening of the facial appearance will maximize the facial esthetic result when the mandible is set back by surgery (see Figure 29.7C–F). If mandibular extractions are required, the second bicuspids are usually removed to minimize retraction of the lower incisors. Class II mechanics, or reverse orthodontics, which accentuate the deformity, are often used to achieve these presurgical orthodontic goals. The increase in negative overjet allows for a normal incisor relationship postsurgically and will reestablish a normal mentolabial soft-tissue contour. Bilateral posterior crossbites evident presurgically are usually resolved with the surgical mandibular setback.

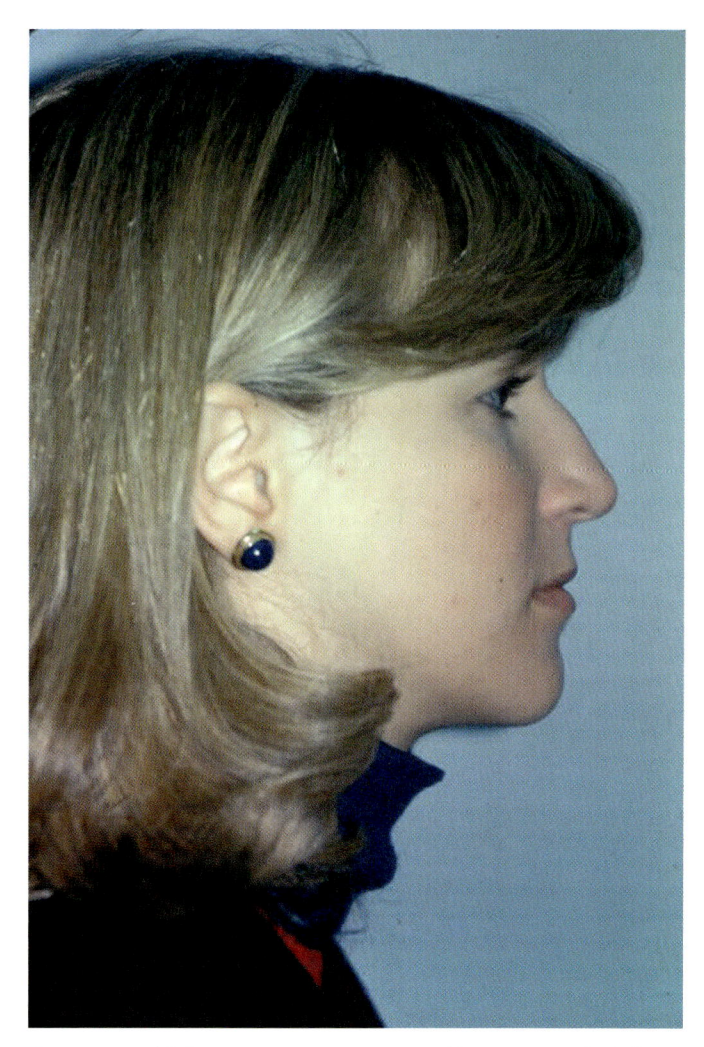

Figure 29.7 (C) Four-year postoperative profile. Surgery included augmentation with cheekbone implants and vertical subcondylar osteotomy (VSO) of the mandible.

At least three variations of prognathism exist. Dentoalveolar prognathism is a horizontal prominence of the lower lip and dentition only. Since the chin is relatively normal in its relation to the upper face, profile prediction tracing of the surgical setback makes the patient appear "chin deficient." Orthodontics alone or alveolar osteotomies are therefore indicated rather than ramus surgery. A transfer of the inferior border may be necessary in bimaxillary prognathism with open bite for graft source and shortening of the facial height (Figure 29.8A and B). Alveolar

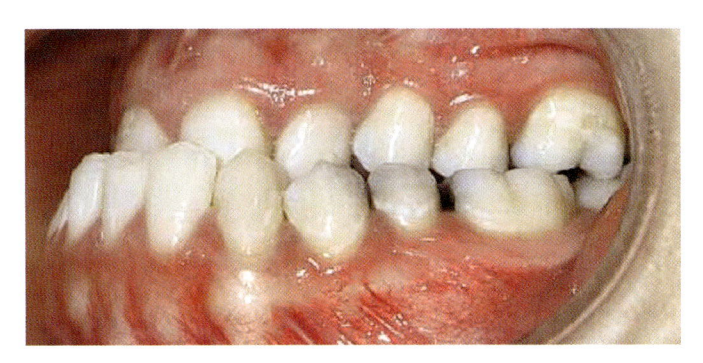

Figure 29.7 (D) Initial pretreatment Class III malocclusion.

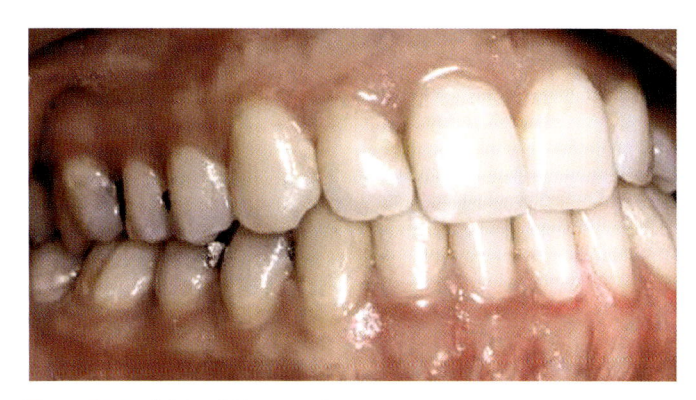

Figure 29.7 (E) Final Class I occlusion.

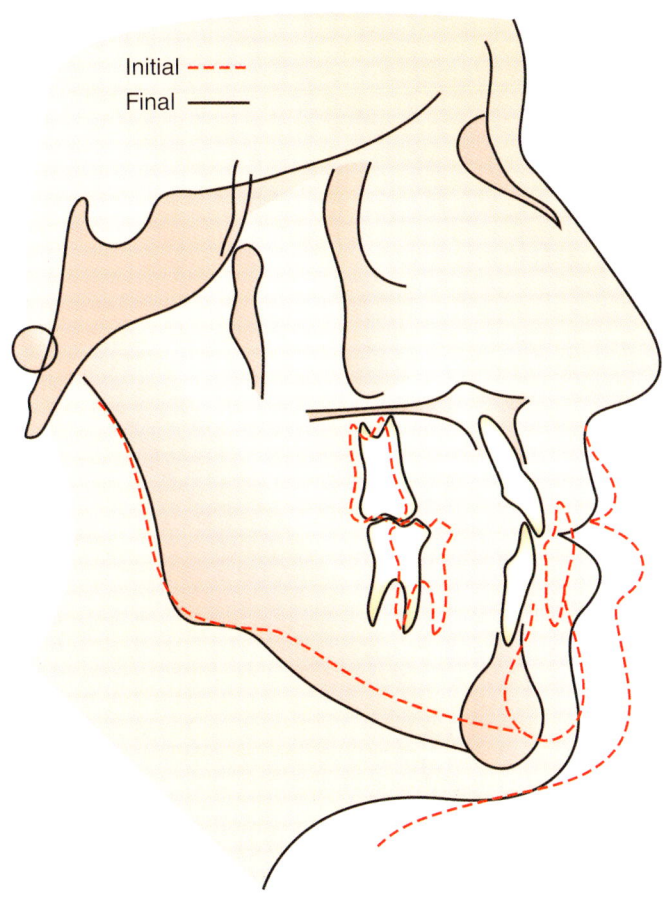

Figure 29.7 (F) Pretreatment and final tracing 4 years after surgery.

osteotomies are usually stabilized using splints without IMF. Pseudo or false prognathism is a relative expression of mandibular horizontal excess secondary to a horizontal or vertically deficient maxilla. Correction of the maxillary midfacial deficiency will often obviate the need for mandibular surgery. The diagnosis and treatment are discussed in the section on maxillary deficiency. Prognathism may also be unexpressed in patients with VME. The features of true prognathism become evident when the maxilla is moved superiorly to a normalized position and the mandible autorotates upward and forward.

Surgery for correction of most prognathic cases consists of intraoral osteotomies in the ramus—vertical subcondylar, inverted "L," or sagittal split type. Occasionally, a body osteotomy is indicated. The intraoral VSO or vertical ramus osteotomy (VRO) is performed through a mucosal incision lateral to the midpoint of the anterior border of the ramus extending down to the vestibule opposite the first molar. Subperiosteal reflection of the lateral surface of the ramus and very limited posterior border reflection allow for placement of special retractors. A slightly curved oblique osteotomy is performed with oscillating saws from the anterior sigmoid notch to the angle of the mandible, avoiding the lingual area. The mandible is set back by overlapping of the ramus with the condylar segment (Figure 29.9A–C). The segments are rigidly fixated. Direct wire

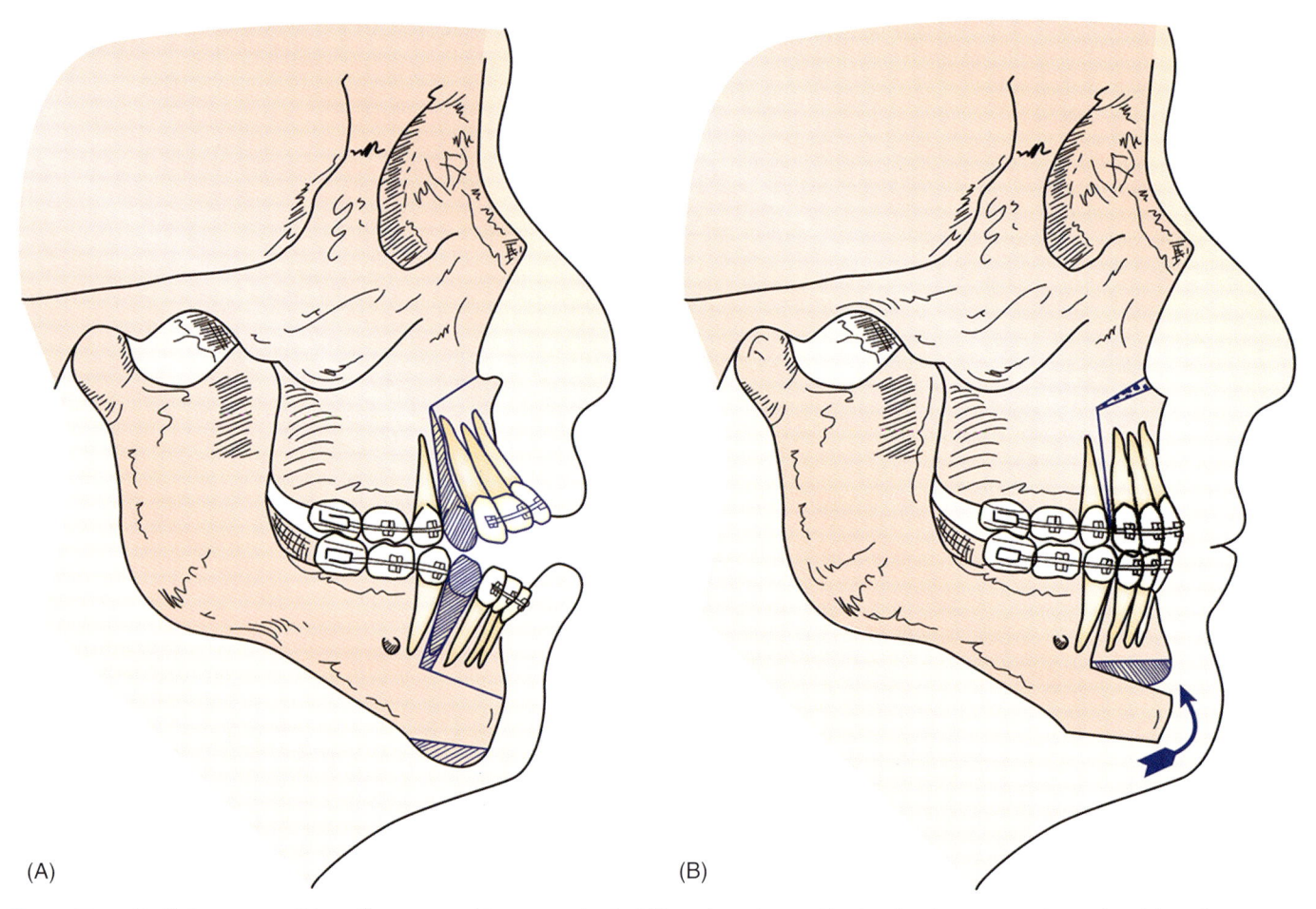

Figure 29.8 (A, B) Correction of bimaxillary prognathism, excessive facial length, and open bite by alveolar osteotomies and excision of inferior border.

fixation is sometimes used if bone apposition is questionable or condylar sag is apparent. Intermaxillary fixation with wires or elastics is necessary for 6–8 weeks if rigid fixation is not used. Relapse in the form of a Class III open-bite condition is seen if excessive soft tissue is detached from the condylar segment or if inadequate bone contact occurs between segments. Injury to the inferior alveolar nerve is possible but uncommon. Sensory disturbance associated with vertical ramus osteotomy varies from 0% to 70% with a mean of 9%. The results are usually quite satisfactory with the VRO, a procedure used for over 55 years extraorally and for over 45 years intraorally.

The inverted "L" osteotomy, a modification of the VRO that maintains the coronoid process, is indicated when the ramus of the mandible is lengthened at surgery to close an anterior open bite with prognathism. Bone blocks are wedged along the horizontal cut to maintain the normal condyle–fossa relation. The sagittal split osteotomy, also used for correction of prognathism with or without an open bite, is more frequently used for mandibular deficiency, and the technique is described in the "Mandibular deficiency" section.

The body ostectomy is indicated in unusual and very specific cases of prognathism sometimes seen with open bite that is not attributable to excessive maxillary growth or deep bites. If orthodontics and ramus surgery cannot produce an acceptable Class I occlusion and correct a posterior molar crossbite, a body ostectomy may be indicated. The anterior segment is repositioned according to the ostectomy cut, which may be triangular, rectangular, or stepped. The inferior alveolar nerve may require repositioning to perform the ostectomy. Injury to the nerve during this procedure is possible. Fixation of the segments is with wires or bone plates along the inferior border (Figure 29.10A–C). Mandibular prognathism combined with maxillary deformities such as VME or others may result in extreme deformities requiring surgical correction in both jaws (Figure 29.10C–E).

Mandibular deficiency

In mandibular deficiency, or retrognathism, the soft-tissue characteristics are manifested primarily in the profile view (Figures 29.11A and B and 29.12A–D). There will be a short or normal facial height, a deep or normal labiomental sulcus, horizontal deficiency of the lower lip and chin, but a sometimes adequate chin contour. The maxilla may be normal or slightly protrusive, depressing the lower lip. When the patient protrudes the mandible to a Class I posture, the relative protrusion of the maxillary teeth disappears and the profile view improves. From the frontal view, only the deep mentolabial fold may be apparent (see Figure 29.12A), although often there is evidence of mentalis

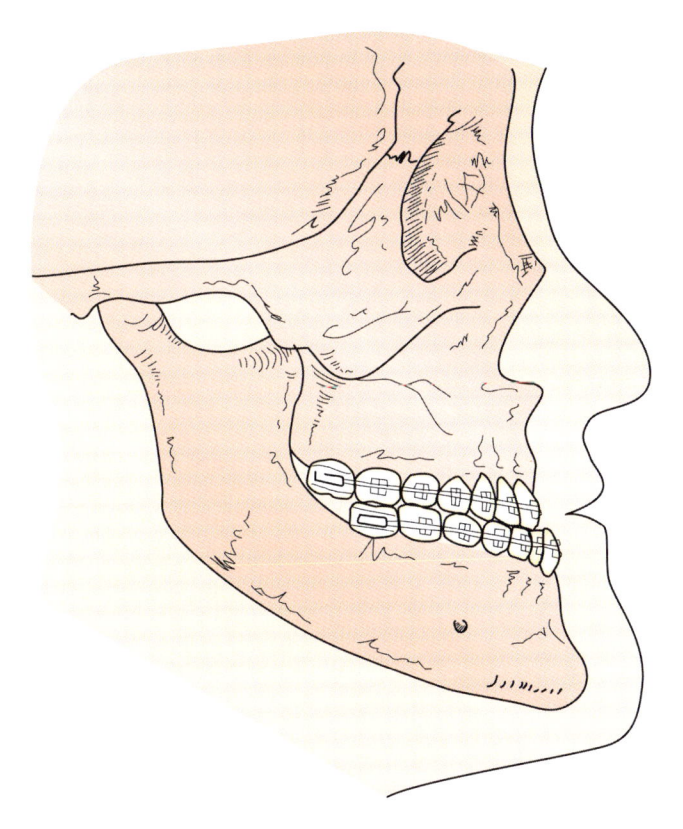

Figure 29.9 **(A)** Profile of hard and soft tissues in classic mandibular prognathism with Class III malocclusion.

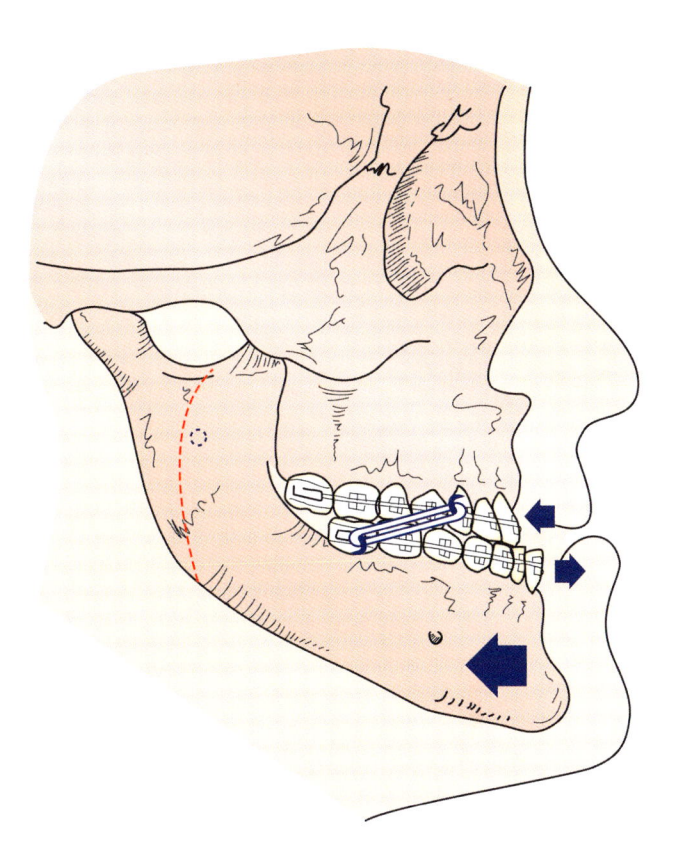

Figure 29.9 **(B)** Preoperative orthodontic tooth movement reverses dental compensations, produces correct inclination of incisors, and worsens facial appearance so that mandibular setback maximizes esthetic results. Note the outline of the proposed VSO.

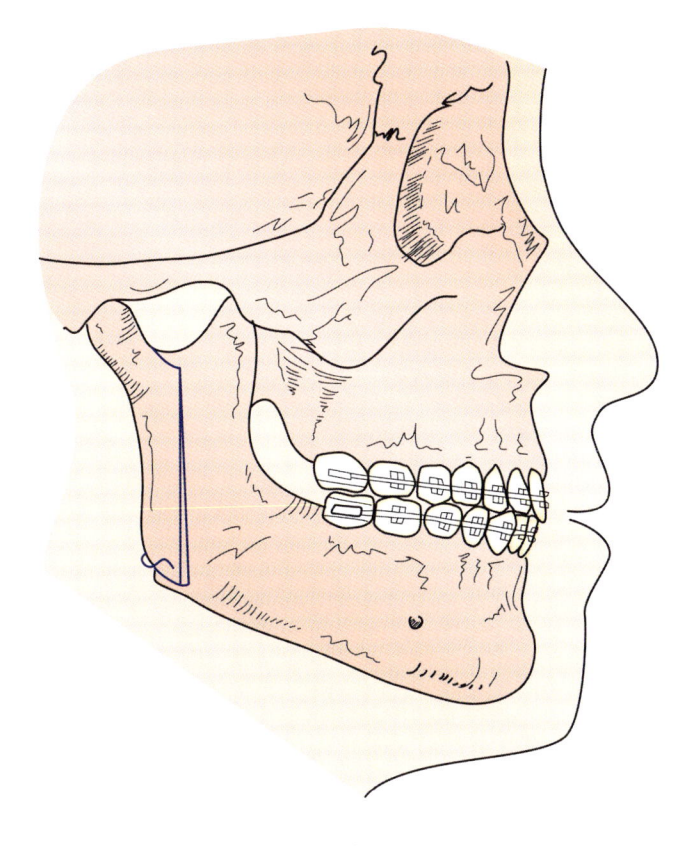

Figure 29.9 **(C)** Postoperative position of mandible and Class I occlusion following VSO.

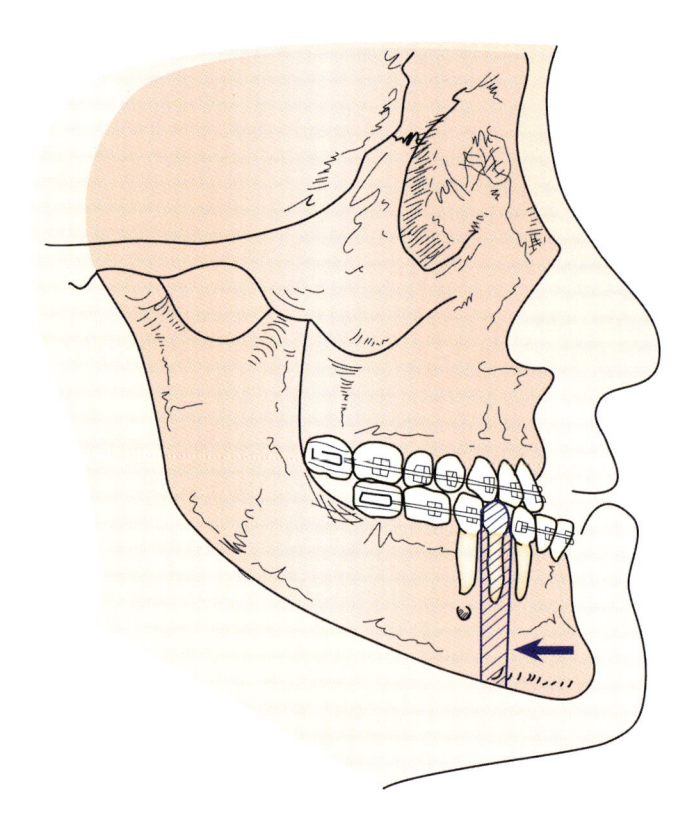

Figure 29.10 **(A)** Correction of mandibular prognathism by body ostectomy through the first premolar site.

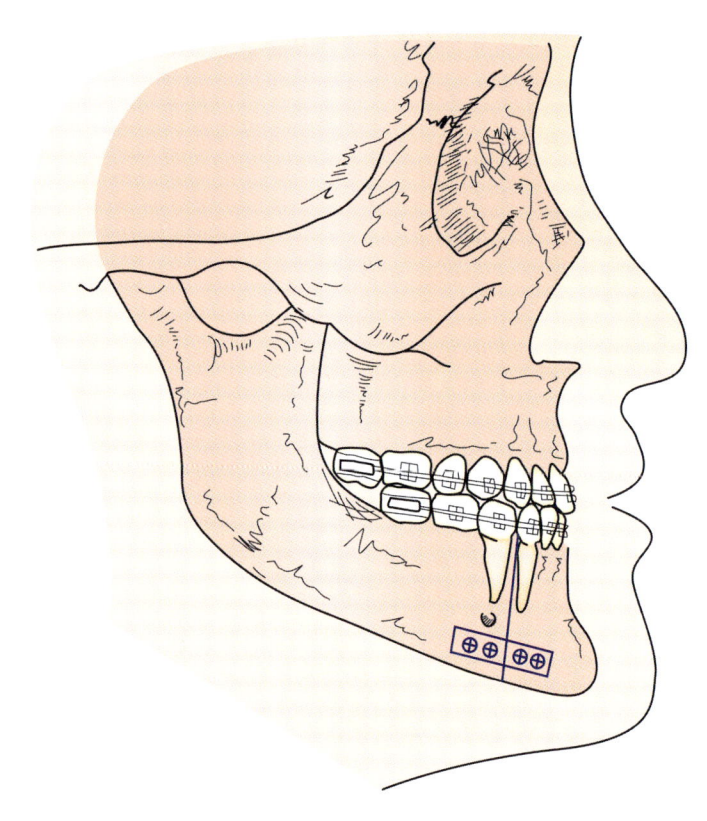

Figure 29.10 **(B)** Postoperative stabilization of the mandible with bone plates.

strain. Cephalometrically, the ANB angle will be increased, the SNB and facial angles will be decreased, and the lower incisors will be protrusive. In Class II, Division 2 types, the maxillary incisors will be retrusive. Dentally, there is an increased overjet, a deep impinging overbite, Class II cuspid and molar relationships bilaterally, and a narrow maxillary arch with transverse discrepancy when the mandible is moved forward.

Orthodontic reversal of dental compensations is necessary to position the teeth over basal bone. The severely flared lower incisors often seen in these cases require lower first premolar bicuspid extractions to achieve significant uprighting. If the horizontal position of the upper incisors is satisfactory, the maxillary second bicuspids may be extracted to exaggerate the Class II molar relationship and minimize the retraction of the maxillary incisors. Seldom are these cases treated with extractions only in the lower arch since Class III molar relationships rarely function well in the occlusal scheme. Class III mechanics are used to retract and upright the lower incisors to the proper axial relationship (see Figure 29.11A). The reciprocal effect of the elastics on the maxillary arch will preclude retraction of the upper incisors, accentuate the overjet, and facilitate maximal surgical advancement of the mandible for improved facial esthetics.

It is preferred to presurgically level the lower arch, although in Class II, Division 2 cases the leveling of the exaggerated curve of Spee, which usually accompanies these types, may be quite difficult. Bite plates are often used to facilitate the leveling. Crowding in the upper arch is usually resolved once the upper incisors have been flared forward to their proper relationship.

Class II cases with an acceptable transverse relationship preoperatively may develop posterior crossbites after mandibular advancement. These cases may require significant preoperative maxillary orthodontic expansion or provisions for concomitant surgical expansion of the maxilla.

All surgical procedures for correcting Class II deformities are directed at correcting the majority of horizontal changes with mandibular osteotomies and vertical changes with maxillary osteotomies. Maxillary procedures are as described for VME. The sagittal splitting osteotomy of Obwegesser is by far the most frequently used and time-honored procedure for correction of mandibular deficiency with and without open bite and limited facial asymmetry (see Figure 29.11B). The intraoral incision is similar to that used in the VSO procedure. Soft tissue is detached on the medial surface of the ramus and lateral surface of the body but not the lateral ramus surface. Medial ramus and lateral body cortical cuts are joined with an osteotomy cut along the anterior border of the ramus and external oblique ridge. Splitting of the mandible is performed with wide, thin osteotomes and gentle prying. Visualization of the inferior alveolar nerve prior to final separation is key to avoid injury to the nerve. Detachment of the medial pterygoid muscle usually allows full advancement. When anterior border wiring is used to approximate segments, 6 weeks of IMF are usually adequate because of the large area of cancellous bone apposition. More commonly, rigid fixation with bone screws allows for immediate movement of the mandible; however, patients must still be maintained on a liquid diet for several weeks. Temporary anesthesia of the inferior alveolar

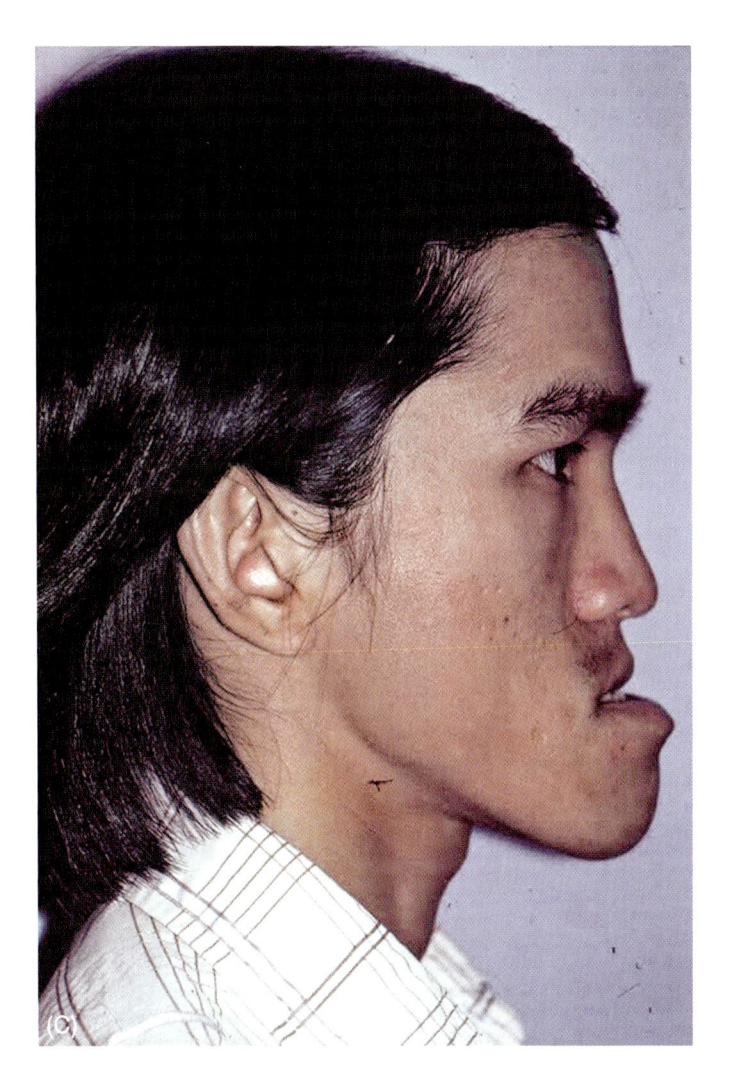

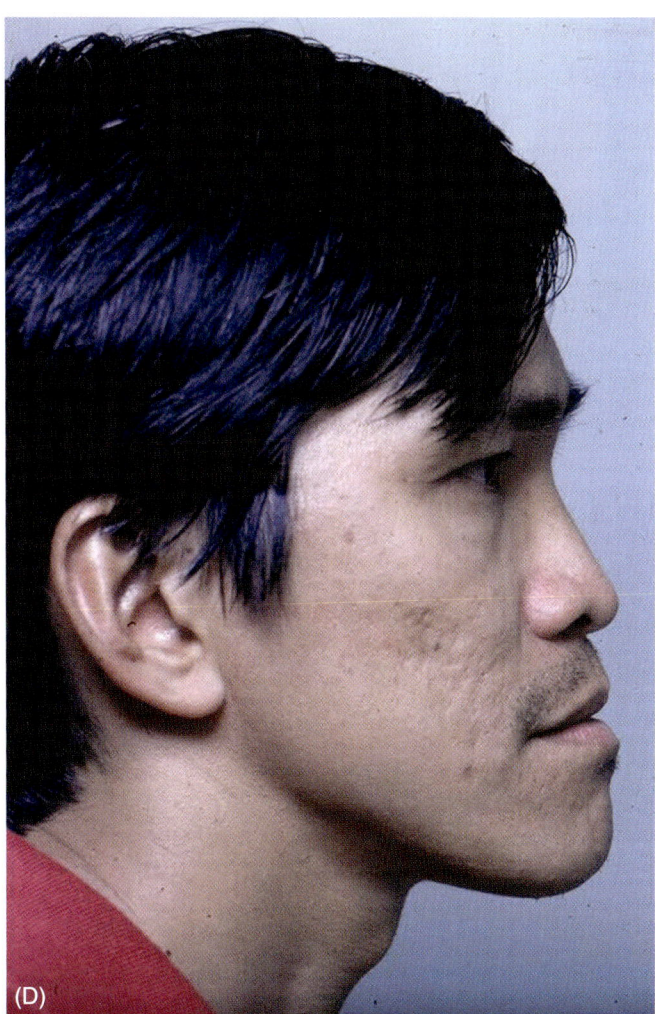

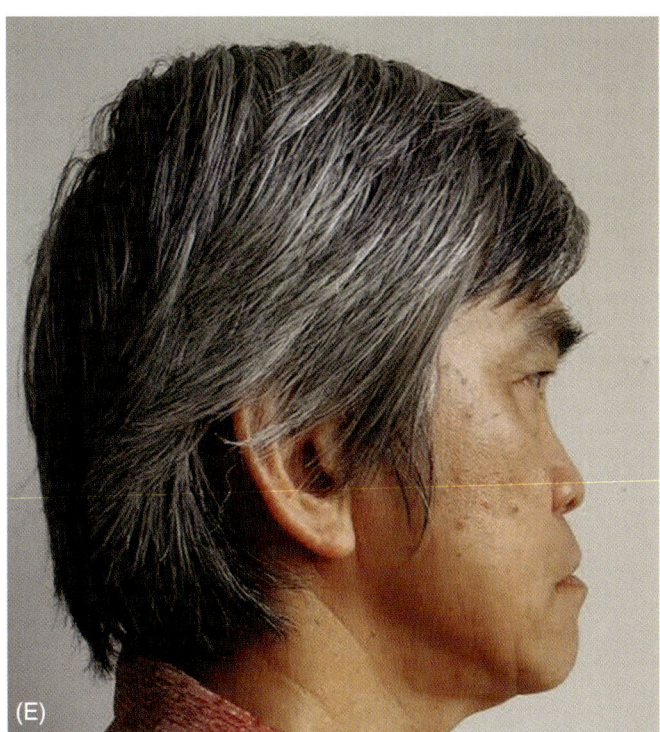

Figure 29.10 **(C)** Presurgical and **(D)** 5-year postsurgical correction of severe mandibular prognathism and maxillary deficiency by body ostectomy of the mandible (setback) and Le Fort I osteotomy of the maxilla (advancement). Postoperative stabilization of the mandible with bone plates. **(E)** The 40-year follow-up.

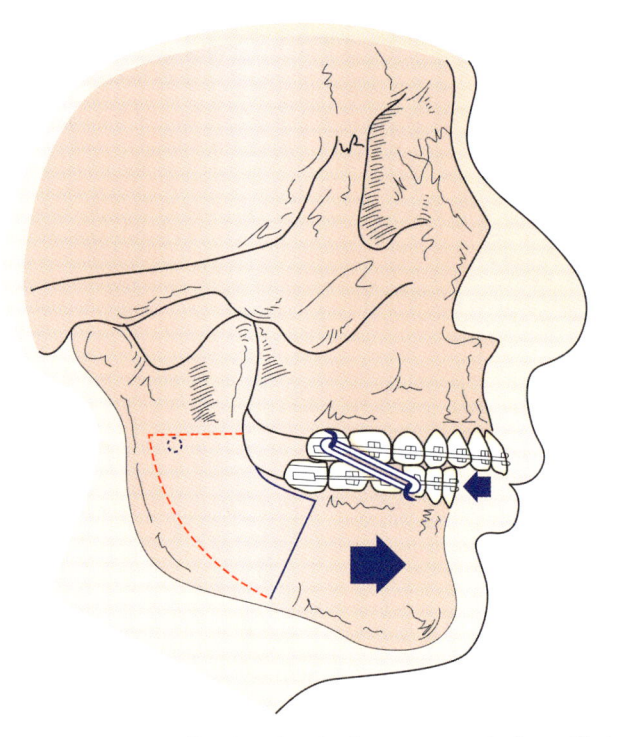

Figure 29.11 **(A)** Profile of hard and soft tissues typical of mandibular deficiency or retrognathism and Class II malocclusion. Preoperative orthodontic treatment reverses dental compensation by uprighting the lower incisors. This permits maximum advancement of the mandible by surgery. Note the outline of the proposed sagittal split osteotomy.

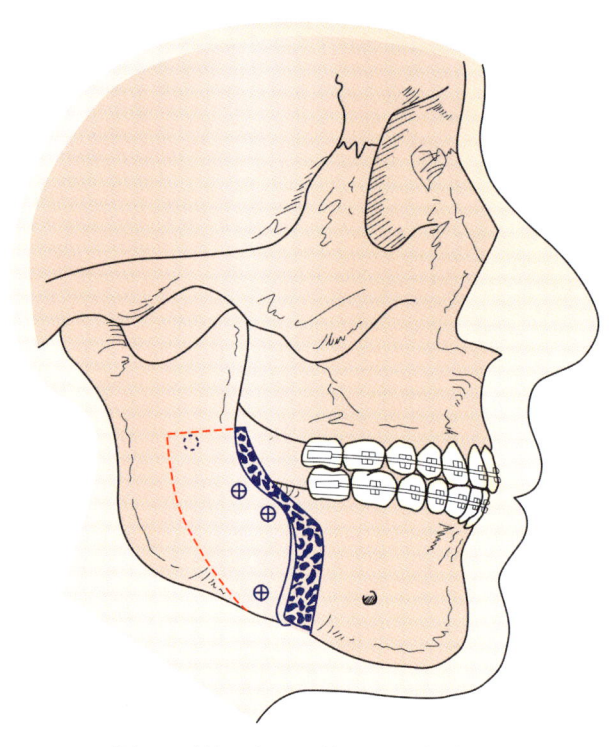

Figure 29.11 **(B)** Mandible advanced by sagittal split osteotomy and stabilized by rigid fixation bone screw technique. Intermaxillary fixation is not required.

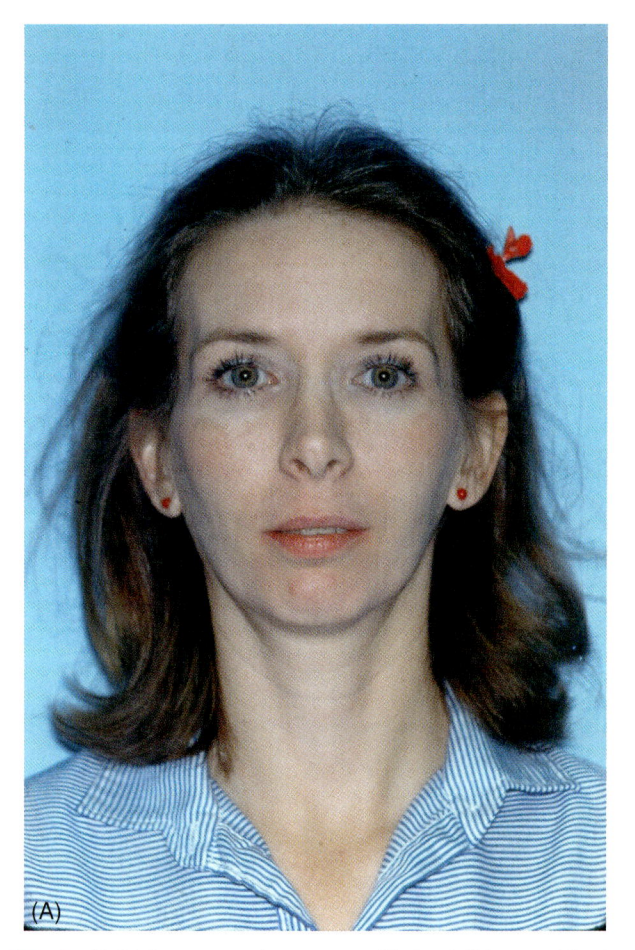

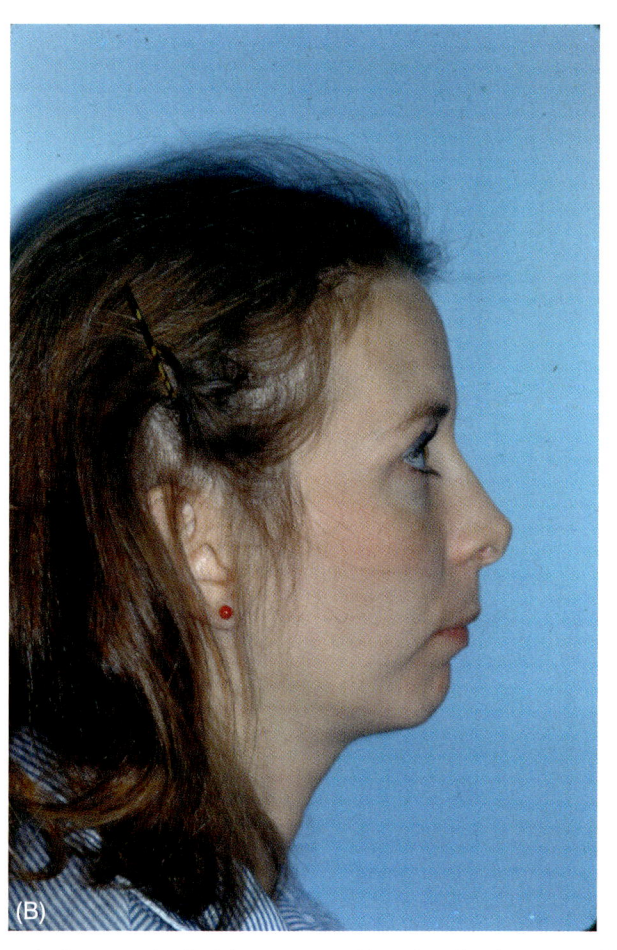

Figure 29.12 **(A, B)** Correction of severe mandibular deficiency with microgenia. Preoperative facial appearance. Note that the chin is retruded and deficient in contour.

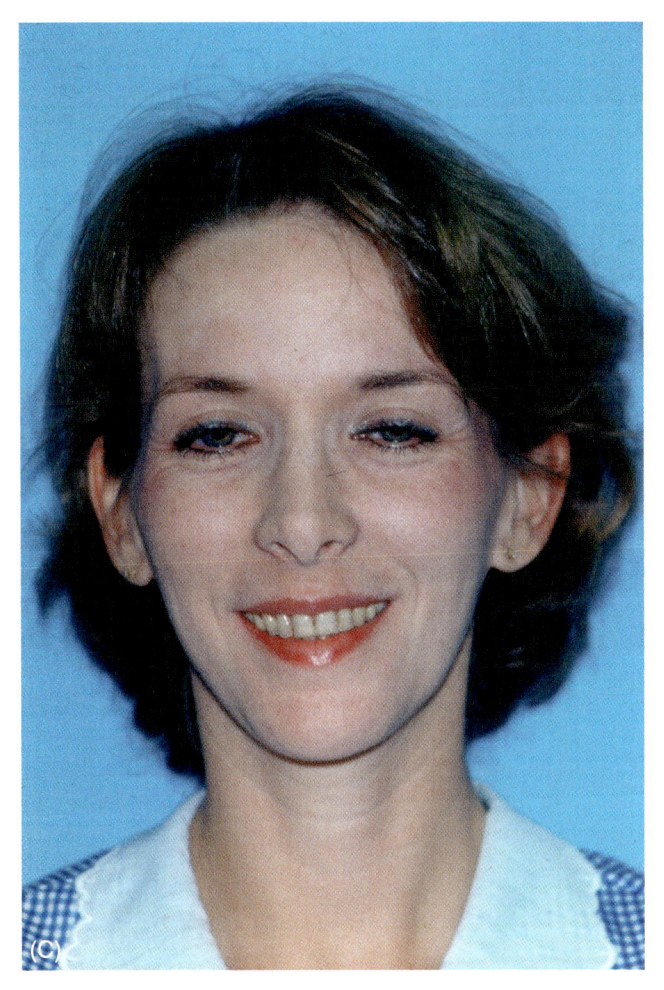

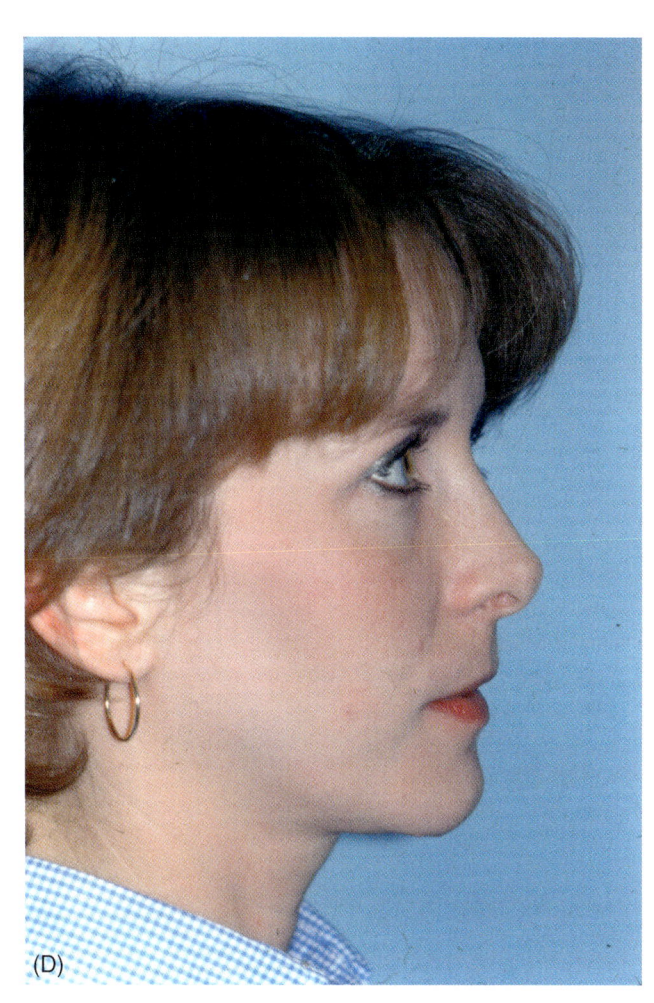

Figure 29.12 **(C, D)** Postoperative facial appearance following advancement of the mandible and chin by sagittal split osteotomy and chin implant.

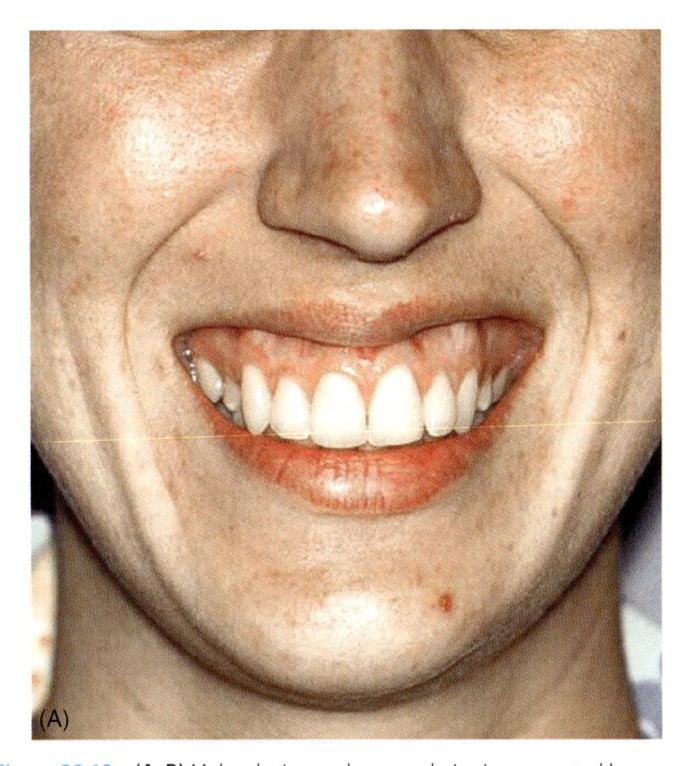

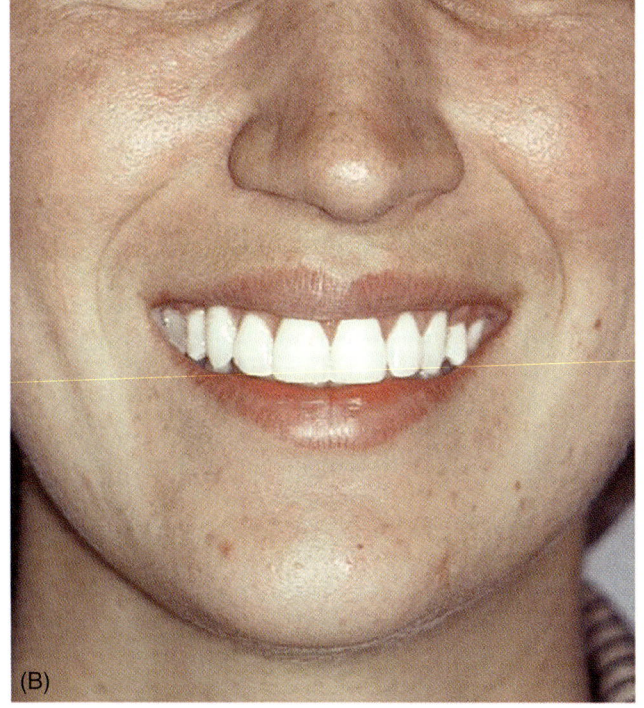

Figure 29.13 **(A, B)** Malocclusion and exposed gingiva corrected by superior repositioning of the maxilla with Le Fort I osteotomy.

nerve is frequent, but, fortunately, permanent anesthesia is infrequent. Sensory disturbance associated with sagittal splitting osteotomy varies from 0% to 75% with a mean of 35%. Inappropriate splitting, extensive swelling, and hemorrhage are very infrequent but can occur.

Other procedures, such as "C" or "L" osteotomies, may be performed either intraorally or extraorally. They are, however, reserved for micrognathia, extreme advancement, or other unusual conditions and may require bone grafting. Additional chin advancement by horizontal osteotomy of the symphysis or chin implant for retrognathia or micrognathia is frequently necessary. These procedures are described later.

Maxillary excess

Maxillary excess with a normal mandible rarely occurs as a single entity. It is usually accompanied by mandibular deficiency, mandibular excess, or mandibular asymmetry. The facial soft-tissue characteristics of VME are manifested equally in both the frontal and profile views. The facial features are dominated by a long tapering face with a narrow alar base, increased nasolabial angle, lip incompetence, a highly convex profile, a flat mentolabial fold, and usually a deficient chin. Excessive display of maxillary anterior teeth is seen with the lips at rest, and a "gummy smile" is apparent (Figure 29.13A and B). Cephalometrically, there will be a large increase in the lower anterior facial height and mandibular plane angle and a decrease in posterior facial height. VME occurs with or without an anterior open bite. Horizontal excess or protrusion of the incisors may be seen, and bilateral posterior crossbites are common.

The mandible may be rotated clockwise (down and back) because of VME (Figure 29.14A). When a prediction tracing moves the maxilla superiorly to a normal lip–incisor relationship, the mandible will rotate upward and forward toward a more normal position. If this is not the case, surgery to advance the mandible may also be necessary (Figure 29.14B and C). If VME is accompanied by a normal mandible or mandibular excess, mandibular setback surgery may be necessary to correct a protruding mandible that is rotated forward secondary to maxillary superior positioning.

Although extractions are frequently required to alleviate crowding, it is often desirable to delay extractions in the upper arch until the time of surgery, using the teeth to be extracted to aid in the leveling and alignment of the posterior segments and to preserve the alveolar bony dimensions. By performing segmental osteotomies with a Le Fort I osteotomy, the surgeon can retract and upright protrusive maxillary incisors and expand or advance posterior segments (see Figure 29.14B). If space is required in the arch, the extraction sites should be closed completely preoperatively. The curve of Spee in the lower arch should be leveled completely.

Presurgical orthodontic treatment of VME cases differs greatly from that of prognathic or retrognathic cases. Since the extrusion of teeth via conventional orthodontic mechanics is potentially unstable, mechanics that would produce this effect are avoided in all instances. Intramaxillary mechanics are used extensively, rather than Class II, Class III, or headgear forces, and deliberate care is taken to ensure the preservation of any open bite. Segmental rather than complete arch leveling is necessary in the maxilla to preserve an exaggerated compensating curve or "stepped" occlusion in the canine region (see Figure 29.14B). In those cases in which the maxilla is to be surgically segmentalized and no extractions are contemplated, it is helpful to diverge the dental roots for passage of the surgical saw. Historically, maxillas were segmentalized between the canines and first premolars. With orthodontic support, more osteotomies are performed between the canines and lateral incisors. Since bilateral crossbites often accompany VME cases, it is often preferable to plan for surgical expansion in the posterior segments at the time the osteotomies are performed.

Vertical changes in the maxilla through Le Fort I osteotomy and concomitant vertical and horizontal changes in the mandible by surgery may produce tremendous functional and esthetic results (Figure 29.15A–C). Le Fort I osteotomy of the maxilla is usually performed through a vestibular incision 5 mm superior to the mucogingival junction from the first molar to the first molar. Tunneling beneath the mucoperiosteum to the pterygoid plates and reflection of the nasal mucosa from the floor of the nose allow for osteotomes and air-driven saws to produce osteotomies for down-fracture of the maxilla from pterygoid plates, nasal septum, lateral maxillary, and nasal walls. The amount of bone to be excised is determined from mock surgery and measurements on models mounted on an anatomic articulator. Division of the maxilla in the canine area or between the central incisors allows for a variety of vertical, horizontal, and transverse movements of all segments. Turbinectomy, nasal septal straightening, palatal repositioning, and buccal lipectomies are frequently done to anatomically correct all aspects of VME. An intermediate splint keyed to the unoperated mandible ensures correct superior positioning of the maxilla. Once the maxilla is stabilized with wires or bone plates, mandibular surgery is performed if necessary. The mandible is stabilized with a final splint to the newly positioned maxilla. Intermaxillary fixation is rarely indicated. Rather, light elastics between the maxilla and mandible will correct any minor occlusal discrepancies into the final occlusal splint.

Maxillary deficiency

Maxillary deficiency most commonly associated with other deformities can occur in all three planes of space: anteroposterior, vertical, and transverse. Transverse deficiency or posterior crossbite can be bilateral or unilateral and is most commonly associated with other deformities. The apparent transverse deficiency accompanying true mandibular prognathism is usually resolved with the surgical repositioning of the mandible. Class II deformities usually do not have posterior crossbites until the mandible is advanced into the planned Class I position. Concomitant maxillary posterior segmental osteotomies may be required if palatal expansion is not possible. Many VME cases, especially the open-bite types, have transverse deficiency, which is corrected with segmental Le Fort I osteotomies.

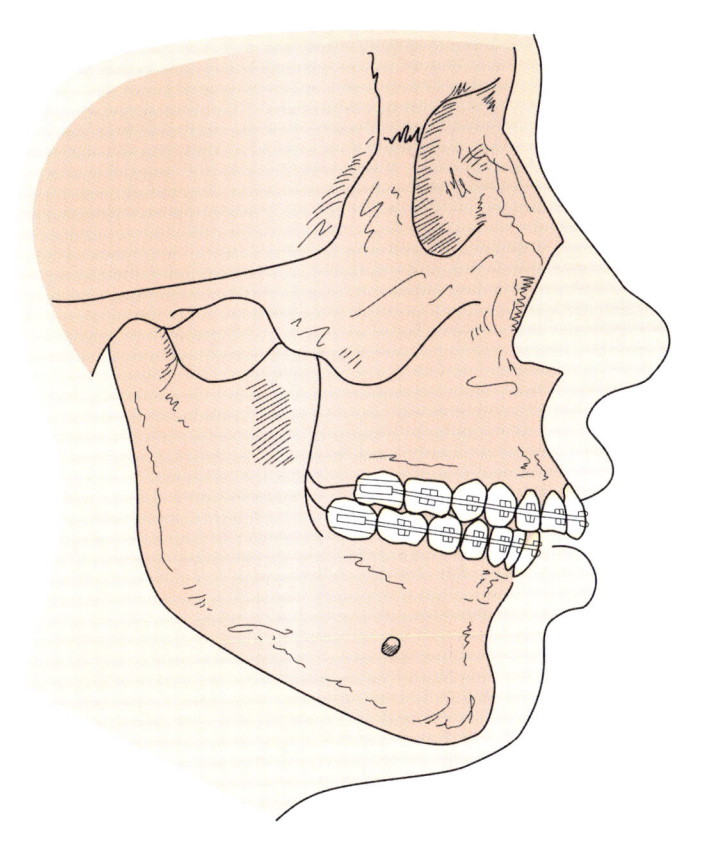

Figure 29.14 **(A)** VME is characterized by excessive exposure of incisors, lip incompetence, mandibular deficiency, and increased anterior facial height.

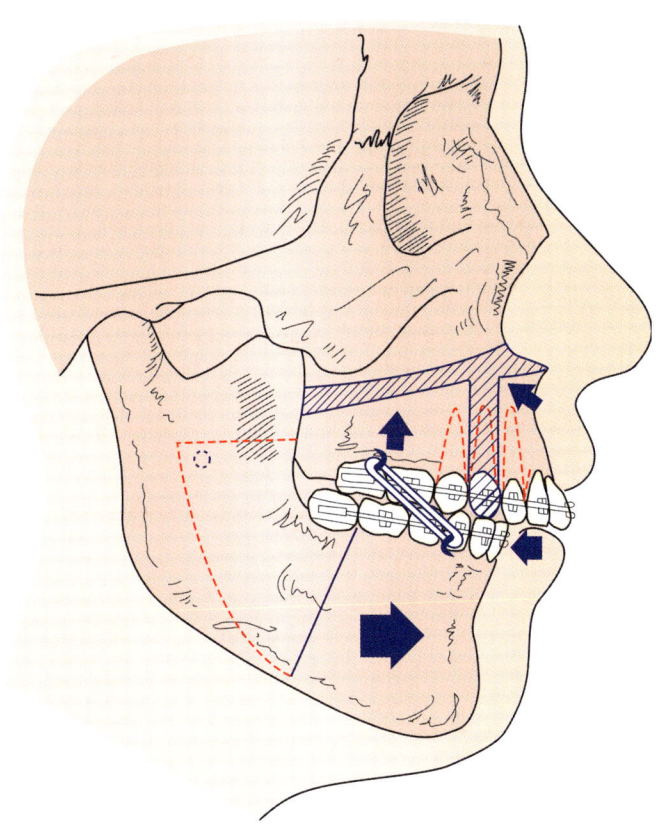

Figure 29.14 **(B)** Preoperative tracing shows orthodontic changes that preserve the deformity by uprighting lower incisors and maintaining the maxillary arch position. Treatment is extraction of maxillary premolars, maxillary and mandibular movement through Le Fort I osteotomy of the maxilla with anterior/posterior splitting, and mandibular advancement by sagittal split osteotomy.

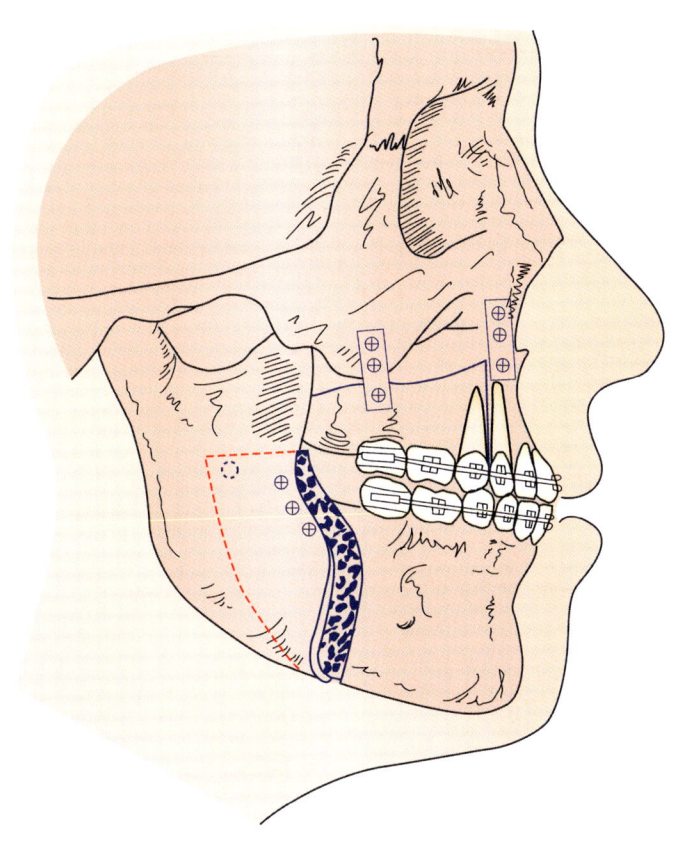

Figure 29.14 **(C)** Stabilization of maxilla and mandible by rigid fixation—bone plates and screws.

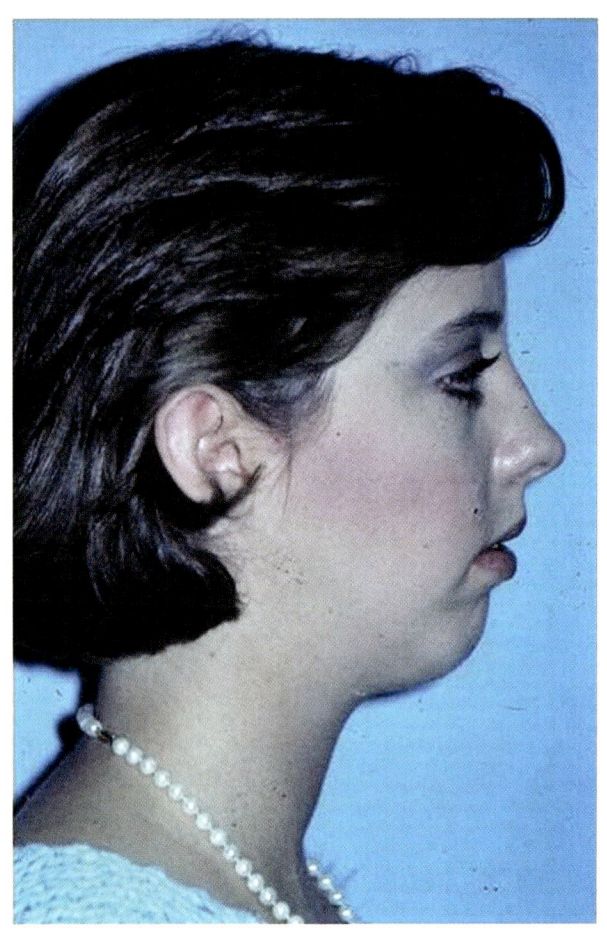

Figure 29.15 **(A)** Severe convex dentofacial deformity with VME, mandibular deficiency, and Class II malocclusion. Preoperative profile with relaxed lips shows true amount of lip incompetence.

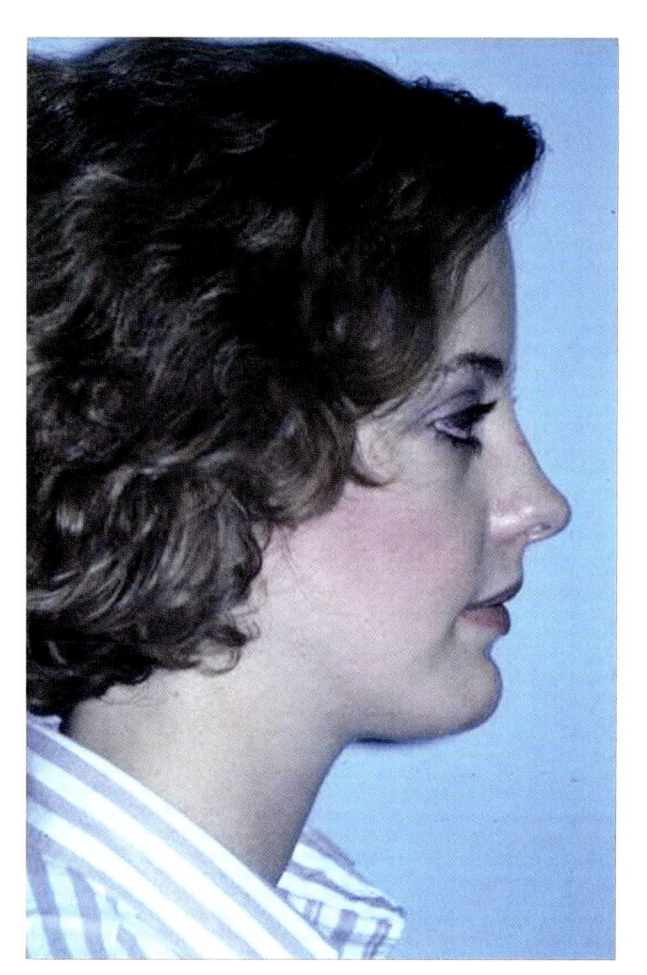

Figure 29.15 **(B)** Three-year postoperative profile following orthodontic treatment, superior repositioning of the maxilla by Le Fort I osteotomy, advancement of the mandible by sagittal split osteotomy, and an alloplastic cheekbone and chin implant.

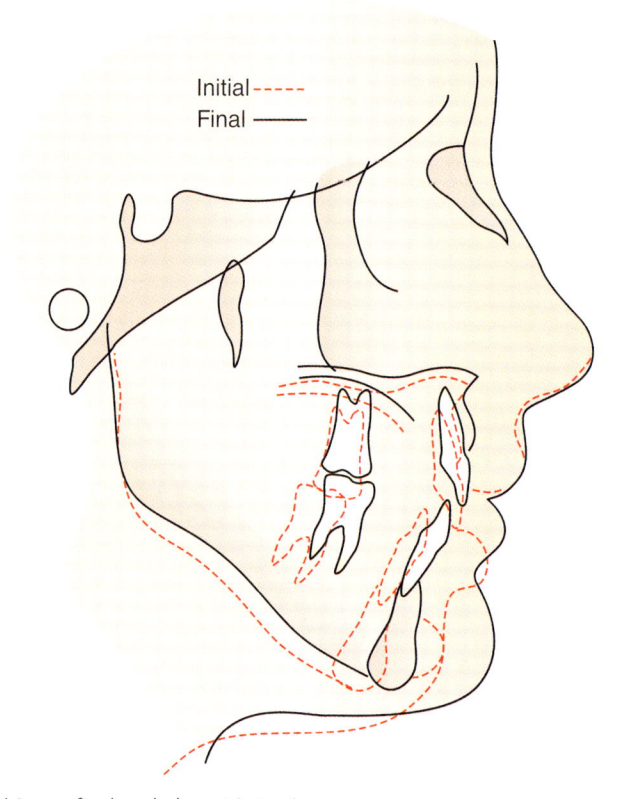

Figure 29.15 **(C)** Initial pretreatment and 3-year final cephalometric tracing.

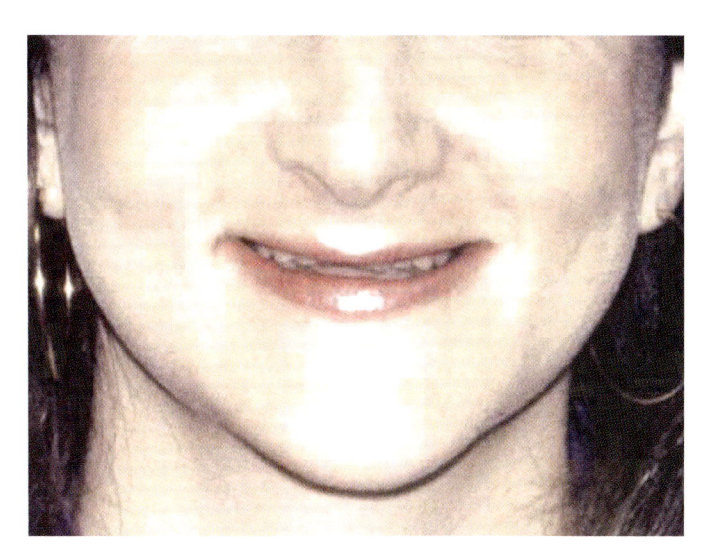

Figure 29.16 **(A)** Vertical maxillary deficiency corrected by inferior repositioning of the maxilla (downgrafting) with Le Fort I osteotomy and autogenous iliac crest bone graft. Preoperative frontal view demonstrates decreased facial length and hidden maxillary incisors on smiling.

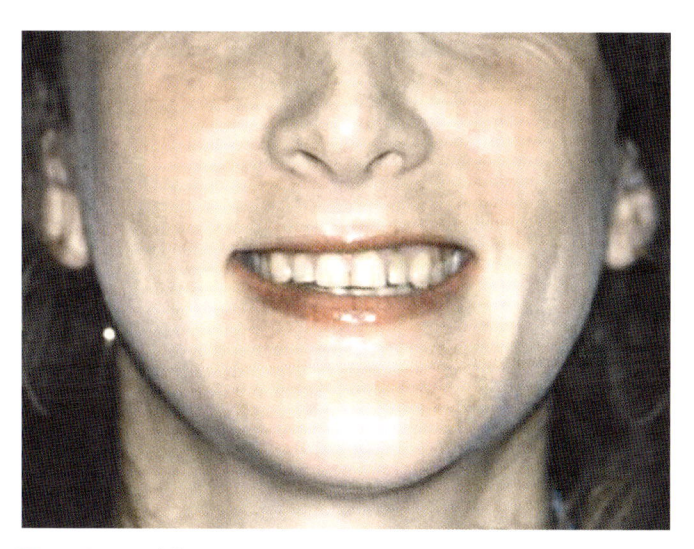

Figure 29.16 **(B)** Postoperative view demonstrates increased facial length and exposure of maxillary incisors.

Vertical maxillary deficiency usually has the appearance of an edentulous patient not wearing an upper denture (Figure 29.16A and B). The soft tissue will appear squashed, with the teeth in occlusion, and the mandible may appear to be prognathic. With the mandible in the normal rest position, significant freeway space is seen, and a more normal profile is observed. Cephalometrically, the SNA will be normal, the SNB may be increased, the mandibular plane may be decreased, and anterior facial dimensions and the ANB will be decreased. The occlusion will vary from borderline Class I to Class III. It is important to note the lack of display of a normal amount of the maxillary incisor with the upper lip at rest. The rest position must always be used for diagnosis and treatment planning since smile patterns vary too much and have only limited value. We treat to idealize the incisor shown at rest, not at smile.

Anteroposterior or horizontal deficiency will have a soft-tissue appearance similar to that of true mandibular prognathism. A decreased SNA and ANB and an obtuse nasolabial angle are characteristic. The addition of several wide strips of wax or a cotton sponge under the upper lip may improve the profile. Patients with cleft lip and palate with failure to develop the normal horizontal and vertical positions of the maxilla represent a common type of horizontal maxillary deficiency (Figure 29.17A–D).

Vertical and horizontal maxillary lengthening or advancement through Le Fort I osteotomy can produce dramatic results (see Figures 29.16 and 29.17). Special consideration must be given to methods of stabilization and fixation. In horizontal deficiencies, the bone of the maxilla is characteristically very thin. With advancement, bone contact may be minimal or inadequate. Stable results are obtained with the use of autologous bone from the iliac crest or cortical–cancellous demineralized bone products placed in defects of the lateral maxillary wall and between the posterior maxillary wall and pterygoid plates. Rigid internal fixation with wires or malleable bone plates will produce predictable results without IMF. If simultaneous mandibular surgery is necessary, rigid fixation of the sagittal split osteotomy may also eliminate IMF.

Facial asymmetry

Diagnosis and surgical orthodontic treatment of facial asymmetry such as condylar hyperplasia or hemifacial microsomia is perhaps more difficult, challenging, and dramatic than any other deformity. Variations of asymmetry are common, corrective procedures are less standardized, and, in many cases, much original thought is required. An elaborate preoperative work-up from multiple radiographic views is required to confirm the diagnosis, eliminate uncommon pathology as an etiology, and arrive at a treatment plan.

There is always a certain amount of asymmetry to the face and to the mandible. In many instances, the face, although slightly asymmetric, is attractive, projects warmth, and is an integral part of an individual's character. Pronounced asymmetry, however, has been detrimental to character development and social and economic progress. Equally important, but only recently appreciated, are the functional deficits associated with facial or mandibular asymmetry. Fortunately, correction of form almost always improves function.

It is the dentist's responsibility to seek surgical evaluation of patients for whom restorative dentistry is proposed to correct an asymmetric mandible or maxilla. In more recent times, numerous uncomplicated surgical procedures have produced dramatic improvements in appearance and function for patients formerly considered beyond help. Because of the complexity of the deformity, treatment is individualized and may involve osteotomies, recontouring, and associated soft-tissue surgery.

A classification of asymmetry is necessary for proper diagnosis and treatment (Table 29.1).

Condylar hyperplasia

This is the most common cause of asymmetry, resulting from overproduction or prolonged production of cartilage in the condyle. The usual deformity is an enlarged condyle and

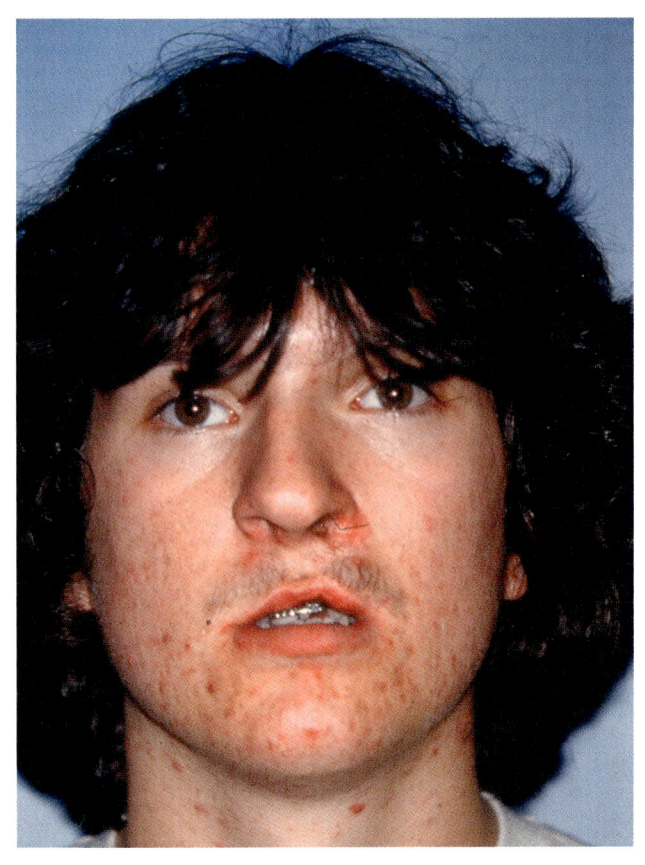

Figure 29.17 **(A)** Vertical, horizontal, and transverse maxillary deficiencies in a patient with cleft lip and palate and severe Class III malocclusion. Preoperative facial appearance.

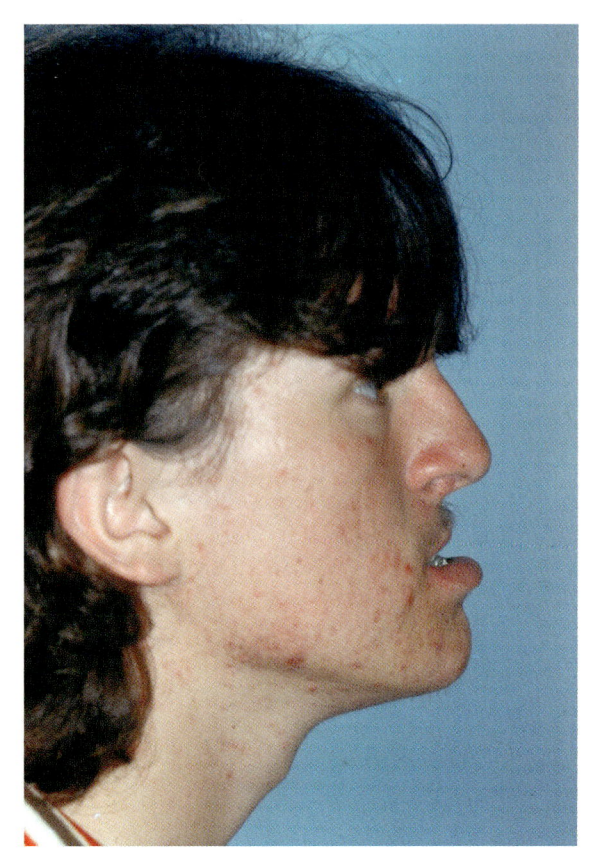

Figure 29.17 **(B)** Profile before surgery following orthodontic treatment to correct dental compensations.

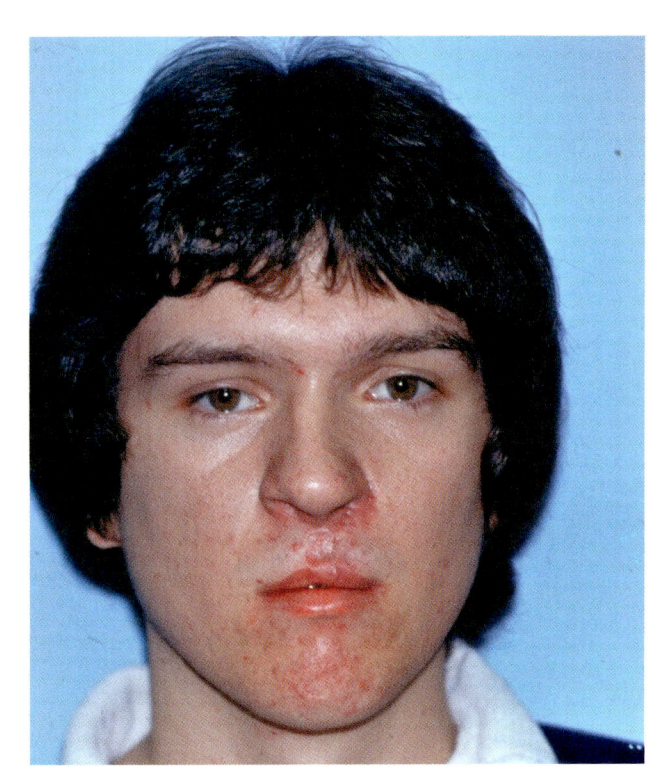

Figure 29.17 **(C)** Postoperative frontal view at 3 years.

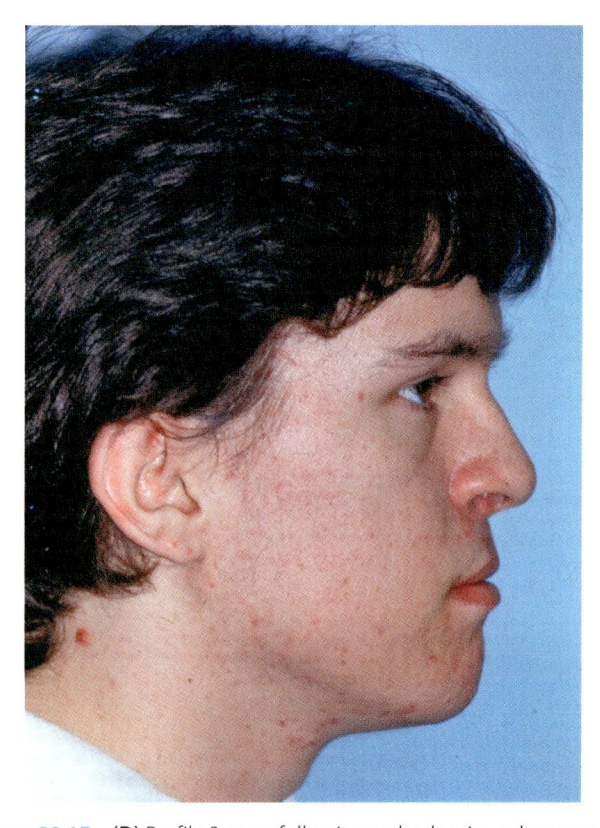

Figure 29.17 **(D)** Profile 3 years following orthodontics, advancement, and expansion of the maxilla by Le Fort I osteotomy with autogenous iliac crest bone graft, closure of oronasal fistula, and secondary repair of the lip.

Chapter 29 Surgical Orthodontic Correction of Dentofacial Deformity

Table 29.1 Classification of Asymmetry

Overdevelopment
Hemihypertrophy (facial)
Condylar hyperplasia
Mandibular hypertrophy (macrognathia)
Deviation prognathism (laterognathia)
Unilateral masseteric hypertrophy
Alveolar (maxillary or mandibular)

Underdevelopment
Hemifacial microsomia
Condylar hypoplasia
Mandibular hypoplasia
Alveolar (maxillary or mandibular)
Treacher Collins syndrome (mandibulofacial dysostosis)

Acquired states of asymmetry
TMJ ankylosis from trauma
Tumors
Infections
Inflammation

elongated condylar neck. The result is an outward bowing of the ramus and the body and a downward growth of the mandible that may produce an open bite on the involved side and a crossbite on the opposite side. If the onset is before puberty, the maxilla grows downward and maintains some degree of occlusion with the mandible. If the onset were late, one would not expect to find a down-growth of the maxilla but instead a developing open bite.

Treatment planning for facial asymmetry involves careful notation of all facial and dental relationships. The facial, chin, and dental midlines are marked (Figure 29.18A). The vertical differences in right to left mandibular inferior borders are noted, including the degree of occlusal plane cant (Figure 29.18B). Bone scans and serial radiographs are helpful to determine remaining condylar growth potential. Photographs, cephalometric analysis, and models mounted on an anatomic articulator aid in treatment planning. Model surgery determines the exact bony movements to be carried out during surgery (Figure 29.18C–F).

As in the case presented, a Le Fort I osteotomy is performed first to achieve normal tooth–lip esthetics and a level maxilla with correct positioning in all directions. Ramus osteotomies and possible condylectomy follow maxillary surgery.

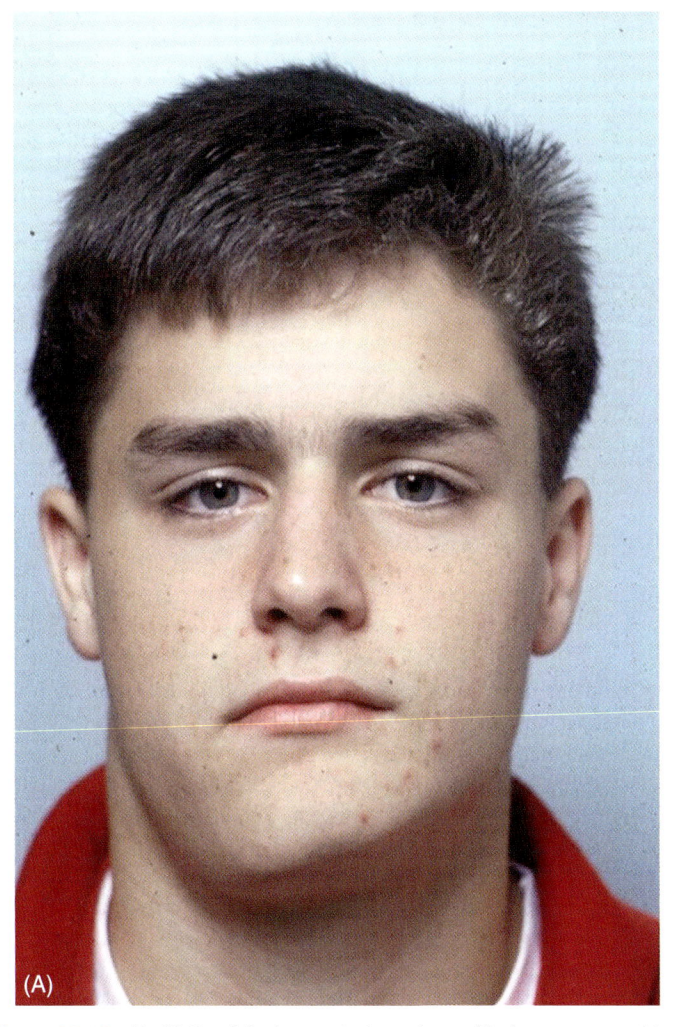

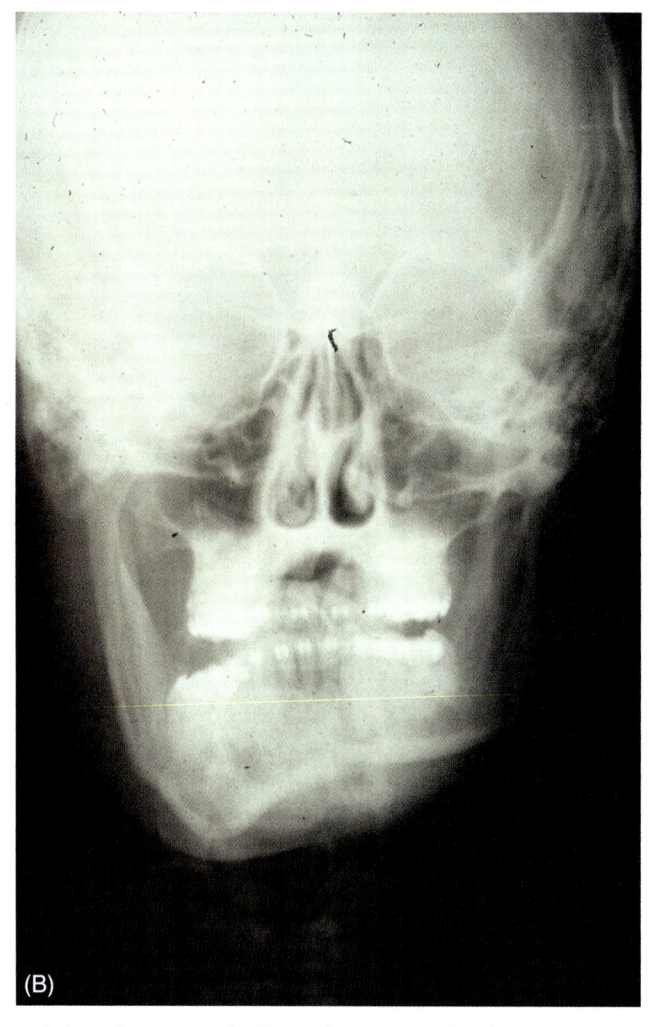

Figure 29.18 (A, B) Condylar hyperplasia and mandibular macrognathia, frontal view of patient and radiograph. Note grossly enlarged right condyle and enlarged inferior border of mandible producing severe facial asymmetry and malocclusion.

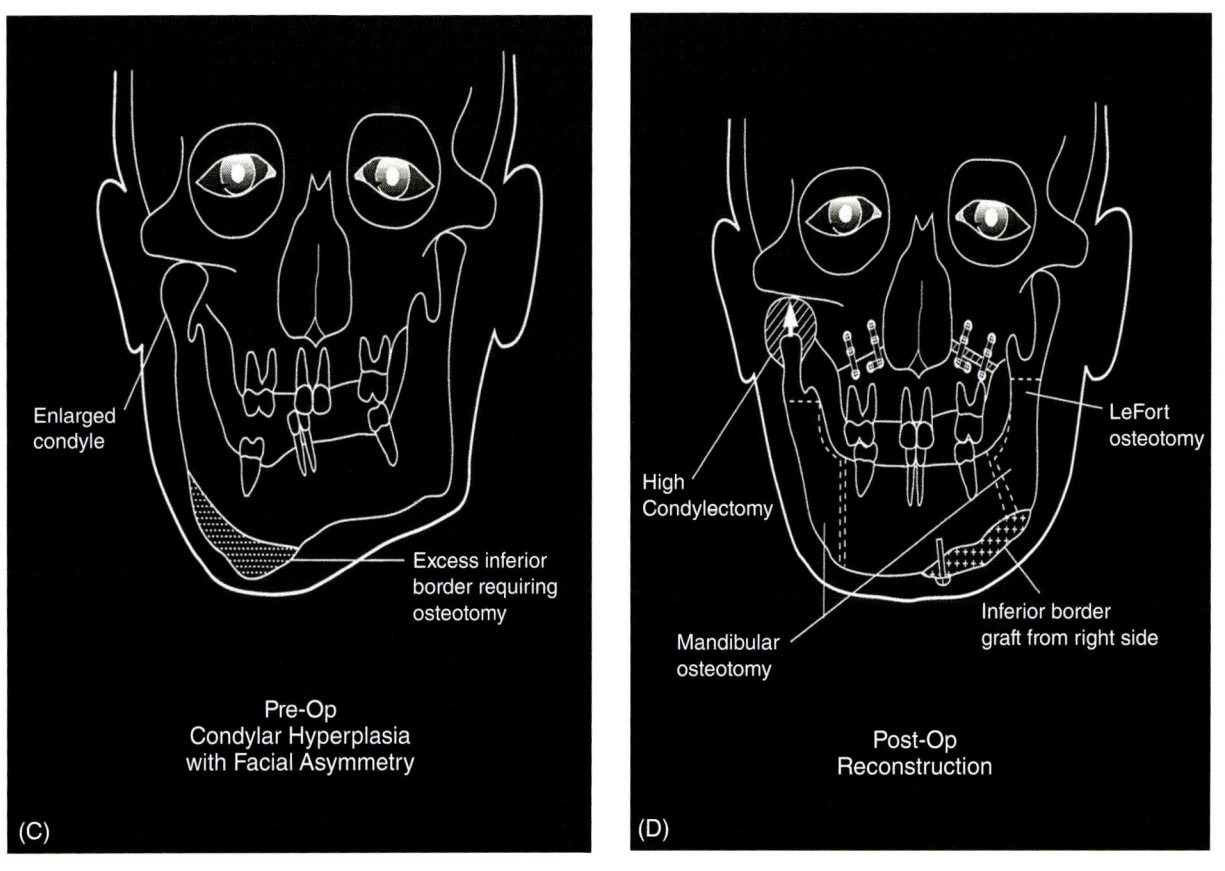

Figure 29.18 **(C, D)** Frontal view cephalometric drawings showing preoperative asymmetry findings **(C)** and multiple operative procedures to obtain postoperative reconstruction symmetry **(D)**.

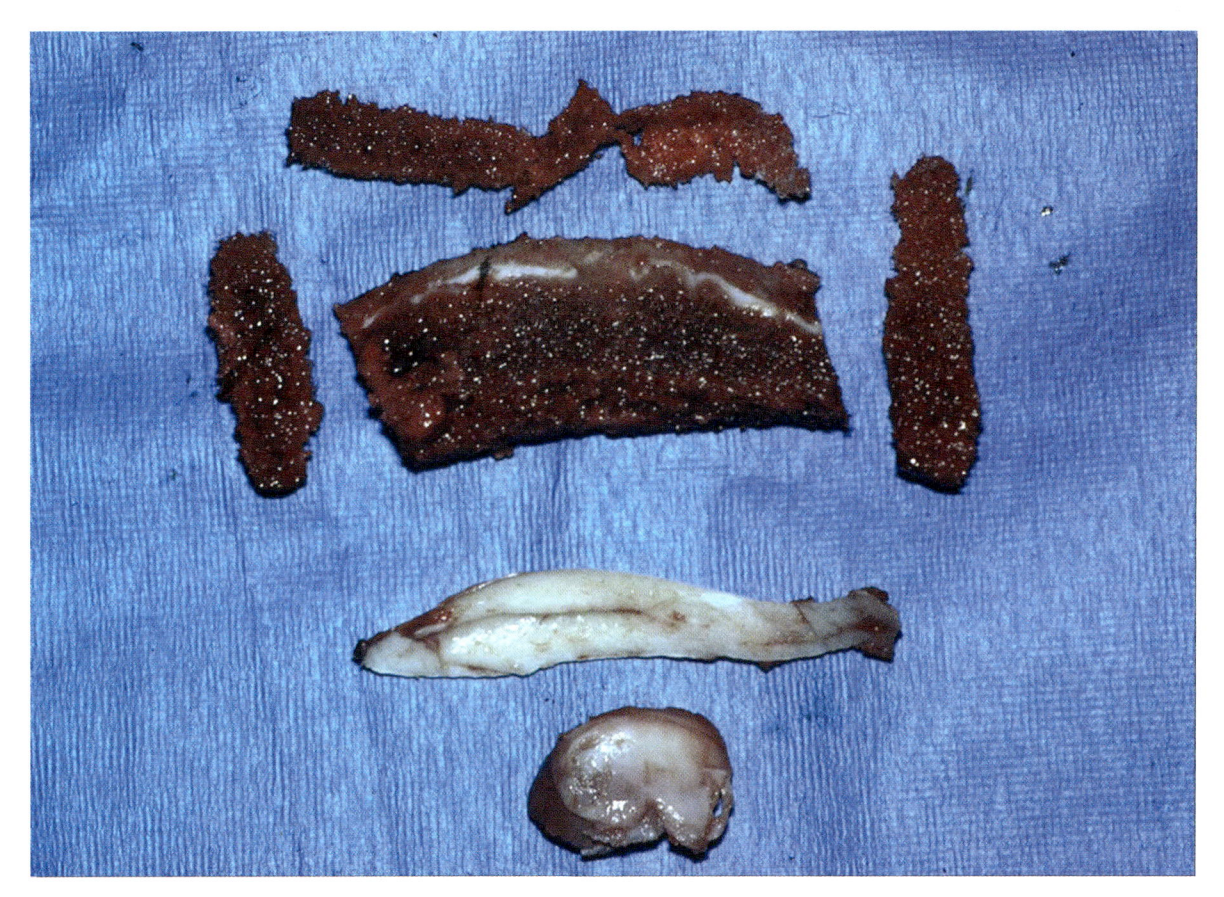

Figure 29.18 **(E)** Bone graft from iliac crest used to downgraft left maxilla. Patient's right excess inferior border of mandible was transferred to left side. Removal of right condyle shortened right side of face.

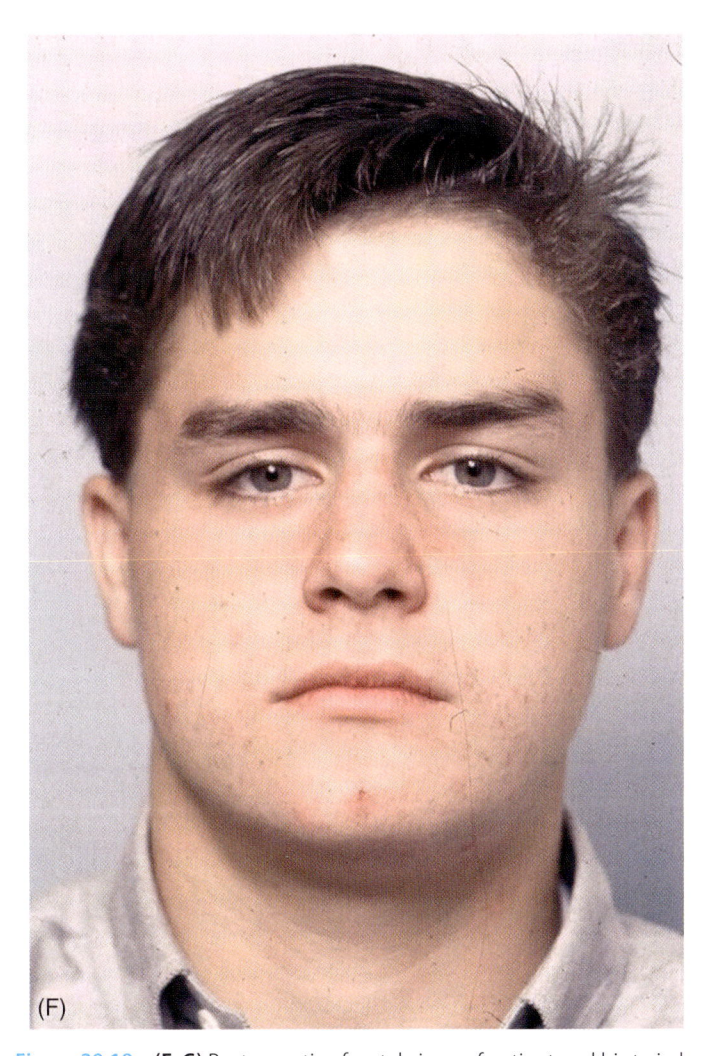

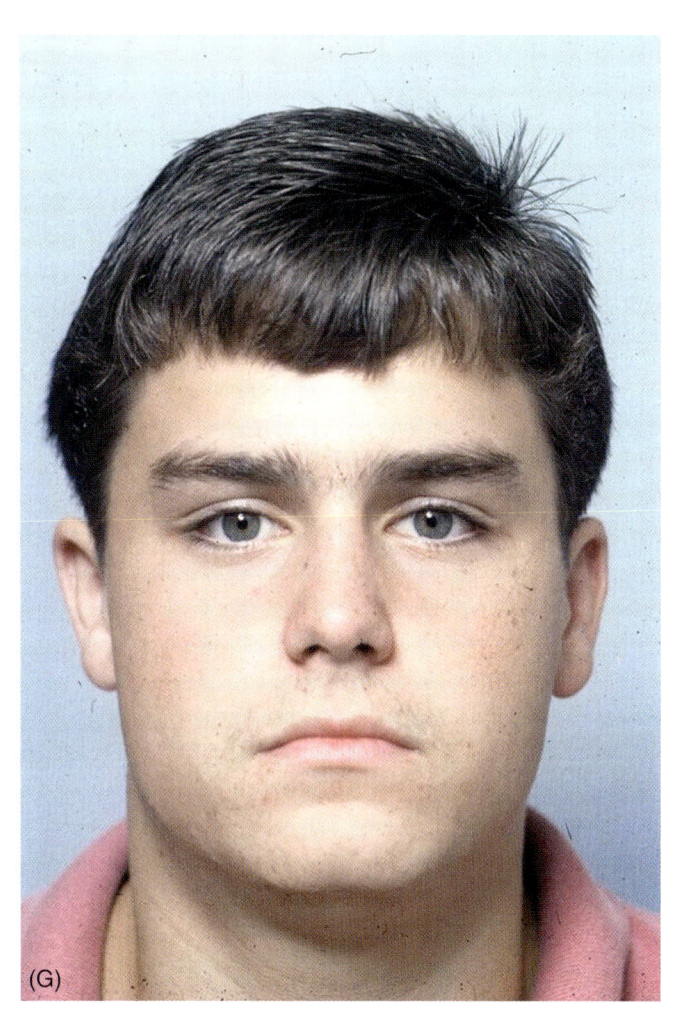

Figure 29.18 (F, G) Postoperative frontal views of patient and his twin brother.

A condylectomy may be indicated in cases of hyperplasia and hypertrophy where additional growth is anticipated and pain and dysfunction are noted. Otherwise, a subcondylar osteotomy is used on the side being shortened, and a sagittal split, or "L" osteotomy with graft, is used on the side being lengthened. (Figure 29.18A–G). Inferior border leveling by ostectomy and genioplasty by sliding horizontal osteotomy may be necessary in severe cases. Facial onlay procedures with alloplasts or tissue transfer are also used to refine symmetry.

Hemifacial microsomia

This is the most common cause of asymmetry, which occurs as a result of failed mandibular condyle growth. It is a distinct unilateral entity within the group of syndromes that encompass failure of growth of derivatives of the first and second branchial arch. It is postulated that stapedial artery hemorrhage in utero leads to a loss of functional matrix responsible for the normal formation of several anatomic structures (most notably ramus, glenoid fossa, and external ear). The extent of the deformity ranges from mild mandibular asymmetry to severe hypoplasia of the mandible and facial skeleton and overlying soft tissues on the affected side. The skeletal defects of hemifacial microsomia with vertical facial shortening are classified according to the morphology of the ramus and temporomandibular articulation. These deformities may be limited to hypoplasia of the ramus and glenoid fossa or may include nearly complete absence of these structures, including the external ear. The lack of mandibular development restricts maxillary growth on the affected side, and this produces upward occlusal plane canting. Alterations in orbit and zygoma position and size are common in severe cases. The chin becomes displaced to the affected side with Class II malocclusion. Once the occlusion is surgically and orthodontically corrected, hard- and soft-tissue asymmetric problems frequently require secondary grafting or implant procedures (Figure 29.19A–K).

Distraction osteogenesis

Distraction osteogenesis is a surgical technique in which there is an osteotomy created and the two segments are progressively moved apart. The procedure consists of an osteotomy, a latency period, a distraction device activation period, a consolidation period, and a bony remodeling period.

Distraction has been established as a predictable method for maxillary and mandibular bone elongation, with generation of bone in the distraction site. This is the result of slow pulling apart of the bone edges with an external or internal fixator that

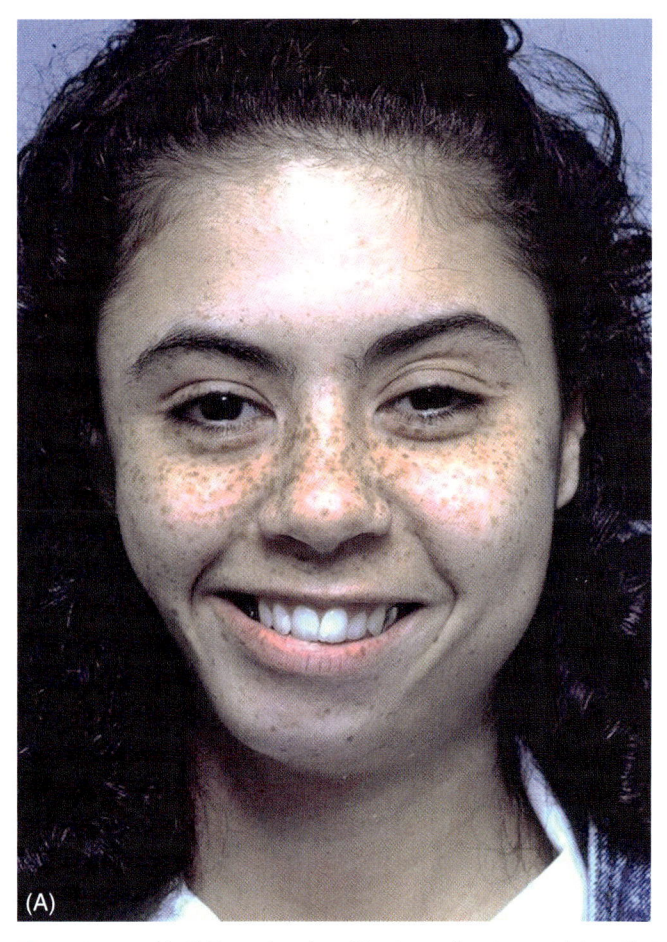

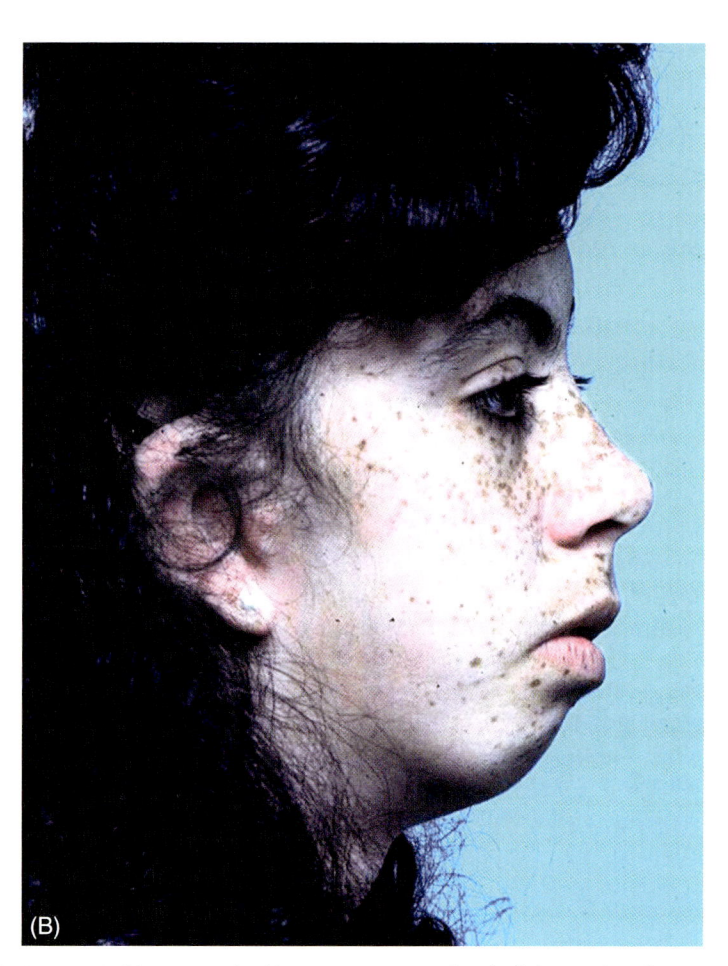

Figure 29.19 (A, B) Frontal and profile views of patient with hemifacial microsomia. Missing ear had been reconstructed with abdominal graft as a child. Today, missing external ears are more esthetically reconstructed using skull-placed dental implants to support a prosthetic ear. Note severe retrognathia of mandible with facial asymmetry.

mechanically creates a gap in which new bone generates between the two edges. Mandibular distraction osteogenesis is indicated when severe mandibular retrognathia or micrognathia is present. Mandibular advancements of 10–20 mm are difficult to perform with a sagittal split osteotomy. Acute mandibular lengthening of 10–20 mm requires significant stripping and stretching of the musculature and soft tissue attached to the mandible, with an increased chance of skeletal relapse. Distraction osteogenesis techniques allow gradual soft-tissue adaptation, and proliferation in response to mandibular lengthening. The distraction process, or callus manipulation, occurs at a rate ranging from 0.5 to 2 mm a day. The rate will depend on the age of the patient and the type of osteotomy. The gold standard for clinical distraction osteogenesis is 1 mm a day, divided into two or four activations per day. The distance of distraction is determined by the amount of skeletal and occlusal change desired. Transoral activation arms are typically removed under local anesthetic and/or sedation at the completion of the distraction.

The consolidation period in adults should be a minimum of 3 months and can be extended up to 6 months as needed.

Devices can be intraoral or extraoral, and there are numerous advantages and disadvantages of each. The main advantage to the intraoral devices is that the device is located under the soft tissue and socially preferred by the patients. Disadvantages include the device cannot perform three-dimensional corrections, less control of vector lengthening in relation to the extraoral devices, and a second operation for device removal is required.

The most striking feature of distraction osteogenesis is the significant distance of lengthening that can be achieved with new bone formation.

Surgically assisted orthodontics

Corticotomy-assisted orthodontic treatment can offer several unique options to address the limitations of traditional orthodontic treatment in adults. A review of the literature in this surgically assisted technique reveals several distinct advantages. These include a reduced treatment time, enhanced expansion, differential tooth movement, increased traction of impacted teeth, and improved postorthodontic stability. Corticotomy has been described in orthopedics dating back to the early 1900s. Köle introduced a surgical procedure involving both osteotomy and corticotomy to accelerate orthodontic tooth movement, based on the concept that teeth move faster when the resistance exerted by the surrounding cortical bone is reduced via a surgical procedure. Köle further explained that the reduced resistance

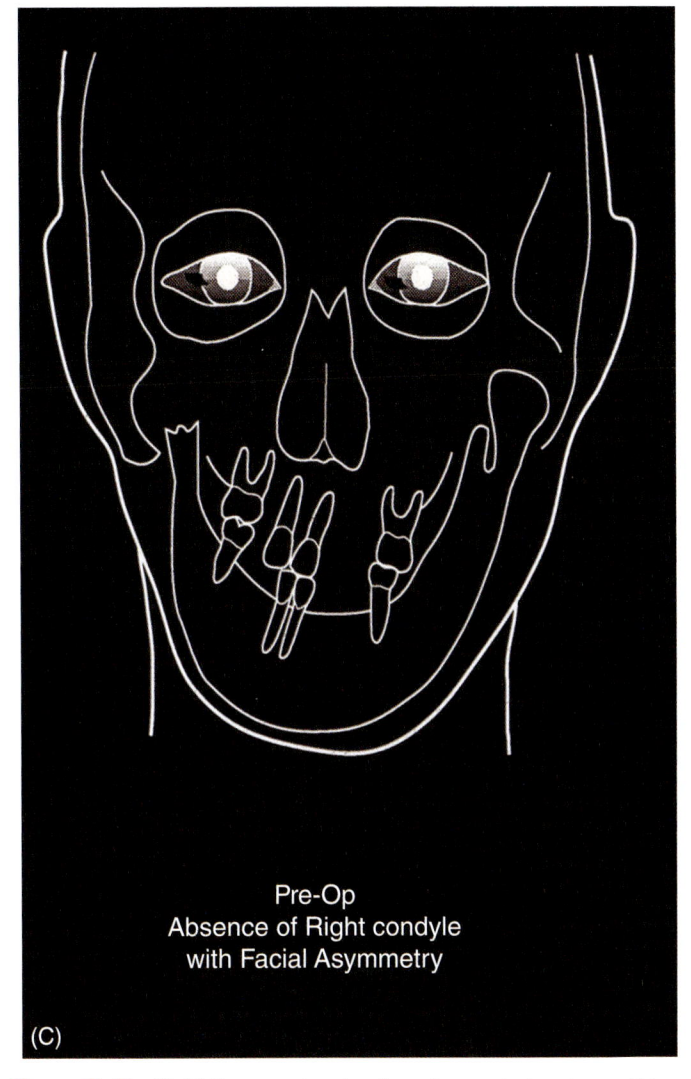

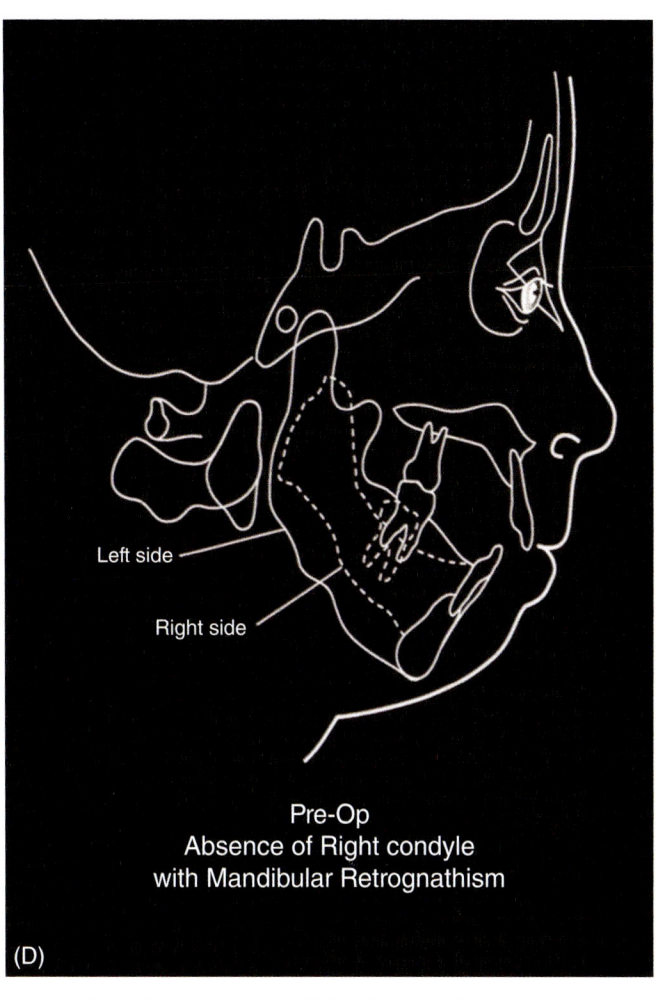

Figure 29.19 (C, D) Preoperative drawings demonstrate retrognathia, missing condyle, and malocclusion with facial asymmetry.

enhances an en bloc movement of the entire alveolar cortical segment, which is connected by softer medullary bone, including the confined teeth, when exposed to orthodontic forces. Frost found a direct correlation between the severity of bone corticotomy and/or osteotomy and the intensity of the healing response, leading to accelerated bone turnover at the surgical site. This was designated as "regional acceleratory phenomenon," which was explained as a temporary stage of localized soft- and hard-tissue remodeling that resulted in rebuilding of the injured sites to a normal state through recruitment of osteoclasts and osteoblasts via local intercellular mediator mechanisms involving precursors, supporting cells, blood capillaries, and lymph.

The accelerated osteogenic orthodontics (AOO) technique described by Wilcko is as follows: full-thickness flaps are reflected labially and lingually using sulcular releasing incisions. Vertical releasing incisions can be used, but they should be positioned at least one tooth away from the "bone activation." Flaps should be carefully reflected beyond the apices of the teeth to avoid damaging the neurovascular complexes exiting the alveolus and to allow adequate decortication around the apices. Selective alveolar decortication is performed in the form of 0.5 mm cuts into the cortical bone, combined with selective medullary penetration to enhance bleeding. This poses little threat to tooth vitality and makes AOO much safer than the osteotomy technique, in which cuts extend into the medullary bone around the teeth that are to be moved. Adequate bioabsorbable grafting material is placed over the injured bone. Flaps are then repositioned and sutured into place. Sutures should be left in place for a minimum of 2 weeks. Tooth movement should start 1 or 2 weeks after surgery. Unlike conventional orthodontics, the orthodontic appliance should be activated every 2 weeks until the end of treatment after periodontal AOO. There are several indications in which this surgical technique can be offered to patients: resolve crowding and shorten treatment time, accelerate canine retraction after premolar extraction, enhance postorthodontic stability, facilitate eruption of impacted teeth, facilitate slow orthodontic expansion, molar intrusion, and open bite correction.

There are certain limitations to this technique. Patients with poor periodontal health or gingival recession are not

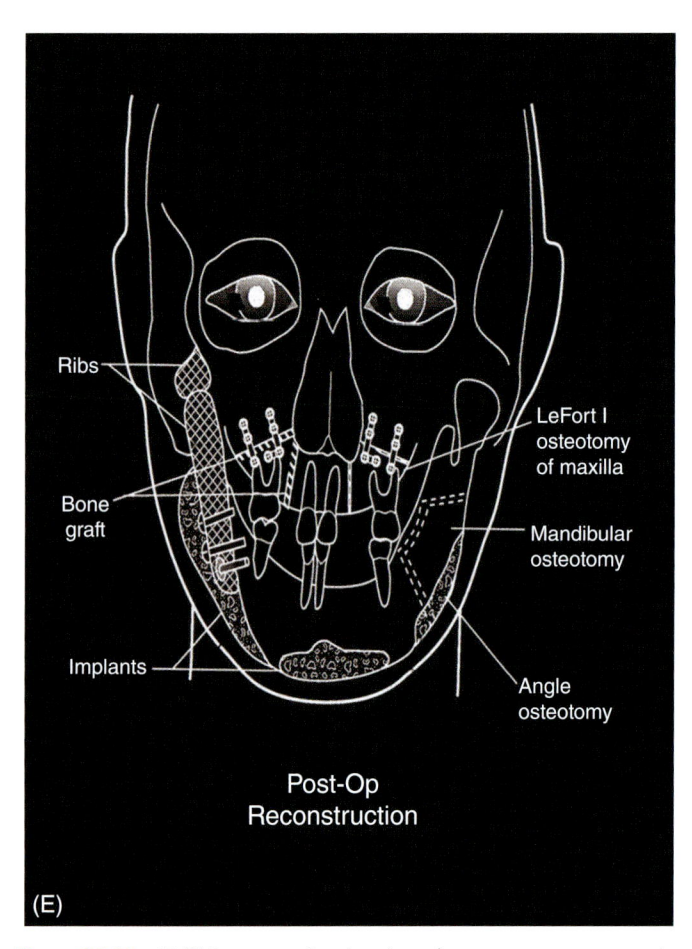

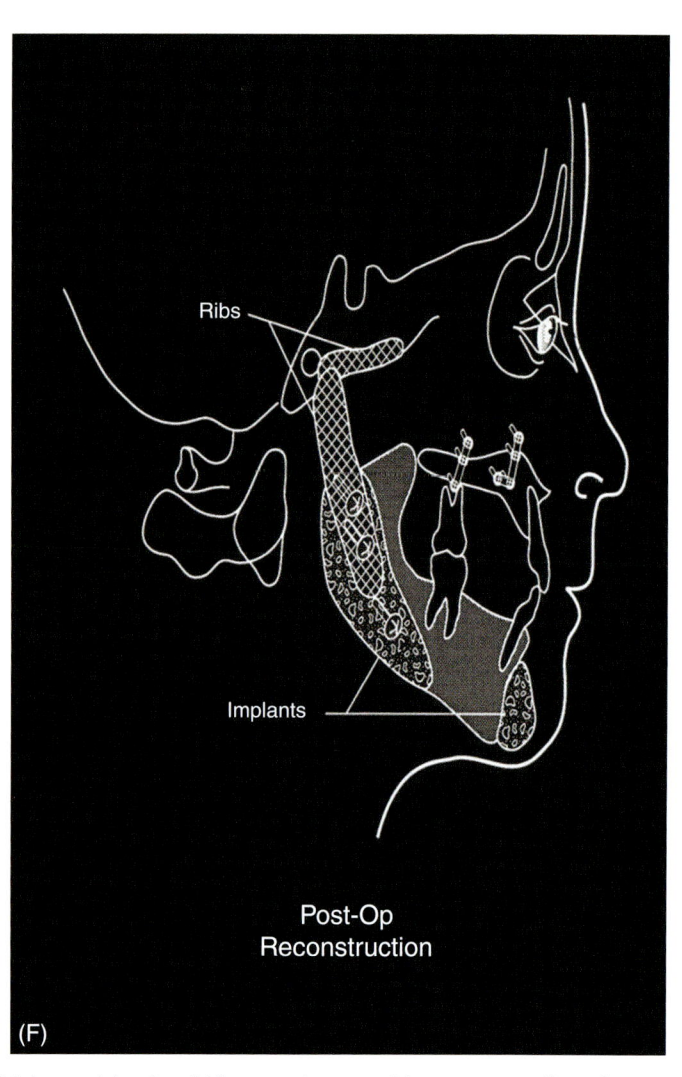

Figure 29.19 **(E, F)** Postoperative drawings demonstrate reconstruction of right condyle, glenoid fossa, and ramus with autogenous rib graft, left mandibular osteotomies, Le Fort I osteotomy of maxilla with bone graft to level and lengthen the right maxilla, and multiple chin and facial implants.

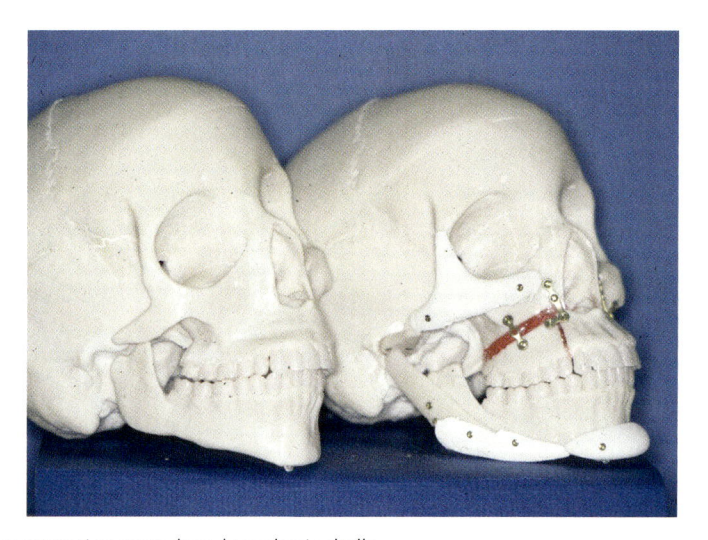

Figure 29.19 **(G)** Deformity and reconstruction reproduced on plastic skulls.

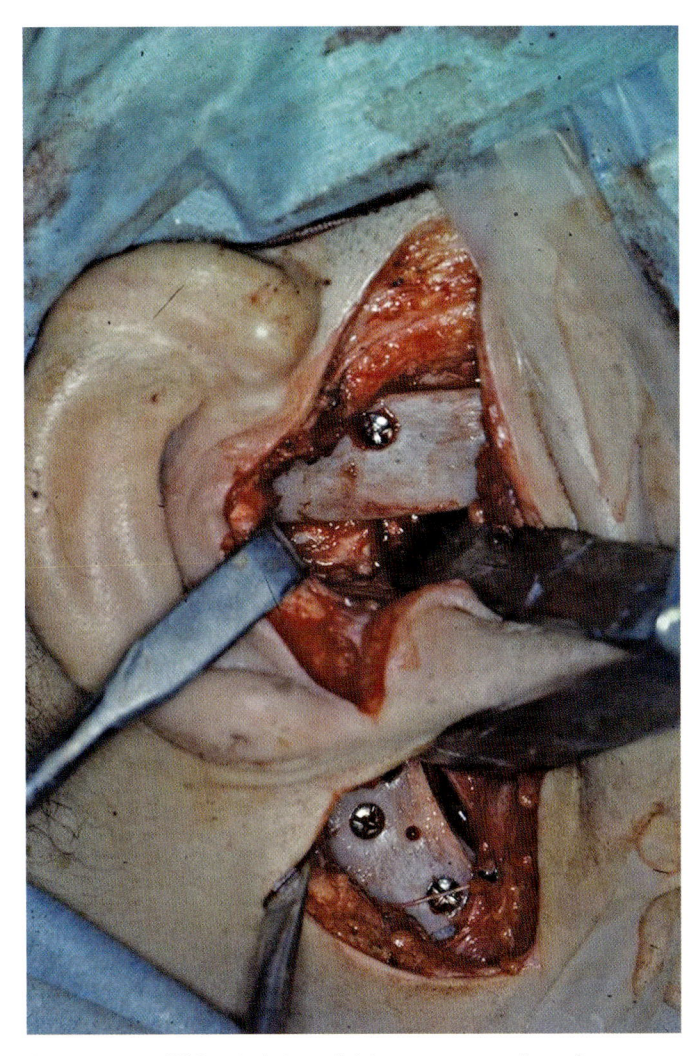

Figure 29.19 **(H)** Surgical view of right autogenous rib graft to restore fossa, condyle and deficient ramus.

appropriate candidates. Complications of AOO include slight interdental bone loss and loss of gingival attachment. There have also been reports of hematomas along with the expected postoperative swelling and pain.

Adjunctive hard- and soft-tissue procedures

The most common adjunctive procedure performed at the time of orthognathic surgery is genioplasty (chin reshaping). Other procedures commonly performed simultaneously include rhinoplasty, septoplasty, onlay augmentation, submental lipectomy/liposculpture, buccal lipectomy, platysmaplasty, lip augmentation, reduction cheiloplasty, V–Y lip advancement (to lengthen the upper lip), and alar cinch (to narrow the alar base).

Osteotomies and alloplastic implant augmentation are commonly employed when facial contour deficit exists in the presence of a normal occlusion or when maxillary or mandibular surgery to correct malocclusion fails to satisfy esthetic requirements. When properly performed, both the osteotomy and alloplastic augmentation are quite stable. Chin contour correction by an osteotomy is usually performed through an intraoral vestibular incision. Horizontal augmentation or advancement of a deficient chin occurs with a sliding horizontal osteotomy of the symphysis (Figure 29.20), a chin implant, or a combination thereof for extreme deformity. The chin is pedicled to the genioglossus and geniohyoid muscles to maintain blood supply, and direct wiring or plating stabilizes the segment. The soft-tissue augmentation change is at least 70% of the amount of bone advancement (Figure 29.21A–D).

If excessive vertical dimension exists, a wedge of bone may be removed. Likewise, a short chin may be lengthened by interposing bone or hydroxylapatite blocks. Prominent and excessively long chins may be reduced by chin shaves but are more accurately corrected by reverse sliding of the symphysis with a horizontal osteotomy and/or ostectomy of excess bone.

Alloplastic implants used for mandibular, facial, and cranial augmentation most commonly employed today include silicone rubber (i.e., Implantech, Ventura, CA), porous polyethylene (i.e., Medpore, Porex Surgical, Newnan, GA), and expanded polytetrafluoroethylene (i.e., Gore-Tex, W.L. Gore and Associates, Flagstaff, AZ). These materials are preformed to fit particular anatomic areas and can be trimmed and/or recontoured. They are placed subperiostally through intraoral incisions and secured with sutures, wires, or bone screws. Chin and cheekbone augmentations with alloplast are very commonly used to enhance the surgical treatment of dentofacial deformities (see Figures 29.7C, 29.15B, and 29.21D).

Role of orthognathic surgery in treating obstructive sleep apnea

Obstructive sleep apnea (OSA) has come to the forefront as a major public health concern. Researchers are continuously finding different ways in which interrupted or lack of sleep is detrimental to our health, mostly through inflammatory effects and a decrease in the body's natural ability to repair inflammatory damage during sleep. Altered sleep affects the cardiovascular, pulmonary, renal, endocrine, and vascular systems in general and all systems in specific manners that create multiple health issues. Probably the most obvious effect is on the brain with daytime sleepiness, altered cognitive abilities, and increased risk of stroke. OSA is characterized by repeated pauses or obstructions in breathing, usually combined with snoring. This leads to fragmented sleep and decreases in oxyhemoglobin saturation, both damaging to all body systems. The incidence of OSA has been estimated to be as high as 90 million Americans. Almost half of individuals above the age of 40 snore, and the incidence of sleep apnea in those individuals is at least 17% of men and 15% of women. Although obesity is given as the cause of the majority of OSA cases, a significant percentage of individuals have an anatomic predisposition to airway collapse due to retrusive jaws and relative decreased space for the tongue.

Although the primary medical treatment of OSA is the use of continuous positive airway pressure (CPAP), appropriate dental treatment can be just as important. Dental practitioners need to recognize existing dental skeletal patterns as well as future effects of orthodontic treatment, either of which may be detrimental to the patient's airway health. A seemingly innocuous four bicuspid

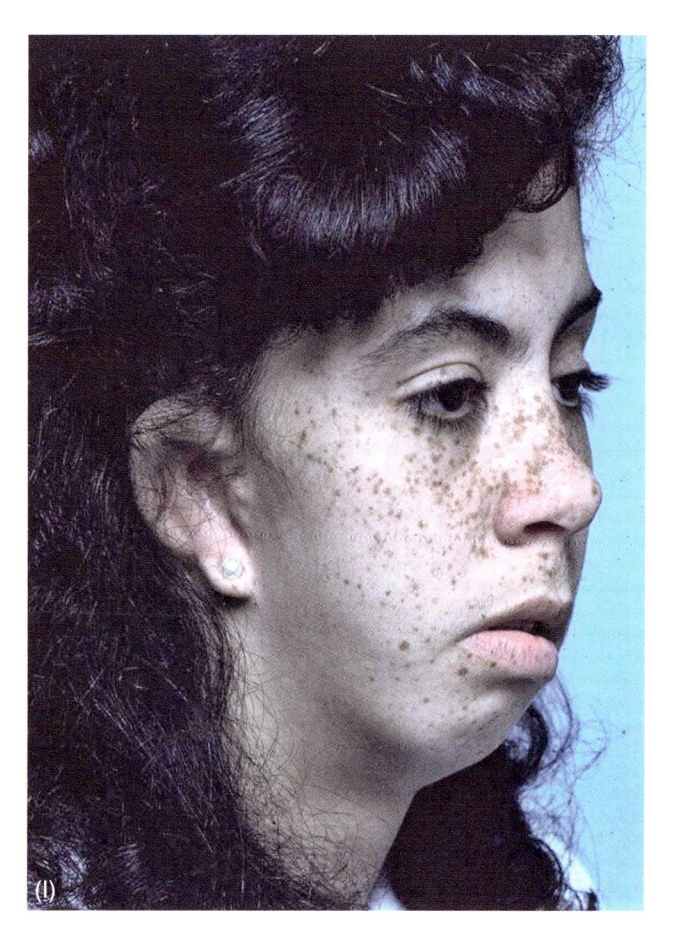

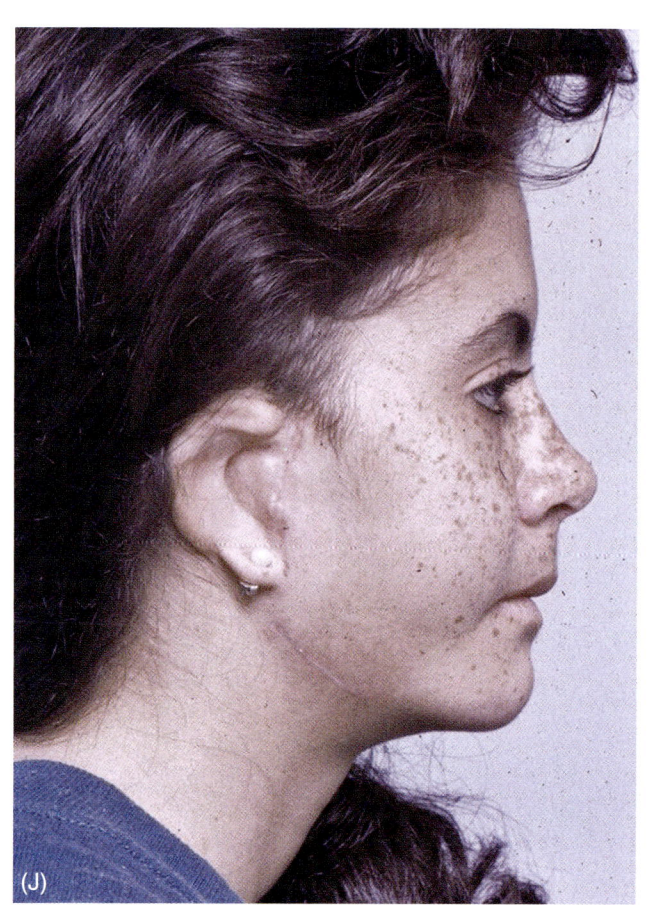

Figure 29.19 **(I, J)** Preoperative and postoperative profiles.

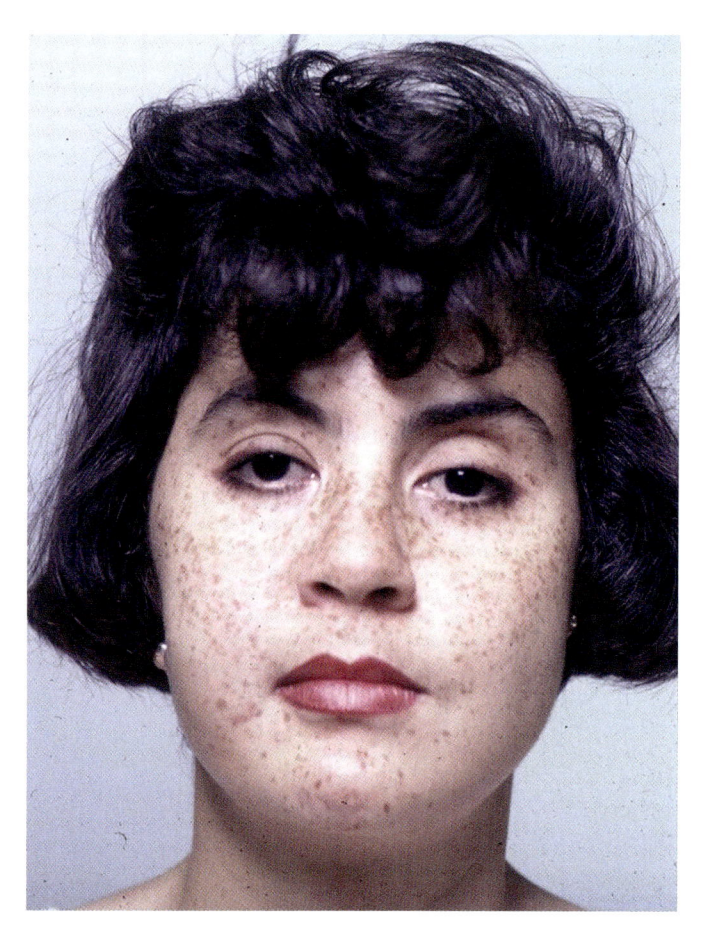

Figure 29.19 **(K)** The 10-year frontal view of face.

Figure 29.20 Tracing advancement genioplasty by intraoral sliding horizontal osteotomy of the symphysis.

extraction to camouflage a Class II or III malocclusion or a surgeon's failure to not minimize a mandibular setback are examples of adverse consequences when that patient reaches their 40s or 50s. The facial skeleton provides much of the support for the upper airway and, as such, orthodontic treatment that reduces the upper airway space should be a concern as the patient ages. As doctors, the rule of *primum non nocere*, or first do no harm, has to be considered when undertaking procedures that decrease the volume of the upper airway space.

The use of concepts and procedures learned from orthognathic surgery has recently become a promising treatment for individuals affected by OSA. In orthognathic surgery, the surgeon uses maxillary and mandibular osteotomies to effect a change in the patient's facial skeleton to improve masticatory function, speech, and appearance. In orthognathic surgery or telegnathic surgery to treat OSA, the surgeon uses these procedures to increase the posterior airway space, increase space for the tongue, and in 97–98% of the patients cure OSA. Since OSA has become such a large public health concern, and many patients tolerate CPAP poorly, options such as oral repositioning devices and orthognathic surgery have become valid alternatives to cure OSA. Compliance is a large problem with CPAP, and even some oral repositioning devices; therefore, mandibular/maxillary advancement orthognathic surgery can be a life-saving procedure for many individuals.

Although orthognathic surgery often simultaneously corrects OSA and produces a pleasing esthetic/occlusal change, orthognathic surgery for the treatment of OSA has a defined purpose and may have a potentially different outcome than orthognathic surgery used for the correction of a craniofacial deformity alone. If a middle-aged patient with OSA has an underlying craniofacial deformity, many will have a facial skeleton with cephalometric norms. The general idea in orthognathic surgery to cure OSA is to pull the facial skeleton and the tongue away from the posterior pharyngeal wall; thus, some patients will look as if their lower face is too prominent. This gives some middle-aged patients the appearance as if they have had a face lift, and is thus aesthetically pleasing. Other patients will look abnormal. The thought process has to be altered to consider that the surgery is being done not for appearance improvement but rather to cure the patient of a deadly malady.

Figure 29.22A illustrates the changes that occur in a normocephalic male that decrease the posterior airspace. The illustration projects how aging increases the length of the soft palate from negative-pressure snoring and irritation. This, combined with relative increases in tongue size and excess fat, results in the creation of the conditions favorable for the development of OSA.

Figure 29.21 **(A)** Preoperative frontal view of patient with chin deficiency.

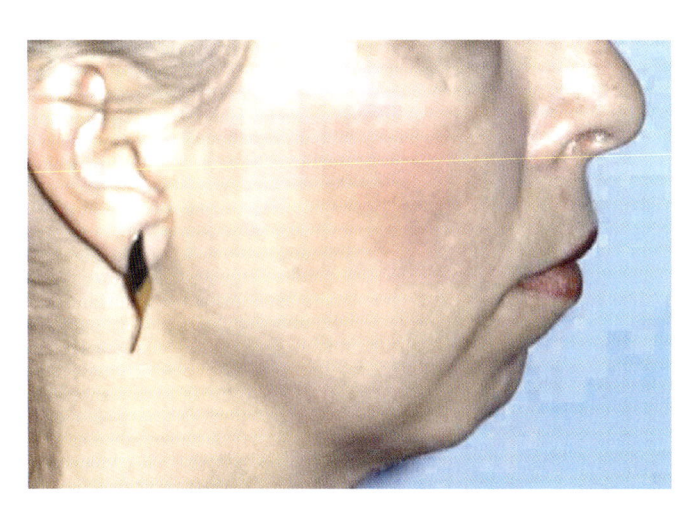

Figure 29.21 **(B)** Preoperative profile appearance.

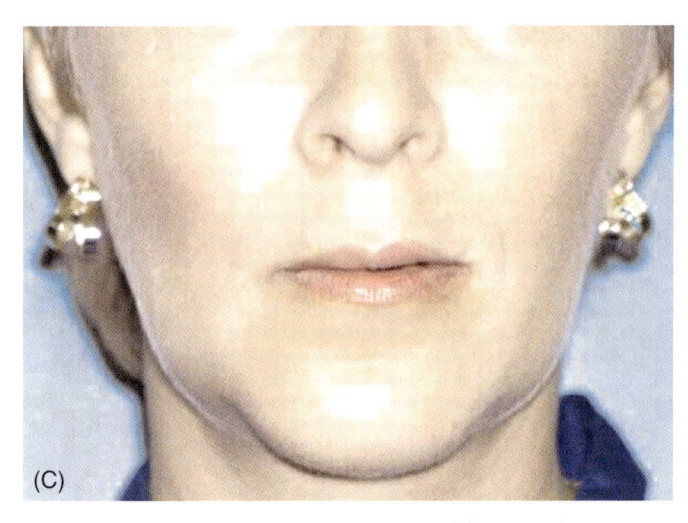

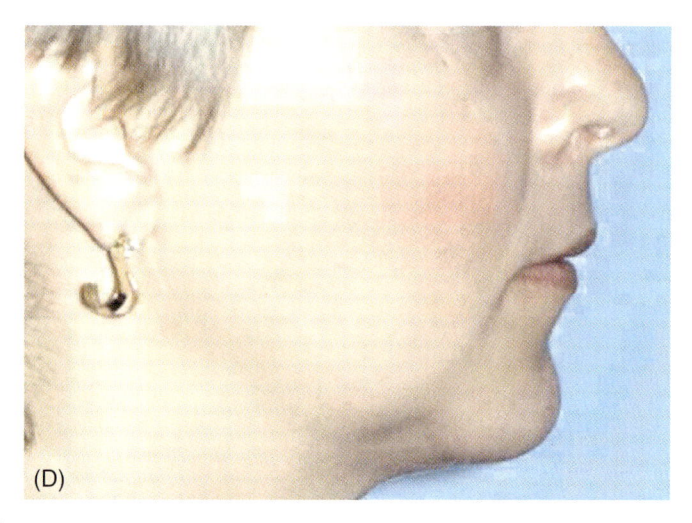

Figure 29.21 (C, D) Postoperative appearance following advancement of the chin with sliding horizontal osteotomy and chin implant placed over advanced chin.

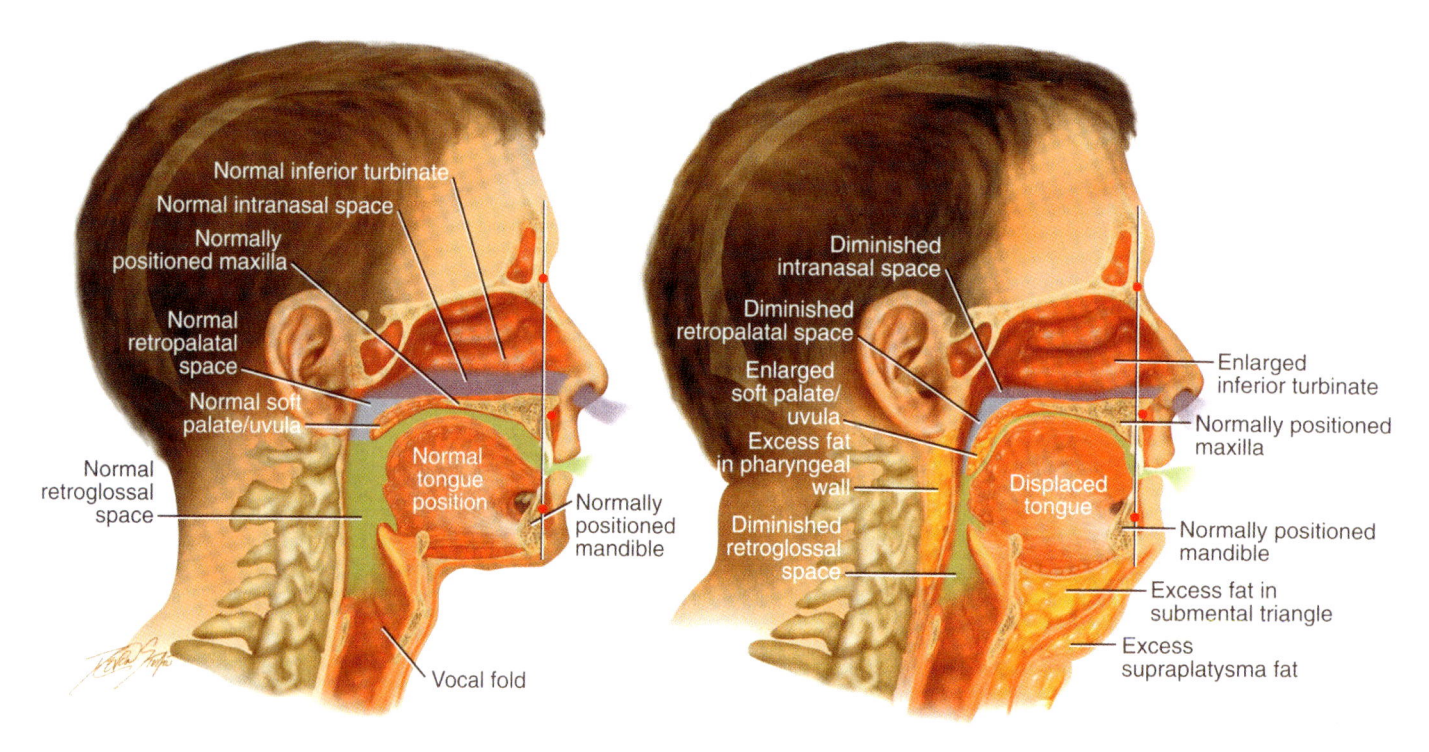

Figure 29.22 (A) Illustration of the changes that occur in a normocephalic male that decrease the posterior airspace. *Source:* Figure courtesy of Dr Jeffrey C. Posnick, *Orthognathic Surgery. Principles and Practice.* 2014. Published by Saunders, an imprint of Elsevier Inc. Chapter 26, Figure 26-1, page 995.

Figure 29.22B illustrates how a patient with a preexisting hypoplastic mandible predisposes a patient for OSA and how maxillomandibular advancement surgery can effect a change that is not only esthetically pleasing but is beneficial to the patient's health as it makes positive effects on the airway space.

Figure 29.22C illustrates a necessary maxillomandibular advancement to correct OSA in a middle-aged man with a short face jaw growth pattern and a harmonious occlusion.

The usual workup involves obtaining a polysomnogram (sleep study) to determine the severity of OSA. Patients with apnea–hypopnea index (AHI) per hour of above 20 with oxygen desaturations below 90% are candidates for maxillomandibular advancement if their symptoms dictate and they are unable or unwilling to use CPAP. In addition to the polysomnogram, a cephalometric workup which may include software that can measure and detect the area of greatest constriction is used to plan the surgery. Most practitioners aim for a 10 mm advancement with a counterclockwise rotation of the maxillomandibular complex. Such large advancements may necessitate impaction of the anterior maxilla to prevent too much tooth show but also add to the desired counterclockwise movement.

Surgical cures of OSA are considered if the AHI can be lowered to below 5. Many patients begin with AHIs of above 80, and a reduction of the AHI to below 15 is considered a success but not a cure.

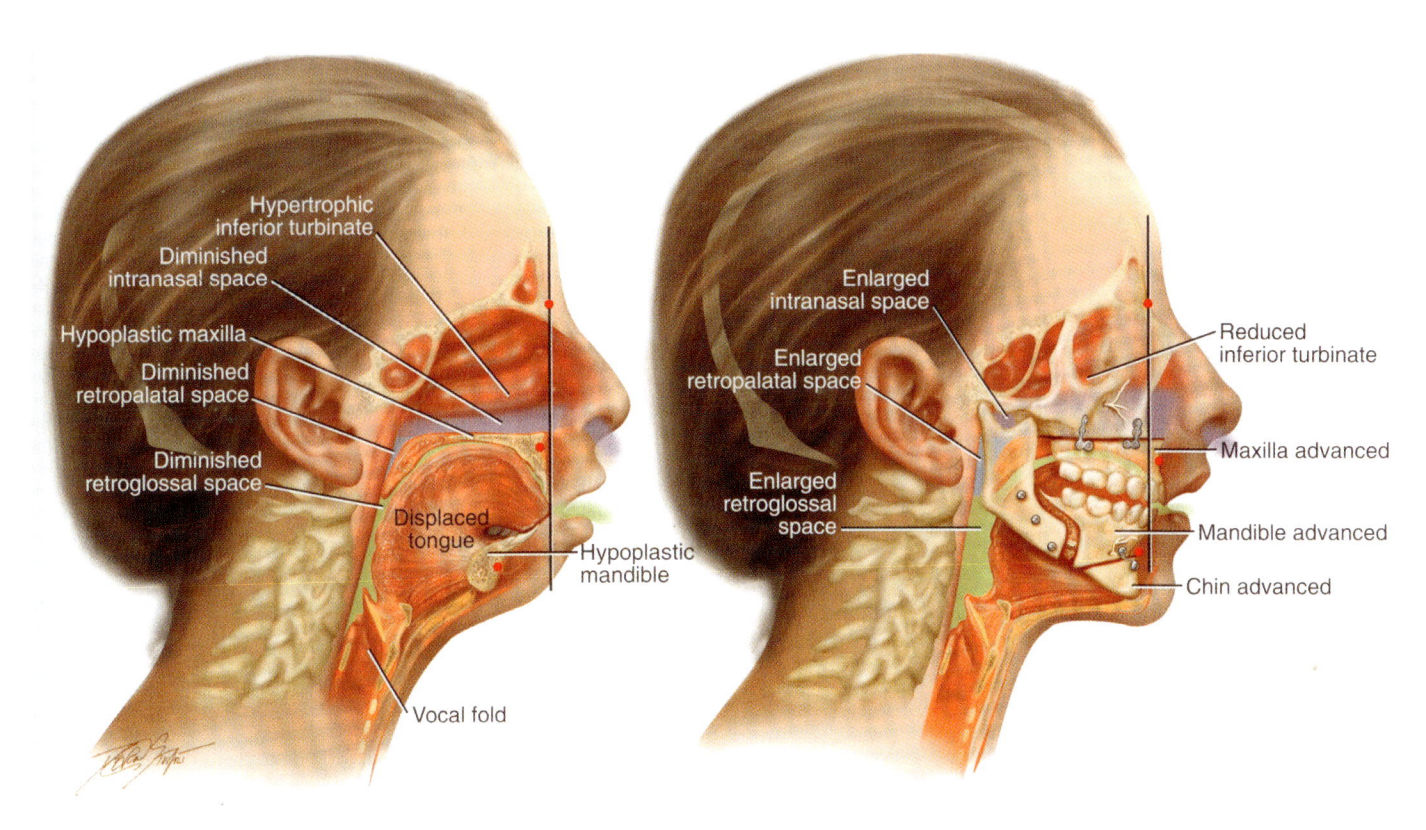

Figure 29.22 **(B)** Illustration of how a patient with a preexisting hypoplastic mandible predisposes a patient for OSA. *Source:* Figure courtesy of Dr Jeffrey C. Posnick, *Orthognathic Surgery. Principles and Practice.* 2014. Published by Saunders, an imprint of Elsevier Inc. Chapter 26, Figure 26-2, page 997.

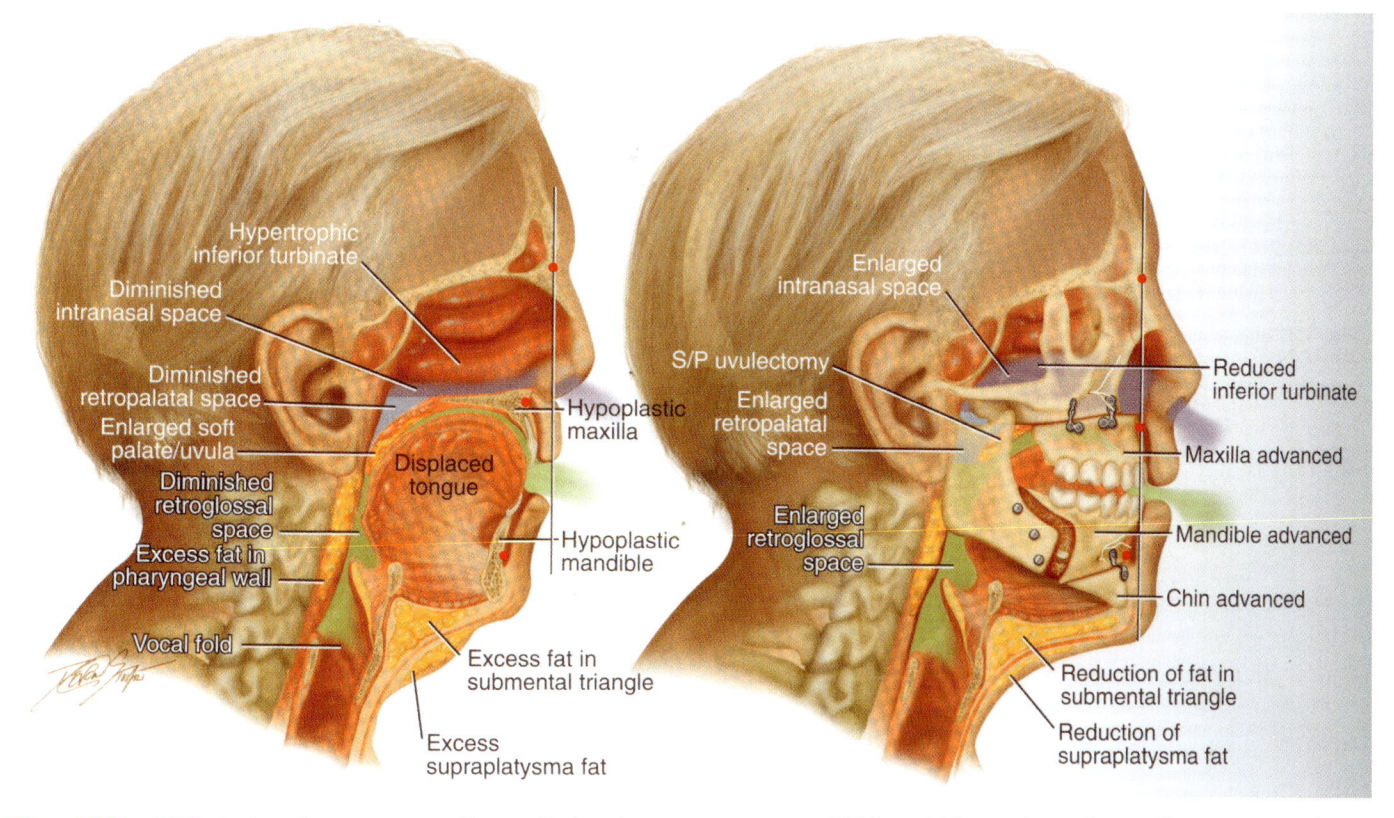

Figure 29.22 **(C)** Illustration of a necessary maxillomandibular advancement to correct OSA in a middle-aged man. *Source:* Figure courtesy of Dr Jeffrey C. Posnick, *Orthognathic Surgery. Principles and Practice.* 2014. Published by Saunders, an imprint of Elsevier Inc. Chapter 26, Figure 26-3, page 998.

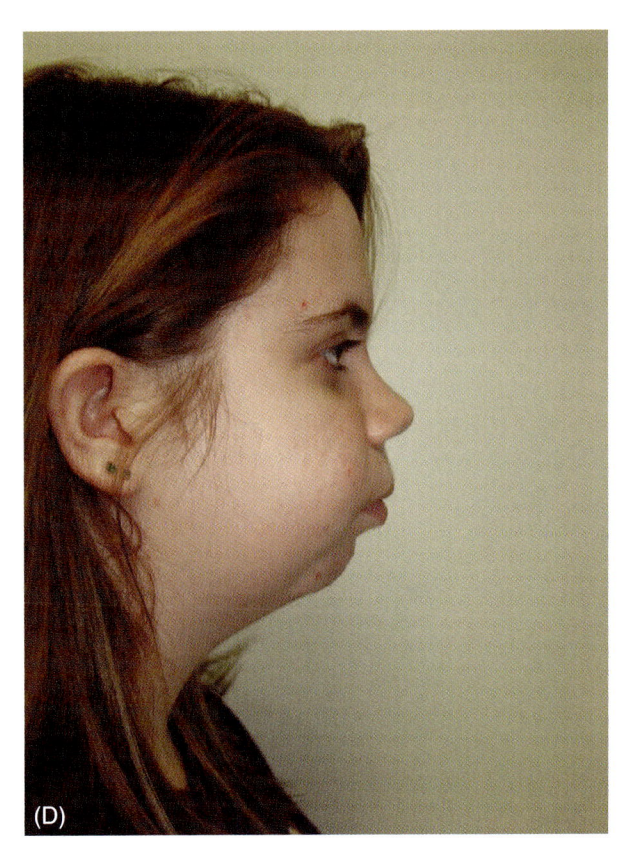

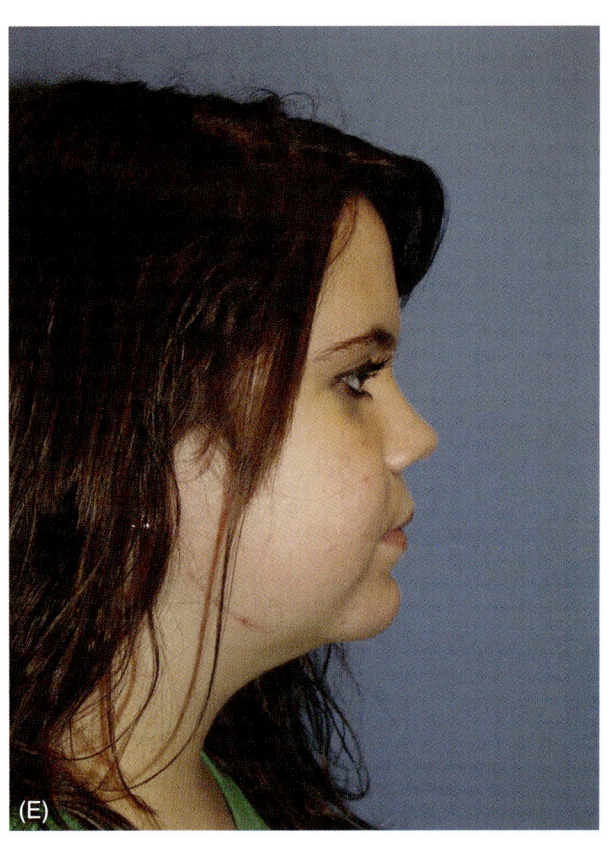

Figure 29.22 **(D)** This 18-year-old female had OSA as a result of severe juvenile rheumatoid arthritis which had produced severe bilateral resorptions of condyles. **(E)** Her maxilla was advanced 6 mm and her mandible 15 mm, along with a 7 mm chin advancement genioplasty. A good esthetic and functional result was achieved that cured her OSA.

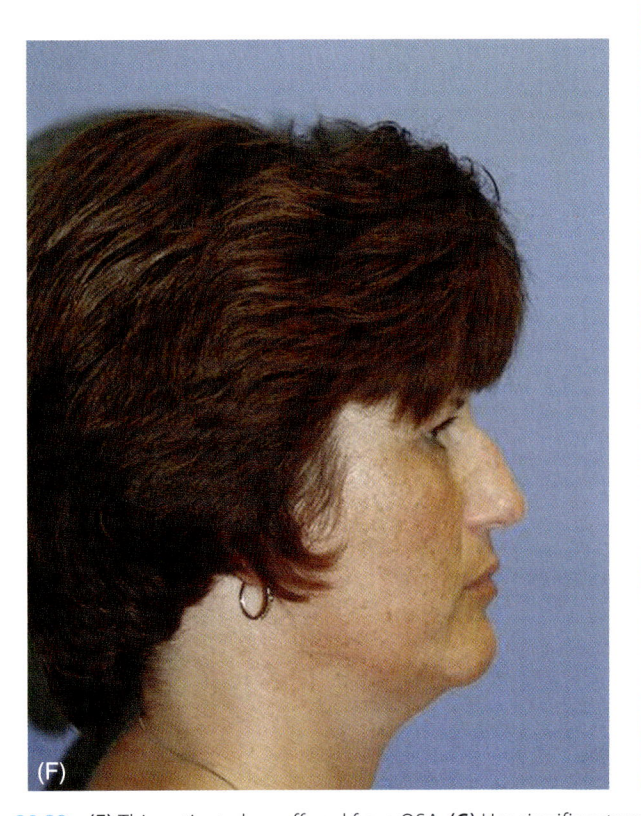

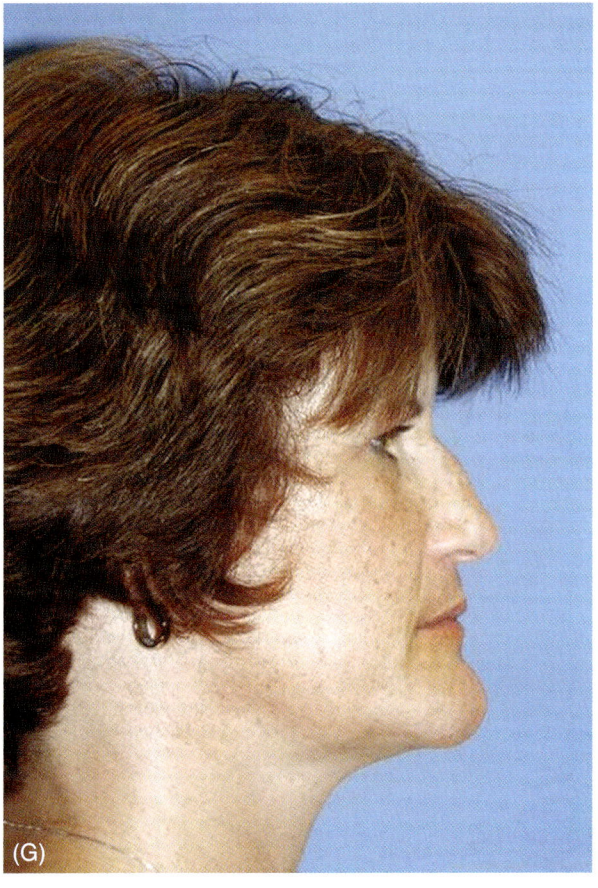

Figure 29.22 **(F)** This patient also suffered from OSA. **(G)** Her significant mandibular advancement cured her OSA, and although the chin protruded excessively, she was nonetheless very pleased.

The patient in Figure 29.22D and E achieved an OSA cure with esthetic improvement via maxillomandibular advancement, while the patient in Figure 29.22 F and G achieved OSA cure from maxillomandibular advancement at the expense of a too prominent lower face. She was nevertheless pleased.

Additional resources

Bays RA, Bouloux GF. Complications of orthognathic surgery. *Oral Maxillofac Surg Clin* 2003;15(2):229–242.

Bell WH, ed. *Modern Practice in Orthognathic and Reconstructive Surgery*. Philadelphia, PA: WB Saunders; 1992.

Bell WH, Jacobs JD, Quejada JG. Simultaneous repositioning of the maxilla, mandible, and chin. Treatment planning and analysis of soft tissues. *Am J Orthod* 1986;89:28–50.

Carlotti AE Jr, Aschaffenburg PH, Schendel SA. Facial changes associated with surgical advancement of the lip and maxilla. *J Oral Maxillofac Surg* 1986;44:593–596.

Carlotti AE Jr, Schendel SA. An analysis of factors influencing stability of surgical advancement of the maxilla by the Le Fort I osteotomy. *J Oral Maxillofac Surg* 1987;45:924–928.

Crawford SD. Class II division 1 history of TMJ trauma—maxilla and mandible orthognathic surgery. *Orthod Rev* 1988;2:18–25.

Ellis E III. Bimaxillary surgery using an intermediate splint to position the maxilla. *J Oral Maxillofac Surg* 1999;57:53–56.

Epker BN. *Esthetic Maxillofacial Surgery*. Philadelphia, PA: Lea & Febiger; 1994.

Epker BN, Stella JP, Fish LC, eds. *Dentofacial Deformities: Integrated Orthodontic and Surgical Correction*. St. Louis, MO: Mosby; 1995.

Fonseca RJ. Oral and maxillofacial surgery. In: Betts NJ, Turvey TA, eds. *Orthognathic Surgery*, Vol. 2. Philadelphia, PA: WB Saunders; 2000.

Frost HM. The regional accelerated phenomenon. *Orthop Clin N Am* 1981;12:725–726.

Gallagher DM, Bell WH, Storum KA. Soft tissue changes associated with advancement genioplasty performed concomitantly with superior repositioning of the maxilla. *J Oral Maxillofac Surg* 1984;42:238–242.

Gao YM, Qiu WL, Tang YS, Shen GF. Evaluation of the treatment for micromandibular deformity by distraction osteogenesis with submerged intraoral device. *Chin J Dent Res* 1999;2:31–37.

Hiranaka DK, Kelly JP. Stability of simultaneous orthognathic surgery on the maxilla and mandible: a computer-assisted cephalometric study. *Int J Adult Orthodon Orthognath Surg* 1987;2:193–213.

Köle H. Surgical operation on the alveolar ridge to correct occlusal abnormalities. *Oral Surg Oral Med Oral Pathol Oral Radiol Endod* 1959;12:515–29.

Lapp TH. Bimaxillary surgery without the use of an intermediate splint to position the maxilla. *J Oral Maxillofac Surg* 1999;57:57–60.

Major PW, Philippson GE, Glover KE, Grace MG. Stability of maxilla downgrafting after rigid or wire fixation. *J Oral Maxillofac Surg* 1996;54:1287–1291.

Manna LM, Berger JR. Technique for vertical positioning of the maxilla after Le Fort osteotomy. *J Oral Maxillofac Surg* 1996;54:652.

Masui I, Honda T, Uji T. Two-step repositioning of the maxilla in bimaxillary orthognathic surgery. *Br J Oral Maxillofac Surg* 1997;35:64–66.

Posnick JC. Craniofacial dysostosis. Staging of reconstruction and management of the midface deformity. *Neurosurg Clin N Am* 1991;2:683–702.

Posnick JC, Tompson B. Modification of the maxillary Le Fort I osteotomy in cleft-orthognathic surgery: the unilateral cleft lip and palate deformity. *J Oral Maxillofac Surg* 1992;50:666–675.

Posnick JC, Tompson B. Modification of the maxillary Le Fort I osteotomy in cleft-orthognathic surgery: the bilateral cleft lip and palate deformity. *J Oral Maxillofac Surg* 1993;51:2–11.

Rosen HM. Segmental osteotomies of the maxilla. *Clin Plast Surg* 1989;16:785–794.

Schendel SA, Williamson LW. Muscle reorientation following superior repositioning of the maxilla. *J Oral Maxillofac Surg* 1983;41:235–240.

Schwestka R, Engelke D, Kubein-Meesenburg D, Luhr HG. Control of vertical position of the maxilla in orthognathic surgery: clinical application of the sandwich splint. *Int J Adult Orthodon Orthognath Surg* 1990;5:133–136.

Shetty V, Caridad JM, Caputo AA, Chaconas SJ. Biomechanical rationale for surgical–orthodontic expansion of the adult maxilla. *J Oral Maxillofac Surg* 1994;52:742–749.

Song HC, Throckmorton GS, Ellis E III, Sinn DP. Functional and morphologic alterations after anterior or inferior repositioning of the maxilla. *J Oral Maxillofac Surg* 1997;55:41–49.

Sperber GH. *Craniofacial Development*. Hamilton, ON: BC Decker; 2001.

Stanchina R, Ellis E III, Gallo WJ, Fonseca RJ. A comparison of two measures for repositioning the maxilla during orthognathic surgery. *Int J Adult Orthodon Orthognath Surg* 1988;3:149–154.

Sullivan SM. Isolated inferior repositioning of the maxilla, with or without bone grafting, is a very unstable orthognathic procedure which is confirmed by these surgeons' results. *Aesthetic Plast Surg* 2000;24:72–75.

Turvey TA. Simultaneous mobilization of the maxilla and mandible: surgical technique and results. *J Oral Maxillofac Surg* 1982;40:96–99.

Vu HL, Panchal J, Levine N. Combined simultaneous distraction osteogenesis of the maxilla and mandible using a single distraction device in hemifacial microsomia. *J Craniofac Surg* 2001;12:253–258.

Wessberg GA, O'Ryan FS, Washburn MC, Epker BN. Neuromuscular adaptation to surgical superior repositioning of the maxilla. *J Maxillofac Surg* 1981;9:117–122.

Wilcko WM, Ferguson DJ, Bouquot JE, Wilcko MT. Rapid orthodontic decrowding with alveolar augmentation: case report. *World J Orthod* 2003;4:197–205

Wilmot JJ, Barber HD, Chou DG, Vig KW. Associations between severity of dentofacial deformity and motivation for orthodontic–orthognathic surgery treatment. *Angle Orthod* 1993;63:283–288.

Zarrinkelk HM, Throckmorton GS, Ellis E III, Sinn DP. Functional and morphologic alterations secondary to superior repositioning of the maxilla. *J Oral Maxillofac Surg* 1995;53:1258–1267.

Zaytoun H, Phillips C, Terry B. Long-term neurosensory deficits following transoral vertical ramus and sagittal split osteotomies for mandibular prognathism. *J Oral Maxillofac Surg* 1986;44:193–196.

PART 6
ESTHETIC PROBLEMS OF SPECIAL POPULATIONS, FACIAL CONSIDERATIONS, AND SUPPORTING STRUCTURES

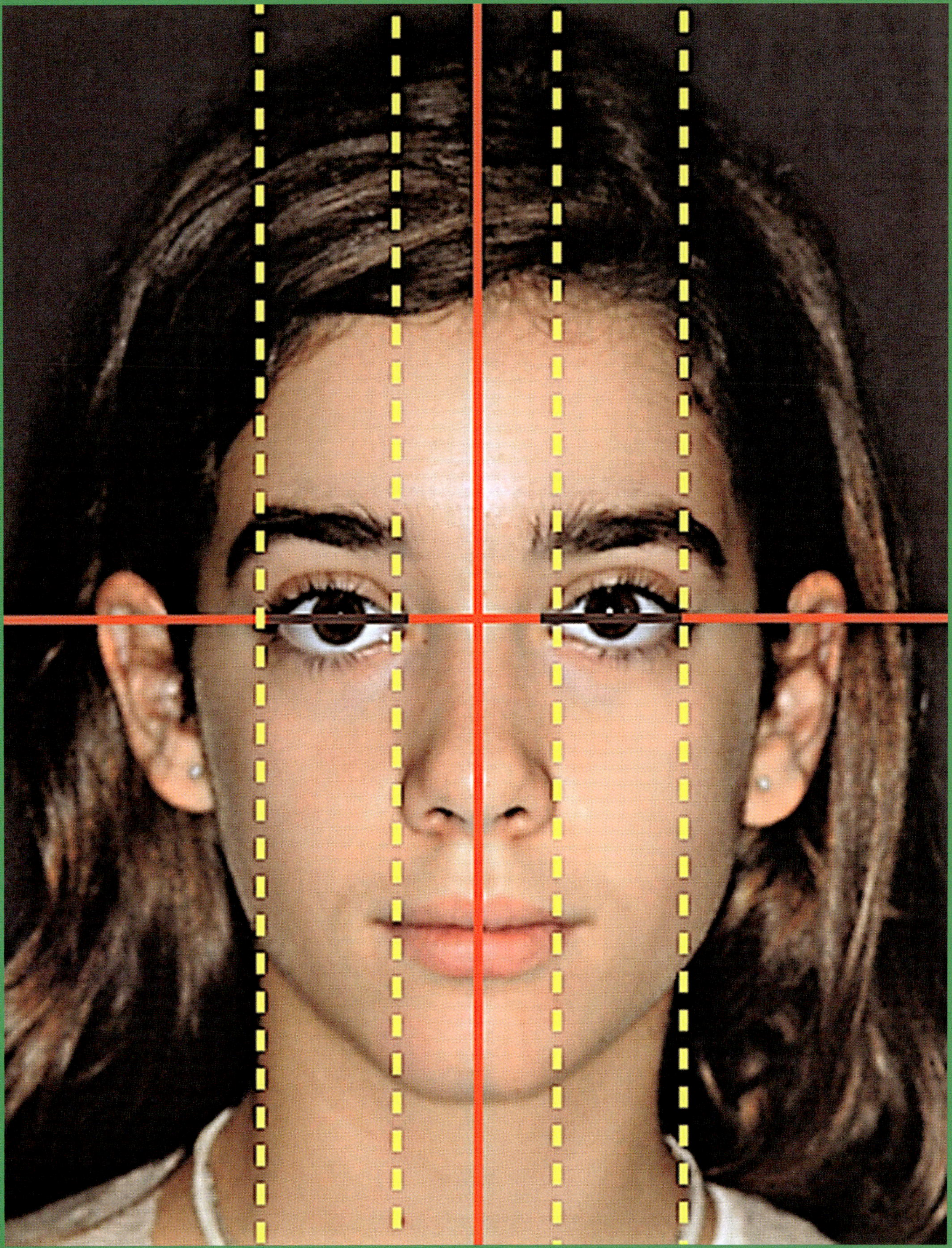

Chapter 30 Pediatric Dentistry

Claudia Caprioglio, DDS, MS, Alberto Caprioglio, DDS, MS, and Damaso Caprioglio MD, MS

Chapter Outline

Materials and techniques	970
Glass ionomers and modified ionomer cements	970
Compomers	970
Ozone therapy	971
Laser-assisted pediatric dentistry: minimally invasive treatment	971
Laser–tissue interaction	971
Hard tissue removal: absorption and laser ablation	971
Adhesion to erbium-lased tooth structure	972
Soft-tissue applications	973
Esthetic dentistry: operating procedures	973
Procedure	973
Nursing bottle syndrome and/or tooth loss due to caries and/or to dental trauma	979
Patient with multiple agenesis: ectodermal dysplasia	982
Trauma management in primary dentition and in the first phase of mixed dentition	983
Application of lasers in dental traumatology	984
Traumatic injuries to hard dental tissue and pulp	984
Traumatic injuries to the periodontal tissues	985
Injuries to developing teeth	986
Case studies of trauma	986
Facial harmony in pediatric dentistry: esthetic keys	1005
Cephalometrics and soft tissue analysis	1005
Esthetic reference parameters in children	1006
Frontal view: symmetry between different parts of the face	1007
Profile view considerations	1008
The future	1010

To quote Jean Cocteau, "A defect of our body, if corrected, can improve our soul," or, to paraphrase an old Jewish saying, "He who gives a smile to a child gives a smile to the world."

In the period that spans the end of deciduous and the beginning of early mixed denition, the esthetics and harmony of the dental arches are determined by physiological changes in the teeth and the presence of diastemas, a correct canine relationship, and a correct occlusal plane. The occlusion of the primary dentition should be considered a biological unit with specific esthetic, functional, and skeletal characteristics, and the main role of the pediatric dentist is to monitor its evolution throughout childhood and adolescence.

The pediatric dentist's duty is actually twofold: to perform preventive and/or conservative dentistry and also to apply the space management techniques necessary to ensure an optimal morphofunctional outcome.

To allow a modern, dynamic approach to pediatric dentistry, close interaction between the dentist, parents, and child is crucial. Furthermore, the chosen approach, methods, and timing of application are more likely to be correct if the child is first seen very early on, at 2–3 years of age. Children are naturally fearful of new experiences, and in the case of dental treatment this fear is linked not only to the technology used—high-tech instruments are involved—but also to cultural, environmental, and psychological factors. Thus, a correct psychological approach is essential to gain the child's trust and cooperation, which are necessary for successful treatment.

The goal of pediatric dentistry is to educate both children and parents about clinical prevention (fluoride use, pit and fissure sealants) and tertiary prevention (the limiting of complications and restoration of optimal conditions).[1,2] The common objective is tissue preservation: new techniques and instruments such as digital radiology with low radiation emission, diagnostic lasers, dental operative microscope, minimally invasive therapy (ozone therapy, air abrasion, and laser micropreparation) allow a stress-free approach and are very effective treatment options.[3]

Materials and techniques

Therapeutic strategies used in the primary dentition must be based on careful evaluation of the physiological state of the deciduous tooth and of the likely efficacy of the treatment. A careful diagnostic workup must be performed to arrive at an accurate prognosis. Furthermore, pulp and periodontal lesions of the primary dentition differ from those of the permanent dentition, and a poor awareness of the available pulp treatment options may result in insignificant therapeutic improvements, and thus treatment failures and, consequently, unnecessary additional treatment procedures and use of materials. The reader is advised to consult the literature for more detailed information on this aspect.[4–6]

The currently available materials for the restoration of teeth in primary and mixed dentition are briefly described here.

The introduction of light-cured composite resins has changed clinical pediatric dentistry. These materials are, indeed, welcome treatment options that address both esthetic and functional issues. Their advantages are their considerable hardness, high rigidity, and high resistance to compression. However, these materials are very technique sensitive and can show marginal infiltrations, reduced wear resistance, polymerization contractions, surface roughness, and discoloration.

Composite resins are the materials of choice to restore anterior teeth, the recommended ones being microfilled hybrid composite resins. More research into these materials has led to considerable improvements, particularly in traumatology, and thus to the possibility of achieving tooth fragment reattachment. This, in turn, has allowed dentists to exploit true biological restorations to achieve a good anterior guide, improved resistance to wear, and higher color stability in the follow-up years.[7,8]

Composite resins can be used for Class I and II restorations of posterior teeth, where etching time is an extremely important factor.[9] Furthermore, the use of a glass ionomer cement as a cavity base and reconstruction of the tooth by applying the incremental technique and using a rubber dam have been found to reduce the wear index and improve cavity adhesion. Marginal adaptation is, instead, influenced by the kind of polymerization (direct or incremental).[10]

Glass ionomers and modified ionomer cements

These materials first appeared in the early 1970s. They are composed of a powder, a calcium–fluoride–aluminum silicate glass, and a liquid, generally a polyacrylic or polymaleic acid. Considering their capacity to bond with dentin, fluoride-leaching properties, and high resilience, these materials have proved to be useful in the treatment of caries lesions in primary molar teeth.

Resin cements are the most popular and most routinely used cements in dentistry. The main dental cements available for stabilizing porcelain-fused-to-metal, all-ceramic, or all-metal restorations include resin-modified glass ionomer (RMGI) cements, resins requiring a separate self-etching bonding agent, resins that incorporate a self-etching primer, and resins used with total-etch bonding systems.[11] Although these materials have a higher percentage of failure than amalgam (33% versus 20%), and although they lack abrasion resistance, translucence, and multiple color choices, they nevertheless offer great advantages: minimal destruction of sound tooth tissue and less use of local anesthetic.

RMGI cements are polymerizable materials whose resin compound also improves fracture resistance. They are recommended for Class I and II restorations in primary teeth, which typically do not last beyond 3 years. RMGIs are associated with little or no tooth sensitivity postoperatively, form a natural chemical bond with the tooth structure, offer moderate strength compared with other cements, release fluoride ions, are relatively insoluble in oral fluids, and have demonstrated positive in vitro clinical characteristics.[12,13]

Compomers

Introduced in the early 1990s, compomers are materials made from mixed composite resins with an acid modification; therefore, they are more similar to composite resins than glass ionomers. They do not have improved characteristics of resins, but they are easy to handle, which reduces operating times and makes them a good option for restorations. In a study that evaluated and measured compression resistance, flexion resistance, microhardness, and surface roughness of three different compomers, the values obtained were compared with those of a composite resin and an RMGI cement. The flexion and compression resistance values and the microhardness of the compomers tested were found to be higher than those of the cement but lower than those of the composite resin, whereas no significant differences in surface roughness values were reported.

Compomers demonstrate the following properties:

- good adhesion to dental tissues (a dentinal adhesive is used instead of acid etching);

- easy handling, enhanced by the possibility of incremental polymerization;
- a reduced marginal fissure due to their property of absorbing water during hardening;
- a good fluoride absorption-release system;
- an acceptable range of colors and brightnesses that allows good esthetic results, albeit not quite comparable to those of composite resin.[14]

Thanks to the availability of these dental restorative materials, the pediatric dentist can apply preventive treatments and perform early conservative therapy and, in the most severe cases, restore function and improve esthetics. Improved treatment techniques, better materials, and a heightened awareness of the benefits of preventive dentistry are together allowing more predictable results based on achievement of the postulates of successful pediatric dentistry:

- optimal esthetic restoration;
- elimination of infection, inflammation, and pain;
- maintenance of the arch perimeter length;
- stimulation of alveolar growth.

There are also alternative treatment solutions that exist based on other means of cavity excavation, namely ozone therapy and laser therapy.

Ozone therapy

Ozone is a strong oxidizing agent, present in nature as triatomic oxygen (O_3). Rich in energy but with a very unstable structure, O_3 has a very effective and rapid oxidizing action. It also has a strong disinfecting power and an effective antibacterial activity, also on cariogenic bacteria. Ozone therapy is able to disinfect the treated area and to induce biofilm acid proteins lysis. Despite the use of rotary instruments, anesthesia is not required during pediatric treatments using this technology; because the carious dentin is sterilized, it does not need to be removed. Ozone therapy is useful for treating fissure, root, and cervical caries, for Class V restorations, and for desensitizing carious cervical tooth substance. The ozone generated is delivered by a multilumen tube and special handpiece with a silicon single-use cup; a hermetic seal must be obtained, and application time ranges from 10 to 60 s.[15,16]

Laser-assisted pediatric dentistry: minimally invasive treatment

Laser technologies are alternative methods that sometimes complement and sometimes replace traditional techniques; various applications, using different laser wavelengths, are possible on both soft and hard tissues.

Although this is not the place for a detailed discussion of the physical basis of laser therapy, it should nevertheless be remembered that the various wavelengths interact in different ways with the different chromophores (hemoglobin, water, hydroxyapatite) contained in the target tissues (mucous membranes, gingiva, dental tissue); thus, treatments are influenced by the optical affinity and absorption coefficients of the tissues for each particular wavelength. This issue is still debated in the literature; indeed, with various wavelengths advocated for hard tissue removal, there continues to be certain heterogeneity with regard to recommended laser parameters and power densities. Erbium lasers (Er:YAG and Er,Cr:YSGG) are the most efficient for cavity preparation and, when the parameters are right, they have low thermal side effects.

Although there is clearly a great need for "gold standards," these would be difficult to establish in practice, given the variety of laser parameters (pulse repetition rates, amount of cooling, energy delivered per pulse, and types of pulse, etc.) and the existence of target tissue-related factors that also influence the interaction (i.e., whether the target tissue is healthy enamel, decayed enamel, or dentin, and the extent of its (de)mineralization).

Laser–tissue interaction

Laser light (laser energy) may interact with the target tissue in four different ways, depending on its optical properties:

- It may be absorbed by the target tissue. The amount that is absorbed depends on certain characteristics of the tissue, such as pigmentation and water content, and on the laser wavelength and emission mode.
- It may be transmitted through the tissue (transmission is the opposite of absorption). This has no effect on the target tissue. This phenomenon is highly dependent on the wavelength of the laser light.
- It may be reflected from the tissue surface (reflection). This, too, has no effect on the target tissue. A caries-detecting laser device (DIAGNODENT®-kavo) uses reflected light to measure the amount of sound tooth structure. Two types of reflection are described: specular and diffuse.
- It may be scattered. Scattering weakens the intended energy and possibly produces no useful biological effect.

Hard tissue removal: absorption and laser ablation

Hard tissue laser ablation exploits a series of biophysical properties, such as wavelength, energy density, and pulse duration of the laser radiation, as well as the properties of the tissue (tissue interaction). The laser energy must be absorbed by the target to achieve tissue removal, which, in this context, is the primary beneficial effect of laser energy. The goal of dental laser applications is to optimize this photobiological effect.

The lasers used in dentistry to remove hard tissue are those belonging to the erbium family. Both the solid-state Er:YAG laser (2940 nm) and the Er,Cr:YSGG laser (2780 nm) have a high affinity for water and hydroxyapatite. This explains their effectiveness when working on enamel, dentin, and bone.

The energy is transferred to the target tissue through a handpiece attached to an articulated arm or an optical fiber. The handpieces used in dentistry may be contact-free (noncontact) or contact, straight, or angled. Erbium lasers can be regulated by the operator, who can adjust pulse energy (millijoules), frequency (hertz or pulses per second), and duration (long, short, very short), the air–water spray, and the size of the focal spot (increased: focused mode; decreased: defocused mode). Various studies and clinical reports have shown that the laser, often used as an alternative to rotary instruments in pediatric restorative dentistry, offers an added measure of safety and new scope for minimally invasive interventions even in the treatment of very young children. Overall, it is better accepted than traditional techniques.[15,17]

The mechanisms underlying tooth structure removal, which is based on the principle of ablation or decomposition of biological materials, are photochemical, photothermal, and plasma mediated.

Currently, laser removal of tooth substance is based on the principle of thermal ablation: laser energy is coupled into the irradiated material by an absorption process that yields a rise in temperature. A shockwave is created when the energy dissipates explosively as a volumetric expansion of the water contained in the hard tissue. This process is called *cavitation*. Efficient conversion of this incoming energy into a temperature increase depends on the presence of an absorptive component in the irradiated material. All dental hard tissues contain water; water molecules in the target tissue become superheated, an explosion occurs, and, in turn, the tooth structure and/or caries is ablated.

Laser removal of tooth substance generates a characteristic popping sound. The free-running pulse-mode provides the maximum power to facilitate the explosive expansion; with an adequate amount of water spray, thermal pulp damage can be avoided; temperature rises up to 3–5 °C. The Er,Cr:YSGG laser system generates a loud snapping sound even when used in a noncontact mode; it is an effect termed "plasma decoupling" of the beam with a hydrokinetic cutting. The microexplosion of the water molecules removes the decayed dental hard tissue (mechanical effect); however, because the water contained in the decayed hard tissue evaporates rapidly, the healthy tissue is conserved (thermal effect).[18]

With these technologies, it is essential to use the correct parameter settings to prevent structural alterations and/or pulp reactions and preserve the integrity of the cells. Enamel treated with correctly set lasers appears chalky, without carbonization, and with the characteristic lava-flow appearance: grooves, flakes, shelves, and sharp edges are all features more indicative of microexplosions than of melting; other features are open prisms and dentin with open tubules and a difference in the mineral thickness between peritubular and intertubular dentin.

The clinical applications of erbium lasers range from prevention to conservative treatment of primary and permanent teeth (immature and mature) affected by superficial (tooth enamel hypoplasia, mild discolorations) or deep lesions.

Pediatric laser treatment generally offers the following advantages:

- minimum invasiveness;
- selectiveness and effective cleansing;
- less (or no) anesthesia;
- positive psychological impact.[3,19]

Adhesion to erbium-lased tooth structure

The adhesion of composite to lased surfaces continues to be a controversial topic. Many authors have reported that adhesion to laser-ablated or laser-etched dentin and enamel of permanent teeth is lower than adhesion to surfaces treated conventionally (with rotary preparation and acid etching). Studies stress the importance of energy output and of avoiding substructural damage, the need for standardized laser energy outputs for different tooth substrates, and the need to acid etch both dentin and enamel, even after laser conditioning and in primary dentition.

Although Er:YAG laser ablation creates a smear-layer-free dentin surface, acid etching nevertheless seems to be necessary to expose any dentin collagen that is needed to allow hybridization with the bonding agent. The term "laser etching," used several times in the laser literature, refers to the laser-induced modification of the tooth surface at lower fluence; a more appropriate term would be "laser conditioning." Recrystallization of the dentinal apatite possibly with the formation of an additional phase of calcium phosphate results in vitrification. The degree of vitrification inevitably depends on the amount of laser energy the dental substrate is subjected to, given that the phenomenon is induced by the production of heat. It has been reported that Er:YAG laser irradiation reduces the carbon-to-phosphorus ratio and leads to the formation of more stable and less acid-soluble compounds that can hamper the chemical adhesion of ionomer cements and the activity of etching and conditioning products. A more acid-resistant surface was found after Er:YAG laser treatment in enamel; this feature also seemed to be present in peritubular dentin. On lasing at subablative energy densities, it emerged that temperature induces loss of carbonate; carbonate loss begins at 100 °C and becomes more intensive at 700 °C. Complete carbonate loss is reached at around 1000 °C (melting point). Chemical alterations may also appear on laser-irradiated dentin after application of subablative Er:YAG laser energy densities: degradation, loss of H_2O, and an increase of OH were reported. In addition, factors such as pulse duration, output energy, and water cooling have been seen to influence the chemical composition of the Er:YAG-lased dentin substrate. The excessive heat that can be generated during cavity preparation may cause denaturation of the collagen network and a decrease in dentin permeability. The importance of energy output cannot be understated, and there is clearly a need to establish relevant gold standards for optimal enamel and dentin preparations, as well as for conditioning.

The bond strengths of the currently favored three-step etch-and-rinse adhesives and of the two-step etch-and-rinse adhesives used in Er:YAG-lased cavities are higher than those of the newer self-etching systems. The current data on the bond strengths associated with the use of laser systems on enamel and dentin surfaces suggest that it is better to avoid using these systems and that acid etching of lased surfaces is still to be preferred.

Glass ionomers are auto-adhesive materials that bond to dental tissue through combined micromechanical and chemical mechanisms. The Er:YAG laser creates a rough surface that could favor this material retention. Data on the tensile bond strength of glass ionomer cements in association with laser dentistry are very scarce. All studies on microleakage in association with glass ionomer cements, both pure and resin-modified, showed that these materials failed to prevent microleakage, regardless of whether the tooth substance was lased or prepared with a high-speed handpiece. Furthermore, it was demonstrated that leakage at the gingival margin was, in both cases, higher than at the occlusal enamel margins.

Soft-tissue applications

The laser as a means of removing diseased oral tissue and treating lesions of the oral mucosa has specific applications in the field of pediatric dentistry. All laser wavelengths with optical affinity for hemoglobin and water (the chromophores contained in gingival tissue and the oral mucosa) can be used for these applications; argon, KTP, diode, Nd:YAG, and CO_2 lasers are useful for soft-tissue cutting, vaporization, and decontamination. Also, because of their excellent coagulating and haemostatic actions, they are also ideal for vascular lesions. The Er,Cr:YSGG and Er:YAG lasers are also effective for these applications owing to the good absorption of their wavelengths by the water contained in the gingival tissues and mucosa, but they provide less effective bleeding control. The use of an air–water jet delivered through the handpiece of the erbium laser allows a clean incision and vaporization of the soft tissues with a limited increase in temperature; furthermore, the absence of peripheral necrotic tissue makes it possible to carry out very accurate biopsies.

Many authors agree on the advantages offered by laser applications for the treatment of soft tissues: these lasers are quick and easy to use, reduce the use of local anesthesia, allow excellent control of bleeding during incision making, provide effective decontamination, allow the use of sutureless techniques, and result in postoperative healing by second intention, which is often asymptomatic due to the laser's decontaminating, antalgic, and biostimulant effects; there is, therefore, also less need for analgesic anti-inflammatory medications.

Lasers are suitable for the following procedures:

- soft-tissue surgery (gingivectomies, gingivoplasties, surgical cutting, removal of foreign bodies, frenectomies, operculum cutting);
- treatment of periodontal defects;
- socket decontamination;
- biostimulation;
- treatment of labial herpes, oral aphthosis, hemangiomas, fibromas, papillomas, epulis, mucocele, eruption problems, or dentigerous cysts.

The use of lasers, with different wavelengths, is well documented in adult endodontics, but few studies have been conducted in the field of pediatric endodontics. Lasers in endodontics are indicated for pulp capping, pulpotomy, and root canal disinfection.

The PubMed library indexes several studies that investigate laser performance in maintaining pulp tissue vitality. Different devices, and thus different laser wavelengths and parameters, are used in these studies. A common feature was the low level of laser power applied (0.5–1.0 W), delivered in a defocused mode, preferably using a low repetition rate or superpulsed mode.[20]

Esthetic dentistry: operating procedures

Over the past 15 years, composite resins have been revolutionized. Their adhesion, polish, and esthetics have improved so much that they are now the best restoration material for anterior teeth damaged by caries or trauma, direct or indirect. One of the undeniable merits of this kind of restoration is the "reversibility" of the treatment, which allows it to be redone when necessary.

Procedure

Step 1: Carefully evaluate the tooth shape and the position of the contralateral tooth, so as to plan the reconstruction.

Step 2: Choose the color of the restoration, as the subsequent isolation with a rubber dam will not allow an accurate assessment of this aspect.

Step 3: Isolate the area and remove the carious lesion, taking care to conserve as much healthy tooth tissue as possible.

Step 4: Laser preparation. The erbium family of lasers can provide effective thermomechanical ablation of tooth tissues without side effects on surrounding tissues, removing the smear layer, opening and cleansing dentinal tubules, and effecting decontamination.

Step 5: Reconstruction. Ensure modeling is as precise as possible to reduce chair time and improve the final esthetic outcome.

Step 6: Finishing. It is sometimes possible to use a flame-shaped diamond bur to reproduce the microanatomy of the rather irregular enamel surface. The finishing phase is completed by using disks of different granulometry and rubber polishers.

Step 7: Remove the rubber dam and evaluate the results. Next, polish the interproximal areas with pop-on disks and abrasive strips, taking care not to remove the contact point. Then, polish the other areas of the buccal face using rubber cups and polishing pastes with decreasing particle size.

Step 8: Color check. After initial dehydration, the tooth regains its original color. Note that chromatic evaluations should be postponed to the subsequent visit.

Clinical case 30.1: Preventive resin restoration in a 7.2-year-old

Problem

This 7.2-year-old female had a Class I carious lesion in tooth #3. The cavity shape and size are determined by the extent of the carious process; nevertheless, it is important to treat the patient with minimum preparation.

Treatment

Erbium lasers, in accordance with the concept of microdentistry, allow considerable sparing of tissue. The preparation is extended to the surrounding sulcus, thereby obtaining a sealed preventive resin restoration. The use of restorative materials (flow composite or glass ionomer cement) is combined with sealing of the sulcus (Figure 30.1).

(Output energy 150 mJ to 10 Hz for enamel, 100 mJ to 10 Hz for dentin—SMART 2940 PLUS/DEKA.)

Result

A good esthetic outcome with effective decontamination and tissue conditioning thanks to the highly selective action of the laser beam and the removal of only decayed tissue that ensured minimum tissue loss (Figure 30.2).

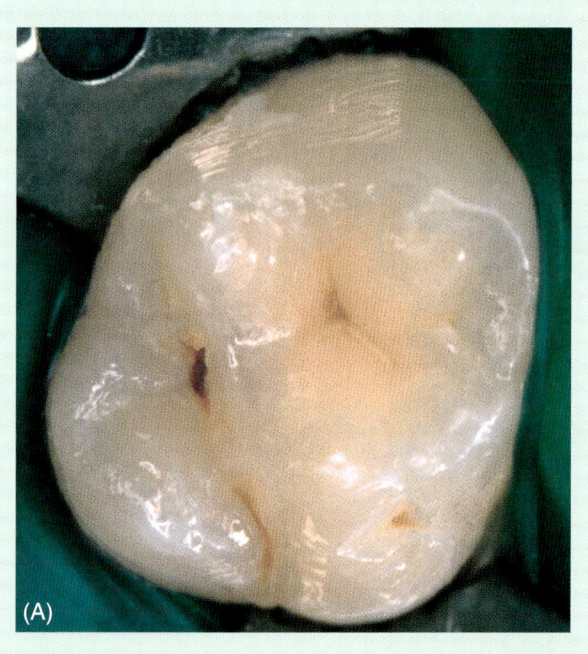

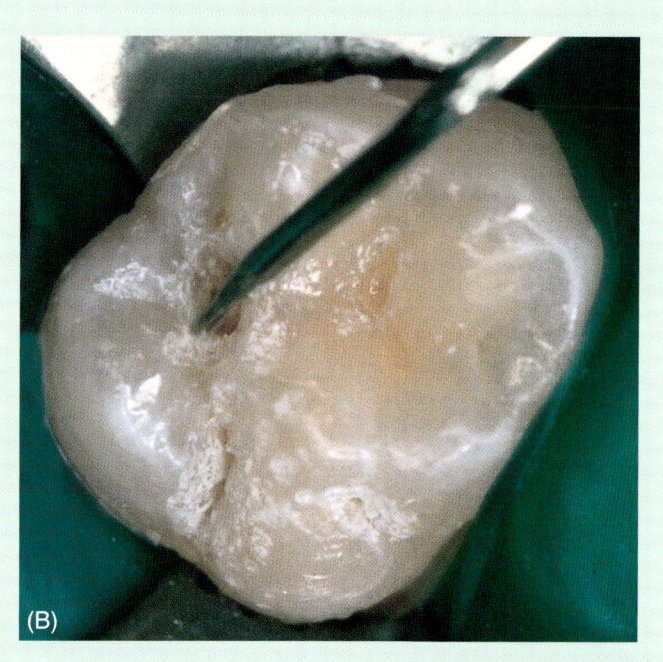

Figure 30.1 Class I carious lesion of tooth # 3 (**A**). Minimally invasive laser-assisted preparation and manual removal of softened tissue (**B**).

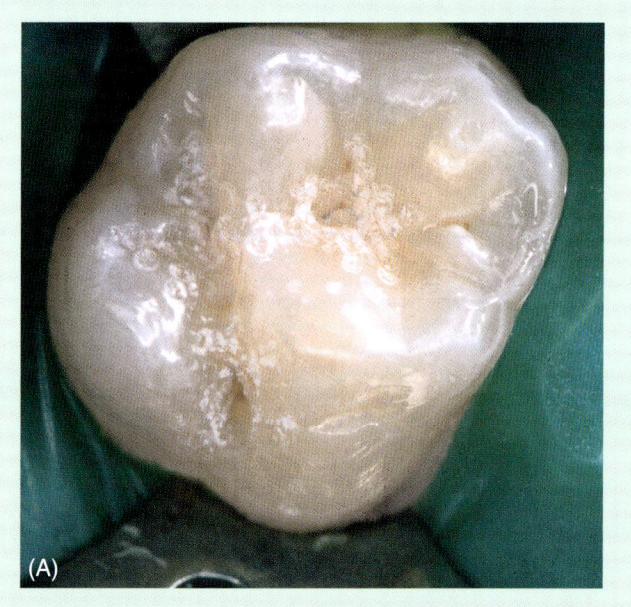

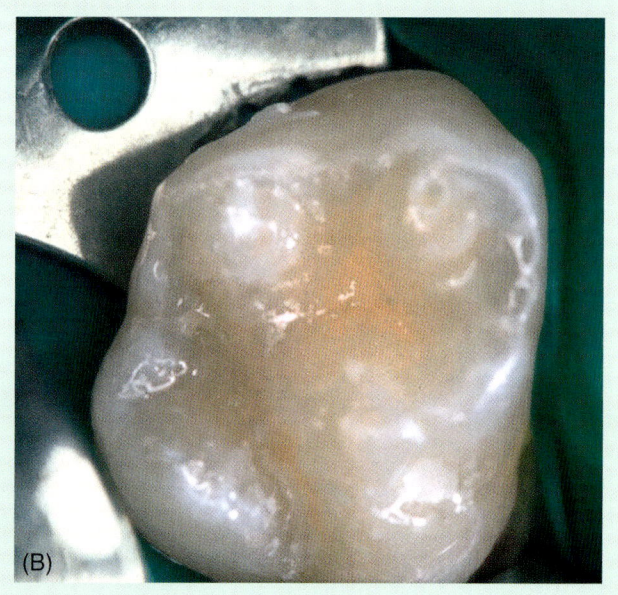

Figure 30.2 Occlusal view before acid etching (**A**) and final restoration of the palatal site with flow composite resin and application of a pit and fissure sealant to the occlusal site (**B**).

Clinical case 30.2: Amelodentinal dysplasia

Problem

This 8.1-year old female had amelodentinal dysplasia of preventively sealed tooth #14. We needed ensure minimum tissue loss and a conservative approach in a young patient at risk of decay.

Treatment

Enamel or amelodentinal dysplasias, often described as complications of dental traumas, or simply regarded as nonpathological structural abnormalities, are clinical situations in which the esthetic aspect is of paramount importance, even in young children. Laser-assisted therapy is an easy approach allowing good compliance. It is also more economic than other prosthetic therapies and provides a good esthetic outcome with minimum tissue loss. In this case, the hypoplastic area is removed working at low wattage and low output rates, leaving a cratered and extremely irregular surface with a very chalky appearance (Figure 30.3).

Result

Close re-creation of the often quite irregular microanatomy of this young patient's teeth, thanks to the procedure chosen: etching and application of adhesive bonding, use of more opaque composite materials, manual finishing of margins, and polishing (Figure 30.4).

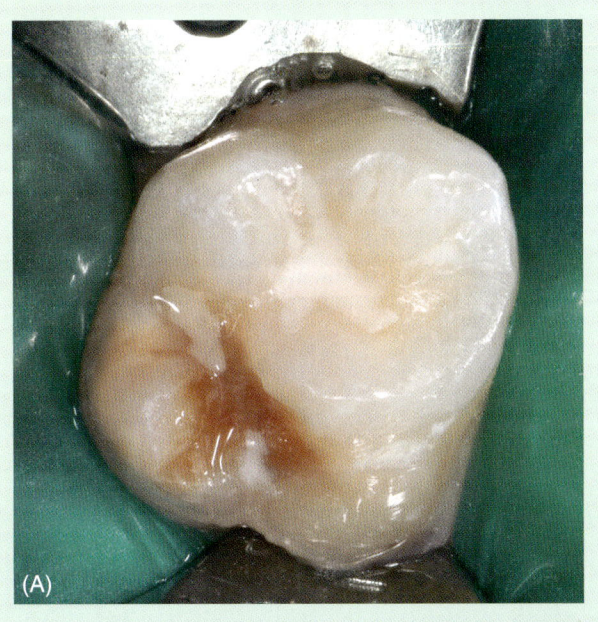

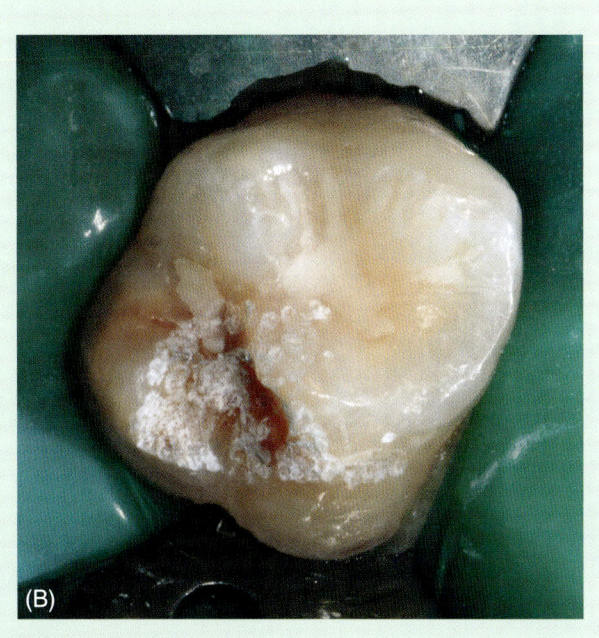

Figure 30.3 Amelodentinal dysplasia of tooth #14 **(A)** which is prepared with an Er:YAG laser **(B)**.

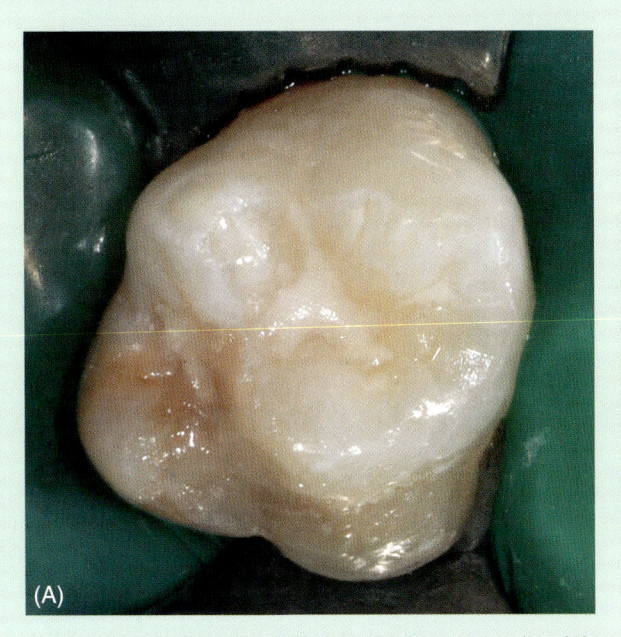

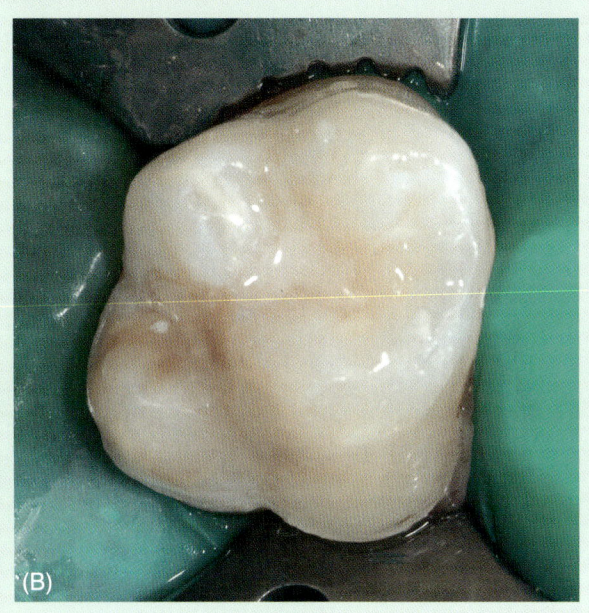

Figure 30.4 Laser preparation guarantees minimum tissue loss **(A)** and a good esthetic final outcome **(B)**.

Clinical case 30.3: A 6.2-year-old male with extensive cavities

Problem

This 6-year-old male patient with interproximal caries of tooth L was not compliant. It was necessary to raise the patient's tolerance threshold through an effective ablation of hard tissue involving no mechanical trauma and reduced or no use of anesthetics.

Treatment

Erbium lasers bring about rapid evaporation of the water contained in decayed tooth enamel and dentin and have an effective ablative effect on hard tissues. Providing the correct parameters are adhered to, structural alterations and/or pulp reactions can be prevented and postoperative complications are reduced (Figures 30.5 and 30.6).

There are several important anatomical ultrastructural differences between permanent and deciduous teeth at the level of enamel and dentin. The enamel prisms of deciduous teeth, unlike those of permanent teeth, do not show an orderly spatial organization. The large superficial crystals are irregular due to posteruption maturation, and the enamel is often aprismatic, which explains why deciduous teeth are more opaque. The aprismatic enamel is more frequently found at the interproximal, vestibular, and oral aspects of the crown. Moreover, the enamel of primary teeth is less mineralized and more porous.

As regards the dentin, the main differences between permanent and deciduous teeth concern the size and number of the dentinal tubules. Operating parameters have to be reduced when working on enamel and dentine of primary teeth, depending on the water and mineral composition of these tissues.

Result

The restoration achieved the esthetic objective and restored normal function and anatomy (Figure 30.7).

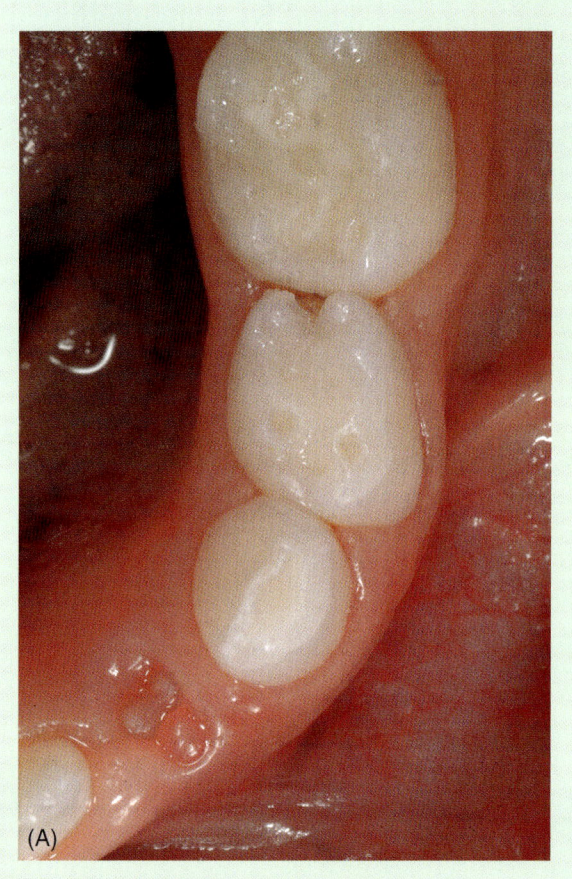

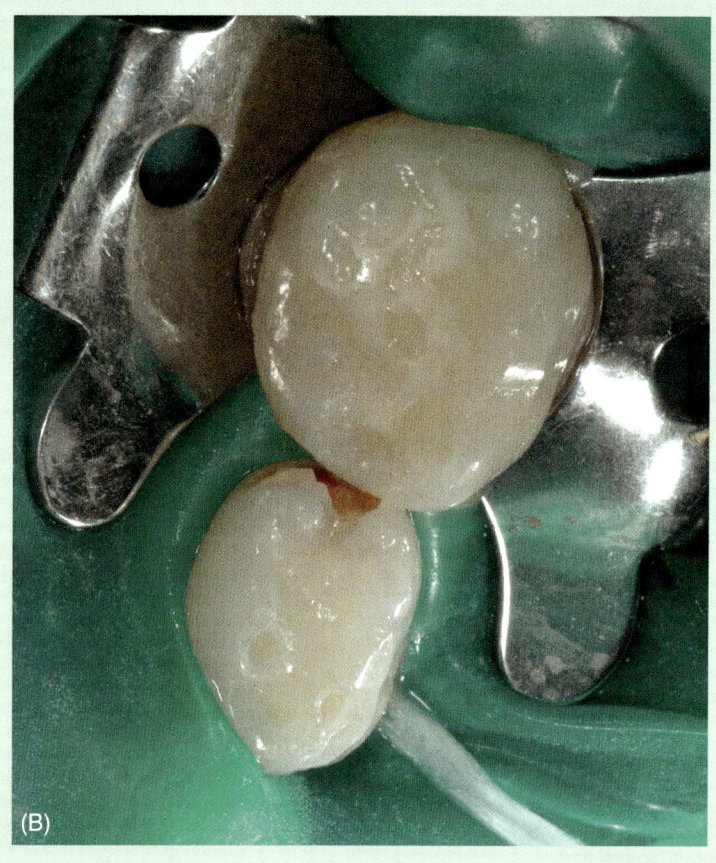

Figure 30.5 Interproximal lesion of tooth L in a very young patient of 6.2 years (**A**). Rubber dam isolation (**B**).

Chapter 30 Pediatric Dentistry

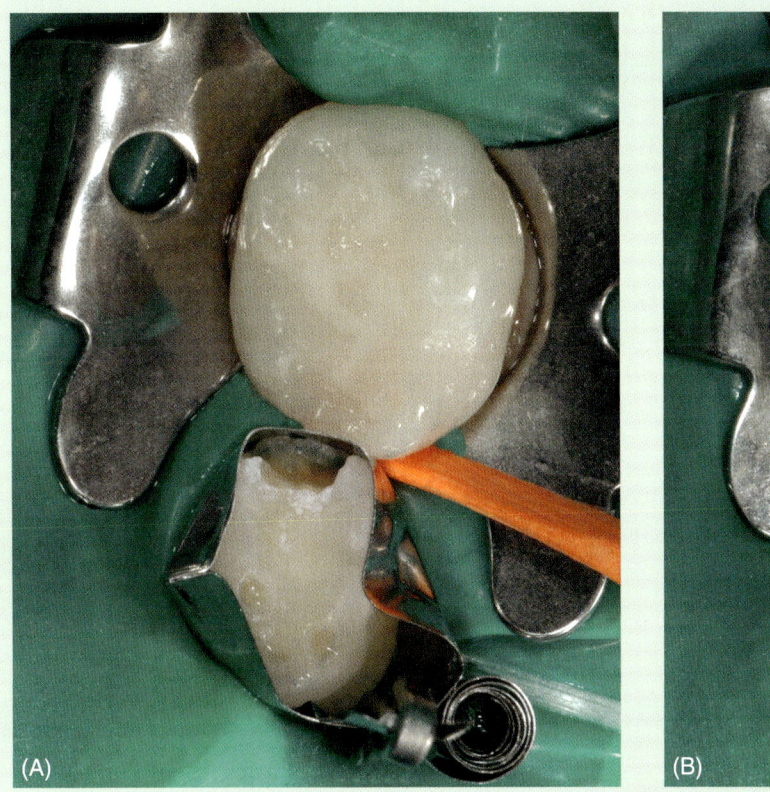

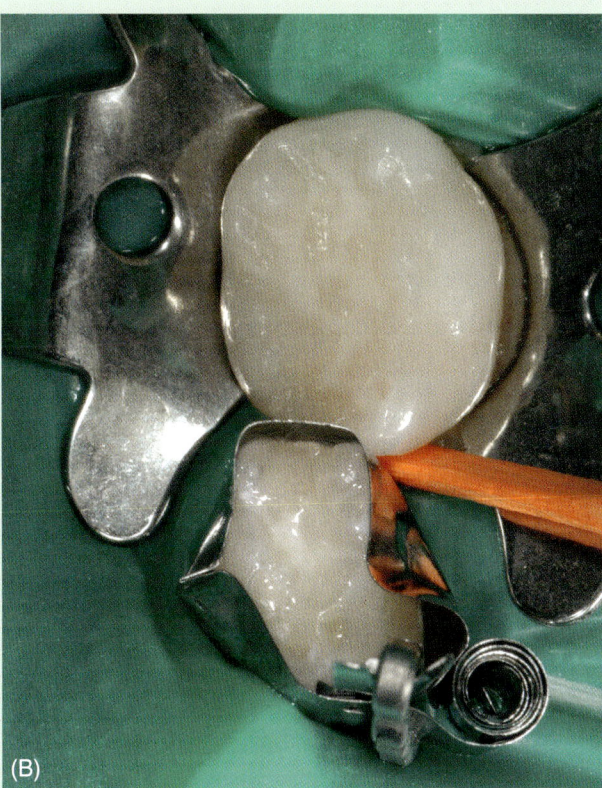

Figure 30.6 Initial preparation with an erbium laser **(A)**. Enamel and dentin are etched, rinsed and dried. The bonding agent is applied **(B)**.

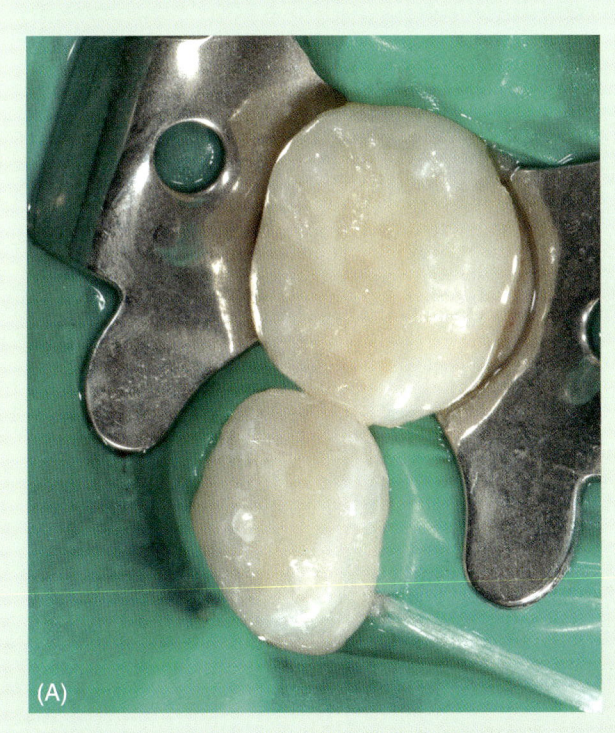

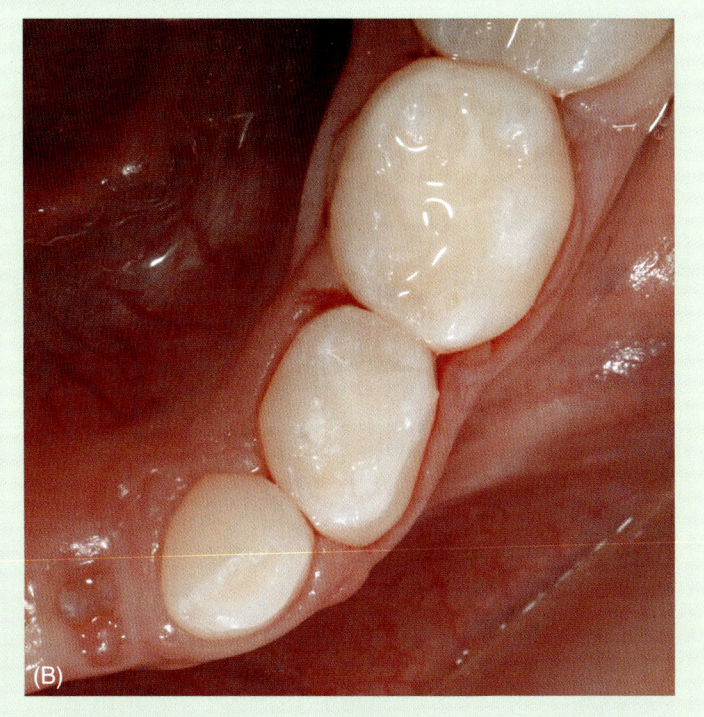

Figure 30.7 A thin layer of flow composite resin is placed and the restoration is completed **(A)**. Final outcome after finishing and polishing **(B)**.

Clinical case 30.4: Enamel hypoplasia

Problem

An 8.4-year-old male patient had severe and diffuse enamel hypoplasia and poor oral hygiene. Surface structure and texture needed restoration with a minimally invasive cavity preparation (Figure 30.8).

Treatment

Ablation of the decayed tissue using an Er:YAG laser. Clinical cases confirm that an acceptable ablation speed and safe procedure can be obtained using lower pulse rates and moderate energy levels (Figure 30.9).

Result

Restoration of morphology and color through the anatomical layering technique. The restoration is built up with one to two layers of dental material (opaque) of the same hue, but with different chroma (the first labial layer having the highest saturation) and a layer of enamel material (translucent). Finishing and polishing with different polishing disks and rubber polishers. A highly reflective surface gloss may be obtained using an abrasive polishing paste (Figure 30.10).

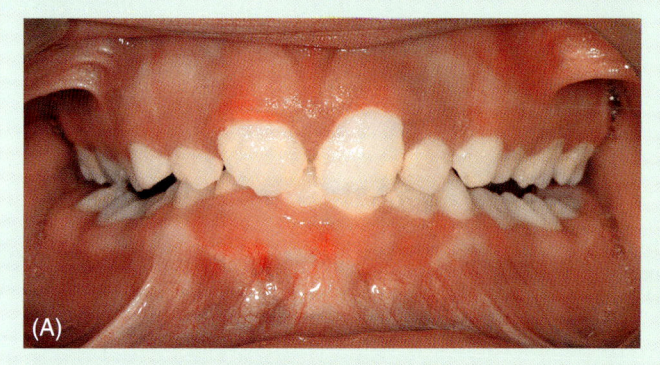

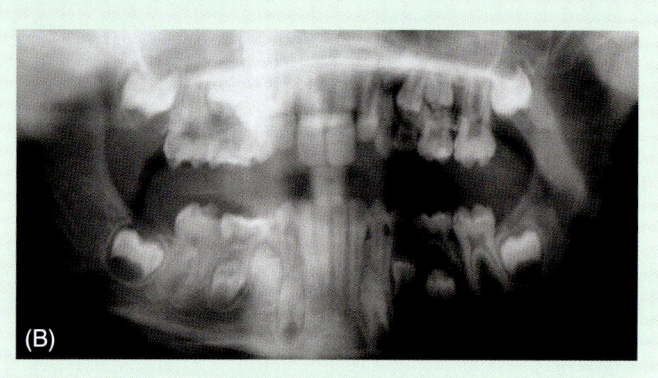

Figure 30.8 Severe enamel hypoplasia in a young patient with poor oral hygiene (**A**). Orthopantomograph (**B**).

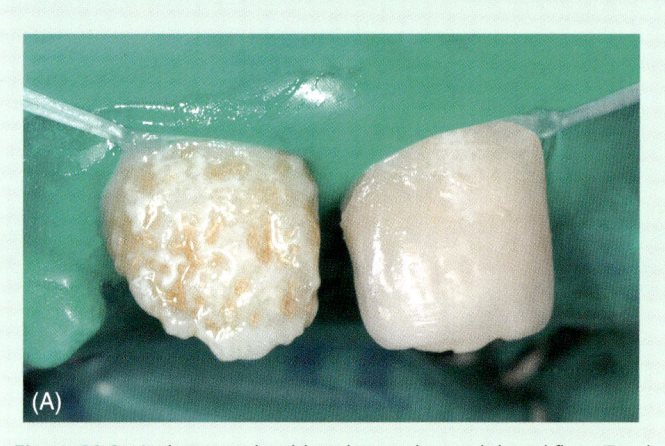

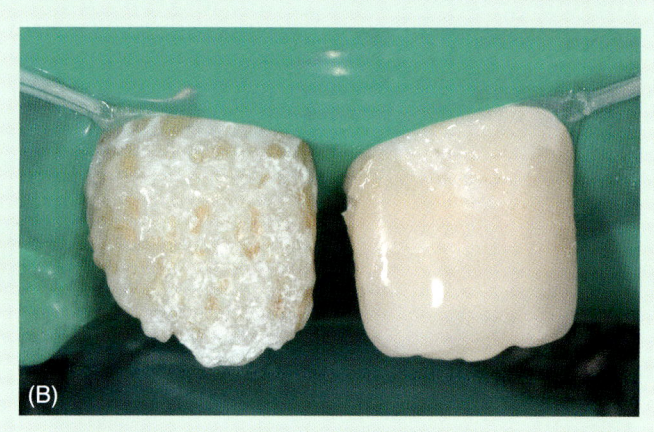

Figure 30.9 Isolation with rubber dam and waxed dental floss. Tooth #9 had already been restored. Postoperative view of tooth #8 (**A**) after laser ablation. Labial view after water rinse and air drying (**B**).

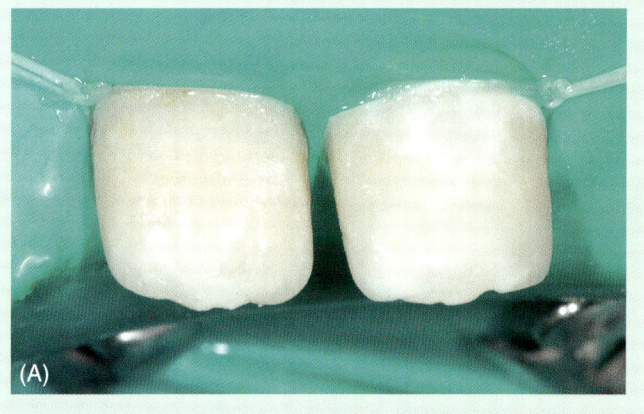

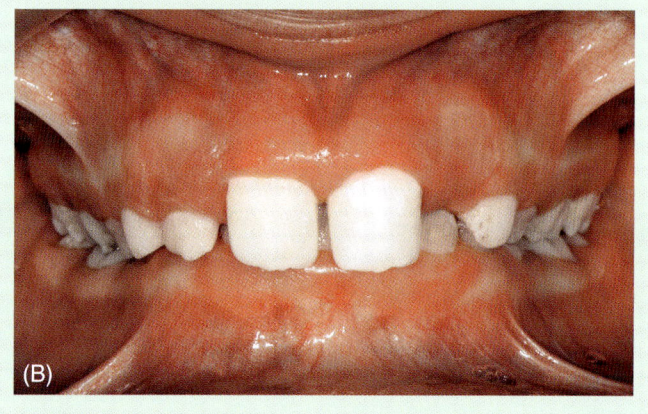

Figure 30.10 After application of the dentin bonding system, a thin layer of flow resin composite is applied (**A**). Color and morphology are restored by the anatomical layering technique (**B**).

Nursing bottle syndrome and/or tooth loss due to caries and/or to dental trauma

Early childhood caries

Early childhood caries (ECC), also known as baby/nursing bottle syndrome, is a particularly severe and rapidly destructive manifestation of dental caries whose main cause is the excessive and prolonged use of infant feeding bottles containing sugary drinks or even unsweetened milk, especially during nighttime when the flow of saliva is greatly reduced.

The clinical signs of ECC range from initial enamel demineralization to complete destruction of the crowns. The area usually affected is the vestibular surface of the anterior teeth, from where it rapidly spreads to the rest of the teeth.[21,22] According to the literature, the prevalence of the condition ranges from 1% to 12% in the industrialized world to more than 70% in developing countries and in the weaker sections of the population, even in wealthy countries. Given the risk of loss of one or more anterior teeth due to these deep caries lesions, this disease can have serious consequences. The most critical teeth are the maxillary incisors and, in relation to the dental eruption sequence, the first primary molars.

When children present with chronic and recurrent fistulas and abscesses, tooth function becomes limited. Radiographic investigation and clinical examination frequently show an infectious necrosis of the pulp in an advanced phase. The affected teeth are extracted (if endodontic restoration is not possible), and a pediatric prosthetic appliance is constructed. It is important to be aware that correct space management and maintenance are necessary to ensure normal evolution and eruption of the permanent teeth and improved esthetics and speech.[4]

The possible complications associated with ECC include infectious and systemic pathologies, such as focal disease; locally, there may develop follicular and radicular cysts and hypolasia of the permanent teeth; orthognathodontic complications are related to possible loss of the canine guide, loss of space with dentoalveolar disharmony of the permanent teeth, and also loss of vertical dimension leading to alteration of the profile; functional complications can arise as a result of alterations of the mandibular kinematics, phonetic function, and swallowing; and finally, esthetic problems linked to the loss of teeth can arise, especially at the front.

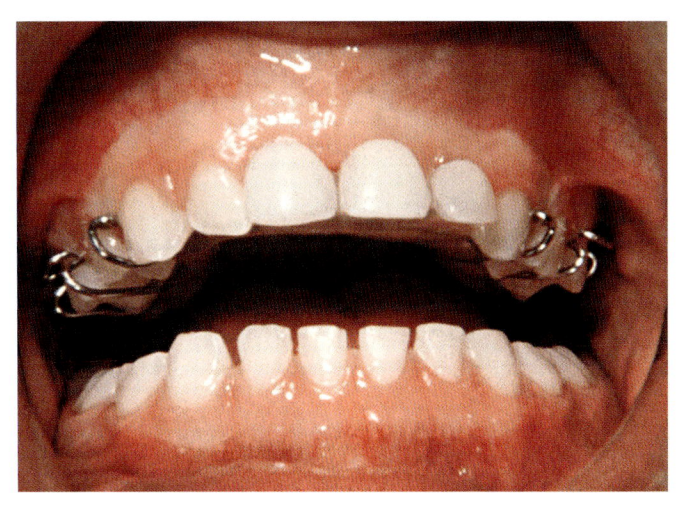

Figure 30.11 A pedodontic removable prosthesis is placed to restore frontal tooth loss due to ECC.

This form of caries is often treated by extraction of many or all the primary teeth, not only because of the severity of the lesions but also because the very young age of the patients makes them unsuitable candidates for long and complex conservative treatments with uncertain outcomes.

Clinical prevention of ECC includes:

- preventive therapies—behavioral–educational, alimentary and oral hygiene care, fluoride therapies;
- esthetic and functional recovery (tertiary prevention).

Pedodontic prostheses

Pedodontic prostheses (also used in cases of trauma and/or tooth agenesis) are removable appliances that can offer a simple, safe, and efficient therapeutic solution, not least because they can reduce the orthodontic treatment time. Recourse may be had to these prostheses when the child and its parents are collaborative and providing precise clinical conditions are met (relating to the tooth class, available space, and subject's health, both general and oral) (Figure 30.11).

Clinical case 30.5: A 3.9-year-old male with advanced caries and loss of teeth

Problem
Rampant caries, loss of the lower anterior teeth, and advanced caries in the posterior teeth. Tooth T was extracted.

Treatment
Restoration of teeth K and L with composite resins. Replacement of T with a resin tooth. Use of a pedodontic prosthesis to maintain the anterior space, preserve the vertical dimension, and avoid supereruption of the upper anterior teeth (Figure 30.12).

Result
Good functional restoration and achievement of the desired psychological result, with lasting benefits. The patient has undergone periodic (yearly) checkups.

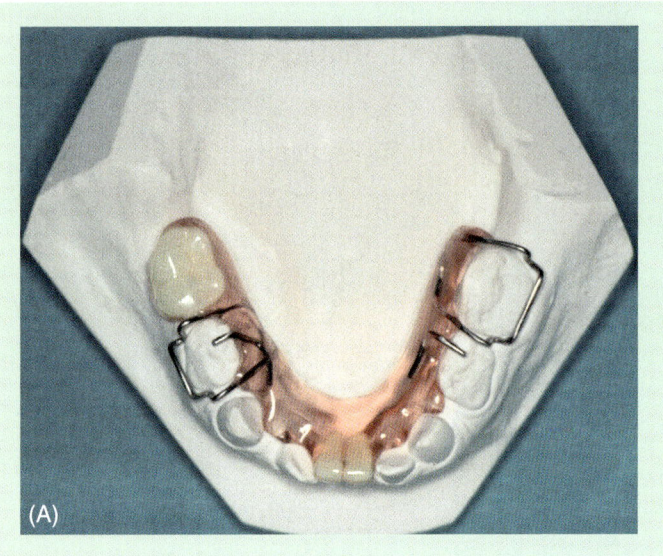

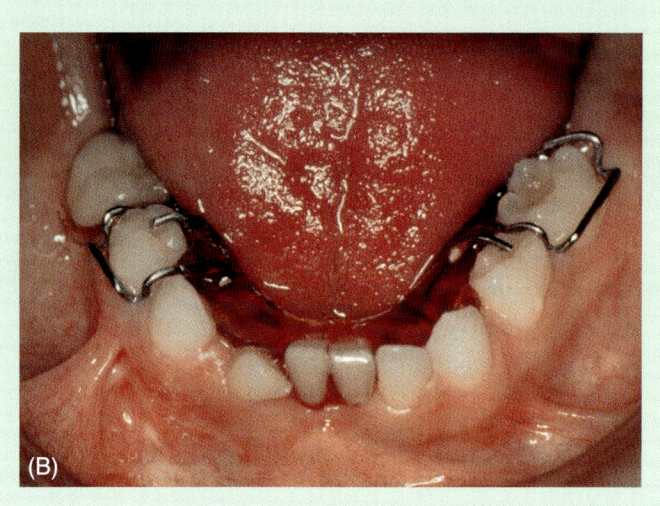

Figure 30.12 Plaster model of a 3.9-year-old patient. A removable space maintainer is designed **(A)** and placed in the lower arch **(B)**.

Clinical case 30.6: Severe trauma and loss of teeth in a 7.4-year-old

Problem

Severe trauma to the anterior region and loss (exarticulation) of teeth #8 and #9. Extrusion and internal root resorption (undiagnosed) due to previous trauma to tooth #25 (Figure 30.13).

Treatment

A complete orthodontic assessment to evaluate criteria for interceptive orthodontics (e.g., direction of growth and skeletal discrepancies).

Use of a function regulator (Bionator) with replacement of the anterior teeth to obtain sagittal correction with restoration of normal neuromuscular function and structure. Application of a lingual arch as a space maintainer (Figures 30.14 and 30.15).

Endodontic treatment of tooth #25 with $Ca(OH)_2$.

Result

Good functional restoration with good esthetic and psychological results. Interceptive orthodontic treatment was performed to improve alveolar growth, preserve vertical dimension, and avoid supereruption of the lower anterior teeth. Over the coming years, different orthodontic and endodontic treatments allow achievement of the final result (Figures 30.16 and 30.17).

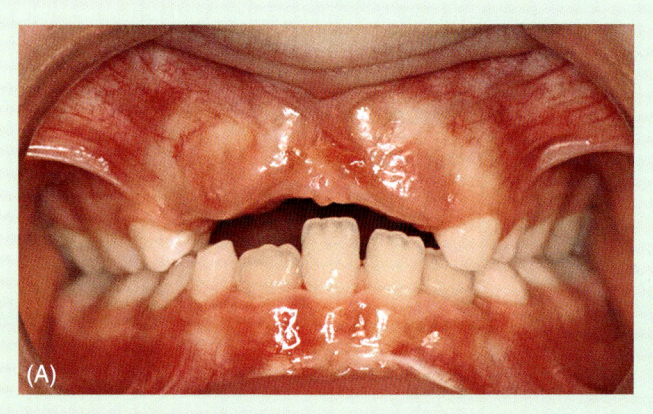

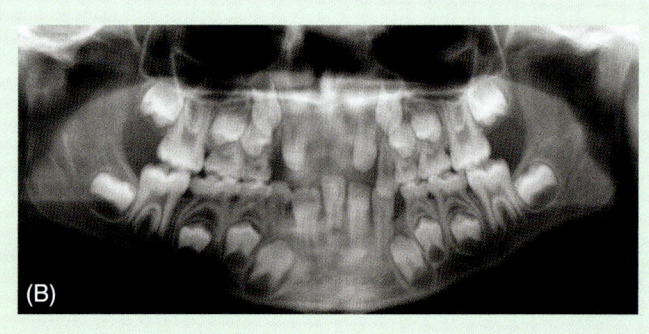

Figure 30.13 Frontal teeth loss due to trauma and extrusion of the lower right central incisor **(A)** Orthopantomograph **(B)**. Note the internal root resorption of tooth #25.

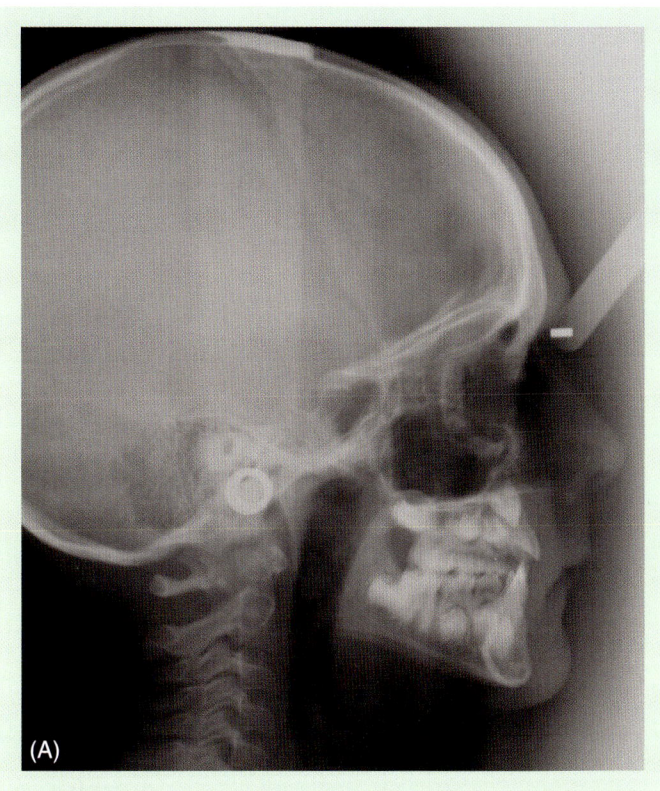

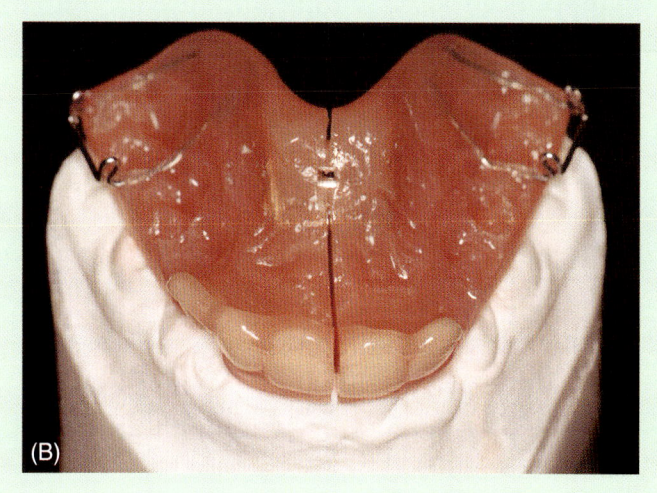

Figure 30.14 Lateral teleradiograph **(A)**. Functional appliance (Bionator) **(B)**.

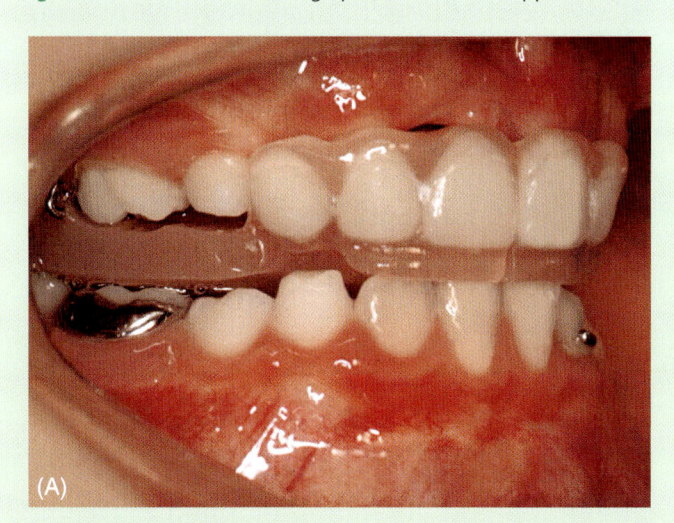

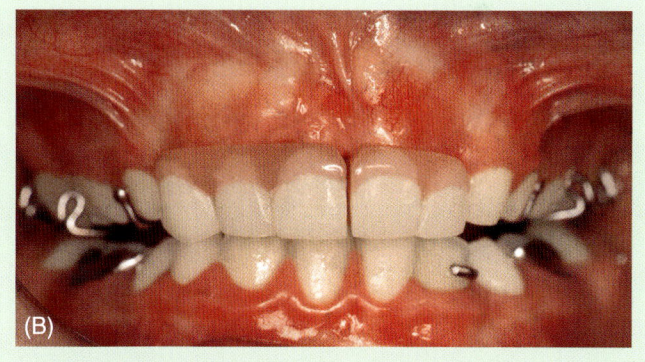

Figure 30.15 Intraoral view of the removable appliance **(A)**. A lingual arch is applied to the lower arch **(B)**.

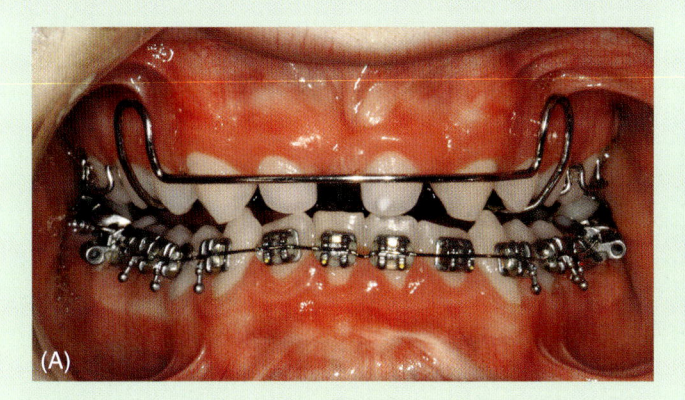

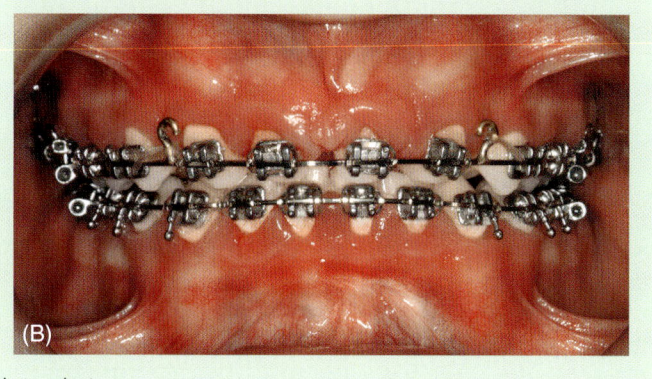

Figure 30.16 **(A, B)** Different orthodontic treatments phases to detail the occlusion.

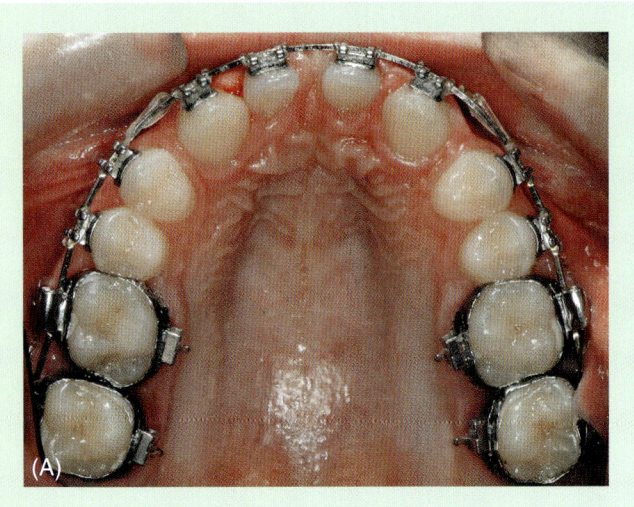

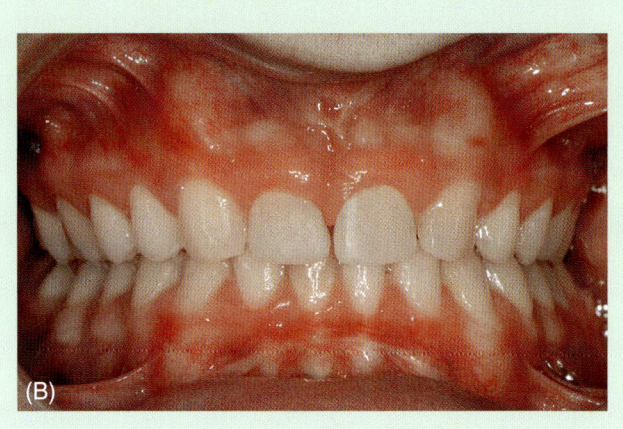

Figure 30.17 Occlusal view before debonding **(A)** and at the end of the treatment with coronoplasty of teeth #7 and #10. Frontal intraoral view: the patient at 14 years of age **(B)**.

Removable space-maintaining appliances offer considerable advantages: they can determine orthodontic movements and can help to prevent orofacial muscle imbalance and/or harmful sucking habits, such as finger, thumb, or lip sucking. Furthermore, they can be modified as the patient grows, improving the esthetics and thus reducing psychological problems. On the downside, their volume can make them uncomfortable for the young patient; they also need periodic checks and high patient and parental cooperation. In addition, they may be more prone to breakage than fixed appliances.[23]

Patient with multiple agenesis: ectodermal dysplasia

Congenital absence of teeth is common, occurring sporadically or with a hereditary component. The presence of conical teeth is frequently associated with absence of the corresponding teeth on the opposite side of the arch. There exist over 120 syndromes of the head and neck manifesting with missing teeth. In these conditions, the important aspect is not so much the number of missing teeth but which teeth are absent.

Clinical case 30.7: Ectodermal dysplasia

Problem

A 5.2-year-old made with ectodermal dysplasia characterized by multiple agenesis, fine, sparse hair with shaft abnormalities, dry skin, frontal bossing, maxillary hypoplasia, and lips showing little of the vermilion margin (Figure 30.18A and B).

Ectodermal dysplasia refers to a group of inherited disorders involving the ectodermally derived structures (hair, teeth, nails, skin, and sweat glands). The most common expression is the hypohidrotic X-linked form.

Treatment

Treatment of this condition aims to provide adequate function, maintain the vertical dimension, and improve esthetics. Ideally, treatment should begin as early as possible, depending on

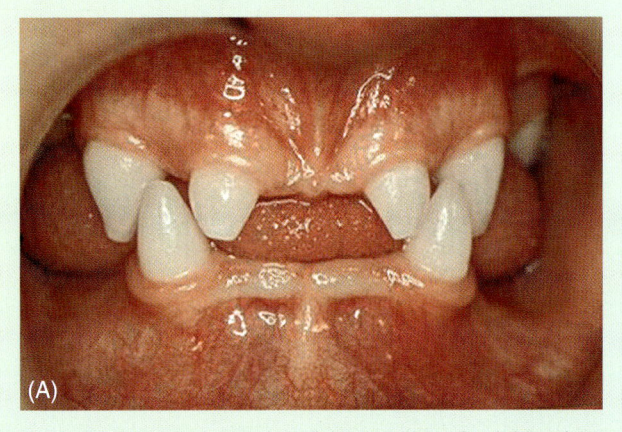

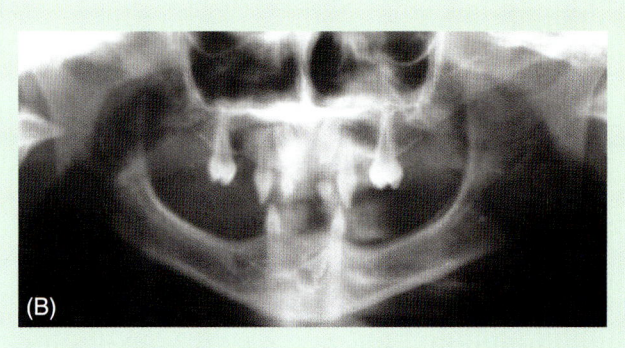

Figure 30.18 Typical appearance of the dentition of a child with ectodermal dysplasia **(A)**. Panoramic radiograph; note the conical-shaped teeth and also the large number of missing teeth **(B)**.

the child's compliance. Partial dentures can be applied; acid-etch composite buildups of conical teeth can be performed, similar to surgical exposure of impacted teeth; orthodontic adjustment of spaces can be carried out over the following years (Figure 30.19).

Result

Achievement of normal speech development and increased self-acceptance thanks to treatment with removable prostheses, modified during the child's growth to improve his smile (Figure 30.20).

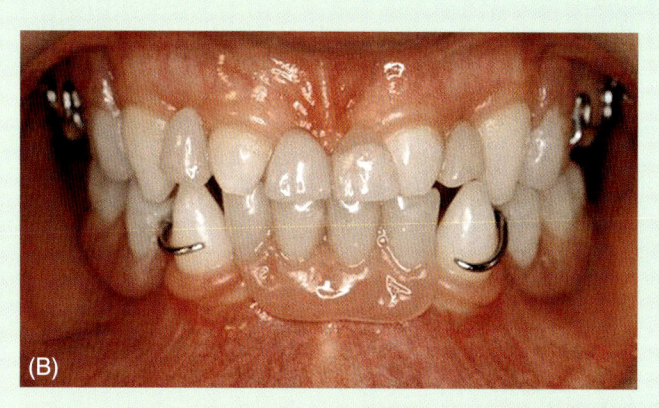

Figure 30.19 (A, B) Young children tolerate dentures with Adam's cribs (and/or ball retainers), which provide ideal retention around primary molars.

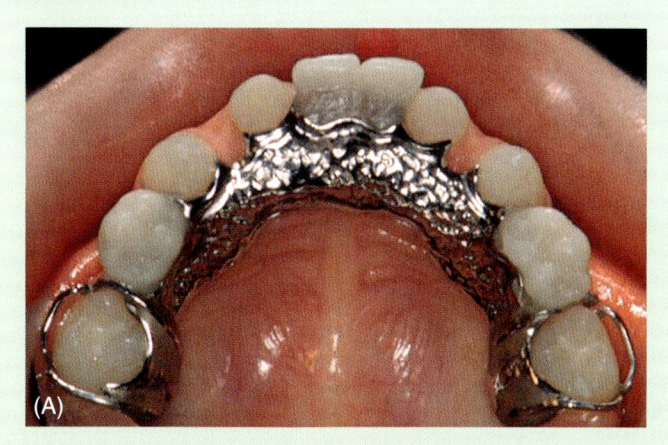

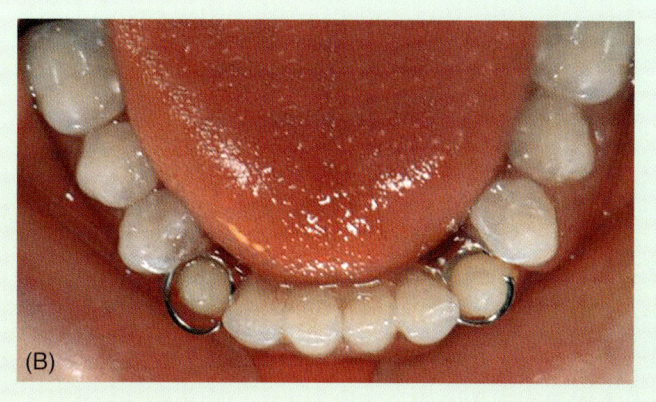

Figure 30.20 (A, B) Removable space maintainers in a growing patient.

The major conditions associated with oligodontia include ectodermal dysplasia, clefting, Down's syndrome, chondroectodermal dysplasia (Ellis–van Creveld syndrome), Reiger syndrome, incontinentia pigmenti, and orofacial–digital syndrome (types I and II).

Trauma management in primary dentition and in the first phase of mixed dentition

Trauma is a frequent event seen in pediatric dentistry. Furthermore, it is often very difficult to establish accurately the extent and severity of the traumatic injury, manage the initial treatment of the acute phase, and plan the long-term follow-up. Dental traumas, like dental caries, are true emergencies and demand an accurate diagnosis to save teeth, restore the function of the dental arches, improve the oral esthetics, and avoid complications.

As dental trauma is a high-incidence pathology, effective preventive measures need to be taken to reduce its effects and also the complications that can arise in young patients. Thus, it is crucial to develop and implement effective prevention and information campaigns targeting the general public. The aims of such campaigns should be to reduce trauma-related functional, esthetic, and biological damage to the orofacial area and to raise awareness of the problem among patients and practitioners, thereby making it possible to reduce sequelae, avoid unnecessary treatment procedures, and provide the biological basis for healing after injury.[24]

In particular, the most effective preventive measures include timely orthodontic correction to reduce increased overjet; early correction of habits such as finger, thumb, and lip sucking, and abnormal swallowing; use of a mouthguard to protect permanent teeth during sporting activities; and accurate initial diagnoses and timely treatments, both of which are essential in guaranteeing a correct initial therapeutic approach, avoiding overtreatment, and preventing long-term sequelae.

Application of lasers in dental traumatology

Careful dental history taking and a thorough clinical examination are the basis of an accurate diagnosis. The use of specific standardized charts is recommended to save time and ensure an exhaustive assessment. Every phase, both pre- and posttreatment, must be fully documented through radiographic and photographic examinations and pulp vitality tests, as this will make it easier and quicker to monitor the evolution of the clinical case at subsequent visits and to compile a full medico-legal report, which is often required during and at the end of dental trauma treatment.

Pulp testing in dental trauma is a controversial issue, and different tests have been proposed. Laser Doppler flowmetry is a promising new method of diagnosing the state of pulp revascularization; however, it is still in the experimental phase and not yet available for general use.

Thanks to their characteristic versatility, the Er:YAG and Er,Cr:YSGG lasers can be applied to both hard and soft tissues and are thus indicated in the treatment of dental traumas. Other technologies indicated for the treatment of these injuries are the KTP, Nd:YAG, diode, and CO_2 lasers (Table 30.1).

In the absence of randomized clinical studies of traumatic dental injuries and laser-assisted therapy, we here describe our own clinical experience and aim to stimulate more extensive scientific research in this field.

Traumatic injuries to hard dental tissue and pulp

Uncomplicated and complicated crown fractures

Crown fractures involve the enamel and dentin; complicated crown fractures also expose the pulp. The examination should start with cleansing of the injured area and a careful examination to detect any pulp exposure. An X-ray and vitality tests should be performed; sometimes there is accompanying damage to the soft tissue, in which case it is necessary to look for tooth fragments in tongue, lips, and oral mucosa.

The availability of modern bonding agents and laser technology has revolutionized our clinical practice.

Treatment with erbium lasers

Erbium lasers can give good results, reducing postoperative discomfort and sensitivity as well as allowing minimally invasive dentistry.[15] Laser cavity preparation is closely related to a series of different variables. Fluence, power density, and pulse length, as well as the laser beam angle, focus mode, and amount of air–water jet delivered, are all factors that can cause substructural damage to the dentin. A final conditioning at low wattage on both dentin and enamel is advisable. Acid etching on lased dentin and enamel produces uniform results, eliminating the thin layer of substructural damage, exposing the collagen fibers, and creating a substrate for the formation of the hybrid layer; acid etching turns Silverstone class 2 and 3 enamel into class 1 enamel, allowing better composite adaptation.[25] The action of erbium lasers on hard tissues and pulp is extremely precise and leaves the treated surfaces cleansed and sterilized. The temperature increases during treatment, already minimal, can be decreased by water-spray cooling. Thanks to the various effects of these lasers, they exert a bactericidal action, do not produce a smear layer, open the dentinal tubules, and promote the formation of a hybrid layer; they can be used to perform the whole therapeutic procedure: excavation, coagulation of the exposed pulp (if necessary), pulpotomy, or pulpectomy. Another feature is their very superficial thermal effect, as a result of which the necrotic zone is likely to be very small.

In crown fractures, many dentinal tubules are exposed: between 20,000 and 45,000 in just $1\,mm^2$ of dentin. These open tubules are a pathway for bacteria and thermal and chemical irritants, which can cause pulp inflammation; erbium lasers are effective for removing organic material, smear layer, and can achieve a bactericidal effect, but the Nd:YAG and diode lasers also exert an effective decontaminating action. The capacity of the erbium laser to fuse and seal the dentinal tubules (to depths of up to $4\,pm$) can result in a reduction of the tissues' permeability to fluids, and thus of dentinal hypersensitivity.

Another structural change induced by these lasers is vitrification. This phenomenon can be very useful because it increases dental hardness and thus hard tissue resistance to acid remineralization and to dental abrasion.

Treatment with Nd:YAG and diode lasers

The Nd:YAG and the diode lasers exert a beneficial therapeutic action in direct traumas. These lasers, exploiting their photothermal effect, can be used to treat both pulp and dentin. They can be applied:

- to treat dentinal hypersensitivity;
- to perform indirect or direct pulp capping;
- to remove endodontic material;
- to treat infected root canals.

Table 30.1 Classification of Lasers

Hard and soft tissues	Er:YAG 2940
	Er,Cr:YSGG 2780
Soft tissues	KTP 532
	Argon
	Diode 810, 940, 980
	Nd:YAG 1064
	CO_2 10600
Low-level lasers	Helium neon 635
	Diode 810
	KTP 532

The CO_2 laser, instead, has a purely thermal effect on the tissue: 90–95% of the energy it delivers is absorbed by a fine tissue layer and transformed into heat. It is indicated for:

- pulp capping (following dentin fracture);
- pulpotomy (following crown or root-crown fractures);
- surgical cutting (e.g., to remove a tooth fragment embedded in the lip or oral mucosa).

Lasers have been proposed for pulpotomy, and one study favorably compared CO_2 laser treatment to formocresol for pulpotomy in primary teeth, recording a survival rate ranging from 91% to 98%. Other studies reported that the superpulsed mode produced markedly higher success rates than the continuous-wave mode. During this procedure, attention must be paid to the energy applied. Low energy delivered in defocused and pulsed or superpulsed mode guarantees good superficial coagulation and good decontamination, thereby helping to maintain the vitality of the residual pulp in pulp capping applications.

In view of the characteristic anatomy of the dental root apex and the penetration depths of near-infrared lasers, particular care must be taken when applying laser energy in primary root canals for root canal cleaning and disinfecting procedures.[26]

Crown fracture and root fracture

Crown fractures, unlike root fractures where the fracture is located entirely within the alveolus, cannot be expected to heal. In these cases, the coronal fragment is usually removed and the subsequent treatment should focus primarily on the possibility of using the remaining fragment. In the case of a superficial fracture without pulp exposure, it is recommended to remove loose fragments, smoothing the rough subgingival fracture surface and covering the exposed dentin. When the residual coronal fragment comprises one-third or less of the clinical root, pulpectomy and root canal filling are advocated, again after the removal of any loose fragments. The fracture surface must be exposed using a gingivectomy or osteotomy procedure, and this is followed by prosthetic restoration.

Laser-assisted therapy can be useful not only in coronal fragment restoration but also in supporting tissue surgery and endodontic therapy (gingivoplasty, gingivectomy, crown lengthening).[27] Lasers work effectively in these soft-tissue procedures as they easily incise, cut, ablate, and reshape soft tissue with no or minimal bleeding; furthermore, they are less painful and have a bactericidal effect. Lasers with deeply penetrating wavelengths (Nd:YAG and diode) produce a thicker coagulation layer than those with superficially absorbed ones (CO_2–erbium). With the former, the technique is similar to electrosurgical tissue removal.

Treatment factors such as optimal repositioning and flexible splinting have a positive influence on healing, as do immature root formation, lower age, and less displacement of the coronal fragment. If a splint is used, which may even be an esthetic orthodontic splint (ceramic brackets), it must be kept in situ for several weeks at least.

It is also worth noting that the use of an Nd:YAG laser can make bracket removal procedures atraumatic; furthermore, the intrapulp temperature increases induced by this laser are lower than those generated when using conventional high-speed instruments. Therefore, the laser-assisted procedure is safer, quicker, and more comfortable than the traditional approach.[28]

Traumatic injuries to the periodontal tissues

Nd:YAG and diode lasers uses are as follows:

- decontamination of the alveolus following a traumatic avulsion;
- treatment of a periodontal defect following a dental luxation or subluxation;
- microgingival surgery for the treatment of a traumatic dental injury;
- gingivectomy and gingivoplasty;
- surgical cutting (e.g., to remove a tooth fragment).[19]

Indirect dental traumas are lesions to the dental supporting structures, in particular, the alveolar bone, the periodontium, frenum, and lips. The Nd:YAG and diode lasers have a beneficial therapeutic action in such injuries. Indeed, these lasers have a decontaminating as well as a biostimulating and a reparative effect; they eliminate the need for sutures, allow good and rapid healing by second intention, and reduce patient discomfort. Finally, they also exert an appreciable analgesic effect on both hard and soft tissues.

Both the diode laser and the Nd:YAG laser are used in oral surgery, the former in continuous or pulsed mode and the latter always in pulsed mode but with different pulse amplitudes. The increase in temperature generated by these lasers has an excellent thermostatic effect. Furthermore, in all luxation injuries, the bactericidal and detoxifying action of lasers (Er:YAG, Nd:YAG, diode, and argon) makes it possible to achieve favorable conditions for the attachment of periodontal tissue. Laser decontamination and/or photobiomodulation (cutaneous and subcutaneous tissue irradiation) can be exploited for tissue repair and for pain relief.

Even though helium–neon lasers were initially used ($\lambda = 632.8$ nm), the ones in use today are the semiconductor diode type ($\lambda = 830$ or 635 nm).

The water absorption coefficient of the wavelengths used in low-level laser therapy (LLLT) is reduced, and the beams are able to penetrate both soft and hard tissues from a distance of 3–15 mm.

LLLT has a number of applications in dentistry, both on soft tissues (biostimulation of lesions, aphthous stomatitis, herpetic lesions, mucositis, pulpotomy) and at the neural level (analgesia, neural regeneration, temporomandibular pain, postsurgical pain, dental pain during orthodontic treatment).

In short, LLLT stimulates tissue repair processes and, influencing a large number of cell systems, can also produce a series of benefits on inflammatory mechanisms (antalgic, biostimulating, anti-inflammatory effects).[29–31]

The use of LLLT, or soft laser therapy, can ensure a nontraumatic introduction to dentistry. There is a large body of literature on this topic even though, methodologically and in terms of doses, there is still considerable difference of opinion.

Nd:YAG, diode, and KTP lasers can also be used as an alternative approach in nonvital bleaching.[32] Lasers are being used increasingly in gingival and dental surgery, where they are taking the place of electrosurgical techniques. The CO_2 laser, in particular, is used for surgical cutting (e.g., to remove tooth fragments from lips or oral mucosa).

Injuries to developing teeth

Disorders of permanent teeth caused by traumatic injuries to primary teeth can be divided into two groups according to the type of dental trauma (direct or indirect). The prevalence of these disorders ranges from 12% to 69%, depending on the study; avulsion and intrusive luxations are injuries associated with very high rates of developmental complications.[24]

Laser-assisted therapy can be useful in:

- enamel discoloration—treatable with the erbium laser;
- circular enamel hypoplasia—treatable with the erbium laser;
- ectopic eruption—treatable with surgical exposure or soft-tissue laser surgeries (all the wavelengths of the near–medium and far infrared spectrum).

Case studies of trauma

Although we acknowledge the importance of guidelines, the need for information and prevention programs, the following case studies do not include reference to classifications, clinical examinations, medical history, or special investigations, although these are absolutely essential for comprehensive treatment planning. For the sake of brevity, our goal is to describe several clinical trauma cases in which cooperation between the pedodontist and the orthodontist led to a good esthetic and functional outcomes.

Clinical case 30.8: Fracture of anterior teeth in an 8.3-year-old

Problem

Uncomplicated enamel–dentin crown fracture of the left upper central incisor with an immature apex. The tooth fragment was not available. The tooth had been protected with $Ca(OH)_2$ (Figure 30.21).

Treatment

Following routine clinical, instrumental, and radiographic examinations, treatment of the surface was with an Er:YAG laser without anesthesia. Decontamination of the dentin.

After etching and rinsing, definitive composite restoration at a low operating temperature and with minimum tissue loss (Figure 30.22).

Result

Restoration of the anterior guide and correct reproduction of the biting edge in a single-sitting, minimally invasive procedure. Minimal discomfort for the patient during treatment, thanks to reduced sensitivity (Figure 30.23).

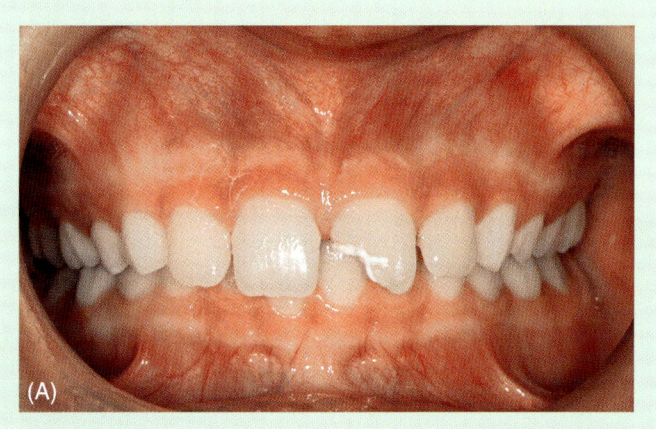

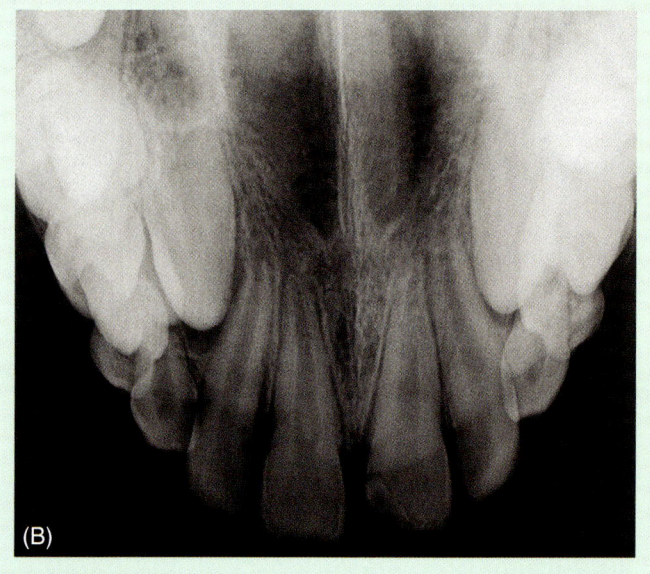

Figure 30.21 Deep but uncomplicated crown fracture of tooth #9 (**A**) and control X-ray (**B**). The tooth had previously been protected with $Ca(OH)_2$.

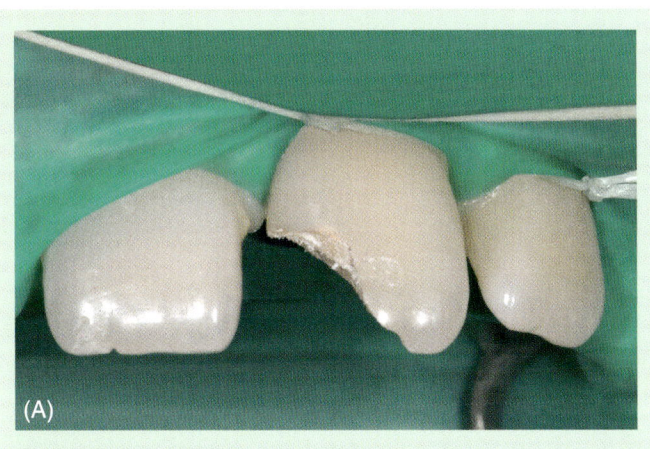

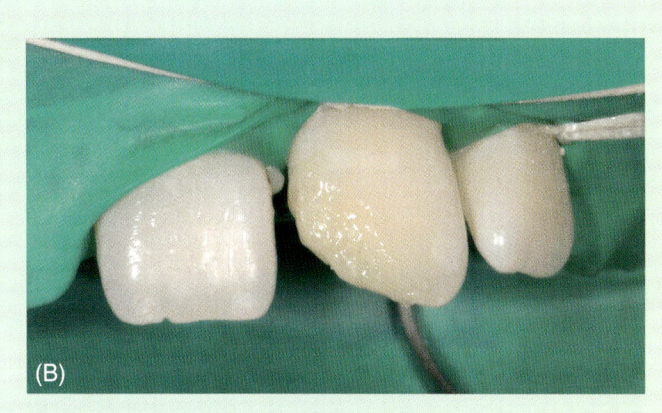

Figure 30.22 Rubber dam isolation and a minimally invasive treatment, performed with an erbium laser **(A)**. Application of enamel–dentin system **(B)**.

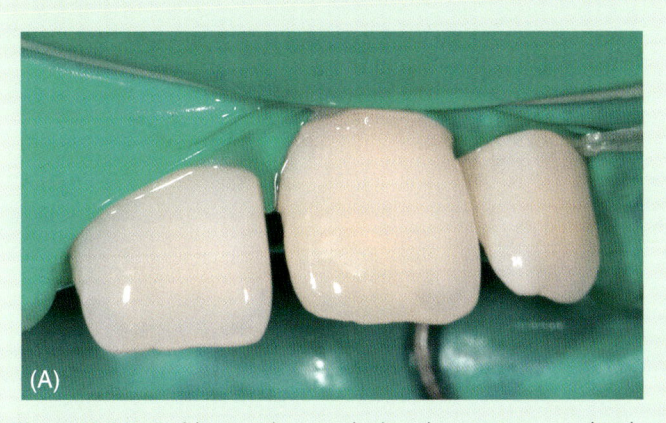

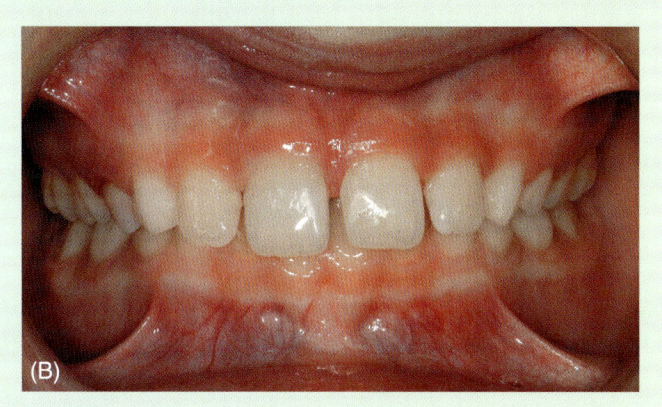

Figure 30.23 Building up the incisal edge; this part is covered with a thin layer of enamel material **(A)**. Finishing the restoration with abrasive disks and rubber polishers. Final appearance after rubber dam removal **(B)**.

Clinical case 30.9: Unacceptable result of treatment in trauma injury in a 19-year-old

Problem

Unacceptable result (incorrect morphology and lack of color) 11 years after treatment for traumatic dental injury with crown fracture of tooth #8. No retreatment between baseline and 11 years (Figure 30.24).

Treatment

Minimally invasive laser preparation of tooth surface using an Er:YAG laser after isolation with a rubber dam. Treatment with the anatomical layering technique; to imitate the facial dentin surface, an opaque dental material is

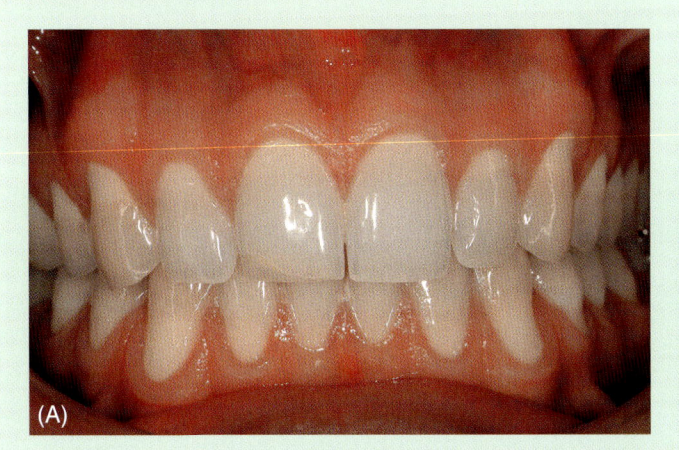

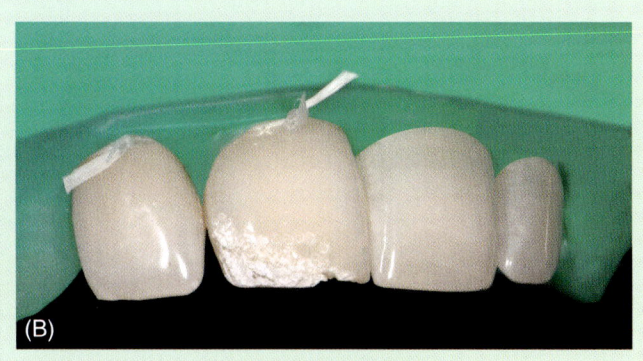

Figure 30.24 Preoperative view **(A)**. Enamel and the previous resin restoration are treated with an Er:YAG laser **(B)**.

applied (first layer) and then a thin layer of enamel material (translucent) (Figure 30.25).

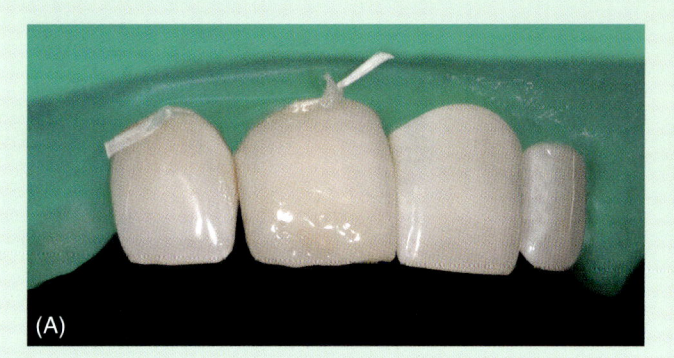

Result
Perfect restoration of morphology and color.

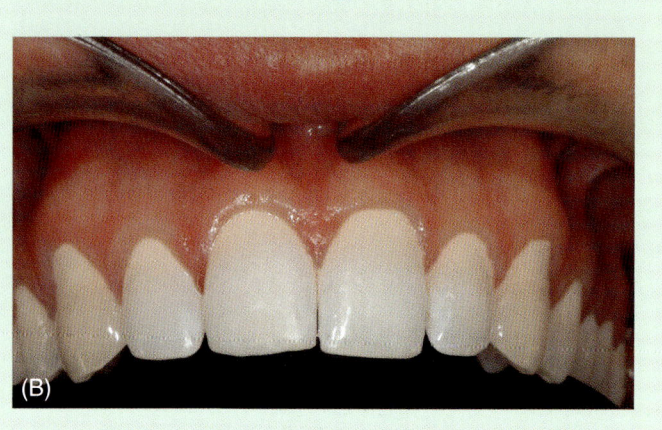

Figure 30.25 To reproduce the facial dentin surface an opaque material is added **(A)**. Final appearance after rubber dam removal **(B)**.

Clinical case 30.10: Discoloration of tooth due to previous subluxation injury in a 20-year-old

Problem
Discoloration of tooth #9, due to a previous subluxation injury. Almost complete obliteration of the root canal (Figure 30.26).

Treatment
Nonvital dental bleaching using the KTP laser (λ= 532 nm) with a red gel as source of activation. After prophylaxis with paste

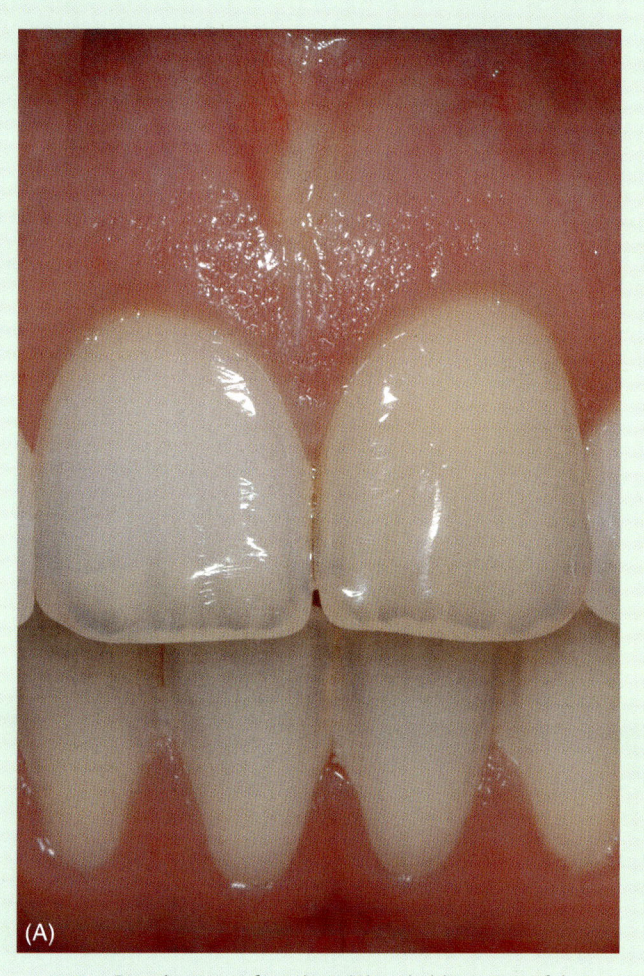

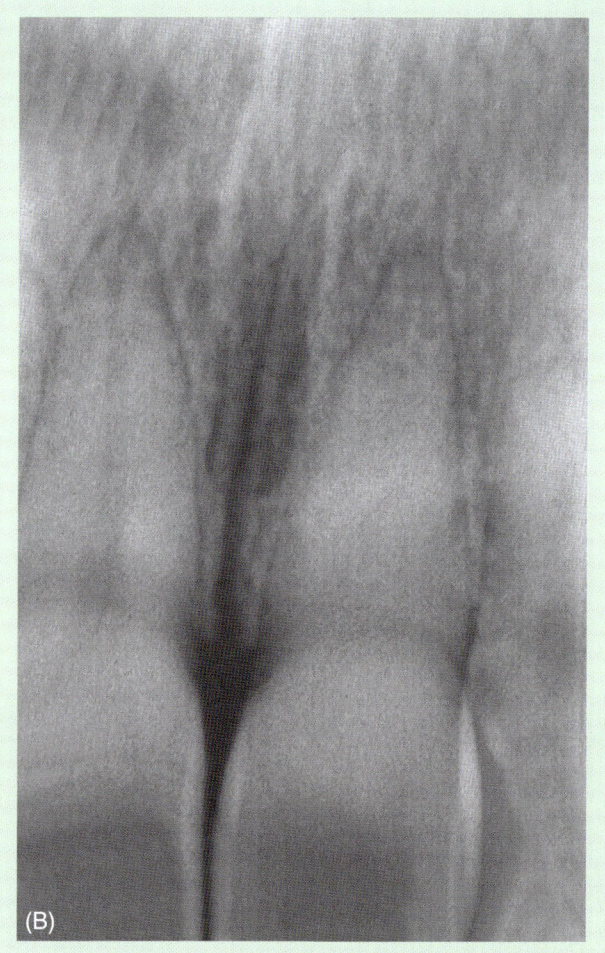

Figure 30.26 Discoloration of tooth #9 **(A)** and obliteration of the root canal due to a previous subluxation injury. Control X-ray **(B)**.

and water, photographs are taken to record the initial color. Application of a gingival barrier on gingiva and the interproximal area. Several cycles (bleaching procedure repeated two or three times) during a single sitting. Orange protection goggles were needed (Figure 30.27).

Result

Very effective outcome of laser-assisted dental bleaching with no morphological or chemical effects on the enamel, and no thermal effects on the pulp (Figure 30.28).

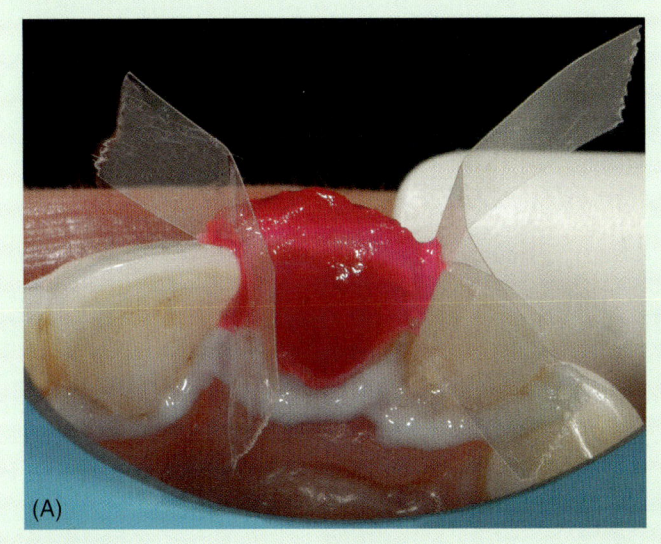

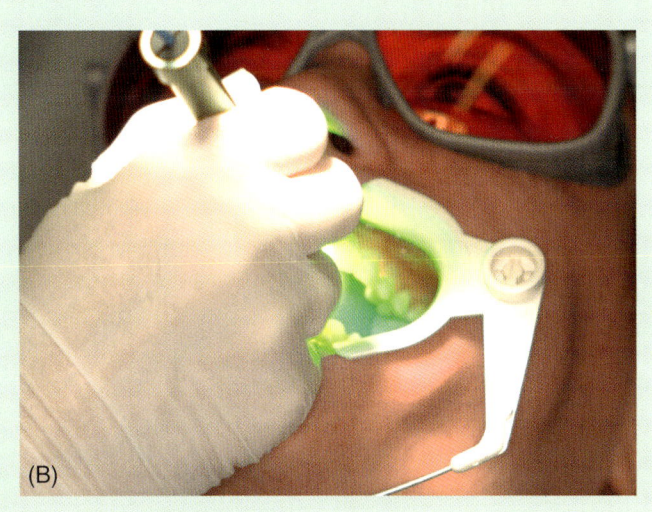

Figure 30.27 A gingival barrier is applied prior to bleaching with a KTP laser. Red gel is applied on the buccal and palatal surfaces **(A)**. KTP irradiation **(B)**.

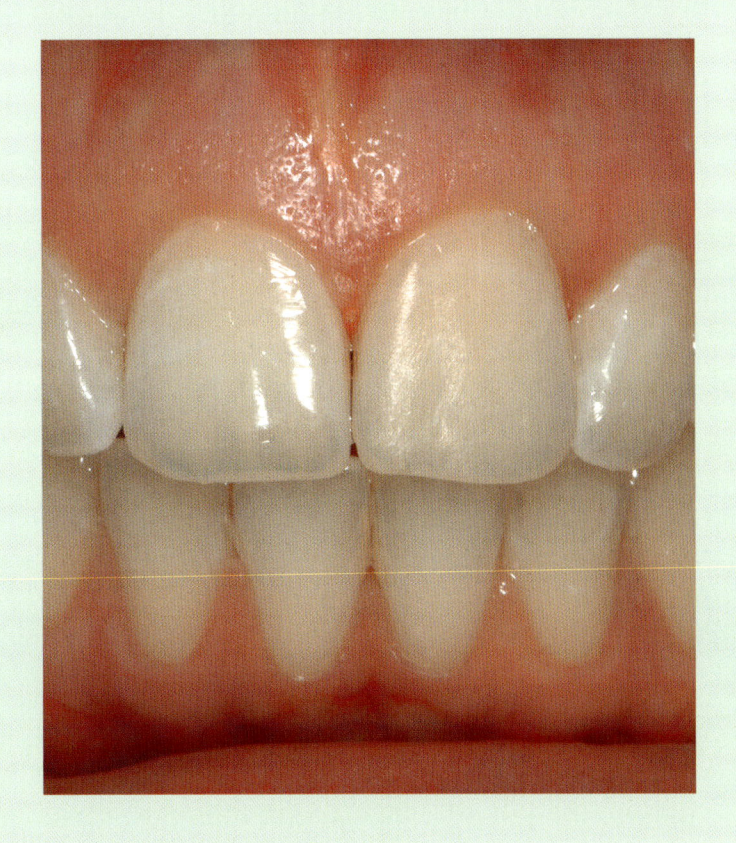

Figure 30.28 Final result.

Clinical case 30.11: Severe intrusive luxation with complicated crown fracture in an 8.2-year-old

Problem

Abscess and pain 30 days after trauma. Severe intrusive luxation with complicated crown fracture of immature tooth #8 that had not been treated. Uncomplicated fracture of tooth #9 that, instead, had been reconstructed. Class II malocclusion with mandibular retrusion. The patient came to our attention after 30 days (Figures 30.29 and 30.30A).

Treatment:

Endodontic treatment of tooth #8 using $Ca(OH)_2$ (Figure 30.30B). Soft-tissue treatment with an Nd:YAG laser. Application of an orthodontic splint to align the upper frontal group and the incisor. Follow up until the end of mixed dentition (Figures 30.31, 30.32, and 30.33). Subsequently, orthodontic treatment of both arches to obtain good alignment and correct tipping (Figures 30.33 and 30.34). Endodontic treatment of tooth # 9 (Figure 30.35B and C).

Result

Dyschromia of the two upper frontal teeth at the end of the orthodontic therapy (Figure 30.35A). Therefore, to improve the patient's smile, nonvital laser-assisted dental bleaching with a KTP laser was performed, and both upper incisors were restored with composite resin to achieve better esthetics (Figure 30.36).

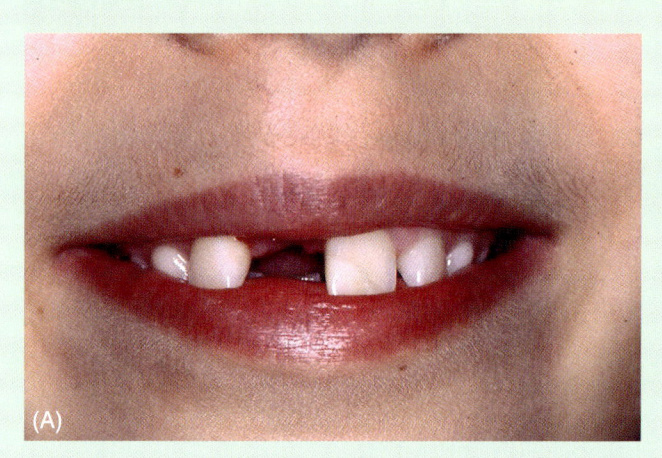

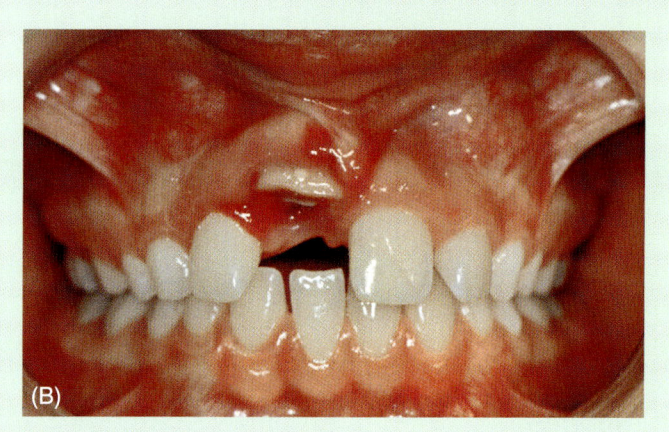

Figure 30.29 A very young patient **(A)** with a severe luxation injury with a complicated enamel dentin fracture of tooth #8 (not treated) and an uncomplicated crown fracture of tooth #9, which was reconstructed **(B)**.

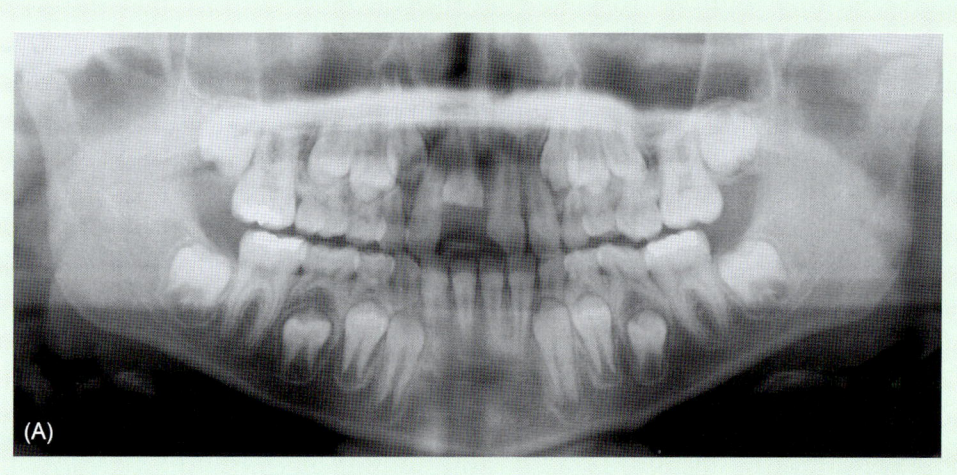

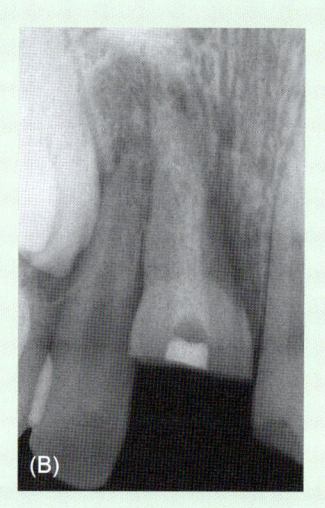

Figure 30.30 Orthopantomograph **(A)** and preliminary endodontic treatment of tooth #8 using $Ca(OH)_2$ **(B)**.

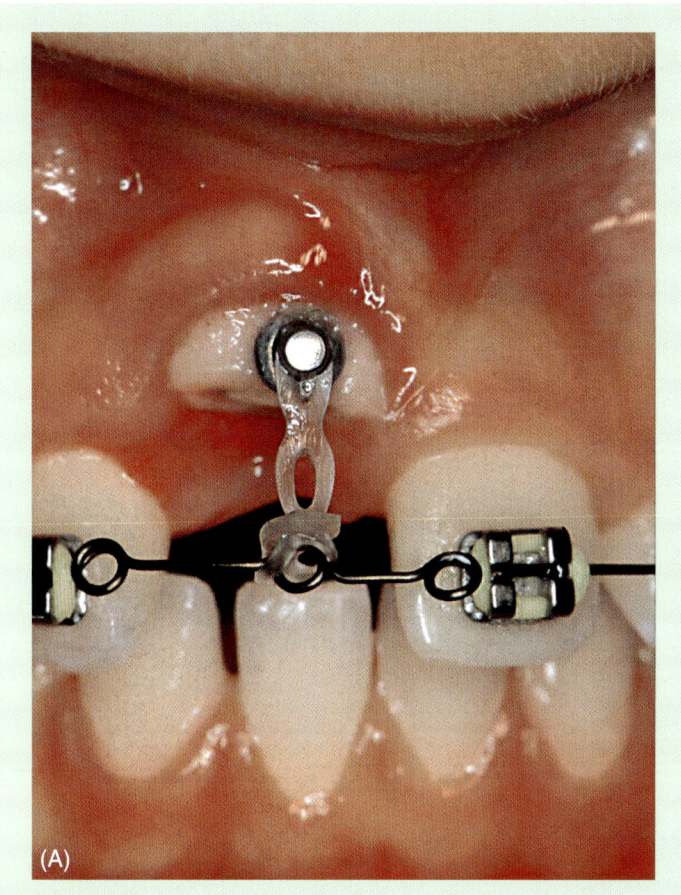

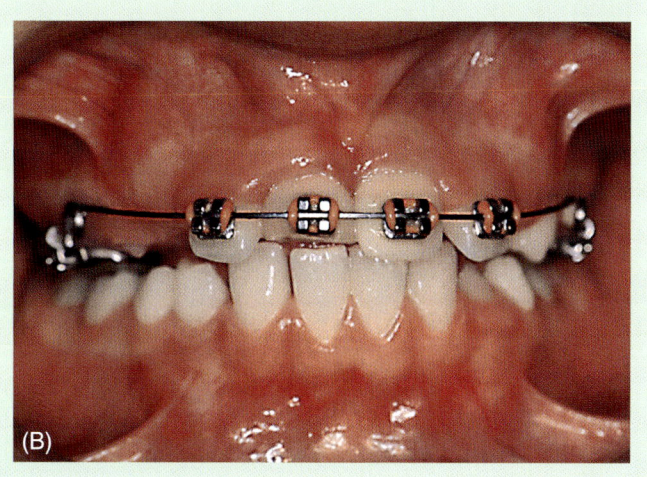

Figure 30.31 Orthodontic splint to extrude the tooth **(A)** and final alignment **(B)**.

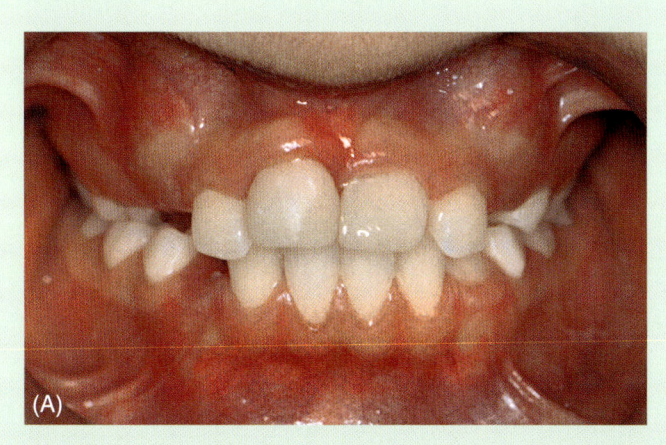

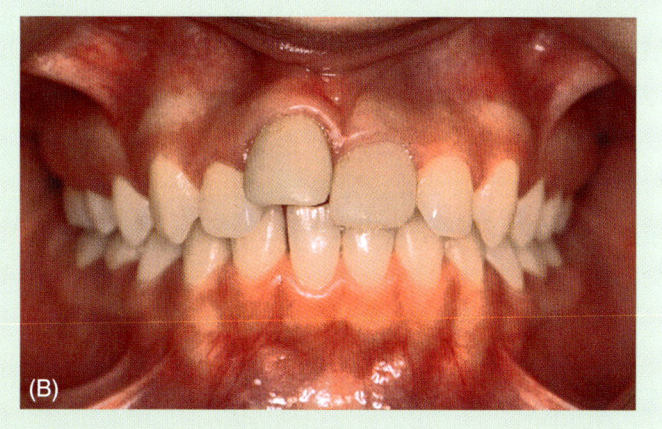

Figure 30.32 A composite restoration was carried out **(A)** and the patient was followed up to the end of the mixed dentition period **(B)**.

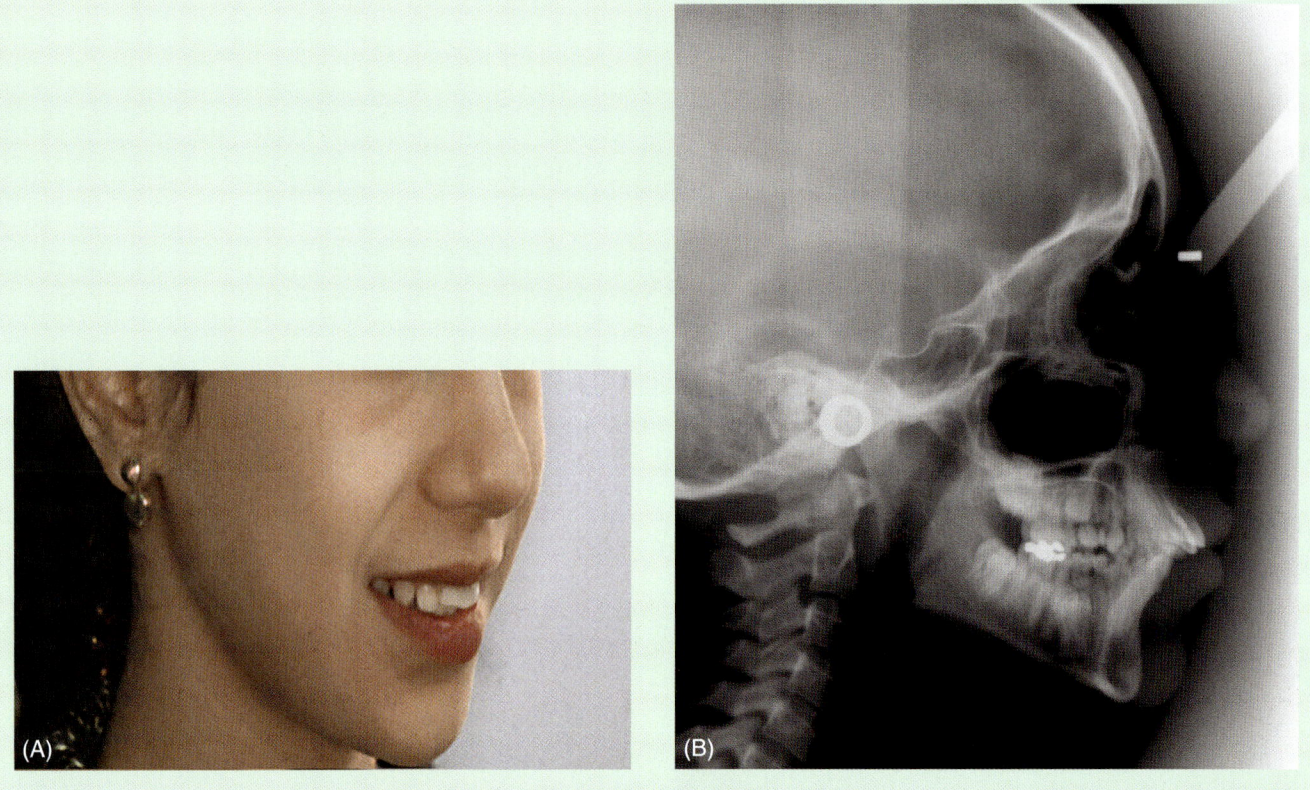

Figure 30.33 The patient at 12.6 years of age **(A)** and a lateral teleradiograph **(B)**.

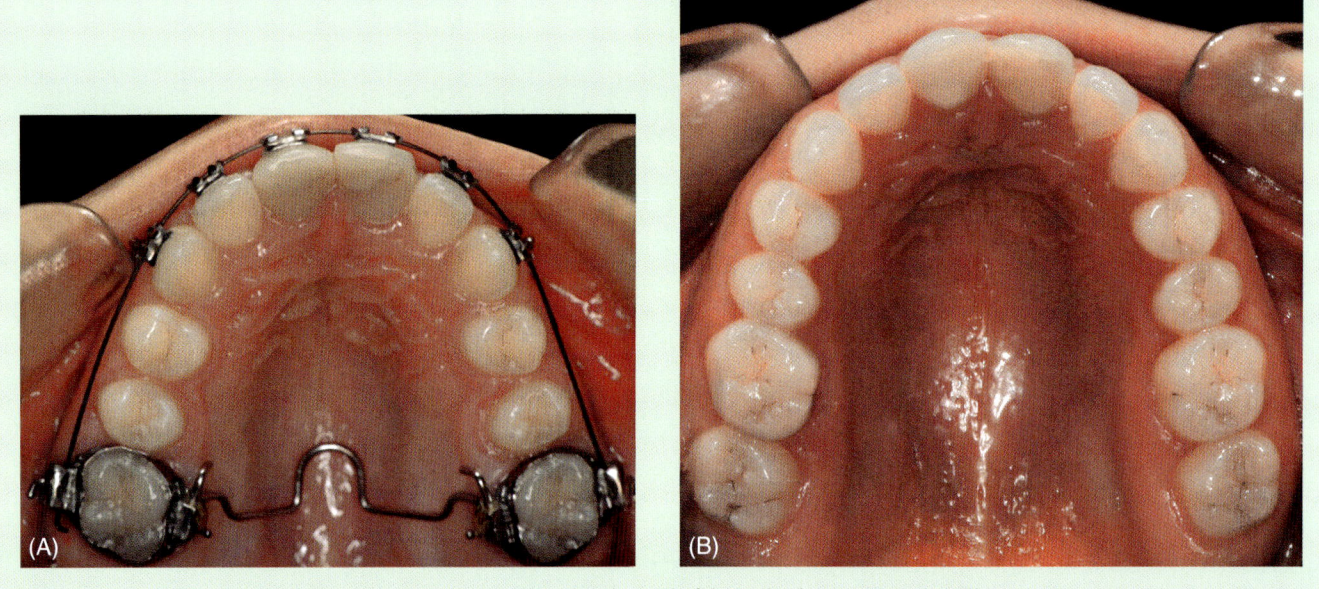

Figure 30.34 Occlusal view of the upper arch during **(A)** and at the end of the orthodontic treatment **(B)**.

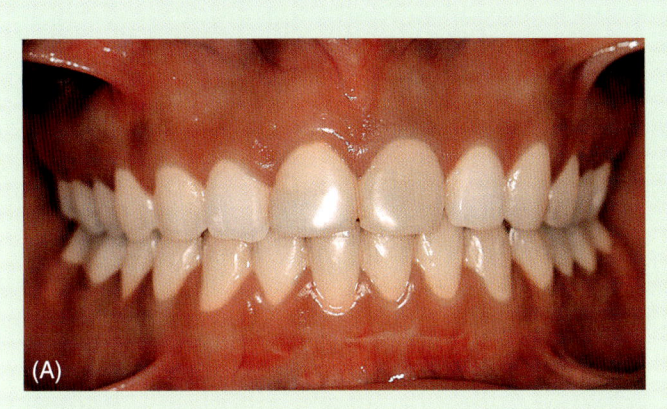

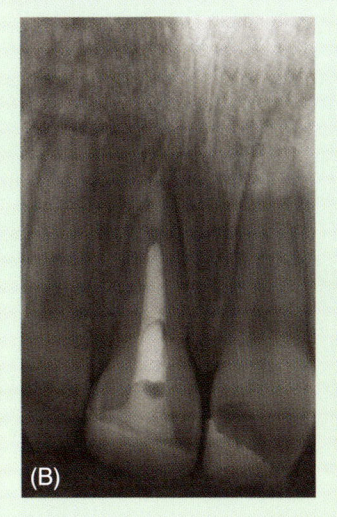

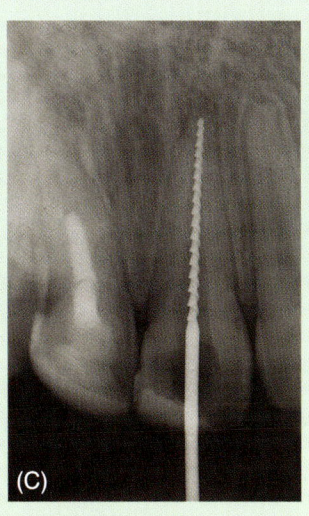

Figure 30.35 Frontal view of occlusion at the end of the therapy; the esthetic result is limited by teeth discoloration **(A)**. Definitive endodontic treatment of both upper central incisors. Control X-rays **(B, C)**.

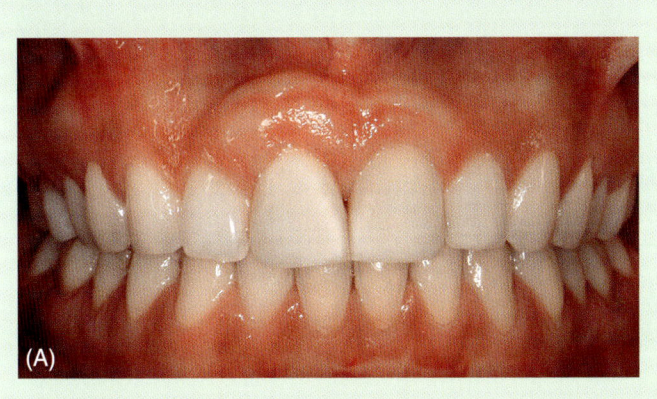

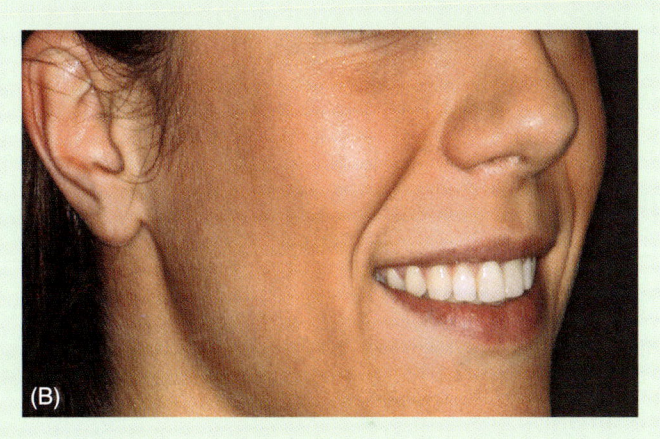

Figure 30.36 A KTP laser bleaching and definitive composite restorations were carried out to improve esthetics **(A)**. The patient's smile 15 years after the traumatic injury **(B)**.

Clinical case 30.12: Luxation injury in a 7.8-year-old female

Problem

Luxation injury of teeth #8 and #9, with lip pain and edema and bleeding (Figure 30.37A and B).

Treatment

Soft diet and oral hygiene instructions. LLLT (at a dose of 3–4 J) within 4 days to treat pain, swelling, and inflammation and to promote tissue repair with deep tissue penetration.

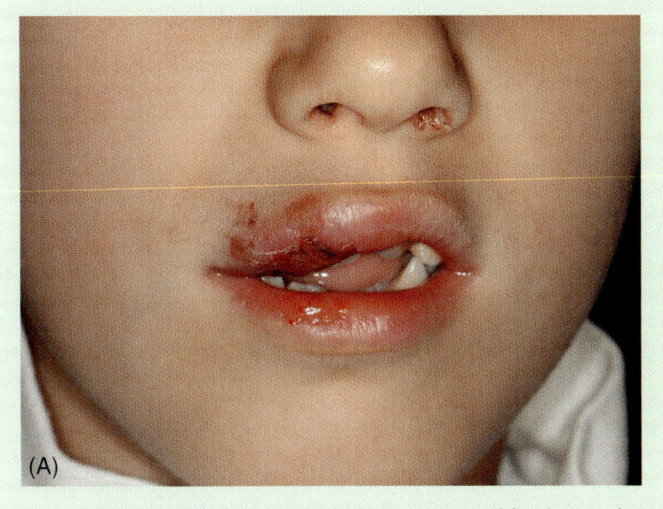

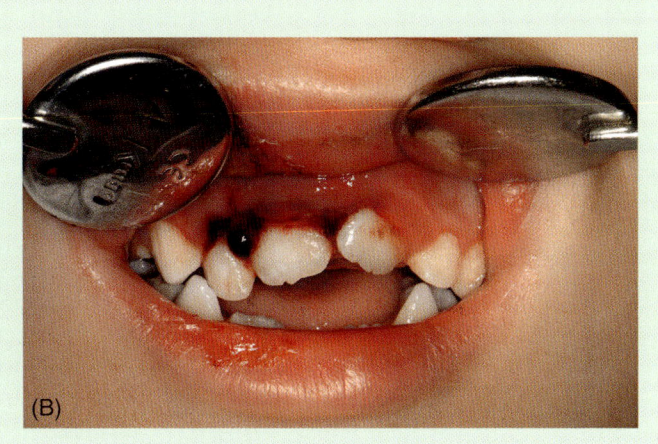

Figure 30.37 **(A, B)** An injury to supporting tissues: bleeding and pain are present.

Result

Biostimulation of soft tissues and lips led to greatly improved wound healing thanks to faster epithelization and collagen deposition (Figure 30.38).

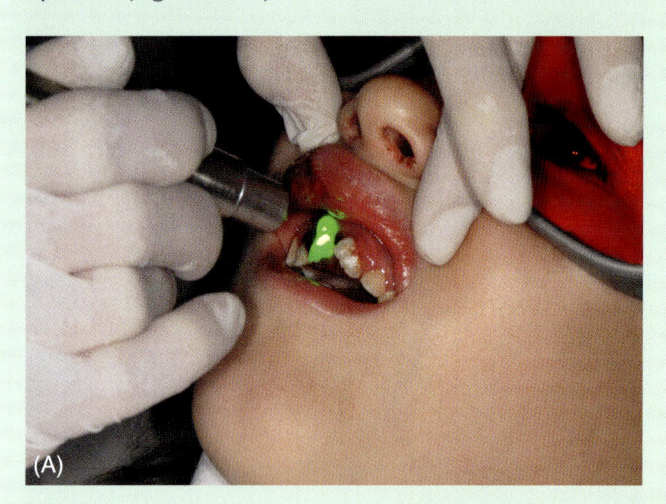

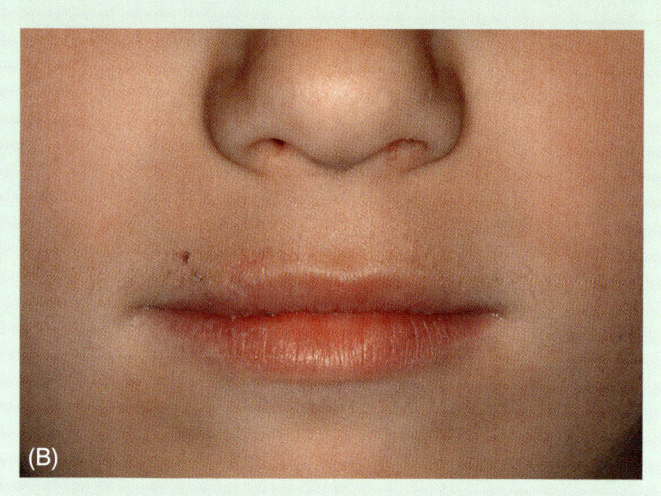

Figure 30.38 (A, B) A KTP laser is used to decontaminate the inflamed area and to exploit the laser's antalgic and biostimulating action, thereby improving positive outcome and reducing complications.

Clinical case 30.13: Discolored frontal upper incisor due to previous trauma in a 19-year-old

Problem

Discolored frontal upper incisor due to a previous trauma and desire to improve esthetics (Figure 30.39).

Treatment

Careful diagnostic wax-up (it is recalled that a well-planned and well-executed diagnostic wax-up is essential to ensure good communication with both the patient and the laboratory). Preparation of teeth for porcelain laminates. Fabrication of temporary restorations from a matrix formed over the diagnostic wax-up (Figure 30.40A).

Result

Satisfactory color correction using porcelain laminates (Figures 30.40B and 30.41).

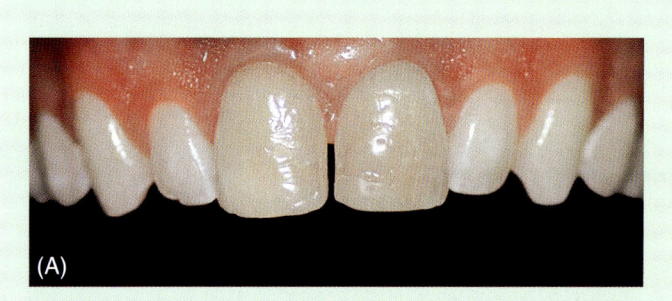

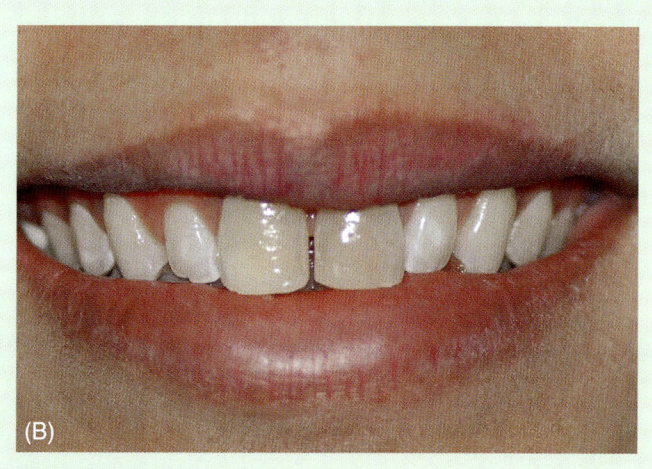

Figure 30.39 (A, B) Discoloration of teeth #8 and #9 due to a previous traumatic injury.

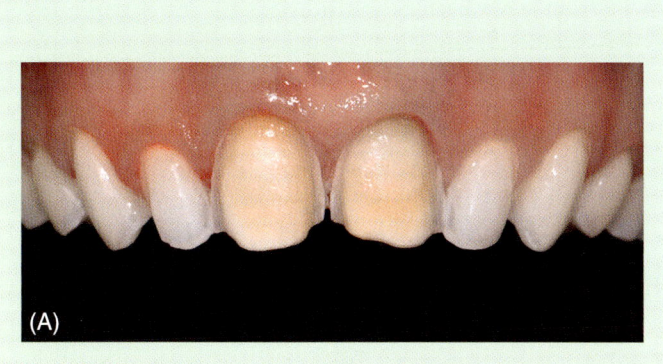

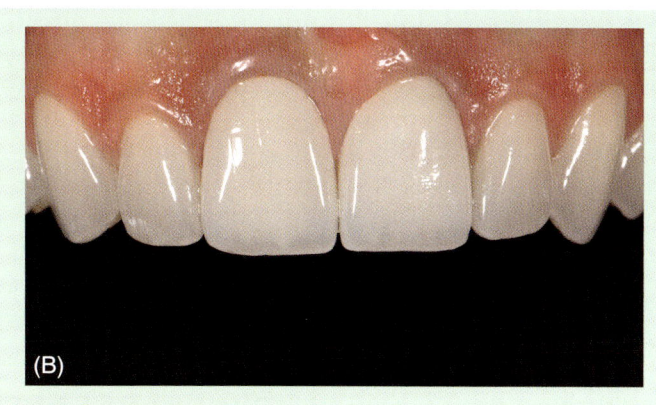

Figure 30.40 Teeth are prepared **(A)** and porcelain laminates are placed **(B)**.

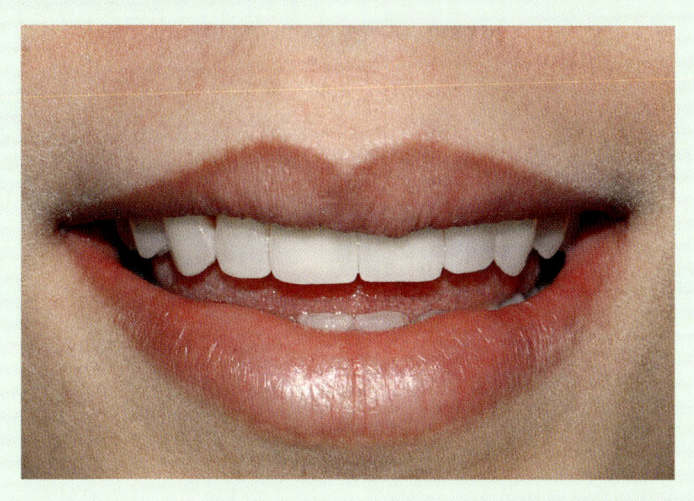

Figure 30.41 Post-treatment smile.

Taking into account several fundamental concepts as well as new therapeutic trends that focus on shape resetting for improved esthetics and harmony of the dental arches, the approach used is to balance the arch symmetrically and monitor the eruption of the first permanent molar (tipping, uprighting) to prevent mesialization of the first lower molars. Next, a correct dentoskeletal analysis, cephalometric study, and careful evaluation of the means and materials must be done before formulating a diagnosis and logical prognostic evaluation. Finally, the application of orthodontic brackets to primary teeth has a number of advantages that must be considered. These include reduced risk of demineralization; the possibility of good anchorage, which decreases the reaction counterforce; and the reduction of acid-etching time and problems associated with the removal of orthodontic brackets.

The dentist can perform several different treatments:

- slicing of the primary cuspids and/or primary second molars;
- placement of a lip bumper on the primary second molars;
- symmetrical balancing of the arches following premature loss or extraction of the primary cuspid;
- uprighting of the first permanent molars.[23]

Particularly prominent among the fundamental concepts of pediatric dentistry is the need to obtain correct evolution of the arches, as well as to treat any irregular condition.[33,34] The first primary molars are the ones that, during eruption, determine the first proprioceptive reflexes on the transverse plane. Compared with the second primary molars, however, their role and maintenance are of secondary importance. Indeed, the second primary molar plays a strategic role, its presence being essential to guide the eruption and articulation of the first permanent molars. The restoration and preservation of the posterior primary teeth are vital to maintaining the arch length and eliminating the risk of mesial drift of the permanent molars.

Arch length and arch anatomy can be modified by:

1. Tooth crowding, or loss of space (unilateral or bilateral). This may be associated with different conditions: premature extractions because of caries, tooth loss in traumatic events, ectopic eruptions, impactions, transpositions, ankylosis, agenesis, microdontia, or supernumerary teeth.
2. Habits such as oral breathing, sleep apnea syndromes, and thumb sucking. Patients with harmful oral habits usually present with a reduction of transverse (cross) diameters, as well as the loss of one or more primary molars, which could lead to a further collapse of the arch.
3. Presence of a malocclusion—Class II with an increased overjet and/or overbite or Class III with an anterior crossbite and/or posterior crossbite and/or open bite.[6,35]

The pedodontist, often working with the orthodontist, must perform a careful analysis of the dentition. The goal is arch harmony and a good balance between function, arch form, and oral tissue conditions.

Optimal space maintenance therapy is based on preservation of the primary molars until natural exfoliation. Dental education and improved prevention have reduced the number of children who develop malocclusion because of premature loss of primary teeth. This has indeed become one of the most controllable causes of malocclusion. When posterior teeth are damaged or lost, pediatric crowns for grossly damaged teeth, space maintainers (fixed or removable appliances), or esthetic posterior restoration techniques can be used to maintain arch length.

Interproximal caries in primary teeth, due to the different thickness of the enamel and dentin, can more easily extend to the pulp, making endodontic therapy necessary. In this context, compomers and composite resins are the materials of choice on account of their easy handling, reduction of tooth preparation, reasonable wear properties, good esthetics, and fluoride-leaching properties.

Clinical case 30.14: Agenesis of teeth in a 14-year-old male

Problem

Agenesis of teeth #7 and #10. Alignment of dental arches and closure of spaces after treatment with a fixed orthodontic appliance; the cuspids need reshaping to improve esthetics (Figure 30.42).

Treatment

Placement of a rubber dam to maintain isolation during a multiple bonding procedure. Etching of the cuspid surfaces, followed by restoration with composite resin (Figure 30.43).

A diagnostic wax-up and computer imaging may help the patient to appreciate the anticipated result.

Result

The final result can be seen in Figure 30.44. Greatly improved smile (well proportioned and more attractive) after a single-sitting procedure.

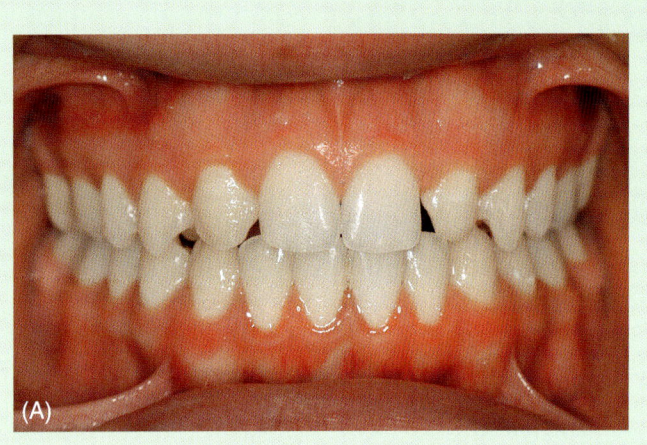

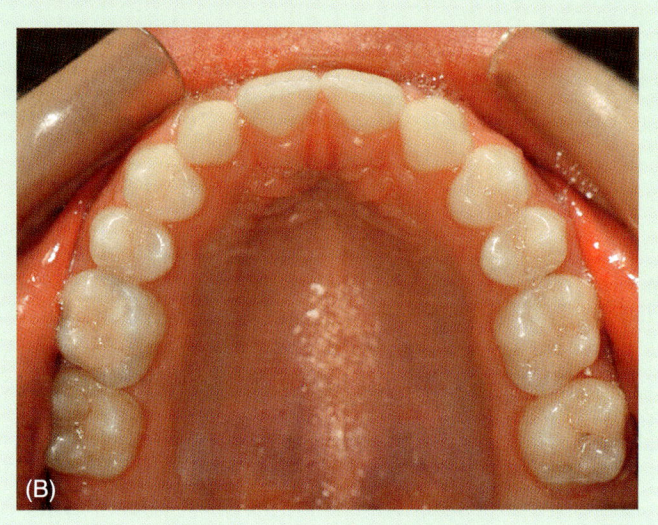

Figure 30.42 The patient after the orthodontic treatment; teeth #7 and #10 are missing. Frontal (A) and occlusal (B) views.

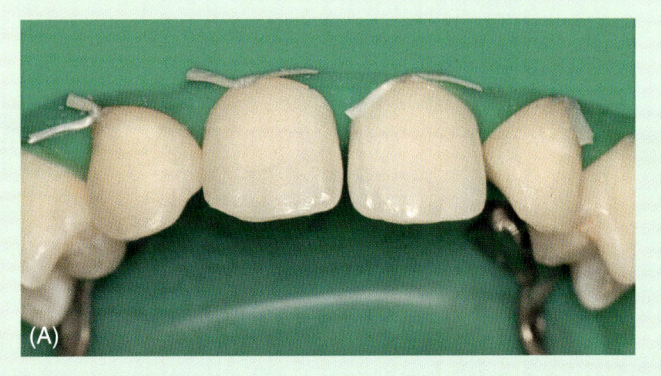

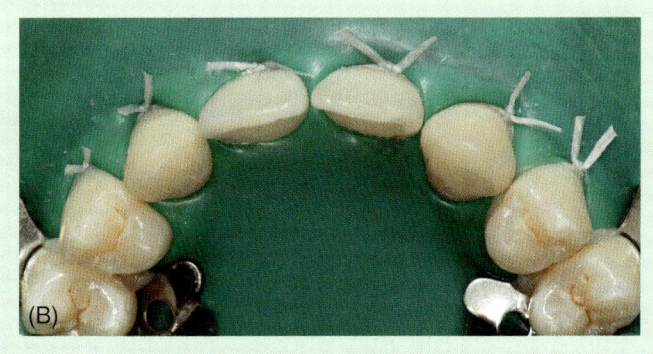

Figure 30.43 (A, B) Placement of a rubber dam to maintain isolation during a resin bonding procedure to reshape cuspids as laterals.

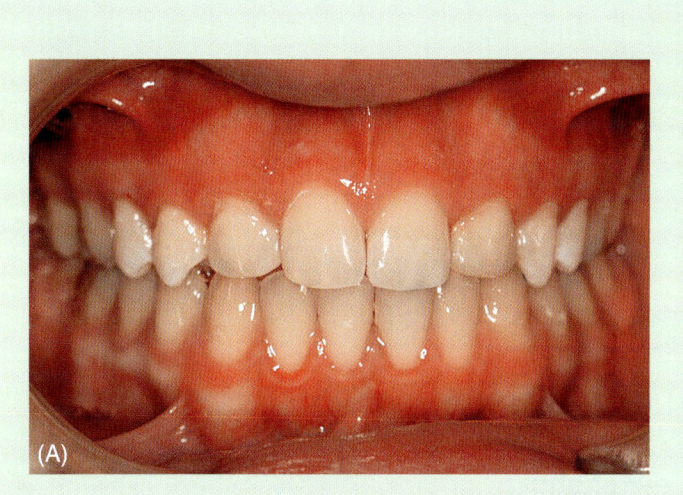

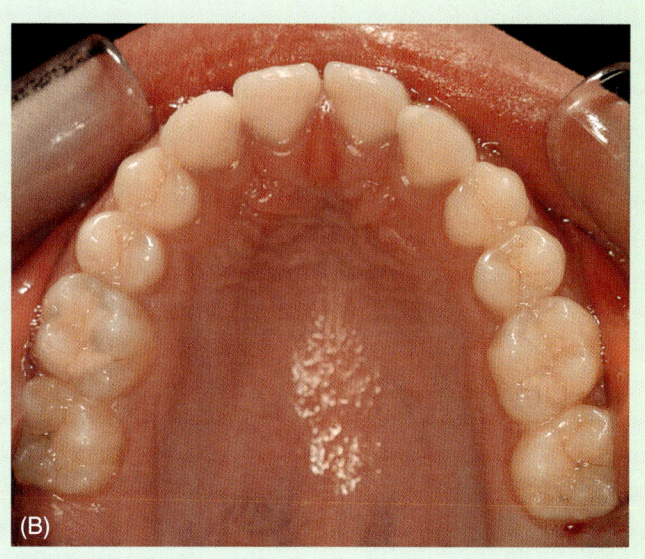

Figure 30.44 The final result after coronoplasty. Frontal **(A)** and occlusal **(B)** views.

Clinical case 30.15: Inclusion of tooth and crowding in a 12.7-year-old female

Problem

Inclusion of tooth #6 and minor crowding of the lower arch after phase 1 interceptive orthodontic treatment. Ortho surgery for guided eruption not indicated due to the tooth position (Figures 30.45 and 30.46).

Treatment

Transplantation of the tooth (vital) after orthodontic space preparation in the upper arch and lower arch alignment. Extraction and immediate repositioning of tooth #6 after avulsion of C and the creation of a new alveolus. Fixation of the cuspid, first by suturing and later by splinting with an orthodontic appliance. Control of tooth vitality by thermal and electrical tests and by X-ray examination during the orthodontic treatment (Figures 30.47, 30.48, 30.49, and 30.50).

Result

Successful esthetic outcome in a patient with a variety of problems (Figures 30.51 and 30.52).

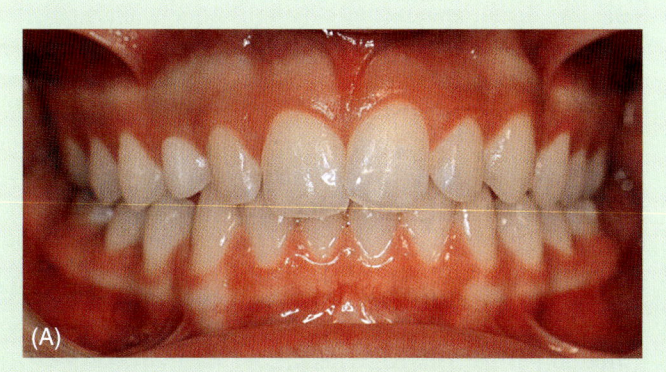

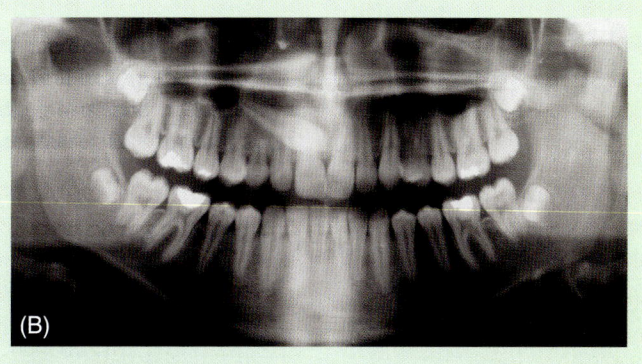

Figure 30.45 Frontal view: note the retention of tooth #6 **(A)** and orthopantomograph **(B)**.

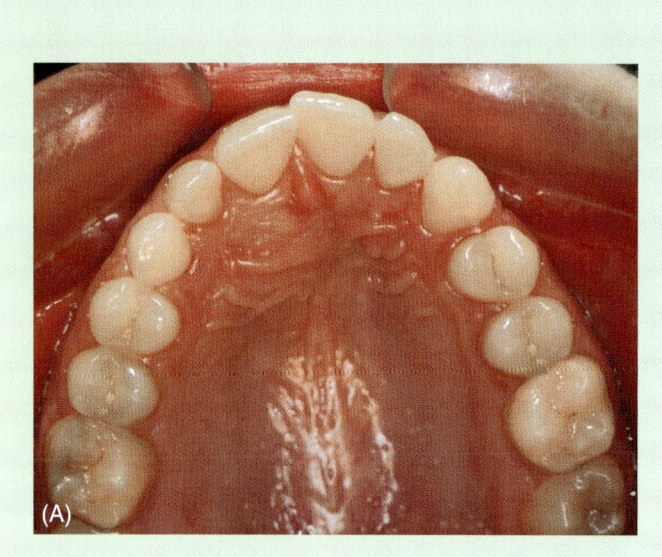

Figure 30.46 Occlusal view **(A)** and occlusal control X-ray **(B)**.

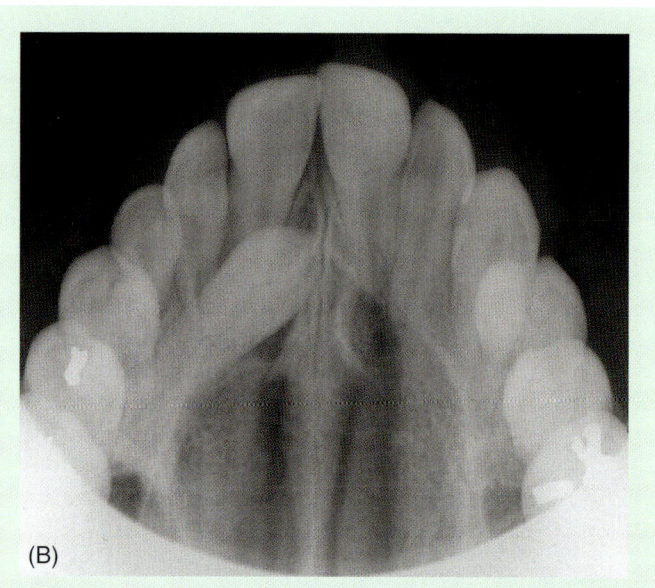

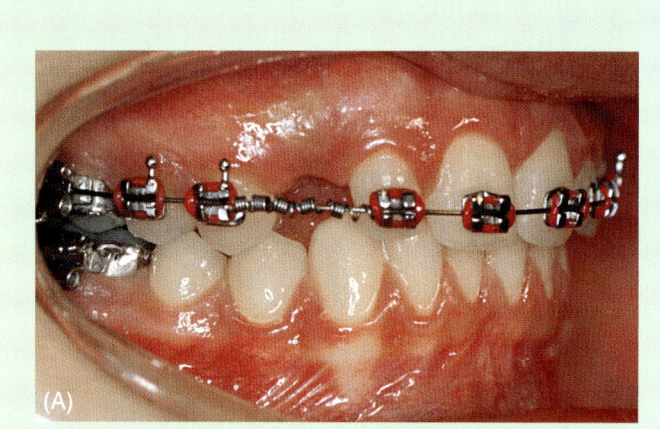

Figure 30.47 Orthodontic space preparation **(A)** and control X-ray before autotransplantation **(B)**.

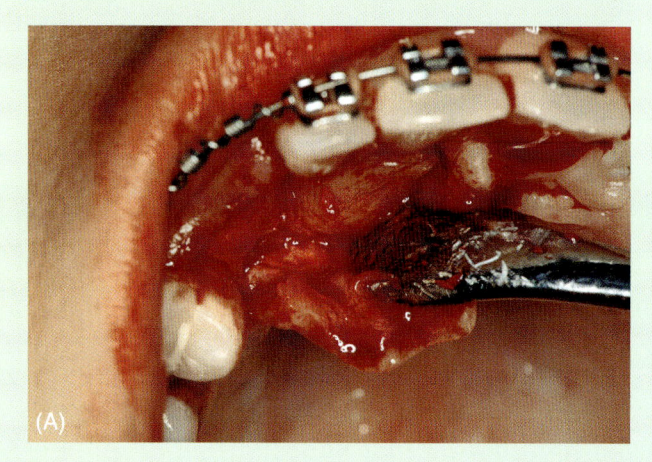

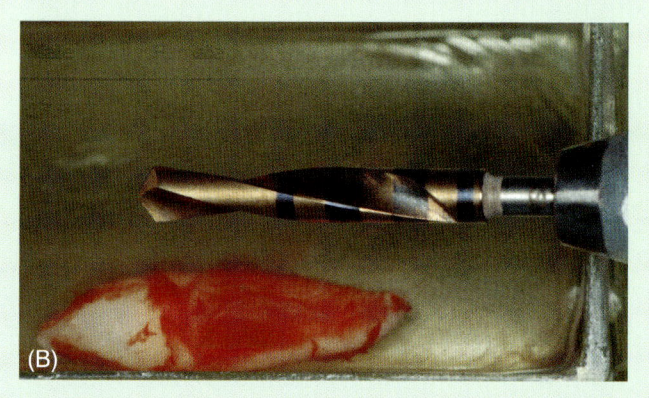

Figure 30.48 Surgical tooth exposure **(A)**. Tooth #7 is extracted and conserved in saline solution until transplantation **(B)**.

Chapter 30 Pediatric Dentistry

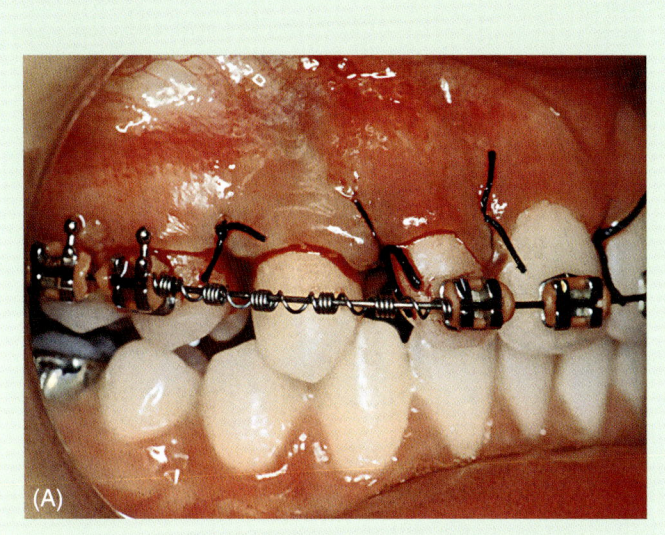

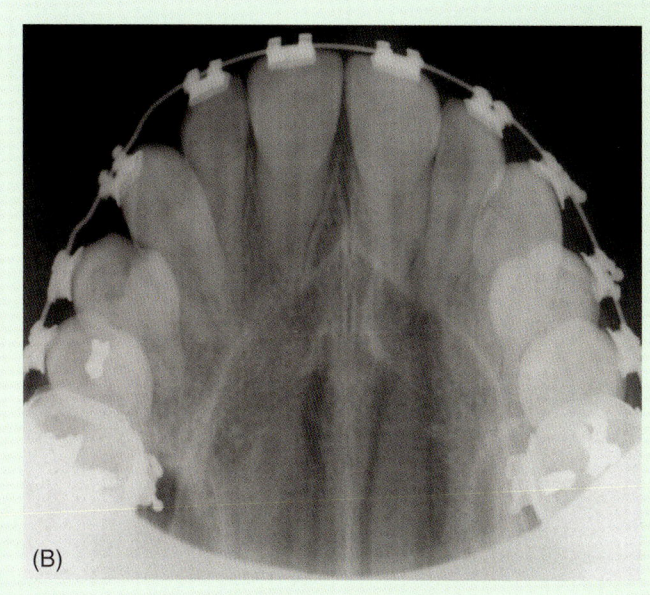

Figure 30.49 The tooth is inserted in the alveolus created **(A)**. Control X-ray **(B)**.

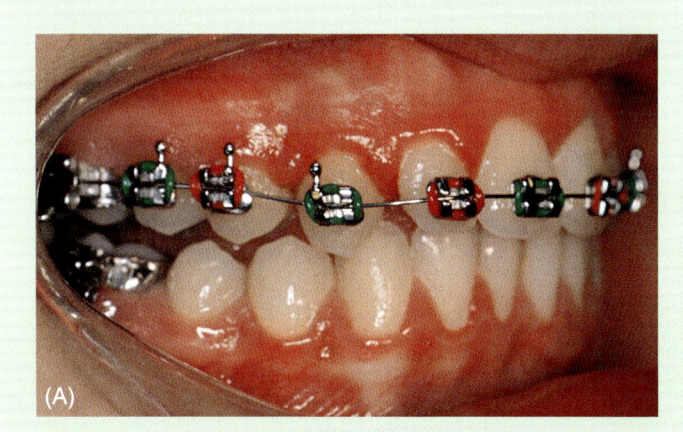

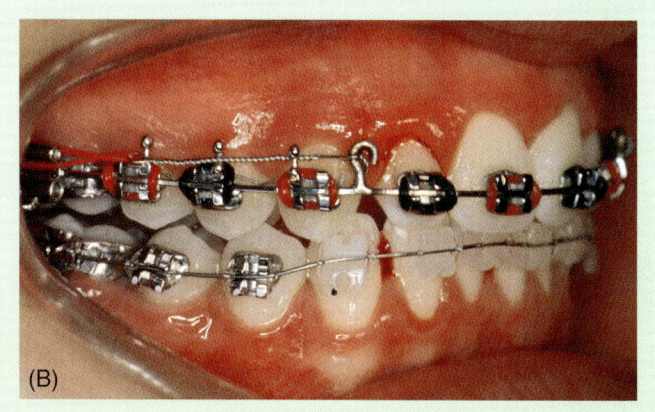

Figure 30.50 **(A, B)** The patient during different orthodontic treatment phases.

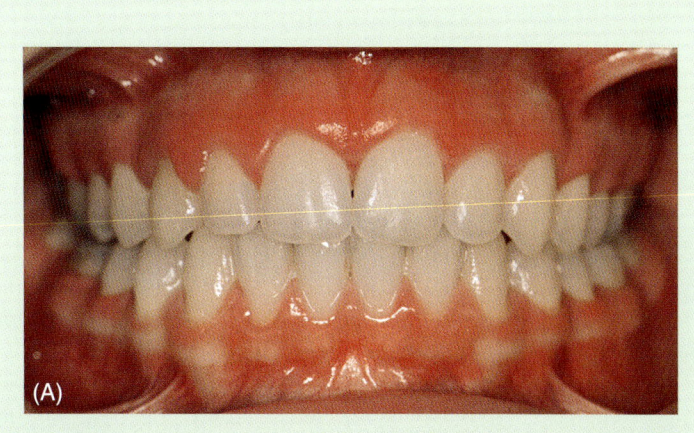

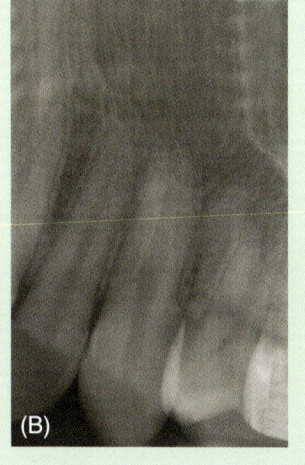

Figure 30.51 The patient at the end of the treatment. The transplanted tooth #6 is vital **(A)**. Control X-ray **(B)**. A very good balance and good esthetics are achieved.

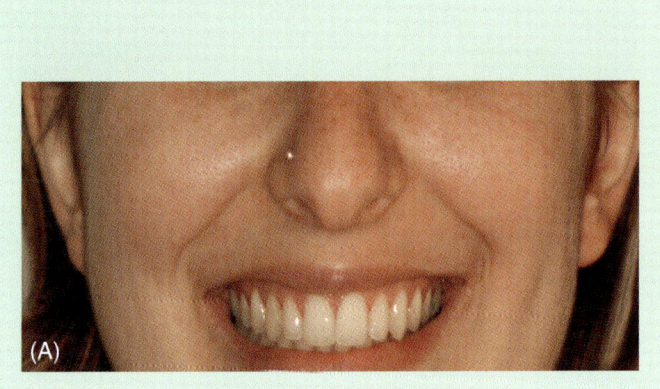

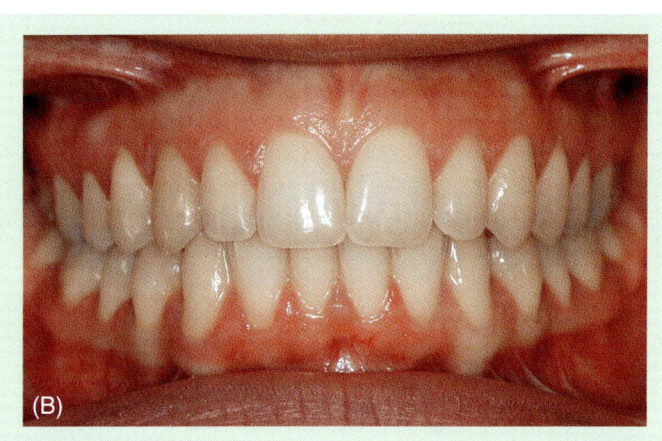

Figure 30.52 The patient's smile **(A)** and frontal intraoral view **(B)** 10 years later.

In such patients who may present, for example, included teeth, drifting, crowding, and malocclusion, the intervention of several dental disciplines is required. As dental professionals, we should try to form groups of practitioners specializing in different areas who can all participate in a patient's diagnostic workup to ensure a successful esthetic outcome.

Clinical case 30.16: Supernumerary (double) tooth in a 9.2-year-old male

Problem

A supernumerary (double) tooth in place of the central upper left incisor (tooth #9) (Figure 30.53). This anomaly manifests itself as a structure resembling two teeth that have been joined together. In the anterior region, the anomalous tooth usually has a groove on the buccal surface and small cut in the incisal edge. X-rays are necessary to determine whether there is a union (fusion) of the pulp chambers. Fusion exists when two teeth are joined at the level of the pulp and dentin. There are usually two root canals, as in this case (Figure 30.54).

Treatment

Surgical separation and extraction of the fused supernumerary tooth; application of a fixed orthodontic appliance to the maxillary arch to align the arch and close the anterior diastema.

Subsequently, restoration of the incisal margin and the interproximal area of tooth #9 to improve esthetics and gingivoplasty to improve gingival margins. Monitoring of the tooth by vitality testing and X-ray examinations (Figures 30.55, 30.56, 30.57, and 30.58).

Result

Good morphofunctional recovery and an esthetic result that satisfied the patient, achieved through the teamwork of several specialists (Figures 30.59 and 30.60).

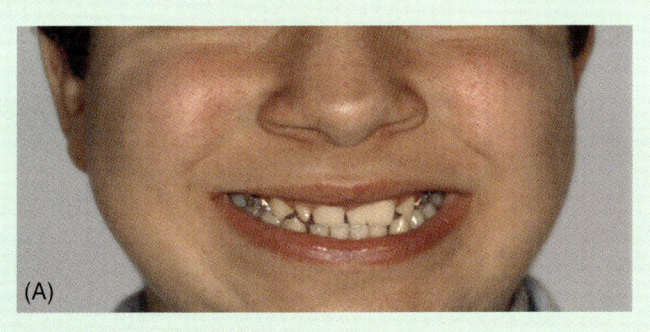

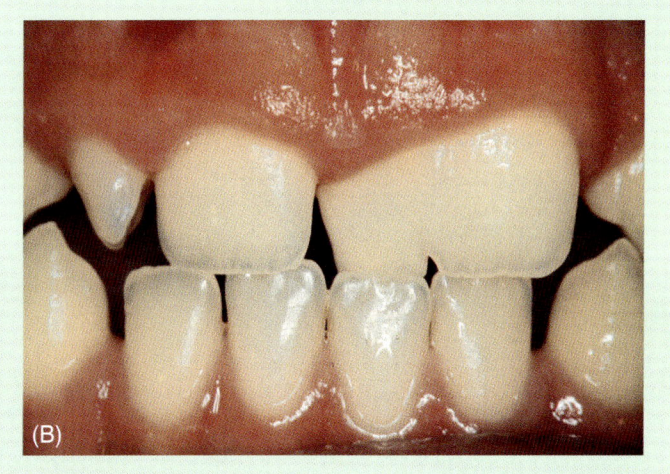

Figure 30.53 A double tooth in place of the central upper left incisor. The patient's smile **(A)** and intraoral frontal view **(B)**.

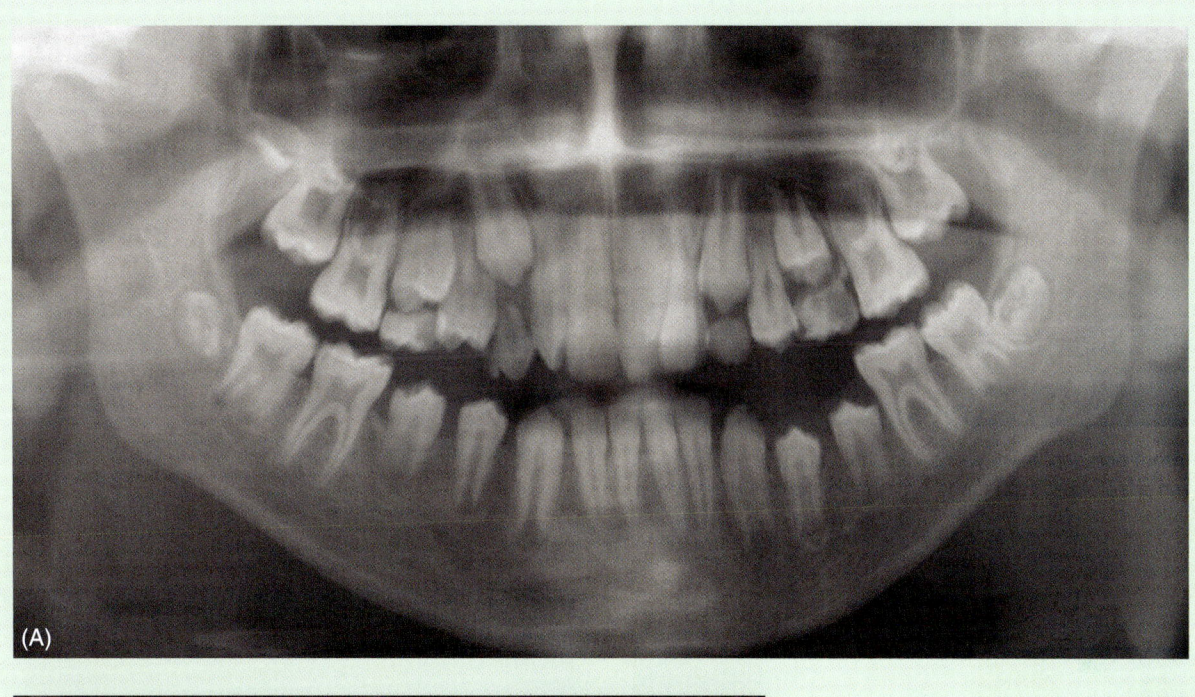

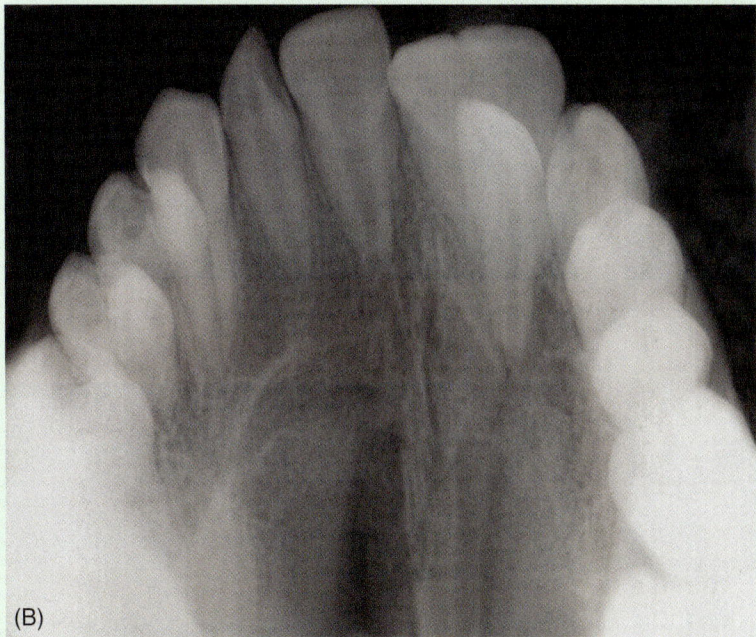

Figure 30.54 Initial orthopantomograph **(A)** and control X-ray **(B)**.

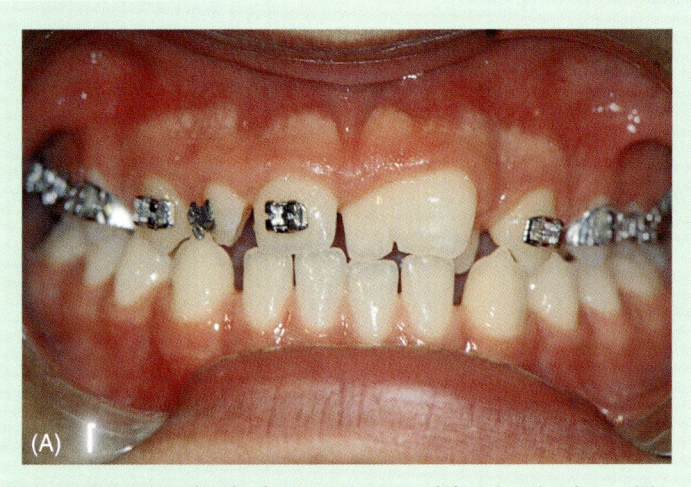

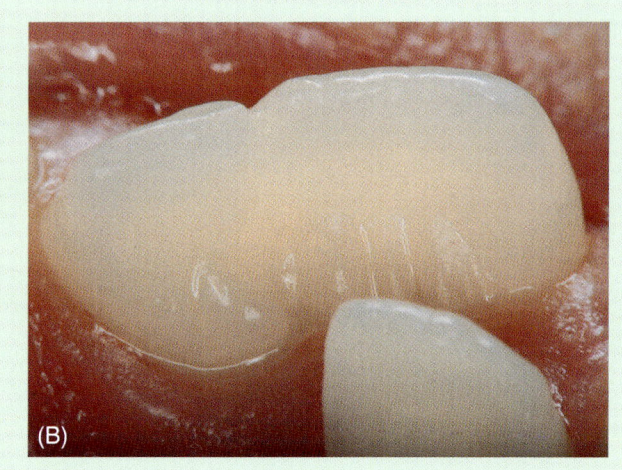

Figure 30.55 Initial orthodontic preparation (A) and occlusal view (B).

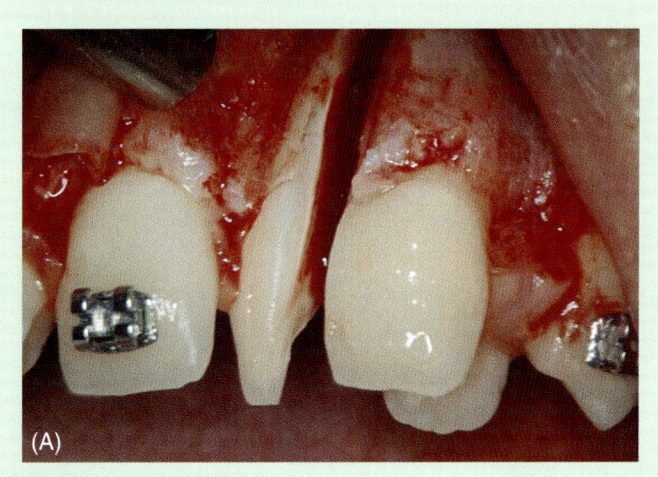

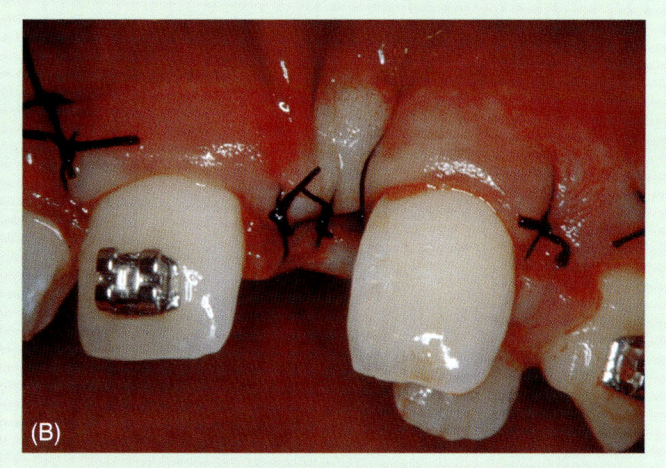

Figure 30.56 The fused supernumerary tooth is surgically separated (A) and extracted (B).

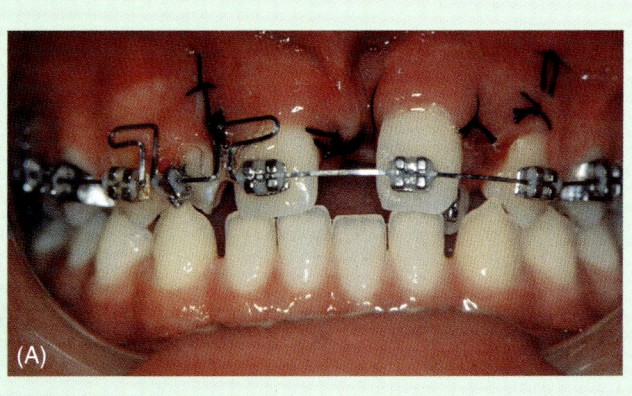

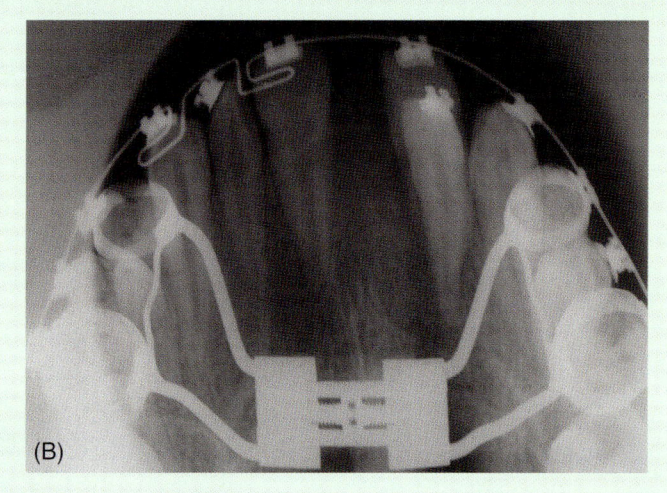

Figure 30.57 Immediately after surgery a rapid palate expander is placed (A). Control X-ray (B).

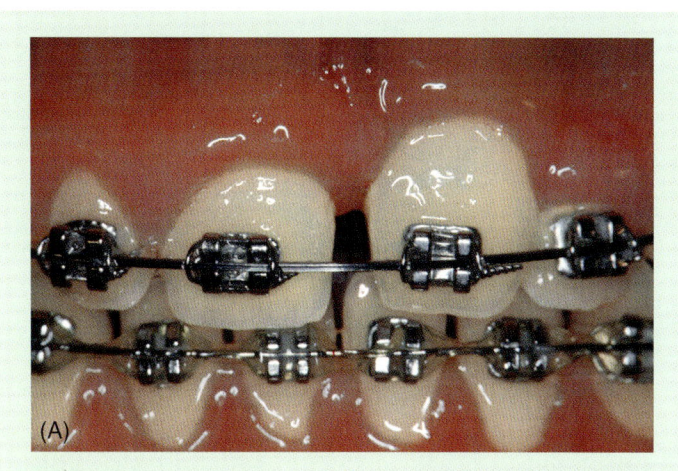

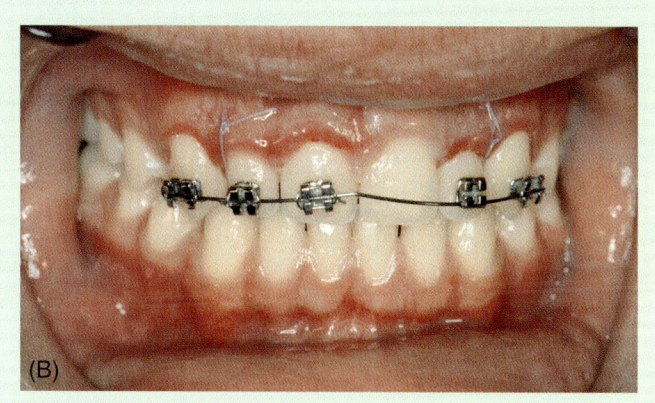

Figure 30.58 Orthodontic treatment phase to align teeth and close the anterior diastema **(A)**. Prior to bracket removal, a gingivoplasty procedure is performed **(B)**.

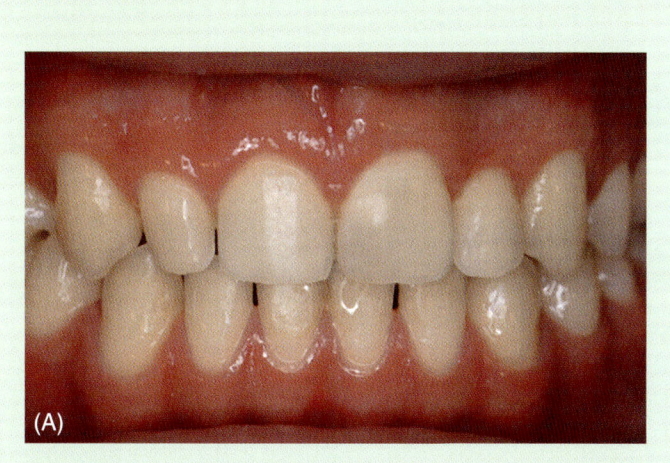

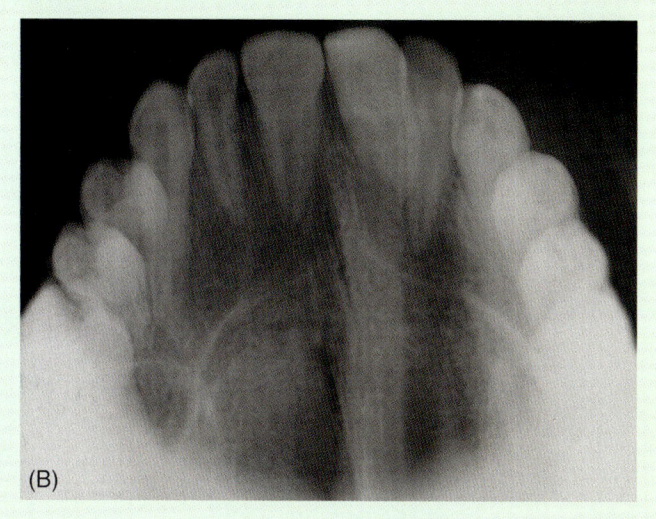

Figure 30.59 The patient's occlusion at the end of the treatment; note that the gingival margins of the central incisors are level **(A)**. Post-treatment control X-ray **(B)**.

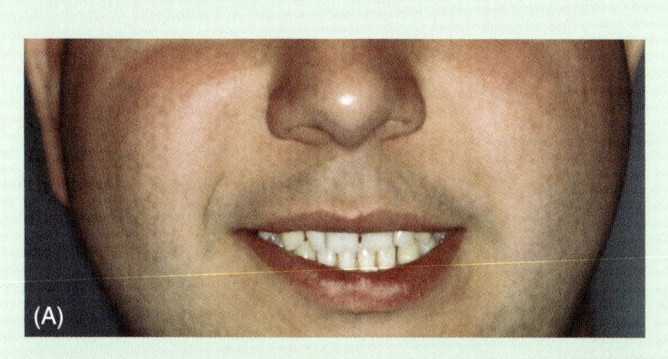

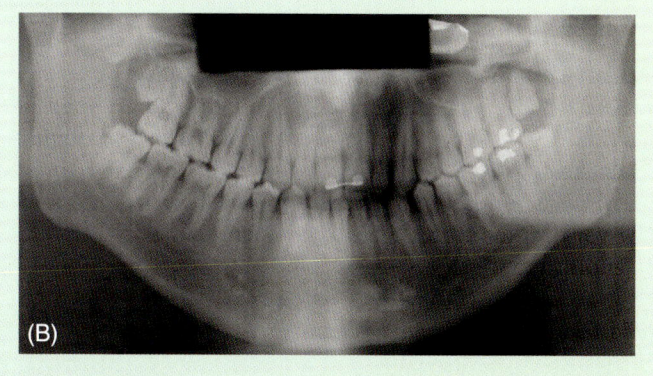

Figure 30.60 The patient 10 years after the end of the treatment **(A)**. Orthopantomograph; notice that tooth #9 is still vital **(B)**.

Clinical case 30.17: Patient with an open bite

Problem
Severe dentoalveolar open bite caused by thumb sucking (Figure 30.61).

Treatment
Two-phase orthodontic treatment: use of a functional appliance to reduce open bite followed by use of a fixed orthodontic device to improve arch morphology and occlusal function (Figures 30.62 and 30.63).

Result
Successful two-phase orthodontic treatment resulting in arch balance and improved esthetics and health of oral tissues. Greater self-confidence and well-being, thanks to the improved smile (Figure 30.64).

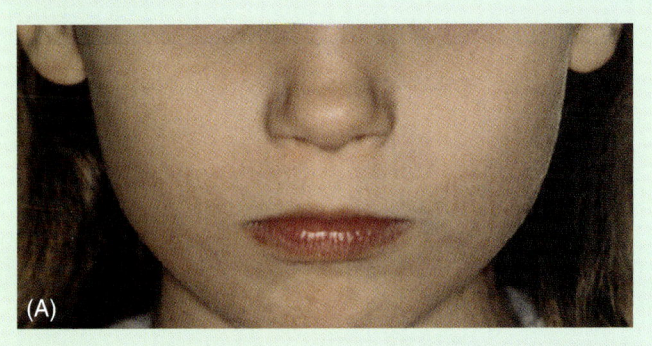

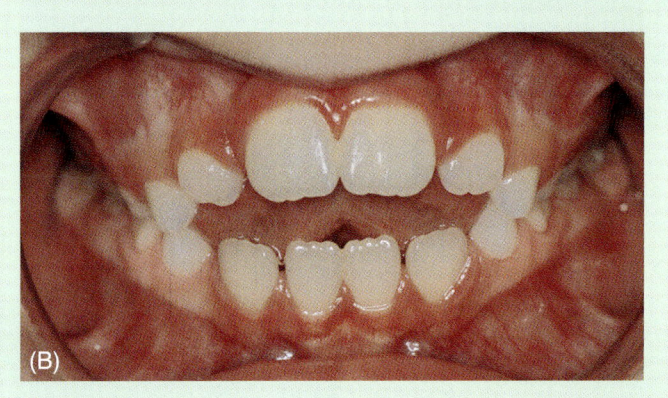

Figure 30.61 A young patient (A) with a severe dentoalveolar open bite from thumb sucking (B).

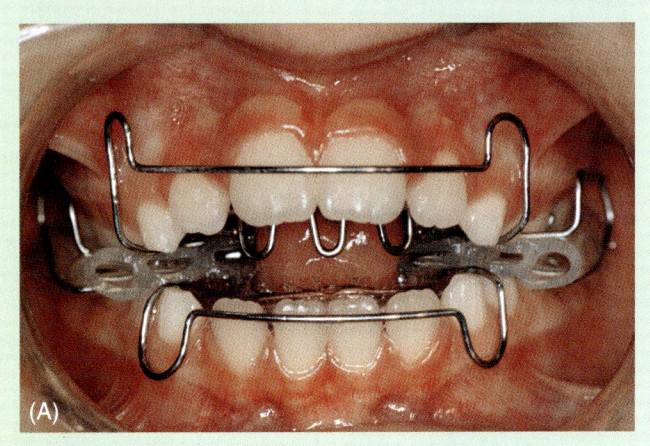

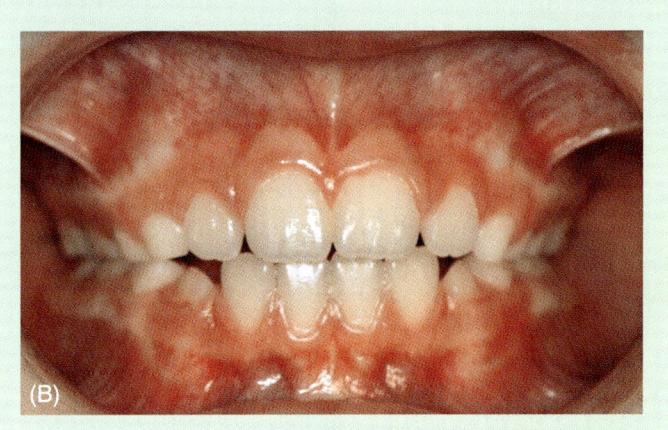

Figure 30.62 The patient was treated with a functional regulator worn for a period of 1 year (A). Frontal view after interceptive orthodontics (B).

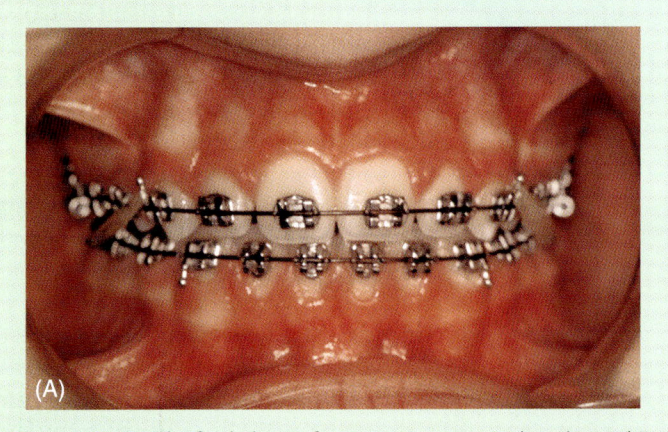

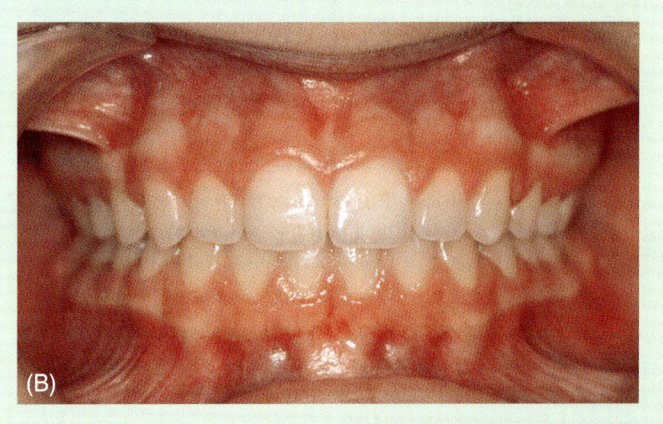

Figure 30.63 The final phase of treatment to correct the relationship of the front teeth in the vertical plane (A). The patient at the end of the treatment (B).

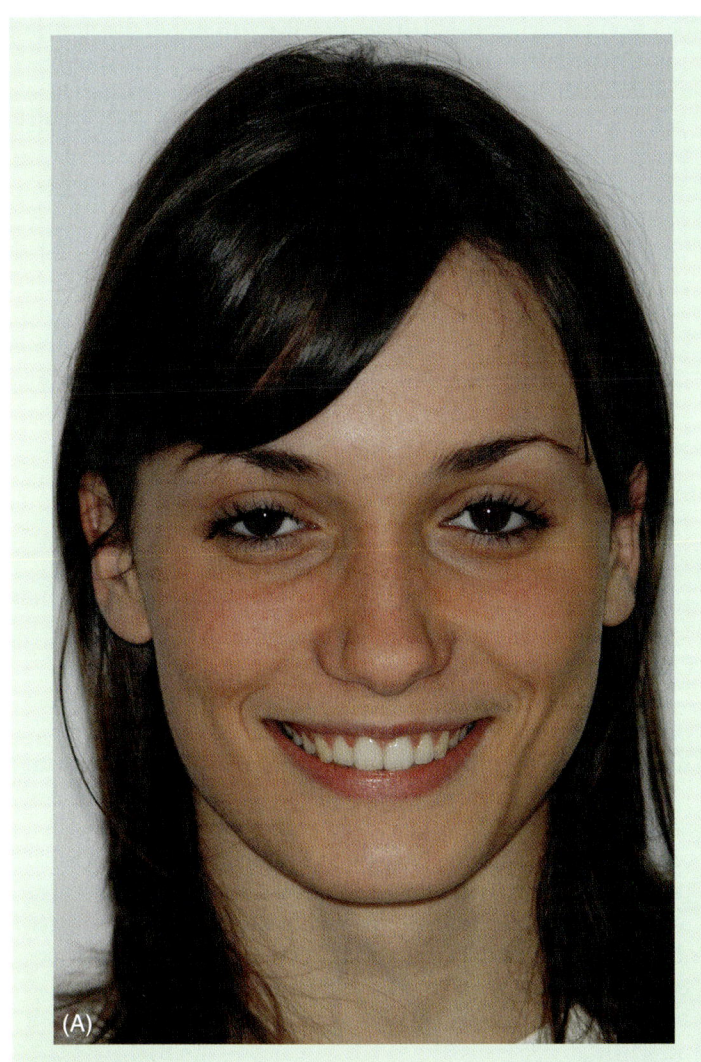

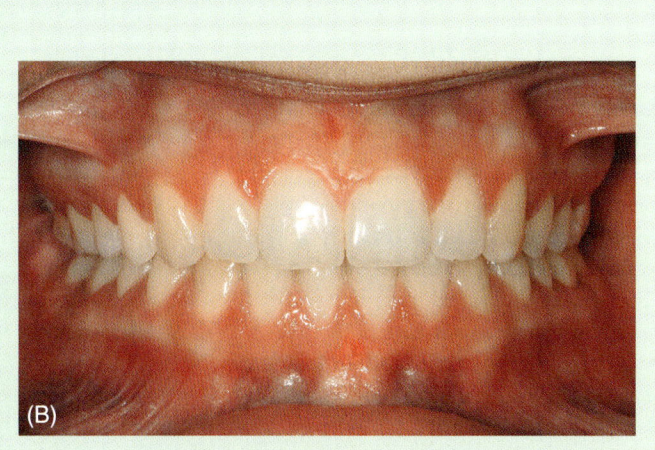

Figure 30.64 The patient's face **(A)** and the frontal view **(B)** after 10 years.

Facial harmony in pediatric dentistry: esthetic keys

The concept of "beauty" has always been subjective. With regard to individual facial esthetics, many attempts have been made over the centuries to establish what constitutes the golden section or divine proportion. In spite of all these efforts at standardization, each age and every century has brought its own esthetic canons, just as each individual may have their own esthetic ideals. However, our society is continuously creating new trends and ideals of beauty to which people aspire. Over the past few decades in the Western world, an individual's appearance has assumed much more importance and become essential in establishing self-image. Ultimately, it contributes to success in all aspects of professional and social life. For this reason, many branches of medicine that have an esthetic component are continuing to research and improve their techniques. One such discipline is orthognathodontics, which is extending its field of activity from the smile to the entire face of the patient.

As Goldstein says, "The way you see yourself and think others see you has a great deal to do with the way you feel about yourself. A charming smile can open doors; our own self-image is the key to our happiness."[6,36]

Cephalometrics and soft-tissue analysis

Several authors have shown that orthodontic treatment, including orthognathic surgery, can improve facial harmony. Traditional cephalometrics, based on angular and linear measurements of the patient's soft and hard tissues, have proven to be less than reliable for achieving correct diagnoses and satisfactory esthetic results. It suffices to say that no cephalometric analysis has universal appeal. Most cephalometric analyses use intracranial skeletal plans as a reference. On the basis of the assumption that facial esthetics, harmony, and facial balance are achieved through the achievement of specific dental and bone parameters, diagnosis and proposed treatments are based on these plans. However, many authors now agree that a careful analysis of the soft tissue is needed as well. Thus, cephalometrics now includes studies and measurements also involving soft tissues using the usual teleradiographies of the skull in norma lateralis or the photographic records of the patient in lateral view or, more rarely, in frontal view.

Good functional occlusion that complies with the usual skeletal parameters does not always correspond to an esthetically pleasing facial balance. The soft tissues covering the skeleton of the face can make dentoskeletal analysis an unreliable means of assessing facial harmony. (In other words, if the lips are not well balanced and closed at rest, facial dysmorphosis can be present even in the absence of dentoskeletal alterations.) According to Blanchette et al., the soft tissues have a tendency to mask discrepancies of the bone base (maxilla and mandible); thus, it is suggested that we find thinner soft tissues in subjects with a low-angle facial type and thicker soft tissues in those with a high-angle type.[36] This perhaps explains why Ferrario et al. found significant correlations between skeletal class and soft tissues[37] and why Burnstone et al. argued that no dentoskeletal standard can reliably predict the final esthetics of the face.[38]

The goal of an orthodontic treatment should be the achievement of good functional occlusion along with appealing dentofacial esthetics, maintaining the integrity of the dentoperiodontal tissues. Now several practitioners have started to focus on study of the face rather than the skeleton of the patient. Therefore, the transition has been from a diagnostic system, which can be defined as "centrifugal"—that is, it starts from the skeleton and goes outward—to a "centripetal" system, which instead begins with an analysis of the soft tissues to establish the corrections that are needed at the level of the hard tissues. Arnett and Bergman[39] and Ayala's[40] cephalometric analyses visually evaluated the facial contour of patients' soft tissue exclusively in a natural position, both frontal and lateral views, to arrive at a diagnosis and treatment plan.

Esthetic reference parameters in children

All the existing diagnostic systems based on the analysis of soft tissues are designed for use in adults, particularly candidates for orthognathic surgery. The purpose of this section is to propose a method of analysis for determining esthetic reference parameters reliable for the face of the child (in the different stages of their growth), which may, in turn, be useful for creating a clinical alternative to cephalometric analysis of the soft tissues. Moreover, this method could integrate and complement the usual cephalometric analysis, allowing the clinician to achieve not only esthetic facial harmony but also a good balance.

Holdaway, after analyzing the different methodologies used in different studies to evaluate the harmony of soft tissues in adults, selected reference parameters and data that should be useful and

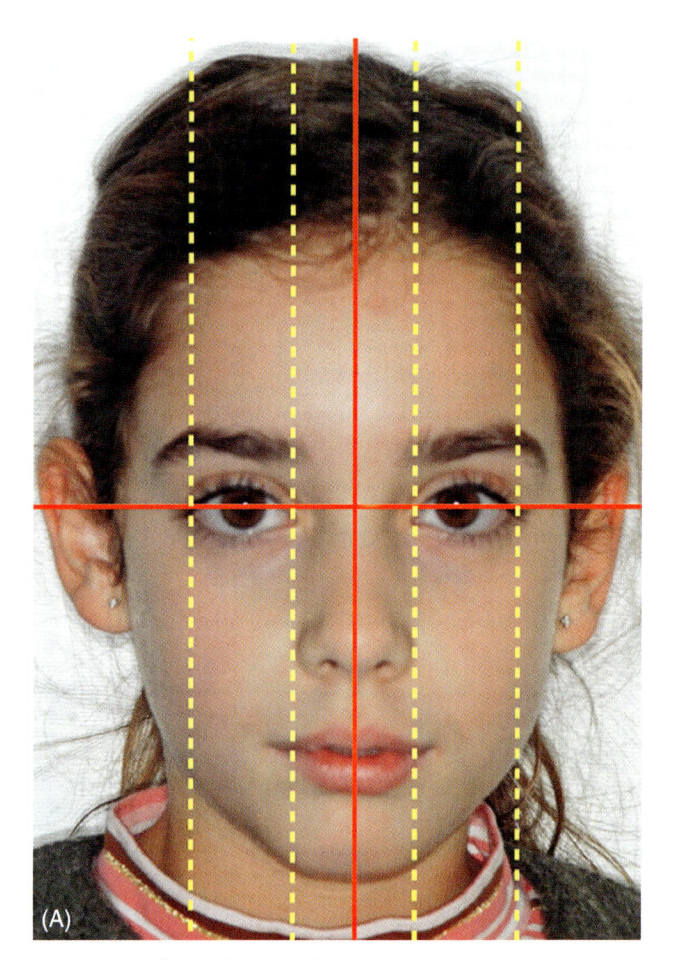

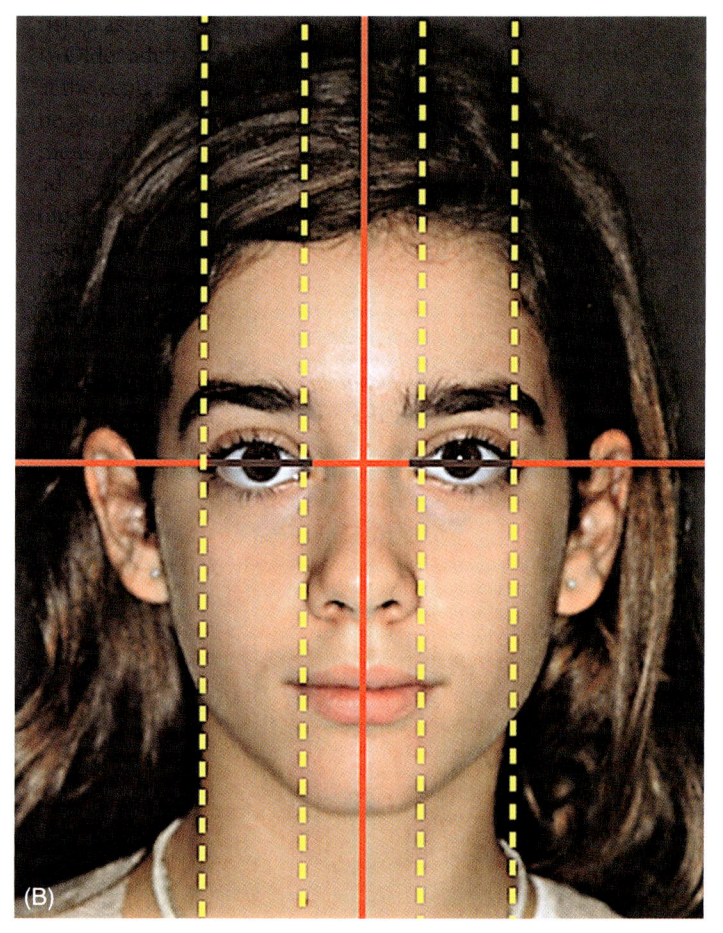

Figure 30.65 **(A, B)** These children's faces appear to be in perfect symmetry.

reliable when evaluating growing patients.[41,42] These parameters and data were subsequently modified to take into account patterns of craniofacial growth. At birth, for example, the splanchnocranium is considerably underdeveloped compared with the neurocranium. Furthermore, the mandible is the least developed part of the lower third of the face and, compared with the rest of the face, tends to grow more and for a longer period of time. Moreover, a precise growth sequence exists in both the maxilla and the mandible. This has been defined as the completion of growth in the three planes of space: growth is completed first in width, then in length, and then in height. The transverse growth of both bones (including the width of the dental arches) tends to be complete before the pubertal growth peak and is influenced little by growth variations occurring during adolescence.[37,43]

Sagittal growth of the two maxillae continues into puberty. In girls, it stops almost immediately, on average between 14 and 15 years of age. In boys, it does not usually stop before 18 years of age. In both sexes, vertical growth of the maxillae and face continues for longer than growth in length. In view of these considerations, canons of esthetic evaluation have been adapted to growing patients. The selected reference parameters are not able to predict linear measures as the growing patient, unlike the adult, cannot have fixed values.[27,43]

Frontal view: symmetry between different parts of the face

As in adults, the child's face (Figure 30.65) must show perfect symmetry, with the eyes, ears, and mandibular angles placed at the same height.

Correct distance between the eyes, nose, and lips

The 1 : 1 ratio between the width of the lips and the distance between the inside margins of the irises (Figure 30.66) remains valid. However, the child's nose base should be smaller than the intercanthal distance, as it will grow considerably.

Middle to lower facial third ratio

The parameters that are reliable in adults cannot be the same as those that are reliable in children (Figure 30.67). As previously stated, the neurocranium grows earlier than the splanchnocranium; therefore, the middle third of the face develops before the lower third. Accordingly, the lower third should be smaller than the middle and upper thirds. Indeed, when the lower third of the face develops earlier, it is a matter of particular concern, being indicative of excessive growth in a vertical direction. These considerations are inversely proportional to the patient's age.

Figure 30.66 Correct distances between the eyes, nose, and lips.

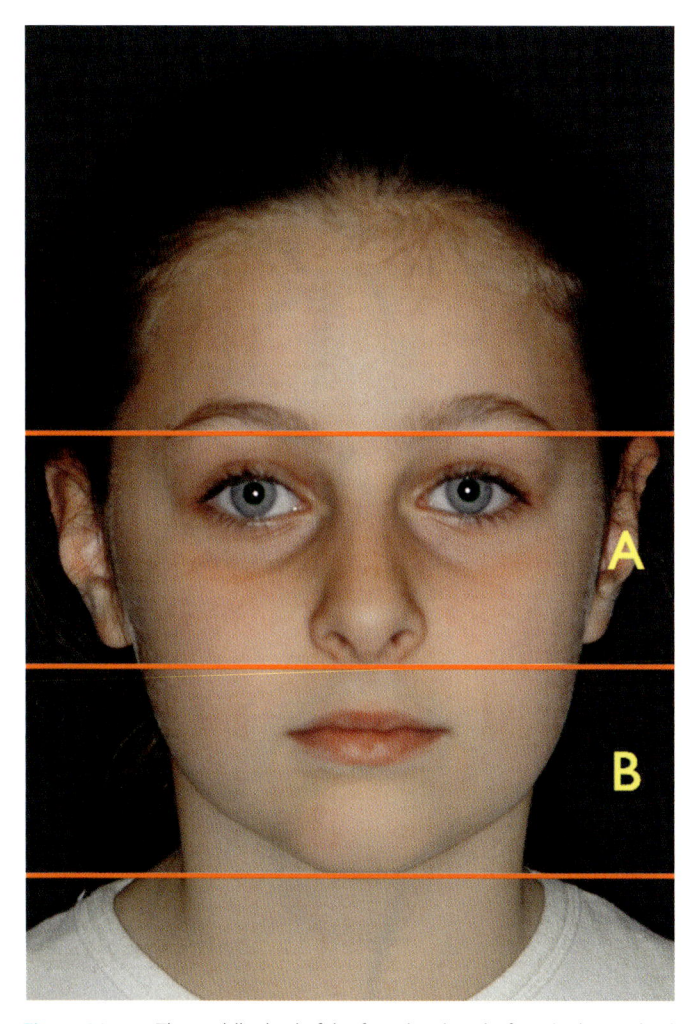

Figure 30.67 The middle third of the face develops before the lower third.

Ratio for esthetic balance

This is the division of the face by a symmetry line passing through the glabella, nasal tip, midpoint of the upper lip, midpoint of the chin, and suborbital line. The ideal trichion (Tr)–menton (Me)/zygion angle (ZA), the ZA ratio, which is 1.35 in the adult male and 1.3 in the adult female, should be lower in the adolescent, who will grow more vertically than widthwise (Figure 30.68). Therefore, the value will start from about 1 in younger subjects, increase gradually during growth, and ultimately reach normal (adult) reference values.

- Tr: the point of the hairline in the midline of the forehead. In early childhood, this landmark may be difficult to identify because of an irregular or indistinguishable hairline.
- ZA: the most lateral point of each zygomatic arch. It is identical to the bony zygion of the malar bone.
- Me (chin): the lowest median landmark on the lower border of the mandible.

Sclera exposure

Excessive exposure of sclera, the firm white fibrous membrane that forms the outer covering of the eyeball, implies a developmental deficit of the middle third of the face. If this sign is present and accompanied by other symptoms, such as oral breathing with a narrow pointed nose, reduced transverse diameters of the upper maxilla with crossbite, and, dentally, upper arch crowding with a tendency to cuspal inclusion, a skeletal Class III with maxillary hypoplasia is present.

Incisal exposure

In children, when teeth can be exfoliating or erupting, there are no reliable reference points for this parameter. However, if, when smiling, a considerable quantity of marginal gingiva is exposed, then excessive facial anterior vertical growth or excessive maxillary protrusion could be present.

Lip closure without tissue strain

Over time, all soft tissues tend to relax; therefore, it is acceptable for a young subject, compared with an adult, to have a slightly shorter upper lip and, hence, moderate lip incompetence. However, this should not persist beyond the age of 7–8 years.

Profile view considerations

Skeletal convexity from the zygomatic area to the interlabial gap

Because in children the lower facial third develops ahead of the middle third, children can be expected to have a more convex cheek profile than an adult (Figure 30.69).

It is to be noted that, in a child, a curve indicating a trend to high-angle mandibular growth is alarming.

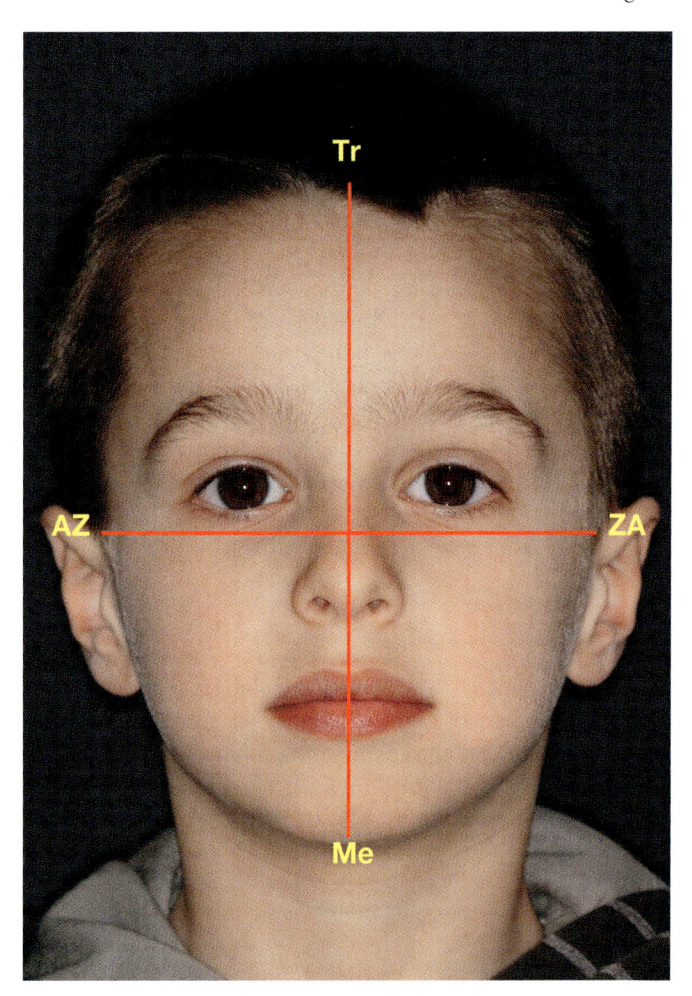

Figure 30.68 The ratio for esthetic balance.

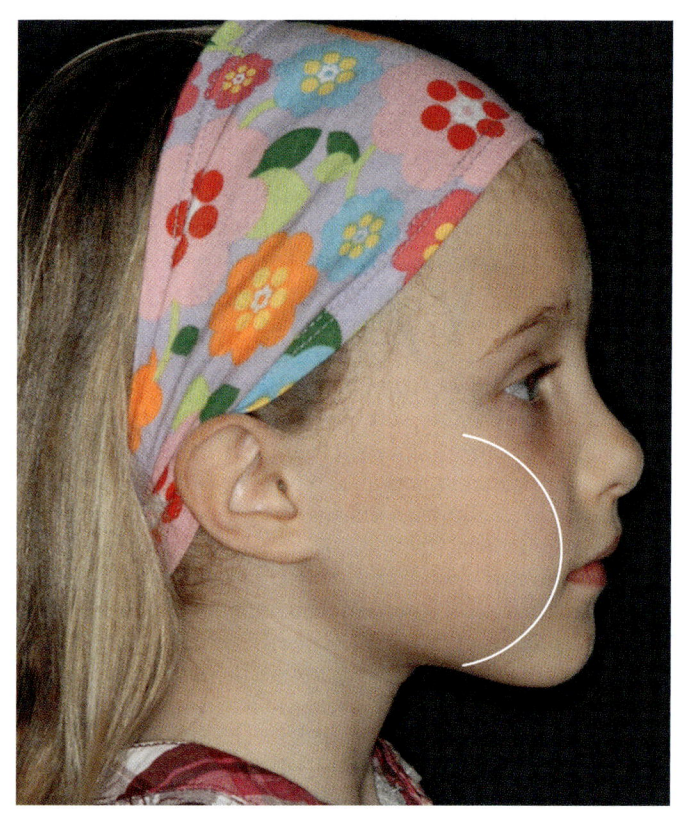

Figure 30.69 In children, the cheek profile is more convex than in adults.

Nose prominence

This is measured from the subnasal to the pronasal parts of the nose (i.e., from the point at which the columella merges with the upper lip in the midsagittal plane to the most prominent anterior point of the nose). This distance, which normally ranges from 16 to 20 mm in adults, will obviously be smaller in children (Figure 30.70). It is important to note that a prominent nose is generally a contraindication to extractive treatment.

The shape of the nose must also be considered. Indeed, the tip of the nose tends to move down and forward with growth. Therefore, it is obvious that a convex nose shape in a child will worsen considerably as they grow. Conversely, the prognosis is better in children with a concave or flat nose shape. In these cases, it is also very useful to observe the parents. In fact, the eyes and nose are the somatic features of the face that show the highest level of heredity.

An increased nasolabial angle must not be considered an absolute contraindication to a protocol of serial extractions, but only as one of the clinical factors to be taken into account when evaluating the case.

Lip curvature

Both the upper and lower lips must show a slight curvature, with concavity pushing forward. A very marked labiomental sulcus in a child may indicate a sagittal mandibular and maxillary vertical deficit, and thus that the child will have a low-angle facial type (Figure 30.71). Alternatively, the total absence or disappearance of this sulcus may indicate sagittal and vertical mandibular development involving both planes and, therefore, a high-angle facial type. High-angle subjects are able to camouflage dentoskeletal Class III components and low-angle subjects Class II components, improving the dental compensations that are present in such cases.

Nasolabial angle

The nasolabial angle can be more open in the child because the tip of the nose grows lower. Generally, in adults, soft tissues generally tend to relax and become less toned. For this reason, it is acceptable for a young patient to have a slightly short strained upper lip and a smile with up 3–4 mm of gingival exposure.

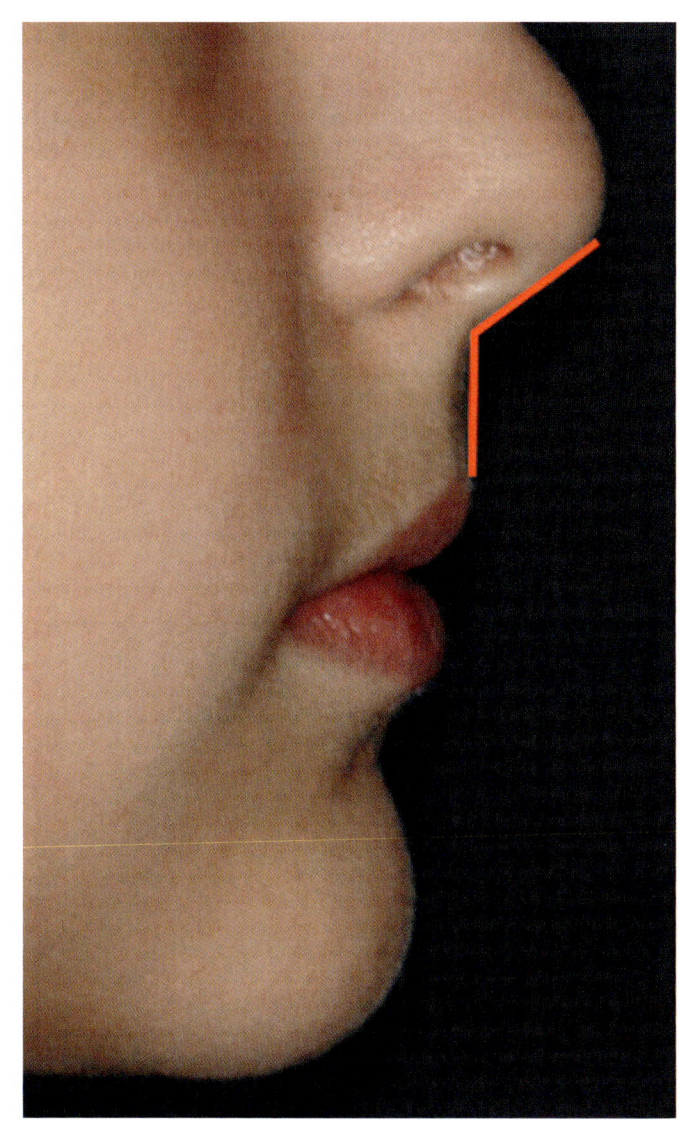

Figure 30.70 The nose prominence (subnasal–pronasal).

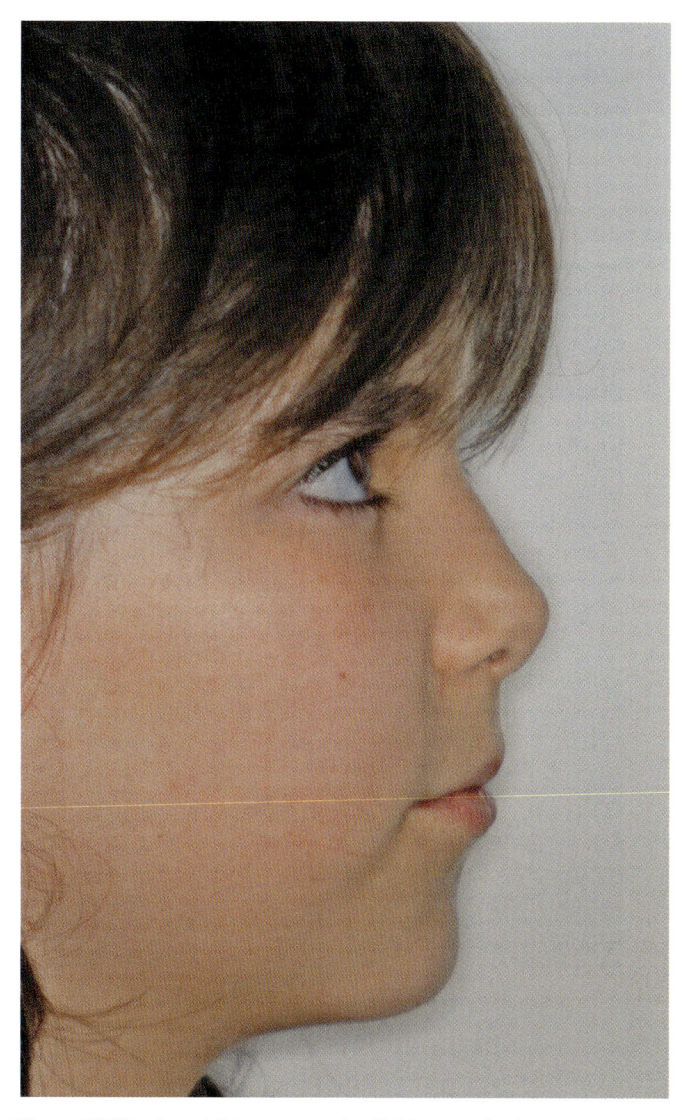

Figure 30.71 In a child, a very marked labiomental sulcus may indicate a sagittal mandibular and maxillary vertical deficit.

Correct ratio between the submental area and the lower facial third

This ratio, NTP–Gn/Sn–Gn, whose normal value in adults is about 0.8, will be higher in children even though the mandible still has to develop in length. There are two reasons for this: the lower third of the face will continue to develop in height and the chin–neck contour is modest in children. Therefore, the usual value in the young patient ranges between 1 and 1.2. Lower values indicate a hypomandible; conversely, higher values indicate a hypermandible.

- NTP, nose tip point.
- Gn, gnathion: a point corresponding to the midpoint between the anterior (pogonion) and inferior (menton) points of the bony chin.
- Sn: subnasal.

The skeletal type of the patient is also a factor to take into consideration. For example, a decrease in the normal value of this ratio in an obese child and an increase in an athletic, long-limbed child are to be expected.

The future

The esthetic measurements and treatments that are available and deemed reliable for adults cannot be considered so for children. There is a real need for new and reliable data that may provide the basis for reviewing and modifying the well-worn cliché of the ideal face (facial proportions) of the Caucasian population during growth. Existing esthetic analyses need to be adapted to growing patients in a way that takes into account the predictable craniofacial growth stages and processes.

Once we are familiar with the craniofacial growth mechanism and the different factors determining it, then it will be possible to reduce the need for orthopedic–orthodontic treatments. True esthetic orthodontics may, in combination with effective pediatric esthetic dentistry, become a protocol for obtaining true facial esthetics and balance.

As Goldstein proposed in the previous edition of *Esthetics in Dentistry*, esthetics is the fourth dimension of dentistry, along with biological, physiological, and mechanical dimensions. Esthetic balance is increasing in importance because, in the 21st century, there is greater cultural awareness of the keys to attractiveness of the face and smile and, in general, of physical appeal. Esthetic harmony is synonymous with skeletal, dental, and neuromuscular harmony and temporomandibular joint harmony.

The fundamental concept is that esthetics in pediatric dentistry lay the foundations of esthetics in adulthood and will thus become an area attracting growing interest in the decades ahead. In the setting of clinical pediatric dentistry, esthetic considerations are increasing in frequency and importance. The pedodontist must work in close cooperation with the orthodontist to apply correct preventive or early interceptive orthodontic and esthetic principles.[44] This close cooperation can reduce treatment times and costs and increase long-term stability because space management will also reduce the need for extractions. It is imperative to appreciate that esthetic harmony can boost psychological health and self-confidence, thereby improving an individual's interpersonal relationships.

References

1. Hiiri A, Ahovuo-Saloranta A, Nordblad A, Makela M. Pit and fissure sealants versus fluoride varnishes for preventing dental decay in children and adolescents. *Cochrane Database Syst Rev* 2006;(4):CD003067.
2. Karjalainen S. Eating patterns, diet and dental caries. *Dent Update* 2007;34(5):295–298, 300.
3. Olivi G, Genovese MD, Caprioglio C. Evidence-based dentistry on laser pediatric dentistry: review and outlook. *Eur J Paediatr Dent* 2009;10(1):29–40.
4. American Academy of Pediatric Dentistry Clinical Affairs Committee-Pulp Therapy Subcommittee; American Academy of Pediatric Dentistry Council on Clinical Affairs. Guideline on pulp therapy for primary and young permanent teeth. *Pediatr Dent* 2008–2009;30(7 Suppl):170–174.
5. Fuks AB. Pulp therapy for the primary dentition. In: Pinkham JR, Casamassimo PS, Fields HW Jr, et al., eds. *Pediatric Dentistry: Infancy through Adolesence*, 4th edn. St. Louis, MO: Elsevier Saunders; 2005:375–393.
6. Goldstein RE. *Change Your Smile*, 2nd rev. edn. Carol Stream, IL: Quintessence; 1988:22.
7. Burgess JO, Walker R, Davidson JM. Posterior resin-based composite: review of the literature. *Pediatr Dent* 2002;24(5):465–479.
8. Yengopal V, Harneker SY, Patel N, Siegfried N. Dental fillings for the treatment of caries in the primary dentition. *Cochrane Database Syst Rev* 2009;(2):CD004483.
9. Ribeiro CC, Baratieri LN, Perdigao J, et al. A clinical, radiographic, and scanning electron microscopic evaluation of adhesive restorations on carious dentin in primary teeth. *Quintessence Int* 1999;30(9):591–599.
10. Assis CP, Moyses MR, Teixeira HM, et al. Fatigue limits for composite restorations with and without glass ionomer cement liners. *Gen Dent* 2009;57(5):485–489; quiz 490–491, 535–536.
11. Christensen GJ. Why use resin cements? *J Am Dent Assoc* 2010;141:204–206.
12. Duque C, Negrini Tde C, Hebling J, Spolidorio DM. Inhibitory activity of glass-ionomer cements on cariogenic bacteria. *Oper Dent* 2005;30(5):636–640.
13. Wisithphrom K, Murray PE, About I, Windsor LJ. Interactions between cavity preparation and restoration events and their effects on pulp vitality. *Int J Periodontics Restorative Dent* 2006;26(6)596–605.
14. De Souza Costa CA, Teixeira HM, Lopes do Nascimento AB, Hebling J. Biocompatibility of resin-based dental materials applied as liners in deep cavities prepared in human teeth. *J Biomed Mater Res B Appl Biomater* 2007;81(1):175–184.
15. Keller U, Hibst R, Geurtsen W, et al. Erbium:YAG laser application in caries therapy. Evaluation of patient perception and acceptance. *J Dent* 1998;26(8):649–656.
16. Lynch E, Smith E, Baysan A, et al. Salivary oxidising activity of a novel anti-bacterial ozone-generating device. *J Dent Res* 2001;80:1178.
17. Hibst R. Lasers for caries removal and cavity preparation: state of the art and future directions. *J Oral Laser Appl* 2002;2:203–212.

18. Moritz A. *Oral Laser Application*. Berlin: Quintessence; 2006:258–277.
19. Martens LC. Laser-assisted pediatric dentistry: review and outlook. *J Oral Laser Appl* 2003;3(4):203–209.
20. Caprioglio C, Vitale MC. Pediatric dentistry. In: Caprioglio C, Vitale MC, eds. *Lasers in Dentistry: Practical Textbook*. Bologna: Martina; 2010:84–104.
21. De Grauwe A, Aps JK, Martens LC. Early childhood caries (ECC): what's in a name? *Eur J Pediatr Dent* 2004;5(2):62–70.
22. Guzman-Armstrong S. Rampant caries. *J Sch Nurs* 2005;21(5):272–278.
23. Caprioglio C. Pediatric dentistry in interceptive orthodontics. In: Caprioglio D, Levrini A, Lanteri C, et al., eds. *Interceptive Orthodontics*. English translation by C Caprioglio, A Caprioglio, R Spena. Bologna: Martina; 1999:97–107.
24. Andreasen JO, Andreasen FM, Andersson L. *Textbook and Colour Atlas of Traumatic Injuries to the Teeth*, 4th edn. Copenhagen: Munksgaard; 2007.
25. Caprioglio C, Caprioglio A. Dental trauma in children. In: Vitale MC, Caprioglio C, eds. *Lasers in Dentistry: Practical Textbook*. Bologna, Italy: Martina; 2010:105–138.
26. Soares F, Varella CH, Pileggi R, et al. Impact of Er,Cr:YSGG laser therapy on the cleanliness of the root canal walls of primary teeth. *J Endod* 2008;34(4):474–477.
27. Sarver DM. Principles of cosmetic dentistry in orthodontics: part 1. Shape and proportionality of anterior teeth. *Am J Orthod Dentofacial Orthop* 2004;126:749–753.
28. Caprioglio C. Lasers in dental traumatology. *Laser* 2010;2:12–18.
29. Weber JBB, Pinheiro ALB, Oliveira FAM, Ramalho LMP. Laser therapy improves healing of bone defects submitted to autologus bone graft. *Photomed Laser Surg* 2006;24:38–44.
30. Pinheiro ALB, Pozza DH, Oliveira MG, et al. Polarized light (400–2000 nm) and non-ablative laser (685 nm): a description of the wound healing process using immunohistochemical analysis. *Photomed Laser Surg* 2005;25:485–492.
31. Tunér J, Hode L. *Laser Therapy: Clinical Practice and Scientific Background*. Tallin: Prima Books AB; 2004.
32. Dostalova T, Jelinkova H, Koranda P, et al. Optical properties and surface structure comparison of tooth whitening using laser system and chemicals action agents. In: Rechmann P, Fried D, Henning T, eds. *Lasers in Dentistry IX*. Proceedings of SPIE 4950. Bellingham, WA: SPIE Press; 2003:37–45.
33. Pinkam JR, Casamassimo PS, Fields M, et al. *Pediatric Dentistry: Infancy Through Adolescence*. Philadelpha: WB Saunders; 1994.
34. Profitt W, Fields HW Jr, Ackerman J, et al. The etiology of orthodontic problems. In: *Contemporary Orthodontics*, 2nd edn. St. Louis, MO: Mosby; 2000:105–138.
35. American Academy of Pediatric Dentistry. Guideline on the management of the developing dentition and occlusion in pediatric dentistry. *Pediatr Dent* 2005–2006;27(7 Suppl):143–155.
36. Blanchette ME, Nanda RS, Currier FG, et al. A longitudinal cephalometric study of the soft tissue profile of short- and long-face syndromes from 7 to 17 years. *Am J Orthod Dentofac Orthop* 1996;109:116–131.
37. Ferrario VF, Sforza C, Serrao G. et al. Reliability of soft tissue references for anteroposterior measurement of dental bases. *Int J Adult Orthodon Orthognath Surg* 1998;13:210–216.
38. Burnstone CJ, James RB, Legan H. Cephalometrics for orthognathic surgery. *J Oral Surg* 1978;36:269–278.
39. Arnett WG, Bergman RT. Facial keys to orthodontic diagnosis and treatment planning. Part I. *Am J Orthod Dentofac Orthop* 1993;103:299–312.
40. Ayala M. Estetica facciale. In: *Atti congresso SIDO*, Roma, 2/12/99.
41. Holdaway RA. A soft-tissue cephalometric analysis and its use in orthodontic treatment planning. Part I. *Am J Orthod* 1983;84:1–28.
42. Holdaway RA. A soft-tissue cephalometric analysis and its use in orthodontic treatment planning. Part II. *Am J Orthod* 1983;88:279–293.
43. McNamara L, McNamara JA, Ackerman MB, Baccetti T. Hard and soft tissue contributions to the esthetics of the posed smile in growing patients seeking orthodontic treatment. *Am J Orthod Dentofacial Orthop* 2008;133:491–499.
44. Sabri R. The eight components of a balanced smile. *J Clin Orthod* 2005;39:155–167.

Additional resources

Ackermann MB, Ackermann JL. Smile analysis and design in the digital era. *J Clin Orthod* 2002;34:221–234.

Andreasen JO, Andreasen FM. *Textbook and Colour Atlas of Traumatic Injuries to the Teeth*, 3rd edn. Copenhagen: Munskgaard; 1994.

Bass NM. The esthetic analysis of the face. *Eur J Orthod* 1991;13:343–350.

Berkman MD, Goldsmith D, Rothschild D. Evaluation–diagnosis–planning. The challenge in the correction of dentofacial deformities. *J Clin Orthod* 1979;13:526–538.

Cameron AC, Widmer RP, eds. *Handbook of Pediatric Dentistry*. London: Mosby-Wolfe; 1997.

Caprioglio C, Olivi G, Genovese MD. Pediatric laser-assisted dentistry: a clinical approach. *Laser* 2011;1:8–15.

De Moor RJ, Delmé K. Laser-assisted cavity preparation and adhesion to erbium-lased tooth structure: part 1. Laser-assisted cavity preparation. *J Adhes Dent* 2009;11:427–438.

De Moor RJ, Delmé K. Laser-assisted cavity preparation and adhesion to erbium-lased tooth structure: part 2. Present-day adhesion to erbium-lased tooth structure in permanent teeth. *J Adhes Dent* 2010;12:91–102.

Flores MT, Andreasen JO, Bakland LK, et al. Guidelines for the evaluation and management of traumatic dental injuries. *Dent Traumatol* 2001;17:1–4.

Glendor U. Epidemiology of traumatic dental injuries—a 12 year review of the literature. *Dent Traumatol* 2008;24(6):603–611.

Goldstein RE. *Esthetics in Dentistry*. Philadelphia: JB Lippincott, 1976.

Goldstein RE, Parkins FM. Air-abrasive technology: its new role in restorative dentistry. *J Am Dent Assoc* 1994;125:551–557.

Harris R, Nicoll AD, Adair PM, Pine CM. Risk factors for dental caries in young children: a systematic review of the literature. *Community Dent Health* 2004;21(1 Suppl):71–85.

Holan G, Eidelman E, Fuks AB. Long-term evaluation of pulpotomy in primary molars using mineral trioxide aggregate or formocresol. *Pediatr Dent* 2005;27(2):129–136.

Kitchens DH. The economics of pit and fissure sealants in preventive dentistry: a review. *J Contemp Dent Pract* 2005;6(3):95–103.

McDonald RE. *Dentistry for the Child and Adolescent*. Mosby; 1982.

Olivi G, Genovese MD. Effect of Er:YAG laser on enamel: SEM observations. *J Oral Laser Appl* 2007;7(1):27–35.

Overloop K, Blum R, Verheyen P. Esthetic dentistry with smart bleach: an overview of clinical cases. *J Oral Laser Appl* 2001;(2):129–134.

Park YC, Burstone CJ. Soft-tissue profile—fallacies of hard-tissue standards in treatment planning. *Am J Orthod Dentofac Orthop* 1986;90:52–62.

Queimat MA, Barrieshi-Nusair KM, Owais AI. Calcium hydroxide vs mineral trioxide aggregates for a partial pulpotomy of permanent molars with deep caries. *Eur Arch Paediatr Dent* 2007;8(2):99–104.

Sarver DM. The importance of incisor positioning in the esthetic smile: the smile arc. *Am J Orthod Dentofacial Orthop* 2001;120:98–111.

Sarver DM, Ackermann MB. Dynamic smile visualization and quantification: part 1. Evolution of the concept and dynamic records of smile capture. *Am J Orthod Dentofacial Orthop* 2003;124:4–12.

Sarver DM, Ackermann MB. Dynamic smile visualization and quantification: part 2. Smile analysis and treatment strategies. *Am J Orthod Dentofacial Orthop* 2003;124:116–127.

Smallridge J. UK National Clinical Guidelines in Paediatric Dentistry. Use of fissure sealants including management of the stained fissure in first permanent molars. *Int J Paediatr Dent* 2010. doi: 10.1111/j.1365-263X.2009.01035.x.

Staele HJ, Koch MJ. *Kinder und Jugendzahn heilkunde*. Köln: Ärzte-Verlag Grubtl; 1996.

Steiner CC. Cephalometrics in clinical practice. *Angle Orthod* 1959;29:8–29.

Tweed CH. Indications for the extraction of teeth in orthodontic procedure. *Am J Orthod Oral Surg* 1944–1945;42:22–45.

Wylie GA, Fish LC, Epker BN. Cephalometrics: a comparison of five analyses currently used in the diagnosis of dentofacial deformities. *Int J Adult Orthodon Orthognath Surg* 1987;2:15–36.

Worms FW, Spiedel TM, Bevis RR, Waite DE. Post-treatment stability and esthetics of orthognathic surgery. *Angle Orthod* 1980;50:251–273.

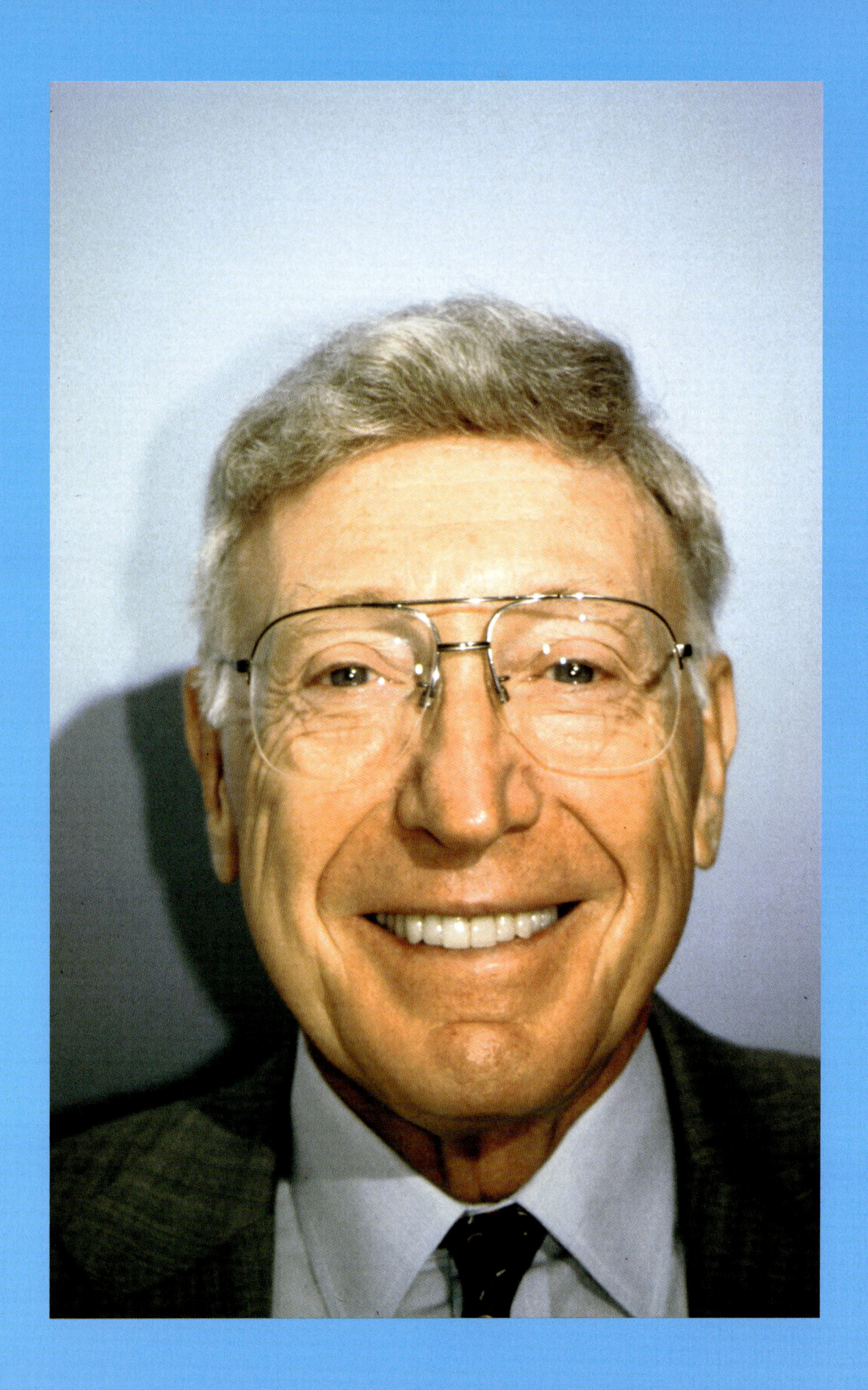

Chapter 31 Geresthetics: Esthetic Dentistry for Older Adults

Linda C. Niessen, DMD, MPH, MPP, Ronald E. Goldstein, DDS, and Maha El-Sayed, BDS, DMD, MS

Chapter Outline

Demographics: an aging population	1015
From baby boomers to baby zoomers	1016
The mature esthetic dental consumer	1017
Chronic illness and esthetic dental care	1020
Medical/dental history and oral examination	1022
Prevention and risk assessment	1023
Maintaining oral health in older patients	1023
Caries management by risk assessment	1024
Treatment planning in the older patient	1024
Managing other chronic illness and sequencing of procedures	1024
Imaging in decision-making process	1025
Financing	1025
Esthetic dental consultation and facial surgery	1025
Esthetic dental procedures for older adults	1025
Vital tooth bleaching	1025
Cosmetic contouring and bonding	1025
Orthodontics	1029
Periodontal therapy	1029
Laser-assisted new attachment procedure	1029
Prosthodontics, endodontics, and implants	1030
The nursing-home or assisted-living resident	1036

How old would you be, if you didn't know how old you are?

(Satche Paige)

In 2011, the world's population reached 7 billion. While the world's population has exploded in the past 50 years, birthrates are not up, longevity is. As life expectancy increases, a global aging boom is occurring. This aging trend is transforming patient populations in dental offices throughout the world. Older adults, like their middle-age children, want to look and feel their best. More and more are recognizing that they are not healthy without good oral health and they want to benefit from all the advances dentistry has to offer. This chapter discusses the esthetic oral health needs of older adults. It reviews the demographics of a global aging society and the expectations they bring to the dental office. It discusses the effects of systemic illnesses on oral health, the importance of prevention at any age, and the diagnosis and treatment planning when providing esthetic dental services to older adults.

Demographics: an aging population

The world is aging. Today, the population ≥60 years old is estimated to be 680 million, or 11% of the world's population. By 2050, this number is expected to grow to 2 billion, or 22% of the world's population.[1] The populations of both Europe and Japan are predicted to remain the oldest populations in the world. Although China and India have a lower percentage of their population over age 60, the size of their older population is growing rapidly and reflects more older adults than in the United States. Table 31.1 lists a sample of countries and the percentage of their populations over age 65.[1] Germany and Japan lead the world, with over 20% of their population over age 65 years, compared with only 13% in the United States (or 35 million people). By 2030, this percentage is expected to increase to 20% in the United States. South America and Africa have a far lower percentage of older adults, but these countries are seeing their populations age as well.

In 1900, the average life expectancy in the United States was 47.3 years. By the year 2010, the average life expectancy at birth had increased to 78 years.[2] The increasing life expectancy at birth has resulted from improved infection control, public health advances, and improvements in medical and surgical treatment. Healthier lifestyles and improved medical care are enabling those reaching age 65 to live even longer. Table 31.2 lists the remaining life expectancies for United States' adults aged 65 and older by gender and race.[2] For each age group until 85 years old, women outlive men and white Americans outlive African Americans. For the groups ages 85 and older, the trends reverse and African American men and women live longer than their white counterparts. At age 65, American adults can expect to live on average 19.3 years, or about 20% of their lives, in the retirement years. Regardless of age, adults want to make the most of their remaining years.

Goldstein demonstrated the benefits of esthetic dentistry as an important health service in a paper over two decades ago.[3] Goldstein and Niessen later expanded that concept to identify important benefits and issues to consider when providing esthetic dentistry for older adults.[4] Since that time, esthetic dentistry has become a well-accepted part of dental care. Adults of all ages have experienced the benefits that esthetic dental services can provide to their overall health. The older adult in Figure 31.1A–O benefited from extensive esthetic dental treatment, including orthodontia.

From baby boomers to baby zoomers

Individuals born between 1946 and 1964 (known as the baby boomers in the United States) are fueling concern about aging in the United States. This group, comprised of 76 million people in the United States, represents almost 30% of the US population.[5] In 2011, the first of the baby boomers reached age 65. These baby boomers are redefining what it means to be old. If you frequent a health club, spa, or ski resort these days you are likely to be a part of this group, causing some to rename them from the "baby boomers" to the "baby zoomers." Perhaps more significant than their sheer numbers, is their educational

Table 31.1 Aging Throughout the World

Country	Estimated Population >65 Years in 2017 (%)
Australia	16.1
Canada	18.3
China	10.8
Costa Rica	7.8
Germany	22.1
India	6.2
Japan	27.9
Mexico	7.0
Peru	7.4
Russia	14.3
Sweden	20.1
Ukraine	16.3
United Kingdom	18.0
United States	15.6
Uruguay	14.3

Source: Adapted from CIA World Factbook.[1]

Table 31.2 Remaining Life Expectancies: Adults Aged 65 Years and Older in the United States

Age in 2012 (Years)	Total (Years)	White (Years)		African American (Years)	
		Male	Female	Male	Female
65	19.3	17.9	20.5	16.2	19.5
70	15.6	14.4	16.5	13.2	15.9
75	12.2	11.2	12.9	10.4	12.6
80	9.1	8.3	9.7	8.0	9.3
85	6.6	5.9	6.9	6.0	7.2
90	4.6	4.1	4.8	4.5	5.2
95	3.2	2.8	3.3	3.5	3.8
100	2.3	2.0	2.3	2.6	2.8

Source: US National Center of Health Statistics.[2]

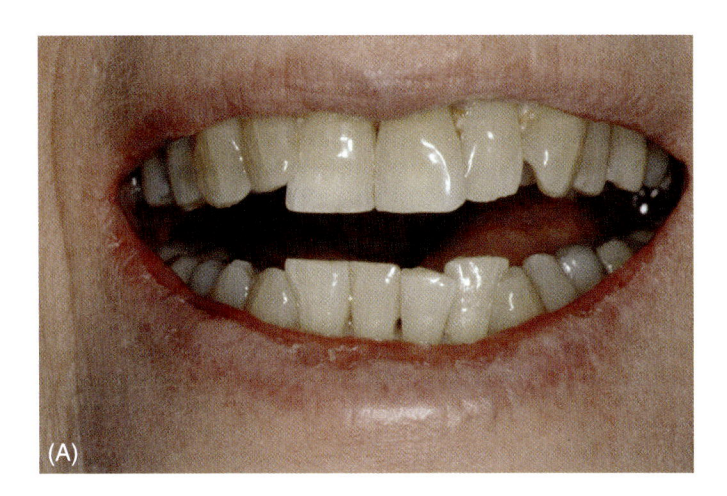

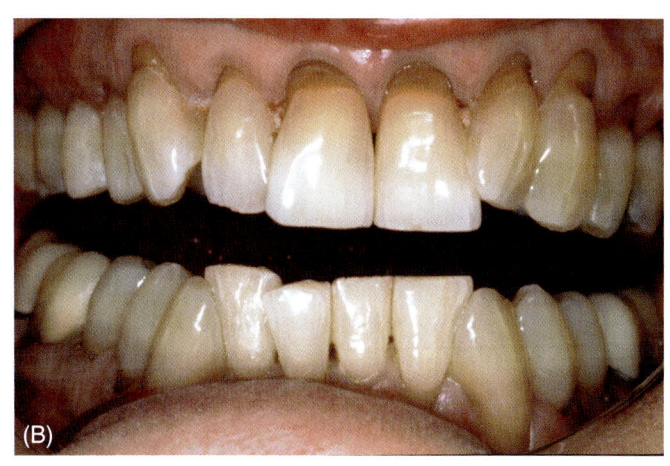

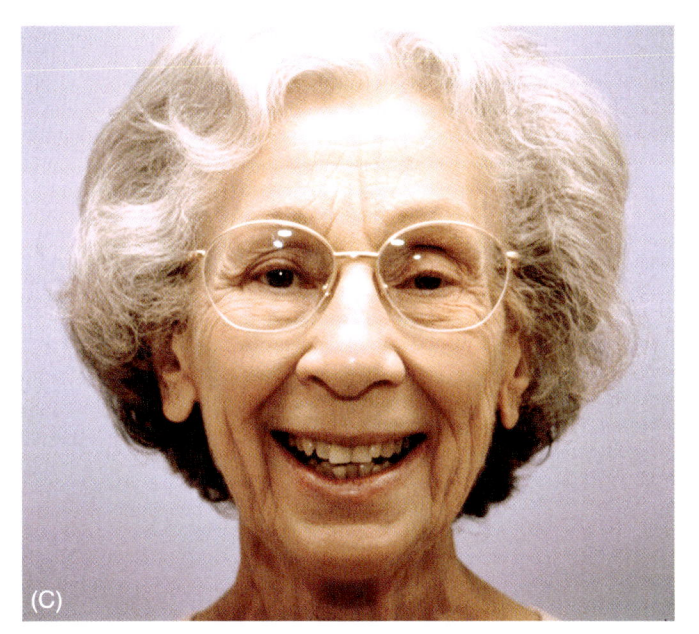

Figure 31.1 (A–C) This 76-year-old lady presented for treatment after a lifetime of dissatisfaction with her crowded teeth.

attainment. Twenty-five percent of this group has a college education. They are demanding, service-oriented, and expect high quality in their goods and services. In addition, they expect to look their best and are working hard to defy the aging process.

From a dental perspective, the baby boom generation represents the first to have benefited from widespread community water fluoridation and preventive dentistry programs. As adults, they are the first group to benefit from widespread workplace dental insurance. This combination of preventive services as children and dental care as adults is resulting in their being the first generation to reach 65 years old with a virtually intact natural dentition.[6] Unfortunately, most are not aware that their health insurance coverage will shift to Medicare when they retire, and they will likely lose their dental insurance benefits. Only select Medicare Advantage programs provide dental care as part of their insurance coverage. Recently, the American Association of Retired Persons has begun to sell an individual dental insurance policy, available when an employee retires or loses workplace dental insurance.

The mature esthetic dental consumer

Today's baby boomers and their parents have experienced the benefits of esthetic dentistry in their lives. They have straightened, whitened, and bonded their teeth as adults. It is anticipated that they will continue to invest in themselves. Their oral health goals will include keeping their teeth healthy, attractive, and functioning. Additionally, they will want to erase the effects of aging on their dentitions to improve their appearance.

Our colleagues in the marketing arena have described baby boomers as "the new health care consumers." These new health care consumers are characterized as more aggressive, demanding, and self-directed in their health care. They use the internet for health information, and are rapidly becoming consumers of social media, joining Facebook and Twitter to stay informed as well as connected with friends and family. The internet has leveled the information playing field, so to speak, between health professionals and consumers. With virtually all professional journals now online, health professionals and consumers can

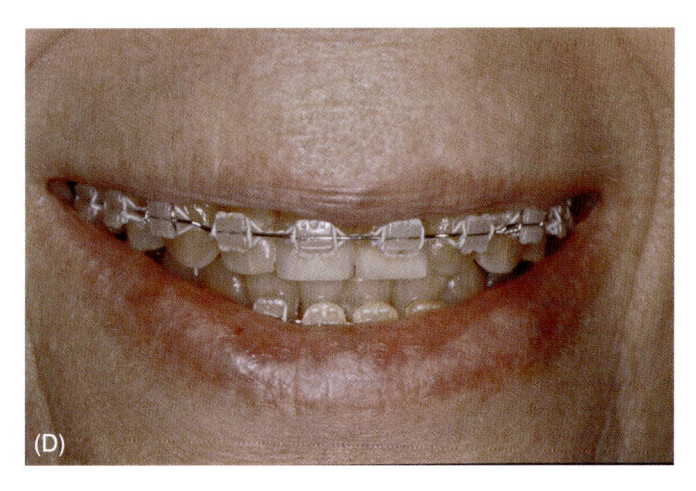

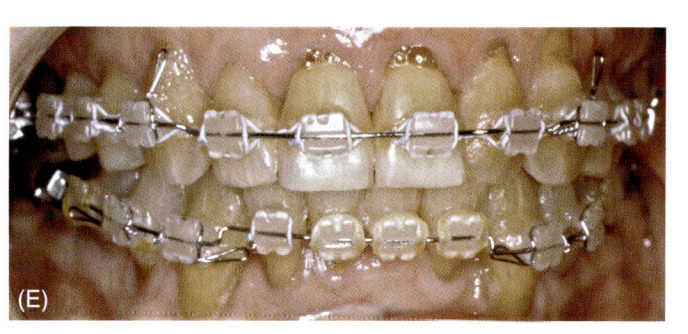

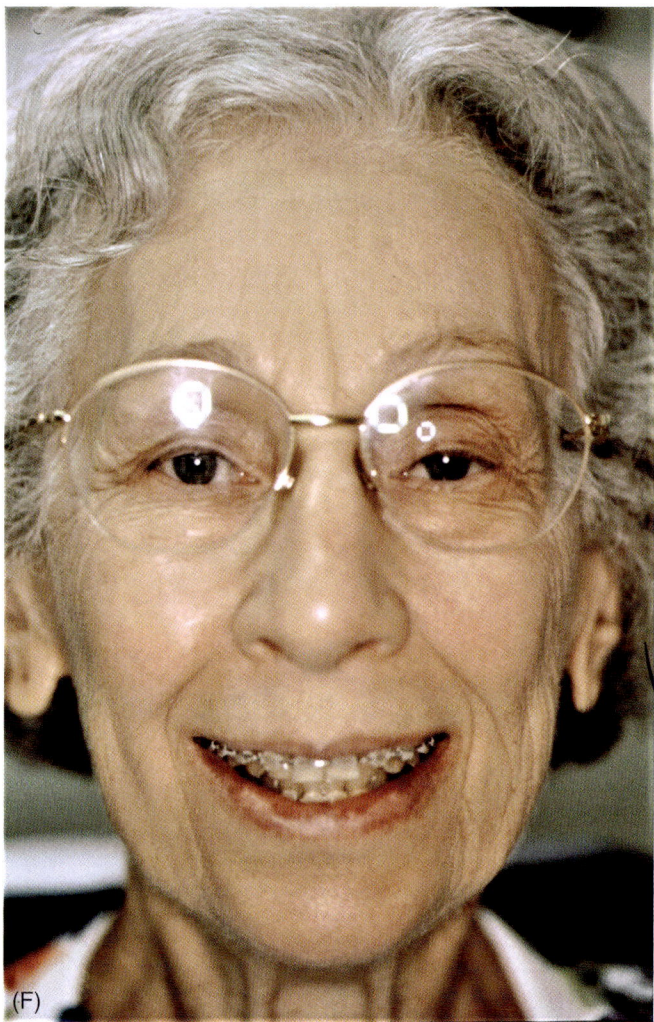

Figure 31.1 (D–F) Tooth-colored brackets were applied because their esthetic appearance gave the patient the confidence to smile during treatment.

be informed about new scientific advances simultaneously. In addition to online health journals, new internet health sites are added every day that serve as a source of health information, treatment options, and clinical trial sites. Chat rooms and blogs with consumers having various health conditions have developed and provide general information and support. Websites are now evaluating dentists or offering coupons for dental services. The internet will continue to expand its role as an intermediary between patients and health professionals for information and access to care, including dental care. While the internet is expanding access to health information, research continues to demonstrate the linkages between oral diseases and systemic

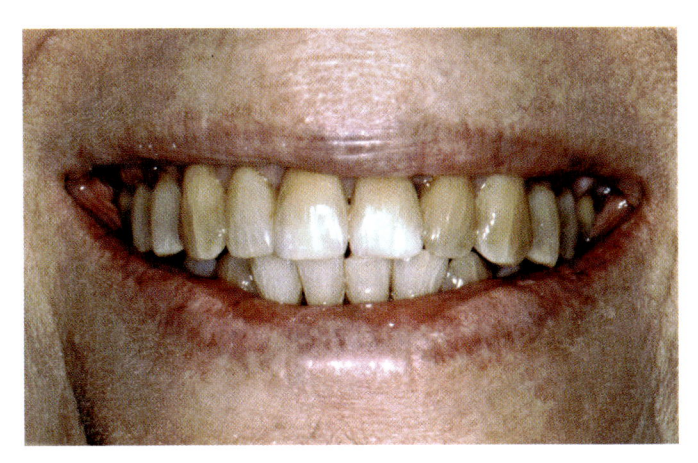

Figure 31.1 (G) After the removal of the orthodontic appliances, the teeth are much straighter but still discolored.

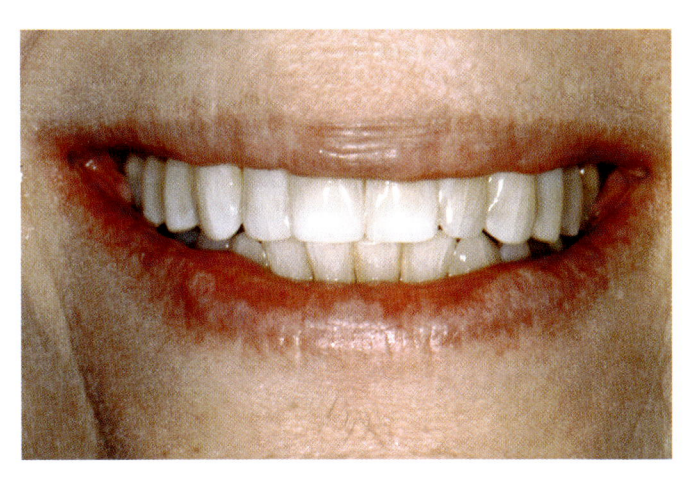

Figure 31.1 (H) After restorative treatment featuring tooth-colored restorations and bleaching, the patient has the smile she has always wanted.

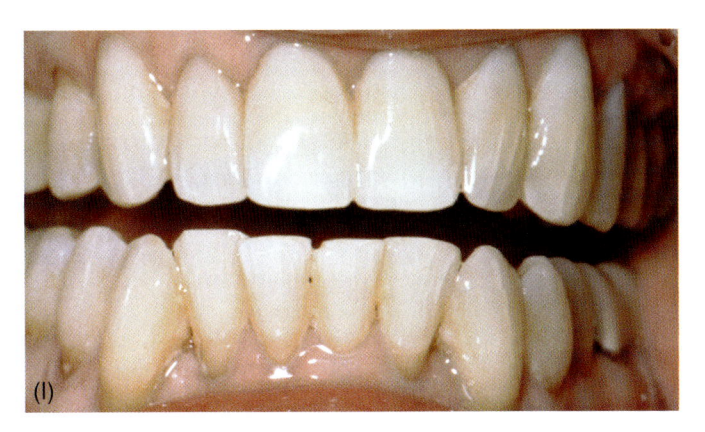

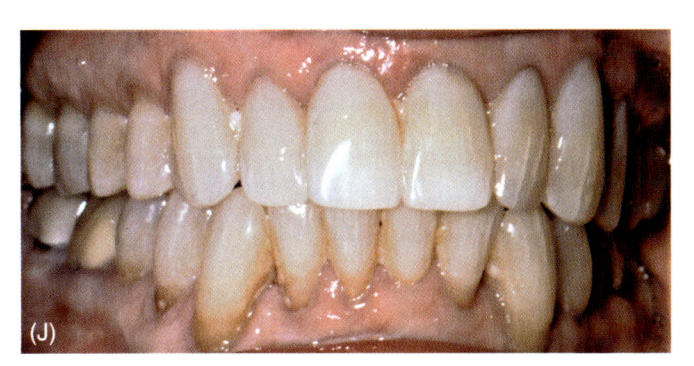

Figure 31.1 (I, J) Note that the formally eroded cervical areas have better contour and will deflect food particles better.

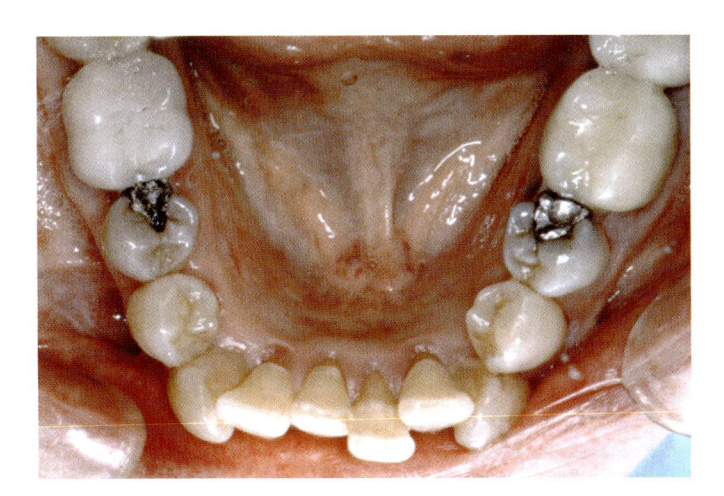

Figure 31.1 (K) Note the crowding of the mandibular anterior teeth.

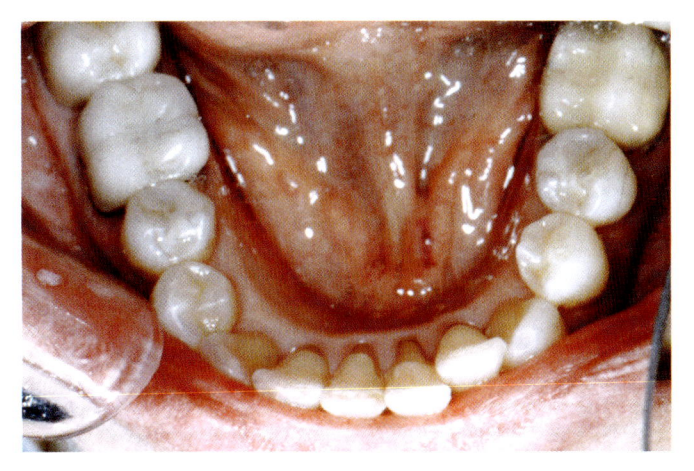

Figure 31.1 (L) The teeth are less crowded, and the new tooth-colored restorations have been placed.

illnesses, most notably the link between periodontal disease and cardiovascular disease and stroke.[7,8] The Surgeon General's Report on Oral Health, *Oral Health in America*, reinforces the message that general health and oral health are related.[6]

Older adults understand better than younger adults that dental health is more than just healthy teeth. It is also the ability to speak, smile, chew, and swallow comfortably. Dental health has become oral health. Patients who receive esthetic dental services readily appreciate this concept of oral health. The ability to smile confidently and the improved self-esteem will continue to drive the demand for esthetic dental services by older adults, particularly as baby boomers age.

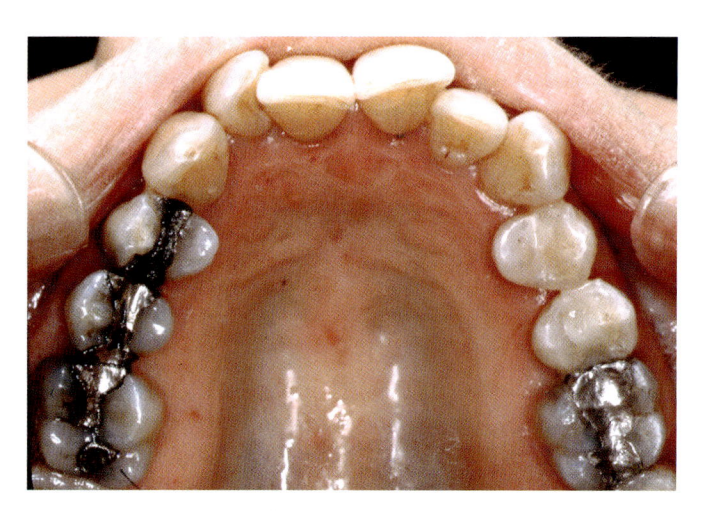

Figure 31.1 (M) The maxillary arch shows anterior crowding and defective amalgam restorations.

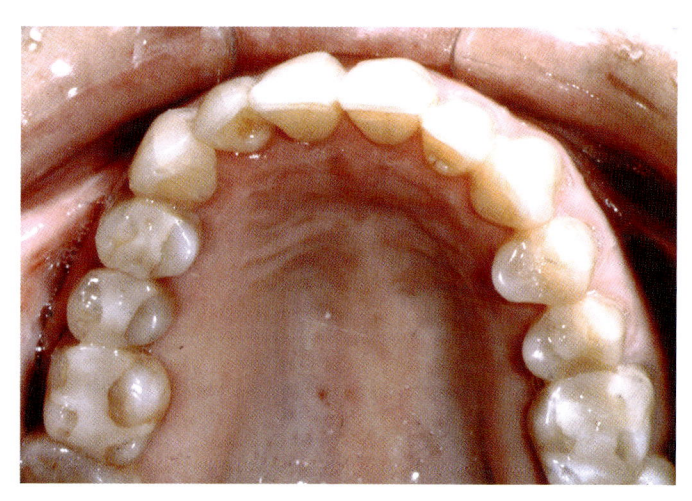

Figure 31.1 (N) Following 12 months of orthodontic treatment, the patient's amalgam restorations were replaced with posterior composite resin.

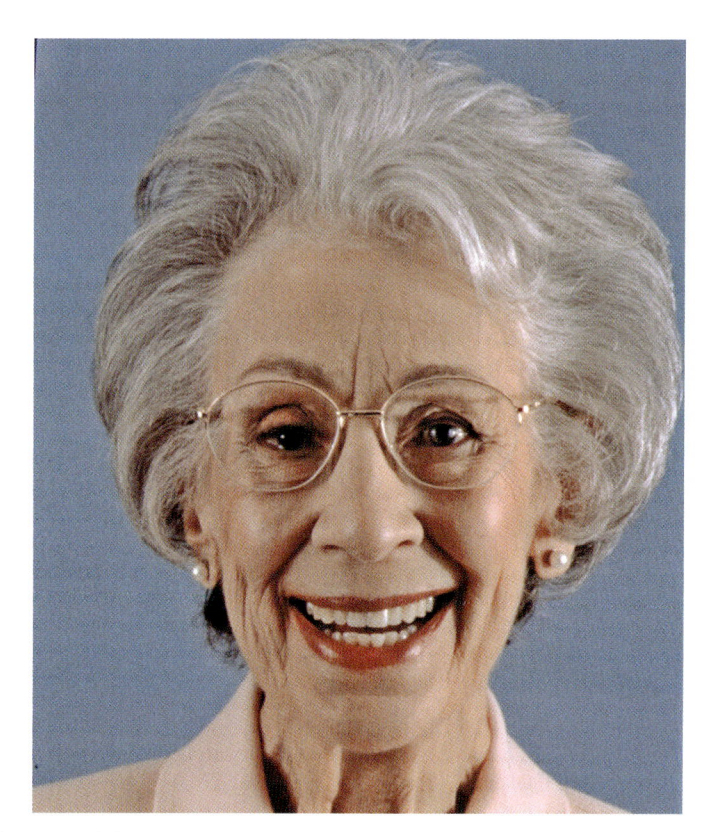

Figure 31.1 (O) Interdisciplinary therapy including orthodontics, periodontics, and restorative dentistry combined to produce this attractive result 2 years following the initiation of treatment in this now younger looking 78-year-old lady.

Data in the United States show an increased use of esthetic services by older adults.[10] Plastic surgery has become less expensive and more readily available for adults of all ages, and dental treatment has become a routine part of facial plastic surgery. Individuals who may be contemplating plastic surgery, such as facelifts, liposuction, or laser skin resurfacing, are also contemplating a smile makeover (tooth whitening to eliminate darkened teeth, crowns or veneers to correct shortened clinical crowns, and/or orthodontics to correct malpositioned teeth) as part of their plastic surgery options. This smile makeover, or "instant facelift" as it is being called, may last 20–25 years, unlike the plastic surgery changes that may last for only 5–10 years.

Chronic illness and esthetic dental care

With aging comes an increase in chronic diseases. Middle-age adults, nicknamed the "sandwich generation," are finding themselves caring for their adolescent children and aging parents. As one reaches the eighth and ninth decades of life, maintaining

Clinical case 31.1: A 57-year-old patient with "ugly smile" receives orthodontics and composite resin bonding

This 57-year-old patient's chief complaint was she had an "ugly smile." Her bruxing had worn away the enamel, shortened her teeth, and decreased her vertical dimension, resulting in an aging appearance. Her treatment plan consisted of full mouth reconstruction to restore her vertical dimension with posterior maxillary and mandibular crowns. Conservative composite resin bonding restored the anterior teeth. As a result of her exceptional home care, she maintained her dental health for 24 years until she died at 80 (Figure 31.2A–H).

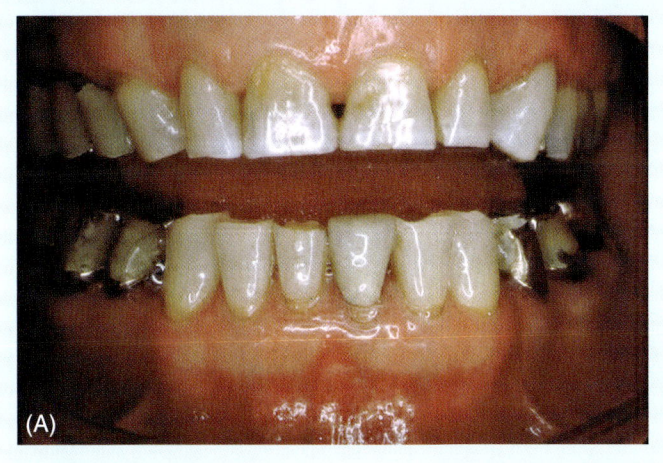

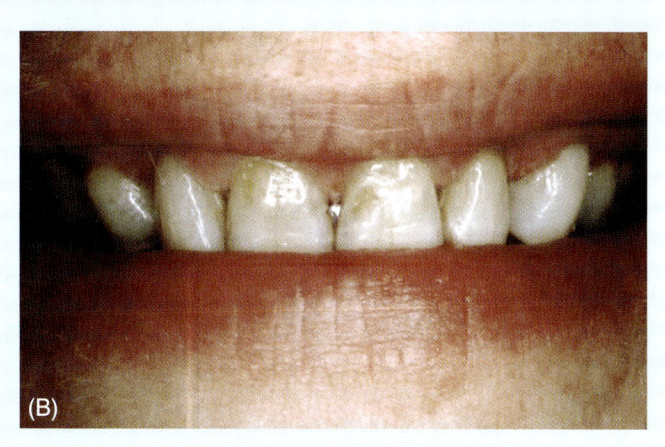

Figure 31.2 **(A, B)** This 57-year-old woman had worn down her posterior teeth so much that she was traumatizing the anterior teeth, which had also worn considerably.

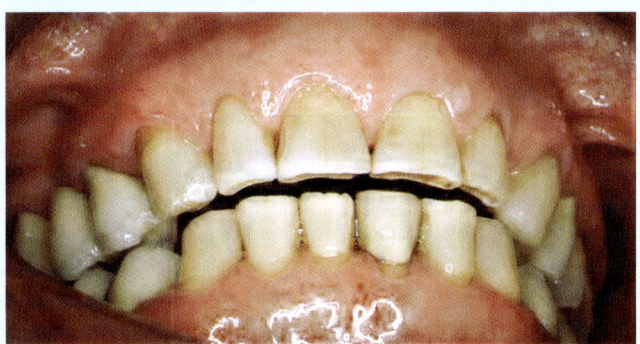

Figure 31.2 **(C)** Treatment crowns to restore vertical dimension were constructed for the patient to wear to determine if she would tolerate the new occlusal position.

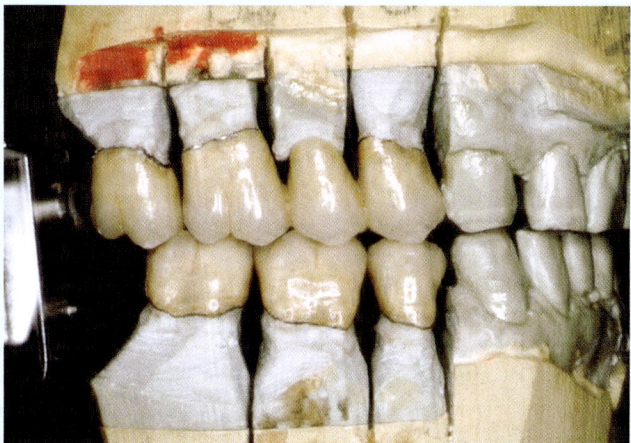

Figure 31.2 **(D)** After three comfortable months of wearing temporary crowns with an increased vertical dimension, final metal-ceramic crowns were constructed for the posterior teeth.

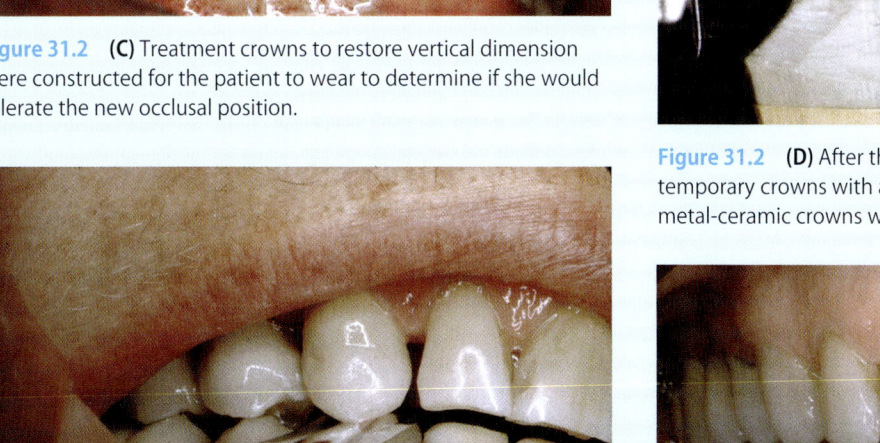

Figure 31.2 **(E)** Artus strips (5/10,000 inch thick) were used to make sure the occlusion was perfect. Note sufficient open space for composite resin bonding to be able to lengthen the maxillary anterior teeth.

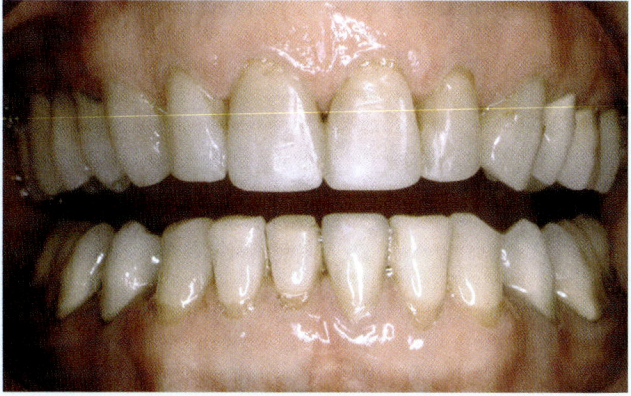

Figure 31.2 **(F)** The maxillary anterior teeth were next bonded with a hybrid composite resin. Note the increased length.

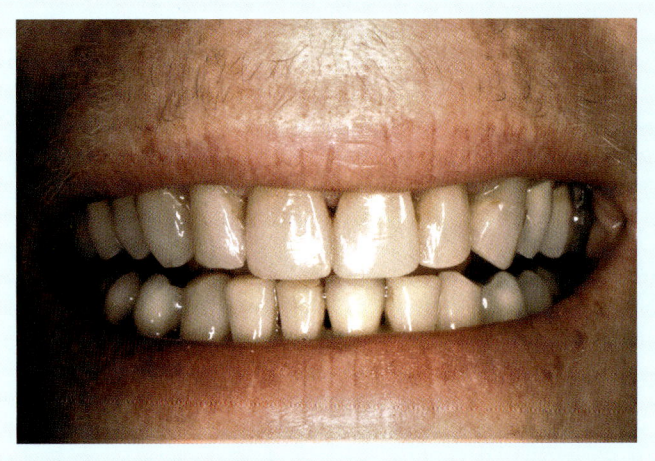

Figure 31.2 **(G)** The final smile helped to create a younger-looking smile line, which lasted for 24 years due in part to the exceptional home care performed by the patient.

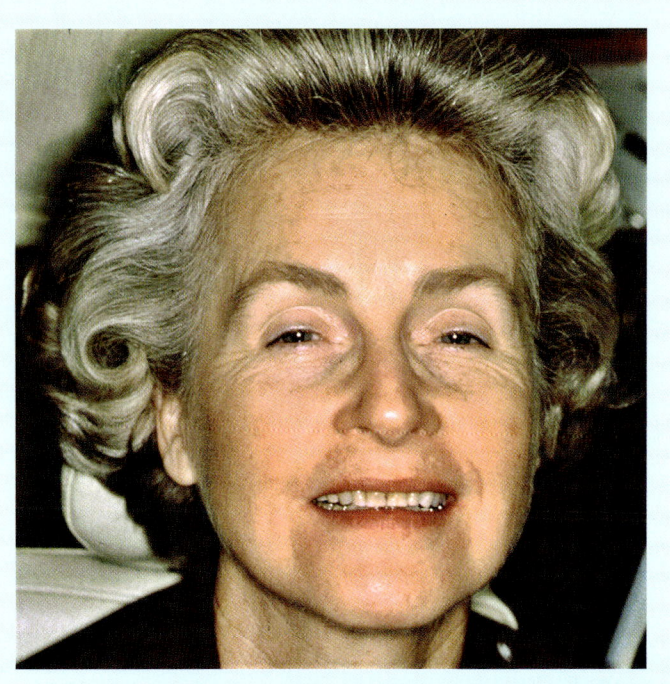

Figure 31.2 **(H)** The combined approach of posterior crowns and anterior bonding greatly improved this patient's smile, her appearance, and self-confidence. Reproduced with permission from Quintessence Publishers.[9]

Table 31.3 Most Common Chronic Conditions in Older Adults

All Ages	Age ≥75 Years
Sinusitis	Arthritis or other musculoskeletal
Arthritis	Heart or circulatory
Orthopedic	Diabetes
Impairments	Vision
Hypertension	Lung
Hay fever	Hearing impairments

Source: Adapted from Centers for Disease Control, National Center for Health Statistics[11] and Summer[12] (based on National Academy on an Aging Society analysis).

oral health in the face of multiple chronic diseases and declining health may become a greater challenge.

Table 31.3 lists the common chronic conditions for individuals of all ages and for those age 75 and older.[11,12] Whereas arthritis affects 28% of 45–74-year-olds, it affects over 50% of adults over age 65.[13] Although these chronic conditions may occur in middle age, they may not cause disability or limitation of activities until over age 65. Data from the National Health Interview Survey in the United States found that 34% of 65–74-year-olds and 45% of those 75 and over reported some limitation in activities because of chronic conditions.[11,12]

Older adults who visit their dentist may be taking a variety of medications for these various chronic conditions. Thus, the recording and interpreting of the medical history and medication history will often require more time in older adults. These chronic illnesses may also necessitate more frequent consultations with the patient's physicians. Patients with cardiac conditions, orthopedic problems, or on anticoagulation therapy are just a few of the examples of systemic illness for which a physician consultation may be warranted. These systemic conditions may make maintaining any esthetic dentistry more difficult. Patients should be advised that their systemic conditions could affect their oral health.

Even the best dentistry can break down quickly in the absence of oral hygiene self-care and the presence of multiple risk factors, such as dry mouth (xerostomia) and a highly refined carbohydrate diet. Patients undergoing esthetic dental services who are about to enter a nursing home or assisted-living facility should be assessed for factors that will increase their risk of oral diseases, such as dementia, stroke (which may cause the loss of ability to use the dominant hand), or medications that cause dry mouth. Once these risk factors are identified, aggressive preventive therapies must be initiated to avoid dental diseases and breakdown of previous dental work.

Medical/dental history and oral examination

The history and physical examination for older adults will clearly require more time and result in more positive findings than for younger adults. In addition to the routine esthetic questions, it is important to ask each patient what their personal goals are for oral health. Does the patient expect to lose any teeth to caries or periodontal disease? Is the patient willing to implement preventive measures to avoid tooth loss? These questions will assist the dental team in understanding the patient's plans and expectations for oral health and whether such plans and expectations are realistic. Clearly, the patient with 7–8 mm of probing depths on posterior teeth that are mobile and who would be devastated to lose any teeth may not have realistic expectations given the current level of oral disease present. The sooner this situation is identified, the sooner the dental team can assist the patient in understanding and accepting what goals are realistic. Questions about the importance of esthetics and the patient's smile will help the patient and dental team understand the patient's self-concept and how esthetic services may affect it. This line of questioning, although not traditional, can result in greater patient understanding and, ultimately, in obtaining the patient's consent for an esthetic procedure.

Esthetic oral health services are not contraindicated for patients with chronic diseases. However, both the dentist and patient must fully understand the effects that one's systemic diseases and medications will have on dental care and subsequent home care. A patient taking nifedipine for hypertension is still a candidate for porcelain veneers but must understand that the medication will increase the susceptibility to plaque-induced marginal gingivitis.

The medical history plays an increasing role in the treatment planning of older adults. The most common chronic diseases seen in older adults include heart disease, arthritis, diabetes, osteoporosis, and senile dementia. Medical conditions must be identified, and the stability of the patient's health status assessed. A patient who has had their hip joint replaced within the past 6 months will require greater assessment and perhaps a consultation with their orthopedic surgeon compared with a patient who had a hip replacement over five 5 years ago and has no other comorbidity.[14] Medical history forms should provide an area for comments on the stability of a patient's medical condition. A medical history form that asks "Do you have heart disease?" with a yes or no answer will not provide the dental team with sufficient information to gauge the status and the stability of the patient's health. The medical history must include an assessment of both the patient's prescription and over-the-counter medications. Studies have shown that salivary flow does not decrease naturally with age; however, the absence of saliva does put a patient at much greater risk for both coronal and root caries.[15]

As part of the oral examination, a patient's salivary flow should be assessed.[16] Salivary flow is much more likely to decrease as a result of multiple medication use. Over 400 medications are estimated to decrease salivary flow.[17] Other medications have been shown to affect oral tissues; for example, nonsteroidal anti-inflammatory medications can cause oral ulcerations, and antihypertensive and antiseizure medications can induce gingival overgrowth. Tests are currently available to assess salivary flow, pH, and buffering capability of saliva.

Providing esthetic dental services for healthy 65-year-olds should not prove difficult for dental practitioners. Rather, the challenge will come when that 65-year-old becomes an 85-year-old with heart disease, stroke, arthritis, chronic obstructive pulmonary disease, and/or Alzheimer's disease. The patient who has invested significant time and money in one's oral health will find the maintenance of the esthetic dentistry investment more difficult if they become frail and medically, mentally, or physically compromised. This scenario represents an opportunity for dental professionals to take a leadership role in both patient education and the education of nursing home staff, families, caregivers, and other health-care professionals about oral health for compromised patients. Health professionals need to understand that oral health does not have to decline simultaneously with a decline in physical or mental functioning.

The oral examination, like the patient's medical and medication history, may take more time than with younger patients. Older adults will continue to be at risk for caries, both coronal and root caries, periodontal disease, occlusal disorders, and oral soft tissue lesions. A thorough oral examination with complete imaging studies will insure that the correct diagnoses are made prior to the development of the treatment plan.

Prevention and risk assessment

Prevention is not just for kids anymore. Preventive therapies must be an integral part of the treatment planning for esthetic dental care.[18,19] By including a comprehensive preventive plan as part of the overall esthetic treatment plan, the unspoken message the dental team conveys to patients is that the team believes in the patient's future. That future is one of oral health, not oral disease. Patients with diabetes may be at increased risk for periodontal disease.[20] New strategies for at-home or in-office therapies can help patients lower their risk for gingivitis and/or periodontal infections prior to esthetic dental treatment. Antimicrobial rinses should be used for individuals at risk of gingivitis. New bacterial monitoring tests are available and may be necessary for individuals particularly at high risk for caries or periodontal disease.

Oral cancer occurs more commonly in older adults, particularly in those who use tobacco and drink alcohol.[21] However, about 25% of oral cancer cases today demonstrate no risk factors, suggesting that an oral cancer examination in every adult patient is a critical part of their dental care. Older adults should be questioned about their interest in quitting tobacco, and smoking cessation counseling should be provided for patients who are interested in discontinuing tobacco use. Do not assume because a patient has been smoking for ≥50 years that they are unwilling to quit. Studies have shown that dental professionals are as effective as their health professional counterparts in getting their patients to quit tobacco.

Maintaining oral health in older patients

Esthetic dentistry for any patient is not successful if it cannot be maintained. As with any dental treatment, maintenance of the oral cavity with appropriate home care is critical to the success and longevity of the dental treatment. A preventive program serves as an integral part of every treatment plan. It must be based on a patient's oral and medical conditions, risk factors, and, especially, the physical and mental ability to perform adequate home care. Oral health education, particularly regarding self-care, remains a staple in the preventive plan for patients of every age. Family members and caregivers play a critical role in maintaining oral health, particularly in the medically and physically compromised older adult. The dental team should not be shy about inviting family and caregivers to assist in the daily oral care for a patient who has become incapacitated and can no longer perform their own oral care.

Older adults with severe arthritis or neurological illnesses like stroke or dementia, will find that oral self-care is more difficult. They may require assistance from a caregiver to make oral self-care easier. Educating patients, caregivers, and family members how to make daily toothbrushing and interproximal cleaning easier will be time very well spent by your dental hygienist.

Caries management by risk assessment

The medical history and oral examination will provide an insight into the risk factors that will affect the oral health of older adults. Patients with low salivary flow rates, a low oral pH, or whose saliva does not have an adequate buffering capability will be at increased risk of root or coronal caries.[15] Caries management by risk assessment (CAMBRA) provides an approach to prevent dental caries in patients of all ages.[22] CAMBRA forms are downloadable through the American Dental Association website (www.ada.org) and CAMBRA helps patients understand their risk factors for dental caries. Once the risk factors are identified, a preventive plan can be developed to help patients lower their risk for caries, prior to any significant restorative or esthetic dental care. The preventive plan can include topical fluorides, provided as gels or fluoride varnishes, to prevent caries in adults.[23] Higher level fluoride toothpastes (5000 ppm) are available for home use, and new products are available to insure that sufficient calcium and phosphates ions are available to help remineralize the enamel or dentin of teeth. Professional and home-use neutral sodium fluoride gels or rinses to prevent root caries or recurrent caries should be prescribed for patients who are considered at high risk, such as patients with decreased salivary flow or impaired dexterity.[24,25] Salivary substitutes may also assist patients with oral dryness to provide comfort and improve oral tissue cleansing by the tongue.

Treatment planning in the older patient

Treatment plans should be based on the patient's needs and wants, not their age. Do not assume that older adults do not care about their appearance. Even grandmother and grandfather want to look their best for the family wedding photos!

Options for esthetic dental care are readily available for those in their 70s, 80s, and 90s just as they are for those much younger. However, with increasing life expectancies, treatment planning the 40-year-old esthetic dental patient requires a life cycle approach. Patients of all ages should be informed that esthetic dentistry does not last forever and procedures will likely need to be repeated at some point as the dental materials age and wear or the oral tissues change in relation to the face.

Older adults in the United States are seeking orthodontic treatment in record numbers to correct long-standing malocclusions and improve their oral function. It should not be assumed that the 78-year-old woman is not interested in whitening her teeth, replacing her worn amalgam restorations with new tooth-colored filling materials, or investing in her smile. When treatment planning older adults, give them the opportunity to "say yes." Older adults have seen their children and grandchildren benefit from modern techniques and new dental materials, and they are interested in benefiting from these same procedures.

Older patient attitudes will vary considerably. Often during the interview, patients will provide clues about their motivation for seeking dental care, particularly esthetic dental services. For some, function and overall health will be the motivating factors in maintaining good oral health; for example, removing oral infection may be the key determining factor. Others may feel that looking good is important to overall quality of life and will have no problem with spending resources for improving their smile. If a restoration needs replacement or the patient requires a new restoration because of caries, ask the patient if they are interested in an esthetic restoration.

Identifying the chief complaint is important when caring for any patient. For older adults seeking esthetic dentistry, it is important to understand precisely what they like and dislike about their appearance as well as their expectations for such treatment. They have lived many years with their smile and often know exactly what they want to change. It is critical for the dentist to assist the patient in articulating one's goals clearly.

Older adults presenting for esthetic dental care may often arrive at the dental office with an adult "child" as a caregiver. It should not be assumed that the adult child is the decision maker. The treatment plan should be addressed to the older adult, and if the older adult needs assistance with the decision making, allow the older adult to ask advice from the adult child. For the patient who may be medically or physically compromised, the individual's ability to cooperate with the dental treatment must be assessed. The appointments must be timed for the patient's comfort.

Managing other chronic illness and sequencing of procedures

Systemic illnesses can affect oral health, and the dental team must educate patients and their families to recognize these changes. Clearly, chronic medical conditions and medications can affect oral health and increase the risk for oral diseases. Because older adults may be managing chronic diseases, esthetic treatment may be delayed due to an acute exacerbation of a chronic illness. The patient with hypertension who suffers a stroke and requires rehabilitation for 3–6 months will have dental treatment interrupted. When dental treatment resumes there will be additional, special medical considerations; for example, if the patient is now taking anticoagulants, this will require monitoring of the international normalized ratio to ensure that bleeding is not a problem during dental treatment. Similarly, a patient with heart disease may undergo cardiac surgery. delaying dental treatment. In this case, it would be prudent to have a consultation with the cardiologist prior to resuming treatment. This may require more time for you and your team, but the patient will appreciate this concern and effort in communicating with the physician.

Sequencing esthetic dental treatment for older adults will be similar to that for younger and middle-aged adults. Caries control and periodontal therapy may be necessary prior to definitive esthetic treatment. Also, consultations with dental specialists may be required, depending on the nature of the patient's oral diagnoses; consultations with the patient's physicians may be required, depending on the patient's medical diagnoses.

Imaging in decision-making process

An accurate diagnosis is the most important first step in providing any esthetic dental service. In the final analysis, *no* treatment is better than the *wrong* treatment. In the words of Hippocrates, "First, do no harm." For individuals unsure about the decision to pursue esthetic dental treatment, imaging can play an important role in assisting the patient to understand how their smile can be altered. Imaging can assist both the patient and dentist in understanding what can be accomplished with esthetic dentistry. Dentists should be wary of the patient who says "I've hated my dental work all my life. I'll be pleased with whatever you do." It is important to find out the exact specifics of what the patient does not like about their teeth and what they expect. On careful questioning and the use of an intraoral camera and/or imaging, the dental team can usually identify the cause(s) of concern and gain insights for potential treatment options.

Informed consent requires that the patient be presented with treatment options. Imaging can assist the patient in understanding the problems and the potential options for treatment. By demonstrating the overall changes and specific changes on each tooth, the patient will understand the goal of each dental procedure and how it contributes to the overall result. For patients who are having difficulty making a decision to pursue esthetic dentistry, imaging gives them the opportunity to share a photograph of the planned results with friends and family, and get feedback that will help them make a decision.

Financing

Financing esthetic dental services will most frequently be out-of-pocket. Although some patients over age 65 may still have dental insurance as part of their employment retirement package, most dental insurance does not reimburse for elective esthetic services. Dental care provided for the treatment of the teeth and/or supporting tissue is generally not reimbursed under Medicare, although more Medicare Advantage plans are including a dental benefit. In some cases, adult children may be willing to incur the cost for esthetic dental services if their parents are not comfortable or able to spend money on themselves for esthetic dental care.

Esthetic dental consultation and facial plastic surgery

Esthetic dentistry can be a part of an overall appearance makeover. New treatment approaches have made facial plastic surgery more affordable and accessible to patients. For a patient considering facial surgery, the consultation with the dentist regarding smile enhancement should occur prior to the facial surgery to maximize the final facial esthetics. In some cases, interdisciplinary dental care such as orthodontics, periodontics, and prosthodontics may be required to achieve the best result and will take several months to accomplish.

Patients, as well as plastic surgeons, should be educated as to the benefits of consulting with a dentist prior to any esthetic surgery procedures. The reasons for this include the following: (1) creating a younger-looking smile may be sufficient to please the patient so that plastic facial surgery may not be necessary or less surgery may be required; (2) oral pathology, such as caries or severe periodontal disease subsequent to facial surgery, may compromise the esthetic surgical result; (3) esthetic dental services provided after facial surgery may involve the use of lip and cheek retractors, and any excessive stretching of the facial tissue is contraindicated during the initial healing phases. If esthetic dental services are provided after facial surgery, patients may perceive the use of retractors as contributing to "new" wrinkle development that the plastic surgery had removed. Oftentimes, these wrinkles were present prior to the dental treatment, but the patients did not notice them until after the dental procedures. When treating a patient who has had plastic facial surgery, the patient should be photographed in repose and smiling close up and full face without make-up to record any existing facial wrinkling prior to dental treatment.

Esthetic dental procedures for older adults

Vital tooth bleaching

Teeth darken and become more yellow as they age. Teeth also tend to take on stain throughout the enamel and cementum surfaces (characterization, as it is euphemistically called). With the trend toward whiter teeth, it is not at all surprising to find patients of all ages requesting tooth-lightening procedures.

Vital tooth bleaching performed either in the office or at home has been demonstrated to be effective in older adults. Since aging tends to darken teeth in the yellow color range, this color range achieves the best results with vital tooth-whitening procedures. In-office and at-home whitening with trays work equally well. Products containing 10–35% peroxide have been shown to work in mature adults. The main determinant is whether the patient desires the whitening results immediately or can wait longer for the at-home whitening agents to begin to work. In older adults, sensitivity does not appear to occur as frequently as in younger patients. This is thought to be due to the gradual receding of the pulpal tissue with age. If a patient has anterior teeth with prominent microcracks, they should be advised of these cracks and monitored carefully to ensure that there is no streaking in the whitened teeth.

Cosmetic contouring and bonding

The teeth of people over 60 years often exhibit the wearing away of hard tissue by erosion, abrasion, or parafunctional habits such as bruxism. Shortened anterior teeth, particularly in the maxilla, result in less of the teeth being seen when one talks or smiles. This shortening of teeth in the maxilla contributes significantly to an older appearance. As hard tissues wear away, patients will lose vertical dimension, resulting in the mandible becoming more anteriorly positioned. The reverse, the so-called "long-in-tooth" phrase that Shakespeare used to describe the aging process, results from periodontal disease.

With age, one shows less of the maxillary teeth and more of the mandibular teeth. The patient at age 50 who wishes to change only the color or shape of the maxillary teeth by age 60 may be requesting similar changes in the mandibular teeth. Both of these age-related changes can add years to an individual's appearance and inhibit oral function. However, esthetic dental treatment can easily transform the patient's appearance, in effect turning back the clock on the aging process.

Cosmetic contouring provides an excellent introduction to esthetic dentistry for patients who are unsure about making significant changes in their smile. It also provides a lower cost option

Clinical case 31.2: Whitening procedure for a 72-year-old patient

The 72-year-old woman in Figure 31.3A believed that her smile made her look older than she felt. Her teeth were whitened using an in-office 35% hydrogen peroxide solution. The result of whitening on her maxillary teeth is seen in Figure 31.3B. In-office whitening procedures provide a more immediate result when patients do not want to take the time for at-home whitening process and waiting several weeks/months for results or have already tried home whitening but had difficulty complying with the daily regimen. Patients should be advised that they will require touch-up treatments after the initial whitening procedures.

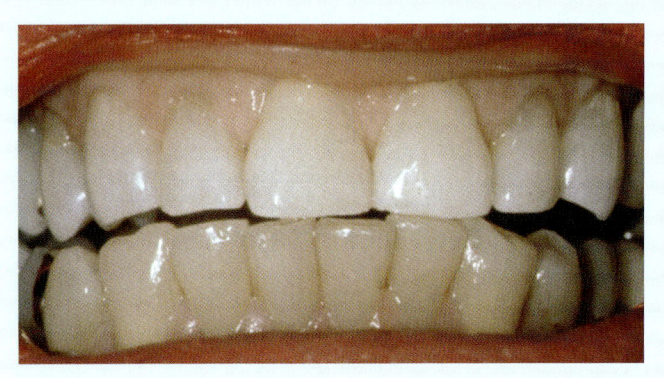

Figure 31.3 (A) This 72-year-old woman felt that the color of her teeth aged her smile.

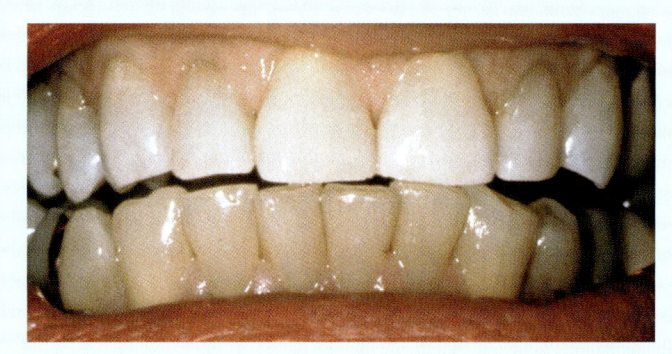

Figure 31.3 (B) After an in-office bleaching procedure on her maxillary teeth, the patient was pleased with her lightened color.

Clinical case 31.3: A 74-year old with cosmetic contouring

The 74-year-old woman in Figure 31.4 was dissatisfied with her smile but was not sure if she wanted considerable changes made. Her chief concern was that she did not like the cant in her upper teeth (Figure 31.4A). Cosmetic contouring of the maxillary arch was done to straighten the appearance of the upper right side to be more symmetrical (Figure 31.4B).

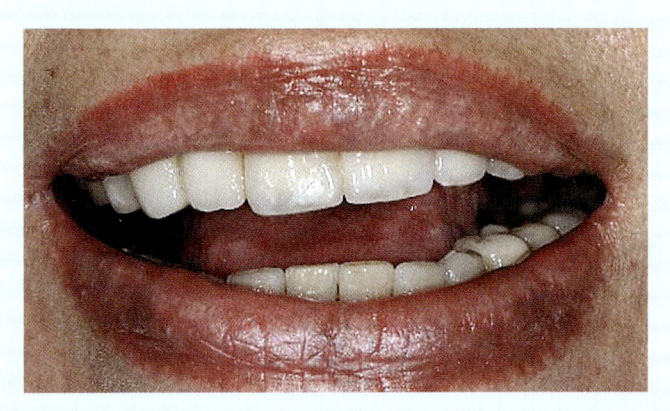

Figure 31.4 (A) This 74-year-old woman was dissatisfied with the appearance of her teeth.

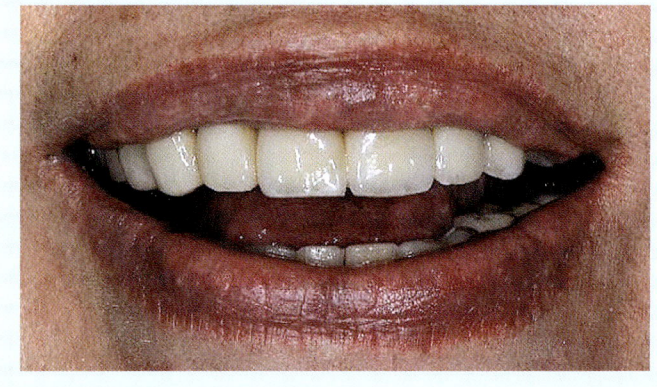

Figure 31.4 (B) Cosmetic Contouring was done on both maxillary and mandibular incisors to make the teeth appear straighter and eliminate the cant.

Clinical case 31.4: Cosmetic resin bonding

The patient in Figure 31.5A and B did not like the appearance of her front teeth and felt that her maxillary central incisors were too dark and too short. Cosmetic resin bonding was chosen as the treatment of choice because of the immediacy of the result. Figure 31.5C and D shows how the teeth were both lightened and lengthened to provide a younger-looking smile line.

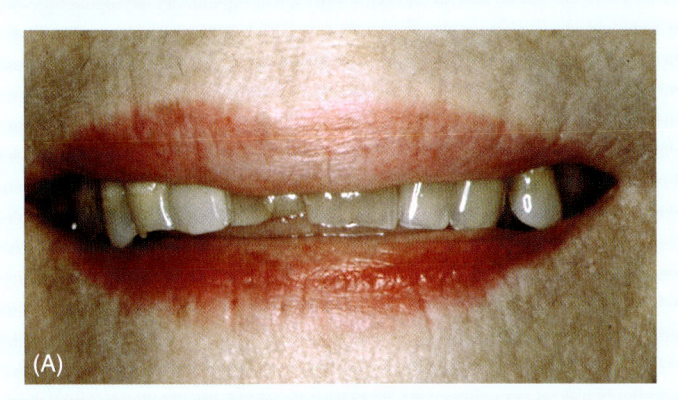

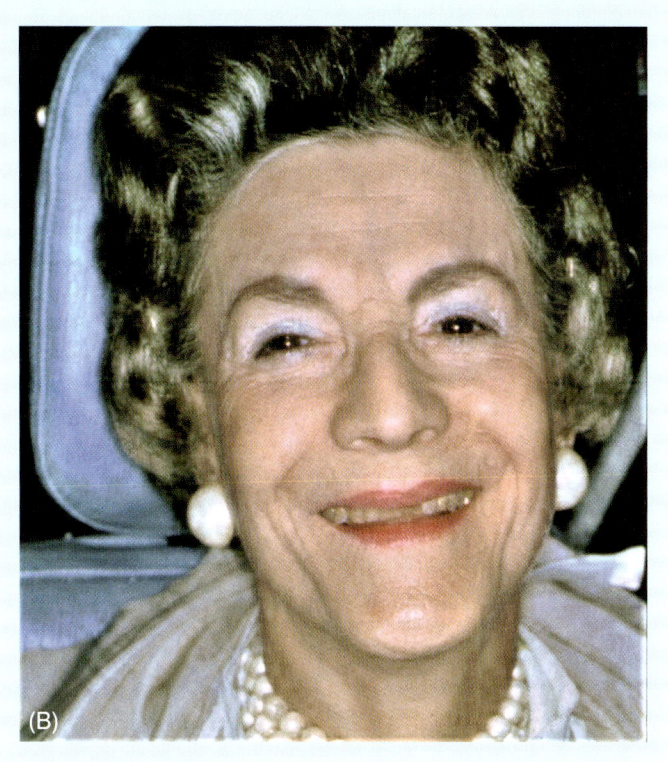

Figure 31.5 (A, B) This 78-year-old lady had shortened and darkened maxillary central incisors. Reproduced with permission from Quintessence Publishers.[9]

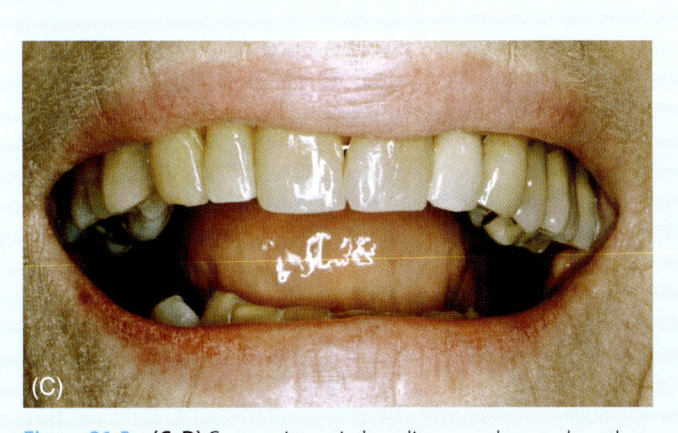

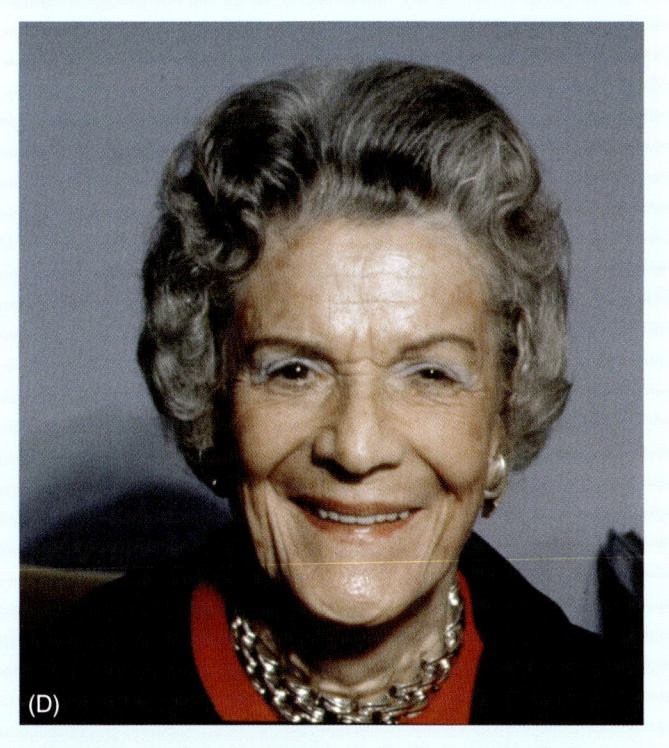

Figure 31.5 (C, D) Composite resin bonding was done to lengthen and lighten the central incisors. Reproduced with permission from Quintessence Publishers.[9]

for those patients with limited financial resources. Bonding with composite resin is a particularly useful esthetic technique for the mature adult. With minimal preparation, the tooth or teeth can be altered to achieve an esthetic result. Bonding also enables the dentist to easily repair chipping and fractures that occur in the teeth of older adults. Although manufacturers have made cosmetic shades lighter to reflect the increasing range of whiter shades of bleached teeth, older patients may require darker composite shades to restore erosion or root caries. Currently, when a patient needs a restoration on a tooth darker than existing composite shades, the dentist may need to use modifiers to make the restoration more natural in appearance and blend with the surrounding teeth. An overlay technique or partial veneer can be used when a spot match is not possible.

Clinical case 31.5: Patient's wife motivated 65-year-old husband to pursue esthetic dentistry

A 65-year-old did not care much about his smile, but his wife thought his smile made him look much older. She encouraged him to have esthetic dentistry by telling him that she would not kiss him until his smile improved. Figure 31.6A and B shows the worn and discolored central incisors and the crowded lower anterior incisors. Figure 31.6C shows cosmetic contouring of the lower incisors. Figure 31.6D and E illustrates the completed esthetic improvement following composite resin bonding of the central incisors.

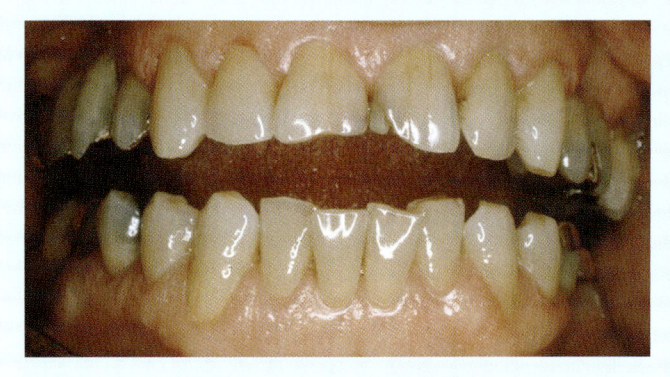

Figure 31.6 (A) This 65-year-old man displayed worn, discolored maxillary central incisors with a fractured anterior composite restoration on tooth #9.

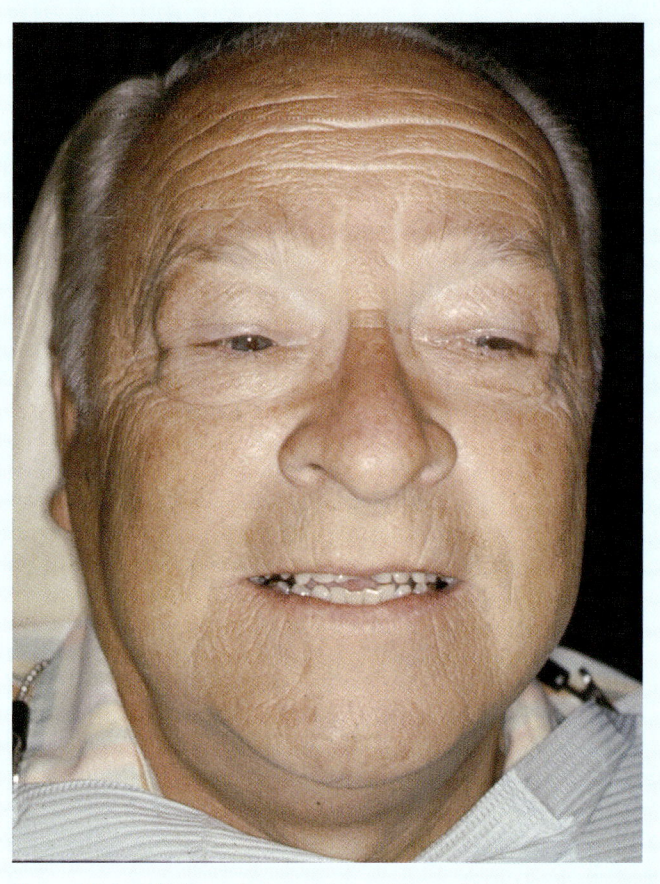

Figure 31.6 (B) The patient avoided smiling to hide his worn, discolored, and fractured central incisors.

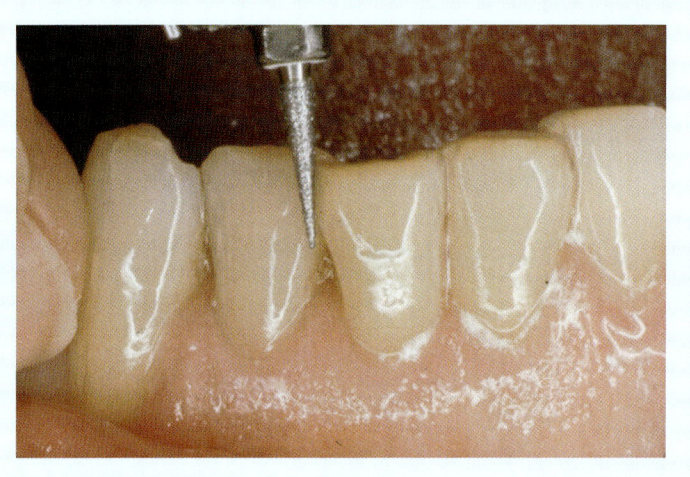

Figure 31.6 (C) Cosmetic contouring of mandibular incisors.

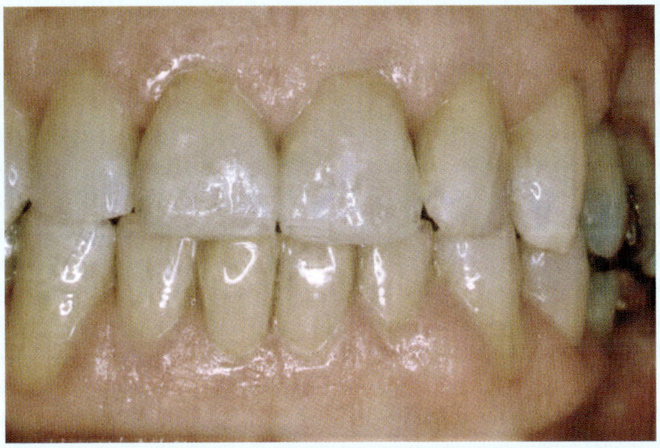

Figure 31.6 **(D)** The view after composite resin bonding of his central maxillary incisors.

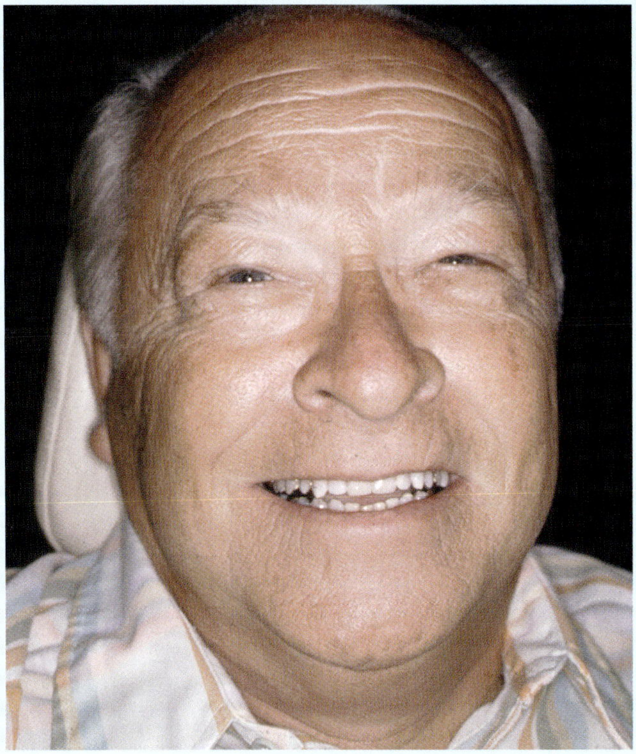

Figure 31.6 **(E)** Note how much younger looking and happier the patient is following his esthetic dental treatment.

Orthodontics

Research has shown that teeth can be repositioned successfully at any age. Orthodontics should always be considered as an option in cases of facial–dental arch discrepancies. Often, orthodontics is the most conservative treatment option to improve malocclusion. It is a mistake to assume that the older adult would not be willing to invest the time or money in orthodontics as a treatment option. Clear aligners have made tooth movement more desirable in patients of all ages. For adult orthodontic patients with missing teeth or insufficient numbers of teeth for orthodontic anchorage, dental and orthodontic implants are being used to assist with the necessary support. Orthodontically repositioning teeth may prevent the need for more aggressive crown and bridge coverage. In baby boomers who may not have as many restored teeth as the previous generation, preserving the natural enamel through orthodontics may be preferable to removing enamel and dentin for crowns or veneers. The orthodontics may also be less costly in the long run than the prosthodontic procedures.

Periodontal therapy

Esthetic dental procedures require a foundation of good periodontal support. Periodontal tissues frame the teeth and need to be healthy and in harmony with the smile. Age is not a contraindication for periodontal plastic surgery or periodontal surgery of any type. Nonsurgical scaling and root planning often form the basis of periodontal treatment. Antimicrobial therapies provide an adjunct for treating localized periodontal infections. New periodontal regeneration procedures are providing older adults who have lost periodontal bone support with options for retaining teeth.

Esthetic surgery, whether periodontal or oral surgical, should be offered to the older adult if surgery provides the best option for an esthetic result. Frequently, interdisciplinary therapy is necessary to achieve the most esthetic result.

Laser-assisted new attachment procedure

One periodontal procedure that may be useful for geriatric patients is the laser-assisted new attachment procedure (LANAP). This conservative technique can avoid periodontal surgical techniques and can make a significant difference in both bone and tissue health. Figure 31.10A shows significant mesial and distal bone loss on an elderly woman. Dr Peter Rubelman, periodontist in Miami, Florida, reported that the lady was 82 years old and a smoker. The osseous defect on the molar probed to 10 mm, and post-LANAP it was 4 mm (Figure 31.10B). Atlanta periodontist Dr Maurice Salama achieved similar success around anterior implants. Even bone loss around implants may be helped with the LANAP procedure. Figure 31.10C shows extensive bone loss around an implant. Figure 31.10D shows significant bone growth around the implant at 6 months. So, being conservative can make a difference, and it may well be worth trying to save both teeth and implants.

Clinical case 31.6: A 70-year-old received bonding, but retained diastemata

A 70-year-old man was unhappy with his look because of worn enamel on his lower incisors, but felt his maxillary diastemas were an integral part of his personality and look (Figure 31.7A and B). He requested bonding to improve the appearance of his lower teeth, but did not want correction of the diastemata. The result of the composite resin bonding of the mandibular incisors is seen in Figure 31.7C.

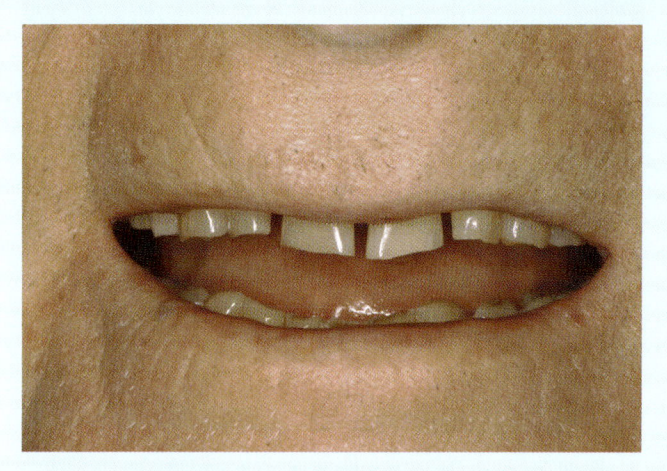

Figure 31.7 **(A)** This 70-year-old man was unhappy with the look of the worn enamel on his mandibular incisors but felt that his maxillary diastemas were an integral part of his personality.

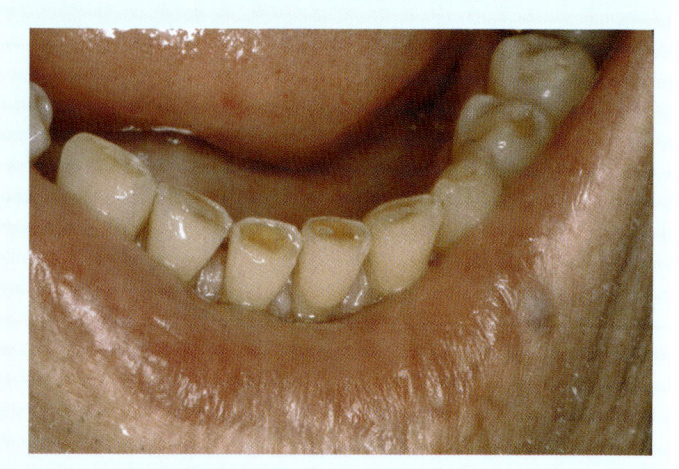

Figure 31.7 **(B)** The extent of tooth loss due to bruxism.

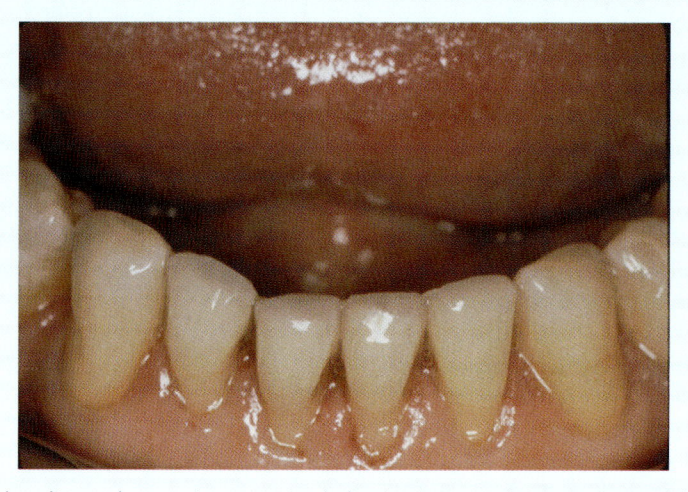

Figure 31.7 **(C)** Composite resin bonding and cosmetic contouring helped to improve the appearance of the mandibular anterior incisors.

Prosthodontics, endodontics, and implants

Prosthodontic procedures can restore the function and esthetics of an aging, worn dentition. Prosthodontic treatment may last longer than composite resin bonding. Often, the bonding procedures serve to introduce the patient to how esthetic dentistry can improve their smile at a lower cost. Later, when it needs to be redone, the patient may opt for the long-lasting, more expensive prosthodontic procedures.

Endodontics procedures are also not contraindicated in older adults. However, since dental pulps decrease in size with age, endodontics can be more difficult in older adults than in younger adults with larger pulp chambers. Consultation with an endodontist can assist the dentist in performing these procedures successfully.

Porcelain veneers are by far one of the most effective and yet conservative methods to achieve an esthetic result, especially when eight or more teeth are involved. If the patient's goal is to improve their smile, the dentist should first note how many teeth are involved in this smile improvement. Generally, the patient should smile to their fullest, and then which of the posterior teeth shows at the corner of the mouth can be noted. Sometimes, it may be a second molar. If so, the esthetic result the patient desires will not be achieved if only eight teeth are included in the treatment plan.

Clinical case 31.7: A 56-year-old patient orthodontics and cosmetic resin bonding, and 24 years later

A 56-year-old woman was unhappy with her smile and for health reasons wanted to correct her malocclusion (Figure 31.8A). In addition, she was also dissatisfied with her appearance and opted for tooth-colored brackets (Figure 31.8B). The teeth were repositioned in 18 months. The patient maintained her newly esthetic dentition with regular use of retainers. Figure 31.8C demonstrates the effectiveness of long-term orthodontics in this photo taken 24 years after initial orthodontics and cosmetic resin bonding.

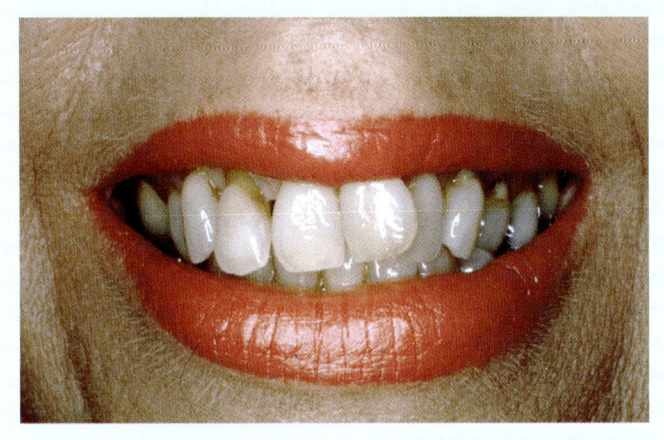

Figure 31.8 **(A)** This 56-year-old woman was unhappy with her malpositioned teeth and was willing to undergo orthodontic treatment. Reproduced with permission from Quintessence Publishers.[9]

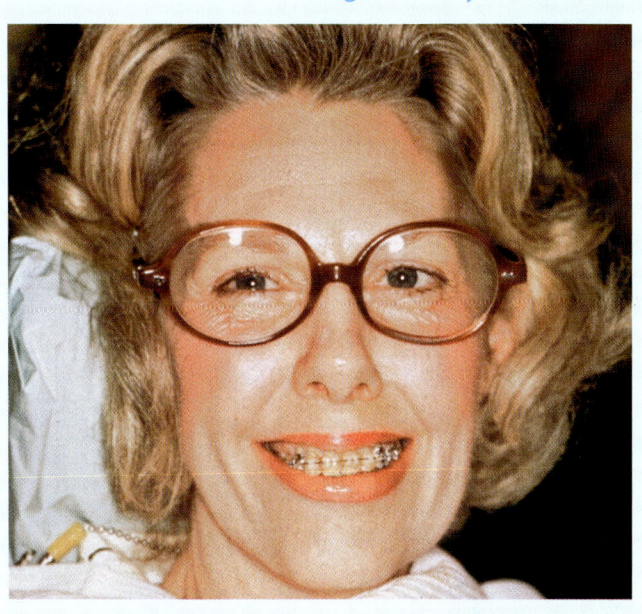

Figure 31.8 **(B)** Tooth-colored brackets were applied because of her concerns about her appearance during treatment. Reproduced with permission from Quintessence Publishers.[9]

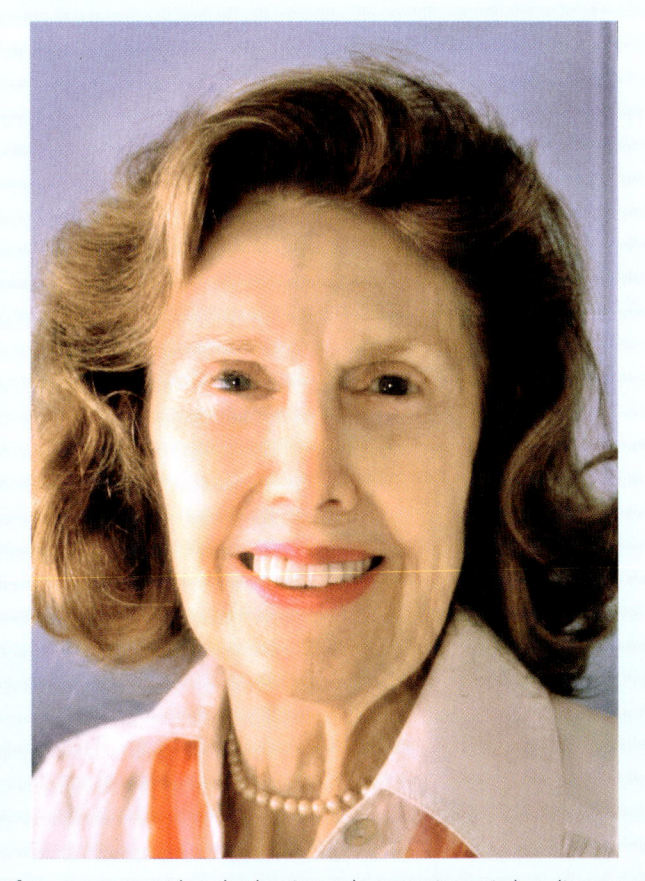

Figure 31.8 **(C)** Twenty-four years after treatment with orthodontics and composite resin bonding, as well as regular use of retainers, shows effective esthetic treatment. Reproduced with permission from Quintessence Publishers.[9]

Clinical case 31.8: Younger-looking smile achieved with periodontal surgery and porcelain veneers and posterior crowns/inlays

Figure 31.9A shows an older man with discolored and worn teeth and irregular gingival margins that contributed to his unattractive smile. He requested a younger-looking smile. His treatment plan consisted of periodontal surgery to improve the gingival contours and porcelain veneers plus posterior crowns and inlays. Figure 31.9B and C shows the final result with lighter teeth and improved tooth shape and arch alignment.

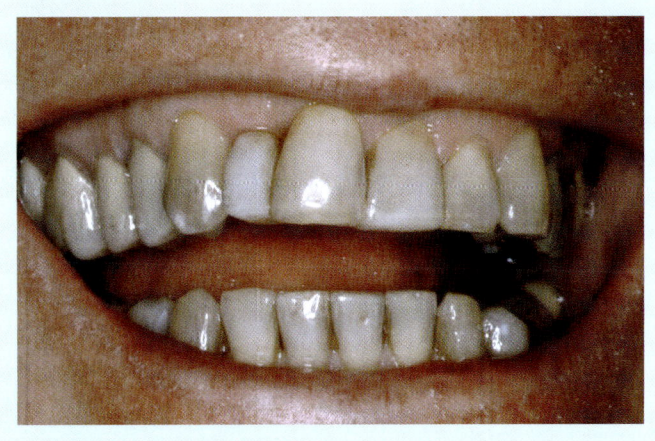

Figure 31.9 (A) This chief executive officer had discolored and worn teeth and irregular-looking gum tissue, resulting in an aged smile. Reproduced with permission from Quintessence Publishers.[9]

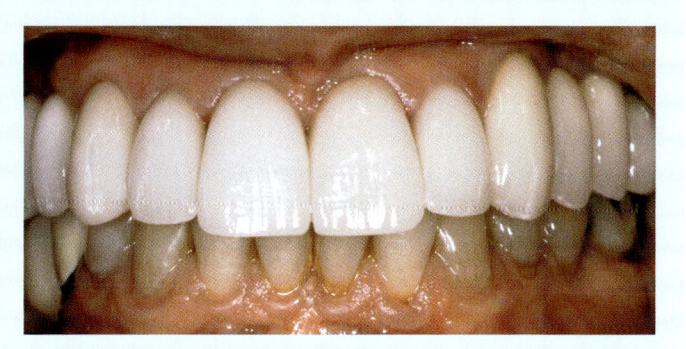

Figure 31.9 (B) After cosmetic periodontal surgery, during which the gingiva was cosmetically and functionally improved, five porcelain laminates were placed, as well as posterior crowns and inlays.

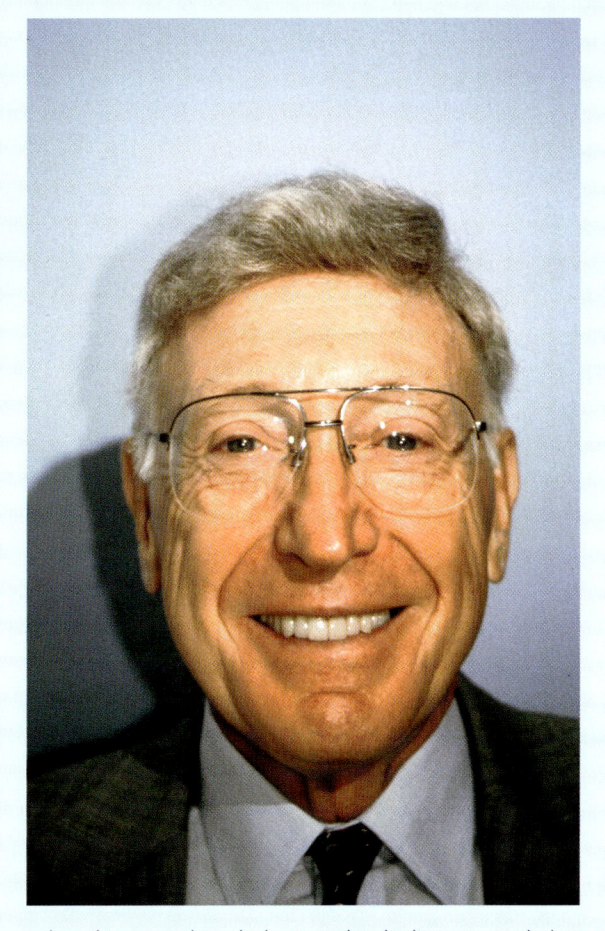

Figure 31.9 (C) The result was lighter teeth and improved tooth shape and arch alignment to help create a younger-looking smile. Reproduced with permission from Quintessence Publishers.[9]

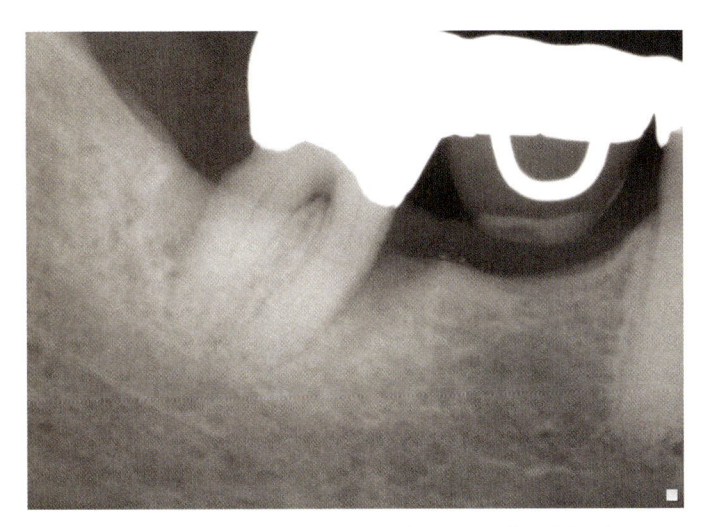

Figure 31.10 (A) This X-ray shows significant mesial and distal bone loss in an 82-year-old woman.

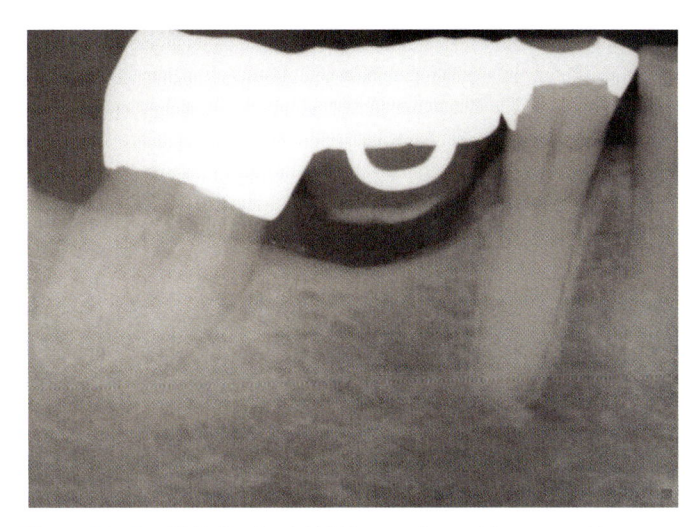

Figure 31.10 (B) Following LANAP procedures, this post-op X-ray shows a significant amount of bone growth.

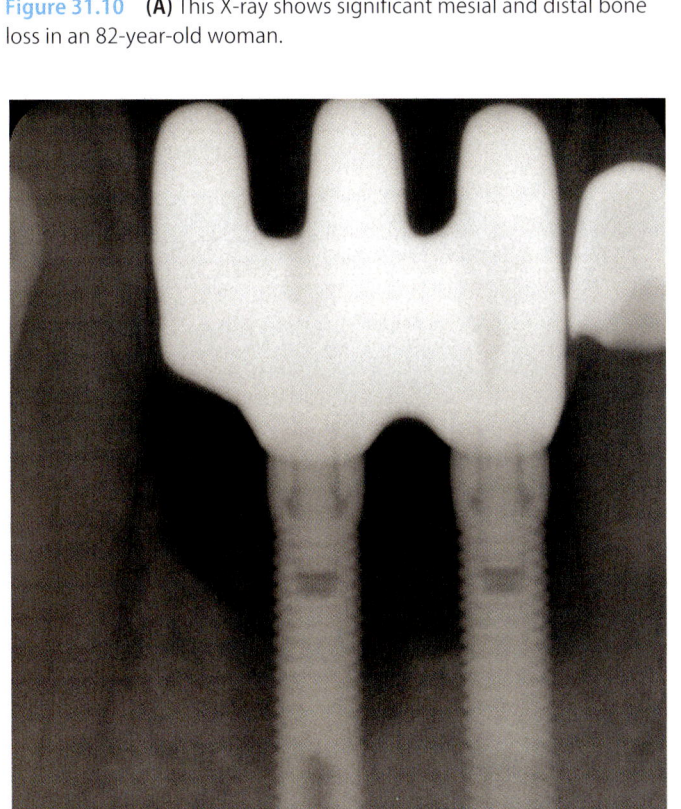

Figure 31.10 (C) This X-ray reveals extensive bone loss around an implant.

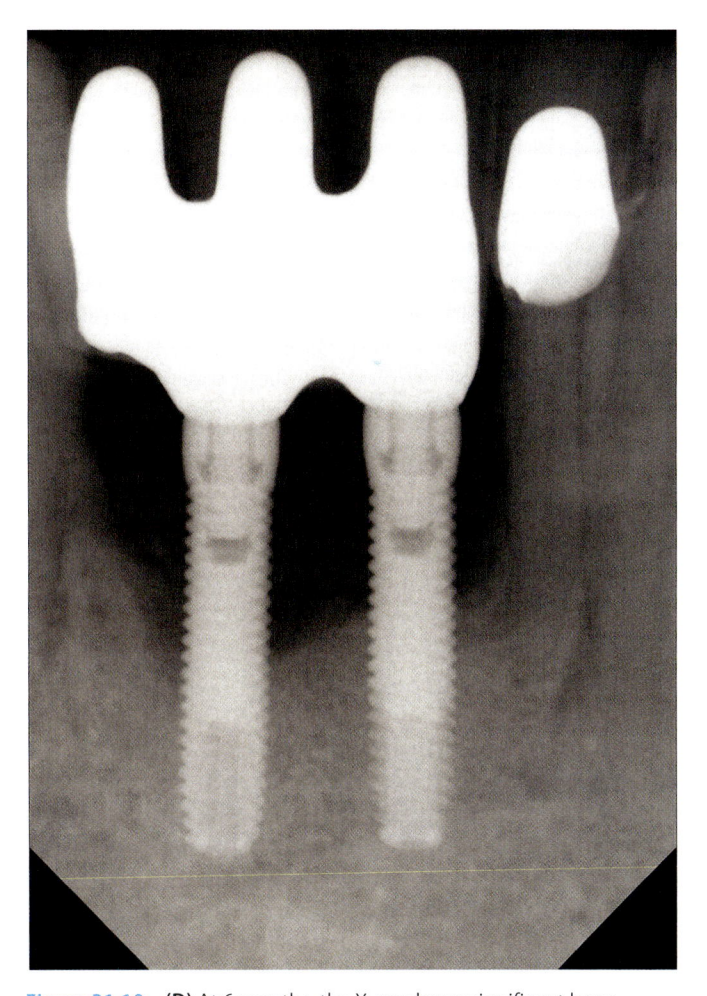

Figure 31.10 (D) At 6 months, the X-ray shows significant bone growth around the implant.

Since the upper lip line varies considerably in older adults, this assessment will be critical to achieving an esthetic result pleasing to the patient. The most artificial result occurs when only the six anterior teeth are restored in a lighter shade, with 8 or 10 teeth showing when the patient smiles. The unrestored posterior teeth now appear even darker than before and detract from the anterior teeth. The result is a false-looking smile on the older adult.

If the patient cannot afford to include 10 or 12 teeth in the treatment plan, consider bleaching the posterior teeth first to see if you can avoid laminating all of the teeth. The opposite arch should be whitened so that the entire smile will look as natural as possible.

As patients age, they tend to show more mandibular teeth and less maxillary teeth. Most patients often request the esthetic dental treatment for their maxillary teeth only, feeling that people will not see their lower teeth. However as patients age, mandibular teeth play a greater role in their smile and esthetic appearance. Where possible, it is critical to educate patients who are seeking esthetic dental treatment to include their mandibular teeth in any esthetic dental treatment plan.

Porcelain restorations of all types offer the ability to retain their color over the years and not darken with age as the natural dentition does. Porcelain veneers can also be used to reshape teeth that show loss of interdental papillae. Newer, low-fusing porcelains are showing considerably less wear to opposing teeth than the high-fusing porcelains. This is particularly important for middle-aged patients (e.g., age 50) undergoing esthetic dental treatment with a 30-year remaining life expectancy. When the patient requires complete oral rehabilitation, the full crown remains the restoration of choice. It can be expected to provide a greater functional life than bonding. It can be combined with porcelain veneers to accomplish an esthetic result. In many cases of bite problems that require an esthetic solution, the full crown, rather than porcelain onlays, will offer the most occlusal support against fracture.

Age and dysfunctional habits can contribute to severe wear over the years. Figure 31.11A and B demonstrates evidence of bruxism in an 86-year-old woman who had been advised to wear a bite guard when she was in her mid-50s. She disappeared from the practice and returned 30 years later demonstrating severe wear, loss of vertical dimension, loss of masticatory function, and temporomandibular joint pain and dysfunction. Additionally, she was embarrassed by her smile. Her treatment plan consisted of temporary crowns and bridges to restore vertical dimension and comfort. She was subsequently treated months later with fixed prosthodontics using metal–ceramic restorations (Figure 31.11C). She regained much of her self-confidence, as well as masticatory function, following the esthetic reconstruction of the maxillary arch (Figure 31.11D) and planned to restore the lower arch.

Fixed and removable prosthodontics can be used to improve appearance and function. The 78-year-old patient in Figure 31.12A and B showed severe wear on his upper and lower incisors, which compromised his smile line. He also had

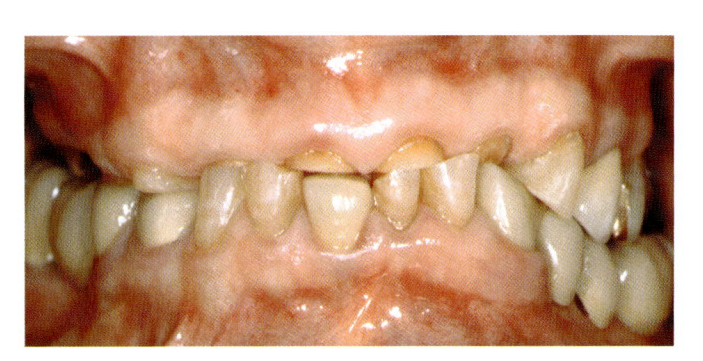

Figure 31.11 **(A)** This lady presented with a severe bruxism habit that resulted in virtually no maxillary anterior teeth showing at rest or when smiling.

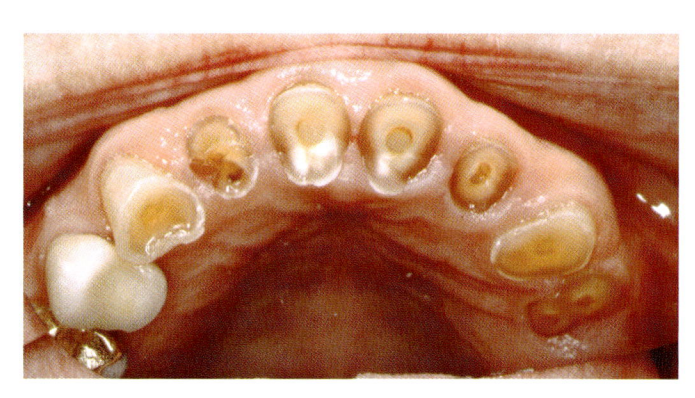

Figure 31.11 **(B)** Although she was advised more than 30 years previously to wear a night guard, she chose not to do so.

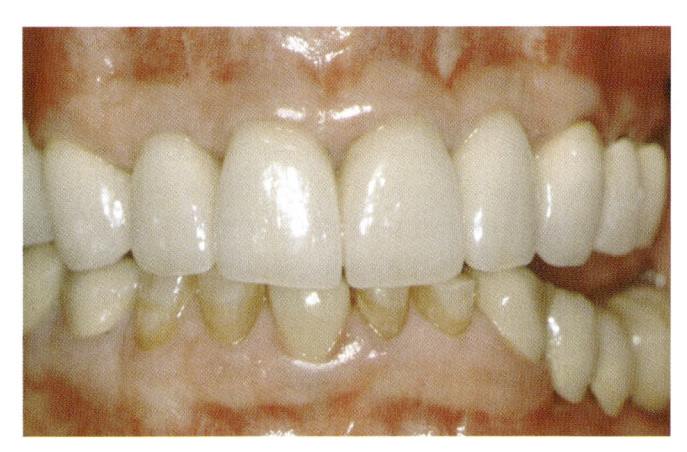

Figure 31.11 **(C)** Crown lengthening followed by prosthodontic reconstruction helped to recreate her smile. The next step is for her to rebuild the mandibular arch.

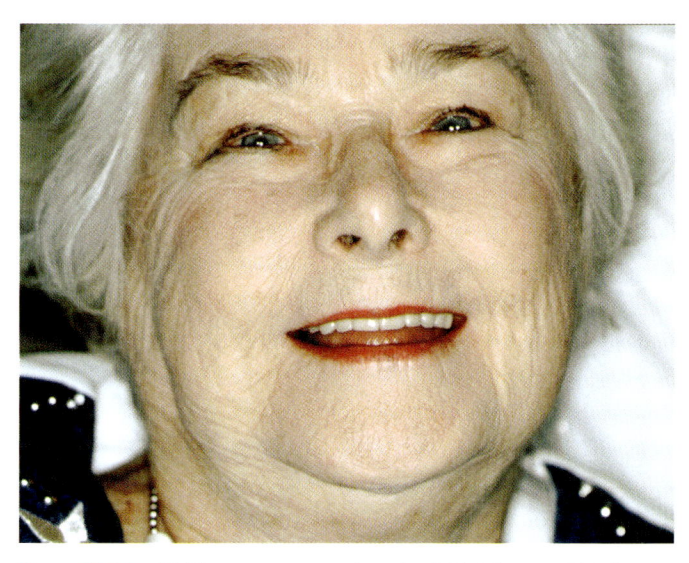

Figure 31.11 **(D)** The reconstructed teeth of this 88-year-old lady now enhance her smile.

multiple missing teeth. He was president of a large company and felt that he looked older than his actual years because his smile did not show any teeth. His treatment plan included crowns on his remaining natural teeth and a maxillary precision attachment removable partial denture. The final result shows both improved appearance and function (Figure 31.12C).

Although esthetic dental treatment for older adults may require an interdisciplinary team approach of general dentists and specialists, families may also be involved in helping patients understand the need for dental treatment. Figure 31.13A–C shows a 75-year-old woman who presented with severe root caries and moderate periodontal disease. Her daughter, who disclosed that her mother was difficult to please, referred her. The daughter was very supportive of her mother receiving dental treatment; however, her mother was initially not interested. The mother did not think that the esthetic aspect of dentistry was important. During consultation with the dentist, the mother was informed of the infection in her mouth and the potential effect that this could have on her future health and functionality. The patient consented to have the maxillary arch restored with fixed prosthodontics. She refused to accept treatment for her mandibular teeth, preferring to use her existing partial denture. Figure 31.13D and E shows the final result after periodontal and prosthodontic treatment. Although the patient was not particularly grateful to have the dental treatment, her family was thrilled to have her caries and periodontal disease treated and the esthetic appearance improved. The patient lived with her esthetically improved appearance for an additional 13 years.

Implant treatment is increasing in older adults, and is expected to increase further as implants have become the treatment of choice for replacement of a single missing tooth. Research has shown that outcomes with implant prosthodontics are as successful in older adults as in younger adults.[26] Implants remain a viable option for older adults who wish to replace their missing teeth with a more "tooth-like" approach. Age, in and of itself, is not a contraindication to implant therapy. Dental implants have been placed successfully in patients of all ages, including older adults. Many older adults are trading their complete dentures for implant-supported prostheses. A traditional mandibular complete denture provides considerable more retention and stability when four implants (either traditional or mini-implants) are placed in the mandible. Implant therapy requires a team approach with excellent communication between the surgical and the prosthodontic teams. Contraindications for dental implants relate more to an individual's medical

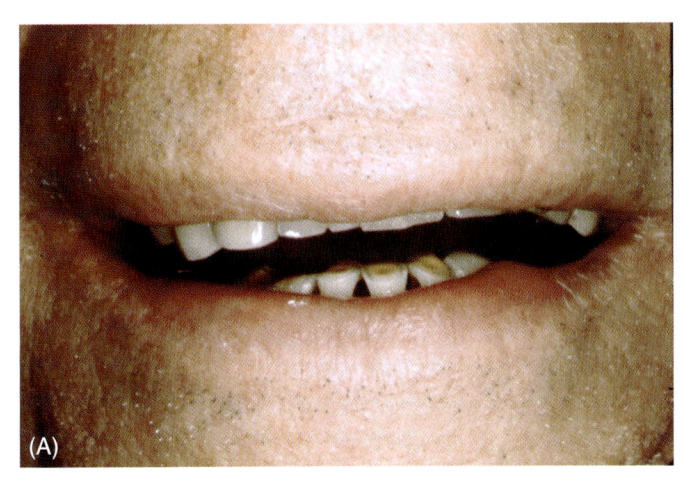

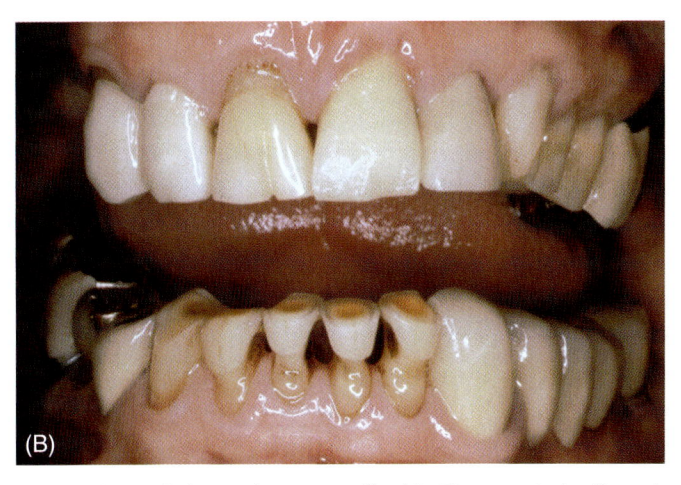

Figure 31.12 (A, B) This 78-year-old man had worn down his maxillary and mandibular teeth during the course of his life. This negatively affected his smile line.

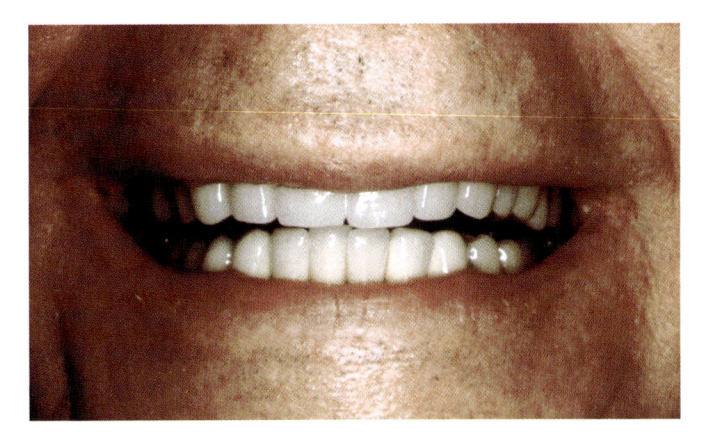

Figure 31.12 (C) All of the maxillary and mandibular teeth were crowned, and a precision attachment partial denture was made to improve both function and esthetics.

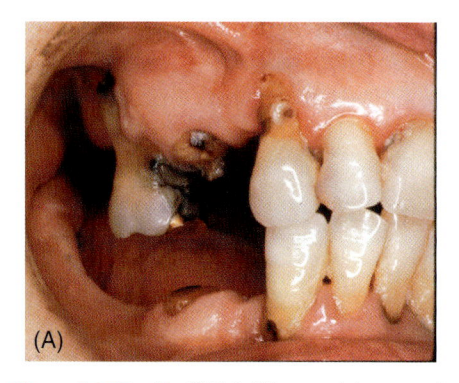

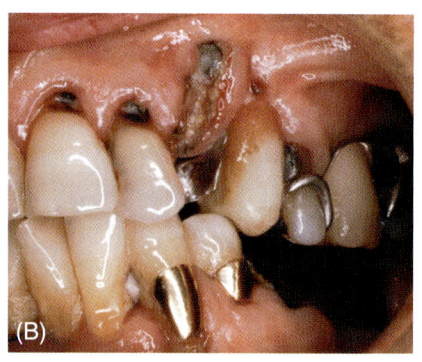

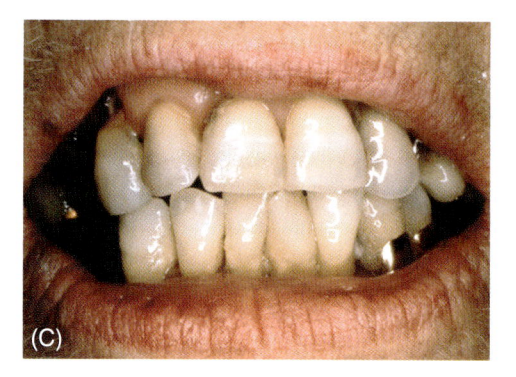

Figure 31.13 (A–C) This 75-year-old woman had severe root caries and moderate periodontal disease.

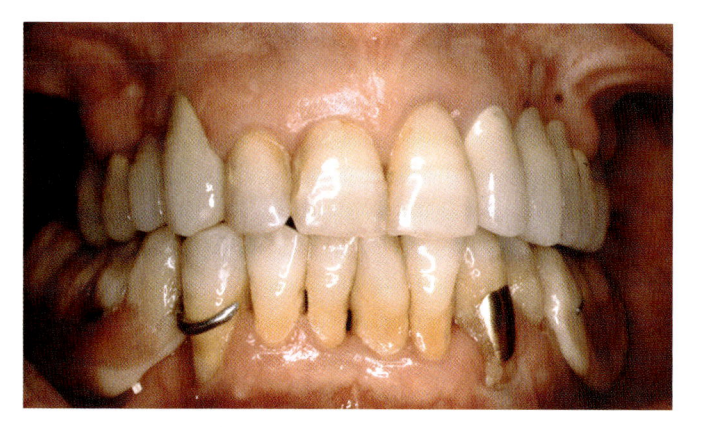

Figure 31.13 (D) Although this woman stated that she would "just as soon have her teeth extracted," she was motivated to have both periodontal and prosthodontic treatment.

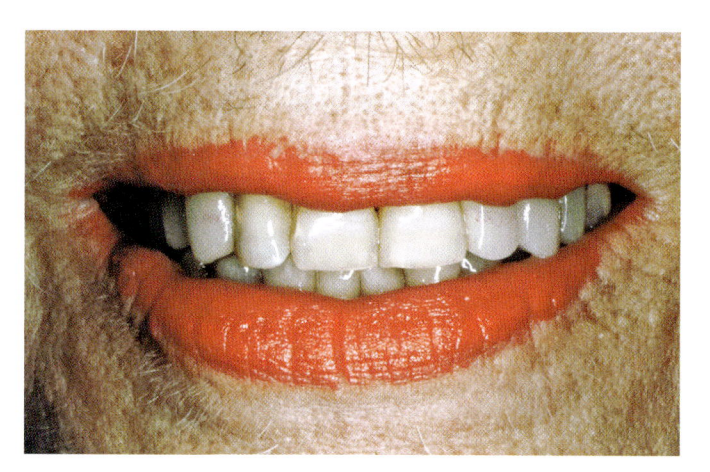

Figure 31.13 (E) The patient's smile after esthetic dental treatment shows how much improved her dental and oral health, as well as her smile are.

condition (e.g., uncontrolled diabetes) than one's age. See the examples in the clinical cases described in Figures 31.14, 31.15, 31.16, 31.17, and 31.18.

The nursing-home or assisted-living resident

The increase in the oldest-old has led gerontologists to define a concept of active life expectancy. Active life expectancy refers to that portion of life in which one can perform the activities of daily living with little or no help. Scientists have estimated that although a 65-year-old man may have an average of 16 years remaining life expectancy, three of those years may be periods of dependency, in which the individual requires some type of care.[2,11] Dependency results from the disabilities caused by long-standing chronic illnesses. Older adults often require more care from their children, family, or unrelated caregivers. Some may also need nursing home care.

In the United States, only 5% of the population over age 65 resides in a nursing home. However, adults over age 65 have a one-in-four chance of spending some time in a nursing home. The most frequent scenario is that of the older woman living alone who falls and fractures a hip. She is hospitalized to have the hip surgically repaired and then may enter a nursing home for months of rehabilitation therapy. More recently, as people age, they consider the concept of assisted living before severe problems arise. Thus, they avoid abrupt change when something adverse does occur. However, good or even adequate home care for them remains a problem.

The probability of residing in a nursing home increases with advancing age and is greatest for those with dementia. In the United States, over 50% of nursing home residents carry a diagnosis of dementia. Data on the oral health needs of nursing home residents in Ohio found that fulfillment of patients' dental needs was declining.[27] The authors hypothesized that patients and their families are delaying entry into the nursing home, opting instead to care for the family member for as long as possible in their home. During this period of home care, dental appointments are often overlooked as the family struggles to meet the care needs of their family member.

Dental care for residents of nursing homes in the United States remains woefully inadequate.[28] Oral health care in most nursing homes is virtually nonexistent. Studies have shown that education of the nursing staff can help improve the daily oral care and the ability to recognize the oral problems of the residents.[29] As baby boomers care for their aging parents and/or make difficult decisions regarding nursing home placement, they may become aware of the lack of essential health care services in nursing homes and demand improvements for the family members. (One can only hope that they demand improved oral hygiene care.)

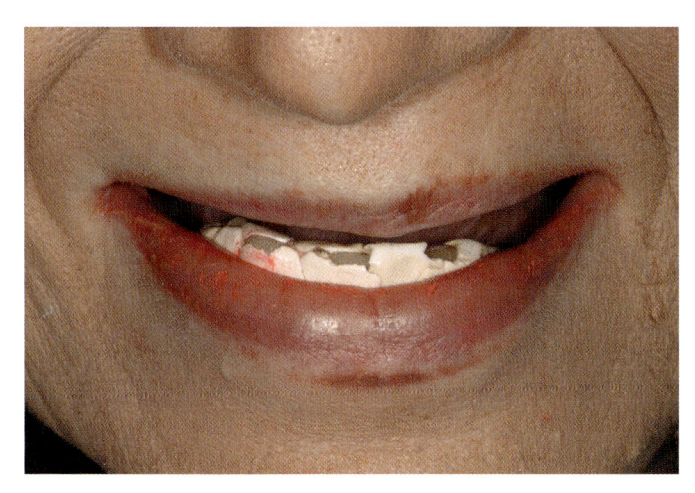

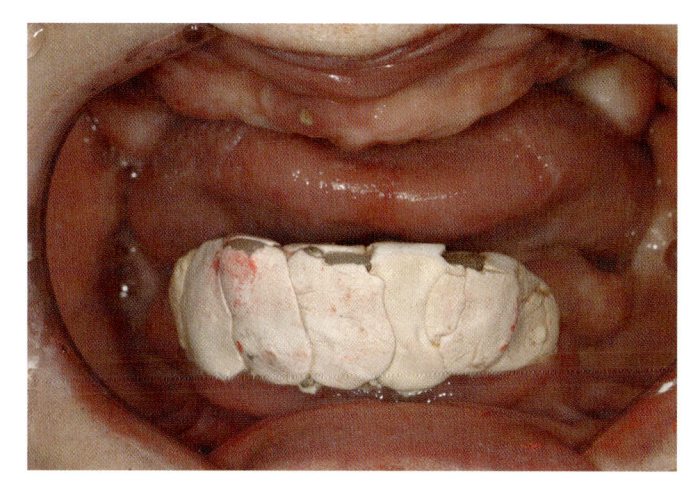

Chapter 31 Geresthetics: Esthetic Dentistry for Older Adults

Figure 31.14 (A, B) A 72-year-old woman was forced to face her dental problems and fears after years of neglect prior to hip replacement surgery. She had only residual roots in the maxilla, onto which she was balancing an old porcelain-fused-to-metal bridge. Her lower teeth had advanced caries and periodontal disease, which she was covering up with over-the-counter dental temporary filling.

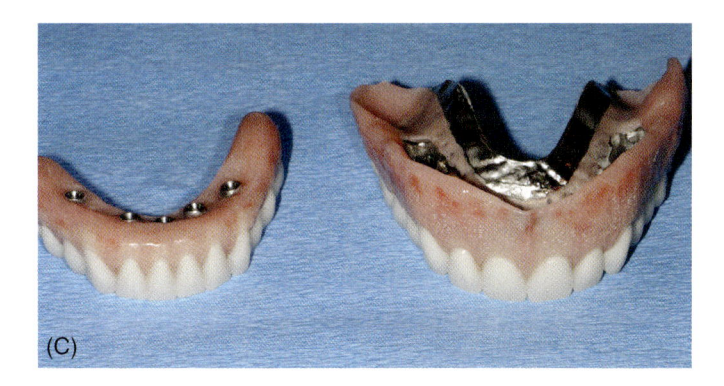

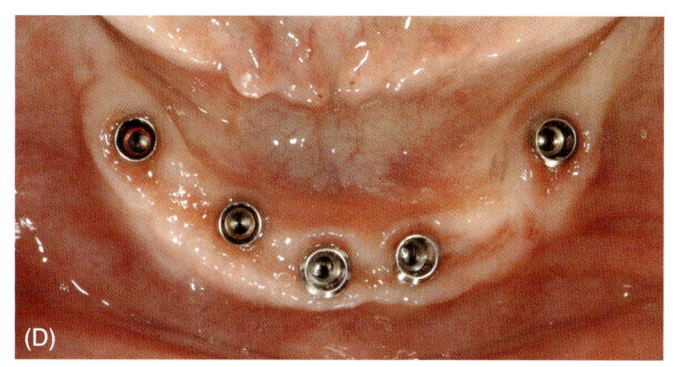

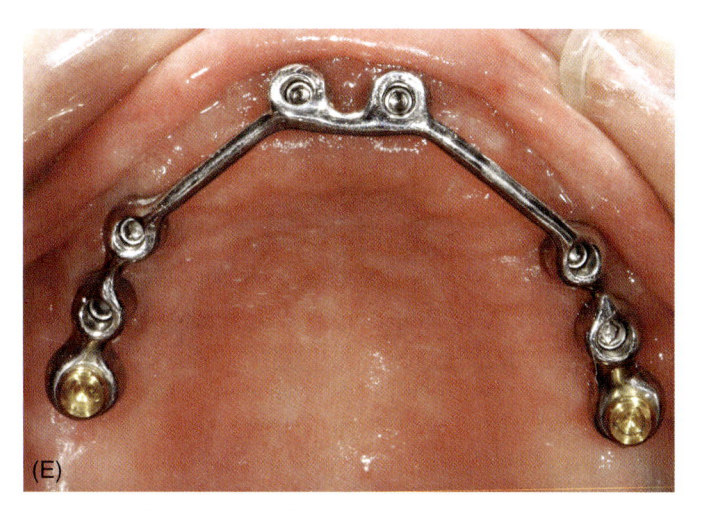

Figure 31.14 (C–E) After extracting her nonrestorable remaining dentition, she was transitioned into treatment dentures. Six maxillary and five mandibular implants were placed and prostheses fabricated: maxillary bar overdenture and mandibular screw-retained hybrid prosthesis.

Patients who have spent considerable time and money for esthetic dental services should not enter a nursing home only to have the lifetime of restorative and esthetic dentistry become undermined by root caries or periodontal infection. The opportunity for dentistry lies in advocating for a change in the standard of oral health care for nursing-home residents. If residents can have their sight and hearing needs met, their oral health needs should be accepted as an important part of their health care needs, particularly given the amount of time that residents spend using their oral cavity to swallow, smile, eat, and, especially, to communicate. These are surely important activities in the life of a nursing-home resident.

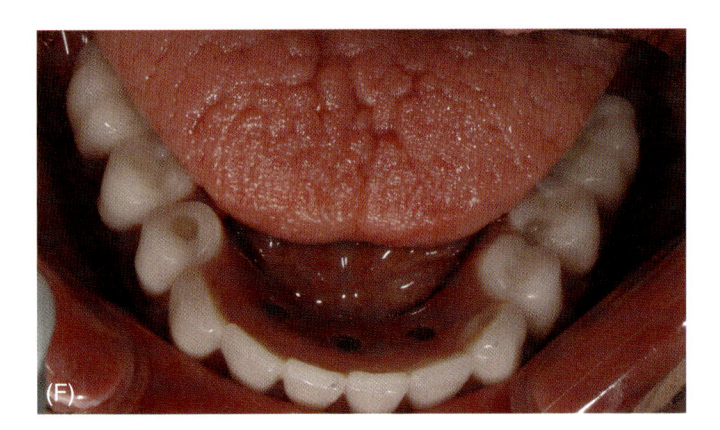

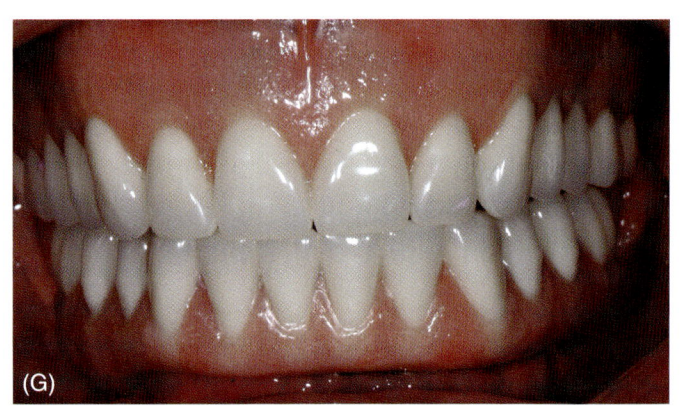

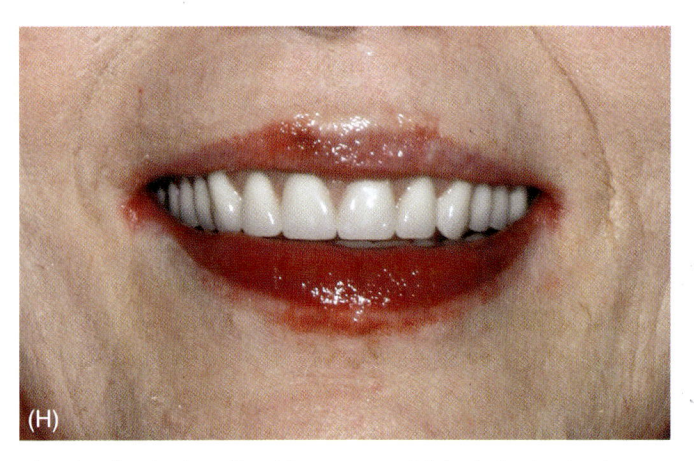

Figure 31.14 **(F–H)** This patient's functional and esthetic oral health were reestablished after having been severely compromised for many years. The patient is maintained on a strict 2- to 3-month hygiene schedule.

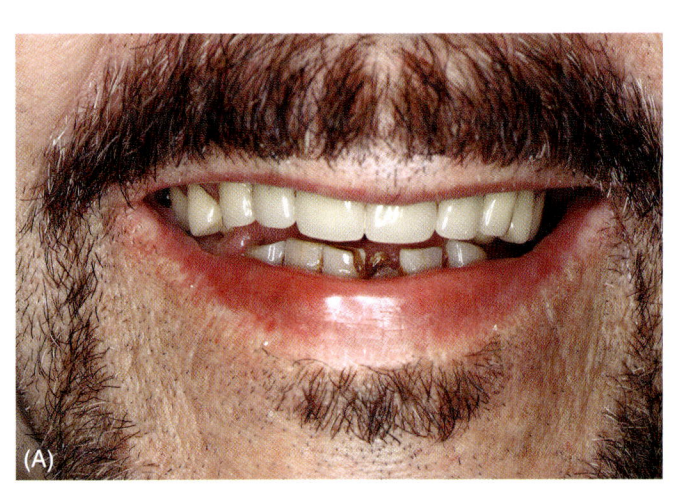

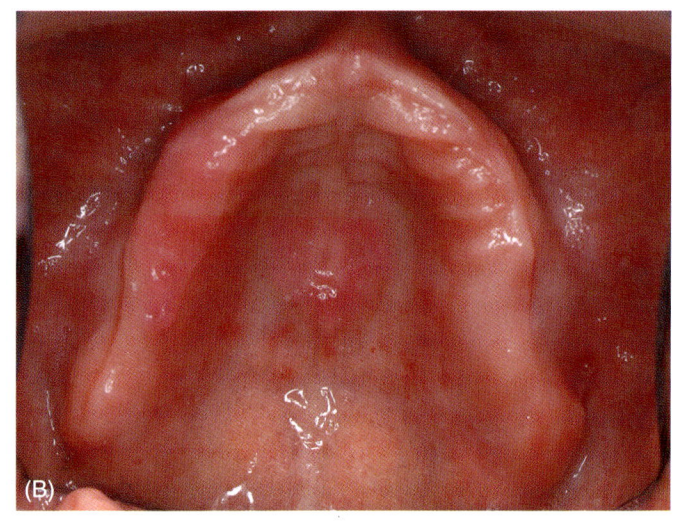

Figure 31.15 **(A, B)** A 65-year-old executive administrative assistant was unhappy with his dental esthetics and function. He had been a maxillary complete denture wearer for several decades. Note the uneven occlusal plane and reverse smile line of the maxillary denture.

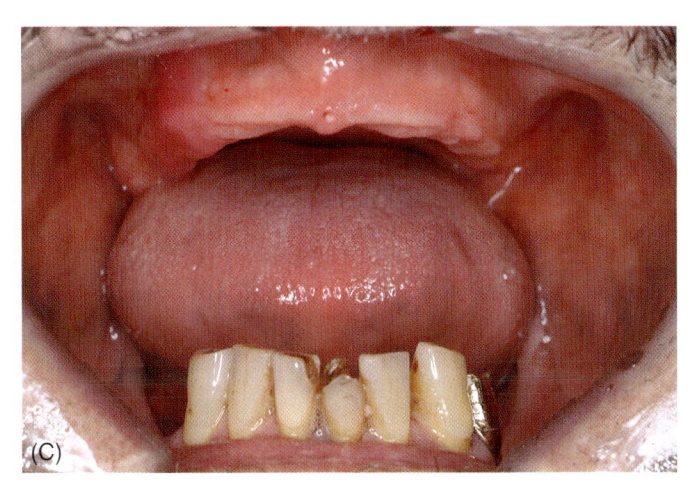

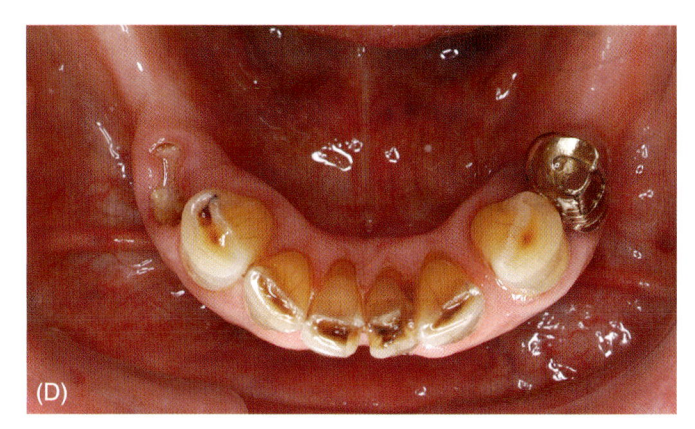

Figure 31.15 **(C, D)** The remaining lower teeth had advanced caries and periodontal problems.

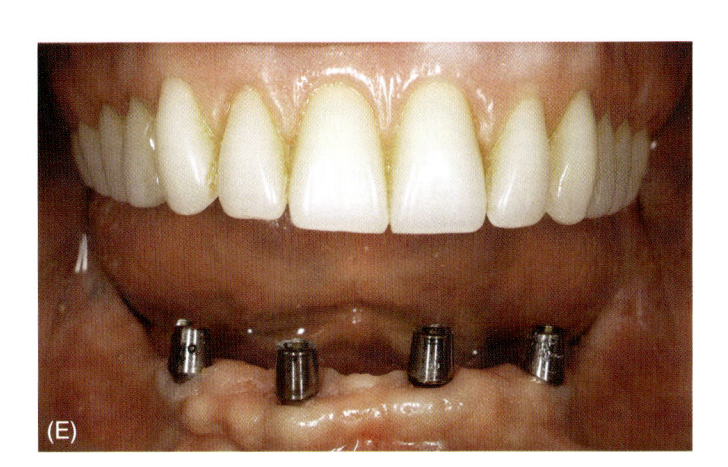

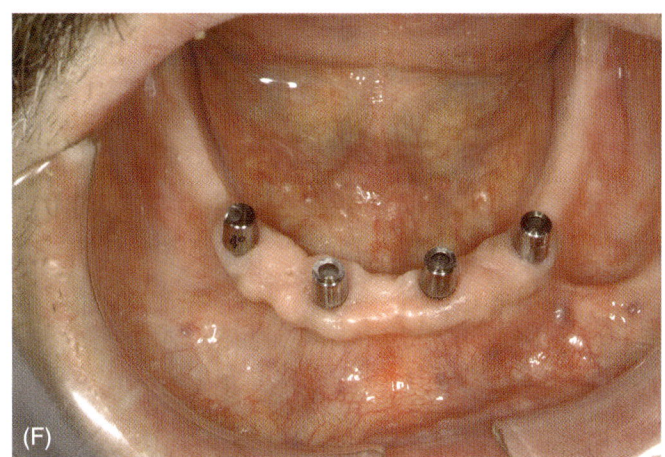

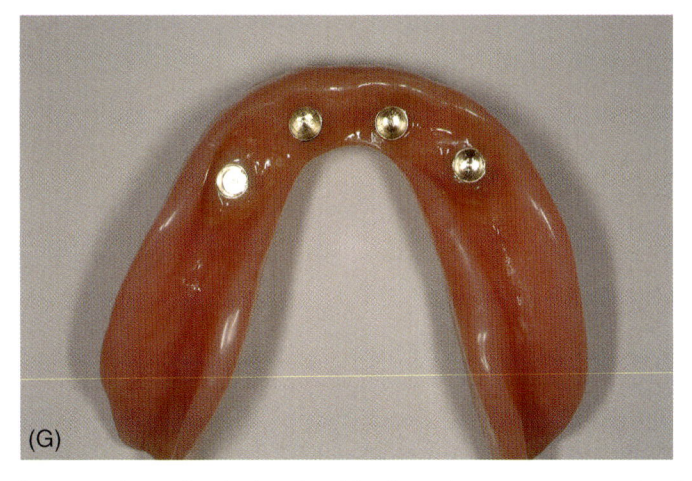

Figure 31.15 **(E–G)** Four Ankylos implants were immediately placed and SynCone abutments connected and four SynCone gold caps were immediately integrated into a previously fabricated immediate lower denture.

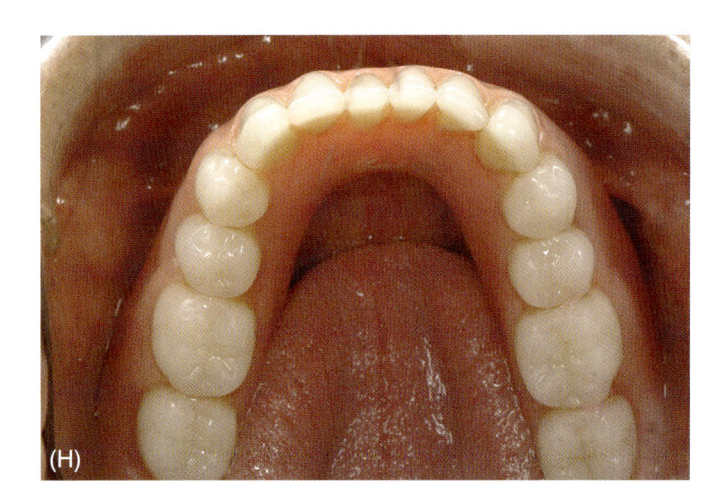

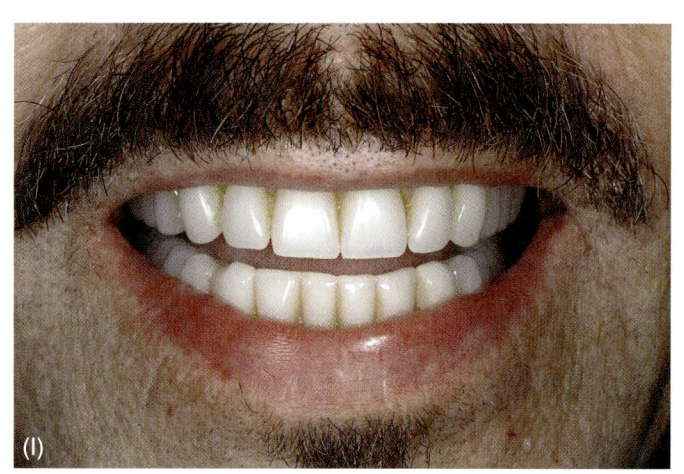

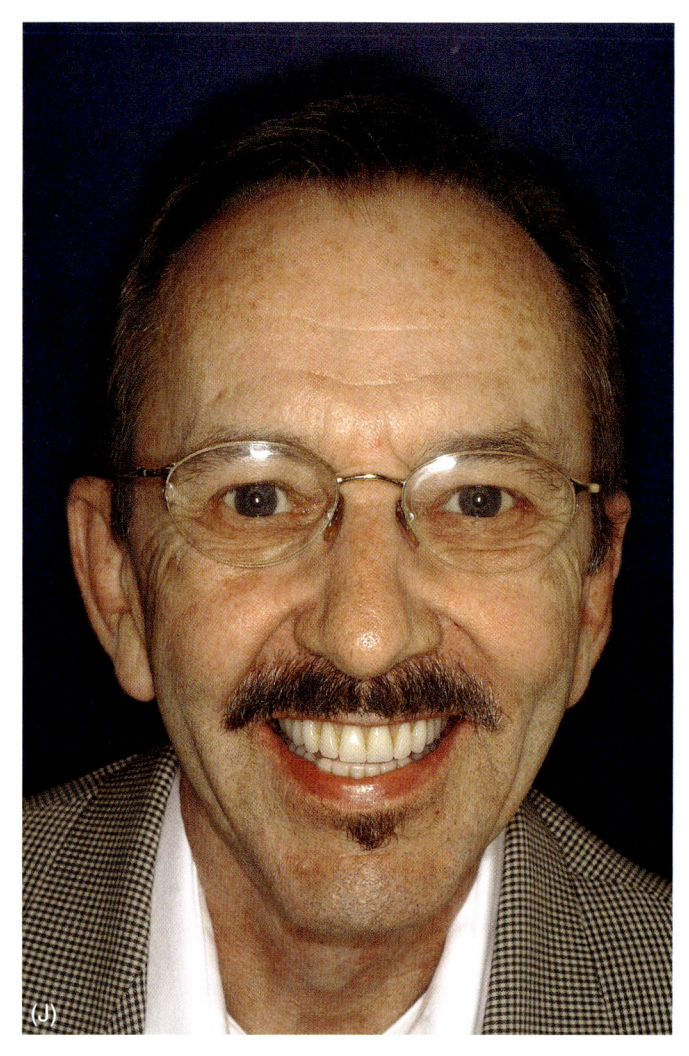

Figure 31.15 (H–J) The patient's facial esthetics and dental health and function have been restored with improved fit and retention.

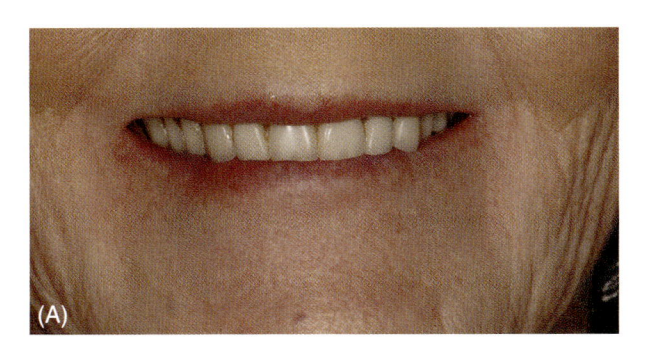

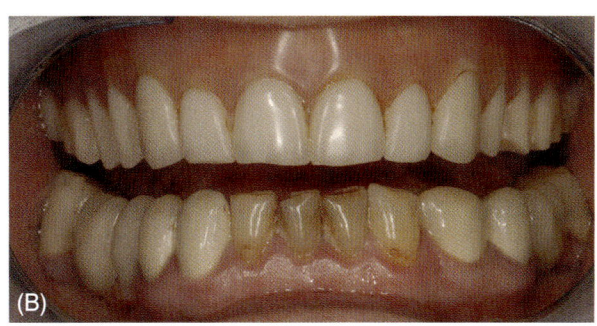

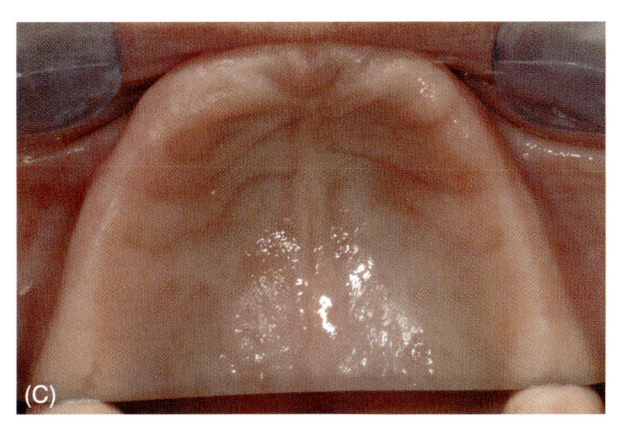

Chapter 31 Geresthetics: Esthetic Dentistry for Older Adults

Figure 31.16 **(A–C)** After three decades of being edentulous, this 72-year-old woman wanted to replace her maxillary full denture and lower bridges with implant-retained prostheses in a desire to improve her overall dental esthetics.

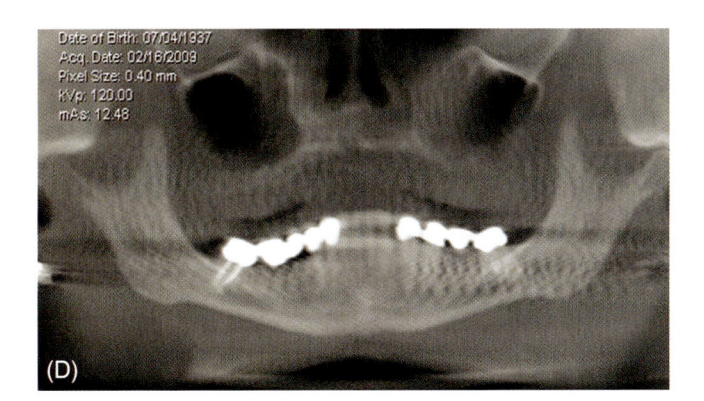

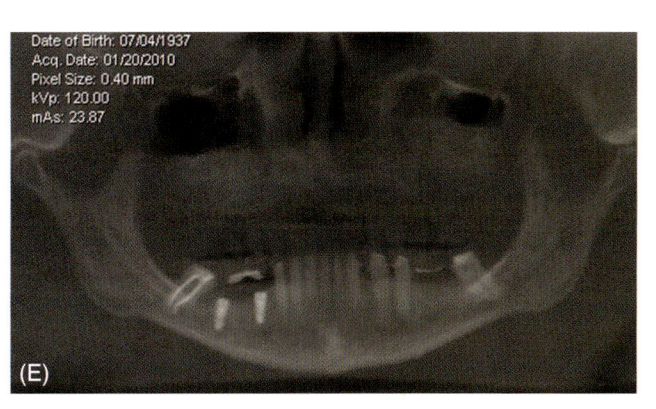

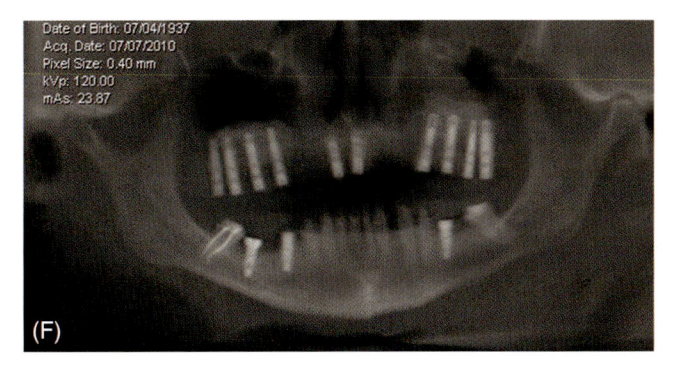

Figure 31.16 **(D–F)** Panoramic CBCT renderings showing before, during and after surgical treatment. Her initial clinical and radiographic evaluations revealed insufficient bone for maxillary implants without extensive grafting and reconstructive surgeries. There were no health, time, or financial restrictions.

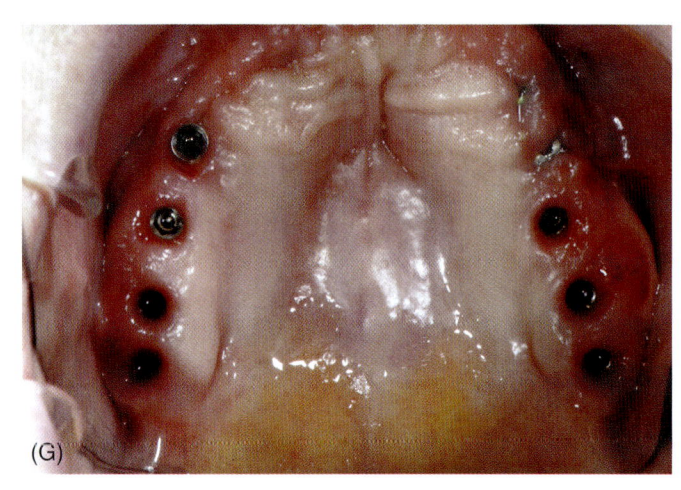

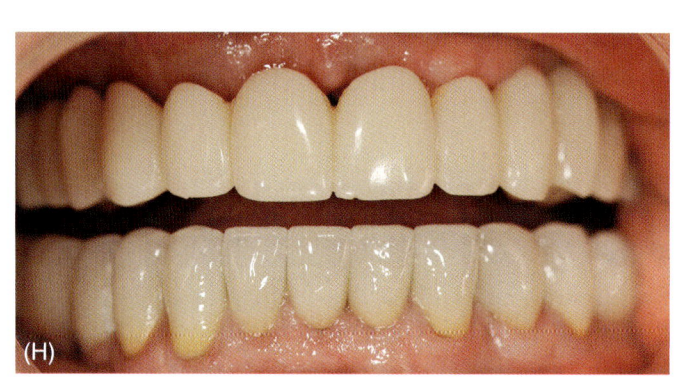

Figure 31.16 **(G, H)** Sequential surgery included bilateral sinus floor augmentation (Figure 30.16E), followed by implant placement in posterior right and left maxilla, and mandibular right and left edentulous spaces. Immediate loading of these implants in a maxillary screw-retained provisional bridge was performed.

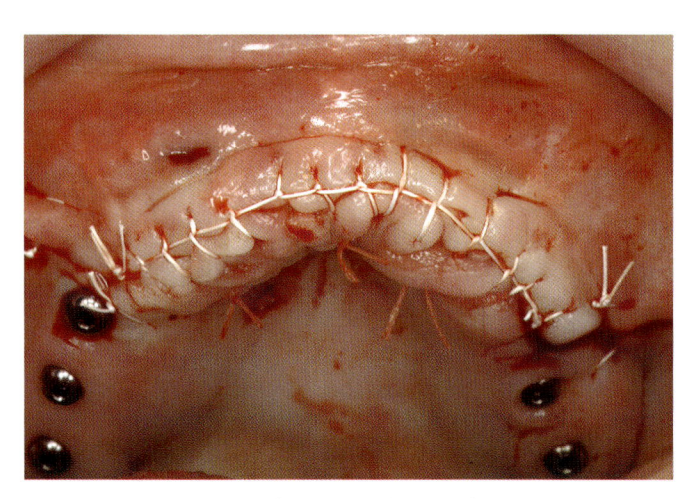

Figure 31.16 **(I)** Later, implants were placed in the anterior maxilla with simultaneous bony ridge augmentation.

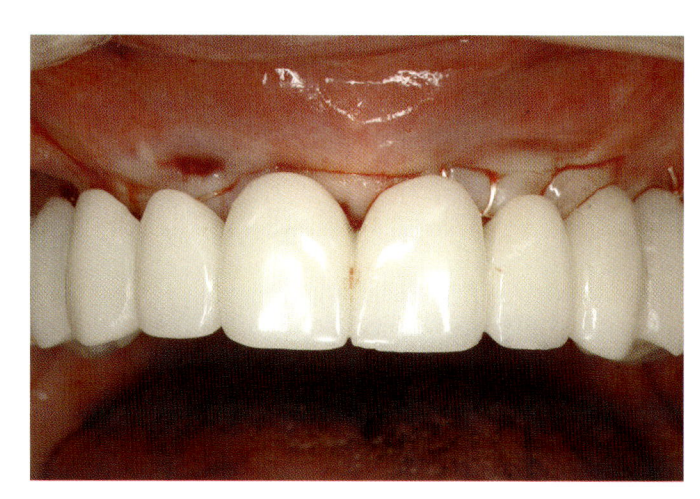

Figure 31.16 **(J)** The aforementioned immediate temporary bridge was placed.

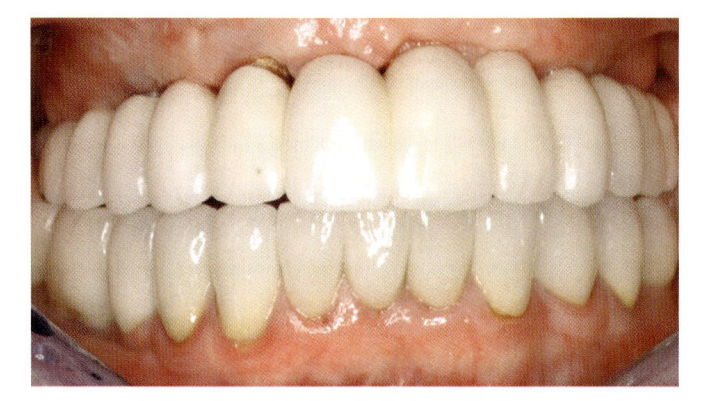

Figure 31.16 **(K)** The final maxillary ceramo-metal implant fixed bridge was seated along with mandibular single natural teeth and implant crowns.

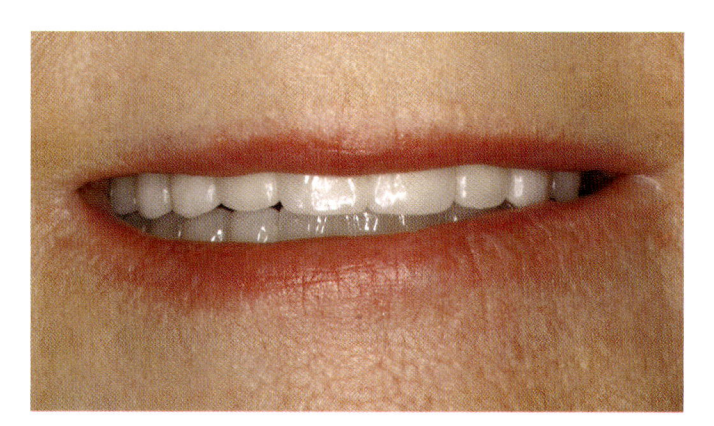

Figure 31.16 **(L)** The patient was extremely pleased with the esthetic and functional treatment outcome and later pursued plastic surgery interventions to further enhance her facial esthetic and more youthful appearance.

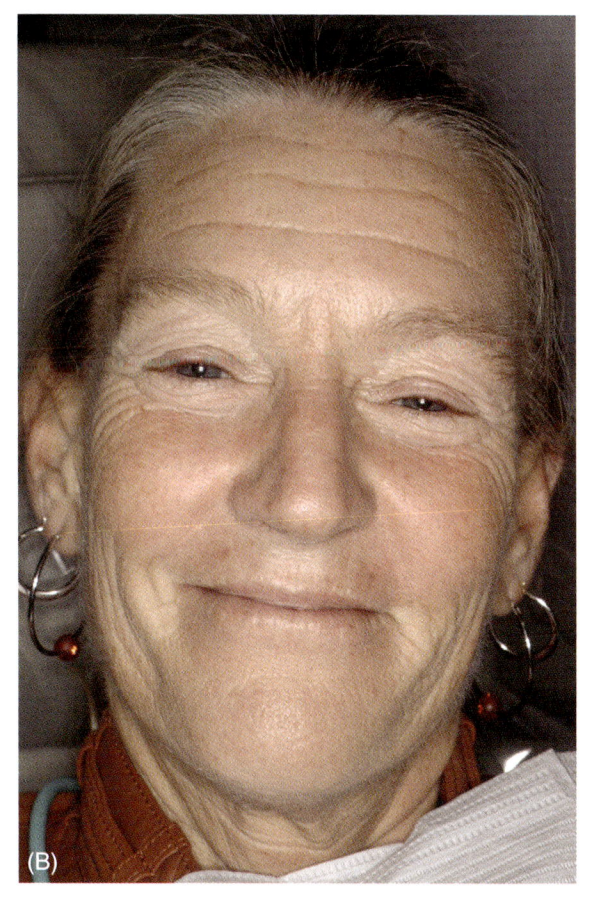

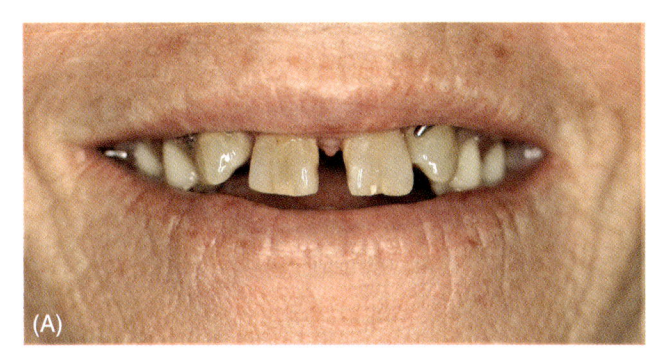

Chapter 31 Geresthetics: Esthetic Dentistry for Older Adults

Figure 31.17 **(A, B)** This 60-year-old female was avoiding dental visits and treatment due to her extreme dental fears and anxiety.

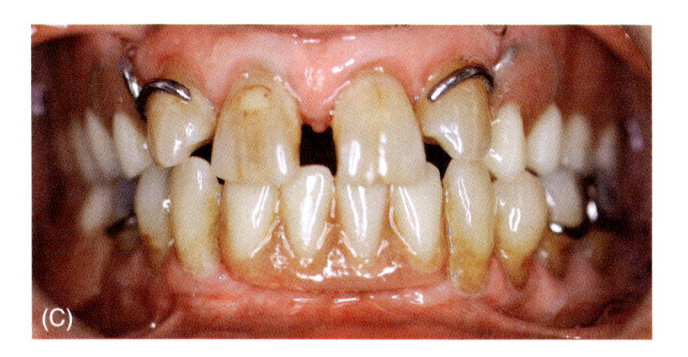

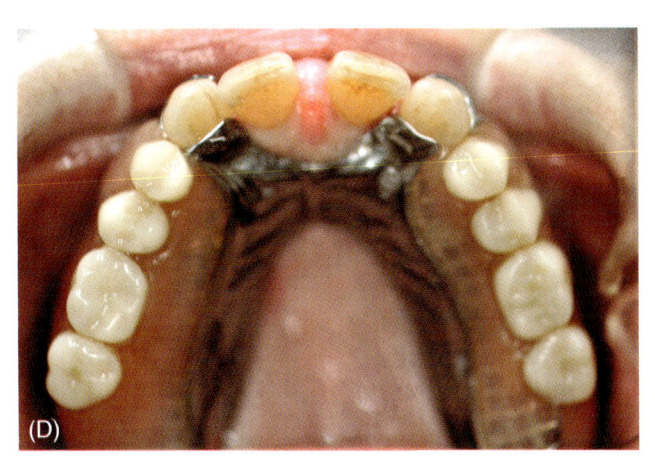

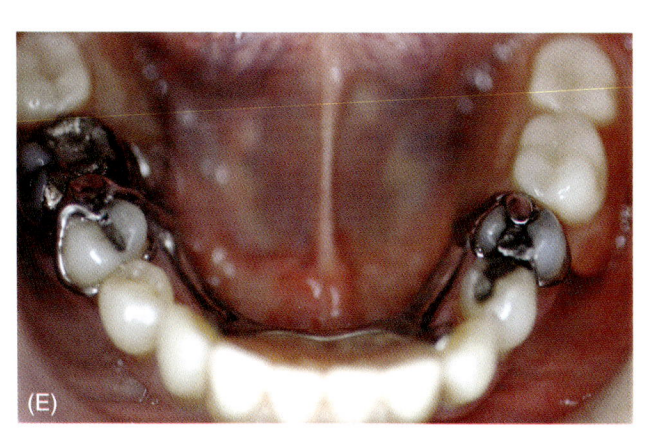

Figure 31.17 **(C–E)** The patient had congenitally missing maxillary lateral incisors, large diastemas and flaring in her anterior maxillary teeth. In addition, she was missing all of her posterior maxillary teeth and mandibular incisors and all-but-one periodontally compromised molar #30.

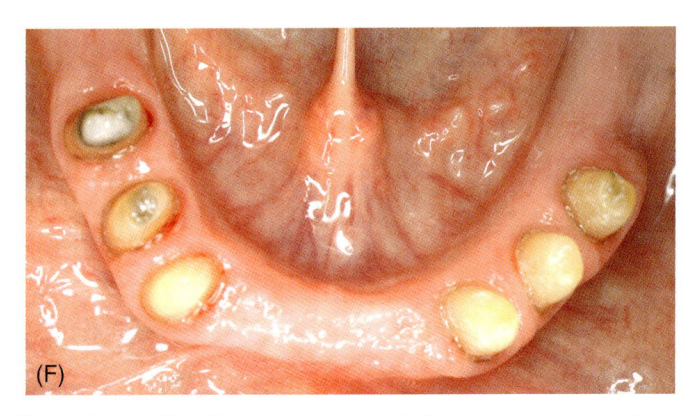

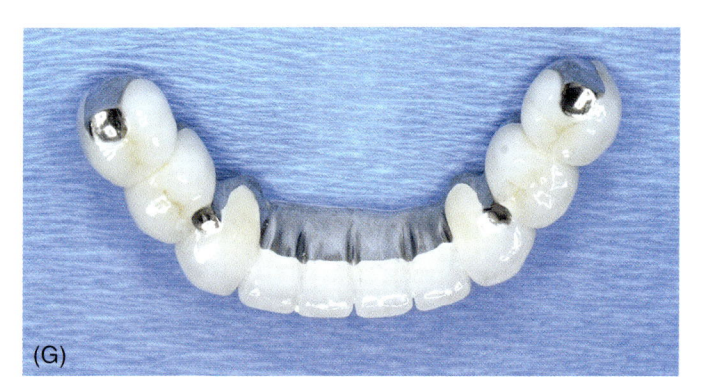

Figure 31.17 **(F, G)** The mandibular rehabilitation included extraction of a nonrestorable molar (#30) and preparation of lower right and left canines and premolars for a fixed bridge replacing the lower incisors. Note the metal rests as a contingency plan for a removable partial denture to replace her mandibular molars.

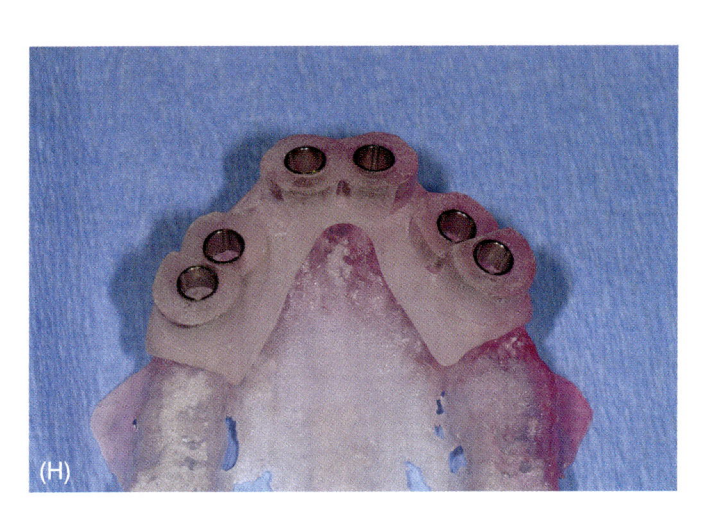

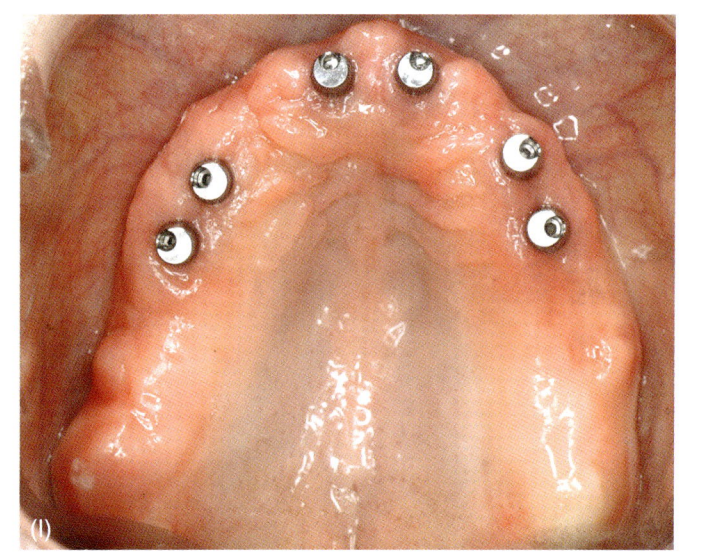

Figure 31.17 **(H, I)** A surgical guide was derived from cone beam computed tomography imaging and utilized in her implant surgery. The maxillary treatment included computer-aided design/manufacture surgical treatment planning and guidance for extraction of teeth #6, #8, #9, and #11 and placement of six Ankylos implants.

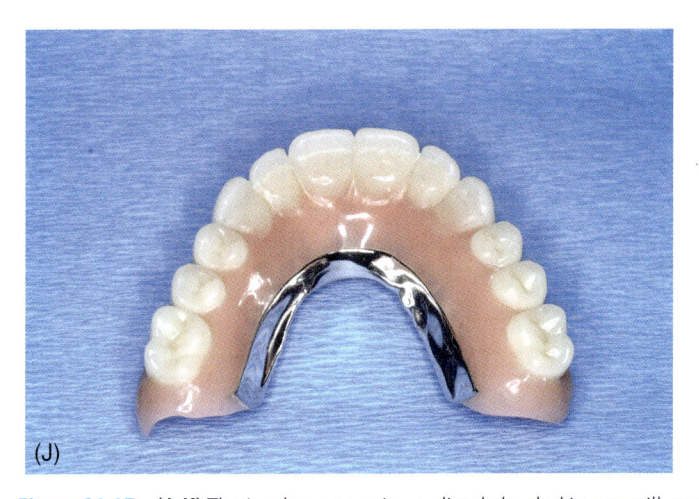

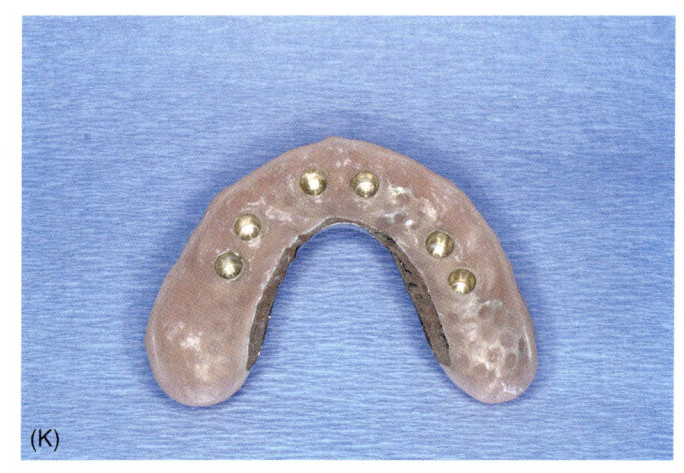

Figure 31.17 **(J, K)** The implants were immediately loaded in a maxillary treatment denture. Upon osseointegration, a final SynCone overdenture was fabricated.

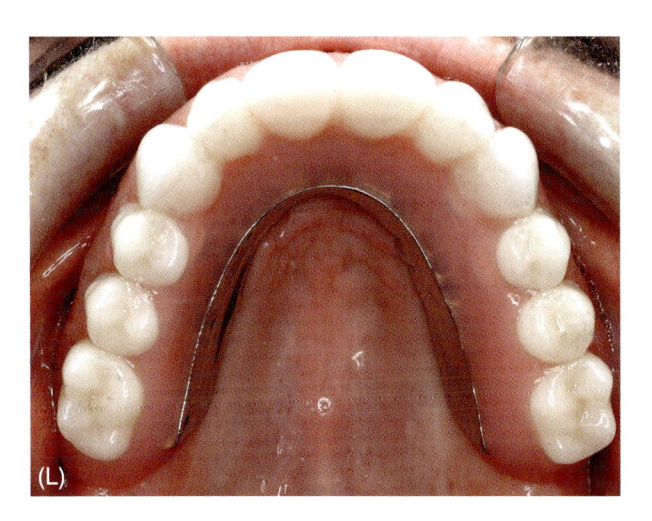

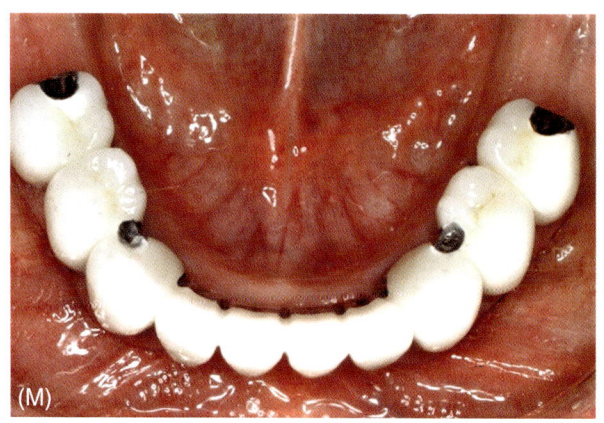

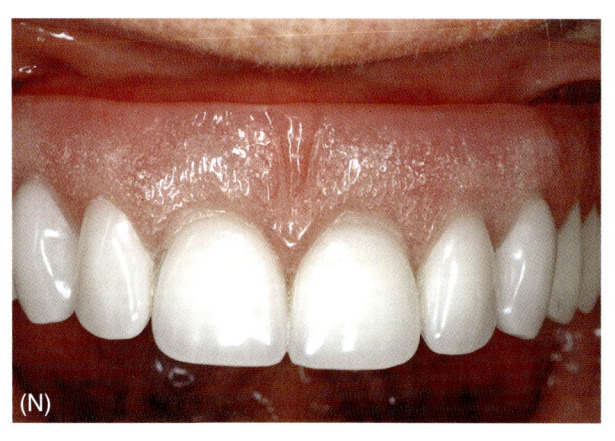

Figure 31.17 **(L–N)** The patient's final treatment has restored not only her dental function and esthetics, but her trust in the dental profession.

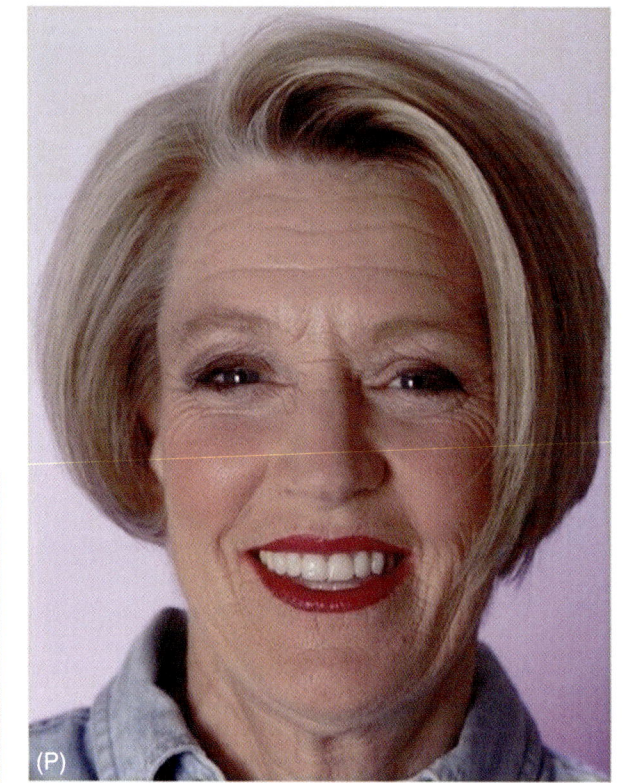

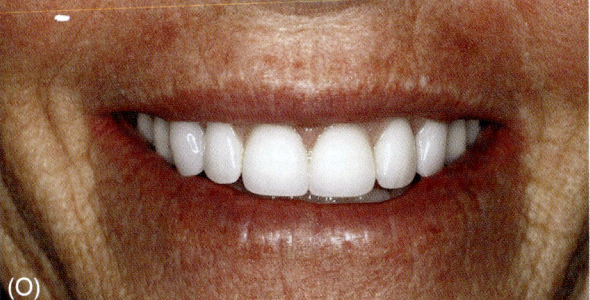

Figure 31.17 **(O, P)** Six years later, the patient remains in great dental shape and among the most pleasant, compliant, and regular dental patients. The dramatic result she received is a true measure of the difference in quality of life that esthetic prosthetic dentistry can help provide.

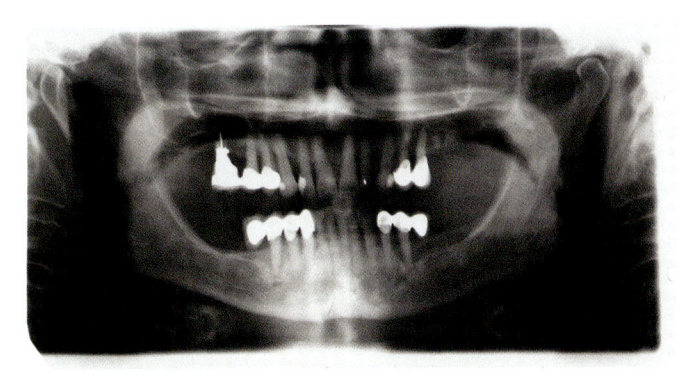

Figure 31.18 **(A)** A 75-year-old female patient presented with advanced periodontal disease and loose failing dentition.

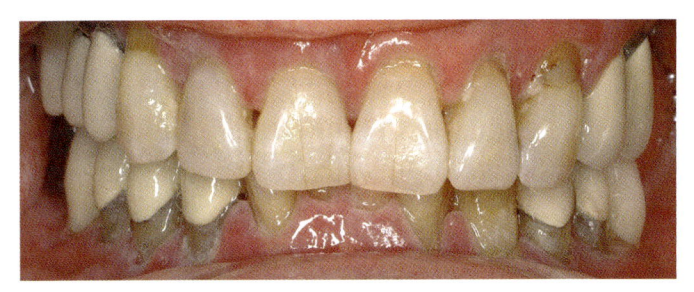

Figure 31.18(B) New patient photos show the advanced attachment loss and inflammation. Clinical examination revealed dental caries and mobility.

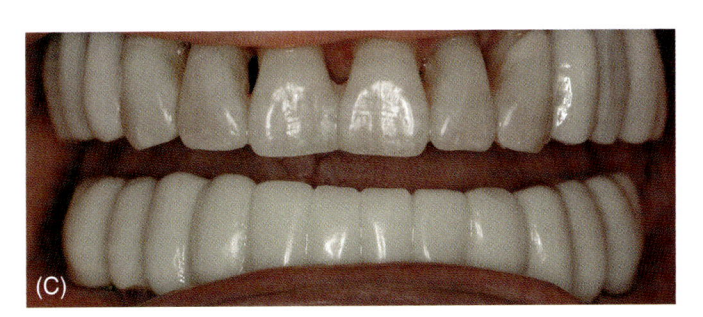

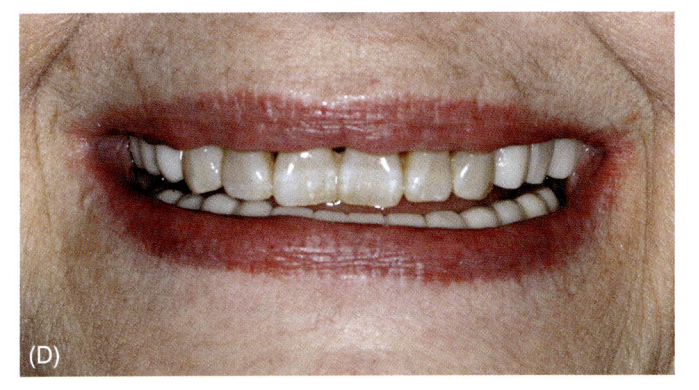

Figure 31.18 **(C, D)** After sequential surgeries, extraction of lower teeth with immediate implant placement and immediate provisionalization, bilateral sinus lift, and eventual implant placement and provisionalization. Full lower, upper right, and upper left posterior implant-retained provisional bridges.

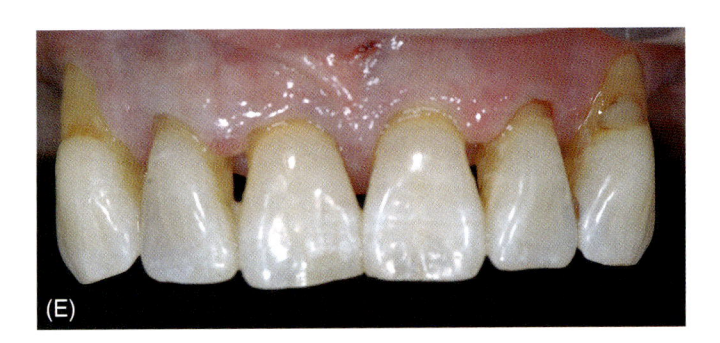

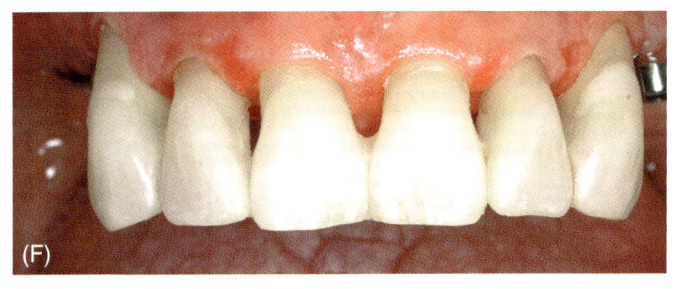

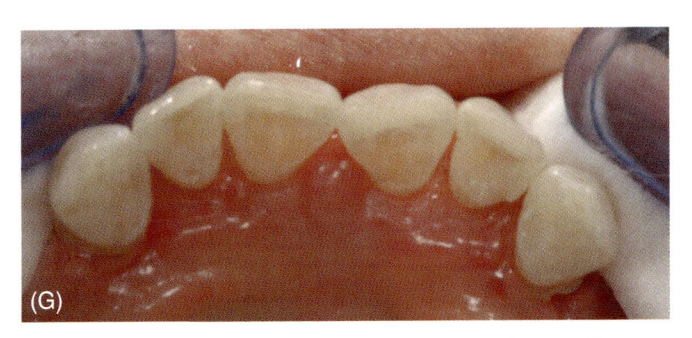

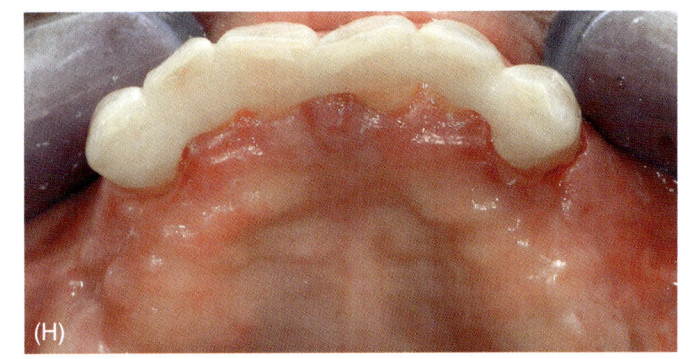

Figure 31.18 **(E–H)** The decision was made to retain her maxillary anterior teeth until her maxillary posterior implants are restored, and eventually be replaced with implants as well. However, after periodontal therapy, replacement of old composite resin restorations as well as a lingual bonded retainer were completed, it was decided to retain her maxillary anterior teeth due to their improved prognosis.

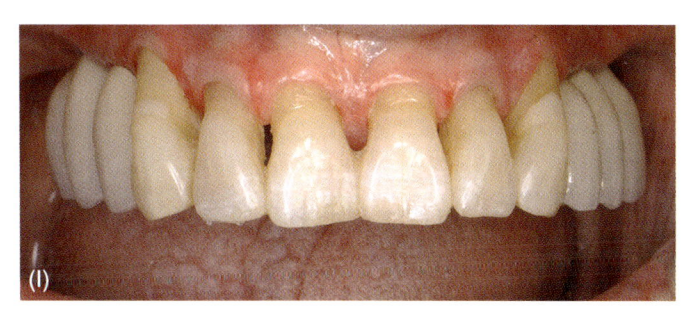

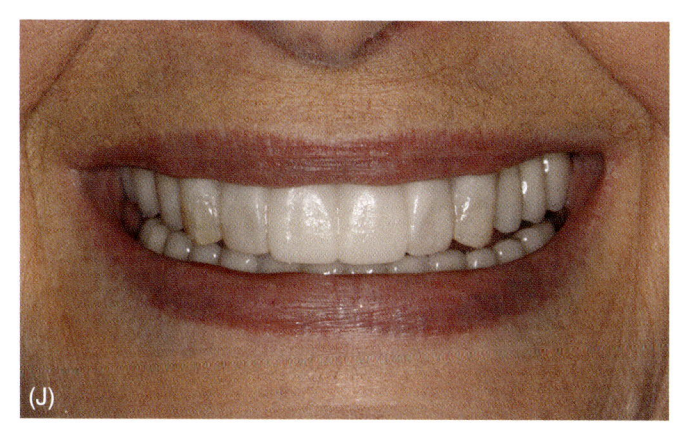

Figure 31.18 (I, J) After seating full mandibular and maxillary posterior final implant ceramo-metal crowns and bridges and despite bleaching her maxillary front teeth, the patient inquired about improving their esthetics as well. A trial smile was performed based on an updated diagnostic wax-up. The teeth have been stable periodontally and the patient was extremely compliant with home care and frequent periodontal maintenance recalls. A change in treatment plan was made from extraction and implant placement to splinted porcelain-fused-to-metal crowns.

Conclusion

There are few things in a dental practice that can be more satisfying than helping a patient to obtain the best esthetic appearance possible; it can be just as important to work toward that goal when the patient is elderly. Although it may be the family and friends who enjoy seeing their loved one look and feel their best, ultimately it is the older individual who has the most to gain with enhanced esthetics and function. Esthetic dentistry has the potential to contribute greatly to improving the oral health and quality of life of older adults. Americans now have the potential to enjoy a lifetime of oral health rather than suffer from a lifetime of oral diseases. The desire to feel good and look healthy is not limited by age.

The new procedures, materials, and techniques that have provided an esthetic revolution in dentistry will provide older Americans with improved quality of life, greater self-esteem, and a lifetime of oral function. Patients should be given the opportunity to learn how esthetic dentistry can improve the quality of their life at any age. Even in the nursing home, life revolves around speaking, smiling, eating, and socializing—all functions of the oral cavity. An esthetic smile is an asset at any age and in any venue.

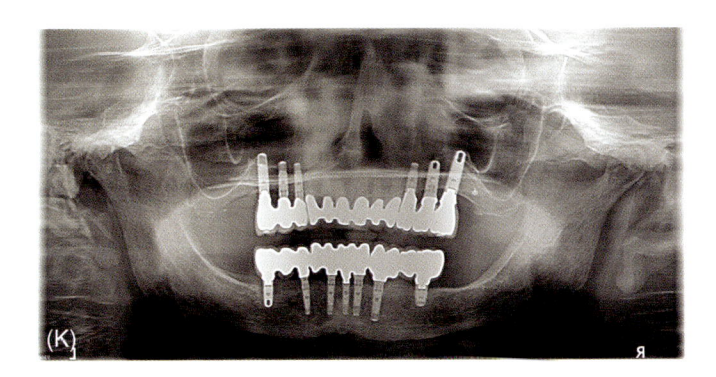

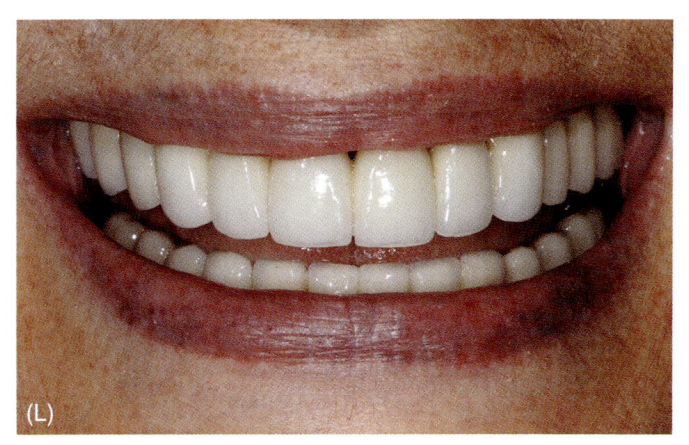

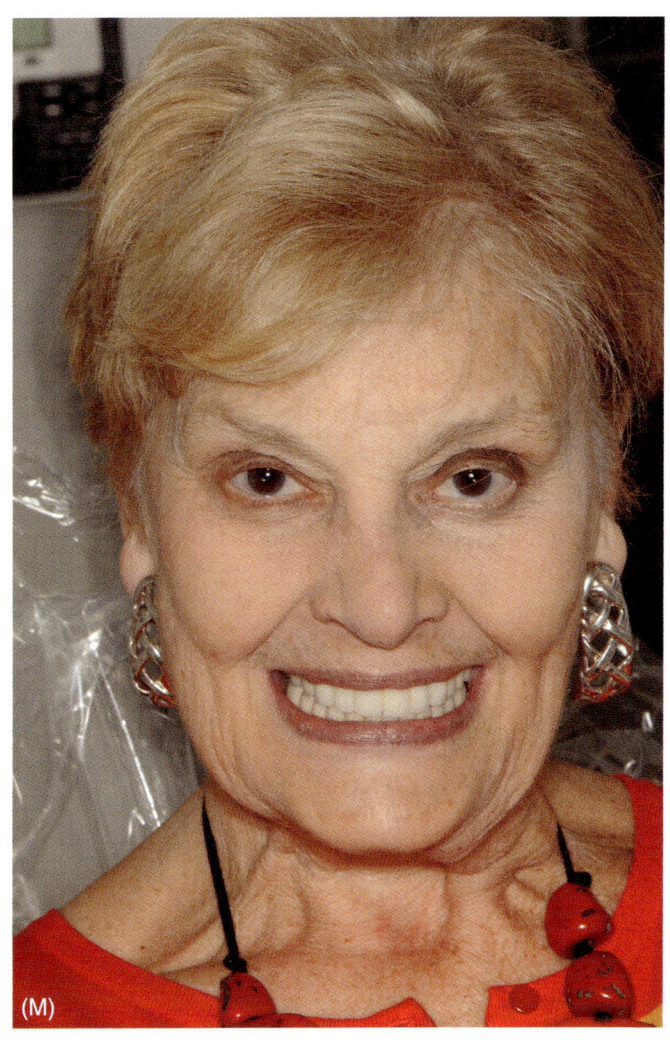

Figure 31.18 (K–M) Over 2 years after treatment completion, the patient continues to be compliant, healthy and happy with her treatment delivered.

References

1. *CIA World Factbook*, 2003–2011. https://www.cia.gov/library/publications/download/index.html (accessed November 3, 2017).
2. Arias E, Heron M, Xu J. United States life tables, 2012. *National Vital Statistics Reports*, vol. 65, no. 8, November 28, 2016.
3. Goldstein RE. Esthetic dentistry: a health service. *J Dent Res* 1993;72:641–242.
4. Goldstein RE, Niessen LC. Issues in esthetic dentistry for older adults. *J Esthet Dent* 1998;10:235–242.
5. U.S. Bureau of the Census. *Statistical Abstract of the United States, 2012*. Washington, DC: Government Printing Office; 2012.
6. National Institutes of Health. *Oral Health in America: A Report of the Surgeon General*. Washington, DC: Government Printing Office; 2000.
7. Beck JD, Offenbacher S. Systemic effects of periodontitis: epidemiology of periodontal disease and cardiovascular disease. *J Periodontol* 2005;76(11 Suppl):2089–2100.
8. Wu T, Trevisan M, Genco R, et al. Periodontal disease and risk of cerebrovascular disease. *Arch Intern Med* 2000;160:2749–2755.
9. Goldstein RE. *Change Your Smile*, 3rd edn. Carol Stream, IL: Quintessence; 1997
10. American Society for Aesthetic Plastic Surgery. *2010 Statistics in Cosmetic Surgery* (April 4, 2011). www.cosmeticplasticsurgerystatistics.com (accessed November 3, 2017).
11. National Center for Health Statistics. *Health, United States, 2011*. Hyattsville, MD: NCHS; 2011.
12. Summer L. *Chronic Conditions: A Challenge for the 21st Century*, Vol. 1. Washington, DC: National Academy on an Aging Society; 1999.
13. Prevalence of doctor-diagnosed arthritis and arthritis-attributable activity limitation-United States, 2007–2009. *MMWR Morb Mortal Wkly Rep* 2010;59(39):1261–1265.
14. Sollecito TP, Abt E, Lockhart PB, et al. The use of prophylactic antibiotics prior to dental procedures in patients with prosthetic points. *JADA* 2015;146(1):11–16.
15. Fontana M, Zero DT. Assessing patients' caries risk. *J Am Dent Assoc* 2006;137(9):1231–1239.
16. Fox PC. Differentiation of dry mouth etiology. *Adv Dent Res* 1996;10:13–16.
17. American Dental Association. *Xerostomia (Dry Mouth)*. www.ada.org/en/member-center/oral-health-topics/xerostomia (accessed November 28, 2017).
18. DeSpain B, Niessen LC. Health promotion and disease prevention for patients seeking esthetic dental care. Part I. Strategies for health promotion. *J Esthet Dent* 1995;7(5):189–196.
19. Niessen LC, Gibson G. Oral health for a lifetime: preventive strategies for the older adult. *Quintessence Int* 1997;28(9):626–630.
20. Mealey BA, TW Oates. Diabetes mellitus and periodontal diseases. *J Periodontol* 2006;77:1289–1303.
21. National Cancer Institute. *Cancer Stat Facts: Oral Cavity and Pharynx*. www.seer.cancer.gov/statfacts/html/oralcav.html (accessed November 3, 2017).
22. Featherstone JDB, Domejean-Orliaguet S, Jensen L, et al. Caries risk assessment in practice for age 6 through adult. *J Calif Dent Assoc* 2007;35(10):703–713.
23. American Dental Association Council on Scientific Affairs. Professionally applied topical fluoride: evidence-based clinical recommendations. *J Am Dent Assoc* 2006;137(8):1151–1159.
24. Gibson G, Jurasic MM, Wehler CJ, Jones JA. Supplemental fluoride use for moderate and high caries risk adults: a systematic review. *J Public Health Dent* 2011;71:171–184.
25. Tan HP, Lo ECM, Dyson JE, et al. A randomized trial on root caries prevention in elders. *J Dent Res* 2010;89(10):1086–1090.
26. Bryant SR, Zarb GA. Outcomes of implant prosthodontic treatment in older adults. *J Can Dent Assoc* 2002;68(2):97–102.
27. Strayer M. "Catching up" with the problem of homebound care. *Spec Care Dent* 1998;18:52–57.
28. Gift HC, Cherry-Peppers G, Oldakowski RJ. Oral health care in US nursing homes, 1995. *Spec Care Dent* 1998;18:226–233.
29. Lin CY, Jones DB, Godwin K, et al. Oral health assessment by nursing staff of Alzheimer's patients in a long term care facility. *Spec Care Dent* 1999;19:64–71.

Additional resources

Curtis D. Are we doing enough for the geriatric patient? *Int J Prosthodont* 2016;29(2):111–112.

DeVisschere L, Van Der Putten GJ, deBaat C, et al. The impact of undergraduate geriatric dental education on the attitudes of recently graduated dentists towards institutionalized elderly people. *Euro J Dent Educ* 2009;13:154–161.

Eymard AS, Douglas DH. Ageism among healthcare providers and interventions to improve their attitudes toward older adults: an integrative review. *J Gerontol Nurs* 2012;38:26–35.

Goldstein RE. Diagnostic dilemma: to bond, laminate, or crown. *Int J Periodont Restor Dent* 1987;87(5):9–30.

Goldstein RE. Esthetic principles for ceramo-metal restorations. *Dent Clin North Am* 1988;21:803–822.

Goldstein RE. Finishing of composites and laminates. *Dent Clin North Am* 1989;33:305–318.

Goldstein RE, Feinman RA, Garber DA. Esthetic considerations in the selection and use of restorative materials. *Dent Clin North Am* 1983;27:723–731.

Goldstein RE, Garber DA, Schwartz CG, Goldstein CE. Patient maintenance of esthetic restorations. *J Am Dent Assoc* 1992;123:61–66.

Goldstein RE, Garber DA. Goldstein CE, et al. The changing esthetic dental practice. *J Am Dent Assoc* 1994;125:1447–1457.

Kassebaum NJ, Bernabe E, Dahila M, et al. Global burden of untreated caries: a systematic review and metaregression. *J Dent Res* 2015;94:650–658.

Niessen, LC. Geriatric dentistry in the next millennium: opportunities for leadership in oral health. *Gerodontology* 2000;17(1):3–7.

Niessen LC and DeSpain B. Health promotion and disease prevention for patients seeking esthetic dental care. Part II. Clinical strategies for prevention of oral diseases. *J Esthet Dent* 1996;8(1):3–11.

Niessen LC, Gibson G. Aging and oral health for the 21st century. *Gen Dent* 2000;48 (5):544–549.

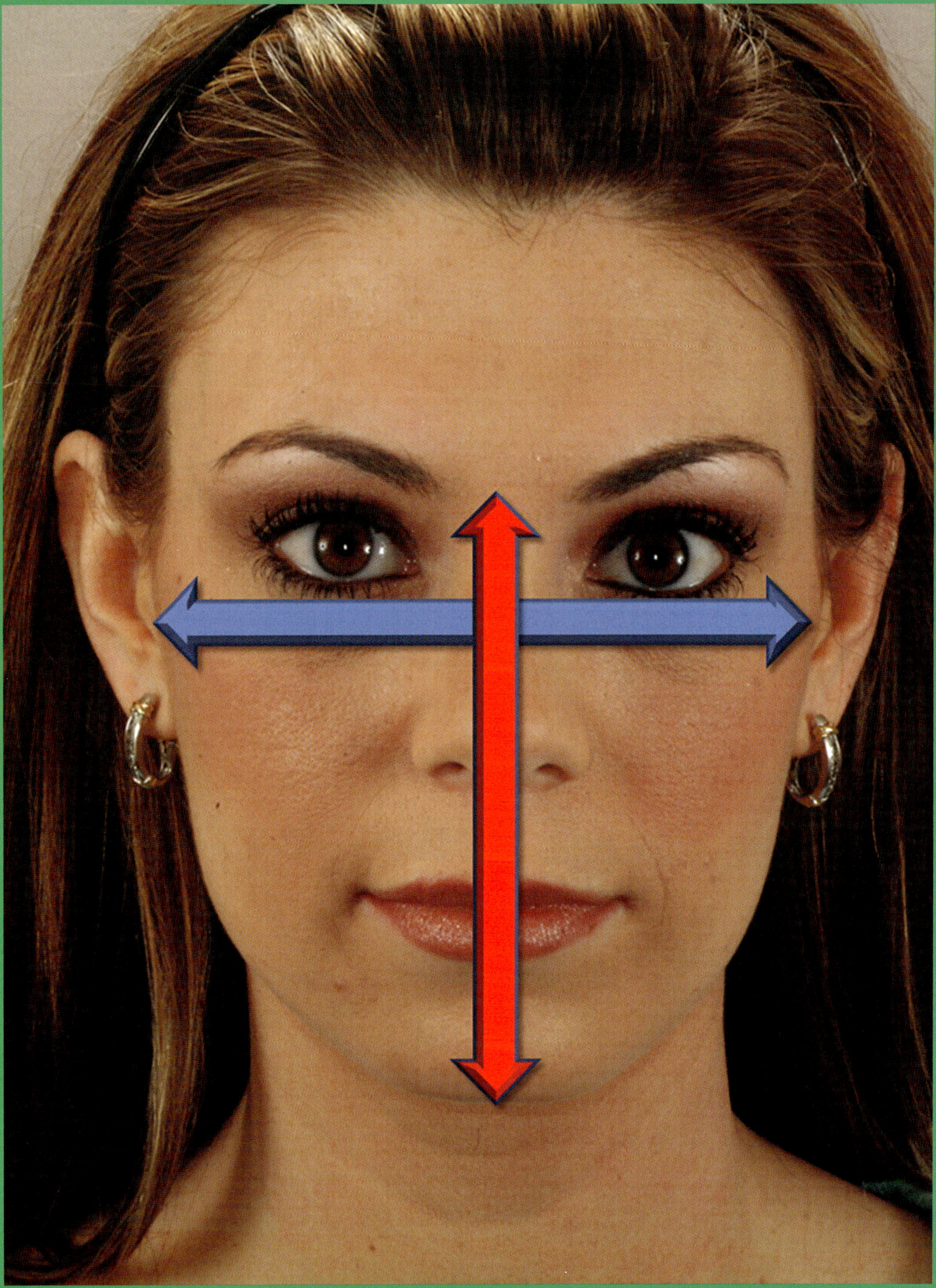

Chapter 32 Facial Considerations: An Orthodontic Perspective

David Sarver, DMD, MS

Chapter Outline

An esthetic approach to evaluation: enhancement of appearance	1051	Macroesthetic evaluation of the face: profile view	1063
Diagnosis and treatment planning in three dimensions: face, smile, and teeth	1052	Macroesthetics and smile dimensions	1068
		Pitch, roll, and yaw	1072
Technology and facial imaging	1056	Clinical case study	1076
Dentofacial analysis: clinical examination	1057	Macroesthetic analysis	1076
Vertical facial proportions	1057	Miniesthetic analysis	1078
		Microesthetic analysis (teeth)	1078
Macroesthetic evaluation of the face: oblique view	1062	Orthodontic–surgical treatment	1079

An esthetic approach to evaluation: enhancement of appearance

While we teach our children that we should not judge a person by their looks, the reality is that the world often judges based on personal appearances. While patients may walk in our offices seeking to correct their bite, the reality is that most are seeking a complete enhancement of the appearance, including dentition, occlusion, their smile, and face, which will greatly affect their self-image and how others perceive them.

The primary focus of cosmetic dentistry focuses on the presentation of the teeth and surrounding smile framework. Contemporary dentistry broadens the esthetic analysis of the patient to include facial form and proportions. We refer to the facial esthetic portion of orthodontic diagnosis and treatment as enhancement of appearance.[1] It is important to analyze the morphologic form of the face, the overlying soft-tissue envelope, and the underlying facial skeleton integrated with the dentition to fully understand comprehensive dentofacial diagnosis. Patients who seek orthodontic and cosmetic dental treatment do so to improve their quality of life,[2] both for functional improvement and enhancement of appearance. To achieve both ideals—occlusion and facial esthetics—is the challenge. When discussing the need for treatment with our patients, occlusal discrepancies require treatment for preservation of dentition and long-term stable occlusion, but to treat only the occlusion treats only half of the patient. Likewise, treating only the esthetic component equally treats only half of the patient.

While the focus in the past has been in using cephalometric analysis as a significant determinant in treatment planning, today our focus is primarily based on soft-tissue assessment with the goal of achieving the necessary skeletal and dental changes to achieve both functional and esthetic enhancement. Conceptually and operatively, the orthodontist and surgeon must try to visualize the desired solution to the specific problem and then assess how a given solution will positively and equally negatively impact the various components. The concept of facial optimization involves the preservation of as many positive elements as possible, while harmonizing those elements that fall short of the esthetic and functional needs of the patient.

Diagnosis and treatment planning in three dimensions: face, smile, and teeth

A systematic analysis of all the facial components, both anatomically static and functionally dynamic, will lead to a greater appreciation of the subtleties of the interaction of each of the facial elements and how each can be appropriately managed through a unified treatment approach.[3,4] Our approach to diagnosis and treatment planning includes three major areas: the face (macroesthetics), smile (miniesthetics), and teeth (microesthetic). These serve as a framework for systematic evaluation of the esthetic needs of each particular patient (Figure 32.1).[5,6] This framework is a departure from the traditional approach based on models and, in the case of orthodontics, cephalometric values. Dental students will remember being taught about the importance of cephalometrics in orthodontic diagnosis, but today's approach is increasingly focused on the clinical examination and quantification of the patient's facial presentation. This leads all disciplines of dentistry and medicine to analyze facial esthetics in a more homogeneous fashion. Our functional goals of occlusion (Class I, overbite, overjet, etc.) still remain in place, but are evaluated in the context of an expanded dentofacial analysis.

1. **Macroesthetics** encompasses the face in all three planes of space. Examples of macroesthetic appearance issues include a long face, a short face, lack of chin prominence, and other facial features.
2. **Miniesthetics** focuses primarily on the smile framework. The smile framework is bordered by the upper and lower lips on smile animation and includes such assessments of excessive gingival display on smile, inadequate gingival display, inappropriate gingival heights, and excessive buccal corridors.
3. **Microesthetics** includes assessment of tooth proportion in height and width, gingival shape and contour, black triangular holes, tooth shade, and other dental attributes.

The goal of esthetic treatment planning is the improvement of negative attributes, while preserving those attributes that are deemed favorable. Traditional treatment planning focused on generating a problem list and pursuing solutions for each problem without regard for potential negative changes to the patient's existing positive attributes. For example, a classic orthodontic treatment of overjet reduction and Class I cuspid relations in a patient with a skeletal Class II mandibular deficiency would be removal of the maxillary first premolars to make space for retraction of the maxillary anterior teeth. While this satisfies the functional and occlusal problem, it may result in profile flattening and an unfortunate effect on overall facial appearance (Figure 32.2A and B). In contrast, a comprehensive esthetic treatment integrates the components of soft-tissue–skeletal analysis with static–dynamic assessment in three dimensions and the

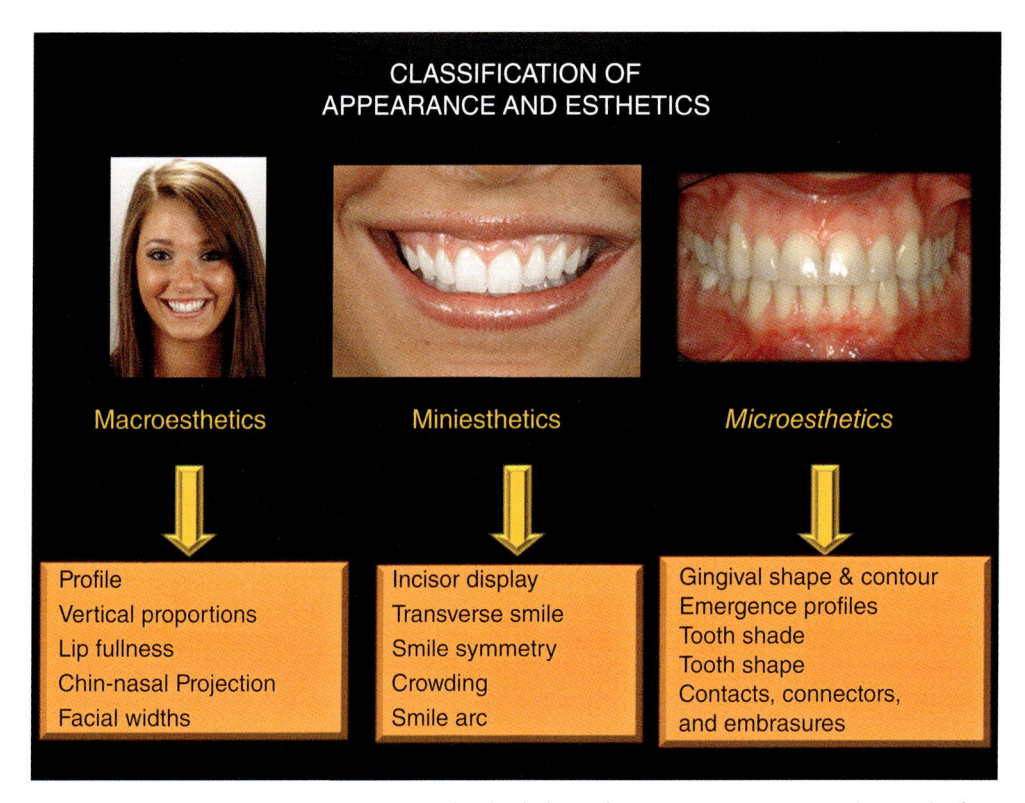

Figure 32.1 Diagnosis and treatment planning of appearance can be divided into three major areas: macroesthetics (the face), miniesthetics (the smile), and microesthetics (the teeth and gingiva).

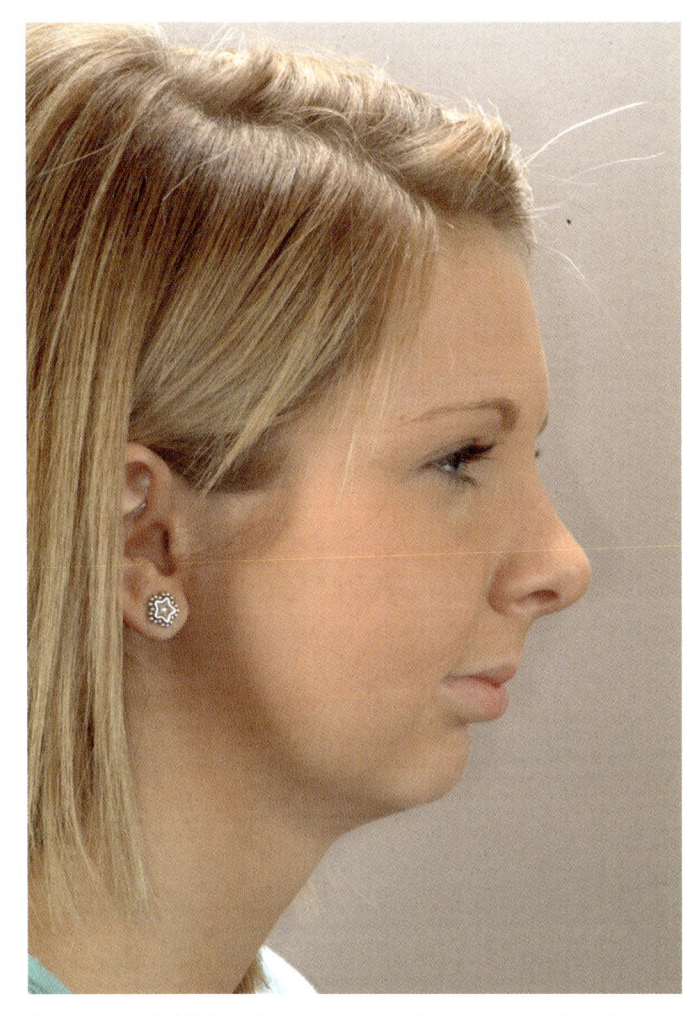

Figure 32.2 (A) This patient was treated for her severe Class II malocclusion through extraction of maxillary first premolars for incisor retraction and overjet reduction. Because the skeletal mandibular deficiency was not addressed, the malocclusion was corrected, but the esthetic outcome was compromised.

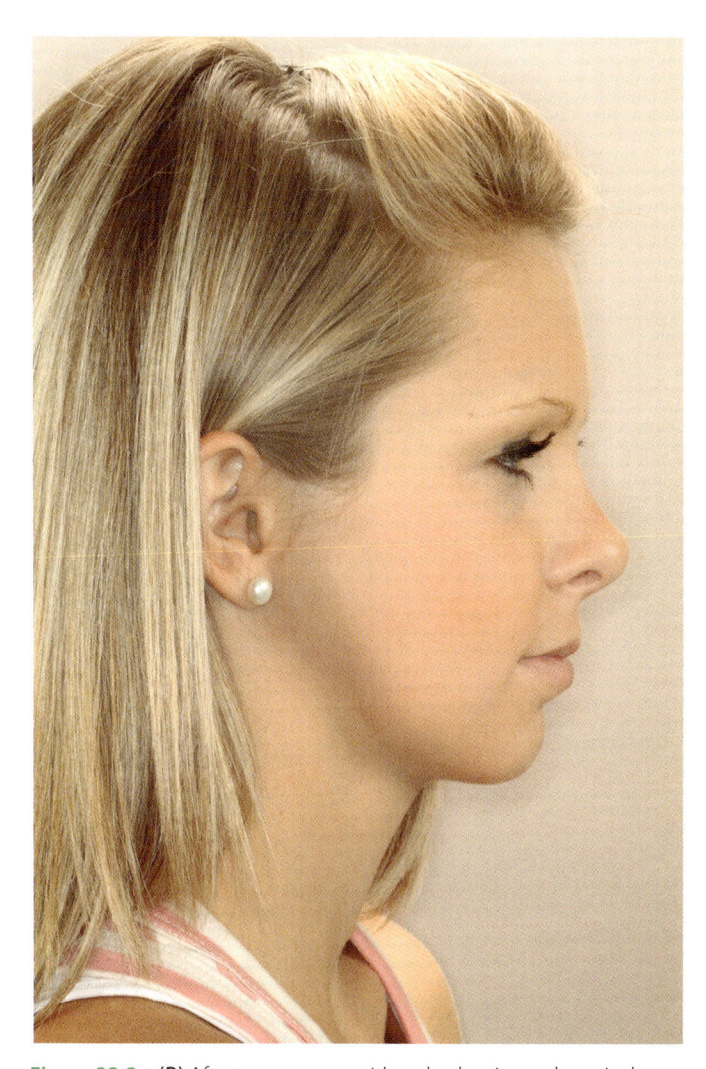

Figure 32.2 (B) After retreatment with orthodontics and surgical bimaxillary advancement, her profile has greatly improved.

positive and negative impact of any one component on another (Figure 32.3). The starting point for the macroesthetic examination is the frontal perspective and is the focus of this chapter.

Macroesthetic evaluation of the face: frontal view

A contemporary analysis of the frontal face needs to go beyond simple categories when defining positive as well as negative attributes that should be considered in the treatment plan. Figure 32.4 and Table 32.1 illustrates the facial landmarks that will be used in the description of the dentofacial analysis.

Excellent imaging naturally infers high-quality care. Quality photographs are an important component in analysis and documentation of the patient's face and serve multiple purposes:

- to allow the clinician to visualize the patient's features and clearly determine the direction of treatment;
- documentation for medicolegal purposes;
- for use in treatment plan presentation to our patients.

For ideal photographic representation of the face, the recommendation is that the camera be positioned in the "portrait" position to maximize use of the photographic field (Figure 32.5). If the camera orientation is in "landscape view", the photo captures too much unneeded background and detracts from the image by diminishing the size of the face (Figure 32.6).

The following facial photographs are recommended as the expected routine for each patient.[7]

Frontal view

The patient assumes a natural head position and looks straight ahead into the camera. Four types of frontal photographs are useful:

- **Frontal at rest** (Figure 32.7). If lip incompetence is present, the lips should be in repose and the mandible in rest position.
- **Frontal view with the teeth in maximal intercuspation, with the lips closed**, even if this strains the patient. This photograph serves as clear documentation of lip strain and its esthetic effect, and the lips-together picture is recommended in patients who have lip incompetence. If lips-apart posture

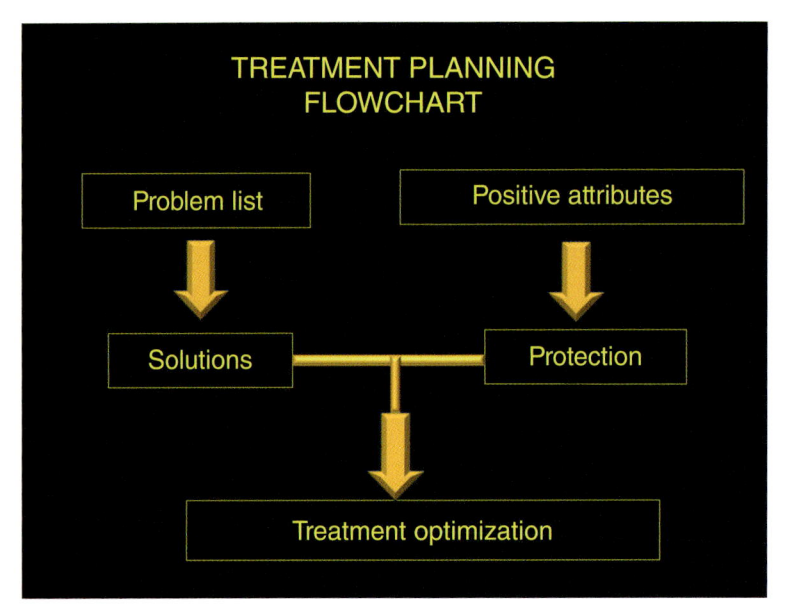

Figure 32.3 Contemporary diagnosis integrates the components of soft-tissue–skeletal analysis with static–dynamic assessment in three dimensions and an understanding of the positive and negative impacts of any one component may have on another.

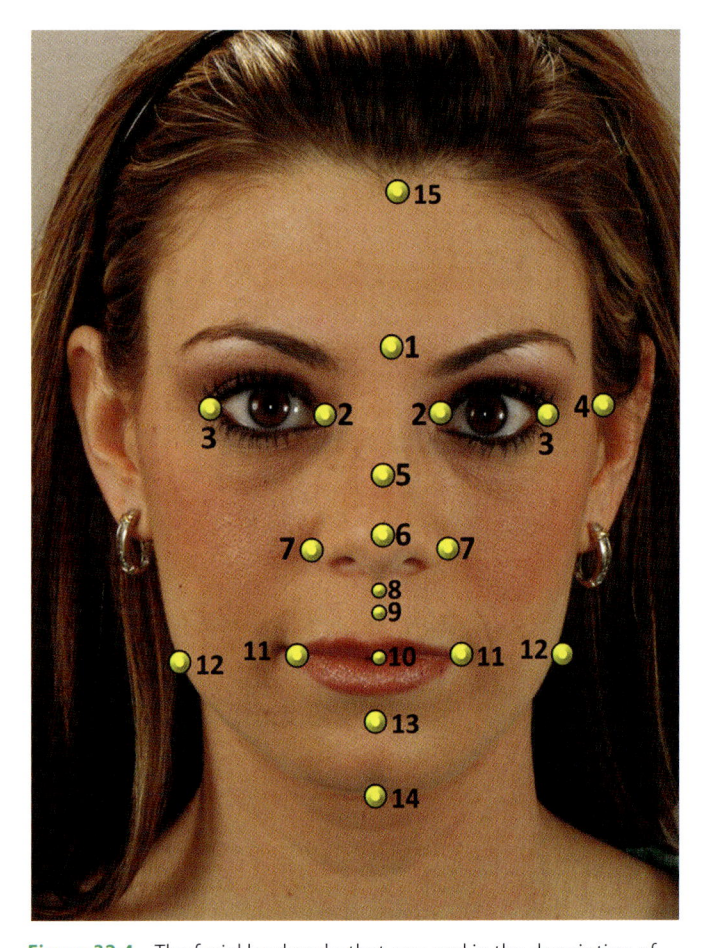

Figure 32.4 The facial landmarks that are used in the description of the dentofacial analysis.

Table 32.1 Frontal Soft-Tissue Points

Glabella	The most anterior aspect of the forehead as it progresses inferior into the nose
Inner canthus	The medial conjunction of the upper and lower eyelids
Outer canthus	The lateral conjunction of the upper and lower eyelids
Zygoma	The outermost aspect of the zygomatic prominence
Mid dorsum	The midpoint of the bony nasal dorsum
Nasal tip	The midpoint of the nasal tip
Alar base	The most lateral aspect of the ala of the nose
Base of nose	The intersection of the nasal columella with the upper lip
Mid philtrum	The midpoint of the philtrum
Inferior philtral tubercle	The most inferior limit of the philtral projection or tubercle of the upper lip
Outer commissure	The lateral conjunction of the upper and lower lips
Gonial angle	The point at the intersection of the posterior ramus and body of the mandible
Labiomental sulcus	The deepest curvature of the lower lip
Menton	The most inferior point of the chin
Trichion	The hairline

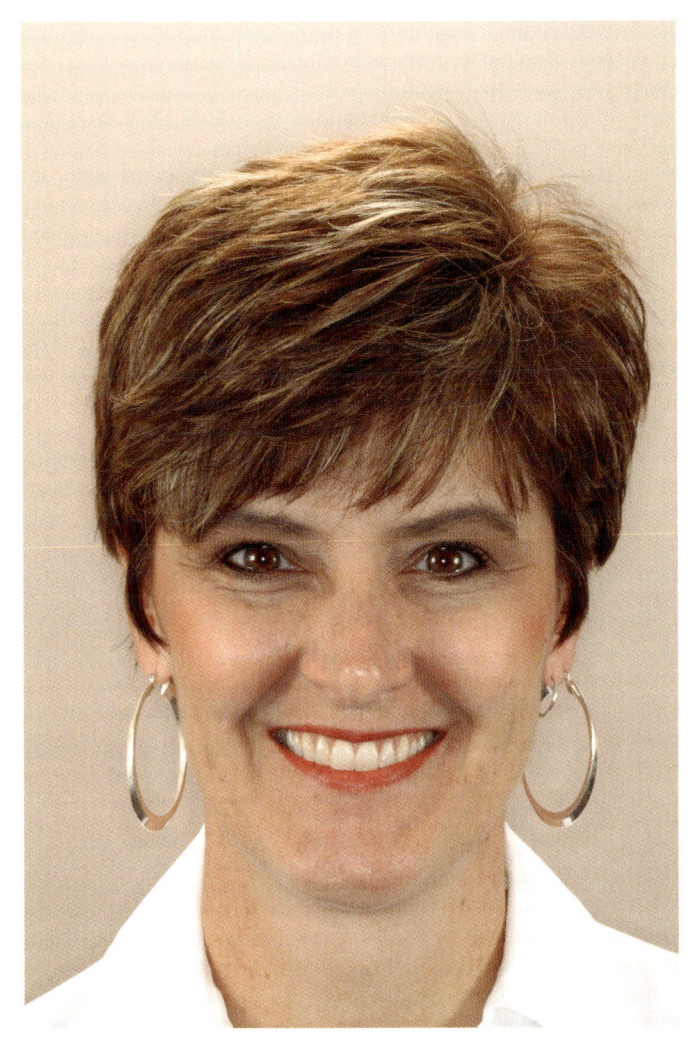

Chapter 32 Facial Considerations: An Orthodontic Perspective

Figure 32.5 For ideal photographic representation of the face, the recommendation is that the camera be positioned in the "portrait" position.

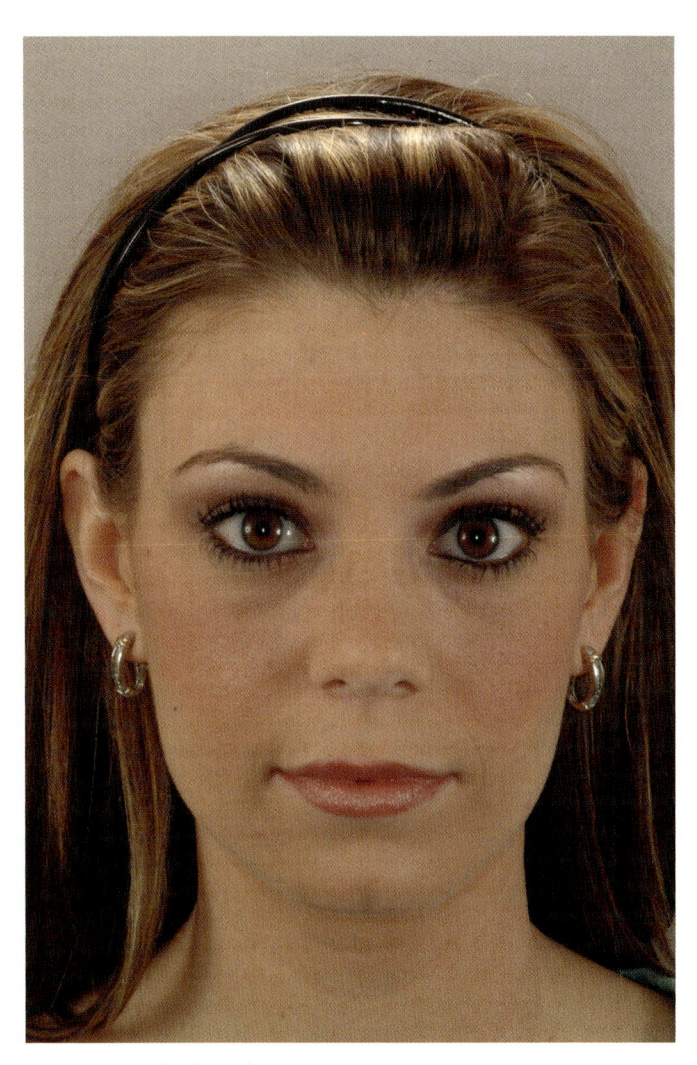

Figure 32.7 The frontal at rest image.

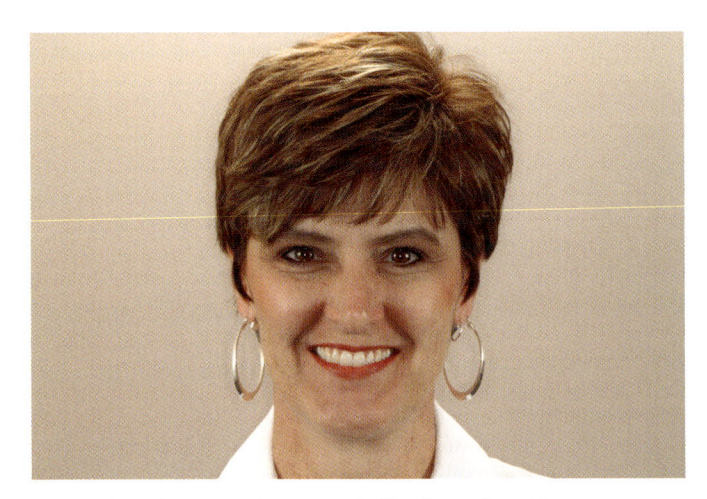

Figure 32.6 Orienting the camera in "landscape" position captures much of the background. This is not only unneeded, but detracts from the image by diminishing the size of the face in the picture.

is present, then an unstrained image is also recommended. The reason for this image is to allow visualization of the philtrum–commissure height relationship, etiologic in the differential diagnosis of excessive gingival display on smile.

- **Frontal dynamic (smile)** (Figure 32.8). As described in more detail later in this chapter, the smile can vary with emotion. A patient who is smiling for a photograph tends not to elevate the lip as extensively as a laughing patient. The smiling picture demonstrates the amount of incisor show on smile (percentage of maxillary incisor display on smile) and any excessive gingival display. The still image of the smile can be variable. If you think about it, we squeeze off a picture that is about 1/125 of a second duration in a process that has a start and a finish (from the lips together through the smile animation back to the lips being together).

Oblique view (three-quarter, 45°)

The patient is posed in natural head position looking 45° to the camera, including the following three views:

- **Oblique at rest** (Figure 32.9). This view is valuable for examination of the midface and is particularly informative of midface deformities, including nasal deformity. We should

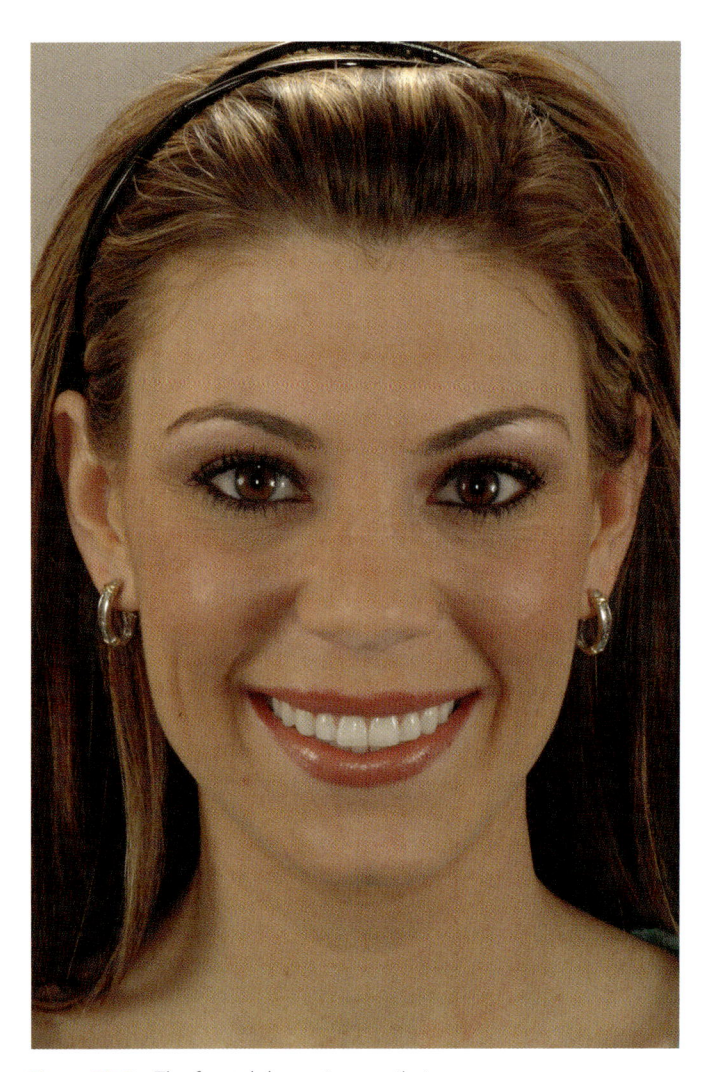

Figure 32.8 The frontal dynamic or smile image.

through those means and it aids the visualization of both incisor flare and occlusal plane orientation. A particular point for observation is the anteroposterior cant of the occlusal plane.

In the most desirable orientation, the occlusal plane is consonant with the curvature of the lower lip on smile (the smile arc). Deviations from this orientation that should be noted as potential problems include a downward cant of the posterior maxilla, an upward cant of the anterior maxilla, or variations of both. In the initial examination and diagnostic phase of treatment, visualization of the occlusal plane in its relationship to the upper and the lower lip is important.

Profile view

The profile photographs also should be taken in a natural head position. The most common method used for positioning the patient properly is to have the patient look in a mirror, orienting the head on the visual axis. The picture boundaries should emphasize the areas of information needed for documentation and diagnosis. My recommendation is that the inferior border be slightly above the scapula, at the base of the neck. This position permits visualization of the contours of the chin and neck area. The superior border should be only slightly above the top of the head, and the right border slightly ahead of the nasal tip.

The inclusion of more background simply adds unneeded information to the photograph. Some clinicians prefer that the left border stop just behind the ear, whereas others prefer a full head shot. Under any circumstance, the hair should be pulled behind the ear to permit visualization of the entire face.

Two profile images are beneficial:

- **Profile at rest** (Figure 32.11). The lips should be relaxed. Lip strain is illustrated better in the frontal view, so a profile photograph with the lips strained in closure is unnecessary.
- **Profile smile** (Figure 32.12). The profile smile image allows one to see the angulation of the maxillary incisors, an important esthetic factor that patients see clearly and orthodontists tend to miss because the inclination noted on cephalometric radiographs may not represent what one sees on direct examination.
- **An optional submental view** (Figure 32.13). Such a view may be taken to document mandibular asymmetry. In patients with asymmetries, submental views can be particularly revealing.

Technology and facial imaging

It is possible to use computer software to calibrate images for quantification and measurement. If we know the dimensions of an object in the field of view, we can use it to calibrate the image, and then measure any dimension we are interested in. For example, on the computer screen, we can digitize the width of one of the central incisors, which allows calibration of the image. The clinician can then measure and calculate the height/width ratio and proportionality of the anterior teeth. Carrying this technology forward, it is also possible to utilize a digitizing module to

recognize that persons are not seen just on profile or from the front, so the three-quarter view is particularly valuable in assessing the way a patient's face is more often viewed by others. This view also reveals anatomic characteristics that are difficult to quantify but are important esthetic factors, such as the chin–neck area, the prominence of the gonial angle, and the length and definition of the border of the mandible. The view also permits focus on lip fullness and vermilion display. For a patient with obvious facial asymmetry, oblique views of both sides are recommended.

- **Oblique on smile** (Figure 32.10). There are diagnostic limitations of plaster casts, virtual models, and, as far as we are concerned, virtually all static records because they do not reflect the relationships of the teeth to the lips and surrounding soft tissue, especially in evaluation of the smile.[8,9] Often, in clinical practice, a patient or parent will ask why the teeth appear flared, and they do a credible job of illustrating what they are seeing by holding their hands next to the child's face to make sure that we see it too. This observation is often not discernible on the models or on the cephalogram, but is readily observable on the patient. The oblique view of the smile reveals characteristics of the smile not obtainable

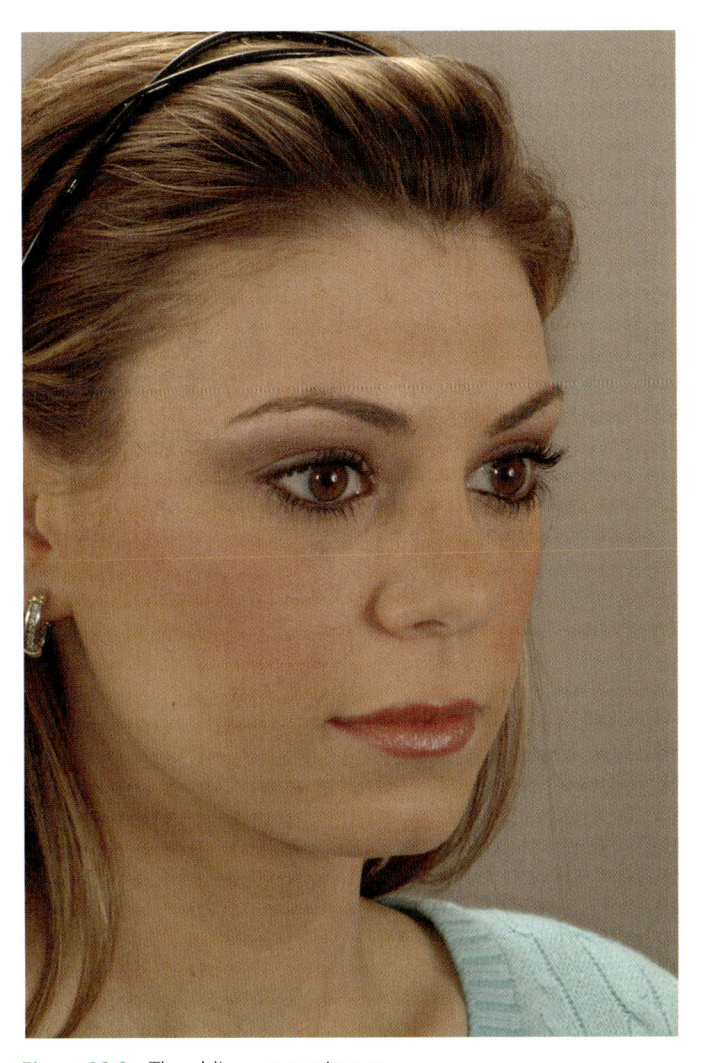

Figure 32.9 The oblique at rest image.

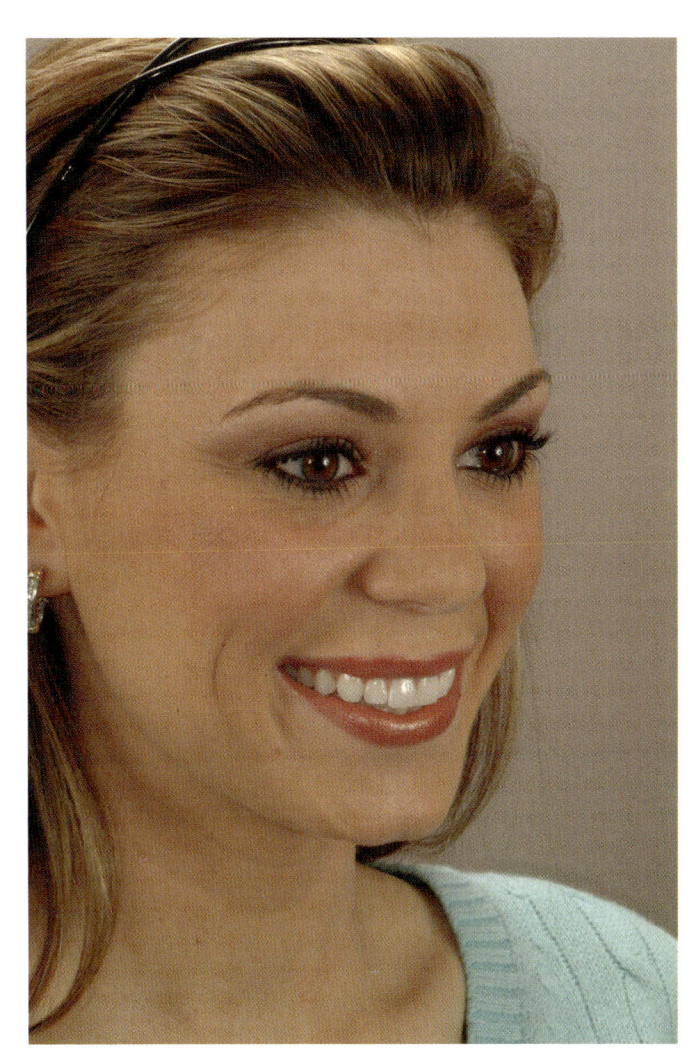

Figure 32.10 The oblique on smile image.

digitize the points of the face, smile, and teeth and have the ratios calculated automatically.

Three-dimensional facial mapping is also possible in today's clinical and research environment (Figure 32.14A and B). The images are obtained with a special type of camera that provides a nonradiographic image and which can be rotated on the computer screen for further analysis. It is also possible to calibrate and measure these images as well.

Dentofacial analysis: clinical examination

The direct clinical examination is critical to successful esthetic and functional dentofacial diagnosis. The systematic approach to looking at every element of the face and smile and measuring them can virtually lead us to the correct diagnosis. The progression of the examination we recommend is as follows.

Vertical facial proportions

The ideal face is vertically divided into equal thirds by horizontal lines adjacent to the hairline, the nasal base, and lower border of the chin[10] (Figure 32.15). Orthodontic and surgical/orthodontic treatment is usually concentrated with the lower facial third. Measurement of the upper face can often be difficult with the variability in identification of landmarks such as the location of the hairline. In the ideal lower third of the face, the upper lip makes up the upper third, and the lower lip and chin compose the lower two-thirds (Figure 32.16). Disproportion of the vertical facial thirds may be a result of many dental and skeletal factors, and these proportional relationships may help us define the contributing factors related to vertical dentofacial deformities.

Facial index

While transverse and vertical relationships comprise the major components of the frontal examination and analysis, the proportional relationship of height and width is far more important than absolute values in establishing overall facial type. In cosmetic dentistry, it is well established that attractive teeth tend to have certain proportions, and the same is true in faces. The *facial index* is defined as the ratio of facial width to facial height (Figure 32.17) using a line from zygoma to zygoma for the width measurement and nasion to

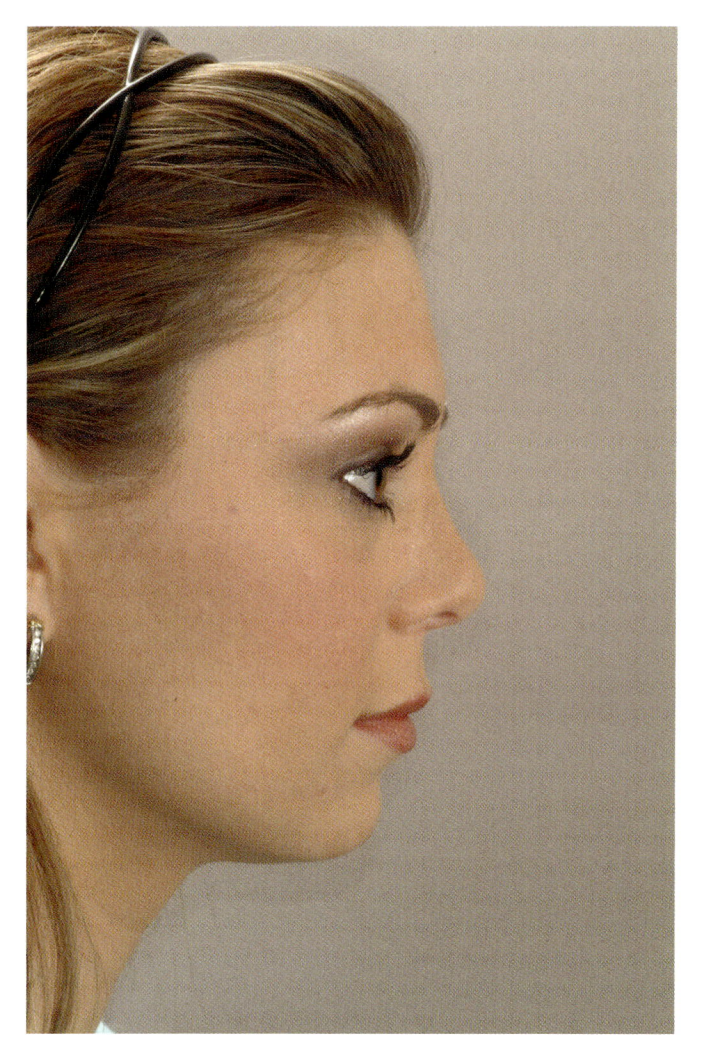

Figure 32.11 The profile at rest image.

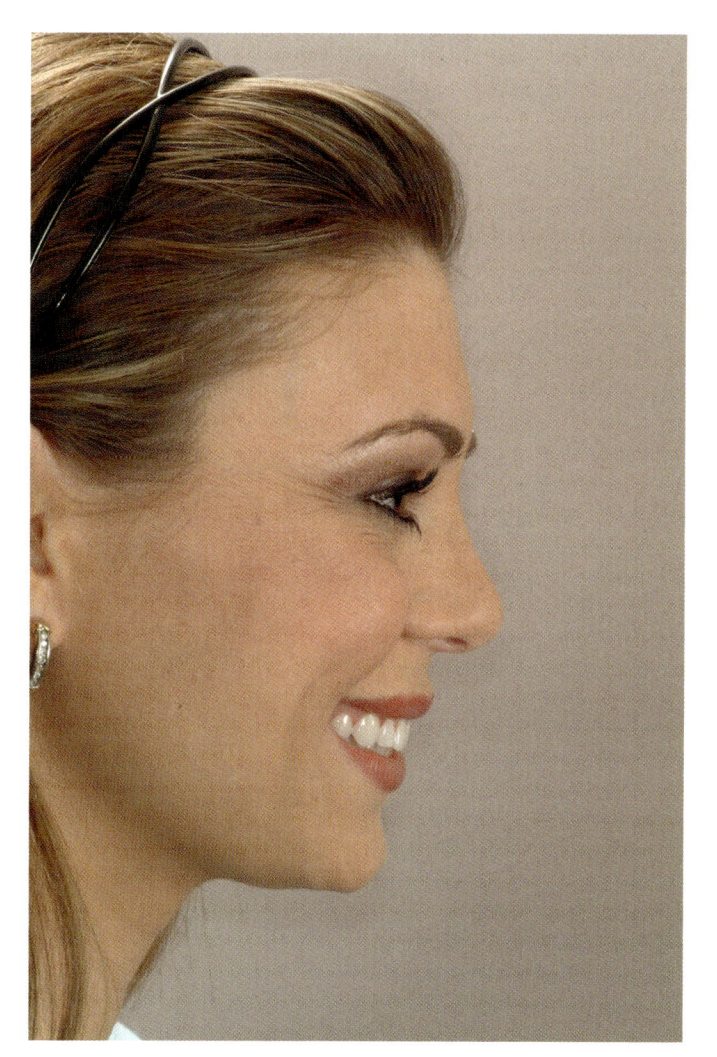

Figure 32.12 The profile smile image.

midsymphysis for the facial height. Farkas and Munro[11] report that the average facial index for males is 88.5% and for females is 86.2%. The classic frontal analysis categorizes faces as either mesocephalic (normal facial heights), brachycephalic (short lower face), or dolichocephalic (long lower face) (Figures 32.18, 32.19, and 32.20). The differentiation between these facial types has to do with the general proportionality of facial width to facial height, with brachycephalic faces being broader and shorter in comparison with the longer and narrower dolichocephalic faces.

Facial taper

Another way to view facial proportionality is the comparison of the zygomatic width and the intergonial width, which can be referred to as the *facial taper*.[12] While studies are currently establishing normative values, Figure 32.21 demonstrates the facial taper of a proportional face. A dramatic example of the esthetic improvement associated with changes in facial taper as a result of orthognathic surgery can be viewed in Figure 32.22A and B. The patient presented with diminished middle third and a square facial taper pattern. Her skeletal pattern was the determinant of her facial pattern, so an orthodontic–orthognathic approach to treatment was indicated. After orthodontic preparation, the patient underwent maxillomandibular surgery to rotate the lower face in such a way as to increase the lower face and steepen the mandibular plane. Even though the width was not changed with the surgical procedure, the face appears to be narrower from the increase in vertical height and resulting change in facial taper.

Transverse facial proportions: the rule of fifths

The assessment of the transverse components of facial width is best described by the rule of fifths.[7] This method describes the ideal transverse relationships of the face. The face is divided sagittally into five equal parts from helix to helix of the outer ears (Figure 32.23). Each of the segments should be one eye distance in width.

The middle fifth of the face is delineated by the inner canthus of the eyes. A vertical line from the inner canthus should be coincident with the alar base of the nose. Variation in this facial fifth could be due to transverse deficiencies or excesses in either the inner canthi or alar base. For example, hypertelorism in craniofacial syndromes can create disproportionate transverse facial esthetics.

A vertical line from the outer canthus of the eyes frames the medial three-fifths of the face, which should be coincident with the gonial angles of the mandible. Although disproportion may be very subtle, it is worth noting since our treatments can positively change the shape or relative proportion of the gonial angles.

The outer two-fifths of the face are measured from the lateral canthus to lateral helix of the ear, which represents the width of the ears. Unless this abnormality is part of the chief complaint, prominent ears are often a difficult feature to discuss with the patient because laypeople only recognize its effect on the face in severe cases. However, studies clearly indicate that large ears are judged by laypeople to be one of the most unesthetic features, particularly in males. Otoplastic surgical procedures are relatively atraumatic and can dramatically improve facial appearance. These procedures can be performed on adolescents and adults, as is illustrated in Figure 32.24A and B.

Another significant frontal relationship is the midpupillary distance, which should be transversely aligned with the commissures of the mouth.[8] Although this is considered the ideal transverse facial proportionality, there is little that can be done therapeutically to correct this disproportion, except in craniofacial synostosis such as Apert syndrome.

Nasal anatomy in the transverse plane should also be assessed through proportionality. The width of the alar base should be approximately the same as the intercanthal distance, which should be the same as the width of an eye. If the intercanthal distance is smaller than an eye width, it is better to keep the nose slightly wider than the intercanthal distance. The width of the alar base is heavily influenced by inherited ethnic characteristics.

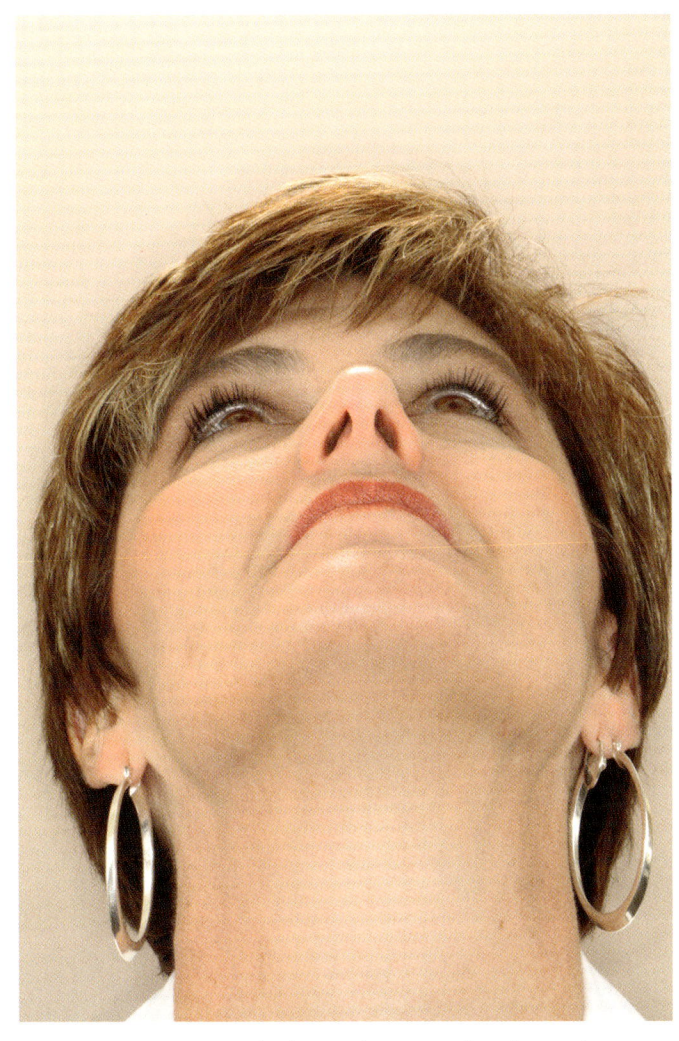

Figure 32.13 An optional submental view may be taken to document mandibular asymmetry.

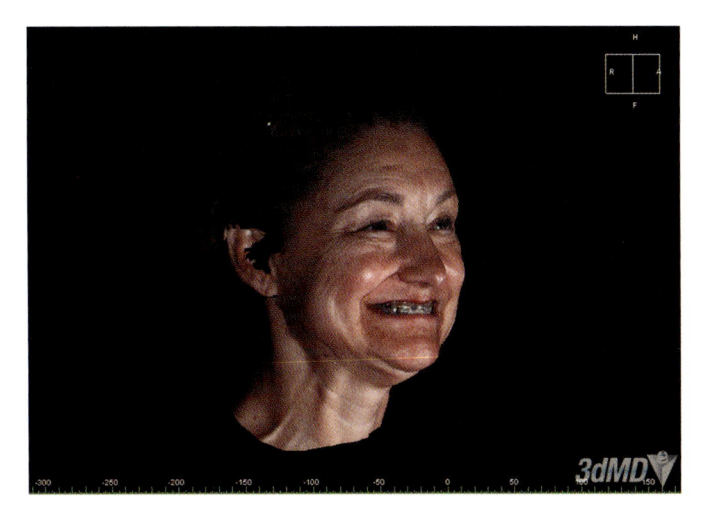

Figure 32.14 (A) Three-dimensional facial mapping is also possible in today's clinical and research environment. The images are obtained with a special type of camera that provides a nonradiographic image which can be rotated on the computer screen for further analysis. It is also possible to calibrate and measure these images as well. This is of a patient prior to orthognathic surgery.

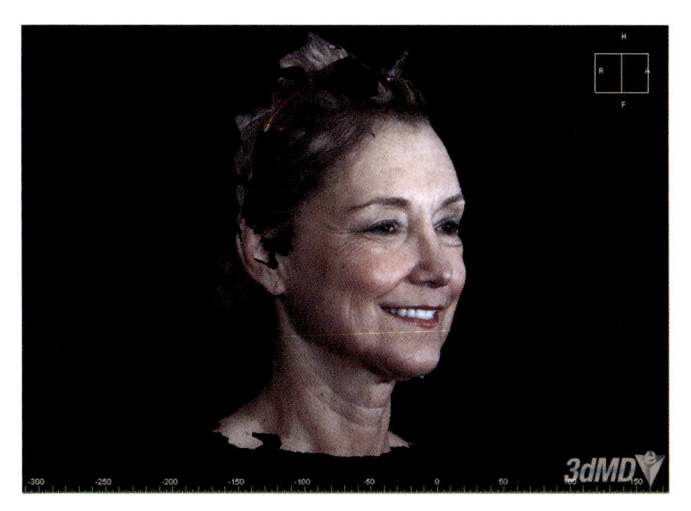

Figure 32.14 (B) The three-dimensional facial map after orthognathic surgery and veneers (3dMd, Atlanta, GA).

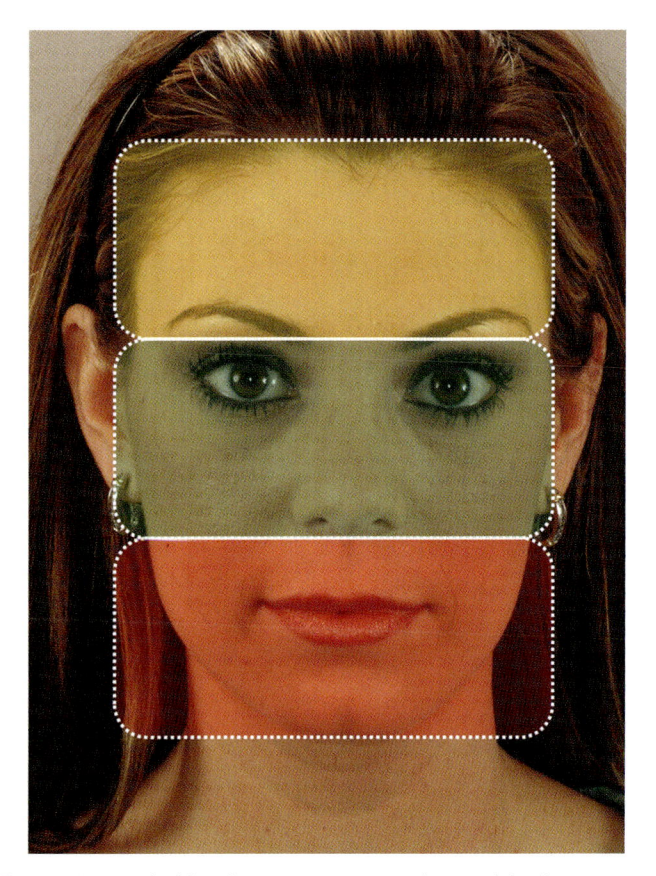

Figure 32.15 Ideal facial proportions in equal vertical thirds.

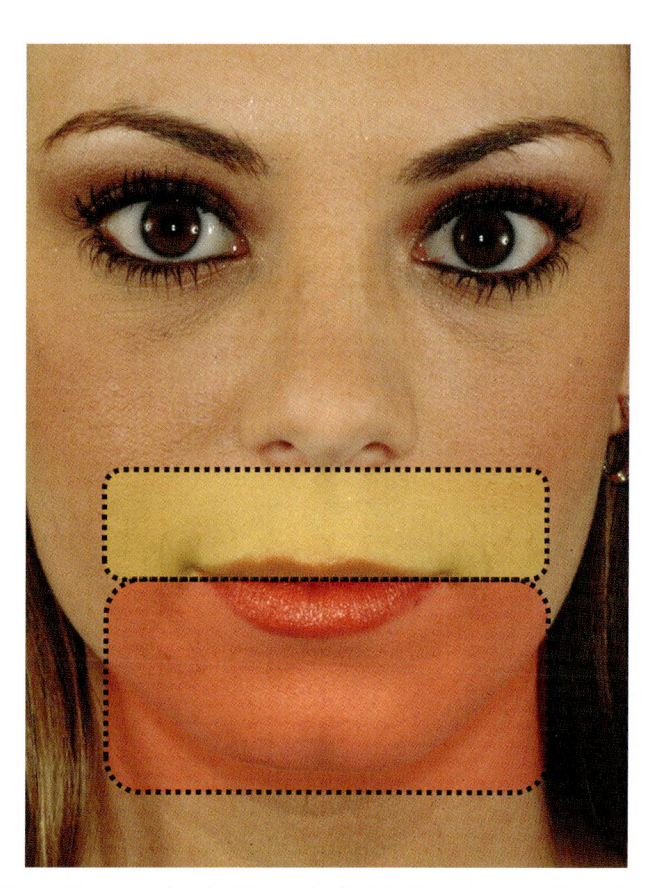

Figure 32.16 In the ideal lower third of the face, the upper lip makes up the upper third, and the lower lip and chin compose the lower two-thirds.

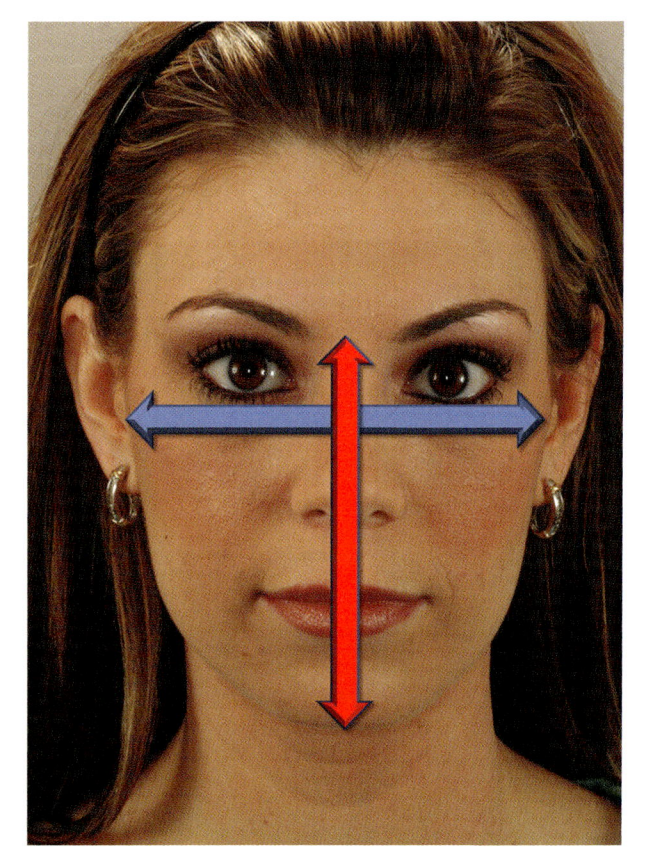

Figure 32.17 The facial index is the ratio of facial width to facial height using a line from zygoma to zygoma for the width measurement and nasion to midsymphysis for the facial height.

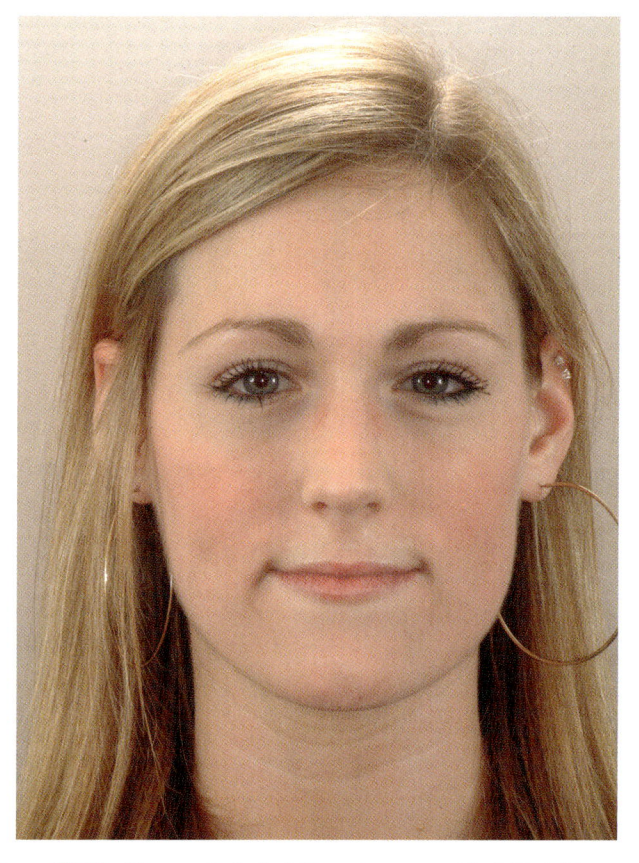

Figure 32.18 Mesocephalic facial form has normal facial heights.

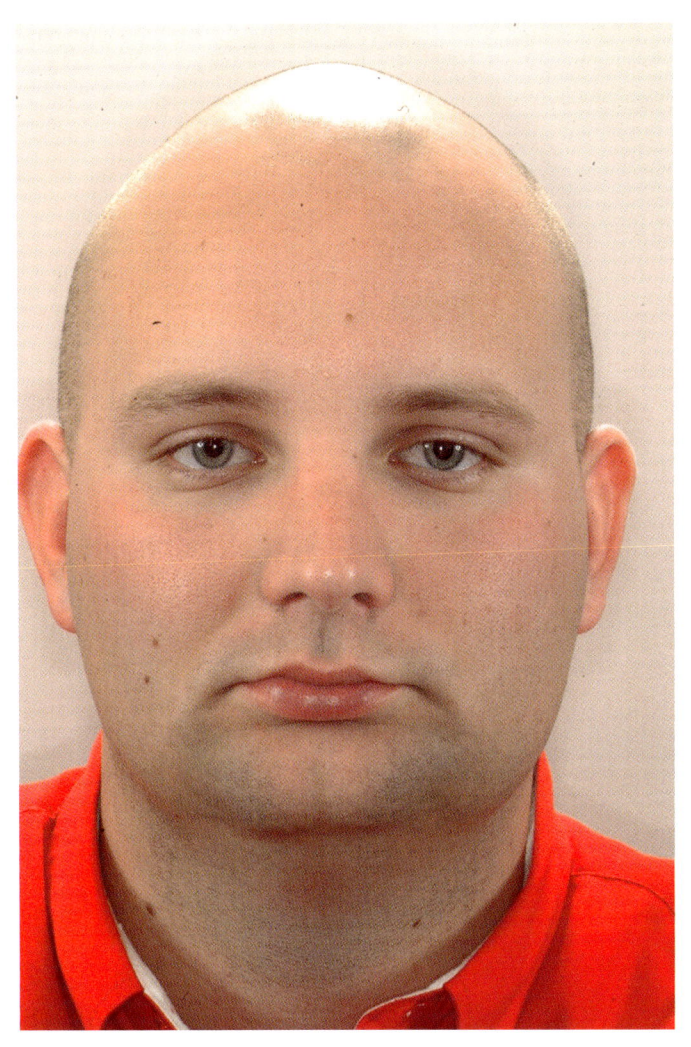

Figure 32.19 Brachycephalic facial form is characterized by a short, square lower facial third.

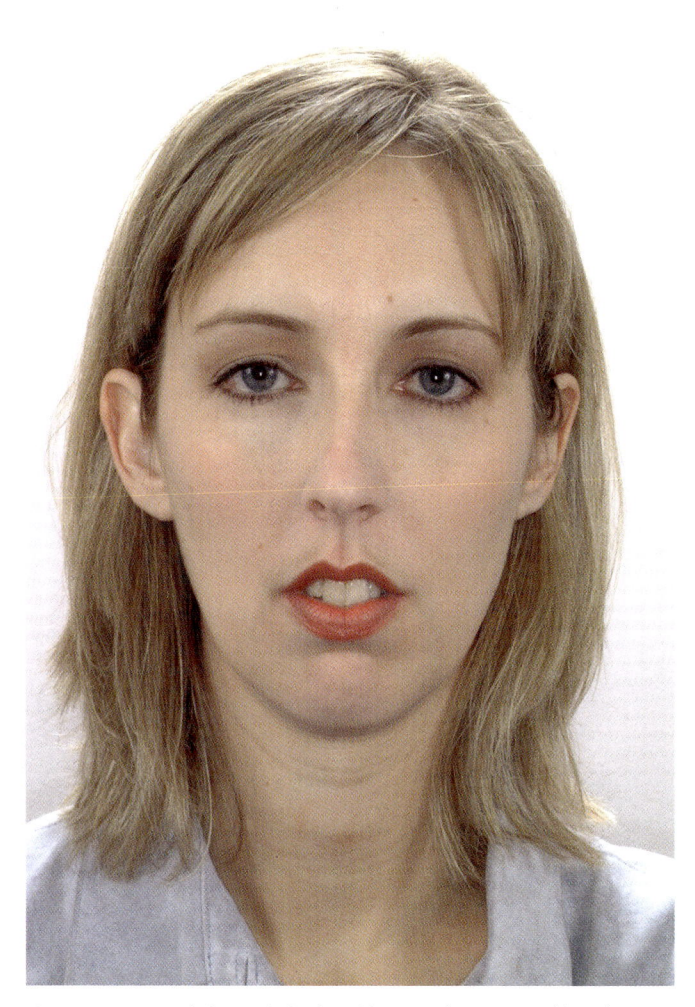

Figure 32.20 Dolichocephalic facial form is characterized by a long, narrow lower facial third.

Facial asymmetry

Facial asymmetry is traditionally assessed in the frontal plane; however, asymmetry occurs in all three planes, and the rotational aspect is described in the "Macroesthetics and smile dimensions" section describing the concepts of pitch, roll, and yaw.

Nasal tip to midsagittal plane
The patient's head should be elevated slightly to better visualize the nasal tip in relation to the midsagittal plane (Figure 32.25). This is evaluated first to reduce the risk of treating the maxillary midline to a distorted nose.

Maxillary dental midline to midsagittal plane
The maxillary dental midline should be evaluated relative to the midsagittal plane. This is best visualized by identifying the peaks of the upper vermilion border of the lips that correlate to the philtral columns, which correlate to the midsagittal plane. In this way, we can readily see the maxillary dental midline in relation to the midsagittal plane as demonstrated in Figure 32.26. A discrepancy could be due to either dental factors or skeletal maxillary rotation. Maxillary rotation is a rarely occurring clinical finding and is usually accompanied by posterior dental crossbite.

Mandibular asymmetry with or without functional shift
Mandibular asymmetry is suspected when the midsymphysis is not coincident with the midsagittal plane. An important diagnostic factor is whether a lateral functional shift is present secondary to a functional shift of the mandible due to crossbite. When the patient is manipulated into centric relation, a bilateral, end-to-end crossbite usually is present, and as the patient moves their teeth into full occlusion they must choose a side to move their mandible into maximum intercuspation. This lateral shift is indicative of true mandibular asymmetry, but of a narrow maxilla resulting in a functional shift of the mandible.

True mandibular asymmetry is suspected when, in closure into centric relation, no lateral functional shift occurs. The truly asymmetric mandible may be due to an inherited asymmetric facial growth pattern or a result of localized or systemic factors. A thorough history of traumatic injuries and a review of systems of the patient will help ascertain potential etiologies of true mandibular asymmetry.

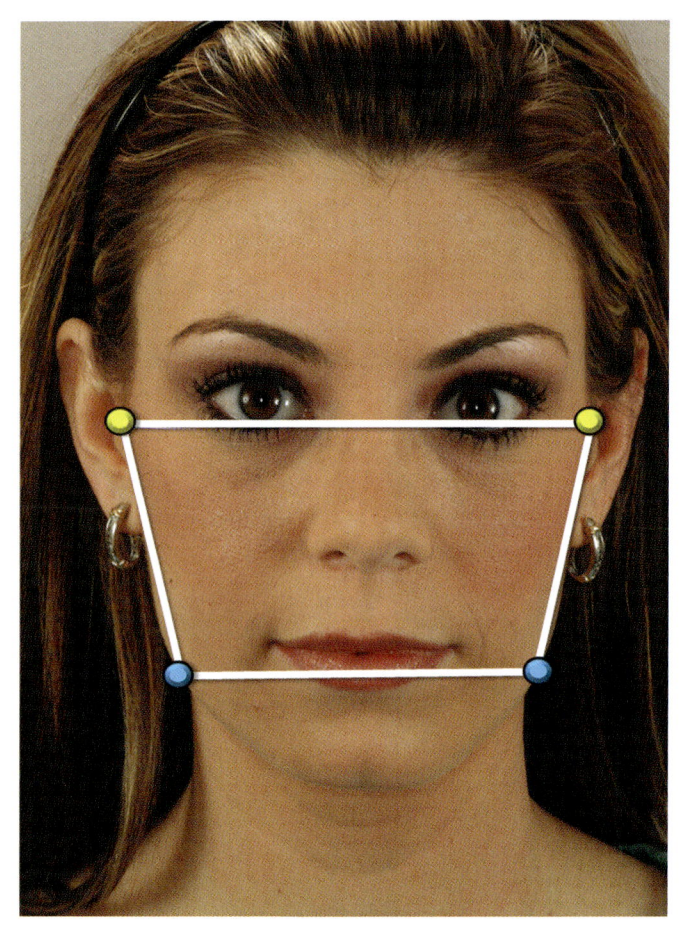

Figure 32.21 The facial taper of a proportional face.

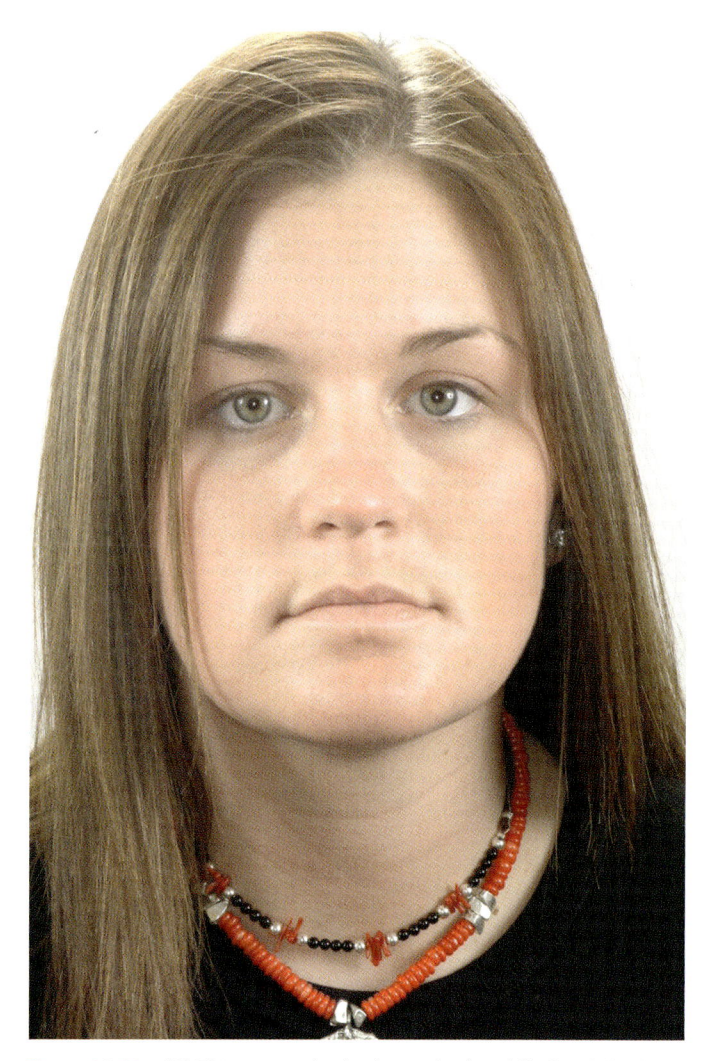

Figure 32.22 **(A)** This patient had a diminished middle facial third and a square facial taper pattern.

Chin asymmetry

Facial asymmetry in some cases may be limited to the chin only. If the systematic evaluation of facial symmetry has dental and skeletal midlines and vertical relationships of the maxilla normal and lower facial asymmetry is noted, then the asymmetry may be isolated to the chin. Measurement of the midsymphysis to the midsagittal plane is a logical indicator of chin asymmetry, but the parasymphyseal heights should also be measured when chin asymmetry is suspected (Figure 32.27A–D).

Maxillomandibular asymmetry

Mandibular asymmetry is often accompanied by maxillary compensation, which is reflected clinically by a transverse cant of the maxilla. This means that evaluation of mandibular deformity should now include the possibility of maxillomandibular deformity, which is described later in this chapter. Transverse tilting of the maxilla may be detectable cephalometrically but is most evident during the macroesthetic examination. The patient in Figure 32.28A is an excellent example. Her smile was characterized by a transverse cant, with the left side of the maxilla significantly lower than the right. The submental view (Figure 32.28B) reflects the chin point (menton) placed to the left of midsagittal plane, with the right mandible longer than the left. The maxilla has compensated during growth for the mandibular asymmetry, resulting in the severe asymmetry of her smile (Figure 32.28C). Correction was achieved by surgical leveling of the maxilla and mandibular surgery, resulting in excellent symmetry (Figure 32.28D and E).

Macroesthetic evaluation of the face: oblique view

The oblique view in the macroesthetic examination affords the clinician another perspective for evaluating the facial thirds. In the upper face, we may view the relative projection of the orbital rim and malar eminence. Orbital and malar retrusion is often seen in craniofacial syndromes. Cheek projection is evaluated in the area of the zygoma and malar scaffold. Skin laxity and atrophy of the malar fat pad in this area may actually be a characteristic of aging, and therefore seen in the older orthognathic population. There is evidence[13] that this loss of midfacial support may be attributed to decreased skeletal volume as well the soft tissue changes. The midfacial area can be described as deficient, balanced, or prominent. Nasal anatomy, which was

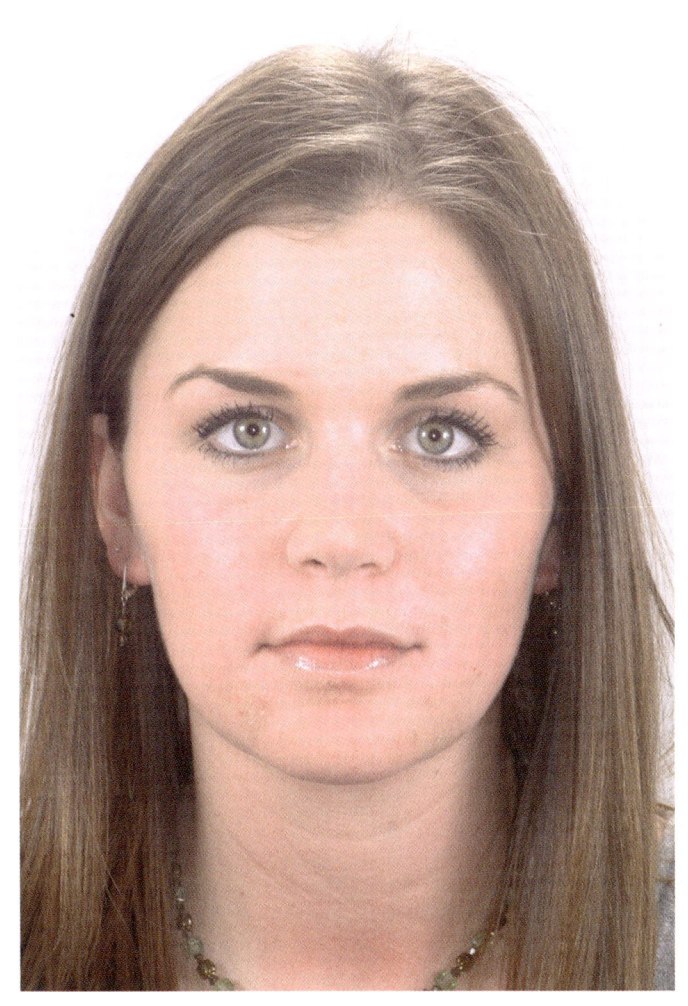

Figure 32.22 **(B)** Maxillomandibular surgery was designed to improve the facial taper and facial height.

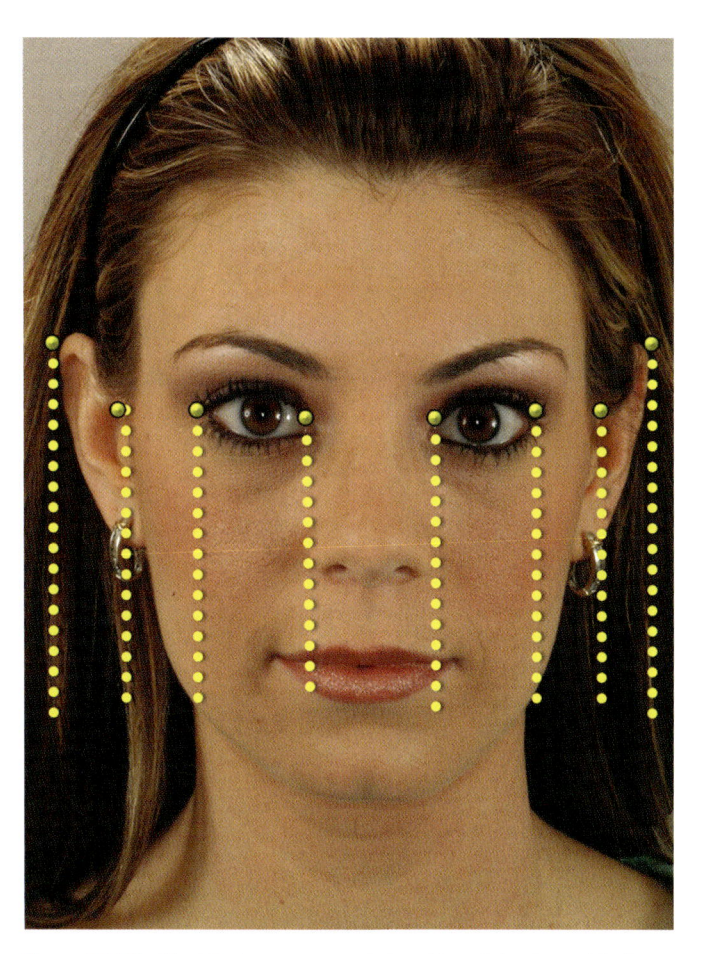

Figure 32.23 The ideal transverse relationships of the face with the face divided sagittally into five equal parts (the width of the eye) from helix to helix of the outer ears.

described in the frontal examination, may also be characterized in this dimension.

Lip anatomy is also examined in the oblique and lateral views. The philtral area and vermilion of the maxillary lip should be clearly demarcated. The height of the philtrum should be noted as short, balanced, or excessive. Vermilion display should be termed as excessive, balanced, or thin.

The relative projection of the maxilla and mandible can be assessed in the oblique view. Midface deficiency can result in increased nasolabial folding, relaxed upper lip support, and altered columella and nasal tip support.

One of the greatest values of the oblique view is visualization of the body and gonial angle of the mandible as well as the cervicomental area.[14] The patient in Figure 32.29 illustrates a desirable definition of the chin–neck anatomy where the gonial angle is well delineated and defined, with a moderately acute angle. The patient in Figure 32.30 has a dolichofacial skeletal pattern with a steeper mandibular plane, not as esthetically pleasing as the previous illustration. The patient in Figure 32.31 demonstrates a brachyfacial skeletal pattern with a very acute gonial angle and short lower face.

Macroesthetic evaluation of the face: profile view

The last view in the macroesthetic examination is the profile perspective. Natural head position is essential for accurate evaluation of profile characteristics.[15–18] The patient should be instructed to look straight ahead and, if possible, into their own image in an appropriately placed mirror. The visual axis is what determines "natural head position." The classic vertical facial thirds also apply in profile view. An assessment of lower facial deficiency or excess should be noted. Figure 32.32 and Table **32.2** illustrate the landmarks used in describing the soft-tissue profile.

Maxillary and mandibular sagittal position can be described by means of facial divergence. The lower third of the face is evaluated in reference to the anterior soft-tissue point at the glabella. Based on the position of the maxilla and mandible relative to this point, a patient's profile will be described as straight, convex, or concave, and either anteriorly or posteriorly divergent. Figure 32.33 illustrates the anterior facial plane formed from lines connecting the glabella to the base of the nose (subnasale) and the chin point.

The nasolabial angle describes the inclination of the columella in relation to the upper lip. The ideal nasolabial angle should be

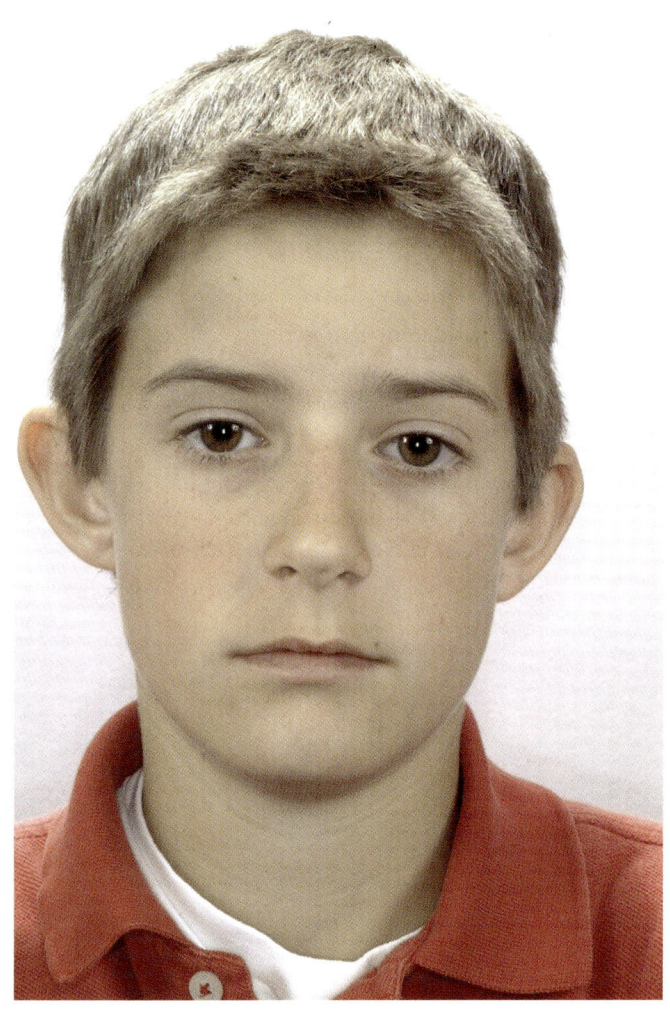

Figure 32.24 **(A)** The young patient had disproportionate width of the outer facial fifth because of his ear prominence.

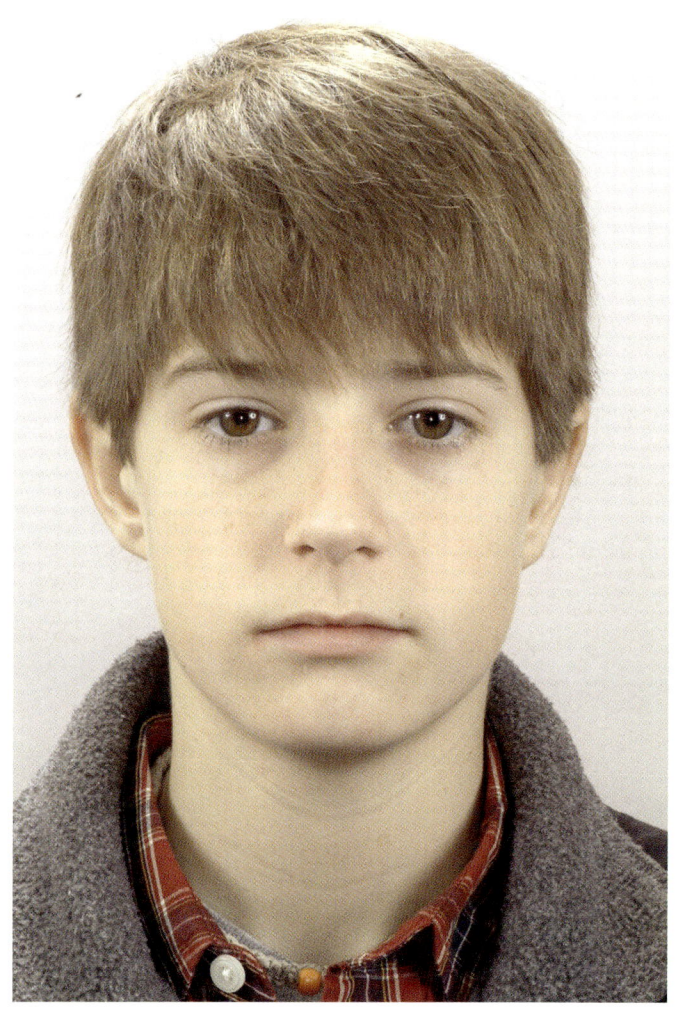

Figure 32.24 **(B)** Otoplasty was performed to improve his appearance.

in the range of 85–105° (Figure 32.34). The nasolabial angle is determined by several factors: (1) the anteroposterior position of the maxilla to some degree; (2) the anteroposterior position of the maxillary incisors; (3) vertical position or rotation of the nasal tip, which can result in a more obtuse or acute nasolabial angle; and (4) soft-tissue thickness of the maxillary lip that contributes the nasolabial angle, where a thin upper lip favors a flatter angle and a thicker lip favors an acute angle. The patient in Figure 32.35A demonstrates the severe maxillary dentoalveolar protrusion and its effect on the nasolabial angle. Because of her protrusion, she had a severe Class II malocclusion with 9 mm of overjet, resulting a very acute nasolabial angle. We elected to treat her through removal of maxillary first premolars and maximum retraction of the maxillary anterior teeth, reducing overjet, upper lip support, and improved nasolabial angle and esthetic lip balance (Figure 32.35B).

While the nasolabial angle is largely influenced by the hard-tissue structures, the nose itself should also be evaluated for possible inclusion in the problem list or attributes. The nasal tip elevation can be established as the position of the nasal tip relative to a perpendicular to the line from the glabella to the chin point at the base of the nose (Figure 32.36). Nasal projection is a description of the nose in height from the glabella to the base of the nose (subnasale) and length by nasal tip to the alar base (Figure 32.37).

Lip projection (Figure 32.38) is a function of maxillomandibular protrusion or retrusion, dental protrusion or retrusion, and/or lip thickness. The description of lip projection should include pertinent information from any of the aforementioned sources. For example, a patient with lower lip protrusion may be maxillary (midface) deficient with dentoalveolar compensation including flared incisors and a thin maxillary vermilion display, or simply may have a thick lower lip that appears protrusive.

The patient in Figure 32.39A had a large maxillary midline diastema as a result of distal drift of the centrals because of

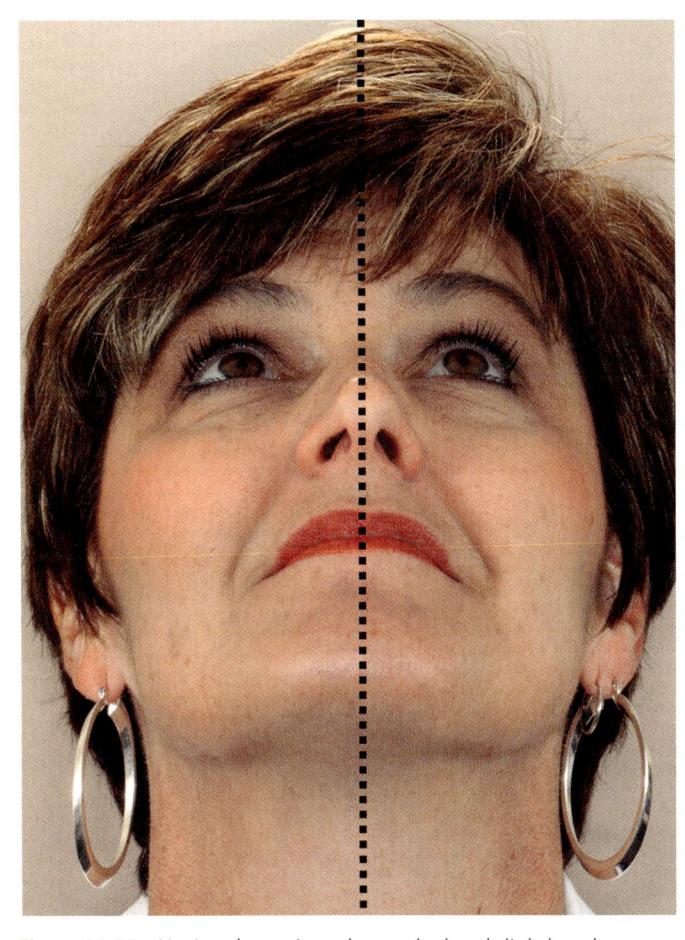

Figure 32.25 Having the patient elevate the head slightly to better visualize the nasal tip in relation to the midsagittal plane provides the best view to evaluate the position of the nasal tip.

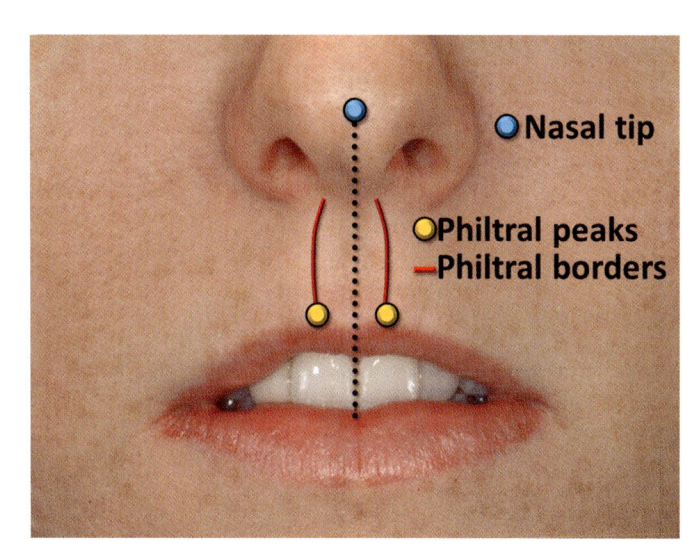

Figure 32.26 The maxillary dental midline is best visualized by its relation to the peaks of the upper vermilion border of the lips that correlate to the philtral columns.

congenitally missing lateral incisors. Conventional wisdom would dictate to orthodontically move the centrals together to close the diastema and create space for implants for prosthodontic restoration of the missing laterals. However, her macroesthetic evaluation (Figure 32.39B) demonstrated marked bidental protrusion with excessive lip projection in relation to the nose and chin. Our treatment plan reflected the global treatment approach of macro–mini–micro by removing lower first premolars for space to retract the lower incisors to reduce protrusion. The maxillary space was also closed posteriorly and the cuspids reshaped and lateralized (Figure 32.39C), thus eliminating the need for implants. The final profile (Figure 32.39D) had a significant improvement in lip protrusion and facial balance.

The labiomental angle (Figure 32.40) is defined as the fold of soft tissue between the lower lip and the chin and may vary greatly in form and depth. The clinical variables that can affect the labiomental fold include:

1. Lower incisor position, where upright lower incisors tend to result in a shallow labiomental angle because of lack of lower lip projection, whereas excessive lower incisor proclination deepens the labiomental fold.
2. Vertical height of the lower facial third, which has a direct bearing on chin position and the labiomental fold. Diminished lower facial height will usually result in a deeper labiomental fold (just as in the overclosed full denture patient), whereas a patient with a long lower facial third has a tendency toward a flat labiomental fold.
3. Mandibular deficiency with associated dental compensation may produce lower lip eversion, excessive vermilion display, and a pronounced labiomental sulcus because of the compensatory proclination and procumbency of the lower incisors.

The patient in Figure 32.41A had a severe Class II malocclusion with a deep bite and severe overjet; compare this with the final occlusion idealized (Figure 32.41B). His frontal facial pattern (Figure 32.41C) was characterized by a short lower facial with soft-tissue redundancy due to vertical overclosure, resulting in a deep labiomental sulcus. His profile (Figure 32.41D) reflected his severe mandibular deficiency with eversion of the lower lip because of his overjet and position of the maxillary incisors between his upper and lower lips. After surgical orthodontic treatment with mandibular advancement and facial lengthening, the vertical facial proportions were more appropriate (Figure 32.41E) and esthetic, and the labiomental sulcus improved as a result of the increased facial height and elimination of overjet. The final profile was also more balanced (Figure 32.41F).

Chin projection is determined by the amount of anteroposterior bony projection of the anterior, inferior border of the mandible, and the amount of soft tissue that overlays that bony projection. In the adolescent, the amount of chin is directly correlated to the amount of mandibular growth that occurs, because the chin point itself is borne on the mandible as it grows anteriorly.

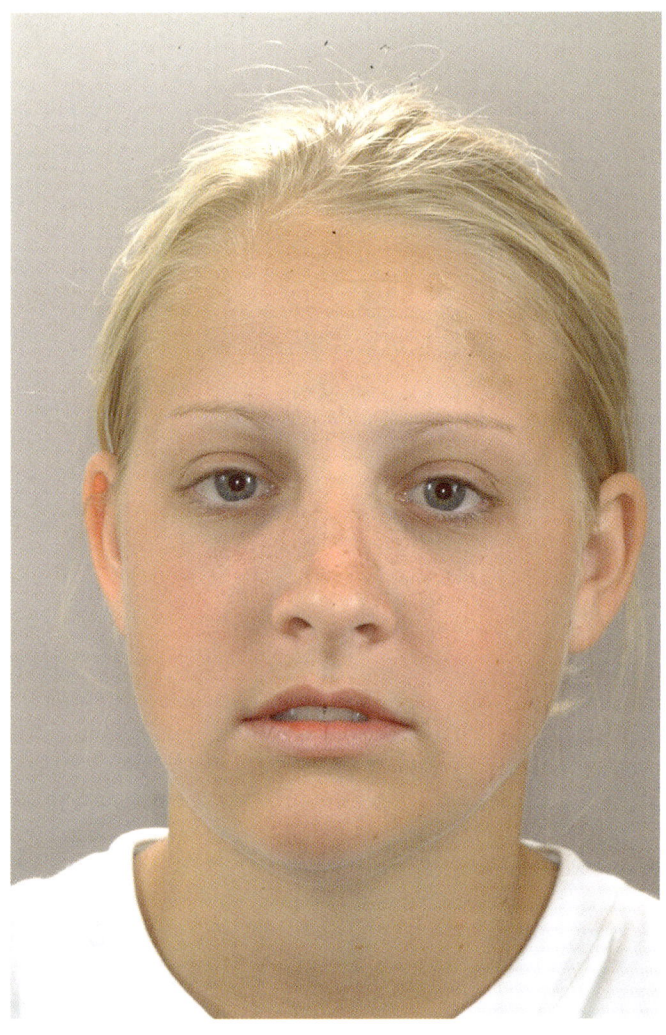

Figure 32.27 **(A)** This patient had a facial asymmetry, but the clinical examination and quantification leads us to the correct diagnosis as to its etiology.

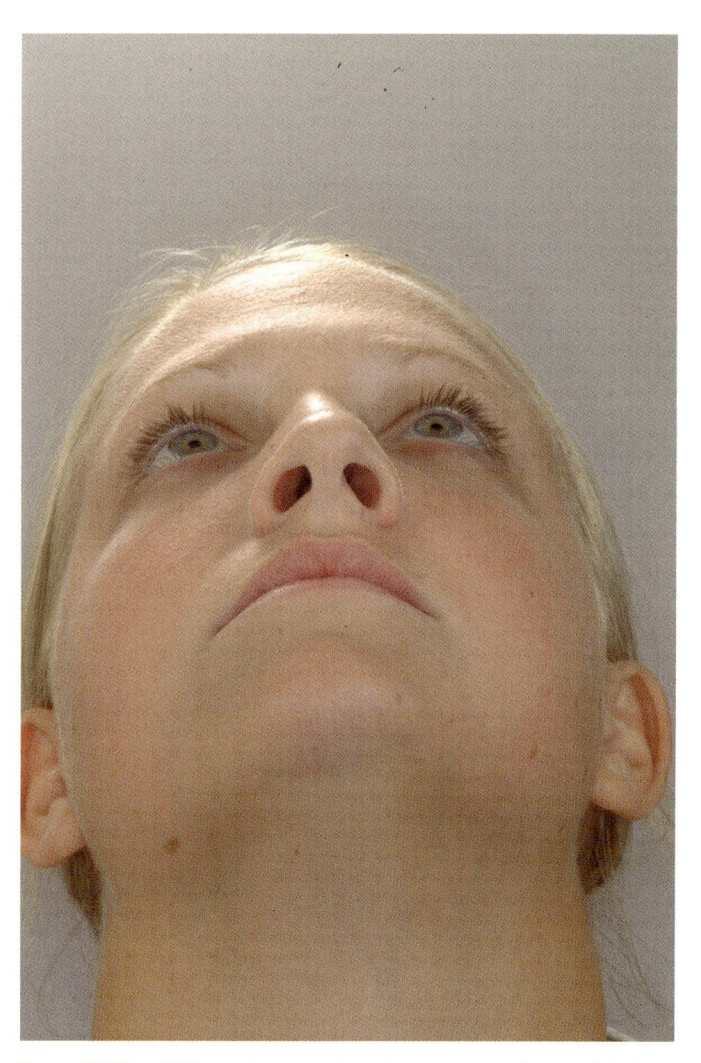

Figure 32.27 **(B)** The submental view demonstrates the nasal tip is to the left, but the midsymphysis is on to the midsagittal plane.

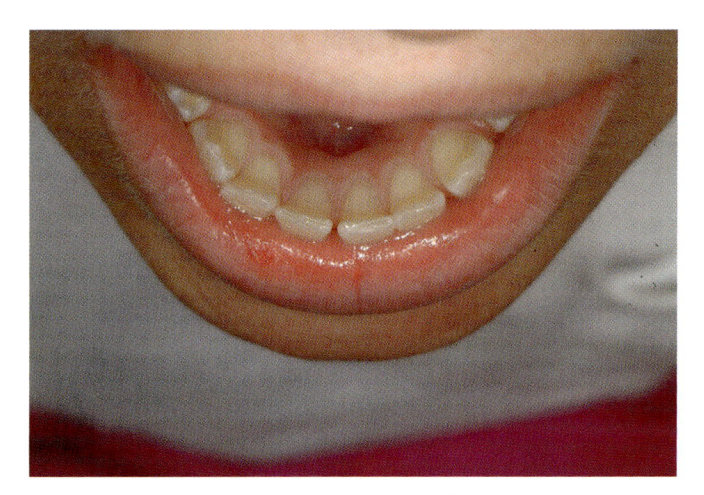

Figure 32.27 **(C)** This view demonstrates the lower dental midline slightly to the right of the midsymphysis.

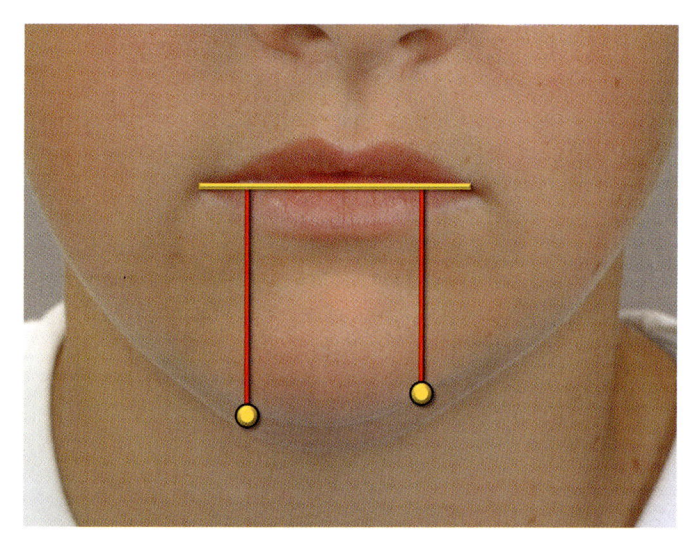

Figure 32.27 **(D)** More careful examination reveals the right parasymphysis was longer than the left, thus leading to the impression of facial asymmetry.

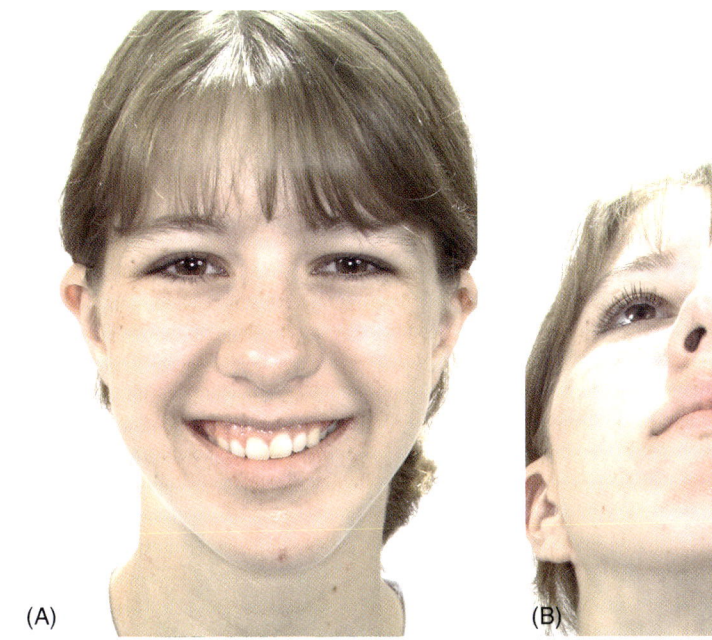

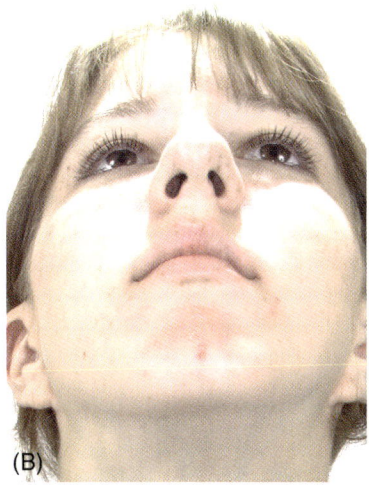

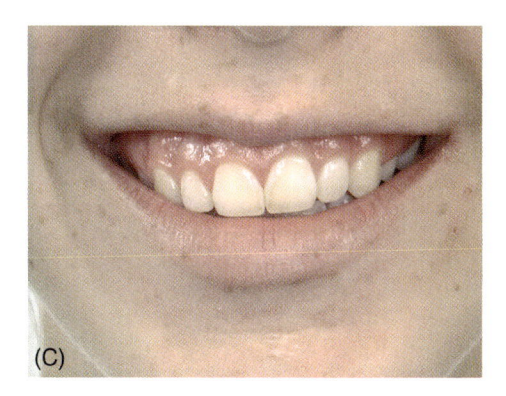

Figure 32.28 **(A)** This patient's smile had an undesirable transverse cant with the left side of the maxilla significantly lower than the right. **(B)** The submental view reflects the chin point (menton) placed to the left of the midsagittal plane, with the right mandible longer than the left. **(C)** The maxilla has compensated during growth for the mandibular asymmetry, resulting in the severe asymmetry of her smile.

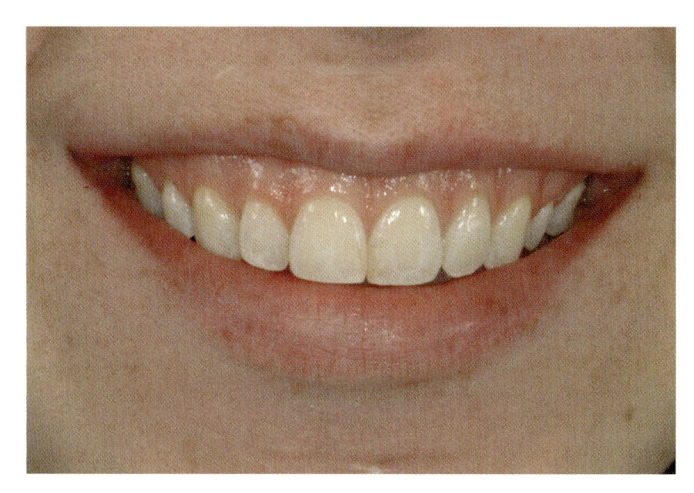

Figure 32.28 **(E)** The close-up smile after surgical leveling of the maxilla reflected excellent smile symmetry.

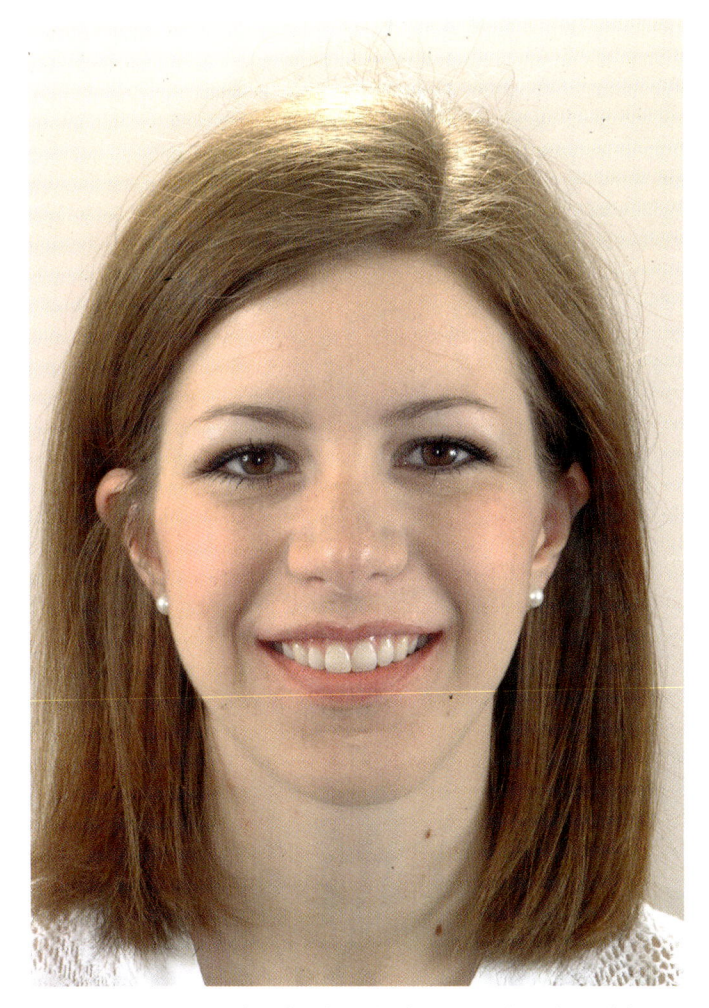

Figure 32.28 **(D)** The final facial result after surgical leveling of the maxilla and mandibular surgery to correct the mandibular asymmetry.

The angle between the lower lip, chin, and R point (the deepest point along the chin–neck contour) should be approximately 90°. An obtuse angle often indicates (1) chin deficiency, (2) lower lip procumbency, (3) excessive submental fat, (4) retropositioned mandible, and (5) low hyoid bone position.

Another important measure in this area is the chin–neck length and chin–neck angle (Figure 32.42). The angle, also termed the cervicomental angle, has been studied extensively in plastic surgery and orthognathic literature. Studies report that a wide range of normal neck morphology exists, and that the cervicomental angle may vary between 105° and 120°, with gender being a major consideration. Age of the patient must be considered with regard to this area. Soft-tissue "sag" due to the loss of skin elasticity during aging is a major cause of change in the

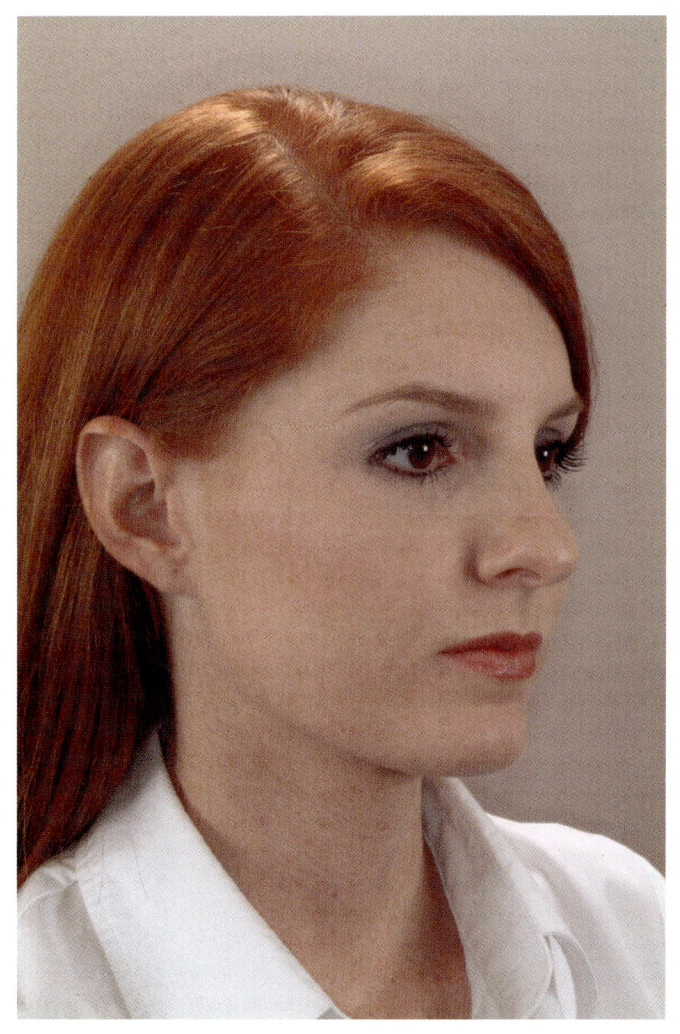

Figure 32.29 This patient has a desirable definition of the chin–neck anatomy with the gonial angle well delineated and defined, and with a moderately acute angle.

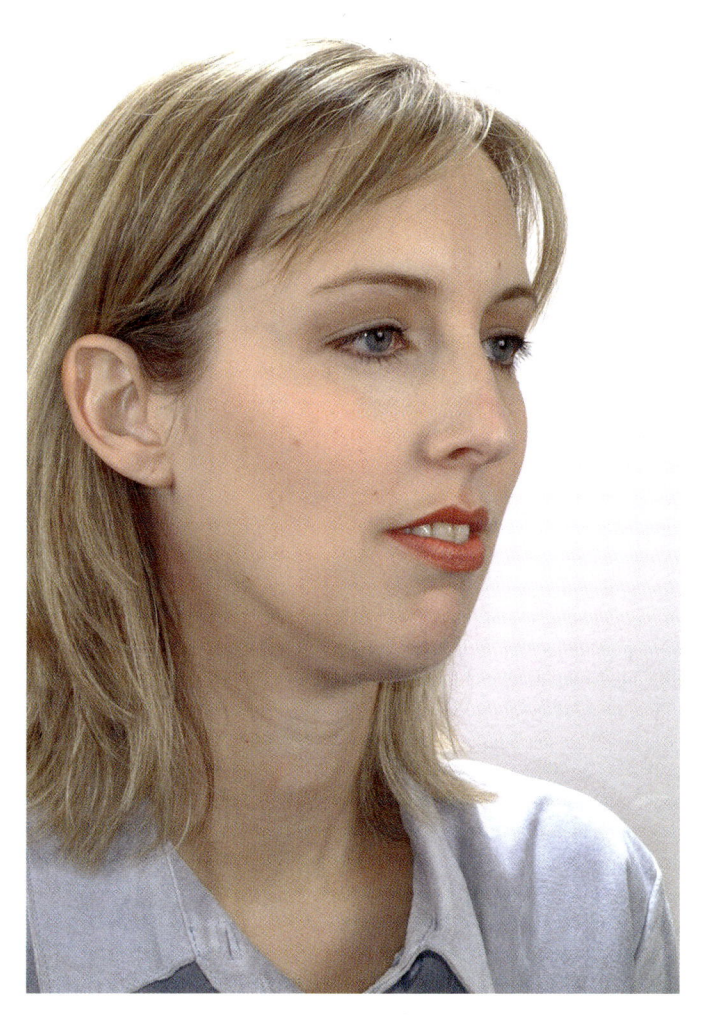

Figure 32.30 This patient has a dolichofacial skeletal pattern with a steeper mandibular plane, which is not as esthetically pleasing as the previous illustration.

cervicomental region. Weight gain is another important factor in the morphology of this area, as is the anatomical position of the hyoid bone. The patient in Figure 32.43A was treated as an adolescent to a very nice Class I occlusion. Her frontal vertical facial proportions were a bit long in the lower face, with lip incompetence a result of the long lower face, and a short maxillary lip length. Because of her vertical maxillary excess and short philtrum, her smile was too gummy (Figure 32.43B). Her profile (Figure 32.43C) was very convex with a marked unattractive chin–neck length and obtuse cervicomental angle. The submental area was a result of (1) down and back rotation of the mandible because of the vertical maxillary excess, (2) mandibular deficiency, (3) lack of chin projection, (4) excessive submental fat deposition, and (5) an unfavorable platysmal muscle morphology.

Her treatment plan was designed to surgically superiorly reposition the maxilla to reduce the lower facial height and decrease the excessive gingival display on smile. V–Y cheiloplasty and rhinoplasty were also performed simultaneously to improve the lip length and nasal esthetics. In addition, advancement of both the maxilla and mandible was planned to increase lower facial projection, thus improving the chin–neck length and cervicomental angle. Further enhancement included submental fat removal and platysmal lift (resection of the platysmal muscle to tighten the gonial and neck soft tissues). Her final smile (Figure 32.43D) was greatly improved, as was her profile (Figure 32.43E).

Macroesthetics and smile dimensions

Smile asymmetry may also be due to soft-tissue considerations, such as an asymmetric smile curtain. In the asymmetric smile curtain, there is a differential elevation of the upper lip during smile, which gives the illusion of transverse cant to the maxilla. This smile characteristic emphasizes the importance of direct clinical examination in treatment planning the smile, since this soft-tissue animation is not visible in a frontal radiograph or reflected in study models. It is not well documented in static photographic images, and is documented best in digital video clips.

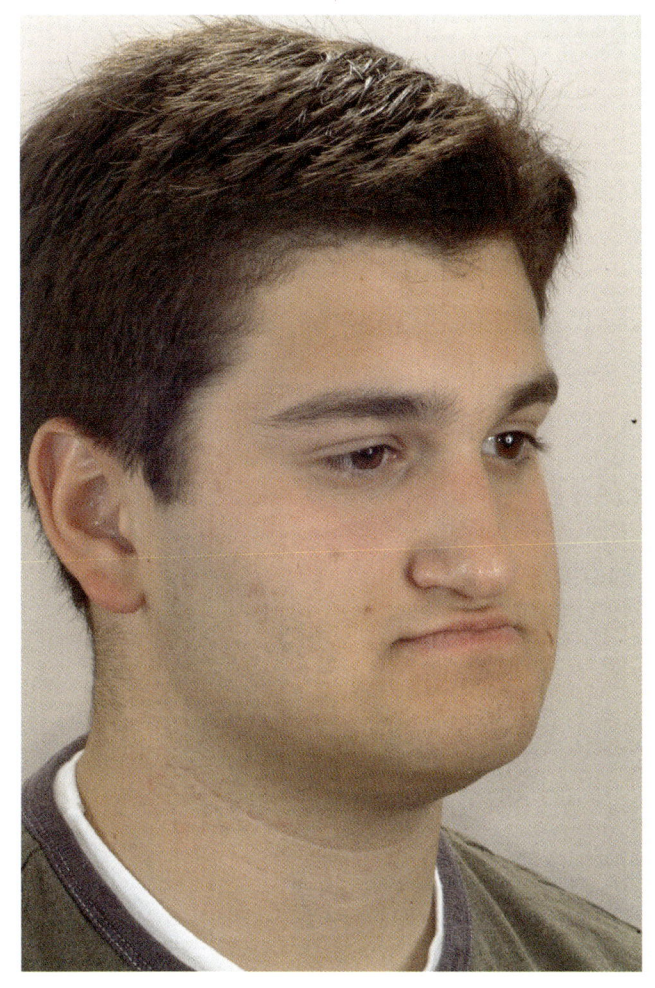

Chapter 32 Facial Considerations: An Orthodontic Perspective

Figure 32.31 This person demonstrates a brachyfacial skeletal pattern with a very acute gonial angle and short lower face.

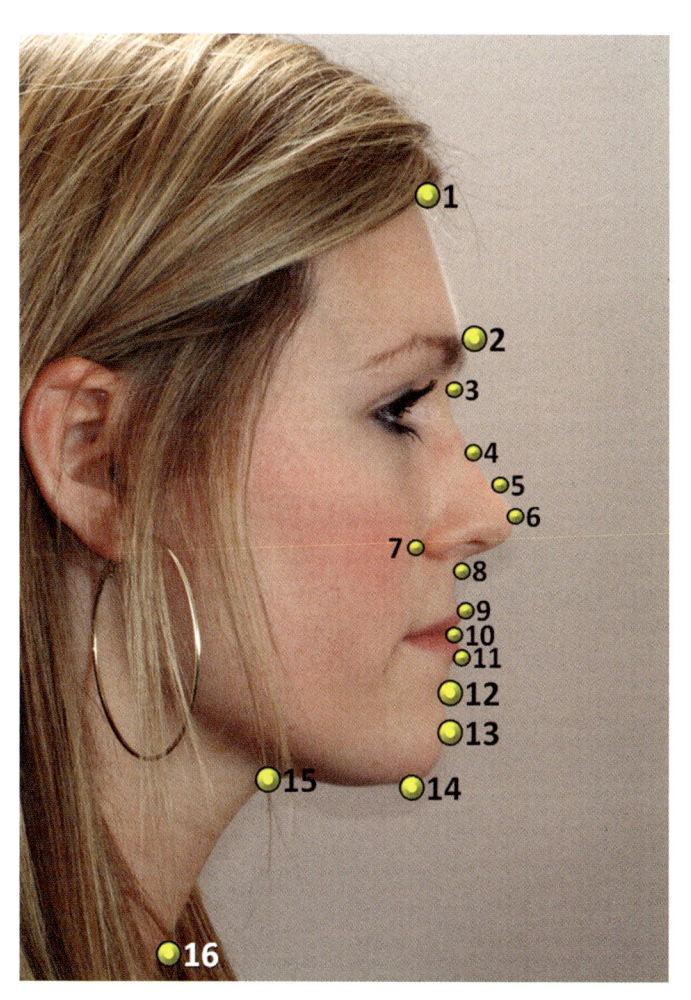

Figure 32.32 The landmarks used in describing the soft-tissue profile.

Table 32.2 Profile Soft-Tissue Points

Trichion	The hairline
Glabella	The most anterior aspect of the forehead as it progresses inferior into the nose
Radix (soft-tissue nasion)	The deepest point on the profile between glabella and the nasal dorsum
Mid dorsum	The midpoint of the nasal dorsum
Supratip break	The junction of the nasal dorsum and the nasal tip cartilage
Nasal tip	The most anterior point of the nose
Alar base	The most distal aspect of the ala at the base of the nose
Base of nose	The intersection of the nasal columella with the upper lip
Upper lip anterior limit	The most anterior point of the upper lip
Lip junction	The intersection of the upper and lower lips
Lower lip anterior limit	The most anterior point of the lower lip
Labiomental sulcus	The deepest curvature of the lower lip
Chin point	The most anterior point of the chin
Menton	The most inferior point on the base of the chin
Reflex point	The deepest point on the curvature of the neck
Base of neck	The intersection of the neck and the sternal complex

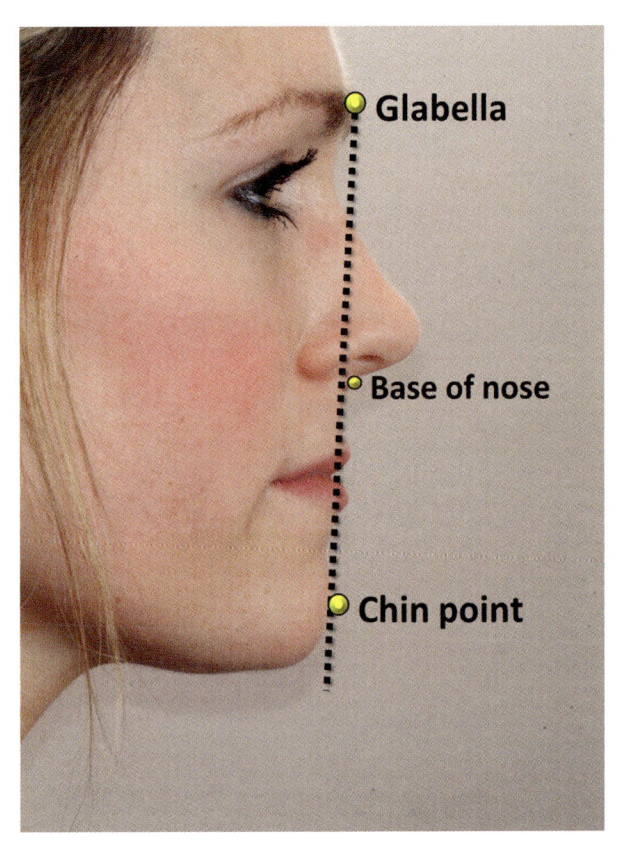

Figure 32.33 The anterior facial plane is formed from lines connecting the glabella to the base of the nose (subnasale) and the chin point.

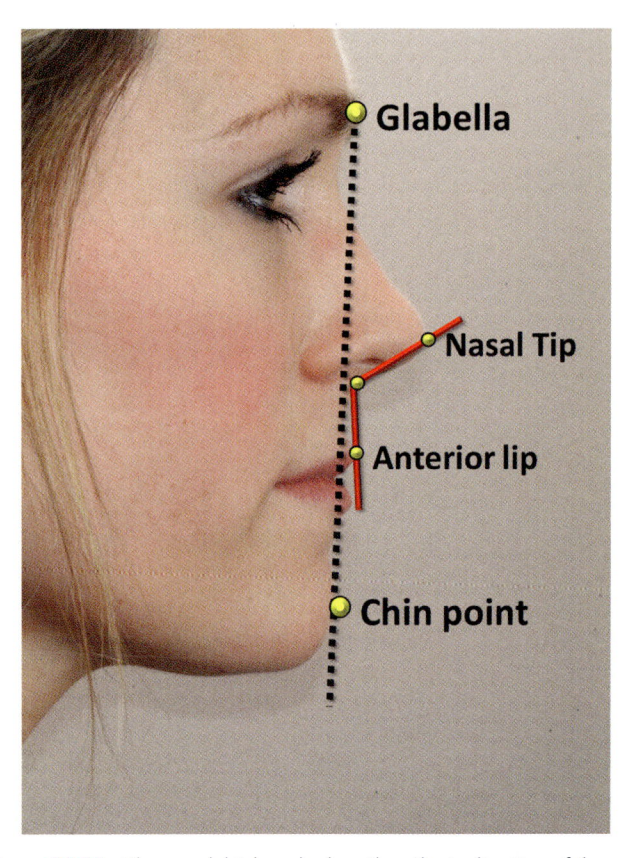

Figure 32.34 The nasolabial angle describes the inclination of the columella in relation to the upper lip. The ideal nasolabial angle should be in the range of 85–105°.

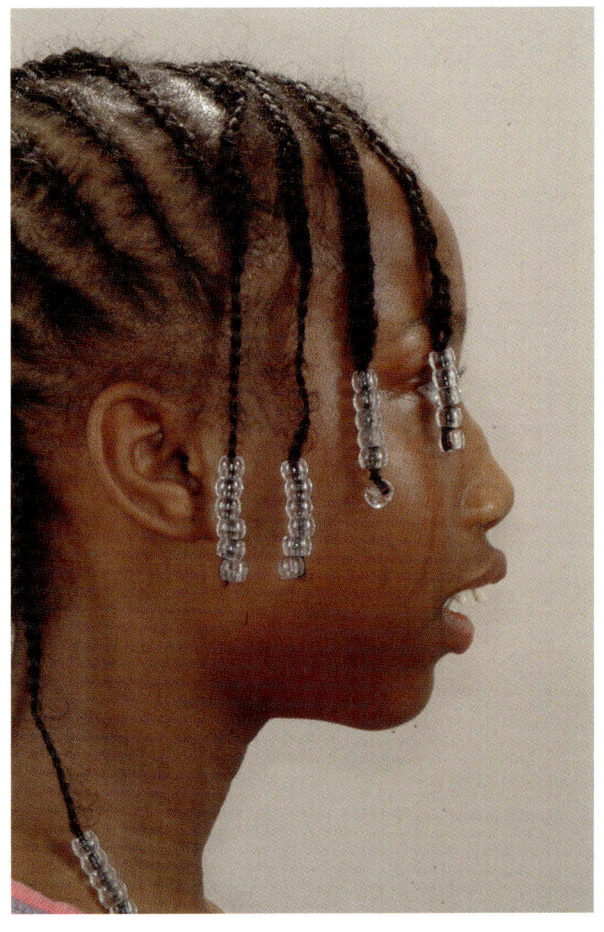

Figure 32.35 **(A)** This young patient had a severe maxillary and dental protrusion with a very acute nasolabial angle.

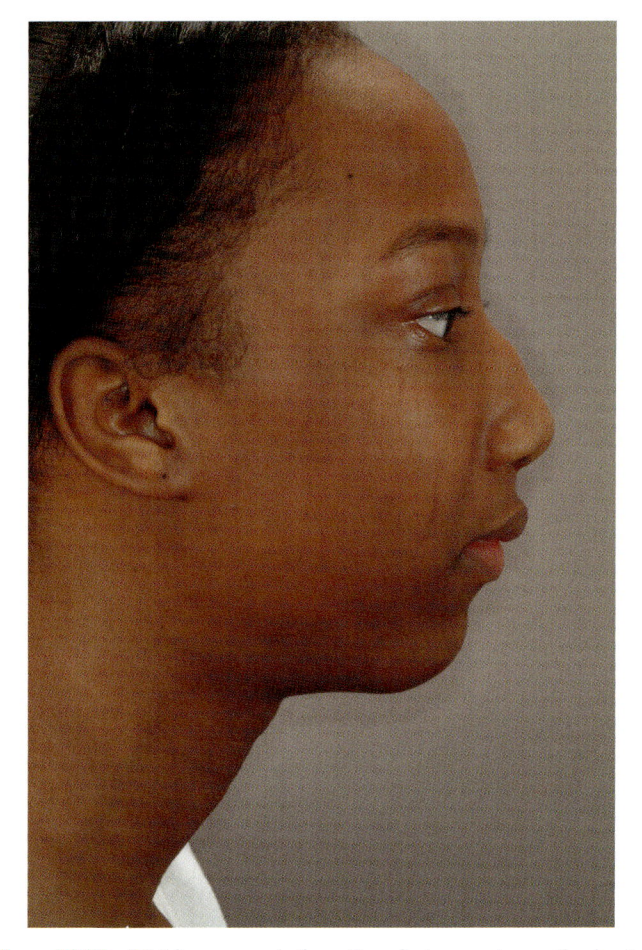

Figure 32.35 **(B)** After removal of maxillary first premolars, orthodontic treatment retracted the maxillary anterior teeth, resulting in a more favorable nasolabial angle.

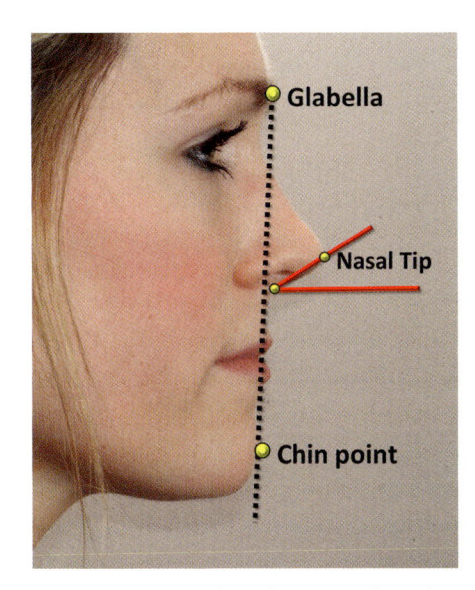

Figure 32.36 Nasal tip elevation reflects the position of the nasal tip relative to a perpendicular to the line from the glabella to the chin point at the base of the nose.

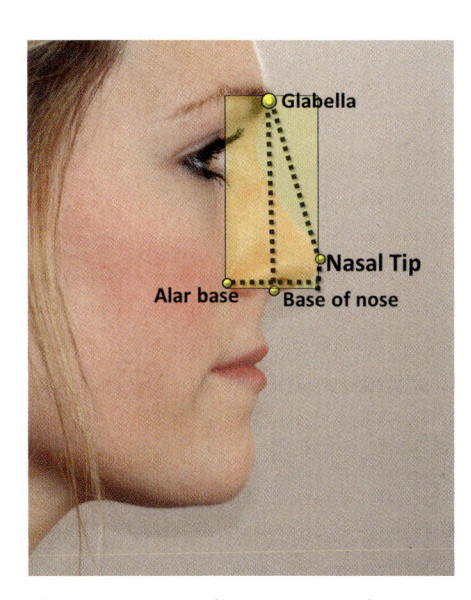

Figure 32.37 Nasal projection is a description of the nose in height from glabella to the base of the nose (subnasale) and length by nasal tip to the alar base.

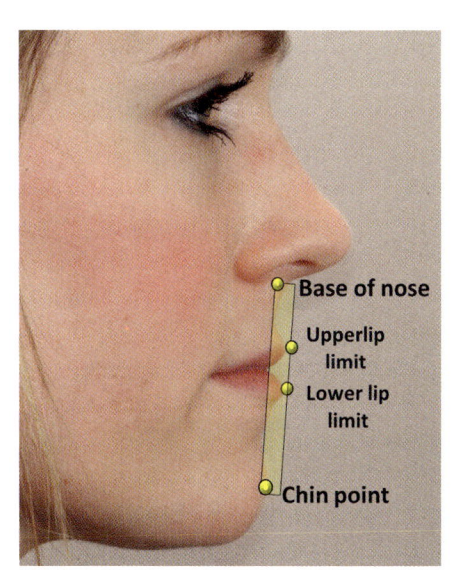

Figure 32.38 Lip projection is a function of maxillomandibular protrusion or retrusion, dental protrusion or retrusion, and/or lip thickness and can be measured from the base of the nose and the chin point to establish its position in relation to those structures.

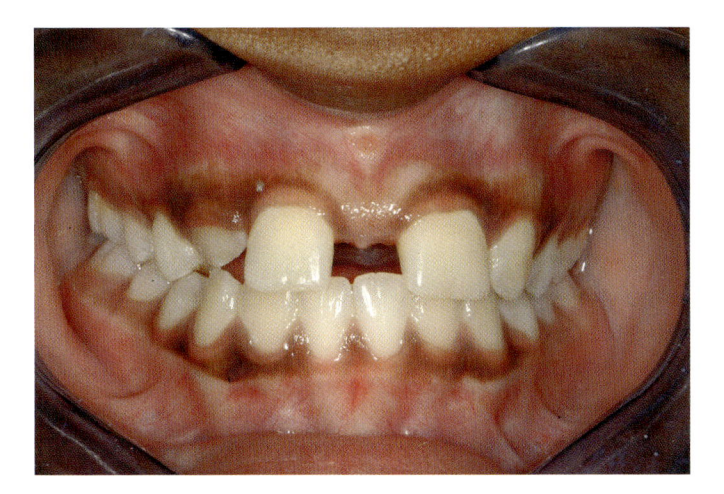

Figure 32.39 **(A)** A young girl was congenitally missing both maxillary lateral incisors with a very large maxillary diastema. A normal option to consider would be to close the diastema and place implants and crowns for restoration.

Transverse cant of the maxilla can be due to (1) differential eruption and placement of the anterior teeth and (2) skeletal asymmetry of the skull base and/or mandible resulting in a compensatory cant to the maxilla. Intraoral images or even mounted dental casts do not adequately reflect the relationship of the maxilla to the smile. Only frontal smile visualization permits the orthodontist to visualize any tooth-related asymmetry transversely.

The smile arc is defined as the relationship of the curvature of the incisal edges of the maxillary incisors, canines, premolars, and molars to the curvature of the lower lip in the posed social smile.[19, 20] Figure 32.44 demonstrates that the ideal smile arc has the maxillary incisal edge curvature parallel to the curvature of the lower lip upon smile. We have expanded that definition to

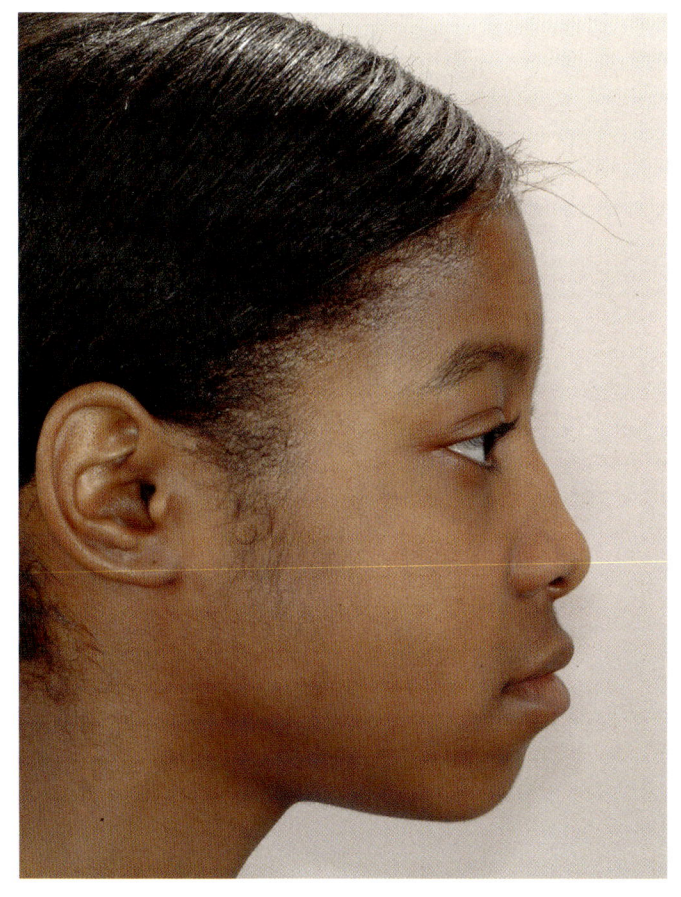

Figure 32.39 **(B)** She had marked lip projection secondary to her severe bidental protrusion.

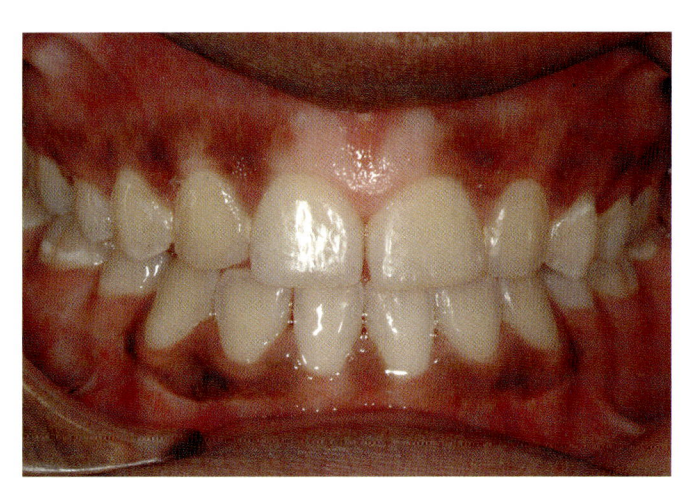

Figure 32.39 **(C)** We elected to extract lower first premolars to make space for protrusion reduction and close all the maxillary space.

include the occlusal plane as being parallel to the curvature of the lower lip upon smile, and the term consonant is used to describe this parallel relationship. A nonconsonant or flat smile arc is characterized by the maxillary incisal curvature being flatter than the curvature of the lower lip on smile. In spite of the professional interest only being a recent phenomenon, recent

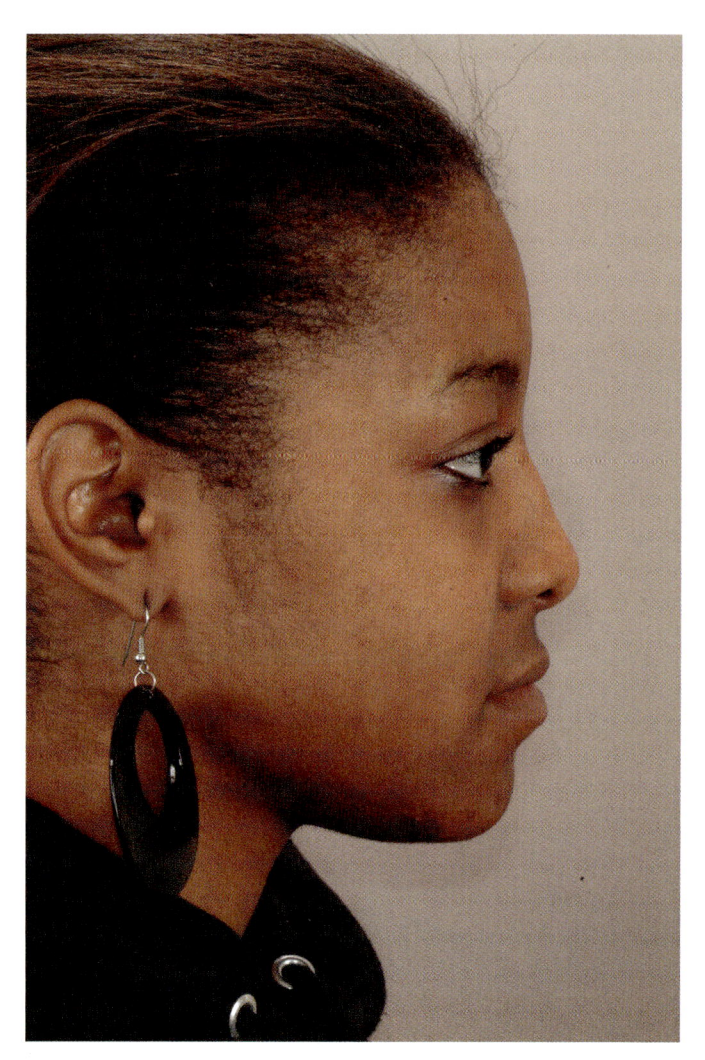

Figure 32.39 **(D)** The final profile was greatly improved, with the need for implants eliminated.

studies reveal that laypeople assess the smile arc as the most important feature in an ideal smile.[21] Early definitions of the smile arc were limited to the curvature of the canines and the incisors to the lower lip on smile because smile evaluation was made on the direct frontal view. But we prefer the oblique view since it reflects other issues that may affect the smile arc, like tilt of the occlusal plane, supereruption of maxillary incisors, and so on.

Pitch, roll, and yaw

Our analysis up to this point has focused on three of the six attributes needed to describe the position of the dentition in the face and the orientation of the head. Simple Class I, II, and III classifications do not adequately reflect the complexities of the craniofacial complex since the concept came from Angle over 100 years ago as the first classification system regarding tooth occlusion. A more complete description is necessary to describe the position of an airplane in space: translation (forward/backward, up/down, right/left), which must be combined with rotation about three perpendicular axes (yaw, pitch, and roll) and is analogous to our effort to describe the orientation of the

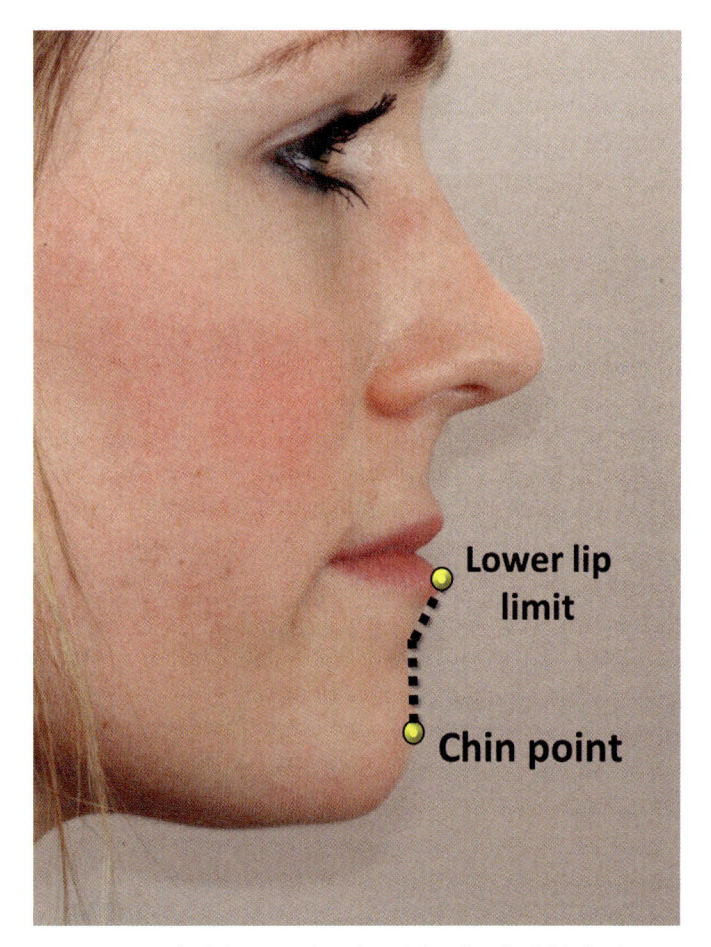

Figure 32.40 The labiomental angle is defined as the fold of soft tissue between the lower lip and the chin and may vary greatly in form and depth.

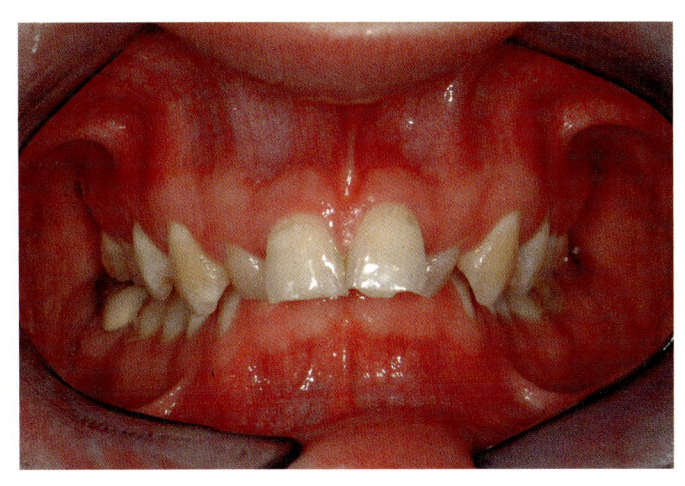

Figure 32.41 **(A)** This patient had a severe Class II malocclusion with a deep bite and severe overjet.

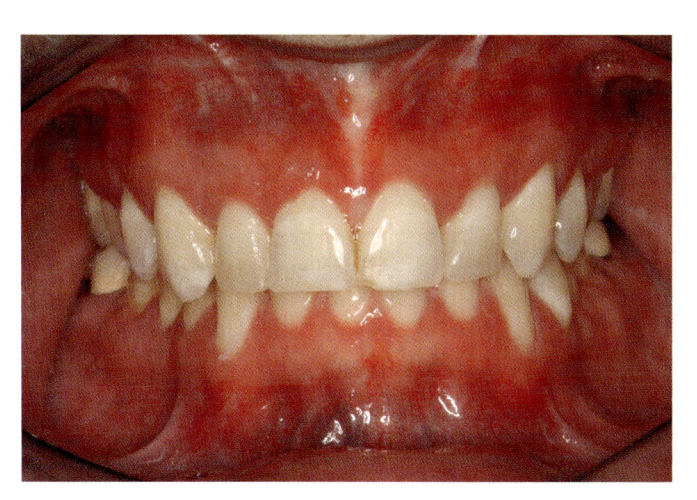

Figure 32.41 **(B)** The finished intraoral shows ideal overbite/overjet.

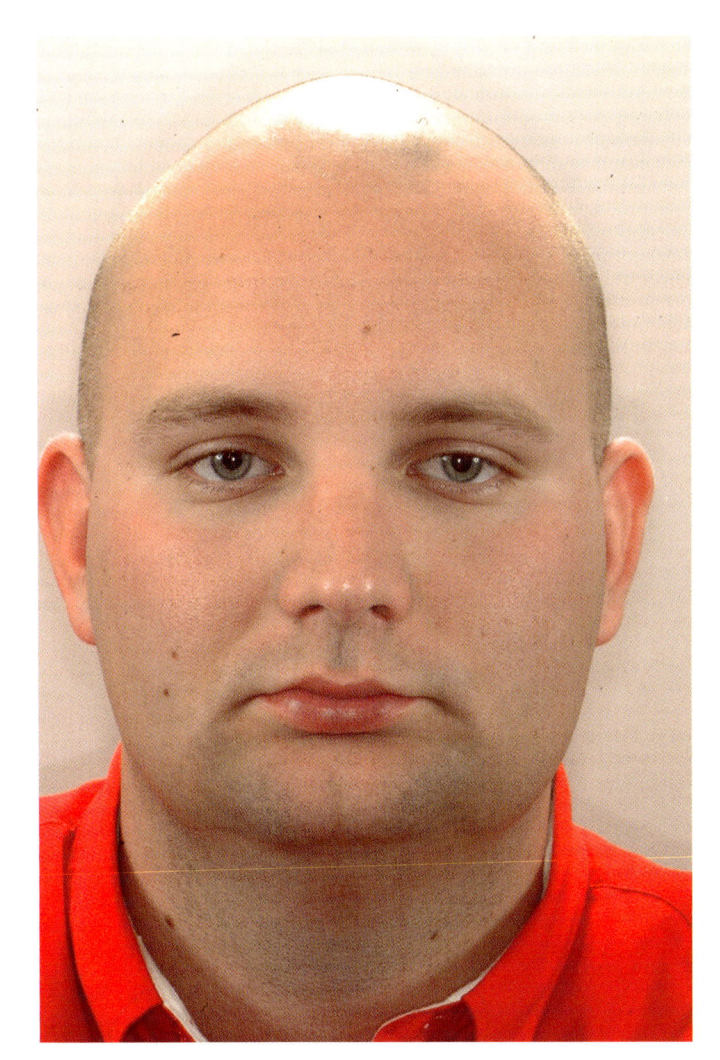

Figure 32.41 **(C)** His facial pattern had a short lower facial with soft-tissue redundancy.

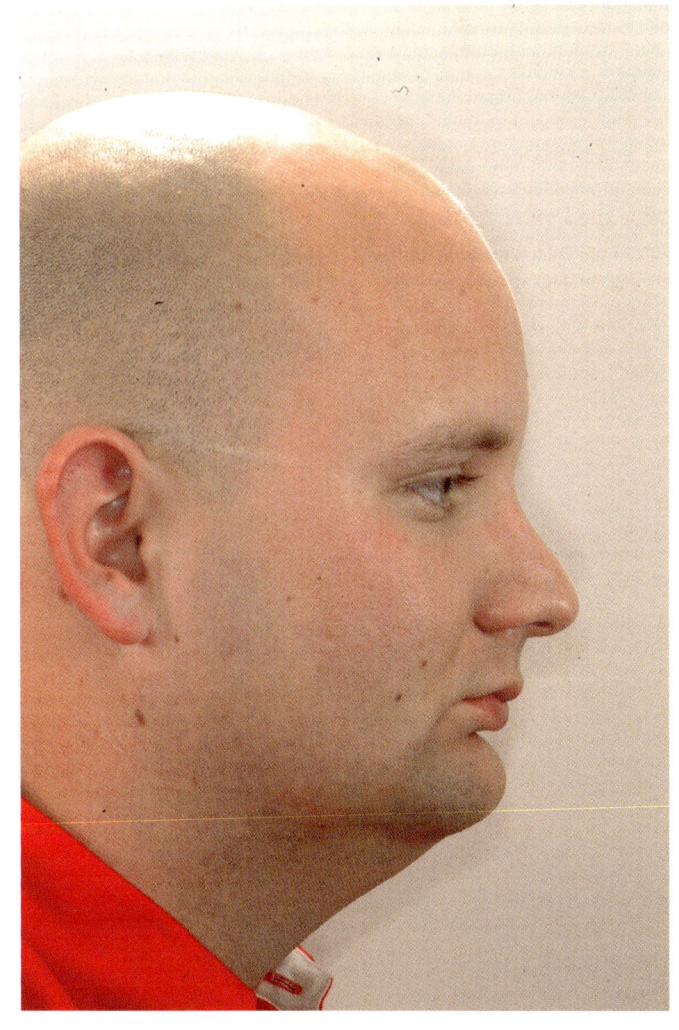

Figure 32.41 **(D)** His profile was mandibular deficient with lower lip eversion resulting in a deep labiomental sulcus.

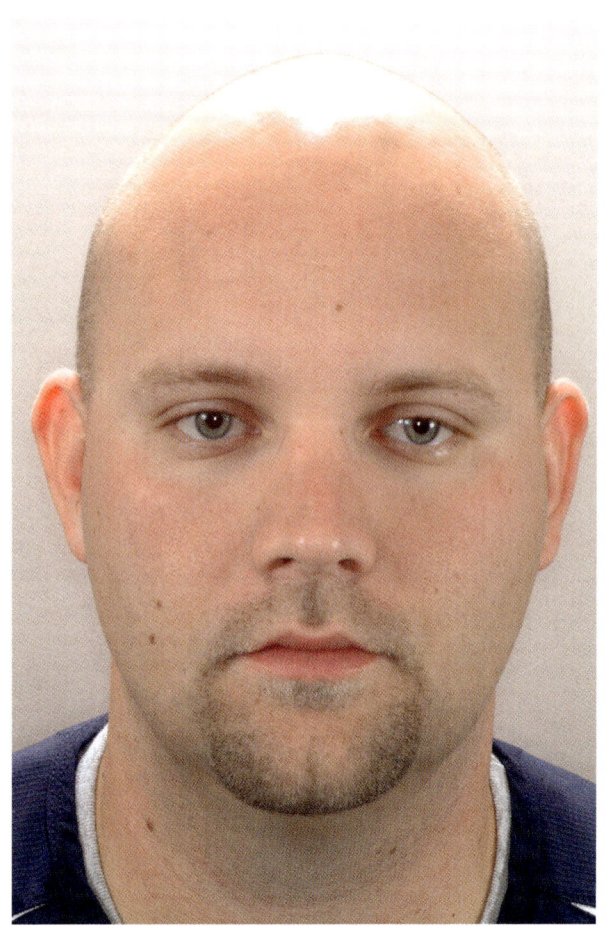

Figure 32.41 **(E)** After orthodontic preparation, the malocclusion was corrected with mandibular advancement, increasing the lower facial height and correcting the overjet.

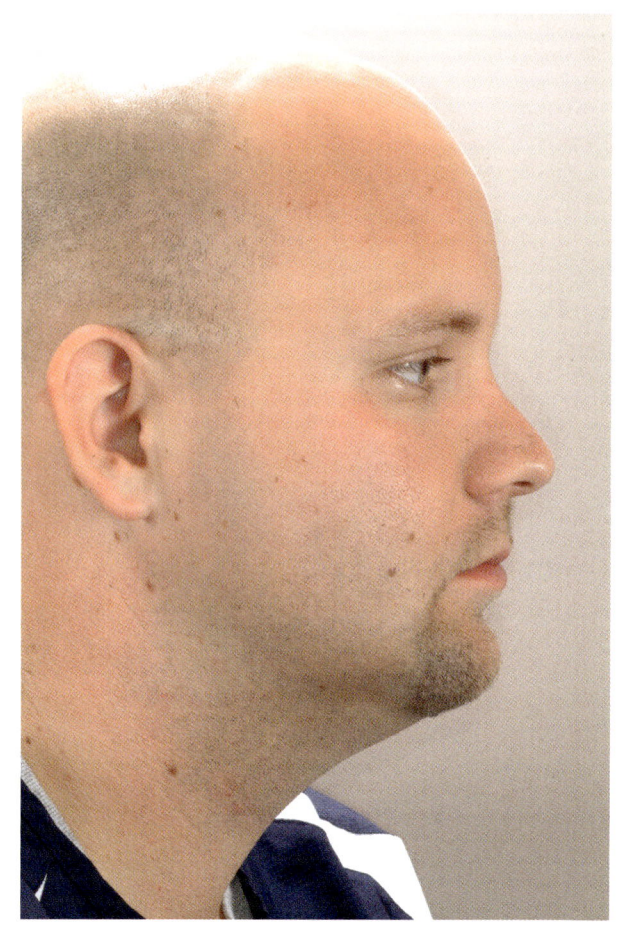

Figure 32.41 **(F)** The final profile with a more balanced profile and facial proportions.

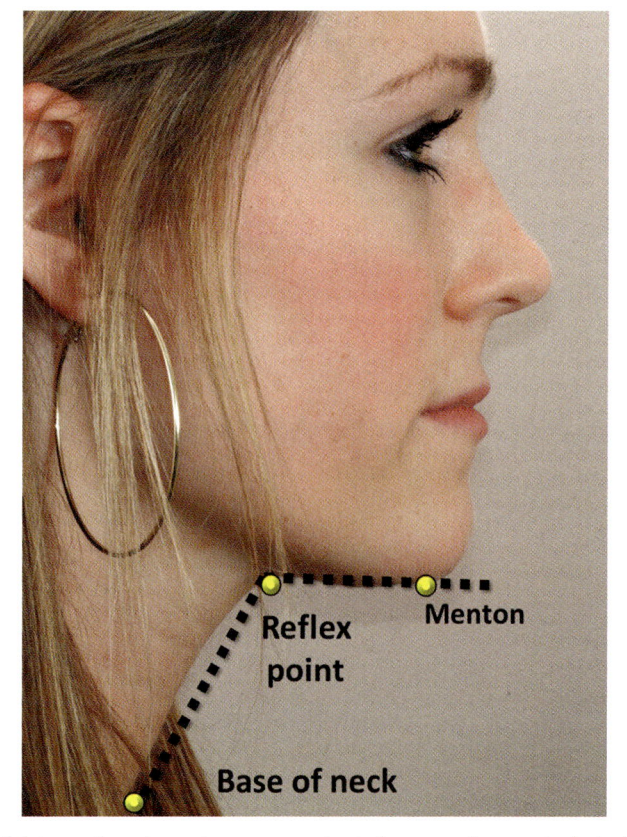

Figure 32.42 The chin–neck length and chin–neck angle are important esthetic features often not included in the esthetic assessment of a patient's dentofacial evaluation. Chin–neck length is from the reflex point to the chin point, and cervicomental angle is measured from the chin point to the reflex point to the base of the neck.

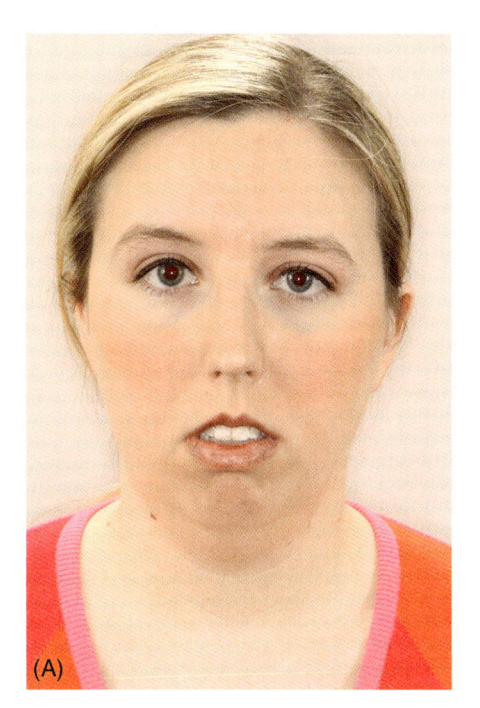

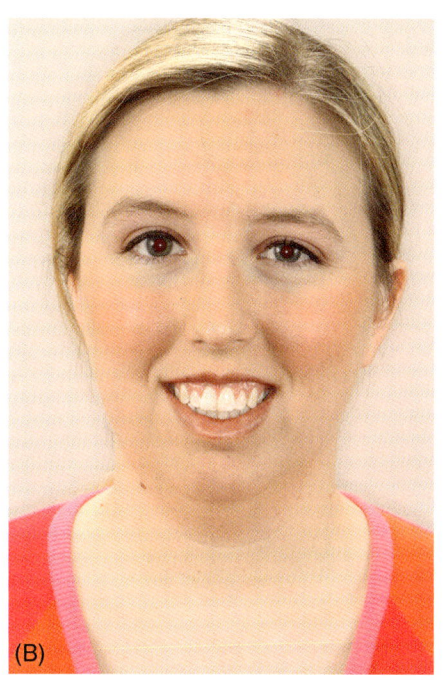

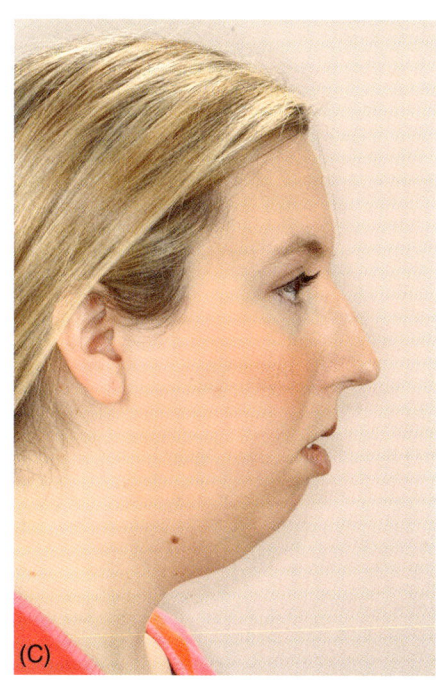

Figure 32.43 **(A)** This patient was treated as an adolescent to a very nice Class I occlusion. Her frontal vertical facial proportions were long in the lower face, with lip incompetence a result of the long lower face and a short maxillary lip length. **(B)** Because of the vertical maxillary excess and short philtrum, she exhibited excessive gingival display on smile. **(C)** Her profile was very convex, with a markedly unattractive chin–neck length and obtuse cervicomental angle.

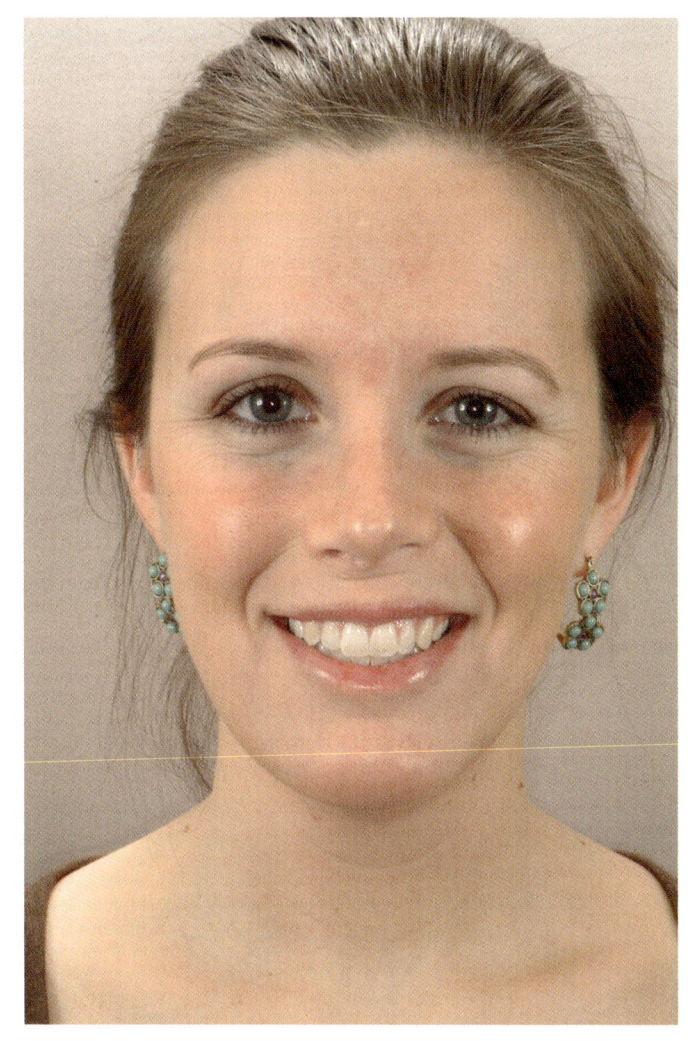

Figure 32.43 **(D)** After orthodontic surgical treatment with maxillary impaction and V–Y cheiloplasty, the facial proportions and smile were greatly enhanced.

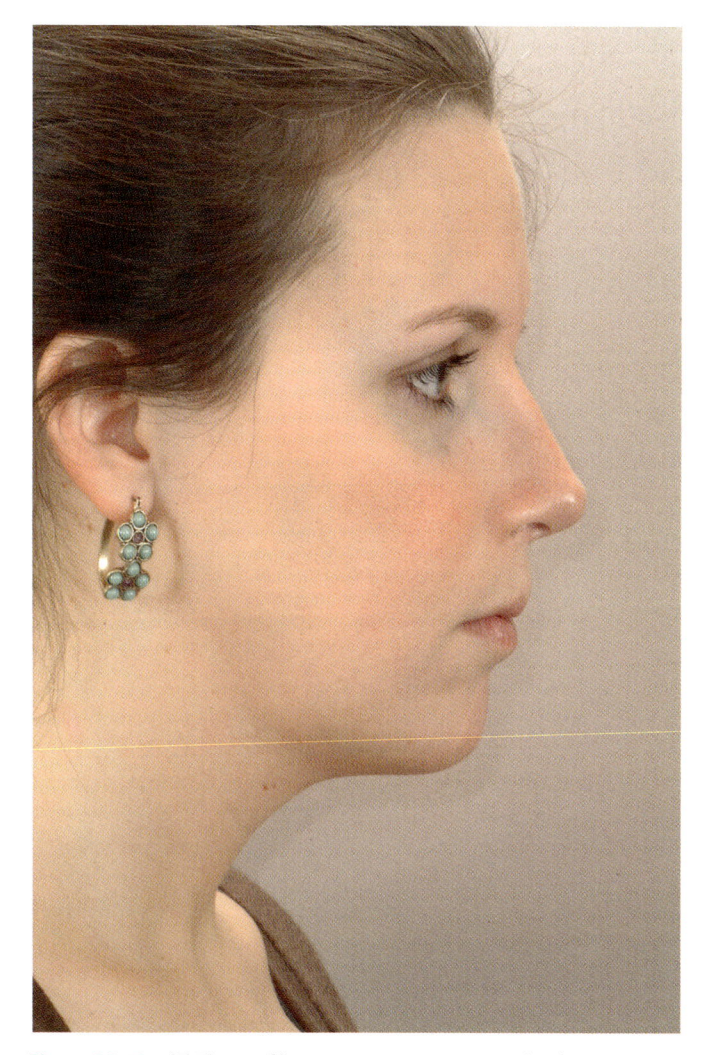

Figure 32.43 **(E)** The profile improvement was a result of bimaxillary advancement, chin advancement, submental fat removal, and platysmal lift.

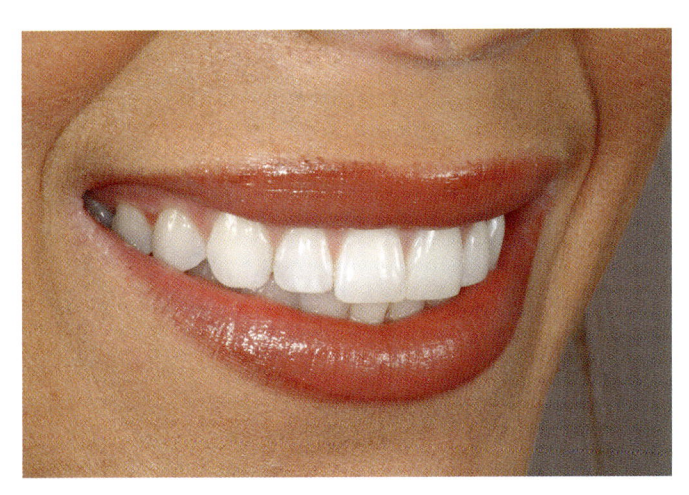

Figure 32.44 The ideal smile arc is defined as where the maxillary incisal edge curvature and occlusal plane are parallel to the curvature of the lower lip upon smile.

dental and skeletal relationships. The introduction of the rotational axes in the description of dentofacial deformities adds precision of the description and, consequently, facilitates development of the problem list (Figure 32.45).[22]

Clinical case study

A 19-year-old patient was referred by her general dentist for improvement in the appearance of her smile. She had a combination of esthetic and functional issues that required an interdisciplinary combination of orthodontics, orthognathic surgery, and plastic surgery.

Macroesthetic analysis

At rest she had the following attributes (Figure 32.46):

- a short lower facial third relative to facial width;
- a wide alar width relative to the intercanthal distance;
- slightly downturned and deep commissures;
- diminished lip support and vermillion display.

Our patient's facial proportions were characterized by a short lower face (often associated with vertical maxillary deficiency) with inadequate lip support for a 19-year-old. She was referred by her dentist for evaluation of her smile esthetic presentation (Figure 32.47) with spacing present and lack of tooth display on smile. The profile (Figure 32.48) provided an important clue: it was concave with a Class III appearance. Her profile was concave with an acute nasolabial angle, and her chin point is anterior of the forehead and base of the nose. The upper lip is also behind the lower lip. Her chin–neck length is adequate, but chin–neck angle slightly obtuse, particularly for a 19-year-old female.

Proclined or flared-appearing incisors can be either dental or skeletal in origin, which makes the correct diagnosis and appropriate treatment even more challenging. How do we make the determination as to the underlying etiology of the incisor proclination? We have previously described a more complete method

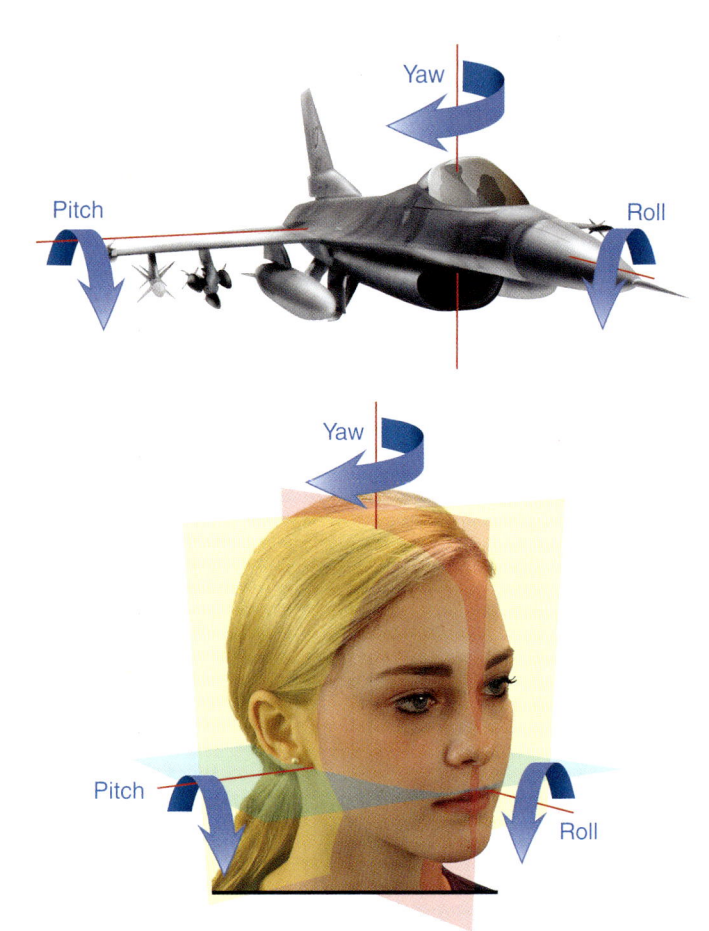

Figure 32.45 Simple Class I, II, and III classifications simply do not adequately reflect the complexities of the craniofacial complex. The introduction of the three rotational axes (pitch, roll, and yaw) in the description of dentofacial deformities adds precision of the description and, consequently, facilitates development of the problem list. This schematic demonstrates the visualization of the face and skeleton in terms of pitch, roll, and yaw. *Source*: Ackerman JL et al.[22]

of craniofacial morphology by describing the concepts of pitch, roll, and yaw to define the facial skeletal pattern. The macroesthetic evaluation is important to leading us to the correct diagnosis.

The Angle classification was inadequate since it describes only the anteroposterior position of the teeth and was never intended to define jaw relationships. In this case, using the Angle classification, we tend to think in terms of the mandible being too large or the maxilla too small. Therefore, our plan most likely would involve movement of the maxilla forward or the mandible back. The concept of pitch, roll, and yaw was intended to emphasize this deficiency in descriptive potential. While her midface was deficient relative to the mandible, the overall skeletal pattern really represented a counterclockwise pitch of the lower face. This is best visualized on the oblique view (Figure 32.49). By facilitating our visual evaluation of the spatial orientation of the maxillary and palatal occlusal planes on smile (Figure 32.50), the oblique view is important in distinguishing the skeletal incisor flare problem from the dental one.

As part of the macroesthetic analysis, the smile was evaluated in the context of its fit and proportion with the overall facial

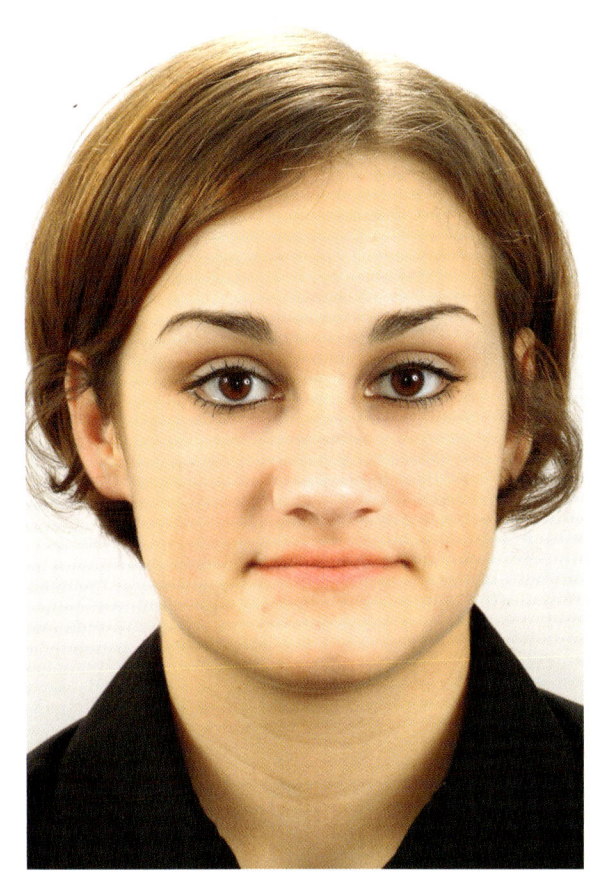

Figure 32.46 This 19-year-old patient had concerns about her overall appearance.

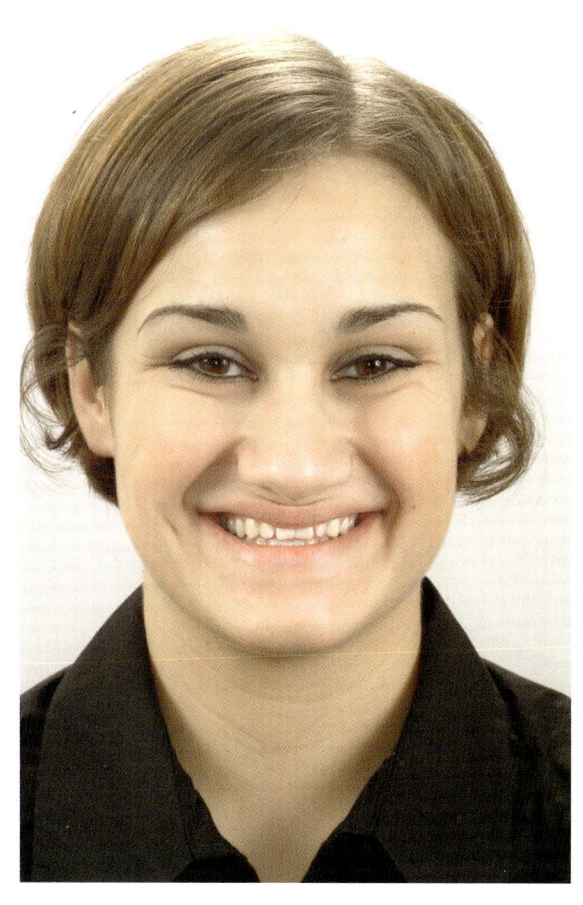

Figure 32.47 Referred by her dentist for smile evaluation, spacing was noted in addition to a lack of tooth display on smile.

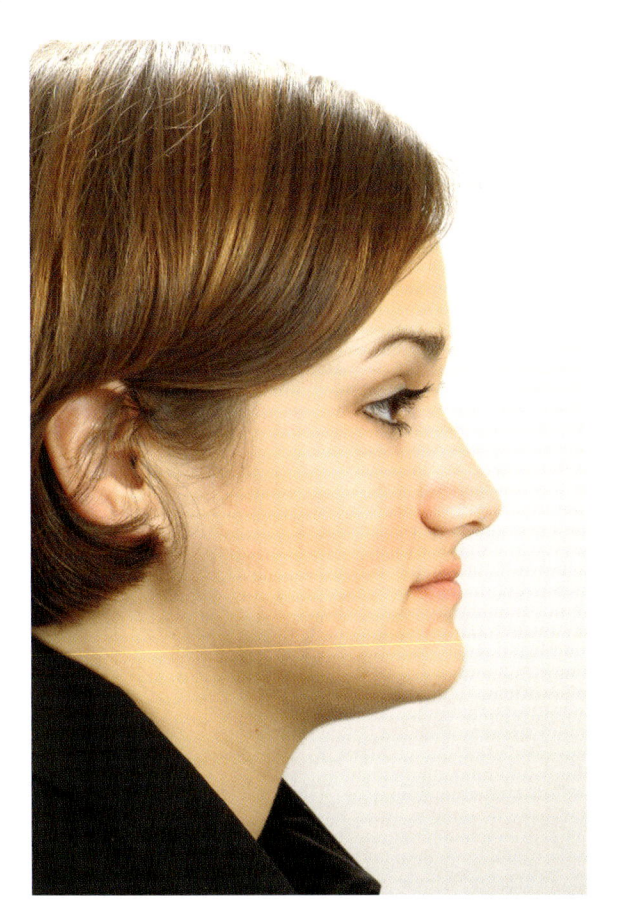

Figure 32.48 The profile was concave, and, in terms of the Angle classification, we tend to call it a "Class III" profile. The Angle classification is a dental system of classification and was never intended to describe skeletal relations.

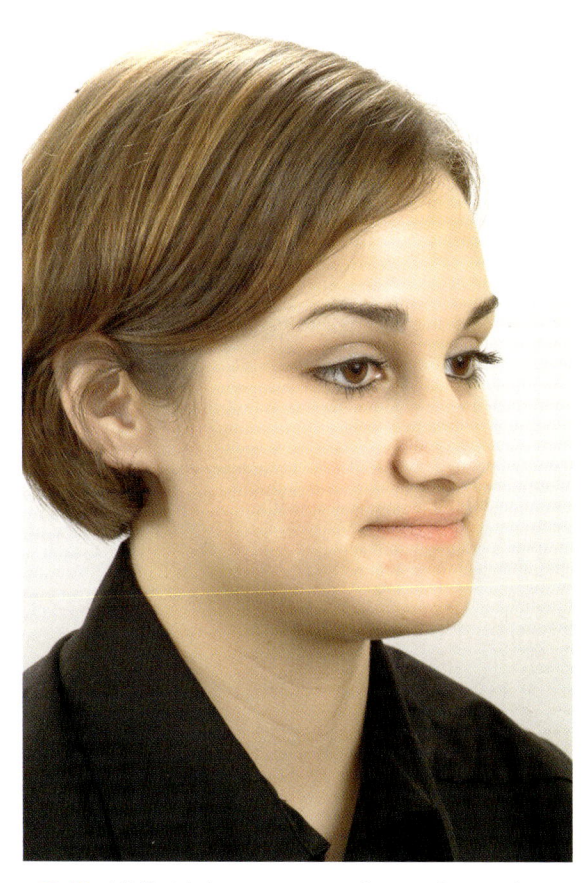

Figure 32.49 Midfacial characteristics such as inadequate lip support are best visualized on the oblique facial view.

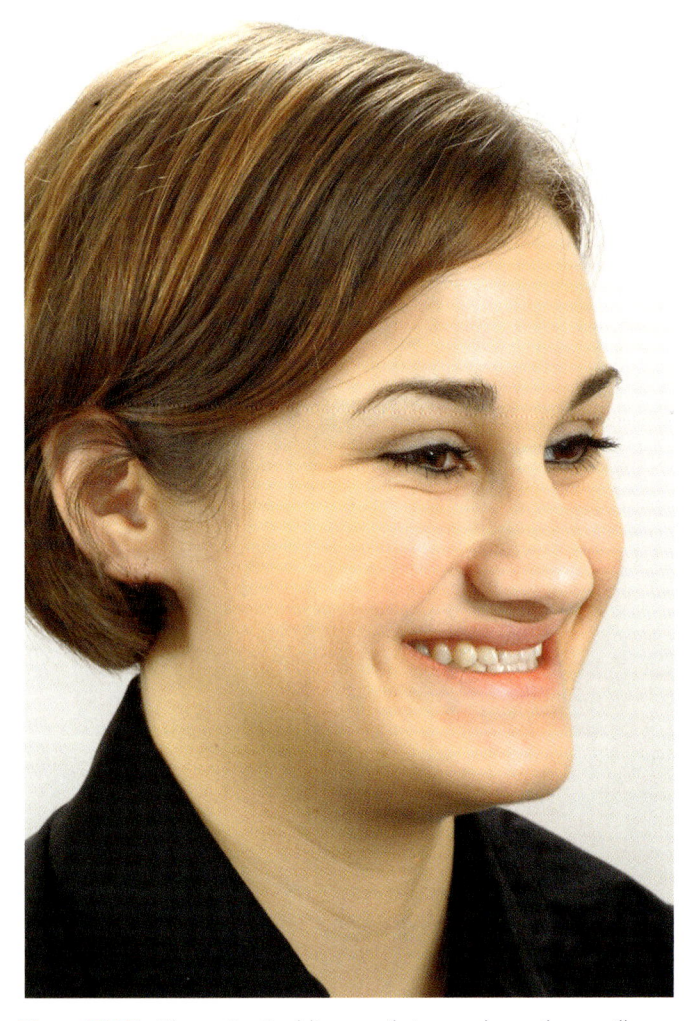

Figure 32.50 The patient's oblique smile image shows the maxillary occlusal plane is flatter than the mandibular plane, a view we can realize without cephalometric radiography.

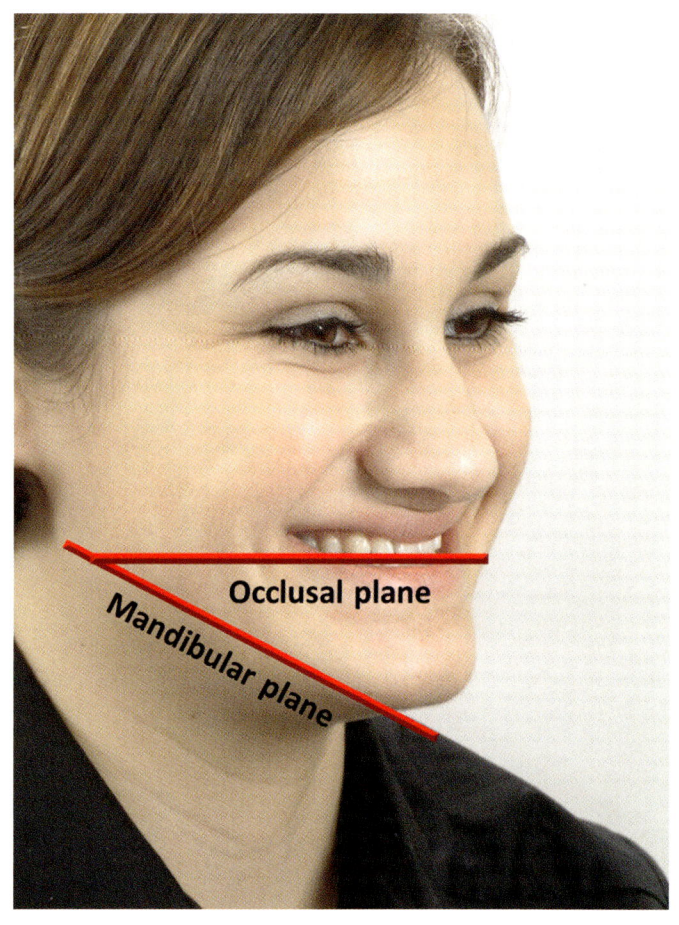

Figure 32.51 The oblique smile picture gives us a good recognition of her interocclusal relationships, and also the "pitch" of her maxillary occlusal plane relative to the Frankfort and mandibular planes.

dimension. On smiling, the patient did not show all of her upper teeth. (Her smile characteristics will be discussed in more depth in the miniesthetic assessment.) In evaluation of her oblique resting relationship, the lack of lip support is even more evident, as is the midfacial characteristics of a low nasal tip, nasal projection, and lack of nasal definition. In Figure 32.51, her oblique smile picture gives us a good recognition of her interocclusal relationships and also the "pitch" of her maxillary occlusal plane relative to the Frankfort and mandibular planes. Her smile retracts the lips, and retracts the nasal tip, accentuating the facial flatness. Her occlusal plane has a counterclockwise pitch to ideal. In other words, the occlusal plane and palatal plane are flatter than the mandibular plane compared with the more ideal example in Figure 32.52.

Miniesthetic analysis

The frontal close-up smile (Figure 32.53) revealed many quantitative and measurable aspects of her smile. On clinical examination, we measured zero incisor display at rest, 5 mm of maxillary incisor display on smile, and her maxillary incisor crown height was 10 mm. These measurements virtually lead us to our orthognathic surgical plan in order to achieve ideal incisor display. If the amount of incisor display on smile is 5 mm and crown height is 10 mm, then the anterior downgraft of the maxilla would equal 5 mm to expose the entire upper incisor on smile.

As a result of the vertical and rotational skeletal pattern, her anterior tooth display on smile was only 4 mm, with the crown height measured at 10 mm. Her smile arc was also nonconsonant, or flat.[5–9] The oblique smile images (Figure 32.54) reflect the flare of the maxillary incisors as a result of the counterclockwise positioning of the maxillary occlusal and palatal planes.

Microesthetic analysis (teeth)

The shape of the maxillary incisors and gingival contour were within normal limits.

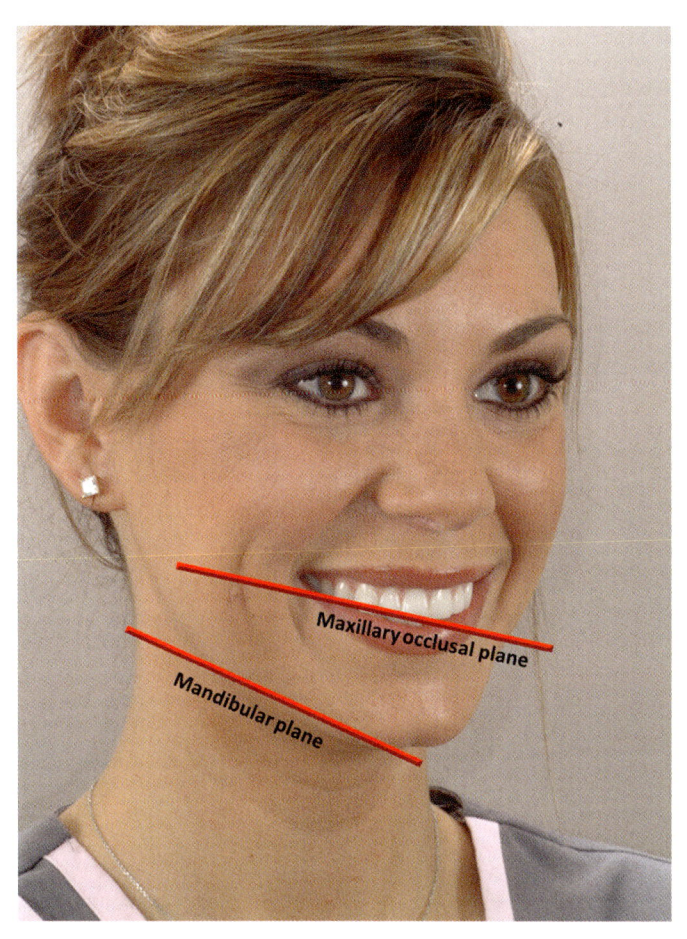

Figure 32.52 In a patient with ideal facial and smile esthetics, the maxillary occlusal plane and mandibular plane are more divergent and closer to ideal.

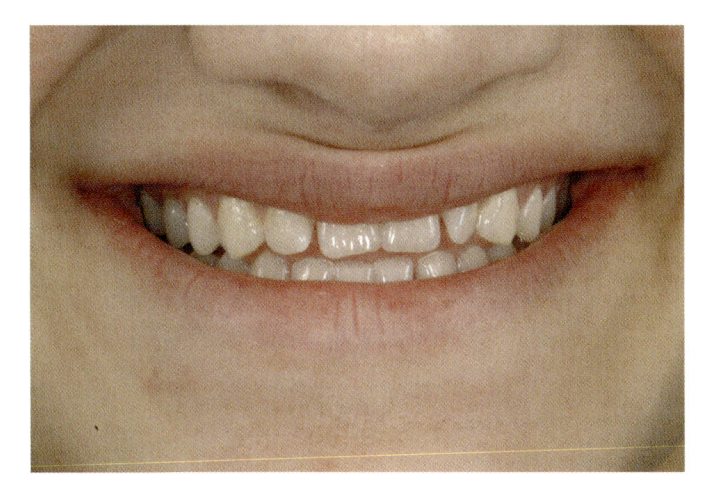

Figure 32.53 Anterior tooth display on smile was only 4 mm, central incisor crown height 10 mm, and a flat or nonconsonant smile arc.

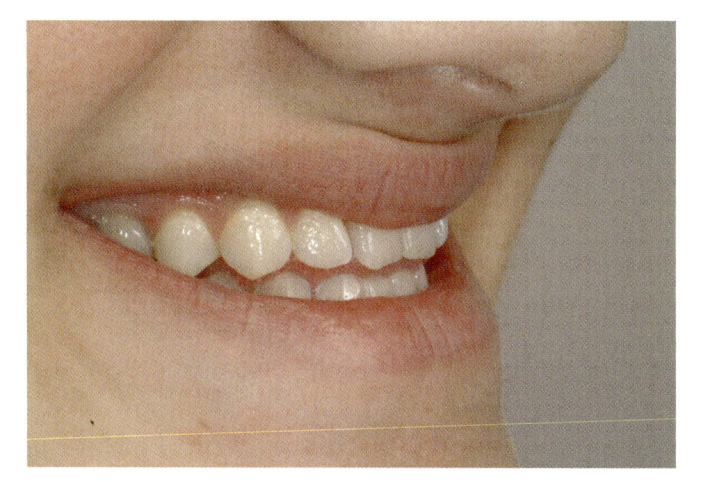

Figure 32.54 The oblique smile image reflects the flare of the maxillary incisors as a result of the counterclockwise positioning of the maxillary occlusal and palatal planes.

Orthodontic–surgical treatment

Our treatment started with orthodontic preparation for a surgical plan of maxillomandibular occlusal plane rotation in a clockwise direction.[10–12] The surgery was planned with the synergistic concepts of macro- and miniesthetics in mind. So the surgical phase of treatment will be presented in a stepwise fashion to illustrate the cause and effect aspect of the quantification of our clinical examination and resulting plan. The surgical treatment plan consisted of both orthognathic and soft-tissue surgery (Figure 32.55).

The maxillary osteotomy

The surgical plan starts with the ideal vertical and anteroposterior placement of the maxillary incisors. This concept is certainly not different from contemporary esthetic dental planning, in which placement of the maxillary incisor is of paramount importance. A Le Fort I osteotomy of the maxilla was performed with anterior downgraft, thus changing the pitch of the maxilla. The amount of anterior downgraft was determined as follows:

- only 5 mm of maxillary incisor was displayed on smile;
- the incisor crown height was 10 mm;
- therefore, the anterior maxilla was downgrafted 5 mm to attain full incisor display on smile.

The maxillary downgraft of the anterior maxilla was planned to increase the amount of incisor display on smile. Downgraft of the anterior maxilla would additionally steepen the occlusal and palatal planes, which would offer a better match of the curvature of the maxillary dental arch to the curvature of the lower lip on smile (improving the consonance of the smile arc). The anterior maxillary vertically lengthening would also result in a compensatory downward movement of the mandible, which would increase the lower facial height, thus improving the facial proportions.

Because of the diminished lip support, maxillary advancement was also planned. And since the occlusal plane was to be changed, mandibular surgery through bilateral sagittal split osteotomy was also required.[23] Advancement of the mandible was planned:

1. To keep the posterior occlusion in contact. As the anterior maxilla moves inferiorly, the mandible must rotate opened, with loss of occlusal contact in the posterior. The mandibular ramus osteotomy allowed the body of the mandible to rotate concomitantly with positioning of the maxilla.
2. To advance the mandible in addition to the maxillary advancement. This would increase lip support, preventing rotation of the chin point posteriorly, resulting in a more obtuse chin neck angle and shorter chin neck length.

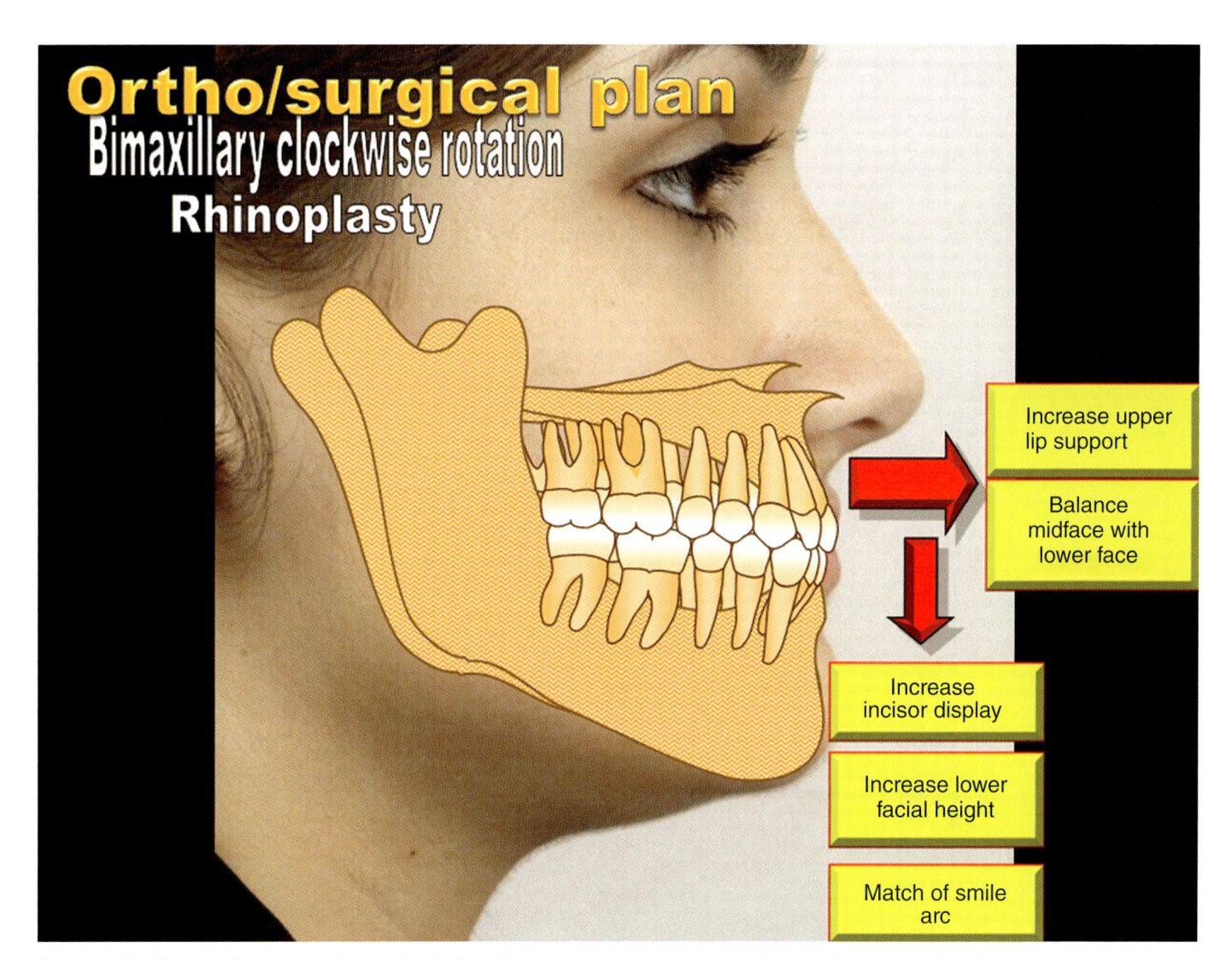

Figure 32.55 The overall treatment plan consisted of maxillary advancement with anterior downgraft to increase facial height, lip support, incisor display on smile, and to tip the occlusal plane to improve the smile arc. The mandibular osteotomy rotated the mandible clockwise in response to the new maxillary position.

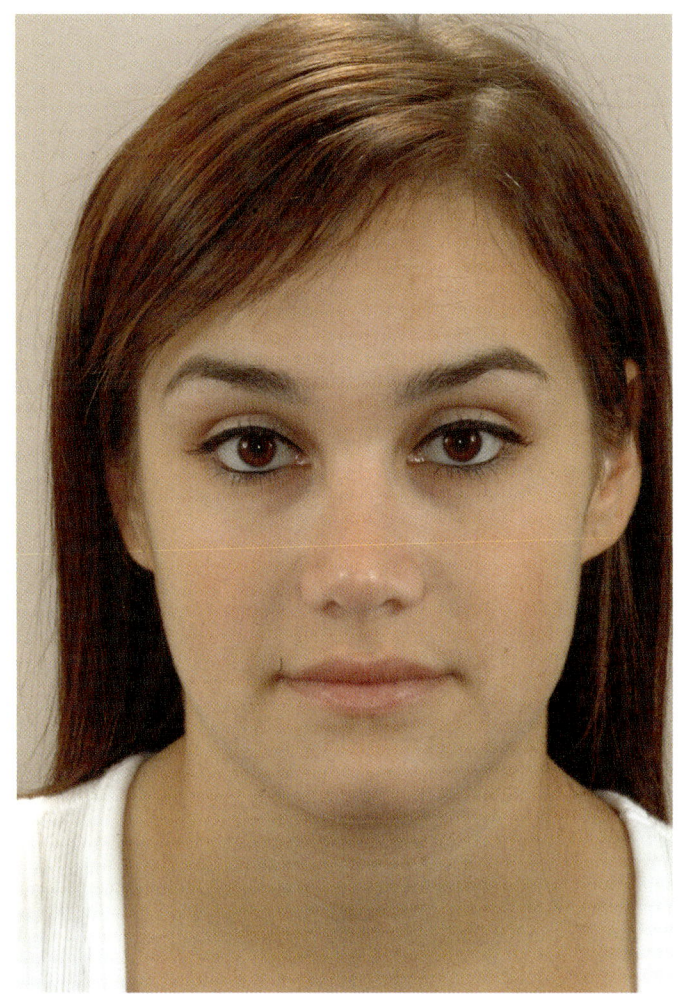

Figure 32.56 The final frontal facial appearance was much more youthful and appealing, and the facial dimensions were more appropriate and the advancement of both jaws greatly enhanced resting lip support.

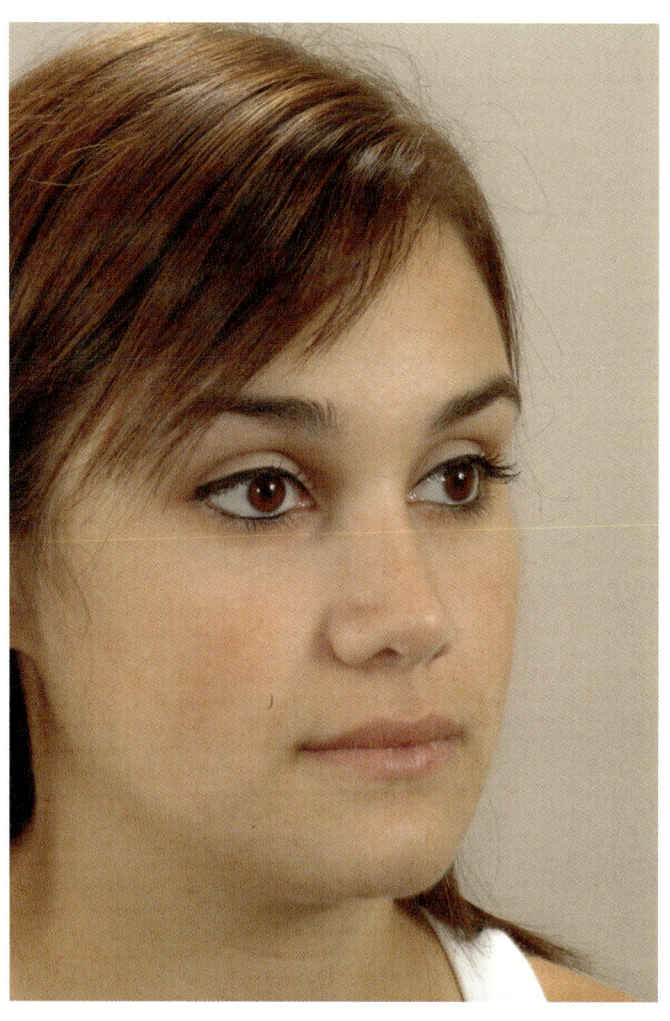

Figure 32.57 The oblique image demonstrates the esthetic refinement and enhancement of the nose and midface with maxillary advancement and rhinoplasty.

Rhinoplasty

The expected changes of the nose as a result of the maxillary surgery were an increase in tip projection, deepening of the supra-tip depression, tip rotation, and alar base widening. Thus, in consultation with the plastic surgeon, a simultaneous rhinoplasty was planned[24] to counter these effects and a V–Y cheiloplasty to increase her lip length.

The rhinoplasty was performed simultaneously with the osteotomies.[13–23] The purpose of the rhinoplasty was twofold:

- Because her nose was already wide and maxillary advancement would cause further widening of the nasal base, the rhinoplasty was indicated so the esthetics of the midface were not compromised by the orthognathic surgery.
- Rhinoplasty was indicated to improve the overall esthetics of her face.

Since the greatest risk for the patient undergoing jaw surgery is the anesthesia, performing the rhinoplasty at the same time did not present any increased risk. Our philosophy is to maximize the risk/benefit ratio of every procedure. Consequently, there was no increased risk, but a greatly increased benefit to the patient's overall appearance in performing rhinoplasty.

Final results

The final facial appearance was much more youthful and appealing and the facial dimensions were more appropriate (Figure 32.56). There is significant improvement in all three components of her esthetic appearance with the increase in lower facial and dramatic increase in vermillion display and lip display. The oblique image (Figure 32.57) demonstrates the esthetic refinement and enhancement of the nose and midface with maxillary advancement and rhinoplasty. The rhinoplasty was successful in narrowing the base of the nose, as well as the refinement of the dorsum and tip, giving her a continuation of the brow into the dorsum and tip. The advancement of both jaws greatly enhanced resting lip support, and anterior downgraft of the maxilla resulted in full incisor display on smile Figure 32.58). The smile arc was enhanced by tipping the curvature of the anterior sweep of the maxillary teeth to better match the curvature of the lower lip (Figure 32.59). The final

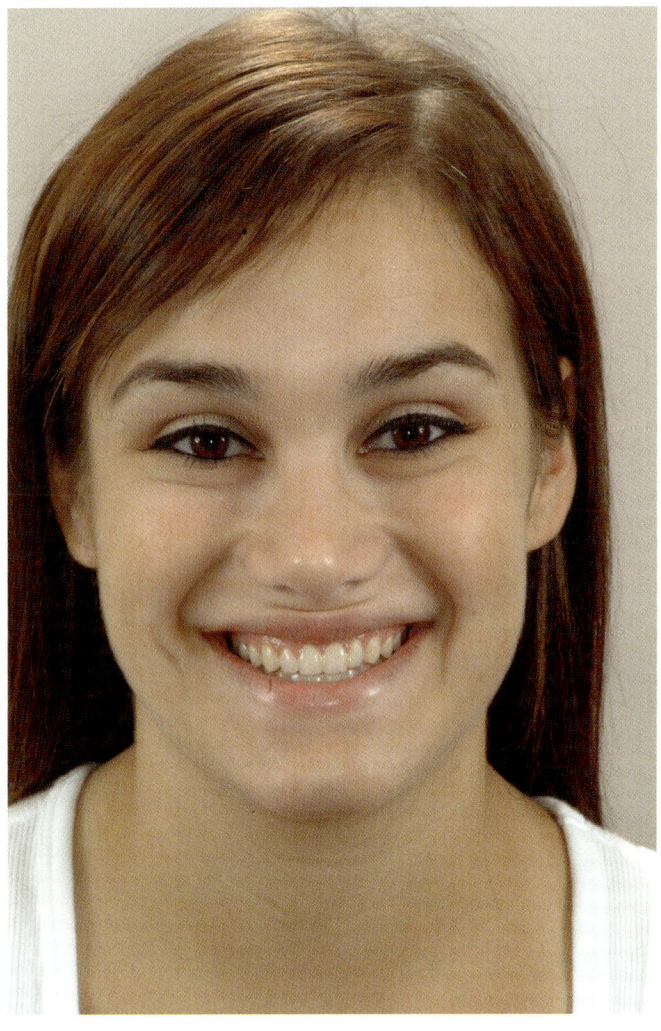

Figure 32.58 The advancement of both jaws greatly enhanced resting lip support, and anterior downgraft of the maxilla resulted in full incisor display on smile.

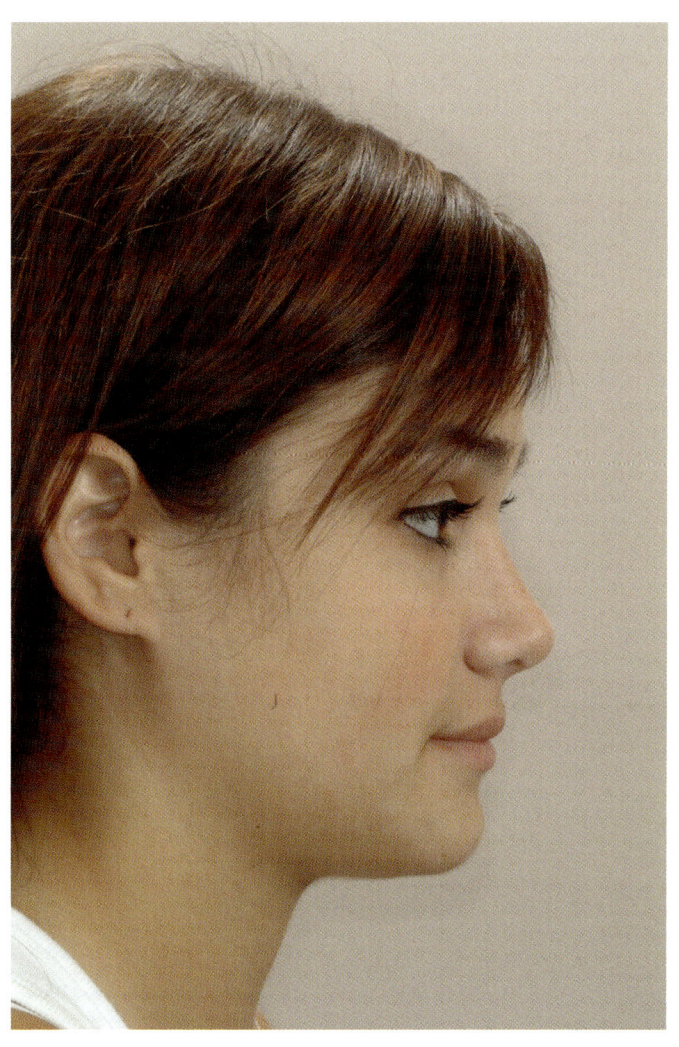

Figure 32.60 The final profile was much more esthetic, with anteroposterior balance of the maxilla and mandible along with improved facial proportions.

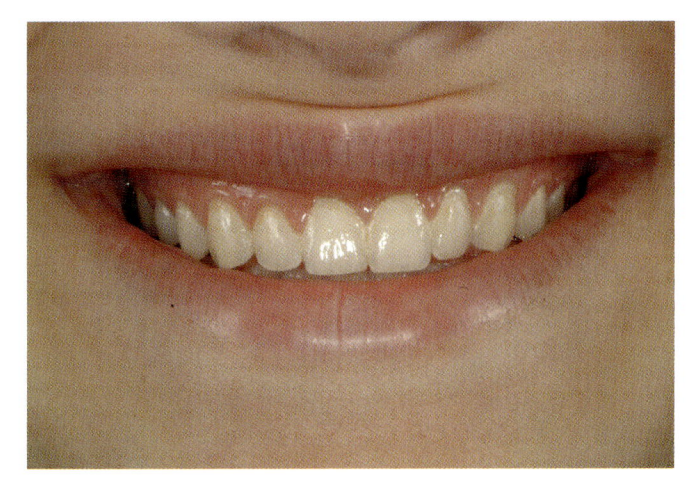

Figure 32.59 The smile arc was enhanced by tipping the curvature of the anterior sweep of the maxillary teeth to better match the curvature of the lower lip.

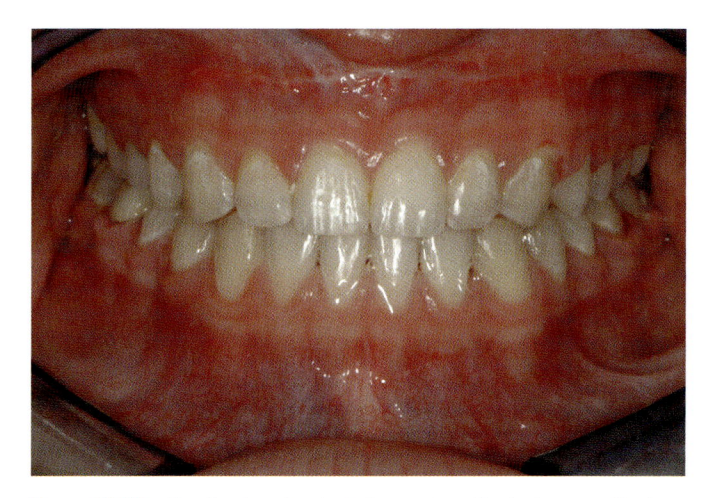

Figure 32.61 The final occlusal photographs reflected an excellent occlusal outcome.

profile was much more esthetic, with anteroposterior balance of the maxilla and mandible along with improved facial proportions (Figure 32.60). The final occlusal photograph is shown in Figure 32.61. The frontal smile underwent remarkable changes that occur with increase in incisor display. The overall results were much more youthful in appearance, which is of paramount importance in facial rejuvenation.

Acknowledgements

I would like to express a special thanks to Marc Ackerman for his significant contribution to a previous version of this chapter, entitled "Database acquisition and treatment planning" by Marc B. Ackerman, DMD and David M. Sarver, DMD, MS. In: Miloro M, Ghali GE, Larsen P, Waite P, eds. *Peterson's Principles of Oral and Maxillofacial Surgery*, 2nd edn. BC Decker; 2004.

References

1. Ackerman MB. *Enhancement Orthodontics: Theory and Practice*. Copenhagen: Blackwell Munsgaard; 2008.
2. Mazur A, Mazur J, Keating C. Military rank attainment of a West Point class: effects of cadets' physical features. *Am J Sociol* 1984;90:125–150.
3. Sarver DM. *Esthetic Orthodontics and Orthognathic Surgery*. St. Louis, MO: Mosby; 1997.
4. Sarver DM, Flax H. Interview with David Sarver, D.M.D., M.S. *J Cosmet Dent* 2007;23(3):126–134.
5. Sarver DM. *The Art and Science of Appearance and the Smile*. Monograph for the 2003 Moyer's Symposium. Ann Arbor, MI: The University of Michigan; 2004.
6. Sarver DM. Soft-tissue-based diagnosis and treatment planning. *Clin Impressions* 2006;14(1):21–26.
7. Sarver DM, Ackerman MB. Dynamic smile visualization and quantification and its impact on orthodontic diagnosis and treatment planning. In: Romano R, ed. *The Art of the Smile-Integrating Prosthodontics, Orthodontics Periodontics, Dental Technology, and Plastic Surgery*. Chicago, IL: Quintessence; 2005;99–139.
8. Ackerman JL, Proffit WR, Sarver DM. The emerging soft tissue paradigm in orthodontic diagnosis treatment planning. *Clin Orthod Res* 1999;2:49–52.
9. Sarver DM, Ackerman JL. About face—the re-emerging soft tissue paradigm. *Am J Orthod Dentofac Orthoped* 2000;117:575–576.
10. Powell H, Humphreys B. *Proportions of the Esthetic Face*. New York: Thieme Stratton; 1984.
11. Farkas LG, Munro JR. *Anthropometric Facial Proportions in Medicine*. Springfield, IL: Charles C. Thomas; 1987.
12. Sarver DM, Jacobson RS. The aesthetic dentofacial analysis. *Clin Plast Surg* 2007;34(3):369–394.
13. Pessa JA. The potential role of stereolithography in the study of facial aging. *Am J Orthod Dentofacial Orthop* 2001;119:117–120.
14. Sommerville JM, Sperry TP, BeGole EA. Morphology of the submental and neck region. *Int J Adult Orthod* 1988;3:97–106.
15. Moorrees CFA, Kean MR. Natural head position, a basic consideration for the analysis of cephalometric radiographs. *Am J Phys Anthropol* 1958;16:213–234.
16. Lundström A, Lundström F, Lebret LM, Moorrees CF. Natural head position and natural head orientation: basic considerations in cephalometric analysis and research. *Eur J Orthod* 1995;17(2):111–120.
17. Cooke MS. Five year reproducibility of natural head posture: a longitudinal study. *Am J Orthod Dentofacial Orthop* 1990;97:489–494.
18. Dvortsin DP, Ye Q, Pruim GJ, et al. Reliability of the integrated radiograph-photograph method to obtain natural head position in cephalometric diagnosis. *Angle Orthod* 2011;81(5):889–894.
19. Sarver DM. The smile arc—the importance of incisor position in the dynamic smile. *Am J Orthod Dentofacial Orthop* 2001;120:98–111.
20. Hulsey CM. An esthetic evaluation of lip–teeth relationships present in the smile. *Am J Orthod* 1970;57(2):132–144.
21. Ker AJ, Chan R, Fields HW, et al. Esthetics and smile characteristics from the layperson's perspective: a computer-based survey study. *J Am Dent Assoc* 2008;139(10):1318–1327.
22. Ackerman JL, Proffit WR, Sarver DM, et al. Pitch, Roll, and yaw: describing the spatial orientation of dentofacial traits. *Am J Dentofac Orthop* 2007;131(3):305–310.
23. Burstone CJ, Marcotte MR. The treatment occlusal plane. In: *Problem Solving in Orthodontics: Goal-Oriented Treatment Strategies*. Chicago, IL: Quintessence Publishing Co.; 2000:31–50.
24. Sarver D, Rousso D. Plastic surgery combined with orthodontic and orthognathic procedures. *Am J Orthod Dentofacial Orthop* 2004;126(3):305–307.

Additional resources

Sarver DM, Ackerman MB. Dynamic smile visualization and quantification: Part I. Evolution of the concept and dynamic records for smile capture. *Am J Dentofac Orthop* 2003;124;4–12.

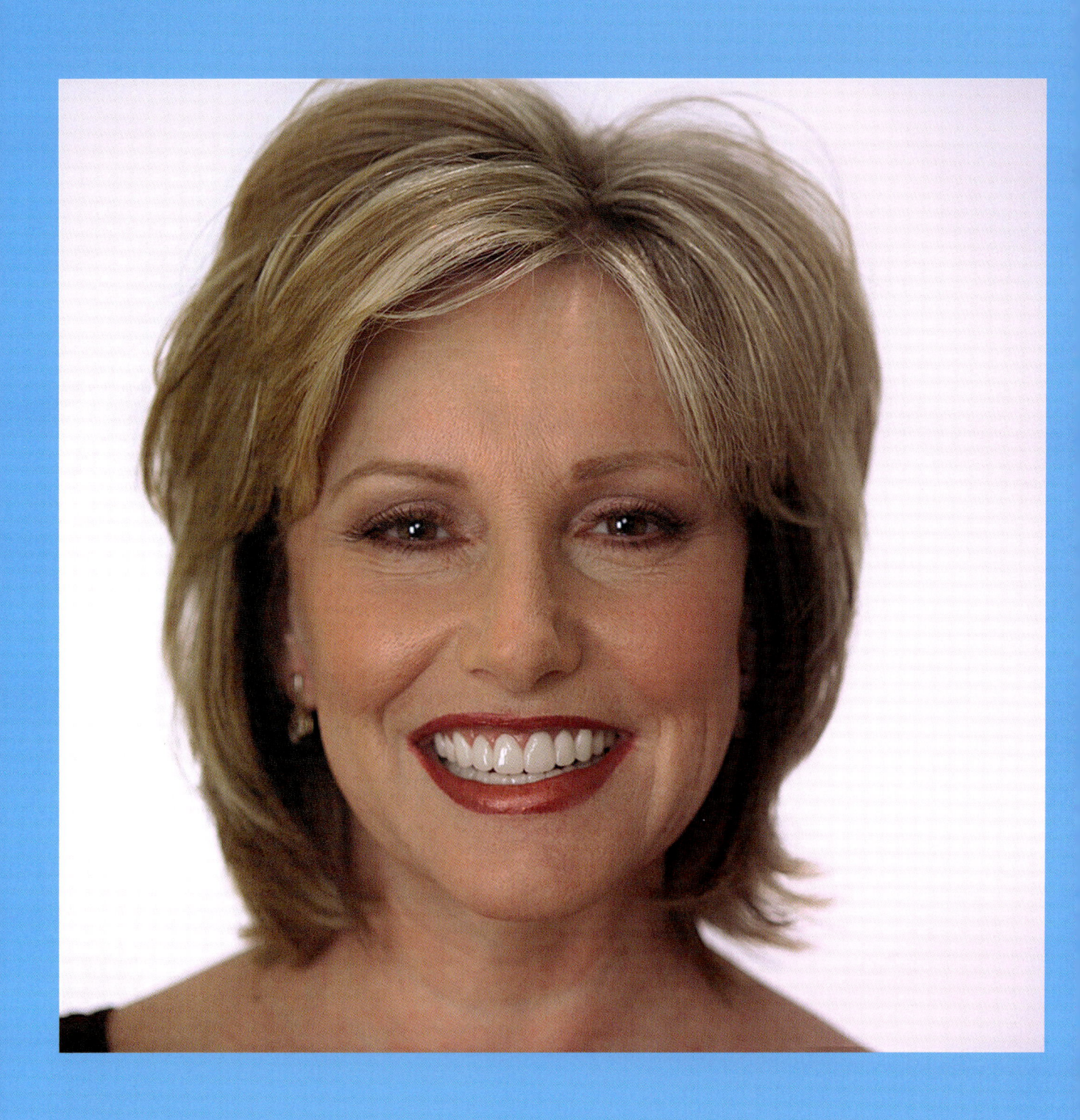

Chapter 33 Facial Considerations in Esthetic Restorations

Ronald E. Goldstein, DDS and Bruno P. Silva, DMD, PhD

Chapter Outline

Importance of facial diagnosis	1086
Facial expressions	1088
Facial asymmetry	1089
Facial midline	1090
Asymmetry location	1094
Esthetic relevance of facial symmetry	1094
The golden proportion	1095
Facial analysis	1097
Facial analysis: frontal view	1098
Facial reference lines	1098
Vertical facial proportions	1101
Nasal tip and facial midline	1104
Maxillary dental midline and facial midline	1104
Chin and facial midline	1107
Incisal plane and interpupillary line	1107
Lip symmetry	1111
Lip length	1112
Lips at rest position and interlabial gap	1113
Closed lip position	1113
Facial analysis: oblique view	1113
Facial analysis: profile view	1113
Profile angle	1113
Nasolabial angle	1114
Lip position and projection	1115
Ridge replacement	1118
Tooth position	1118
Labiomental angle	1118
Dentofacial analysis	1119
Tooth exposure at rest	1119
Incisal edges and the lower lip	1120
Smile line	1122
Papilla display during smiling	1124
Smile width	1125
Buccal corridors	1125

Esthetics and beauty have been studied and discussed for thousands of years. Although in years past it may have been taboo to even speak about the possibility that your patient may eventually want or need facial plastic surgery, such is not the case today. In fact, if your patient's are in need of orthodontic therapy to improve their appearance or if they need you to rebuild the smile to reduce the appearance of aging, let them know the advantage, and sometimes necessity, of having the dental treatment completed before any other facial surgery is planned.

The concept of esthetics is defined as "the philosophical discipline that studies beauty and art." It is a very broad concept, subjective and ambiguous. Hegel stated: "Beauty as the essence of imagination and perception cannot be an exact science."[1] Modern dentistry cannot be based merely on subjective concepts; predictable results are required instead. Multiple studies have tried to determine the objective and esthetic criteria that are associated with a beautiful and attractive smile.

Ronald E. Goldstein's Esthetics in Dentistry, Third Edition. Edited by Ronald E. Goldstein, Stephen J. Chu, Ernesto A. Lee, and Christian F.J. Stappert.
© 2018 John Wiley & Sons, Inc. Published 2018 by John Wiley & Sons, Inc.

The sum total of this phenomenon is that esthetic dentistry must adopt a new paradigm for the concept of treatment planning for a patient. The science is so dramatic and the outcomes are so revolutionary that the traditional concepts of treatment planning for a patient who wants to look forever young are obsolete. The art and science of esthetic dentistry is becoming central to building the foundation on which all other treatment modalities must emerge to satisfy the ever increasing desire of agelessness.

Visual perception is just as important for the esthetic evaluation as the visual examination is for the clinical examination.[1,2] Therefore, understanding the processes that are involved in the perception of beauty will help clinicians in the esthetic diagnosis process. The perception process involves the organization and integration of sensorial data by the intellect. A response is triggered in the intellect based on previous experiences or dogmas, which are interpreted subconsciously. The area of the brain responsible for perception is not located in the cognitive region. Rather, it is located in the subconscious or primitive side, called the limbic system, where instincts are believed to reside. This limbic system most strongly perceives the visual cues of balance, symmetry, and proportion, and therefore defines beauty objectively[3] (Figure 33.1).

While artists need inspiration, clinicians cannot seat the patient in the dental chair and wait for inspiration to appear. Dental professionals need scientific methods, diagnosis, and protocols.[3] Even art is taught via principles and tenets, leaving the rest to the creativity of the artist. Yet, when the human body is the canvas, there is little room for such creativity, save for in the development and utilization of various techniques. Different types of tissue interact in a smile: teeth, lips, gums, and skin. The smile then interacts with the remaining facial structures to be seen as a whole entity. Numerous dental-related studies have analyzed the smile in efforts to discover which characteristics make it more or less attractive to establish objective clinical criteria to guide the restorative dentist, which will be discussed thoroughly in this chapter.

Importance of facial diagnosis

Kokich et al.[4] were one of the first to study the perception of the esthetic discrepancies of the smile. They established the levels of recognition for the different types of esthetic discrepancies for both dentists and laypeople. Since then, diverse studies have focused on the esthetic alterations, mainly by laypeople representing the patients seeking dental treatment.[3–9] Most of these studies showed pictures of a smile alone, having eliminated other

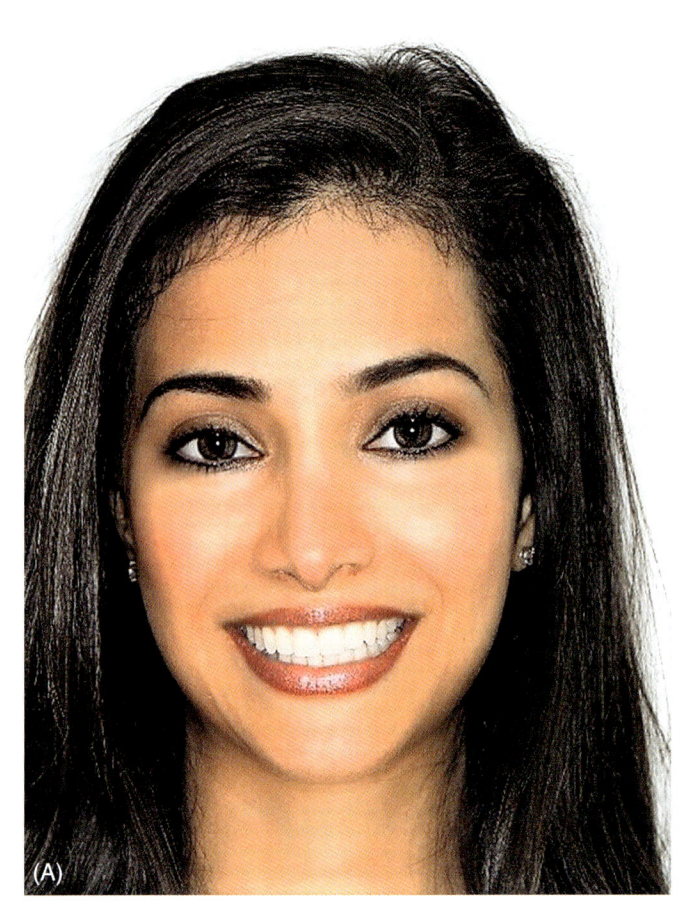

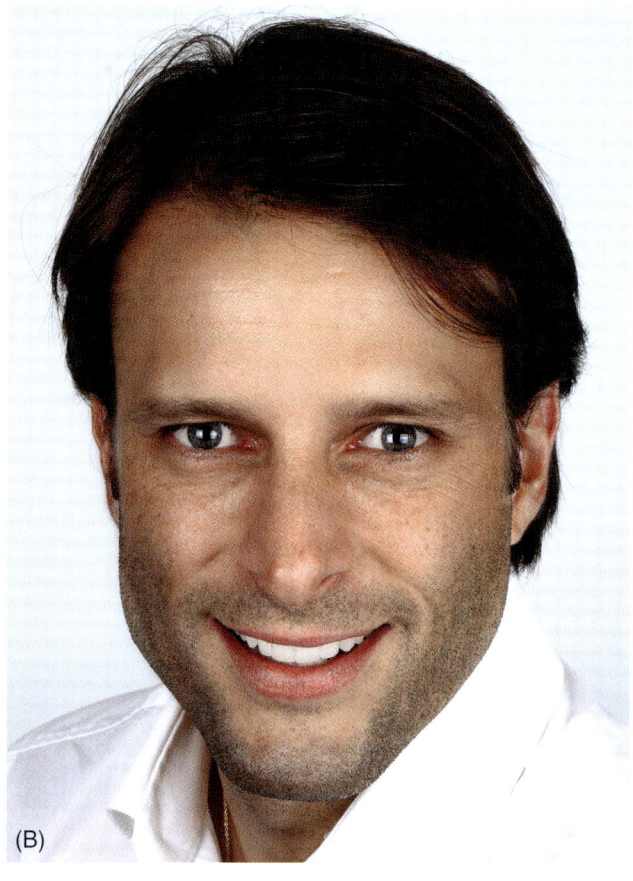

Figure 33.1 Human perception of what is considered beautiful resides in the subconscious, and is based in a larger part on balance, symmetry, and proportion. Here are examples of both female **(A)** and male **(B)** faces that have been judged as "beautiful."

surrounding facial structures to avoid superfluous factors that could potentially confuse or bias the observer.[4–6,8] However, elimination of the surrounding facial structures creates an artificial perception. We rarely see a smile segregated and apart from the face. Lombardi[10] established the principles of visual perception as they apply to denture esthetics. One principle was that "isolation" is improbable and that the mind is constantly observing, analyzing, processing, and interpreting the relationship "in between" objects (Figure 8.5).

Teeth are framed by the lips to create the smile, which is then framed by the face. All of this gives a global expression to the gesture of smiling. We cannot ignore the role that some facial structures play in the overall perception of the smile. Beyer and Lindauer[7] published an investigation about the impact that different facial structures have on the esthetic perception of midline discrepancies. He concluded that facial structures and their deviations affect the way observers perceive smile esthetics. However, too many variables existed in the Beyer and Lindauer[7] study and they were unable to reach conclusions regarding how different facial structures can influence or interfere with our perception of the smile.

Currently, our field is limited not only by the degree of visual detail that some conservative treatments require but also by our postural working position. We have a tendency to sit too close to and hunched over the patient, which neutralizes our ability to best frame the facial composition. It is necessary to step back from our routine treatment position, because shortening the distance to more than that of a social conversational position will reduce the visual examination field to a dentofacial perspective instead of an overall viewpoint that would help diagnose a facially directed esthetic evaluation (Figure 33.2A and B). Therefore, patients are asked to stand close to a neutral-colored background wall to take full facial photographs. Studying these two different dimensional views allows us to clearly visualize facial discrepancies (Figure 33.3A and B). The subtleties of the interaction of the different facial elements associated with the smile can be better appreciated when a systematic analysis of all the different facial components is

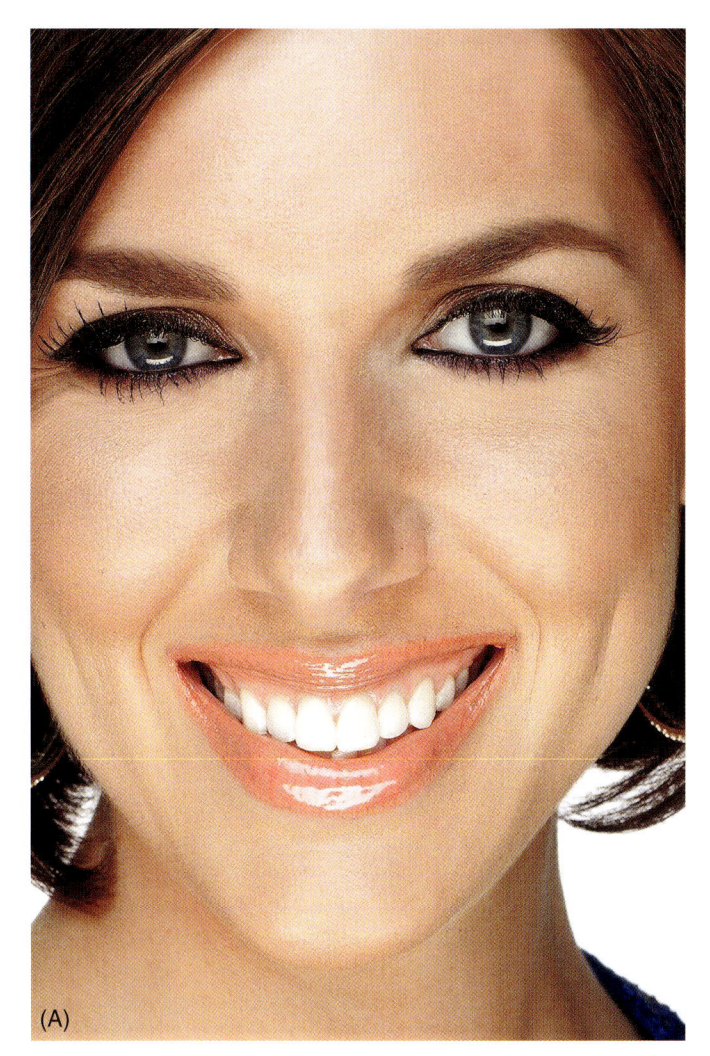

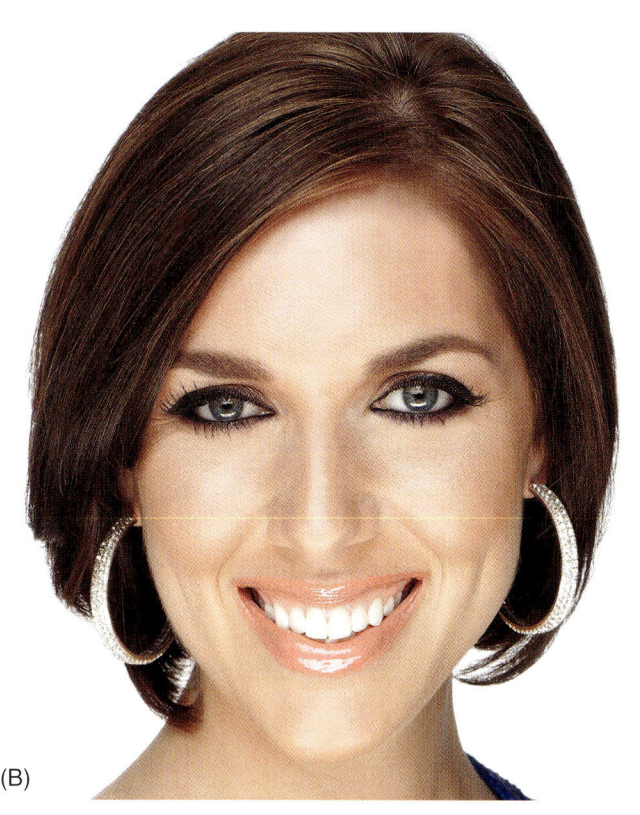

Figure 33.2 **(A, B)** The distance at which we view a person's face affects our judgment. For instance, note how the close-up photo results in a lack of ability to accurately evaluate balance and proportion, which can affect smile design.

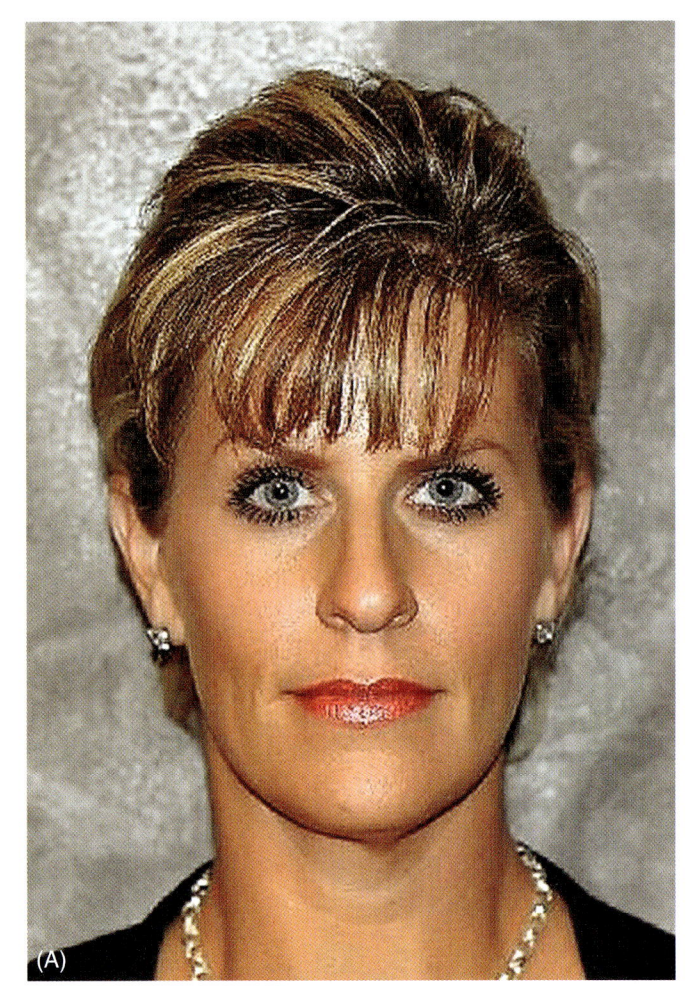

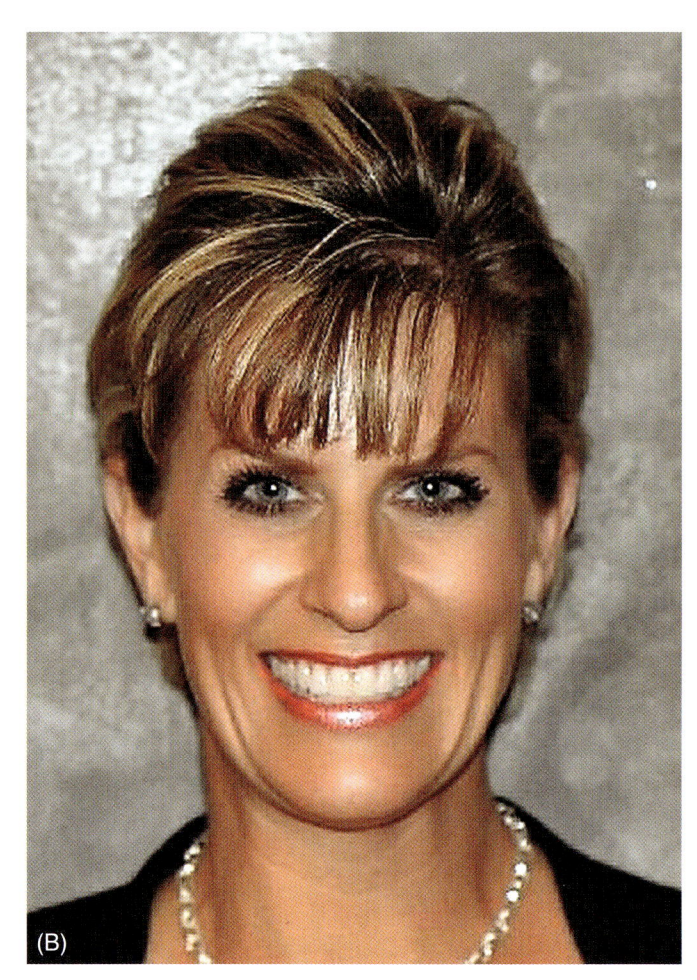

Figure 33.3 **(A, B)** Looking at the face directly in our traditional dental treatment position does not allow for an accurate, facially directed esthetic evaluation. A two-dimensional digital photograph of the face makes it easier to view facial discrepancies and silhouette form. A neutral background for these photos is preferred.

performed, inclusive of the static and the functionally dynamic smile.[11]

When a patient presents with an esthetic problem or complaint, avoid the mistake of diagnosing only the particular tooth or teeth in question. The teeth should always be kept in perspective with the entire smile, and the smile in perspective with the total face. Only then can a comprehensive diagnostic evaluation be presented to the patient. This does not mean that every patient with a discolored or fractured tooth is a candidate for an extended analysis of facial form and diagnosis. On the contrary, the objective is to fulfill the patient's goal of looking as good as they want to. Most patients will want to look their ultimate best, whereas others will want to improve only one isolated tooth to achieve the appearance they are comfortable with.

Generally, patients demanding esthetic restorative treatment do so to improve confidence within themselves and outward appeal to others, allowing an overall enhanced quality of life. In addition, a long-term stable occlusion must be acquired, and treatment of any occlusal discrepancies must be done to preserve the dentition. Despite teaching children to look for inner beauty, the reality is that perception is formulated on physical appearance and presentation. Although some patients may wish to correct their occlusion to improve function, most patients seek treatment to improve the appearance of their dentition, occlusion, smile, and face. There is a general consensus regarding the importance of the role that occlusion plays in mid- and long-term restorative dentistry. But treating only the occlusion would be like treating one small part of the puzzle, not unlike a patient who only seeks a pleasing smile. The challenge lies within trying to integrate the function and esthetics of the smile into the total facial composition.[11]

Facial expressions

The dentist is in the best position to diagnose abnormalities that can alter facial expressions. Certain people typically have tense or sad expressions. Reverse smile lines, abnormalities in the teeth or lips, or wrinkles in the mouth can contribute to such expressions. Wrinkles around the mouth and other lip problems could be corrected by plastic surgery, lip filler, injections such as Botox®, or improved with makeup. The dentist should be aware of the types of corrections that can be accomplished by the generalist or more appropriately by specialists in prosthodontics or related fields such as plastic or orthognathic surgery.

Certain patients will appreciate the fact that you have both an understanding of and a working relationship with plastic surgery. True interdisciplinary therapy encompasses both dental and medical specialists, especially when it concerns the patient's need to look and feel better about their total appearance. The question is how to approach the subject of plastic surgery without offending the patient. The best way is to include the term in normal conversation about a possible problem. For instance, if the patient has a nose that severely deviates from the midline and the patient expects the dental restoration to correct the intraoral midline, the response could be as follows: "I can correct the jaw midline to line up with a bisected line from your facial midline to your chin, but it may call more attention to your nose. We may want to get a consultation with a plastic surgeon to see what it would take to correct that as well." Because many times the correction might also include an orthodontist and/or a cosmetic periodontist, you might also say "I work with a great interdisciplinary team of orthodontists, oral surgeons, plastic surgeons, and periodontists and I think it would be wise to at least get a group consultation to explore all the possibilities (and all your alternatives)." Neither suggestion is offensive and does show your concern for the patient to get the very best esthetic result. Remember, the most a patient can say is "I am not interested," and you can document the fact that you did give your patient the option.

Esthetic dental procedures can change facial expression and frequently alter one's personality. Many times, when a patient with an unhappy appearance receives an esthetic smile transformation, a favorable change in personality occurs. They may say that they smile more because they are proud of their teeth, when in reality their self-image has improved and their personality has assumed the associated positive traits.

Facial asymmetry

Symmetry is one of the main concerns in esthetics.[1,2,5,10,12–17] Symmetry refers to the regularity in the organization of forms and objects. Some consider symmetry and balance to be related, while others highlight the differences between them.[1,2] The importance of symmetry increases the closer the midline or center is approached. When we enhance midline symmetry, the transition between hemispheres is smoother; the closer we get to the midline, the easier it becomes to identify asymmetries.[2,18]

Symmetry can be horizontal or vertical when it refers to a line as the image on a mirror, or radial when it refers to an axis. Horizontal symmetry is psychologically predictable and comfortable, but it tends to be monotonous.

Few naturally possess a completely symmetrical face. But a face does not have to be symmetrical to be considered beautiful. In fact, several winners of beauty contests, as well as movie and TV stars, have asymmetrical faces, based on our inspection of over 1000 photographs (Figure 33.4A and B).

As observers, we wish to see objects that form a composition in a stable position, as the human eye is conditioned by expectations based on previous experiences.[1,10,12] The human being is externally considered as two symmetrical parts. By definition, this would imply the existence of a mathematically equal image of both right and left facial halves. However, these statements are not categorical, as the symmetrical theory is affected by

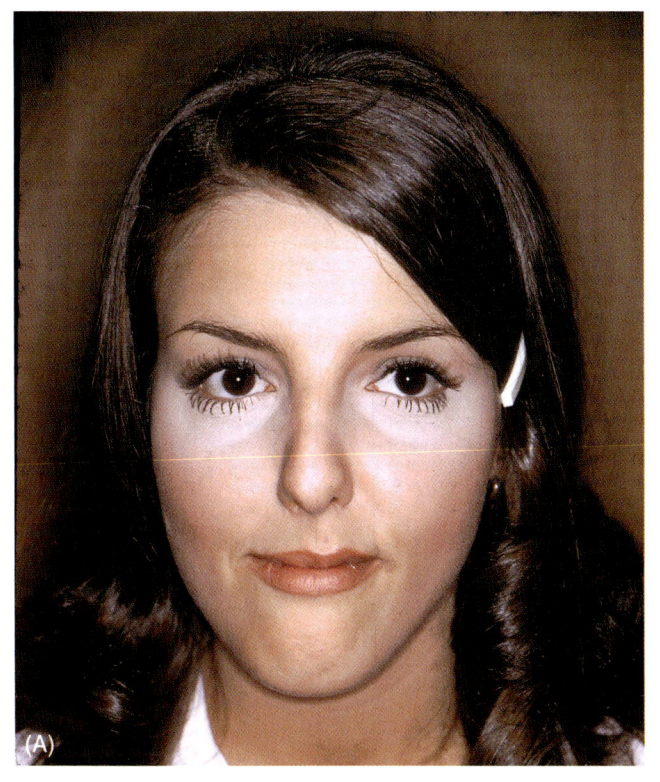

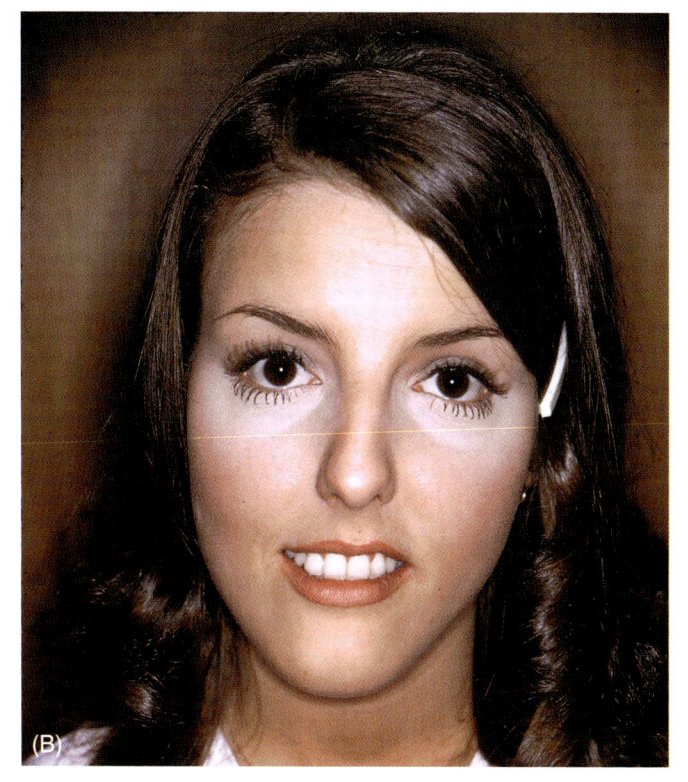

Figure 33.4 (A, B) A two-dimensional photograph makes it easier to diagnose facial asymmetry, which is important for smile design.

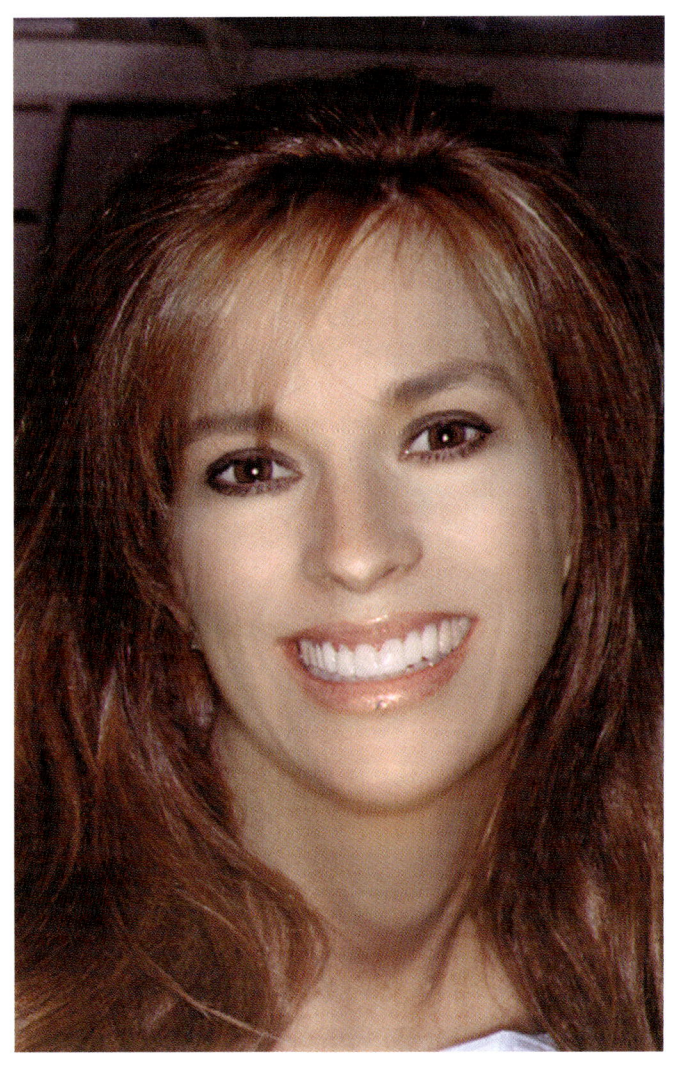

Figure 33.5 Although this model was judged as the most beautiful by a major magazine, she pointed out to Dr Goldstein how asymmetrical her face was.

can be a deviated nose or chin, but more than likely it will be something related to the smile. It is extremely important to communicate in a positive manner any facial deviation you find. Failure to do so may well cause serious problems later on when restorations do not satisfy the patient's quest for a perfectly symmetrical result, when, in actuality, obtaining symmetrical perfection was never possible to begin with. Trying to explain this fact after having placed restorations becomes a defensive tactic, which may create difficulties in having the patient understand the possible limitations of the esthetic results. Therefore, the patient's space asymmetry will result in improvement, but still be a compromise from what they may envision. It is crucial to have the patient understand this in treatment planning. Furthermore, it is always a good idea to state this fact in a written document signed by both clinician and patient.

Facial midline

To analyze facial symmetry, one must first and foremost know how to establish the facial midline. Because of the existing differences between both facial halves, the facial midline is hardly defined as a precise geometrical division. This can explain the differences found when defining this parameter: a vertical line through the forehead, the septum, the dental midline, and the chin;[2] a vertical imaginary line bisecting the nasion, subnasal, pogonion, trichion, and pronasale points;[15] a vertical line through the glabella, nose, philtrum, and the chin's extremity;[30] and a vertical line through the philtrum when the pupils are in line with the natural posture of the head.[31,32]

The definition of the facial midline can be extremely controversial; it is quite difficult to draw a line based on unclear anatomical spots such as the "nose," "forehead," "septum," and "chin," although these definitions can be found in the literature, which somehow explains the difficulty in defining this parameter. We agree that a vertical line through the philtrum, when the pupils are in line with the natural posture of the head,[31,32] seems to be the best way to define the facial midline for a diagnostic purpose (Figure 33.6A). However, they suggest that the most important parameter might not be finding the exact landmarks that define the midline of a geometrically irregular shape such as the face. Rather, it may be understanding the process that our perception uses to establish the hypothetical facial midline, imposed by facial and dentofacial elements, to analyze the apparent symmetry. This hypothetical facial midline can also be called the perceived facial midline and is determined by all facial midline structures, such as the glabella, nose, philtrum, and menton (Figure 33.6B). A line does not need to be expressed to be perceived; it can be suggested by two or three points in a directional movement.[1]

Except in cases of pathology or injury, it is generally accepted that, even when the human face is "symmetrical," one-half does not mirror the other. Renner states "Differences in facial symmetry are due in large measure to differential development of the facial muscles on each side of the face as well as the underlying supportive skeletal structure"[33] (Figure 33.7A–D).

The dominant hemisphere of the brain is thought to strongly influence differences in facial muscle development; the brain is

biological imperfections, some inherent to natural developmental processes and others to the environment.[19]

Facial asymmetry, within certain limits, is not considered to be a pathological condition, despite the nonexistence of objective scientific criteria to differentiate normal and abnormal asymmetries. This judgment generally results from subjective criteria and the harmonic sense of the clinician or technician[19] (Figure 33.5). According to some studies, it is not uncommon to find slight facial asymmetries within a normative population absent of pathology.[13,20-29] The soft tissues disguise the possible skeletal imbalances,[13,26] thereby making skeletal asymmetries that fall below 3% clinically insignificant.[21]

Our approach has always been to first engage the new patient in conversation, hopefully motivating the patient to smile or laugh naturally. Video records can be made with a patient's consent. These dynamic records can help with the diagnosis and also with reminding the dentist of the patient's chief complaint and other small details that can be unnoticed at the first interview. It is recommended to maintain eye-to-eye contact, but to note any negative facial aspect that takes the focus away from the eyes; it

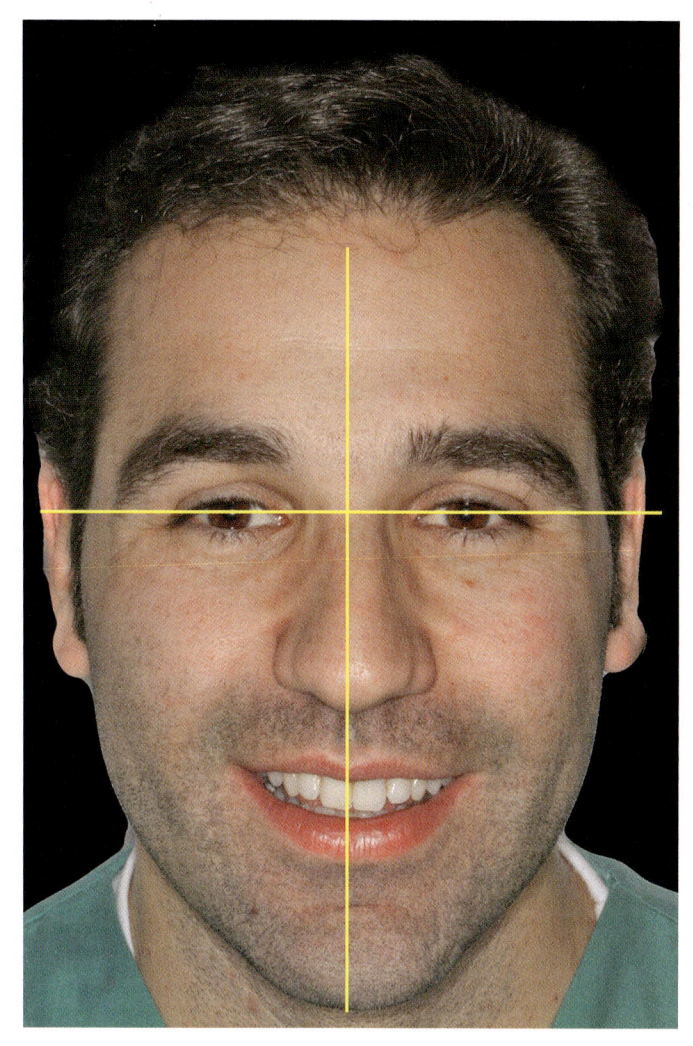

Figure 33.6 **(A)** Facial midline—vertical line through the philtrum when the pupils are in line with the natural posture of the head.

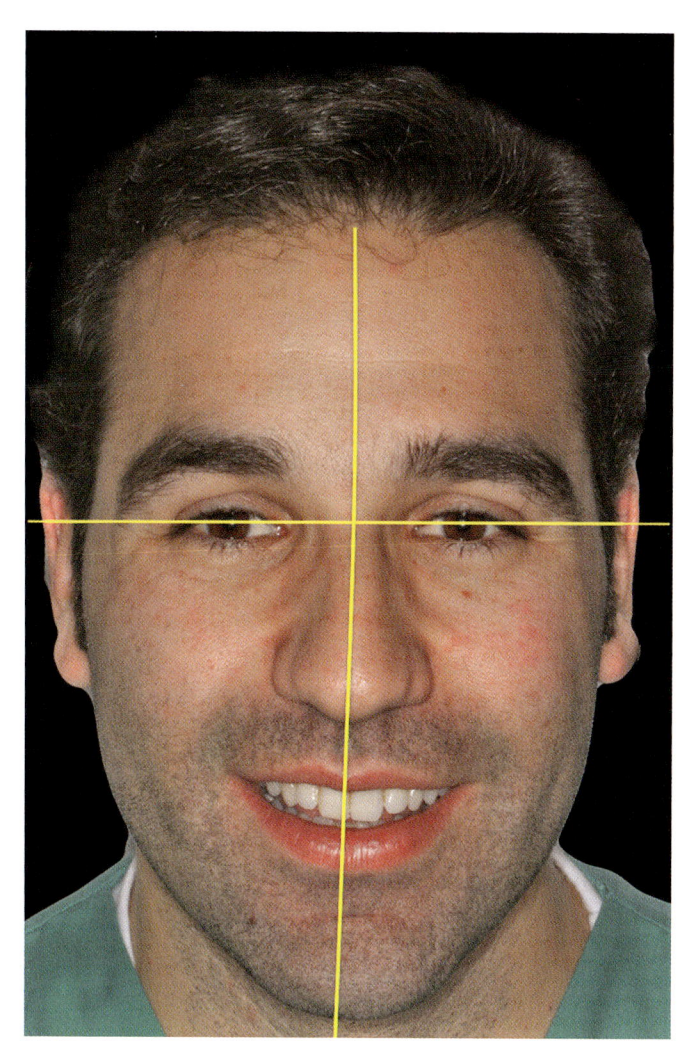

Figure 33.6 **(B)** Perceived facial midline, determined by all facial midline structures, such as glabella, nose, philtrum, and menton.

governed by the principle of contralaterality, with the right cerebral hemisphere controlling the left half of the face, and vice versa. To a great extent, this slightly uneven development creates nuances of expression in an individual and adds interest and uniqueness to a face.

In many individuals, features of the face slant one way or the other and make it difficult to see the true midline in the dentition. Figure 33.8A shows an attractive face where the incisal plane and dental midline are actually canted, but because the nose is deviated, and the interpupillary line in the natural head position is not completely parallel with the horizon, the canting can go unnoticed. An eccentric midline of the teeth is in many cases acceptable and may enhance the illusion of harmonious composition. The midline is important within the overall facial considerations and must be analyzed carefully.

Patients tend to concentrate on the dental arch midline and are quick to think that it is not perfectly aligned. This is because most patients think the facial midline must coincide with the midline on their central incisors. But the true problem is that the appearance of asymmetry can be the fault of any other facial element, such as the lips, philtrum, nose, or chin or arch alignment.

Therefore, it is imperative to diagnose and present to the patient any facial anatomic anomaly or asymmetry that may influence the esthetic result. This can be done using digital photography software, such as Adobe Photoshop®, to analyze face symmetry. Figure 33.8B shows how Adobe Photoshop can be used to align the interpupillary line with the horizontal and to trace reference lines to emphasize canting of the incisal plane and dental midline. The most important factor is having a good facial picture, with the patient standing up with their head in natural position. Long-haired patients should pull their hair back to completely expose both sides of the face so that the picture can be as centered as possible on the face. A striped background helps to establish the relation of the interpupillary line, in patient's natural head position, with the horizon. Tilted pictures can create the illusion of facial asymmetries by exposing more of one side of the face than the other. Figure 33.8C and D shows how a slightly tilted picture to the left side of the patient can lead to a misperception of the incisal canting.

The importance of comprehensive consideration of various facial characteristics, especially in anticipation of anterior restorative procedures, cannot be overemphasized.

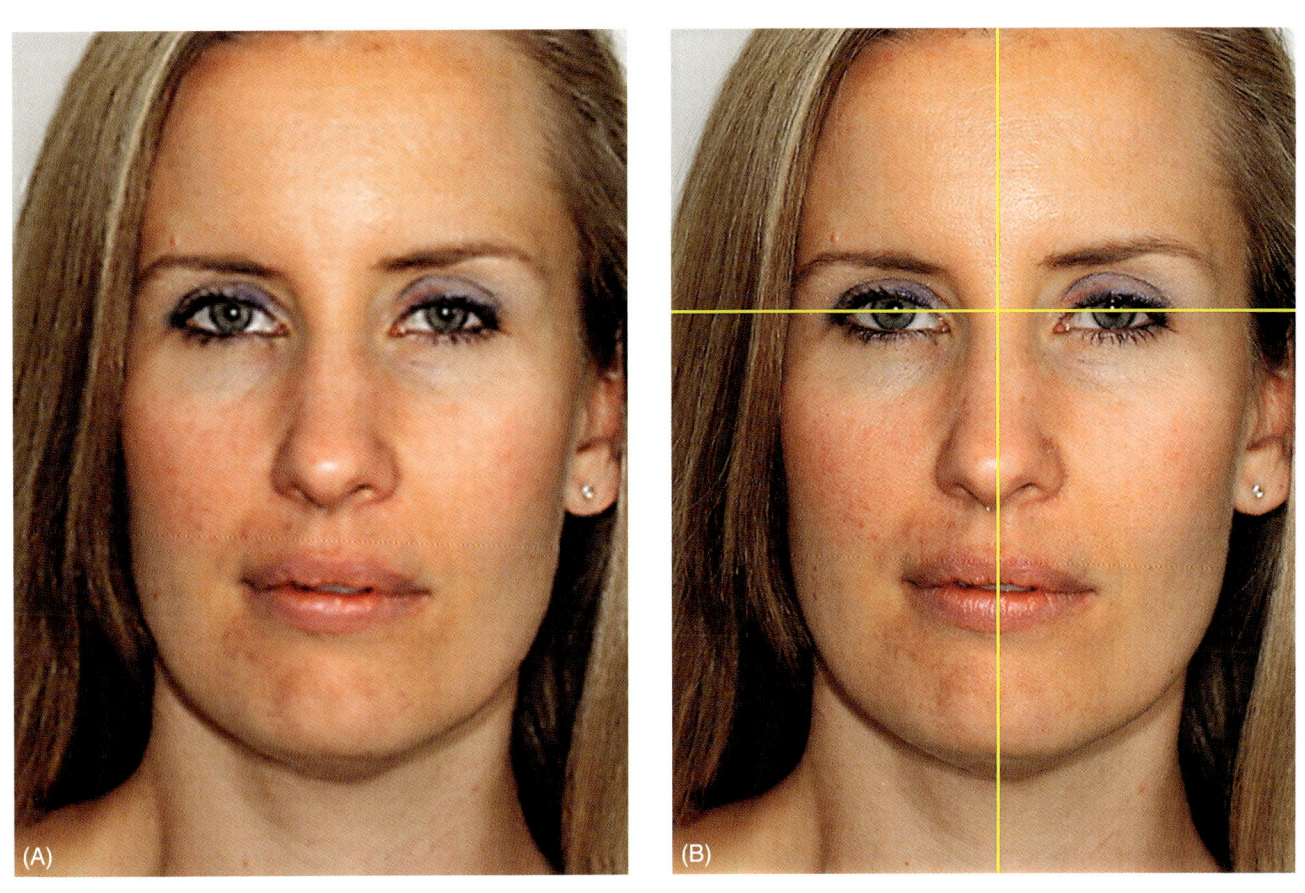

Figure 33.7 **(A, B)** To show that the face is not totally symmetrical, the face was bisected and mirrored to provide perfect symmetry. Studies have shown that perfect symmetry is not as appealing as slight asymmetry.

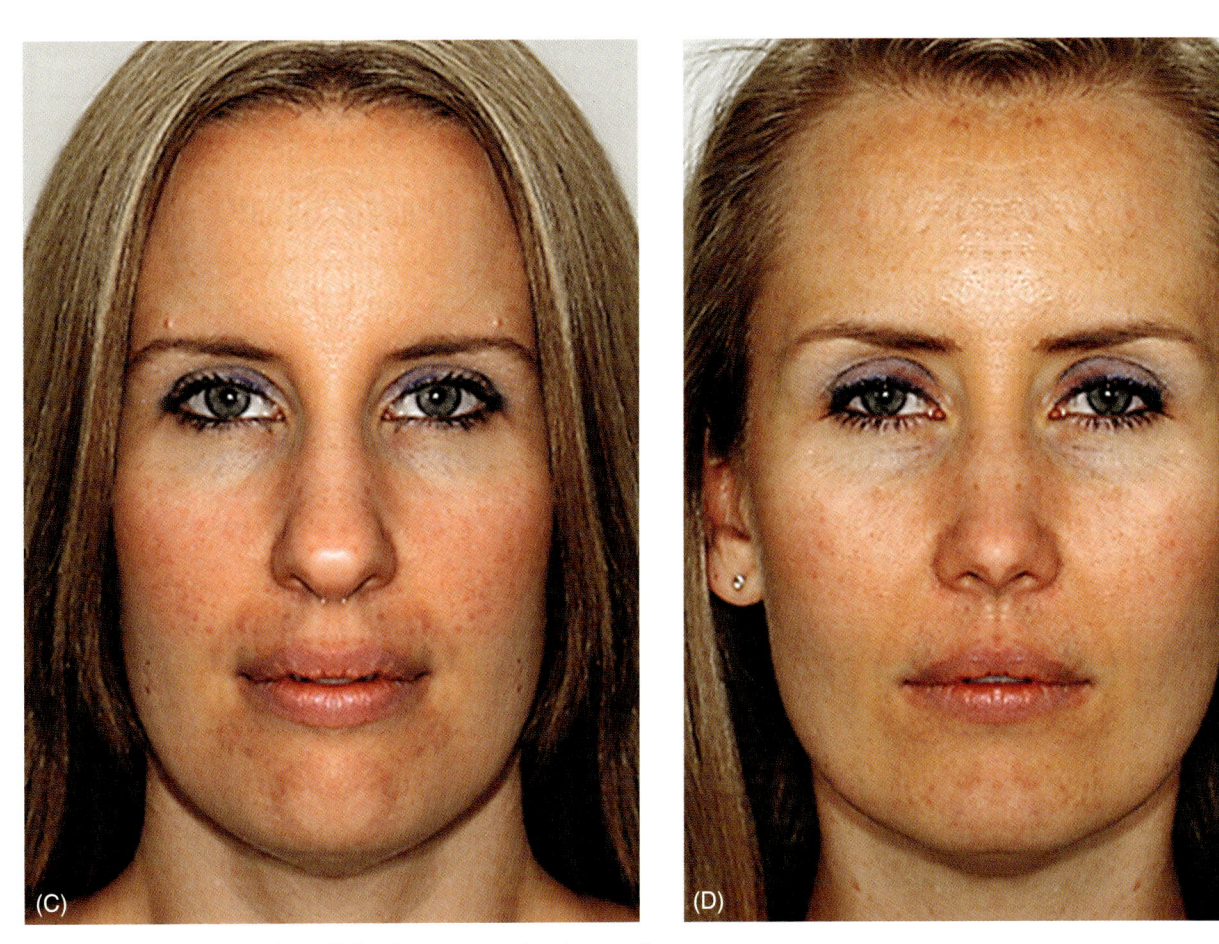

Figure 33.7 **(C, D)** The right side and left side are mirrored to show perfect symmetry.

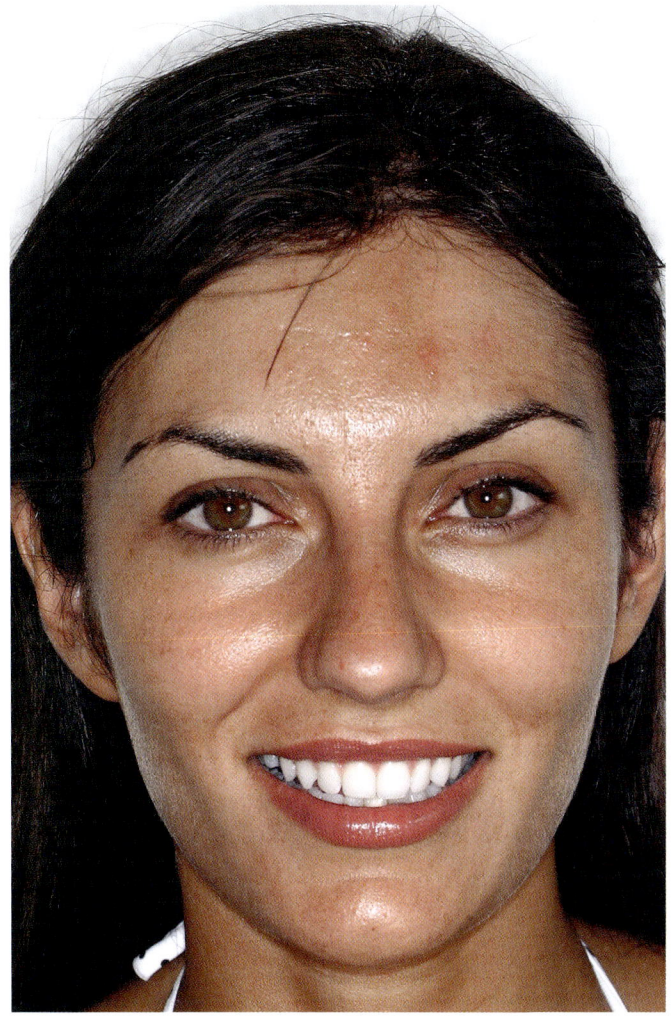

Figure 33.8 **(A)** An attractive face where the incisal plane and dental midline are canted. The nose deviation, and the interpupillary line, in natural head position, is not completely parallel with the horizon; the canted midline and incisal plane can be unnoticed.

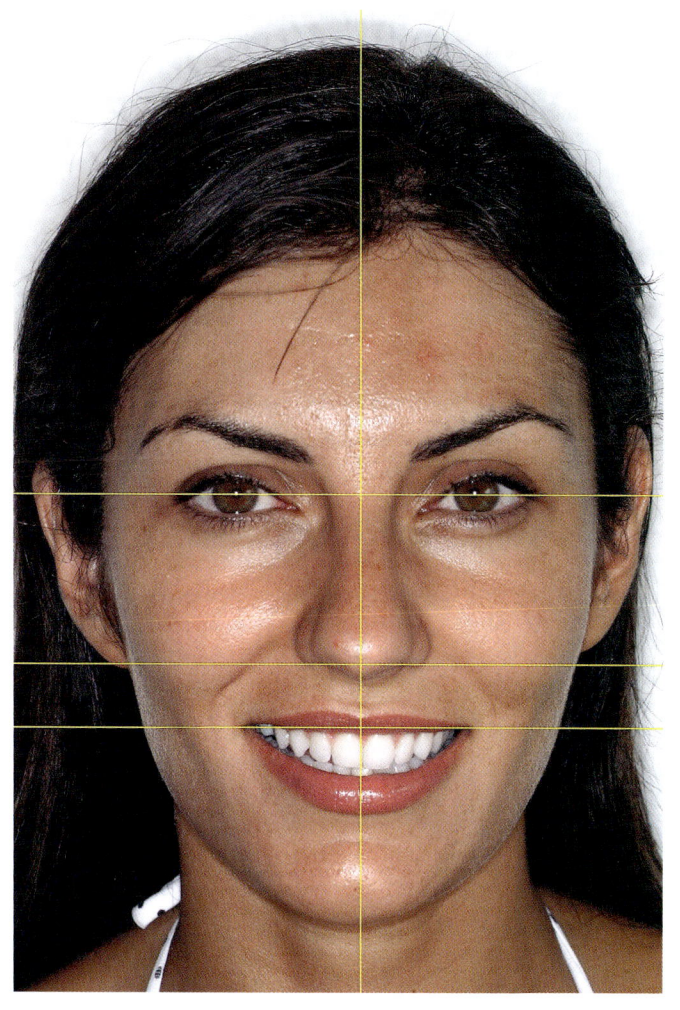

Figure 33.8 **(B)** After aligning the interpupillary line with the horizontal and by tracing some reference lines, using Adobe Photoshop, the incisal plane and dental midline canting are now more evident.

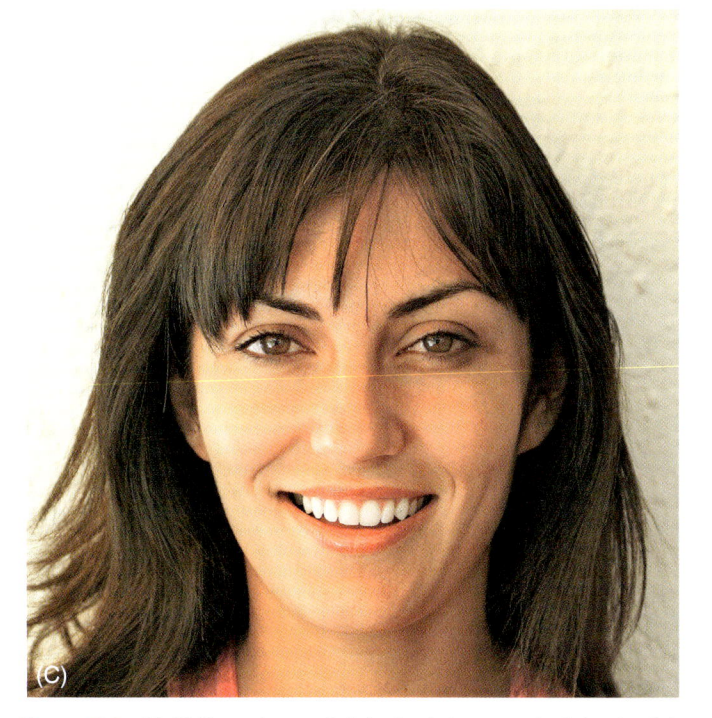

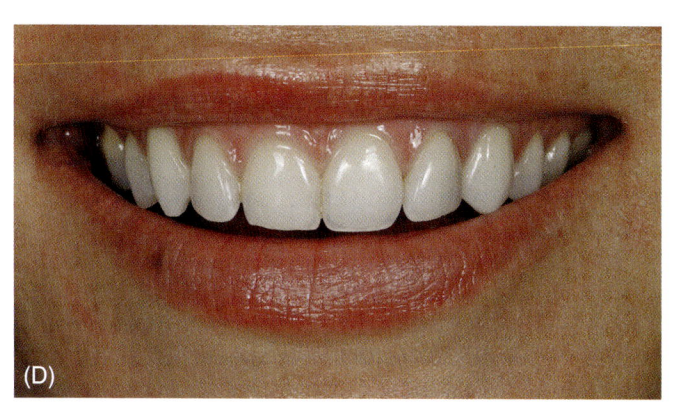

Figure 33.8 **(C, D)** Shows how a slightly tilted picture to the left side of the patient can lead to a misperception of the incisal and dental midline canting.

The midline or vertical division of the face into halves is one aspect often overlooked by the dentist. The relationship between the midline of the face and the midline of the maxillary dental arch can have a definite influence on the composition and harmony of esthetic restorations. In the final analysis, it is of utmost importance to inform patients of any limitations regarding midline discrepancies, so they will not expect perfection in the final result.

The dental midline should be perpendicular to the incisal plane and parallel to the midline of the face (Figure 33.9). Error may occur in slanting the midline formed by the mesial line angle of the central incisors either to the left or to the right. This may result in the illusion of malposition of the teeth or distortion of facial expression. Figure 33.10A–D shows a patient whose naturally slanted midline was acceptable to her, but her chief complaint was that her lateral incisors did not show when she spoke, giving the illusion that she had no teeth. Full porcelain crowns were placed on the lateral incisors to create a fuller smile and speaking line.

The maxillary centrals and cuspids were reduced proximally to allow normal-sized lateral incisors to be placed. Because the midline deviation was of no concern to the patient, no correction was indicated, and even with a deviated midline the patient has an attractive smile.

On the other hand, a patient may request a midline correction. For example, the 23-year-old woman in Figure 33.11A and B presented with a deviated midline and incisal wear. The patient was extremely concerned about her unattractive smile because she was an entertainer. A measurement of the true midline showed a diagonal deviation to the left (Figure 33.11B), and the incisal wear had produced what appeared to be an arch deformity. Because the patient wanted an economic immediate result, composite resin bonding was selected (Figure 33.11C and D). Figure 33.11E and F shows graphically how the esthetic transformation was accomplished.

True arch deformity can also be visually improved with a combination of periodontal cosmetic surgery consisting of crown raising. Next, restorative treatment could include ceramic veneer or full crown restorations (Figure 33.12A–D).

Asymmetry location

In the literature we find relevant differences in the asymmetry degree that can be found on different facial areas. Several studies agree that the gonion is one of the facial landmarks where the face presents greater asymmetry.[13,15,34] One of the explanations for this fact is the functional response to an asymmetric chewing action.[35–37]

In 2001, Ferrario published a three-dimensional investigation stating that the tragion, gonion, and zygyon points were the facial paired landmarks with greater asymmetries, whereas the endocanthi had the least asymmetries.[34] The nasal tip or pronasale was the most asymmetric point out of the ones placed on the midline, and this asymmetry was greater in males than in females; the same difference between sexes was noted with the pogonion (Figure 33.13).

The most recent research using three-dimensional methods tends to highlight the middle third of the face as showing greater asymmetry, although the most asymmetric points registered in this third are the tragion, gonion, and zygion, which are distant from the facial midline. However, the most asymmetrical point located on the midline was the pronasale (Figure 33.13).

Esthetic relevance of facial symmetry

Facial symmetry was suggested as a stability frame of development that can even be relevant when choosing a partner in human beings.[38] Numerous articles state there is a positive relationship between facial symmetry and beauty.[38] However, some recent investigations found that symmetrical faces are still classified as the most attractive when only one of the halves is presented.[38] This suggests that it is not because of the symmetry but because symmetrical faces usually have characteristics (that are not identified) that make them more attractive or esthetic.[38,39] Tarnow et al. implied there is a strong relationship between the tenets of beauty in a smile and the parallelism between reference

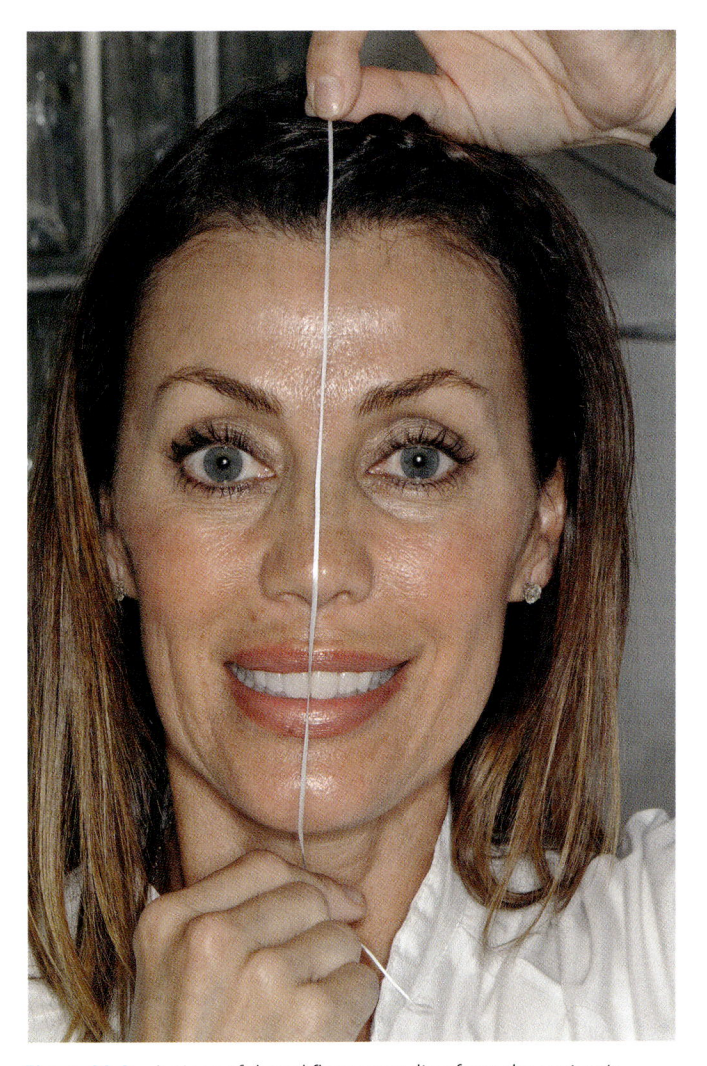

Figure 33.9 A piece of dental floss extending from the patient's forehead to their chin helps both the patient and practitioner visualize the dental and facial midlines.

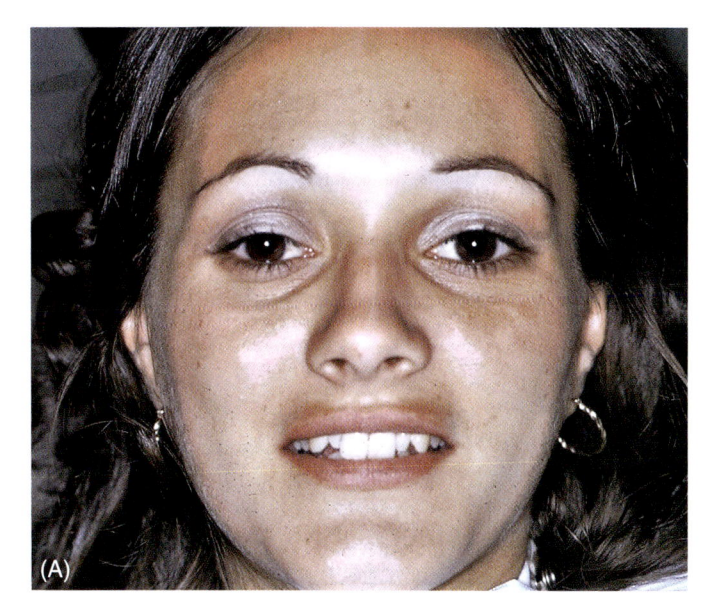

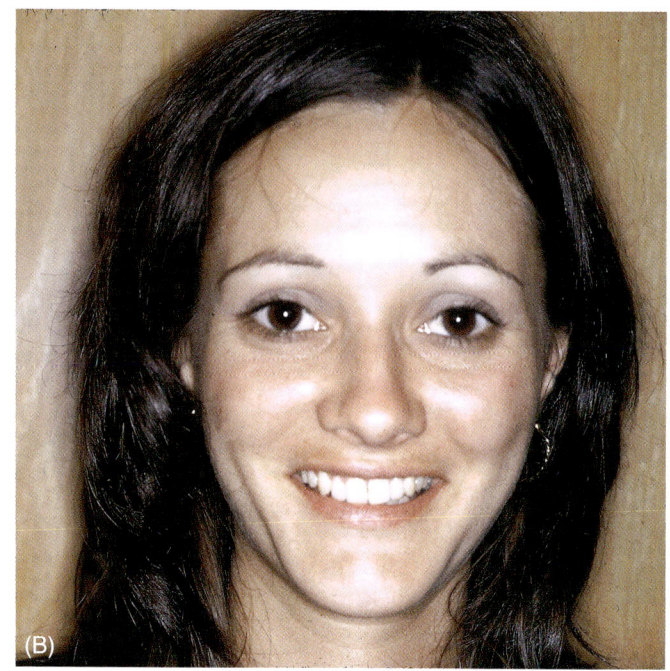

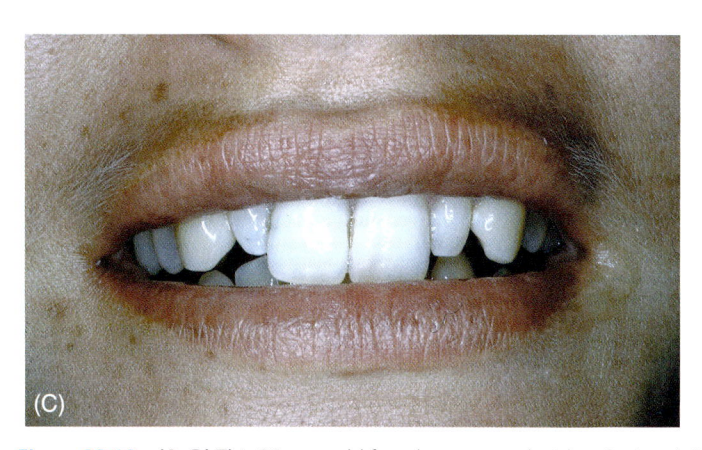

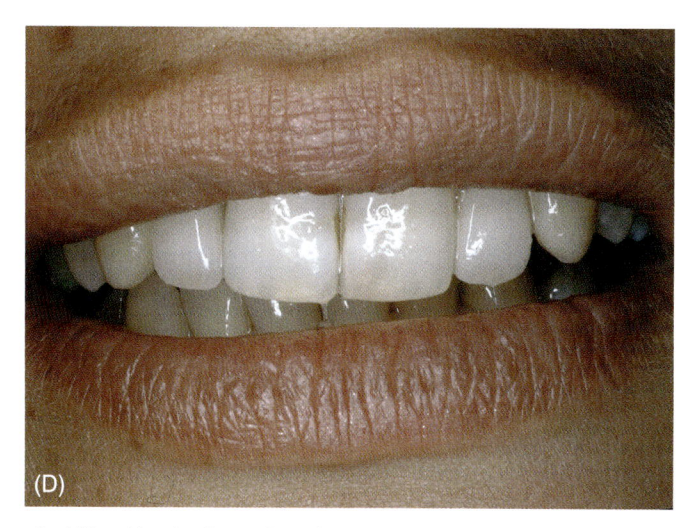

Figure 33.10 **(A–D)** This 26-year-old female presented with a deviated dental midline. Her chief complaint, however, was that her lateral incisors did not show during speech. (A, B) Full porcelain crowns were placed on the lateral incisors to create a fuller smile and speaking line. Since the midline deviation was of no concern to the patient, no correction was indicated (C, D).

lines and the teeth with the facial midline.[15] Symmetry should be the ultimate goal, not so much to achieve it but to get close to it. The focus should be placed on similar and differing parts of the face and compared with concepts of esthetic guidelines. Similar disharmonies can be brought to smile design. For example, bolder and slightly misaligned teeth will blend with a face that is noticeably asymmetrical. Strict symmetry in a smile may appear beautiful in a very symmetrical face but unnatural in a very asymmetrical face.[15] These imperfections were named "perfect imperfections" by Gebhard,[40] who considers that these tenets are important in creating diversity, naturality, and unique attractiveness in a smile design.

According to Springer et al.,[41] symmetry is one of the characteristics of an esthetic and attractive face, but there are exceptions to this rule (Figure 33.7A and B). Under some circumstances, symmetry can be completely unacceptable from an esthetic point of view. Several publications[42–44] demonstrate that an asymmetrical face is rated better from an esthetic standpoint versus a completely symmetrical face, which would be obtained artificially by joining two same right or left halves of the face (Figure 33.7C and D). This can be explained by horizontal symmetry, which is psychologically predictable and tends to be monotonous because diversity is missing to catch the observer's attention.

The golden proportion

Since the days of ancient Greece, beauty and numerical values have been closely associated, specifically in regard to the theory of proportions, which applies and implies arithmetic. The

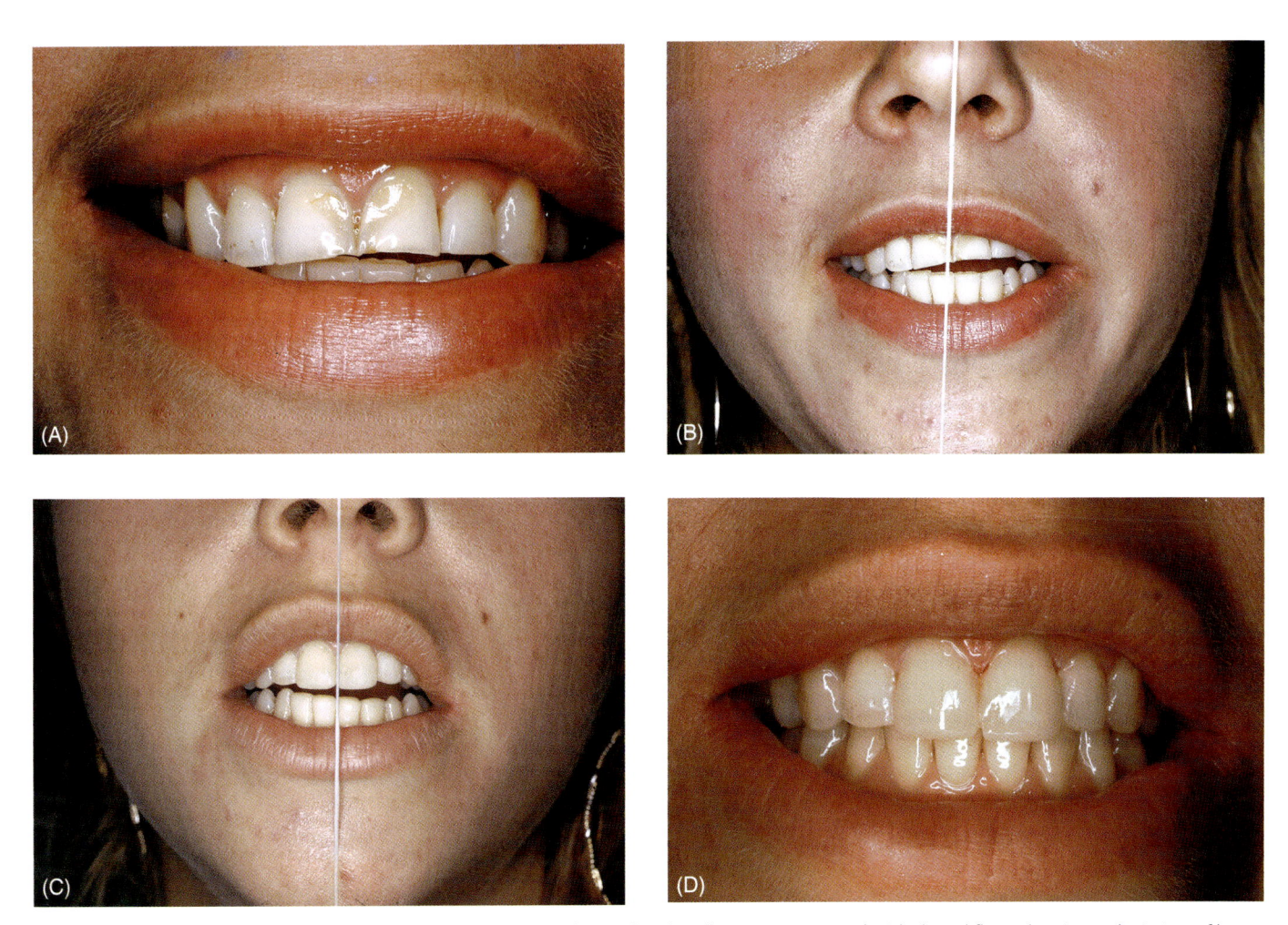

Figure 33.11 **(A–D)** This 23-year-old wanted to improve her smile. Her facial midline was measured with dental floss, showing a deviation of her dental midline diagonally to the right. The midline deviation and worn smile line were corrected with direct resin bonding on three of the maxillary anterior teeth.

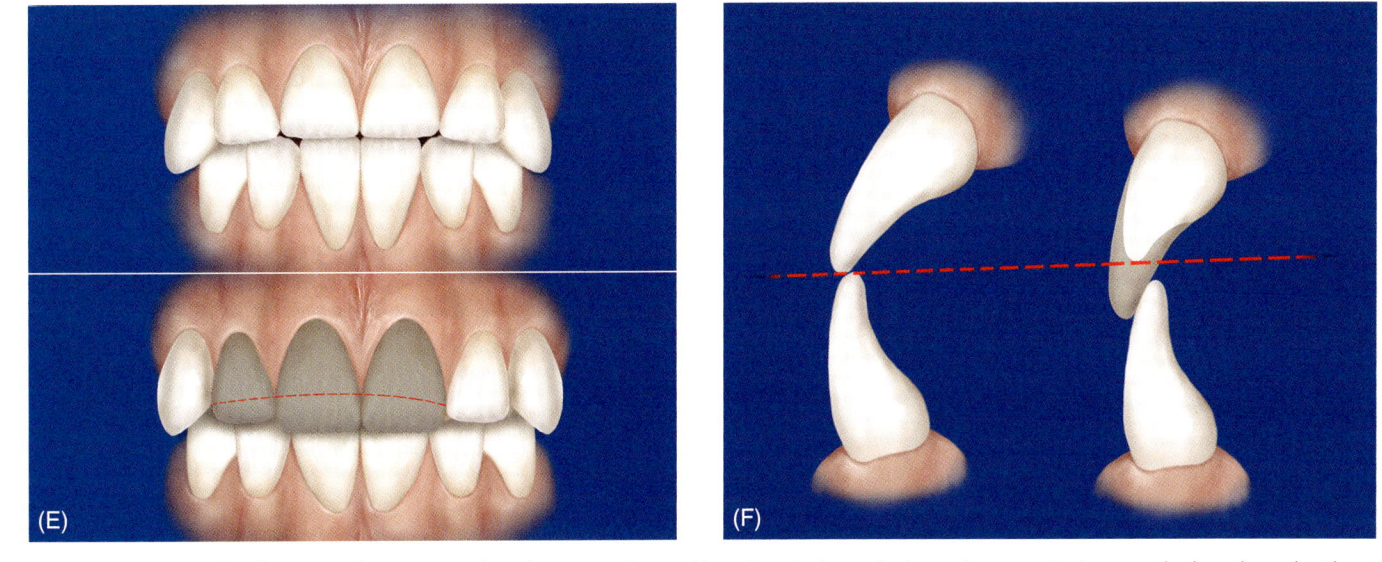

Figure 33.11 **(E, F)** This illustration demonstrates how by contouring and beveling the lower incisors, the upper incisors can be lengthened without altering their protrusive relationship.

concept of perceived beauty corresponds to the harmony of proportions. Applying mathematics to the arts as a new objective criterion of evaluation led to generations of philosophers and mathematicians attempting to find a formula to express beauty.[3,45]

The Greek civilization was concerned about finding methods for craftsmen and artists to quantify beauty and reproduce it in a predictable way. Their aim was to discover a simple arithmetic formula to represent harmony and beauty. This led to Pythagoras in 530 BC trying to find a mathematical answer to what was beautiful and ugly, and the result was the golden proportion. The "golden rule" or "golden proportion" used the number 1.618 as the "perfect" proportion and subsequently applied this to all fields of art and esthetics, including dentistry[3,45,46] (see Chapter 9). According to this rule, animated or unanimated objects that followed this ratio possessed an inherent beauty.

The beauty of flowers and faces was identified with characteristics that agreed with the ratio 1.618. Architects and sculptors of ancient times exploited the golden proportion to create buildings, such as the Pantheon in Athens and classical statues. Many artists also used this proportion to create masterpieces, such as Piero della Francesca and his *Baptism of Christ*. Plato claimed that other proportions or recurrent ratios could also show beauty. He disqualified the pretensions of the Pythagoras concept of beauty without answering the universality of the golden number.[2]

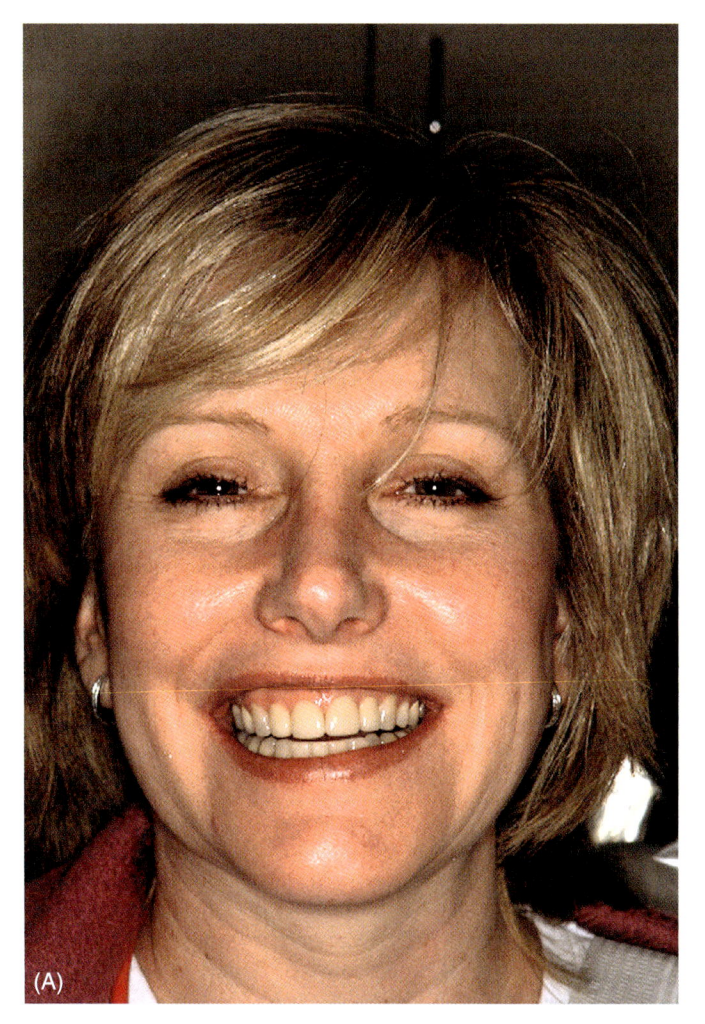

Studies on human facial morphology revealed a polar growth center in the base of the sphenoid. The growth registered around this point seemed to display proportion radially. Around this point the structures grew less than more distant ones, to keep the proportionality of the face in a three-dimensional context. Several facial and dental structures and landmarks have shown consistency in golden progressions. Examples are the width between the inner canthus to the nose ala; the length of the philtrum cupid's bow to the base of nose's columella, and the vertical height of upper and lower lip combination; and the lower and upper central incisor width, and the apparent width of six anterior maxillary teeth from a frontal perspective. Although, if all animals and plants were to obey this ratio we would be surrounded by clones. However, in the animal world, if some characteristics do not show standard dimensions, beauty may be compromised. What is the reason behind this disparity? To create diversity and individuality, the recurrent proportions or ratios are more important than a specific ratio (see Chapter 9).

Nowadays, the idea of beauty resulting from a combination of ratios/average proportions and individual subjective sensibility inherent to a determined space and time seems more acceptable. The beauty of the dentofacial composition strongly depends on the presence of several ratios and elements that are connected to structural or biometric beauty; this also applies to tooth arrangements (Figure 33.14).

Facial analysis

A systematic facial and dentofacial analysis protocol should be adopted on a routine basis, to avoid misdiagnosing any situation that can compromise the overall esthetic outcome. Generally speaking, the full face may be divided into vertical halves, left and right, and into horizontal thirds: (1) the superior third, composed of the forehead and hair; (2) the middle, containing the eyes, nose, zygomatic region, and ears; and (3) the inferior, comprising the lips, cheek, and chin. For Caucasian patients, the facial horizontal thirds are approximately equal, and the midline bisects the face between the eyes from forehead to chin (Figure 33.15).

In clinical practice, the standard records include digital photographs, radiographs, and mounted or unmounted study

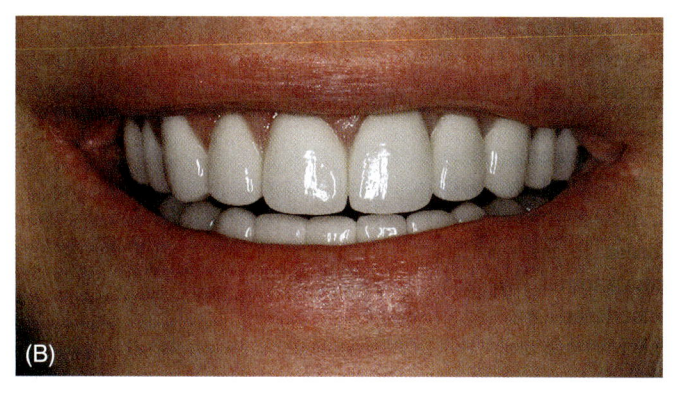

Figure 33.12 **(A)** This patient has a deviated arch form. **(B)** The deviated arch was corrected by periodontal and restorative procedures, see page 1098.

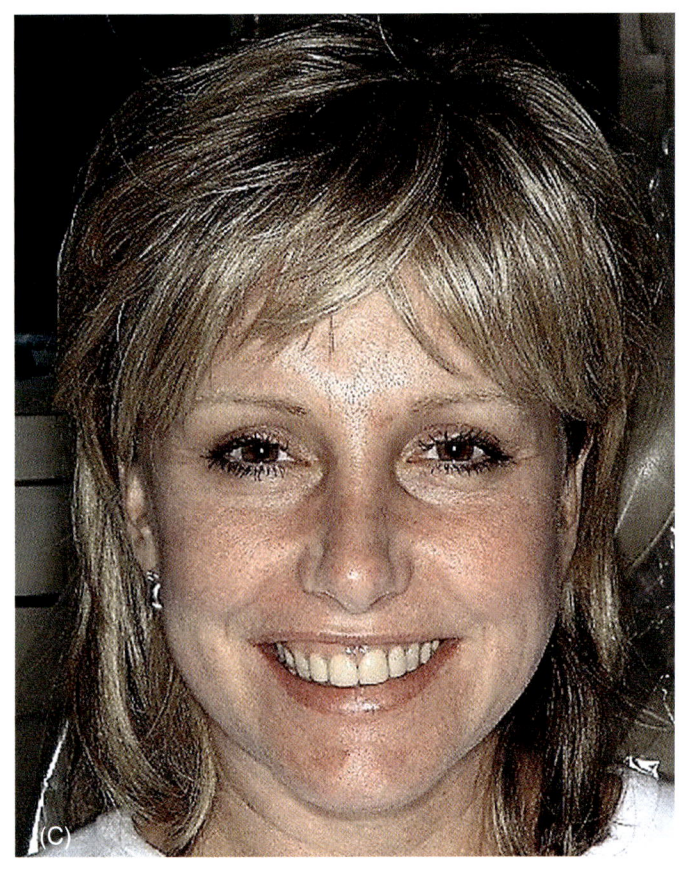

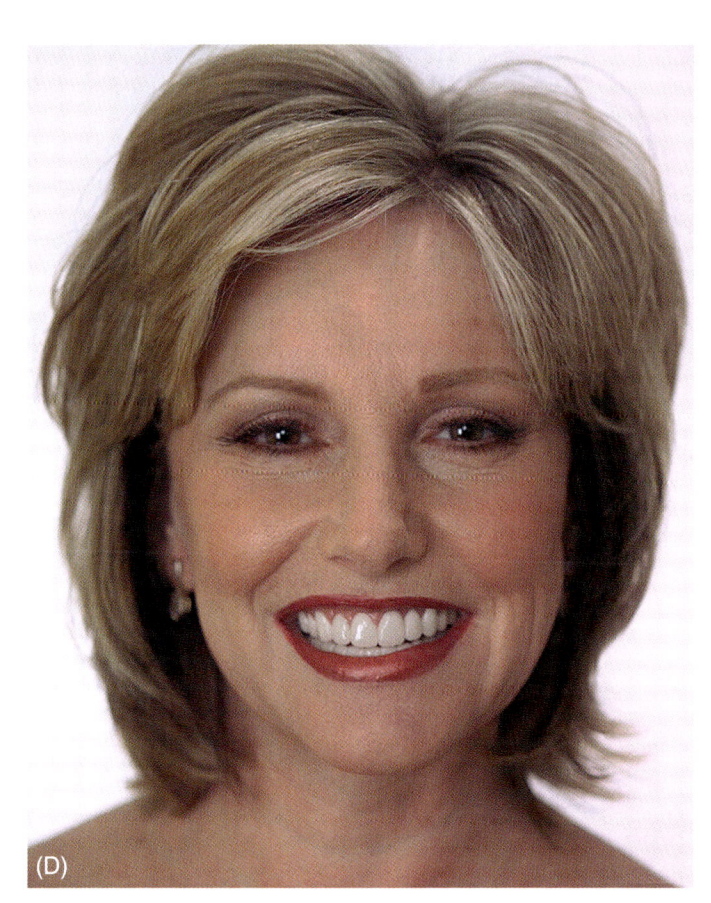

Figure 33.12 **(C, D)** Cosmetic periodontal surgery consisted of crown raising followed by brighter looking all-ceramic crowns in much better alignment that helped to improve her smile and facial beauty.

models. The most used facial images include frontal at rest, frontal smile, and profile at rest 1 : 1 images, which do not provide enough diagnostic information as they do not contain enough information for three-dimensional visualization and quantification.[11] A complete facial analysis requires more records and perspectives: profile smiling, facial oblique 45° smiling for both sides, close-up frontal smile, and close-up oblique 45° smile for both sides. In addition to these static records, contemporary smile analysis also requires dynamic records. Digital technology allows clinicians to record anterior tooth display during speech and smiling. The video record should also be taken in the frontal position and another in an oblique view.

Before proceeding to a detailed facial analysis, it is important to differentiate between the posed smile and the spontaneous smile. Posed smiles have been used for a long time in esthetic assessments for their reproducibility, but current video graphic and computer technologies allow us to perform other diagnostic assessments.

Posed smiles can be influenced by the individual's skills and emotional background. Patients that are either embarrassed by their appearance or that suffer from dental phobia will display a learned or an inhibited smile by hiding the teeth with the lips, hands, or changing the head position. Van der Geld et al.[47] studied the vertical and transversal characteristics of a posed and spontaneous smile and came to the conclusion that maxillary lip-line heights during spontaneous smiling were significantly higher than during posed smiling. Compared with spontaneous smiling, tooth display in the molar area during posed smiling decreased by up to 30% along with a significant reduction of smile width. During the posed smile, the mandibular lip-line heights also changed and the lower teeth were covered more by the lower lip than during the spontaneous smile.[47]

Facial analysis can be divided into two major components: facial analysis and dentofacial analysis. Facial analysis looks into relations of the smile with the other major facial structures, and dentofacial analysis pays attention to the teeth with the surrounding facial structures located on the lower third of the face.

Facial analysis: frontal view

For the frontal analysis, the patient should be with the head in the natural position, allowing the patient to sit or stand upright in front of the observer; this is the optimal position to evaluate the frontal plane.[30] Faces can be classified as mesocephalic, brachycephalic, or dolichocephalic by the classic frontal analysis, the difference being in the facial width to facial height general proportions. Brachycephalic faces are broader and shorter in comparison with dolichocephalic, which are longer and narrower (Figure 33.16).[11]

Facial reference lines

Reference lines are defined by points or structures that are taken into account during the perception process to find out if an esthetic composition is harmonically distributed. The reference

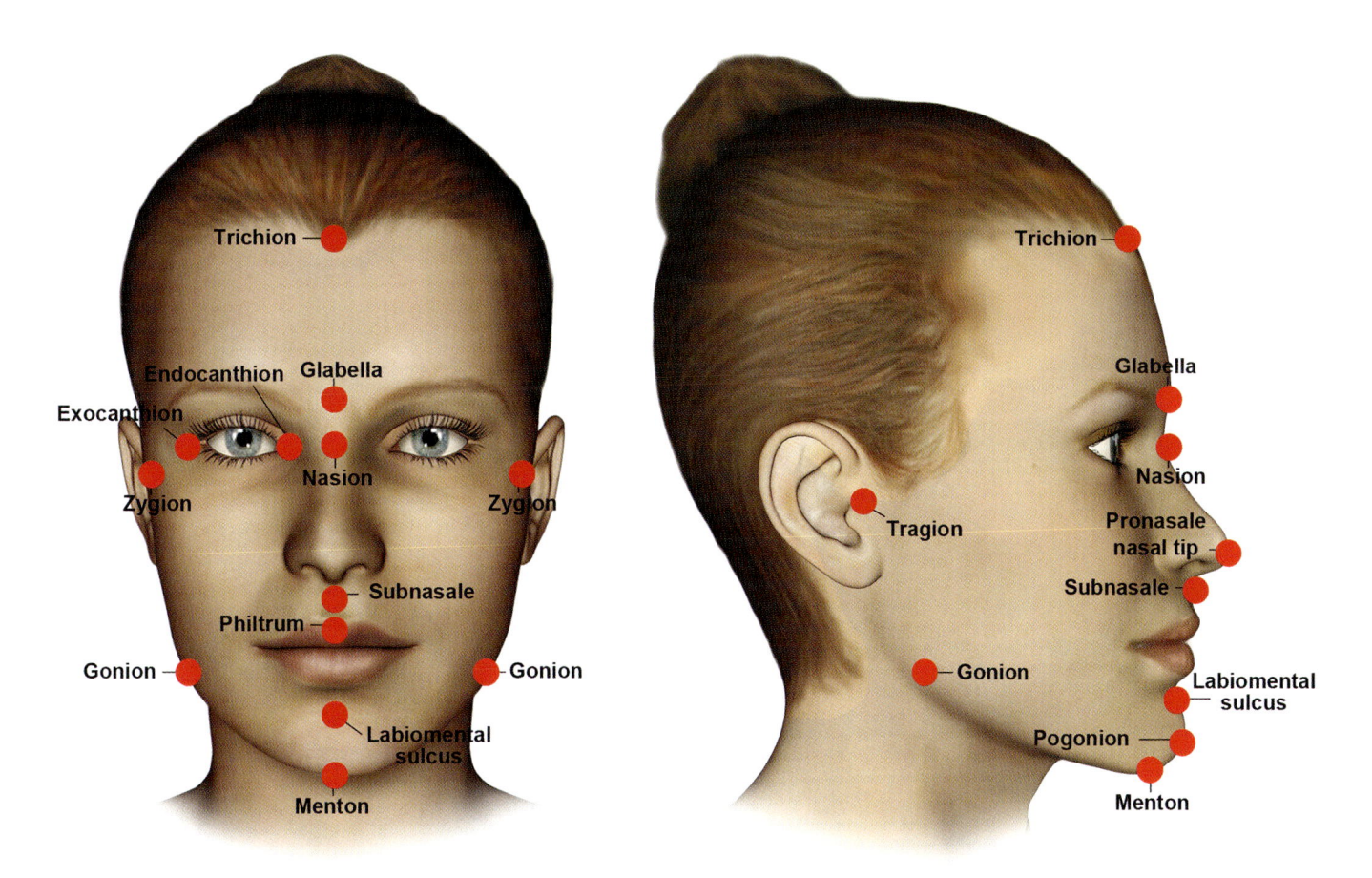

Figure 33.13 Frontal and profile facial landmarks associated with identifying facial asymmetry.

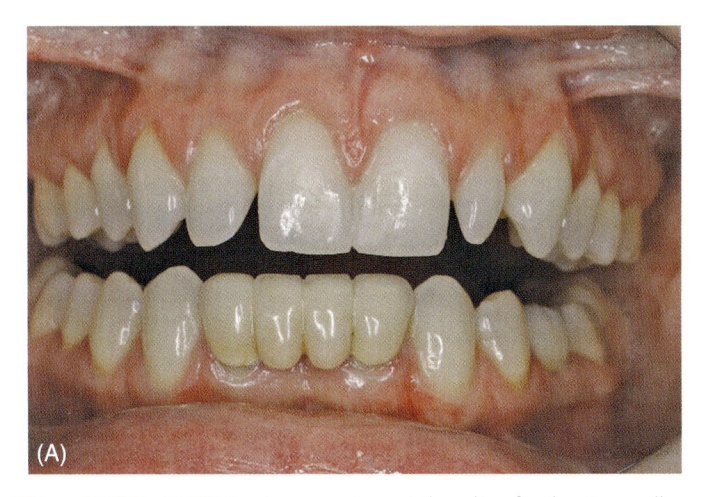

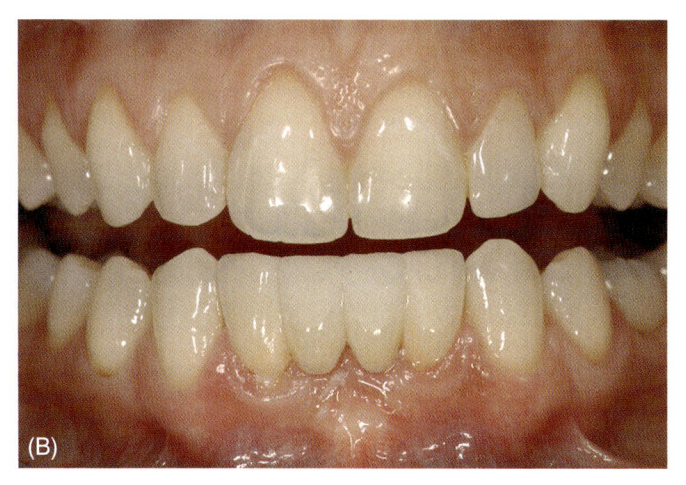

Figure 33.14 (A, B) Direct composite resin bonding for the six maxillary anterior teeth was chosen to restore this young lady's too narrow incisors. The final result demonstrates more appropriately sized teeth with more harmonious proportions.

lines of facial and dentofacial compositions are considered one of the key factors of biological and structural beauty.[2] Remember that a line does not need to be expressed to be perceived; it can be suggested by two or three points in a directional movement.[1]

When we look at a face in the frontal plane, our brain considers multiple reference lines. The most important reference lines in the frontal plane are the interpupillary line and the facial midline. These two lines define a "T," which works as the dorsal spine of the whole facial architecture.[10,12] All the facial structures should be parallel or perpendicular to one of these lines. When artists start drawing a face, they first establish a "T." In an esthetically attractive face, the interpupillary line is also parallel to other horizontal reference lines, such as the commissural line, inter-ear line, lip line, and the eyebrow lines[12,31,32,48] (Figure 33.17).

The most harmonic relation between two lines is parallelism; attraction originates from the general sense of parallelism and symmetry between facial characteristics, but it does not need to

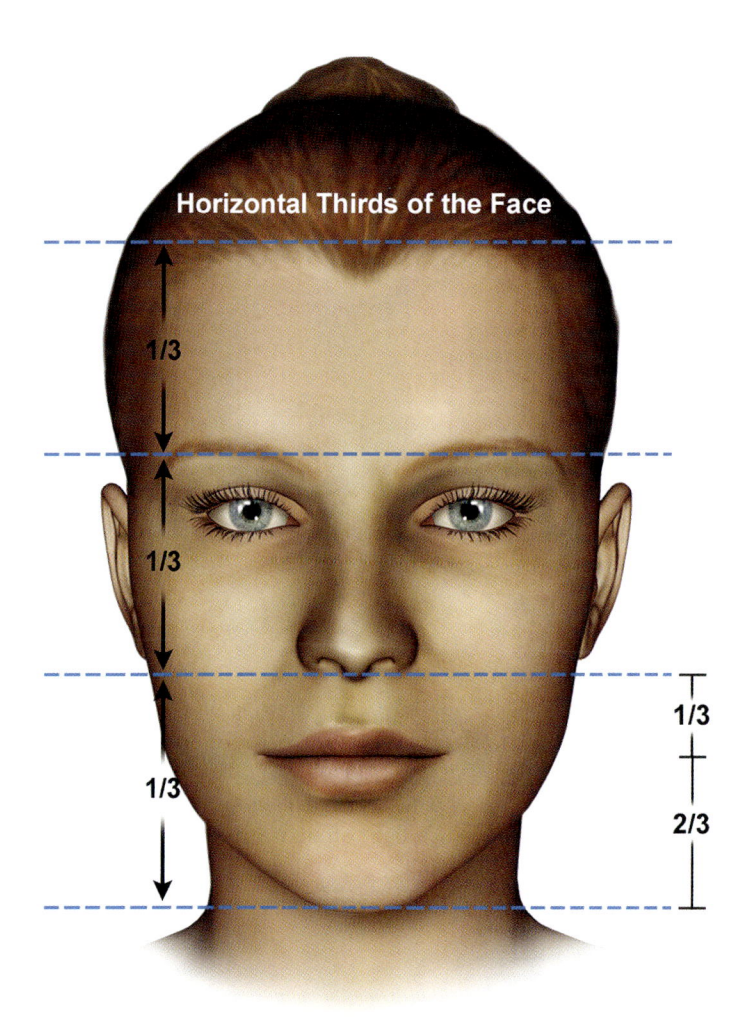

Figure 33.15 In Caucasian patients, the facial horizontal thirds are approximately equal.

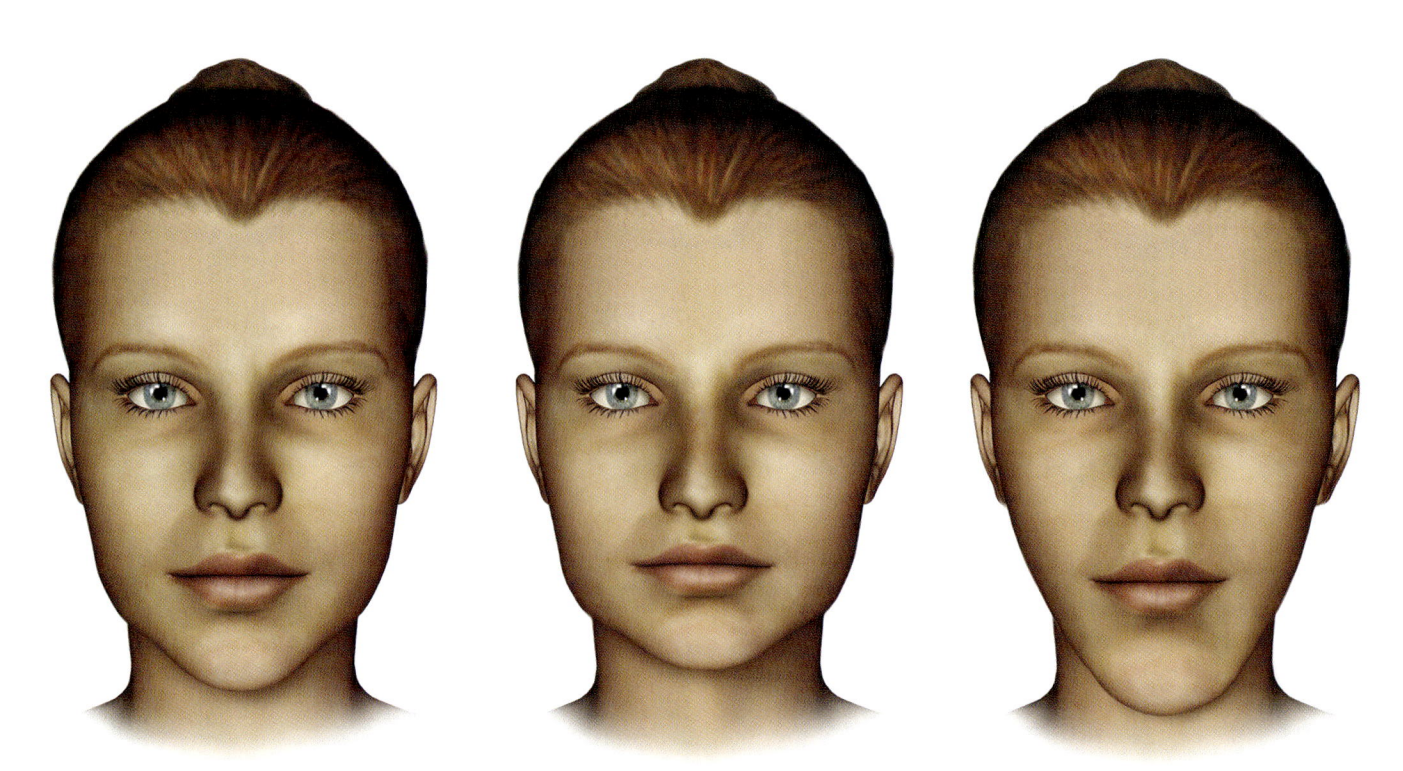

Figure 33.16 The first (leftmost) face, demonstrating equal facial thirds, is classified as mesocephalic. The middle face is more square, with the lower third being diminished in proportion, which is classified as brachycephalic. The face on the right is typical of one that is dolichocephalic, which indicates a larger lower facial third.

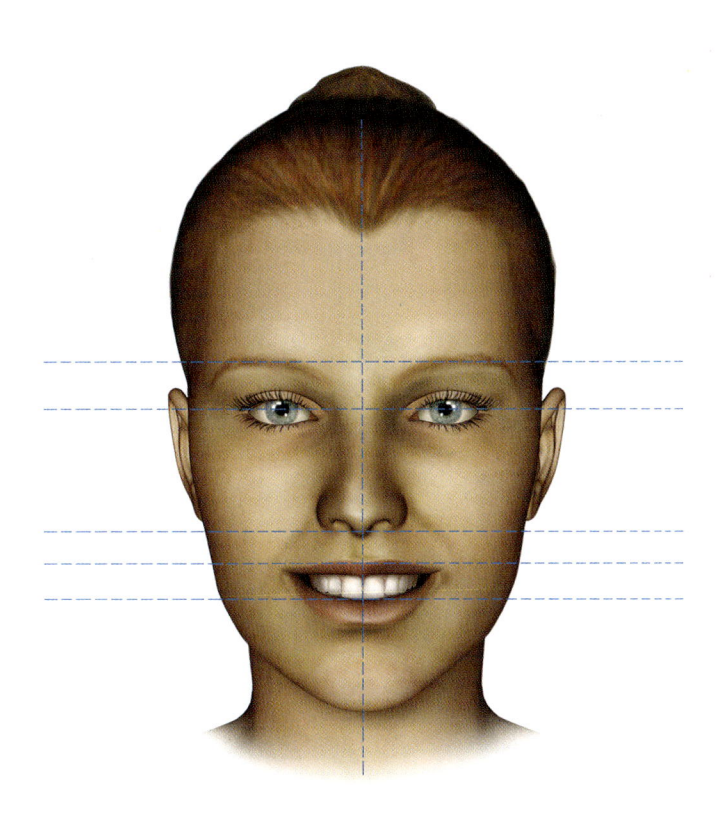

Figure 33.17 Looking at the face from a frontal view, facial reference lines help define dentofacial proportions. The "T" that is formed by the interpupillary line and the facial midline is of utmost importance.

be strictly from parallelism. Most people have nonevident inclinations that require little or no correction. The irregularities created by slight inclinations can cause some tension within the related structures and may need partial fixing, or, if the patient is very demanding, even total correction might be possible.[12] But, which inclinations are the ones that really matter in terms of esthetics? Several authors[2,4,10,12] suggest that axial inclination of the dental midline is esthetically unacceptable for it does not respect the parallelism rule. Midline shifting is considered less important provided that it is parallel to the facial midline. It was observed in a perceptional study with 196 lay subjects that asymmetric deviations of some facial midline structures, such as the nose tip and chin, modify how the dental midline canting is perceived. They found that when the dental midline was canted in the same direction as nose tip and chin the esthetic ratings were higher than when the canting was opposite the nose and chin deviation (Figure 33.18A and B).[49] The same rule was observed for the dental midline shift (Figure 33.19A and B).[50]

This implies that because some facial structures such as nose and chin frequently present asymmetries, the perceived facial midline is not always perpendicular to the horizontal, and mild inclinations of the dental midline are allowed without breaking the esthetic harmony, provided the parallelism among facial elements is preserved (Figure 33.8A). We believe that the same rule can be applied to interproximal contacts.

The lips work as curtains regulating the degree of dental exposure, both during resting and smiling. They are arguably the most dynamic structure in whole face. The labial commissures define a very important horizontal reference line known as the commissural line (Figure 33.17). Besides the commissural line, there are other labial reference lines that are used to evaluate teeth exposure of maxillary teeth at rest. During smiling, these lines will also determine the amount of gingival exposure. Incisal edges of the maxillary teeth define another reference line: the incisal curve. According to Tjan et al.,[51] this line is parallel to the lower lip in 85% of the population. Golub[52] established that one of the most significant facial juxtapositions is the dental midline being perpendicular to the interpupillary line; it centers the smile on the face. The hypothetical midline, or the one imposed by the elements of the facial and dentofacial composition and the perpendicularity with the horizontal reference lines, guarantees the presence of segregation forces, a fundamental requirement for esthetic approval.[1,12,52] To conclude, it can be said that multiple lines can help us understand the human face, and achieving a balance between symmetry and harmony is required in any technique.[18]

Vertical facial proportions

The optimal facial proportion generally follows the facial thirds concept, which divides the face vertically into three equal parts.[1,11] Artists and orthodontists generally agree upon the concept of using facial thirds to evaluate beauty. More attractive faces display optimal balance when these proportions are present.[53,54] The upper third is defined by an imaginary line parallel to the horizontal that crosses the hairline (trichion) and another one that passes through the midbrow; the middle third goes from the midbrow to the subnasale region, and the lower third is the area between the subnasale and the menton's soft tissues. The ideal lower third can be further divided in thirds, with the upper lip being the upper third and the lower lip and chin representing the lower two-thirds[11] (Figure 33.15). There are several skeletal causes behind disproportions among vertical facial thirds, and analyzing the proportional relationships can aid in diagnosing the different factors involved in vertical facial deformities.[11] Measuring the upper third can often be difficult because of the variability in landmarks such as the location of the hairline (trichion). The 1 : 1 proportion between the middle and the lower thirds should not be used as a determining factor when undertaking facial height changes. This is because the degree of incisor exposure and the interlabial gap (see Chapter 32) in the lower third play a much more important role when assessing balance.[31] If the lower third height is larger than the upper two-thirds and the patient cannot close the lips without strain (Figure 33.20A and B), the esthetic proportion of the face as a whole can be restored by surgically modifying the patient's alveolar height and/or vertical dimension[55] (Figure 33.21A–C).

The aging process is greatly noticeable in the lower third of the face, which presents an excellent opportunity to rejuvenate a patient's looks. During the normal aging process, facial and masticatory muscles undergo degrees of atrophy and associated fibroses of their fibers and tendons. This shortens the working length of the face and manifests in sagging and wrinkling of the face. Premature aging of the face can be brought on by repeated overexposure to the sun as well as habits such as cigarette smoking. Especially damaging to a youthful appearance is the early

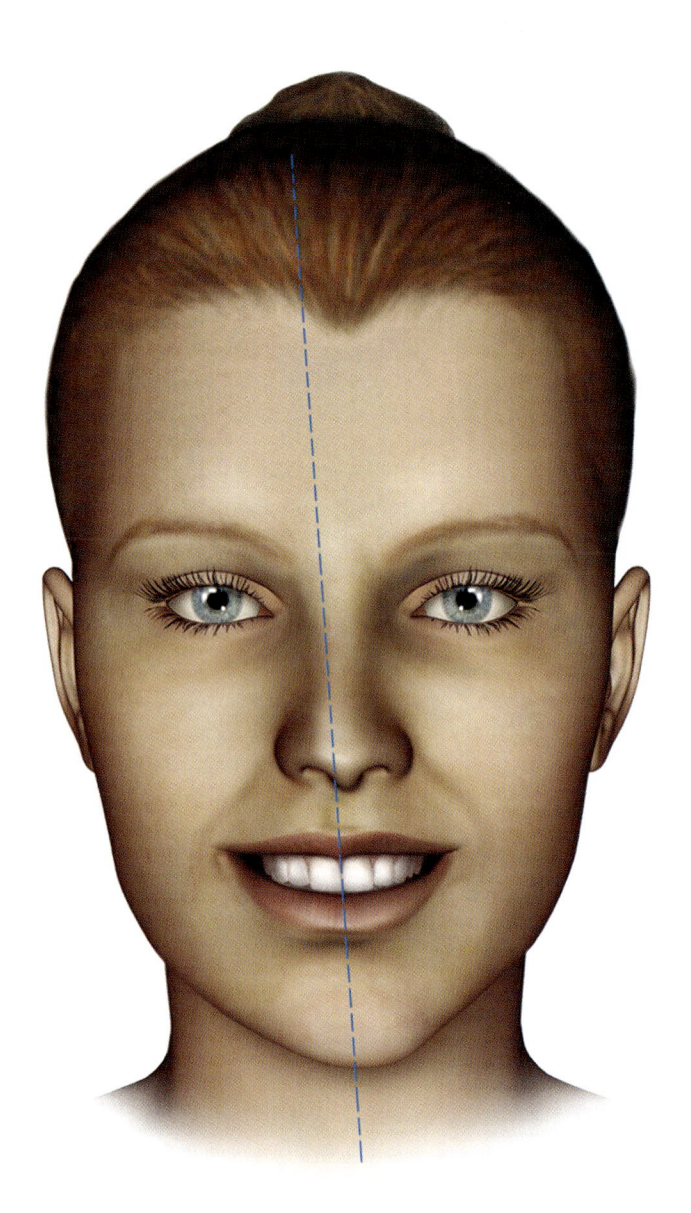

Figure 33.18 (A) When the dental midline is canted in the same direction as the nose and chin, some harmony and parallelism are maintained.

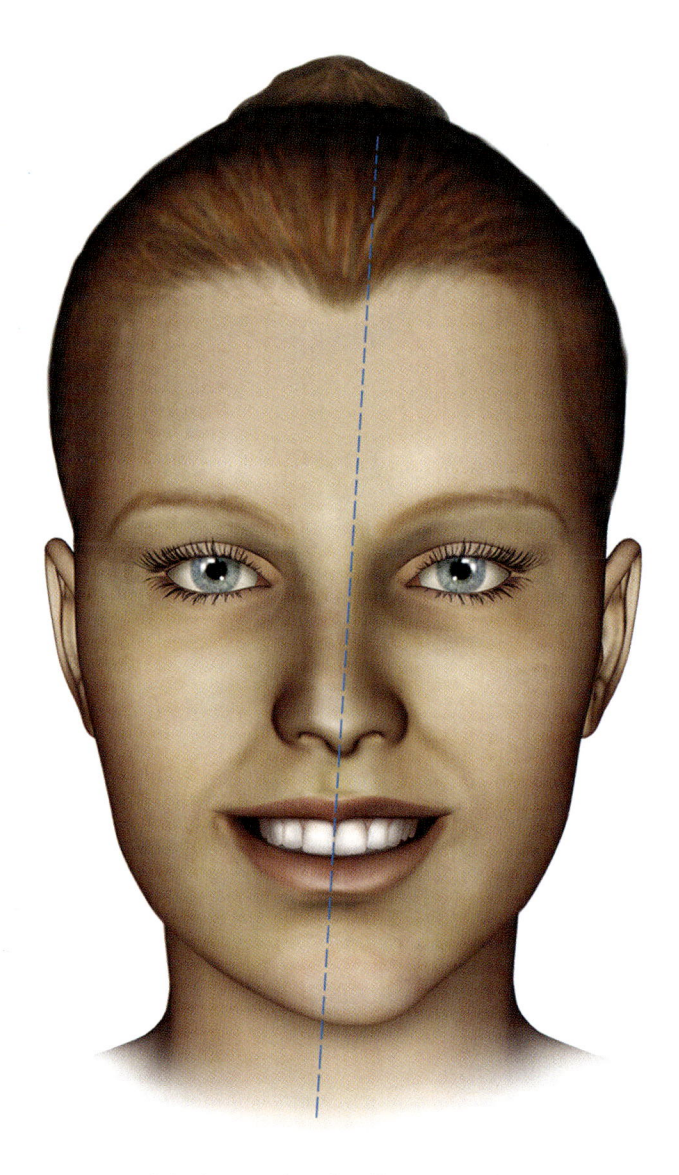

Figure 33.18 (B) When the dental midline is canted in the opposite direction of the nose and chin, harmony and parallelism are disrupted.

loss of the dentition, which eventually results in the partial or total resorption of alveolar bone, and leads to the "overclosed" or "collapsed" appearance associated with advanced age (Figure 33.22A–I).

A reduced facial lower third can be caused by tooth wear with loss of vertical dimension or by undereruption of the posterior teeth.[56] In some cases, increasing the vertical dimension can improve facial beauty,[57-60] but it is considerably difficult to achieve large changes in facial lower third height and dramatically transform facial proportions while preserving a correct occlusal relationship.[61,62] When the vertical dimension is increased or decreased, the overjet is also significantly altered; for each 3 mm vertical change in the anterior teeth there is approximately a 2 mm horizontal change in an anterior–posterior dimension, modifying the overjet (Figure 33.23). Therefore, attempting to increase the vertical dimension by 9 mm will result in a 6 mm increase in overjet, making it almost impossible to obtain a correct occlusal relationship unless the patient was initially in Class III occlusion. This is also the reason why it is extremely difficult to correct facial proportions when the lower third height is increased and the vertical dimension needs to be reduced (see Figure 33.24A–D).[61]

Research shows dentists were unable to see the difference in esthetics when discrepancies were caused by vertical dimension changes of 2, 4, and 6 mm. Gross found that until vertical dimension changes reach 8 mm, dentists could not assess the difference in facial features.[61] The reason behind this is that, although VDO is normally evaluated with teeth contacting, most everyday activities are done with teeth apart and thus facial proportion is not affected.[61,62]

The frontal view of the lip position at rest can also be evaluated to assess the vertical dimension and its impact on the face's lower third height; this position should create an optimal facial proportion.[63] At times, closure from this rest position to

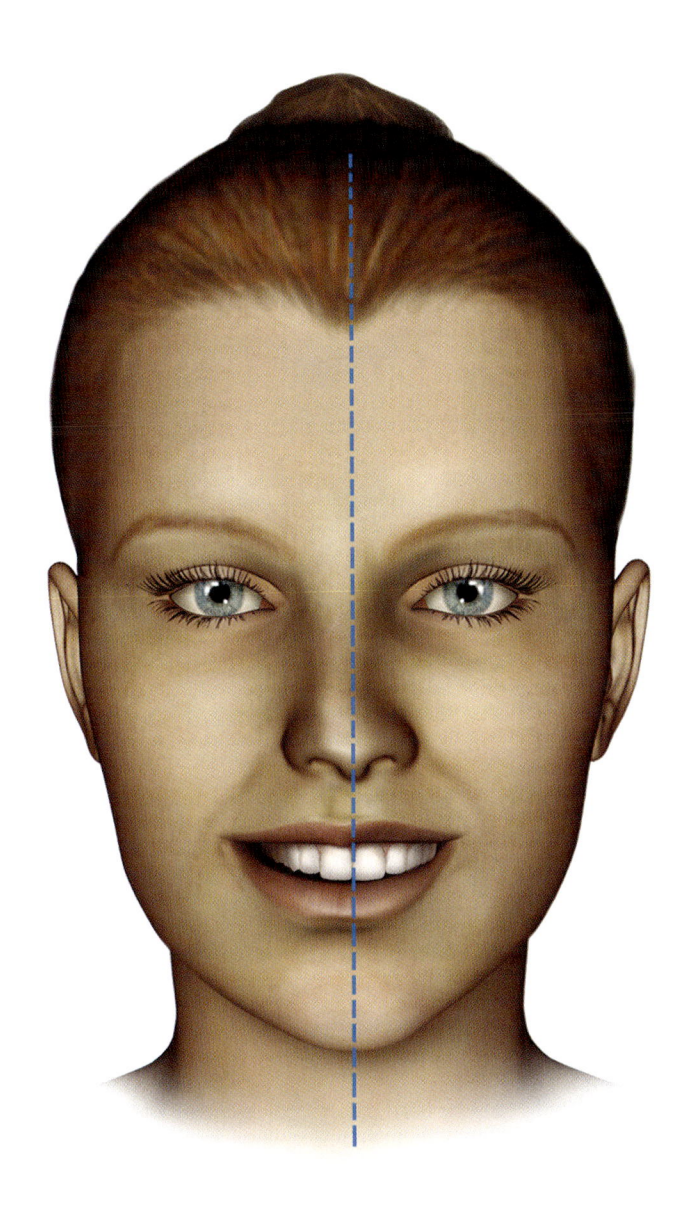

Figure 33.19 (A) This illustration shows how the dental midline is shifted approximately 2 mm in the same direction as the nose tip and chin. Dental midline shifts in the same direction as the facial midline maintain some harmony.

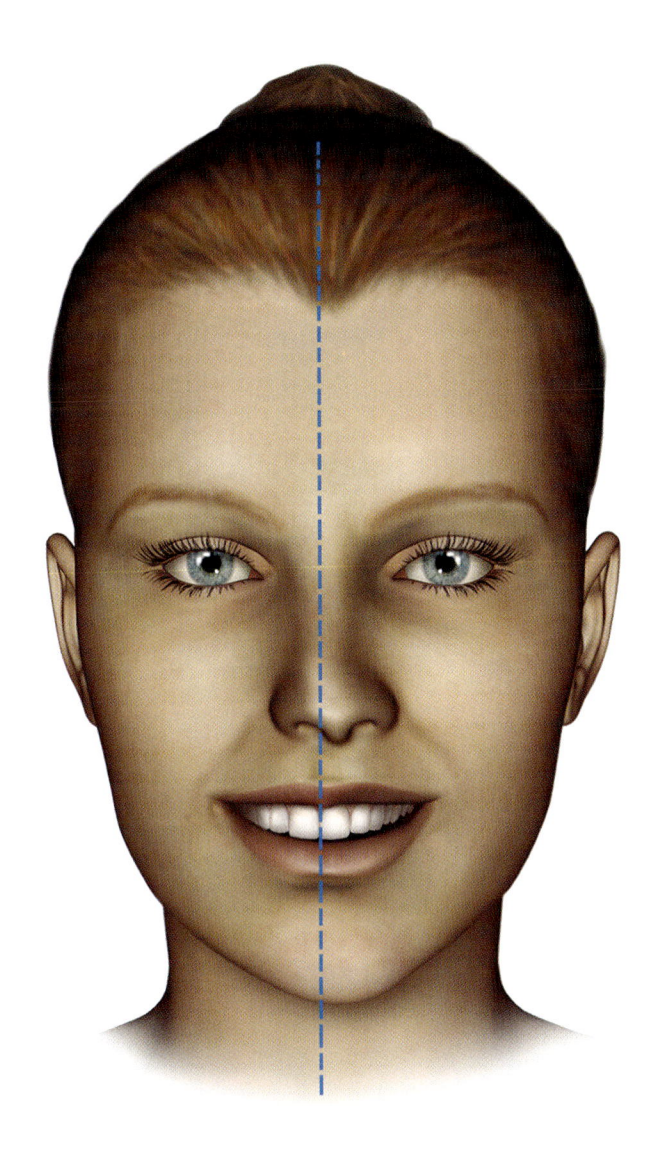

Figure 33.19 (B) When the dental midline is shifted approximately 2 mm in the opposite direction as the nose and chin, harmony is disrupted.

maximum intercuspation reveals a significant decrease in facial height and is esthetically unpleasing due to reduced labial visibility and increased labiomental sulcus depth.[64] This generally indicates an inadequate vertical position of either the maxillary or mandibular occlusal planes. These should also be evaluated with pictures and videos; therefore, picture series in frontal view should include rest and maximum intercuspation positions.

Ideally, there should be minimal effect on facial height and, thus, facial esthetics when the patient closes from the vertical dimension of rest to maximum intercuspation.[11] Usually, when there is a significant difference between these two positions, patients appear to have one of two conditions: deep bite associated with vertical maxillary deficiency and mandibular retrusion (Class II malocclusion)[31] or reduced VDO due to either one of the previously mentioned conditions: significant wear, loss of posterior support due to tooth loss, or undererupted posterior teeth.[63] A composite or acrylic overlay can be placed on the lower back molars (without previous etching) to allow the patient to occlude slightly closer to the vertical dimension of rest; the vertical dimension change and its effect on esthetics and comfort can then be assessed. For further evaluation, a composite overlay can be used to mount the diagnostic casts on an articulator with the new vertical dimension and to do a diagnostic wax-up of the proposed changes. If the mounted casts reveal that altering the teeth to improve facial or dental esthetics would compromise the patient's dentition either biologically or structurally, a multidisciplinary treatment approach should be taken (restorations alone should not be used to treat this case, and orthodontics and orthognathic surgery should be considered).

Clinically, there are many ways of either restoring or altering vertical dimensions in patients. Either fixed or removable temporary restorations can be constructed to provide the planned vertical opening. Perhaps the safest way to make sure your patient will be comfortable with the new opening is to have the

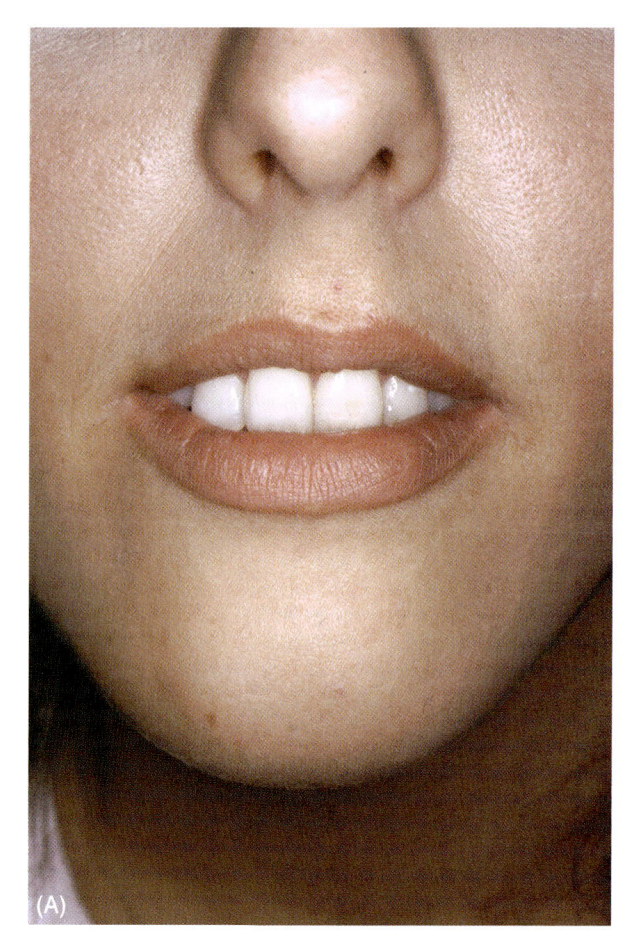

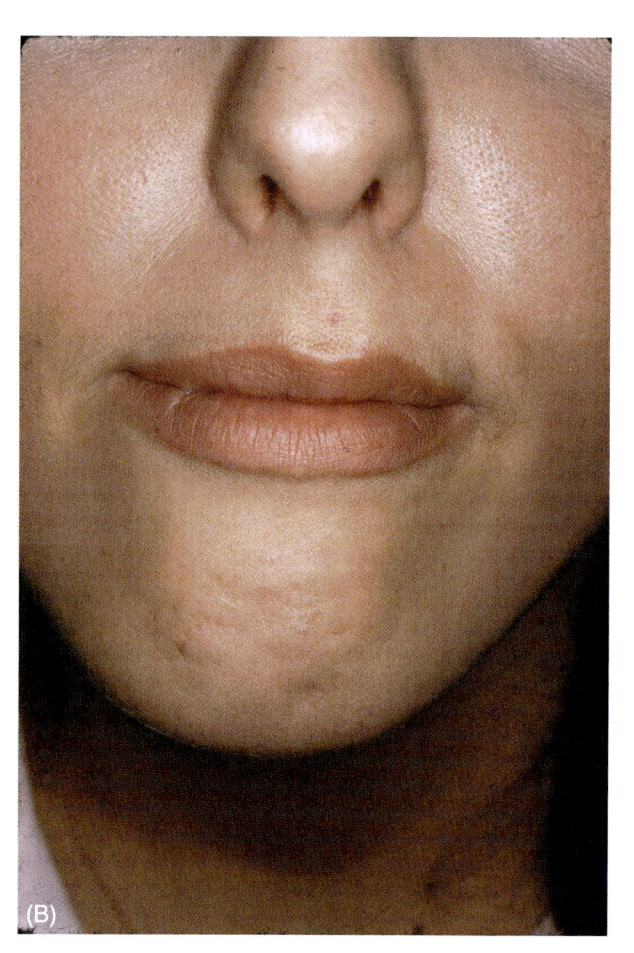

Figure 33.20 (A, B) Because of this patient's long, narrow face, she shows muscular strain when trying to close.

patient wear their temporary restorations for 3 months, followed by an extended time in final temporaries once the teeth are prepared. In addition, the anterior teeth can be temporarily bonded with composite resin to also provide the patient with a trial smile so they can approve your esthetic smile design. When there are perceptible abnormalities that bother the patient, such as skeletal asymmetries, a referral may be made to an oral and maxillofacial specialist.[63] Nothing can be done dentally to affect structural changes to the upper two-thirds. Decreased lower-third height cases due to undererupted posterior teeth should be referred for orthodontic treatment. These teeth are minimally affected by wear, so restorative treatment alone to increase the vertical dimension would create an unfavorable crown-to-root ratio; it is also possible to cause unnecessary damage to the teeth by preparing them.[56]

Nasal tip and facial midline

According to Ferrario's three-dimensional study,[65] the nasal tip is the most asymmetric midfacial point. The nasal tip position should be assessed beyond the frontal view with the patient's head slightly elevated.

The relation of the nasal tip with the facial midline, philtrum, and dental midline should be registered to reduce the risk of treating the dental midline to a distorted nose. Further studies need to be done to obtain further conclusions about the role that the nasal tip and other midfacial structures play on dental esthetic perception.

Maxillary dental midline and facial midline

The relation between the maxillary dental midline and the midfacial plane should be evaluated in terms of parallelism between them and also to the horizontal plane. Some discrepancies could be caused by dental factors such as missing teeth and crowding or by skeletal maxillary rotation.

A dental symmetrical arrangement is considered a key factor in an esthetically attractive smile[10,19,51,66–68] because patients can easily identify a wrongly positioned midline.[2,19] This idea was accepted into dental practice, albeit without scientific evidence to support it.[9] It was not until the late 1990s when the first studies attempting to quantify midline shifts identifiable by both laypeople and oral health professionals were published. Owens et al.[48,69] concluded that dental midline deviations from the line bisecting the interpupillary line were found in 30% of the population without racial and sex differences; this was subdivided into 22% to the left side and 8% to the right. Miller and Jamison[17] found a 25% midline deviation.

The published studies concluded that a dental midline shifting from the facial midline over 2 mm was easily identified and considered to be hardly esthetic by most people, regardless of their dental education.[7,8] However, some investigations brought up very different results, such as those by Kokich et al.[4] and

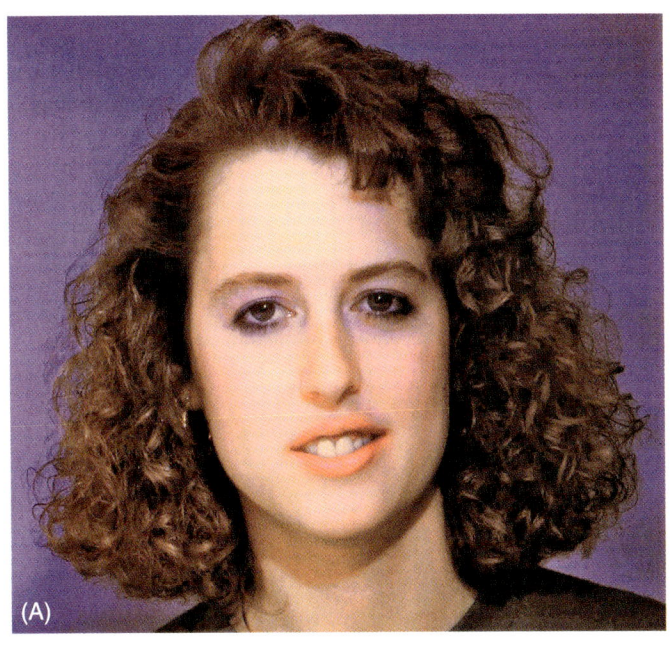

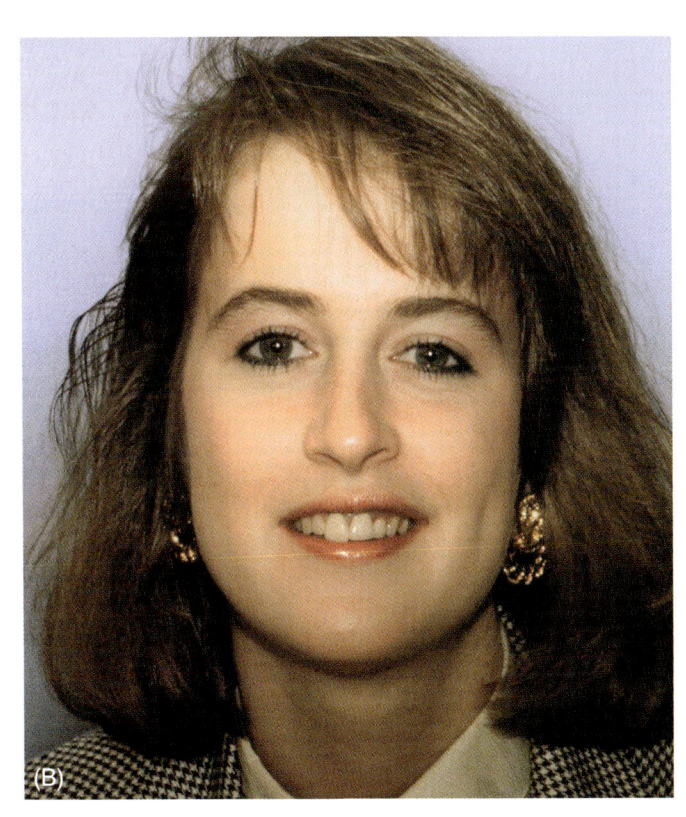

Figure 33.21 **(A, B)** In a dolichocephalic face, the lower third is often increased due to a vertical maxillary excess. This problem can be handled by surgically modifying alveolar height and vertical dimension. Now she is a good candidate for restorative esthetic dentistry. (Orthognathic surgery performed by Louis Belinfante.)

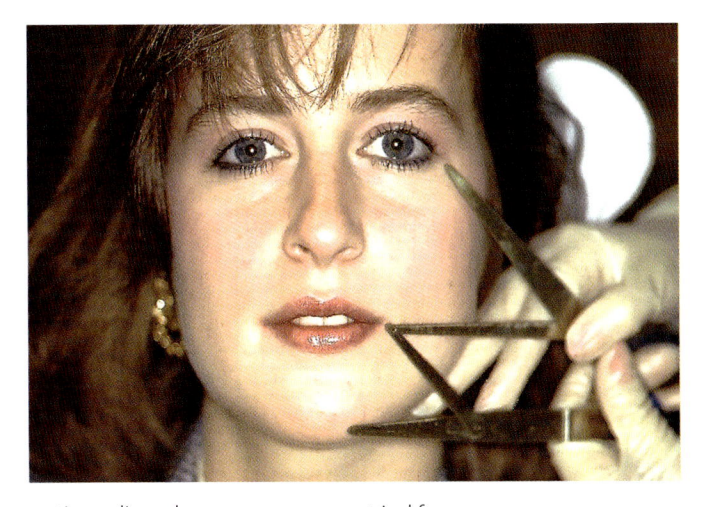

Figure 33.21 **(C)** Note how the golden proportion caliper shows a more symmetrical face.

Pinho et al.,[70] who considered that a 4 mm shifting had no impact on the esthetic appearance as judged by a layperson. However, there was a significant difference between the results obtained in these studies. The main difference was that while the 2 mm threshold studies used facial photographs evaluating the entire facial composition, those that obtained higher thresholds used photographs of the two lower facial thirds evaluating the dentofacial composition without taking the eyes, nose, and chin into account. This emphasizes the importance of taking a step back from the traditional dentofacial assessment and a step toward a facially oriented/comprehensive esthetic analysis. Slight inclination of the dental midline does not respect parallelism to the facial midline and is thus considered unattractive, tending to create a degree of visual tension.[2,4,10,12] Frush[71] argued that canting of the dental midline was significantly more critical than its shifting. This means that the inclination of the dental midline is more easily detectable than its deviation, even if it keeps parallelism to the facial midline.[12]

The aforementioned perceptual study came to the conclusion that a 3.5° dental midline cant was easily detected; furthermore, when the dental midline was canted in the same direction as the nose tip and chin, the esthetic ratings were

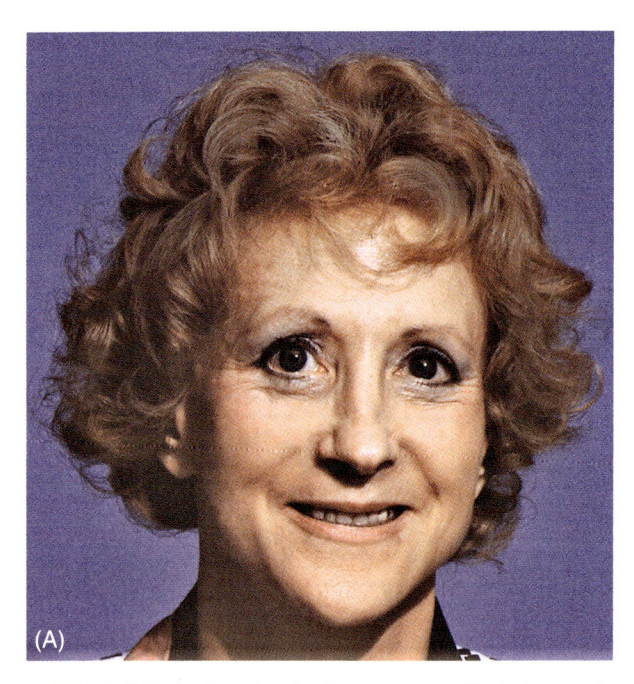

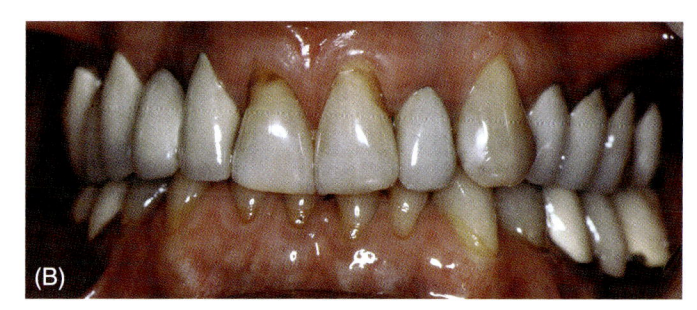

Figure 33.22 **(A, B)** This patient had temporomandibular joint pain related to her collapsed bite and lack of stable posterior contacts. Although she had a rehabilitation completed in another country, it was determined that her bite had been overclosed.

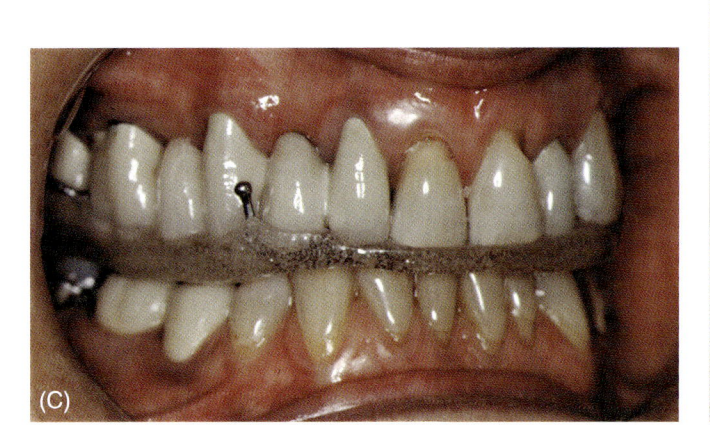

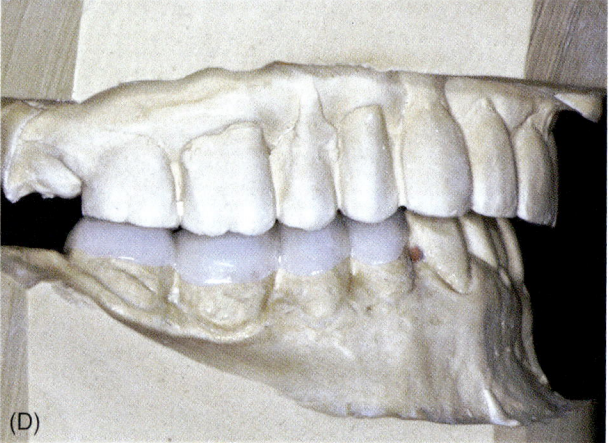

Figure 33.22 **(C)** The occlusion was tested with a full-coverage removable appliance for 3 months. **(D)** Two four-unit overlays were worn for 3 months to see whether the new posterior occlusion achieves the desired comfort and stability.

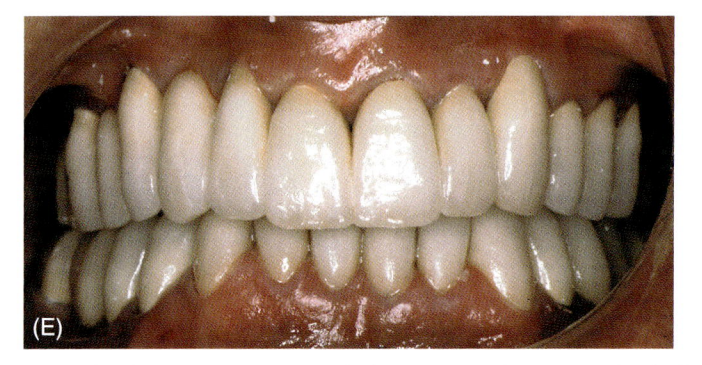

Figure 33.22 **(E)** The final maxillary and mandibular restoration consisted of ceramo-metal crowns and porcelain veneers.

higher than when the canting was in the opposite direction of the nose and chin deviation (Figure 33.18A and B). This means that each case should be evaluated individually because each face is unique. Moreover, these numbers should not be taken as thresholds of recognition that can be applied to everyone. What seems clear is that some facial structures can have an impact on the perception of some midline discrepancies and thus cannot be neglected during the esthetics diagnosis.

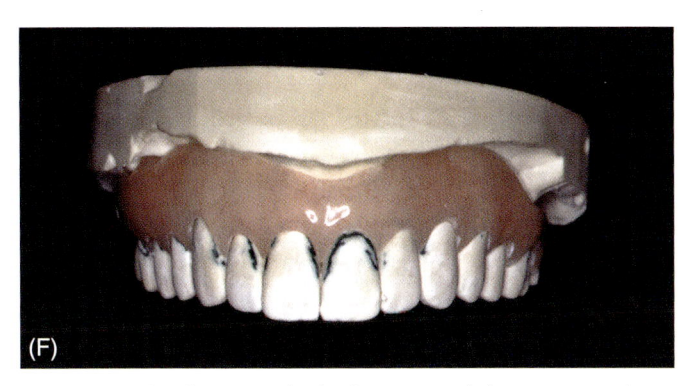

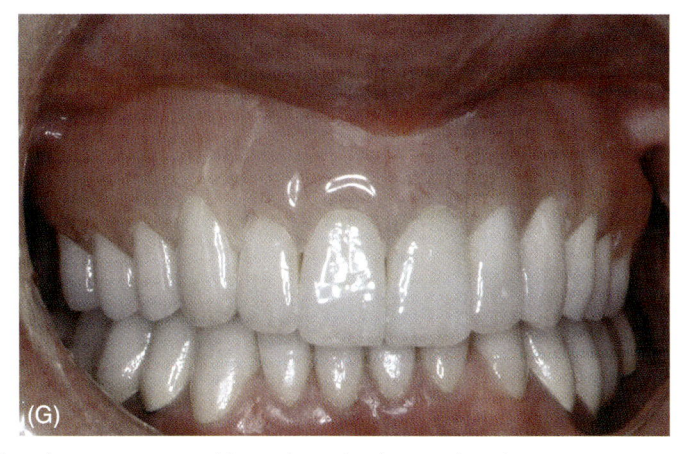

Figure 33.22 **(F–G)** Because the final restoration left open gingival interdental spaces, a removable acrylic artificial gingival appliance was constructed. The removable gingival appliance helped to better proportion the size of her teeth.

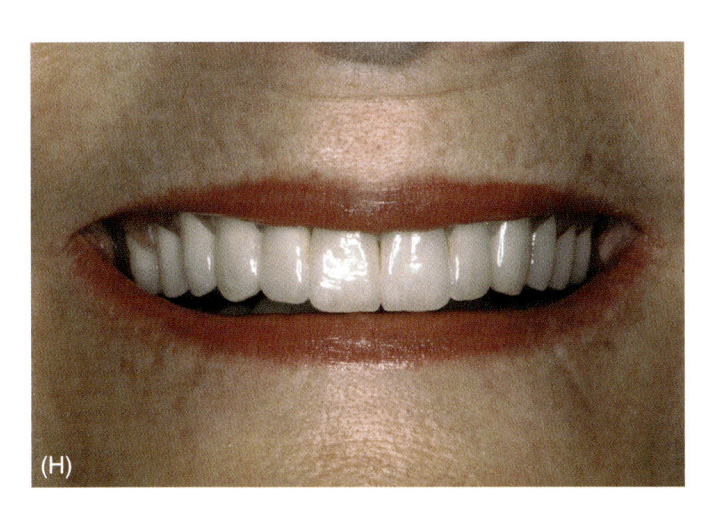

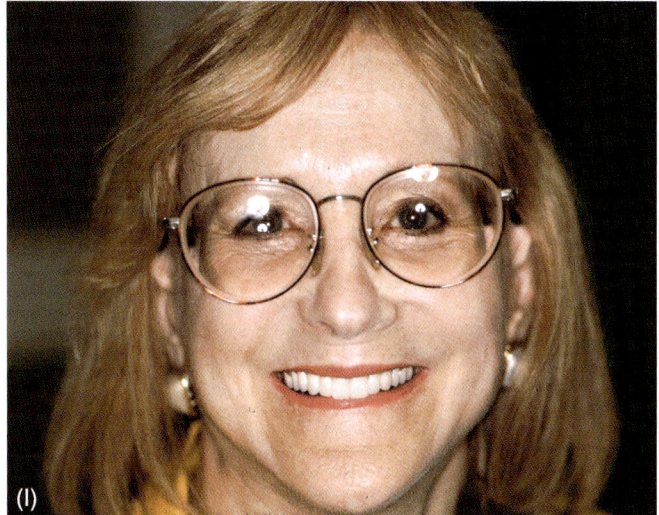

Figure 33.22 **(H–I)** Since the patient lived in a different state, it took considerable time for her to complete her therapy. Nevertheless, the patient felt the final functional teeth result was well worth the extra time and effort involved.

Chin and facial midline

Facial asymmetry can often be limited to the chin. If systematic analysis of facial symmetry reveals normal dental and skeletal midlines and vertical relationships of the maxilla but a lowered facial asymmetry, the asymmetry could possibly be isolated to the chin. Our opinion is that the chin's impact on the perceived facial midline and smile esthetics, as a midfacial structure, is smaller than the nose's tip; nonetheless, the chin cannot be neglected.

Incisal plane and interpupillary line

The incisal plane is a virtual plane that touches the incisal edges of the maxillary incisors and the tips of the cuspids in a frontal view. In this frontal plane, it can also be called the plane of occlusion. The perpendicularity of the incisal plane with the facial midline creates segregation forces that make the mouth the dominant element of the face. It is possible to evaluate the inclination of the incisal plane through a frontal full-smile facial photograph or, to be more precise, through a frontal cephalometry. Taking digital photographs with the half or three-quarter facial view just above the eyes can be very helpful.

Clinically, the interpupillary line usually is the reference line used to evaluate the orientation of the incisal plane, the gingival margin plane, and the maxilla.[12,48] Many facebow transferring systems use this horizontal reference line to relate the position of the maxilla to the cranial base; this is generally done when creating new occlusal guidances and planes of reference. Imbalances or disharmonies between the horizontal facial planes are possible and should be recognized and noted, such as the inter-ear line, interpupillary line, commissural line, and/or the horizontal line of reference.[18] Make sure you evaluate your patient in their natural head position. The best method is to have your patient either sitting straight or standing in front of a striped background with the stripes accurately demarcating the horizontal plane.

A lack of parallelism between the interpupillary line and the horizontal plane should be noted in the early stages; otherwise the facebow registration will be done using an arbitrary plane. This would directly affect the orientation of both the horizontal and vertical planes of reference of the future smile line.[18] If the natural head position is not parallel with the interpupillary line and the horizontal plane, and if the commissural line is parallel to the horizon, the commissural line should be considered as the horizontal plane of reference (Figure 33.25). If this is not corrected when transferred to the articulator, such discrepancies will show in the midline and horizontal planes, resulting in restorations that do not adhere to the principles of parallelism. Yet, if the interpupillary and commissural lines are parallel to one another but not to the horizontal plane, they can still be used as the horizontal plane of reference (Figure 33.26).

To sum up, if the interpupillary and commissural lines are not parallel to one another nor to the horizontal plane, the situation should be discussed with the patient to analyze their individual horizontal plane of conformity to the facial structures. Figure 33.8A–C shows a patient with an attractive smile who presents an interpupillary line not parallel with the commissural lines. However, the incisal plane is parallel to the commissural line, which makes the teeth appear harmonious inside the lip frame. Furthermore, the entire smile fits with the facial asymmetries, making the whole facial expression look very compatible in a natural posed smile.

In these cases, further stages are required to relate the smile to the horizontal plane. First, record the smile with the teeth and lips and reproduce it in the articulated cast to determine the soft-tissue reference. Second, relate the facebow transfer with a bite registration containing a horizontal element that would line up with the horizon. Third, adjust the provisional restorations intraorally to acquire a smile plane that is parallel to the horizontal. Fourth, use cross-mounted interchangeable casts of the provisional restorations with working casts.[18]

Another common mistake is canting the facebow while mounting it. This frequently occurs because the ear plugs of the facebow are positioned on soft tissue, which allows enough small movement to introduce a small cant of 1–2° on the incisal plane. There are two ways to avoid this problem. The first is to make a picture of the patient with the mounted facebow, which allows for detection of any cant and subsequent correction if needed. Another way is to use the digital facebow concept (see Chapter 4), which uses a calibrated and standardized frontal picture and a couple of reference points to mount the upper cast on the articulator according to the real horizontal plane determined from the picture (Figure 33.27A–D).

Some studies show that normal individuals with no pathology can present an average inclination of the occlusal plane in the frontal plane between 2.15° and 2.4°; this was without significant discrepancies between sexes.[20] Evaluating the incisal plane is

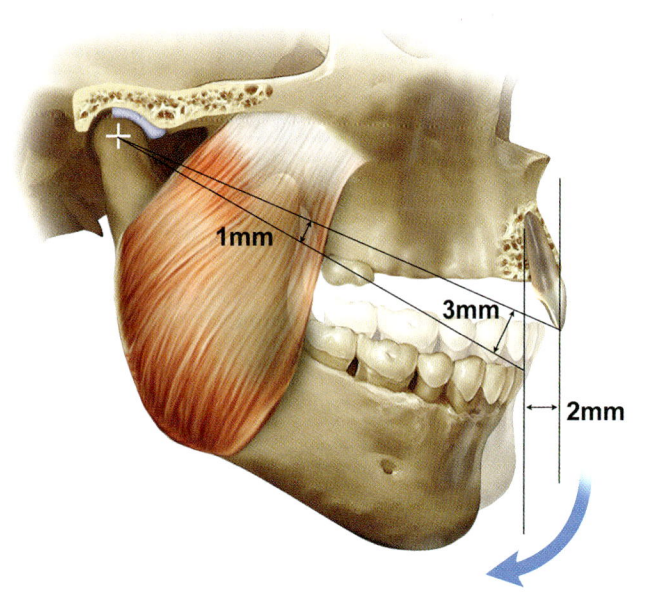

Figure 33.23 Increasing the vertical dimension of occlusion (VDO) by 3 mm in the incisal area means opening approximately 1 mm in the molar region (a 3 : 1 ratio). This 3 mm anterior opening also causes approximately 2 mm of horizontal change in overjet anteroposteriorly (a 3 : 2 ratio).

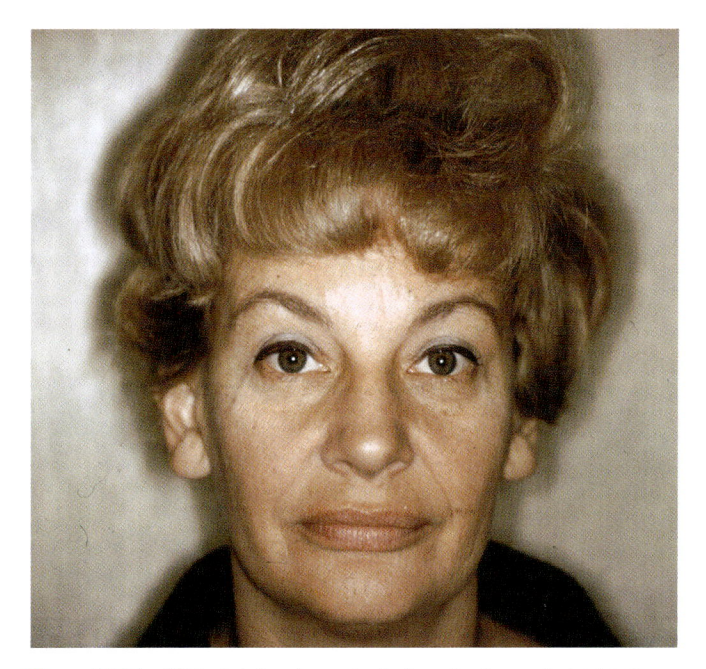

Figure 33.24 **(A)** In this brachycephalic face, the lower facial third was diminished due to severe wear and malocclusion (deep overbite).

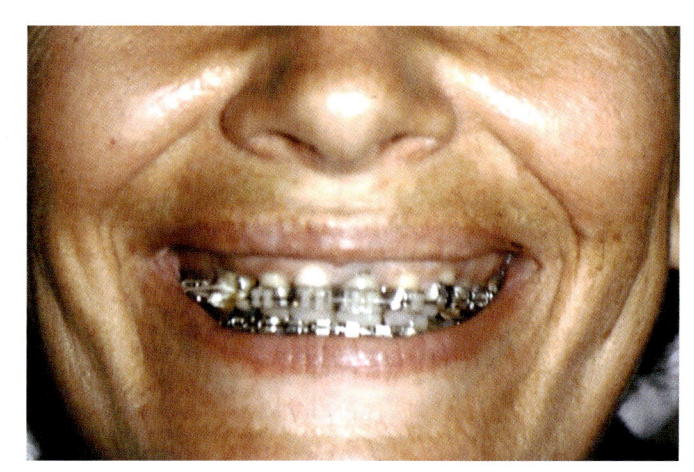

Figure 33.24 **(B)** Orthodontic treatment before final restoration improved the interocclusal relationship, allowing for better esthetics and function.

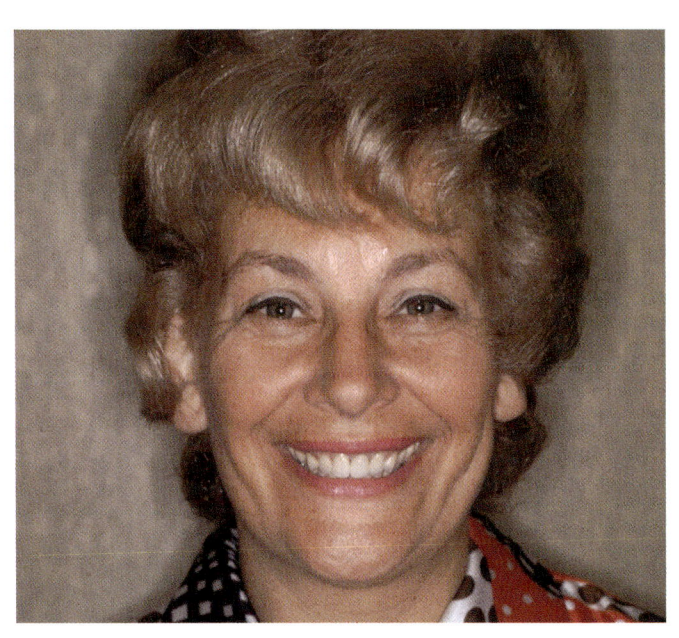

Figure 33.24 (D) Final full coverage restorations gave the patient the function and smile that she was hoping for.

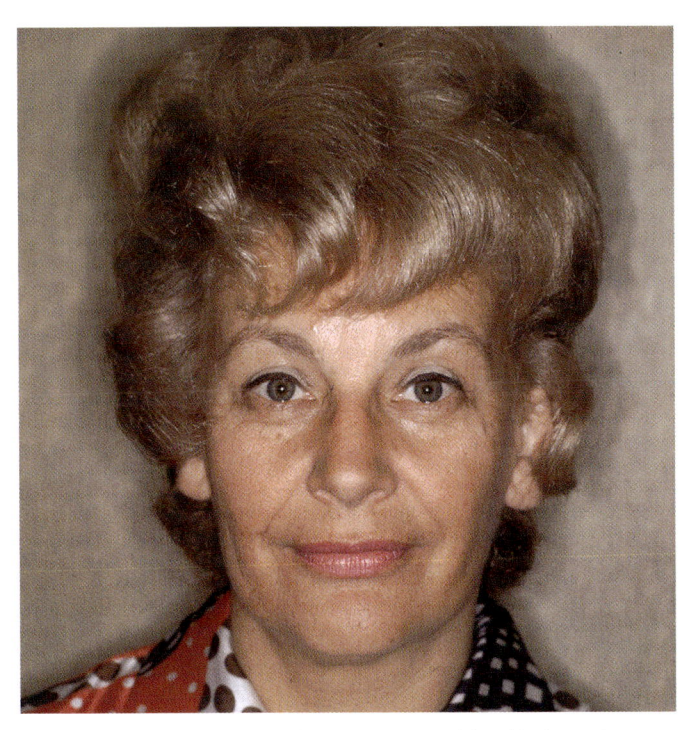

Figure 33.24 (C) Increasing the VDO improved facial balance. In more extreme cases, it may be difficult to achieve large changes in the lower third by only increasing the VDO.

important in patients with clear facial asymmetries, but also in apparently normal individuals needing extensive dental treatment. Padwa et al.[20] were the first to quantify the inclination of the plane of occlusion in the frontal plane identifiable by both laypeople and dentists. He reached the conclusion that a layperson can identify occlusal plane angulations greater than 4° in

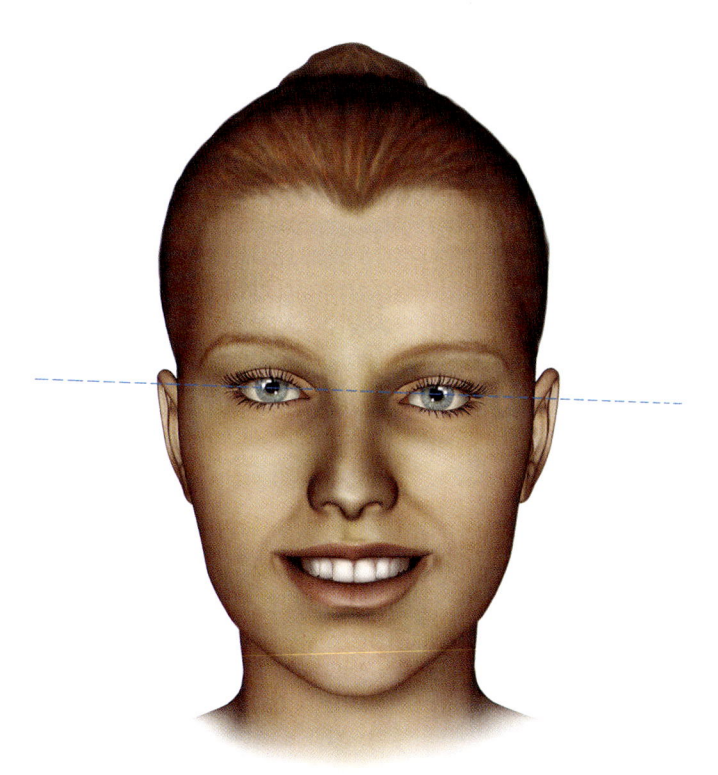

Figure 33.25 Postural head position reveals a lack of parallelism between the interpupillary line and the horizontal plane (horizon). In this situation, a facebow that parallels the interpupillary plane will result in a canted smile line. Instead, if commissural line is parallel to the horizon it should be used as the plane of reference. This must be diagnosed before treatment planning the case, so the maxillary cast can be mounted and waxed up to match the desired reference plane.

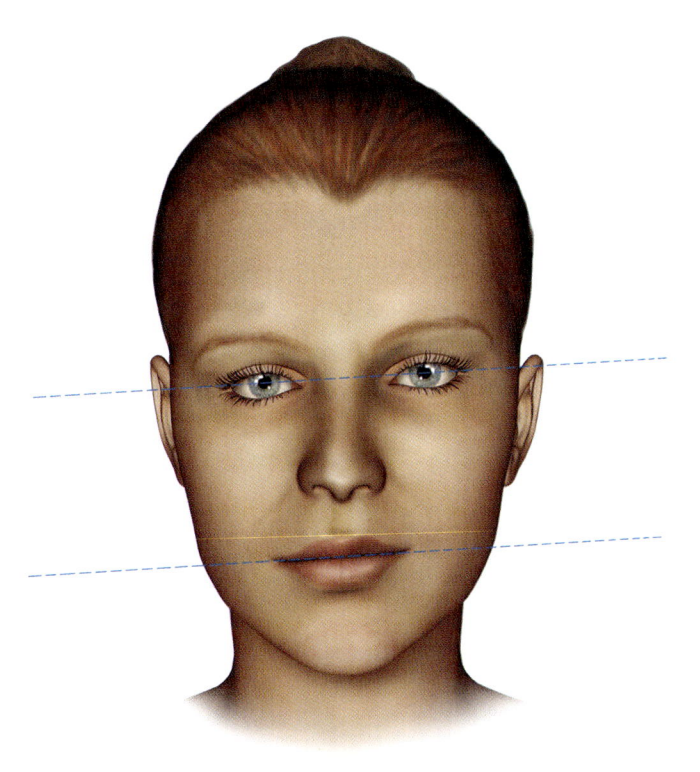

Figure 33.26 In this illustration, interpupillary and commissural lines are parallel to one another, but not parallel to the horizontal. In this situation, a thorough pretreatment diagnosis must be completed to determine the optimal plane of reference.

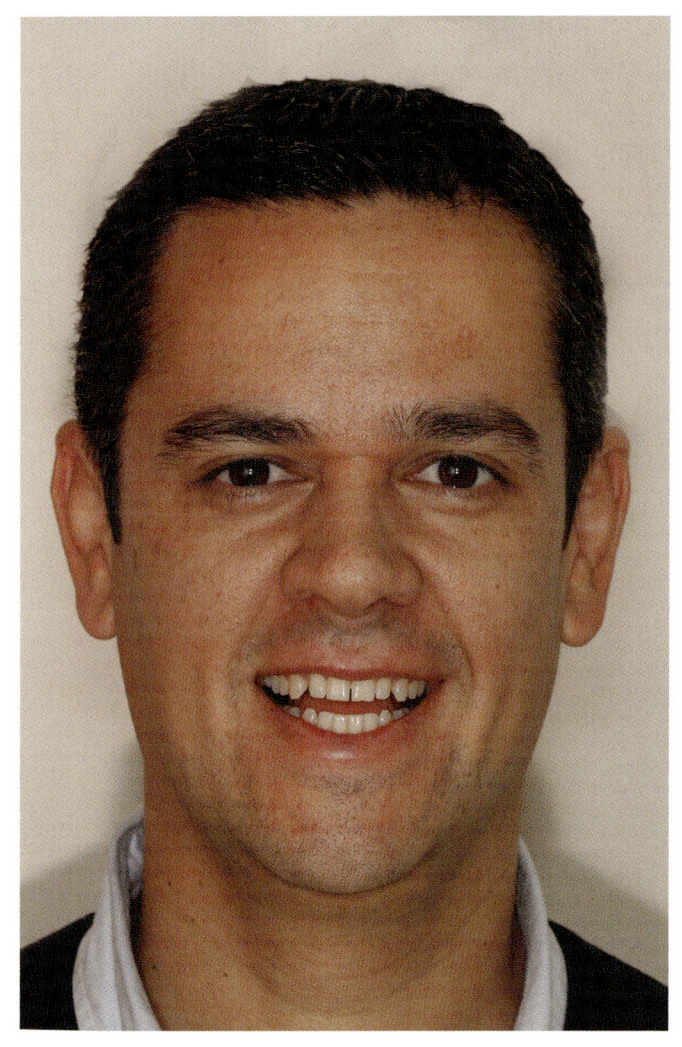

Figure 33.27 **(A)** Facial frontal picture is oriented according with the natural posture of the head. Two parallel and horizontal lines can be drawn crossing the pupils and the teeth.

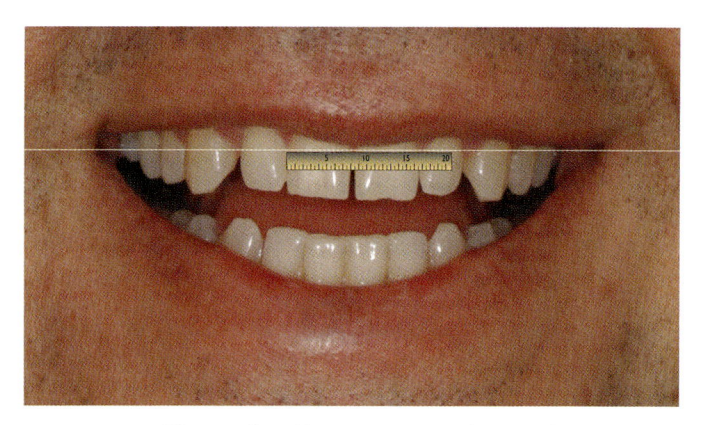

Figure 33.27 **(B)** Dentofacial frame is cropped from the facial picture. A digital ruler is calibrated according to the width from the distal to the distal of the two centrals according to what was measured with a caliper in the stone cast.

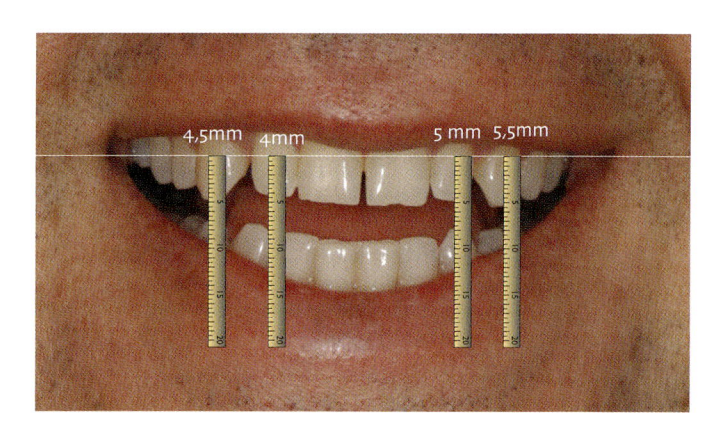

Figure 33.27 **(C)** The digital ruler is now ready to measure the distance from the incisal edges to the horizontal plane in three or four different reference points.

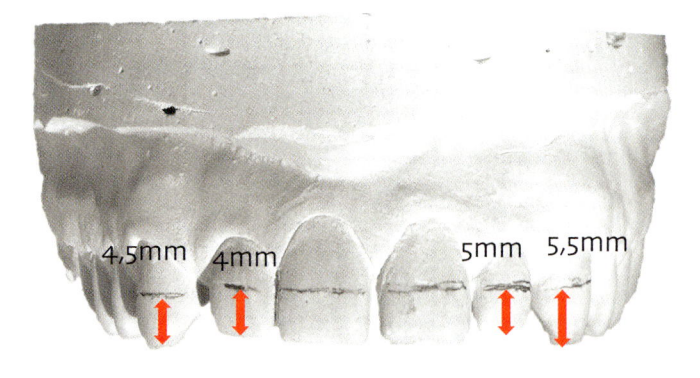

Figure 33.27 **(D)** The points are now transferred to the cast model allowing to the trace line (the real horizontal plane, determined from the facial picture). Now the model is ready to be transferred according with this plane.

90% of cases; this was such the case with 98% of the experts (Figure 33.27E–I). The reported difference between laypeople and expert observers was not statistically significant, which suggests that the clinical identification of occlusal canting depends on the canting degree rather than necessarily on the dental qualification of the observer. According to Padwa et al.'s conclusions,[20] over 50% of the population can recognize an occlusal inclination of just 2°, and apparently symmetric patients can have an occlusal canting that ranges from 0° to 2.4° (Figure 33.27E–I).[20] Finally, it must be noted that transverse tilting of the maxilla is generally accompanied by mandibular asymmetry.

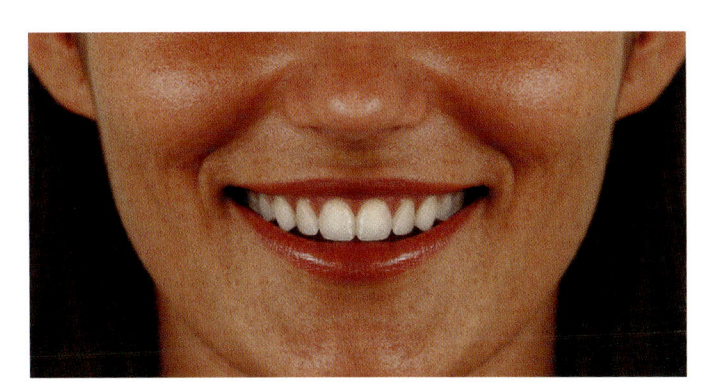

Figure 33.27 (E) Incisal plane parallel with the horizontal plane.

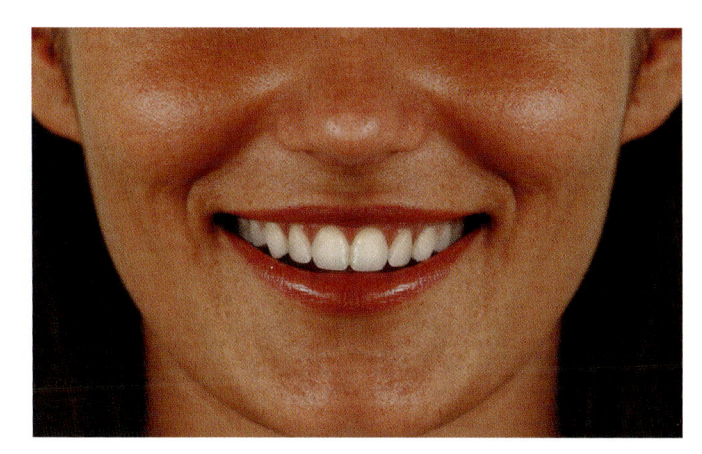

Figure 33.27 (F) Incisal plane cant 2°.

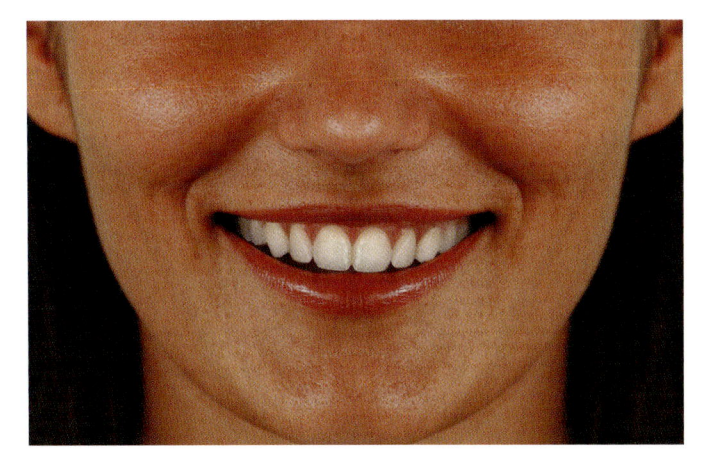

Figure 33.27 (G) Incisal plane cant 3°.

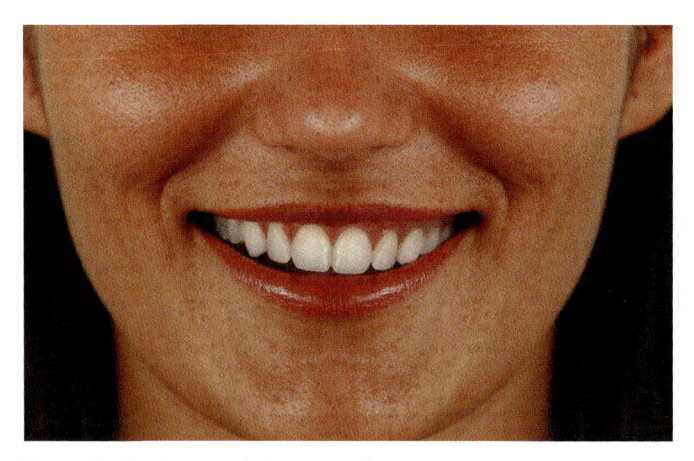

Figure 33.27 (H) Incisal plane cant 4°.

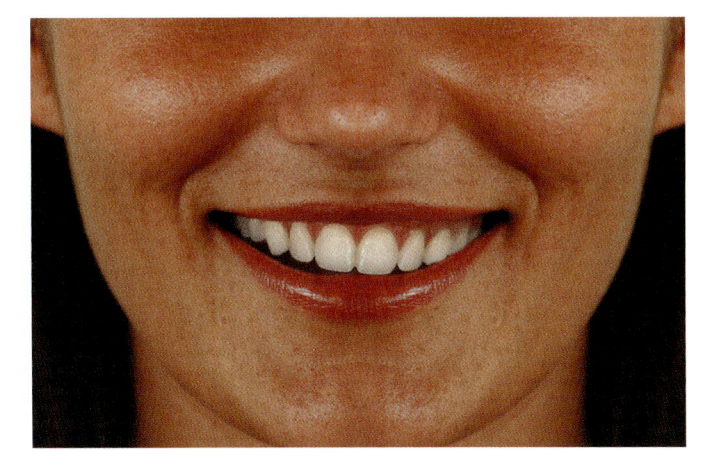

Figure 33.27 (I) Incisal plane cant 5°.

Lip symmetry

Lip symmetry should be assessed while in both rest and function. It is relatively common to find completely symmetric lips when at rest that lose their symmetry when they perform functions like smiling. These situations are much more frequent nowadays with the increased popularity of Botox or other esthetic lip treatments. These asymmetries are often unesthetic due to the irregular tooth exposure between the right and left sides (Figure 33.28A and B).

Attention should be drawn to labial commissures that do not have the same height, as they will cause one of the main facial reference lines, the commissural line, to be canted. This must be diagnosed from the beginning to avoid using the wrong horizontal reference plane. As was said before, these cases require further steps and discussion with the patient to analyze their individual horizontal plane of conformity to the facial structures. In some cases, it may be appropriate to take the commissural line as a reference point while maintaining the parallelism of the incisal curve with the lip frame, as long as harmony with the other facial structures is not broken (Figure 33.8A–D). In other cases, the interpupillary line, or even a mean between both reference lines, is more indicated. In summation, each case should be individually assessed and supplemented by a good diagnostic wax-up with a mock-up, which immensely aids both clinician and patient in making a decision.

Another phenomenon is the rising of the lip higher on one side than on the other upon smiling (Figure 33.28A and B). This particular patient, however, could use much less lip coloring—or a lighter shade—to deemphasize the mouth. The arch of the lip on the left side should not be accentuated. Rather, coloring should be applied straight across to make the arch much less noticeable.

Lip irregularities combined with arch asymmetry can compound any esthetic restoration. Thus, it is absolutely essential to communicate the problem to the patient so that they thoroughly understand the nature of the deformity and the best options available to correct it. If there are no favorable options available,

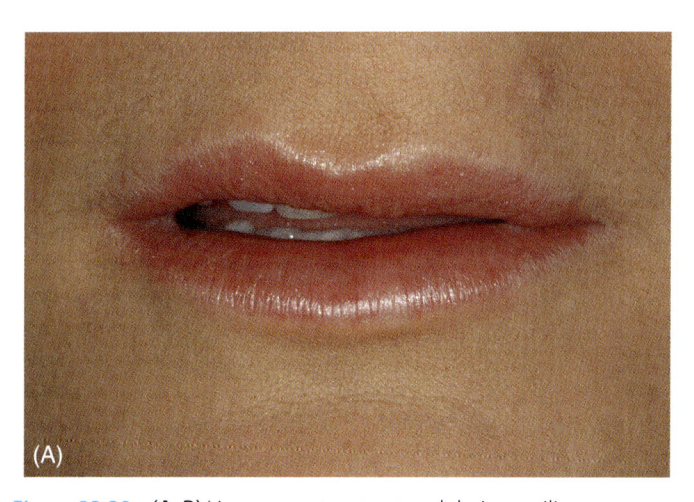

Figure 33.28 (A, B) Lip asymmetry at rest and during smiling.

then it is important to let your patient know to what degree you can help them. The result will obviously be an esthetic compromise, and there should be no surprises at the end of the treatment. This is definitely the time to plan one or more methods to let the patient know what to expect. This can be done via esthetic imaging, a pretreatment trial smile, and/or a treatment trial smile. The first two are preferred, since a different option can be easily presented if the patient is not satisfied with the proposed treatment plan. The rule "no treatment is better than the wrong treatment" definitely applies here.

Excess mucosal tissue can make the mouth unattractive (Figure 33.29A); scar tissue can also create an unattractive lip line (Figure 33.29B). Both conditions are treatable by plastic surgery. Patients with this condition should make the eyes the focal point of the face and deemphasize the mouth, achievable by using little or no lip coloring and more eye makeup (Figure 33.29C).

Be sure to carefully document every detail you explain to your patient, as well as everything your patient tells you. This is a good indication for a consultation to be recorded using video so that there can be no misunderstanding about what is and is not promised or even implied.

Lip length

The lengths of the upper and lower lips can aid in establishing a differential diagnosis between an anatomically short upper lip and a vertical maxillary excess. To accurately assess lip length,

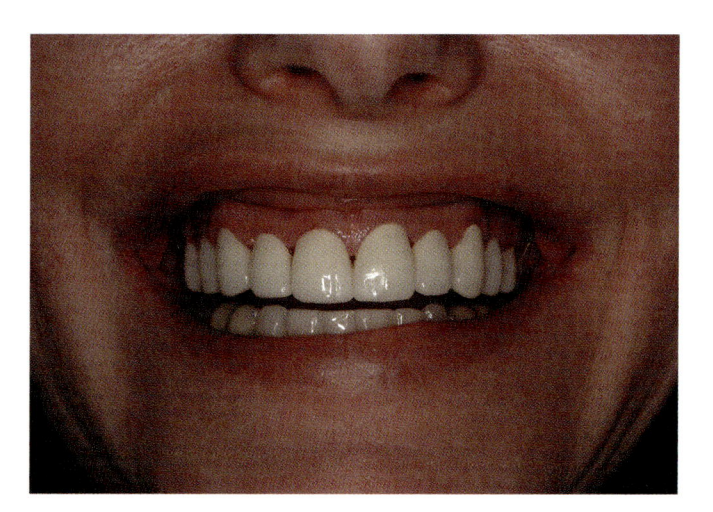

Figure 33.29 (A) Excess mucosal tissue on the patient's lip detracts from her smile.

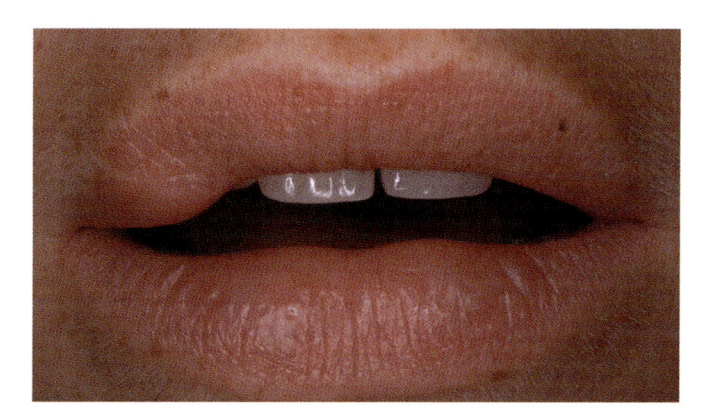

Figure 33.29 (B) Scar tissue shows how it affects the lip line.

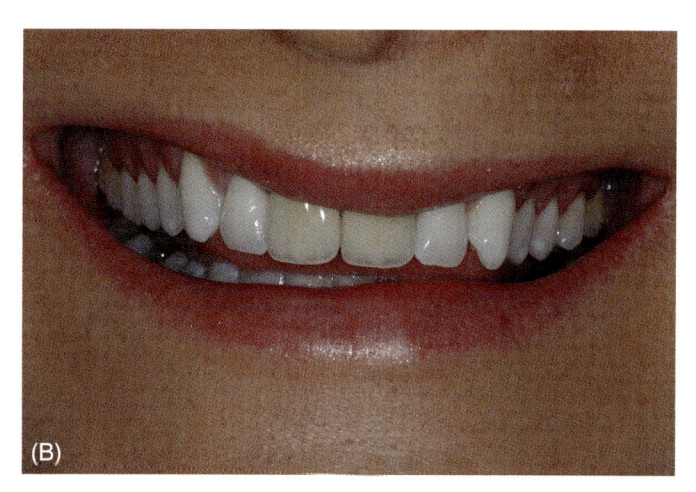

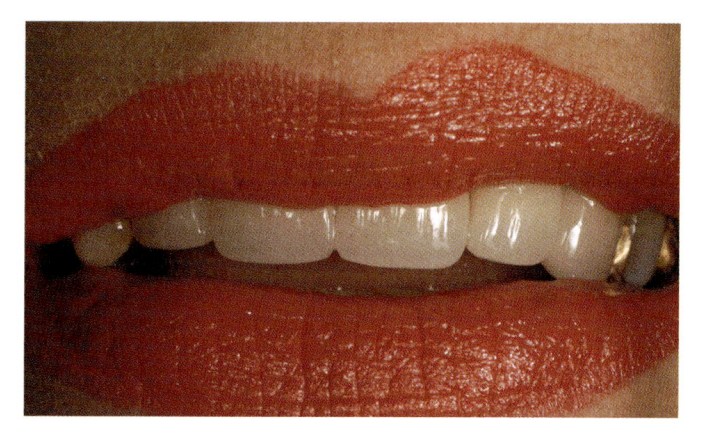

Figure 33.29 (C) An asymmetric lip line affects the appearance of the smile. In this case, the lady would help her appearance if she altered the height of her lipstick.

the lips must be at rest without tooth contact. The lips should be measured separately in a relaxed frontal position. The normal length from the subnasale to the upper lip in a young adult is between 19 and 22 mm.[31] An upper lip of 18 mm or less is considered to be short and is generally accompanied by increased incisor exposure and an interlabial gap with a normal lower facial height.[31] This should not be confused with vertical maxillary excess, where the interlabial gap, incisor exposure, and lower third facial height are increased.[31]

The lower lip is measured from the superior border of the lower lip to the soft-tissue menton point, and it normally measures 38–44 mm. The normal ratio of the upper to lower lip is 1 : 2.[31] The association between an anatomic short lower lip and a Class II malocclusion is frequent and can be verified measuring the lower anterior dental height on the cephalometry (lower incisor tip to hard-tissue menton; women 40 ± 2 mm, and men 44 ± 2 mm).[31] A difference should be made between an anatomically short lower lip and a short lower lip secondary to posture when the upper incisors interfere with the lower lip; this is generally associated with a Class II deep overbite. The plastic surgery procedure known as a genioplasty can be performed to lengthen an anatomic short lip.

Lips at rest position and interlabial gap

The interlabial gap with lips at rest should be 1–5 mm (the distance between the inferior edge of the upper lip and the superior edge of the lower lip). Women usually tend to show a larger gap than men. The interlabial gap may be larger in situations where there is an anatomic short upper lip, vertical maxillary excess, and/or a mandibular protrusion with an open bite due to cusp interferences.[63] A decreased interlabial gap is found with vertical maxillary deficiency, anatomically long upper lip, or mandibular retrusion with a deep bite. In any of these cases, the restorative dentist cannot do much to change the interlabial gap.

Closed lip position

To improve the diagnostic patterns and to be able to detect disharmonies between skeletal, dentition, and soft-tissue length, it is necessary to thoroughly understand the closed lip position. Increased mentalis muscle contraction, lip strain, and alar base narrowing are observed when the vertical dimension is increased far from what is recommended; this can also happen in cases with vertical skeletal excess (Figure 33.21A–C), anatomic short upper lip, and some cases of mandibular protrusion with an open bite. Lip redundancy can be found when patients have lost vertical occlusion; it can also be associated in some cases of mandibular protrusion with a deep bite.

Facial analysis: oblique view

The oblique view provides information that is not obtainable on the frontal view about spatial relations between the maxilla and mandible in a facial three-dimensional context. The occlusal plane can sometimes be canted anteroposteriorly and therefore not be consonant with the inner curvature of the lower lip.

Lip anatomy should be analyzed from both an oblique and a profile view. The height of the philtrum should be noted as short, balanced, or excessive, and the vermillion display can be easily evaluated from this view as excessive, balanced, or thin. This perspective adds valuable data about how teeth relate with perioral tissues at rest and in function (see "Dentofacial analysis" page 1119). Therefore, pictures and video should also be taken in both left and right oblique views, approximately at 45°. This is important to do because in most social encounters we only briefly look at people's faces from a frontal perspective. However, the rest of the time we socialize from different oblique angles.

Facial analysis: profile view

Profile analysis is conducted while the head is in its natural position.[11,30,31,56,64] The patient should be instructed to look straight ahead, possibly looking for their own image in a mirror. The natural head position can be checked using the Frankfort plane (the most inferior orbit point with external auditory meatus) as reference; usually this plane makes an 8° angle with the horizontal.[64]

Profile angle

The facial profiles are evaluated based on the relative sagittal position of the maxilla and mandible with the glabella. The angle formed by the glabella, subnasale, and soft-tissue pogonion allows the appraisal of general harmony of the lower third.[11,30,31,56,64] Class I dental and skeletal relationships present an angle range of 165–175° with a slightly convex facial plane. Class II angles are less than 165°, giving a greater convex appearance. Those characteristics of Class III are greater than 175° and show a concave relationship of these three points.[30,31] Class II angulation includes maxillary protrusion (rare), vertical maxillary excess (common), and mandibular retrusion (common). Class III relationship includes maxillary retrusion (common), vertical maxillary deficiency (rare), and mandibular protrusion. Several studies have analyzed the profile differences among races[48] and have found that North Europeans tend to show posterior divergence while Native Americans frequently present anterior divergence.[48]

In order to produce a more comfortable intercuspation position, it is crucial to first establish a differential diagnosis of a Class III VDO (due to skeletal relationship) or a pseudo-Class III (secondary to dental interference or lack of posterior teeth) which leads to an anterior mandibular rotation. Some patients with loss of VDO can exhibit a concave profile that resembles a skeletal Class III relationship for the same reason as a pseudo-Class III: the anterior rotation of the mandible into maximum intercuspation. In these cases, restoring the VDO will decrease the overbite and increase the overjet as the mandible rotates back to centric relation, creating space for lengthening the teeth. This can be clinically checked before treatment using a composite resin mock-up and assessment of phonetics, occlusion, and facial esthetics (Figure 33.30A–D).

Excessive convex and concave facial profiles cannot be changed restoratively. Patients who seek esthetic treatment to change these conditions should be referred to an orthodontist or an oral surgeon.

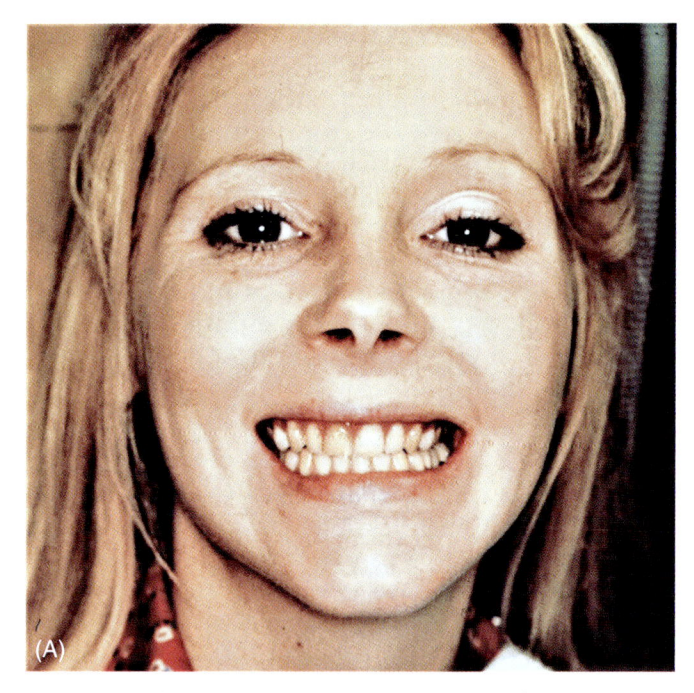

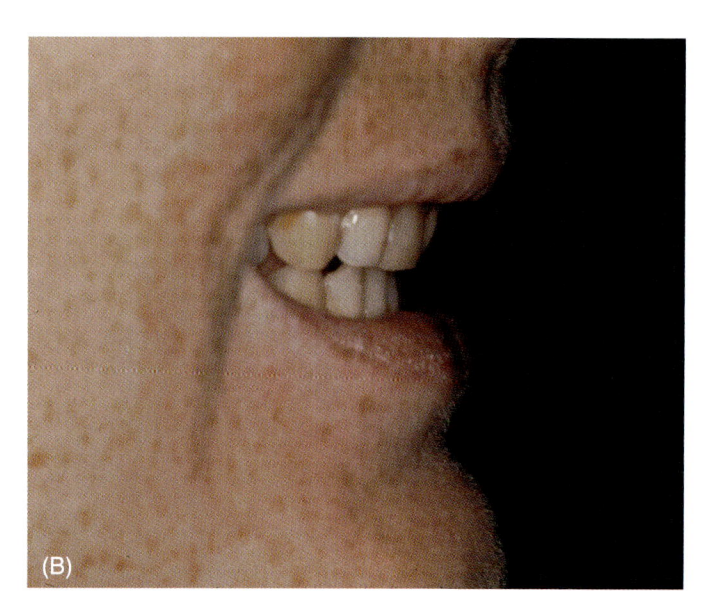

Figure 33.30 (A, B) This young lady had a convex profile complicated by her lingually slanted maxillary interiors.

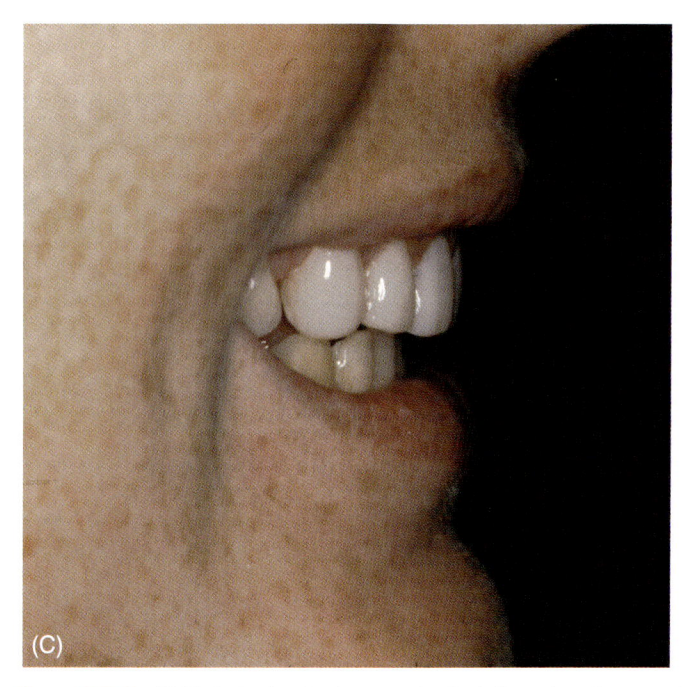

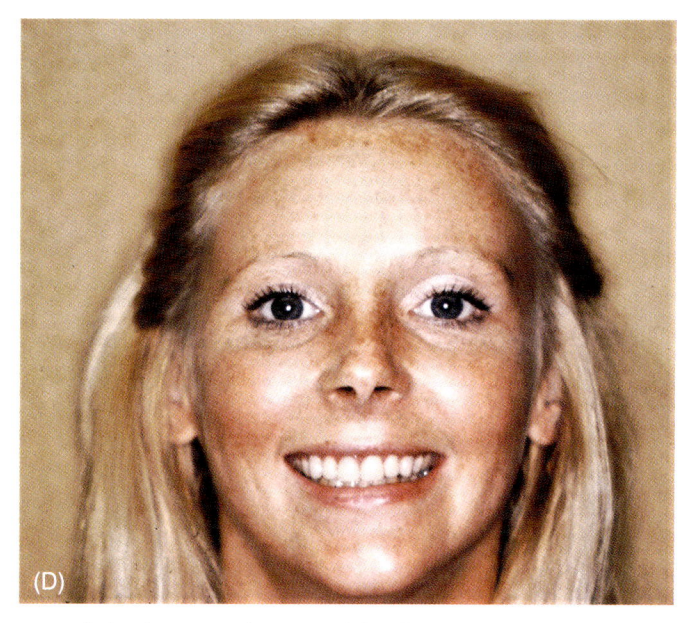

Figure 33.30 (C, D) Orthodontic therapy plus final direct-bond composite veneers helped improve the patient's facial appearance.

Nasolabial angle

Figure 33.31 shows the nasolabial angle, formed by connecting the columella to the subnasale and upper lip anterior point. It allows for the evaluation of the lip position on a sagittal plane and also gives some information about skeletal and dental relationships. There are significant sex differences: female patients usually show a more obtuse angle (100–105°) than males (90–95°). Some authors have found significant differences between Caucasians (who presented mean values between 102° and 110°) and Koreans (93°), Chinese (92°), and African Americans (90°), who presented significant inferior values for the nasolabial angle.[48]

Restorative dentistry alone can have a slight effect on the nasolabial angle and lip position because both are determined by several factors: the anteroposterior position of the maxilla, anteroposterior position of the maxillary incisors, vertical position or rotation of the nasal tip, and soft-tissue thickness of the maxillary lip, which contributes to the nasolabial angle. Restorative

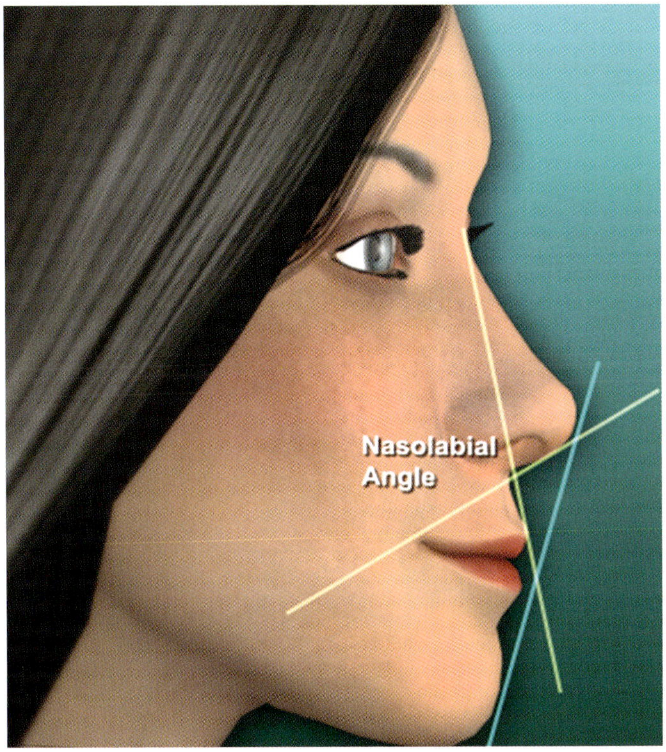

Figure 33.31 The nasolabial angle is formed by connecting columella to subnasale and upper lip anterior point. It allows the evaluation of the lip position on a sagittal plane, and also gives some information about skeletal and dental relationships.

dentistry can only change one factor: the anteroposterior tooth position. It is important to know that the lower half of the upper lip is supported by alveolar bone and by the gingival two-thirds of the maxillary incisors; this means that the incisal third and the incisal edge position have a minimal effect on lip position.

The patient's profile, nasolabial angle, and lip position can suggest the size/dominance of maxillary anterior restorations. If the maxilla is prominent and the nasolabial angle is less than 85°, or the profile is convex, consider using smaller and less dominant anterior restorations to naturally balance the esthetic convexity of the patient's profile.[64] On the contrary, more dominant anterior restorations can have an esthetic impact on concave profiles.[64] Whereas orthognathic or plastic surgery combined with orthodontics is usually the ideal treatment, orthodontics plus lighter shaded direct composite resin bonding can make an improved facial appearance (Figure 33.30A–D).

Orthodontic and orthognathic treatments are the only means to achieve major lip repositioning. Plastic surgery can be used to fill out lip contour and decrease the nasolabial angle or to correct an inferior border of the nose that gives an abnormal nasolabial angle. In an esthetic face, the inferior border of the nose is canted slightly above the horizontal from the base of the nose to the tip. In circumstances where the nose tip cants downward below the horizontal, changes to the nasolabial angle may be desired, in which case plastic surgery is the appropriate treatment.

A profile dominated by a disharmonious nose shape or size can seriously limit esthetic improvement by dental intervention, and therefore should be evaluated for correction by the plastic surgeon. However, there are patients who prefer the strong influence of the shape of their nose; thus, any change in the arch alignment may negatively alter the facial balance. In this situation, the patient must be thoroughly informed about all the treatment possibilities and variances. Figure 33.32A–C shows the profile of a young lady who was concerned about her slightly protruding porcelain laminates but who liked the shape of her nose. Although orthodontic treatment would ordinarily be the choice of correction, computer imaging revealed that her nose would be out of proportion to her face after orthodontic correction. Unless she had both the teeth and nose treated, she would be better off without any correction.

Lip position and projection

The esthetic nature of the face is such that the lips play a major role. Lip position not only controls facial expression but also influences the beauty of the face. Several factors influence the appearance of the lips. To begin with, the size of the lips can influence the patient's perception of the selected tooth shade. For instance, when patients with very large thick lips speak or smile slightly, there is a shadow created by the lip that can make a light tooth appear darker. This also means it is imperative to know if a patient with thin lips has any desire to have the lips enhanced. If so, suggest a lighter shade than you would normally do and let the patient know why.

People display their teeth in four basic ways when they smile. They may show only their maxillary teeth, only their mandibular teeth, both, or neither. To restore esthetics, it is important to attempt to preserve or restore the patient's best smiling position. The appearance of the entire face is affected by lip position. For example, the relative prominence of the chin can be influenced by lip position. If the lower lip protrudes, the prominence of the chin is diminished. The converse is also true. If the lower lip is retrusive, the chin appears more prominent. The prominence of the nose is affected in the same way, but by the position of the upper lip. The patient may have acquired abnormal lip mannerisms in speaking or smiling for any of the following reasons: in an attempt to hide bad teeth, because of a collapsed bite, or because of lost or reduced occlusion or other type of malocclusion. These habits affect how the teeth are viewed and may not disappear, even with complete occlusal rehabilitation (Figure 33.33A–F). Patients may also develop unnatural occlusal relationships to hide a retrusive or rather asymmetrical jaw. They develop these detrimental habits because they either consciously or unconsciously see improved facial shape by doing so; furthermore, it is not uncommon to find temporomandibular joint problems in these patients.

Sagittal lip position can be esthetically evaluated using one of the published reference lines[3,12,30,31,42,44,64] (Figure 33.33G). "The relationship of the lips relative to these lines can be helpful in the diagnosis and treatment planning of the position of anterior teeth and the alveolus. The use of these lines will demonstrate if the lips are anterior or posterior to the ideal, giving an indication as to the positioning of the underlying teeth and alveolus. Lips that appear anterior to the reference lines generally require retraction of the teeth and/or the alveolus."[56]

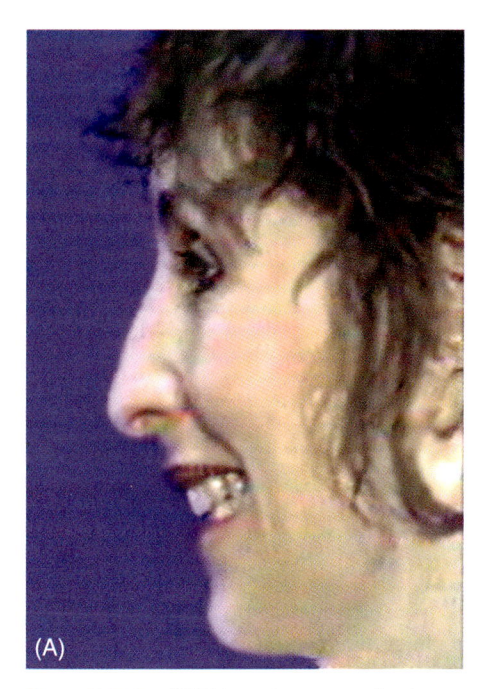

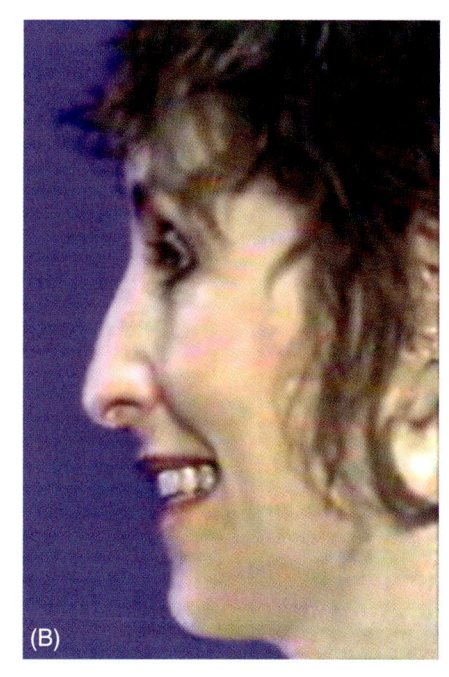

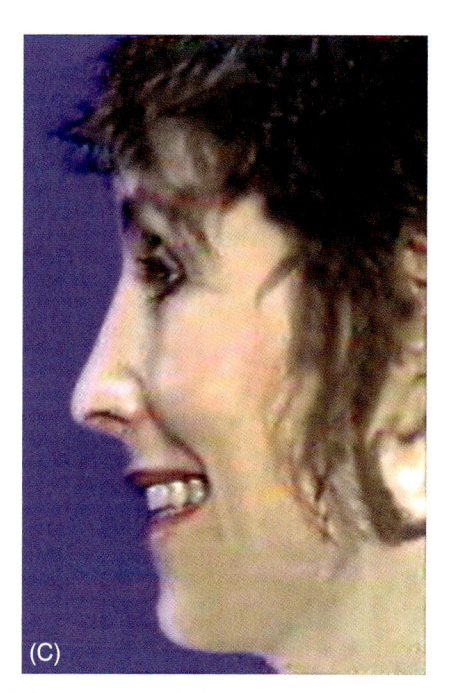

Figure 33.32 **(A)** This patient wanted to have porcelain veneers to build out her teeth, but was advised the veneers would be too thick unless orthodontic treatment was done before. **(B)** This image shows the patient that if orthodontic therapy was done it would make her nose disproportionate to her face. **(C)** Unless the patient was willing to commit to surgical correction of the nose along with orthodontic intervention, she would be better off without the orthodontic change. This photo shows the patient what the combined orthodontic, veneers, and surgical correction to her nose would look like. Since she loved her "Roman-shaped" nose, she declined any treatment.

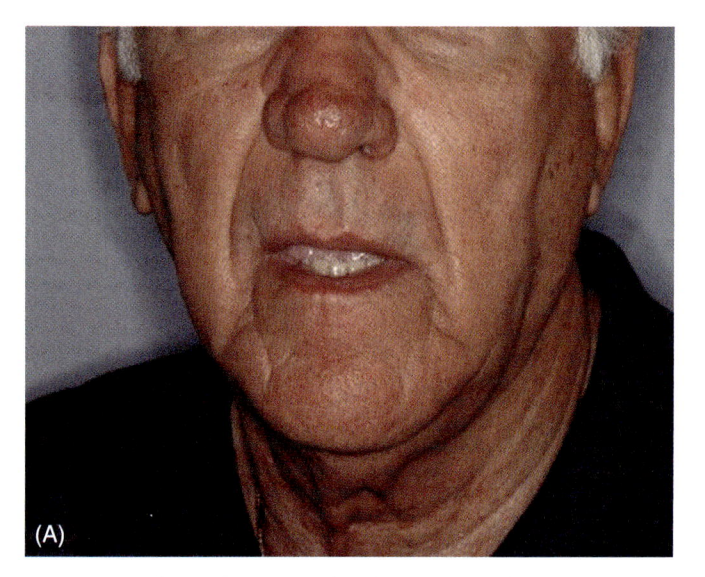

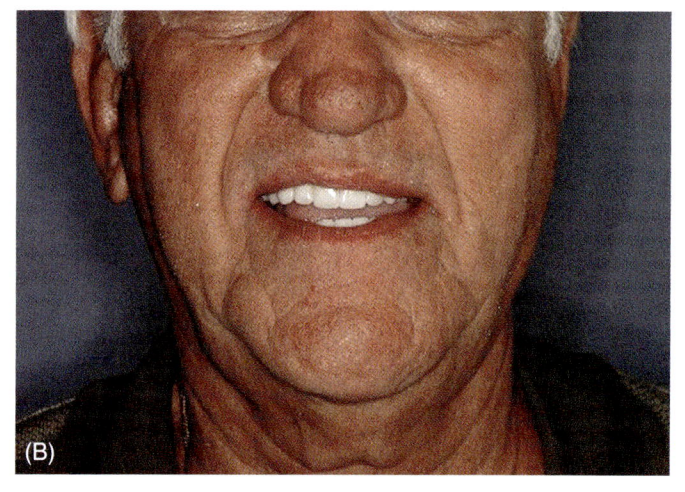

Figure 33.33 **(A, B)** This patient developed a habit of hiding his upper teeth when speaking or smiling in order to hide his Class III occlusion plus discolored and failing dental treatment.

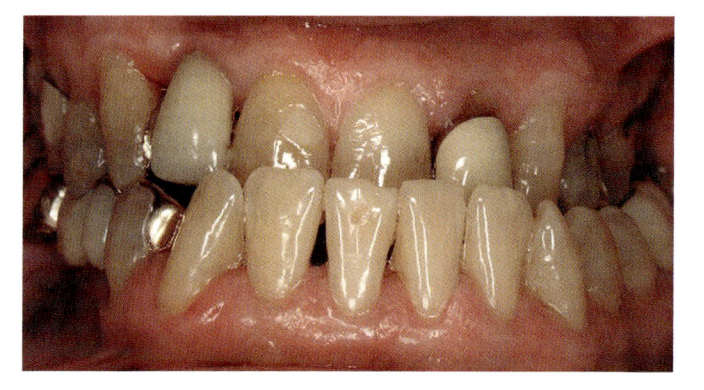

Figure 33.33 **(C)** Since the patient declined orthodontic or surgical treatment, a full mouth rehabilitation was required to stabilize function and improve esthetics.

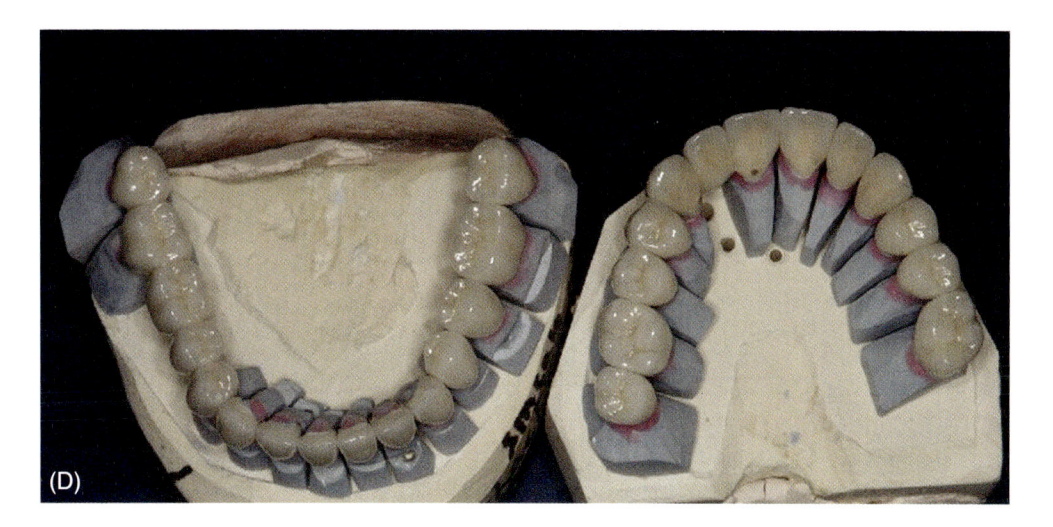

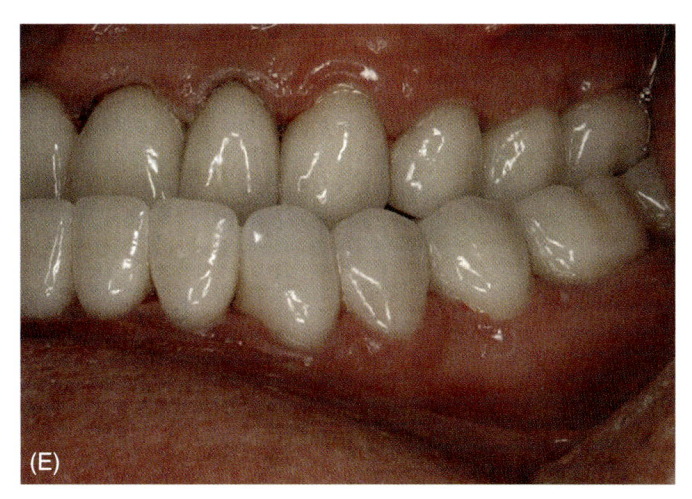

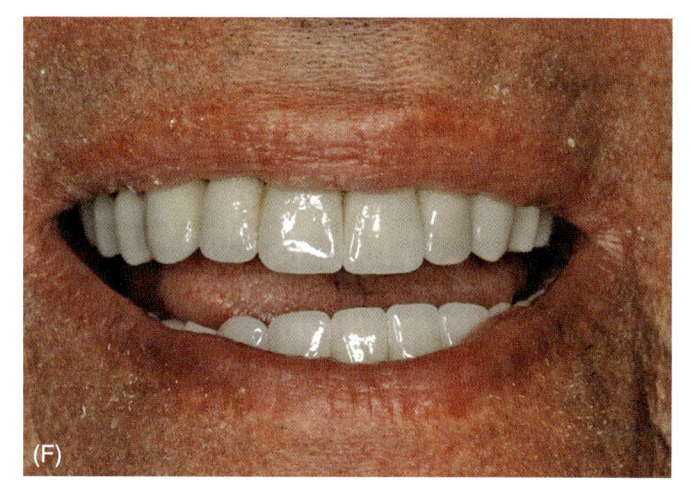

Figure 33.33 (D–F) With his new restorations, over time he grew more comfortable and was able to smile and speak with confidence.

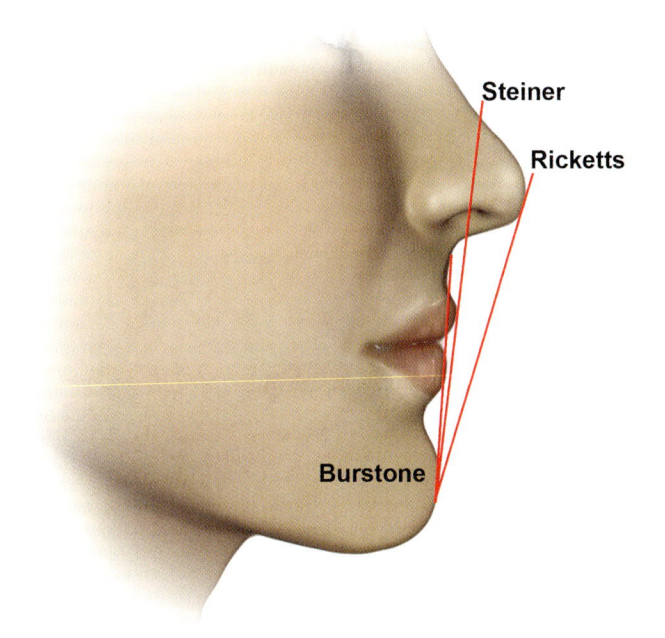

Figure 33.33 (G) Sagittal lip position can be esthetically evaluated using one of the published reference lines suggested by Ricketts, Steiner, and Burstone.

Ricketts[42] established the E-plane from the nasal tip to the chin, where in an ideal profile the upper lip should be 4 mm from this plane and lower lip 2 mm.[3,12,30,64] We recognized that significant differences may exist between sexes. Recent research[48] studied this relationship among different races and reached the conclusion that the majority of races studied (Japanese, Chinese, Korean, Hispanic) obey the Ricketts principle. However, Caucasians have shown a particularly different mean distance from the E-plane: 7.5 mm for the upper lip and 5.2 mm for the lower. Furthermore, African American lips are usually found to be anterior to the E-plane and the lower lip is more prominent than the upper lip: 0.3 mm and 2.9 mm anterior to the E-plane respectively. According to Steiner, the upper and the lower lip touch the line that connects the nose midpoint to the chin.[43] Finally, Burstone[44] established that the upper and lower lip should be 3.5 mm and 2.2 mm respectively farther from the line that connects the subnasale point to the pogonion point.

In cases where the lips seem excessively posterior to these lines, advancement of the maxilla or mandible may be required, and a referral to the orthodontist or the maxillofacial surgeon should be considered.[56] As mentioned previously, some authors argue that, in 70% of cases, lip support comes from the cervical two-thirds of the maxillary incisors. In addition, the upper lip position is determined by tooth position instead of incisal edge positioning.[72]

Ridge replacement

The location of the alveolar ridge contributes to lip support and facial appearance. Most facial deformities stem from malformations of alveolar processes, which can cause malpositioning of the teeth, lips, and cheeks. If the alveolar ridge is in a protruded or anterior position that makes the lip overextend, the removal or loss of a tooth will not provide an esthetic solution. A prominent alveolar ridge can interfere with the esthetics of any anterior restoration because the patient will show too much gingival tissue, resulting in an unpleasant smile, even if all teeth are present. In this situation, any fabricated anterior restoration will usually be prominent and noticeable. When correcting a ridge deformity, orthodontic treatment or orthognathic surgery may also be necessary to successfully create an esthetically balanced appearance.

Just as the protruded ridge causes a problem, so does the retrusive ridge. Early tooth loss can also cause ridge resorption over a period of years. When this occurs, the position of teeth in a prosthesis becomes important. It may be necessary to position the teeth anterior to the ridge to gain good lip support. Alternatively, it may be necessary to position the teeth in a labial inclination, depending on the relationship of the anterior teeth to the lips. Adequate lip support is essential to compensate for the retruded position of the ridges and the subsequent facial profile around the area of the oral cavity. Figure 33.34 shows the labial inclination of the maxillary anterior teeth that achieves an esthetic lip position in the Class III patient.

A major alternative treatment for ridge resorption is ridge augmentation surgery. Several types of surgical procedures can be attempted. The ridge should be viewed from two perspectives: horizontal and vertical. Horizontally, it is rather facile to see where the ideal ridge position should be. Much harder to see is the "trench-like" deformity left by tooth extraction that can best be seen by looking from the incisal aspect. Both deformities can be repaired through ridge augmentation (see Chapter 37).

Tooth position

Relative tooth position in the arch is a determinant of lip position. A change in the teeth—occlusion, type, size, position, or vertical or horizontal overlap—may alter the facial appearance. A dramatic example is one of a patient who cannot close their lips when the teeth are at rest or in centric relation or severe protrusion (Figure 33.4A and B).

The relationship between the upper and lower lips is also influenced by the degree of overjet and overbite. Excessive overjet can make the lips protrude. Excessive overbite can contribute to the loss of vertical facial height, collapse of the lips, and wrinkling around the corners of the mouth.

Labiomental angle

Defined by the curve of soft tissue between the lower lip and the chin, the labiomental angle can vary greatly in form and depth.[11,31] The mandibular sulcus contour can be affected by the

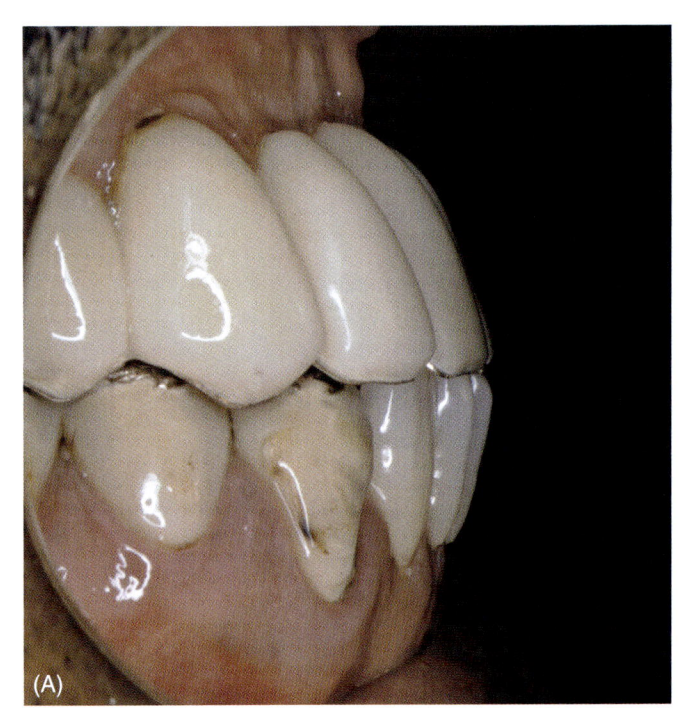

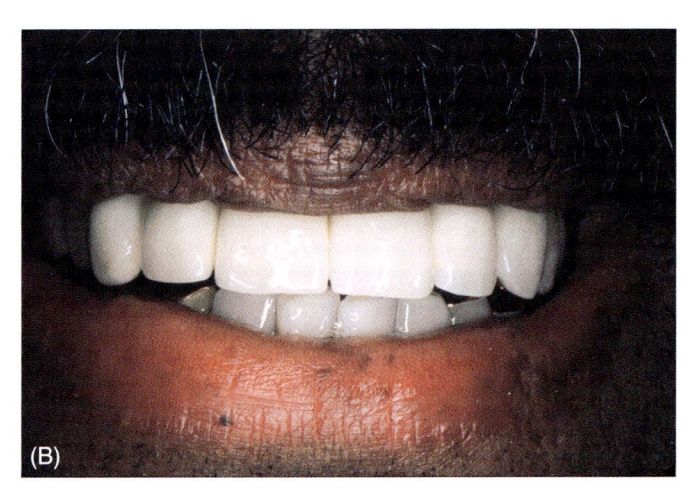

Figure 33.34 **(A, B)** In this gentleman's dental rehabilitation, a labial inclination of the maxillary incisors makes up for a deficient alveolar ridge. This provides lip support, as well as an esthetic relationship between the maxillary and mandibular dentition. However, other surgical and orthodontic treatments should also be considered when treatment planning a case such as this.

lower incisor position and lower facial height.[11] Upright incisors will result in a shallow labiomental angle due to the lack of lower lip support; on the contrary, excessive proclination of lower incisors will deepen the contour. If the lower facial height is decreased for any of the aforementioned reasons, the result will usually be a deeper labiomental fold.[11]

Dentofacial analysis

The relationship between the incisal edges of the upper incisors, the lower and upper lips, and the gingival margins of the maxillary incisors is a key feature of facial esthetics. The natural postural head position should also be used in dentofacial analysis.

Tooth exposure at rest

The amount of tooth exposure at rest should be evaluated from a frontal view with the patient standing in an upright position. The mandible should be at rest, lips slightly apart in the rest position, and teeth not touching. Sometimes it is difficult getting the patient into the rest position while being able to take a good picture. For this reason, video is definitely the best method to evaluate how the patient gets into rest position in a completely natural matter. A rehabilitation plan involving tooth position references that have been lost requires considerations of the upper and the lower lips and the incisor exposure as reference points.

The incisor exposure at rest is one of the main factors that can be used to determine incisal edge position. This will be determined by considering the age and sex of the patient, the length and curvature of the upper lip, and the clinical crown length.[73] The average anatomic crown length values for the maxillary central incisor are 10.5 ± 1 mm.[74] A central incisor that can be seen when smiling but not at rest will give the appearance of an older face (Figure 33.35A–B).

Vig and Brundo[75] demonstrated how the degree of dental exposure is a dynamic element throughout life. The clinician should be aware that the amount of maxillary teeth exposure at rest decreases throughout life, while mandibular teeth exposure increases. Vig and Brundo[75] studied the relationship between the incisor exposure through resting lips with aging and came to the conclusion that time is a major factor on the amount of this exposure. The average 20-year-old exposes 3.5 mm of the maxillary incisors and none or very little of the mandibular teeth. The muscles and perioral tissues become increasingly lax with age, reducing the amount of maxillary incisors displayed and increasing the visibility of the mandibular incisors. The laxness starts

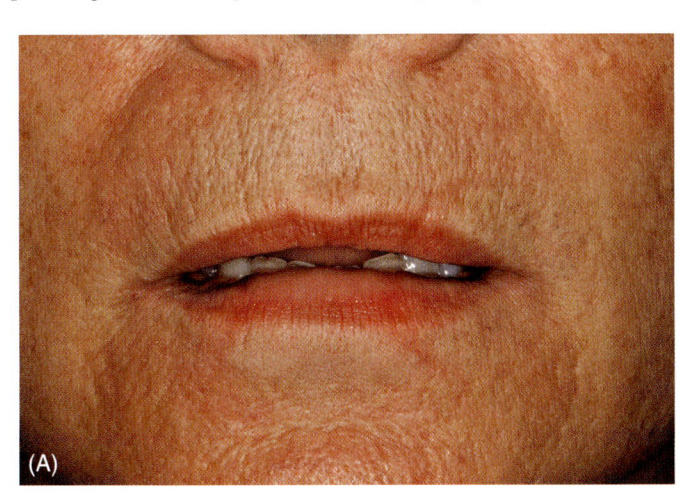

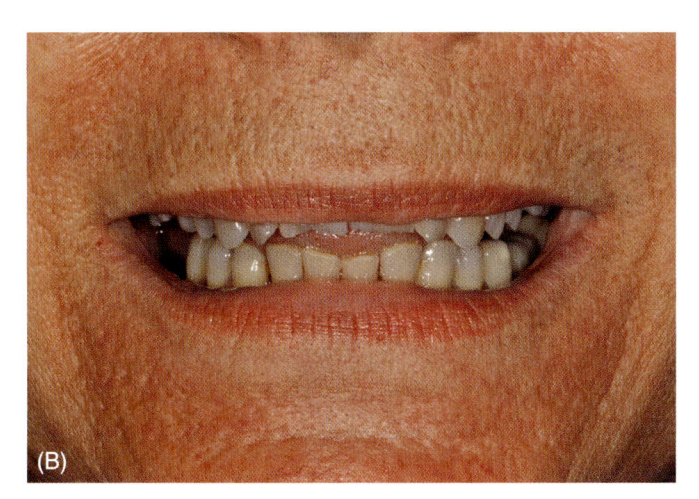

Figure 33.35 **(A–B)** Reduced visibility of the maxillary incisors both at rest and smiling due to extreme tooth wear.

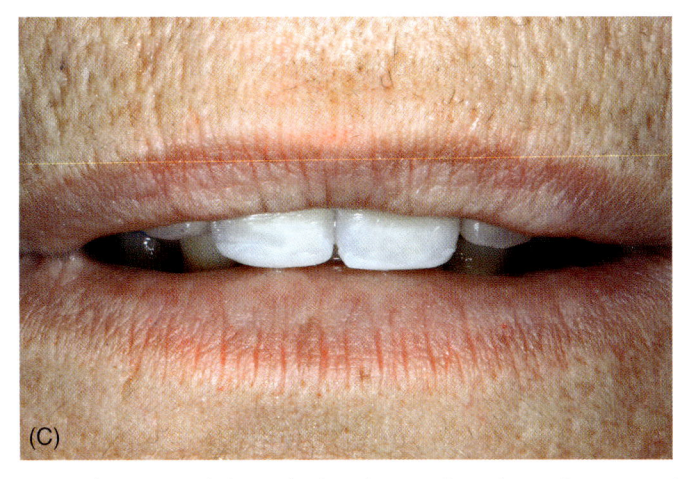

Figure 33.35 **(C)** Quick direct composite mock-up on teeth (#8 and #9), without etching the teeth to assess the incisal edge lengthening esthetically and functionally (phonetics).

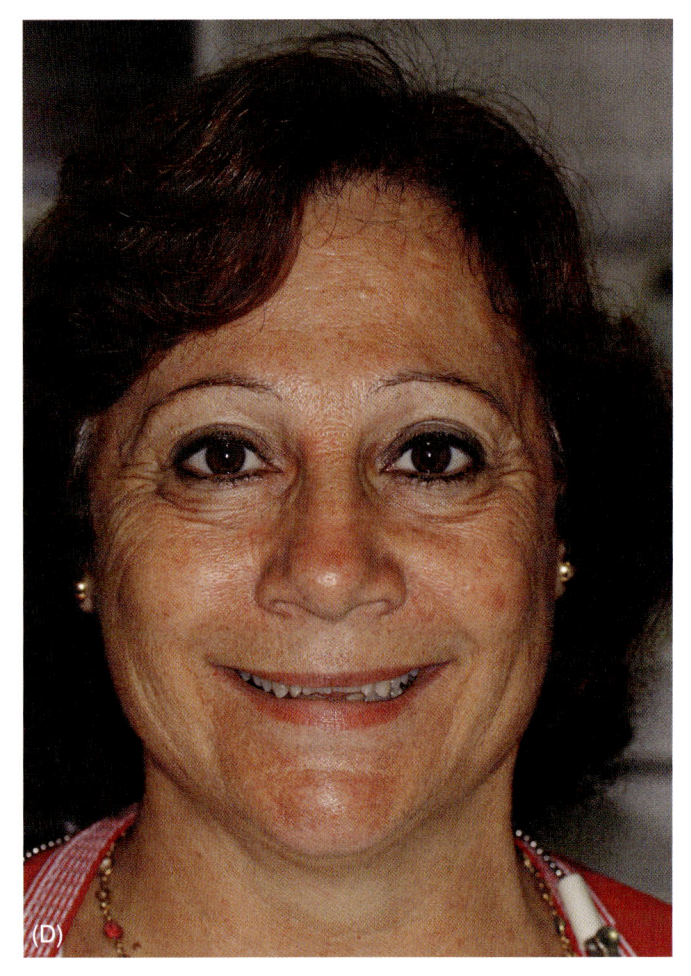

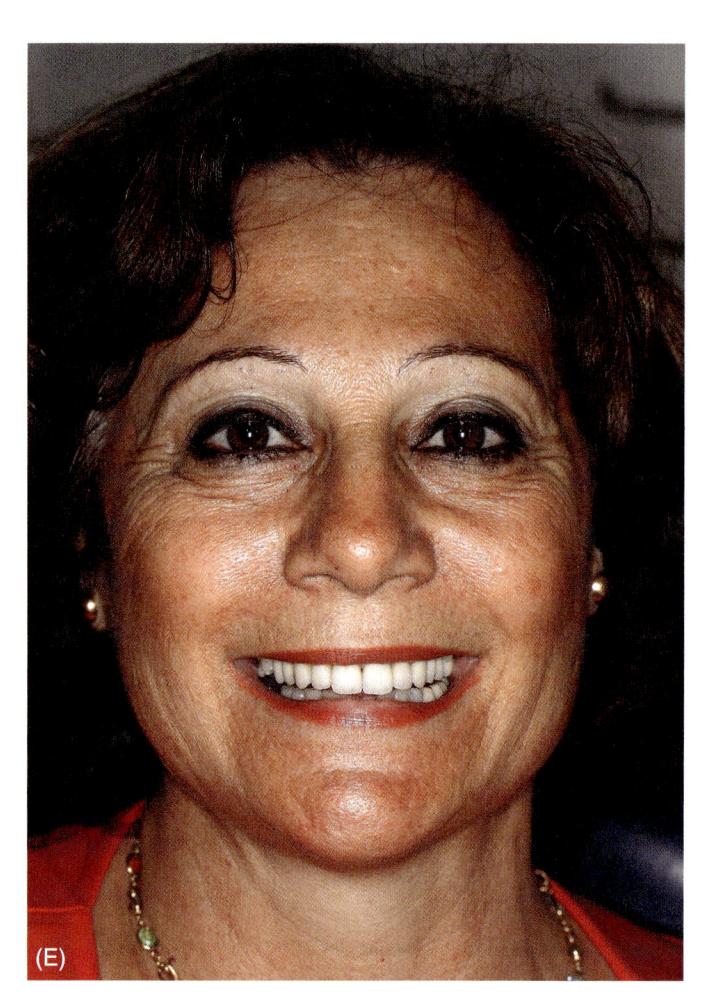

Figure 33.35 **(D–E)** Comparing the before smile on this patient, it is easy to see why she was so pleased with her new look.

around the age of 30–40 years, causing the maxillary incisor exposure average to decrease to less than half. Afterward, the maxillary incisor exposure is further reduced 0.5 mm on average for each decade, such that by the age of 70 years they are no longer visible.

Dickens et al.[76] conducted a study demonstrating that the heights of both the philtrums and the commissures increase with time and lead to a decreased display of teeth with increasing age. Furthermore, the philtrum's lengthening rate is greater than that of the commissure's; this is the responsible factor for flattening the "M" that is characteristic of the vermillion border of the upper lip in older patients compared with young people (Figure 33.35I and J).

Different conditions can reduce the amount of incisors shown at rest, such as excessive wear. The compensatory eruption that occurs in some patients suffering from incisal attrition is not fast enough to compensate for the loss of tooth structure, leading to a reduced visibility of the maxillary incisors both at rest and smiling (Figure 33.35A–B). In these situations, plan on a quick direct composite mock-up on teeth #8 and #9. This must be done without etching the teeth to esthetically and functionally assess the incisal edge lengthening (phonetics) (Figure 33.35C). Photographs and videos should be done in both frontal and oblique perspectives; and if the patient is comfortable and esthetics are favorable, the incisal edge index registration can be done with polyvinyl siloxane putty. The lab technician can easily transfer the preset incisal edge position by repositioning the index on the mounting casts before starting the diagnostic wax-up. The final result can be seen in Figure 33.35D–H.

The delayed eruption of the maxillary permanent incisors due to early loss of the primary maxillary incisors (As and Bs) before the complete development and eruption of the permanent teeth (generally due to caries or trauma) can allow the mandibular incisors to overerupt. This supereruption creates an unfavorable edge-to-edge occlusal position and a reduced maxillary incisor exposure.

Finally, the anterior teeth exposure can also be affected by the length and thickness of the upper lip, with longer and thicker lips reducing the tooth exposure.

Incisal edges and the lower lip

The relationship between the incisal edges of the maxillary anterior teeth and the lower lip, in both a posed and spontaneous smile, is another reference that can be used to determine the incisal edge position anteroposteriorly and midfacially. Attention

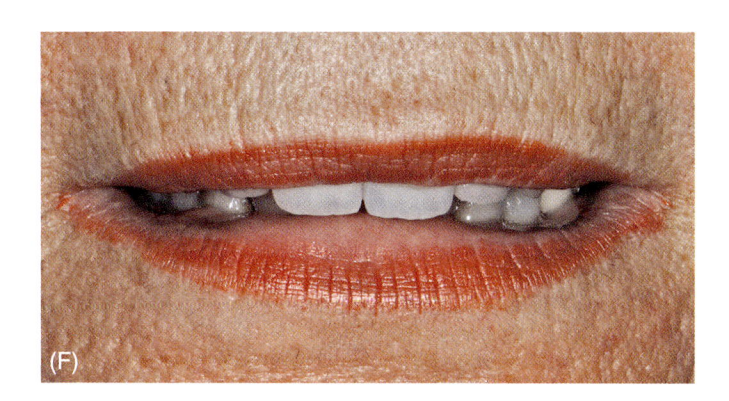

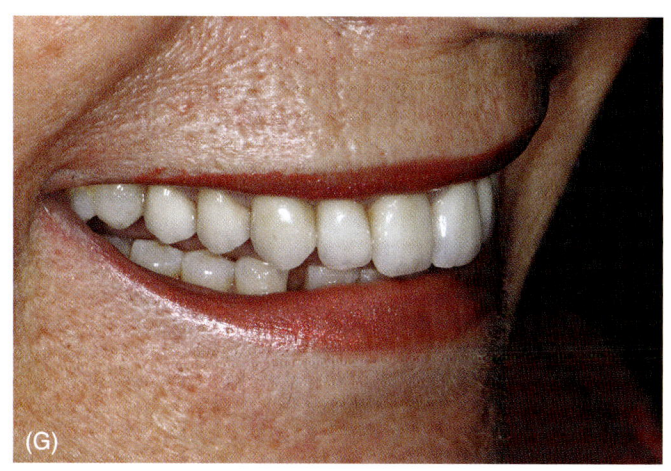

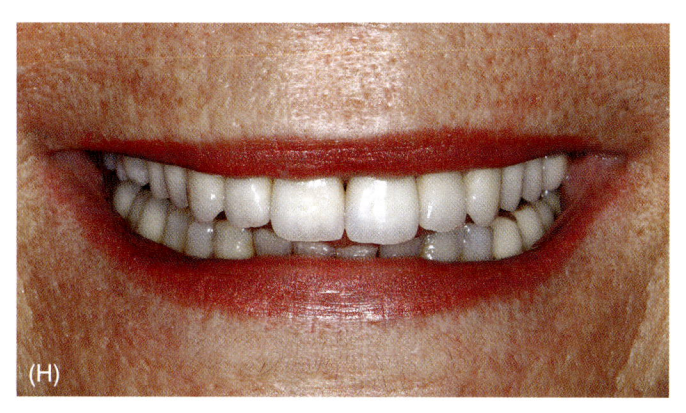

Figure 33.35 (F–H) Upper arch rehabilitation was performed, with a small increase of VDO, to restore the incisal curve, tooth exposure at rest, and smiling, giving the patient a much younger look.

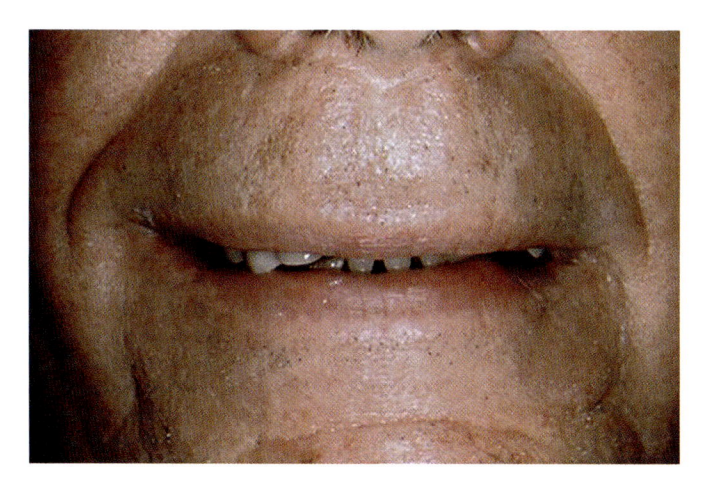

Figure 33.35 (I) This 78-year-old man's smile illustrates a decreased display of teeth, resulting in an older-looking appearance.

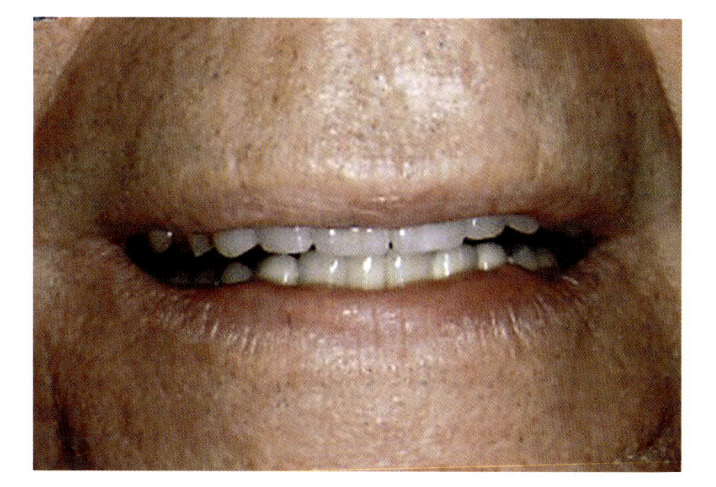

Figure 33.35 (J) Restoration consisted of restoring vertical dimension and lengthening his maxillary teeth that resulted in a much younger look.

should be made when taking photographic records to evaluate this parameter; this is because sometimes patients force a posed smile by placing the lower lip against the incisal edges, giving the illusion that there is no space between them. As such, the clinician should evaluate this parameter while talking with the patient to make an accurate diagnosis. Dynamic records should be taken in frontal, oblique, and profile perspectives to allow a sufficiently three-dimensional evaluation of this parameter.

From the frontal perspective of a smile, the maxillary incisal curve (defined by the incisal edges of the maxillary incisors) and the buccal cusp tips of the posterior maxillary teeth inscribe a convexity that follows the inner curve of the lower lip. Tjan et al.[51] found that parallelism between the upper incisal curve and the lower lip existed in 85% of the population, while Owens et al.[69] found 74% in an interracial study with no race or sex differences.

Frush[71] first described the reverse smile line (when the cuspids drop lower than the incisors) as being unattractive. White ivory wax was used to show the patient the proposed result. In this case, four full porcelain crowns were constructed to correct the problem (Figure 33.36A–C).

In other situations it may be possible to cosmetically contour the cuspids and the posterior teeth to lessen, or even eliminate, the reverse smile. The best approach is to use a black alcohol marker (Masel) and black out the areas of the teeth that could be contoured. Next, take a digital full-face picture with the patient smiling; then erase the marker and add composite or wax to lengthen the maxillary anterior teeth to their ideal position. Finally, take another digital full-face picture to compare the two treatment possibilities on the monitor; this will help the patient determine which treatment option would be most desired (Figure 33.37A–C).

Excessive incisal abrasion can flatten the maxillary incisal curve, or in more severe cases reverse this curvature. The esthetic result would be a reverse incisal curve, or a reverse smile line, where the canines stand out as the dominant smile element, giving an aggressive and older look to the facial expression. Figure 33.35I and J shows a patient with a reverse smile line due to a combination of attrition and erosion. The canines stand out upon smiling, making the smile less attractive. No tooth exposure at rest was observed, and visibility of the maxillary incisors at smiling was reduced. Upper arch rehabilitation was performed with a small increase of VDO to restore the incisal curve and tooth exposure, ultimately giving the patient a much younger look. Besides abrasion, an anterior open bite can cause loss of symmetry between the incisal curve and lower lip. A differential diagnosis should be made at the first stages to help plan the treatment.

As mentioned before (see "Lip symmetry" section), the lower lip is not always symmetric. In these cases, note that the inner curvature of the lower lip should not be used as a reference line for incisal curvature in the restorations.

Many authors suggest that the maxillary canines should come very close to touching or should actually touch the lower lip when smiling. Furthermore, the maxillary incisors should come about 2–4 mm short from touching the lower lip inside the vermillion border.[11] In their research about the position of the incisal curve relative to the lower lip, Tjan et al. reported that 47% of the population showed the maxillary anterior teeth touching the lower lip, 35% showed them not touching, and 17% had the incisal edges completely covered by the lower lip.[51] Tjan et al. used posed smile photographs; we believe that these results could change dramatically if they were to use dynamic records with spontaneous smiling. According to Van der Geld et al.,[47] the teeth are less covered by the lower lip when a person smiles spontaneously than when the smile is posed. He also concluded that, from an esthetic point of view, the differences between a spontaneous and posed smile were the most relevant for anterior mandibular teeth.

Smile line

The smile line refers to the position of the inner border of the upper lip during smiling, and thereby determines the tooth and gingival exposure. The smile line can be divided into three

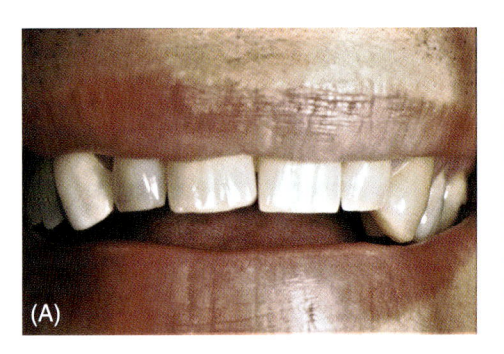

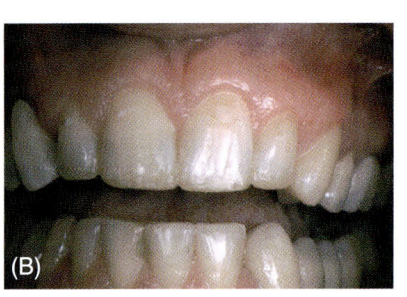

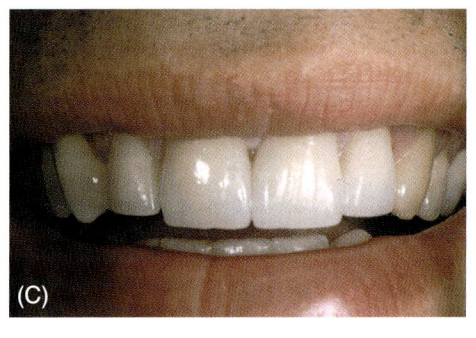

Figure 33.36 **(A)** This man had a reverse smile line with the cuspids much longer than the lateral and central incisors. **(B)** Ivory wax is added to the incisal edges so the patient can see how added length to the maxillary central and lateral incisors improved the smile. **(C)** Four porcelain crowns plus new posterior restorations helped provide a more attractive smile line.

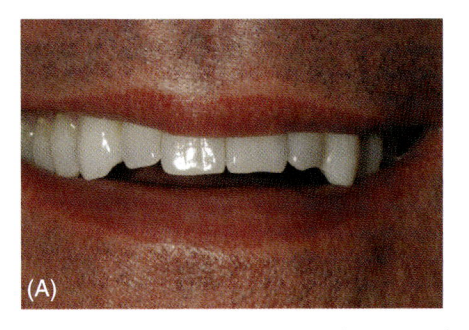

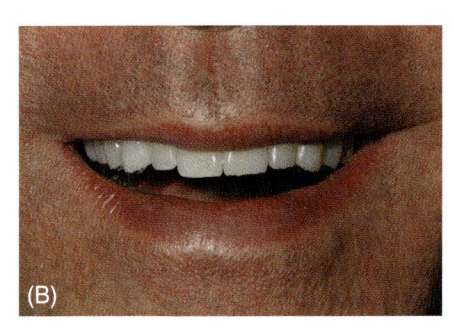

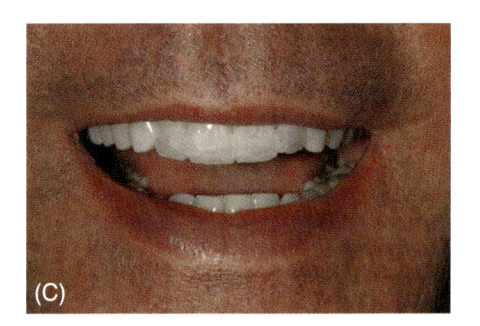

Figure 33.37 **(A)** This man wanted to correct his reverse smile line. **(B)** A Masel alcohol marker was used to show what the smile would look like if the teeth were contoured. **(C)** Ivory-colored wax was added to show what the smile would look like if the teeth were lengthened to correct it.

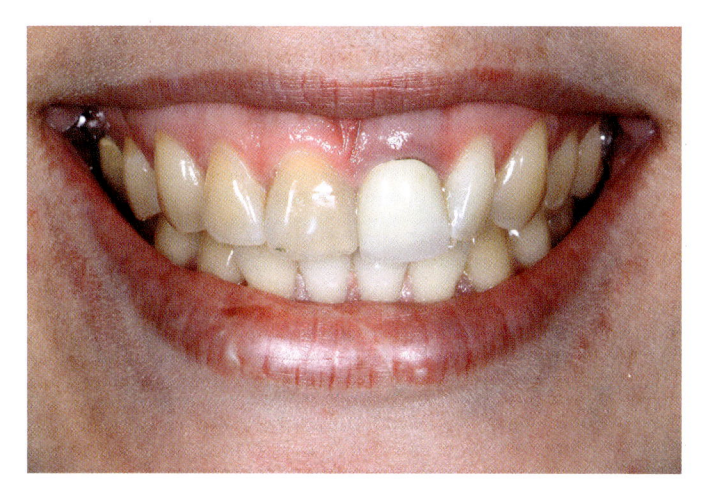

Figure 33.38 **(A)** Example of a high lip line.

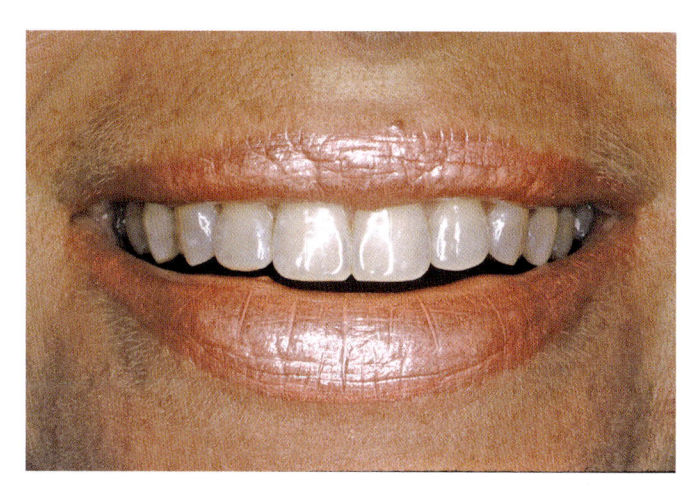

Figure 33.38 **(B)** This smile illustrates a medium lip line.

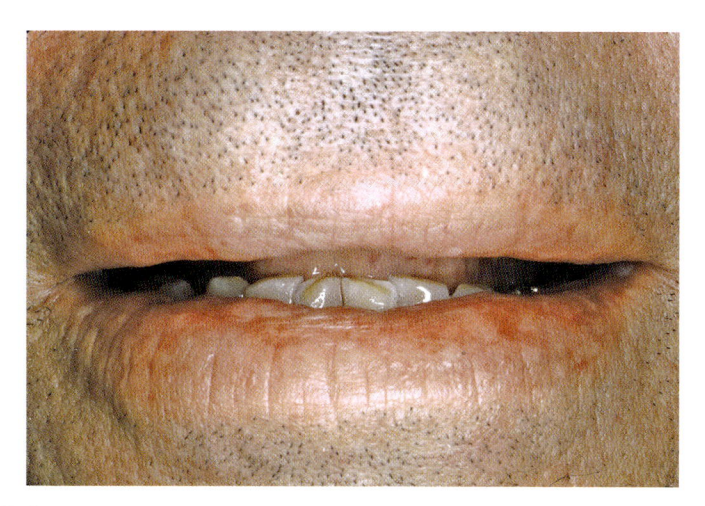

Figure 33.38 **(C)** Example of a low lip line.

categories: a high smile line, when the clinical crown and gingiva of the anterior maxillary teeth are exposed (Figure 33.38A); an average smile line, when 75–100% of the clinical crown length of the maxillary anterior teeth are exposed in addition to the gingival embrasures (Figure 33.38B); and a low smile line, when the clinical crown display of anterior maxillary teeth is less than 75% of their length, and little or no maxillary teeth are exposed (Figure 33.38C).

Authors seem to agree that the most esthetically pleasing smile should not show more than 3 mm of gingiva.[56,64] Tjan et al. found that 10.5% of subjects had a high smile line, whereas 69% presented an average smile line, and 20.5% a low smile line. Significant differences were found between sexes: women presented twice as high a smile line than men did.[51] These findings were confirmed later by Owens et al.,[48] who found significant differences in gingival display between races: African American and Caucasians presented the greatest amount of gingival tissue exposure. However, we believe that these findings could change dramatically if dynamic records had been taken instead and, according to Van der Geld et al.'s conclusions, the prevalence of a high smile line would be much greater.[47]

A "gummy" smile, or excessive gingival display, consistent with a high smile line, may be considered an unesthetic characteristic by many patients. "The decision as to whether the amount of gingival display is an esthetic problem for which treatment is desirable is a personal choice."[11] This condition can have multiple etiologies, which should be identified early on: altered eruption, incisal attrition with compensatory eruption, and vertical maxillary excess. The diagnosis of vertical maxillary excess can be confirmed by facial analysis that shows any of the following: a long lower face, lip incompetence, or excessive incisor display at rest and smiling. These patients should be referred to an orthodontist and a maxillofacial surgeon. Altered eruption can be diagnosed by probing the facial bone crest, and crown lengthening can be done if necessary in these situations. A differential diagnosis between passive and active altered eruption must be done before periodontal surgery.

When discolored or nonvital teeth must be restored, a high smile line can pose the greatest difficulty (Figure 33.38A). If the gingiva recedes following placement of a veneer or full crown, the darkness of the root will be revealed, displeasing the patient. Another esthetic failure can result if the cervical margin of an anterior tooth is above the matching tooth in the quadrant; therefore, cosmetic periodontal treatment becomes much more important in the case of a patient with a high lip line.

If the patient has a so-called short upper lip and a high smile line, it is sometimes possible to shorten the teeth and raise the gingival level. However, if enough attached gingiva is present, gingivoplasty or gingivectomy may provide some improvement.

A true long or low smile line may be seen in Figure 33.40. When a patient has this type of smile line, it is possible to use any dental procedure without showing the cervical margin of the teeth. The patient may complain about not showing teeth, which can be remedied by orthodontics, bonding, veneers, crowns, or some other type of restorative procedure to lengthen the teeth. Figure 33.39A–D shows correction of this problem in a patient who needed full mouth reconstruction. In this case, the vertical dimension was restored and the incisors were lengthened through a combination of orthodontics and full mouth reconstruction of both arches. Note the improved smile line in Figure 33.39C.

Individuals with incisal wear can give the appearance of a low smile line. Figure 33.40 shows a patient with a short upper lip complicated by mandibular prognathism. In this case, the incisal level of the lower arch could have been adjusted when the mandibular reconstruction was performed to improve the facial appearance. Figure 33.33A and C shows the appearance of a low lip line in a Class III patient. A low lip line can be caused by a bad habit, such as a conscious attempt to hide an unsightly oral condition, leading to the development of muscle control into an unconscious response. Even after this disagreeable condition has been corrected, it will take additional time and reassurance before this bad habit can be broken so that the patient can have a relaxed smile.

Finally, the loss of tooth structure is physiologic, and is a natural consequence of aging and wear. In physiologic tooth structure loss, vertical dimension is maintained by modeling of the alveolar bone (compensatory eruption) and the facial height remains constant. If the tooth loss is excessive, there is a high probability that the facial height will decrease due to the loss of VDO.[77]

Papilla display during smiling

Hochman et al.[78] studied the interproximal papillae exposure when smiling. This seems to be a critical issue to consider during the diagnosis in any esthetic restorative procedure. This research evaluated subjects with ages ranging from thirties to those in their eighties. The conclusion was that 91% of subjects showed interproximal gingiva when smiling. One of the most interesting

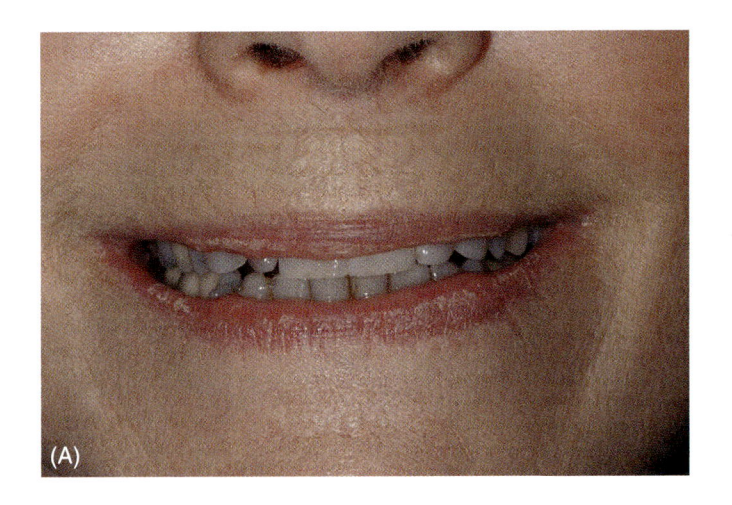

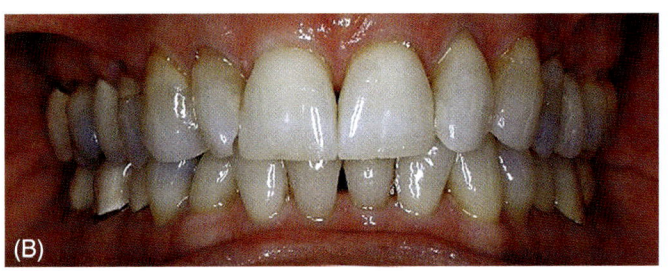

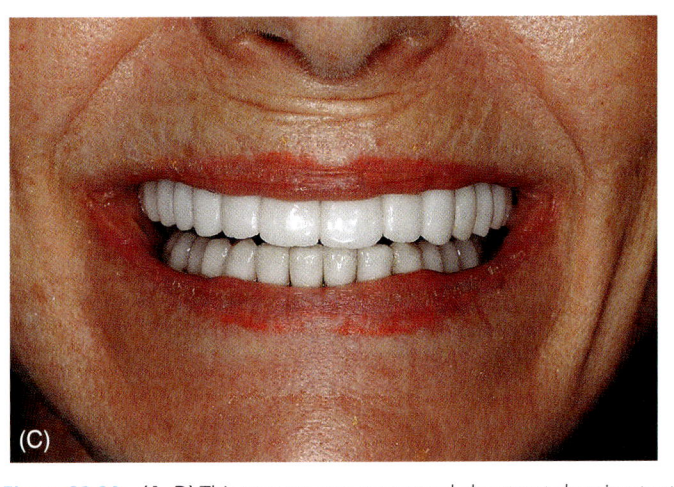

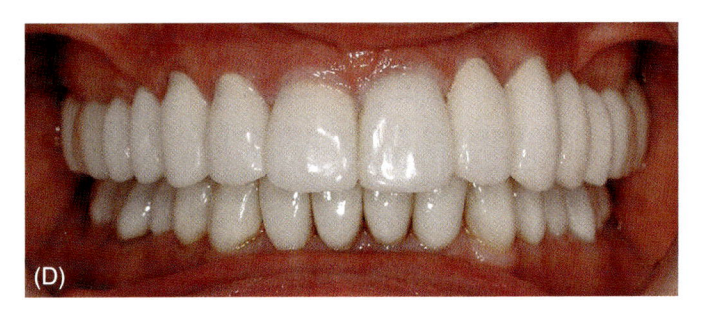

Figure 33.39 **(A–D)** This woman was concerned about not showing teeth when she smiled, as well as their dark color. There was insufficient tooth display due to her low lip line. A combination of orthodontic treatment and a full reconstruction of her upper and lower arches with a brighter tooth shade achieved the esthetics she desired.

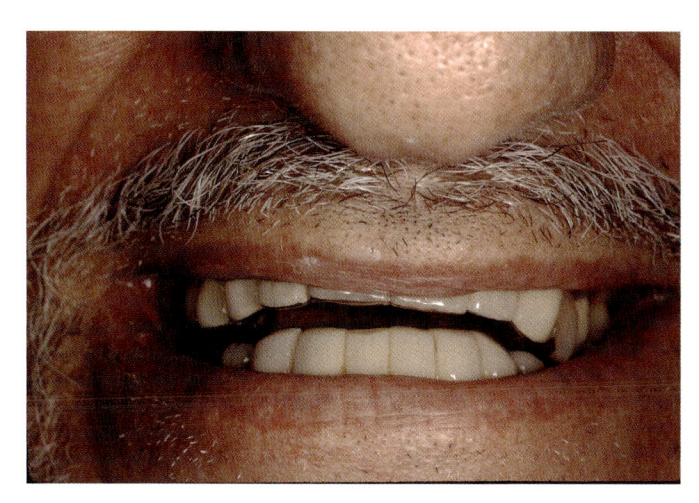

Figure 33.40 This patient had incisal wear and a short upper lip, complicated by mandibular prognathism. His smile could have been significantly improved if the mandibular teeth had been contoured at the time of his lower arch reconstruction.

findings of this study is the high prevalence (87%) of individuals with a low smile line who also displayed interdental papillae upon smiling. Clinically, this means that, even when treating adult patients with medium or low smile lines, the interdental papillae should be considered during the diagnostic and treatment planning process. This can make the difference between natural- and esthetic-looking restorations, versus artificial ones with increased interproximal contact surfaces between the teeth.

Smile width

Smile width refers to the number of teeth displayed in a smile and is directly related to arch form. A narrow or collapsed arch usually results in a narrow and unattractive smile; orthodontic and, possibly, surgical intervention are required to correct this. The smile width is determined by different factors: arch form, intercommissure length, facial muscle tone, and position of the buccal surfaces of the posterior upper teeth. Clinically, in posterior crown preparations, the margin location can be an esthetic issue when treating broad arches. The smile width is especially important when treating discolored teeth, as a misdiagnosis can lead to unesthetic situations. Sometimes the esthetic impact of a narrow arch can be reduced by building out the surfaces of premolars with bonding, veneers, or crowns (Figure 33.41A and B). Tjan et al.[51] has reported the number of teeth displayed in a smile: 7% of people show the six anterior teeth, 48% the six anterior and first premolars, 41% the six anterior and first and second premolars, and 4% the first molar. Van der Geld et al.[47] came to the conclusion that the posterior tooth display increased around 30% from a posed to a spontaneous smile. This can be explained by a significant reduction in intercommissure length in posed smiles compared with spontaneous smiles. We believe that the numbers reported by Tjan et al. could change if the spontaneous smile and the oblique prospective are evaluated instead of the posed smile.

Buccal corridors

The term buccal corridor was initially added by Frush to dental terminology in the late 1950s.[71] The buccal corridor refers to the dark space (negative space) created between the commissures of the mouth and the buccal surfaces of the maxillary posterior teeth that can be seen during a smile. Buccal corridors and smile width depend on the same factors and are inversely related. As the smile width decreases, the buccal corridors increase. Any discrepancy between the values (color) of the premolar and six anterior teeth can increase the darkness and prominence of the buccal corridors. A small amount of darkness is always present in esthetically pleasing smiles, although it can be increased in several situations, as described earlier. The absence of negative space due to, for example, overcontoured crowns has an unesthetic effect on changing the natural smile progression, creating an artificial look. Thus, attention should also be made not to obliterate the buccal corridors (refer to Figure 36.11C and D).

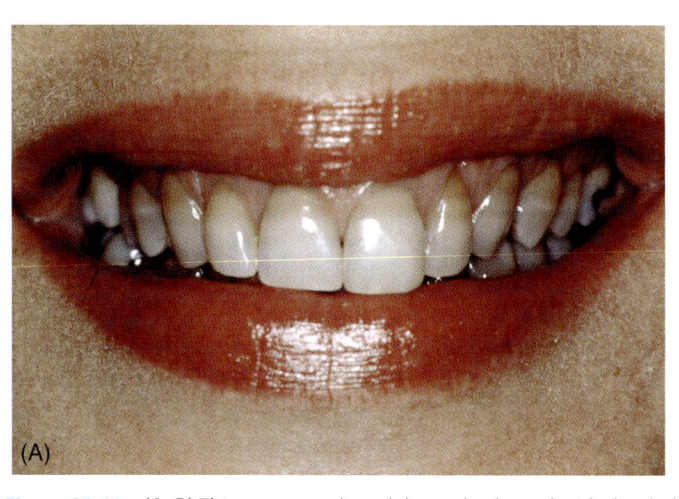

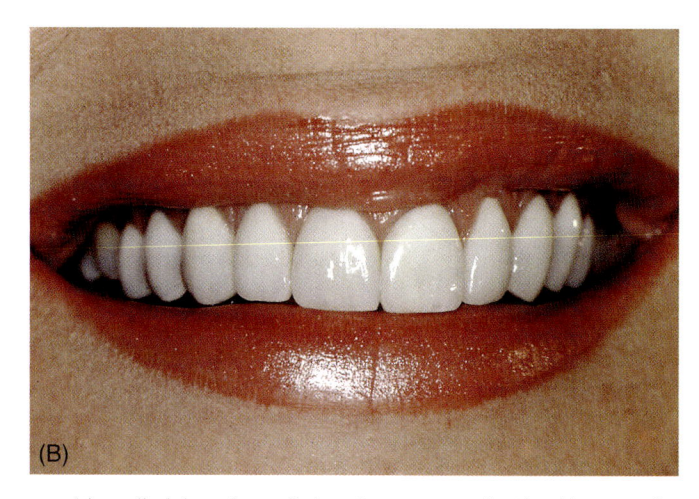

Figure 33.41 **(A, B)** This actress and model was displeased with the dark spaces (she called them "caves") that she saw on each side of her mouth when she smiled. The solution to this cosmetic problem involved building out both the front and back teeth with lighter-colored porcelain veneers. Lighter-colored teeth appear to stand out, whereas darkly stained teeth appear to recede.

Conclusion

Treatment planning a new patient may appear at first glance to be routine, especially if you have had years of clinical experience. However, your next new patient could be your first esthetic failure, which can be extremely stressful as well as costly. The reason? Failure to adequately spend the time to evaluate the various aspects covered in this chapter. Never take anything for granted. Even if your patient states they just want four anterior teeth crowned or veneered, the reality is it may not provide the patient with what they envision esthetically. Instead, the more you analyze and become aware of how all the facial considerations can affect your result, the greater your chance for esthetic success.

References

1. Rufenacht C. *Principles of Esthetic Integration*. Chicago, IL: Quintessence; 2000:63–166.
2. Rufenacht C. *Fundamental of Esthetics*. Chicago, IL: Quintessence; 1990:11–93.
3. Abad DS, Roldán AL, Bertomeu IG, et al. Percepción de la estética de la sonrisa por diferentes grupos de población. *Rev Esp Prot Estomatol* 2008;10(4):323–331.
4. Kokich VO Jr, Kiyak HA, Shapiro PA. Comparing the perception of dentists and laypeople to altered dental esthetics. *J Esthet Dent* 1999;11:311–324.
5. Kokich VO, Kokich VG, Kiyak HA. Perceptions of dental professionals and laypersons to altered dental esthetics: asymmetric and symmetric situations. *Am J Orthod Dentofacial Othop* 2006;130:141–151.
6. Jornung J, Fardal O. Perceptions of patient's smiles: a comparison of patients' and dentists' opinions. *J Am Dent Assoc* 2007;138(12):1544–1553.
7. Beyer JW, Lindauer J. Evaluation of dental midline position. *Semin Orthod* 1998;4:146–152.
8. Ker AJ, Chan R, Fields HW, Beck M, Rosentiel S. Esthetics and smile characteristics from the layperson's perspective: a computer-based survey study. *J Am Dent Assoc* 2008;139(10):1318–1327.
9. Johnston CD, Burden DJ, Stevenson MR. The influence of dental to facial midline discrepancies on dental attractiveness ratings. *Eur J Orthod* 1999;21:517–522.
10. Lombardi RE. The principles of visual perception and their clinical application to denture esthetics. *J Prosthet Dent* 1973;29:358–382.
11. Sarver D, Jacobson RS. The aesthetic dentofacial analysis. *Clin Plast Surg* 2007;34(3):369–394.
12. Chiche GJ, Pinault A. *Esthetics of Anterior Fixed Prosthodontics*. Chicago, IL: Quintessence; 1994:13–30.
13. Peck S, Peck L, Kataja M. Skeletal asymmetry in esthetically pleasing faces. *Angle Orthod* 1991;61:43–47.
14. Lindauer SJ. Introduction. *Semin Orthod* 1998;3:133
15. Ferrario VF, Sforza C Miani A Jr, Serrao G. A three-dimensional evaluation of human facial asymmetry. *J Anat* 1995;186:103–110.
16. Singer BA. Principles of esthetics. *Curr Opin Cosmet Dent* 1994:6–12
17. Miller EL, Jamison HC. A study of the relationship of the dental midline to the facial midline. *J Prosthet Dent* 1979;41:657–666.
18. Tarnow D, Chu S, Kim J. *Aesthetic Restorative Dentistry: Principles and Practice*. Mahwah, NJ: Montage Media Corp; 2007.
19. Bishara SE, Burkey PS, Kharouf JG. Dental and facial asymmetries: a review. *Angle Orthod* 1994;64(2);89–98.
20. Padwa BL Kaiser MO, Kaban LB. Occlusal cant in the frontal plane as a reflection of facial asymmetry. *J Oral Maxillofac Surg* 1997;55:811–816.
21. Lu KH. Harmonic analysis of the human face. *Biometrics* 1965;21:491–505.
22. Shah SM, Joshi MR. An assessment of asymmetry in the normal craniofacial complex. *Angle Orthod* 1978;48:141–148.
23. Alavi DG, BeGole EA, Scheicer BJ. Facial and dental arch asymmetries in Class II subdivision malocclusion. *Am J Orthod Dentofacial Orthop* 1988;93:38–46.
24. Pirttiniemi P. *Association of Mandibulofacial Asymmetries, With Special Reference to Glenoid Fossa Remodeling*. Oulu, Finland: University of Oulu; 1992.
25. Ferrario VF, Sforza C Miani A Jr, Serrao G. Dental arch asymmetry in young non-patient subjects evaluated by Euclidean distance matrix analysis. *Arch Oral Biol* 1993;38:189–194.
26. Ferrario VF, Sforza C, Miani A Jr, Tartaglia G. Craniofacial morphometry by photographic evaluations. *Am J Orthod Dentofacial Orthop* 1993;103:327–337.
27. Williamson EH, Simmons MD. Mandibular asymmetry and its relation to pain dysfunction. *Am J Orthod* 1979;76:612–617.
28. Pirttiniemi P, Kantomaa T, Lathela P. Relationship between craniofacial and condyle path asymmetry in unilateral cross-bite patients. *Eur J Orthod* 1990;12:408–413.
29. Shmid W, Mongini F, Felisio A. A computer-based assessment of structural and displacement asymmetries of the mandible. *Am J Orthod Dentofacial Orthop* 1991;100:19–34.
30. Rifkin R. Facial analysis: a comprehensive approach to treatment planning in aesthetic dentistry. *Pract Periodont Aesthet Dent* 2000;12(9):865–871.
31. Arnett GW, Bergman RT. Facial keys to orthodontic diagnosis and treatment planning. Part I. *Am J Orthod Dentofacial Orthop* 1993;103:299–312.
32. Arnett GW, Bergman RT. Facial keys to orthodontic diagnosis and treatment planning. Part II. *Am J Orthod Dentofacial Orthop* 1993;103:395–411.
33. Renner G: Reconstruction of the lip. In: Baker SR, Swanson NA, eds. *Local Flaps in Facial Reconstruction*, St. Louis, MO: Mosby; 1995:370.
34. Ferrario VF, Chiarella S, Ciusa V, et al. The effect of sex and age on facial asymmetry in healthy subjects: a cross-sectional study from adolescence to mid-adulthood. *J Oral Maxillofac Surg* 2001;59:382–388.
35. Burke PH. Stereophotogrammetric measurement of normal facial asymmetry in children. *Hum Biol* 1971;43:536–548.
36. Ercan I, Ozdemir ST, Sigirli D, et al. Facial asymmetry in young healthy subjects evaluated by statistical shape analysis. *J Anat* 2008;213:663–669.
37. Haraguchi S, Iguchi Y, Takada K. Asymmetry of the face in orthodontic patients. *Angle Orthod* 2007;78(3):421–426.
38. Penton-Voak IS, Jones BC, Little AC, et al. Symmetry, sexual dimorphism in facial proportions and male facial attractiveness. *Proc Biol Sci* 2001;268(1476):1617–1623.
39. Scheib JE, Ganestad SW, Thornhill R. Facial attractiveness, symmetry and cues of good genes. *Proc Biol Sci* 1999;266(1431):1913–1917.
40. Gebhard W. A comprehensive approach for restoring esthetics and function in fixed prosthodontics. *Quintessence Dent Technol* 2003;26:21–44.
41. Springer IN, Wannicke B, Warnke PH, et al. Facial attractiveness: visual impact of symmetry increases significantly towards midline. *Ann Plast Surg* 2007;59(2):156–162.

42. Ricketts RM. Planning treatment on the basis of the facial pattern and an estimate of its growth. *Angle Onthod* 1957;27:14–37.
43. Weickersheimer PB. Steiner analysis. In: Jacobson A, ed. *Radiographic Cephalometry*. Carol Stream, IL: Quintessence Publishing; 1995:83–85.
44. Burstone CJ. Lip posture and its significance in treatment planning. *Am J Orthod* 1967;53:262–284.
45. Ahmad I. Anterior dental aesthetics historical perspective. *Br Dent J* 2005;198:737–742.
46. Preston JD. The golden proportion revisited. *J Esthet Dent* 1993;5(6):247–251.
47. Van der Geld P, Oosterveld P, Berge SJ, Kuijpers-Jagtman A.M. Tooth display and lip position during spontaneous and posed smiling in adults. *Acta Odontol Scand* 2008;66:207–213.
48. Owens EG, Goodacre CJ, Loh PL, et al. A multicenter interracial study of facial appearance. Part 1: a comparison of extraoral parameters. *Int J Prosthodont* 2002;15:273–282.
49. Silva BP, Jimenez-Castellanos E, Stanley K, et al. Layperson's perception of axial midline angulation in asymmetric faces. *J Esthet Restor Dent* 2017; in press. 10.1111/jerd.12347
50. Silva BP, Jiménez-Castellanos E, Martinez-de-Fuentes R, et al. Perception of maxillary dental midline shift in asymmetric faces. *Int J Esthet Dent* 2015;10:588–596.
51. Tjan AH, Miller GD, The JG. Some esthetic factors in a smile. *J Prosthet Dent* 1984;51(1):24–28.
52. Golub J. Entire smile pivotal to teeth design. *Clin Dent* 1988;33–43.
53. Naini FB, Moss JP, Gill DS. The enigma of facial beauty: esthetics, proportions, deformity, and controversy. *Am J Orthod Dentofacial Orthop* 2006;130:277–282.
54. Philips E. The classification of smile patterns. *J Can Dent Assoc* 1999;65:252–254.
55. Bell WH, ed. *Modern Practice in Orthognathic and Reconstructive Surgery*. Philadelphia, PA: Saunders; 1992.
56. McLaren EA. Rifkin R. Macroesthetics: facial and dentofacial analysis. *J Calif Dent Assoc* 2002;30(11):839–846.
57. Kois JC, Phillips KM. Occlusal vertical dimension: alteration concerns. *Compend Contin Educ Dent* 1997;18(12):1169–1177.
58. Tallgren A. Changes in adult face height due to aging, wear and loss of teeth and prosthetic treatment. *Acta Odontol Scand* 1957;15(Suppl. 24):1–122.
59. Atwood DA. A cephalometric study of rest position of the mandible, part I. *J Prosthet Dent* 1956;6:504–519.
60. Dahl BL, Krogstad O. Long-term observations of an increased occlusal face height obtained by a combined orthodontic/prosthetic approach. *J Oral Rehabil* 1985;12:173–176.
61. Spear FM. Approaches to vertical dimension. *Adv Esthet Interdiscip Dent* 2006;2(3):2–14.
62. Gross MD, Nissan J, Ormianer Z, et al. The effect of increasing occlusal vertical dimension on face height. *Int J Prosthodont* 2002;15:353–357.
63. Sarver DM, Ackerman MB. Dynamic smile visualization and quantification: part 2. Smile analysis and treatment strategies. *Am J Orthod Dentofacial Orthop* 2003;124:116–127.
64. Fradeani M. *Esthetic Rehabilitation in Fixed Prosthodontics, Volume 1 Esthetic Analysis: A Systematic Approach to Prosthetic*. Chicago, IL: Quintessence Publishing; 2004:47–59.
65. Ferrario VF, Sforza C, Poggio CE, Tartaglia G. A three-dimensional evaluation of facial asymmetry. *J Oral Maxillofac Surg* 1994;52:1126–1132.
66. Laurence J, Lowentein L. The midline: diagnosis and treatment. *Am J Orthod Dentofac Orthop* 1990;97:453–462.
67. Brisman AS. Esthetics: a comparison of dentists and patients' concepts. *J Am Dent Assoc* 1980;100:345–352.
68. Hulsey CM. An esthetic evaluation of lip-teeth relationships present in the smile. *Am J Orthod* 1970;57:132–143.
69. Owens EG, Goodacre CJ, Loh PL, et al. A multicenter interracial study of facial appearance. Part 2: a comparison of intraoral parameters. *Int J Prosthodont* 2002;15:283–288.
70. Pinho S, Ciriaco C, Faber J, Lenza MA. Impact of dental asymmetries on the perception of smile esthetics. *Am J Orthod Dentofacial Orthop* 2007;132:748–753.
71. Frush J. *Swissdent Technique and Procedure Manual*. Los Angeles, CA: Swissdent Corp.; 1971.
72. Sarver DM. The face as determinant of treatment choice. In: McNamara JA Jr, Kelly KA, eds. *Craniofacial Growth Series Vol. 38: Frontiers of Dental and Facial Esthetics*. Ann Arbor, MI: University of Michigan; 2001:19–54.
73. Gürel G, ed. *The Science and Art of Porcelain Laminate Veneers*. Quintessence; 2003:246.
74. Chu SJ. Range and mean distribution frequency of individual tooth width of maxillary anterior dentition. *Pract Proced Aesthet Dent* 2007;19:209–215.
75. Vig RG, Brundo GC. The kinetics of anterior tooth display. *J Prosthet Dent* 1978;39:502–504.
76. Dickens S, Sraver D, Proffit W. Changes in frontal soft tissue dimensions of the lower face by age and gender. *World J Orthod* 2002;3:313–332.
77. Chu SJ, Karabin S, Mistry S. Short tooth syndrome: diagnosis, etiology, and treatment management. *J Calif Dent Assoc* 2004;32(2):143–152.
78. Hochman MN, Chu SJ, Tarnow DP. Maxillary anterior papilla display during smiling: a clinical study of the interdental smile line. *Int J Periodontics Restorative Dent* 2012;32(4):375–383.

Additional resources

Ahmad I. Anterior dental aesthetics: facial perspective. *Br Dent J* 2005;199:15–21.

Alneuda MD, Rodrigues Farias AC, Bittencourt M. Influence of mandibular sagittal position on facial esthetics. *Dent Press J Orthod* 2010;15:87–96.

Borod JC, Caron HS, Koff E. Asymmetry of facial expression related to handedness, footedness, and eyedness: a quantitative study. *Cortex* 1981;17(3):381–390.

Borod JC, Koff E, White B. Facial asymmetry in posed and spontaneous expressions of emotion. *Brain Cogn* 1983;2(2):165–175.

Chu S. A biometric approach to predictable treatment of clinical crown discrepancies. *Pract Proced Aesthet Dent* 2007;19(7):401–409.

Corman L. *Nouveau Manuel de Morpho-psychologie*. Paris: Stock Plus; 1981.

Corner BD, Richtsmeier JT. Morphometric analysis of craniofacial growth in *Cebus apella*. *Am J Phys Anthropol* 1991;84:323–342.

Dane S, Ersoz M, Gumustekin K, et al. Handedness differences in widths of right and left craniofacial regions in healthy young adults. *Percept Mot Skills* 2004;98:1261–1264.

Edwards N. Re: "A critical review of visual analogue scales in the measurement of clinical phenomena". *Res Nurs Health* 1991;14(1):81.

Farkas LG. *Anthropometry of the Head and Face*, 2nd edn. New York, NY: Raven Press; 1994:103–111.

Farkas LG, Cheung G. Facial asymmetry in healthy North American Caucasians. Anthropometric study. *Angle Orthod* 1981;51:70–77.

Ferrario VF, Sforza C, D'Addona A, et al. ANB skeletal types correlated to facial morphology: Euclidean distance matrix analysis. *Int J Adult Orthodon Orthognath Surg* 1993;8:181–190.

Ferrario VF, Sforza C, Miani A Jr, Tartaglia G. Human dental arch shape evaluated by Euclidean-distance matrix. *Am J Phys Anthropol* 1993;90:443–456.

Ferrario VF, Sforza C, Miani A Jr, Tartaglia G. Maxillary versus mandibular arch form differences in human permanent dentition assessed by Euclidean distance matrix analysis. *Arch Oral Biol* 1994;39:135–139.

Ferrario VF, Sforza C, Pizzini G, et al. Sexual dimorphism in the human face assessed by Euclidean distance matrix analysis. *J Anat* 1993;183:593–600.

Flores-Mir C, Silva E, Barriga MI, et al. Layperson's perception of smile aesthetics in dental and facial views. *J Orthod* 2004;31:204–209.

Franklin RG Jr, Adams RB Jr. The two sides of beauty: laterality and duality of facial attractiveness. *Brain Cogn* 2010; 72:300–305.

Johnson PF. Racial norms: esthetic and prosthodontics implications *J Prosthet Dent* 1992;67:502–508.

Kales P, Diyarbakirli S, Tan M, Tan U. Facial asymmetry in right and left handed men women. *Int J Neurosci* 1997;91(3–4):147–159.

Kim HS, Kim IP, Oh SC, Dong JK. The effect of personality on the smile. *J Wonkwang Dent Res Inst* 1995;5:299–314.

Lele S. Some contents on coordinate-free and scale invariant methods in morphometry. *Am J Phys Anthropol* 1991;85:407–417.

Lele S, Richtsmeier JT. Euclidean distance matrix analysis: a coordinate-free approach for comparing biological shapes using landmark data. *Am J Phys Anthropol* 1991;86:415–427.

Lele S, Richtsmeier JT. On comparing biological shapes: detection of influential landmarks. *Am J Phys Anthropol* 1992;87:49–95.

Levine JB. Esthetic diagnosis. *Curr Opin Cosmet Dent* 1995:9–17.

Melnik AK. A cephalometric study of mandibular asymmetry in a longitudinally followed sample of growing children. *Am J Orthod Dentofacial Orthop* 1992;101:355–366.

Newton JT, Prabhu N, Robinson PG. The impact of dental appearance on the appraisal of personal characteristics. *Int J Prosthodont* 2003;16:429–434.

Patzelt S. Schaible L. Stampf S. Kohal, R. Software-based evaluation of human age: a pilot study. *J Esthet Rest Dent* 2015;27:100–106.

Proffitt WR, Ackerman JL. Diagnosis and treatment planning in orthodontics. In: Garber TM, Swain BF, eds. *Orthodontics: Current Principles and Techniques*. St. Louis, MO: Mosby; 1985:67.

Ras F, Habets LL, van Ginkel FC, Prahl-Andersen B. Three-dimensional evaluation of facial asymmetry in cleft lip and palate. *Cleft Palate Craniofac J* 1994;31:116–121.

Richardson ER. Racial differences in dimensional traits of the human face. *Angle Orthod* 1980;50:301–311.

Salehi P, Oshagh M, Aleyasin Z, Pakshir H. The effects of forehead and neck position on esthetics of class I, II, III profiles. *Int J Esthet Dent* 2014;9:412–424.

Sarver DM, Ackerman MB. Dynamic smile visualization and quantification: part 1. Evolution of the concept and dynamic records for smile capture. *Am J Orthod Dentofacial Orthop* 2003;124:4–12.

Severt TR, Proffit WR. The prevalence of facial asymmetry in the dentofacial deformities population at the University of North Carolina. *Int J Adult Orthod Orthognatic Surg* 1997;12:171–176.

Shaner DJ, Peterson AE, Beattie OB, Bomforth JS. Assessment of soft tissue facial asymmetry in medically normal and syndrome-affected individuals by analysis of landmarks and measurements. *Am J Med Genet* 2000;93:143–154.

Smith WM. Hemispheric and facial asymmetry: gender differences. *Laterality* 2000;5:251–258.

Thomas JL, Hayes C, Zawideh S. The effect of axial midline angulation on dental esthetics. *Angle Orthod* 2003;73:359–364.

Tole N. Lanjnert V. Kovacevic D. Spalj, S. Gender, Age, and psychosocial context of the perception of facial esthetics. *J Esthet Restor Dent* 2014;26:119–130.

Viana PC, Kovacs Z, Correia A. Purpose of esthetic risk assessment in prosthetic rehabilitations with gingiva-shade ceramics. *Int J Esthet Dent* 2014; 9;480–488.

Vig PS, Hewit AB. Asymmetry of the human facial skeleton. *Angle Orthod* 1993;104:337–341.

Woo TL. On the asymmetry of the human skull. *Biometrika* 1931;22:324–352.

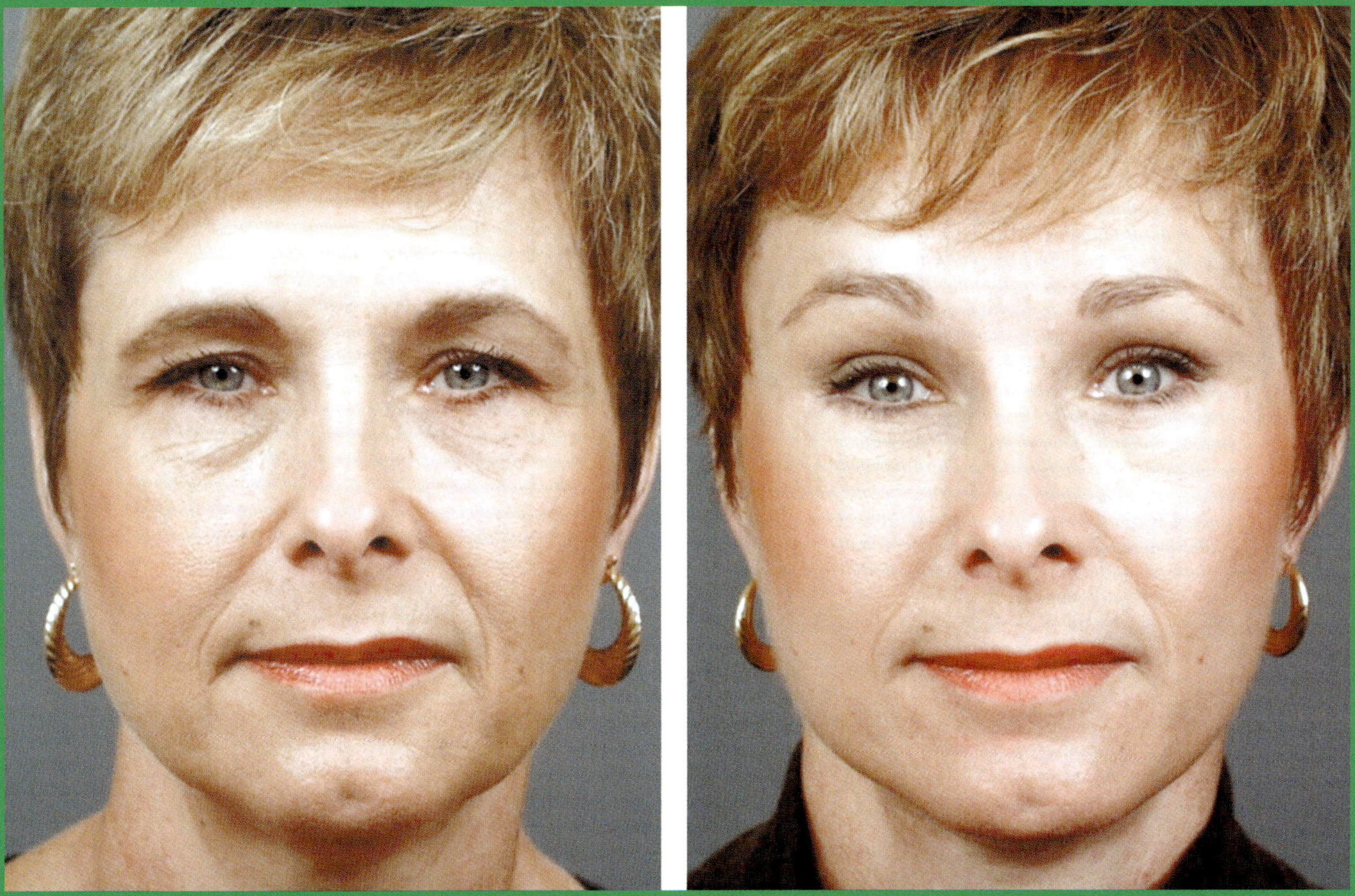

Chapter 34 Plastic Surgery Related to Esthetic Dentistry

Foad Nahai, MD, FACS and Kristin A. Boehm, MD, FACS

Chapter Outline

Upper face	1132	Genioplasty	1137
Browlift	1132	Rhytidectomy	1137
Blepharoplasty	1132	Nonsurgical	1137
Midface	1133	Neurotoxins	1137
Midface lift	1133	Soft tissue fillers	1137
Rhinoplasty	1134	Facial resurfacing	1140
Lower face	1137	Patient safety	1140

Although there are individual preferences as to what constitutes beauty, it seems almost universally accepted that society values a youthful face. Alterations in normal facial anatomy, be it post-traumatic, congenital, or secondary to aging, can have negative social and psychological repercussions for the individual affected. Having a balanced facial physique is inherently important in developing social interactions, maintaining self-confidence, and even securing gainful employment. By creating facial harmony, esthetic surgery procedures have become important adjuncts in restoring patient self-esteem and functionality.

Beauty is subjective, and there is no single formula that defines facial beauty. The concept of facial esthetics is a complex one involving interplay between underlying skeletal framework, soft tissues, and external anatomic structures. Although no single measurement, reference line, or angle completely translates to an esthetic ideal, there are some fundamental features that optimize outward appearance. The concept of balance from one side to the other is one such feature. While some asymmetries individualize a face, they should be minor enough to not disfigure or draw attention. Notions of harmony and proportion are important. Even, flowing curves from the upper to lower face create a harmonious, pleasing profile. Neonatal features, such as large eyes, small nose, round cheeks, and smooth skin, are usually deemed attractive.

Several medical specialties are involved in enhancing facial appearance. Esthetic dentistry focuses on the mouth, with the intent to optimize the quality of the teeth and smile. Altering the jaw and dentition invariably influences nearby structures and becomes intimately related to other procedures affecting facial form. There are numerous plastic surgery procedures that, although not specifically related to the mouth, have a definite relationship to cosmetic dentistry. A variety of both surgical and nonsurgical procedures exist to address the eyelids, nose, cheeks, chin, and neck. Esthetic plastic surgery, therefore, becomes an appropriate complement to esthetic dentistry, and often a combination of both yields optimal results.

To understand the range of surgical techniques available is to understand specific changes in the face as they occur over time.

Erroneous assessment of facial features and the anatomy underscoring those traits may lead to inappropriate treatment and a disappointed patient. A comprehensive approach requires analysis of the face according to the upper, middle, and lower thirds. By evaluating these areas in an orderly fashion and taking into account the patient's personal desires, the plastic surgeon formulates a comprehensive plan to achieve desirable results.

Upper face

Browlift

The brow is usually arched with smooth, taut skin constituting the forehead. Over time, the skin from the hairline to the eyebrows can sag, causing drooping of the brows and skin redundancy in the upper eyelid area. Particularly along the outer portion of the brow, this can lead to hooding and an aged appearance reducing eye size. Muscles in the forehead and between the brows contract in an attempt to elevate the skin, resulting in horizontal and vertical forehead wrinkles. A browlift procedure releases this sagging tissue, resuspends it, and secures it in its newly elevated position. This can be achieved either through a series of small incisions located in the hair-bearing scalp, or through an incision located just behind the anterior hairline.

In either case, scars are usually well camouflaged. The procedure may require general anesthesia, and recovery time averages a week or two secondary to both pain and periorbital bruising. Browlift procedures lift the eyebrow arch, minimize skin redundancy along the upper eyelid region, and smooth out the etched wrinkles that are seen between the brows and in the central forehead. The procedure is often combined with eyelid surgery (Figure 34.1A–D).

Blepharoplasty

Predictable changes occur in the periorbita over time. At the most superficial level, thin eyelid skin is subject to actinic damage and becomes wrinkled or "crepey." Retaining ligaments lose their consistency and weaken, with resultant sagging of skin and cheekbone complexes. The orbital septum, which normally contains the lower eyelid fat pads, relaxes, allowing herniation of the fat and appearance of lower lid "bags." In the lateral canthal region, the lateral canthal tendons elongate and loosen, producing a downward slant to the corners of the eyes (Figure 34.2).

These aging changes are surgically addressed with an upper and lower lid blepharoplasty (Figure 34.3). In the upper lid region, an incision is hidden along the natural upper lid crease. Through this, excess skin is removed and a sharp crease is defined and pretarsal or "eye shadow" space is recreated.

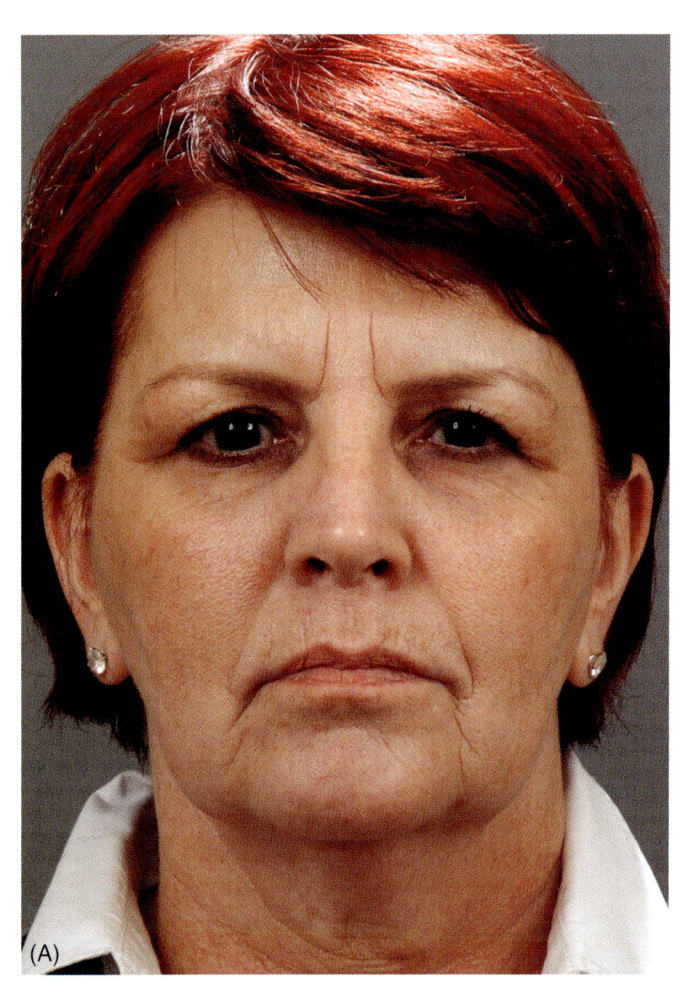

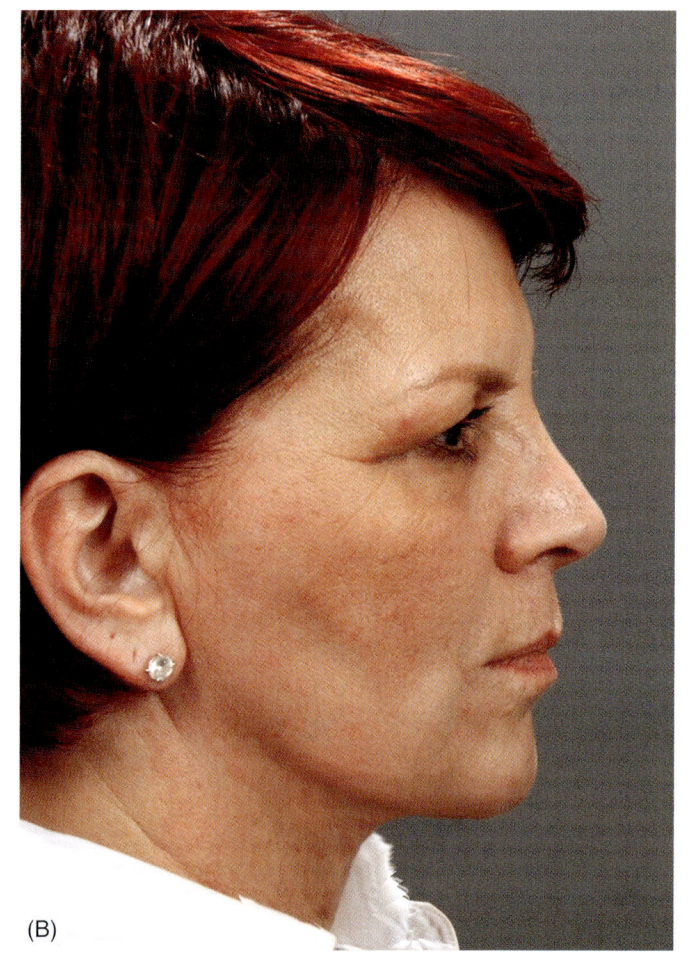

Figure 34.1 **(A, B)** Anteroposterior and lateral views of the patient prior to brow and eyelid surgery.

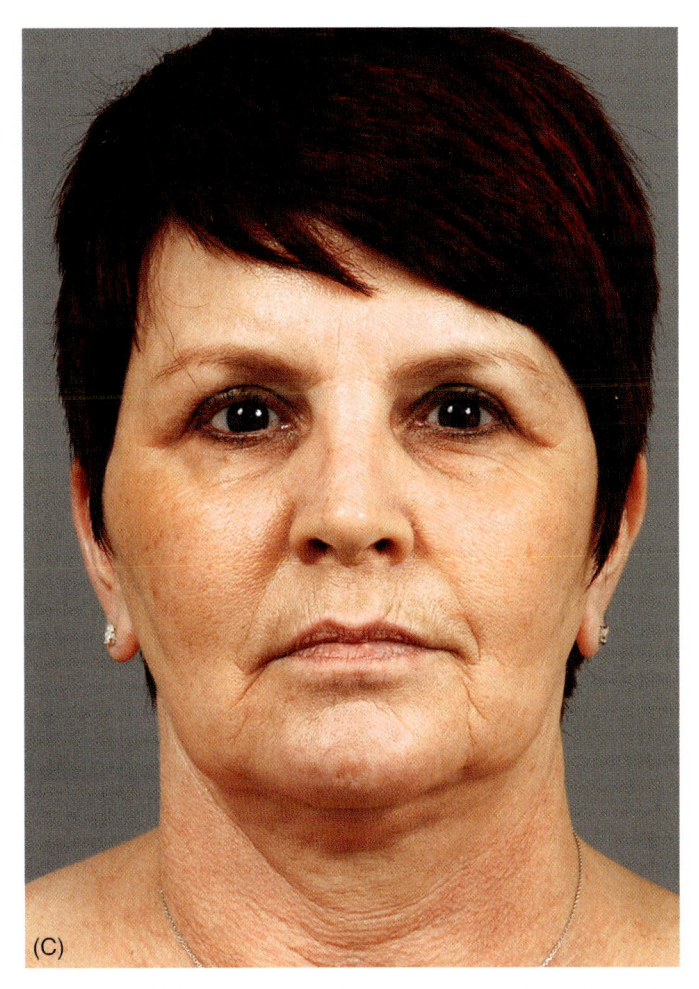

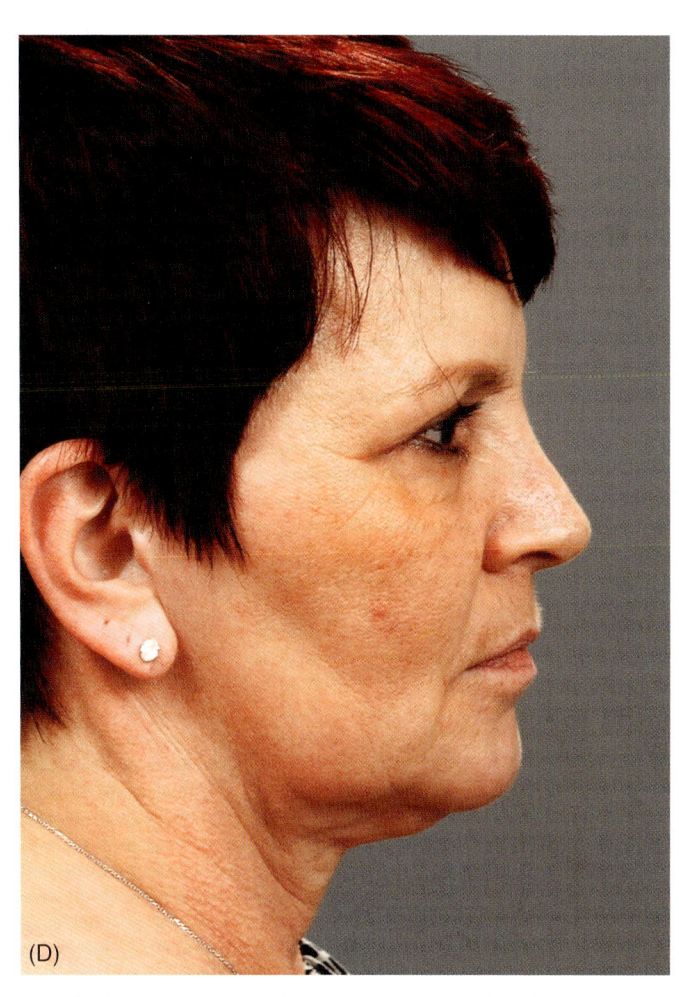

Figure 34.1 (C, D) Same patient after undergoing endoscopic browlift and upper lid blepharoplasty. Note the decreased hooding of the brow, which helps to open up the upper eyelid region and recreate a pretarsal space. The glabellar frown lines have also been substantially softened by the procedure.

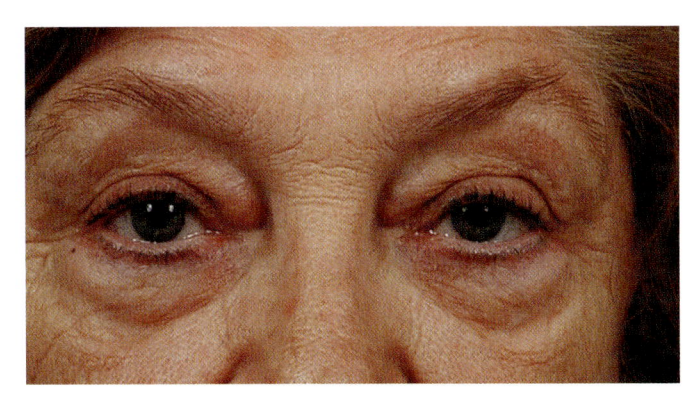

Figure 34.2 Typical changes in the eyelid region, including redundant upper lid skin, prominence of the upper and lower lid fat pads, and loss of the normal upslant along the lower eyelid margin.

Similarly, along the lower lid, an incision is made just below the lash margin. Through this, skin is elevated and redraped, and prominent fat pads are contoured or trimmed. Additionally, the lax canthal tendons can be tightened with either a canthopexy or canthoplasty. This positions the lower lid tightly to the globe at the level of the lower limbus, reestablishing a positive canthal tilt, or upward slant to the corner of the eye.

In most cases of upper blepharoplasty only, local or monitored anesthesia care suffices. General anesthesia is usually more appropriate for patients undergoing quad blepharoplasty. While not terribly painful, there is often a fair amount of postoperative ecchymosis and swelling that can take 14 days or more for resolution. There may also be a transient period of dry eyes, necessitating ocular lubricants. Patients are typically advised to refrain from strenuous activity for 4 weeks following surgery (Figure 34.4A–D).

Midface

Midface lift

Recently, there has been an expanding appreciation for the changes that occur in the malar region. In youth, the cheek is characterized by a smooth convexity from the lower lid to the area below the infraorbital rim. With aging, the midface musculature and malar fat pad descend. This is accompanied by volume loss, which has a deflationary effect and exacerbates midface descent. The result is loss of cheekbone prominence and lengthening of the distance between the lower eyelid and cheek.

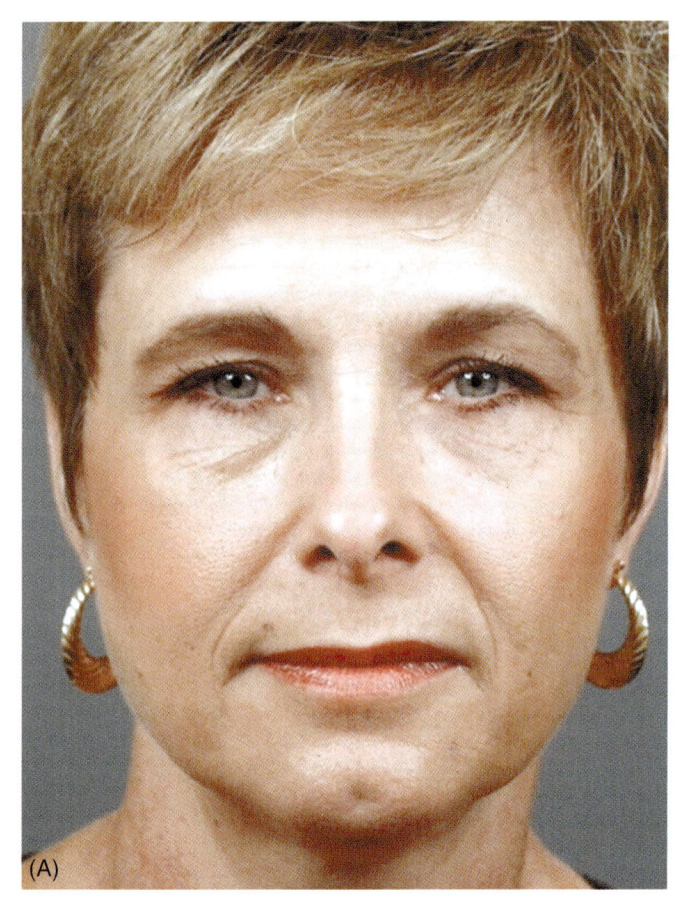

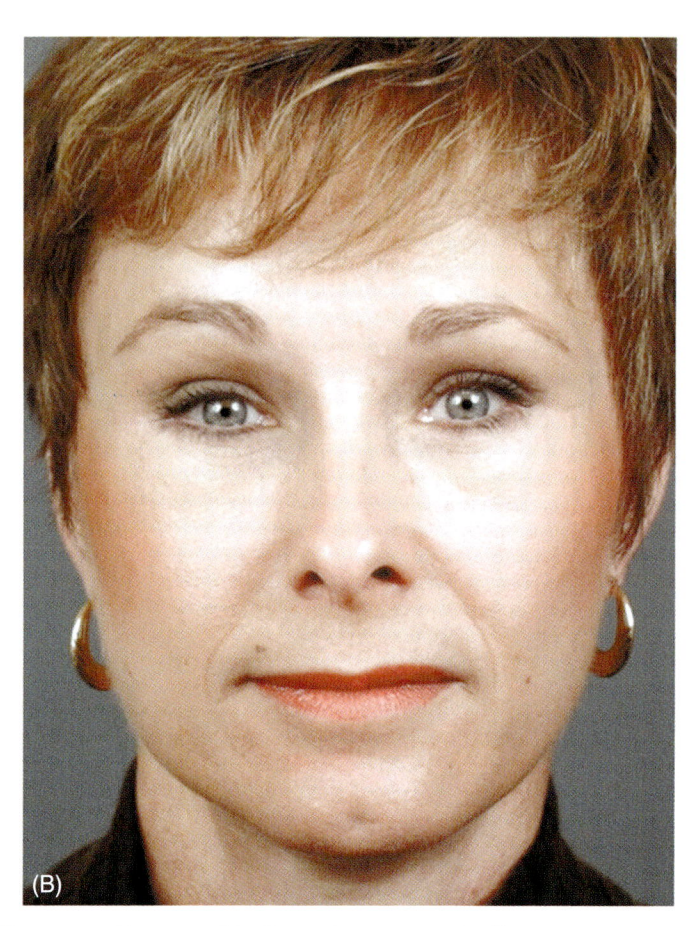

Figure 34.3 **(A)** This middle-aged woman has laxity of her brows, and puffy upper and lower eyelids. She underwent a minimally invasive (endoscopic) brow lift combined with upper and lower eyelid surgery. **(B)** After the operation she has a much more alert and less tired look and the puffiness of the eyelids has been improved. *Source:* Nahai 2011 from *The Art of Aesthetic Surgery: Principles.* Reproduced with permission of Taylor and Francis Group LLC.[1]

Hollowing occurs in the infraorbital region with development of tear troughs and nasojugal grooves. The nasolabial fold deepens as soft tissues push downward against the relatively fixed nasolabial retaining ligaments (Figure 34.5A and B).

A midface lift reverses these changes by releasing midface soft tissues and vertically elevating them to restore a natural lid–cheek junction. The result is correction of nasojugal grooves, restoration of malar projection, and softening of the nasolabial lines. The technique involves a subciliary incision, subperiosteal dissection from the inferior orbital rim to the lower border of the malar bone, with elevation and suspension of the mobilized malar soft tissue complex over the infraorbital rim. Lateral canthal fixation in the form of a canthopexy or canthoplasty is essential to reestablish lid tone and counteract the cicatricial forces of midface descent that can occur in the early postoperative period. A midface lift is performed under general anesthesia and can be combined with other surgical procedures to correct changes in the upper and lower face.

Rhinoplasty

There is a wide variability as to what constitutes an esthetic nose. A pleasing nose is influenced by gender, race, skin quality, and the dimensions of other facial features. Typical ideals include a straight and midline nasal dorsum, a refined tip with defined nasal tip points, smooth alar contours without flaring, and a nasolabial angle of 90–95° in men and 95–100° in women.

More so than these specifics, rhinoplasty strives to reshape the nose so that it is in balance with other facial features and to correct nasal irregularities. Possible intraoperative changes can include modifications to the width of the nose at the bridge or base. Techniques exist to remove bony humps often seen on profile. A rhinoplasty can incorporate steps to contour the nasal tip such that it is narrow and slightly upturned. Nostril reshaping may also be performed for wide or flaring nostrils.

Rhinoplasty surgery is typically done under general anesthesia. Incisions are made across the columella, the tissue between the nostrils, as well as intranasally. The soft tissues are elevated off of the nasal framework. This combination of bony and cartilage structures can then be appropriately contoured to achieve desired results.

Recovery includes a 7–14-day period of bruising and nasal congestion. Dressings can include both an external nasal splint and intranasal packing. Swelling can persist for several weeks, but changes should be noticeable after the first week or so. Any need for revisions is delayed for a significant period of time, usually a minimum of 1 year, to allow full resolution of swelling and stability of form (Figure 34.6).

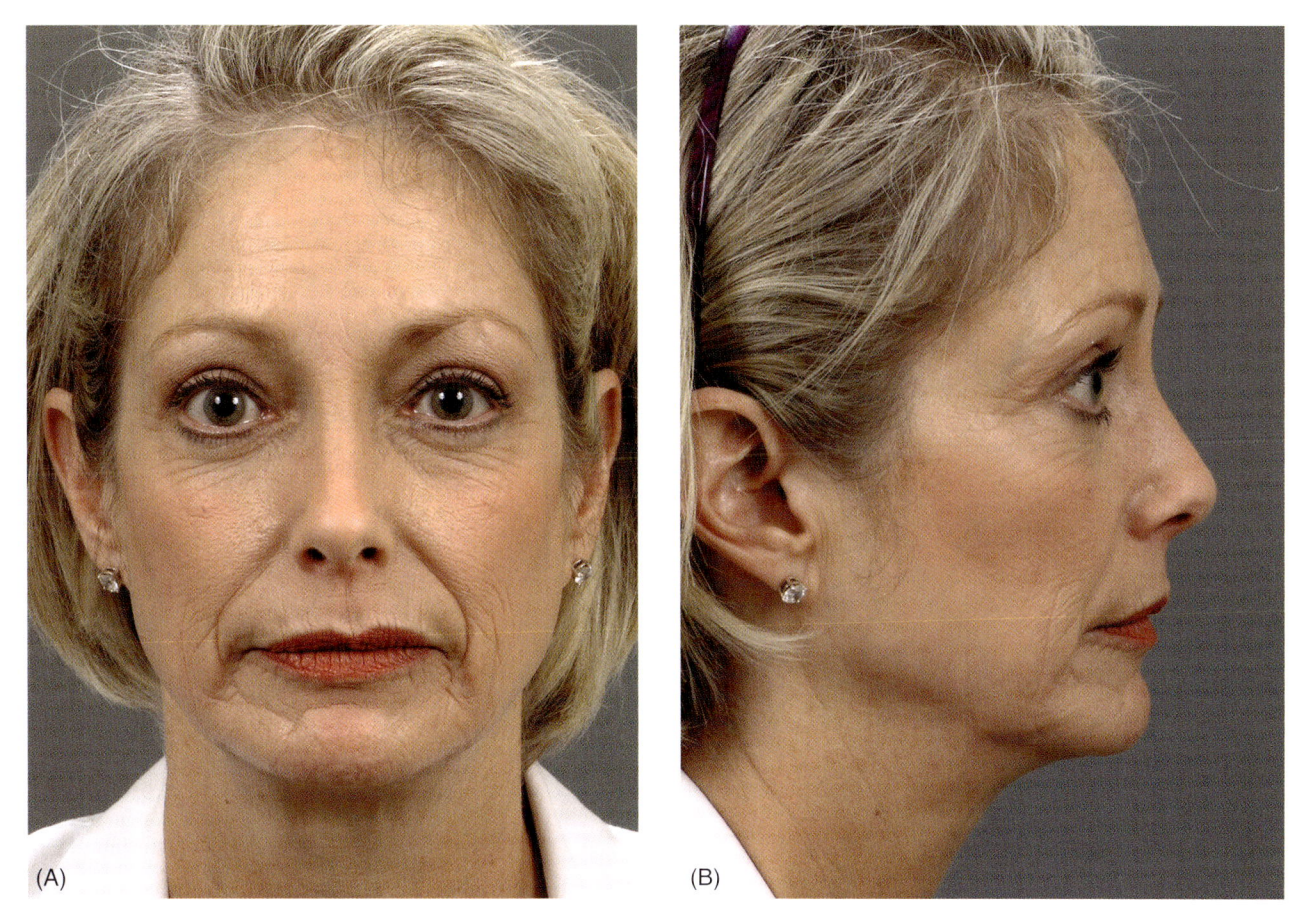

Figure 34.4 **(A, B)** A 58-year-old patient with evidence of lower lid skin laxity and rhytids.

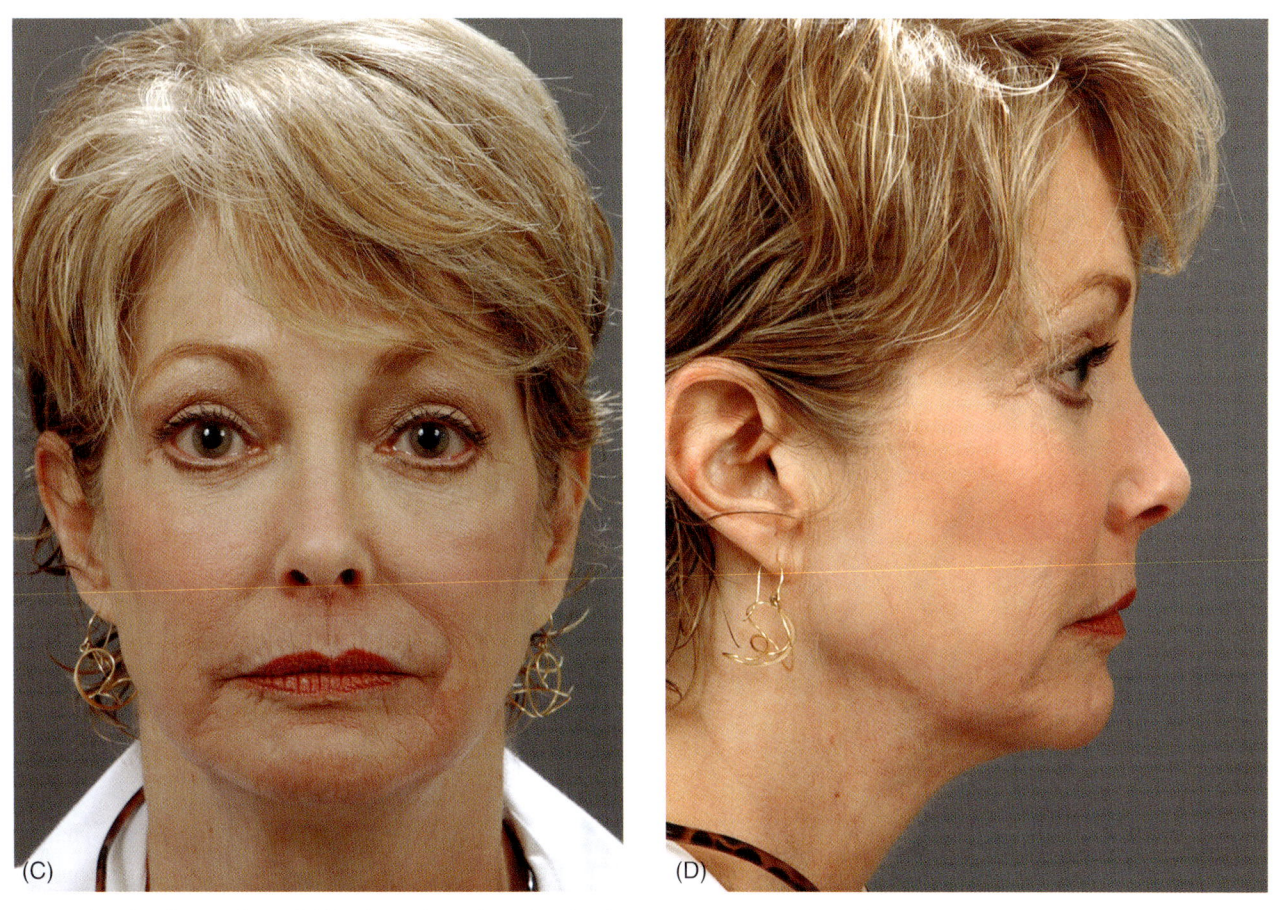

Figure 34.4 **(C, D)** Following lower lid blepharoplasty, the infraorbital region is now smooth and the lower lid position is maintained.

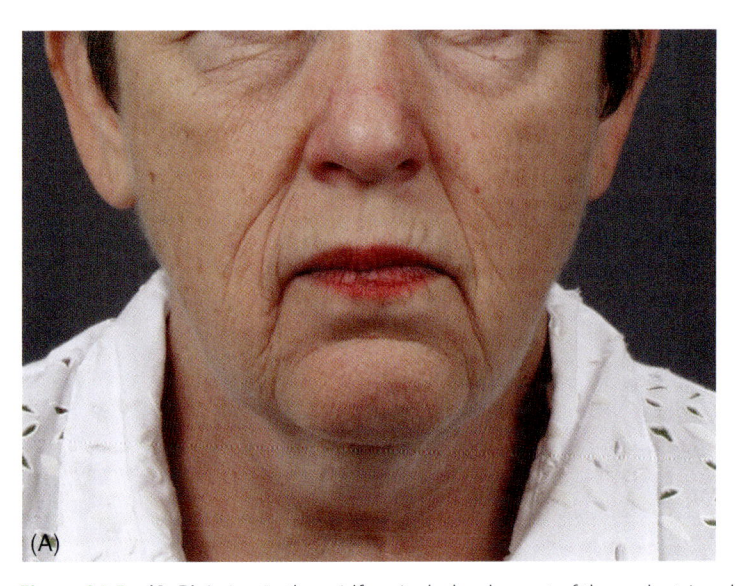

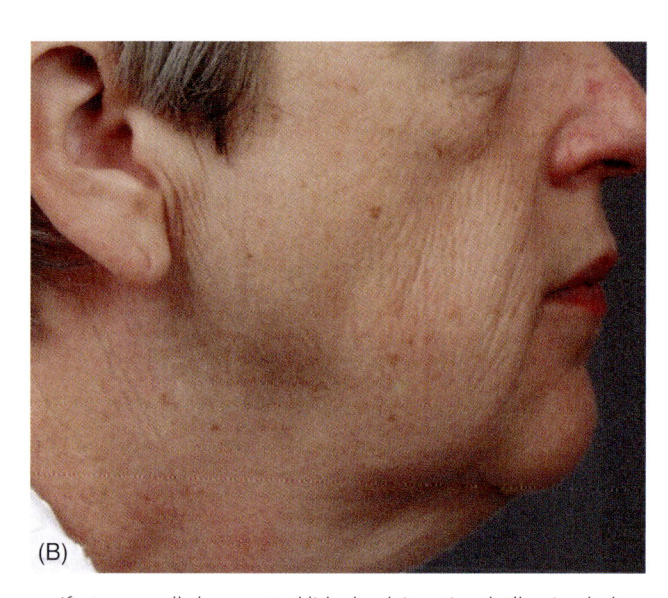

Figure 34.5 **(A, B)** Aging in the midface includes descent of the malar triangle, manifest as a well-demarcated lid–cheek junction, hollowing below the lower lid, loss of cheekbone prominence, and formation of a nasolabial fold. The step off between the lower lid region and the upper cheek is clearly apparent on the lateral view.

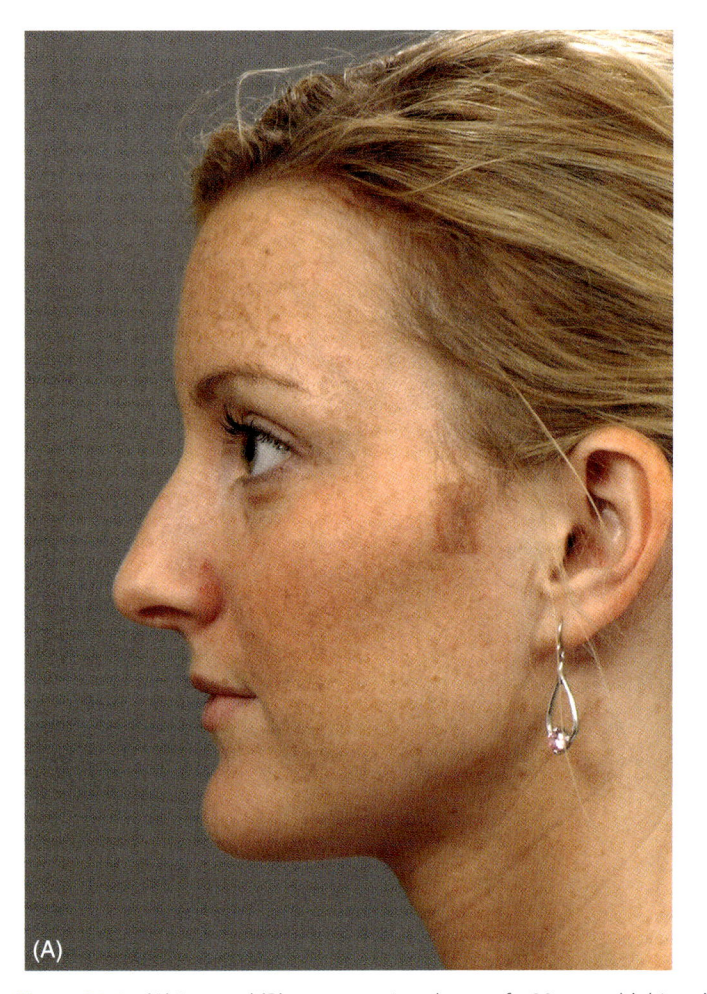

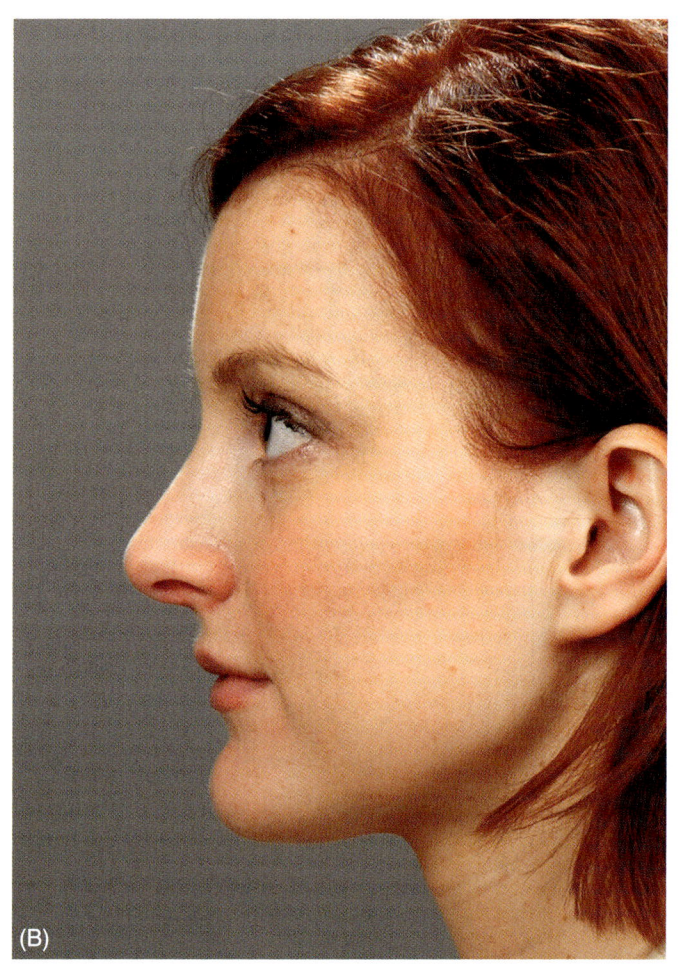

Figure 34.6 **(A)** Pre- and **(B)** postoperative photos of a 29-year-old rhinoplasty patient. The procedure has elevated her nasal tip and refined the slope of the nasal dorsum.

Lower face

Genioplasty

There is an inherent and proportional relationship between the nose and the chin, and in combination they strongly influence the facial profile. Typically, the nose, lips, and chin are in alignment on side or profile view. A common finding seen in rhinoplasty patients is that of a concurrent receding chin or microgenia. The chin is recontoured with insertion of a chin implant, through an intraoral or submental incision. Alloplastic implant augmentation is excellent for minor deficiencies. In situations requiring more significant advancement, an osseous genioplasty can be performed. The approach for a genioplasty is either intraoral or an external submental incision. Recovery time averages 1 week or more.

Rhytidectomy

In youth, the skin of the lower face is firmly draped over the lower mandibular border and submental soft tissues. Changes usually start in the fourth and fifth decades. Although externally viewed as loose, redundant skin, the true etiology of lower facial aging is attenuation of the supportive fascial layers. The superficial musculoaponeurotic system envelops the facial mimetic muscles and is contiguous with the platysma overlying the neck muscles. In the process of facial aging, these structures become subject to gravity and downward-pulling vectors. Retaining ligaments, which normally maintain the skin over the bony periosteum, relax over time. Clinical manifestations of these processes include jowling across the mandibular line, marionette and nasolabial line formation, and loose skin across the anterior neck with an obtuse cervicomental angle (Figure 34.7).

A rhytidectomy, or facelift, addresses these changes not only by excising redundant skin, but more importantly by tightening the underlying connective tissue layers in the face and neck. By elevating and plicating these layers with sutures, sagging facial tissues are resuspended. Midface descent, ptotic jowls, and neck laxity are corrected and fixed at the deeper tissue level. Skin is redraped on this foundation and trimmed in the temporal scalp and along the anterior and posterior aspects of the ear. With tension directed toward the deeper layers and away from the skin, the result is a more natural, well-contoured look with less of a "windswept" appearance and "operated look" (Figure 34.8).

A drain is placed and removed within the first few days postoperatively. Patients are maintained in a removable chin strap to counteract swelling and facilitate skin retraction. Neck flexing should be minimized and blood pressure is well controlled to prevent hematoma formation. Recovery in terms of pain, swelling, and bruising ranges from 1 to 2 weeks.

Nonsurgical

The long-standing gold standard for achieving significant and durable changes in facial appearance is surgery. Injectable, nonsurgical treatments are recent options. According to the American Society for Aesthetic Plastic Surgery 2015 statistics, over 6.6 million injectable procedures were performed in 2015.[2]

Although in most cases the results achieved with injectables are temporary and require repeat treatment, there are other advantages that make them highly appealing alternatives or, in some cases, adjuncts to surgery. Treatments are performed with or without local or topical anesthesia in an office setting. Recovery time is brief, with the most notable sequelae being the possibility of several days of bruising. Results are often immediate without incurring surgical scars. Cost is reasonable and much less than surgical procedures, but the cost is accumulative. For patients with medical comorbidities that preclude surgery, there is usually no contraindication to facial injections.

Neurotoxins

Most facial wrinkles are the result of underlying muscle activity. This is particularly true in the upper face, where dynamic muscles result in expression lines commonly known as "frown lines" between the eyebrows, "crows feet" around the eyes, and transverse forehead lines. Neurotoxins limit hyperactive muscle activity with softening of wrinkles and furrows. By eliminating muscle contractions, neurotoxins improve the appearance of established wrinkles and prevent the development of new ones. These injections may also be therapeutic in cases of facial asymmetry, such as facial paralysis, where treating muscle imbalance improves overall facial appearance. Results of neurotoxin injections typically manifest 2–7 days after treatment. Duration of results can vary from individual to individual but is most commonly in the 3–4 months range.

Soft tissue fillers

Facial hollows and depressions are the stigmata of aging, trauma, and occasionally surgery. The last two decades have seen a surge in techniques and products to fill facial wrinkles and augment folds. Dermal fillers are designed to restore volume, whether to a wrinkle line, a larger area, or a specific structure. Traditionally, fillers have been injected in the area around the nose and mouth, but more recently the areas for treatment have expanded. Fillers improve the nasolabial folds that arc from the alar base of the nose to the mouth and the marionette lines that extend from the corner of the mouth to the chin. Filler volume can also camouflage depressions such as the prejowl sulcus along the mandibular border, posttraumatic scars, or irregularities following rhinoplasty. They can enhance shape and definition when injected into the lips. Temporal hollowing, under-eye tear troughs, and malar volume depletion may also be treated with dermal fillers, resulting in some improvement and restoration of convexity. Fillers can also be used to enhance otherwise normal structures where volume and fullness are desired. Lip augmentation and cheekbone definition are examples of this (Figure 34.9).

There are a variety of fillers available, varying in chemical composition, duration, and applicability. Some are temporary, lasting in the region of 6 months, some are longer lasting, in the region of 2 years, and others are permanent. Not every filler is appropriate for every facial region. An experienced injector is well versed in assessing the facial contours, determining what product will be most efficacious, and utilizing injection techniques that minimize the risk of complications.

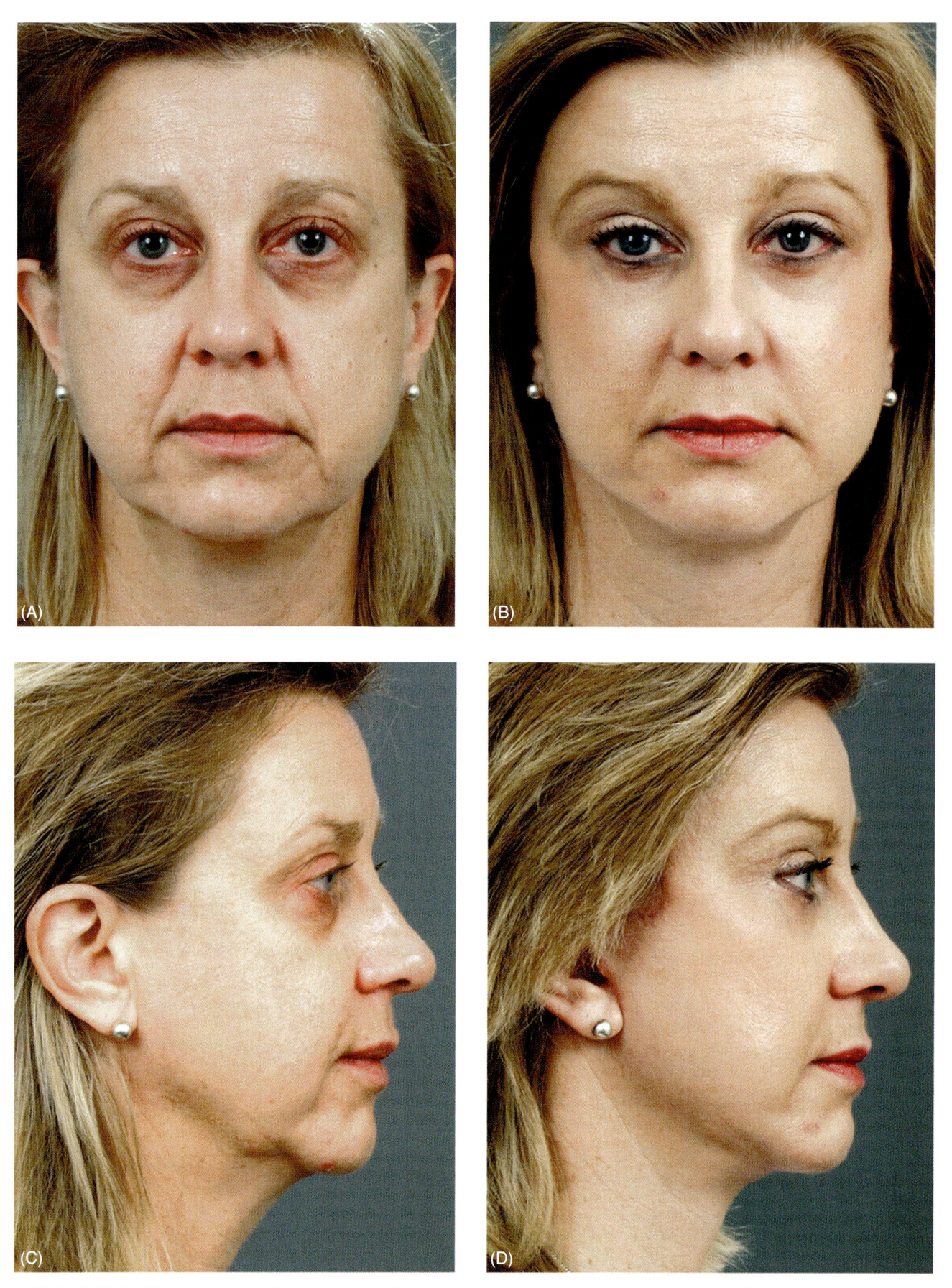

Figure 34.7 **(A, B)** This 56-year-old patient has age-associated changes in her brows, around the eyes, cheeks, jaw line, and neck. She underwent a minimally invasive (endoscopic) brow lift, upper and lower blepharoplasty and full face and neck lift. **(C, D)** Postoperatively she looks refreshed and less tired. Note the softening of the lid/cheek junction below the eyes, improvement in the marionette lines, and tightening across the mandibular jawline. *Source:* Nahai 2011 from *The Art of Aesthetic Surgery: Principles*. Reproduced with permission of Taylor and Francis Group LLC.[1]

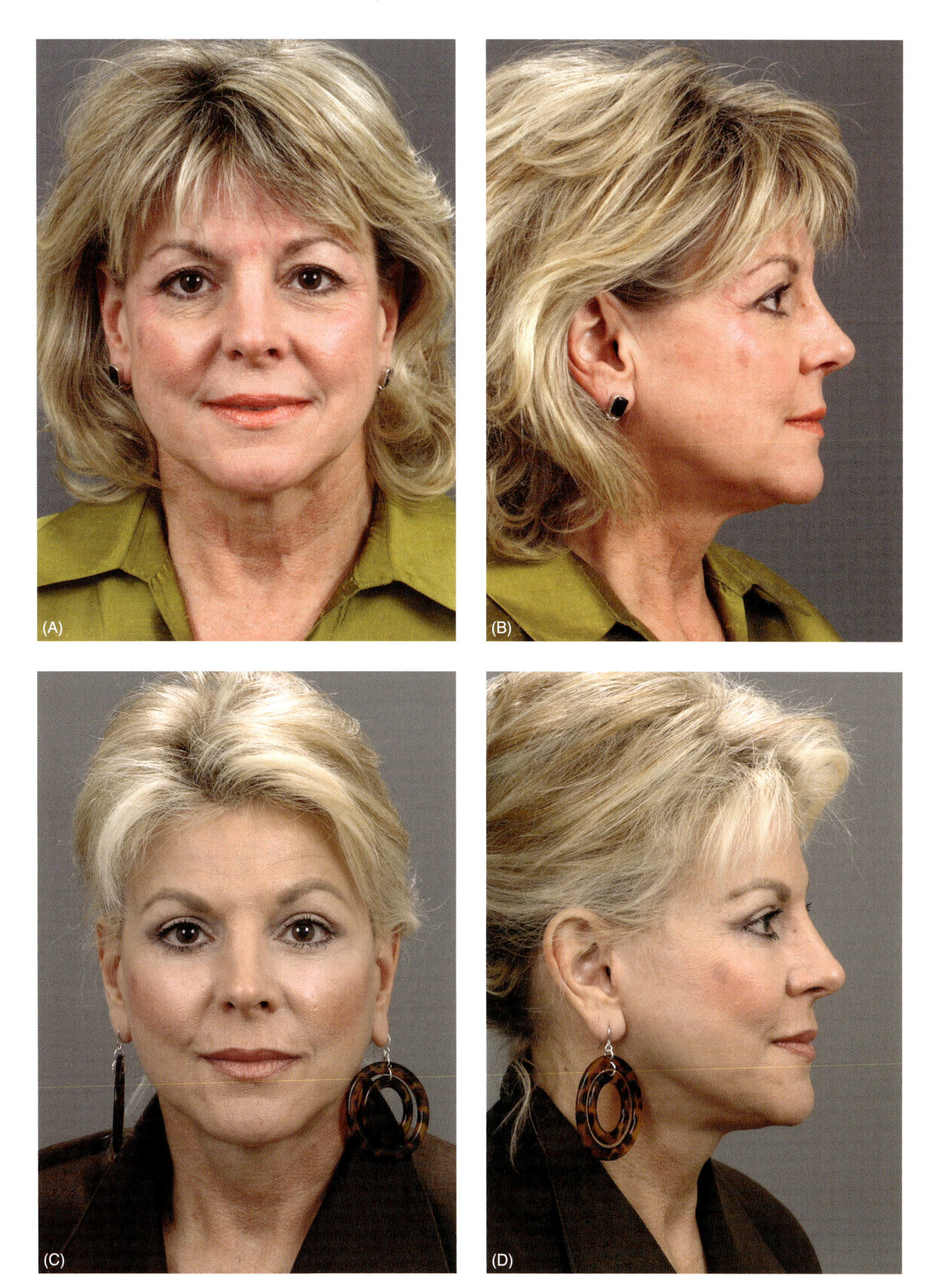

Figure 34.8 **(A, B)** A 58-year-old patient desiring facial rejuvenation. **(C, D)** Patient following rhytidectomy and four-lid blepharoplasty. Patient appears younger without the stigmata of an "operated appearance."

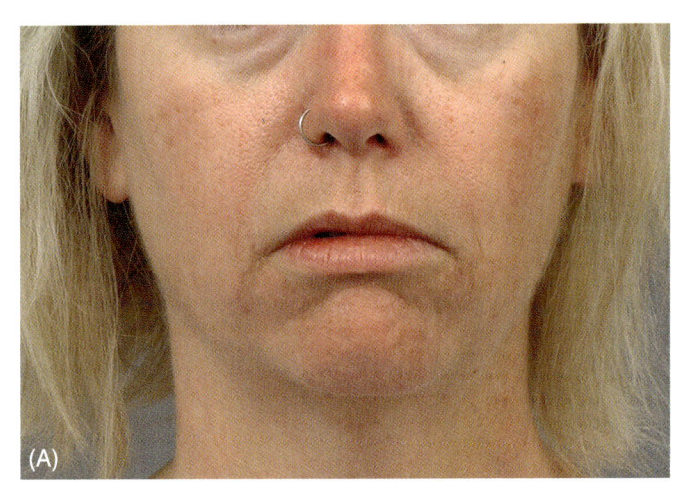

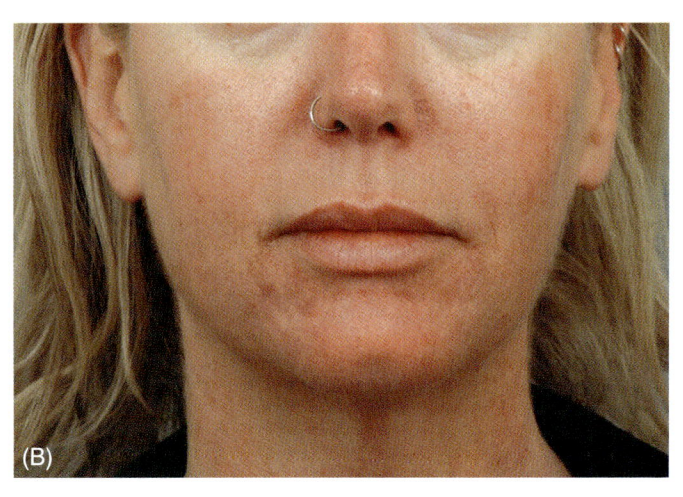

Figure 34.9 (A, B) Patient with soft-tissue fillers placed in her lips and lower face. The volume improves her symmetry and softens her overall appearance.

Facial resurfacing

Facial and neck skin undergo changes as a result of aging and photodamage. Although surgical techniques can correct structural changes that occur over time, they do little to address the textural changes seen in the skin. Deep perioral wrinkles or established crows feet often persist after facial surgery. Clinical improvement in skin quality and appearance is more readily achieved with nonsurgical techniques. Skin resurfacing softens wrinkles, erases sun-induced dyschromia, and tightens skin laxity. Lasers direct thermal energy to replace a damaged dermis with new collagen that results in wrinkle removal and skin tightening. Chemical peels essentially remove outer skin layers to improve irregular pigmentation and soften wrinkles. Dermabrasion remains useful to treat particularly deep or resistant wrinkles, such as "lipstick lines," acne scars, or posttraumatic scars.

Despite being noninvasive in nature, these resurfacing techniques do have some associated recovery time while reepithelialization is occurring. Immediate aftertreatment often involves maintaining skin moisture with occlusive dressings until epithelialization is complete. Long term skin improvement will be enhanced with adoption of a comprehensive skin care regimen and sun avoidance.

Patient safety

Any decision about what plastic surgery may be beneficial begins with an evaluation and consultation by a board certified plastic surgeon with expertise in esthetic surgery and cosmetic medicine. Because state laws permit any licensed physician to call themselves a "plastic" or "cosmetic" surgeon, prospective patients must select their doctor carefully. There are many physicians today practicing esthetic plastic surgery who have received their formal training in another specialty, often a nonsurgical specialty. A board certified plastic surgeon is certified by the American Board of Plastic Surgery (ABPS). ABPS is the only board recognized by the American Board of Medical Specialties to certify physicians in the full range of plastic and reconstructive procedures. To be certified by the ABPS, a physician must have at least 6 years of approved surgical training, including a residency in plastic surgery. They must also pass comprehensive written and oral exams in plastic surgery. A qualified physician is usually a member of a national plastic surgery organization, such as the American Society for Aesthetic Plastic Surgery or the American Society of Plastic Surgeons. With an emphasis on patient safety, the surgeon should be performing procedures in an accredited hospital or outpatient surgery center.

Conclusion

The goal of esthetic plastic surgery is to remodel normal structures to improve appearance. In facial surgery alone, many procedures are available to achieve just this. A skilled plastic surgeon is not only well versed in performing the technical aspects of these operations, but also in preoperatively assessing the possibility of achieving desired results. Accurately setting realistic expectations for the patient becomes a crucial component of achieving postoperative patient satisfaction.

Esthetic plastic surgery remains particularly relevant in the realm of dental esthetics by complementing work that is done to the jaw, teeth, and perioral region. Both disciplines are in constant evolution with the development of new products and techniques to improve outcomes and optimize patient safety. Although it is impossible to predict what innovations may occur in these specialties in ensuing decades, the link between esthetic dentistry and esthetic plastic surgery is a well-forged one that will persist.

References

1. Nahai F, ed. *The Art of Aesthetic Surgery: Principles & Techniques*. Boca Raton, FL; CRC Press; 2011.
2. The American Society of Aesthetic Plastic Surgery. *2015 Cosmetic Surgery National Data Bank Statistics*. https://www.surgery.org/sites/default/files/Stats2015.pdf (accessed November 6, 2017).

Additional resources

Bashour M. History and current concepts in the analysis of facial attractiveness. *Plast Reconstr Surg* 2006;118(3):741–756.

Bauer U. The science of temporary and permanent fillers: an overview of fillers. In: Cohen SR, Born TM, eds. *Facial Rejuvenation with Fillers*. London: Elsevier; 2009:1–10.

Borah GL, Rankin MK. Appearance is a function of the face. *Plast Reconstr Surg* 2010;125(3):873–878.

Goldstein RE. *Change Your Smile: Discover How a New Smile Can Transform Your Life*, 4th edn. Chicago, IL: Quintessence; 2009.

Naini FB, Gill DS. Facial aesthetics: concepts and canons. *Dent Update* 2008;35:102–107.

Pacella SJ, Nahai F, Codner MA. Treatment of the superficial musculoaponeurotic system during minimally invasive surgery. In: Nahai F, Nahai FR, eds. *Minimially Invasive Facial Rejuvenation*. London: Elsevier; 2009:137–153.

Peck H, Peck S. A concept of facial aesthetics. *Angle Orthod* 1970;40:119–127.

Sullivan PK, Hoy EA. Necklift VS. Neck rejuvenation. In: Nahai F, Nahai FR, eds. *Minimially Invasive Facial Rejuvenation*. London: Elsevier; 2009:99–109.

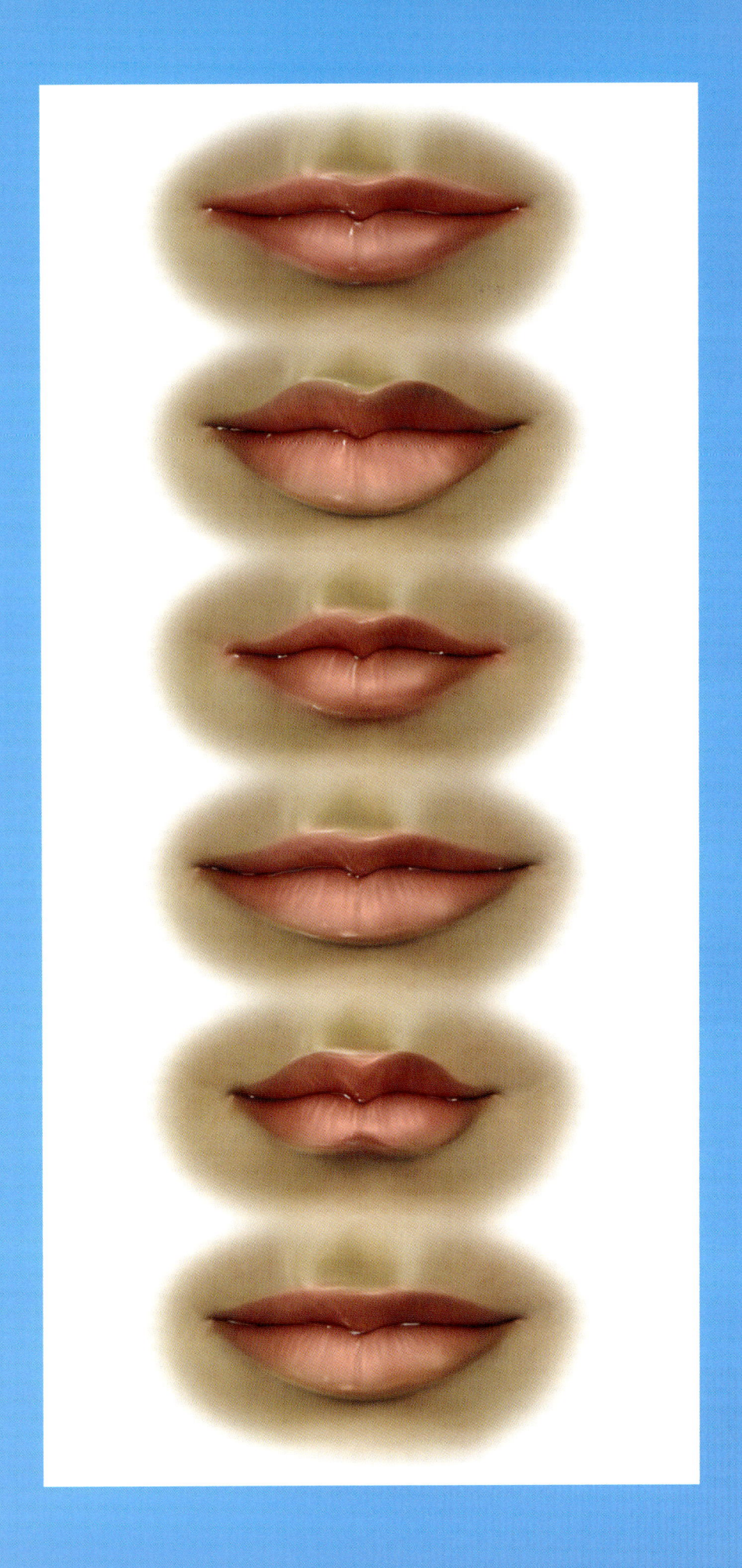

Chapter 35 Cosmetic Adjuncts

Ronald E. Goldstein, DDS, Richard Davis, and Marvin Westmore

Chapter Outline

Facial shape for women	1144	Makeup and color	1149
Principles of esthetics	1144	Corrective makeup and contouring	1149
Hair color	1147	Lip coloring	1150
Facial shape for men	1147	Selecting the right lipstick color	1151
Makeup	1149	Makeup for a disfigured face	1151
Skin care	1149	Makeup for men with disfigurements	1151
Makeup… an illusion	1149		

The main goal of the cosmetologist, makeup artist, hairstylist, and plastic surgeon is the same as the cosmetic dentist: to help the person look their best. What the dentist needs to be aware of is that different facial shapes may require different sizes, shapes, color, and arrangement of teeth to help achieve the best look for that type of face. Thus, a partnership with the professional hairstylist, makeup artist, cosmetologist, or plastic surgeon can play an important role.

Since facial diagnosis plays such an important part in smile design, I have my dental assistants take a full series of digital photographs, including adequate full-face photos as outlined in Chapter 3. The photos are immediately downloaded in the computer, so both my patient and I can study them during the consultation. If I feel that one or more auxiliary facial treatments will improve the overall esthetic outcome, a discussion with the patient will take place during this or the next consultation appointment. I have never had a problem explaining possibilities once my patient asks my advice. In fact, when I plan a full mouth smile makeover, I will frequently include a complimentary "day at one of the best hair salons in Atlanta." Usually, I suggest a new hairstyle and makeup session with the salon. Most patients cannot wait for this day to take place and never let me forget it!

The question most dentists ask me is how can they bring up the subject without insulting the patient? I preempt my discussion with an explanation to the patient that "I design the smile based on how it will look best with your face so I need to know a few things about your future plans. First, do you ever change your hairstyle or are you open to change? And second, are you planning any facial surgery in the future? Your answer may well influence the type of smile design I create."

Obviously, it is wise to discuss cosmetic adjuncts with patients who are really looking for a new smile to help "change their life" or to look much younger. These types of patients generally appreciate my advice and ask who I would refer them to for a makeup artist and plastic surgeon. And if a plastic surgeon is desired, I offer several names I have worked with.

I actually began my study of the topic early on in my career when I examined thousands of male and female faces and even formed the first interdisciplinary esthetics study club that consisted of a plastic surgeon, hairstylist, and makeup artist among other dental specialists. We learned from each other with our biweekly meetings, usually with live patents as well as slide presentations.

The bottom line is the more you study the possibilities of what can be accomplished with plastic surgery, makeup, and hairstyle, the more qualified you will be not only in smile design but also in helping your patients get the most out of their life.

Hairstyling can be a positive asset to enhancing one's appearance. The length and texture of the hair as well as the color and style all have an influence on a person's self-image. A hairstyle frames the face and can minimize or conceal protruding ears or an overly round face as well as a prominent forehead. On the other hand, the hairstyle can draw attention to negative facial features. Thus, a hairstyle can play a major role in the balance and symmetry around the face. Hair design utilizes illusions that not only can enhance the face but also help the dentist achieve a more satisfied patient with their new smile.

The hair design that a person may choose can improve or take away from their overall appearance and the treatment that has been completed on their smile. For instance, an excessively short hair design could be very flattering on a perfect oval or square face but could be unflattering on a long or triangular face. Hair that frames the face can draw attention to specific areas or it can be used to change the area of exposed face to give a more pleasing shape. Care must be taken in determining the hair design, so as to enhance the positive aspects of the face. A hair design that an individual may choose could be determined by many factors: personal desire, lifestyle, ease of care, type of hair (i.e., coarse thin/thick, etc.) current fashion trends, or peer influence.

The most important factor, though, should be the proper balance with the facial features and bone structure. The ideal solution for a dental practice is to seek out a professional hair designer/hairstylist who has a reputation for creating complimentary and flattering hair design for improving esthetic appearance. Websites are usually quite helpful to see just how successful a hairstylist has been with previous clients or models.

A hair designer will work with several different facial shapes, as shown later, but most people fall into five basic facial shapes: oval, round, square, long, heart shape. Ideally, all angles of the face need to be considered when making a hairstyle selection.

Facial shape for women

The ideal illusion most often sought after by stylists is the oval face. To distinguish an oval face, the length of the face should be one and a half times the width, as in Figure 35.1. Oval faces can be the most proportionate, meaning they can wear any kind of cut or style (short, medium long, sharp, and full). There are several styling suggestions for working with an oval face. For example, if the face looks long, having the stylist create bangs across the brow line can break up the length and also add width to the face.

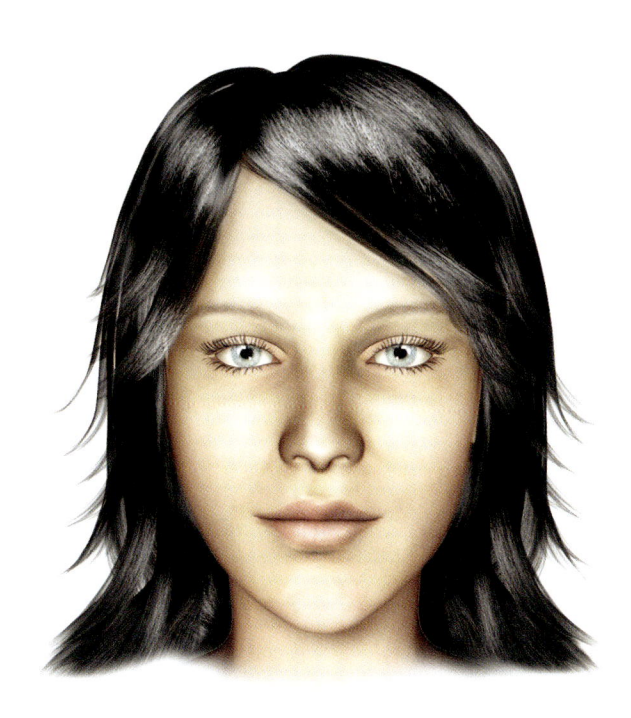

Figure 35.1 This illustration demonstrates how the oval face can look good with most any hair type or style.

Another suggestion is creating a short cut with side swept hair across the forehead which can show off the neck and collarbone. It can also break up a long face.

The round face is as wide as it is long (Figure 35.2A and B). A great design would be a layered cut with a swooping side bang. Avoid super-short designs unless there are longer layers around the face, to keep the face as slim as possible. Another technique is creating a sleek up-style above the ears which will create greater facial definition. This will make the cheekbones appear longer, and with the height it will even out the rounder dimensions. Another suggestion is a pixie cut that can emphasize the cheekbones and eyes. A round face also looks great with an uneven cut which has a mix of different lengths. The face will look slimmer if the hair is side swept across the forehead.

A square face has angular cheeks and jaw (Figure 35.3A). In having a square face, the goal is to play down the strong angular jaw. To soften these features, curls or frayed ends can be added. Layering is another technique the stylist can use. This type of face can also wear a short, spiked look or a long sleek design with soft layers starting around the jawline. A tousled short shag cut with body can deemphasize the square shape of the face (Figure 35.3B).

Principles of esthetics

The heart-shaped face, has a narrow jaw with wider cheek bones, and sometimes a wider forehead (Figure 35.4A–D) This shape may be able to sport shoulder-length hair and long waves. They can also wear shorter hair, but should always have either full or longer bangs swept across to cover the wider forehead. The goal is to emphasize the eyes.

Chapter 35   Cosmetic Adjuncts   1145

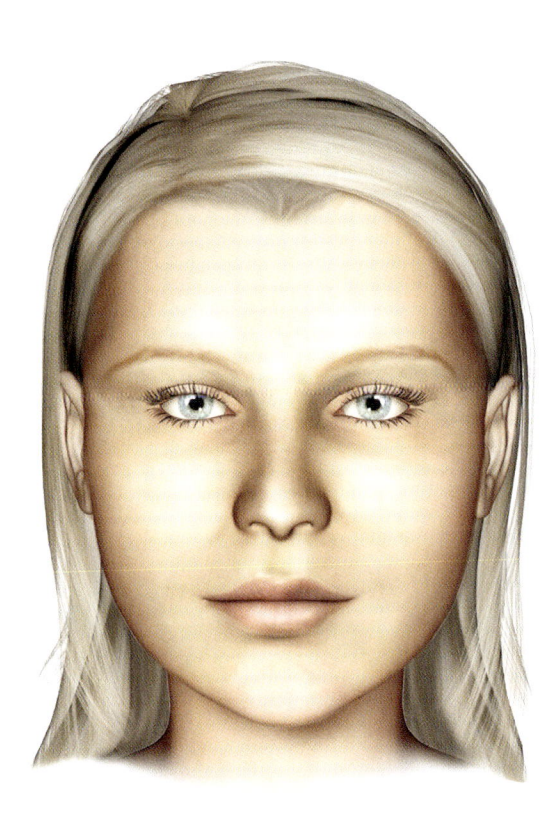

Figure 35.2 **(A)** This illustration of a female with a round face emphasizes the roundness when the hair is pulled back behind the ears.

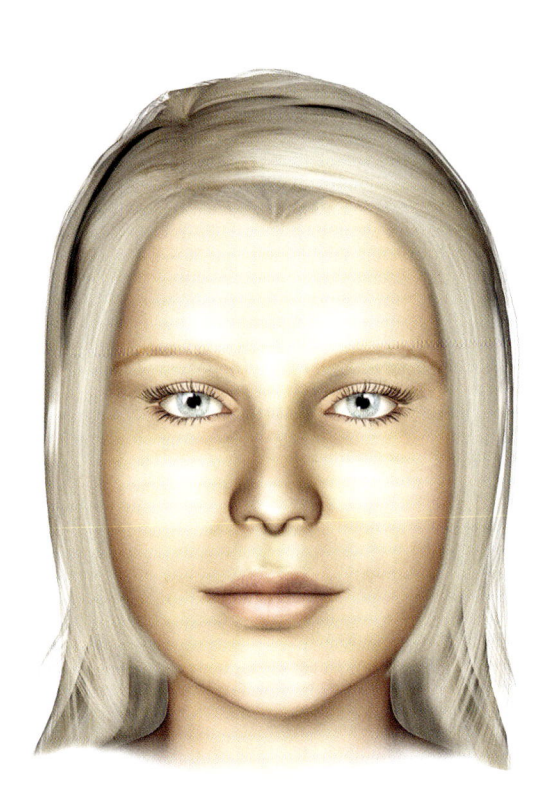

Figure 35.2 **(B)** The face would look slimmer if the hair was pulled over the ears, thus slimming the face.

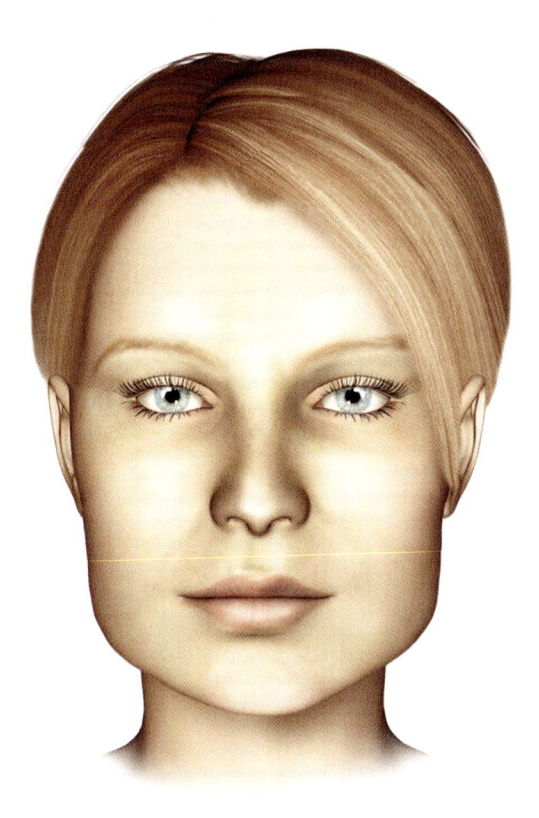

Figure 35.3 **(A)** This illustration shows how the angular jaw contributes to a more square-looking face.

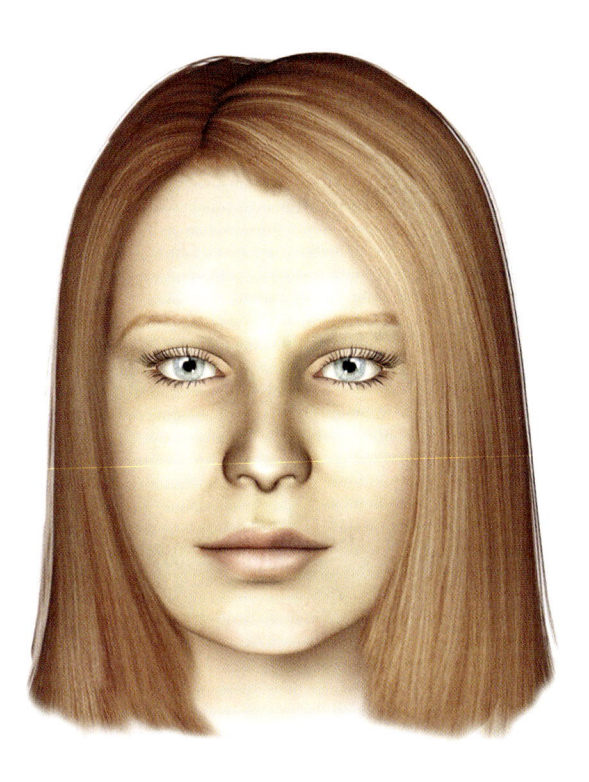

Figure 35.3 **(B)** Note how a hairstyle that covers the angular part of the face helps soften the square look.

(A)

(B)

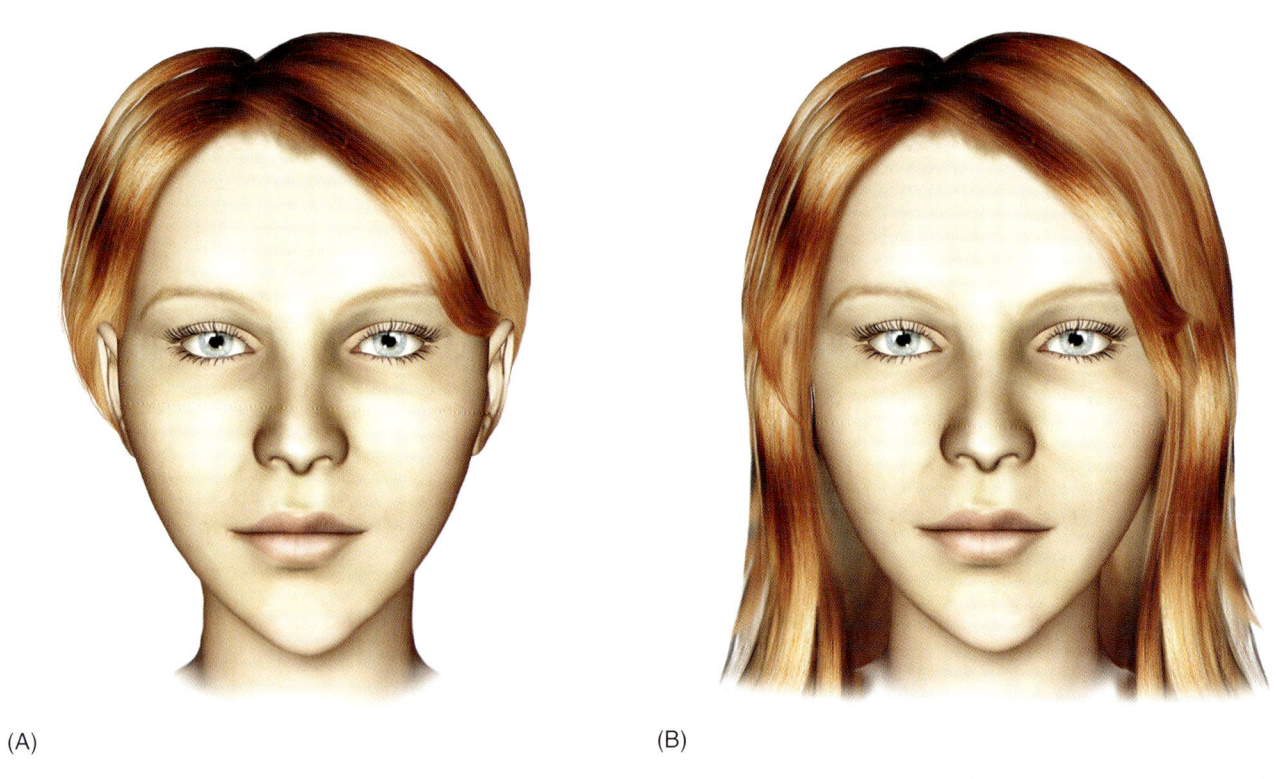

Figure 35.4 **(A, B)** The heart-shaped face calls for masking a wide forehead, plus a better hairstyle, which helps the face appear more oval.

(C)

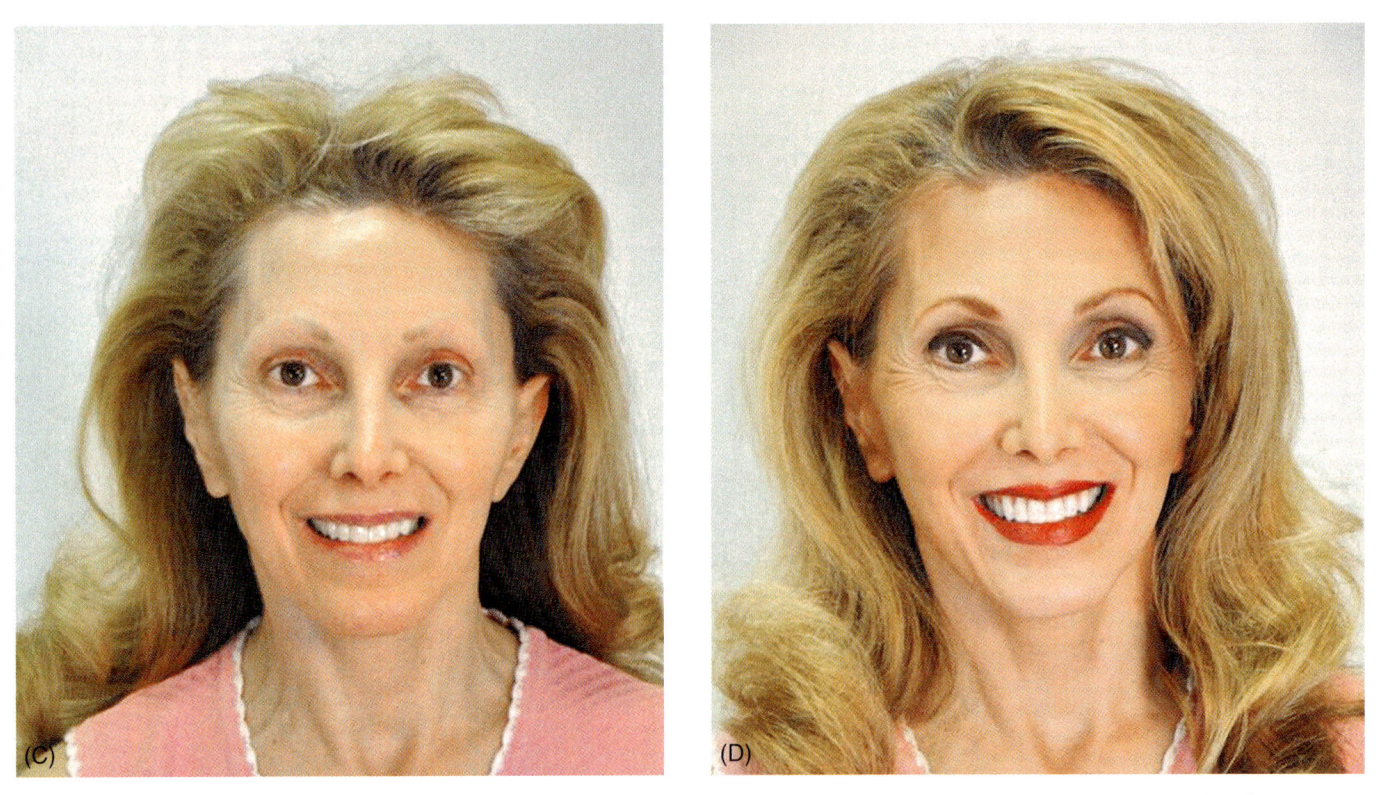

(D)

Figure 35.4 **(C, D)** This woman has a heart-shaped face, so the goal of the makeover was to balance her narrow chin with the width of the upper part of her face. The makeup artist applied a crème foundation lighter than her natural skin tone as a highlight on her chin to diminish its sharpness and softened her forehead and cheek areas with darker shades of powder and blush. The hairstylist gave her long layers to add fullness around her chin line and just a wisp of bangs to give her a more balanced look. (Makeup by Rhonda Barrymore; hair by Richard Davis.) *Source:* Goldstein 2009, from *Change Your Smile*, 4th edition. Reproduced with permission of Quintessence Publishing Co. Inc., Chicago.[1]

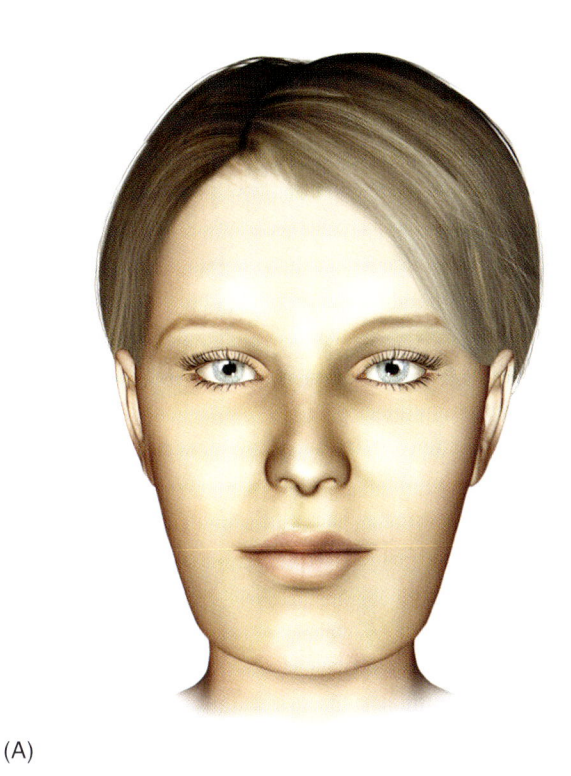

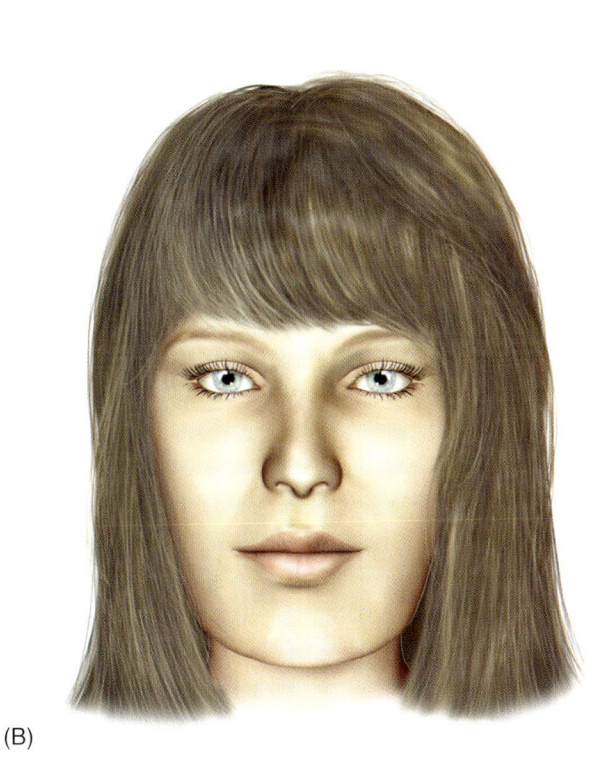

Figure 35.5 **(A, B)** The long face can be masked somewhat by the use of bangs in the hairstyle.

A middle part is one style to avoid because it can appear unflattering.

A long face is similar to a round face but narrower (Figure 35.5). Designs can vary from short, medium, to long. A wedge or graduated short haircut shaping the face would work very well, adding width to the face and adding straight across bangs with a side part.

Other styles that work well are longer layers and designs at the chin or shoulders turning under or with a flip. Stay away from short layers on the top, as this would add height and extend the length of the face more, as well as a middle part.

Hair color

Hair coloring can also be very helpful in creating illusions, or just adding a more youthful look to the face. A woman with gray hair can have an aging appearance if the skin tone is milky white. A short cut can be very attractive, but the majority of the time it will cause an aging effect. In doing a complete new color for this person, the designer should stay one or two shade's lighter than the client's original color. The designer could also decide to add lowlights or highlights if the person has premature gray hair instead of all-over color. These techniques would also benefit a woman with a dull drab color, giving the hair more life and dimension. For a quick fix, a mess-proof marker and mascara-like brushes offer instant gray root coverage between salon visits.

Tooth shade plays an important role when deciding on hair color. A patient with gray hair would look best with bright white teeth. A person with brown hair which is highlighted can make the teeth look more yellow.

Paying attention to lipstick color can also help to downplay yellow teeth or highlight white teeth. For example, a bold red shade will draw attention to white teeth, but make yellow teeth stand out more. On the other hand, a nude color lipstick will draw attention away from yellowed or stained teeth.

Highlights are the use of a lighter shade of color than the natural hair, where lowlights create just the opposite. In addition, highlights of blonde or caramel, or red tones for warmth, can bring life and dimension to the hair as well as frame the face. Natural-looking highlights are a great way to add age-defying definition. In understanding the different shades of hair, just as in makeup, a stylist can hide various flaws in the facial shape and an improved total facial look can be created.

Facial shape for men

Men, as with women, have a need for a hairstyle that works with their facial shape to provide an illusion that will improve their appearance. Men tend to have a hairstyle they feel works best for their chosen profession, as well as what makes them feel comfortable. They may be losing their hair and feel insecure and try to hide the fact, or just wear the style that their spouse, girlfriend, or partner likes best. The kindest advice is to suggest to your patient that he might want to talk to a hair professional to suggest a style that can enhance his new smile. Basic hairstyles for men are somewhat more limiting for them than for women.

Nevertheless, there are ways to help men by emphasizing or deemphasizing the lower part of the face, even though it may be more challenging. The hair design that is chosen can improve or take away from the overall appearance. A man also has a different hair feature that can either enhance or take away his best look: facial hair. If used to enhance the smile, facial hair should be groomed and still work with creating the shape and look of the face (Figure 35.6). The oval shape is versatile, and any hairstyle will enhance it, but the patient needs to be aware of the thickness or thinness of his hair texture on his head. Men with a square face may choose short hair for the conservative look with a little natural height on top or they can wear a longer look that takes away from their strong jaw line. Men with long faces should have hairstyles that show width or fullness on the side. A heart shape face or diamond, as in women, features a more pronounced chin that may also be covered with facial hair. The shape can be changed by slimming the forehead with full bangs, while widening the chin area with a tapered look. Also, a very short cut could also work well.

There are some instances when the dentist is not able to create an "ideal" smile for the patient. Often, the patient has financial considerations and a budget that may limit cosmetic dentistry. In these cases, the hairstylist may want to create illusions with the hair that will draw attention away from the smile. For example, a patient with a high lip line who has chosen to not have gum surgery to raise the gum line may have a "horsey" smile. The hairstylist needs to work with his face to draw the attention to other features, and using hair as a directional guide can work wonders.

Ultimately, both the cosmetic dentist and the hairstylist must consider the shape of the face, bone structure, skin color, eye color, hair texture, and smile before they make changes. A cosmetic dentist who takes a digital photo of a completed patient's face and sends it to the hairstylist with notations would be doing the patient a great service in highlighting areas of the face or mouth that the stylist may have overlooked.

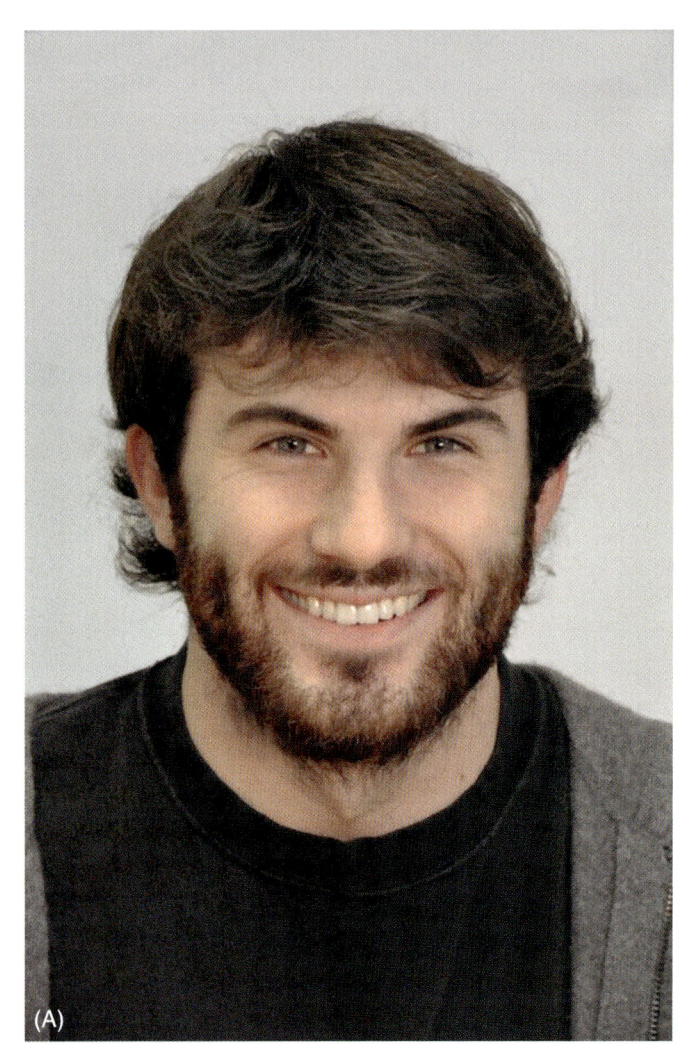

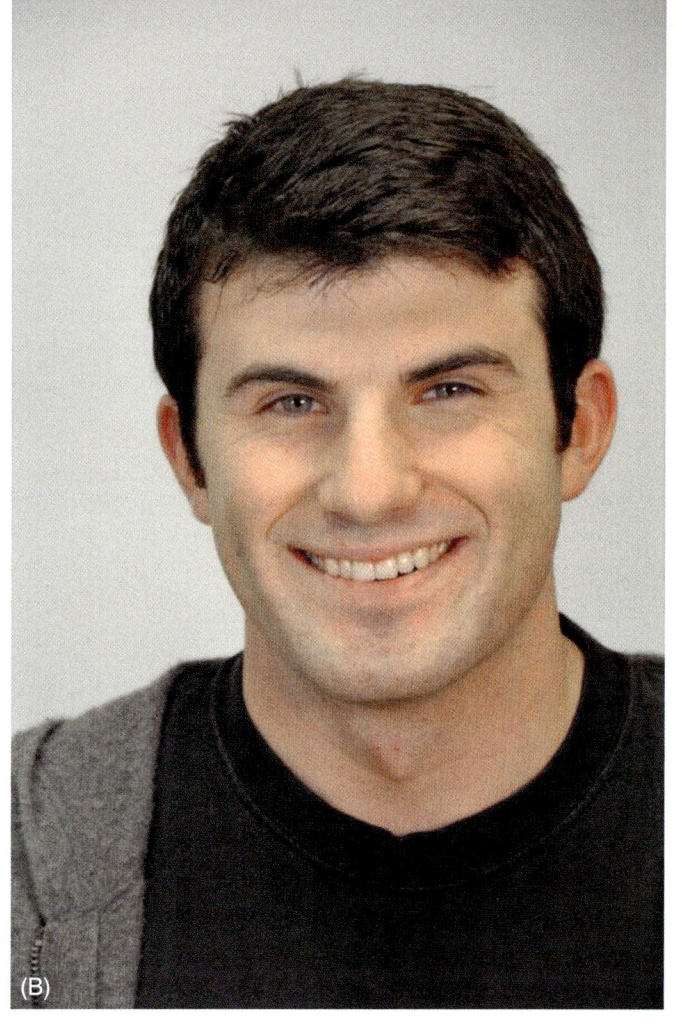

Figure 35.6 (A, B) This young man had allowed his hair to grow while traveling, giving him a "rugged" look. After he shaved and got a much shorter haircut, his look was more updated. (Makeup by Rhonda Barrymore; hair by Richard Davis.) *Source:* Goldstein 2009, from *Change Your Smile*, 4th edition. Reproduced with permission of Quintessence Publishing Co. Inc., Chicago.[1]

Makeup

The quest for an improved appearance has directed the thoughts and actions of mankind since the beginning of time. Today especially, the general public is extremely aware of physical appearance. Society places high value on youth and health and has set up stringent standards for what is attractive, as dictated by trends in fashion, hairstyles, and makeup. Beauty or strength of character is generally mirrored in facial features and hair. The degree to which these features are accented or emphasized will often determine whether one is merely accepted by his or her peers or admired by them. The term "reflective/self-image" is two inseparably connected images. The "outer image" is how others view a person, and the "self-image" is how the individual perceives themselves. Reflective self-image also determines, to a great extent, the level of one's self esteem, and how one thinks others view one. Self-image is a strong determinant of how a person acts and interacts in society. It determines whether one will be confident and aggressive or shy and passive. A positive self-image enables the individual to compete rather than follow the crowd. As a result, concern for one's appearance, seeking realistic self-improvement, is important to improving reflective self-image.

Plastic surgery and cosmetic dentistry have given patients the option of improving their appearance in more permanent ways. These two fields of medical science have tremendously brightened the lives of people they have touched by helping to create self-confidence.

Cosmetics or makeup, used as an adjunct to esthetic dentistry, as well as corrective/esthetic surgery are further aids for the person seeking maximum results in the pursuit of an improved reflective/self-image. The proper use of makeup can be of tremendous help in enhancing facial features and in diminishing or disguising unsightly facial disfigurements. The use of makeup is an art of illusion that uses color and design to help create a balance and style to enhance or define one's appearance. Makeup is temporary; it must be applied daily, but it is extremely effective when properly used to enhance a woman's attractiveness.

Skin care

Proper cleansing, rinsing, and moisturizing are basic to the total facial appearance. Neglect or improper care in and around the mouth can lead to blackheads, scaling skin, chapped lips, and excessively dry skin. It is as important to maintain proper cleansing and moisturizing around this area as it is on the rest of the face.

Makeup… an illusion

It is important to first understand that the purpose of makeup is to balance and enhance one's appearance or to create the illusion of beauty. The face and its features cannot be changed by makeup, but it can help how others look or perceive a sense of attractiveness. However, improper or excessive use of makeup can make an individual look out of step, hard, theatrical, or out of fashion. The proper use of makeup is an art that can be learned.

There are many types and shapes of faces, and each has its own charm. We live in a world of multiple ethnicities, where there is no longer one set of standard face shapes as a guide. Each ethnicity has its own charm. The trick lies in making the most of an individual's nonverbal communication features. We need to forget the shape of the face and concentrate on creating balance and symmetry while defining and decorating the nonverbal communication features, the eyebrows, eyes, and lips/mouth. These three areas carry the weight of the facial reflective/self-image and nonverbal communication.

Makeup and color

Makeup colors should be selected by a professional makeup artist or esthetician that has an in-depth background and knowledge of makeup products and colors that will suit all ethnicities. These makeup color products generally consist of

- foundations, to even the facial skin tones;
- concealers, to diminish or conceal facial skin discolorations;
- powders, to set the foundation and concealer for maximum wearability;
- blushers, to restore the natural flush to the skin or for a fashion statement;
- eyebrow makeup, to color or shape the eyebrows;
- eyeliner, to define the eyelids;
- eye shadow, creates a fashion statement; and
- lip color, to define and shape the lips.

Each ethnicity from light to dark skins has makeup colors that suit their specific skin color, culture, and lifestyle/fashion.

Corrective makeup and contouring

It is common in the field of consumer makeup for cosmetic sales people, makeup artists, and estheticians to recommend a corrective makeup/contouring approach to designing a woman's face. This entails highlighting features to bring them out or shadowing features to diminish them. A common concern among women is the challenge of reducing the appearance of a double chin. Makeup solutions can help correct this problem. When applying makeup to downplay a double chin, start with shadowing below the jawbone and use a darker concealer to blend down as needed. Then, highlight other features, such as the eyes. Start by applying a neutral shade of eye shadow to the lids. Next, use an eyeliner for definition. For a nighttime look, dark liners like brown/black, charcoal/black, or black can add drama. For a fresh awake look, line the lower inner lashes with white or any light color. Curl the lashes and coat them with mascara. In addition, add some glow and color with blush or bronzer on the apples of the cheeks. The final component is adding lipstick. The lips are close to the chin, so choose a color that helps make them look more attractive. The classic red lipstick is usually a good option—especially with bright white teeth—but not all women can pull it off.

Another tip to minimizing the double chin is to show off the neckline. Keeping the neck free of hair will accentuate the neckline and jawline. A tip for long hair is to wear it in a bun, hair clip, braid, or pony tail. A tip for short hair is to have the hair cut above the jawline to draw attention to the cheekbones instead.

- *Foundation*: Foundations are applied to even the facial skin tones. The foundation color should accurately match the client's real skin tone. It should be matched at the jaw line, which is the medium tone of the face.
- *Concealers*: A facial cosmetic concealer can be compared to the opaque layer used to mask a dark tooth or metal. But in cosmetology, it is used to mask blemishes and discolorations on the face. Concealers should match the skin tone to conceal skin discolorations. It should be applied before the foundation, as the foundation will minimize some minor skin discolorations.
- *Powder*: The powder is applied over the foundation and concealer; this will set the makeup, so it will wear longer and not rub off easily. The powder should not be a tinted powder; it should be colorless or color free, so as to not change the color of the foundation that is matched to the skin tone.
- *Blushers*: Even the sheerest foundation will diminish or conceal the natural flesh or blush of the skin. Blusher is used to restore the appearance of the natural flesh or blush. Blusher can also be used as a fashion statement. The enhanced natural blush of the skin gives a more youthful, healthy look to the face.
- *Eye makeup*: The eyes can be the most expressive feature of the face and, as such, attract attention. Made up properly, the eyes can add attractiveness and charm to the face and create the illusion of beauty. Eye makeup can draw attention away from the less attractive facial features and draw attention away from the lower third of the face if the dentist is unable to achieve the desired esthetic dental effect.
- *Eyebrows*: The eyebrows frame the eyes and help create facial expressions, such as happiness, fear, surprise, anger, and friendliness. Proper shaping and application of eyebrow makeup help to frame and focus attention on the eyes.

Lip coloring

Lip coloring brings the face to life. It is the final balancing feature of the face. The mouth/lips are one third of our nonverbal communications/facial expression. The lip color should be selected in harmony with the color of the clothes being worn. The "no mouth" look, extremely light or white lip color, is most unflattering and detracts from the individual's facial features. Lighter lip colors can be used to deemphasize unattractive mouth contours. Too dark a lip color looks hard unless it is color coordinated with wardrobe colors.

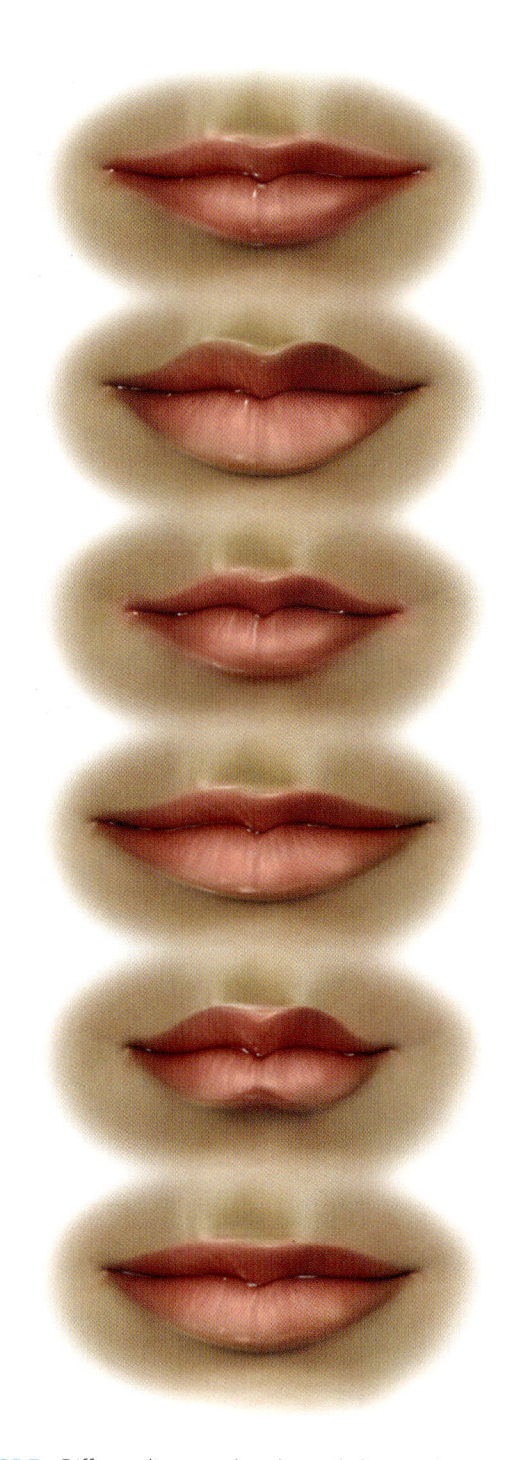

Figure 35.7 Different lips can alter the smile line, so doing a trial smile can help both the patient and yourself see how different tooth shapes and lengths can affect the smile.

Simple yet effective lip contour changes will create a more symmetrically balanced and desirable lip shape. They are outlined in Figure 35.7.

- *Narrow, thin mouth*: Build up the lips by letting the color extend ever so slightly beyond the natural lip line.
- *Large, full mouth*: Add a film of foundation over lips, powder thoroughly to set the lipstick and apply lip color only to area shown. This results in the mouth appearing smaller.

- *Small mouth*: To make fuller, apply a lip liner first to create the shape and then fill in with color.
- *Wide mouth*: Apply color as normal, but stop short at the corners of the lips.
- *Cupids bow*: To minimize the extreme cupids bow, apply lip color slightly outside the lip line and across the top lip, except on the two points where it should be held right to the lip line. To create or emphasize the cupid's bow, carry the color just barely outside the lip line on the two points, but stay on the natural line across the remainder of the upper lip.
- *Restoring the natural lip line*: If the natural lip is incomplete or interrupted (due to an accident or congenital condition), outline the lips with a warm natural colored lip line crayon/pencil. This will create a normal lip shape. Then, fill in with a normal lip color and blend the lip color and lip liner to appear as one.
- *Shape*: Women should never allow the finishing corners of the mouth to droop. To create the illusion of perfect harmony and happiness in the face, always allow these outside corners to finish in a graceful, upward line. Drooping or hanging lines tend to suggest sadness and age. Never make the corners blunt.

Selecting the right lipstick color

SELF Magazine in 2012 featured the article titled "23 lip shades that make your teeth look pearly white."[2] When selecting a color for the lips, *SELF Magazine* offered tips in selecting the right lipstick color. Keep in mind that lipstick colors change with fashion from season to season.

- Shades with strong yellow or orange tones are colors to avoid—these can bring out those same shades in your teeth, making the smile appear duller.
- Do not use nude colors or go too light for the skin complexion—it can make the teeth appear darker in contrast.
- Be careful of deep hues, like purples, because they can reflect on the teeth and also makes the mouth appear darker than it really is.

Makeup for a disfigured face

The diminishing or concealing of minor scars and skin discolorations around the mouth is accomplished with makeup concealers that accurately match the skin tone in the area of need. Some of the mental depression that normally accompanies a disfiguring injury or a congenital skin discoloration can be eliminated with the appropriate makeup.

Makeup for men with disfigurements

Diminishing, concealing, or disguising scars and congenital disfigurements for men are accomplished the same as for a women, minus the eye makeup, blusher, and lip color.

The primary difference is that the concealer and foundation must accurately match the men's skin tone in the area of need. Another element in concealing men's disfigurements that was not discussed in women's makeup is the many skin nuances in a man's face. These nuances are the beard pattern/texture and the pore texture/coloration. The makeup is applied (beard/pore texture color) with a coarse red rubber or a black synthetic sponge in a stippling (patting) motion. Scars that run through a mustache, eyebrow, or beard pattern area can be penciled in with a sharpened eyebrow pencil using hair-like strokes. It is best to use a stick or grease-based cream foundation that matches the men's skin tone, because it is waterproof and wears better when powdered with a color-free setting powder. Any beard pattern or pore texture makeup colors applied after the concealer/foundation must then be repowdered to set them to keep them from smudging. The skin nuances beard color, beard pattern, and texture are found in theatrical makeup but should not be theatrical looking. For men with a facial disfigurement as well as a flush to their complexion or ruddy skin it is recommended that they try to match the nuance of the regular colors of the skin with a color that matches their normal skin. It is unlikely that a man would be able to do this without some professional instruction.

It should be remembered that cosmetics in all its forms is temporary. It is a daily procedure that, when used properly, can and will improve an individual's appearance. An understanding of the proper use of cosmetics enhances anyone's ability to achieve a natural look and can be an important part of the entire esthetic dental treatment plan. When used together, esthetic dentistry and the art of makeup can give a patient an improved enhanced reflective/self-image.

References

1. Goldstein RE. *Change Your Smile: Discover How a New Smile Can Transform Your Life*, 4th edn. Chicago, IL: Quintessence; 2009.
2. Malhotra R. 23 lip shades that make your teeth look pearly white. *SELF Magazine*, February 16; 2012. http://www.self.com/beauty/2012/02/lip-shades-that-make-your-teeth-look-white-slideshow#slide=1 (accessed November 7, 2017).

Additional resources

The ultimate guide to looking younger! *NewBeauty* (Winter 2012). Sandow Media LLC; 2011;102.

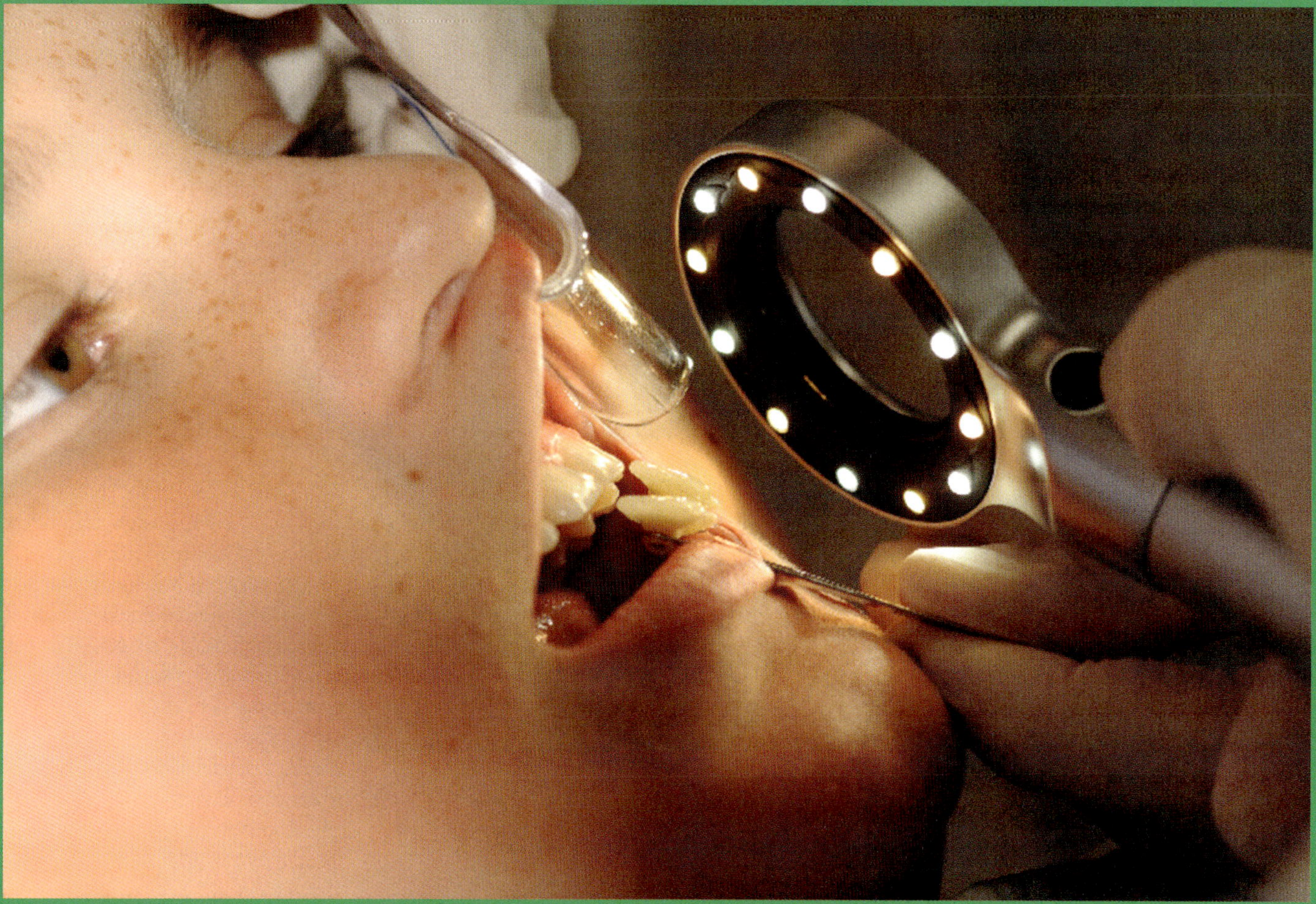

Chapter 36 Esthetic Considerations in the Performing Arts

Ronald E. Goldstein, DDS and Daniel Materdomini, CDT

Chapter Outline

Economic dental procedures	1154	Metal restorations	1169
Cosmetic acrylic stent	1155	Orthodontic treatment	1169
Composite resin stent/splint	1155	Periodontal treatment	1171
Composite resin direct bonding	1155	Prosthetic treatment	1172
Removable porcelain veneers	1155	Temporary measures	1172
Dentures: removable partial or full	1156	Fixed restorations	1173
Overlay dentures	1156	Specific issues for performers	1174
Creating a character with acrylic overlay	1156	Emergency treatment	1176
Checklist for creating a character	1157	Long-distance consultation	1176
Creating a specific character	1159	Summary of important principles for treating performers	1177
Direct composite resin for theatrical makeup	1160	The trial smile: demonstrating using imaging and video and informed consent	1177
General tips for direct composite resin	1161		
Achieving esthetics in natural teeth	1165	Lighting considerations and effects on appearance of the teeth	1178
Suggestions for achieving brighter/whiter teeth	1165		
Cosmetic contouring	1167	The goal: attractive, natural-looking teeth	1178
Composite resin restorations	1167		
Selecting a shade	1168		

Professionals in performing arts, such as in film, television, theater, and modeling, need cosmetic dentistry more than the general public. Whether the performer appears on the movie screen, television, stage, or catwalk, constant public scrutiny is a major part of the job description.

Entertainers in the motion picture industry, having realized that an attractive smile is integral to success, created one of the first demands for esthetic dentistry. Gigantic screens and close-up shots compelled actors with unsightly smiles to seek out the benefits of cosmetic dentistry. In the late 1920s and early 1930s, Dr. Charles Pincus pioneered many techniques, both permanent and temporary, for masking some of the cosmetic problems that became painfully obvious in close-ups. For film actors, the advent of high-definition video and the growth of IMAX cinemas make attractive teeth essential for their careers.

Performers who limit the range of facial expressions to avoid exposing unsightly teeth might never attain their full potential. Success in the entertainment field is tied to the level of confidence about body image. An attractive smile and range of spontaneous facial expressions can contribute greatly to that confidence.

Ronald E. Goldstein's Esthetics in Dentistry, Third Edition. Edited by Ronald E. Goldstein, Stephen J. Chu, Ernesto A. Lee, and Christian F.J. Stappert.
© 2018 John Wiley & Sons, Inc. Published 2018 by John Wiley & Sons, Inc.

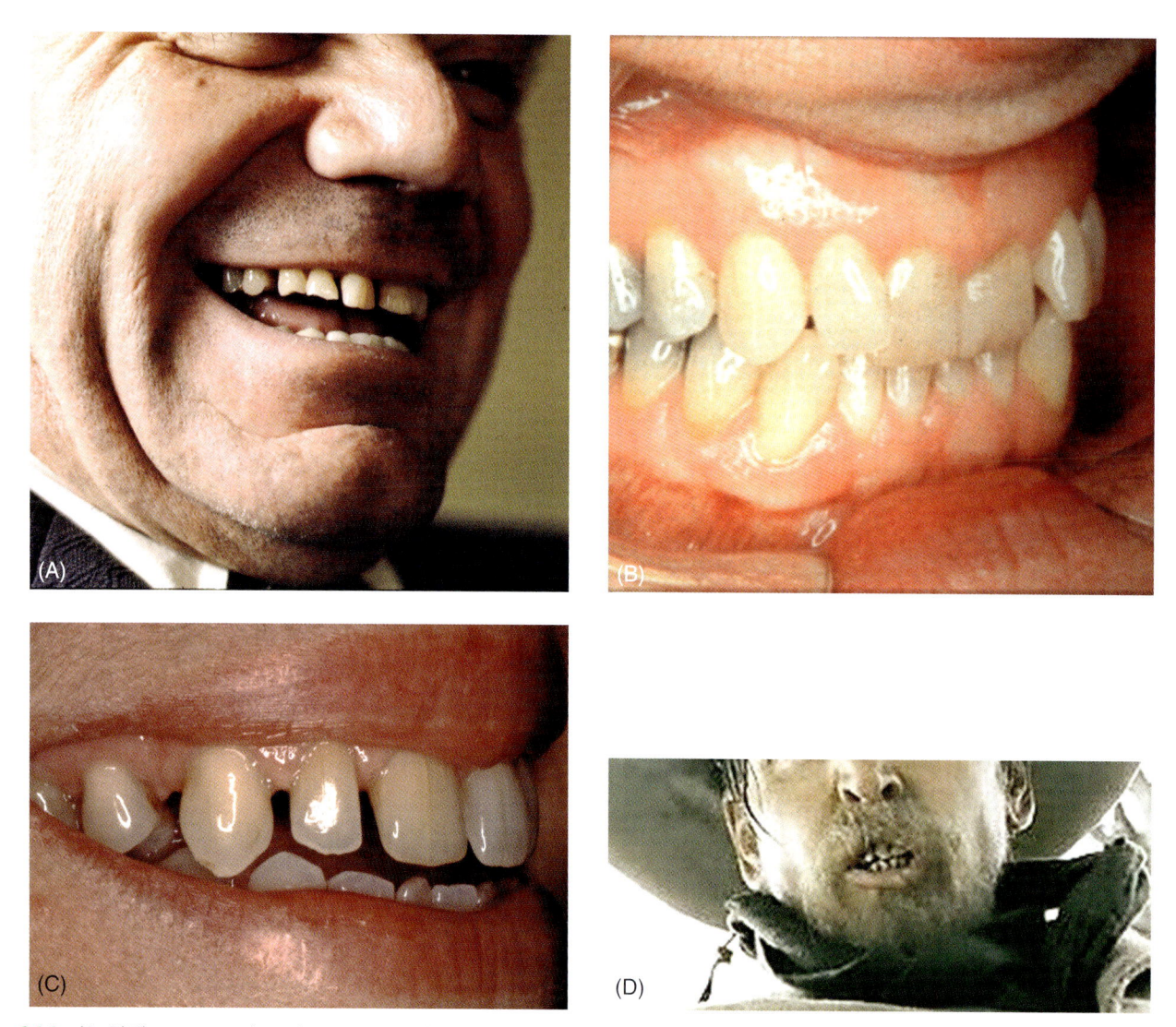

Figure 36.1 **(A–D)** These actors show diastema, incisal wear, and other teeth irregularities that were no obstacles to their success.

There are exceptions, of course. For example, certain actors prefer to retain a natural look, even with something as obvious as diastema. The men in Figure 36.1A–D are film and television actors whose diastemas, incisal wear, and teeth irregularities have certainly been no obstacle to their success. In fact, they have probably contributed to it, and many stage and film performances today require creating a character with bad teeth or other unattractive orthodontic features. In the 2010 film *True Grit*, actor Barry Pepper's broken teeth, which were created for the role, are a key characteristic in his portrayal of a convincing villain.

This chapter will address procedures for creating a character through the use of dental prostheses. However, it must be noted that actors depend on their appearance for their livelihood, and most do not want a permanent alternation in their look. The treatments covered in this chapter should ensure that the actor can revert to their original, recognizable appearance.

The public has long expected performers and models to be attractive, and it is a reasonable assumption that only persons who are naturally attractive would choose such a career. However, this assumption does not hold when the smile is the primary consideration. In 1968, Goldstein produced the first published study of its kind and that evaluated the attitude toward esthetic dentistry among a group with strong interest in physical appearance—beauty pageant contestants. Of the 60 beauty contestants who participated in the study, 90% could have used some esthetic treatment, and an additional 7%, although already considered pleasing to the eye, expressed a desire to enhance their smiles. Only 3% believed they would not have benefited from such procedures. When the candidates were asked how they felt about their appearance, only 20% were satisfied with how they looked, and 28% thought that the condition and appearance of their teeth detracted from their smile and, ultimately, their overall attractiveness.

Economic dental procedures

Because such a large percentage of performers and models barely make a living, they need to understand that not all cosmetic dental procedures are expensive. It is important to remember this during treatment planning so that alternatives to the more costly procedures are included as economic options for esthetic correction and improvement. Note, too, that dental procedures performed on actors and other entertainers may qualify as tax-deductible expenses.

When developing a treatment plan, be sure to view the performer/patient from all angles. Several approaches utilizing both video and photographs will give the patient/performer the opportunity to see what the audience sees. (This approach is discussed further in Chapter 7.) The mouth is essential for expression, and while the mouth muscles can be more expressive than the eye muscles, both muscle groups work together and should be included in the diagnostic evaluation.

Various cosmetic dental procedures have been proved successful for performers and are addressed herein. These procedures are:

- cosmetic acrylic stent
- composite resin stent/splint
- composite resin direct bonding
- removable porcelain veneers
- removable partial dentures
- overlay dentures
- acrylic overlay for theatrical makeup
- direct composite resin for theatrical makeup.

Cosmetic acrylic stent

Many performers need esthetic improvement for their teeth, but some are not willing to reduce perfectly sound tooth structure, which may have to be removed to achieve the desired result. One temporary procedure for photographic purposes is a removable cosmetic stent. This can temporarily hide conditions such as diastema during a performance or photo shoot. In 1978, Bob Hope was the entertainer at the annual Thomas P. Hinman Dental Meeting in Atlanta and showed me the removable splint Dr Pincus had made him to hide his diastema when taking certain photographs or in movies.

Here's how to create a stent: use white wax on a stone model or the patient's mouth to "restore" it to esthetic standards or to create the specific look and process the prosthesis in acrylic. For added stability, the overlay may be worn with an adhesive, although friction alone will usually provide sufficient anchorage (Figure 36.2A–C).

Composite resin stent/splint

Constructing the splint directly in the mouth with composite resin allows complete control over both color and surface characteristics. A thin coating of lubricant can be applied to the teeth before bonding them with composite resin. When the polymerization and finishing procedures are completed, the splint is gently forced off by first letting the patient rinse with water, then teasing off the appliance. Pay careful attention to any undercut areas, because the composite may lock into them. Block out known undercuts, except where you may find some necessary for retention/suction grip before placing the composite resin. This technique works best with diastemas, but it can also be effective when build-out of individual or multiple teeth is required (Figure 36.3A–D).

Composite resin direct bonding

In many situations, the most effective temporary means of achieving cosmetic correction is through the use of composite resin. Stains can be masked, tooth sizes can be altered, and arch alignment can be corrected by bonding teeth without etching enamel.

However, you may need to etch if you cannot easily lock it in by connecting it to adjacent teeth. When the performer has completed a role, the bonding can be removed. Frequently, the correction appears so natural that performers eventually opt for the more permanent treatments that utilize direct bonding or even porcelain veneers.

Temporary bonding also works well in closing diastemas. This procedure is fast and easy, and the fee can be much less than the fee for procedures that require laboratory assistance. Before bonding was available, many dentists used soft, molded wax to hide spaces for photographic purposes. However, the advent of direct-light polymerized composite resins made such procedures obsolete.

The technique is relatively simple. Select the appropriate shade of a microfill composite resin. A microfill is usually used because it can produce the best final luster. If occlusion is a problem, a microhybrid composite resin serves as an alternative. However, a microfill can still be used as the outermost layer to obtain a high polish.

Removable porcelain veneers

The cost of porcelain veneers can be considerable. Therefore, the use of this technique is usually limited to those performers or directors who want the most attractive temporary result without regard for cost. In addition to the laboratory expenses, there are professional time and artistic requirements associated with the construction and temporary placement of the veneers.

The first dentist to use such a technique was Pincus. In 1929, he described the use of temporary porcelain "shells" to immediately improve the screen appearance of certain movie stars. The costs were usually absorbed by the film studios and did not factor in the decision process for the patient. It should be noted that porcelain was basically the only material available at the time for cosmetic dentistry. They were held in with denture paste.

Tooth preparation is not required to construct removable veneers. An impression is taken using polyvinyl siloxane. Then, the veneers are constructed in the laboratory and individually fitted to each tooth. They can be inserted with a temporary, non-hard-setting cement to ensure that the color will remain constant. Another, more temporary, means of attaching the veneer is with soft, sticky wax (Moyco). Performers can be taught how to place the temporary veneers on themselves, but they must obviously be secure enough so as not to come off during the performance.

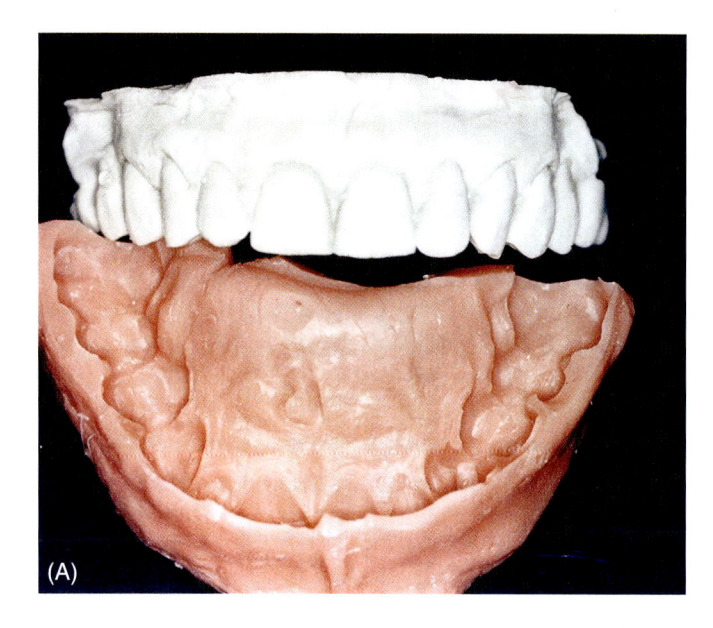

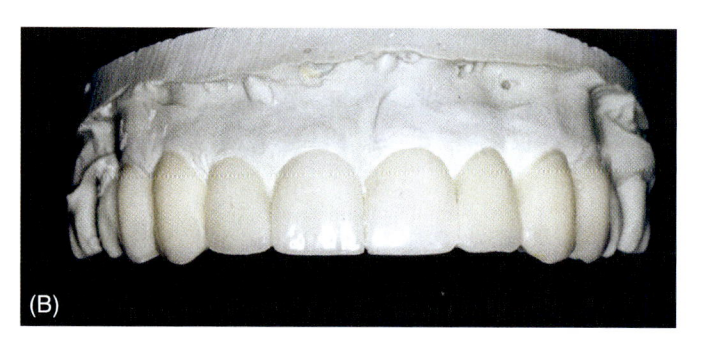

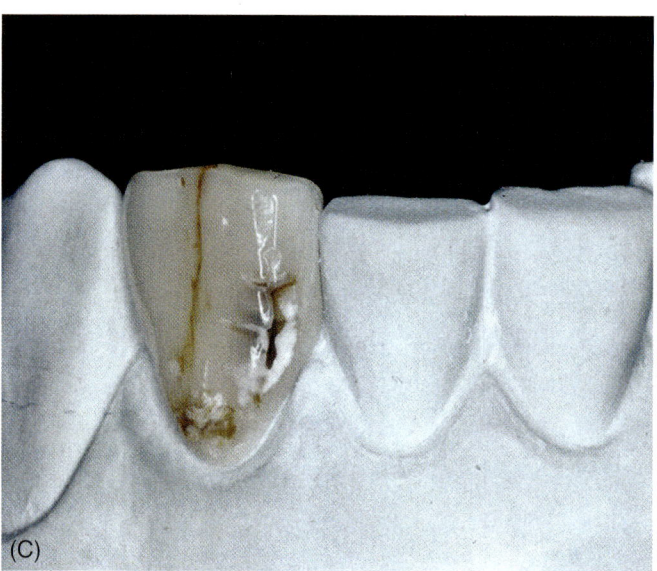

Figure 36.2 **(A–C)** Fred Ward's role in *Miami Blues* required him to "gum" his food. A mouthpiece was made to cover the actor's teeth. After a paper-thin denture fell out of his mouth, veneers were applied over his teeth to make them look like dentures.

Dentures: removable partial or full

It is possible to construct a removable partial denture with the esthetic correction built into the appliance. Spaces can be closed and overlays can even be attached to the partial. Special effects can also be easily built into the acrylic-attached teeth or veneers. The advantage of the removable partial for a performer who wants to alter their appearance is the avoidance of repeat dental office visits and their costs.

Overlay dentures

A full denture is constructed over the existing maxillary natural teeth. The technique involves mounting accurate stone casts on an adjustable articulator and creating a temporary full denture. Because this technique usually requires considerable opening of vertical dimension, there may be restraints on the extent of time this denture can be worn during the day (Figure 36.4).

Creating a character with acrylic overlay

Occasionally, a dentist is called on to create an unattractive, objectionable appearance for theatrical purposes. Character alterations can be achieved with the use of the acrylic overlay. Incorporating stains, various shapes, and arrangements to both teeth and gingiva can contribute to the elaboration of character (Figure 36.5).

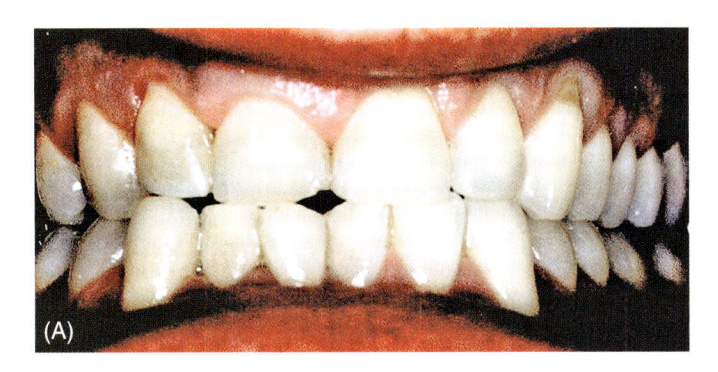

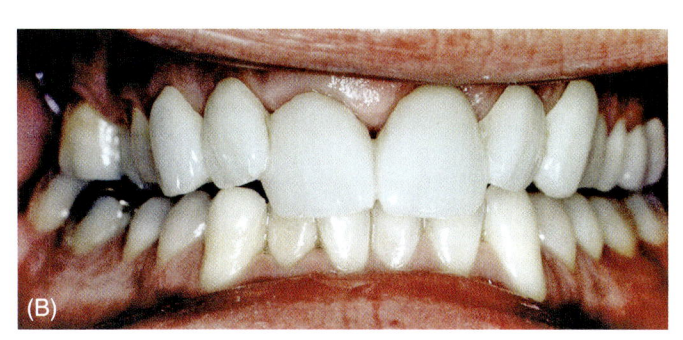

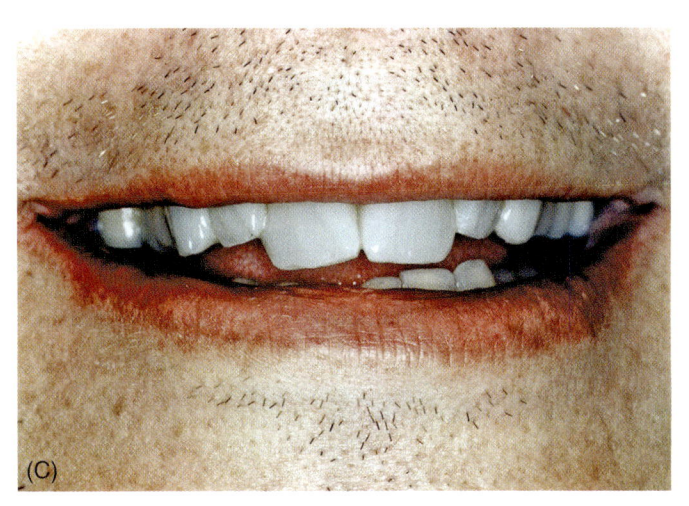

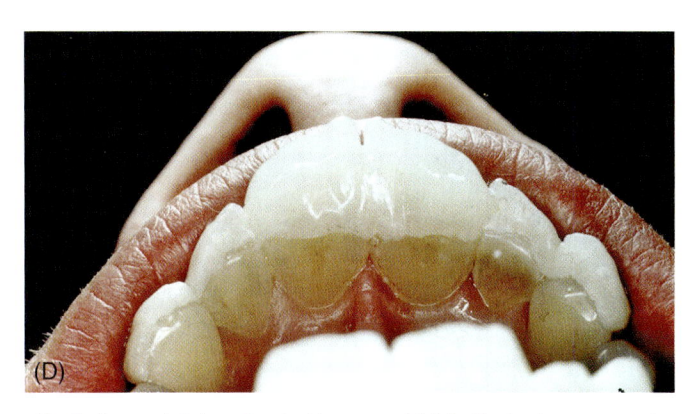

Figure 36.3 **(A–C)** These images show the teeth Jim Belushi wore as a mentally challenged dishwasher in *Homer and Eddie*. Notice how a mouth extension was required to show the actor's teeth. **(D)** Note how the splint was attached to the incisolingual surfaces.

Tips for creating an acrylic overlay are as follows:

1. Make a drawing or sketch of the proposed changes as a guide for the lab technician. Use the shade chart in detail to note stains, shade differences, chipped or fractured teeth, and gingival irregularities.
2. If vertical dimension is to be altered, be careful not to obliterate freeway space. All functional mandibular movement must be accommodated.
3. The patient should be encouraged to allow sufficient time to practice speaking while wearing the overlay. If a speech impediment is desired, the appliance can be constructed to create one. The use of even a handheld video camera can be useful for showing your patient just how they sound and look while wearing the appliance.
4. Provide the patient with clear instructions regarding the care, insertion, and removal of the appliance to avoid breakage.

Acrylic overlays are perfect appliances for the vampire look commonly used in film and television today (Figure 36.6).

Checklist for creating a character

1. Ensure that the patient is in good dental health before beginning treatment.
2. Determine the type of look the performer wants for the character being portrayed. For example, will it be a serious character versus someone who's comical?
3. Coordinate with the director or producer on the look of the teeth before designing the prosthesis on a computer and then fabricating it. Photoshop can be used to virtually modify the teeth and create any desired look. The performer should send a photo of their teeth via e-mail to your dental office and the image can be visually enhanced or modified on the computer. Send the enhanced image to the producer or director to see whether the modification is acceptable.
4. All key people involved must sign off on the image. This means the actor, the producer, the director—anybody who has a say in the end result of how the performer is supposed to look. Again, consider routine communication throughout via e-mail. Even photos and/or video of the performer wearing and speaking with the appliance can be sent via zip files using the Internet.
5. Determine whether the look is temporary or permanent. The initial prosthesis will be made of plastic to test the construction, how well it suits the performer's face, and to determine whether the actor can tolerate wearing and speaking with it. This temporary design can be designed on the computer, but it is essential the performer tests the plastic prosthesis in the mouth and be able to speak comfortably while wearing it. Only then will four or five final prostheses be fabricated for use during the performance.

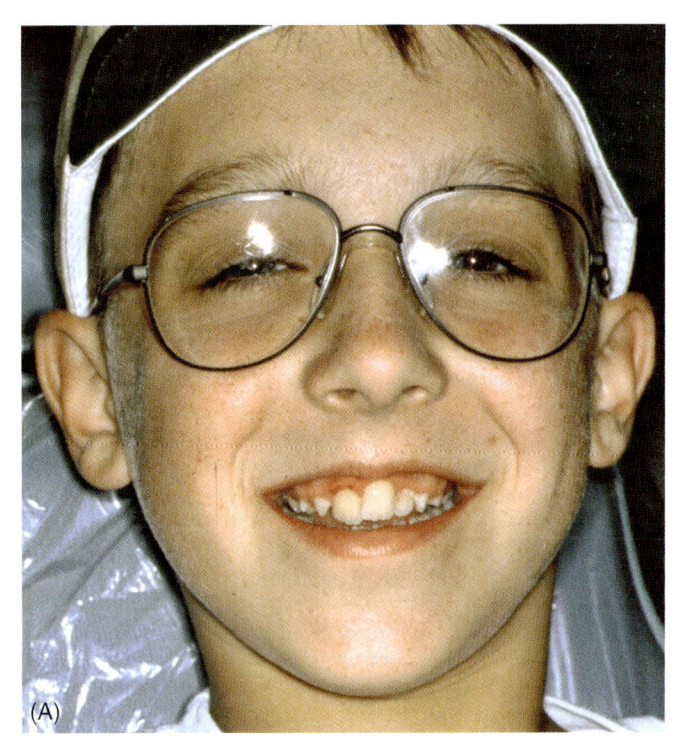

Figure 36.4 **(A)** This 10-year-old actor was chosen to play the part of a boy who gets into two fights and has some of his teeth knocked out (*The War*).

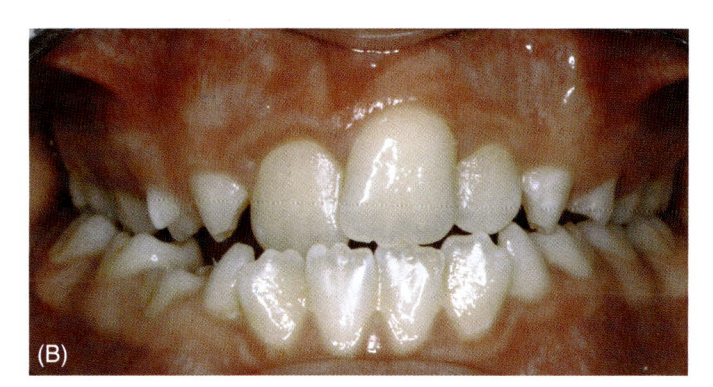

Figure 36.4 **(B)** His severe malocclusion was a major problem in planning the appliance to create the illusion of missing teeth.

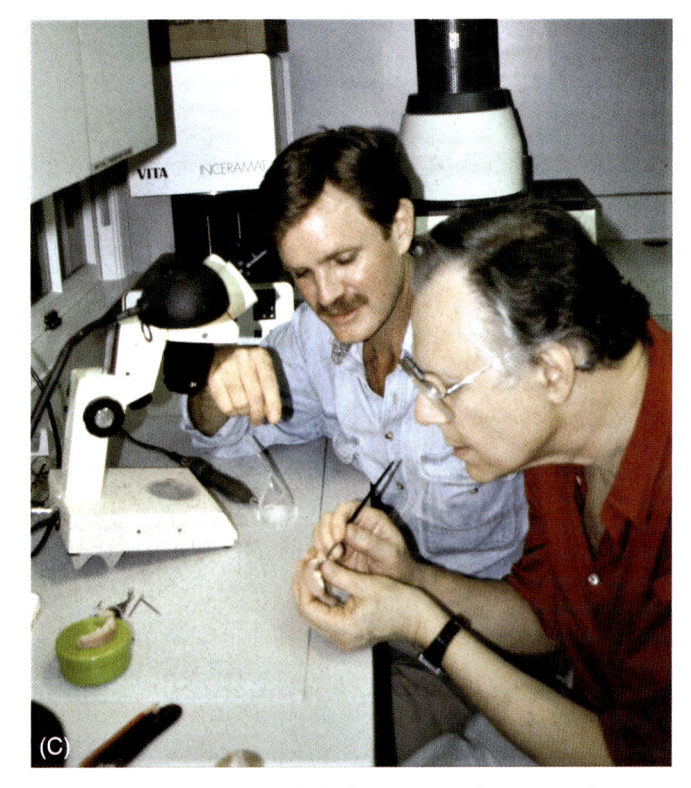

Figure 36.4 **(C)** Working with the laboratory technician, Mark Hamilton, a plan was devised to create several overlay dentures the boy would wear throughout the movie.

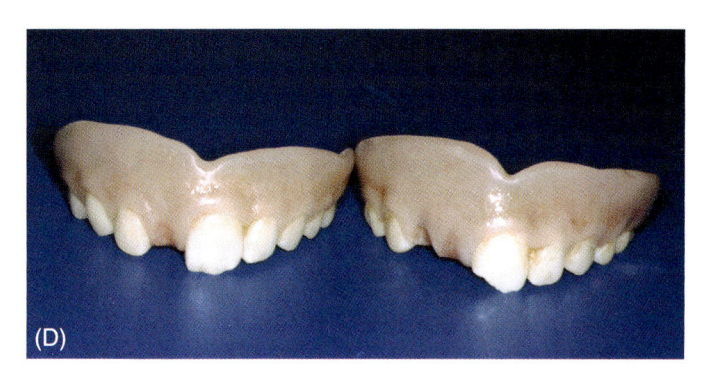

Figure 36.4 **(D)** Multiple appliances were fabricated to show the progression of the character's teeth problems throughout the movie.

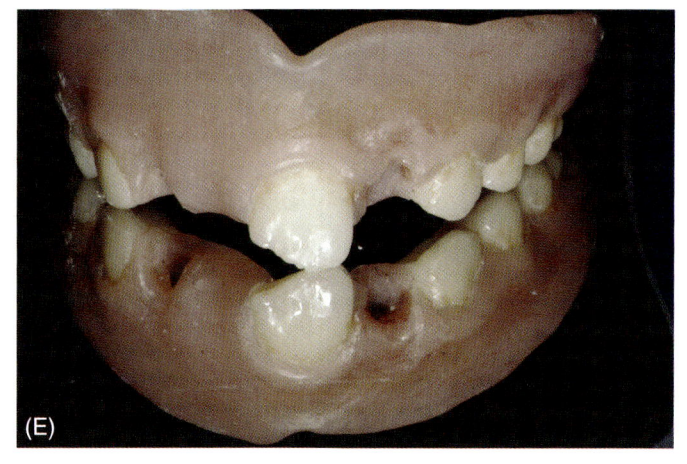

Figure 36.4 **(E)** Note in the mirror view how the tooth sockets were carved out to appear more natural.

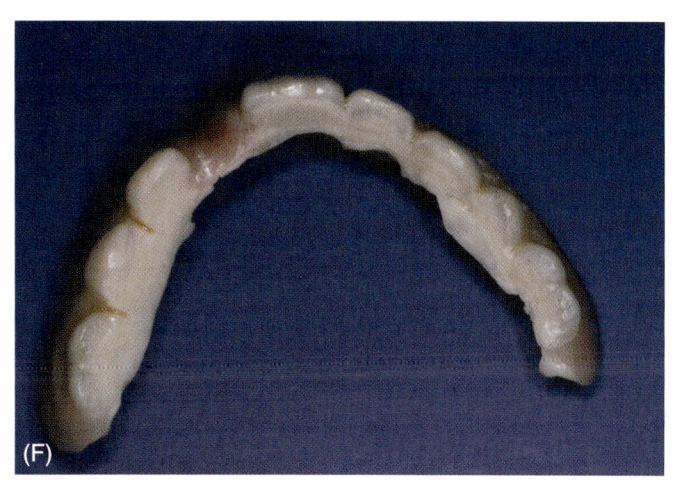

Figure 36.4 **(F)** The first overlay dentures were made, so that they could fit securely over his teeth but also allow him to speak sufficiently.

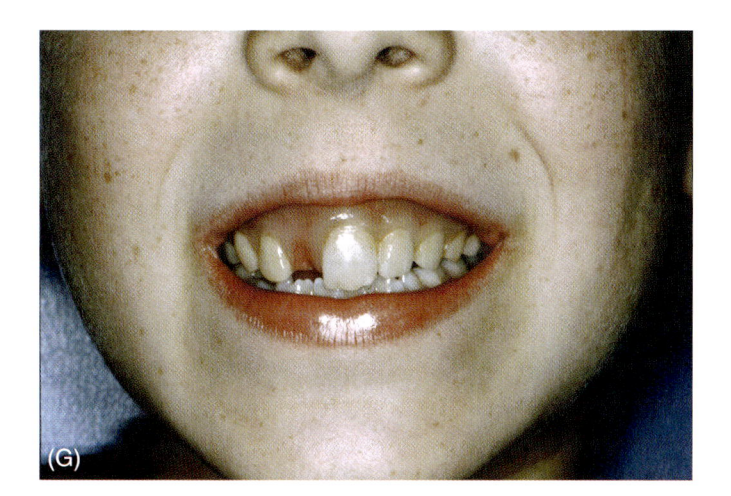

Figure 36.4 **(G)** This was the look after the first tooth was supposedly knocked out. It is very important that the buccal flange be high enough so that when the actor smiles it will look believable.

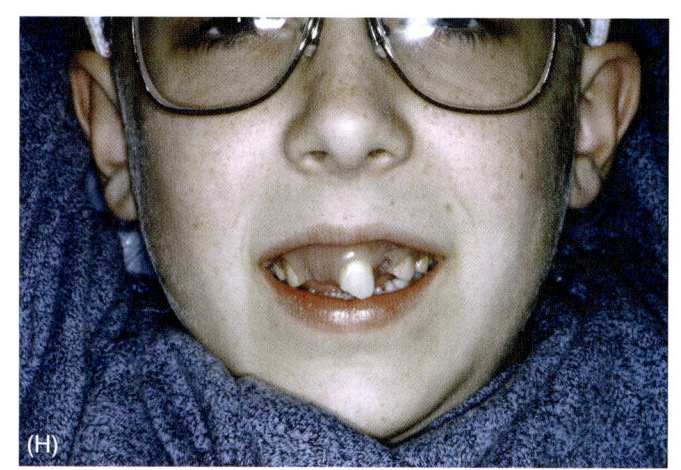

Figure 36.4 **(H)** The final overdenture constructed showed more teeth knocked out plus a fracture on his left central incisor.

6. Know when to say "no" if you believe the procedure could cause future negative effects on the performer's dental health, such as if the prosthesis will cause teeth to move.
7. Charge an hourly rate for the procedure, because this type of work involves trial and error and it is difficult to quote a specific overall fee for a product. Typical time required is 1 week, but the shortest time frame is 1 or 2 days.
8. The most time-consuming work involves creating a whole new facial appearance for a performer, whereas changing the appearance of just the teeth is relatively simple, such as vampire teeth. Treatments that involve altering the performer's facial configuration, the mouth, and the speaking ability are the most challenging. Marlon Brando's use of prostheses in his lower cheeks for *The Godfather* was a good example of this type of treatment.
9. Determine who qualifies as a candidate for this type of dentistry. Price varies, but the average cost is about $300–$750 per hour.
10. Depending on the situation, creating special effects can be time consuming, and amateurish attempts should be avoided. It is important to understand the procedures and the steps taken. You may wish to contact a dentist who has expertise in this area to train and learn how to avoid negative outcomes for the patient and the dentist.

Creating a specific character

In the example shown in Figure 36.7A–H, a major movie producer wanted the actor Richard Kiel's mouth to show abuse and neglect. Compare the actor before (Figure 36.7A) with the final result (Figure 36.7B).

The "heart-of-gold" crown technique was achieved as follows:

1. A stone model was made of the maxillary arch, and a tooth-colored acrylic was applied directly to the prepared model (Figure 36.7C).
2. A controlled-temperature pressure heater hardened the acrylic. A further buildup of acrylic continued until the basic splint was formed in the tooth areas.
3. Tissue-colored acrylic was applied to replicate the gingiva; the acrylic was then hardened in the pressure oven.
4. A heart was carved out of an old piece of shell gold and was added to increase personality to the characterization (Figure 36.7D). It was locked into place on the lateral incisor

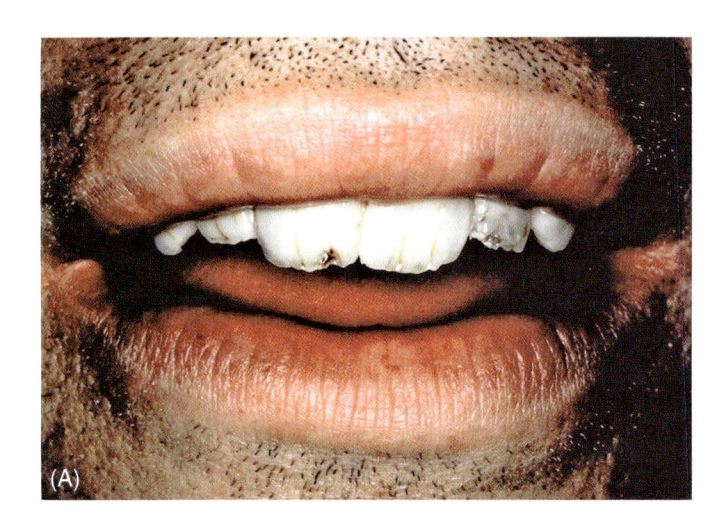

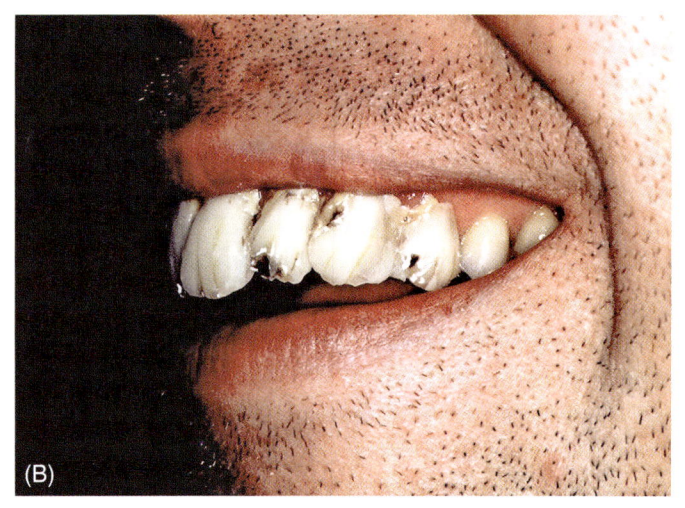

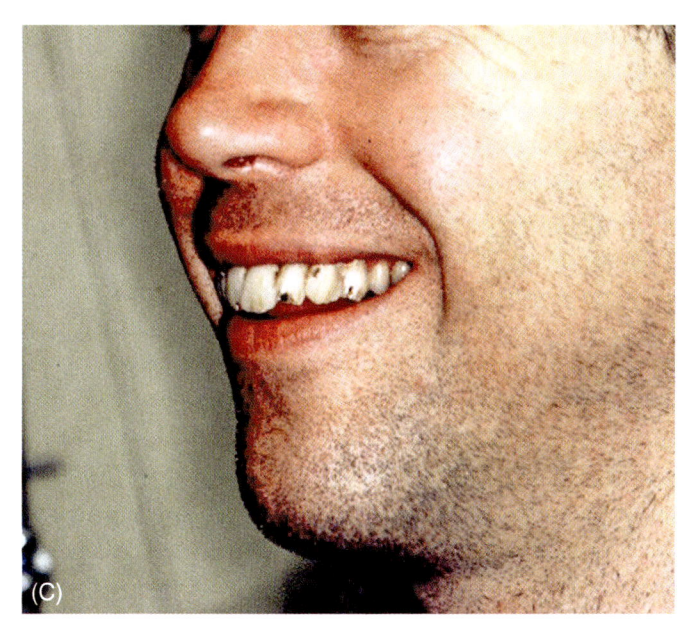

Figure 36.5 **(A–C)** Playing Stalin's projectionist in *The Inner Circle*, Tom Hulse required teeth that showed decay, plaque, stains, and misalignment. These images show the actor's teeth in close-up, side, and full facial views.

by bending the edges, then refinished using brown and green polishing wheels.
5. Additional material was added to the labial gingival area to depict periodontal disease.
6. Gingival erosion, fractured teeth, and other defects were carved into the overlay with a straight handpiece No. 701 bur.
7. Quick-cure resin stains were placed to replicate caries, microcracks, stains, defective restorations, and calculus (Figure 36.7E).

An acrylic or composite overlay would have enough flexibility to allow for careful placement over the natural teeth. Figure 36.7 F shows the lingual view of the overlay. Because the actor was to portray an ex-boxer, a removable appliance was constructed for the mandibular arch (Figure 36.7G) that would pouch-out the cheek to simulate facial disfigurement. The characterization created by makeup and dental changes is shown by the comparison of Figure 36.7A and H.

Occasionally, dentists are called on to create dynamic special effects. As mentioned earlier, for example, a removable prosthesis was made to create a strong prognathous jaw for Marlon Brando's character in *The Godfather*, and maxillary and mandibular appliances were fabricated to give actress Linda Blair a demonic look for her role in *The Exorcist*.

Direct composite resin for theatrical makeup

Although the acrylic overlay is the easier method for creating character, an extremely natural appearance can be achieved with direct composite resin bonding. Stained composite resin restorations are created by applying dark composite material to the enamel. If problems of retention occur, a 0.5–1 mm etch can hold the composite to the teeth. However, there are limitations regarding the length of time the performer can wear it. Direct bonding

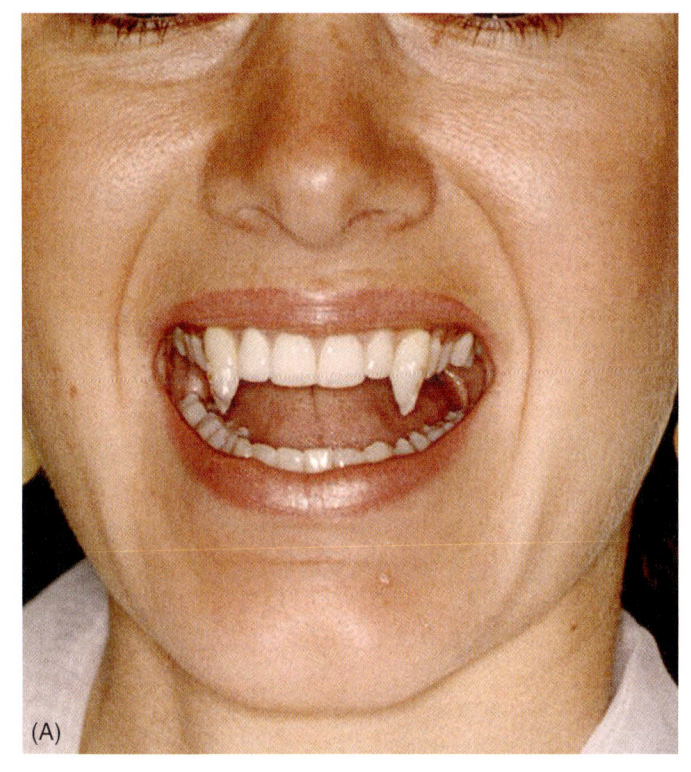

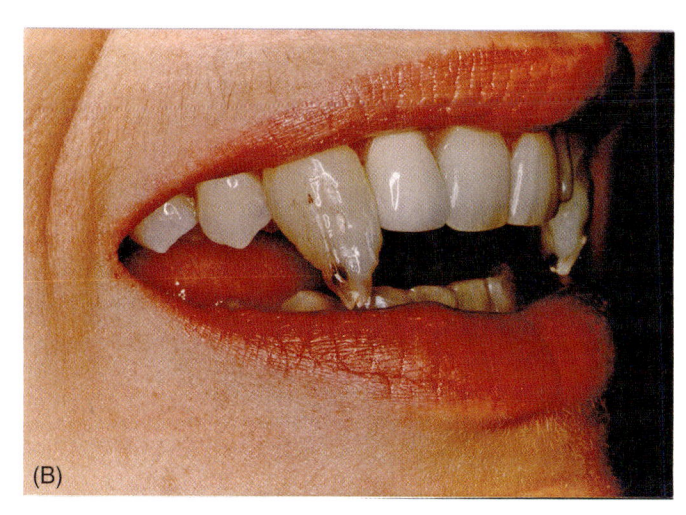

Figure 36.6 **(A, B)** For the film *Vampires*, a new concept was used. An internal passage was created for sucking blood through the teeth.

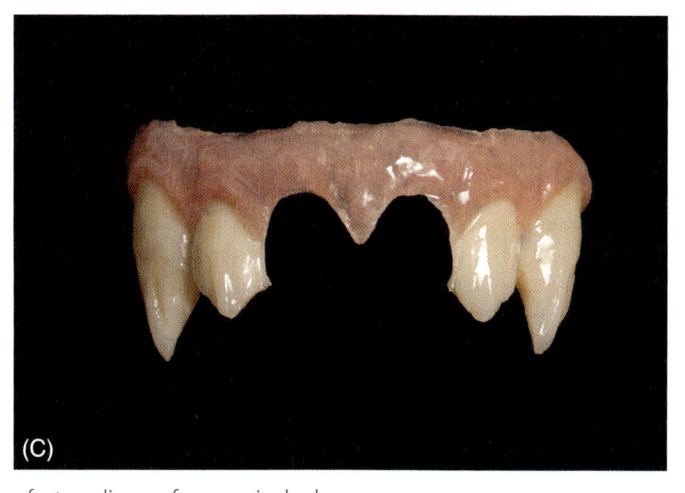

Figure 36.6 **(C)** Acrylic overlays are perfect appliances for vampire looks.

has the disadvantage of requiring a dentist to replace the effect each time it is needed, making this technique especially labor intensive. It should be noted that if the actor does not mind wearing the effect for an extended length of time, it is possible to attach the bonding for that required time frame by extending the etching just slightly to 1.5–2 mm.

General tips for direct composite resin

To create noticeable effects, the following guidelines apply:

1. Overemphasize color change. If you want old restorations to really standout, make the stain about two shades darker than you might have initially anticipated.
2. Tooth form requires careful attention. A realistic effect is believable only if the teeth can withstand close scrutiny. This is especially true in the motion picture industry, where an actor's teeth appear on giant screens.
3. The condition of the gingival tissue should reflect the appearance of the teeth. If you are creating an unattractive prosthesis effect, remember that neglected teeth most likely are surrounded by periodontal disease. An acrylic tissue insert that depicts red and swollen gingiva will further enhance the believability of the characterization (Figure 36.8).
4. Do not stop at the cuspids; include as many teeth as necessary to ensure realism, even with maximum smiling. Rather than creating a cuspid-to-cuspid effect, extend to the bicuspids or

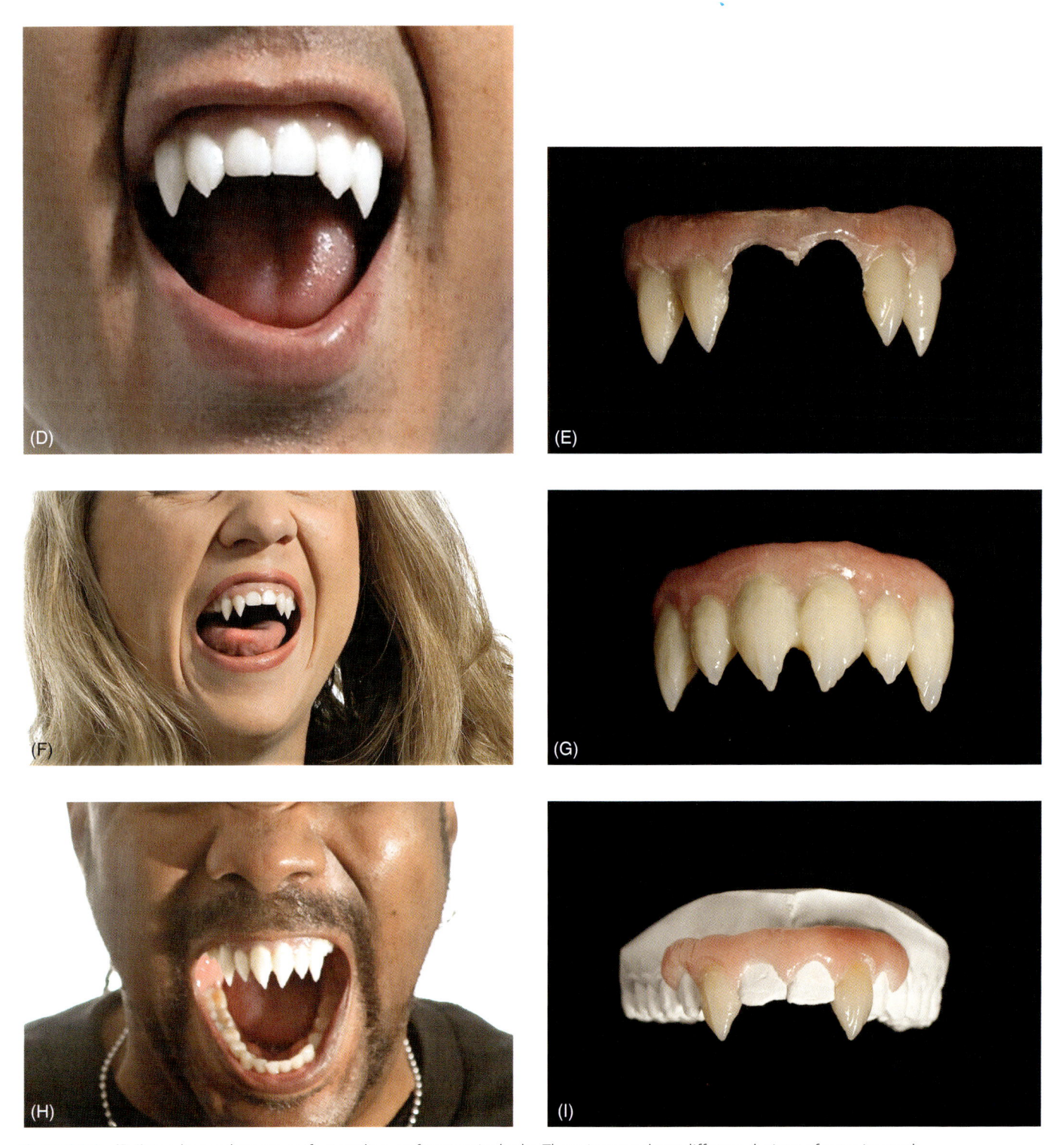

Figure 36.6 **(D-I)** Acrylic overlays are perfect appliances for vampire looks. These images show different designs of vampire teeth.

even the first molar for total realism in the lateral views. Remember, the audience must "buy into" the character's total look.

5. Consider the perspective of the audience. If the actor will be revealing occlusal surfaces during the performance, then these surfaces should be altered as well. A typical example is when the character tips their head back for a "sinister" laugh.

6. Do not neglect the mandibular teeth. Even when only the incisal edges are visible while speaking, if they do not match the maxillary corrections, the desired result will elude you. Furthermore, even straight incisal edges can be bonded or

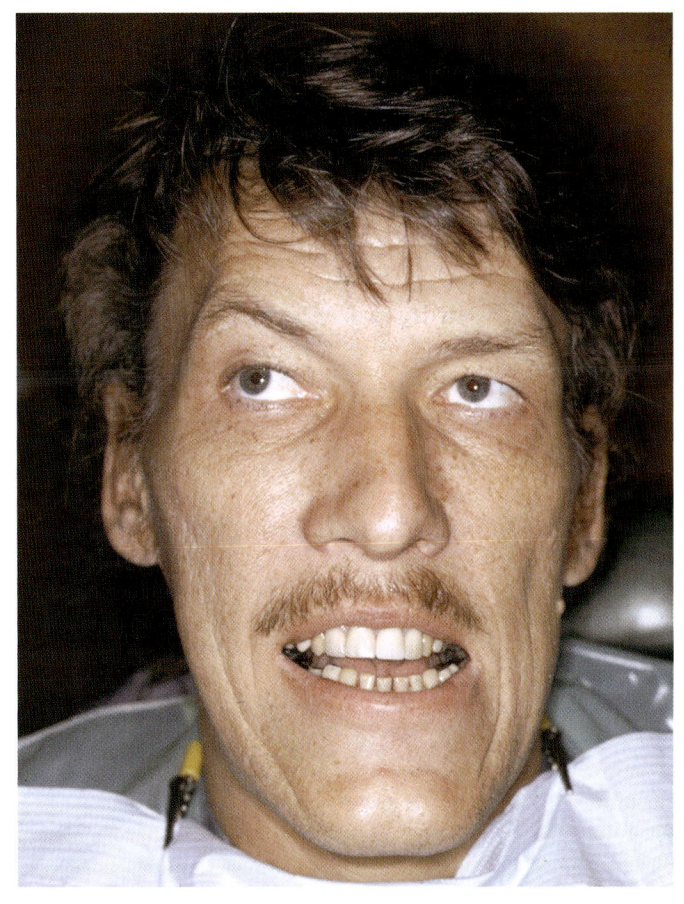

Figure 36.7 (A) Actor's smile and teeth prior to procedure.

overlapped to look crooked. Again, it is advisable to overemphasize the amount of crowding and good color to ensure believability. If orthodontics is selected as the ideal treatment, remember to include cosmetic contouring to achieve ideal straightening (Figure 36.9).

7. Video the performer in character. If possible, record the actor speaking from their script, smiling, and laughing. Include lateral, top, and bottom views. A video like this can be invaluable, not only for planning the extent and type of treatment or correction, but also for demonstrating clearly to the actor or other interested parties the necessity of creating a more complex correction than may have initially been anticipated.

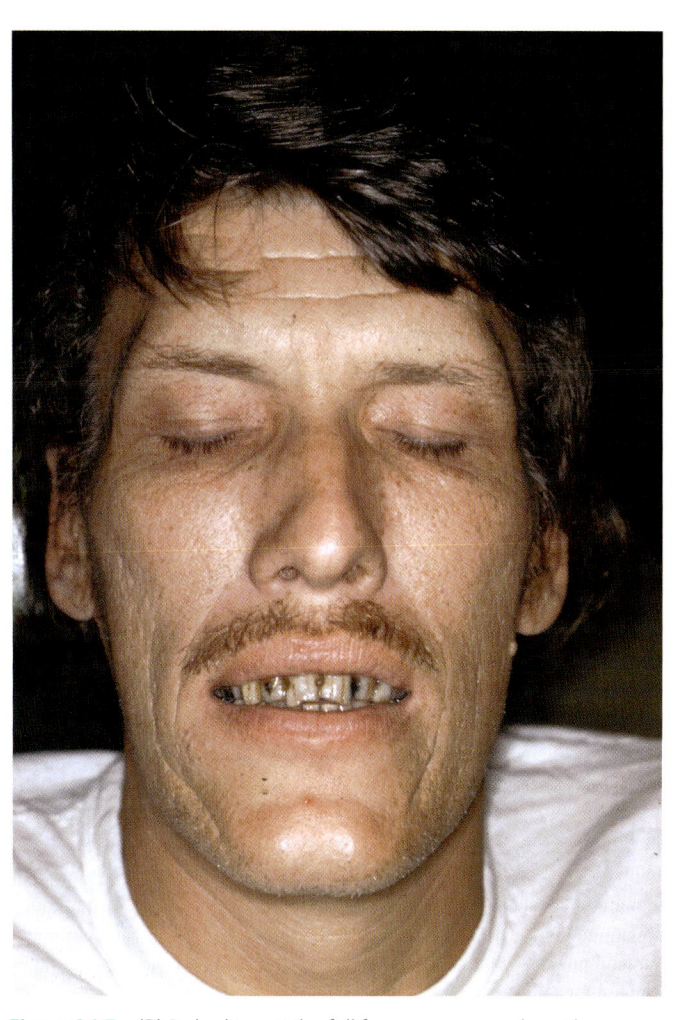

Figure 36.7 (B) By looking at the full face, you can see how the characterization in his teeth accomplished what the director wanted for the appearance of this character.

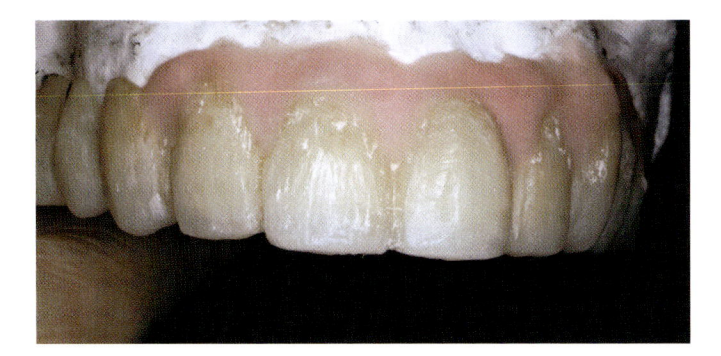

Figure 36.7 (C) A stone model was made of the maxillary arch; tooth-colored acrylic was applied directly to the prepared model.

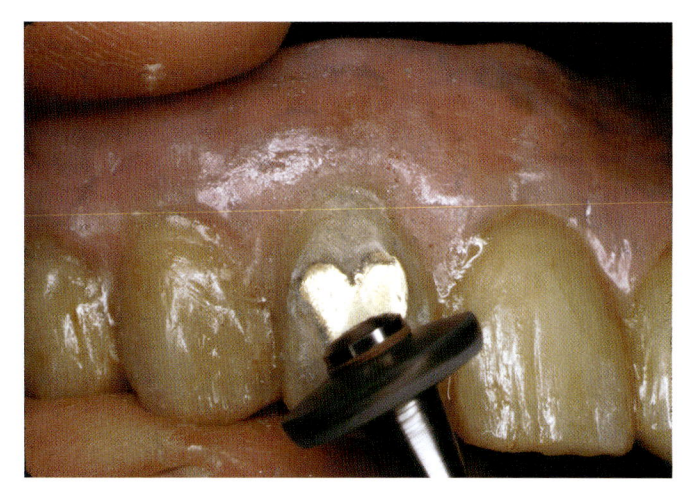

Figure 36.7 (D) A heart was carved out of an old piece of shell gold and added to increase personality to the characterization and locked into place on the lateral incisor by bending the edges.

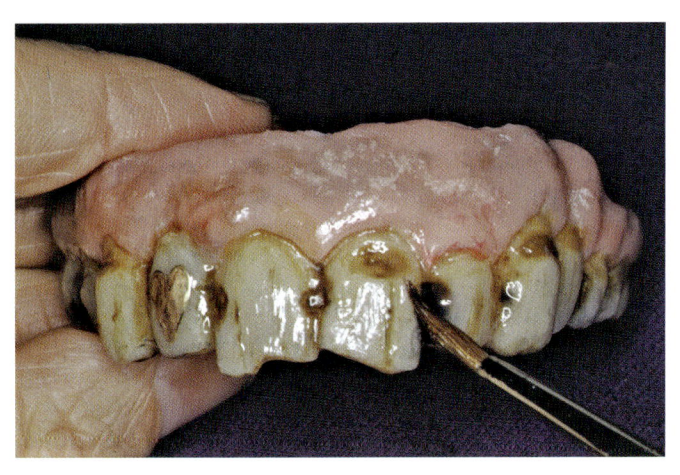

Figure 36.7 **(E)** Additional material was added to the labial gingival area to depict periodontal disease. Other defects were also incorporated into the overlay, followed by quick-cure resin stains to create caries, microcracks, stains, defective restorations, and calculus.

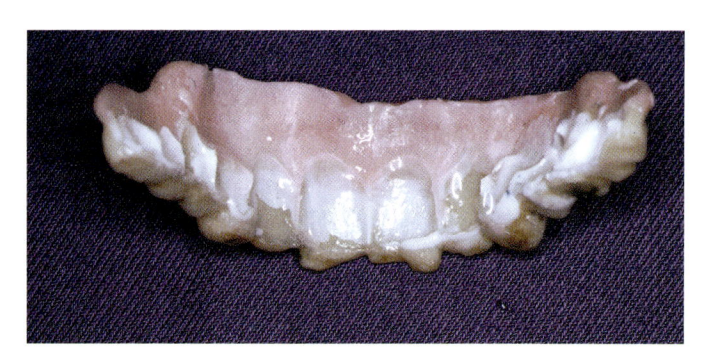

Figure 36.7 **(F)** Looking at the appliance from the lingual view, you can see how the actor would lock it into place.

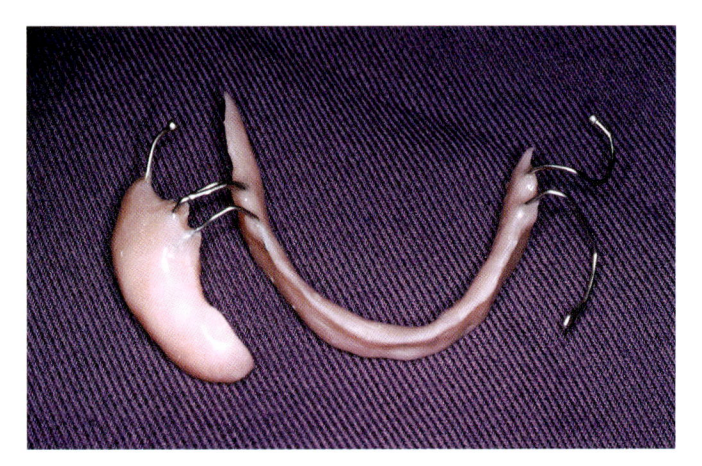

Figure 36.7 **(G)** Because the actor was to portray an ex-boxer, a removable appliance was constructed for the mandibular arch that would pouch out the cheek to simulate facial disfigurement.

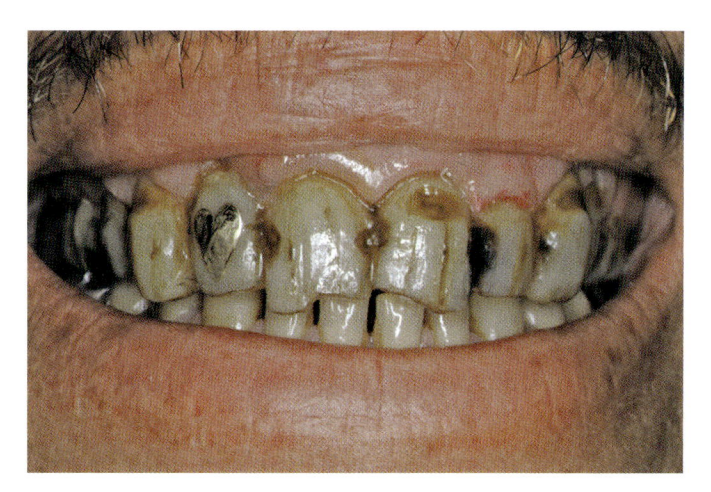

Figure 36.7 **(H)** The characterization created by makeup and dental changes is shown in his smile.

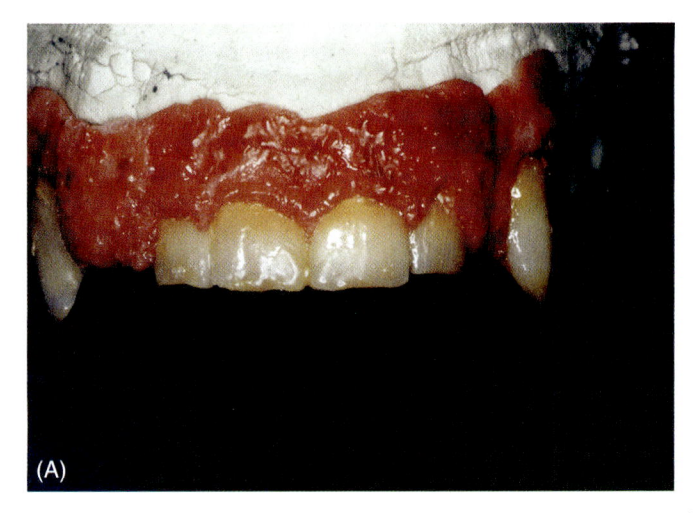

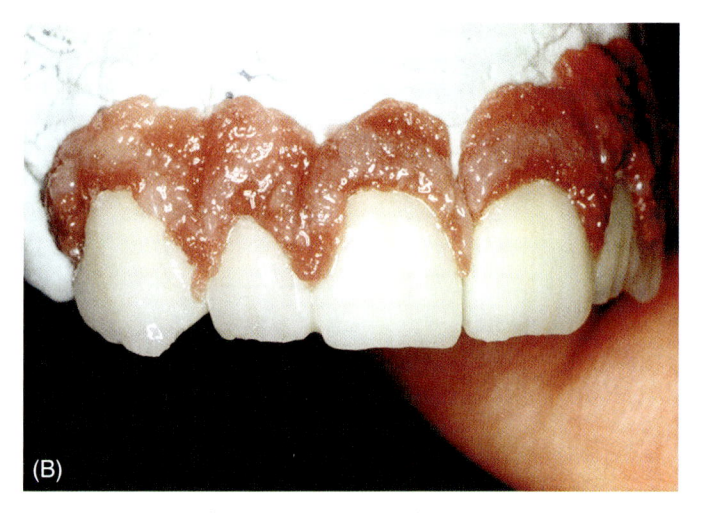

Figure 36.8 For one movie role Nicolas Cage played a half-man and half-ape. **(A)** A prototype of the ape-like teeth and swollen gums that were created for the role. **(B)** Teeth that are more human in appearance.

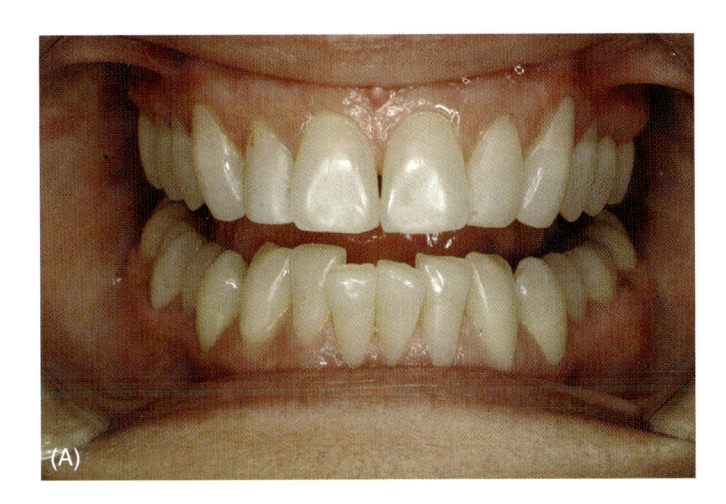

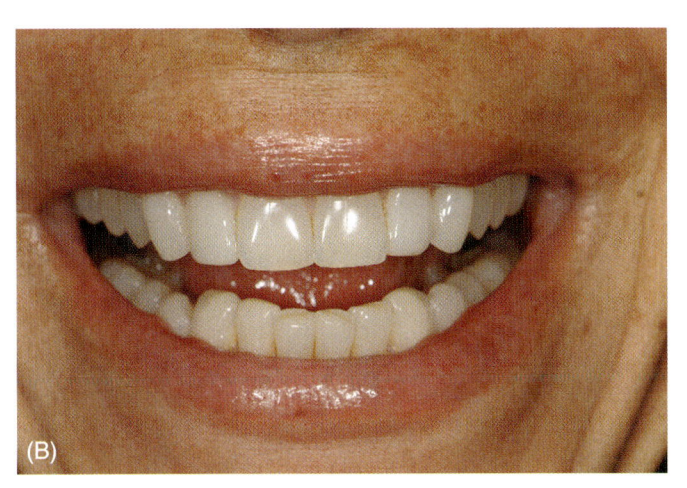

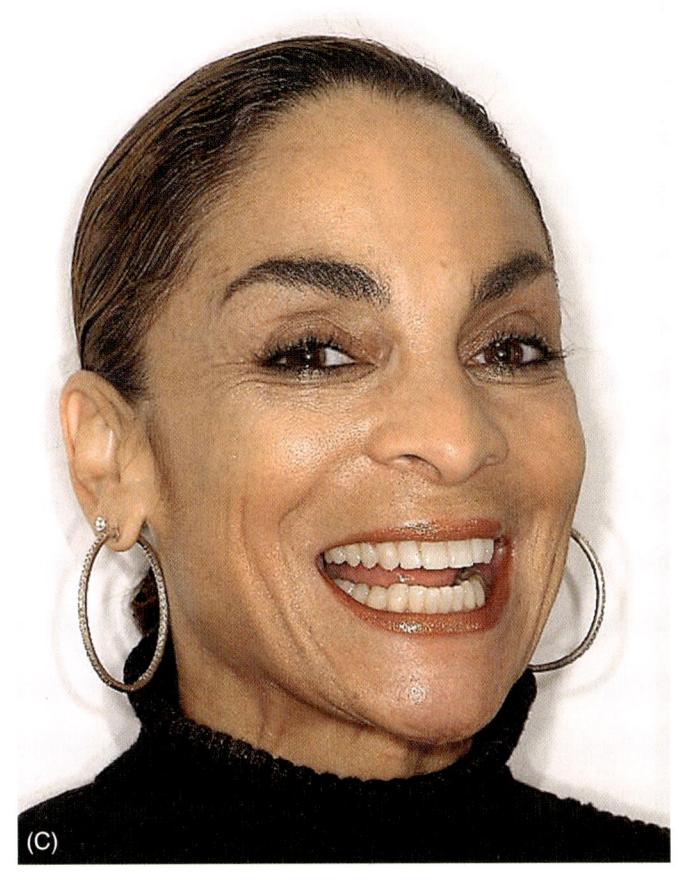

Figure 36.9 (A) As this leading actress's teeth became crowded over time, she wanted to improve her smile. (B) Minor orthodontics, bleaching, cosmetic contouring, and bonding helped to produce a more attractive smile. (C) The actress now shows straighter looking teeth both close up and from a distance on theatrical performance.

Achieving esthetics in natural teeth

Photographic models and film actors place a high value on their appearance and are especially interested in having healthy teeth and gums (Figure 36.10A–E). However, their natural dentition is often poorly arranged, decayed, or stained. In the following we demonstrate how some of these problems may be managed with minimal time and effort required of the patient.

Suggestions for achieving brighter/whiter teeth

Many performers are extremely concerned about the darkness of their teeth and wish to have them lightened. Here are nine suggestions for achieving brighter teeth:

1. After a thorough prophylaxis, pumice the teeth and polish them with tin oxide. Even using impregnated polishing

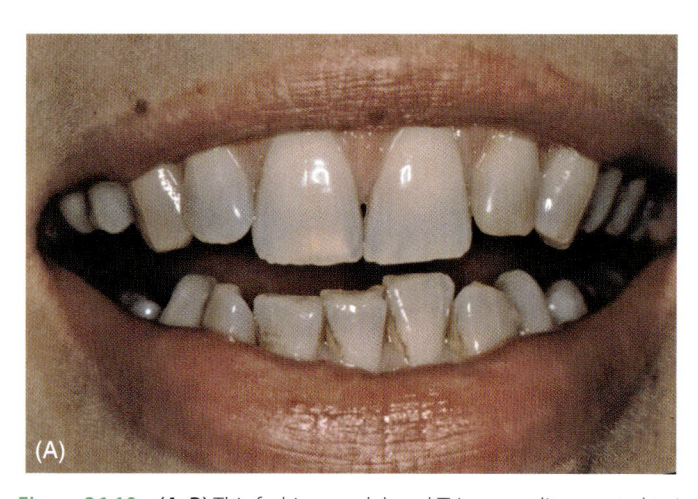

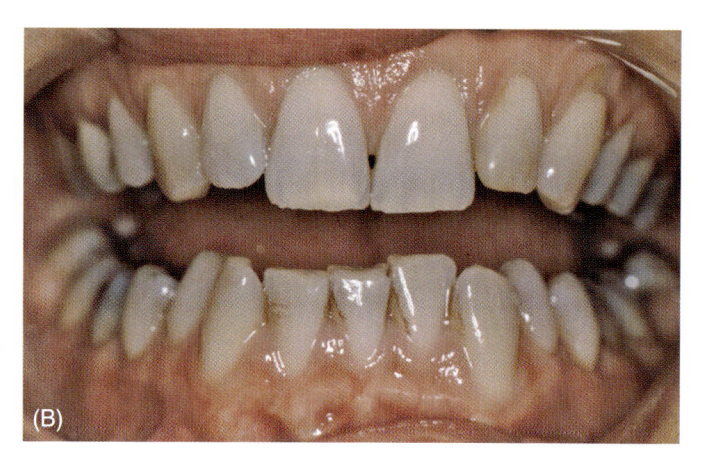

Figure 36.10 **(A, B)** This fashion model, and TV personality, wanted to improve her smile to do photographic modeling as well.

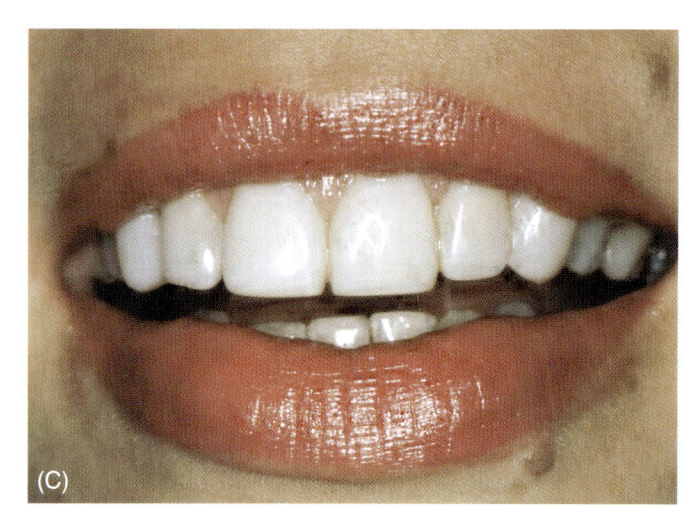

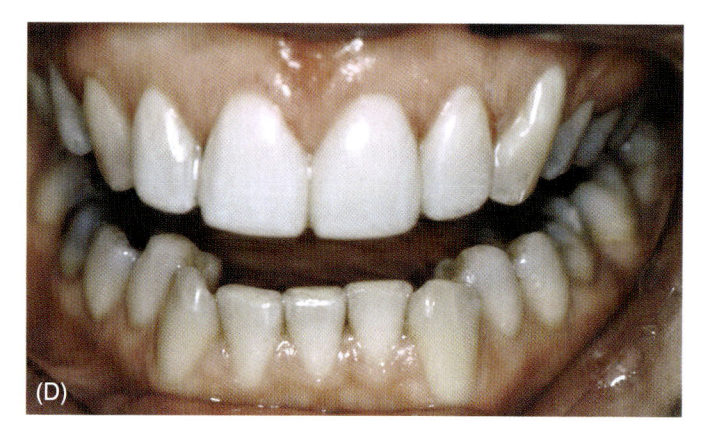

Figure 36.10 **(C, D)** Cosmetic contouring and composite resin bonding instantly improved her smile.

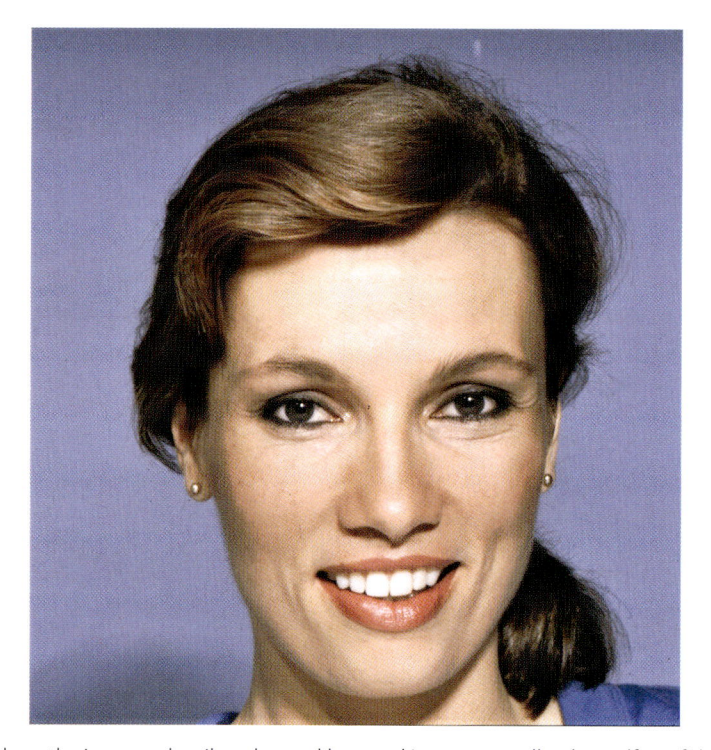

Figure 36.10 **(E)** The final result shows how the improved smile enhanced her total image, as well as her self-confidence.

wheels can create brighter looking teeth because of the increased luster after polishing in this fashion.

2. Use a more abrasive toothpaste than normal to retard further staining.
3. Advise the performer to apply darker shades of makeup so the teeth appear whiter against the darker skin tone.
4. Professionally bleach the natural teeth. However, entertainers vary considerably in their expectations, patience, ability, and willingness to spend time and money for in-office procedures. One alternative is for the patient to bleach themselves, outside of the dental office. Specific techniques can be found in Chapter 12. When bleaching the teeth of entertainers, recommend the "power bleach" as the starting point or even the entire treatment, since busy entertainers may not want the bother with home bleaching.
5. If the patient objects to bleaching, a temporary treatment may be suggested. In these cases, the acrylic cosmetic overlay in a lighter shade than the natural shading of the patient's teeth might be used.
6. Lightening can also be accomplished by bonding a composite resin or porcelain overlay onto the visible teeth. The patient should be informed of the limited life expectancy and of the necessity for periodic replacement.
7. Porcelain veneers offer the most attractive, longest-lasting conservative solution to the problem (Figure 36.11A–E).
8. If the teeth are severely discolored and the patient's demand for esthetics is great, the only satisfactory method of whitening may be the full crown. This should be done when it is the only way to achieve a satisfying esthetic result.
9. If there are maintenance issues associated with any of these procedures, be sure to discuss this before suggesting treatment.

Cosmetic contouring

When the teeth are extremely malposed, and if orthodontia is contraindicated or unacceptable to the patient, cosmetic contouring of the natural teeth may help. Figure 36.10A–E illustrates the effectiveness of cosmetic contouring for a photographic model (see Chapter 11 for technique.)

Because the esthetic result is achieved so quickly, it should always be considered when treating performers. Almost every model or actor should be esthetically evaluated to determine whether cosmetic contouring could enhance their appearance. This noninvasive procedure requires minimal adjustments and minimal time. See Chapter 11.

Composite resin restorations

If the teeth are well aligned, shaped well, and not discolored, the possibility of caries is still present and should be treated esthetically with the use of direct composite resin if trying to save expense and time.

Composite resin can be used to restore most teeth that are seen when speaking, smiling, and laughing. The patient should be informed that these resins must be replaced periodically. Goldstein, in *Change Your Smile*,[1] offers ranges of life expectancy for composite resin restorations and other esthetic treatments for most every cosmetic dental problem. Nevertheless, many patients in the performing arts or modeling consider this treatment as part of their professional expenses. Although composite resin restorations may last longer, the expected life expectancy plus limitations should be explained. Staining is always a possibility, so the patient should be warned of the possibility of early discoloration from cigarettes, tea, coffee, or other causes. However, discolored teeth can be made to look bright again by refinishing them with a 30-blade carbide (ET, Brasseler USA) and air-abrading. Follow this procedure by etching and applying a product such as a low-viscosity, light-cured resin formulation. Only one application of a formulation (BisCover Bisco) is required to create a smooth, polished tooth surface. It may also be necessary to slightly strip the facial surface and re-veneer with a thin layer of brighter polished composite resin.

Composite restorations can be used as both a temporary and a permanent treatment and can be modified to create both good- and bad-looking teeth. Furthermore, composites are an effective method for sculpting different looks, because they can be added directly to the mouth and polymerized.

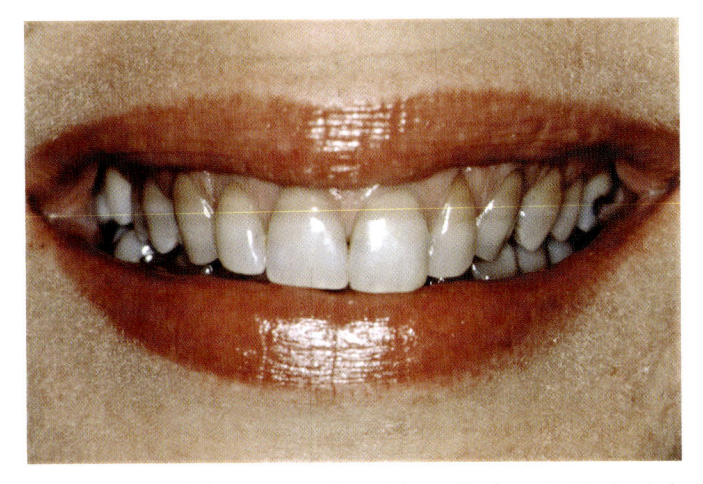

Figure 36.11 (A) This actress and model was displeased with the dark spaces (she called them "caves") that she saw on each side of her mouth when she smiled.

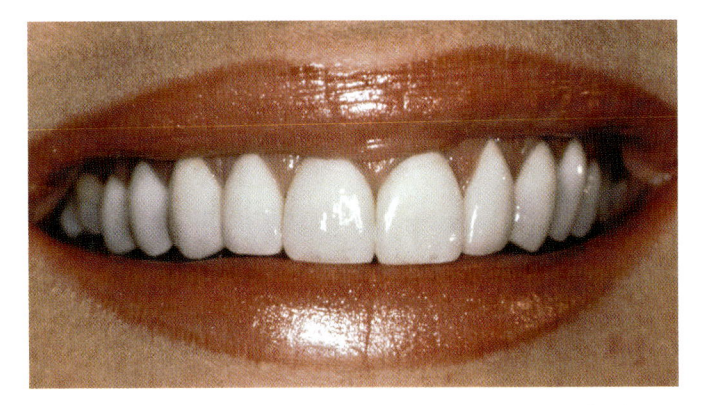

Figure 36.11 (B) The solution to this cosmetic problem involved building out both the front and back teeth with light-colored porcelain veneers.

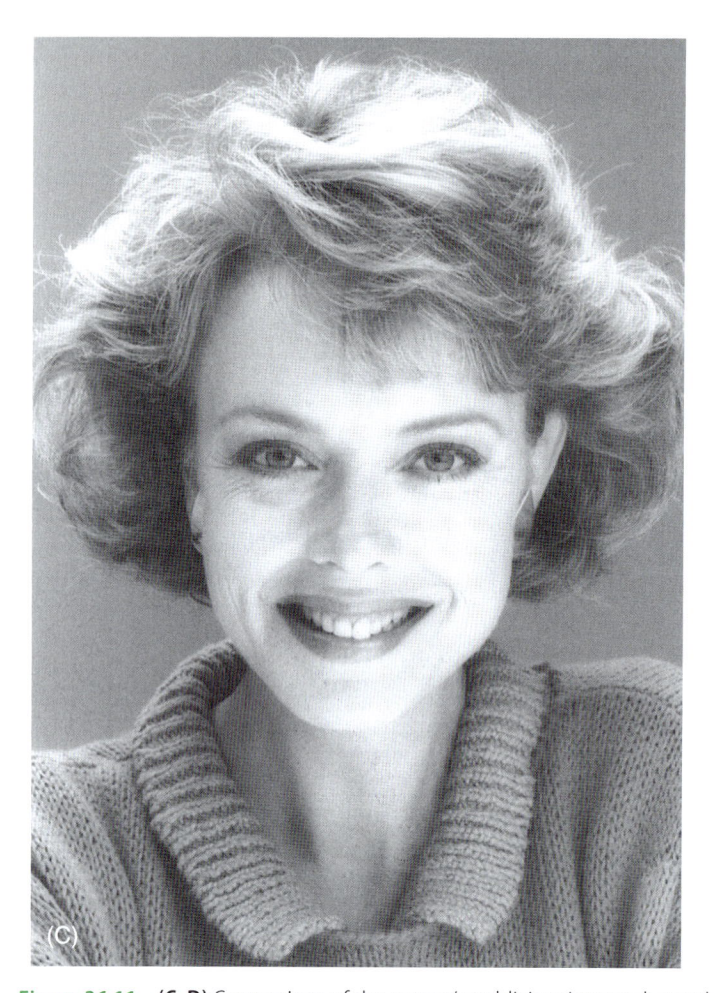

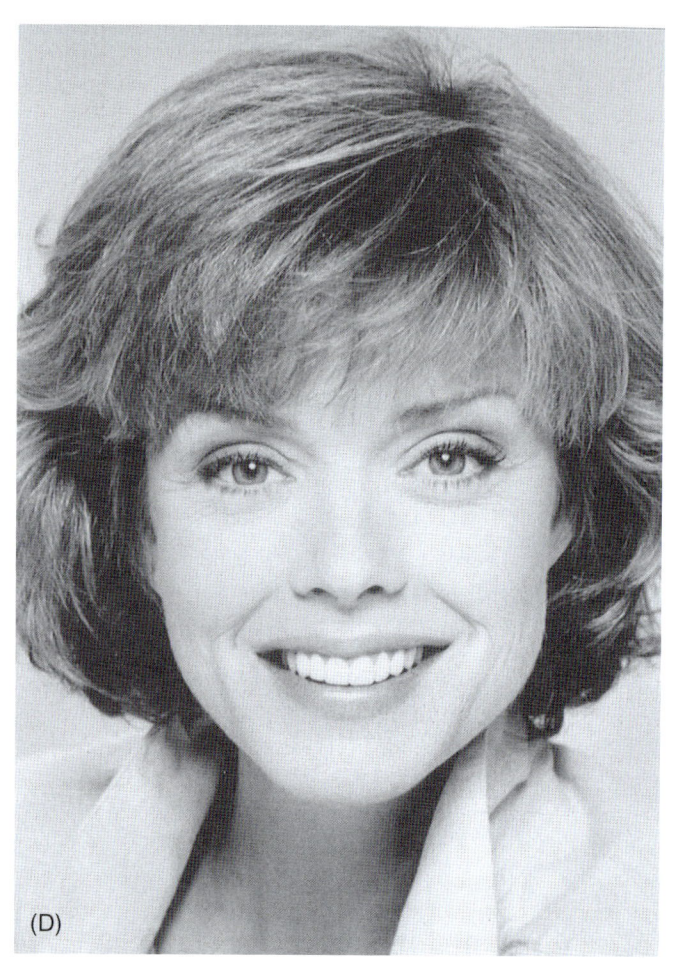

Figure 36.11 (C, D) Comparison of the actress's publicity pictures shows the difference in her smile after a brighter color and widening of the arch through porcelain veneers. *Source*: Images (C) and (D) reproduced with permission of Quintessence Publishing.[1]

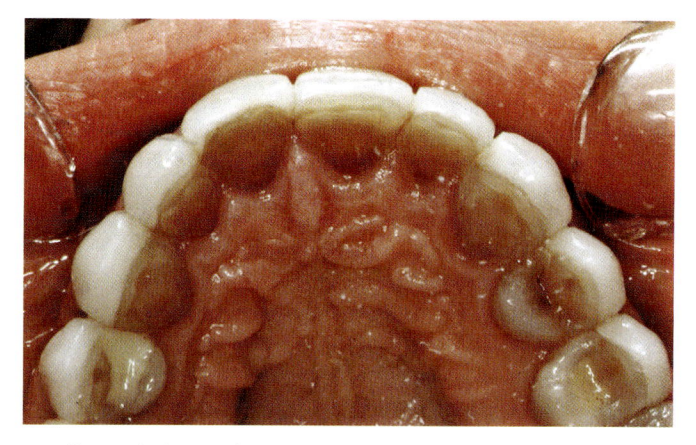

Figure 36.11 (E) It is important to have sufficient thickness of porcelain to be able to mask the underlying tooth color. *Source*: Reproduced with permission of Quintessence Publishing.[1]

Selecting a shade

Choosing the color is probably the most important element in creating a look for a performer's teeth. Color is the most distinctive visual feature for creating a dramatic difference in appearance. Changing the shape of the teeth is not as effective as changing the color because tooth shape is less visible than having one tooth darker than another. For instance, darkened teeth can be seen in the last row of a theater.

Selecting an appropriate shade for an entertainer is one of the most important aspects of the procedure. Generally, there are two treatment options:

1. Select a shade that is perhaps brighter than is normal for nonperforming patients, but which would still appear natural.
2. Defer to the performer's choice of the brightest shade available, regardless of how unnatural it may appear in an off-camera setting.

A possible third choice for performers is a shade just slightly less bright than the second option.

The first choice requires no explanation. The second, however, has roots in cosmetic dentistry lore with an ultrabright shade that bears the initials of the legendary entertainer Phyllis Diller. She had requested the lightest tooth shade available, which at the time was an extra-light hybrid composite. However, after seeing a polymerized direct test shading, Ms Diller said she wanted an even lighter shade. Even though the color already seemed too light, the entertainer insisted that it was not white enough, despite the fact that it was the lightest prepackaged shade then available. The treating dentist (Goldstein) decided to mix white opacifier with the prepackaged shade to create an even brighter shade of white. Containing approximately 75% opacifier, the resulting shade has been called "PD White" ever since. Even now, with bright "bleach shades" of composite resin available, there may be times when you need to use more of the white opacifier to obtain the desired shade.

A color that had previously been considered an embarrassingly bright tooth shade under theater lighting actually looked appropriate on Ms Diller. The heavily textured surfaces of the composite resin used in the procedure also soften the harshness of bright stage lights, a feature that makes for additional appealing results (Figure 36.12).

Metal restorations

Polished amalgams, inlays, onlays, or gold crowns may cause a reflection problem. When these restorations are appropriate or already present, use air abrasion (or micro etcher) to create a dull finish. This procedure can be repeated as necessary.

There is a variation of the aforementioned procedure that can be used to mask an existing gold inlay. The inlay is prepared with about half the occlusal gold removed and covered with tooth-colored composite material. The margins of the cavity preparation are actually covered by a thin edge of gold that bevels back into the body of the inlay. More of the mesial marginal ridge is covered than the distal. The effect of gold inlays that are too visible can be minimized by abrading the surface with air abrasion or microetcher, which puts a satin-like or antique finish to dull the polished metal.

Orthodontic treatment

Problems of malocclusion may present special difficulties to performers because most entertainers travel a great deal and the frequent and necessary adjustments are difficult to arrange. Because appearance is a primary concern, several considerations should be included in the treatment plan.

Whenever possible, try to use "invisible" orthodontic appliances, such as Invisalign, Hawley, or Crozat, because the patient can remove them when performing (Figure 36.13). Ideally, the patient should wear the removable appliance for 24 h a day, although 18–20 h may be acceptable and will ultimately create proper movement. The following photographs illustrate this transformation. The treatment can be completed in five working days using porcelain veneers.

- Always consider Invisalign first, since few people, if any, will be able to tell it is being used. Invisalign is the premier choice of treatment, unless the patient has the time for conventional orthodontics, which would include tooth-colored ceramic brackets.

Figure 36.12 (A) The actress and well-known comedian Phyllis Diller needed a brighter and younger looking smile, especially for her stage performances.

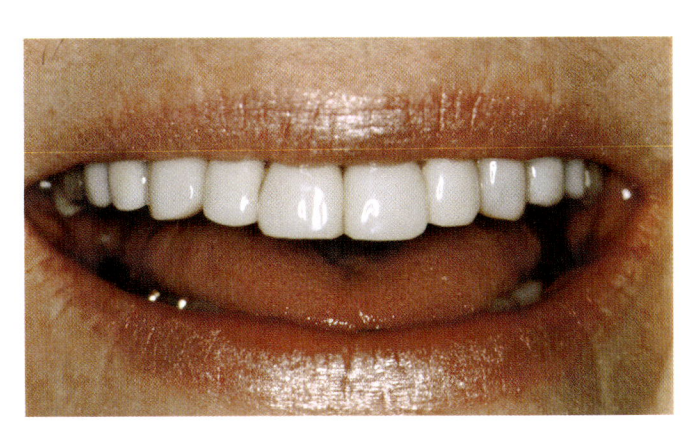

Figure 36.12 (B) The finished appearance consisting of composite resin direct-bonded veneers.

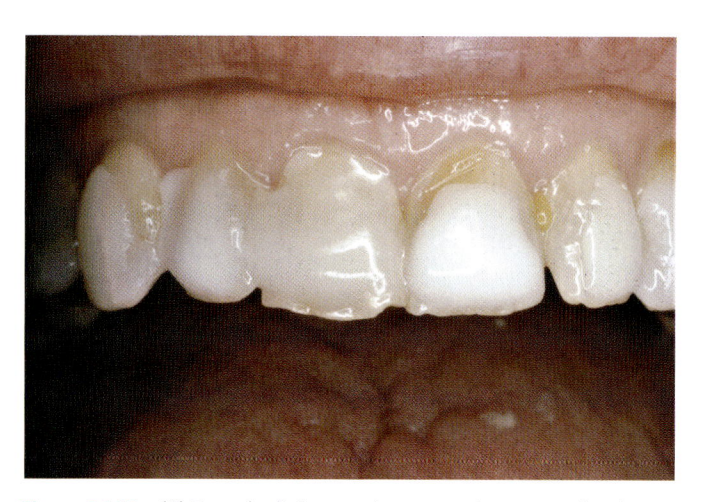

Figure 36.12 **(C)** Even the lightest color composite was not bright enough for the patient, so Dr Goldstein decided to mix opacifier with the brightest color composite.

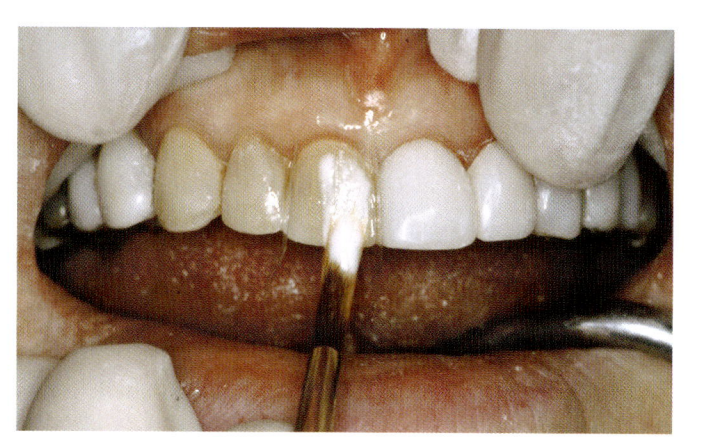

Figure 36.12 **(D)** A white opacifier was applied directly to the etched and polymerized resin before applying the special shade composite resin, termed "PD White" in honor of the patient.

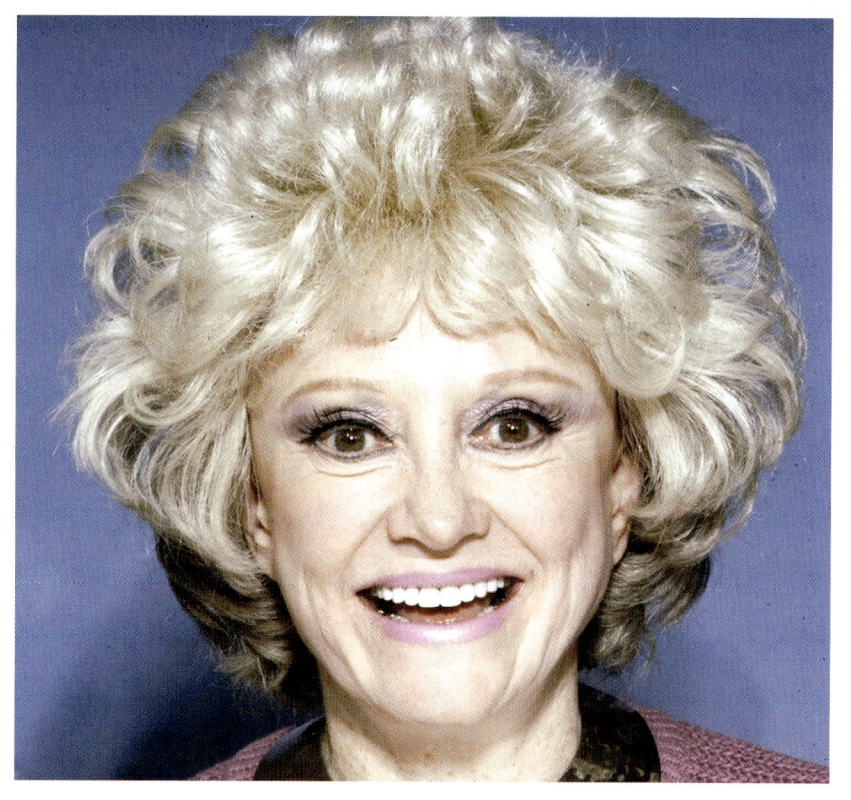

Figure 36.12 **(E)** The final smile was accomplished by bright-colored direct composite veneers, which included lengthening her central incisors to produce a younger-looking smile line.

- If full banding techniques are necessary, recommend that the orthodontist utilizes ceramic brackets on the anterior teeth at a minimum, so that the patient will be able to perform without showing unsightly metal appliances (Figure 36.14).
- If possible, consider the use of lingual, or invisible, braces. It is important to note, however, that there are five problems associated with the use of lingual bands on entertainers:
  - Speech may be affected or impeded.
  - The extraction of one or more anterior teeth may sometimes be required.
  - Frequent adjustments are usually necessary.
  - Lingual bands may be more expensive.
  - Dental visits can possibly interfere with a performer's travel schedule.

With the increasing demand for interdisciplinary therapy, more and more performers have taken advantage of the benefit that orthodontics can bring. This also means there is much less need for a compromise treatment when there are easy orthodontic treatment options available.

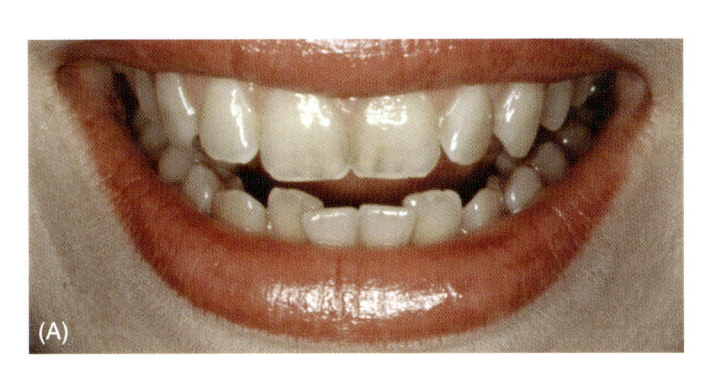

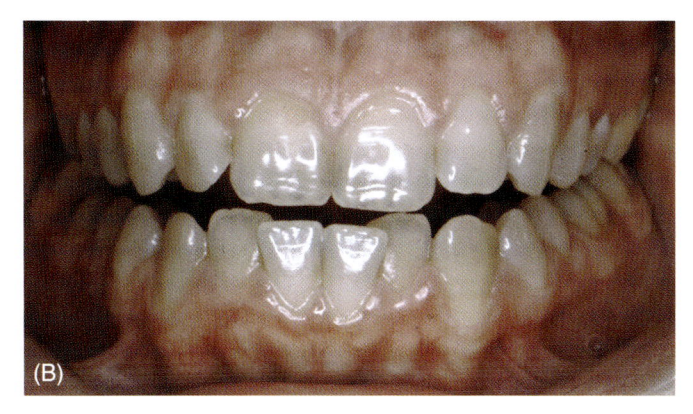

Figure 36.13 (A, B) This performer was concerned about her discolored and crowded teeth.

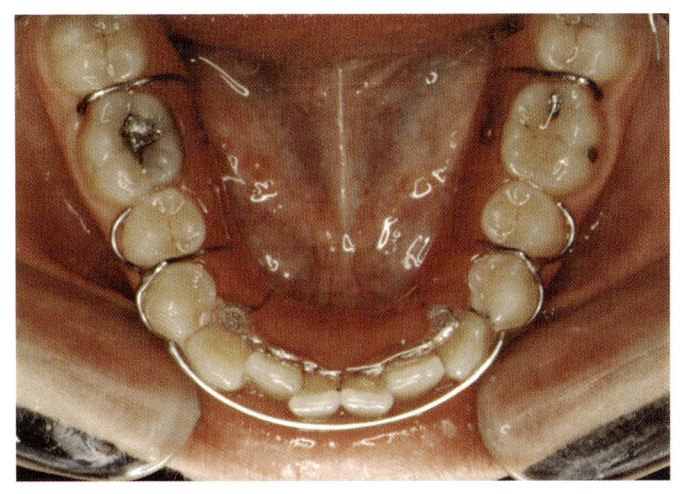

Figure 36.13 (C) A removable Hawley retainer was constructed to reposition her mandibular anterior teeth.

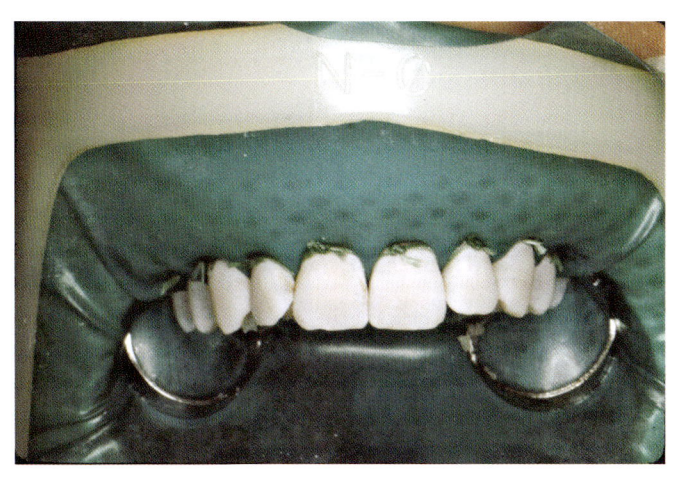

Figure 36.13 (D) The teeth were then bleached in the office with 36% hydrogen peroxide while the lowers were being straightened.

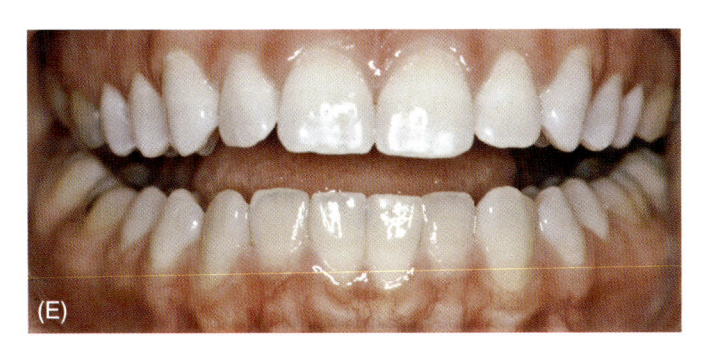

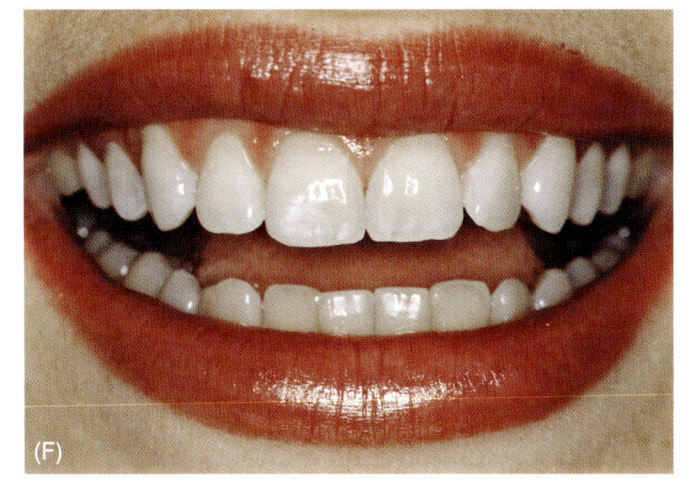

Figure 36.13 (E, F) The final result shows straighter and brighter teeth, producing a more attractive smile.

Periodontal treatment

Given the nature of their profession, entertainers need to look as attractive as possible. Appearance problems, such as a high lip line, can many times be corrected through esthetic periodontal surgery. Teeth should be proportionate to the face; when the gingiva covers too much of the tooth surface, disharmony occurs between teeth and gums. A good example can be seen in Figure 36.15. The actress depicted was unaware of the reason for her unattractive smile. Describing it as "too gummy," she was determined to improve her smile. Computer imaging enabled her to see that lightening her teeth and exposing more of the

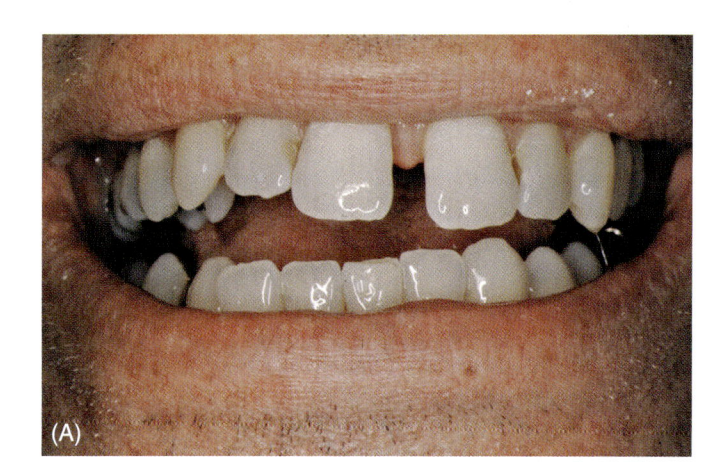

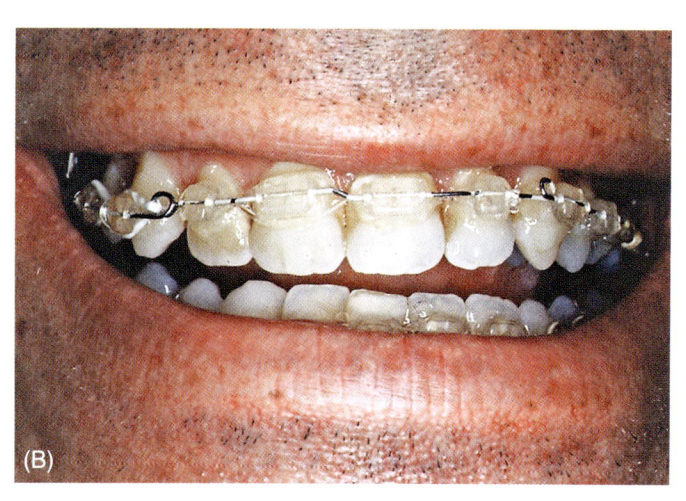

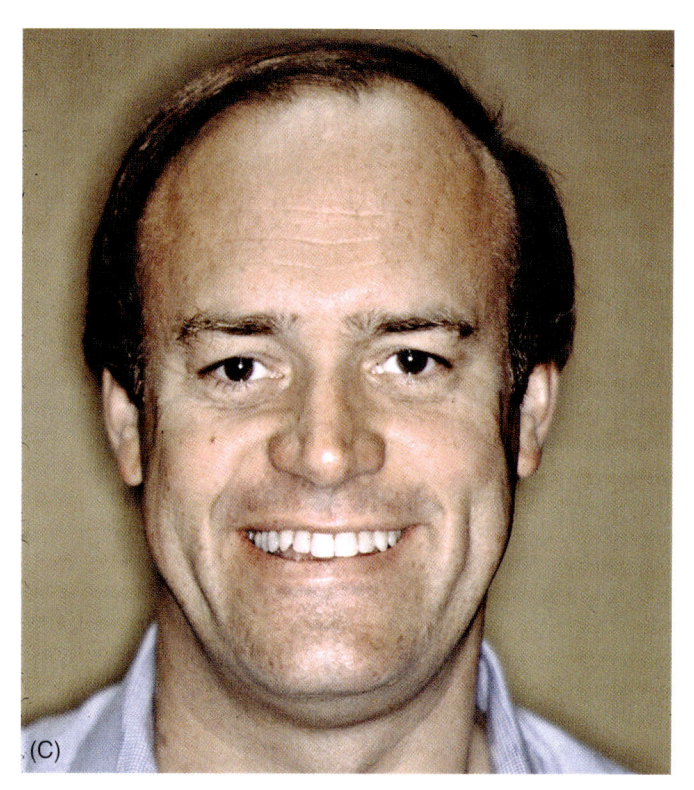

Figure 36.14 (A) This well-known broadcast journalist was concerned about the diastema between his front teeth. (B) Because of his constant appearance on television, ceramic brackets were chosen to help improve his smile and close the space. (C) The final result shows a better looking smile and also helped for more close-up television appearances.

natural tooth structure would accomplish that aim. Therefore, procedures to raise tissue were used, and the teeth were bleached as the finishing touch.

It is important to note that a patient must be in good periodontal health before any type of dental restorative treatment is started. Occasionally, if periodontal surgery is required where restorations are present, unattractive interdental spaces may result. Therefore, consider using laser-assisted new attachment procedure and refer to a periodontist or general dentist who uses this technique. However, if interdental spaces already exist, consider using an acrylic gingival insert or composite resin bonding that will mask the unwanted spaces. Figure 36.16A–E illustrates a combined periodontal, orthodontic, and restorative therapy that transformed the appearance of a young photographic model.

Prosthetic treatment

Temporary measures

A common problem that can detract from an attractive appearance is spacing of the teeth. Because the spaces cannot reflect light, intense lighting reveals spaces as black voids. Irregular spacing can even be more of a problem. Some models have a habit of placing the tongue behind the anterior teeth to mask a

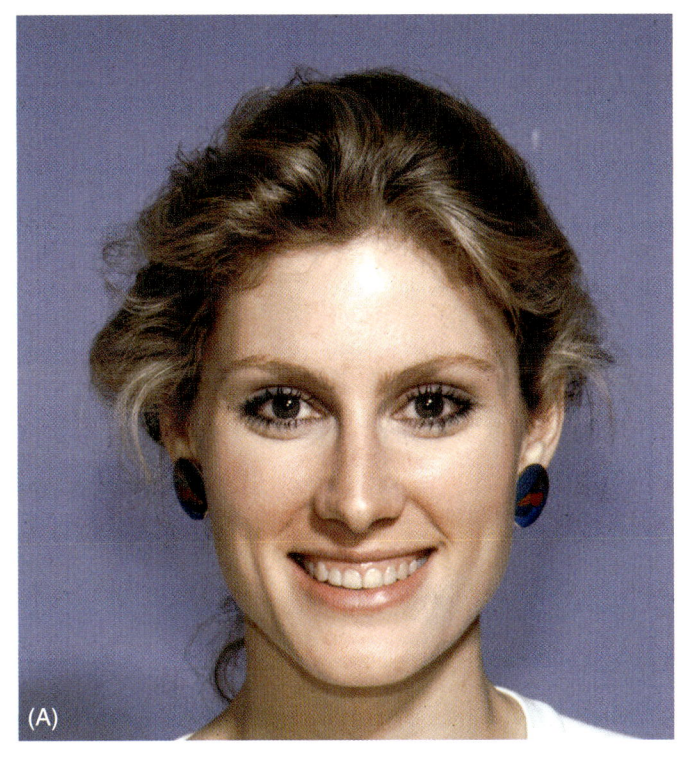

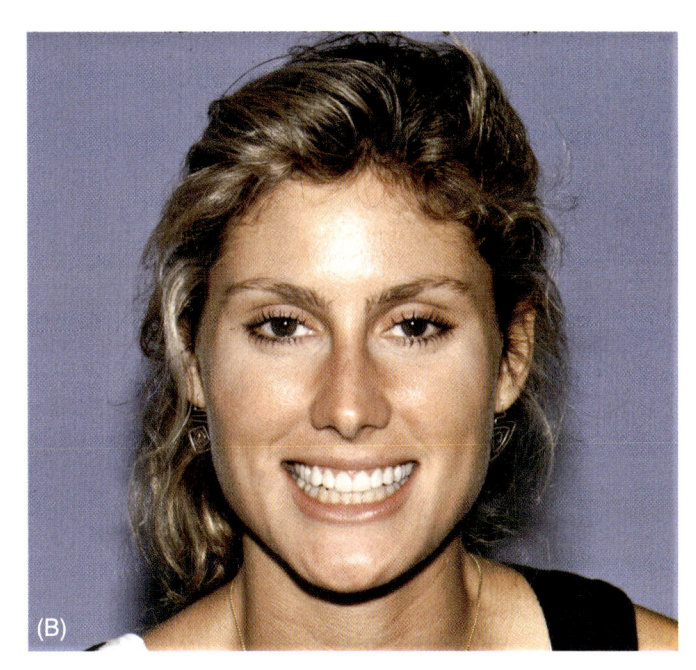

Figure 36.15 **(A)** This part-time actress and model wanted to improve her gummy smile. **(B)** After crown lengthening, bleaching, and composite resin bonding, her smile was improved.

diastema (see Figure 25.5B). The constant pressure from this habit can cause even more space between the teeth. The obvious and ideal treatment includes either orthodontics or restoring with composite resin bonding porcelain veneers or even full crowns if needed. However, two temporary measures can be used when time is a factor. White mortician's wax has been used by some performers to close the gaps during performances or photographic sessions. Composite resin bonding, done with or without etching, can also temporarily close diastemas and should provide the most esthetic result. Clinical case 36.1 illustrates one approach. Other methods of resolving the problem are discussed in Chapter 26.

Fixed restorations

Many performers will require prosthetic restorations to give them a sense of confidence and the best appearance possible. There are special considerations for constructing crowns and fixed partial dentures for performers that may not be discussed elsewhere.

First, most performers work under very strong lighting, and for this reason there are many significant esthetic factors to consider when constructing their prosthetic restorations. Special attention to crown contours, embrasure form, and overall shaping are crucial to creating natural-looking teeth, light reflection, and silhouette form. Variation in incisal lengths is extremely important for performers who want to look younger. Because most performers do prefer a younger look, a youthful smile line

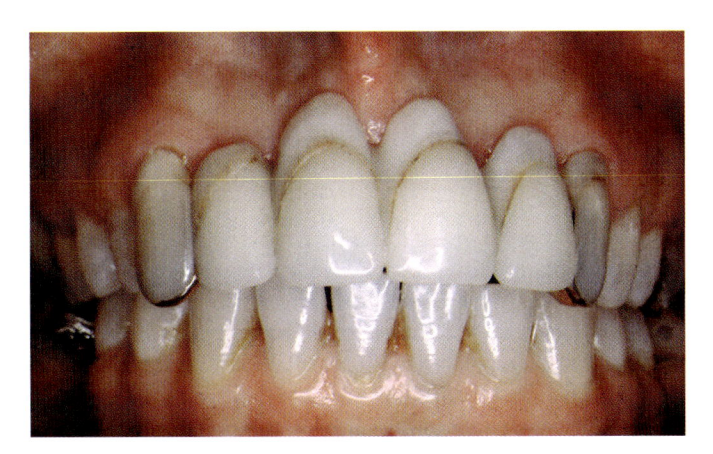

Figure 36.16 **(A)** This runway fashion model was displeased from the poor esthetic treatment received from another dentist and wanted a better smile to do more photographic modeling.

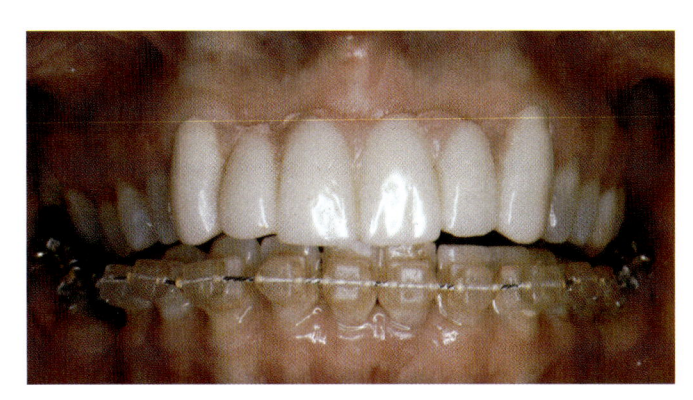

Figure 36.16 **(B)** An immediate six-unit acrylic bridge plus lower ceramic orthodontic brackets were placed to help improve her smile.

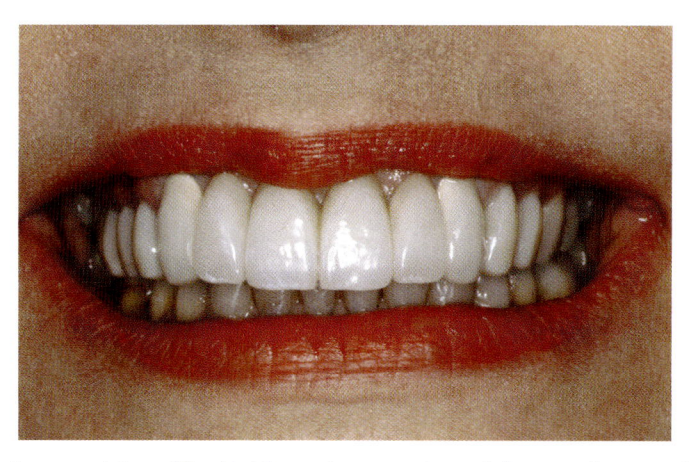

Figure 36.16 **(C)** Final prosthetic restorations, consisting of fixed bridge and crowns, showed absence of symmetrical interdental papilla.

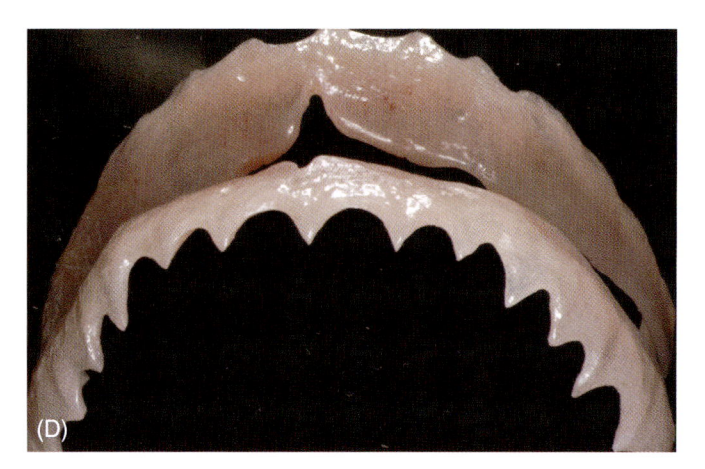

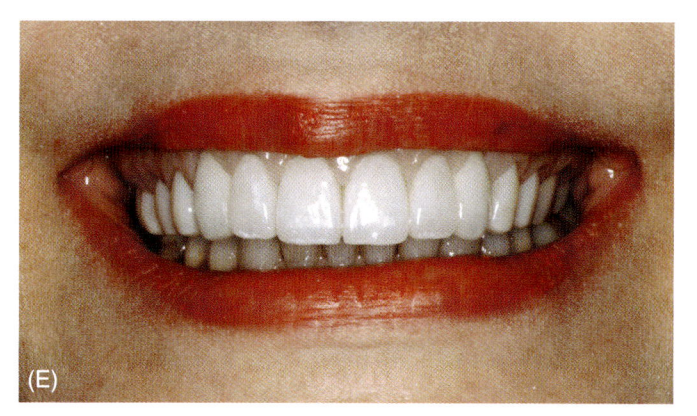

Figure 36.16 **(D, E)** An acrylic gingival tissue appliance was constructed to help provide a more esthetic appearance.

can be created by making the centrals longer than the laterals (Figure 36.18). Shading is also important; teeth that are too light show up just as glaringly as teeth that are too dark.

Specific issues for performers

- *Effects of distance and lighting:* As distance increases, detail is quickly lost in very light or dark teeth. When the teeth are not separated enough, light teeth show up as a solid white band. The appearance of missing teeth can be created when dark shades are used for a patient with heavy lips or when one bicuspid is in linguoversion. Beards and mustaches throw the smile shadow forward, creating an even darker or grayer shadow over the teeth. To balance this effect, use a lighter shade.
- *Treating teeth that are too light or too dark:* There is a tendency for performers to want extremely white teeth. Conversely, if the shade is too dark, it may appear as if teeth are missing. Because entertainers may prefer teeth that are blindingly white, there is little one can do other than use digital photos computer imaging or a very bright trial smile to illustrate to the patient just how unnatural the look can be.
- *Use heavier texture:* This should be done on the labial surface for patients who will be under bright spotlights. This will help break up the reflection of the spotlights.
- *Be careful using yellow in shading:* Too much yellow in shading may give a yellowish-orange cast to restorations that—under some lighting—can make teeth appear unnatural, and much darker.
- *Vary incisal lengths:* Most entertainers want to look more youthful. Therefore, make central incisors longer than the laterals. Creating a greater interincisal distance in anterior teeth, especially veneers or crowns, from 0.5 to 1.5 mm is the range for a younger-looking smile line (Figure 36.18).
- *Open incisal and gingival embrasures:* Anterior restorations will appear as one solid band unless incisal embrasures are opened (Figure 36.18).
- *Do not overbuild porcelain:* Unless you are purposely building out the restorations, avoid making your restorations too bulky. Labial bulk only creates a false appearance to restorations. Be sure to reduce enough tooth structure during the preparation.
- *Add characterization:* Characterization not only increases the "naturalness" of the facial appearance but also prevents light-colored teeth from looking like one continuous unit on

Clinical case 36.1: Immediate closure of diastema with composite resin bonding

Problem

Figure 36.17A–D shows a movie and television actress who wanted a diastema between her upper anteriors closed. She had been using mortician's wax to cover the gap during filming but said that doing so gave her a "spooky" feeling. Also, the patient did not want orthodontics or sound teeth reduced.

Treatment

It was decided to close the space with composite resin. The patient was cautioned that the bond would have to be repaired or replaced periodically. She decided that this was her best solution because this procedure resulted in immediate improvement and did not require tooth reduction.

The first step is to decide which tooth or teeth and surfaces should be included in the treatment. Generally speaking, the distal surface of the tooth closest to the midline is best. Whenever possible, the resin is added mainly to the distolingual surface so as not to make the tooth too wide.

Result

Figure 36.17D shows that the space closure did not make the tooth appear overbuilt because its contact area was carved to the lingual. The biggest problem with this type of restoration is that staining can occur. Patients whose teeth stain easily will usually need to have their restorations refinished more frequently or choose porcelain veneers. Alert the patient that bonding tends to discolor over time. Therefore, polishing or resurfacing will be required.

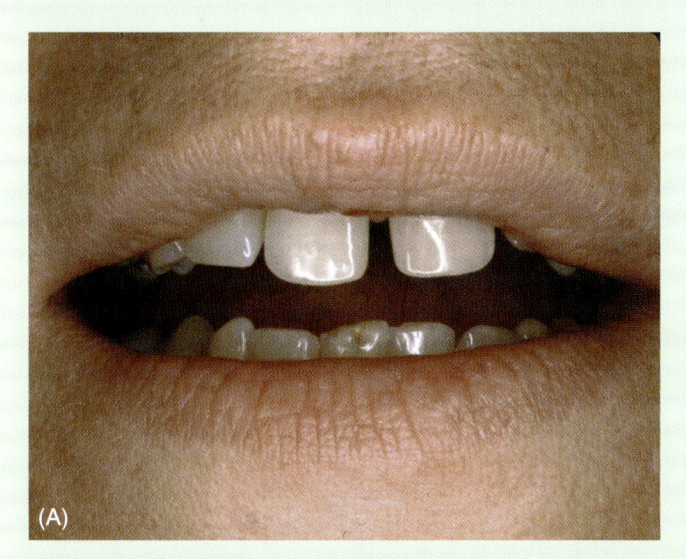

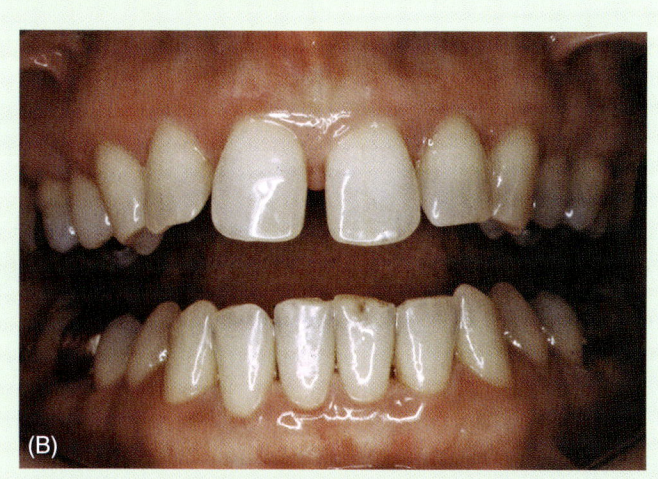

Figure 36.17 (A, B) This actress played the part of a stripper in a movie thriller with her natural teeth, but another movie option came up that required a better looking smile so she wanted her teeth instantly changed.

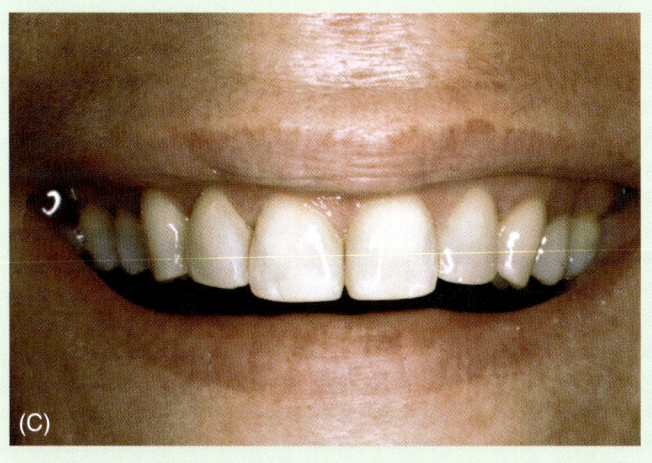

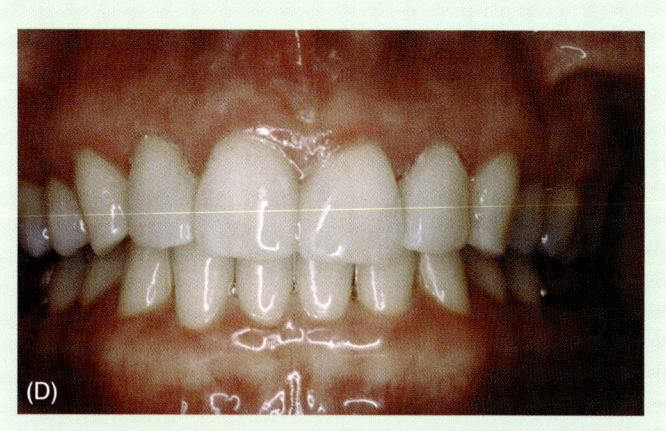

Figure 36.17 (C, D) Direct composite resin bonding was chosen to accomplish diastema closure. Later, if she wanted to return to her diastema, the space could be reopened as necessary.

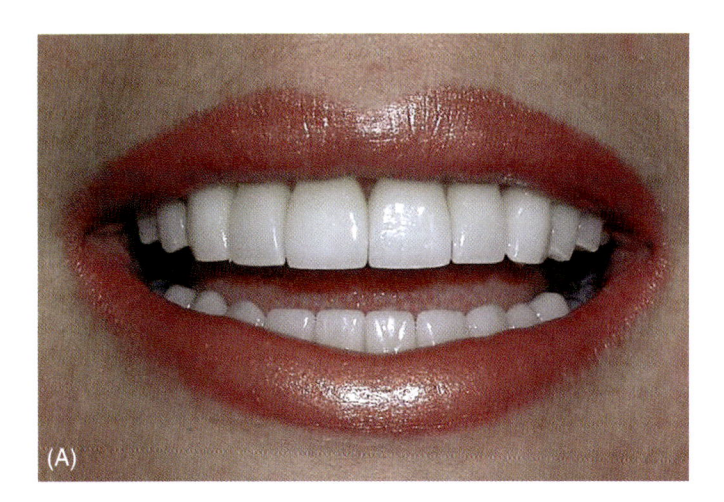

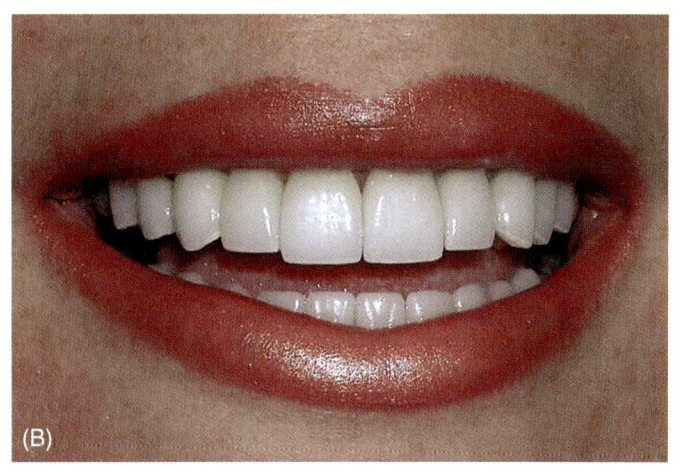

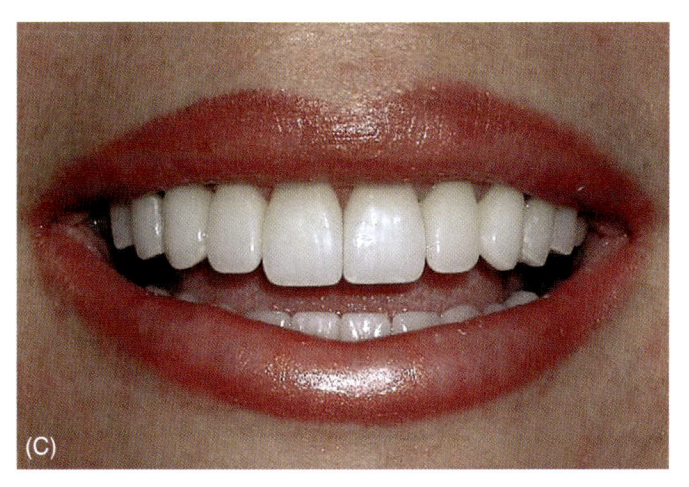

Figure 36.18 (A–C) These frontal smile images from the Loren Library Interactive Smile Style Guide depict three attractive variations for performers looking to improve their smiles. Note the differences in incisal length.

photographic interpretation (see Chapter 8). Incisal translucence can go a long way toward making your restorations look more natural, but make certain your patient will allow you to include it.

Emergency treatment

Entertainers have special requirements when it comes to emergency treatment. A dentist who treats performers must be willing to extend special office time to them because, as the adage says, the show must go on. Performers may require priority attention when they have an emergency. Note, however, that the nature of a performer's dental emergency may not be the same as an emergency for a patient who does not work in the entertainment industry. Given their esthetic needs, entertainers have much more at stake, because their livelihoods depend much more on their appearance than those of a nonperformer do.

Long-distance consultation

Long-distance consultation offers another option for treating traveling performers who need modifications to their appearance. This option taps into dentistry's growing use of computer-assisted design and computer-assisted manufacturing. The use of computer imaging and e-mail can be an effective method for treating an actor on a film shoot, for instance. Once it is approved, the prosthesis can be sent to the location by the following day.

Although many entertainers have high travel expenses and low income, they should not be penalized by inferior treatment. This means extraction is not necessarily the best answer for a tooth that could be preserved and useful for a long time. It may take several years before an entertainer can afford more extensive or expensive treatment. Nevertheless, there is no reason that they should lose a tooth because of cost or time constraints. A more economic treatment plan, perhaps consisting of composite resin bonding or even acrylic or composite resin treatment crowns, could be an excellent interim esthetic compromise. In cases where extraction of an anterior tooth is mandatory, it may be possible to salvage the patient's natural tooth crown for quite a long time. Although ideal treatment might well consist of extraction and an immediate implant, it may be out of the performers budget or even not possible during filming.

Occasionally, entertainers may require removable dentures for a special effect. The patient in Figure 36.19, a comedian, wanted a "comic arrangement." The denture was constructed in the

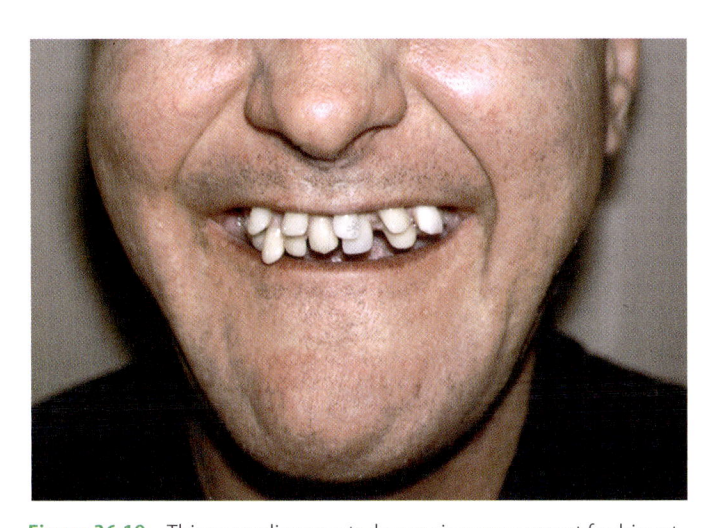

Figure 36.19 This comedian wanted a comic arrangement for his act, so a denture was constructed in the conventional manner but the teeth were widely spaced, in multiple rows placed at random and oversized to create the abnormal effect.

conventional manner, but the teeth were widely spaced in multiple rows at random and made oversized to create the abnormal, comedic effect.

Summary of important principles for treating performers

The trial smile: demonstrating using imaging and video and informed consent

Although the use of esthetic imaging and video can help the performer understand the proposed treatment and the expected result, there is no substitution for a trial smile to make certain the look you propose is also the same as the performer expects (see Chapter 3). If an extremely light shade is desired, be sure to show your patient how the effect of the too-white restorations may look. As seen in the case of Phyllis Diller, some patients will want or need to have a smile with unnaturally light-colored teeth, but

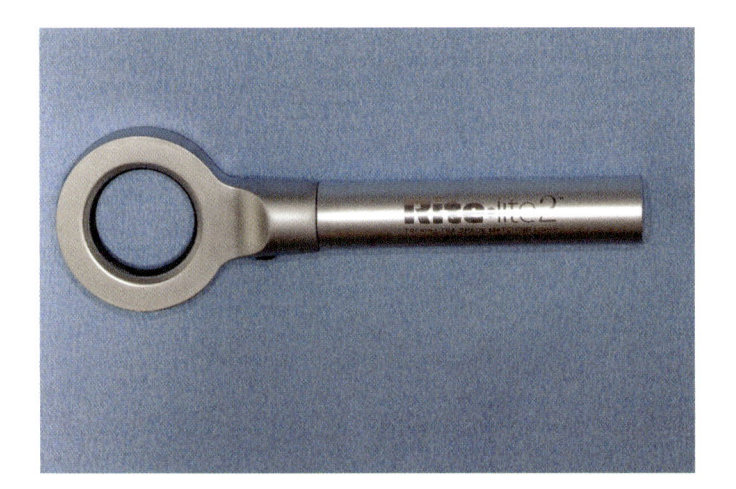

Figure 36.20 **(A)** The Rite-Lite 2 (AdDent) has three sources of light: incandescent, fluorescent, and a combination of both. This way, patients can be tested to make sure the restoration will look good in different environments.

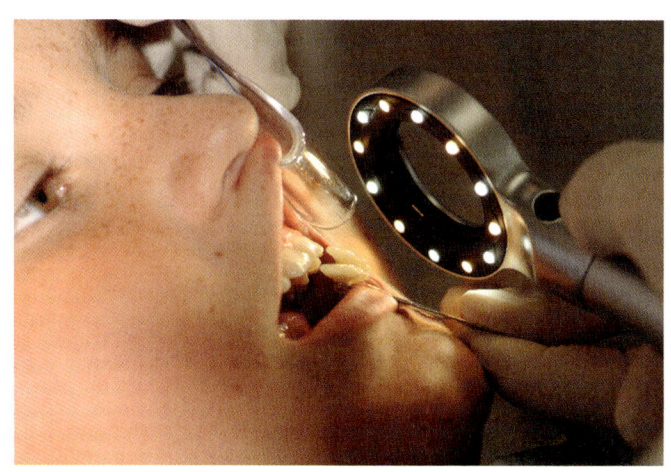

Figure 36.20 **(B)** The light source shown here is a combination of both fluorescent and incandescent light.

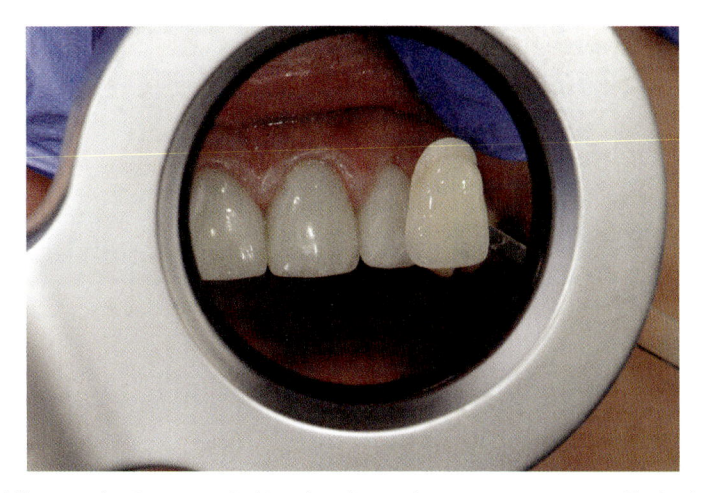

Figure 36.20 **(C)** Note the precise difference the Rite-Lite 2 (AdDent) makes in determining a proposed light shade.

these patients should be urged to at least consider their off-stage appearance. As long as the patient is aware of the expected results and approves it in writing before treatment begins, there should be no surprises. Just make sure you have a well-written, understandable informed consent form (see Chapter 6).

Lighting considerations and effects on appearance of the teeth

Careful consideration of light reflection from studio lighting

The effect of light reflection on the appearance of teeth is an important phenomenon to consider, and anything that modifies the reflection, such as lips, beard, or tongue, must be studied appropriately. Under studio lighting, little difference can be seen in similar shades of the all-ceramic crowns, porcelain-fused-to-metal, porcelain veneers, and composite resin restorations. An acceptable difference may be detectable in acrylic resin splints and sometimes in all-ceramic crowns. Such restorations may appear darker than shades used with the other materials. The goal is to have all these materials blend favorably with natural teeth on screen or in still photographs when the shades are matched under different lighting. Incandescent light is generally used in theatrical plays, video productions, or movie productions. One shade detection light that can be quite helpful is the Rite-Lite 2 (AdDent). This has three light sources that can be seen just by pressing a button on the device (Figure 36.20A–C); the three sources have fluorescent, incandescent, and a combination of both.

Restorations that lack deep depressions in the interproximal contact and shoulder areas lose the appearance of separation between the teeth and will appear as broad bands of white. This problem is sometimes encountered in metal-based veneered restorations, when the opaque metal close to the interproximal surfaces reflects light excessively. Staining can be used to resolve this situation when the embrasures cannot be deepened.

Effects of black lighting

If the performer's porcelain restorations will be seen frequently under black light, porcelain that has a luminous effect should be considered. Although the built-in reflecting quality does not completely mimic the qualities of the natural tooth, it is better than ceramic restorations that do not possess this characteristic.

The goal: attractive, natural-looking teeth

Quality functional and esthetic dental treatment always means maintaining the patient's natural teeth, even if crowning becomes necessary. Extractions and removable or fixed partial dentures should be avoided. An attractive, natural appearance is essential for persons in the performing arts. A dentist with a performer for a patient should have a thorough knowledge of the skills covered in this chapter as well as an awareness of the special needs involved in treating patients who appear in films, television, theater, magazines, and on catwalks.

Reference

1. Goldstein RE. *Change Your Smile*, 4th edn. Hanover Park, IL: Quintessence; 2009.

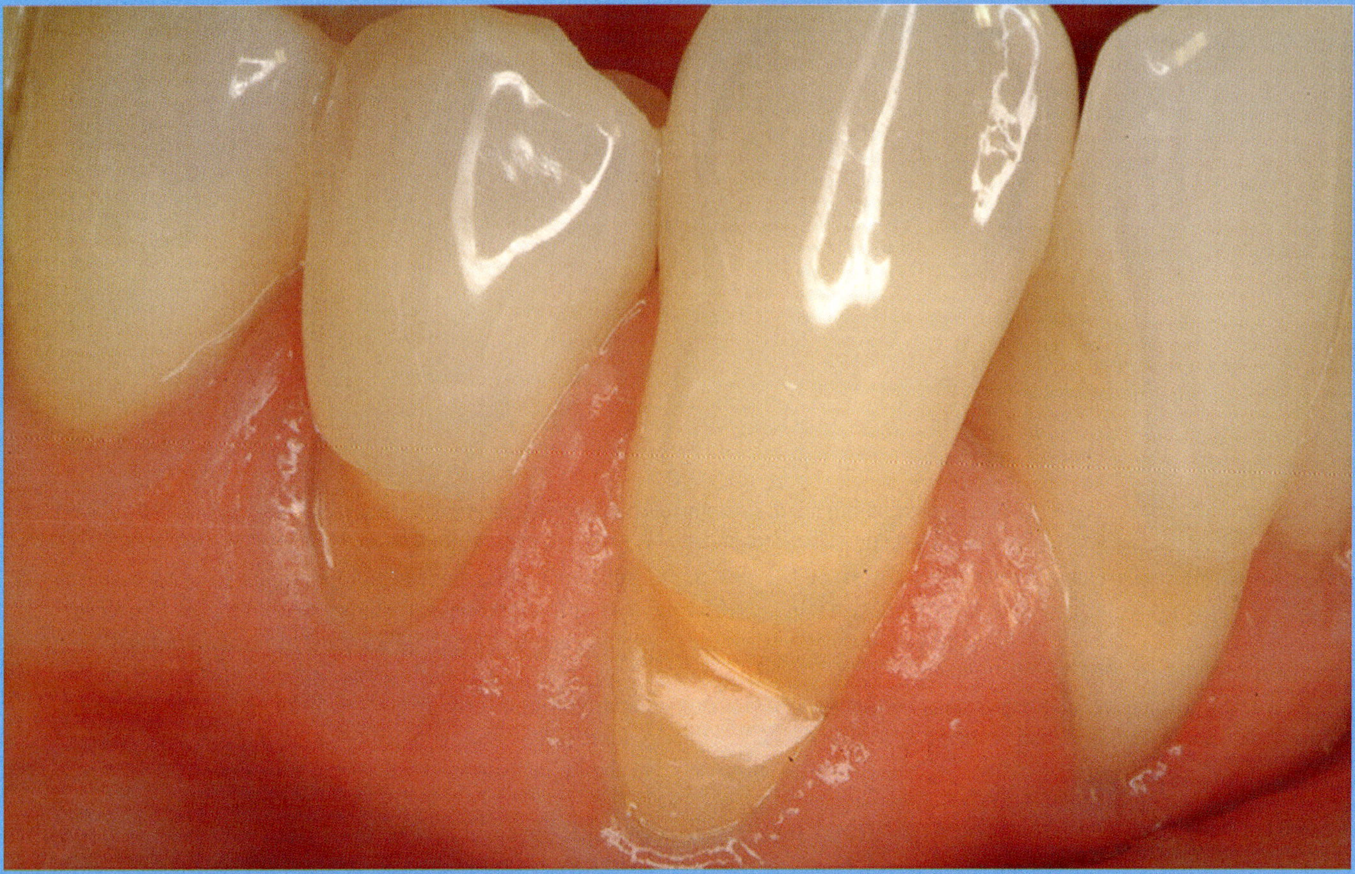
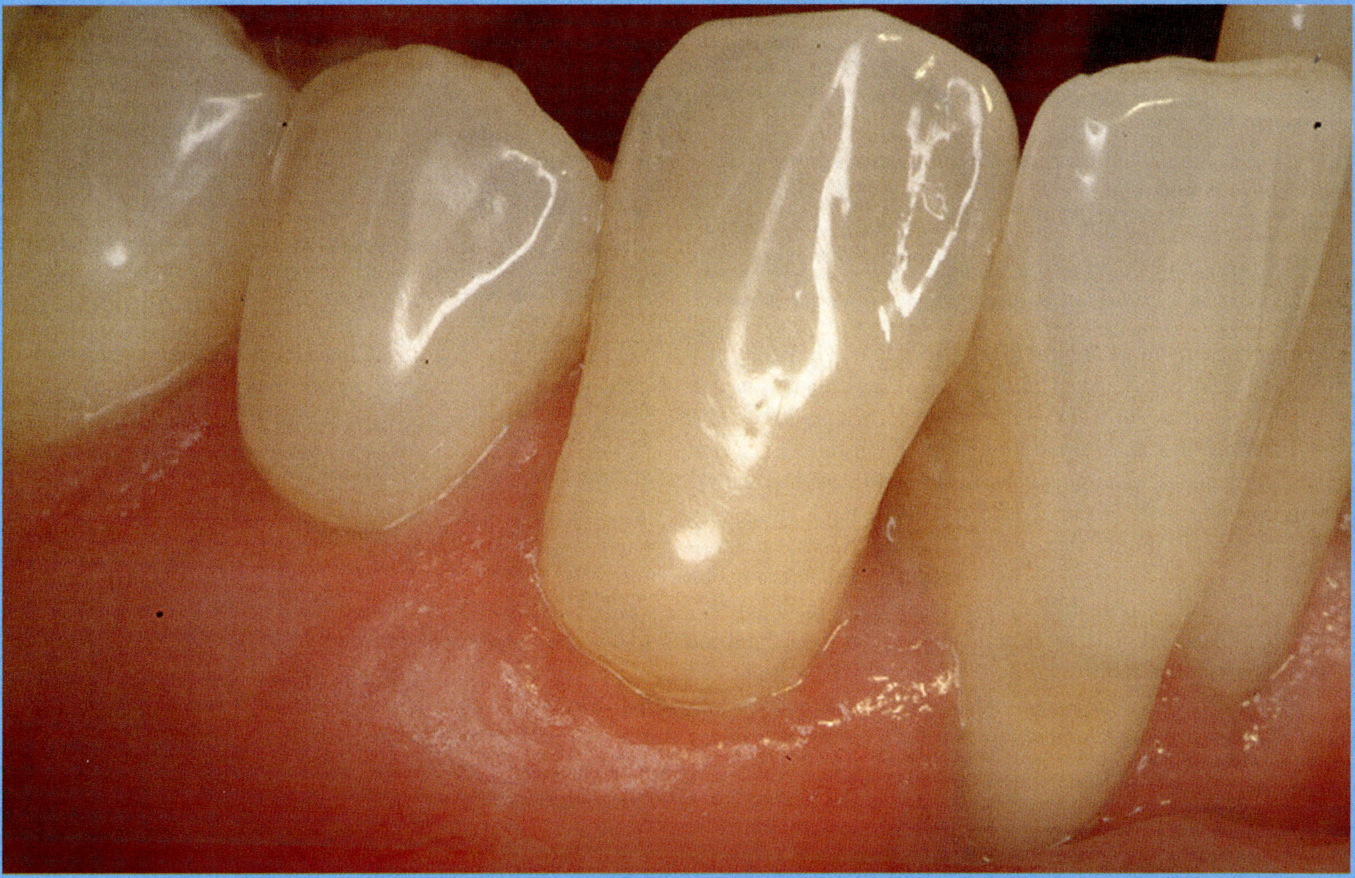

Chapter 37 Periodontal Plastic Surgery

W. Peter Nordland, DMD, MS and Laura M. Souza, DDS

Chapter Outline

Esthetics and function	1181	Other considerations	1194
Microsurgery	1182	Old restorations and root caries	1194
Root coverage	1183	Quality and quantity of donor tissue	1195
Etiology of gingival recession	1184	Grafting over implants	1195
Connective tissue versus allogenic tissues	1184	Restoration of the lost interdental papilla	1195
Indications for gingival augmentation	1185	Multidisciplinary management	1196
Furcation involvement	1185	Surgical technique of papilla reconstruction	1196
Potential for gingival regeneration	1185	Ridge preservation and ridge augmentation	1199
Connective tissue graft surgical technique	1186	Ridge augmentation	1200
Root preparation	1186	Surgical technique	1201
Microincisions and the gingival pouch	1188	Excessive gingival display: esthetic crown lengthening and sculpting	1204
Connective tissue harvesting	1189	Individual's biologic width	1205
Sutures and dressing	1191	Esthetic crown-lengthening surgical procedure	1206
Postoperative instructions and healing	1194		

Esthetics and function

Periodontal plastic surgical procedures have the ability to assist the restorative dentist and patient to achieve beautiful results. Esthetic excellence in restorative dentistry mimics the natural shape and color of the teeth. The final restorative outcome will only be optimal when soft tissue and bone also mimic the natural anatomy. The role of periodontal plastic surgery is to give patients back the natural framing when normal anatomy is deficient or missing. Periodontal plastic surgery should restore color, texture, symmetry, size, and proportion while bringing tissues to an anatomically correct position.[1,2] Surgical results should be predictable and long-lasting with health.

This subspecialty is also meticulously focused on preserving the soft tissue and bone during oral surgical procedures to allow for an optimal esthetic result. This is extremely important, especially when working in the esthetic zone. An aggressive approach during the surgical procedure can disfigure a patient's smile by creating scar tissue, bony defects, papilla loss, and gum recession. Focusing on this goal, it is important that the surgeon minimizes or totally avoids releasing incisions. This is mostly evident in the maxillary anterior region with delicate biotype patients.

The papillary microvasculature has been identified as an end-artery organ with delicate blood supply.[3] Loss of the interdental papilla caused by trauma or periodontitis remains a significant esthetic challenge to dentistry.[4] Once the defect has been created, it can be very challenging to correct. Many clinicians have tried over the years to reconstruct lost interdental papillae around natural teeth; however, a high level of success and predictability have not been achieved.[5-14] Examples showing incision defects are presented in Figure 37.1. A simple surgical tooth extraction can also lead to bone loss and a soft-tissue defect.[15] An anterior collapsed ridge can make it impossible to place an implant in the area and always increases the challenge for the restorative dentist (Figure 37.2). A conservative and delicate approach during a surgical extraction does not always guarantee a good foundation, but will allow for faster healing and less discomfort during the recovery, in addition to a better esthetic result. The likelihood of a severe ridge collapse or soft-tissue defect should be drastically diminished with a delicate microsurgical approach (Figure 37.3).

Microsurgery

When performing microsurgery, small microsurgical instruments can help make the surgical procedure less invasive and less traumatic.[2,16,17] Microsurgical instruments can include microscalpels, microforceps, and miniaturized surgical instruments (Figure 37.4A).[2,17] The use of the surgical dissecting microscope can be helpful to minimize incision size and easily hide incisions.[17] The surgical microscope offers increased illumination and visual acuity to perform procedures with greater precision than with other methods of magnification.[2,17,18]

Microsurgical blades such as the N6900 were developed to allow for atraumatic and undetectable surgical incisions (Figure 37.4B). These scalpels can be modified to provide curves using small bends in the blade and in the shank to allow the

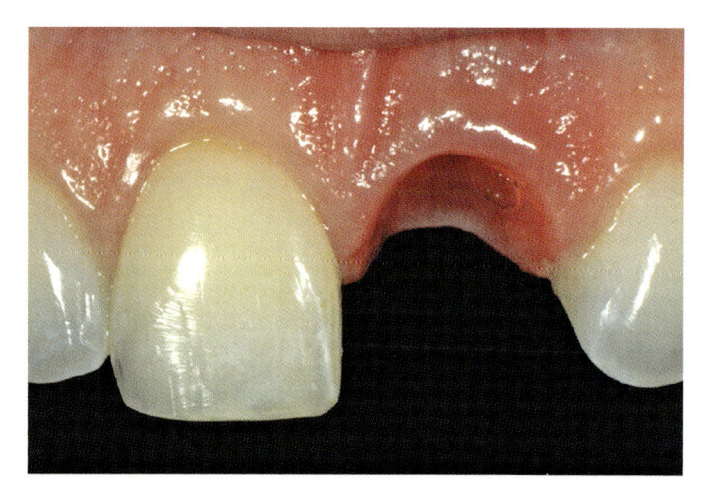

Figure 37.3 All anatomical contours were maintained with a delicate microsurgical approach.

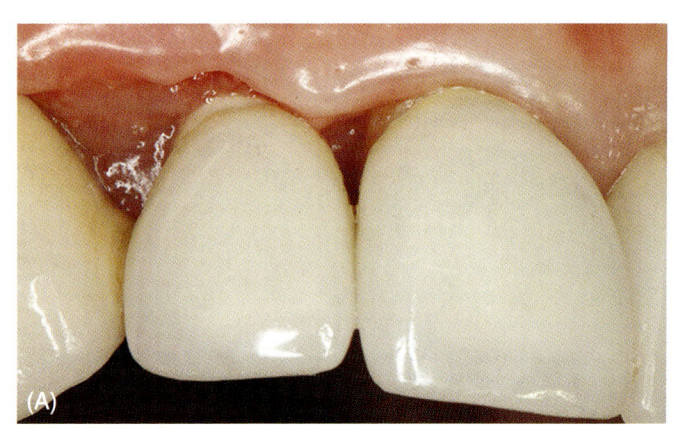

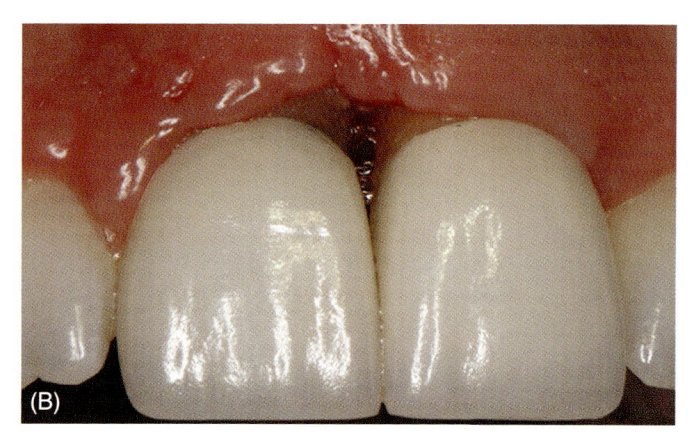

Figure 37.1 (A, B) Previous incisions in the esthetic zone disfigured these smiles.

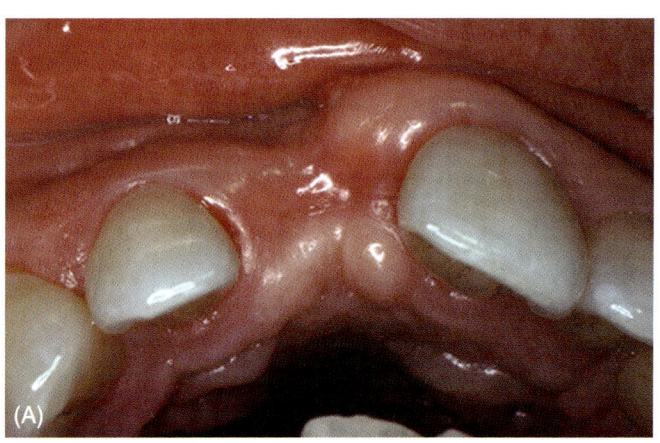

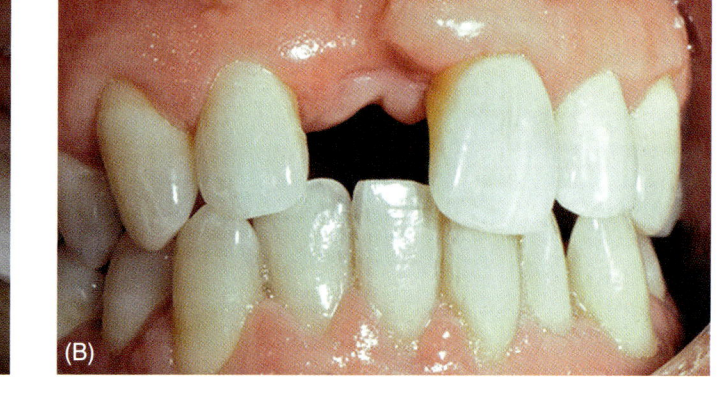

Figure 37.2 (A, B) Photos demonstrating anterior ridge collapse.

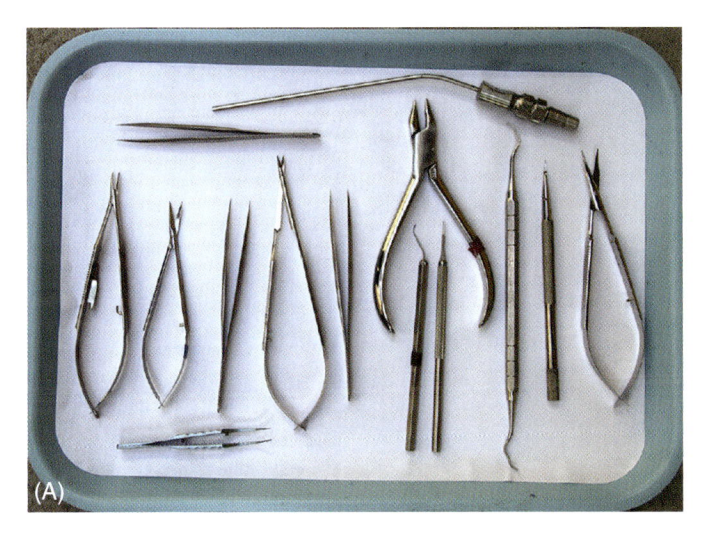

Figure 37.4 (A) Nordland microsurgical kit (Hu-Friedy).

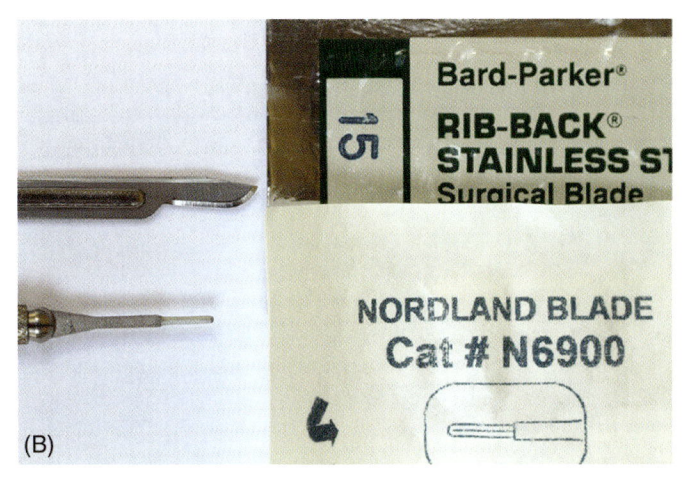

Figure 37.4 (B) A comparison between the microsurgical N6900 and the 15-C blades.

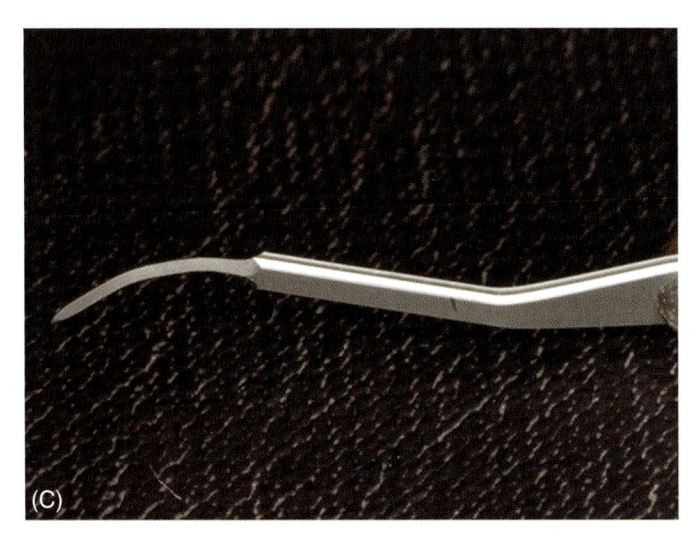

Figure 37.4 (C) N6900 with blade and shank customization.

dissection under papillae or around tori (Figure 37.4C).[17,19] Making curved incisions around obstacles can avoid additional releasing incisions that otherwise might be used to create access, minimizing soft-tissue traumas and defects.[19] In addition, the surgical dissecting microscope and microsurgical instrumentation have allowed the surgeon the capability of fine-tuning surgical procedures.[2,17,20]

Root coverage

The use of the free gingival graft, as described by Sullivan and Atkins in 1968, detailed the use of a very thin graft harvested from the palate.[21–23] Although the free gingival graft could increase the band of attached keratinized gingiva, it did not provide root coverage. Unfortunately, the tissue color and texture would appear different from the native tissues and remain obvious, creating a permanent unesthetic result (Figure 37.5).

A paper by Cole et al. in 1980 demonstrated, with human histology, that new attachment was possible through acid demineralization of the root surface.[24] This encouraged further studies of soft-tissue grafts with acid demineralization to promote root coverage with possible new attachment. In 1982, Miller published the use of a thicker gingival graft that used butt joint incisions, which enhanced vascularity of the thicker graft by including blood supply to the sides of the graft tissue. This technique incorporated the use of acid demineralization to achieve root coverage and potentially new attachment to the root surface.[25] Later in 1985, Miller demonstrated predictable root coverage using a free soft-tissue autograft following citric acid application.[26] The use of subepithelial connective tissue in a pouch was introduced by Langer and Calagna to correct ridge defects.[27] Raetzke adapted the use of a pouch technique to help surround grafted tissue over exposed roots.[28] This further enhanced vascularity and the surgical outcome for root coverage procedures. In that same year, Langer and Langer[29] also published their paper detailing the use of subepithelial connective tissue to achieve coverage. Nordland, in 1989, published a

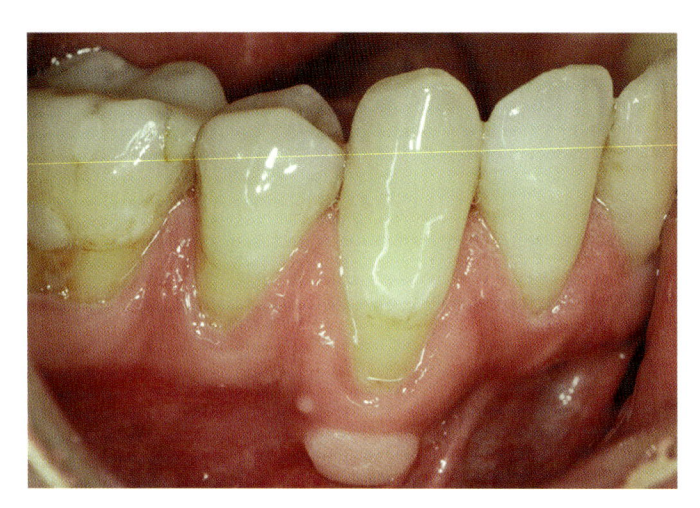

Figure 37.5 Example of an unesthetic free gingival graft result.

technique paper to detail the use of connective tissue, acid demineralization, and envelope recipient bed and envelope donor tissue harvesting to achieve consistent root coverage with the potential for new attachment.[30] In 1994, Allen published the use of a tunneling technique to essentially surround the cells totally with blood supply.[31]

Current techniques, as described by Nordland, take advantage of surrounding the graft almost entirely with blood supply, thereby improving the survivability of all the transplanted cells. Esthetic color blending and natural surface textures are maintained in the recipient area because the surface tissues are unchanged, keeping the original native appearance.[19,20] The Miller classification provides guidelines for predictability of root coverage.[32] It has been shown that periodontal root coverage procedures are highly predictable for Class I and II recessions even when root surface defects are present. Success rates for complete root coverage range from 92% to 99% and are stable over time.[33,34]

Etiology of gingival recession

Several etiologic agents have been recognized to cause gingival recession. Often, the etiology of recession can be multifactorial, and the factors may include the following:

- *Inflammation.*[35] The presence of bacterial plaque and its toxins will cause an inflammatory process in the gingival tissue that may lead to bone loss, attachment loss, and recession as a result.
- *Toothbrushing trauma.*[36] Toothbrush abrasion or other cleaning devices can cause mechanical trauma to the gingival tissue, resulting in recession of the gingival margin. A more modern concern could arise from mechanical electric toothbrush devices.
- *Tooth position.*[37–39] If orthodontic treatment is planned, then a thin band of keratinized gingiva can increase the susceptibility for gingival recession.[37] The tooth position plays a key role determining if gingival augmentation is necessary.[38] Teeth that are moved orthodontically to a prominent position have thinner surrounding bone and thin soft tissue that could make them more prone to trauma and gingival recession. If a tooth erupts out of the bony housing, it could emerge through the alveolar mucosa, thereby lacking attached keratinized gingival protection that could result in future susceptibility to recession.[39]
- *Tooth prominence.* Teeth with prominent crowns or roots will be more affected by mechanical trauma from toothbrushing and food than other less prominent teeth and may also experience a thinning of the overlying bone and gingiva.[40]
- *Prominent frenum.* It is thought that a prominent frenum could exert a pull or tug at the gingival margin and thereby contribute to recession, especially if the frenum extends close to the free gingival margin.[41,42]
- *Dental restorations.* Restorations could traumatize delicate tissues with placement of retraction cord. Prominent margins can contribute to plaque retention, and prominent restorations could push the marginal tissue apically.[43–45]
- *Abfractions.* These have not been shown to create gingival recession directly; however, tooth flexure could promote loss of the crystalline enamel structure, resulting in enamel loss and dentinal exposure.[46–48]

Predisposing factors:

- lack or minimal presence of attached keratinized gingiva;
- delicate biotype (Figure 37.6A and B).

Connective tissue versus allogenic tissues

Allogenic tissue has become popular owing to the unnecessary palatal wound and the unlimited supply of donor tissues, allowing the surgeon to treat many areas of gingival recession in one sitting. The supply of autogenous donor tissue is limited and could require sequential surgical procedures when full mouth treatment is anticipated. There is debate whether connective tissue grafts can increase the amount of attached keratinized gingiva, as shown in Figure 37.7A and B. Using autogenous connective tissue, the grafted tissue can create a cell line that will survive and replenish itself over time. The risk of regression is minimized. Allogenic tissues can thicken the tissue surrounding a tooth; however, their efficacy is questionable long term, compared with the use of autogenous connective tissue graft.[49]

Unfortunately, there have been tissue bank recalls of allogenic tissues used for other purposes, which can create a concern by the anxious patient. Allogenic tissues also add an increase in cost for the material. Allogenic material also has the potential to show through in areas of thin native tissue, especially in delicate biotype patients.

In a study evaluating the histologic composition of connective tissue grafts in humans, Harris found that, even though most connective tissue grafts are not uniform in composition, all grafts were successful in producing root coverage with a mean root coverage of 97.7% in Class I or II defects.[50] Long-term stability of root coverage and esthetic results perceived by patients were significantly better 10 years after connective tissue graft surgery, statistically, than after guided tissue regeneration surgery using bioabsorbable barriers.[51] According to Lee et al.,[52] the connective tissue graft is a predictable method for root coverage and the clinical outcomes gained can be well maintained. Chambrone et al.,[53] in a Cochrane systematic review, evaluated the effectiveness of different root coverage procedures including free gingival grafts, laterally positioned flaps, coronally advanced flaps, subepithelial connective tissue grafts alone or in combination with laterally positioned or coronally advanced flaps, acellular dermal matrix grafts, guided tissue regeneration, and the use of enamel matrix protein in the treatment of recession-type defects and concluded that, where root coverage and gain in keratinized tissue are expected, the use of subepithelial connective tissue grafts appears to have superior results.

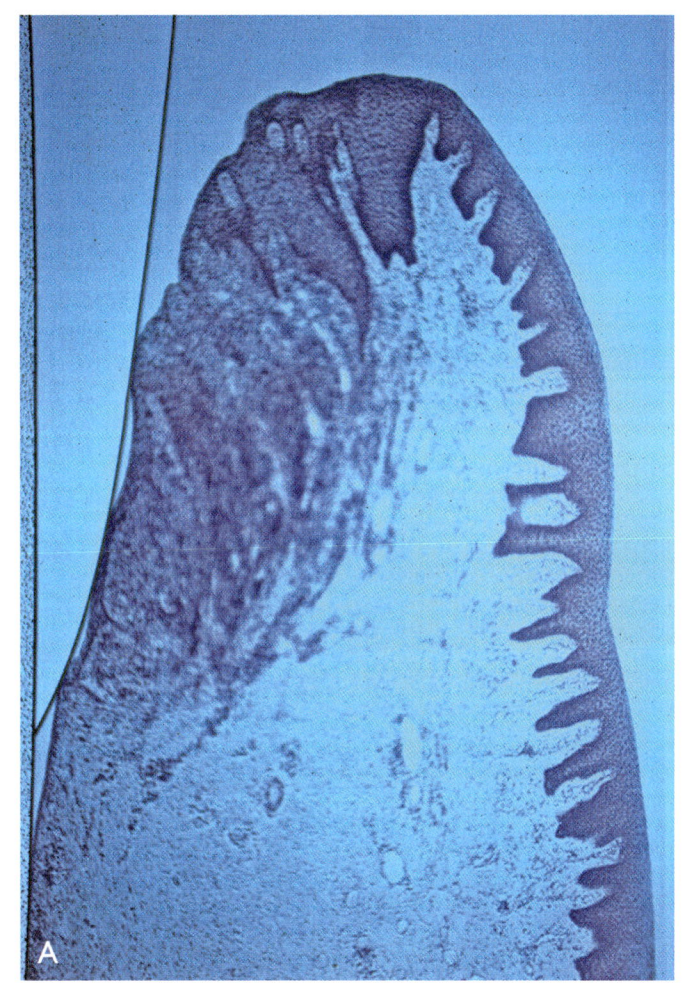

Figure 37.6 **(A)** Histologic image of a thick gingival biotype with inflammation.

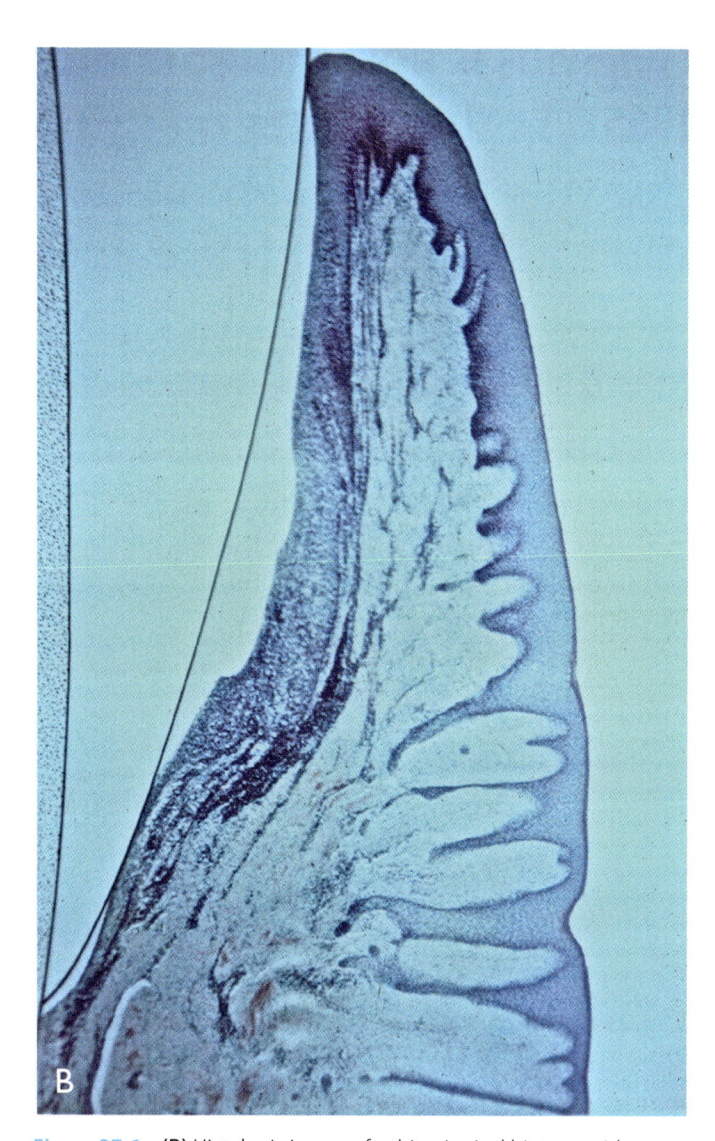

Figure 37.6 **(B)** Histologic image of a thin gingival biotype with inflammation.

Indications for gingival augmentation

The following are indications for gingival augmentation:

- gingival recession with root sensitivity, root caries, cervical class v restorations, or overextended crowns;
- insufficient attached keratinized gingiva, which could make the site more vulnerable to recession;
- correction of gingival tissue asymmetry before planned restorative procedures;
- thin tissue with anticipated facial orthodontic tooth movement.

Furcation involvement

Studies by Nordland et al.[54] have shown that furcation sites do not respond as well to nonsurgical therapy as flat surfaces and interproximal areas do. It is unclear whether gingival augmentation over Grade I or II furcation sites can provide better long-term furcation maintenance; however, the possibility for new attachment is biologically plausible and clinically promising (Figure 37.8A and B).

Potential for gingival regeneration

The addition of a connective tissue graft to cover root surfaces could raise the concern for creation of a periodontal pocket. Minimal probing pocket depth is desirable following root coverage procedures. It is expected that a pocket would be created if new attachment of the grafted soft tissue does not occur. To avoid the creation of a pocket, new attachment is necessary. A landmark study by Cole et al.[24] in 1980 showed for the first time that new attachment in humans was possible. This study used demineralization of the root surface to expose collagen fibers of the root with close re-apposition of the flap, and showed that new attachment could occur. Another study, by Steiner et al.,[55] using all the same steps as Cole, showed that new attachment did not occur without the acid demineralization step.

Because acid demineralization increased the potential for new attachment in humans, clinicians have used this rationale to potentiate new attachment with gingival augmentation. Initially, citric acid was used; however, issues with root resorption were

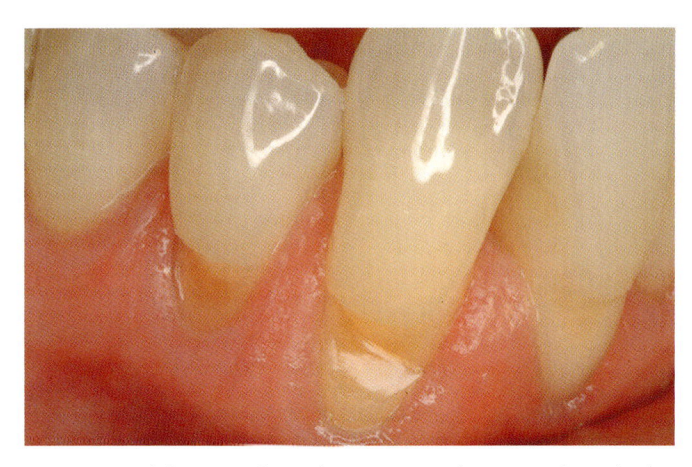

Figure 37.7 **(A)** Pre-op photo shows a minimal amount of attached keratinized gingiva.

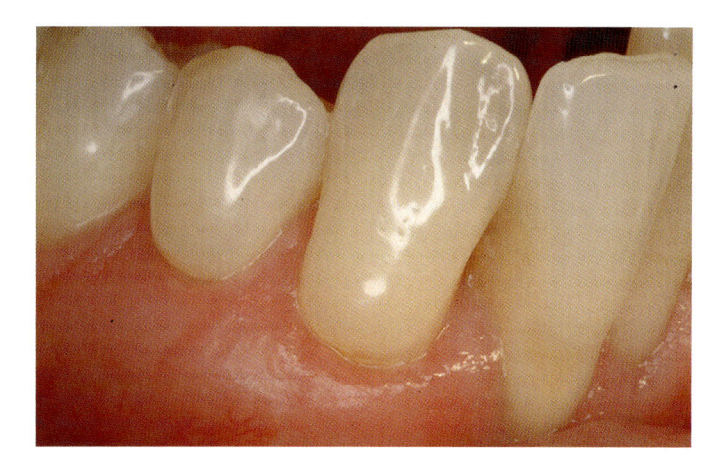

Figure 37.7 **(B)** Post-op photo shows a significant increase in the amount of keratinized gingiva.

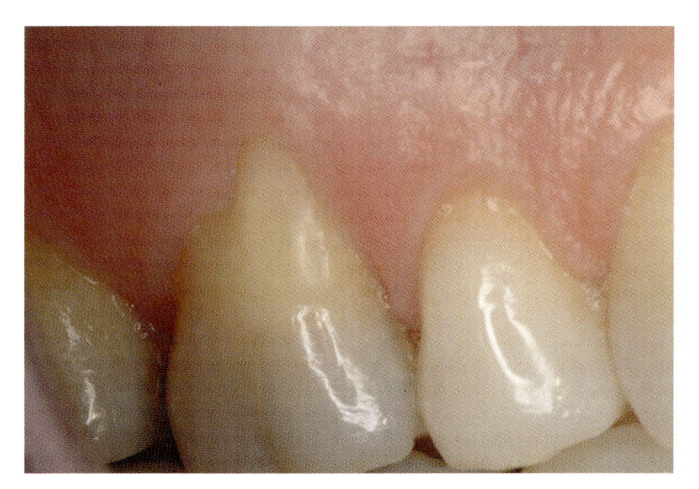

Figure 37.8 **(A)** Pre-op photo of a molar with significant recession and Class I furcation involvement.

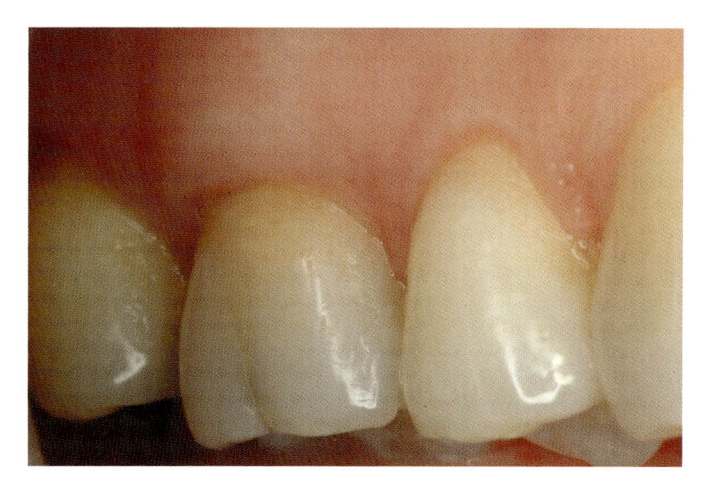

Figure 37.8 **(B)** After connective tissue grafting, root coverage was achieved with an increase in the band of attached keratinized gingiva and minimal probing depth.

reported, and most clinicians now use tetracycline due to its availability and long-term efficacy (e.g., Arestin, Atridox, and Actisite). Block section histology following connective tissue grafting has demonstrated new attachment.[56] Connective tissue root coverage has also been shown to be successful as an alternative to root coverage restorations.[57,58]

Connective tissue graft surgical technique

The patient in Figure 37.9 presents with multiple areas of root exposure, root sensitivity, with minimal or no attached keratinized gingiva.

Root preparation

A thorough debridement of the root surfaces needs to be accomplished. Bacterial endotoxins and calculus are removed using ultrasonic scalers, rotary instruments, and hand instruments. Rotary instruments also help reduce areas of prominent root surfaces and reduce undercuts. Finishing burs of varying sizes can be used to clean the root surfaces and modify root

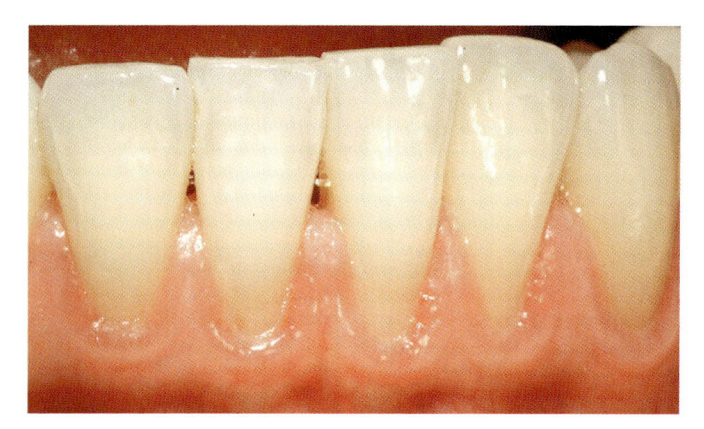

Figure 37.9 This patient presents with multiple areas of root exposure, root sensitivity, with minimal or no attached keratinized gingiva.

prominences (Figures 37.10, 37.11, and 37.12). Undercuts are reduced and flattened. Caries and restorative materials should be removed with the sequential use of finishing burs. Hand instruments are used to smooth and flatten the facial surfaces (Figures 37.13 and 37.14). A 10/11 scaler (G. Hartzell & Son) can

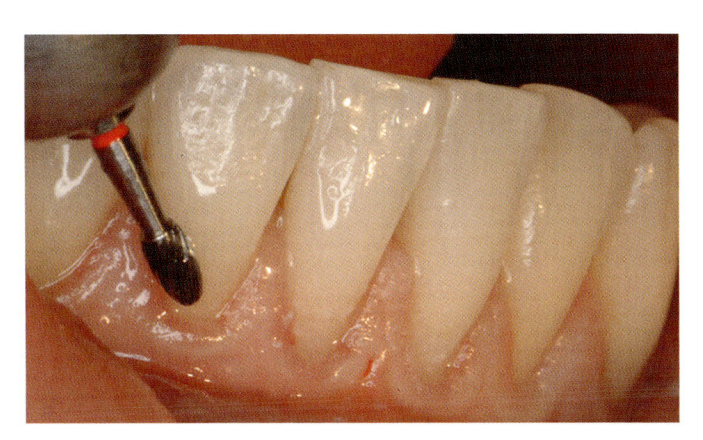

Figure 37.10 Finishing burs of varying sizes can be used to remove old composites, clean the root surfaces, and modify root prominences.

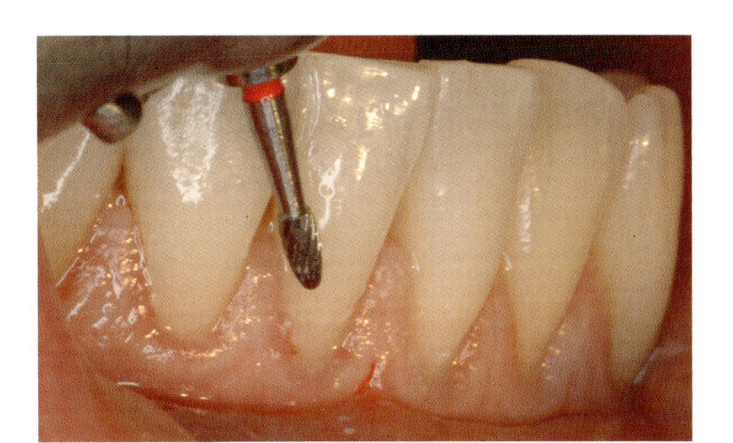

Figure 37.11 A #18 finishing bur is selected to clean the root surfaces and modify root prominences.

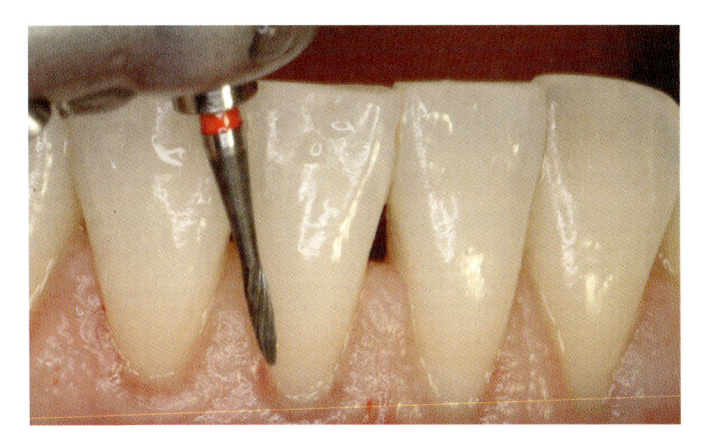

Figure 37.12 A #5 finishing bur is used to extend subgingivally.

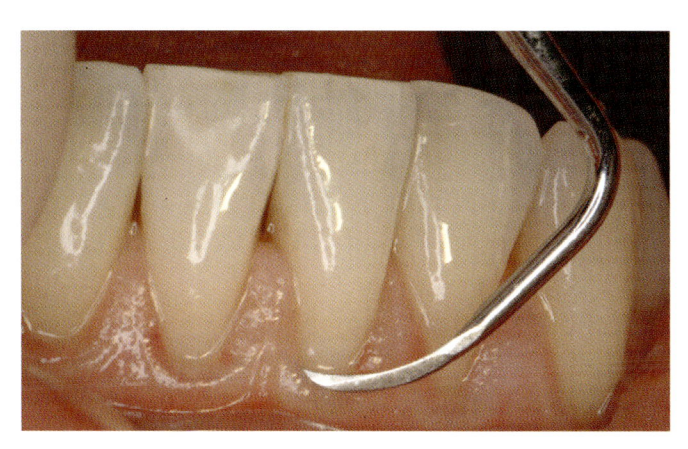

Figure 37.13 A 10/11 scaler (G. Hartzell & Son) can be used to easily reduce prominent line angle contours.

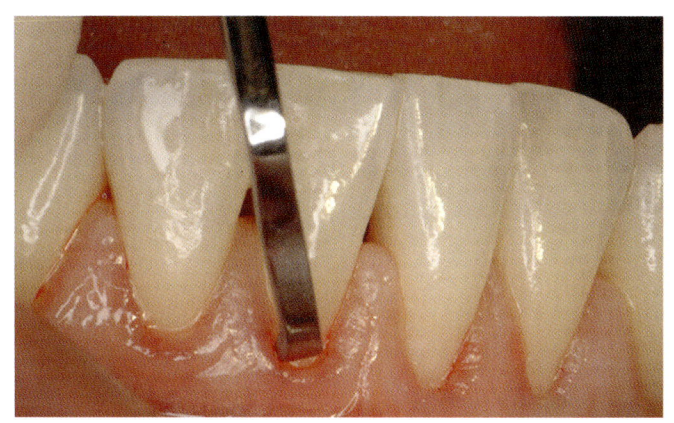

Figure 37.14 Microsurgical instruments have been developed, such as the SPN1 and SPN2 back action micro-chisels (G. Hartzell & Son) for small areas needing root planing and root smoothing.

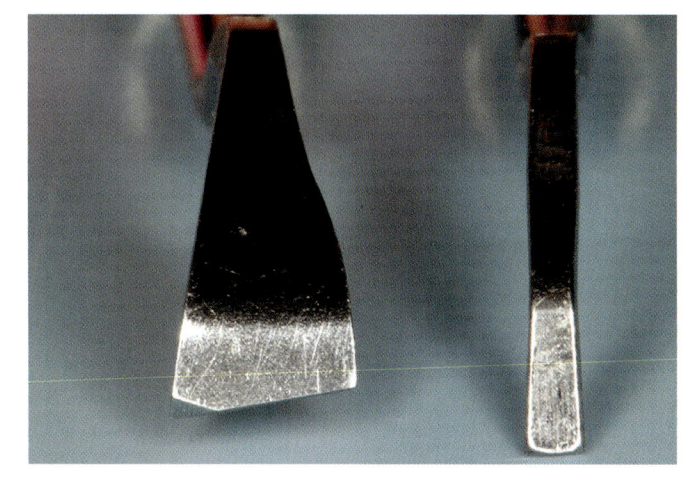

Figure 37.15 The newer and smaller SPN1 (G. Hartzell & Son) is compared to the traditional 13-K.

be used to easily reduce prominent line angle contours (Figure 37.13). Microsurgical instruments are especially helpful when treating small anterior teeth. Special instruments have been developed, such as the SPN1 and SPN2 back action microchisels (G. Hartzell & Son) to achieve accessibility for root planing and root smoothing (Figure 37.14). The newer and smaller SPN1 (G. Hartzell & Son, Figure 37.15) is compared with the traditional 13-K that is too large to access small root surfaces. Traditional hand instruments that are too big for the surgical areas are not recommended for this part of the procedure to avoid any unintentional trauma to the surrounding tissues (Figure 37.16). After the roots are thoroughly debrided,

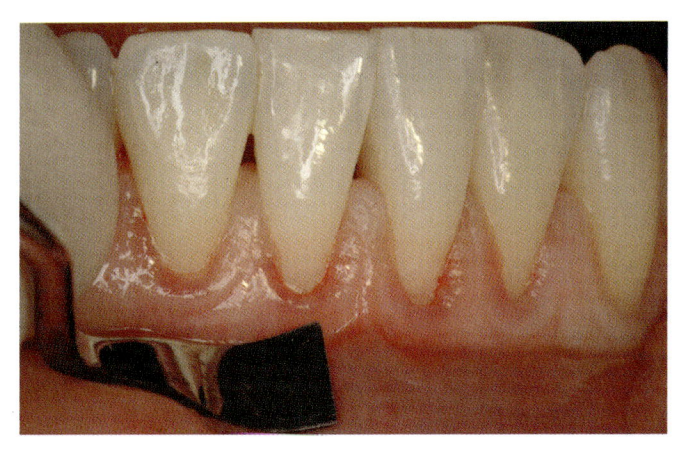

Figure 37.16 Traditional hand instruments that are too big for the surgical areas are not recommended for this part of the procedure to avoid any unintentional trauma to the surrounding tissues.

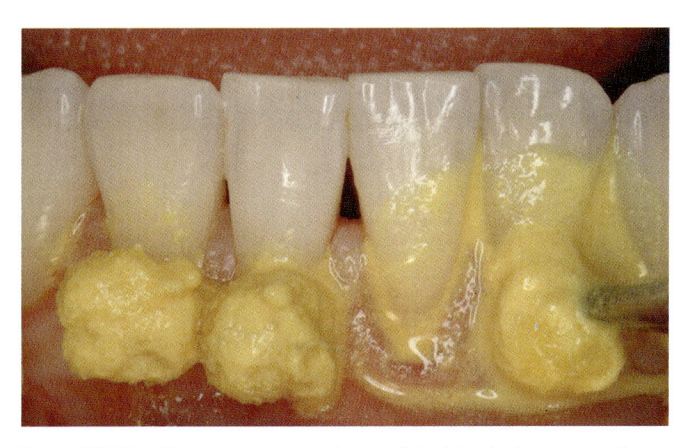

Figure 37.17 After the roots are thoroughly debrided, a tetracycline paste on cotton pellets is applied.

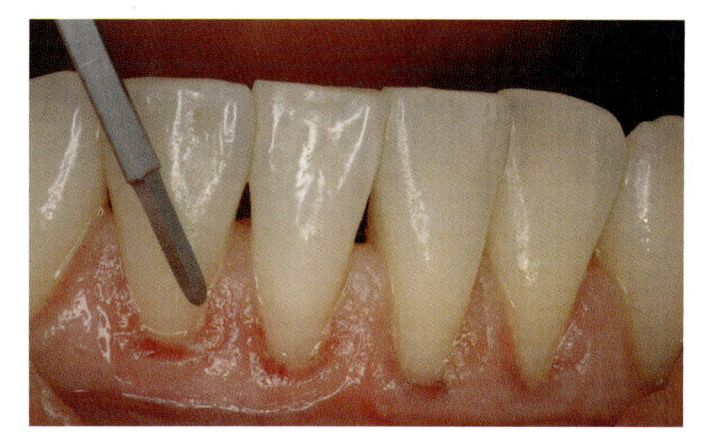

Figure 37.18 An N6900 microscalpel is selected owing to its small size and ability to be customized.

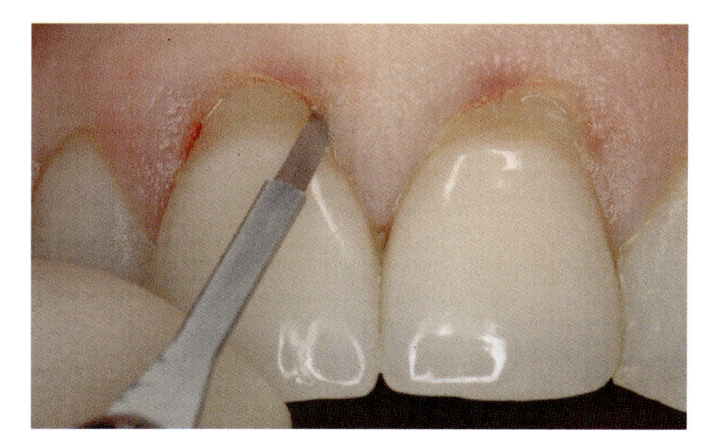

Figure 37.19 The sulcular split-thickness incision extends around the mesial, facial, and distal, even undermining the papillae.

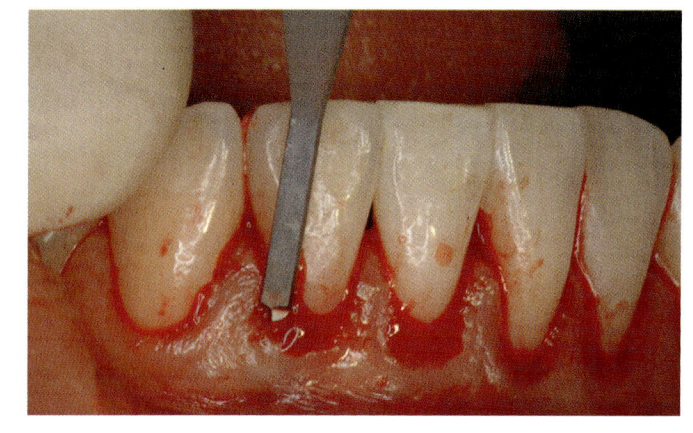

Figure 37.20 The sulcular incision is extended past the mucogingival junction.

a tetracycline paste on cotton pellets is applied for the purpose of demineralizing the root surface and exposing collagen fibers of the root surfaces, thereby encouraging new attachment (Figure 37.17).

Microincisions and the gingival pouch

The N6900 microsurgical scalpel has been specifically developed to create a sulcular incision that can easily penetrate the sulcus with precision and minimal trauma. The sulcular incision is extended around the facial circumference of the tooth and extended past the mucogingival junction (Figures 37.18, 37.19, and 37.20). As the N6900 microscalpel is inserted into the facial sulcus, obstacles are typically encountered, such as changing contours and bony exostoses, creating unseen obstacles. The microsurgical blade can be modified with custom bending to negotiate these challenging contours to allow separation of a split-thickness flap (Figures 37.21, 37.22, 37.23, and 37.24). Orthodontic bending pliers help to create gentle curves with the scalpel and/or shank to achieve individualized and customized surgical incisions (Figures 37.21 and 37.23). Shank modification is helpful when dealing with the mandibular anterior teeth to help move the scalpel handle into a more ideal working position.

Once the surgical incisions have been accomplished through a sulcular incision, it is important to achieve a patent facial tunnel to allow placement of the connective tissue graft. The interdental papillary area can also be undermined to allow for papillary addition, if desired. Undermining the papilla can also help to reduce any bulkiness of the facial tissue and achieve a gradual

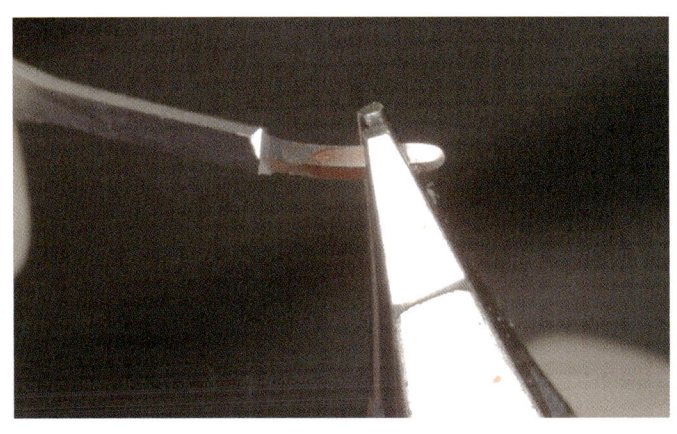

Figure 37.21 The microsurgical blade can be modified with custom bending.

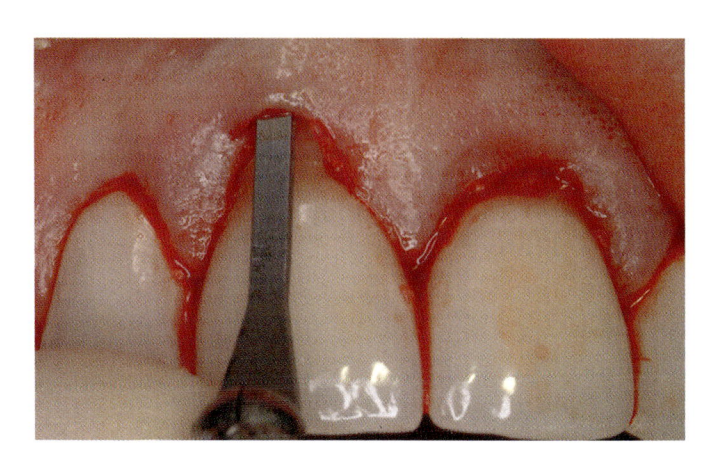

Figure 37.24 Customized scalpel curves allow insertion into the surgical incision to match the individual anatomical contours.

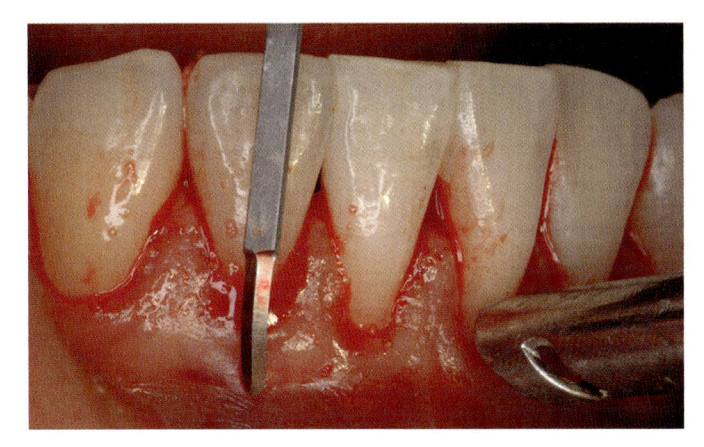

Figure 37.22 The modified microsurgical blade can then negotiate the challenging contours to allow separation of a split-thickness flap.

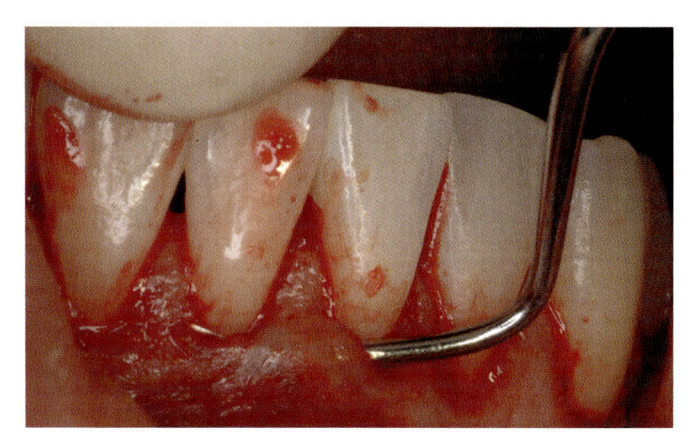

Figure 37.25 A sharpened 10/11 scaler (G. Hartzell & Son) can easily facilitate tunnel patency.

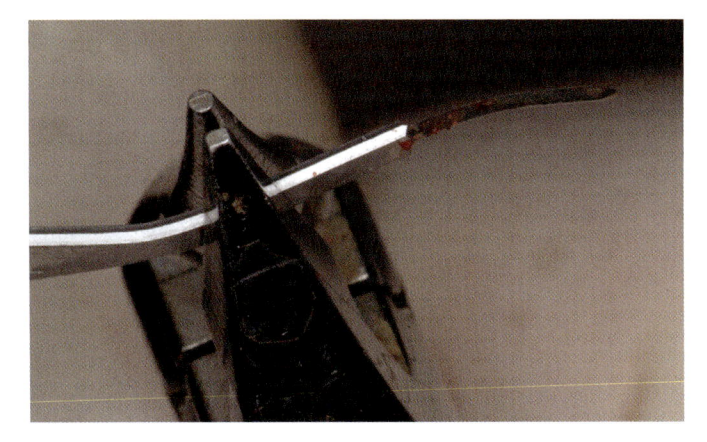

Figure 37.23 The shank of the microsurgical blade can also be bent to conform to surgical needs.

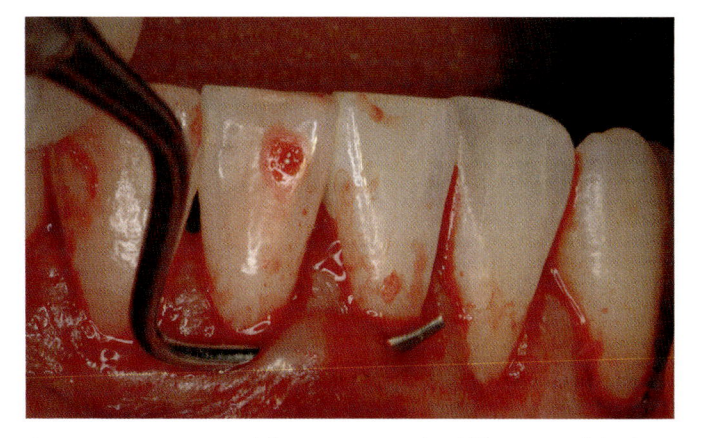

Figure 37.26 Tissue mobility assessment should be accomplished to assure that the new tissue position will meet the desired goals.

blending at the base of the papilla. A sharpened 10/11 scaler (G. Hartzell & Son) can easily facilitate tunnel patency.

Once it has been determined that the tunnel is patent, tissue mobility assessment should be accomplished to assure that the new tissue position will meet the desired goals (Figures 37.25 and 37.26).

Connective tissue harvesting

Specific graft size is determined by measuring the amount of necessary donor tissue with a periodontal probe (Figure 37.27). A connective tissue graft is harvested from the palate using a tunneling approach that allows control of the graft thickness

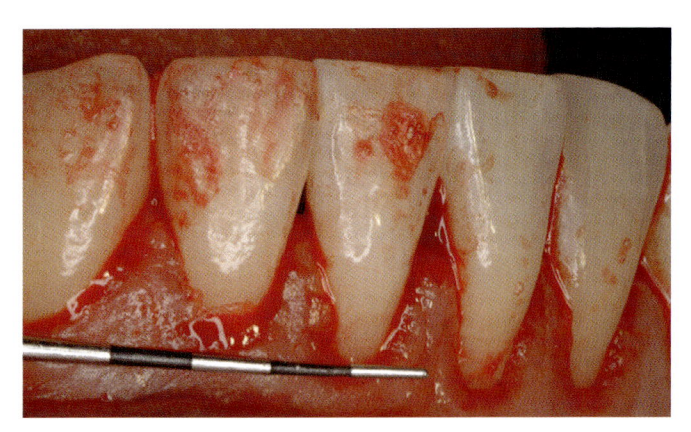

Figure 37.27 Specific graft size is determined by measuring the amount of necessary donor tissue with a periodontal probe.

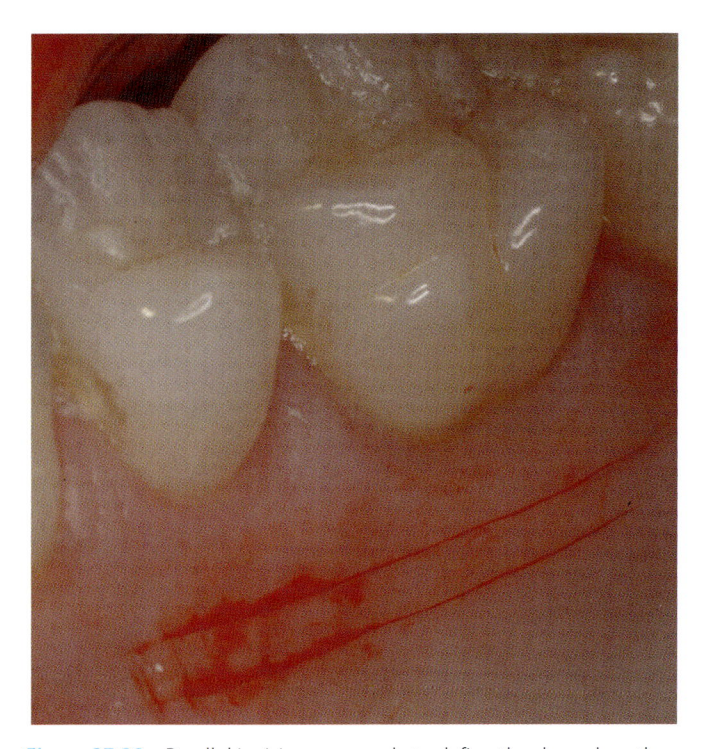

Figure 37.28 Parallel incisions are made to define the donor length and thickness.

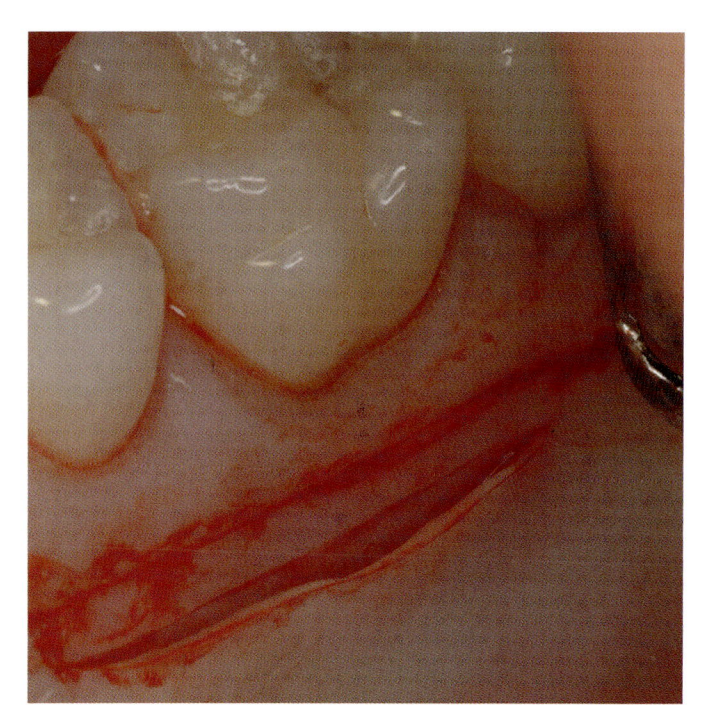

Figure 37.29 A uniform graft thickness is created.

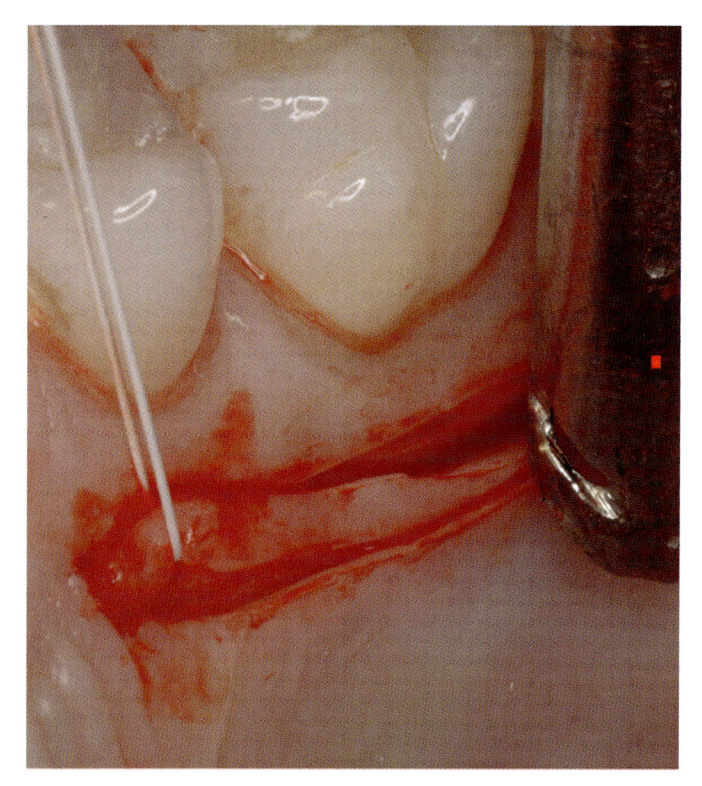

Figure 37.30 A suture is used to secure the donor tissue.

(Figures 37.28 and 37.29). Palatal connective tissue is lassoed with the suture to allow for delicate manipulation and extraction of the desired tissue dimension (Figures 37.30, 37.31, and 37.32).

Removal of the epithelium is important as the epithelium can survive creating potential epithelial cysts or possible folds in the future healing (Figures 37.33 and 37.34). Once the epithelium is removed, it can be reapplied to the palatal wound to create an ideal surface protection and will typically survive to allow ideal healing of the palatal wound (Figure 37.35). Resorbable or nonresorbable sutures can be applied to maintain wound closure (Figure 37.36). Ideally, a palatal stent is fabricated ahead of time to minimize bleeding, and optimize comfort by protecting the donor site from traumatic stimuli (Figures 37.37 and 37.38).

Modification of the connective tissue graft is accomplished by the removal of the epithelium. Any extraneous tissues, such as adipose tissue or mucous glands, are removed.

Beveling the mesial and distal segments of the graft helps to create a smoothly blended result (Figure 37.39). Once the tissue is contoured and modified, it is placed over the site to reconfirm the graft dimensions and thickness (Figure 37.40). The graft is worked into the tunnel to extend under the incisions and is guided into place. Working the tissue through a tunnel can be difficult. A variety of instruments can be used to

Chapter 37 Periodontal Plastic Surgery

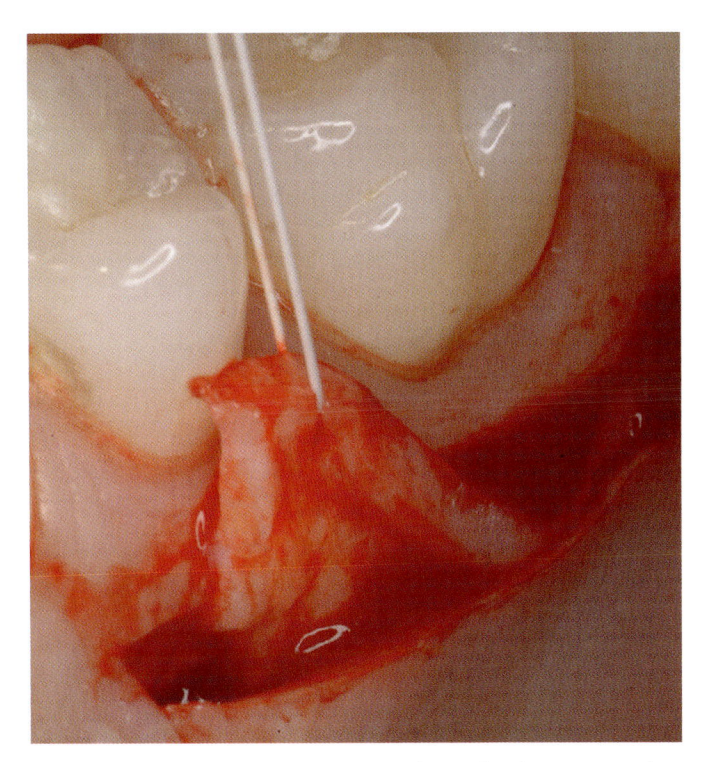

Figure 37.31 Palatal connective tissue is lassoed with a suture and harvested using a light tugging force while sharp dissection elevates the donor tissue.

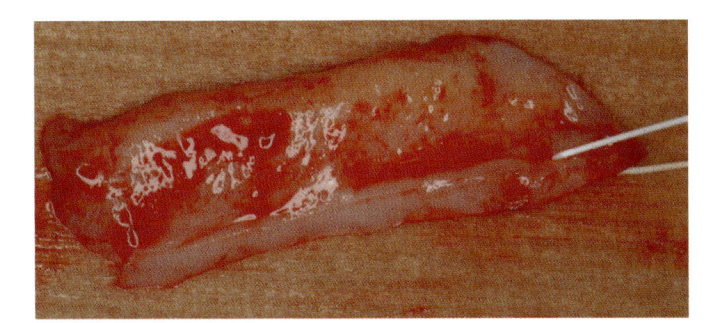

Figure 37.32 Palatal connective tissue is placed on a moistened tongue blade.

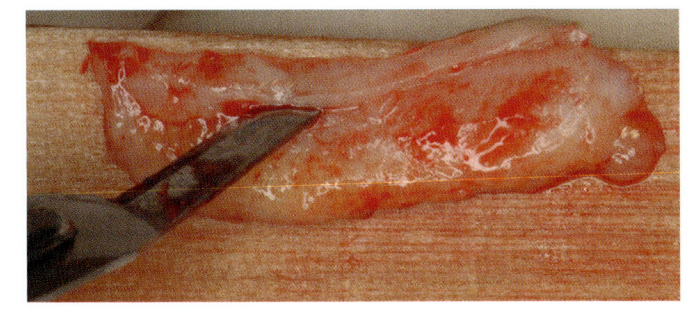

Figure 37.33 The tongue blade provides support for modification of the donor tissue.

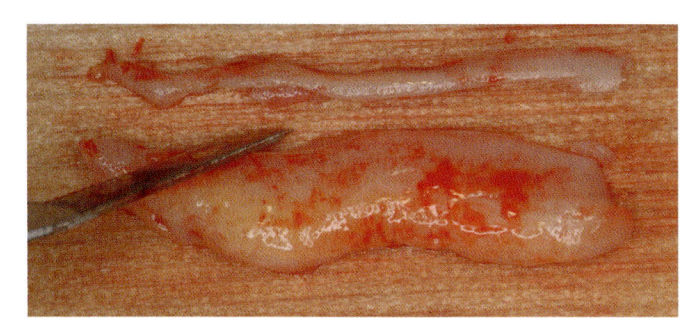

Figure 37.34 The epithelium is removed.

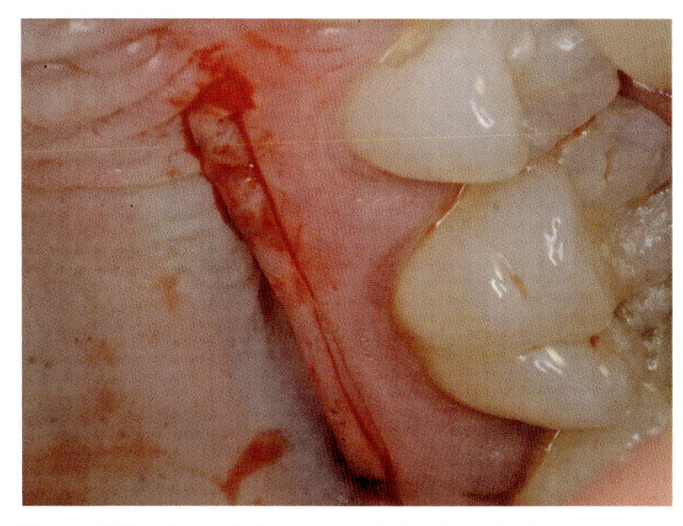

Figure 37.35 The epithelium is reapplied to the palatal wound.

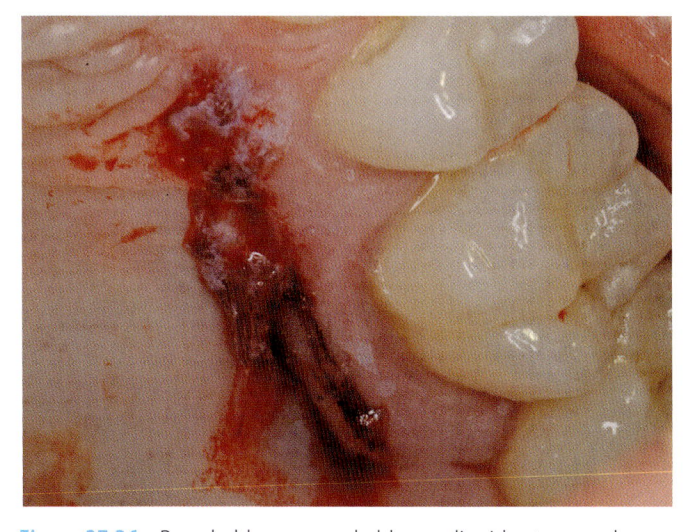

Figure 37.36 Resorbable, nonresorbable, or a liquid suture can be applied to maintain wound closure.

accomplish this task. Sometimes it can be helpful to use a suture to pull the tissue through the tunnel. Typically, only hand instruments, such as 10/11 scaler and periodontal probe, are necessary (Figures 37.41, 47.42, and 37.43).

Sutures and dressing

Sling sutures are used to position the overlying existing tissue and stabilize the connective tissue graft under the flap. Once the connective tissue graft is positioned properly, a suture is placed through the flap tissue and through the underlying graft tissue to position it (Figures 37.44, 37.45, 37.46, 37.47, and 37.48). Generally, it is helpful to suture only two teeth at a time as it will

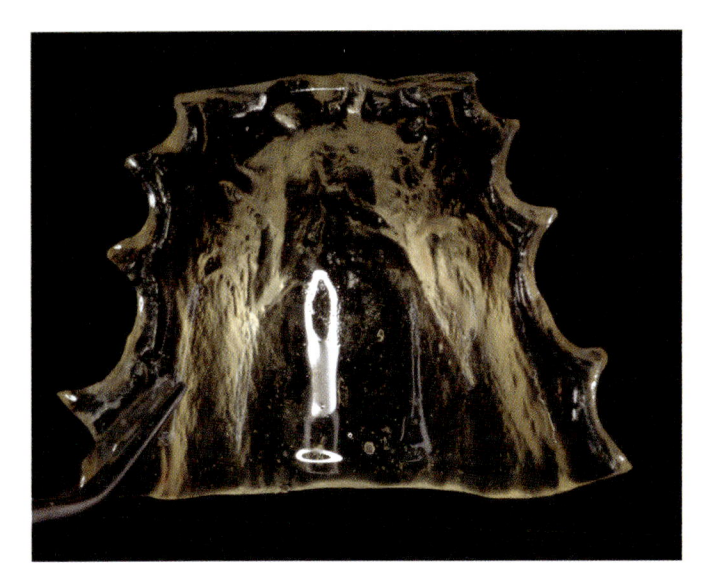

Figure 37.37 A palatal stent.

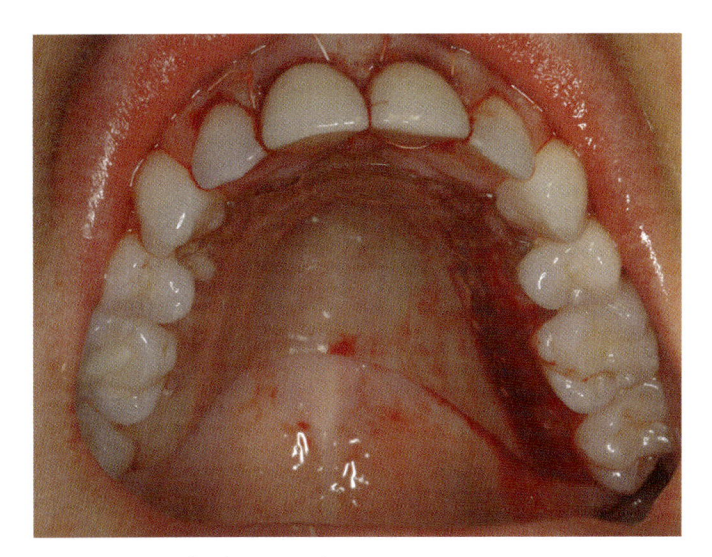

Figure 37.38 Palatal stent in place.

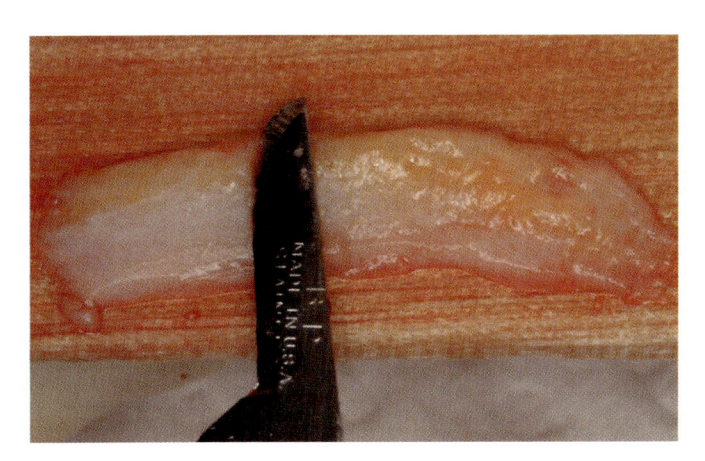

Figure 37.39 Beveling the mesial and distal segments of the graft helps to create a smoothly blended result.

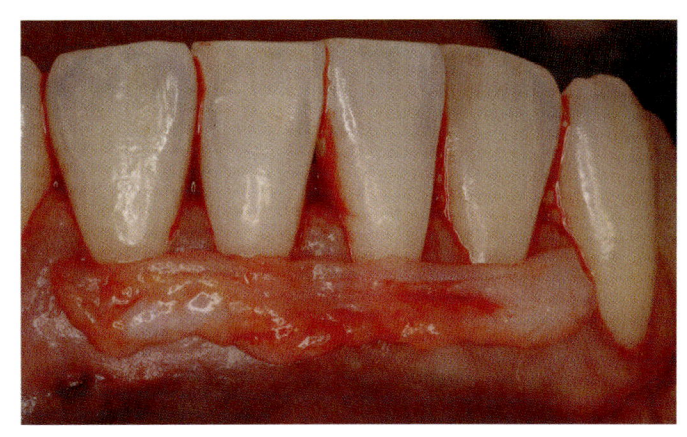

Figure 37.40 Once the tissue is contoured and modified, it is placed over the site to reconfirm the graft dimensions and thickness.

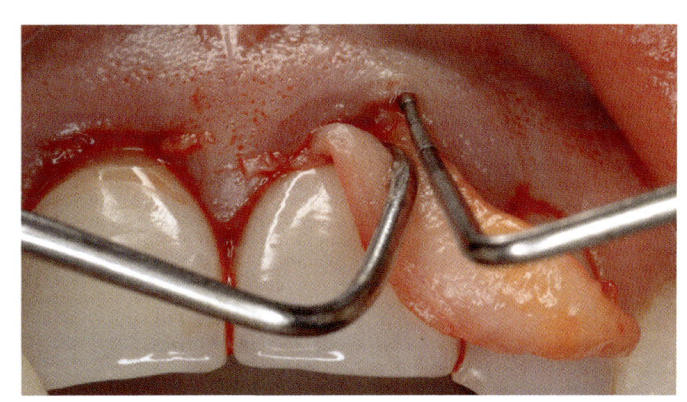

Figure 37.41 The graft is worked into the tunnel to extend under the incisions and is guided into place using 10/11 scaler and periodontal probe.

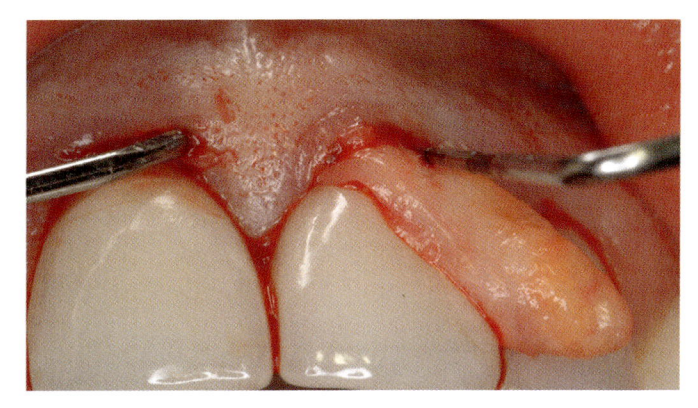

Figure 37.42 The graft is pulled into position.

allow for better control and positioning of the flap with its underlying connective tissue graft. Ideally, the connective tissue graft should be fully covered by the overlying preexisting soft tissue to insure grafted tissue survival; however, this is not always possible. Previous surgical incisions create scarring and can make the release of the tunnel even more difficult. In these cases, additional time and attention need to be given to achieve a patent movable tunnel and overlying tissue.

Chapter 37 Periodontal Plastic Surgery

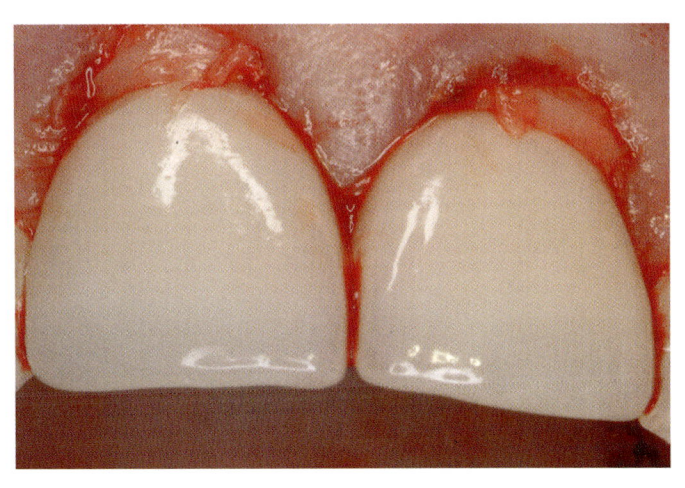

Figure 37.43 The graft is worked into the final position in the tunnel.

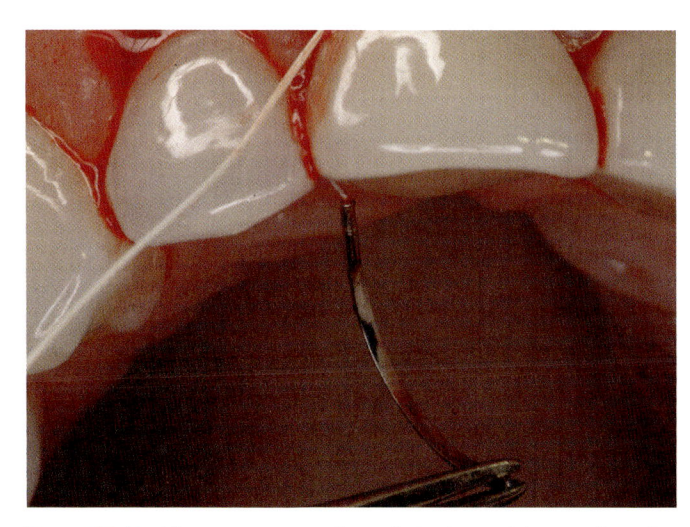

Figure 37.46 The suture passes through the base of the papilla and exits at the base of the palatal portion of the papilla.

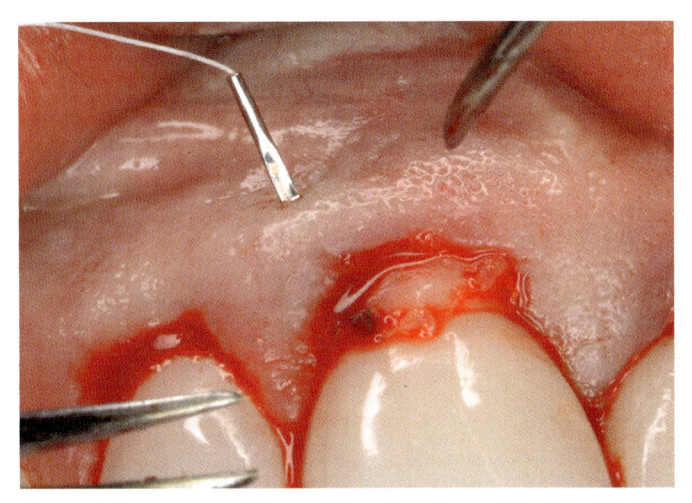

Figure 37.44 A suture is placed through the flap tissue and through the underlying graft tissue to position it.

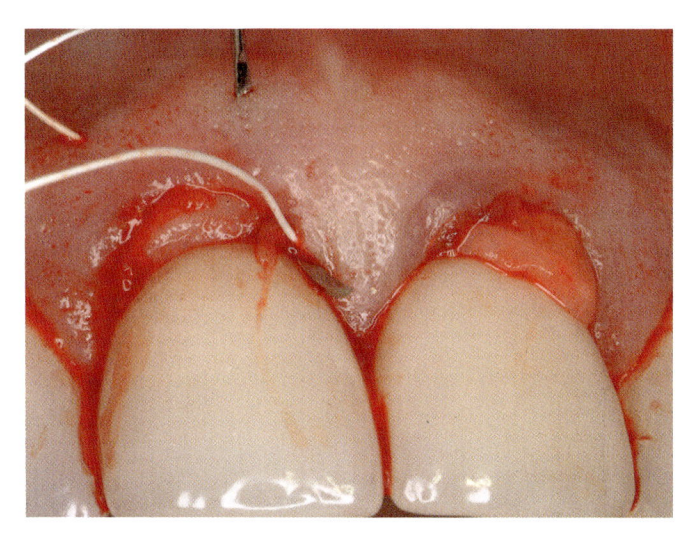

Figure 37.47 The suture is wrapped around the palatal surface of the tooth and re-enters the facial flap at the corresponding line angle.

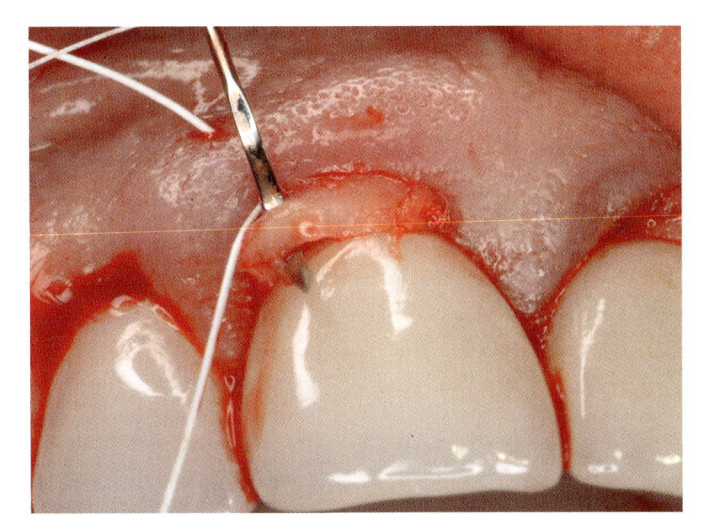

Figure 37.45 The graft was moved out of the tunnel to show how the graft is secured with the suture.

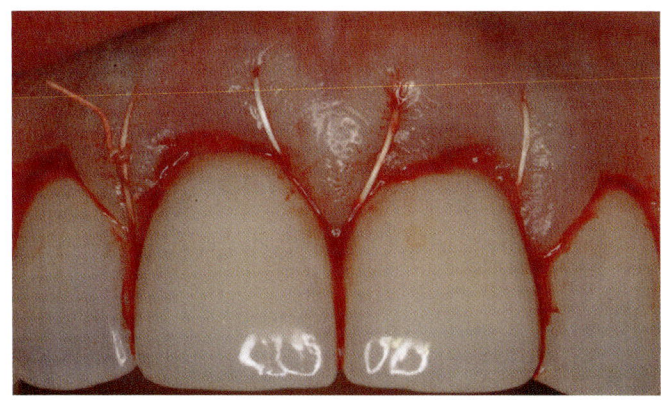

Figure 37.48 The adjacent tooth is treated in a similar fashion using the continuing uninterrupted suture.

Once the soft tissue has been ideally positioned, stabilization with a liquid suture (isobutyl cyanoacrylate) can be helpful (Figures 37.49 and 37.50). A liquid suture can bring wound edges together without typical needle penetration wounds and has been shown to have a minimal inflammatory result compared with conventional sutures.[59] A dissolving dressing can be placed to help the patient avoid trauma during the first few days of healing (Figure 37.51).

Postoperative instructions and healing

The care of the surgical area is extremely important during the first week. The patient should avoid foods that can cause trauma or hot liquids that can stimulate bleeding and increase swelling. Brushing or flossing the surgical site must be avoided. A 0.12% chlorhexidine gluconate rinse should be used during the first 7 days. An anti-inflammatory prescription is recommended to avoid additional swelling that could otherwise compromise surgical healing. The surgical stent should be kept in place for 1 week.

Sutures can be removed in 1 week and oral hygiene instructions are essential to ensure that the patient does not traumatize the area. Many times, the replaced epithelium of the palate heals uneventfully. Reinforcement of oral hygiene techniques is crucial for long-term success. Delicate biotype patients are cautioned against the use of electric toothbrushes that could traumatize the newly grafted tissue. Six to eight weeks of soft-tissue healing is a minimum before restorative procedures can be considered (Figure 37.52).

Other considerations

Old restorations and root caries

Root surfaces with restorative materials and caries can be considered a challenge because they serve as an obstacle for the graft tissue to reattach to the root surface. Even though they can be successfully removed as described earlier, the visualization for such a task can be difficult without magnification. The surgical dissecting microscope is a valuable tool, as it can make

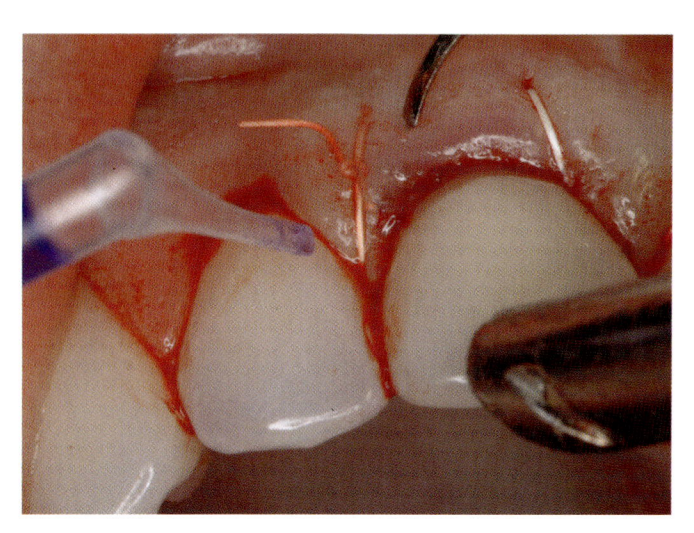

Figure 37.49 A liquid suture (isobutyl cyanoacrylate) is applied with a micropipette.

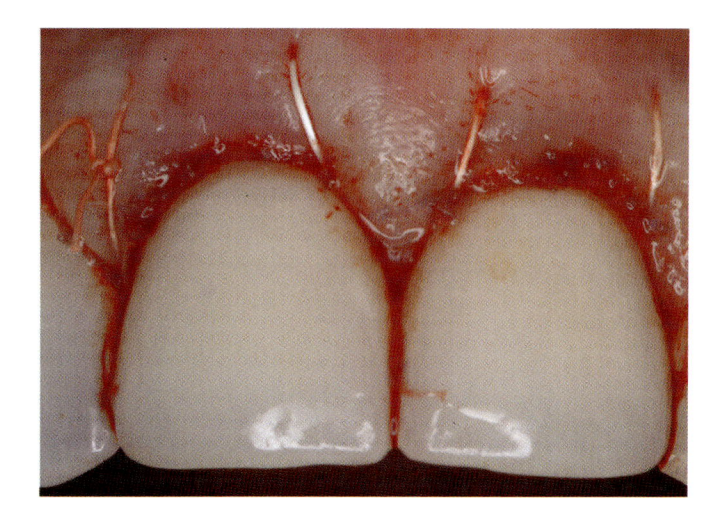

Figure 37.50 Stabilization with a liquid suture (isobutyl cyanoacrylate) insures ideal tissue position and minimal bleeding.

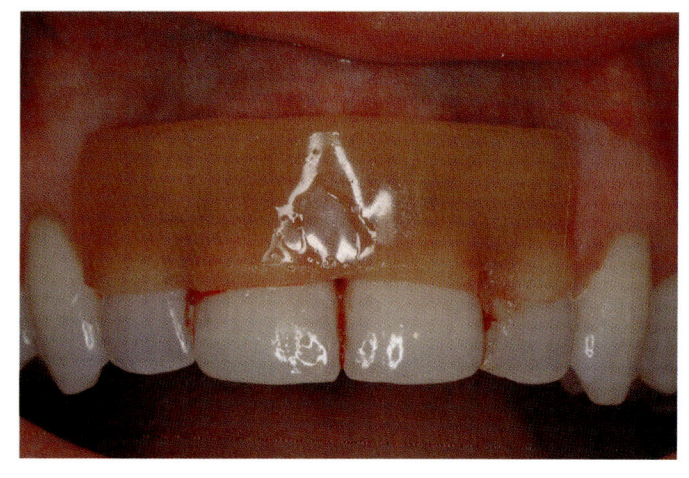

Figure 37.51 Dissolving gelatin dressing in place.

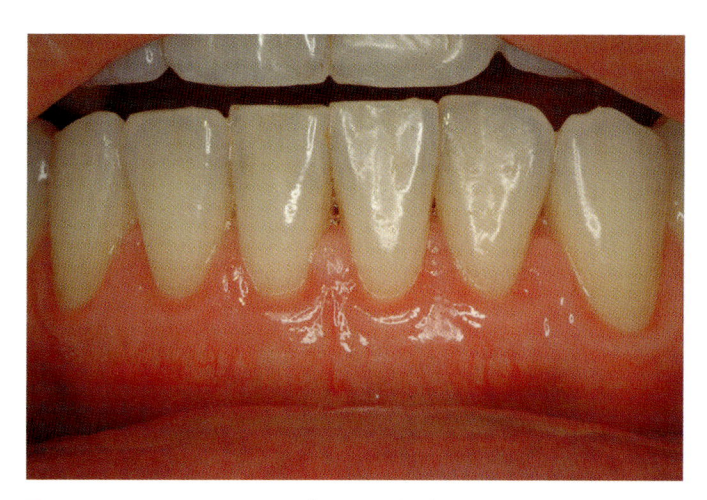

Figure 37.52 Postoperative photograph after 6 weeks.

visualization of tooth-colored restorative materials more obvious and thereby increase the potential for the success of the final result.[17] It has also been shown that once root caries is removed, connective tissue grafting for root coverage is equally predictable as it is to noncarious roots (Figure 37.53A–C).[57]

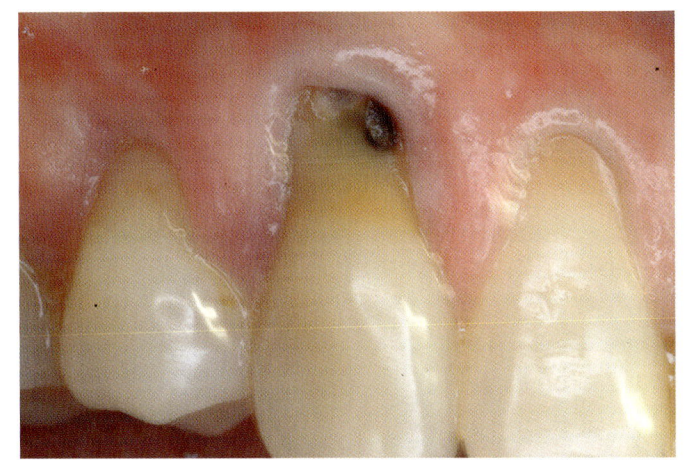

Figure 37.53 (A) Severe carious lesion on the root surface.

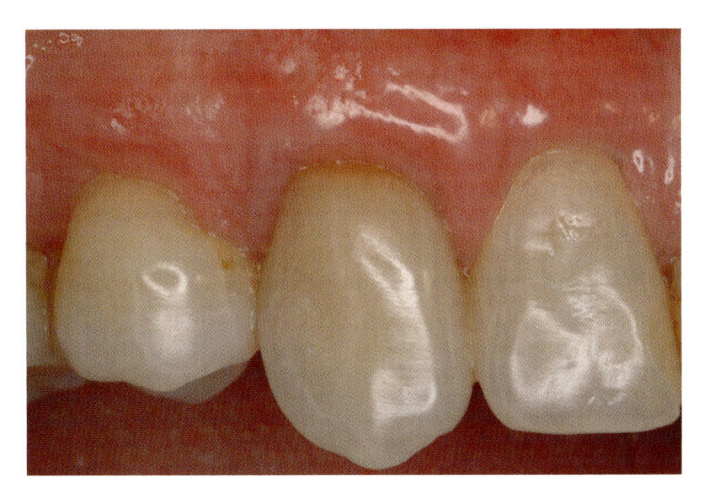

Figure 37.53 (B) Connective tissue graft successfully covered the root surface with minimal probing depth.

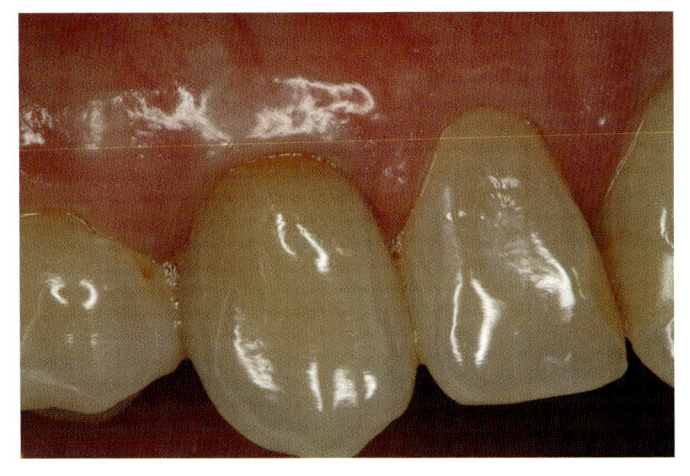

Figure 37.53 (C) Esthetic result well maintained after six years.

Quality and quantity of donor tissue

The quality of the graft tissue to be harvested can vary depending on the patient's biotype and individual tissue thickness. The best quality will be the tissue that is more homogeneous and has a dense fibrous connective tissue composition. It is generally desirable to remove any adipose and glandular tissue from the harvested graft.

When many areas need to be grafted, the amount of available donor tissue can determine how many and which teeth can be treated in the same surgical procedure. The amount of donor tissue available also varies according to the patient's biotype. It has become clear that individuals with thin and delicate gingival tissue, prone to the development of recession, often also present with thin palatal mucosa that might not be suitable for obtaining connective tissue of proper thickness for periodontal plastic surgery.[60] Usually, the quantity and quality of the palatal connective tissue to be harvested can only be assessed precisely during harvesting. If sequential surgical procedures are necessary, harvesting of new tissue should target the healed previous donor site because the healed wound will have a higher percentage of dense fibrous tissue. It is helpful to wait 3 months to assure healing of the palatal wound before reentry.

Grafting over implants

Connective tissue grafting over unesthetic implants can also be accomplished. Ideally, correction of soft-tissue deficiencies should be performed before implant placement. Because the connective tissue graft will not attach to the implant or abutment surfaces, if tissue is added, then the sulcular depth can increase, creating a pocket. The clinician must therefore evaluate exactly how much vertical extension of gingival tissue should be added. The goal is to promote esthetically acceptable tissue contours and gain attached keratinized gingival protection without creating a pocket. The new tissue contours must allow for plaque removal by the patient during daily oral hygiene. Because the soft tissue generally follows the shape of the underlying tooth surface, the final custom abutment and crown should be in place before surgical addition. If coronal tissue positioning is desired, then the prominence of the abutment should be reduced to promote room for the new tissue. After prominences are reduced, the abutment must be thoroughly smoothed and polished to avoid bacterial accumulation in the future (Figure 37.54).

Restoration of the lost interdental papilla

Gingival augmentation of the lost interdental papilla has been very challenging due to the small area in which to work. The vascular supply to this terminal-end organ involves capillary loops, and the dimensions of the area are difficult to negotiate. Conventional surgical techniques are unpredictable due to the small working spaces and limited blood supply to the area.[19]

Many articles have described techniques attempting correction of papillary defects.[5-14] Han and Takei (1996)[5] described the use of a facial approach with a semilunar incision to gain access

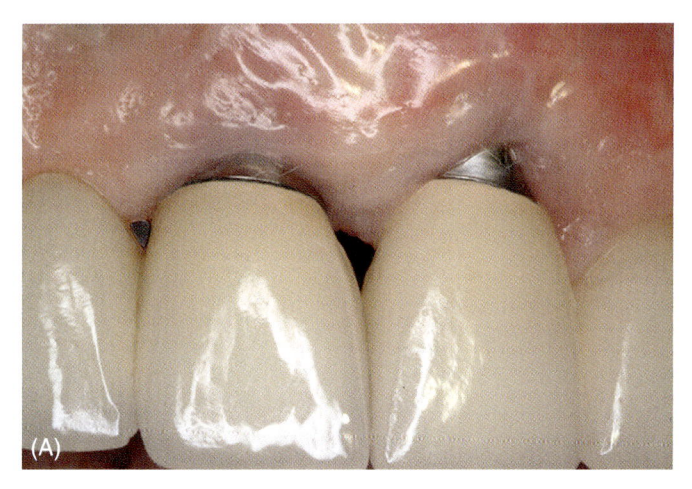

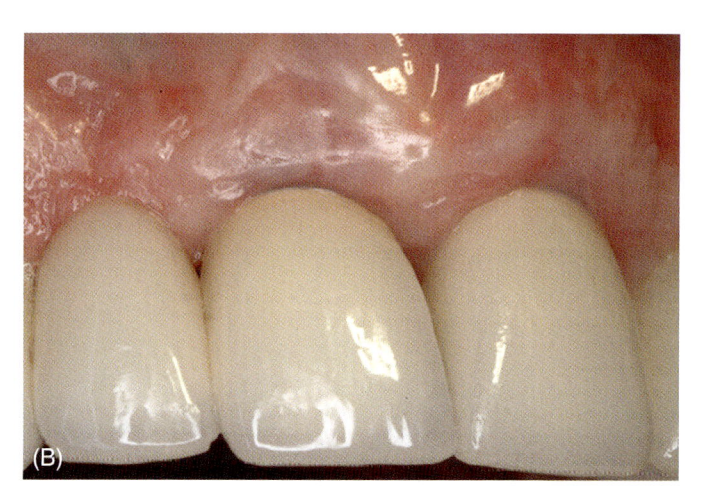

Figure 37.54 (A, B) Connective tissue graft surgery accomplished to cover implants in the esthetic zone.

to the papillary area for augmentation of the papilla. Cortellini et al.[6,7] proposed a simplified papilla preservation flap that requires a releasing incision in the papillary area and placement of a barrier membrane under the surgical site. Azzi and coworkers[8–10] developed techniques to gain access to augment the connective tissue and bone under the deficient papilla; however, these techniques may jeopardize the blood supply due to the use of releasing incisions.

The success of microsurgical techniques is dependent on preservation of blood supply and minimal tension on wound closure.[61] Releasing incisions can also cause trauma to the delicate papillary isthmus and risk unesthetic surgical scarring and wound-edge necrosis. It has long been recognized that reduction or elimination of releasing incisions will improve vascularity to the surgical area and enhance the postsurgical outcome.[19] Tunneling surgical approaches can eliminate the need for releasing incisions.[62] Because of the small dimensions of the area being reconstructed, microscopic magnification and use of microsurgical instruments can be of significant value.[4,17]

Multidisciplinary management

Clinical management of the deficient papilla can be multidisciplinary and involve orthodontic root repositioning and restorative contour modification, in addition to surgical correction.[4] Generally, if a papillary defect was caused by a surgical insult, then surgical addition of soft tissue can be the best choice of treatment modalities.[4] Some important variables which may influence the presence of the papilla include interproximal contact position, root angulation, crown form, and embrasure areas.[63]

Interproximal reduction of crowns and orthodontic root alignment can help to close the embrasure spaces when papillary space is opened during orthodontic correction of overlapped teeth. The management of the embrasure space or "missing papilla" due to malalignment of teeth or orthodontic movement of teeth is discussed in an excellent work by Kurth and Kokich.[63]

Long cylindrical teeth can have a narrow cervical area and contact point located near the incisal edge.[40] To increase the chance for embrasure space closure, it may be advisable to move the contact point apically with restorative procedures.[4] The adjustment of the mesiodistal width of teeth can also be accomplished restoratively, creating a wider crown with the addition of restorative materials and allowing some degree of closure of the embrasure space.[64,65]

When all three treatment modalities are anticipated, it is usually recommended to start first with surgical addition because the access will be the greatest before either orthodontic tooth repositioning or restorative space closure (Figure 37.55).

Surgical technique of papilla reconstruction

Nordland and Sandhu[19] published an article in 2008 that described a microsurgical procedure to position the donor tissue under a deficient interdental papilla. The use of the surgical dissecting microscope and microsurgical instrumentation obtain access under the existing interdental papilla without releasing incisions, increasing the likelihood of donor tissue survival and thereby minimizing trauma, excessive bleeding, scarring, and pain (Figure 37.56A and B).[17,19] It must be noted, however, that this procedure is technique sensitive, and it may not be predictable in everyone's hands.

Defect assessment and root preparation

The classification of the initial preoperative interdental papilla is determined using the Nordland and Tarnow classification scheme (Figure 37.57A–D).[66] The defect is measured preoperatively to establish a baseline to determine just how much tissue gain is achieved. First, the desired gingivoincisal height is measured using a periodontal probe (Figure 37.58). This will determine exactly how much donor tissue volume is needed to be added to the deficient site.

After local anesthesia, root debridement and preparation is accomplished using finishing burs, hand instruments that include the SPN1 and SPN2 chisels, and 10/11 Hartzell scaler (G. Hartzell & Son). Root demineralization and sterilization is performed using tetracycline paste application for 60 s.

Incisions and papillary mobility

A circumferential sulcular incision, using the N6900 microsurgical blade, is made to the crest of bone (Figures 37.59, 37.60, 37.61, and 37.62). This incision also extends circumferentially around the adjacent teeth.

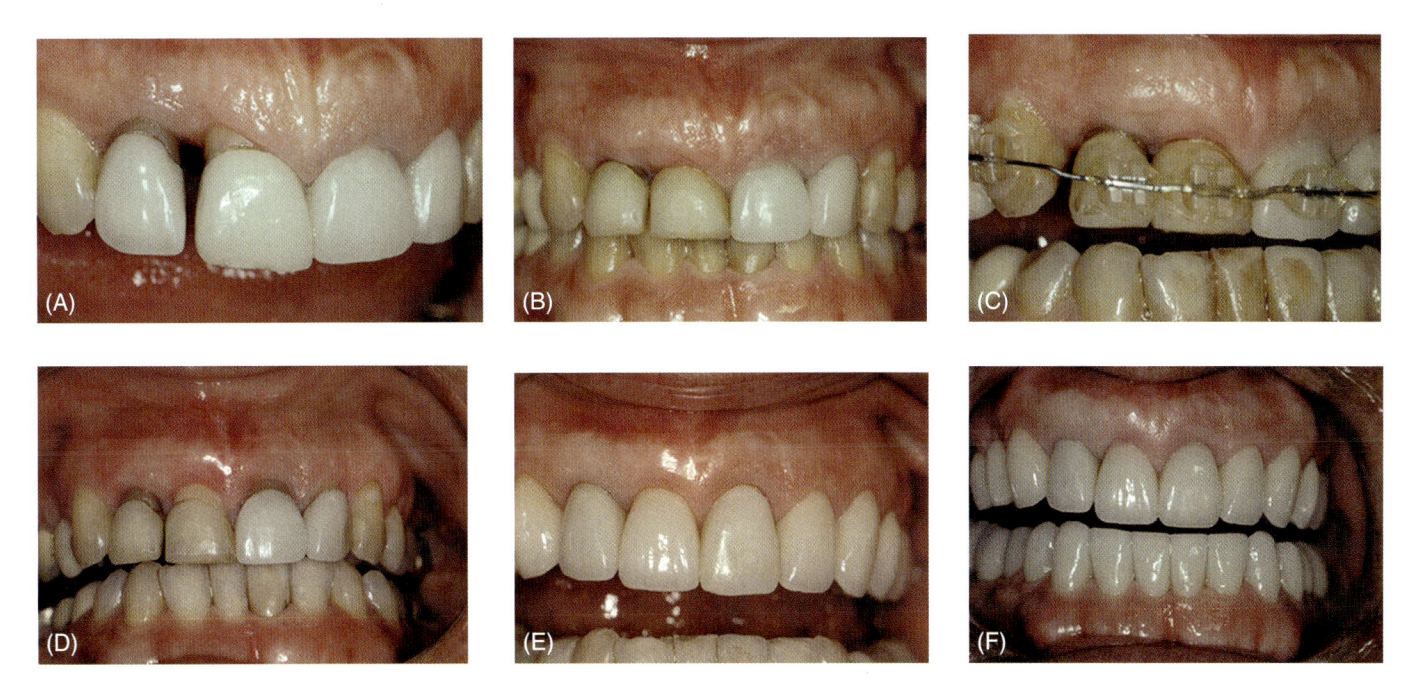

Figure 37.55 Example of a reconstruction of the lost interdental papilla using a multidisciplinary approach. **(A)** Pre-op image showing the defect caused by a surgical mishap. **(B)** Papilla augmentation was performed using connective tissue graft and microsurgical approach. **(C)** Orthodontic treatment assisted the closure of the space. **(D)** Sculpting was also performed to create symmetry and natural contours for the esthetic zone. **(E)** Beautiful porcelain crowns were finally placed, giving the patient a beautiful smile. **(F)** This 13-year follow-up image shows that results were maintained long term.

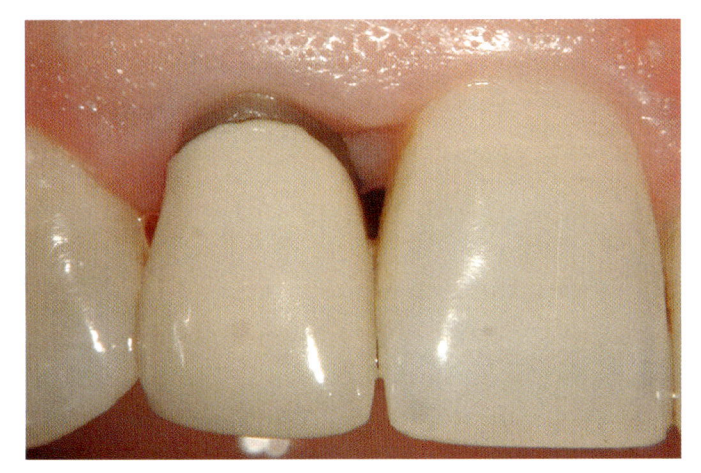

Figure 37.56 **(A)** Pre-op figure showing iatrogenic trauma following a root planing procedure.

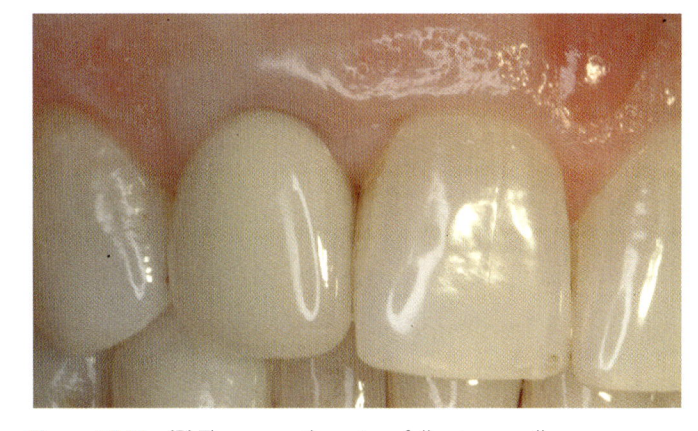

Figure 37.56 **(B)** Three-month post-op following papilla reconstructive surgery and a new crown for tooth #7.

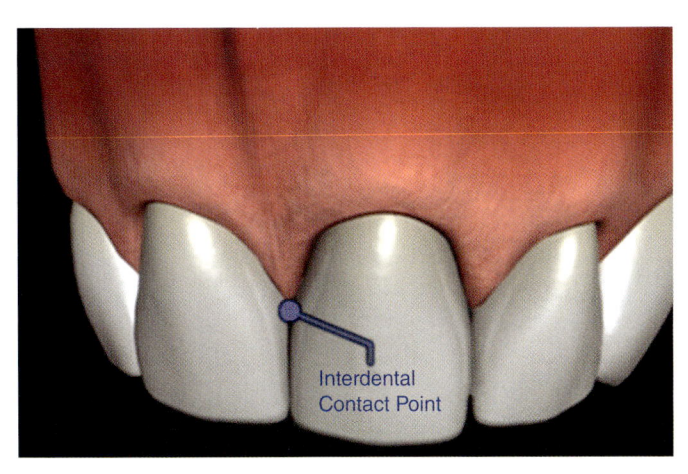

Figure 37.57 **(A)** Papilla within the normal limits.

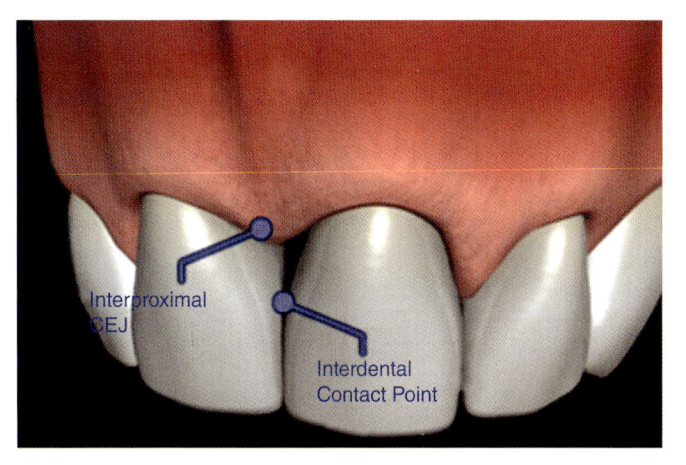

Figure 37.57 **(B)** Class I papilla defect: papilla positioned apically to the contact point but coronal to the interproximal cementoenamel junction (CEJ).

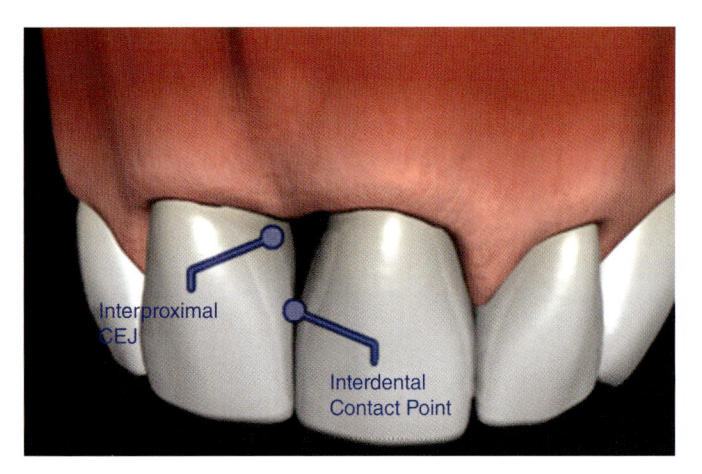

Figure 37.57 **(C)** Class II papilla defect: papilla positioned apically to the interproximal CEJ but coronal to the facial CEJ.

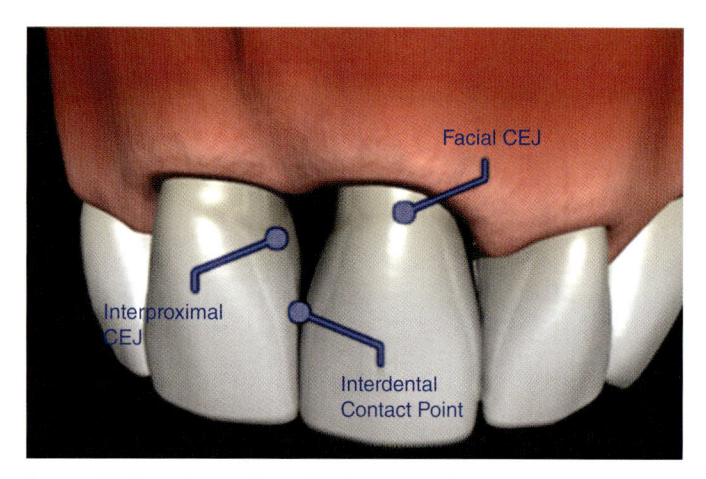

Figure 37.57 **(D)** Class III papilla defect: papilla positioned apically to the facial CEJ.

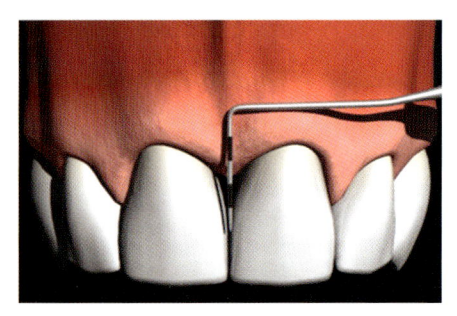

Figure 37.58 The desired gingivoincisal height is measured using a periodontal probe.

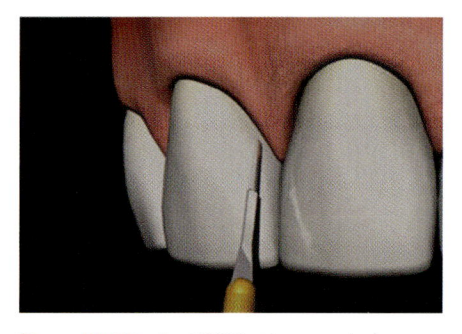

Figure 37.59 An N6900 microsurgical scalpel is used.

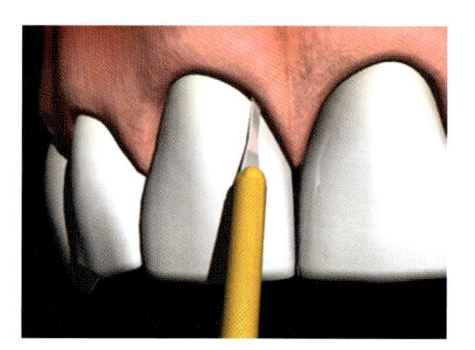

Figure 37.60 The scalpel is inserted into the sulcus.

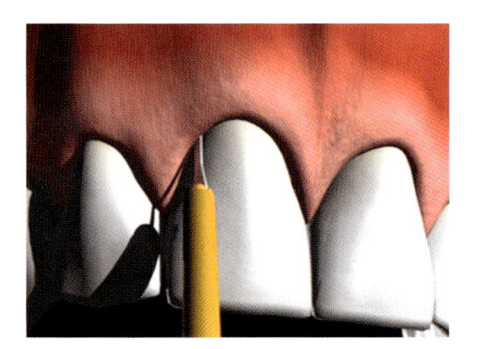

Figure 37.61 A sulcular incision, using the N6900 microsurgical blade, is made to the crest of bone.

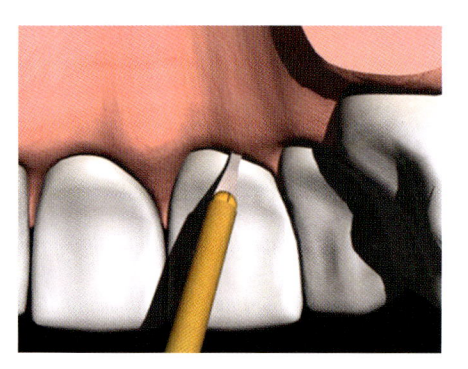

Figure 37.62 The circumferential sulcular incision extends to the facial and palatal bony crest.

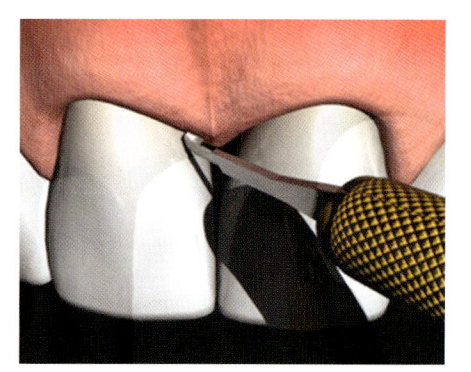

Figure 37.63 Custom modification of the microscalpel allows for complete undermining of the delicate papillary tissue.

The surgical dissecting microscope is used to visualize the morphology of the entire area and will help the surgeon avoid inadvertent severing of the delicate papillary isthmus. Following the minimal circumferential sulcular incision, a split-thickness flap is prepared. Custom modification of the microscalpel allows for complete undermining of the delicate papillary tissue (Figures 37.63 and 37.64). The customization of the microsurgical blade helps to negotiate subtle facial contours of the buccal gingiva and underlying bony contours. This delicate and tedious dissection allows the surgeon to extend the incision past the mucogingival junction. Once the incision extends past the

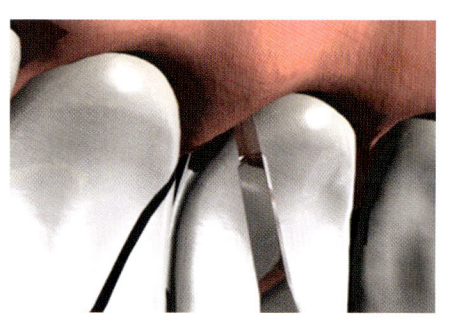

Figure 37.64 Palatal portion of the papilla is undermined.

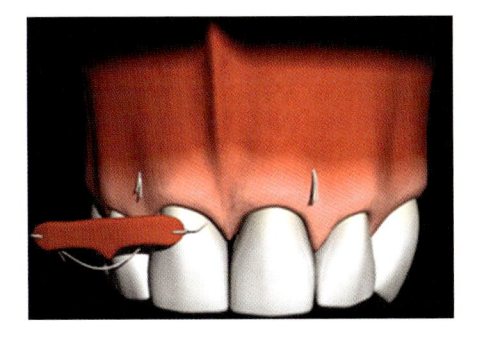

Figure 37.65 Lasso sutures secure the ends of the donor tissue.

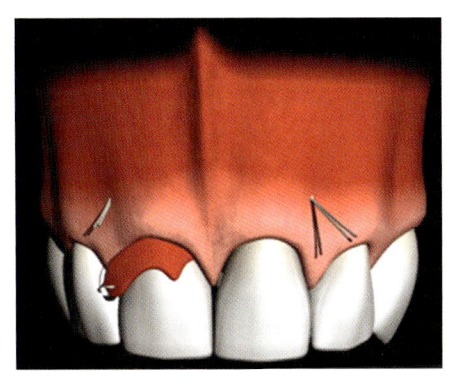

Figure 37.66 Sutures are positioned through the tunnel to gently pull the donor tissue into position.

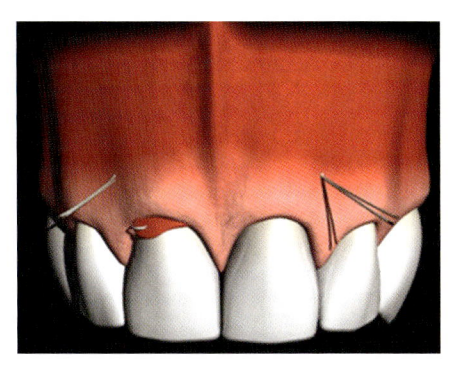

Figure 37.67 After the tissue is positioned the sutures anchor it in place.

mucogingival junction, mobility of the undermined tissue can be achieved. Papillary mobility is essential to allow for the creation of space under the papilla to receive the connective tissue graft.

Harvesting the connective tissue graft

An adequate volume of donor tissue must be procured as determined by the papillary space requirement.[4,19] Bone sounding can be performed to locate donor tissue of adequate dimensions. If a large volume of papillary tissue is required, the maxillary tuberosity will frequently be the donor site of choice because of its fibrous nature and thickness. The graft is shaped to produce the needed papillary dimensions and extends laterally to assist in root coverage, if needed. Often, a papillary shape can be reproduced by harvesting the palatal papillary tissue between the second premolar and first molar as a gingival unit transfer.[67]

Positioning and stabilizing the graft

A "lasso" suture is used to help pull and position the ends of the donor tissue. Sutures are positioned through the tunnel to gently pull the donor tissue into position and anchor it in place. Positioning of the graft under the interdental papilla can be challenging, but it is critical to the success of the procedure (Figures 37.65, 37.66, and 37.67).

Suspensory sutures

Lip musculature and tissue memory can create pressure and tension on the overlying tissue and thereby create a tendency to pull the papillary tissue back to its original position as it heals. To preserve the new papillary tissue position, a "suspensory suture" is used. This suture begins at the base of the papilla and is anchored around the interproximal contact point. The suspensory suture is essential to maintain the new position and height of the papilla. The addition of a composite bonding material at the interproximal contacts of the adjacent teeth can help prevent this suspensory suture from slipping through the interproximal contact. The suspensory suture also maintains the donor tissue under the papilla in its coronal position until the overlying flap has matured at its postsurgery position, thus preventing apical migration or displacement of the graft. If this suture is not used, then retraction of the tissue usually occurs (Figure 37.68).

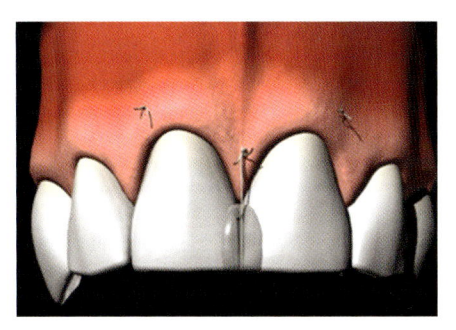

Figure 37.68 A suspensory suture anchors the papillary tissue position.

Postoperative instructions and healing

The care of the surgical area is extremely important especially during the first week. The patient should avoid foods that can cause trauma or hot liquids that can stimulate bleeding and increase swelling. Brushing or flossing the surgical site must be avoided. The mouth should be thoroughly rinsed daily using a 0.12% chlorhexidine gluconate rinse during the first 7 days. An anti-inflammatory prescription is recommended to avoid additional swelling that could otherwise compromise surgical healing.

Most of the sutures can be removed in 1 week. The suspensory sutures should remain in place for at least 2 weeks, and oral hygiene modifications are essential to ensure that the patient does not traumatize the area. Cleaning devices for the interdental area, such as interproximal brushes and triangular toothpicks, should be avoided. Reinforcement of oral hygiene techniques is crucial for long-term success. Six to eight weeks of soft-tissue healing is a minimum before restorative procedures can be considered.

Ridge preservation and ridge augmentation

Ridge defects are a deformity that can occur when the dentoalveolar bone and gingiva collapse after tooth loss.[2,20] Ridge deformities can create esthetic and functional dilemmas for the patient and restorative dentist.[2] Sometimes, patients might not reveal the defect in their smile, and at other times patients psychologically avoid smiling for fear of showing the defect. To provide an acceptable esthetic result, the ridge collapse can be masked, hidden, or corrected. This collapse creates a deformity that can make it challenging for the restorative dentist to develop an esthetic outcome due to the increased space and can also result in less lip support and a prematurely aged appearance.[20]

According to Abrams et al., the loss of an anterior tooth causes a significant deformity 91% of the time.[15] Ridge deformities have both soft-tissue (papilla and attached gingiva) and bony-alveolus components. Soft-tissue deformities can occur when surgical incisions are made in delicate areas (thin gingiva, alveolar mucosa and papillae as shown in Figure 37.1A and B). Deformities of bone can occur following a simple extraction of a tooth, but deformities are even more common if there has been a predisposing factor present such as a thin dentoalveolus, previous endodontic surgery, endodontic failure, iatrogenic bone removal, intentional bone removal to gain access, root fracture, or periodontal bone loss. Pressure atrophy from a removable prosthetic appliance (such as a flipper) can compress the alveolar ridge and allow the collapse of the adjacent papillae.[2] Until periodontal plastic surgical procedures were developed, a ridge deficiency would necessitate the overbuilding of prosthetic tooth structure, prosthetic gingiva, or acceptance of a space that could appear dark. Phonetics could also be affected where the space could allow for passage of air and saliva.[2]

Modern exodontia techniques focus on an atraumatic and conservative approach during a tooth extraction with the placement of a bone graft and a barrier membrane at the time of extraction to minimize bone collapse while maintaining the soft-tissue surroundings.[2] Delicate biotype patients can present with high, thin bone scalloping, making them even more susceptible to bone collapse. Presence of an acceptable bony foundation following extraction does not always provide ideal soft-tissue contours, and soft-tissue augmentation may need to be considered. Along with maintenance of the bony foundation and soft-tissue contour, the interdental papilla also requires careful consideration. If the papillary tissue is unsupported, then it is reasonable to expect it to collapse as well. Papilla preservation can be initiated prior to tooth extraction with interdisciplinary treatment planning. Ideally, the restorative dentist will fabricate an immediate tooth replacement that duplicates the previous tissue support to provide immediate bracing of the papillary tissue. The immediate tooth replacement should be well anchored and cleansable.

Ridge augmentation

If a ridge defect is present, a bridge pontic will be constructed longer than ideal, or if a tooth of normal length is created, then a dark space can show. With either compromise, the result is unnatural and unesthetic. If an implant is planned, a ridge defect will mandate a longer clinical crown.

Ridge augmentation can minimize or eliminate a ridge defect. Independent of the type of tooth replacement, (bridge or implant-supported crown) or the quality of the bony foundation, a ridge augmentation procedure can restore the natural appearance of the gingival contour in the edentulous area. An ideal ridge will mimic the presence of a root prominence, creating an illusion that the tooth is naturally emerging out of the gingival tissue. Ridge augmentation is a periodontal plastic surgical procedure that also helps function by restoring a band of attached keratinized gingival protection for the pontic or implant. In 1982, Langer and Calagna[27] described the use of a subepithelial connective tissue graft to enhance anterior cosmetics in ridge-deficient areas. The correction of ridge deformities as described by Seibert in 1983, used an onlay graft technique, transplanting a thick epithelialized graft from the palate.[68,69] The thick epithelialized graft created a large tender donor site and a thick free gingival graft patch-like appearance that might not mimic the surrounding area. Periodontal plastic surgical refinements have since been developed to reduce patient morbidity, enhance esthetics, and improve predictability (Figures 37.69A and B and 37.70A and B).

This procedure incorporates a microsurgical technique using a connective tissue graft harvested from the palate, creating minimal discomfort and trauma to the patient; and because grafted

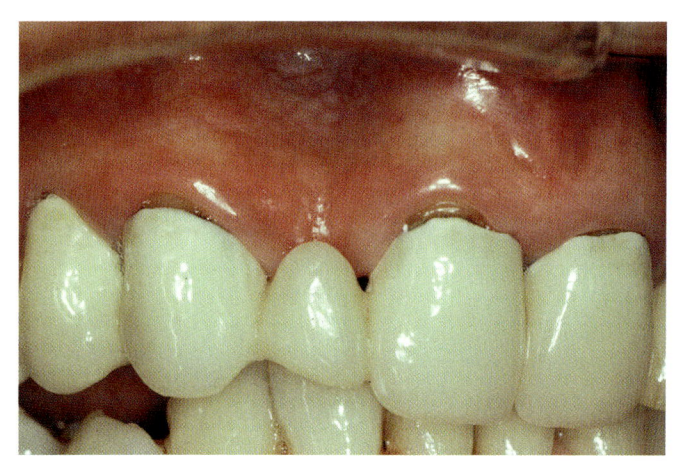

Figure 37.69 **(A)** Patient was unhappy with the ridge collapse in the #7 area.

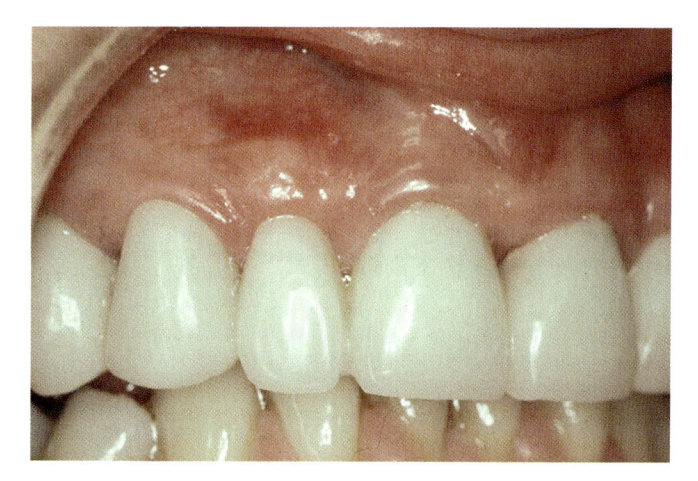

Figure 37.69 **(B)** Ridge augmentation was performed and a new bridge placed.

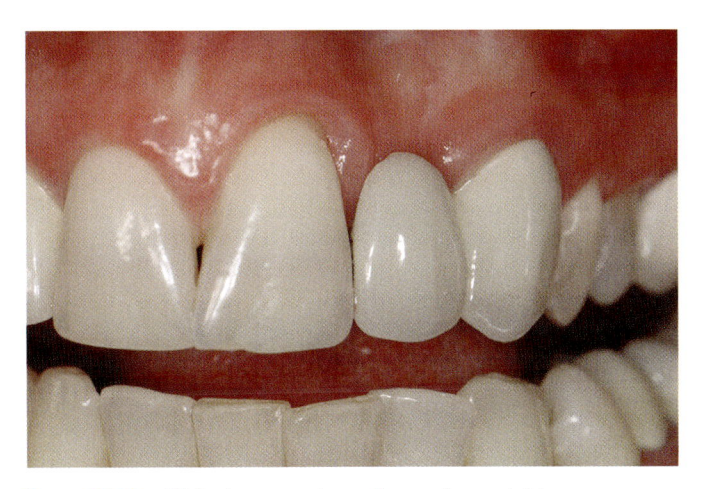

Figure 37.70 (A) Patient experienced recession and ridge collapse on #10.

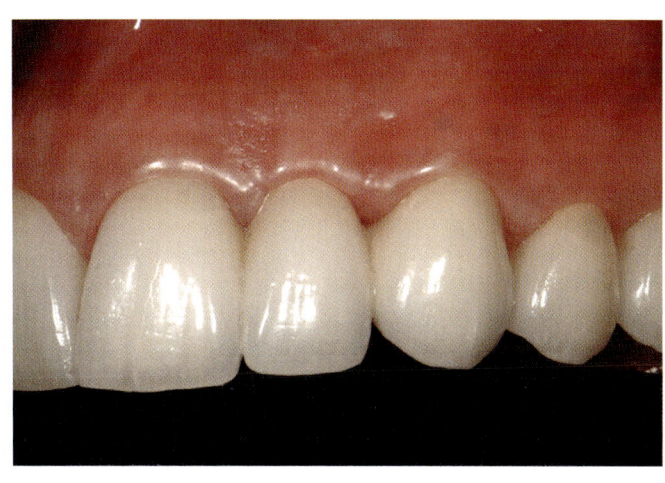

Figure 37.70 (B) Ridge augmentation and root coverage were accomplished, providing natural contours for a new replacement.

tissue cells are surrounded by a vascular supply, the predictability of cell survival is improved. An ovate pontic is used to allow for cleansability, and its placement during the surgery creates a natural tooth emergence. This procedure is covered in a step-by-step fashion.

Indications for ridge augmentation

- Correction of anterior ridge defects.
- Minimal or lack of attached keratinized gingiva at the edentulous site.
- Can be performed following an extraction that has already healed and before the final replacement (implant surgery or final bridge).

Surgical technique

In this example, the patient presents with a preexisting three-unit bridge with a desire to have a normal ridge contour and appearance. She noticed a dark space around her missing tooth, especially evident in photographs. Psychologically, she was self-conscious and hesitated to smile. Her restorative dentist could remake the three-unit bridge and place a longer tooth or consider surgery to replace the missing contour (Figure 37.71).

Provisional bridge

The restorative dentist removed the preexisting bridge and placed a provisional restoration extending from teeth #7, #8, and #9. Once the bridge was removed, a significant amount of calculus was exposed and removed from the abutment teeth (Figure 37.72). The ridge-lap pontic was converted into an ovate pontic using a flowable composite resin of a matching shade (Figure 37.73). The ovate pontic will help reinforce the illusion of a natural tooth growing out of the gingiva and is easily cleansable with flossing.

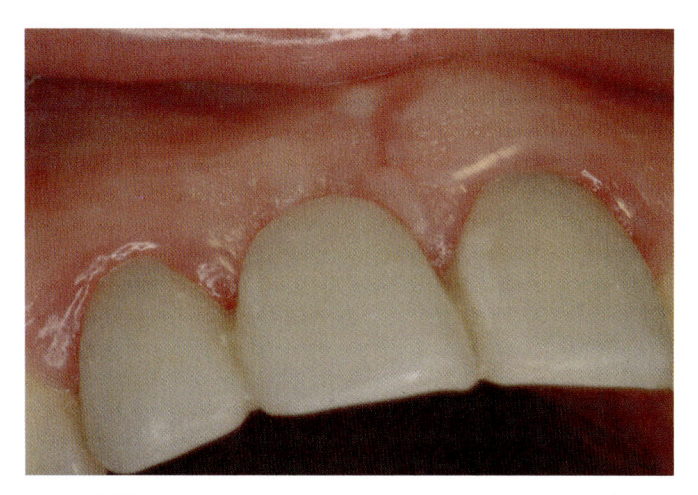

Figure 37.71 Patient presents with a preexisting three-unit bridge with a desire to have a normal ridge contour and appearance.

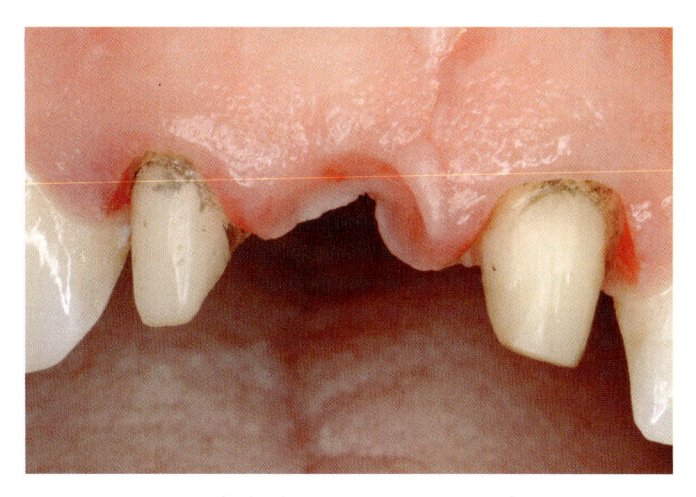

Figure 37.72 Once the bridge was removed, a significant amount of calculus was exposed and removed from the abutment teeth.

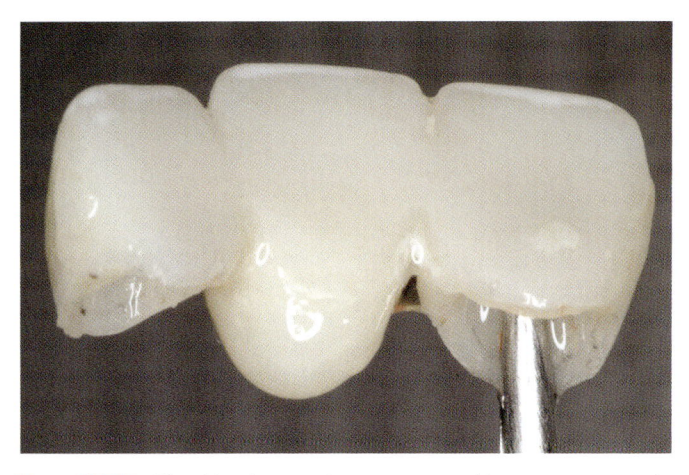

Figure 37.73 The ridge-lap pontic was converted into an ovate pontic.

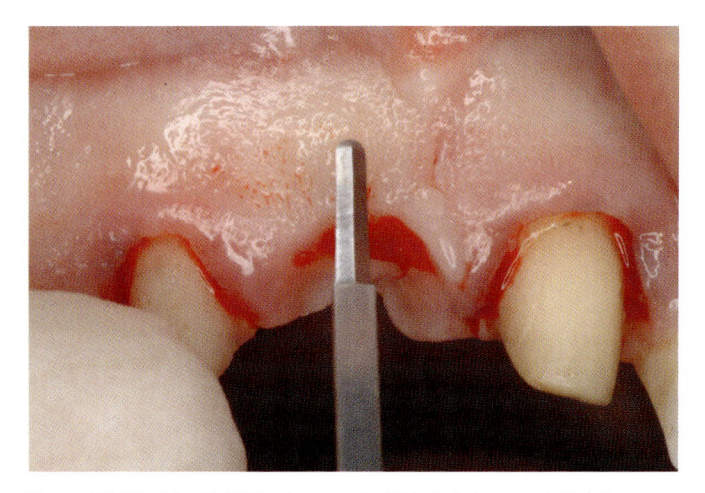

Figure 37.74 The N6900 microsurgical blade is inserted slightly palatal to the future sulcus.

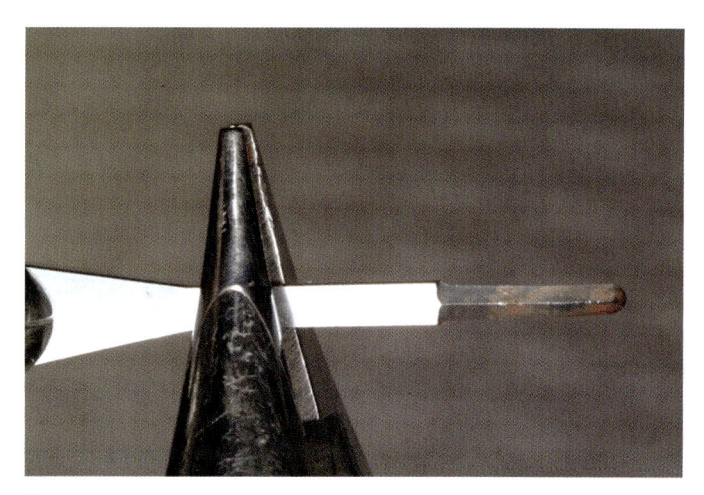

Figure 37.75 The scalpel shank is modified using orthodontic bending pliers.

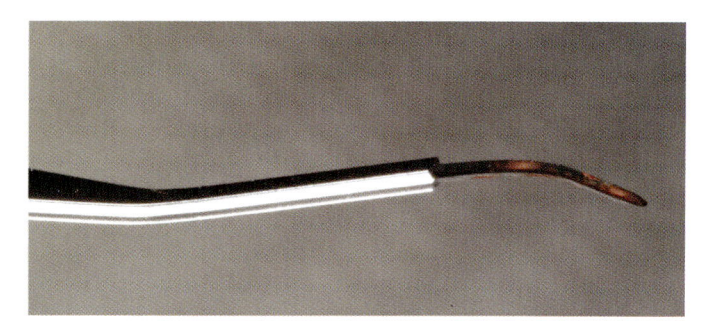

Figure 37.76 The scalpel blade is modified to follow the underlying bony ridge contour.

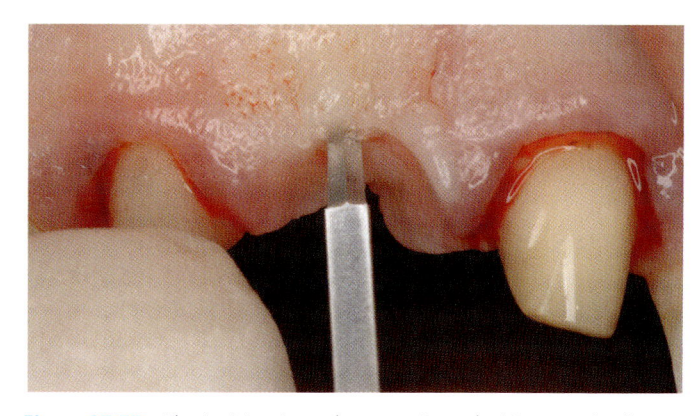

Figure 37.77 The incision is made approximately 1.5 mm palatal to the previous pontic facial location.

Microincision

The N6900 microsurgical blade is inserted slightly palatal to the future sulcus. The scalpel is unmodified initially (Figure 37.74). As the incision is extended deeper, bony contours are frequently encountered and the scalpel blade can be easily modified with orthodontic bending pliers to follow the underlying bony ridge contour. The shank is modified as needed for ease of angulation (Figures 37.75 and 37.76). While performing the soft-tissue dissection, the surgeon can also evaluate the underlying bony contour if implant placement is to be contemplated in the future.

In this case, the former pontic created a small ridge depression, which acted as guide for the initial incision. The incision was made approximately 1.5 mm palatal to the previous pontic facial location (Figure 37.77). The N6900 scalpel is inserted past the mucogingival junction, creating a tunnel in an attempt to recreate a contour that mimics the former tooth root prominence (Figures 37.78 and 37.79). The previous soft-tissue scarring is relieved with the dissection, and tunnel patency was confirmed with the use of a 10/11 Hartzell curette (Figure 37.80). The palatal portion of the pontic receptor site was prepared with the use of a #6 round bur to create a slight depression for the future pontic emergence (Figure 37.81).

Harvesting connective tissue

A connective tissue graft was harvested from the palate that mimicked the conical shape of the previously extracted root to create the illusion of a root prominence. The tissue was harvested using a lasso suture and modified using Le Grange scissors (Figures 37.82 and 37.83). The graft was sutured into location. An initial suture needle penetration was made at the apical extent of the tunnel, then the graft was sutured through its apical end and pulled into the tunnel (Figure 37.84). The graft was

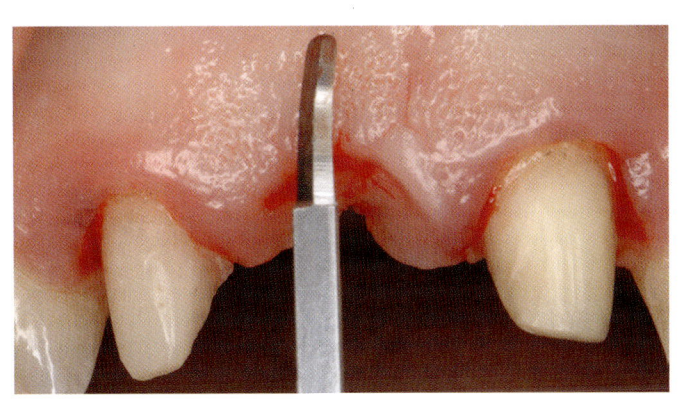

Figure 37.78 The N6900 scalpel contour conforms to the anatomical contour.

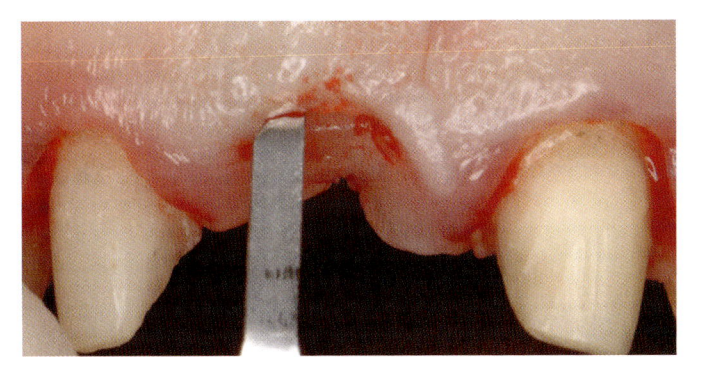

Figure 37.79 The N6900 scalpel is inserted past the mucogingival junction, creating a tunnel in an attempt to recreate a contour mimicking the former tooth root prominence.

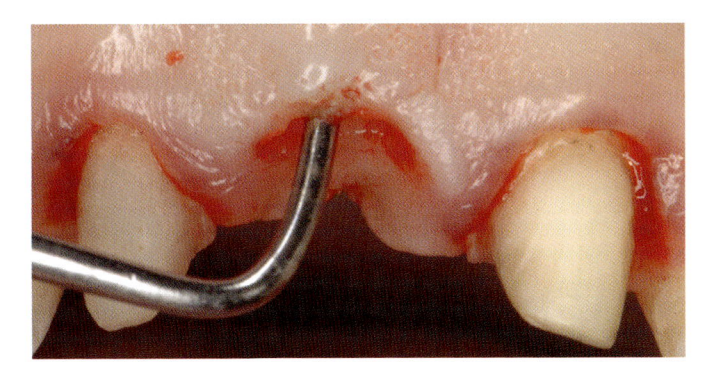

Figure 37.80 The previous soft-tissue scarring is relieved with the dissection, and tunnel patency is confirmed with the use of a 10/11 Hartzell curette.

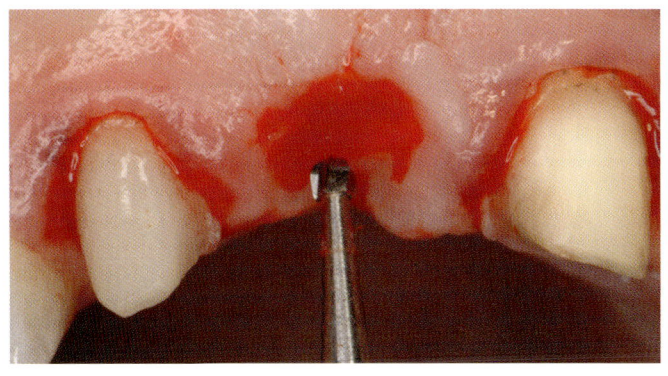

Figure 37.81 The palatal portion of the pontic receptor site is prepared with the use of a large round bur, creating a depression for the future pontic emergence.

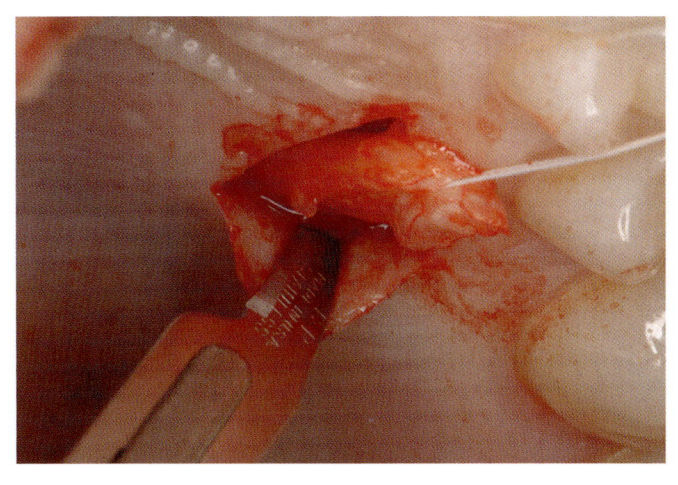

Figure 37.82 A connective tissue graft is harvested from the palate.

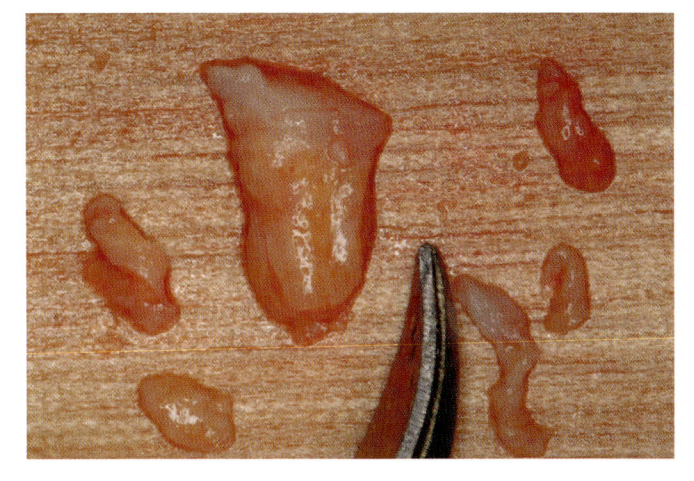

Figure 37.83 Donor tissue is modified using Le Grange scissors to mimic the root contour.

anchored at both ends to assure its position apically and coronally using a Gore-Tex suture (Figure 37.85).

Provisional bridge placement

The pontic was converted into an ovate pontic and the bridge reinserted into position. The pontic should extend at least 2 mm into the tissue and create a sulcus for the new pontic (Figures 37.86 and 37.87). This will create the illusion that the tooth is emerging out of the tissue. The palatal wound was sutured closed and covered by a surgical protective stent.

Postoperative instruction and healing

Postoperative instructions are similar to those described for previous procedures.

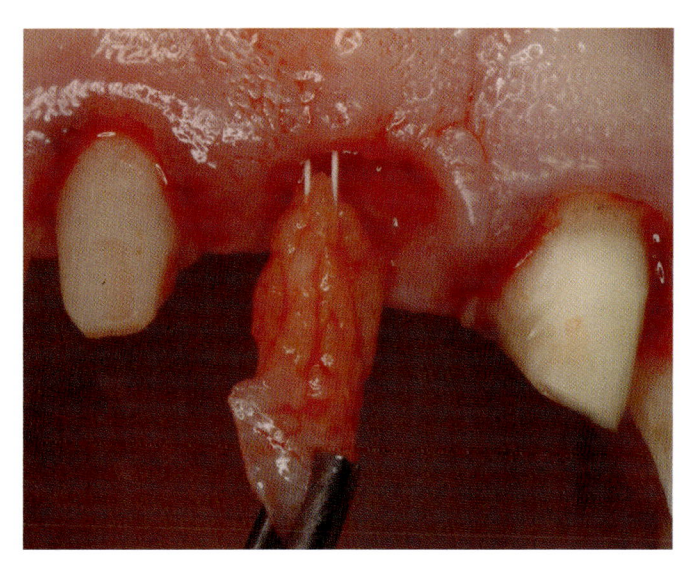

Figure 37.84 The graft is pulled into the tunnel.

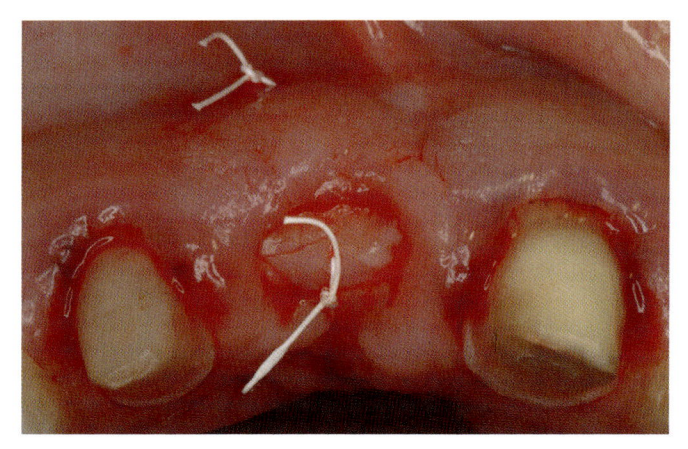

Figure 37.85 The graft was anchored at both ends to assure its position apically and coronally using a Gore-Tex suture.

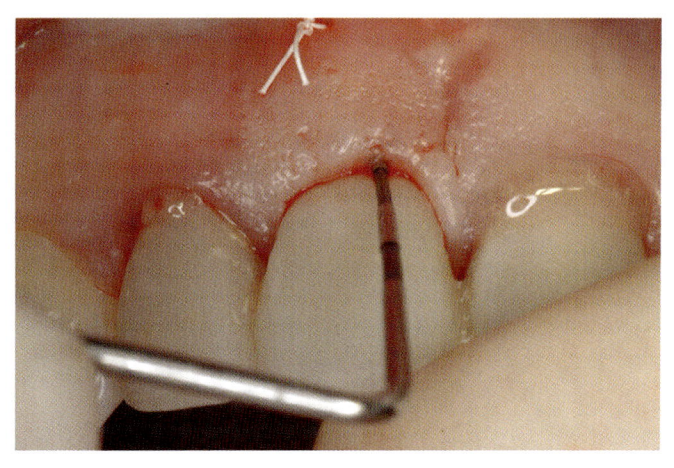

Figure 37.86 The bridge is reinserted into position. The pontic should extend at least 2 mm into the tissue and create a sulcus for the new pontic.

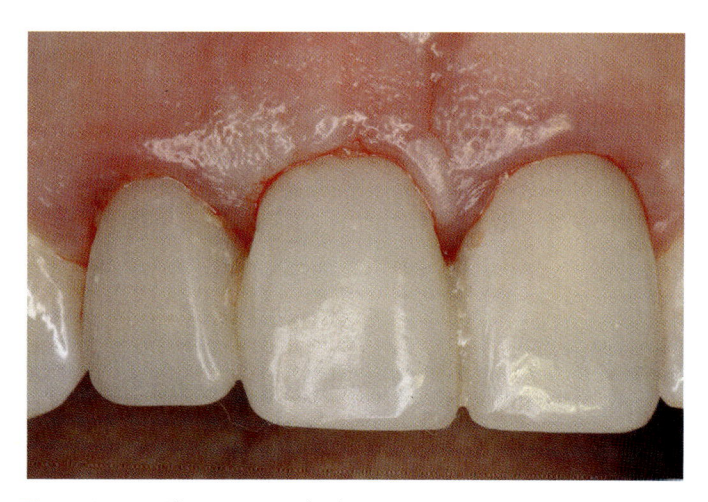

Figure 37.87 The temporary bridge is re-cemented.

Ovate pontic

Ridge-lap pontics have a concavity under the pontic, against the ridge. Unfortunately, the concavity hides bacteria, and inflammatory reactions are found more than 95% of the time.[70] In 1981, Garber and Rosenberg described ovate pontics as esthetically and functionally superior to other pontic designs of the past.[71] The concept of the ovate pontic uses a rounded egg-shaped pontic that allows for a natural-appearing emergence profile and an ease of oral hygiene cleansability.[71] The ovate design is esthetic, cleansable, and promotes a thick healthy periodontium.[72] The pontic should extend 1.5–2 mm below the gingival margin to support the surrounding facial gingiva and the interdental papilla.[2]

Excessive gingival display: esthetic crown lengthening and sculpting

Excessive gingival display, commonly referred to as a "gummy smile," is a description for the situation whereby the patient shows too much gingiva. Commonly in the adult, the gingival margin will be located at or near the CEJ, and normally a patient will show very little if any gingiva over the central incisors when smiling. Three common causes of an excessive gingival display are vertical maxillary excess, excessive alveolar bone, and excessive gingiva.[2] These can occur individually or in combination.[2] Vertical maxillary excess exists if there is an abnormally tall maxilla. In this situation, orthognathic surgery can be considered to move the maxilla to a new level. Orthodontic and oral surgical consultations will determine the ideal position of the maxilla.[2]

When excessive gingiva covers enamel, the sulcus depth will increase, thereby allowing a safe harbor for bacteria and making plaque removal difficult. Osseous resective procedures have been developed to reshape the dentoalveolar architecture to create a more favorable environment for periodontal maintenance and health.[73] Resective periodontal plastic surgery can remove excessive gingiva and bone. If the enamel of the teeth is covered by gingiva and bone, then the smile can be hidden. Microsurgery to remove precise amounts of gingiva

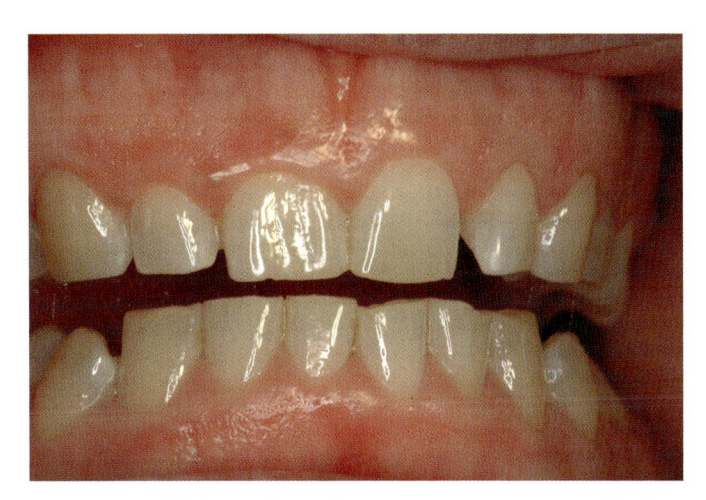

Figure 37.88 **(A)** Pre-op figure showing an excessive gingival display.

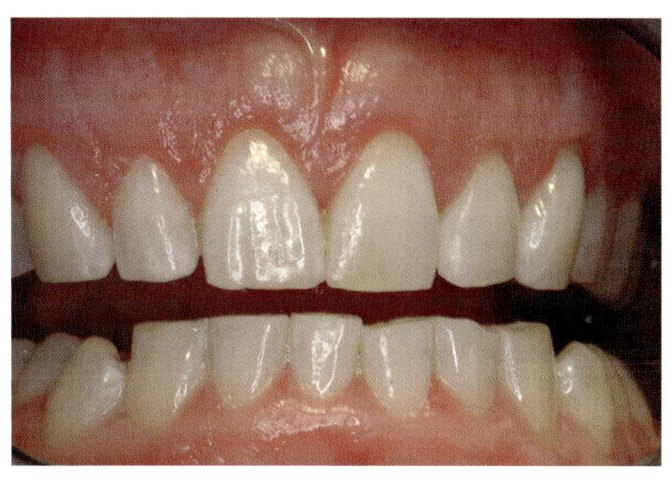

Figure 37.88 **(B)** After an esthetic crown-lengthening procedure, smile was enhanced showing the hidden enamel profile.

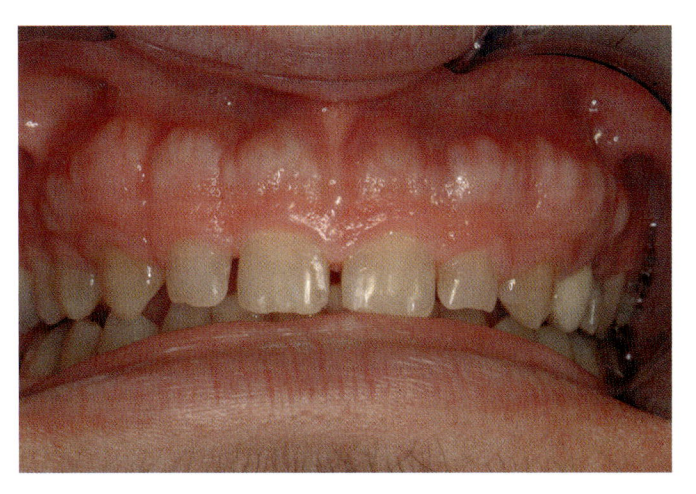

Figure 37.89 **(A)** Pre-op figure showing excessive gingival tissue with excessive underlying bone.

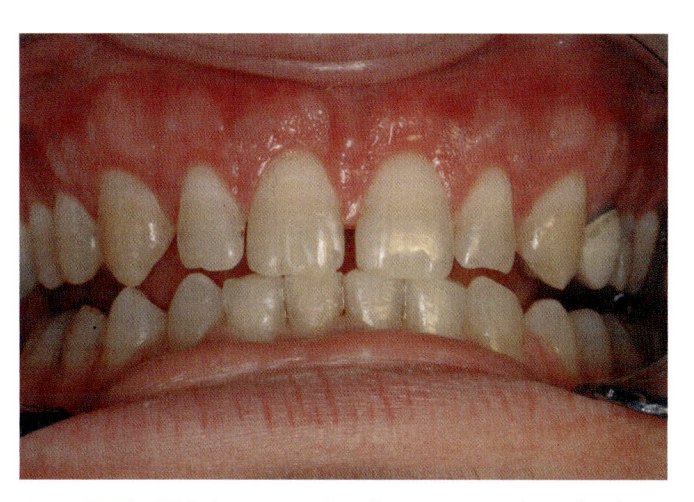

Figure 37.89 **(B)** Esthetic crown lengthening was performed with reduction of the large bony exostoses and soft-tissue sculpting.

and corresponding alveolar bone can show the full enamel profile of the teeth, which usually creates a bigger, brighter smile (Figure 37.88A and B).[20]

Clinical parameters exist detailing esthetic tissue positions of the maxillary anterior arch and may serve as a guideline for a predictable esthetic outcome.[74,75] In the esthetic crown-lengthening surgery, patient biotypes[76] can play a role in the amount of rebound healing of the newly established gingival margin.[77] Individual variation in gingival thickness will modify final tissue healing levels postoperatively. "Thick" tissue biotypes show the greatest tendency to rebound in a coronal direction.[77]

Excessive alveolar bone can affect the overall tissue contour in both height and thickness. Because the full enamel profile is not visible, the anterior teeth will appear short and square. Both bone height and thickness can also vary considerably. If the alveolar bone is abnormally low, incisally positioned or thick, both bone and gingiva must be treated together during surgery (Figure 37.89A and B). Simple use of a laser can raise bone height but will not taper the contour of the bone to the tooth. Because excessive bony contours can predispose a patient toward gingivitis and periodontitis due to an inability to remove bacterial plaque effectively,[73] the recontouring of excessive tissue can provide a functional as well as cosmetic benefit.[2]

Excessive gingiva (gingival hypertrophy) can occur without an excessive amount of underlying bone. In this case, simple excision of the soft tissue without manipulation of the bone can achieve a normal-appearing result.[2]

Individual's biologic width

In a classic study, Gargiulo et al. measured dentogingival anatomy in humans within Orban's four phases of passive eruption. In the case type where the gingival tissue covers the enamel, the distance from the marginal epithelium to the crest of the alveolar bone demonstrated tremendous individual variation.[78] The clinical consensus as to precisely how much bone resection is necessary when planning an esthetic crown-lengthening case is unclear and somewhat controversial. Several authors have suggested surgically removing the periodontal support to an extent, leaving a distance from the level of a planned restorative margin to the level of newly recontoured osseous crest of 2.5–3.5 mm,[79] 3 mm,[80] and 4 mm[81] of the exposed tooth. Unfortunately, not enough research

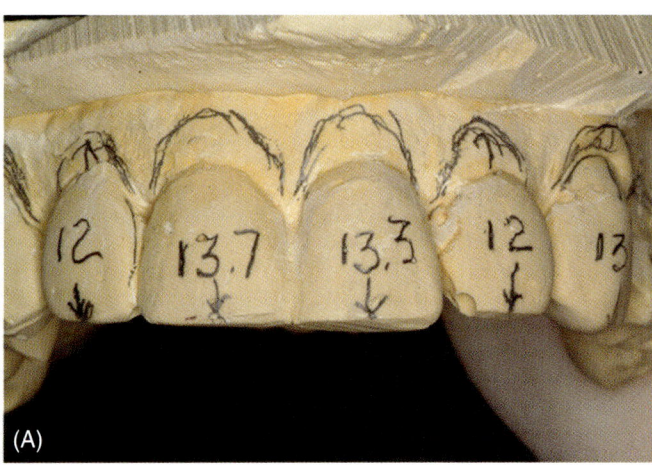

Figure 37.90 **(A, B)** Examples of how to communicate precise desired tissue positions.

#5 – 9.3 mm
#6 –11 mm
#7–9.5 mm
#8–11 mm
#9–11 mm
#10–8 mm
#11–11 mm
#12–8 mm

presently exists to make exacting statements about how much bone should be removed when crown lengthening or sculpting is performed in the esthetic zone.[2] Because there is a great variation in biotypes and biologic widths, a safe guide for bone reduction can consider the patient as having their own "individual biologic width." Clinical observations indicate, for example, that if the soft-tissue reduction is to change 2 mm, then the same 2 mm should be used for bone height modification. This will maintain the "individual's biologic width." Not only should the bone height be modified, but also the bone thickness should be reshaped to create a natural scalloping profile. The thickness and contour are controlled with direct visualization of the bone contour. The use of a laser can reduce height but cannot control bone thickness.

Esthetic crown-lengthening surgical procedure

Before crown lengthening is performed, it is important to have clear communication between the restorative dentist, patient, and surgeon. Precise blueprints of where the future gingival location is desired need to be conveyed. Communication examples could include precise measurements from the incisal edges to the gingival margin, an e-mail, photographs, a mock-up, clear trays, stone models, or whatever communication is necessary to make the request clear to the surgeon (Figure 37.90). Ideally, the restorative dentist will provide a surgical guide based on a mock-up that has been tried in and adjusted on the patient.

Sometimes, sculpting will place the new soft-tissue margin at the CEJ. If the sculpting exposes root dentin, then sensitivity will likely occur if the root is not covered with a restoration. If the restoration is a bonded restoration and extends on to root dentin, the bond will be weakest at that root dentin margin.[82] The restorative dentist must determine if a dentin margin is desired and the patient should be aware of this compromise. Sometimes, root dentin exposure cannot be helped. In this case, precise measurements from the incisal edges are provided by the restorative dentist with considerations for modifications of the tooth shape (e.g., restoration and extension of worn incisal edges) that might be changed with future restorations.

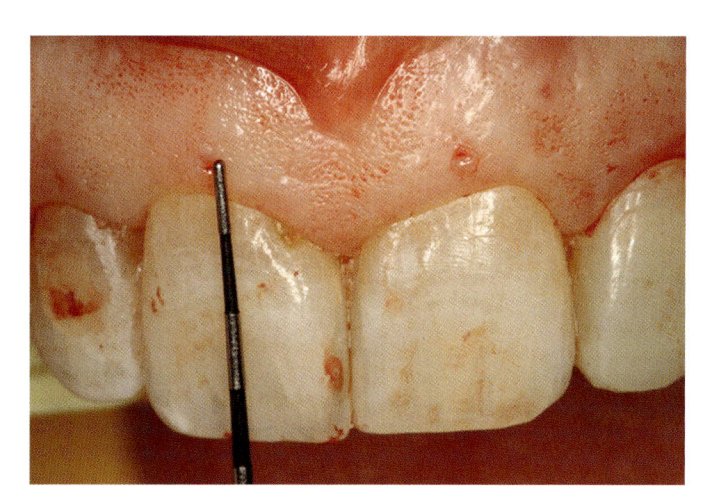

Figure 37.91 Prescribed tissue locations are transferred to the patient, using a periodontal probe and puncture markings at the zenith of the desired soft-tissue location.

Determining the new tissue location

After anesthetizing, prescribed tissue locations are transferred to the patient, using a periodontal probe and puncture markings at the zenith of the desired soft-tissue location (Figure 37.91).

Incisions

After the parabolic peak or zenith has been determined, a scalloped incision is made through the gingiva to the desired level using a 15-C scalpel (Figure 37.92). The incisions should create a papillary design that will meet edge to edge with the future papilla location (Figure 37.93). A sulcular incision is made with the intent to remove the collar of gingival tissue (Figure 37.94). The gingival collar is removed using a sickle scaler (Figure 37.95). Careful attention is paid to the papillary area to create similar incision angles in preparation for future flap replacement without voids or irregularities. The precise replacement of the flap tissue is critical to avoid obvious incision lines, papillary disfiguration, or total papilla loss.

It is important not to thin the papillary epithelium aggressively because it can cause necrosis at the future wound margin.

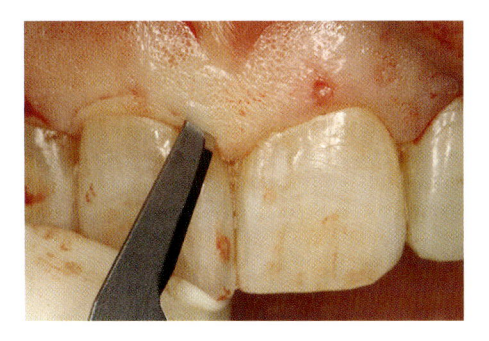

Figure 37.92 A scalloped incision is made through the gingiva to the desired level using a 15-C scalpel.

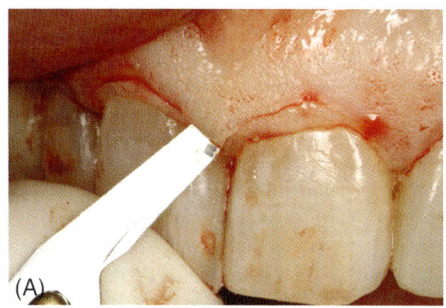

Figure 37.93 (A, B) The incisions should create a papillary design that will meet edge to edge with the future papilla.

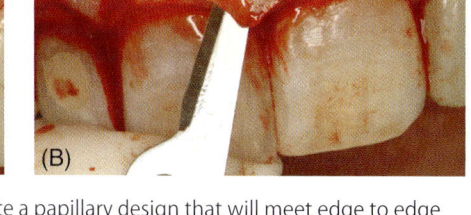

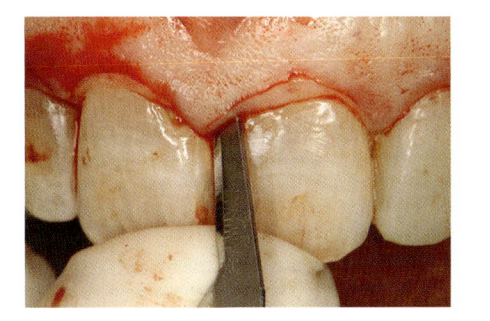

Figure 37.94 A sulcular incision is made with the intent to remove the collar of gingival tissue.

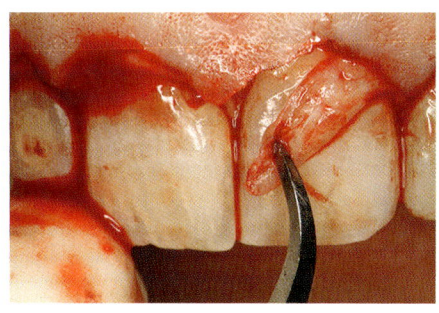

Figure 37.95 The gingival collar is removed using a sickle scaler.

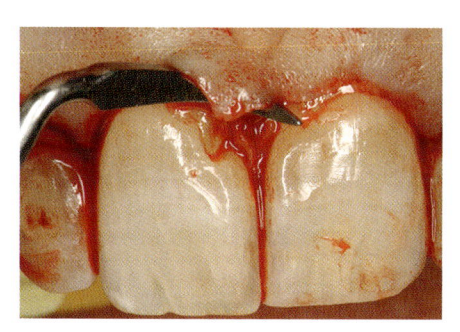

Figure 37.96 A split-thickness incision is used initially to raise the tissue flap delicately.

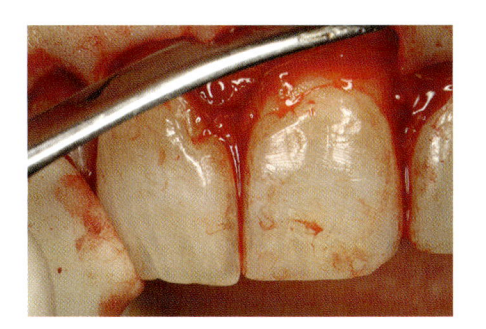

Figure 37.97 The flap is reflected full thickness using a periosteal elevator to visualize the bony contours.

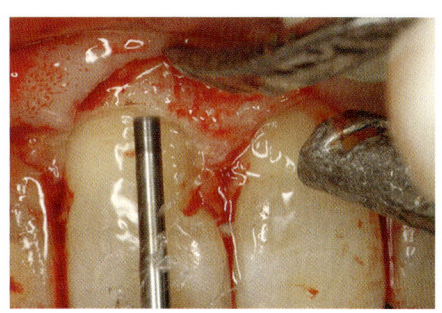

Figure 37.98 End-cutting burs are used for circumferential bone reduction without gouging the root surface.

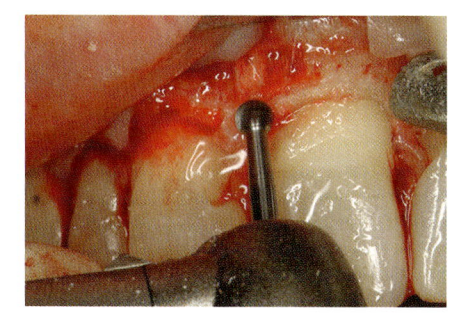

Figure 37.99 A round bur is used to modify any prominence apical and adjacent to the bone reduction areas.

A split-thickness incision is used initially to raise the tissue flap delicately (Figure 37.96). The flap is reflected full thickness using a periosteal elevator to visualize the bony contours (Figure 37.97).

Bone reduction

After achieving adequate visibility of the bony architecture, excessive bony contours are commonly encountered. End-cutting burs allow for circumferential bone reduction without gouging the root surface (Figure 37.98). A round bur can then be used to modify any prominence apical and adjacent to the bone reduction areas (Figure 37.99). Smaller end-cutting burs can reach interproximally to adjust the interproximal bony contours (Figure 37.100). A small round bur is used, ideally with magnification, to blend the osseous contours (Figure 37.101). Varying forms and tooth shapes will affect the tissue position.[40] Sometimes enamel irregularities can be encountered that can also contribute to minor idiosyncrasies in the soft-tissue position. These idiosyncrasies should be taken into consideration with the new desired tissue location. Prominent teeth will require less bony reduction and teeth that are more inset will typically require more aggressive bony contouring. Soft-tissue fiber attachment to the root surface is reduced using small microsurgical hoes SPN1 and SPN2 (G. Hartzell & Son) (Figure 37.102). Fine-tuning of the bone contours is refined using hand instruments (Figure 37.103).

Sutures and final touches

It is extremely critical to realign the wound edges because edge-to-edge incision line apposition will achieve minimal scarring in the delicate and highly esthetic papillary area (Figure 37.104). Delicate individual sutures using a surgeon's knot will help control tissue closure for each individual papilla (Figure 37.105). The soft-tissue position should be reconfirmed once suturing is completed. Minor tissue position modifications can be accomplished using a liquid suture (Figure 37.106). The surgical dissecting microscope can be used to help fine-tune the tissue position. In addition, the use of a laser can perform minor soft-tissue modifications and contour adjustments (Figures 37.107 and 37.108). A surgical dressing is placed to provide protection and stability to the new tissue location during the first week postoperatively. In this case, a surgical dressing, Barricaid (Densply Caulk), has been used (Figure 37.109).

Postoperative instructions and healing

The care of the surgical area is extremely important, especially during the first week. The patient should avoid foods that can cause trauma or hot liquids that can stimulate bleeding and increase swelling. Brushing or flossing the surgical site must be avoided. The mouth should be thoroughly rinsed daily using a 0.12% chlorhexidine gluconate rinse during the first 7 days. An anti-inflammatory prescription is recommended to avoid additional swelling that could otherwise compromise surgical healing.

The sutures can be removed in 1 week. Reinforcement of oral hygiene techniques is crucial for long-term success. Six to eight weeks of soft-tissue healing is a minimum before restorative procedures can be considered (Figure 37.110A and B).

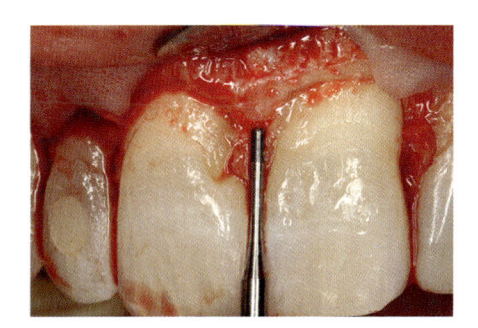

Figure 37.100 Smaller end-cutting burs reach interproximally to adjust the interproximal bony contours.

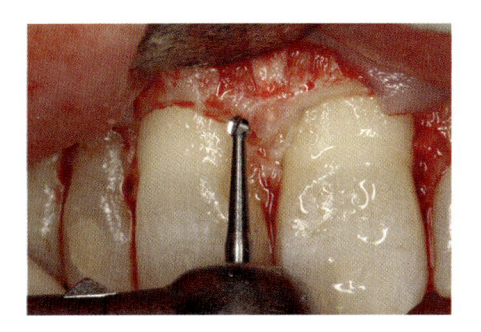

Figure 37.101 A small round bur is used to blend the osseous contours.

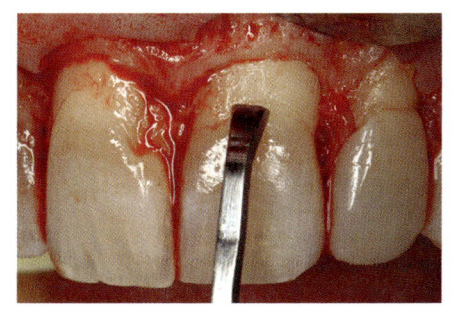

Figure 37.102 Soft-tissue fiber attachment to the root surface is reduced using small microsurgical hoes SPN1 and SPN2.

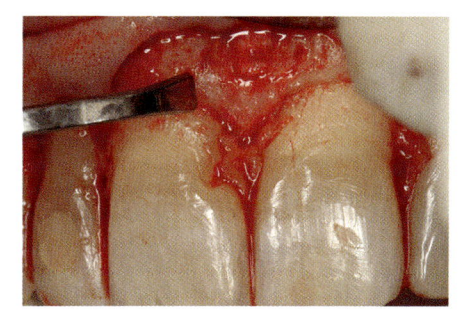

Figure 37.103 Fine-tuning of the bone contours is refined using hand instruments.

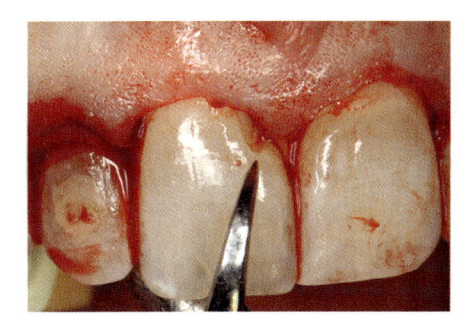

Figure 37.104 Realignment of the wound edges.

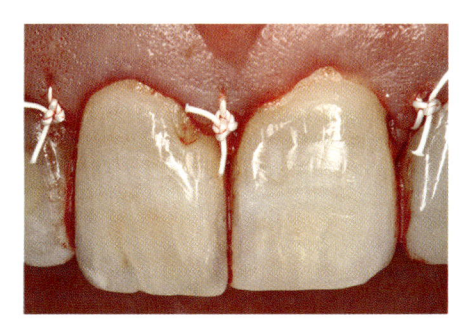

Figure 37.105 Individual sutures using a surgeon's knot.

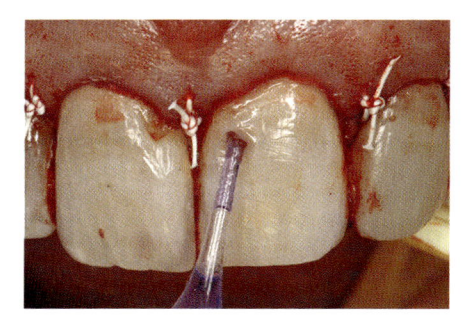

Figure 37.106 Minor tissue position modifications can be accomplished using a liquid suture.

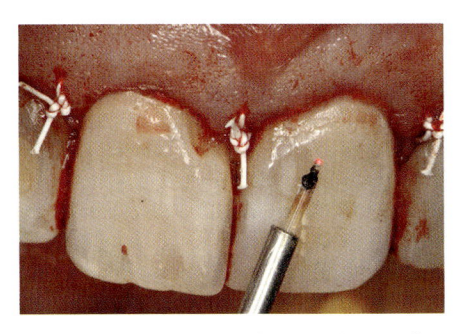

Figure 37.107 The use of a diode laser will perform minor soft-tissue modifications and contour adjustments.

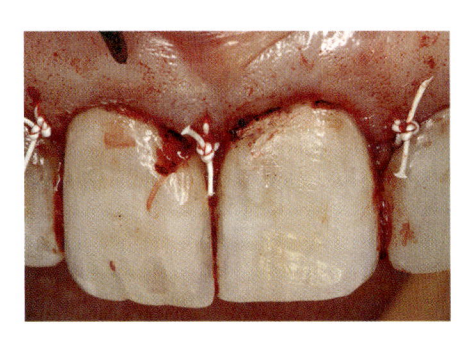

Figure 37.108 The final tissue heights are confirmed.

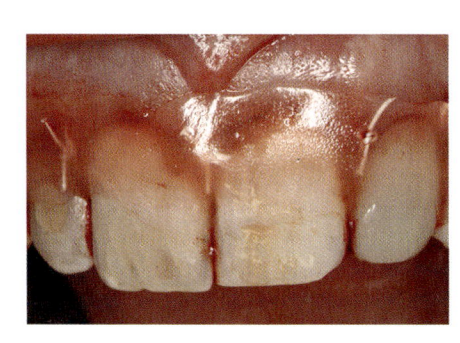

Figure 37.109 Barricaid (Densply Caulk) in place.

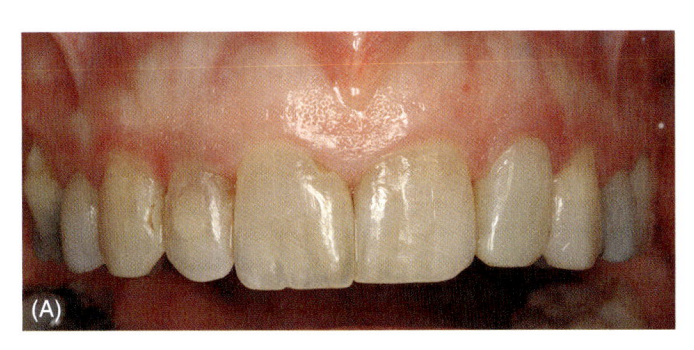

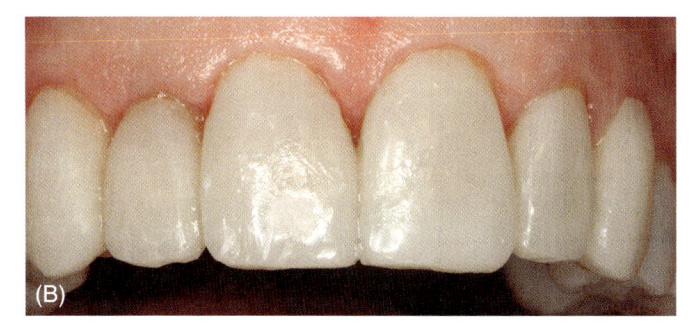

Figure 37.110 **(A)** Pre- and **(B)** post-op figures showing esthetic crown-lengthening procedures. Please note that tooth #10 was bonded to close the space for esthetic purposes.

References

1. Garber DA, Salama MA. The aesthetic smile: diagnosis and treatment. *Periodontol 2000* 1996;11:18–28.
2. Nordland WP. The role of periodontal plastic microsurgery in oral facial esthetics. *J Calif Dent Assoc* 2002;30(11):831–837.
3. Caudil RF, Oringer FJ, Langer B, et al. Esthetic periodontics (periodontal plastic surgery). In: Kornman KS, Wilson TG, eds. *Fundamentals of Periodontics*, 2nd edn. Chicago, IL; Quintessence; 2003:540–561.
4. Sandhu HS, Nordland WP. Interdental papilla reconstruction: classification and clinical management. *Can J Restor Dent Prosthodont* 2010;3:34–38.
5. Han TJ, Takei HH. Progress in gingival papilla reconstruction. *Periodontol 2000* 1996;11:65–68.
6. Cortellini P, Pini Prato GP, Tonetti MS. The modified papilla preservation technique. A new surgical approach for interproximal regenerative procedures. *J Periodontol* 1995;66:261–266.
7. Cortellini P, Pini Prato GP, Tonetti MS. The simplified papilla preservation flap. A novel surgical approach for the management of soft tissues in regenerative procedures. *Int J Periodontics Restorative Dent* 1999;19:589–599.
8. Azzi R, Etienne D, Carranza F. Surgical reconstruction of the interdental papilla. *Int J Periodontics Restorative Dent* 1998;18(5):466–473.
9. Azzi R, Etienne D, Sauvan JL, Miller PD. Root coverage and papilla reconstruction in Class IV recession: a case report. *Int J Periodontics Restorative Dent* 1999;19(5):449–455.
10. Azzi R, Takei HH, Etienne D, Carranza FA. Root coverage and papilla reconstruction using autogenous osseous and connective tissue grafts. *Int J Periodontics Restorative Dent* 2001;21:141–147.
11. Beagle JR. Surgical reconstruction of the interdental papilla: case report. *Int J Periodontics Restorative Dent* 1992;12(2):145–151.
12. Prato GP, Rotundo R, Cortellini P, et al. Interdental papilla management: a review and classification of the therapeutic approaches. *Int J Periodontics Restorative Dent* 2004;24(3):246–255.
13. Van der Velden U. Regeneration of the interdental soft tissues following denudation procedures. *J Clin Periodontol* 1982;9:455–459.
14. Shapiro A. Regeneration of interdental papillae using periodic curettage. *Int J Periodontics Restorative Dent* 1985;5(5):26–33.
15. Abrams H, Kopczyk RA, Kaplan AL. Incidence of anterior ridge deformities in partially edentulous patients. *J Prosthet Dent* 1987;57(2):191–194.
16. Krieger GD, Nordland WP. Aesthetic implant site development, proceedings from 2004 symposium. *The Seattle Study Club J* 2004;8(3):32–36.
17. Schmidt R, Boudro M. *The Dental Microscope: Why and How. Evidence-based Technology and Treatment*. S&B Publishing; 2011:41–57.
18. Belcher MJ. A perspective on periodontal microsurgery. *Int J Periodontics Restorative Dent* 2001;21(2):191–196.
19. Nordland WP, Sandhu HS. Microsurgical technique for augmentation of the papilla: three case reports. *Int J Periodontics Restorative Dent* 2008;28:543–549.
20. Earthman JC, Sheets CG, Paquette JM, et al. Tissue engineering in dentistry. *Clin Plast Surg* 2003;30:621–639.

21. Sullivan HC, Atkins JH. Free autogenous gingival grafts. I. Principles of successful grafting. *Periodontics* 1968;6(3):121–129.
22. Gordon HP, Sullivan HC, Atkins JH. Free autogenous gingival grafts. II Supplemental findings—histology of the graft site. *Periodontics* 1968;6(3):130–133.
23. Sullivan HC, Atkins JH. Free autogenous gingival grafts. 3. Utilization of grafts in the treatment of gingival recession. *Periodontics* 1968;6(4):152–160.
24. Cole RT, Crigger M, Bogle J, et al. Connective tissue regeneration to periodontally diseased teeth: a histological study. *J Periodontal Res* 1980;15:1–9.
25. Miller PD. Root coverage using a free soft tissue autograft following citric acid demineralization. Part 1: technique. *Int J Periodontics Restorative Dent* 1982;2(1):65–70.
26. Miller PD. Root coverage using a free soft tissue autograft following citric acid demineralization, Part III: a successful and predictable procedure in areas of deep wide recession. *Int J Periodontics Restorative Dent* 1985;5(2):15–37.
27. Langer B, Calagna LJ. The sub-epithelial connective tissue graft. New approach to the enhancement of anterior cosmetics. *Int J Periodontics Restorative Dent* 1982;2:22–33.
28. Raetzke PB. Covering localized areas of root exposure employing the "envelope" technique. *J Periodontol* 1985;56:397–402.
29. Langer B, Langer L. Subepithelial connective tissue graft technique for root coverage. *J Periodontol* 1985;56:715–720.
30. Nordland WP. Periodontal plastic surgery: esthetic gingival regeneration. *J Calif Dent Assoc* 1989;17(11):29–32.
31. Allen AL. Use of the supraperiosteal envelope in soft tissue grafting for root coverage. II. Clinical results. *Int J Periodontics Restorative Dent* 1994;14:303–315.
32. Miller PD. A classification of marginal tissue recession. *Int J Periodontics Restorative Dent* 1985;5:8–13.
33. Harris RJ. A comparative study of root coverage obtained with an acellular dermal matrix versus a connective tissue graft: Results of 107 recession defects in 50 consecutively treated patients. *Int J Periodontics Restorative Dent* 2000;20:51–59.
34. Hirsch A, Goldstein M, Goultschin J, et al. A 2-year follow-up of root coverage using sub-pedicle acellular dermal matrix allografts and subepithelial connective tissue autografts. *J Periodontol* 2005;76:1323–1328.
35. Loe H, Anerud A, Boysen H. The natural history of periodontal disease in man: prevalence, severity and extent of gingival recession. *J Periodontol* 1992;63(6):489–495.
36. O'Leary TJ, Drake RB, Jiniden GF, et al. The incidence of recession in young males: relationship to gingival and plaque scores. *Periodontics* 1968;6:109–111.
37. Coatman GW, Behrents RG, Bissada NF. The width of keratinized gingiva during orthodontic treatment: its significance and impact of periodontal status. *J Periodontol* 1981;52:307–313.
38. Dorfman HS. Mucogingival changes resulting from mandibular incisor tooth movement. *Am J Orthod* 1978;74:286–297.
39. Wennström JL, Lindhe J, Sinclair F, Thilander B. Some periodontal tissue reactions to orthodontic tooth movement in monkeys. *J Clin Periodontol* 1987;14:121–129.
40. Olsson M, Lindhe J. Periodontal characteristics in individuals with varying form of the upper central incisors. *J Clin Periodontol* 1991;18:78–82.
41. Whinston GJ. Frenotomy and mucobuccal fold resection used in periodontal therapy. *N Y Dent J* 1956;22:495–499.
42. Friedman N. Mucogingival surgery. *Texas Dent J* 1957;75:358–362.
43. Rodriguez-Ferrer HJ, Strahan JD, Newman HN. Effect of gingival health of removing overhanging margins of interproximal subgingival amalgam restorations. *J Clin Periodontol* 1980;7(6):457–462.
44. Harrison JD. Effect of retraction materials on the gingival sulcus epithelium. *J Prosthet Dent* 1961;11(3):514–521.
45. Ruel J, Schuessler PJ, Malamet K. Effect of retraction procedures on the periodontium in humans. *J Prosthet Dent* 1980;44:508–515.
46. Grippo JO. Abfractions: a new classification of a hard tissue lesion of the teeth. *J Esthet Dent* 1991;3:14–19.
47. Rees JS. The effect of variation in occlusal loading on the development of abfraction lesions: a finite element study. *J Oral Rehabil* 2002;29:188–193.
48. Whitehead SA, Wilson NH, Watts DC. Development of non-carious cervical notch lesions in vitro. *J Esthet Dent* 1999;11:332–337.
49. Harris RJ. A short-term and long-term comparison of root coverage with an acellular dermal matrix and a subepithelial graft. *J Periodontol* 2004;75:734–743.
50. Harris RJ. Histologic evaluation of connective tissue grafts in humans. *Int J Periodontics Restorative Dent* 2003;23:575–583.
51. Nickles M, Ratka-Kruger P, Neukranz E, et al. Ten-year results after connective tissue grafts and guided tissue regeneration for root coverage. *J Periodontol* 2010;81:827–836.
52. Lee YM, Kim JY, Seol YJ, et al. A 3-year longitudinal evaluation of subpedicle free connective tissue graft for gingival recession coverage. *J Periodontol* 2002;73:1412–1418.
53. Chambrone L, Sukekava F, Araujo MG, et al. Root-coverage procedures for the treatment of localized recession-type defects: a Cochrane systematic review. *J Periodontol* 2010;81:452–478.
54. Nordland WP, Garret S, Kiger R, et al. The effect of plaque control and root debridement in molar teeth. *J Clin Periodontol* 1987;14:231–236.
55. Steiner S, Crigger M, Egelberg J. Connective tissue regeneration to periodontally diseased teeth. II. Histologic observation of cases following replaced flap surgery. *J Periodontal Res* 1981;16(1):109–116.
56. Bruno JF, Bowers GM. Histology of a human biopsy section following the placement of a subepithelial connective tissue graft. *Int J Periodontics Restorative Dent* 2000;20:225–231.
57. Goldstein M, Natasky E, Boyan BD, et al. Coverage of previously carious roots is as predictable procedure as coverage of intact roots. *J Periodontol* 2002;73:1419–1426.
58. Nordland WP, de Souza LM, Swift EJ Jr. A connective tissue graft as a biologic alternative to Class V restorations in Miller Class I and II recession defects: case series. *Int J Periodontics Restorative Dent* 2016;36(1):21–27.
59. Javelet J, Torabinejad M, Danforth R. Isobutyl cyanoacrylate: a clinical and histologic comparison with sutures in closing mucosal incisions in monkeys. *Oral Surg Oral Med Oral Pathol* 1985;59:91–94.
60. Muller HP, Eger T. Masticatory mucosa and periodontal phenotype: a review. *Int J Periodontics Restorative Dent* 2002;22:172–183.
61. Burkhardt R, Lang NP. Coverage of localized gingival recessions: comparison of micro- and macrosurgical techniques. *J Clin Periodontol* 2005;32(3):287–293.
62. Zabalegui I, Sicilia A, Cambra J, et al. Treatment of multiple adjacent gingival recessions with the tunnel subepithelial connective tissue graft: a clinical report. *Int J Periodontics Restorative Dent* 1999;19:199–206.
63. Kurth JR, Kokich VG. Open gingival embrasures after orthodontic treatment in adults: prevalence and etiology. *Am J Orthod Dentofacial Orthop* 2001;120(2):116–123.

64. Kokich V. Ecthetics and anterior tooth position: an orthodontic perspective. Part III: mediolateral relationships. *J Esthet Dent* 1993;5(5):200–207.
65. Kokich V. Anterior dental esthetics: an orthodontic perspective, I—crown length. *J Esthet Dent* 1993;5:19–23.
66. Nordland WP, Tarnow DP. A classification system for the loss of papillary height. *J Periodontol* 1998;69:1124–1126.
67. Allen AL. Use of the gingival unit transfer in soft tissue grafting: report of three cases. *Int J Periodontics Restorative Dent* 2004;24:165–175.
68. Seibert JS. Reconstruction of the deformed, partially edentulous ridges, using full thickness onlay grafts. Part I. Technique and wound healing. *Compend Contin Educ Dent* 1983;4(5):437–453.
69. Seibert JS. Reconstruction of deformed, partially edentulous ridges, using full thickness onlay grafts, Part II. Prosthetic/periodontal interrelationships. *Compend Contin Educ Dent* 1983;4(6):549–562.
70. Stein RS. Pontic-residual ridge relationship: a research report. *J Prosth Dent* 1996;16:251–285.
71. Garber DA, Rosenberg ES. The edentulous ridge in fixed prosthodontics. *Compend Contin Educ Dent* 1981;2(4):212–223.
72. Calderon Y, Raviv E, Zalkind M, et al. Esthetic pontic receptor site development: a histologic study in rats. *J Esth Dent* 1995;7(3):95–98.
73. Ochsenbein C. Osseous resection in periodontal surgery. *J Periodontol* 1958;29(Suppl):15–26.
74. Charruel S, Perez C, Foti B, et al. Gingival contour assessment: clinical parameters useful for esthetic diagnosis and treatment. *J Periodontol* 2008;79:795–801
75. Robbins JW. Differential diagnosis and treatment of excess gingival display. *Pract Periodont Aesthet Dent* 1999;11(2):265–272.
76. Seibert J, Lindhe J. Esthetics and periodontal therapy. In: Lindhe J, ed. *Texbook of Clinical Periodontology*. Copenhagen: Munksgaard; 1989:431–467.
77. Pontoriero R, Carnevale G. Surgical crown lengthening: a 12-month clinical wound healing study. *J Periodontol* 2001;72(7):841–848.
78. Gargiulo AW, Wentz FM, Orban B. Dimensions and relations of the dentogingival junction in humans. *J Periodontol* 1961;32(3):261–267.
79. Palomo F, Kopczyk RA. Rationale and methods for crown lengthening. *J Am Dent Assoc* 1978;96:257–260.
80. Ingber JS, Rose LS, Coslet JG. The "biologic width"—a concept in periodontics and restorative dentistry. *Alpha Omegan* 1977;70(3):62–65.
81. Rosenberg ES, Garber DA, Evian CI. Tooth lengthening procedures. *Compend Contin Educ Gen Dent* 1980;1:161–172.
82. Van Dijken JWV, Pallesen U. Long-term dentin retention of etch-and-rinse and self-etch adhesives and a resin-modified glass ionomer cement in non-carious cervical lesions. *Dent Mater* 2008;24:915–922.

PART 7
PROBLEMS OF THE EMERGENCY AND FAILURE

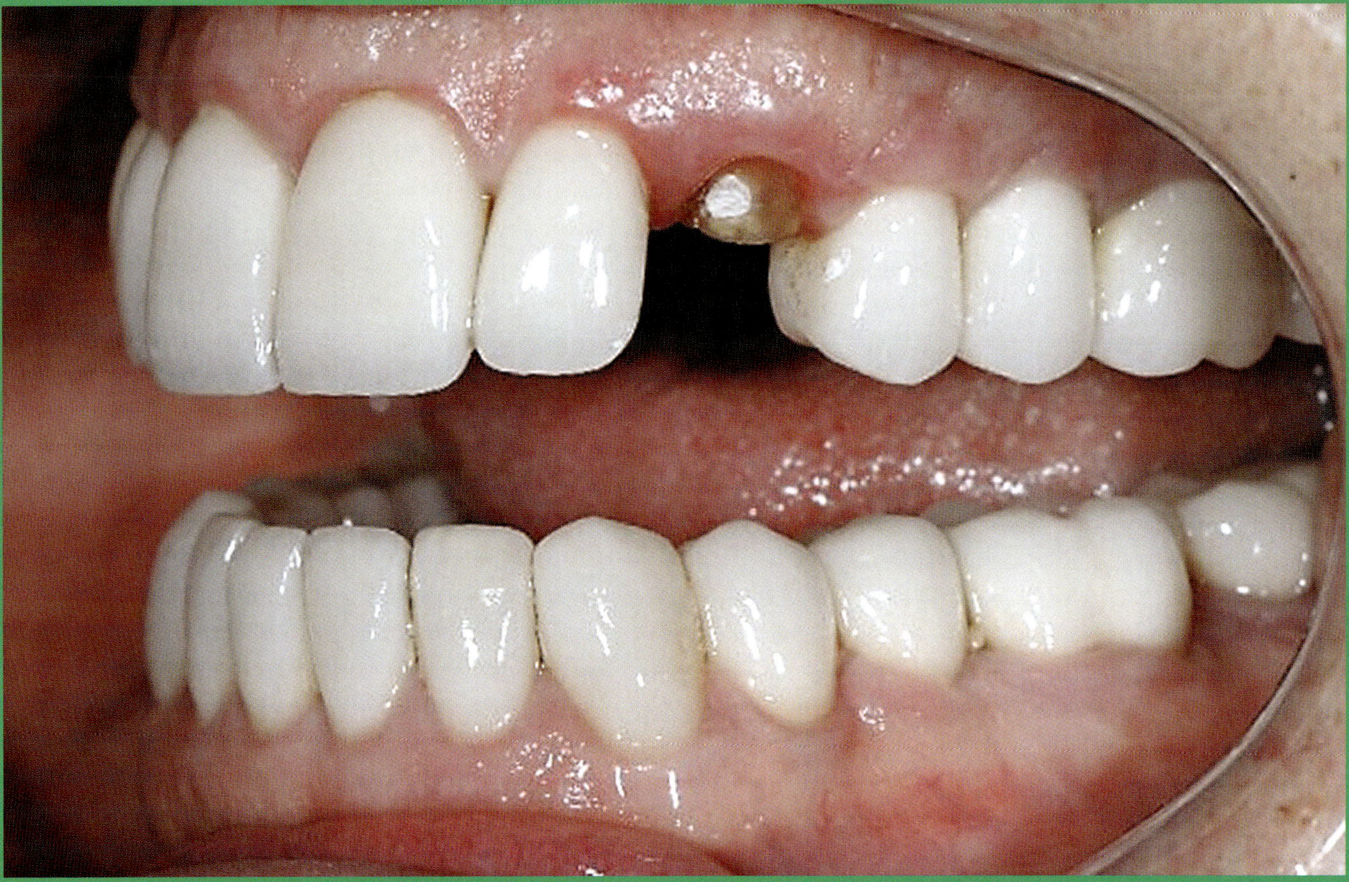

Chapter 38 Esthetic and Traumatic Emergencies

Ronald E. Goldstein, DDS and
Shane N. White, BDentSc, MS, MA, PhD

Chapter Outline

Long-term preservation is the goal	1215	Root fractures	1221
Crown fractures	1216	Luxation injuries	1223
Crown infractions	1216	Avulsions	1223
Uncomplicated enamel and dentin fractures	1216	Fractured restorations	1224
Complicated fractures involving the pulp	1219	Prosthesis fracture, failure, and repair	1231
Crown–root fractures	1221		

The patient who believes they have an esthetic emergency indeed has a real emergency. Psychosocial or life-quality effects are critical to patients. Esthetic and comfort-related issues are particularly important. The perception of a diminution in esthetics, or the psychological trauma associated with loss of a visible tooth, has profound effects on self-image and well-being, comparable to major family life events. Some patients may happily live with a fractured angle of a maxillary central incisor all their lives, whereas others may experience a significant esthetic emergency from a similar event. Perception of unattractive appearance is a major factor in causing patients to present with dental emergencies. Generally, the more severe the injury, the less patients are satisfied with their appearance.

The emergencies discussed in this chapter are primarily those caused by sudden trauma to the dentition. In these cases, the patient is generally seen as soon as possible. Conservative palliative measures are taken when it is not possible to provide more than temporary treatment. Prevention is of paramount importance particularly in athletics, where the use of mouth guards substantially reduces incidence and severity of trauma to the mouth. Dentists have a duty to inform their communities of the need for prevention, urgency, and the correct protocols for managing dental trauma.

Long-term preservation is the goal

The responsibility of the dentist is to facilitate the long-term preservation of the natural dentition, the supporting periodontium and bone, and the surrounding soft gingival tissues. Obviously, some circumstances make this impossible, but this obligation must be remembered when a patient is first seen. Unfortunately, many fractured crowns and roots are extracted when they could have been saved. Not only are precious teeth lost, but consequent changes to the alveolus and gingivae complicate restoration and esthetic replacement. Even if a tooth must be lost, measures can be taken to preserve the hard and soft tissues to facilitate esthetic replacement using an implant. Failure to recognize the need for appropriate multidisciplinary consultation may result in premature tooth, alveolar bone, and soft-tissue loss.

Accurate evaluation of the injury depends on a thorough history (when, where, and how the injury occurred) to make an accurate diagnosis and an optimal treatment plan.[1,2] The medical history should be reviewed for previous injuries and treatment, the general health of the patient, and the presence or absence of pain. Answers to these questions will indicate the nature of the accident, the potential loss of vitality of the injured teeth, the need of prophylactic medication, and the possibility of damage to the supporting structures of the teeth. The possibility of traumatic brain injury must be recognized and appropriate referral made or transportation sought, if necessary. Likewise, the need for a tetanus shot must be assessed. The World Health Organization Classification of Traumatic Injuries to the Dentition, as modified by Jens Andreasen, describes four broad types: luxation injuries to the periodontal tissues, injuries to hard dental tissues, injuries to the supporting bone, and injuries to gingiva and the oral mucosa.[3,4] Traumatic conditions such as avulsion, bony fracture, extrusive and lateral luxation, and root fracture are considered to be acute and demand immediate treatment. Subacute conditions, including intrusion, subluxation, pulpal concussion, and crown fracture with pulp exposure, necessitate treatment within 24 h. Treatment for crown fractures without pulp exposure may be delayed, unless, of course, it presents an esthetic emergency. Useful guidance can currently be found in the online resource "The Dental Trauma Guide" created by Rigshospitalet Denmark and the International Association of Dental Traumatology (https://dentaltraumaguide.org/).

Once the history is obtained, clinical and radiographic examinations determine the extent of trauma. Clinical examination should assess soft tissues, facial bones, teeth and their fractures, mobility, and pulpal status, as well as the periodontium and alveolus. When soft-tissue lacerations are involved, particularly the lips, it is important to ensure that there are no foreign objects or tooth fragments embedded in the tissue. This can be confirmed radiographically, but glass shards or other radiolucent objects may be difficult to identify. The radiographic evaluation may include dislocations, jaw fractures, root fractures, the stage of tooth development, the periodontal ligament space, and the pulp, including its size, conformation, and any resorptive or calcific changes. Periapical films may be made at different angles to provide three-dimensional information. Cone-beam computed tomography may provide useful three-dimensional information in complex cases. An intraoral camera, or even a camera in a mobile phone, can be a valuable diagnostic aid and can record images of the damage.

Follow-up examinations must be planned. Recalls are generally recommended at 1, 2, and 6 weeks, at 3, 6, and 12 months, and at 5 years.[5] Recall examinations must include very careful endodontic evaluations. Sequelae of traumatic injuries include pulp necrosis, pulp canal obliteration through calcific metamorphosis, internal and external root resorption, and ankylosis. The endodontic evaluation includes cold and electrical pulpal vitality tests, percussion, palpation, mobility, periodontal probing, transillumination, and radiographs. Teeth that become more yellow generally have vital pulps that have laid down secondary dentin, whereas teeth that become blue–grey due to infiltration of necrotic blood products into the dentin typically are necrotic, needing root canal treatment. External or internal bleaching can be used, as appropriate. It is important not to overlook esthetic evaluation when treating the emergency patient.

Crown fractures

The majority of esthetic emergencies involve fracture of the clinical crown. In younger patients, this is often due to falls, sports injuries, or other impacts. Automobile accidents, altercations, and contact-sport accidents are common causes of injury in older patients. The upper central incisors are by far the most common teeth to be traumatized. Fractures of the clinical crown are classified as enamel infractions, uncomplicated fractures, or complicated fractures, depending on the degree of tooth involvement.

Crown infractions

Crown infractions are cracks in the enamel that do not involve loss of tooth structure (Figure 38.1A and B). With coronal infractions, the anatomic shape of the tooth is unchanged, and the tooth appears normal radiographically. Fracture or craze lines are evident in the enamel, and are especially apparent with transillumination and intraoral photography. It is important to document infractions in the patient's chart, using photographs of the crack or craze lines present following an injury, to protect the patient especially in cases of insurance or legal liability. Fortunately, most enamel cracks are arrested at the dentinoenamel junction and do not pass into dentin.

If no other injuries are present, the treatment goal is simply to maintain the tooth structure and monitor pulp vitality.[1,5,6] Even though little other signs of injury are evident, impacts may be so great as to cause hemorrhage into the dentinal tubules of the injured tooth and pulpal death. The extent of damage in any injury is evaluated by carful history, examination, endodontic evaluation, and radiography. If the injury is complicated by pulpal hemorrhage, bleaching will be necessary to restore normal color to the tooth. Bleaching techniques for this situation are discussed in Chapter 12. Even if there is no apparent pulpal trauma at the time of the incident, the tooth should still be monitored at follow-up visits for delayed pulpal necrosis.

Uncomplicated enamel and dentin fractures

Uncomplicated crown fractures can involve enamel or both enamel and dentin without involving the pulp chamber. This type of fracture is usually seen on the incisal angles of maxillary central incisors. The prognosis and considerations for uncomplicated fractures involving only enamel are the same as for crown infractions. Treatment for uncomplicated fractures involving only enamel may range from simply smoothing fractured rough edges

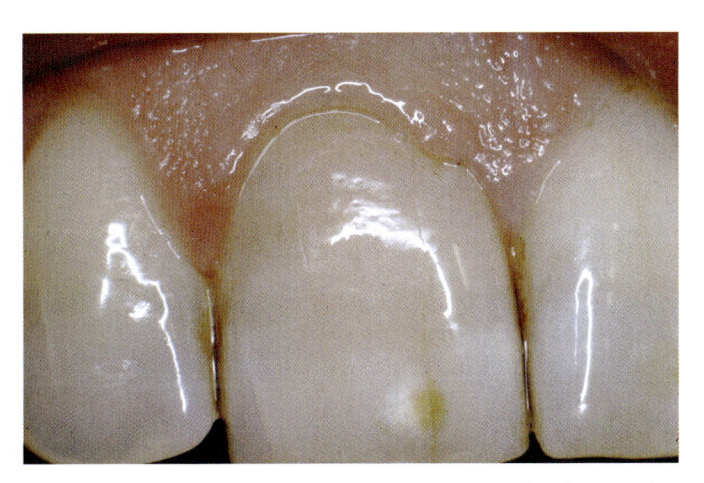

Figure 38.1 **(A)** This patient had a traumatic injury to her front teeth with no loss of enamel. However, it is important to document any craze or fracture lines present in case of any future legal or insurance liability.

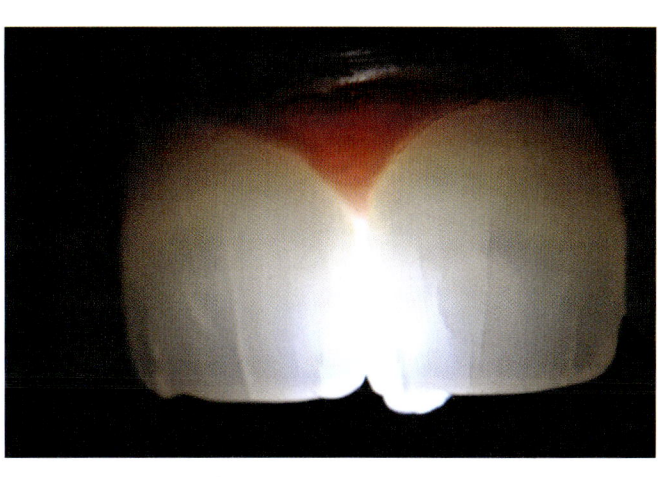

Figure 38.1 **(B)** Transillumination should also be used and photographically documented for the patient. Also, baseline radiographs must be taken to compare against possible future periapical abscess.

and preventing soft-tissue laceration, to placing a conservative-bonded composite restoration[5,6] (Figures 38.2 and 38.3). Parents and patients should be advised that tooth vitality should be monitored.

When injuries involve enamel and dentin, treatment becomes more elaborate.[7-9] Even a minimal amount of traumatically exposed dentin may be quite sensitive to thermal fluctuations, acidic drinks, citrus fruits, and bleaching agents. A great many dentinal tubules connect superficial dentin directly to the pulp. Sometimes, particularly in younger patients, these tubules are patent. Tubules provide a pathway for bacteria, osmotic gradients, and other stimuli to cause pulpal irritation and

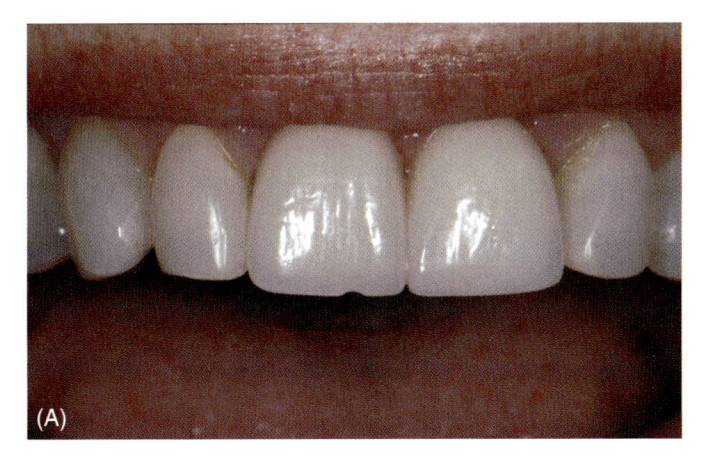

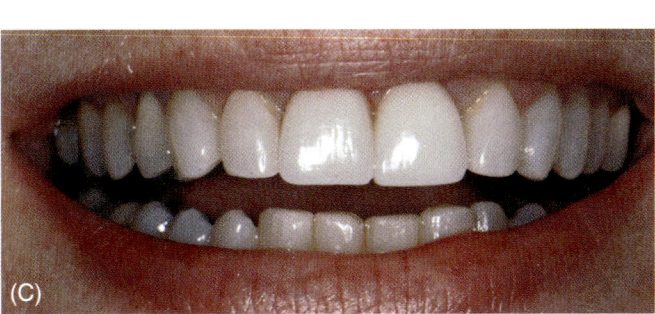

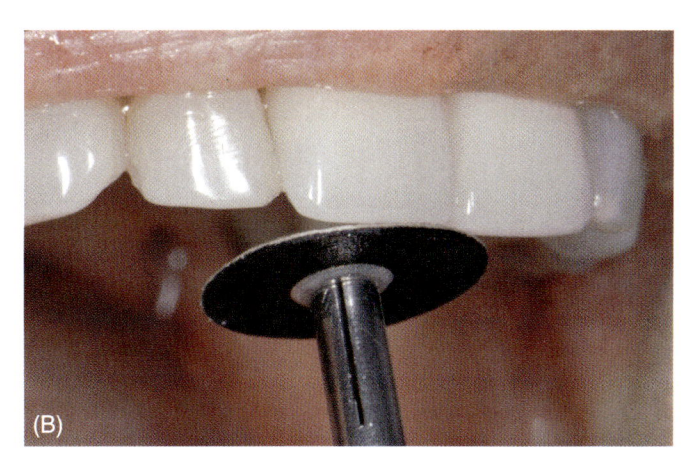

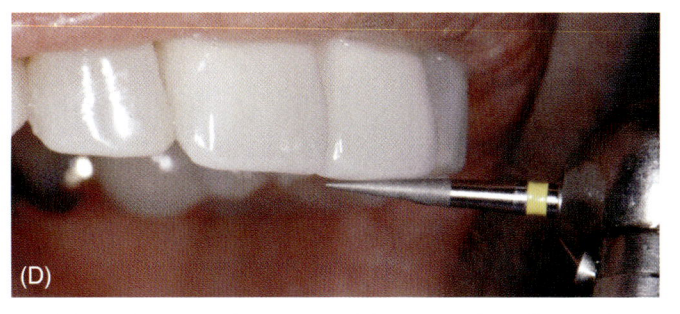

Figure 38.2 (A–D) Accidents involving small chips can many times be contoured depending upon the interincisal distance and its effect on the smile. It is a good idea to let the patient choose between restoring the incisal chip through composite resin bonding versus cosmetic contouring.

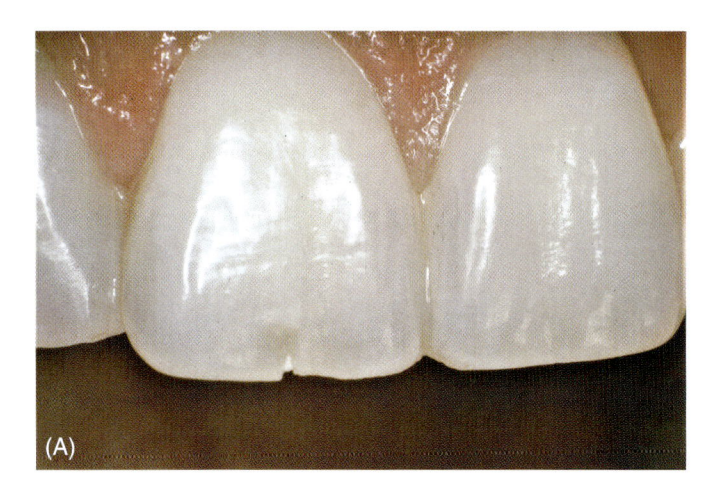

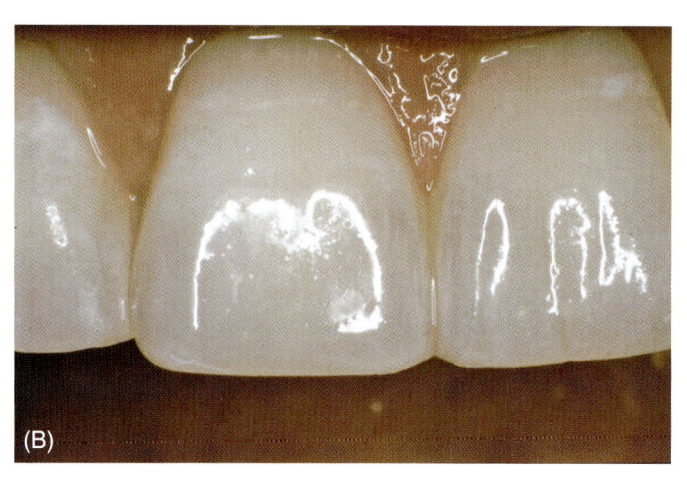

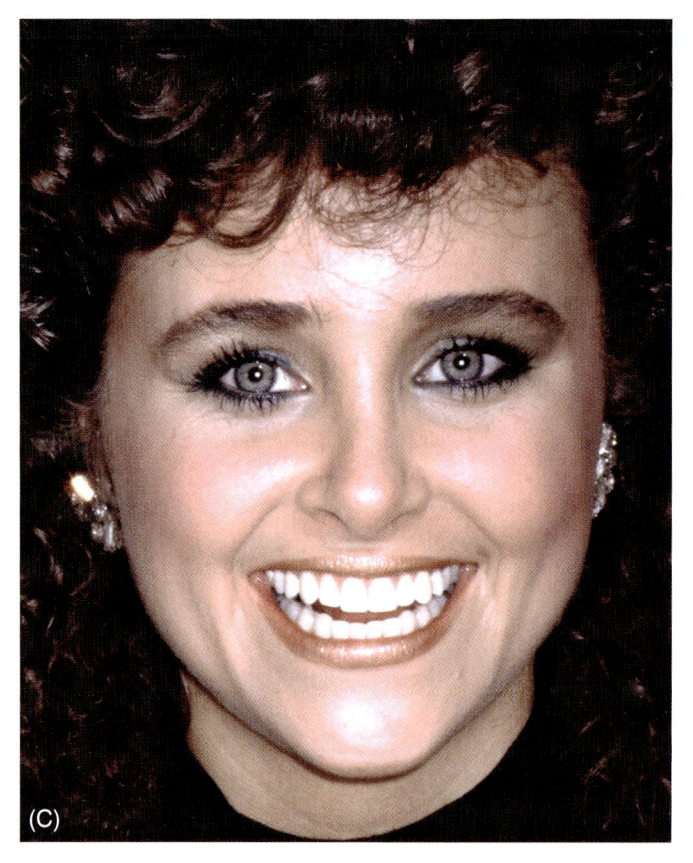

Figure 38.3 (A–C) In this patient, if contouring had been elected, the effect of reducing too much incisal enamel would have altered her smile line. As a result, composite resin bonding was the treatment of choice to restore her smile.

inflammation. Therefore, it is recommended that traumatically exposed dentin, which does not need to be restored or is awaiting restoration, be sealed (e.g., Gluma Desensitizer, Kulzer) to minimize the possibility of symptomatic irreversible pulpitis and pulpal necrosis developing. However, dentin that has become exposed due to gingival recession is more likely to have tubules that have become occluded through an external smear layer, cellular degeneration, or the deposition of secondary dentin.

Most fractures involving dentin necessitate restoration. In the past, a hard setting calcium hydroxide liner was often placed over the deeper dentin. It is now understood that providing an excellent seal to protect dentin from bacteria and their toxic by-products is of paramount importance. Hence, resin-modified glass ionomer bases have become widely used. They seal better than calcium hydroxide liners and have superior physical properties, superior esthetics, and release fluoride. They are also more user friendly than conventional acid–base glass ionomers and may be less likely to cause pulpal irritation. If the dentist chooses, a resin-modified glass ionomer base can be placed over a small calcium hydroxide liner in the area closest to the pulp.

Once the pulp is protected with a desensitizing agent, a hard calcium hydroxide liner, or a resin-modified glass ionomer base, the fractured tooth should receive a bonded composite resin

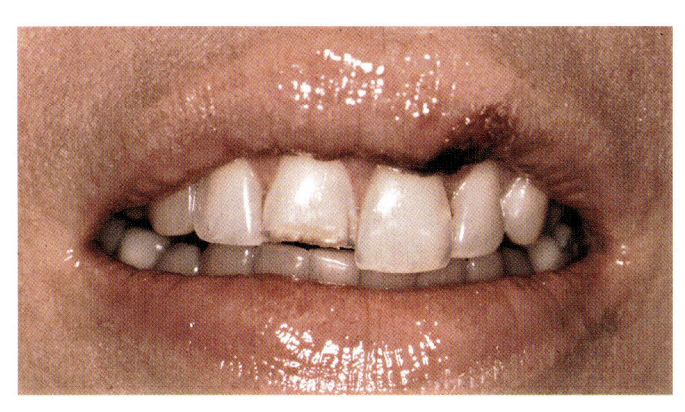

Figure 38.4 (A) Patient presented with fractured right central incisal immediately after an accident.

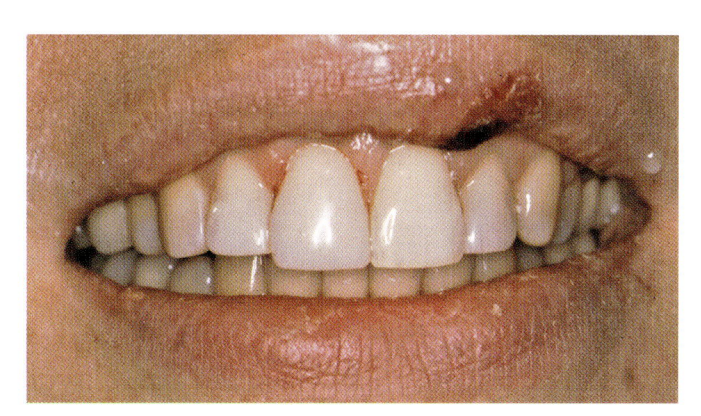

Figure 38.4 (B) Accidents where dentin is exposed are best treated conservatively with as little additional trauma to the tooth as possible. The patient's smile was restored using a resin-modified glass ionomer liner, followed by a combination of a hybrid composite to restore the incisal edge, and a microfill composite for better polish.

restoration (Figure 38.4A and B). This protects the pulp while producing an immediate esthetic result. Alternatively, the fractured coronal fragment may be bonded back into place. This technique, known as fragment bonding, has increased in popularity with improved modern dentinal bonding agents. This procedure has psychological and esthetic benefits, because the restoration will most closely resemble the tooth before the trauma occurred.[7,10–12] The goal of the initial visit with uncomplicated crown fracture is pulpal protection, comfort, and esthetics; the necessity for endodontic procedures will be determined at follow-up.

As for all dental traumas, the patient should be examined at regular intervals, as described earlier. A pulp may be concussed for a week or more after trauma, but then return to normality. Therefore, root canal treatment is generally not initiated until after follow-up examinations and after placement of a restoration that facilitates isolation. Pulpal vitality must be checked regularly. In cases where the root formation had not been completed, the goal is to maintain pulpal vitality as long as possible, so that root formation can be completed. Whether the root is mature or immature, it is very important that a dying or dead pulp be identified before apical pathology has developed. The lesser the magnitude and duration of the pathology, the better the prognosis for root canal treatment.

In most cases, the emergency-bonded composite restoration will be the definitive restorative treatment. Even if root canal treatment is needed, no further restorative treatment will likely be needed, other than closure of the access cavity with another bonded composite restoration. The patient is told that it may last for 3–5 years, but can be repaired and polished as needed. Should a bonded composite restoration be esthetically inadequate, then a conservative porcelain veneer could be placed, even if root canal treatment has been performed. Posts do not strengthen teeth; crown preparation weakens anterior teeth. There is no reason to further reduce the tooth if the patient is pleased with esthetic result.

Complicated fractures involving the pulp

In the permanent dentition, complicated fractures are rarer than uncomplicated fractures. For permanent teeth with mature roots, emergency treatments include direct pulp capping, which will generally need to be followed by root canal treatment; pulpectomy, which will need to be followed by root canal treatment; and root canal treatment at the initial visit.[5,6,9] The best prognosis for a direct pulp cap is for a small traumatic exposure, without contamination, without pain, and which is performed immediately after the traumatic accident, but in the long term the prognosis for pulpal survival in mature teeth is guarded. Rubber dam isolation must be used absolutely for any procedures involving the pulp and is strongly recommended whenever traumatically exposed dentin is encountered or when adhesive procedures are being performed (Figure 38.6A–F).

For permanent teeth with immature roots, the goal is to maintain pulpal vitality through vital pulp therapy or apexogenesis, at least until formation of the entire root has been completed.[1] In this situation, a high or shallow pulpotomy, the Cvek technique, is usually used. The tooth is isolated, and pulpal tissue is gently removed to approximately 2 mm below the exposure using a small water-cooled round diamond bur. The pulp is rinsed with sterile saline, hemostasis is achieved, the clot is gently rinsed away, and a hard calcium hydroxide liner is placed, followed by a glass ionomer or resin-modified glass ionomer base, and then by a bonded composite restoration. Alternatively, MTA (Mineral Trioxide Aggregate, Dentsply) can be placed over the pulp instead of a hard setting calcium hydroxide liner. MTA has advantages in that it can be used in a damp field, seals well against dentin, and is bacteriostatic. However, because it sets slowly, its manufacturer recommends checking at a subsequent appointment prior to restoration. It is likely that quicker setting variants of MTA will soon be introduced. Although traumatized teeth with pulpal exposures should be seen within 24 h, the shallow pulpotomy may still be successful even after a week's exposure.

If the pulp in an immature permanent tooth becomes necrotic, or is already necrotic, then nonvital therapy or apexification is performed.[1,5] The tooth is isolated, carefully and thoroughly debrided, a nonsetting calcium hydroxide paste placed, and a durable provisional restoration made. Nonsetting calcium

Clinical case 38.1

Problem

A 17-year-old student fell while skateboarding and suffered an uncomplicated enamel–dentin fracture of his upper left central incisor (Figure 38.5A). He was not otherwise injured. He located the lost tooth fragment and immediately attended the dentist.

Treatment

Rubber dam isolation was immediately provided. The patient described dentin sensitivity to air and contact by his tongue, but not pain, and requested that local anesthesia not be provided. The fragment and tooth were treated with a multipurpose bonding agent and reunited using a dual-cure resinous cement designed for porcelain veneers. Excess cement was gently trimmed using a multi-fluted carbide finishing bur and then polished using copious water spray.

Result

The patient appreciated the fragment reattachment procedure; he explained that he had a similar accident 3 years before, losing 2 mm from his upper right central incisor (Figure 38.5B). Although that composite restoration had undergone noticeable wear, the patient elected to leave it as is. Given his skateboarding history, the use of a mouthguard was advised.

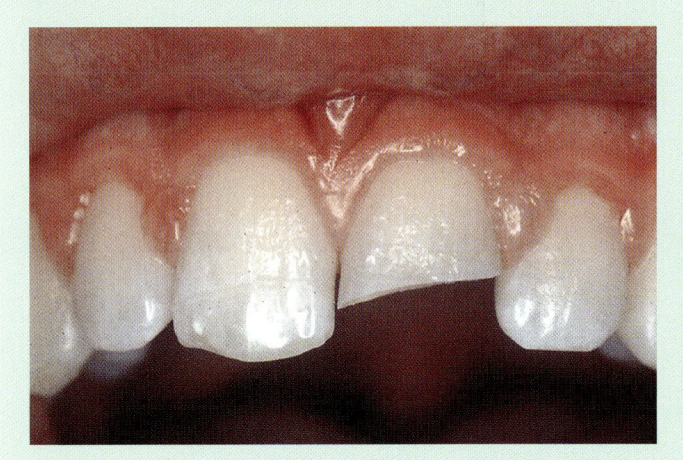

Figure 38.5 (A) This 17-year-old boy fell and fractured his left central incisor while skateboarding. Since it was an uncomplicated enamel–dentin fracture and the patient was able to locate the lost tooth fragment, it was decided to do the most conservative esthetic treatment and reattach the fractured tooth segment.

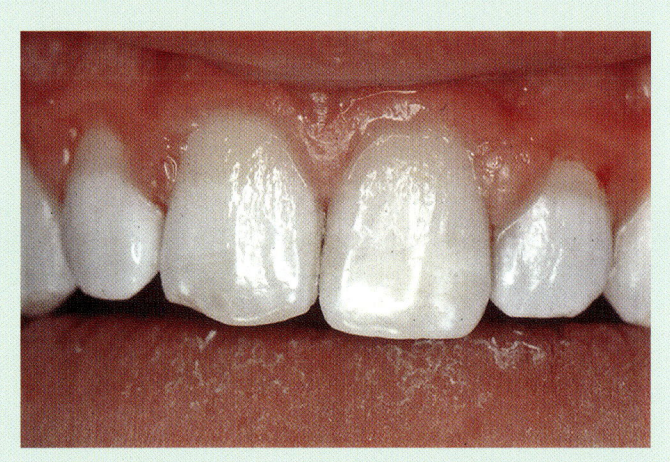

Figure 38.5 (B) The fragment and tooth were treated with a multipurpose bonding agent and reunited using a dual-cure resin cement.

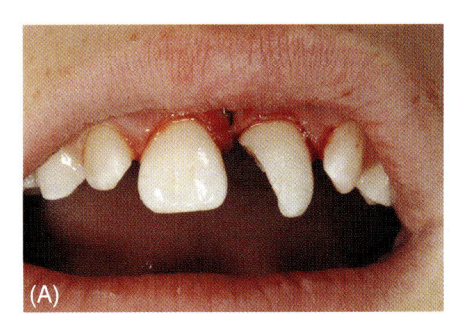

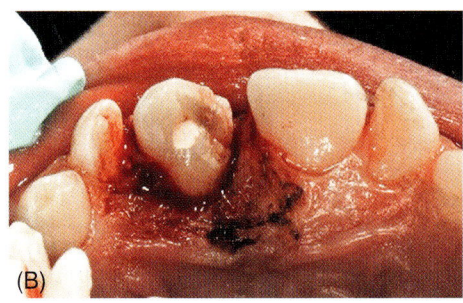

Figure 38.6 (A, B) This 14-year-old boy presented after a fall that fractured the maxillary left central incisor. The patient was referred for endodontics and returned for restoration of the fractured tooth.

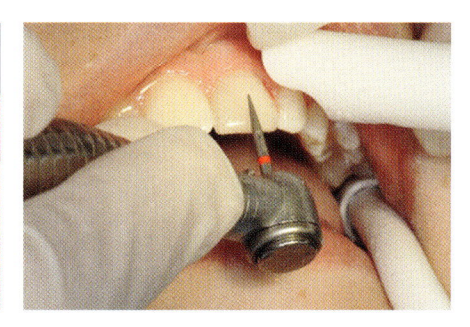

Figure 38.6 (C) Tooth was bonded with composite resin and contoured with a 30-μm diamond (DET-6F, Brasseler USA).

hydroxide paste is bactericidal. Typically, after 3–6 months, a delicate calcific barrier is formed across the root apex, but root formation remains incomplete. Then, the calcium hydroxide is carefully removed, a conventional gutta-percha obturation performed, and the access closed and a definitive coronal restoration made. Alternatively, an apical plug of MTA can be placed after brief placement of calcium hydroxide for 1 week to 1 month, and after setting has been checked a conventional gutta-percha obturation is performed.

In the primary dentition, emergency treatment may include pulpotomy, root canal treatment, or extraction.[1,13,14] If the roots are more than half resorbed, extraction is recommended. If root canal treatment is chosen, a resorbable paste should be used for obturation without gutta-percha or other nonresorbable obturating materials.

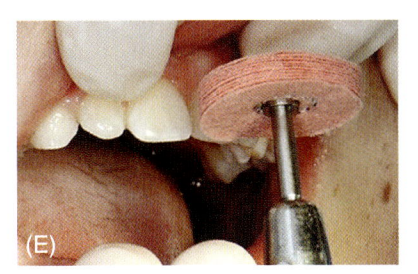

Figure 38.6 (D, E) Final polish was done using abrasive disks (Sof-Lex 3-M) and a polishing wheel (Brasseler USA).

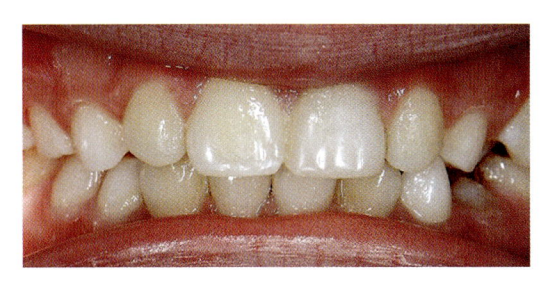

Figure 38.6 (F) Youthful texture surface was incorporated for the most natural look in the final restoration.

As for uncomplicated crown fractures, the conservative-bonded composite is the restoration of choice. Conservative porcelain veneers may be used when extensive destruction has occurred. Posts should be avoided unless there is absolutely no other way to retain the final coronal restoration. Crown preparation should be avoided unless almost all of the coronal tooth structure has been lost.

Crown–root fractures

Crown–root fractures involve enamel, dentin, and cementum.[5,6,9] Careful diagnosis, treatment, and follow-up are necessary even though they only constitute a small proportion of tooth injuries. Anterior teeth are usually injured by direct trauma; posterior teeth are usually injured by indirect trauma. Crown–root fractures may be vertical, horizontal, or oblique; they are often difficult to diagnose visually or radiographically because of their location and orientation. Unless the X-ray beam is almost exactly parallel to the fracture plane, a fracture may not be seen. Fractured tooth and bone fragments may be held in place by the periodontal ligament without any visible displacement and be clinically indiscernible.

Vertical crown–root fractures generally have a very poor prognosis; extraction is often indicated for both primary and permanent teeth (see Chapter 23, Figure 23.14B and C). Some crown–root fractures may be uncomplicated, not exposing the pulp. Uncomplicated crown–root fractures may be managed in the ways described earlier for enamel and dentin fractures. As with other fractures, the pulp should be protected and then the patient should be functionally and esthetically stabilized. Many crown–root fractures are complicated, involving the pulp. Complicated crown–root fractures should receive pulpal management as described earlier for complicated crown fractures involving the pulp. Once the pulp has been treated, the tooth should be temporarily restored until the situation is stable enough to determine a definitive restorative treatment plan. As an interim procedure, loose tooth fragments may be bonded together. Nonrigid splinting to adjacent teeth may be helpful.

Subgingival extension of more than 3 or 4 mm by crown–root fractures requires orthodontic extrusion to expose the fracture surface and allow tooth preparation for full crown or other restorations.[7,15,16] Orthodontic extrusion is preferred to periodontal surgical crown lengthening because the gingival form is preserved. Fractures extending more deeply may require prophylactic root canal treatment, followed by a post and core. Because the restorative prognosis of an endodontically treated tooth is dependent on the bulk of remaining tooth structure, particularly on the height of the remaining dentin stump height, consideration should be given to extraction and replacement using an implant single crown restoration. Likewise, if the crown-to-root ratio is likely to exceed 1 : 1, consideration should be given to extraction and replacement using an implant single crown restoration, which can be seen in Figure 38.7A–H.

Root fractures

Root fractures involve the cementum, dentin, and pulp of injured teeth and represent a small percentage of fractures to permanent teeth.[5,6,9] This type of fracture is rarely seen in deciduous teeth prior to root development. Cementum and dentin are dynamically vital tissues with definite reparative capacities.

Andreasen and Hjortling-Hansen list four types of healing that can occur between the fragments of a root fracture: healing by hard calcified tissue, healing with the interposition of connective tissue, healing with bony interposition, and nonhealing with the interposition of granulation tissue.[17] These are listed in order of most to least favorable prognosis. The first type of healing by hard calcified tissue is the most desirable. In the past, rigid fixation was used for 2–3 months with the aim of healing by bony ankylosis, whereas current approaches use nonrigid splinting for 3–4 weeks for all root fractures with abnormal mobility—except for cervical fractures, when longer periods of up to 3–4 months may be needed—with the aim of preserving the periodontal ligament and avoiding ankylosis.

A wide variety of root fractures occur. If there are no symptoms and no abnormal mobility, then no treatment is indicated. If the coronal segment is mobile, then nonrigid splinting is indicated. If the coronal segment has been displaced, it should be precisely repositioned. If abnormal mobility is present, nonrigid splinting should be used, as already described. It is important to ensure that the tooth is not subjected to occlusal trauma.

A wide variety of pulpal scenarios occur; careful endodontic and radiographic examination and follow-up is critical. Most often, the pulp in both segments remains vital and healthy, and

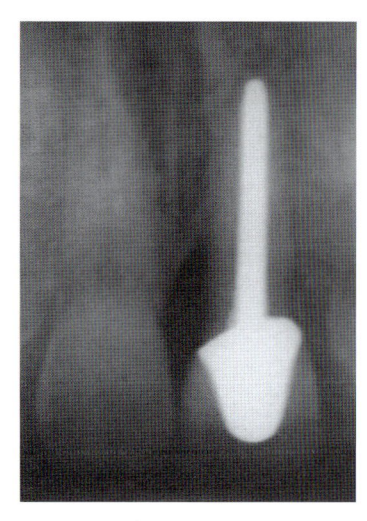

Figure 38.7 (A) This patient fractured his maxillary left central incisor diagonally to the base of the 8 mm mesial defect.

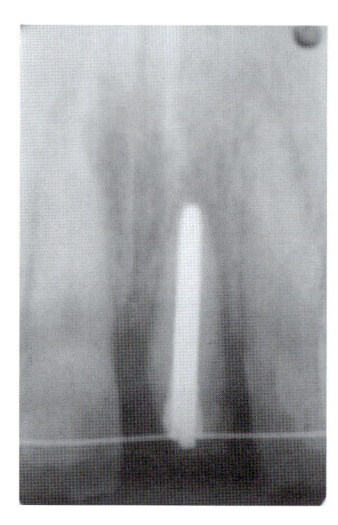

Figure 38.7 (B) The bone defect was corrected through orthodontic extrusion as seen in the above radiograph.

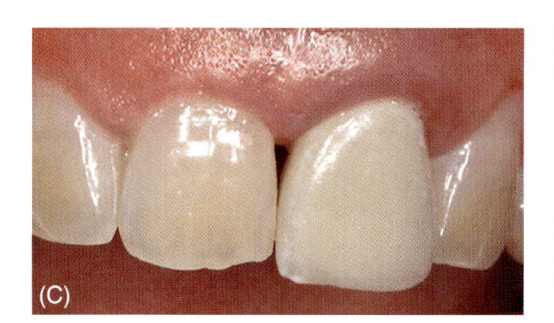

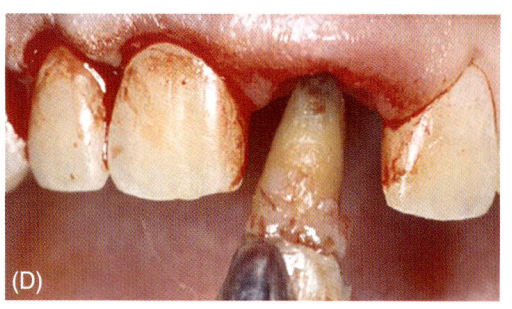

Figure 38.7 (C, D) It is clear to see in these photographs of the patient's anterior incisor how the left central incisor was extruded before extraction.

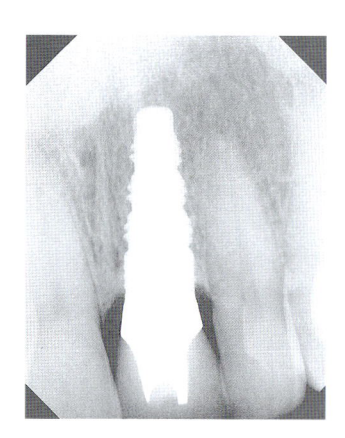

Figure 38.7 (E) This radiograph shows the implant and crown after the crown was seated.

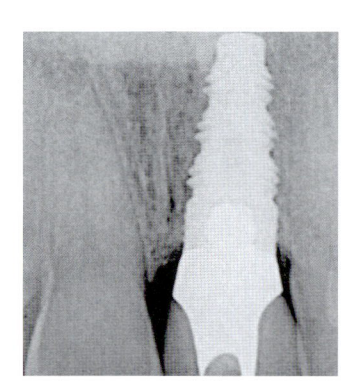

Figure 38.7 (F) Ten years postoperative shows the bone is still stable.

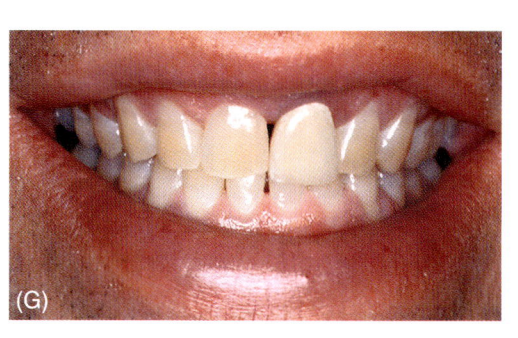

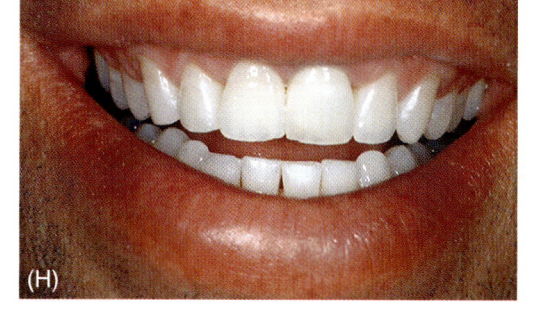

Figure 38.7 (G, H) These before and after photographs show both the functional and esthetic improvement for this young man, who received not only the implant and single crown but also crown lengthening and bleaching.

root canal treatment is not necessary. If both coronal and apical segments become necrotic, both should receive root canal treatment, if possible. If a necrotic apical segment cannot be directly accessed, then the coronal segment should receive root canal treatment and the apical segment should be removed. If the coronal segment becomes necrotic, but the apical segment remains vital, then only the coronal segment needs to receive root canal treatment.

Orthodontic extrusion can be used for root fractures at or near the alveolar crest, but if the crown-to-root ratio is likely to exceed 1 : 1, consideration should be given to extraction and replacement using an implant single crown restoration. In the past, intraradicular splints were sometimes used to unite the coronal and apical segments of fractured roots or to replace the apical fragment and stabilize the tooth.

Primary teeth with root fractures may also be splinted nonrigidly; they can be retained and will usually be shed normally.[13,14] When primary teeth are grossly injured, the coronal fragment should be extracted; but no attempt should be made to retrieve the apical fragment to avoid injuring the succedaneous tooth bud. The apical fragment will eventually be resorbed.[1] Some root-fractured teeth are difficult to diagnose. Others are impossible to save, for which extraction and placement of implant is the treatment of choice.

Luxation injuries

Luxations are injuries to the tooth-supporting structures that result in dislocation or displacement of teeth in the alveolus. They range from concussion to subluxation; extrusive, lateral, and intrusive luxations; and avulsion. The displacement may be vertical or horizontal—a tooth that is displaced by trauma seldom fractures. The patient may complain of a diffuse ache in the affected area or may be free of pain. The injury may cause numbness and accompanying soft-tissue damage. Treatment of luxation injuries depends on the extent of the trauma.[1,5,6] Although many teeth with luxation injuries may need root canal treatment, especially intrusive luxations, others may not; concussions and subluxations rarely need root canal treatment.

Concussion and subluxation involve mild injury to the periodontium; the tooth is tender to touch and biting, but it is not displaced and has normal mobility. The use of a flexible splint for 7–10 days is optional. Follow-up including careful pulpal evaluation is needed. As for all luxation injuries and avulsions, the patient is instructed to have a soft diet, brush with a soft brush after every meal, and to rinse with 0.12% chlorhexidine twice a day for 1 week.

Extrusive luxation is characterized by axial extrusion out of its socket. It is managed by precise repositioning and nonrigid splinting for up to 3 weeks with the same patient instructions outlined directly above. Teeth with mature roots will usually need root canal treatment. Immature teeth will receive periodic recall and careful pulpal evaluation; if they become necrotic, they should receive nonvital therapy or apexification, as described earlier.

Lateral luxation is characterized by lateral displacement, being firmly locked in its new position, and often by an ankylotic metallic tone on percussion. It is managed as for extrusive luxation; but if the marginal bone becomes broken down, the splinting time is increased to 6–8 weeks.

Intrusive luxation is characterized by intrusion into its socket and often by a dull tone on percussion. Mature teeth will almost always need root canal treatment; this is usually delayed until a week or two after the injury. Mature teeth will need orthodontic extrusion or surgical repositioning. Immature teeth generally undergo spontaneous reeruption; they must be closely monitored for pulpal changes or root resorption, which necessitate immediate root canal treatment.

Primary teeth with luxation injuries will generally not need pulpal treatment. Nonrigid splinting is recommended for primary teeth that are mobile after a luxation injury. However, if a primary tooth is significantly displaced, extraction is usually recommended.[13,14]

A splint should be quick to place, not cause any additional trauma, be stable throughout the splinting period, avoid damaging the gingiva or mucosa, facilitate root canal treatment, if needed, and be esthetic. Flexible orthodontic wire, nylon monofilament fishing line (60 lb breaking strain), or other flexible woven polyethylene fibers (e.g., Ribbond) can be used. They are simply point bonded to the facial enamel and must allow physiologic movement. It is important that rigid fixation is avoided so as to reduce the possibility of ankylosis and resorption, and so as to increase the likelihood of periodontal healing.

Two examples of luxation injuries and their treatment follow (Figures 38.8 and 38.9). The patient shown in Figure 38.8A received a luxation injury 24 years ago. He was hit in the mouth when a horse bolted, and the maxillary left central incisor was forced down and lingually into the mouth and the right central incisor was loosened. A tongue depressor was used as the patient bit down, and the teeth were mechanically pushed back into position. No further treatment was performed, and years later the pulps still test vital. (Note the absence of apical pathology in Figure 38.7B.) Clinical case 38.2 was more complex and involved extensive repositioning maneuvers.

Avulsions

A tooth completely avulsed, or exarticulated, from its socket because of injury can be replanted with a relatively good prognosis.[5,18] A clinical examination should be completed to determine if there are crown, root, or alveolar fractures, or obvious contaminants such as soil. The key factors for prognosis are the time outside the socket, the storage conditions, and the stage of root development. Before replantation, the following factors must be checked: presence of gross caries, existing advanced periodontal disease, gross fracture of the alveolar socket, and severe orthodontic crowding.

A good prognosis is achieved when the tooth is replanted within 30 min; the less time out of the socket, just a few minutes, the better. If the tooth was out of the socket for less than an hour,

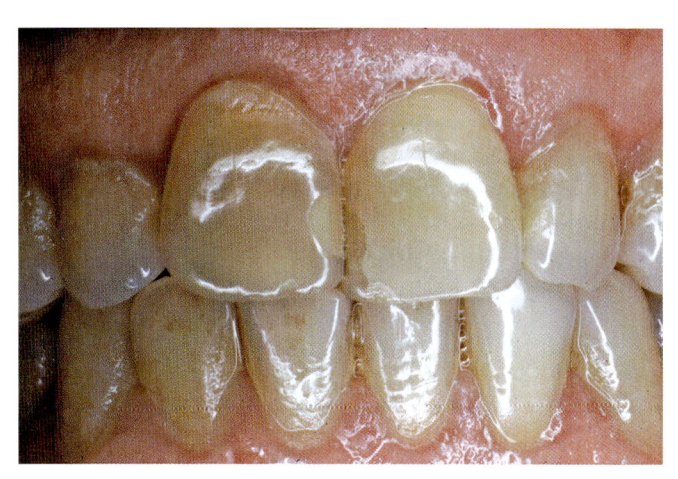

Figure 38.8 (A) Patient presented 24 years later after a luxation injury in which he was hit in the mouth as a horse bolted and caused the maxillary left central incisor to be forced down and lingually and the right central incisor loosened. The teeth were repositioned back into place using a tongue depressor as the patient bit down and no further treatment was performed.

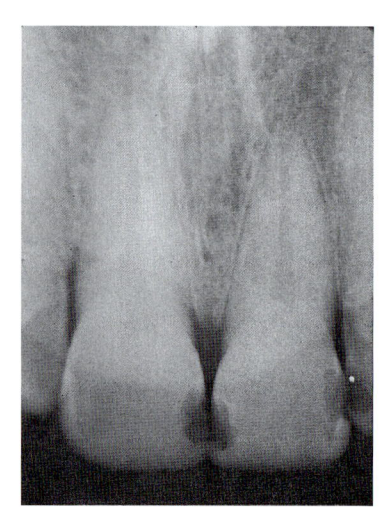

Figure 38.8 (B) Years later, the tooth still tests vital and there were no signs of apical pathology.

root canal treatment is initiated within 7–10 days to prevent external inflammatory root resorption. If the tooth was out of the socket for more than 1 h, little can be done to prevent replacement root resorption. The best prognosis will be when the tooth has been replanted almost immediately, the preferred course of action. Only if the tooth cannot be immediately replanted should it be stored and transported. The order of preference of storage media, from best to worst is: a commercially available purpose-designed storage solution (e.g., Save-A-Tooth), milk, saline, and saliva. Inappropriate nonphysiologic osmolality or pH damages the periodontal ligament cells, making healing less likely. Mature teeth should have root canal treatment initiated within 7–10 days of replantation, after some stability and comfort have been reached, so as to prevent inflammatory root resorption. Immature roots have the best prognosis. Pulpal revascularization is possible. Endodontic treatment is generally avoided. It may take up to 3 months for the return of a normal pulpal response to cold and electric testing. Only if needed should nonvital therapy, or apexification, be initiated, as described earlier.

When replanting an avulsed tooth, hold the tooth by the crown, not by the root, and simply rinse the tooth in saline or under cold running water, taking care not to drop the tooth down a drain. Do not scrub the root or treat it with disinfectants. Replace the tooth in the socket. Verify the position clinically and radiographically. Place a flexible nonrigid splint for 1 week. Suture any gingival lacerations. Prophylactic antibiotics should be prescribed. Arrangements should be made for a tetanus shot, or a booster shot, if the last one was more than 5 years ago. Follow-up appointments should be scheduled (Figure 38.10 A–G).

Reimplantation can also be performed on primary teeth.[13,14] It is a temporary measure, but an excellent method for maintaining space until a more permanent procedure is indicated. Despite the uncertain prognosis, reimplantation is still advisable in children and young people when the jaws have not yet attained maximum growth and development, when a replacement would be difficult, and when the psychological impact of tooth loss might cause irreparable harm.

Fractured restorations

Patients accumulate direct and indirect restorations, composite and amalgam fillings, veneers, onlays, crowns, tooth and implant-supported fixed dental prostheses, and removable prostheses. No matter how well a restoration is made, it has the potential for degradation and complication. Fracture follows only secondary caries as the most common reason for replacement of all types of restorations. Porcelain fracture, just as a fracture of tooth structure or cusp fracture, adjacent to restorations is a common occurrence.[19] Implant-supported crowns appear to have a particularly high incidence of esthetic and prosthetic complications. Recurrent caries makes restoration and tooth fracture more likely; caries must be fully addressed at the time of repair, if repair is even possible (Figure 38.11A–D). Unfortunately, these fractures most commonly occur in visible areas, creating esthetic emergencies.[20] Most fractured restorations are best and esthetically repaired using highly filled hybrid composite resins along with a multipurpose bonding agent, after surface roughening[21] (Figure 38.12A–N).

Although replacement of the prosthesis may ultimately be recommended, patients may need an immediate interim repair (Figure 38.13). Others may not have the time or financial means to replace a restoration or prosthesis at the time of fracture. It is important to stress to the patient that no repair is as strong as the original prosthesis, and it is at a higher risk of failure. Repair of defects to otherwise sound restorations is now widely taught in dental schools around the world. Many authorities favor repair to replacement. Repair can be more conservative of tooth

Clinical case 38.2: Injury involving luxation

Problem

A 28-year-old female was in an automobile accident that crushed the maxillary anterior segment (Figure 38.9A). The maxillary right central incisor was avulsed, and the right lateral and left lateral were fractured. The central incisor was pushed in so far that the patient could not close her mouth.

Treatment

The crushed maxillary right central incisor was repositioned by hand so that the patient could close in normal occlusion (Figure 38.9B). It is important when repositioning teeth or a segment, by hand or instrument, to esthetically align the luxated part. Teeth that were previously rotated can be made straight and then mechanically bonded with composite resin.

The missing tooth was replaced with an acrylic tooth (Figure 38.9C). Since the luxated segment had to be completely splinted, the six anterior teeth were etched to place a strong splinting action across the front. The area was washed and etched with 37% phosphoric acid. Figure 38.9D shows the area when dried and the amount of etching achieved. The entire area was bonded with composite resin, shaped, finished, and glazed (Figure 38.9E). Endodontic treatment was then performed on the left central incisor and three mandibular incisors.

Result

Teeth that are extrusively or laterally luxated in accidents should be repositioned immediately and be nonrigidly splinted to facilitate healing of the periodontium. This way, the patient can function normally until routine dental rebuilding procedures can be performed.

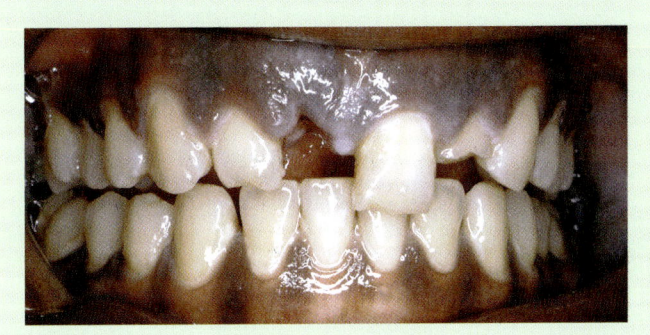

Figure 38.9 (A) A 28-year-old female presented after an automobile accident that caused the maxillary right central incisor to be avulsed, and the right lateral and left lateral were fractured.

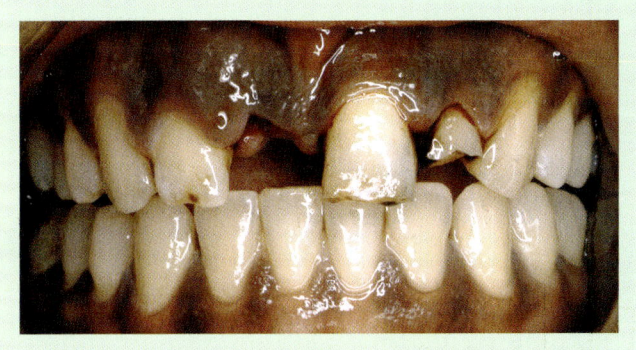

Figure 38.9 (B) The maxillary left central incisor was repositioned by hand, so the patient could close into normal position.

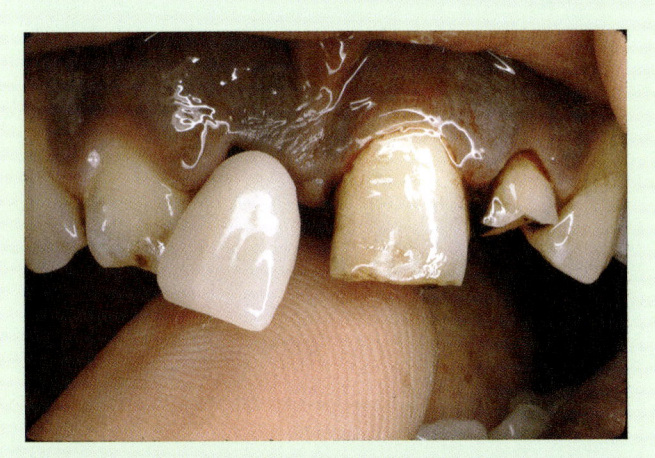

Figure 38.9 (C) The missing tooth was replaced with an acrylic tooth and the luxated segment had to be splinted across the front.

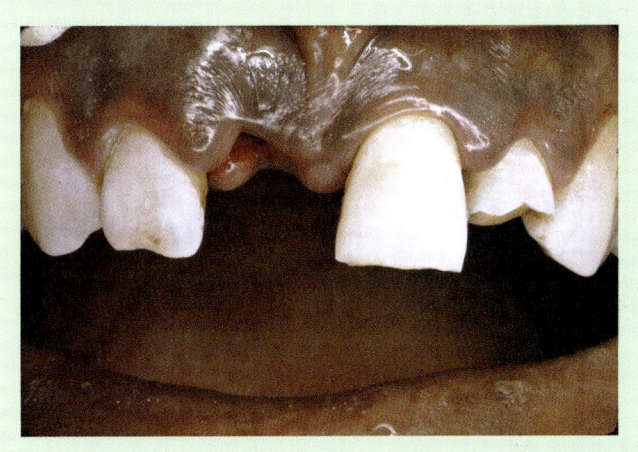

Figure 38.9 (D) The amount of etching achieved is shown when the area is dried.

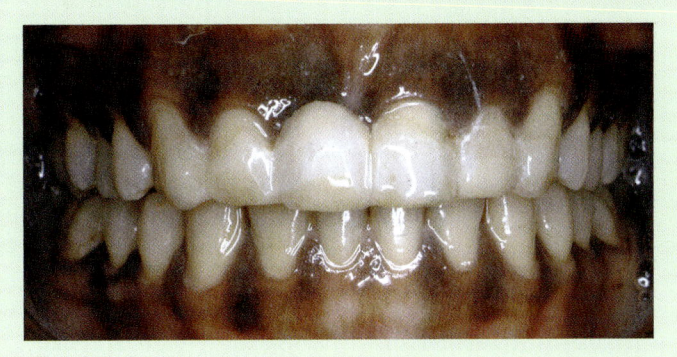

Figure 38.9 (E) The entire area was bonded with composite resin and polished.

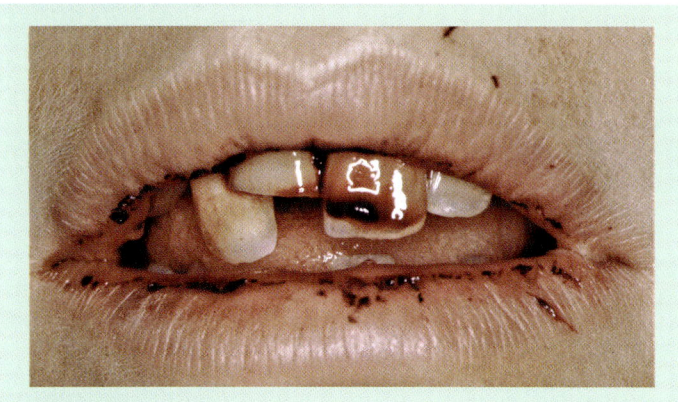

Figure 38.10 (A) A 25-year-old female dental assistant presented for emergency dental treatment after an automobile accident at 1 a.m.

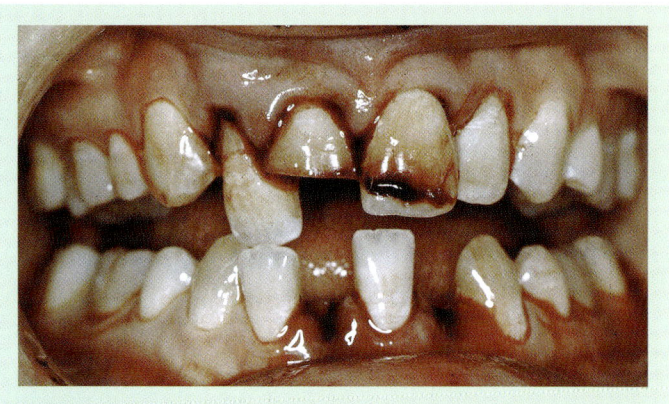

Figure 38.10 (B) The maxillary right lateral incisor plus mandibular right central incisors were avulsed, and the maxillary right central incisor was fractured into the pulp.

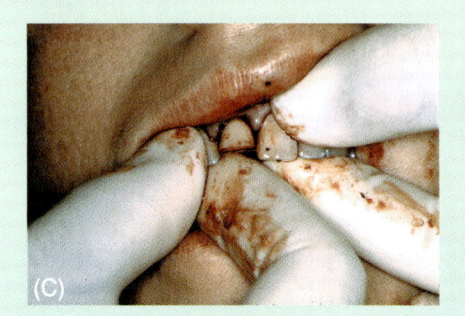

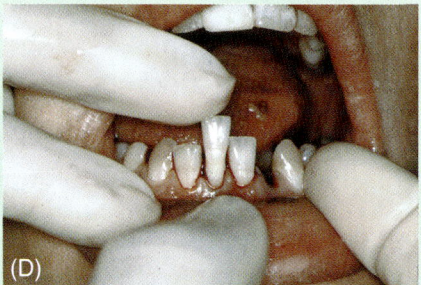

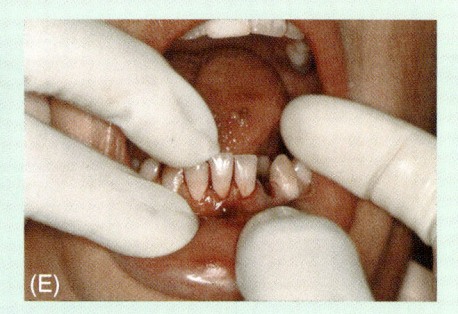

Figure 38.10 (C–E) Following local anesthetic, the avulsed teeth were repositioned back into place.

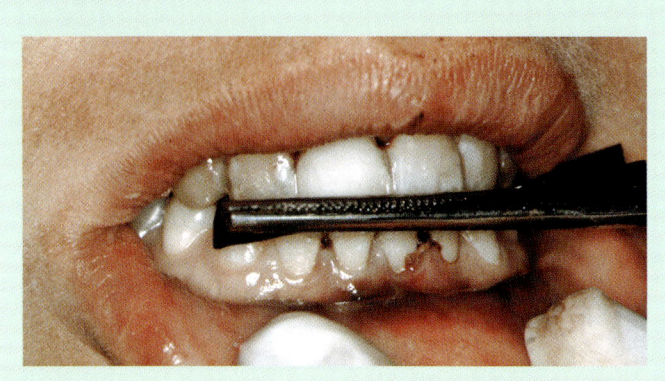

Figure 38.10 (F) After temporary bonding of the maxillary right central incisor, the anterior segments were carefully equilibrated to avoid any occlusal trauma.

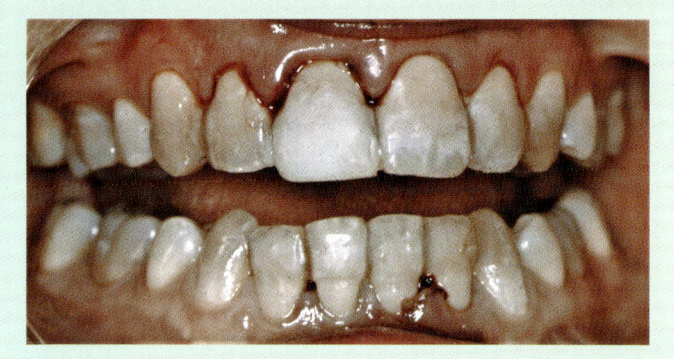

Figure 38.10 (G) The maxillary and mandibular incisors were temporary splinted into place until further treatment could be evaluated.

structure, quicker, less costly, less traumatic, and may not require local anesthesia. Repaired restorations can perform surprisingly well.[20,22]

Small porcelain fractures are most predictably repaired by smoothing and polishing the porcelain. Initial adjustment should be done with a smooth diamond bur with copious water spray (red-band ET diamonds, Brasseler). Afterward, the porcelain should be sequentially polished using coarse to fine porcelain polishers, rinsing between each step.

With larger porcelain fractures, it is usually best to completely replace the restoration. As an interim treatment, direct repairs may be completed to restore esthetics and function. Direct intraoral repair by bonding composite resin to the fractured area is the most common clinical repair technique. For most repairs of restorations, retention comes from micromechanical retention. However, macromechanical retentive and resistance form features are desirable, as long as they do not further compromise adjacent tooth structure or an existing restoration.

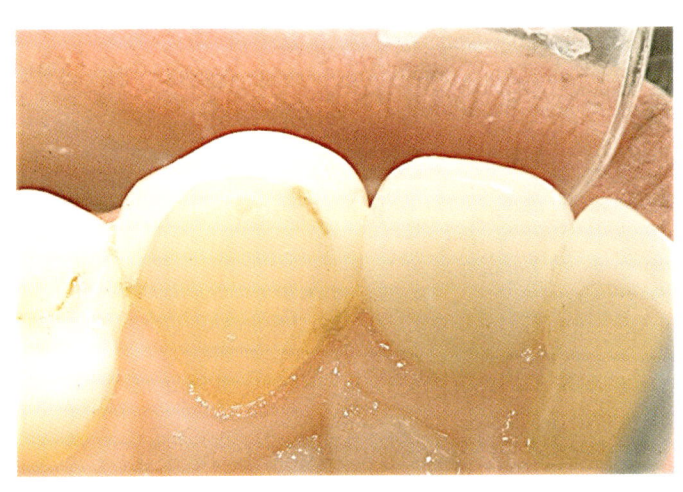

Figure 38.11 (A) Seven years after the placement of porcelain veneers, this patient showed signs of beginning caries at one of the lingual margins.

Several methods can be used to clean and roughen porcelain and other restorative materials. These include roughening using diamond burs, air abrasion using aluminum oxide abrasives, tribochemical silica coating using air abrasion by silica-coated particles (e.g., Coe-Jet Sand), treatment of glassy materials with hydrofluoric acid, treatment of glassy materials with silane coupling agents, treatment of cast metals using tin plating, and the use of multipurpose bonding agents.[20,21,23] Chairside plasma treatments to enhance bonding to a variety of restorative substrates have been studied, but they have not yet been developed for intraoral repairs.

It is clear that a combination of surface treatments produces the strongest bonds[24,25] It is also clear that no single recipe will be optimal for all restorative materials, or even for single class of materials, such as the porcelains or the composites.[26] Air abrasion will effectively roughen most restorative materials: porcelain, composite, base metal alloys, noble metal alloys, gold, titanium, and amalgam.[27] Air abrasion can be used intraorally, and small units are specifically designed for this purpose (e.g., Microetcher, Danville Engineering) but considerable care must be taken to protect airways and eyes. Air abrasion is generally a good first step for most adhesive repair procedures. Air abrasion can be used to create some micromechanical retention on strong all-ceramic core materials without undue damage. Both air

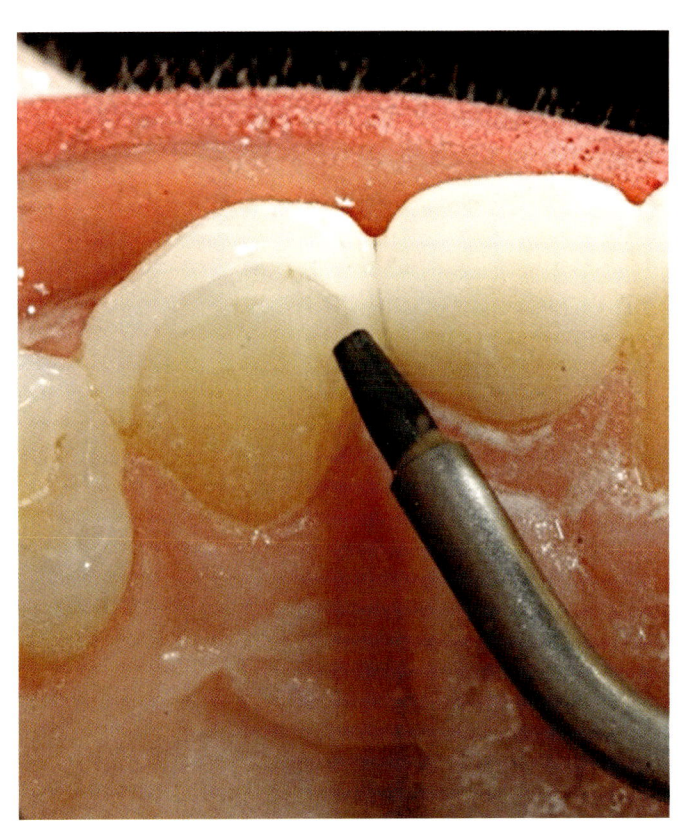

Figure 38.11 (B) Air abrasion was chosen to make the preparation at the lingual margin to both abrade the adjacent porcelain plus avoid any injury to the veneer that might occur if a handpiece and bur were used.

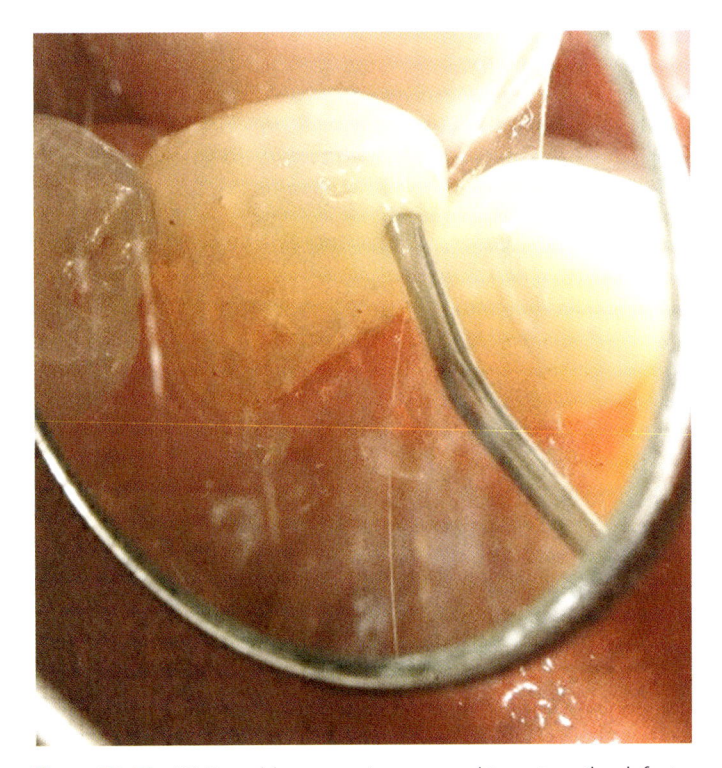

Figure 38.11 (C) Flowable composite was used to restore the defect.

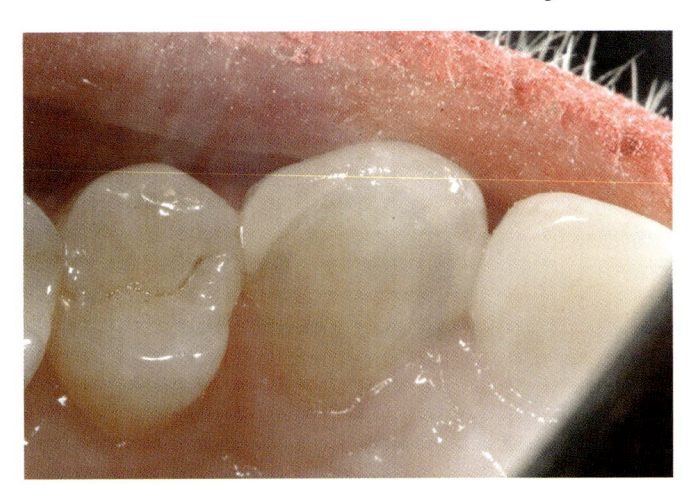

Figure 38.11 (D) The final result shows the margin sealed for restoration longevity.

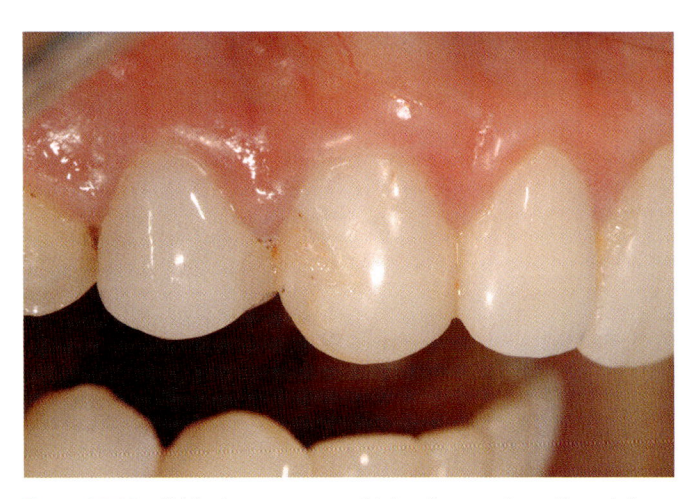

Figure 38.12 (A) Patient presents with her fractured maxillary right cuspid and bicuspid porcelain veneers caused by biting on a porcelain object.

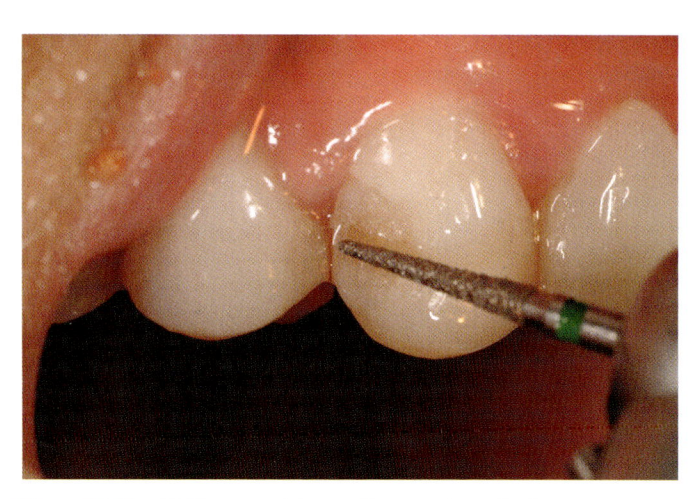

Figure 38.12 (B) The porcelain was first roughened using an extra-coarse diamond bur (AC2, Brasseler USA).

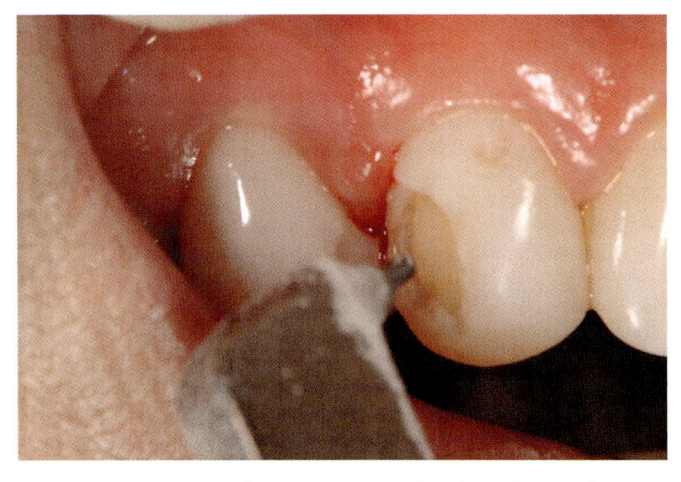

Figure 38.12 (C) Next, the area was treated with air abrasion for maximum micromechanical retention.

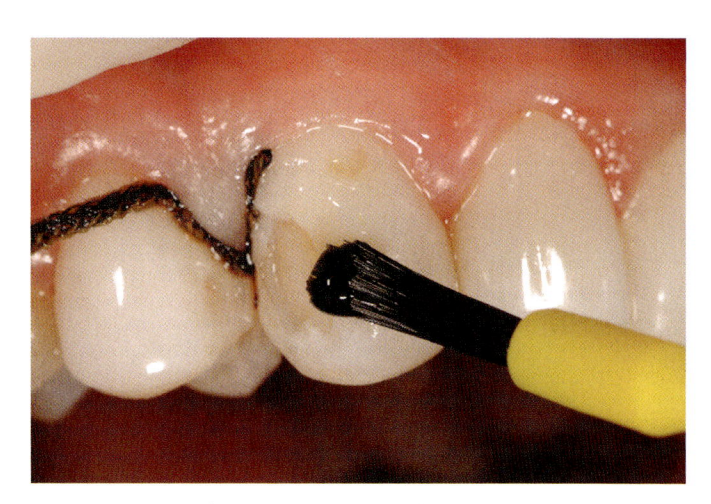

Figure 38.12 (D) The tissue was retracted using cotton cord (Ultradent) to better isolate the area. Hydrofluoric acid 9 (Ultradent) was applied to the porcelain for 90 seconds.

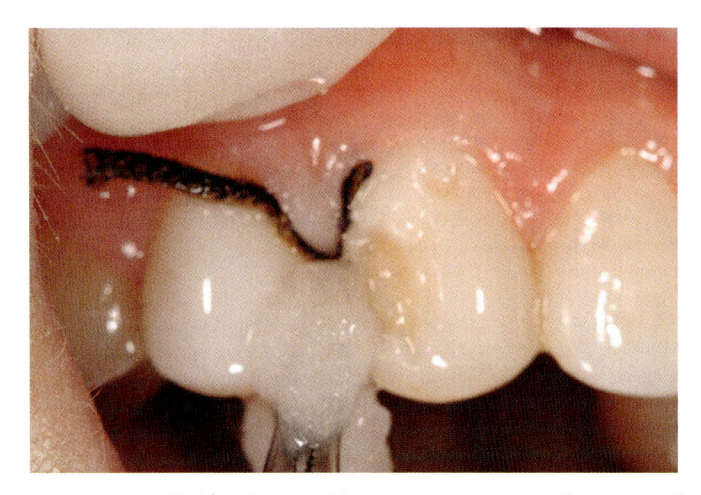

Figure 38.12 (E) After rinsing with water, a wet cotton pellet was used to wipe off any remaining salt deposits.

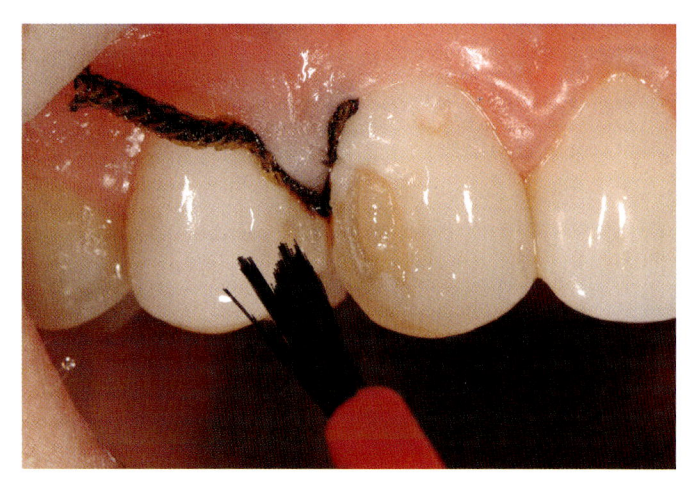

Figure 38.12 (F) Next, 36% phosphoric acid was applied to the dentin and then rinsed.

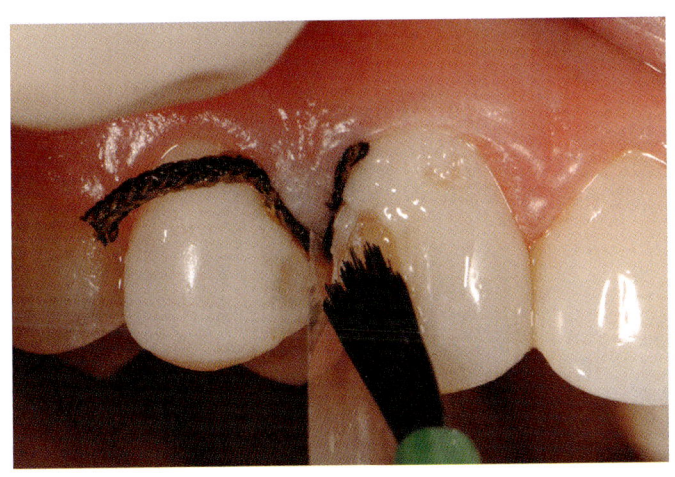

Chapter 38 Esthetic and Traumatic Emergencies

Figure 38.12 (G) Next, bonding resin was applied to both porcelain and tooth structure and polymerized.

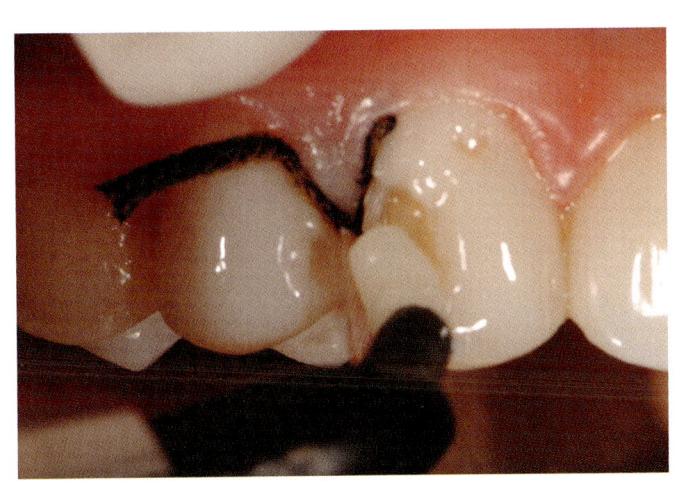

Figure 38.12 (H) For maximum polish, a microfilled composite resin was selected for bonding.

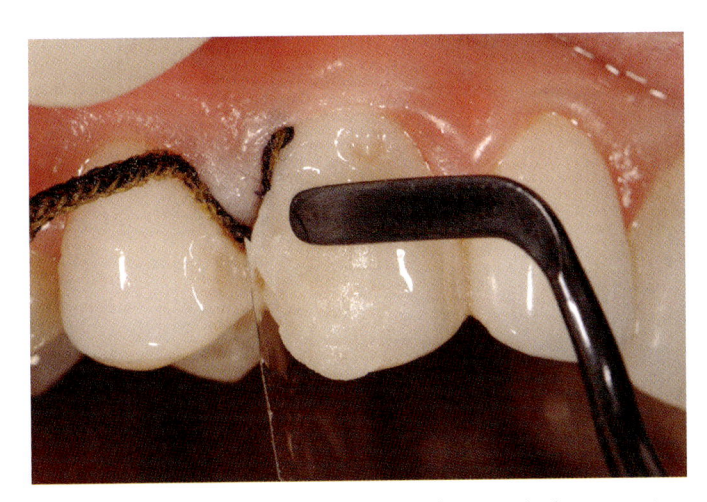

Figure 38.12 (I) A bin-angled Teflon-coated composite instrument (Goldstein Flexi-Thin TNCIGFT4, HU-Friedy) was used for placement and contouring the restoration.

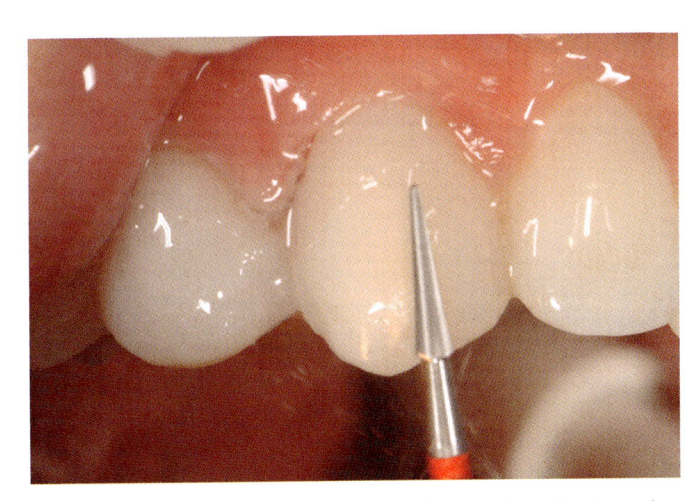

Figure 38.12 (J) An eight-bladed carbide finishing bur (ET6, Brasseler USA) was used to contour and finish the restoration.

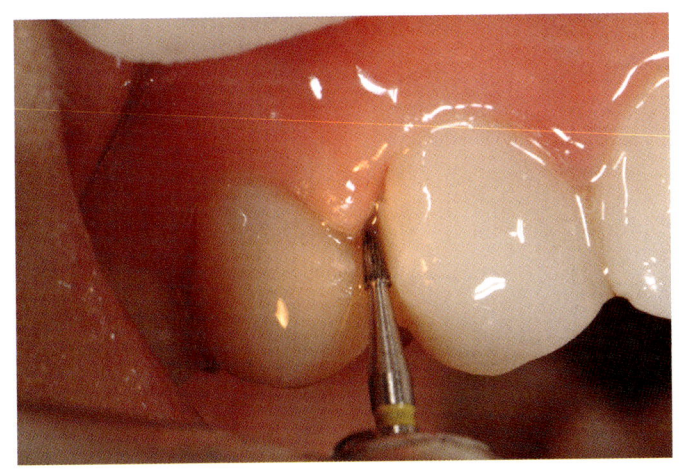

Figure 38.12 (K) A 16-bladed carbide finishing bur (ET4F, Brasseler USA) was used to finish the gingival margins.

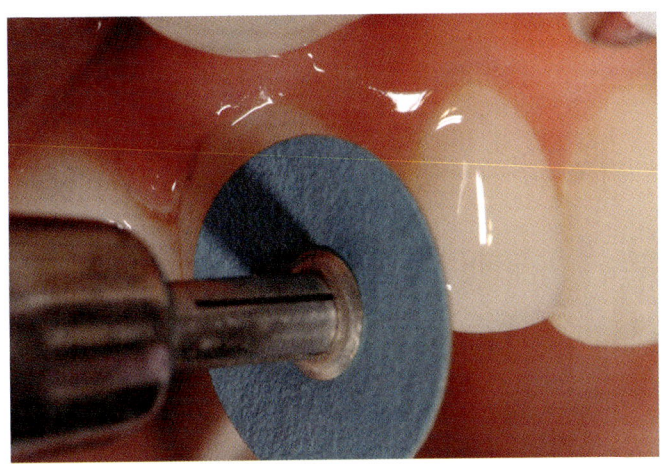

Figure 38.12 (L) A series of four polishing disks (Sof-Lex, 3M) was used for polishing.

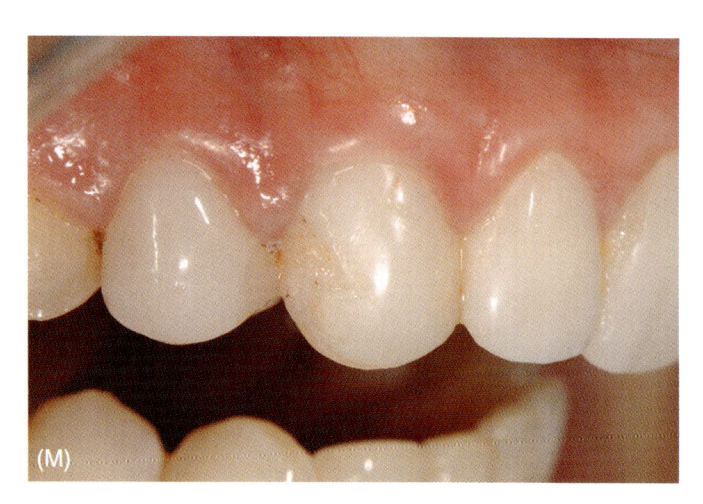

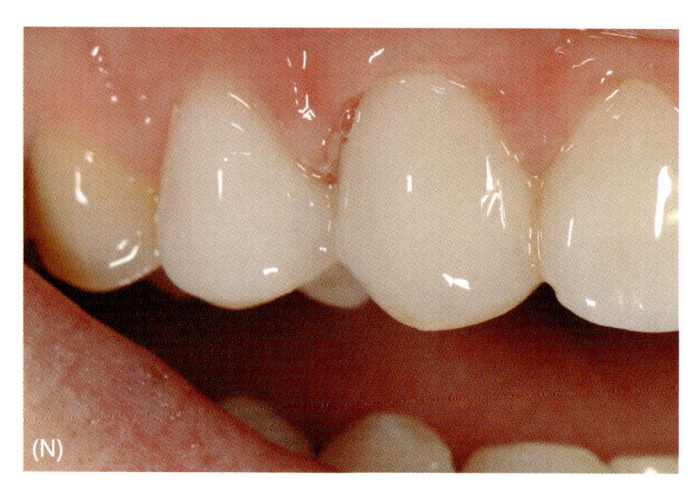

Figure 38.12 (M, N) Note the finish of the microfill composite as it blends in with the porcelain.

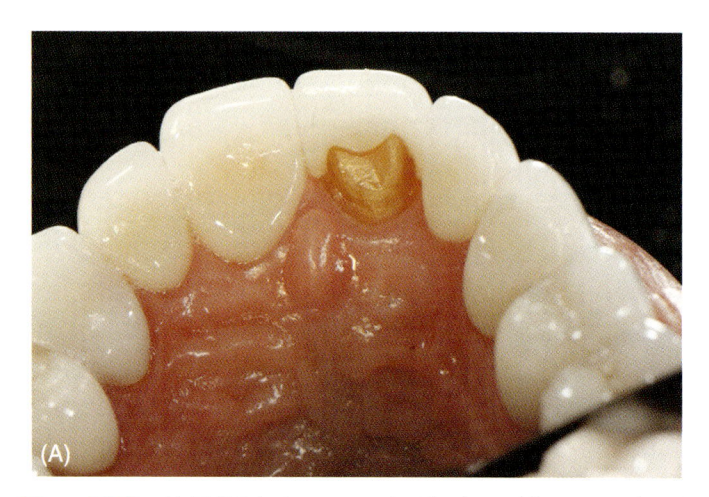

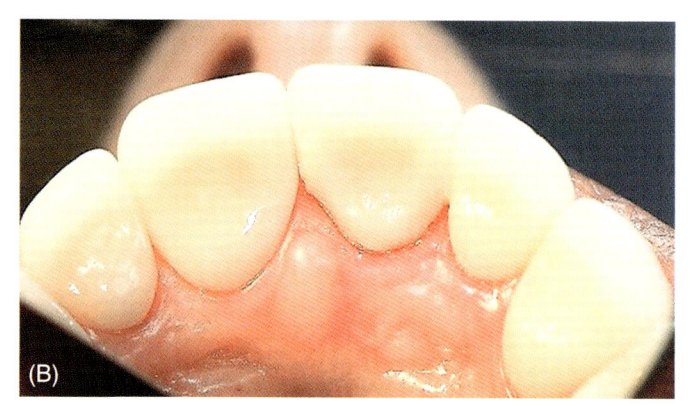

Figure 38.13 (A, B) This lady presented with a lingual fracture on her all-ceramic crown on the left central incisor. Although the crown could be replaced, it was decided to bond the lingual surface with composite resin since there was enough retention of the original crown and facial esthetics would be preserved.

abrasion and tribochemical silica coating have an advantage that they can prepare multiple exposed surfaces at one time.[20]

Hydrofluoric acid gels, at concentrations from 2% to 10%, can be used for 2–5 min to etch and roughen silica-glass porcelains and glass-ceramics, producing strong and durable bonds when multipurpose bonding agents are applied. Hydrofluoric acid is extremely caustic to the soft tissues. Excellent isolation and careful technique are essential if it is to be used intraorally. Gels designed for intraoral use are more amenable to control than the liquids used to prepare indirect porcelain restorations in laboratories. Hydrofluoric acid cannot effectively etch high-strength alumina and zirconia all-ceramic core materials. Hydrofluoric acid should not be used to etch the glassy filler in composite restorative materials because it also damages their resinous matrices, nor should hydrofluoric acid be allowed to contaminate tooth structure. Acidulated phosphate sodium fluoride is ineffective in etching porcelains or composites.

The long-term effectiveness of silane-coupling agents is somewhat controversial. Silane is a dual functional monomer that can react with porcelain and ceramic surfaces as well as with resinous bonding agents. However, silanes tend to lack hydrolytic stability and may be most effective when used in laboratory environments where stability can be attained before they are exposed to the wet oral environments; composites quickly imbibe water in the hours after restorative placement. Nonetheless, the available evidence generally supports the use of silane coupling agents used as adjuncts after air abrasion or etching and before application of a multipurpose bonding.[20,23]

Metals, particularly nonprecious alloys, can be roughened using air abrasion. Tin plating, coating the surface with needle-like crystals, is effective in roughening precious metals. Additional retention can be achieved by roughening and etching adjacent porcelain.

Bonding agents are a key part of the success of any esthetic repair.[28] Opaque masking composites can be applied to exposed metallic surfaces before a layered hybrid composite restoration is placed[29] (Figure 38.14A–D). Fiberglass reinforcement may strengthen large composite repairs. Careful contouring will minimize the amount of finishing needed; thus reducing stresses applied to the new repair.

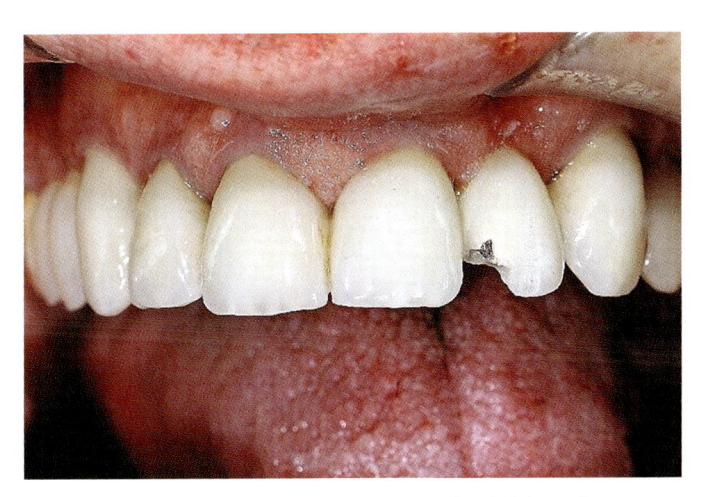

Figure 38.14 (A) This man fractured his maxillary left lateral ceramo-metal crown.

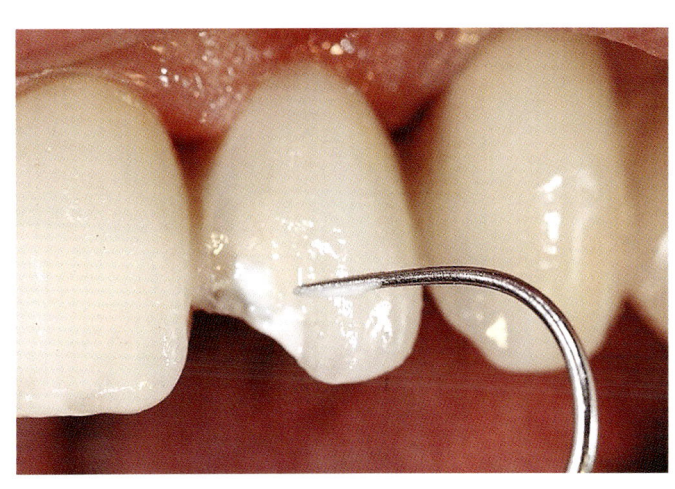

Figure 38.14 (B) After air abrasion, acid etching, Silane and bonding resin, a small amount of white resin opaquer (Cosmedent) was applied and polymerized to mask the exposed metal, followed by a mircrohybrid composite resin to restore the fractured crown.

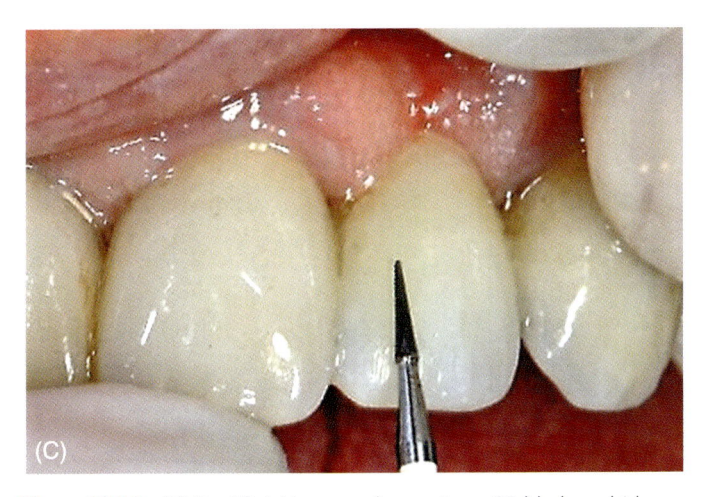

Figure 38.14 (C) Final finishing was done using a 30-blade carbide bur(ET4-UF, Brasseler USA).

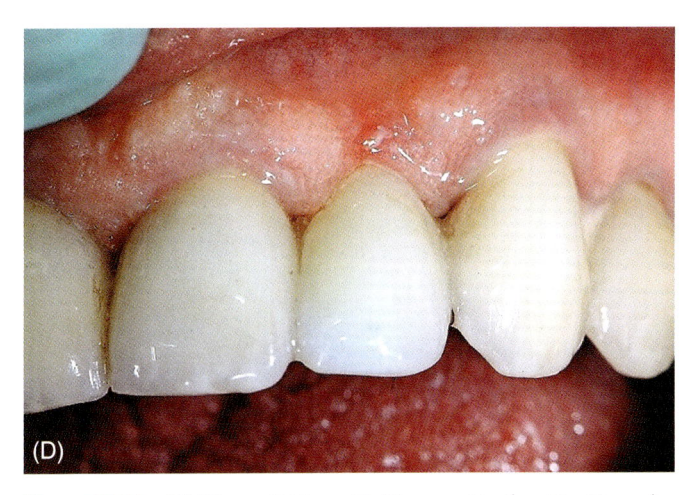

Figure 38.14 (D) After polishing with Diacomp Feather Lite (Brasseler USA) polishers, the crown repair is complete.

Prosthesis fracture, failure, and repair

Fixed, removable, implant-supported, and provisional prostheses also frequently fracture. Many of the direct reparative strategies using bonded composite, described earlier, can be used to address these esthetic emergencies. Indirect reparative veneers or onlays can also be fabricated to replace fractured porcelain or resin;[30] computer-aided design and manufacturing techniques and in-office laboratory support can expedite this approach. Emergency fixed dental prostheses can be formed from fractured natural tooth crowns, failed artificial crowns, or denture teeth held in place by composite resin using polyethylene ribbon (e.g., Ribbond), fiberglass ribbon (e.g., eFiber, Preat Corp.), and orthodontic wires or surgical bars. Debonded resin-bonded bridges can be cleaned, air abraded, and rebonded, but they may be less successful after multiple rebondings. Prefabricated posts can be temporarily retrofitted to displaced crowns (Figure 38.15A–F). Visible-light-cure denture base

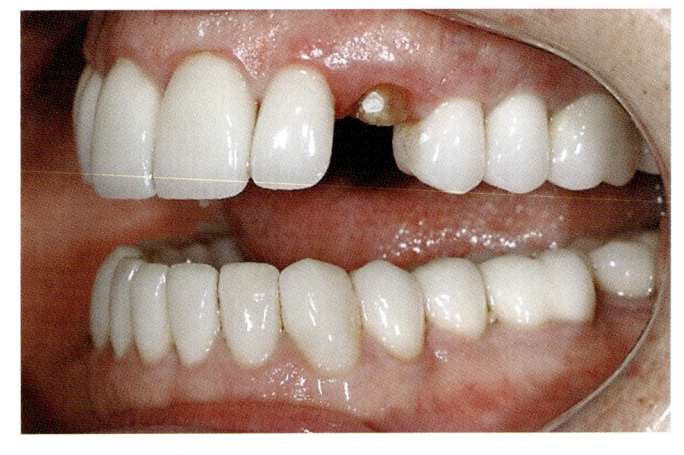

Figure 38.15 (A) This patient fractured his all-ceramic crown and tooth at the gum line. It was decided that the best therapy to try to save his crown would be to retrofit the existing crown to the tooth following endodontic treatment and post placement.

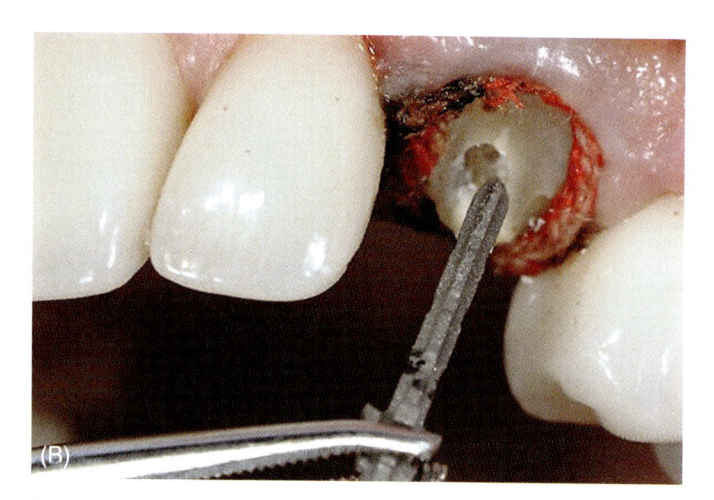

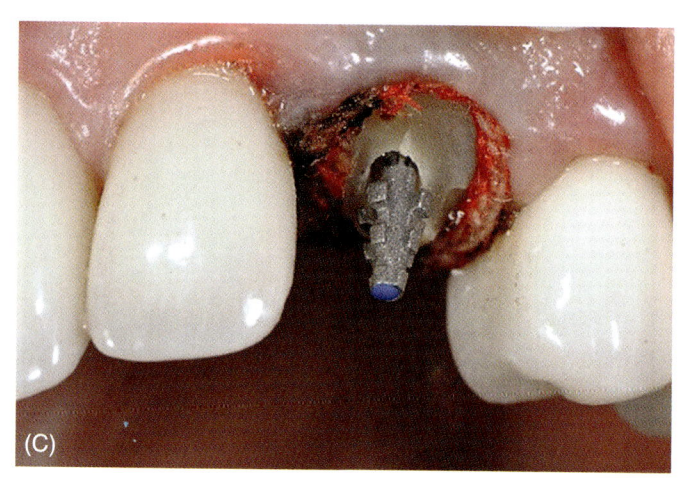

Figure 38.15 (B, C) After tissue retraction, a post canal was prepared and fitted so that the existing crown would fit over the post (Brasseler USA).

materials (e.g., Triad, Dentsply) can be used to make emergency partial dentures or to add to existing prostheses. Lost denture teeth can be replaced using bonded composite. Crowns and pontics from failed fixed prostheses can be added to existing, new emergency, or transitional removable prostheses. Patients should be dissuaded from attempting to repair or recement restorations using superglue. In the case of an esthetic emergency shortly before a social engagement, a dislodged crown or fixed dental prosthesis can be temporarily retained through the application of a little denture adhesive. The patient should be advised to remove the crown after the social engagement, so as to prevent the possibility of its being inhaled or swallowed and to present for care at the dentist's office.

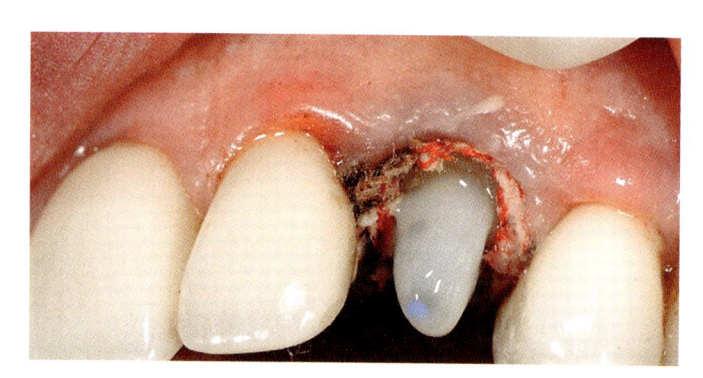

Figure 38.15 (D) After cementation of the post with a resin-modified glass ionomer cement, composite resin was used to build up the tooth for better support and retention of the crown.

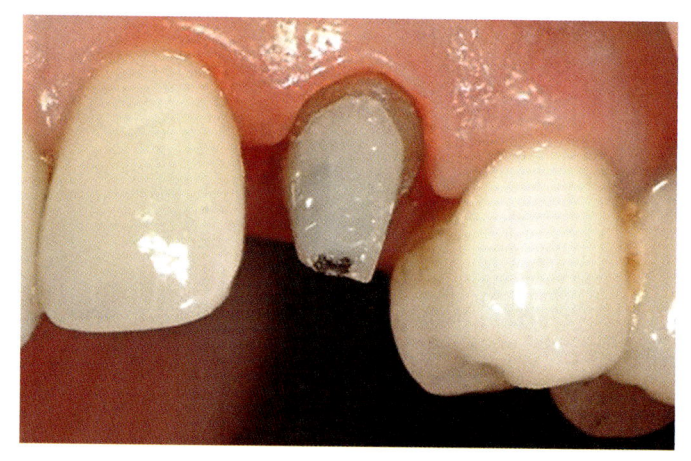

Figure 38.15 (E) A series of adjustments to the buildup was done by continuously trying on the crown until obtaining an acceptable fit.

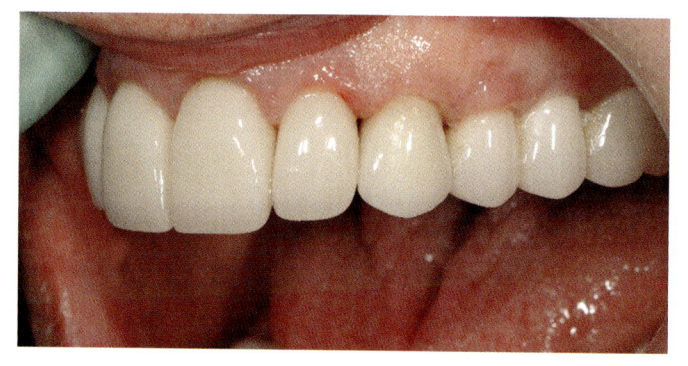

Figure 38.15 (F) The final crown was cemented into place using a resin-modified glass ionomer cement.

Summary

Dentists and patients sometimes incorrectly assume that a tooth fractured beneath the periodontal attachment and within the bone cannot be saved. With proper emergency treatment and surgical and reconstructive techniques, these roots can often be saved for a lifetime. Dentists may assume, again incorrectly, that because of expense or difficulty of treatment, a patient, or their family, would prefer to lose the tooth. As the dentist may not fully appreciate the value placed on a tooth by the individual, the patient should be informed of the options, their advantages and disadvantages, and given the opportunity to decide.

Even though extraordinary measures and a multidisciplinary approach are sometimes required, it may be possible to preserve traumatized teeth and their supporting tissues. A single tooth saved and retained can be far more esthetically pleasing than an artificial replacement. A retained tooth is likely to be less problematic than either a fixed dental prosthesis or an implant. Thus, all possibilities should be considered before a patient is allowed to lose a tooth. Dental care can maintain the integrity, health, and esthetic appearance of the dentition.

References

1. American Academy of Pediatric Dentistry (AAPD) Council on Clinical Affairs. Guideline on Management of Acute Dental Trauma. *AAPD Ref Manual* 2010;32:202–212.
2. Bakland LF, Andreasen JO. Dental traumatology: essential diagnosis and treatment planning. *Endod Topics* 2004;7:14–34.
3. World Health Organization. *Application of the International Classification of Diseases to Dentistry and Stomatology (ICD-DA)*. Geneva, IL: World Health Organization; 1978:88–89.
4. Andreasen JO, Andreasen FM. *Textbook and Color Atlas of Traumatic Injuries*, 3rd edn. Copenhagen: Munksgaard; 1994:151–177.
5. American Association of Endodontists. *The Recommended Guidelines of the American Association of Endodontists for the Treatment of Traumatic Dental Injuries*, revised 9/13. Chicago, IL: AAE; 2013. http://www.nxtbook.com/nxtbooks/aae/traumaguidelines/#/12 (accessed November 8, 2017).
6. DiAngelis AJ, Andreasen JO, Ebeleseder KA, et al. International Association of Dental Traumatology guidelines for the management of traumatic dental injuries: 1. Fractures and luxations of permanent teeth. *Dent Traumatol* 2012;28:2–12.
7. Olsburgh S, Jacoby T, Krejci I. Crown fractures in the permanent dentition: pulpal and restorative considerations. *Dent Traumatol* 2002;18:103–115.
8. Gungor HC, Uysal S, Altay N. A retrospective evaluation of crown-fractured permanent teeth treated in a pediatric dentistry clinic. *Dent Traumatol* 2007;23:211–217.
9. Krastl G, Filippi A, Zitzmann NU, et al. Current aspects of restoring traumatically fractured teeth. *Eur J Esthet Dent* 2011;6:124–141.
10. Badami V, Reddy K. Treatment of complicated crown-root fracture in a single visit by means of rebonding. *J Am Dent Assoc* 2011;142:646–650.
11. Saha SG, Saha MK. Management of a fractured tooth by fragment reattachment: a case report. *Int J Dent Clin* 2010;2:18–22.
12. Macedo GV, Diaz PI, De O Fernandes CA, Ritter AV. Reattachment of anterior teeth fragments: a conservative approach. *J Esthet Restor Dent* 2008;20:5–18.
13. Flores MT, Malmgren B, Andersson L, et al. Guidelines for the management of traumatic dental injuries. III. Primary teeth. *Dent Traumatol* 2007;23:196–202.
14. Needleman HL. The art and science of managing traumatic injuries to primary teeth. *Dent Traumatol* 2011;27:295–299.
15. Heithersay GS. Combined endodontic–orthodontic treatment of transverse root fractures in the region of the alveolar crest. *Oral Surg Oral Med Oral Pathol* 1973;36:404–415.
16. Goenka P, Marwah N, Dutta S. A multidisciplinary approach to the management of a subgingivally fractured tooth: a clinical report. *J Prosthodont* 2011;20:218–223.
17. Andreasen JO, Hjorting-Hansen E. Intraalveolar root fractures: radiographic and histologic study of 50 cases. *J Oral Surg* 1967;25:414–426.
18. Andersson L, Andreasen JO, Day P, et al. International Association of Dental Traumatology guidelines for the management of traumatic dental injuries: 2. Avulsion of permanent teeth. *Dent Traumatol* 2012;28(2):88–96.
19. Pokorny DD. Try-in of completed restoration. *Dent Clin N Am* 1971;15:3.
20. Mjor IA, Gordan VV. Failure, repair, refurbishing and longevity of restorations. *Oper Dent* 2002;27:528–534.
21. Goodacre CJ, Bernal G, Rungcharassaeng K, Kan JY. Clinical complications in fixed prosthodontics. *J Prosthet Dent* 2003;90:31–41.
22. Fernandez EM, Martin JA, Angel PA, et al. Survival rate of sealed, refurbished and repaired defective restorations: 4-year follow-up. *Braz Dent J* 2011;22:134–139.
23. Goldstein RE, White SN. Intraoral esthetic repair of dental restorations. *J Esthet Dent* 1995;7(5):219–227.
24. Ozcan M, Valandro LF, Amaral R, et al. Bond strength durability of a resin composite on a reinforced ceramic using various repair systems. *Dent Mater* 2009;25:1477–1483.
25. Marchack BW, Yu Z, Zhao XY, White SN. Adhesion of denture tooth porcelain to heat-polymerized denture resin. *J Prosthet Dent* 1995;74:242–249.
26. Loomans BA, Cardoso MV, Roeters FJ, et al. Is there one optimal repair technique for all composites? *Dent Mater* 2011;27:701–709.
27. White SN, Yu Z, Zhao XY. High-energy abrasion: an innovative esthetic modality to enhance adhesion. *J Esthet Dent* 1994;6:267–273.
28. Staxrud F, Dahl JE. Role of bonding agents in the repair of composite resin restorations. *Eur J Oral Sci* 2011;119:316–322.
29. Ozcan M, Niedermeier W. Clinical study on the reasons for and location of failures of metal-ceramic restorations and survival of repairs. *Int J Prosthodont* 2002;15:299–302.
30. Kimmich M, Stappert CF. Intraoral treatment of veneering porcelain chipping of fixed dental restorations: a review and clinical application. *J Am Dent Assoc* 2013;144(1):31–44.

Further resource

Padilla RR, Felsenfeld AL. Treatment and prevention of alveolar fractures and related injuries. *J Craniomaxillofac Trauma* 1997;3:22–27.

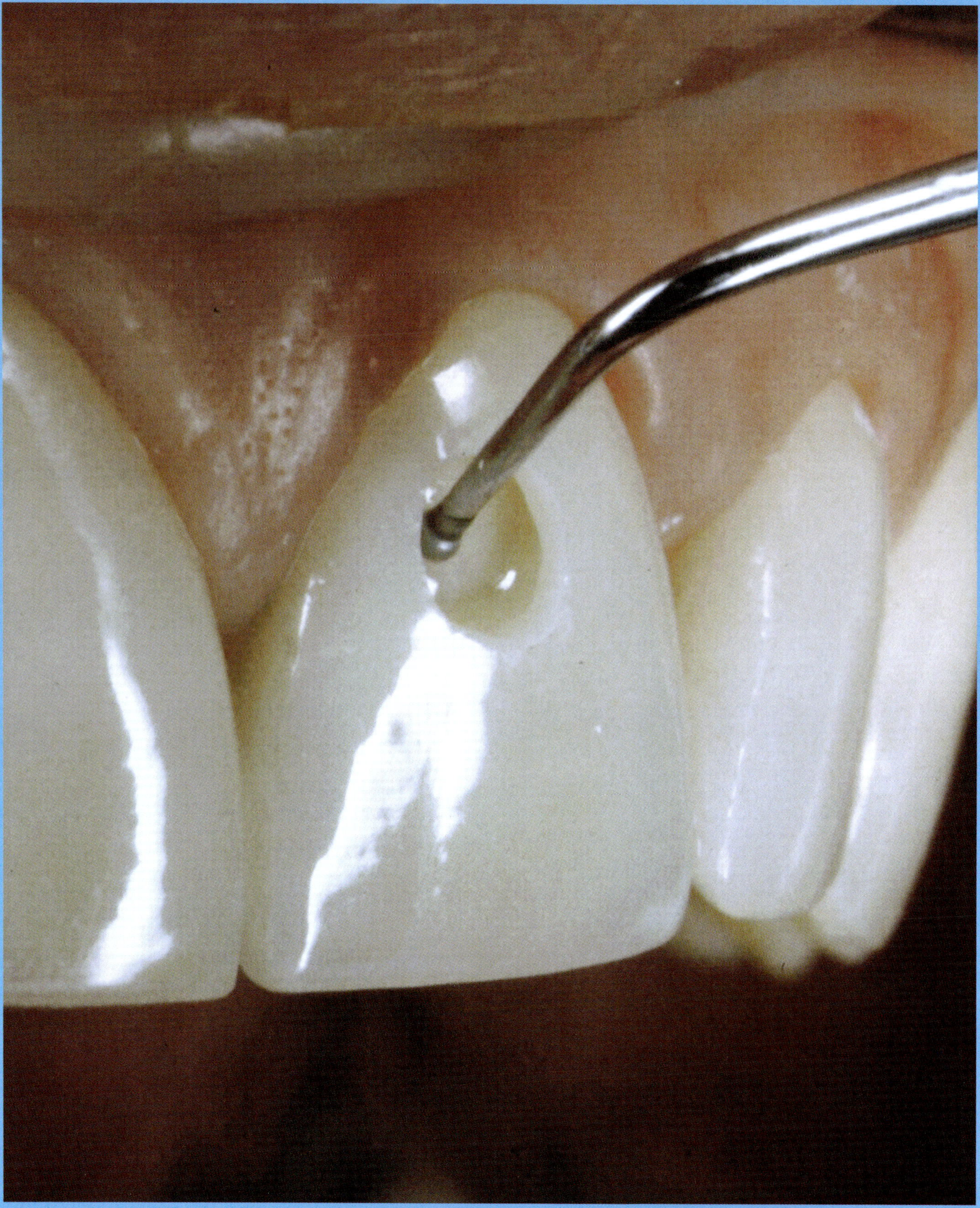

Chapter 39 Esthetic Failures

Ronald E. Goldstein, DDS, Azadeh Esfandiari, DMD, and Anna K. Schultz, DMD

Chapter Outline

Immediate failure	1236	Choice of restoration	1242
Improper crown contours	1236	Compromise when patient rejects repositioning treatment	1243
Unesthetic clasp design	1238		
Incorrect pontic height	1239	Eventual failure: restoration longevity	1244
Failure to alter adjacent or opposing teeth	1239	Problems that cause failure	1244
A compromised treatment plan	1242		

Successful dental treatment is one of the primary objectives of every dentist, and is measured not only by the doctor, but also by the patient; however, what the dentist considers "esthetic" may not be agreed upon by the patient. The inability to fulfill both patient and clinician expectations results in esthetic failure, even in light of long-term retention.[1] It is assumed that if the dentist considers a procedure a "failure" that they will try to rectify the situation; however, many esthetic failures discussed in this chapter were eventually noticed by the patients. It is important to note that the values of the patient, as well as the dentist, are subject to change according to social and cultural norms, as well as dental expertise; therefore, what is accepted as "beautiful" today may seem quite unattractive tomorrow.

Obviously, no dentist wants to fail; however, there are three basic reasons why some dentists fall victim to failure: (1) poor or faulty technique; (2) attempting to manage a case that exceeds the dentist's capability or expertise; and (3) overtreatment.[2]

Poor or faulty treatment is easy to understand, and state boards usually deal with many of these problems. The second reason is more difficult to grasp, because many practitioners think they can solve every patient's problems. One motivating factor in trying to avoid treating a patient who requires skills beyond the dentist's expertise is the issue of cost. Failure in esthetic or restorative dentistry is always costly, both for the patient and the dentist. A realistic and objective analysis at the outset, considering the difficulty in pleasing the patient both esthetically and in function, is paramount. Much stress can be avoided just by understanding one's own capabilities, and perhaps referring a patient to a colleague, who may have the training and experience to more expertly manage a difficult case.

We have seen too many esthetic and functional failures due to overtreatment, involving the dentist placing a full arch of veneers and/or crowns, instead of bleaching, contouring, or orthodontics—any or all of which could have saved the patient a good amount of money. In addition, refraining from overtreatment saves the dentist from potential failure due to future occlusal problems that may need to be solved with orthodontics. Obviously, not all of these types of failures are the fault of the dentist, especially when the patient refuses orthodontics or a recommended treatment.

For the purposes of this chapter, esthetic failure will be divided into three specific types: (1) immediate failure, (2) compromised treatment plan, and (3) eventual failure. These failures could be the result of problems with esthetics, materials, technique, maintenance, or any combination thereof.

Immediate failure

Some restorations fail, from an esthetic standpoint, upon insertion of the restoration. The dentist may have missed the shade completely (Figure 39.1A and B), or they may not have shaped the restorations to match adjacent natural teeth. Perhaps the gingival margins were left exposed and ill fitting, which would eventually cause discoloration and necessitate replacement (Figure 39.1C–E). Regardless of the cause, the result remains a failure upon insertion, and is most often "treatment-induced." The immediate solution to such a failure usually involves remaking the restoration; however, the best solution is obviously prevention—do not let it happen! *Never insert a restoration that you are not completely satisfied with, because the patient may eventually share your dissatisfaction.*

One of the most immediately noticeable signs of failure is discoloration. Intrinsic, extrinsic, and internalized tooth discoloration boast multifactorial etiologies; however, it is interesting to note the etiology of internalized discoloration as a function of the improper use of dental materials. In a 2009 study conducted by the University of Minnesota, it was observed that ferric ions have a very high affinity for hard tooth surfaces. Ferric ions may be found in gingival retraction fluid, most commonly used in the application of impregnated retraction cord by the clinician. Therefore, the unintended etching of dentin by this acidic fluid, in the most commonly used mechanochemical method of soft-tissue management, can result in the absorption of iron into dentin. This causes a black, insoluble, ferric compound to form due to the reaction of iron with the hydrogen sulfide produced by bacteria. This kind of contamination can cause microleakage and the perpetuation of dentinal staining seen under porcelain crowns, creating unesthetic discoloration as a result.[3]

A clinical study reported by the faculty practice group at the University of Minnesota described a 45-year-old woman with four lithium disilicate crowns on her maxillary incisors. The patient's crowns were placed approximately 4 years prior, and the patient had since complained of dark marginal areas around the restorations soon after their placement. Upon evaluation, it was noted that all four incisors showed evidence of black internalized dentinal discoloration, particularly at the shoulder region. A clinician removed the staining by refining the crown preparations and then placed knitted retraction cord soaked in aluminum chloride (Hemodent) to make another impression in order to fabricate four new zirconia-based ceramic crowns. It was observed that when the gingival margin of the preparation extends intrasulcularly, gingival retraction fluid will almost indefinitely contaminate the prepared dentinal surfaces, thereby removing the smear layer and causing microleakage and discoloration, as occurred in this particular patient. To address the problem, the clinician's use of aluminum chloride, as opposed to an iron-containing material, prevented the discoloration from occurring a second time, and the patient has been satisfied with the result since the procedure was completed.[3]

Another classic example of esthetic failure at completion of treatment is seen in Figure 39.2. A previous dentist told this patient that if the crowded lower central incisor were extracted, the remaining teeth would fill the space; however, the patient had the tooth extracted many years ago, and the space never closed. The clinician could have used any number of removable appliances to close this space.

Improper crown contours

One of the most frequent esthetic failures results from a lack of both cosmetic and functional skill in contouring restorations. Such an example of immediate esthetic failure can be seen in Figure 39.3A. The patient originally accepted the dentist's result as the best he could accomplish; however, her friends soon let her know that her smile should look better. From that point on, she hated to smile.

Another example of immediate esthetic and functional failure is shown in Figure 39.3B. The recently placed, overbuilt, posterior porcelain-to-metal crowns not only looked bulky, but also lacked occlusal contours. This patient, who may feel that he or she has achieved an ideal result, may soon find quite the opposite.

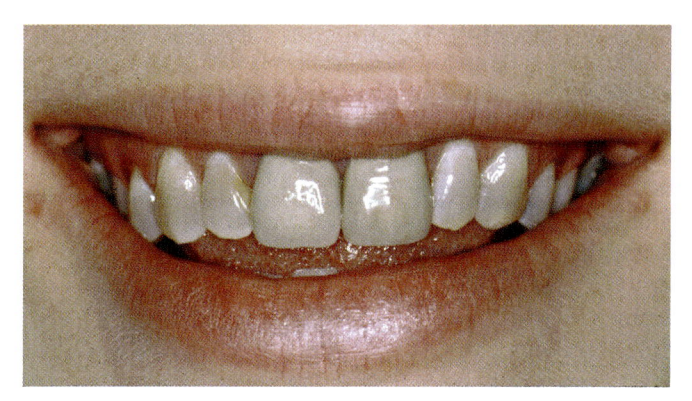

Figure 39.1 **(A)** This 30-year-old woman was dissatisfied with the color of her two front teeth. Although the patient has tetracycline-stained teeth, the attempt to match the patient's shade was a failure.

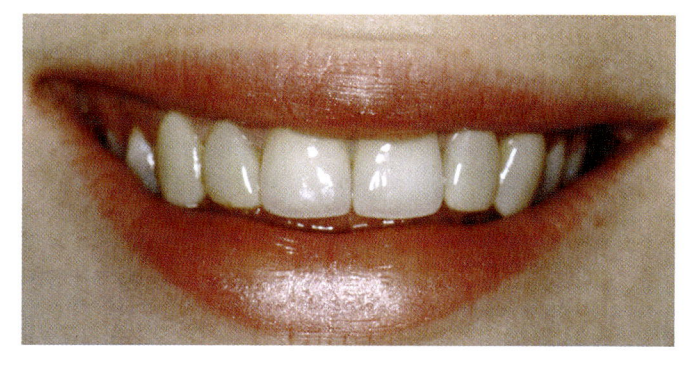

Figure 39.1 **(B)** New crowns with improved shading methods helped enhance this patient's smile.

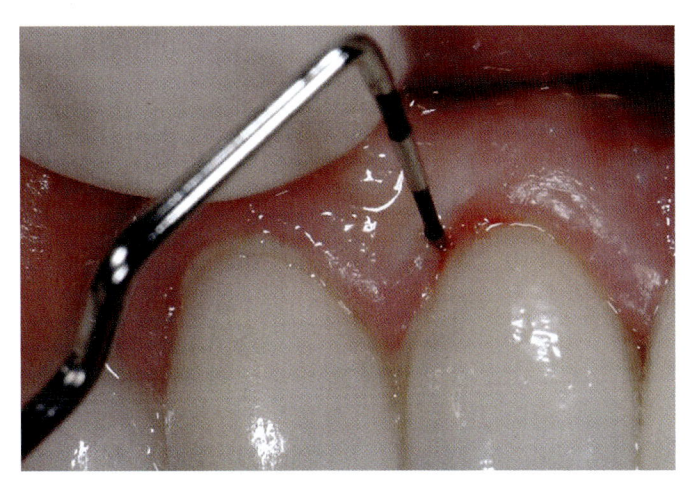

Figure 39.1 **(C)** This patient had 10 porcelain veneers inserted only 7 months before and complained of constant sore gum tissue. Probing of margins showed a poor fit on virtually every veneer. Note exudate around the cervical portion of the right cuspid.

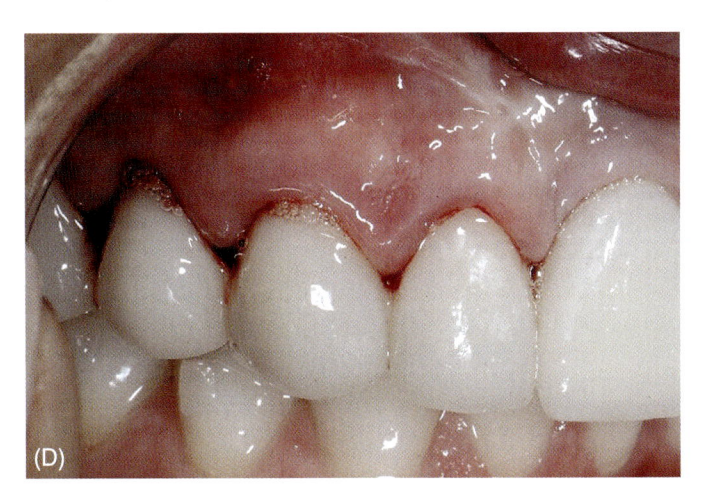

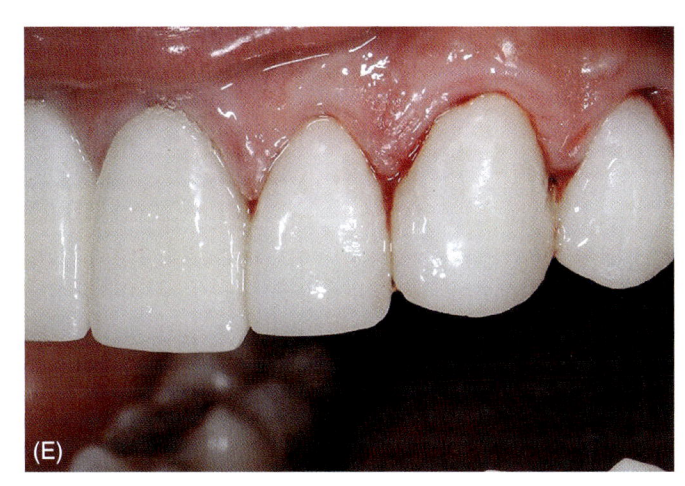

Figure 39.1 **(D, E)** Although the veneers had to be replaced, the first step was to remove as much of the defective margin as possible so that the tissue could begin to heal before veneer replacement.

When basic principles of crown contouring are overlooked, results such as those noted in Figure 39.3C can occur. This ceramometal restoration had only been in the mouth for 2 months, yet it is total failure for the following reasons:

- The porcelain was overbuilt and poorly contoured. Failure to allow for proper embrasures resulted in tissue impingement and gingival hypertrophy (Figure 39.3C and D).
- Unesthetic porcelain contouring, and failure to create adequate incisal embrasures, gave a "straight-across," false appearance.
- There was no variation of depth or shade in the porcelain, resulting in a chalky white and unnatural appearance. Since this patient was a beautiful young model, this unsightly appearance was even more pronounced.
- The dentist failed to create an illusion of separateness. It is important to include both carving and interproximal staining in the fixed restoration in order to create separateness and to avoid a false appearance.
- This young woman was made to look much older when an improper smile line was created. The incisal edge length should have varied to produce a more natural and youthful appearance.
- Lacking feminine crown contours, the result has no personality or appropriate sex characteristics, both of which are so important to an esthetic restoration.

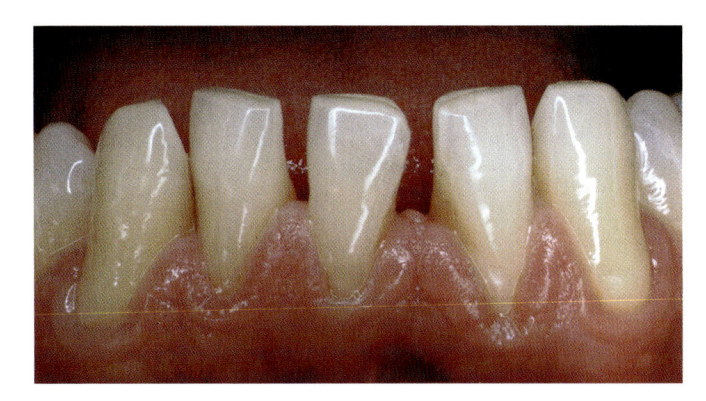

Figure 39.2 In this case, the crowded lower incisor was extracted; however, the remaining teeth never filled the space.

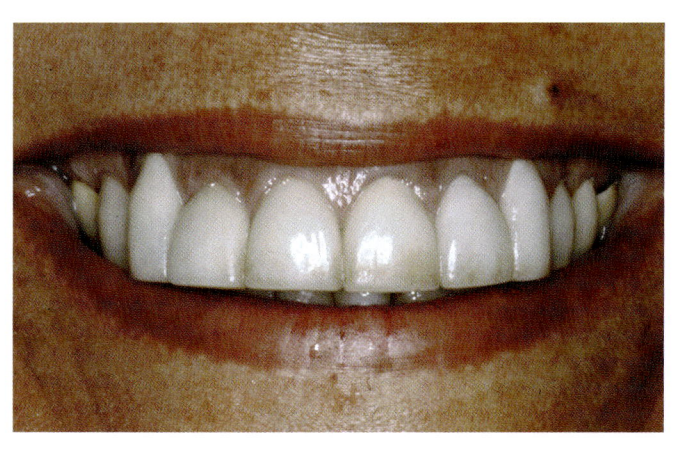

Figure 39.3 **(A)** This woman was embarrassed to smile due to the unesthetic appearance of her restorations placed by her previous dentist. Note the significant widening of the lateral incisors, lack of interincisal distance, and failure to achieve uniform gingival height through cosmetic periodontal surgery.

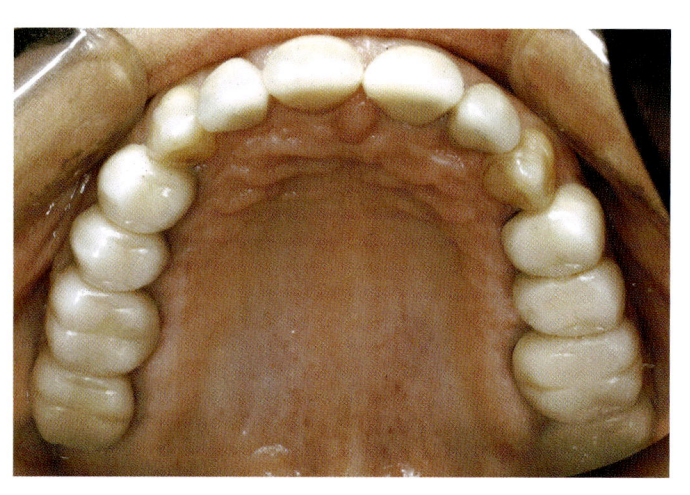

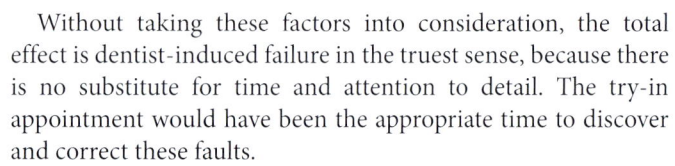

Figure 39.3 **(B)** The overbuilt posterior porcelain-to-metal crowns are not only bulky, but also lack occlusal contours.

Without taking these factors into consideration, the total effect is dentist-induced failure in the truest sense, because there is no substitute for time and attention to detail. The try-in appointment would have been the appropriate time to discover and correct these faults.

If the occlusion is not perfect when crowns are inserted, the teeth may eventually move. Figure 39.4A demonstrates a case in which crowns were inserted too high in occlusion. The dentist told his patient that he would "get used to them," but unfortunately a space developed. After occlusal adjustment and orthodontic repositioning with a removable appliance (Figure 39.4B), two full porcelain crowns were constructed (Figure 39.4C).

The most advantageous time to ensure proper occlusion is prior to placement of the restorations. In the case of a single anterior crown, the restoration should be harmonious with the patient's existing occlusion. If the restoration fractures after placement, the patient's posterior occlusion should be examined and potentially modified to correct the problem; however, if an older patient presents with gross malocclusion evident from the beginning of treatment, and has become well-adapted to this occlusion, it may be more effective to accept this patient's occlusion rather than initiating an extensive occlusal adjustment.[4]

Unesthetic clasp design

Another type of esthetic failure is shown in the case of a poorly designed removable partial denture. An excessive amount of metal, which is evident when a patient smiles, may mean poor clasp design on the removable partial denture. Such a case is

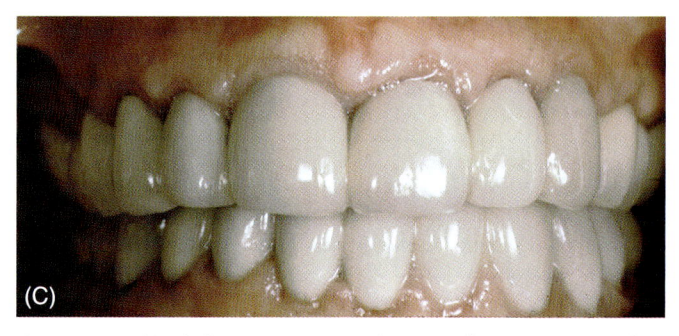

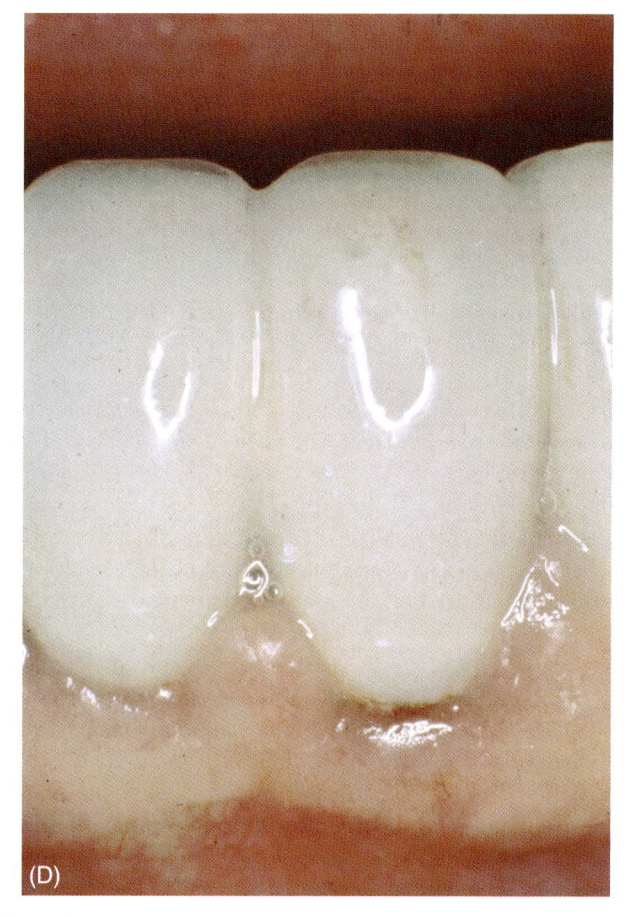

Figure 39.3 **(C, D)** This woman was unhappy with reconstruction done to enhance her smile only 2 months prior. This treatment violated almost all esthetic and functional requirements that the patient assumed would give her a beautiful result.

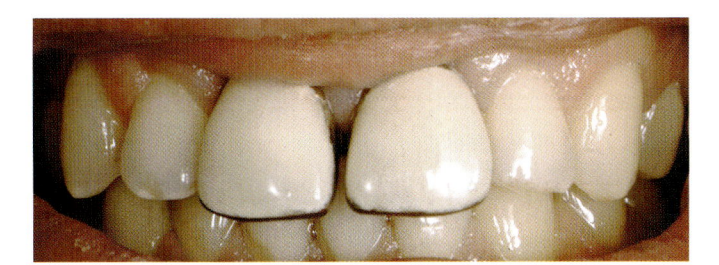

Figure 39.4 **(A)** When his previous dentist inserted this patient's crowns, there was no space between the crowns. Owing to the occlusion not being adjusted properly, eventually the two central incisors moved labially, which resulted in the space. He was told by his dentist that, "he would get used to them."

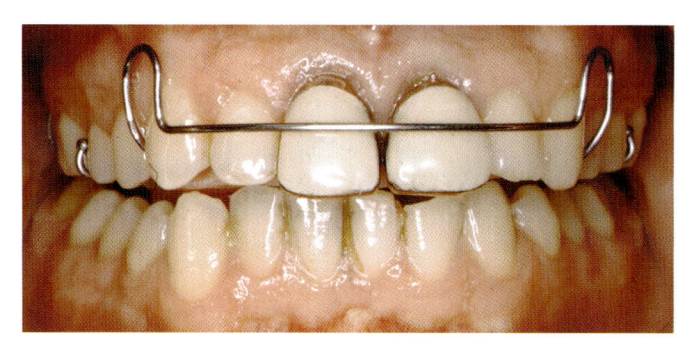

Figure 39.4 **(B)** Orthodontic repositioning by removable appliance. The crowns were replaced.

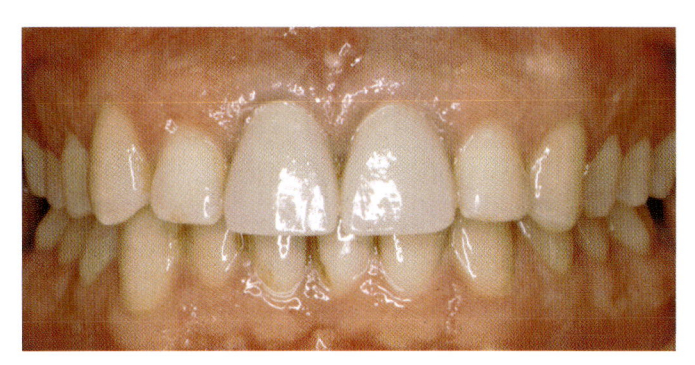

Figure 39.4 **(C)** The final result showed improvement of both proportion and shading.

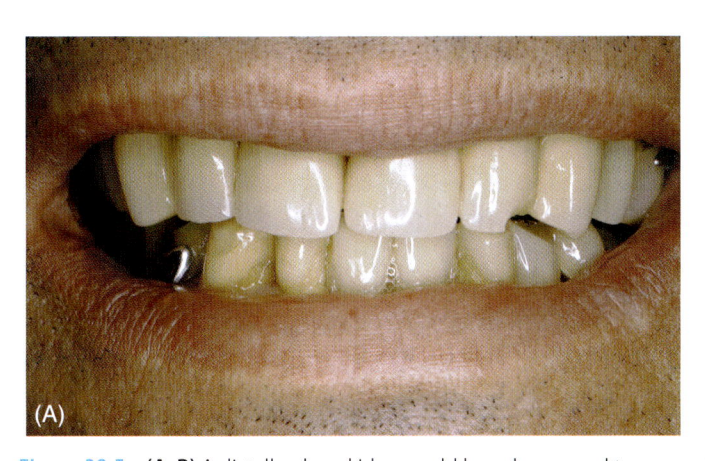

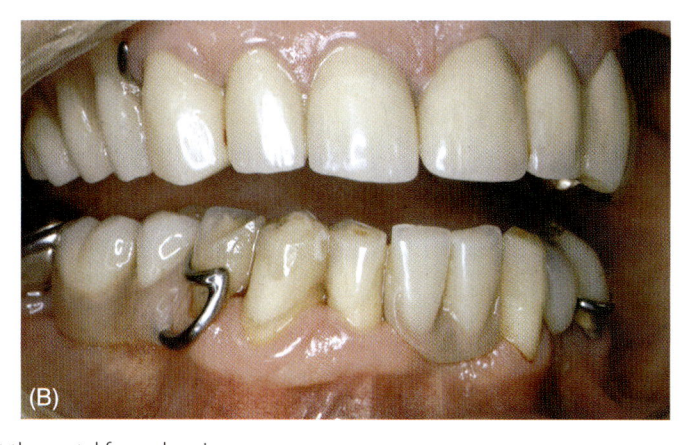

Figure 39.5 **(A, B)** A distally placed I-bar could have been used to prevent the metal from showing.

shown in Figure 39.5A and B. A distally placed I-bar could have been used, or another clasp designed to prevent the metal from showing.

Incorrect pontic height

A basic need in fixed or removable partial denture replacement is symmetrical pontic height. Failure to achieve this symmetry usually results in an unesthetic restoration. Defects of this kind are typically easier to treat if they involve only soft tissue; however, most are usually a combination of both hard- and soft-tissue malformations. The extent of reconstruction depends on the size of the defect and how much of the defect is visible; however, in unesthetic areas, reconstruction may be necessary both to facilitate speech and to prevent excessive salivary outflow.[4] The case in Figure 39.6A–I is an example.

Failure to alter adjacent or opposing teeth

It is important to study adjacent and opposing teeth before planning partial- or full-arch restorations. Cosmetic contouring for extruded or malformed teeth should be completed before fixed restorations are made. If there are esthetic deformities due to tooth position or wear, repositioning or recontouring should be considered. An example of failure to reshape adjacent teeth is seen in Clinical case 39.1 (Figure 39.7A–D).

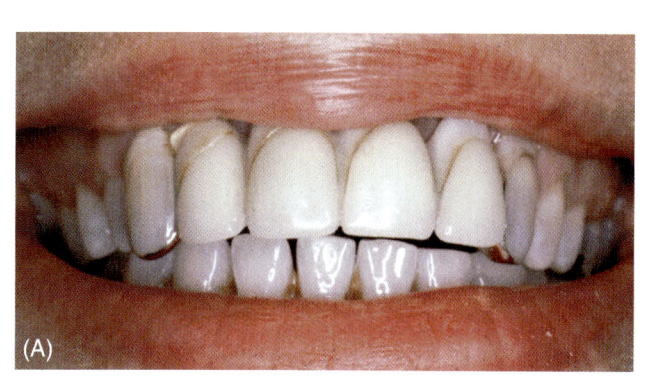

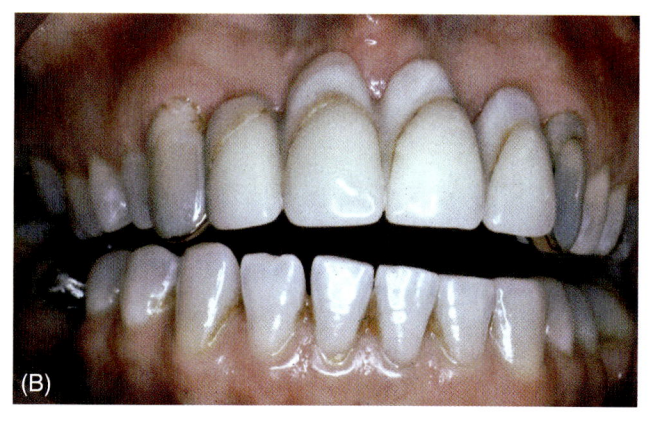

Figure 39.6 **(A, B)** This woman was very concerned about her smile, because she had to hide it for her job as a model.

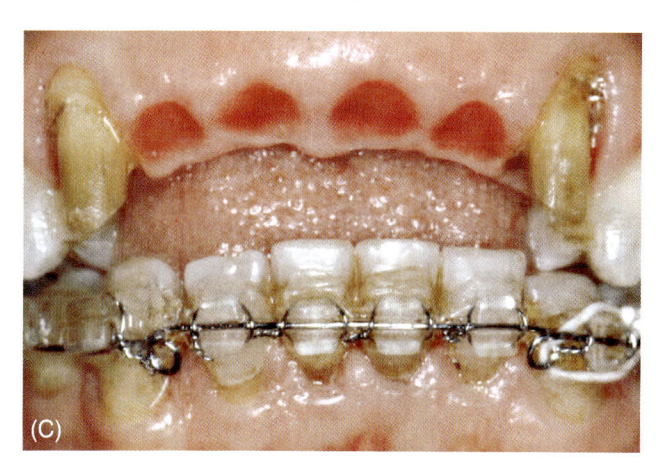

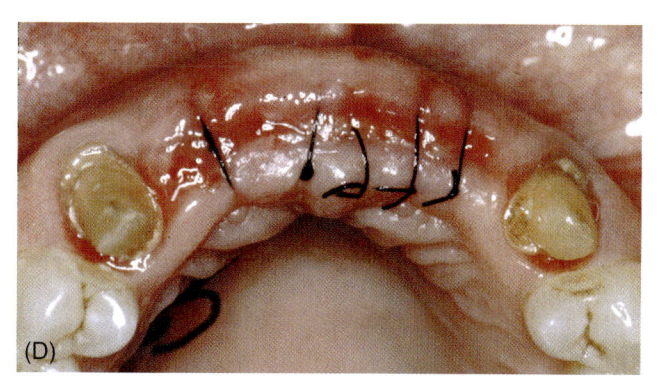

Figure 39.6 **(C, D)** Ridge augmentation was accomplished to improve the pontic area.

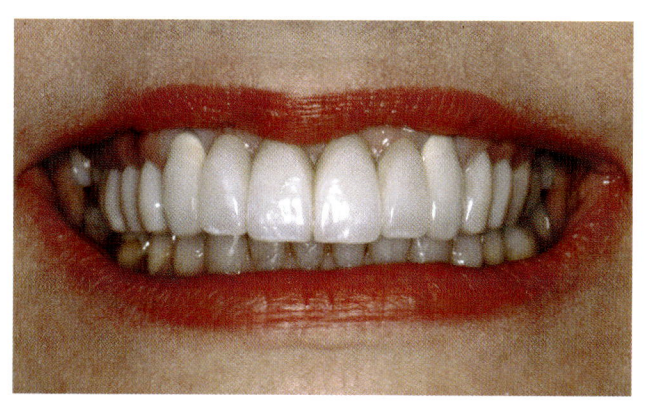

Figure 39.6 **(E)** At the try-in stage, although the gingival height was improved, the esthetic proportions needed improvement.

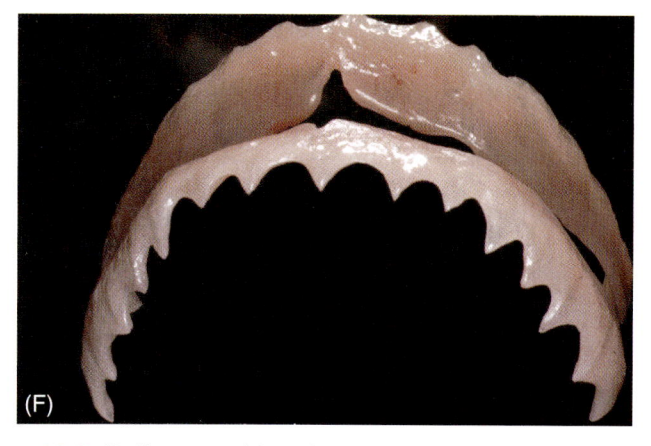

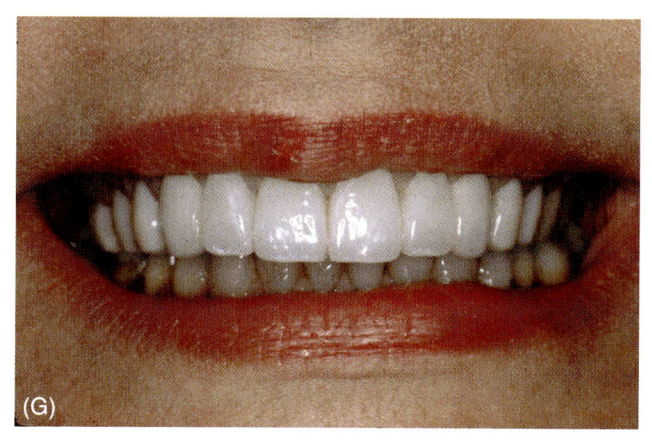

Figure 39.6 **(F, G)** A removable artificial tissue appliance was constructed that could be snapped into place by the patient.

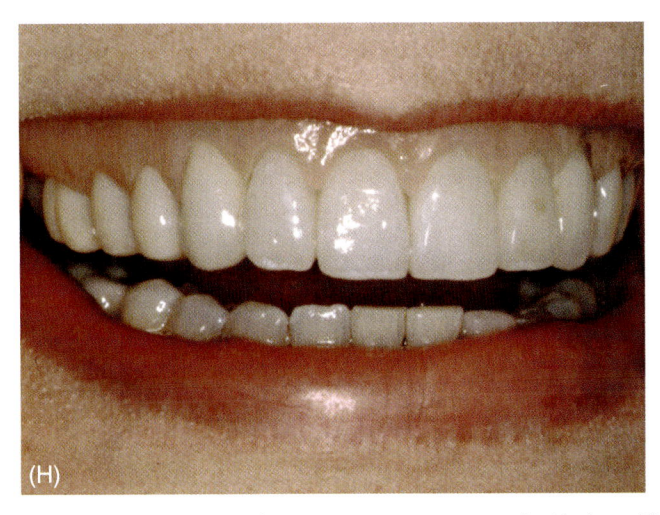

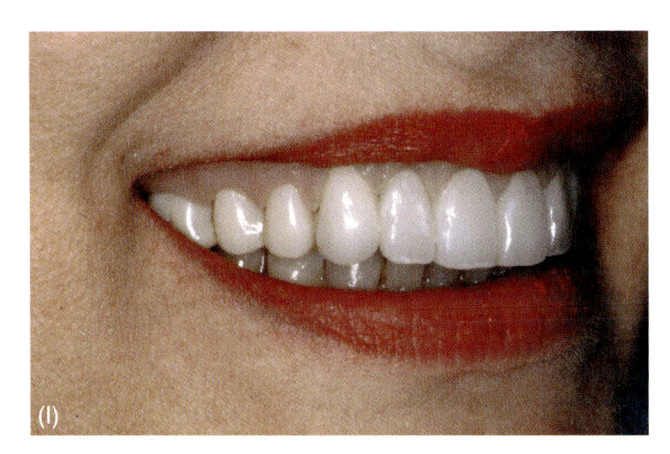

Figure 39.6 (H, I) A more esthetic proportion was created with the artificial tissue appliance, creating a normal crown-to-root ratio, as well as gingival papilla.

Clinical case 39.1: Failure to reshape adjacent teeth

Problem

A 24-year-old female presented with an unattractive porcelain-to-metal crown constructed in labioversion on the maxillary right central incisor (Figure 39.7A). This case is actually a space problem with crowded maxillary incisors. A previous dentist treated this problem by placing the right central in labioversion (Figure 39.7B). Instead of reproportioning the teeth, the dentist made the right central the same size as the left central, and since there was not enough space, the tooth was placed labially. This produced a most unattractive result that displeased the patient, and it contributed to eventual mesial caries on the adjacent central. Lack of embrasures prevented proper cleaning, and a periodontal condition developed. When the patient expressed dissatisfaction, she was told that this was the best that could be done.

Treatment

Teeth that are in labioversion usually reflect more light than others (Figure 39.7A), and unfortunately call attention to themselves. Treatment in this case consisted of cosmetically contouring the adjacent teeth and restoring the right central incisor to the correct position. The key to the success of this case is to correct the acrylic treatment crown (Figure 39.7D); therefore, the lateral and adjacent central incisors were reduced proportionally and recontoured to permit the treatment crown to be positioned correctly. This done, the final crown replaced the temporary crown (Figure 39.7C and D), and the mesial surface of the maxillary left central was treated for caries.

Result

It is possible that the previous dentist suggested orthodontic treatment that the patient refused. Nevertheless, this illustrates poor planning and ignorance of the value of recontouring.

The result shown in Figure 39.7D is a satisfactory treatment alternative to the problem of anterior crowding. It demonstrates a respect for proper crown contours, while emphasizing the importance of adequate gingival embrasures.

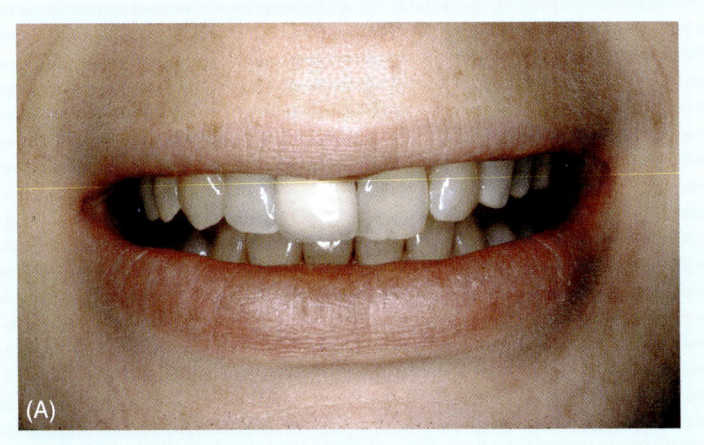

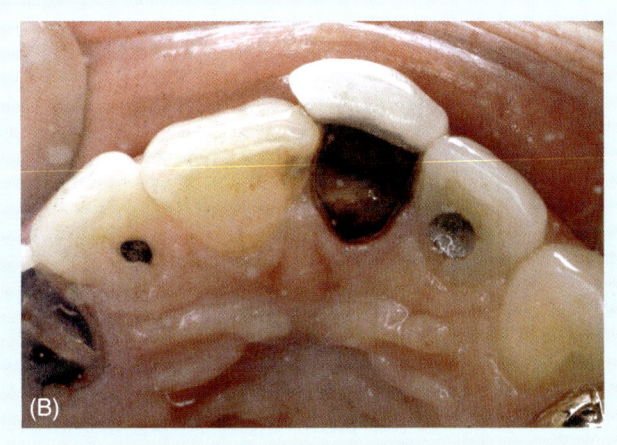

Figure 39.7 (A, B) The dentist who completed the restorative therapy for this patient did not suggest orthodontic treatment and failed to study and alter the adjacent teeth before completing a full crown on the maxillary right central incisor.

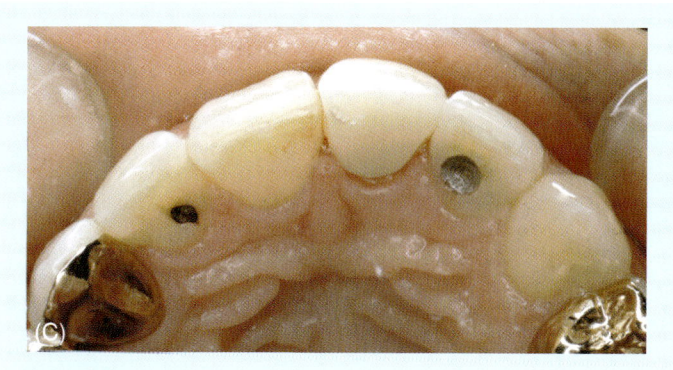

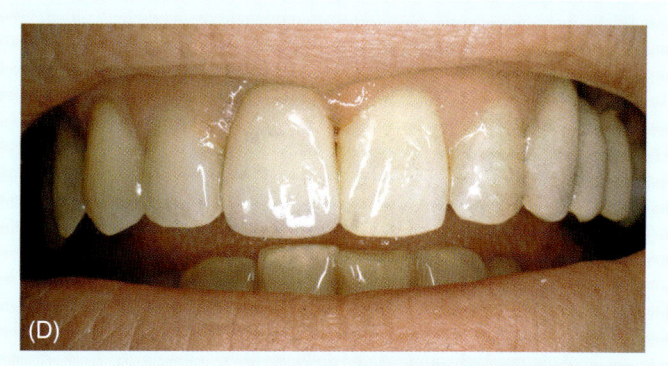

Figure 39.7 **(C, D)** Cosmetic contouring was first done to reproportion the maxillary anterior teeth before replacing the full ceramometal crown with an all-ceramic crown.

A compromised treatment plan

Patients sometimes consider their restorative treatment an esthetic failure, when it is actually the result of a compromised treatment plan. This usually happens when the patient is not fully aware of any treatment limitations. For example, under certain conditions there may not be enough room between abutment teeth to adequately carve and insert teeth of an appropriate size. If the dentist recognizes this problem initially, several alternatives may be possible, including:

- Repreparing the teeth and performing vital extirpation, if necessary, to allow more room.
- Carving overlapping into the restoration to allow for the proper number of teeth.
- Carving one less tooth, but making everything appear symmetrical.
- Contouring adjacent teeth to provide more space.

Regardless of the choice, you must make a compromise and inform the patient, who may view the result as a failure if not forewarned. Sometimes a compromise cannot be avoided in extremely difficult cases, and patients must realize their specific treatment limitations from the outset.

Because of time or financial limitations, patients may impose certain restrictions that make successful esthetic dentistry almost impossible. These limitations, the problems involved, and the reasons for reaching the decision should be documented. Often, all that is necessary is that the limiting conditions be stated in the chart, where the patient signs after approving the treatment plan and estimate.

In cases of financial limitations, oftentimes less expensive treatment may be associated not only with esthetic compromise, but also with longevity. For example, patients who request an inlay in lieu of a crown must understand that, although they may be saving money initially, there may be additional costs associated with their decision in the future. An analysis of indirect restorations performed by Lucarotti and Burke in 2009 demonstrated that crowns outperform other types of indirect restorations, specifically outperforming inlays and veneers. In their study, it was noted that metal crowns, for example, had a reintervention time in excess of 6 years, while inlays involving two or more surfaces displayed reintervention times of less than 3 years. It is of utmost importance that patients fully understand not only the immediate treatment recommendations, but also any potential longevity implications and/or limitations in the future. Patients must be fully informed of all possibilities in the decision-making process.[5]

When an esthetic compromise is necessary, a thorough explanation of the limitations, and the reasons for these limitations, is essential because the patient needs to understand the compromise before treatment begins. Comments on the discussion, and the patient's choice of treatment, should be recorded in the chart, and the patient should also receive a letter documenting this choice. This will serve as a reminder to the patient who may forget the limitations and may consider the treatment of the previous dentist poor. And finally, always have either your dental assistant or treatment coordinator present when these limitations are being discussed.

Choice of restoration

Another issue that is often considered an esthetic failure by the patient is failure of the dentist to discuss the life expectancy of certain restorations. For instance, when patients demand a tooth-colored filling material instead of amalgam or gold, composite resins can be used as a compromise in Class I or II restorations; however, the patient must be informed that these restorations have to be replaced every 3–5 years, lest they consider the restoration an esthetic failure when the time comes. Generally, composite resin failure will be functional rather than esthetic; however, many patients will object to staining that can occur in time with these restorations.

In a study conducted in public dental health clinics in northern Sweden in 2009, the longevity of replaced restorations was evaluated. According to this study, the median ages for replaced restorations of resin composite, glass ionomer cement, and amalgam were 6 years, 11 years, and 16 years respectively, with the most frequently replaced restorations being Class II, followed by Class I and Class IV for resin composite restorations.

This study demonstrates that resin composites, although oftentimes the material of choice for esthetic reasons, are most often replaced for reasons associated with failure. It is also interesting to note that restorations placed in patients with a high caries risk did not last as long as those placed in low-risk patients, regardless of the material used. Additionally, dentists with less experience were more prone to replace restorations than those who had been practicing longer, demonstrating a median longevity of 5 years for replaced restorations completed with more than 5 years professional experience, compared with 4 years for those restorations completed with less experience. Based on this study, it is evident that a portion of these failure statistics could be related to iatrogenic reasons as well.[6]

Many esthetic failures are not easy to remedy. Figure 39.8 shows a case of multiple esthetic problems that are difficult to treat: anterior space limitations and difference in pontic height due to gingival recession of the left central and lateral incisors. Because the patient has a low lip line, treatment can be improved by better proportioning of the anterior teeth. Nevertheless, this case requires complete understanding of patient objectives. A thorough review, including waxed study casts, is needed to find the best esthetic and functional solution.

Compromise when patient rejects repositioning treatment

When the dentist suggests that only repositioning will give an optimal result and the patient rejects such treatment, this must be stated and initialed by the patient in the record. The final esthetic result may not be as pleasing without repositioning. In such cases, the patient often forgets they rejected the dentist's recommended choice of treatment after treatment has been completed. The final restorative treatment plan should thus be considered a "compromised treatment" and the patient made fully aware that they chose the compromise at the outset. Most patients forget that a former dentist ever mentioned any alternatives or warnings of limitations of final esthetic results. An example of this is seen in Figure 39.9. The patient presented with the complaint of two central incisor crowns being too large. When questioned, she at first stated that her previous dentist never suggested orthodontic therapy; however, after extensive discussion, she finally admitted the possibility of this suggestion once being made.

Many esthetic failures may be traced to poor planning. All limiting factors, and the probability of success, must be known

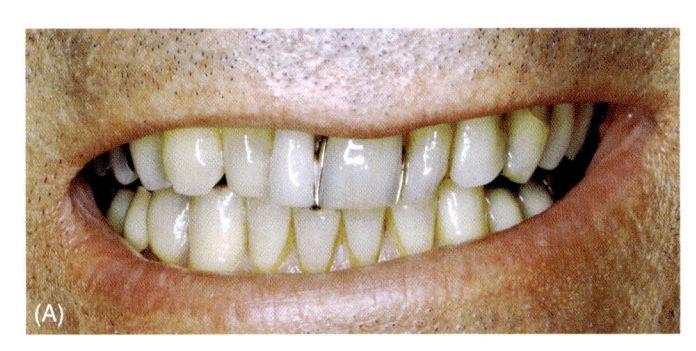

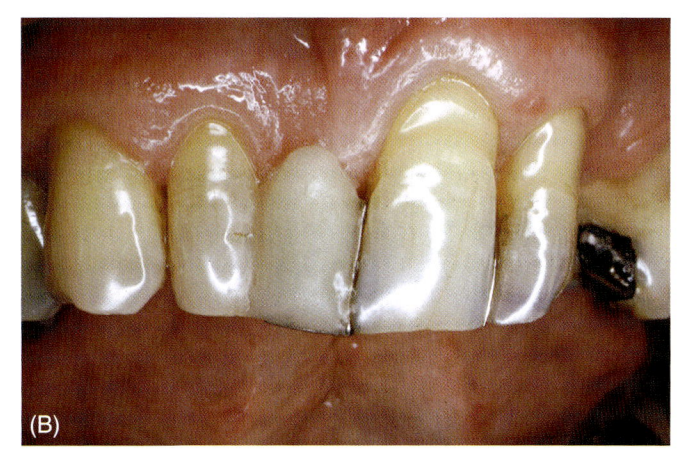

Figure 39.8 (A, B) This man presented with multiple esthetic problems that were difficult to treat: anterior space limitations and difference in pontic heights due to gingival recession of left lateral and central incisors. Here, orthodontics would have been the ideal treatment.

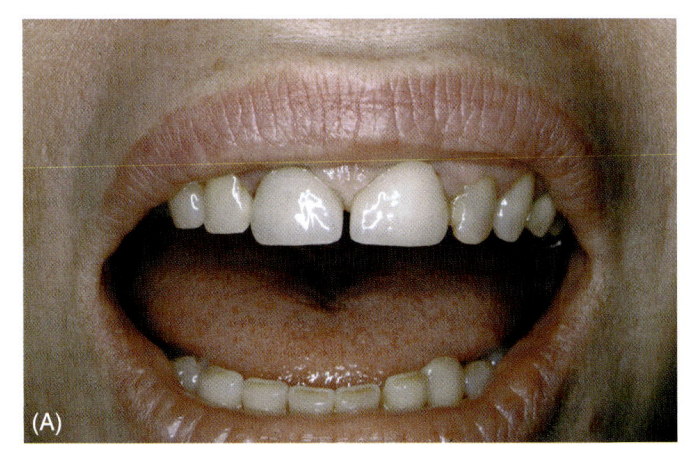

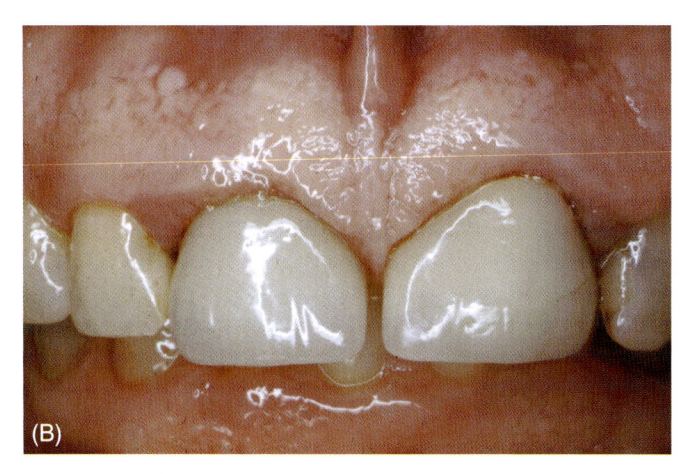

Figure 39.9 (A, B) Although this patient rejected orthodontic treatment, the dentist could have suggested including the adjacent laterals and cuspids, in addition to the centrals, to create a more esthetic result.

before treatment is begun. Checklists, written or mental, should always be used to help determine the various problems and considerations that any one case presents.

Eventual failure: restoration longevity

Few dental treatments last indefinitely—almost every dental treatment has a limited life span. In fact, in a 3-year study of 406 patients by Schwartz et al., it was found that the mean life span for all fixed restorations was 10.3 years.[7] However, more than 20% of the restorations surveyed failed in less than 3 years. A total of 3.3% of these failures were considered by the patient to be esthetic in nature, due either to an excess of visible gold or unesthetic acrylic facings. Almost all restorations eventually need to be replaced; repositioned teeth may continue to move, and even endodontically treated teeth can fracture or become problematic. *Use the word* permanent *with patients only to explain to them that nothing is permanent when it comes to discussing the longevity of any proposed restorations.*

Longevity of a restoration, or the reintervention time, is an important topic to be discussed with patients, especially when considering crowns. A study conducted over a number of years in England and Wales assessed varying crown survival rates. A total of 68% of metal crowns survived 10 years without reintervention, whereas 62% of metal–ceramic crowns survived the same amount of time. If these crowns were to be replaced, 36% of the reinterventions would involve recementing, 17% would involve replacement crowns, 13% would involve direct restorations, 12% would involve root canal treatment, and 19% would involve extraction. This study concludes that all-metal crowns are more successful than both metal–ceramic and all-ceramic crowns.[8]

Although all-metal crowns prove the most successful, they are unfortunately not the most esthetic. A study conducted by Galindo et al. examined the long-term survival of alumina crowns over a 10-year period and found that alumina single-unit crowns had comparable survival rates to those of metal–ceramic crowns. Although certain risk factors, such as bruxism and clenching, must be evaluated on an individual basis, this study supports the use of such restorations in clinical practice.[9]

Some differences in survival rates may be related to esthetic expectations from all-ceramic crowns, as many of these failures could be related to patient and/or clinician dissatisfaction with the appearance of the crown. Regardless, all crowns exhibit reasonable success over the course of 10 years, with the incidence of re-intervention decreasing as the age of the crown increases.[8]

When a patient is dissatisfied, it is usually because they did not understand the treatment limitations. When it becomes necessary to replace restorations, such patients may feel that their previous treatment was inferior, when the opposite may well be true. Thus, always inform the patient as to the life expectancy of all treatment. Generally, it is best to underplay the number of years that any treatment will last, since no one can accurately predict what will happen in any given oral environment.

It is most unfortunate to find patients who have had their entire mouth rebuilt with fixed arch splinting, with great investments of time and money, only to have the reconstruction fail sooner than they thought it should. Few patients ever think that treatment may fail, unless they are thoroughly indoctrinated by the dentist before treatment. Therefore, many of these patients tend to switch dentists, and to seek someone who will assure them that a longer restorative life expectancy can be obtained with different treatment.[10] Generally, the more complex the case, or the longer the span of fixed replacement, the less the life expectancy.[7] A patient who has all of their teeth and healthy supporting bone can likely keep them for life, but they will need restorations replaced from time to time. This is a much easier oral environment to maintain than the patient who is missing many teeth and has weak bone. Such patients must be clearly informed of the limitations of their restorations.

Problems that cause failure

Exposure of margins

Intact margins can be exposed by tissue recession. If the gingival portion of a ceramometal crown contains a small gold collar, eventual exposure of the gold may be considered an esthetic failure by the patient. The purpose of the gold collar should be explained at the onset of treatment, because if the patient objects then some other treatment may be necessary. The patient should also be informed of the potential for this compromised result. It is usually possible to hide the gold collar subgingivally; however, in time, tissue may recede, possibly due to brushing habits or pathological changes in the oral environment. The assumption must be made that the restoration was originally properly contoured at the gingival margin; otherwise, it would be considered an esthetic failure at the outset. If the patient has a high lip line that may potentially show the margin, this must be a consideration in the treatment plan (Figure 39.10A and B).

If a ceramometal crown is being contemplated, an alternate solution would be to use an all-porcelain butt joint, instead of a gold collar, on the labial surface. If the patient has a low lip line that will not expose the margin under normal conditions, you must demonstrate this fact to the patient during examination and treatment planning. Photographs of the patient's smile should be taken for records, with the objective to obtain the widest possible smile for treatment planning purposes. Even all-ceramic crowns can be a problem if the root beyond the ceramic margin is exposed through tissue recession. Again, depending on the lip line, it may not be visible; however, perfectionist patients may well complain, regardless of whether or not their smile line shows the problem area. Therefore, it is critical for you to know your patient and predict just how demanding they can potentially be, so that you can thoroughly discuss any potential problems before your treatment plan is finalized.

Periodontal disease

Poor tissue response to restorations is one of the leading causes of esthetic failure. The probability of success is based on basic functional prosthetic principles; however, the opposite is also true. Improper marginal fit, poor crown contour, and the level of gingival embrasure can all cause gingival hypertrophy and poor tissue response.

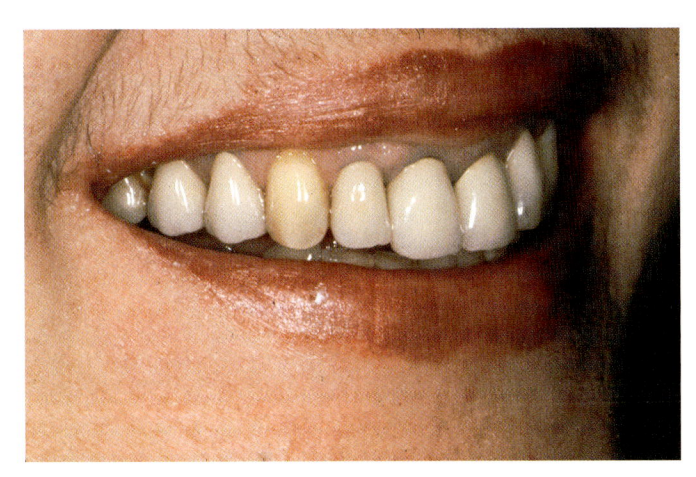

Figure 39.10 **(A)** This patient's high lip line must be taken into consideration when planning anterior restorations that may expose the margins of her crowns.

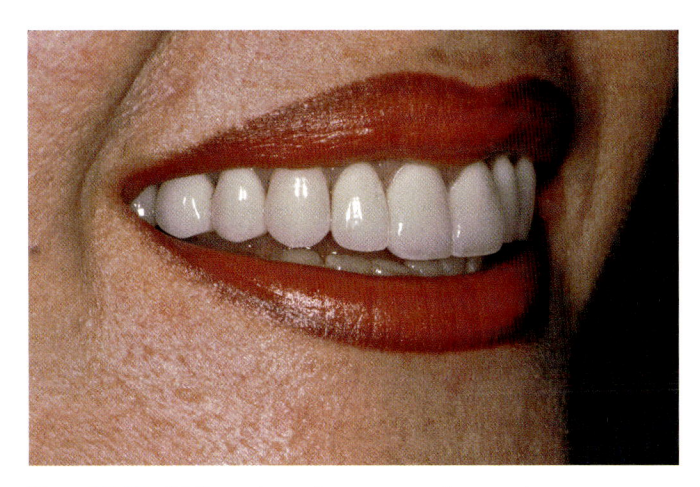

Figure 39.10 **(B)** Since the patient requested a complete treatment plan to improve her smile, crown lengthening plus a combination of porcelain veneers and all-ceramic crowns helped give her the smile she desired.

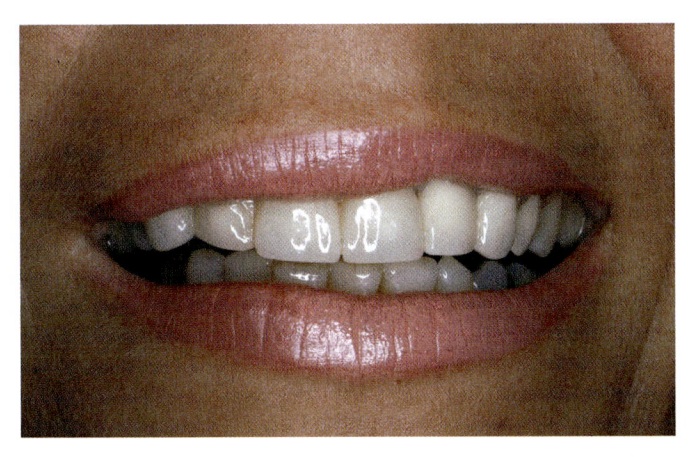

Figure 39.11 **(A)** This woman developed a habit of smiling with the right side of her lip to avoid showing the unesthetic gingival hypertrophy in the upper right posterior quadrant.

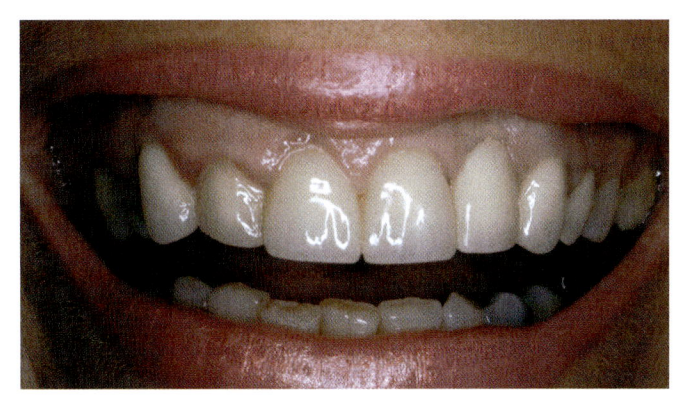

Figure 39.11 **(B)** A natural smile with the patient completely relaxed reveals the unattractive right side of the arch.

Gingival hypertrophy frequently results from improper crown contours and lack of marginal adaptation. The gingiva may grow over the crown, hiding part of the crown and producing an asymmetrical smile. In Figure 39.11A, the patient tries to keep the right side of her lip from rising any higher. This is caused by an asymmetrical hypertrophic reaction of the gingiva (Figure 39.11B). The importance of preventive maintenance for crowns or fixed partial dentures cannot be overstressed.

Patients with short clinical crowns, bulky gingival margins, or localized gingival inflammation due to poorly contoured restorations oftentimes require crown-lengthening procedures to improve appearance. In such cases, it is advantageous to begin with a wide zone of attached gingiva, such that lengthening can be successfully completed without apically positioning the gingival tissues, while still maintaining the zone of attached gingiva. It is most ideal to leave an attached gingival zone of at least 2 mm, although the clinician may have no choice but to apically position the gingival tissues in cases where this zone is found to be too narrow.[4]

In addition to excessive gingival contours, patients may alternatively present with gingival insufficiency. Localized recession might necessitate periodontal surgery instead of extending the margins of the crown, the result of which would be ultimately unesthetic. In cases of gingival insufficiency, try reshaping gingival contours, using either a scalpel or electrosurgery. Such techniques may include coronally and/or laterally repositioned flaps, or palatal autografts, otherwise known as free gingival grafts. The result of such procedures is alleviation of recession and, ultimately, esthetic success.

While soft-tissue defects pose potential problems, esthetic restorations will also fail if supporting bone continues to deteriorate in periodontally involved cases. Patients with periodontal disease should be warned about the possibility of replacement, and an estimate of life expectancy should be given. Prosthetic esthetic failures can occur through no fault of the restoration itself; and if this occurs, either crowns or veneers can be repaired or replaced (Figures 39.12A–E and 39.13A and B).

Recurrent caries

In the Schwartz et al. study,[7] caries accounted for the largest number of failures (36.8%) in fixed restorations, the average life span of which was 11.1 years. Secondary decay can be the result of a multitude of factors, and it is important for the clinician to

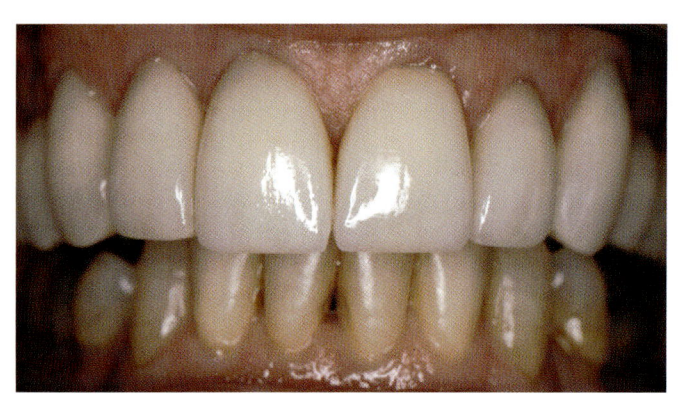

Figure 39.12 (A) This man's previously discolored teeth were masked with porcelain veneers.

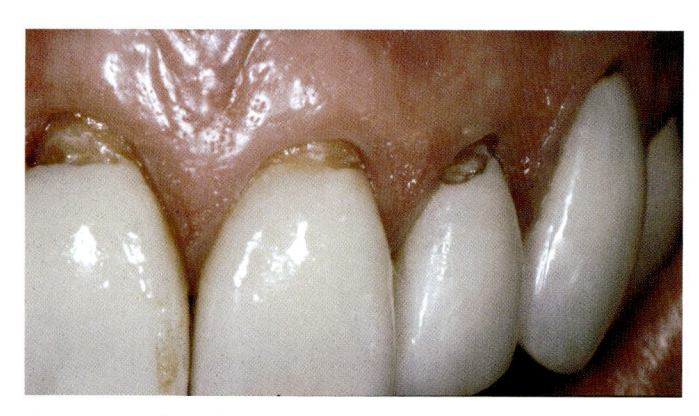

Figure 39.12 (B) A decade later, veneer margins were exposed due to periodontal disease. Since finances were a concern, the patient elected to have the margins repaired, instead of replaced.

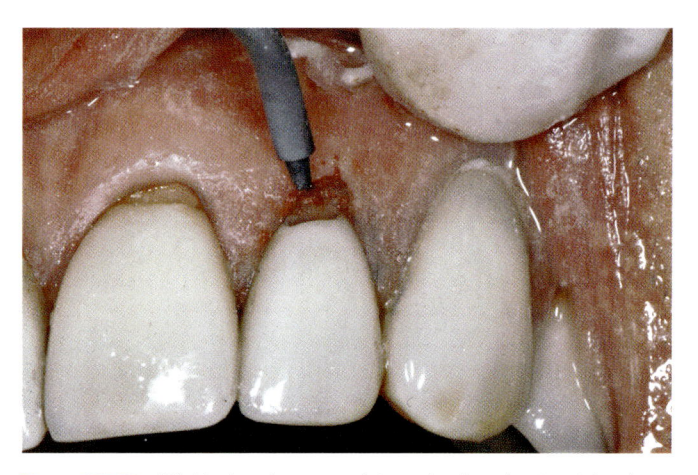

Figure 39.12 (C) Air abrasion, porcelain etch, phosphoric acid etch, silane and microfill composite resin (Renamel..Cosmedent) were used to carefully prepare the root surface, as well as the porcelain.

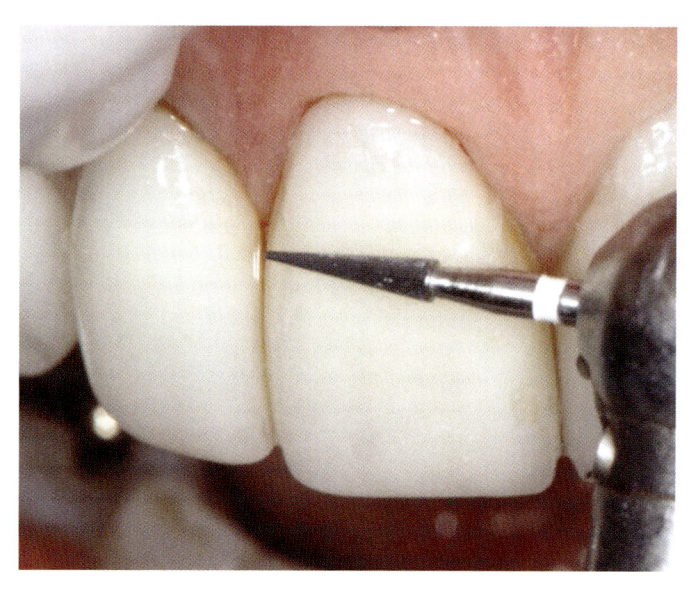

Figure 39.12 (D) A 30-blade carbide bur (ET6UF, Brasseler USA) was used to shape the composite resin for the repair.

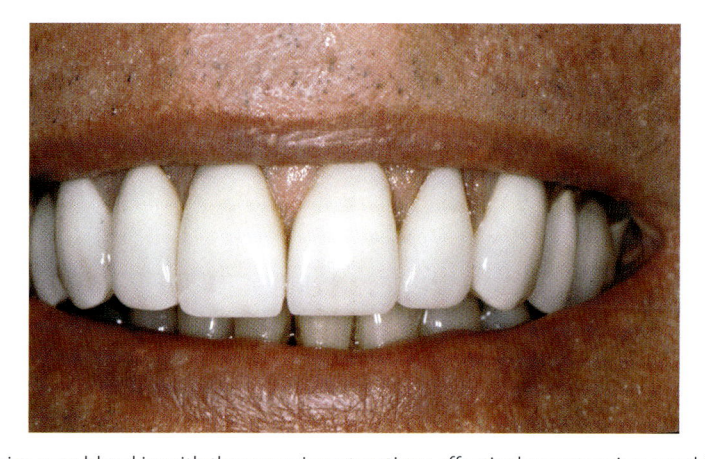

Figure 39.12 (E) The bonded margins now blend in with the ceramic restorations effectively postponing need for replacement.

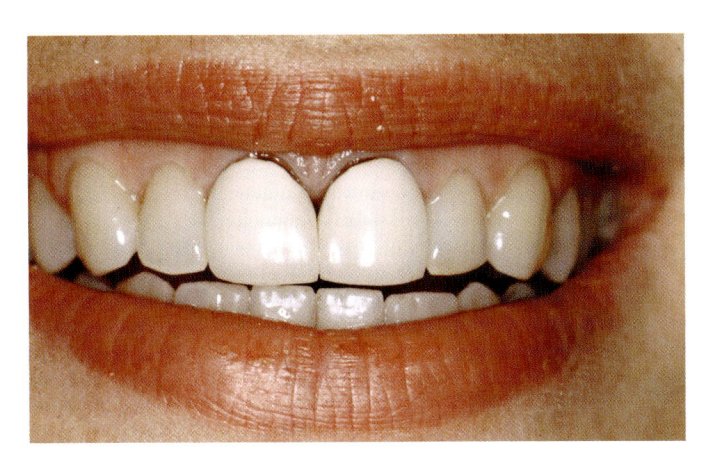

Figure 39.13 (A) This patient was not happy with her exposed margins, even though the crowns lasted for 7 years.

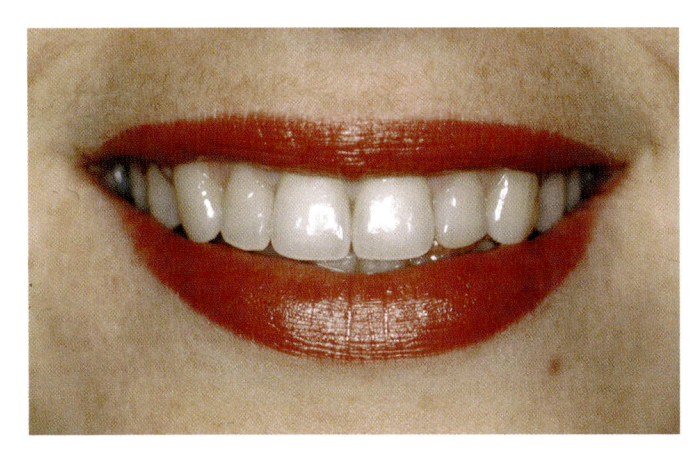

Figure 39.13 (B) The defective crowns were replaced with better-proportioned crowns, following minor orthodontics to reduce the amount of space between the centrals.

understand whether or not maintenance may be feasible from the onset of treatment (Figure 39.14). Based on such factors as the extent of caries, access to the lesion, restorative material used, and the possibility of adequate isolation, caries progression may be arrested through appropriate therapy. Removal of decay, in addition to such prophylactic measures as dietary counseling, fluoride rinse, and consistent reassessment, can better ensure a successful prognosis for the expected lifespan of the restoration.[4]

Regardless of esthetic considerations, failure to control plaque formation, and subsequent caries, can doom the result from initiation of treatment (Figure 39.15A). In order to ensure success, preventive procedures should be routinely instituted before restorative treatment. For example, before fixed restorations are cemented, fluoride should be applied to the abutment teeth. It is especially helpful to continue this process yearly in patients with exposed margins. After restorative therapy, the clinician must continue to review oral disease control measures to avoid plaque formation and recurrent caries (Figure 39.15B). Studies have shown that secondary carious lesion progression is slow (usually 3–5 years), but those who receive acceptable dental prophylaxis tend to demonstrate a decreased rate of progression and, ultimately, an increased rate of success.[11]

It is also advised that a fluoride-containing cement must be considered when cementing restorations in patients prone to dental caries. This is the reason that resin-modified glass ionomer cements have been so popular and, indeed, useful for many years. In our extensive clinical experience with resin-modified glass ionomer cement, only a handful of crowns became

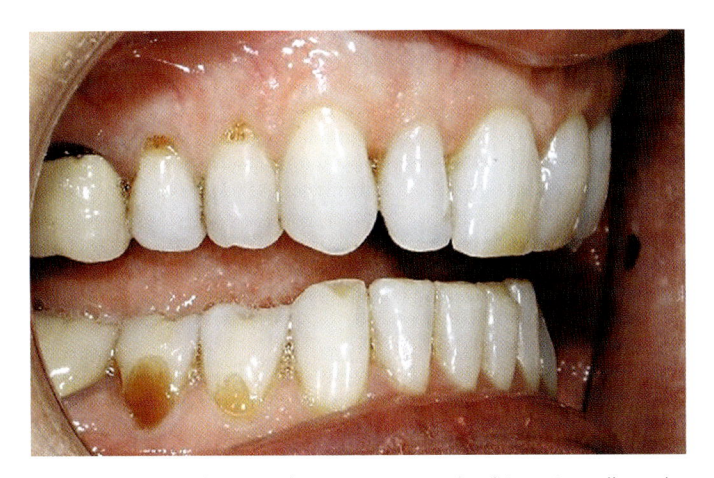

Figure 39.14 Neglect was the main reason why this patient allowed herself to develop recurrent caries under all her restorations.

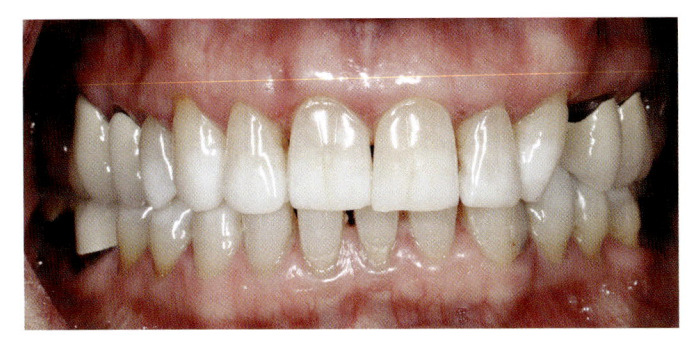

Figure 39.15 (A) This patient presented with recurrent decay around her existing restorations.

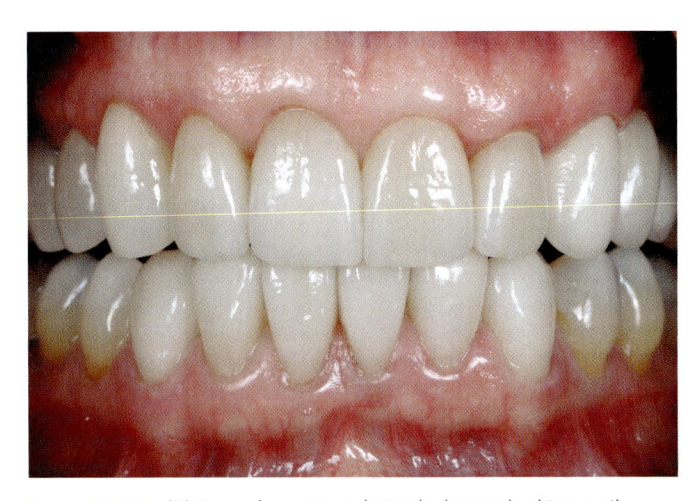

Figure 39.15 (B) Since the patient desired a better-looking smile, full-mouth restorations were fabricated, in addition to replacing the defective restorations.

debonded, and none had caries underneath. As a result, most of our restorations are cemented with resin-modified glass ionomer cement.

Material failure

Porcelain

With material such as porcelain, there is always the possibility of fracture at a later date (Figure 39.16A and B). Although a full porcelain crown is perhaps the most esthetic of fixed restorations, its lifespan is somewhat shorter. Burke and Lucarotti evaluated the long-term success of various kinds of crowns and determined that all-porcelain crowns had the shortest survival rate (48%), compared with 68% survival of full metal crowns over the course of 10 years.[8] Judicious selection of cases where occlusal demands are not too great is necessary.[12] Patients who have habits that put torque on the porcelain, such as bruxism and clenching, will probably have earlier fractures as a result of undue stress on the material. This is especially true if the occlusal

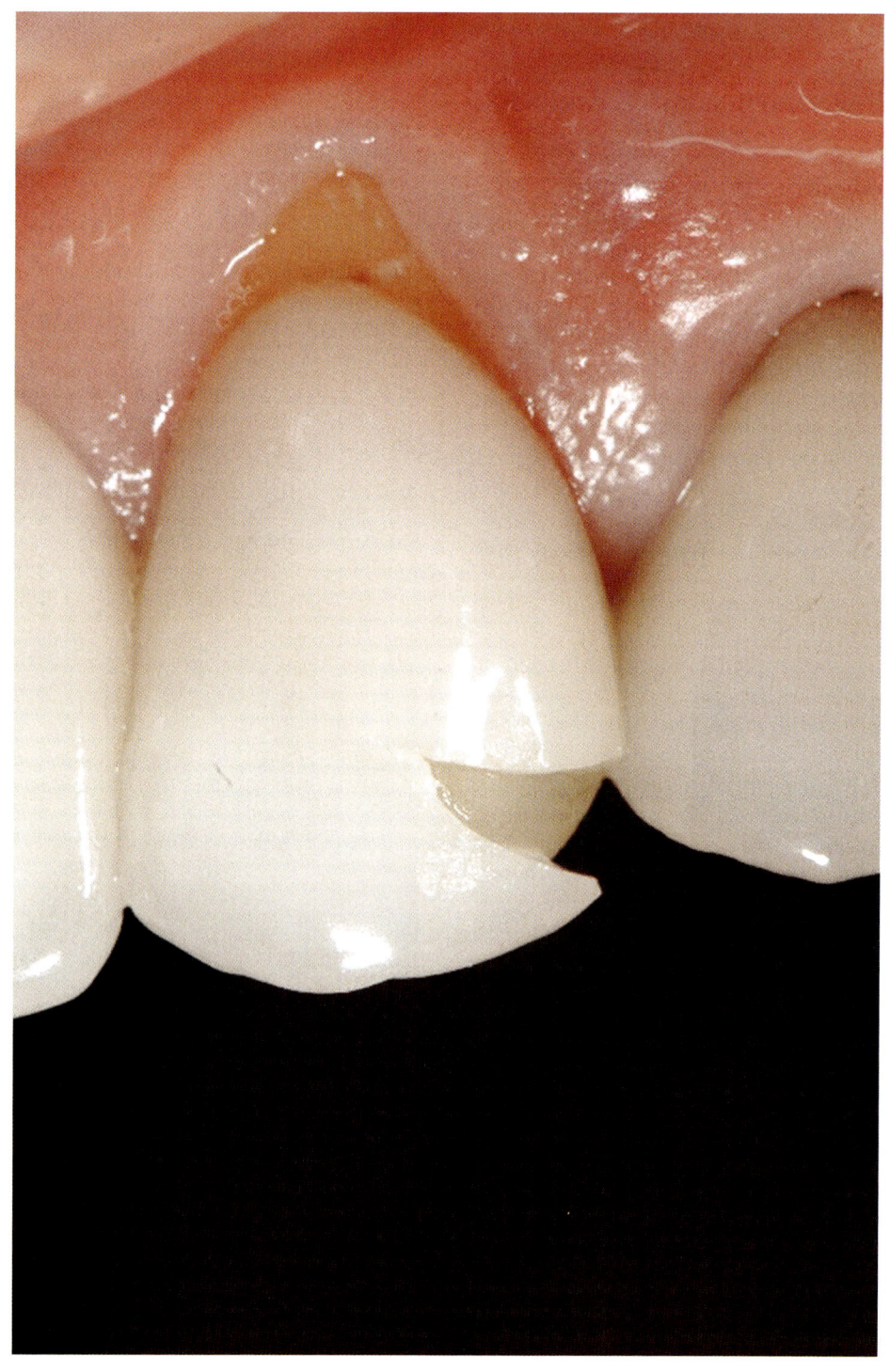

Figure 39.16 **(A)** This patient fractured her porcelain veneer while biting on a foreign object.

surface of the crown is gold and the labial surface is porcelain. Depending on the location of the porcelain-to-metal labial junction, definite problems can exist.

Although the patient's occlusion must be carefully considered when assessing the possibility of porcelain crowns, restorations such as porcelain veneers have been considered to mimic the mechanical behavior of the patient's existing occlusion, so that the biomechanics of the original tooth do not need to be altered. In a study assessing the outcome of porcelain laminate veneers, it was found that 53% of teeth with these restorations survived 10 years without reintervention; however, success rates of 64% and 91% have also been reported in various other studies, a discrepancy that may be attributed to varying operator and patient factors. In this particular study, factors such as patient gender and age were considered most important when assessing the clinical success of these restorations. Findings such as deteriorating periodontal status, reduced posterior support, and/or reduced salivary flow from the use of a variety of medications are all indications for the failure of these restorations due to increasing age[8] (Figure 39.17A–G).

All ceramic

All-ceramic materials with high translucency are preferred in the esthetic zone, and high-strength materials are preferred in the posterior; however, when addressing problems such as discoloration of anterior teeth, higher strength materials may be preferred to mask such problems.[13]

Ceramic crowns and fixed partial dentures also have variable survival rates, depending on the different all-ceramic systems to be used. In a 5-year clinical trial conducted by Larsson and Vult von Steyern, the clinical performances of Denzir® (DZ) and In-Ceram Zirconia® (InZ) two- to five-unit implant-supported all-ceramic restorations were evaluated and compared with one another. The restorations were cemented with zinc phosphate cement onto customized titanium abutments, and were evaluated after 1, 3, and 5 years. At the 5-year follow-up, it was determined that all restorations were in function with both all-ceramic systems; however, 9 of 13 DZ restorations and 2 of 12 InZ restorations exhibited superficial cohesive (or chip-off) fractures. Thus, the results of this study suggest that although the DZ system could not be recommended as a treatment regimen for

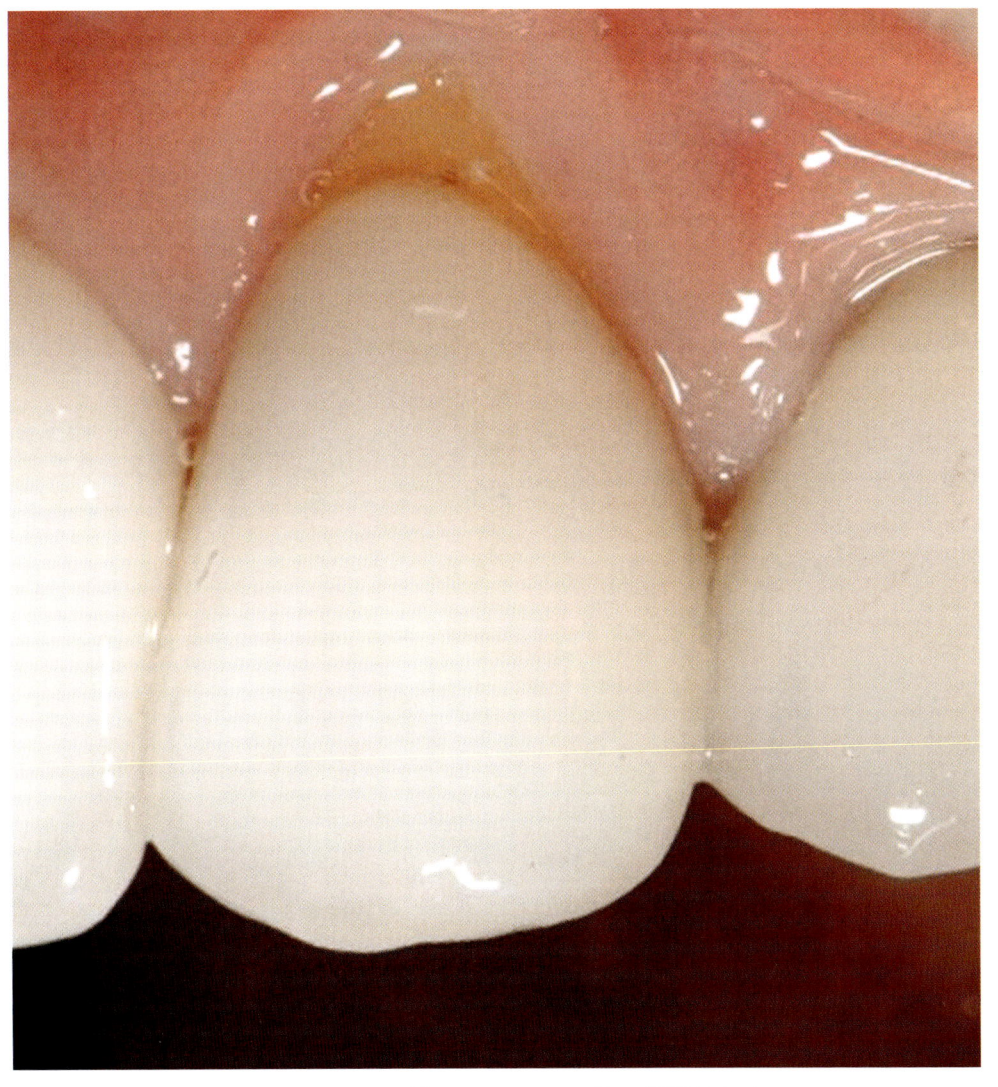

Figure 39.16 **(B)** The fractured area was restored using a microfill composite resin. (Durafill VS, Kulzer).

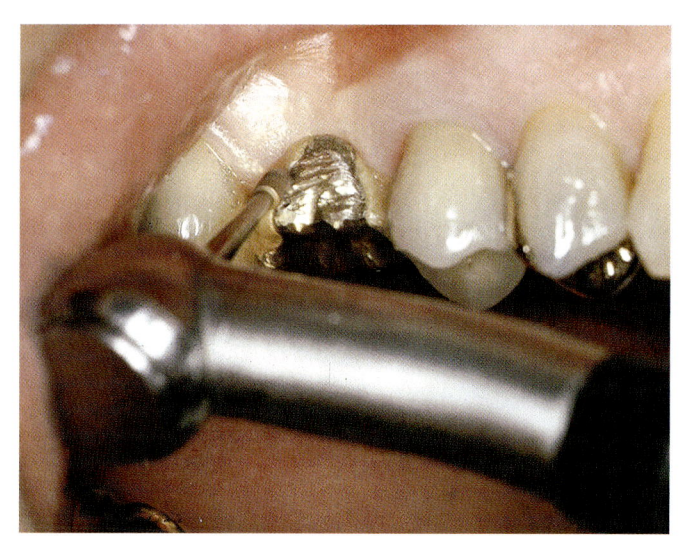

Figure 39.17 (A) This man fractured his maxillary ceramometal bridge and asked if it could be repaired instead of replaced.

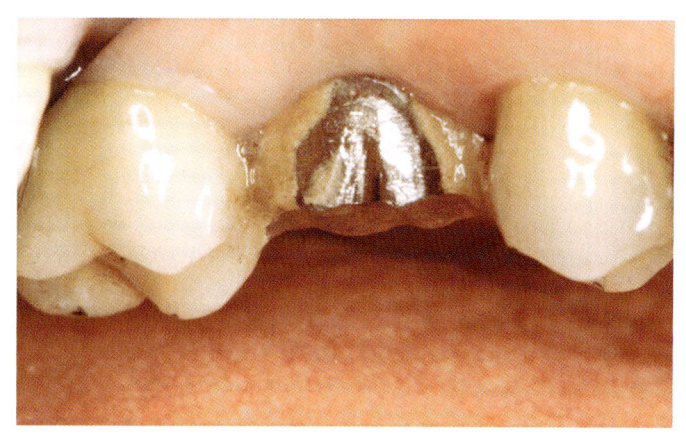

Figure 39.17 (B) The remaining ceramometal pontic was prepared with a taper, so that a new pontic could be constructed.

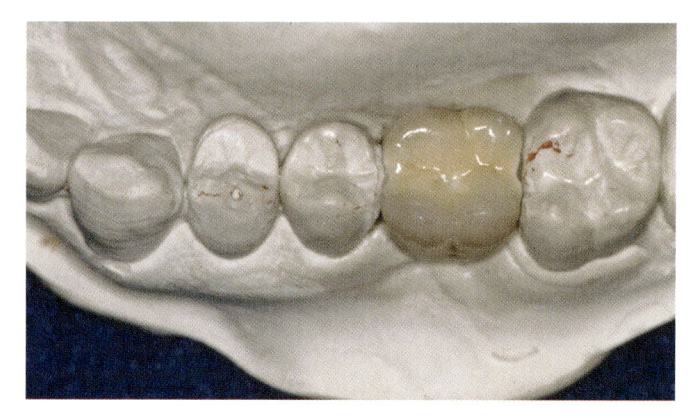

Figure 39.17 (C) An impression was made of the pontic area and a model created, so that a new ceramometal pontic could be constructed.

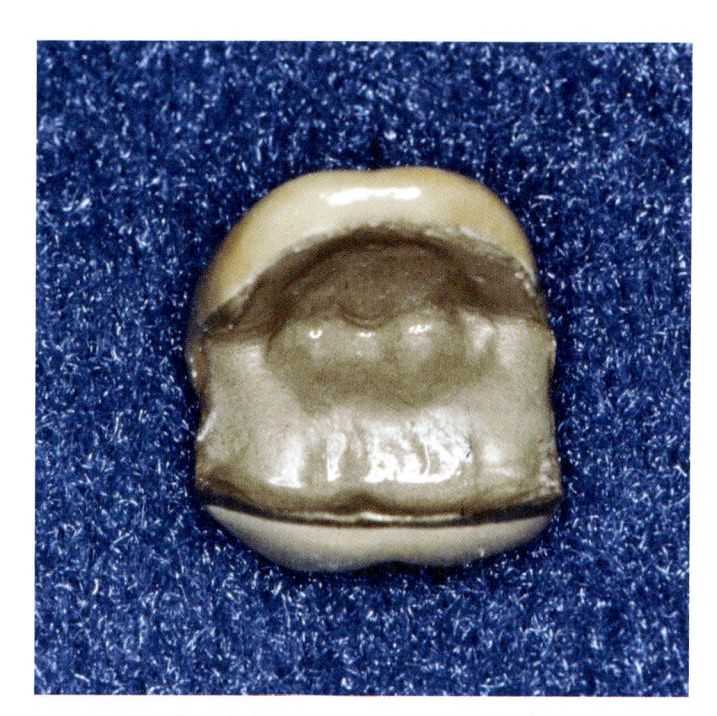

Figure 39.17 (D) This demonstrates the underside of the ceramometal pontic.

this type of restoration, an all-ceramic implant-supported fixed dental prosthesis may be an acceptable treatment alternative.[14]

Fixed-prosthesis frameworks

When evaluating the framework and veneering ceramic possibilities for any case, it is important to note the combinations that produce the best results, so that the longevity of the restoration can be assessed and any errors in material choice avoided. Both ceramometal and all-ceramic fixed prosthetics are susceptible to abnormal or increased occlusal stress, resulting in fracture. Depending on the severity of the stress, it is sometimes possible to repair, instead of replace, the fixed prosthesis (Figure 39.18A–E).

In a clinical study conducted by Christensen and Ploeger, the performance differences between metal, zirconia, and alumina fixed partial denture frameworks were assessed, according to the type of ceramic veneer chosen for each—pressed or layered ceramics.[15] For this study, dentists prepared posterior three-unit fixed partial dentures with 10 different framework/ceramic veneer combinations. The results were as follows: metal frameworks with veneer ceramics had the best clinical performance, followed by zirconia frameworks with veneer ceramics. Of the veneer ceramics, CZR Press veneer ceramic proved to be the best option, mainly because of its leucite-containing and pressed properties. Of all framework possibilities, the alumina frameworks had the most clinically inferior performance.

Composite resin

As in the case of most restorative materials, functional failure usually means esthetic failure. In general, there are five leading causes of failure of in composite resins: (1) marginal leakage, (2) material that is too translucent, (3) esthetic problems in shading, (4) porosity or air pockets, and (5) fracture.

The biggest problem to date with composite resin restorations is marginal leakage, leading to recurrent caries. Depending on such factors as concentration, type, and flexibility of material used, shrinkage stress may preclude restoration contraction, and

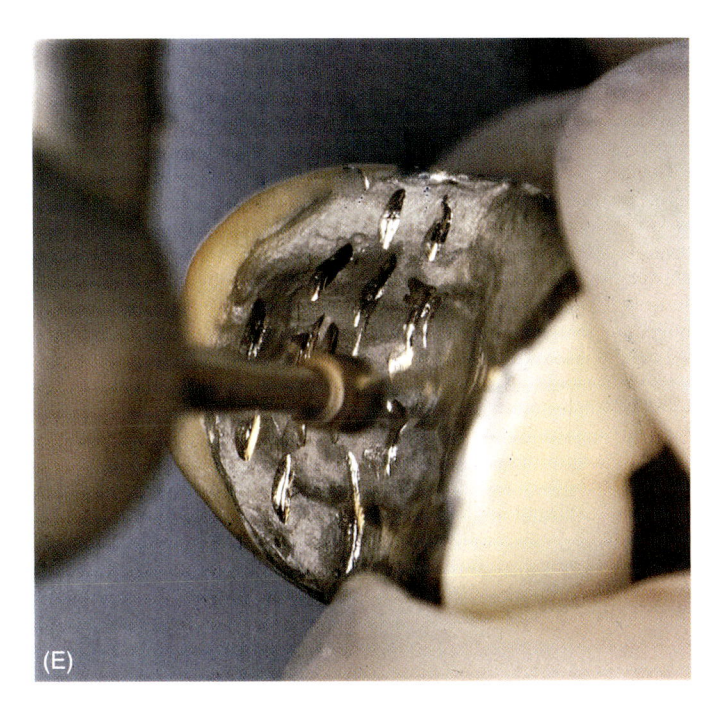

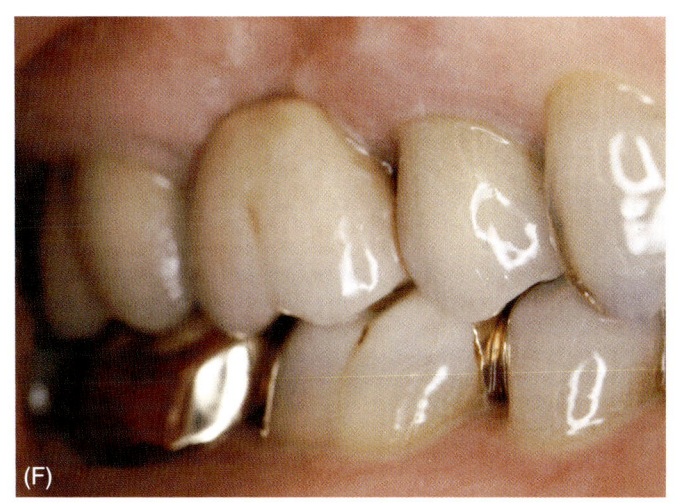

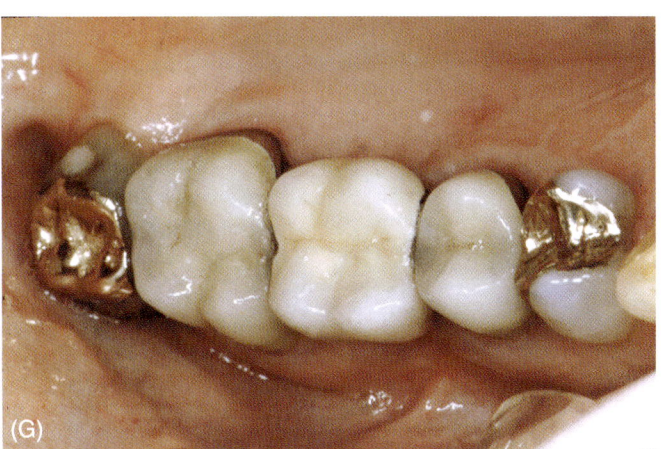

Figure 39.17 **(E–G)** Slight grooves were roughened on the inside to aid in retention of the pontic and cemented into place.

eventually bacterial microleakage, staining, inflammation, and/or caries.[11] The most pronounced clinical symptom is generally discoloration of the resin restoration, with predominance in one particular area of stain, indicating possible caries (Figure 39.19A–C).

In a study by van Dijken and Lindberg, published in 2009, the durability of Class II restorations was assessed over the course of 5 years using two different materials: a low-shrinkage composite and an optimized particle resin composite. It was hypothesized that Class II preparations restored with low-shrinkage composite would be more durable than those restored with the optimized particle resin composite; however, it was concluded that no significant differences existed between the materials, although the low-shrinkage material did prove to last slightly longer, with an annual failure rate of 1.7% compared with 2.4% for optimized particle resin composite. It is notable, however, that shrinkage stress over the course of time manifested itself in the presence of secondary decay, found in both materials. Thus, it may be concluded that secondary decay, regardless of the product used, was the primary reason for failure due to marginal leakage.[11]

While only a small difference between materials was observed, the authors emphasized that the success of these restorations may have been somewhat dependent on technique as well. When conducting their study, an oblique layering technique was employed when possible, intended to reduce the shrinkage effect and configuration factor of the restorations. If such a technique is used, it may be concluded that operator ability, in addition to other factors dependent on the individual patient, may be more important variables to assess when considering durability due to shrinkage, than considerations based on the type of material used.[11]

Another type of esthetic failure with composite is seen in restorations that are too translucent, especially in Class IV restorations. Figure 39.20A and B shows a Class IV restoration that is functionally well done; however, because of a difference in light reflection and translucency between the enamel and the restorative material, the shade variance is apparent.

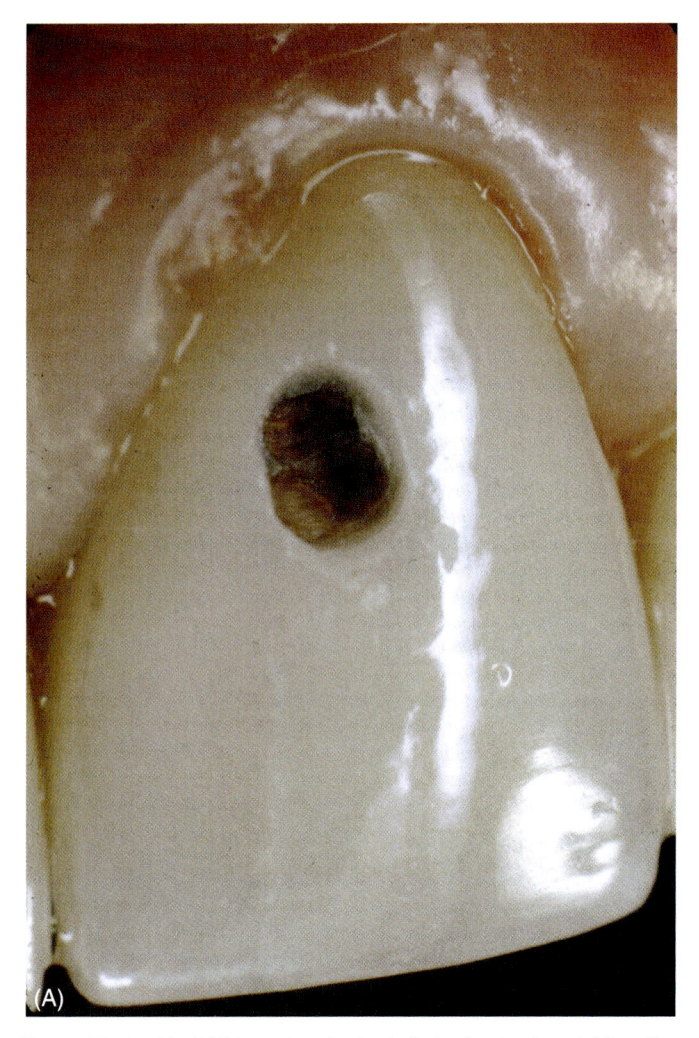

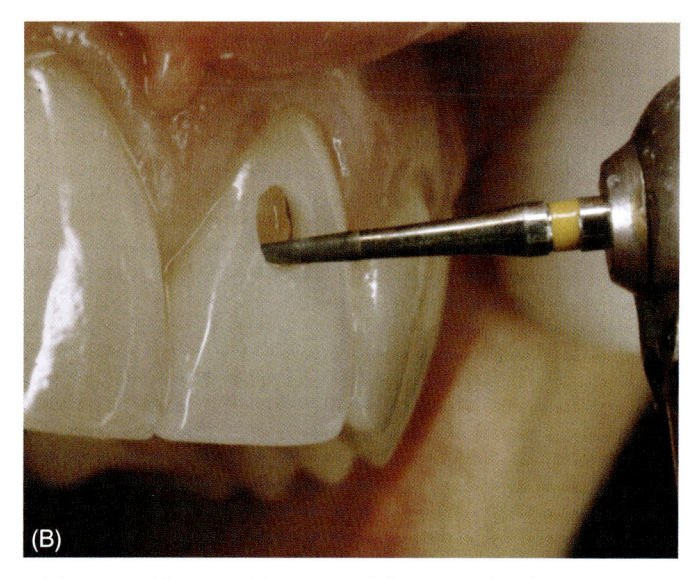

Figure 39.18 **(A, B)** This patient had a dark shadow in the middle of her porcelain veneer. The porcelain was carefully removed in that area to reveal the cause of the discoloration.

Some brands of resin composite are more translucent than others and lack sufficient filler material or opacity to block light. Therefore, use a material that has more opacity, or an opaquing tint, in the restoration for these cases.

A third type of esthetic problem is stain caused by microleakage that occurs at the junction between the restorative material and the margin of the tooth. It can usually be avoided by using a long bevel that involves overlapping of the margin. An example of this type of esthetic problem is seen in Figure 39.21A, which demonstrates a patient with cervical erosion and microleakage on a canine. Figure 39.21B shows the restoration being replaced by using a long bevel. The final result shows how extending the actual margin beyond the bevel allows for easy repair later, if needed (Figure 39.21C).

Another form of composite failure is due to the presence of air pockets or bubbles that attract food, stain, turn dark, and can be due to percolation. In most composites, the catalyst is built into the material, and when it is mixed, a certain amount of evaporation takes place. This sometimes causes the appearance of small air pockets, which could be avoided by careful operative techniques.

A fifth cause of composite resin failure is fracture. The first step in any composite fracture is discovering the reason for the fracture. If the fracture was caused by a patient biting down on a foreign object, such as a fork, then obviously the patient's abusive habit is the cause of fracture, and replacement of the restoration is in order; however, if the patient has another habit (such as clenching or grinding) that causes the fracture, then steps must be taken to control the habit and possibly to adjust the opposing occlusion, demonstrated in Figure 39.22A–F. Even if the patient states that they do not clench or grind their teeth, it has been our experience that, in times of stress, most people unconsciously do so.

Technical failures

Dentists usually assume that laboratory procedures are completed correctly; however, failure occasionally occurs through no fault of the dentist, who must still assume the responsibility and undertake the repair. Unfortunately, patients are not interested in what the laboratory did or did not do. If dentists want to maintain rapport with the public, and specifically with their patients, they must continue to assume such responsibility.

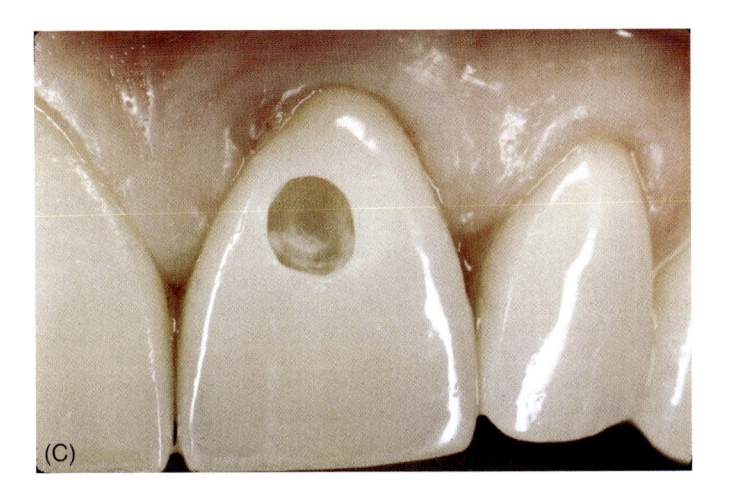

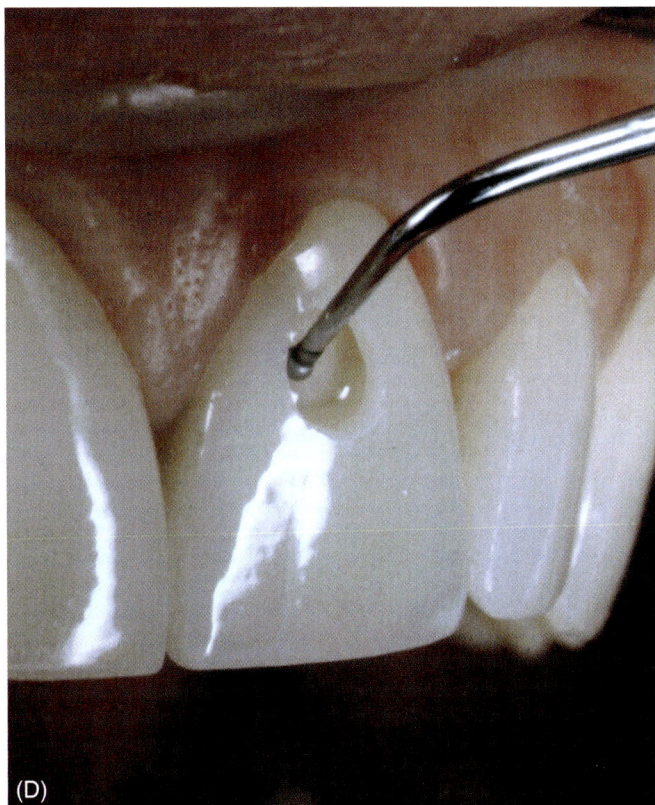

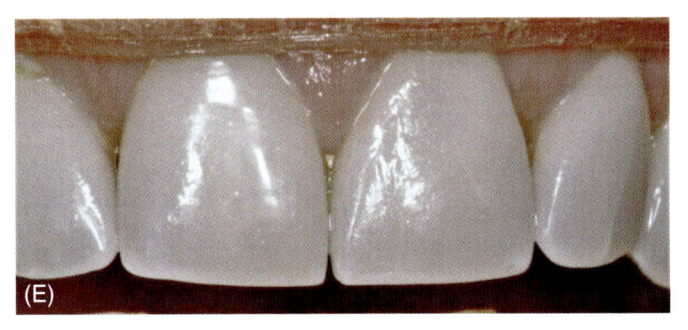

Figure 39.18 **(C–E)** After the final removal of the discolored area, the defect was repaired with microfill composite resin to match the polished surface of the porcelain.

For example, when comparing the probability of failure of three systems of machined zirconia ceramics (Lava, DC-Zirkon, and Cercon) with a zirconia-reinforced aluminum ceramic (In-Ceram Zirconia), it was found that the strength of DC-Zirkon, a postsintered machined yttria-stabilized zirconia (Y-TZP), was higher than that of the other two presintered machined Y-TZPs. The authors found that presintered machined ceramics seem as if they are the better material, because surface flaws that may be created during the milling process are often eliminated after sintering; however, surface grinding of these materials tends to compromise their strength—creating surface cracks, and increasing the size of any remaining defects. In comparison, sintering conducted after machining allows the repair of small cracks and defects, and can allow for maintenance of the inherent properties of the ceramic.[16]

Figure 39.23A illustrates that a void in the metal substructure of a ceramometal crown may result in serious internal stress, producing a fracture when the crown is cemented. The cement is normally displaced in the direction of the arrows; however, the cement applies great pressure on the opaque layer and usually results in the primary fracture area. If the restoration had been a veneer, there would be a chance that the entire facing would pop off without fracturing. A second reason for internal stress to cause fracture is if the dentist removes some of the intaglio metal surface of the crown in attempting to fit the restoration. The dentist should instead use a disclosing material (such as Occlude or other pressure indicator) to indicate areas that need to be adjusted, and adjust the tooth accordingly (instead of the metal) to ensure a proper fit without excessive thinning of the metal. An area of secondary stress may occur if the porcelain coverage is too thin near the bucco-occlusal line, and fracture may occur in this area as well. In any case, the metal should be of consistent thickness, and any voids must be properly repaired, or the crown remade. Stresses may still occur if the metal is thinned beyond its

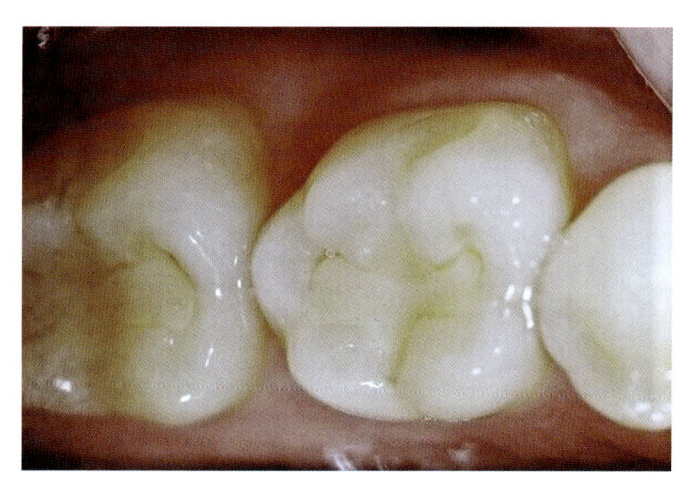

Figure 39.19 **(A)** These composite resin restorations show early signs of microleakage. Note the darker brown stains around the margins.

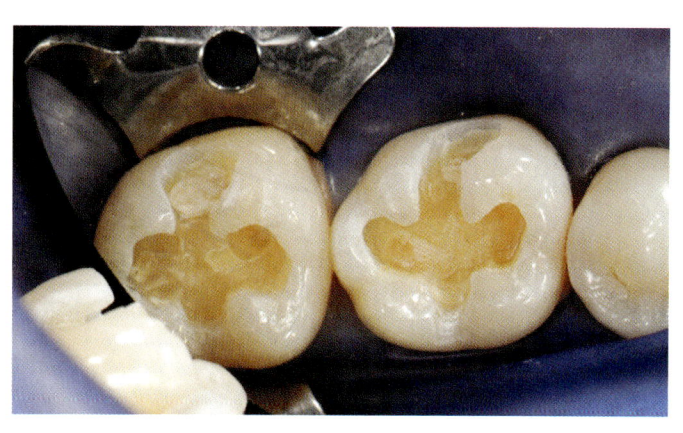

Figure 39.19 **(B)** Although many times it is possible to use air-abrasion and re-seal the margins, if the stained areas are too deep, it is best to replace the entire composite restoration as above.

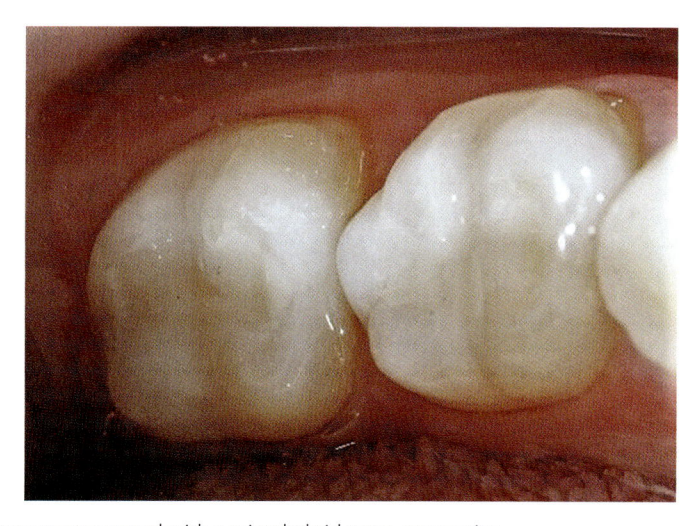

Figure 39.19 **(C)** The final restorations were restored with a microhybrid nano composite.

limits, even though no hole may be present. The clinician must check the thickness with a gauge, and if it is below the specifications it must be refabricated. The main problem is that dentists rarely have the opportunity to examine the metal, unless a metal try-in is arranged (Figure 39.23A).

If porcelain is too thin in the posterior region, owing to improper or inadequate tooth reduction, fracture can occur under occlusal loading. If using a porcelain occlusal surface, a minimum of 2 mm of clearance is required for a ceramometal posterior restoration, to avoid such failure as that shown in Figure 39.23B and C.

As zirconia-based crowns and fixed partial dentures gain popularity, it is important not only to understand clinical errors that might result in fracture, but also to recognize the inherent properties of zirconia that may differ due to the position of teeth, single versus multiple units, and opposing teeth. In a study conducted by Nathanson et al. at Boston University, failure statistics were obtained for zirconia-supported porcelain restorations. Over a period of 2–3 years, the combined total failure rate for porcelain and zirconia restorative systems was 2.8%. Of those failures, 2% were porcelain chips, 0.5% were porcelain fractures, and 0.2% were core fractures; 60% of the failed restorations required replacement.[17] In an additional study conducted by Blatz et al. the clinical survival of posterior zirconia crowns, in particular, was evaluated. When compared to traditional porcelain-fused-to-metal crowns, zirconia crowns did not differ statistically.[18]

According to these studies, zirconia has proven to be a reliable substructure for porcelain veneers; however, it is of utmost importance that clinical and laboratory work be completed satisfactorily to ensure their success. The clinician must ensure adequate reduction, and the lab must ensure that there is a minimal difference in the coefficient of thermal expansion between veneering porcelains and zirconia. Clinicians at the University of Pennsylvania found that, although the bond of veneering porcelain to a zirconia substructure is similar to that of a veneering porcelain bonded to a metal substructure, it is important to ensure that the coefficients of thermal expansion are similar to ensure success.[18]

Four of the leading principles for a successful zirconia restoration include: core integrity, appropriate preparation, marginal ridge support, and anatomical cores. Proper firing temperatures

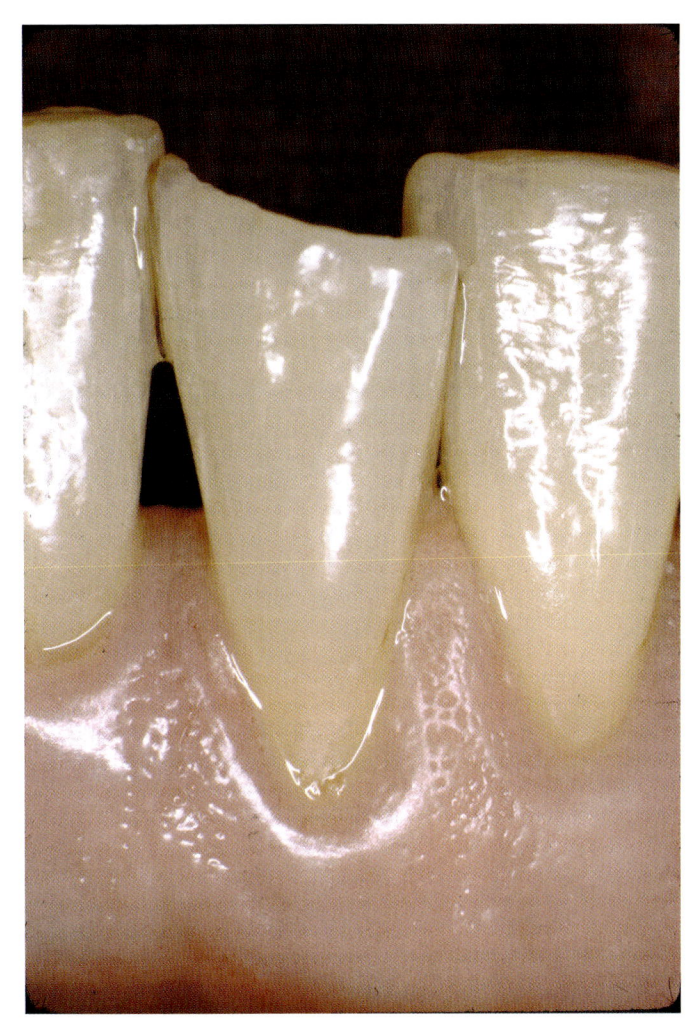

Figure 39.20 (A) This patient presented with an incisal fracture on a lower right anterior tooth.

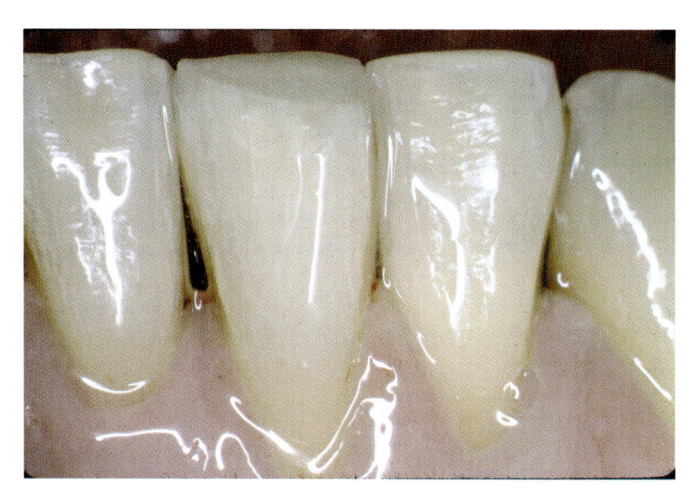

Figure 39.20 (B) Because of the difference in light reflection and translucency between the enamel and the restorative material, the difference in shade is apparent. A more opaque composite is recommended for a more esthetic result.

and appropriate fabrication of the zirconia core are essential to a strong restoration. The teeth to be restored must be adequately reduced to allow room for both the core and the veneering porcelain. There must also be enough core zirconia on the connectors to support occlusal forces, thereby preventing fracture (Figure 39.24A–C). In Figure 39.24D, note the bulk of zirconia also placed over the marginal ridge of the premolar, which would not have been possible without adequate reduction by the clinician. It is also important to remember that however thick the zirconia core may be, it must follow the anatomical contours of the tooth to be restored. Any unsupported zirconia will likely fracture.

If an all-ceramic crown is fractured from occlusal stress and the underlying core material is exposed, it is also important that the wear of enamel opposing a core material be evaluated. If the fracture occurs almost immediately, it is most likely an error of the dentist or laboratory; however, if the exposure of substructure occurs over a longer period of time, the patient's occlusion may have had a more significant impact on the prognosis of the restoration, and it becomes important to evaluate potential solutions for the patient.

In a study published by the *Journal of Dental Research*, the wear of enamel opposing yttrium-oxide-partially-stabilized zirconia core material was evaluated. Researchers found that if the restorations fractured, that zirconia polished with abrasive wheels and diamond polishing paste caused less wear on opposing enamel than did zirconia left as produced. Therefore, if the patient does not wish to completely replace the restoration, this procedure is a viable alternative to extend the lifetime of the restoration and the satisfaction of the patient.[17]

Oftentimes, potential porcelain fracture can be detected by applying occlusal pressure. Figure 39.25 shows a fractured porcelain-to-metal fixed partial denture being evaluated in the mouth. Occlusal pressure from a cotton roll was enough to fracture the inadequately prepared tooth. About 2 mm of clearance is necessary in posterior restorations, to allow space for metal, opaque, and porcelain.

Contaminants

Contaminants are residual essential oils from various solutions: blood, saliva, debris from preparations, and various chemical agents. Many prevent the proper setting of cements and bases; others, such as compounds containing eugenol, inhibit polymerization of restorative resins. Generally, chemical contaminants and tooth debris prevent intimate adaptation of restoratives to the cavity walls and permit unsightly stains to occur, such as those discussed in the event of gingival retraction fluid contamination, leading to the eventual discoloration of dentin and esthetic failure of an anterior crown.

Failure to follow manufacturer's instructions

Manufacturers' instructions include the correct proportions for mixing materials. Many materials have components that, in the wrong proportions, are noxious to vital pulp tissue. These ingredients, if not completely mixed, will not perform optimally, as the finished material will lack homogeneity. In addition, they will not be as strong or as resistant to abrasion, they may be more

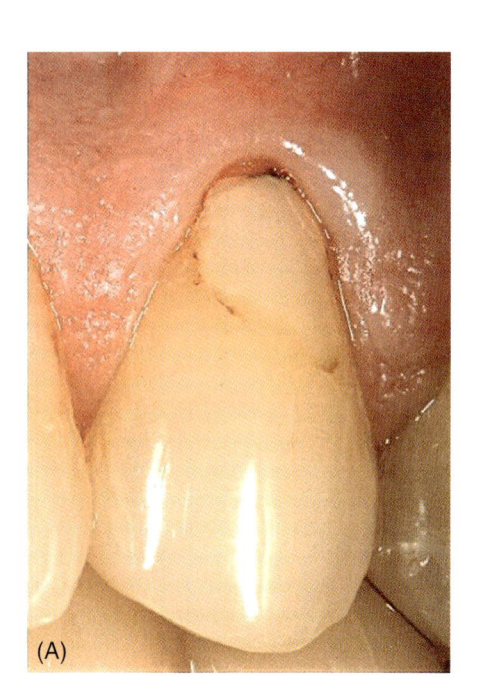

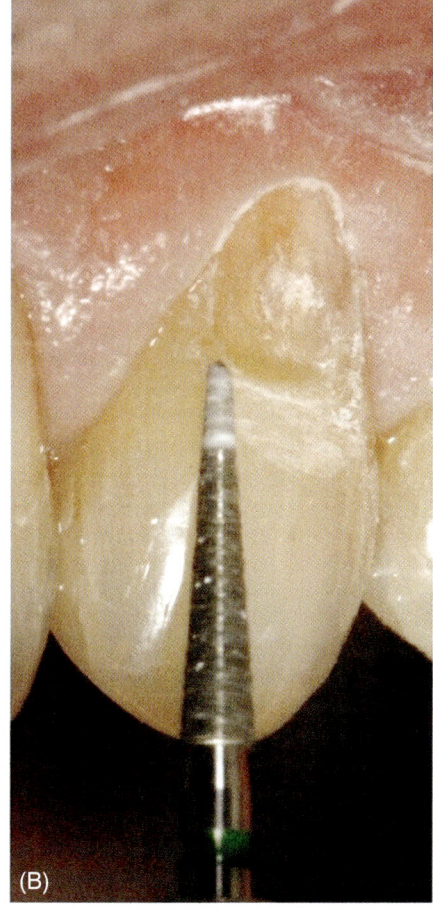

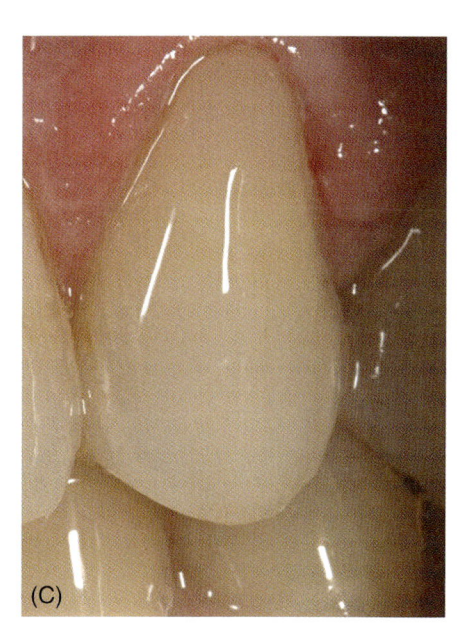

Figure 39.21 **(A)** This patient has microleakage and erosion around a class V on his maxillary left canine. **(B)** A long bevel is placed using the AC2 diamond, (Brasseler USA). **(C)** Final restoration shows the actual margin of the microfilled composite that extends beyond the bevel for ease and later repair, if needed (see Chapter 14 for technique).

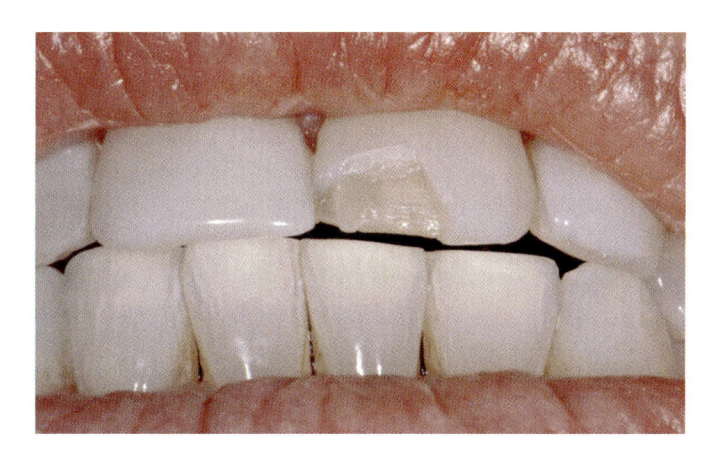

Figure 39.22 **(A)** This patient fractured her left central incisor resin-bonded veneer due to her bruxism habit, uncontrolled during the day.

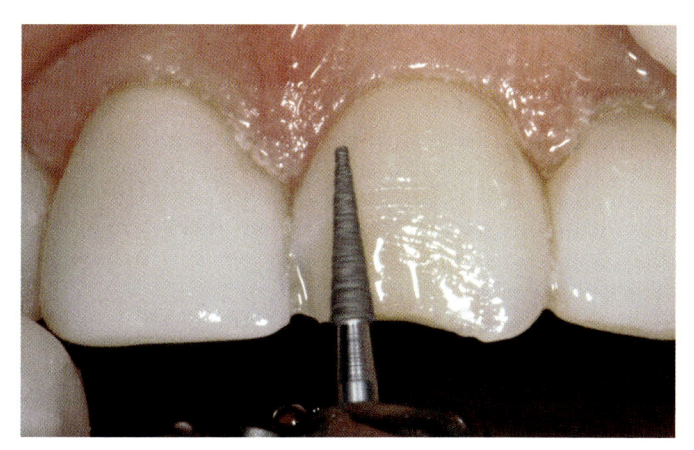

Figure 39.22 **(B)** To repair the Class IV fracture, a long bevel is first placed into the composite resin.

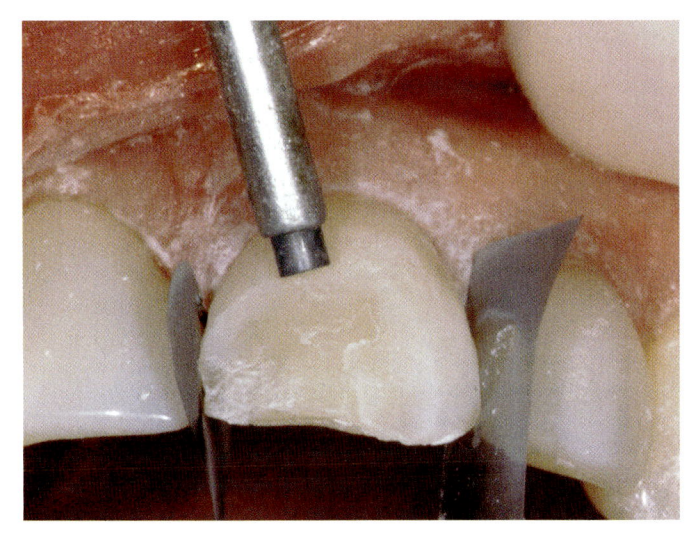

Figure 39.22 **(C)** Air abrasion is then used to prepare any remaining composite on the tooth surface, as well as the restoration itself, for maximum bonding with the new material.

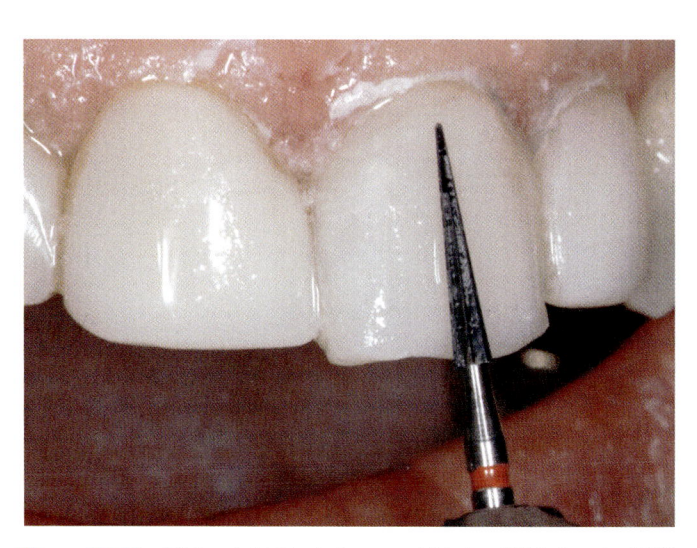

Figure 39.22 **(D)** An eight-blade 9 mm carbide bur (ET 9, Brassler USA) is used to first contour the bonded restoration.

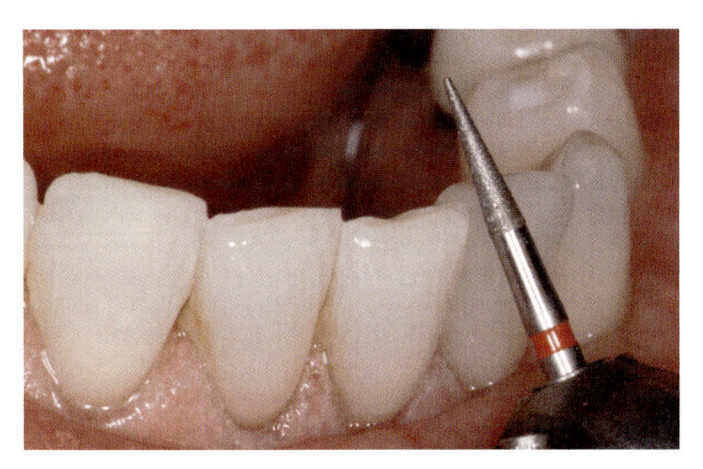

Figure 39.22 **(E)** It is also important to bevel the opposing incisors, to relieve any possible protrusive interference.

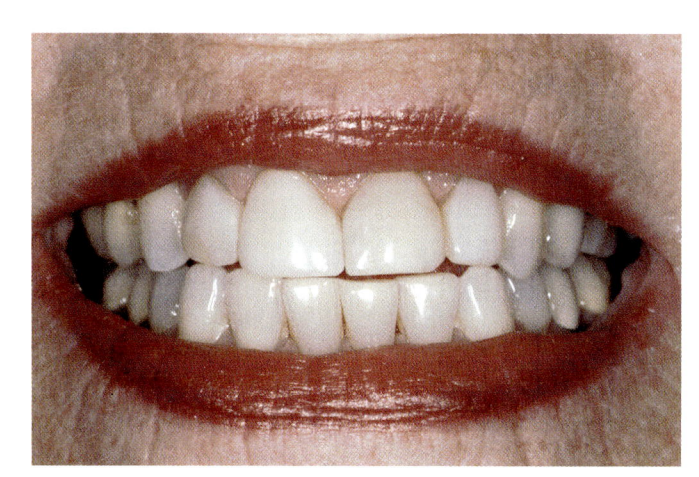

Figure 39.22 **(F)** The final result shows slight spacing, which protected these restorations for many years.

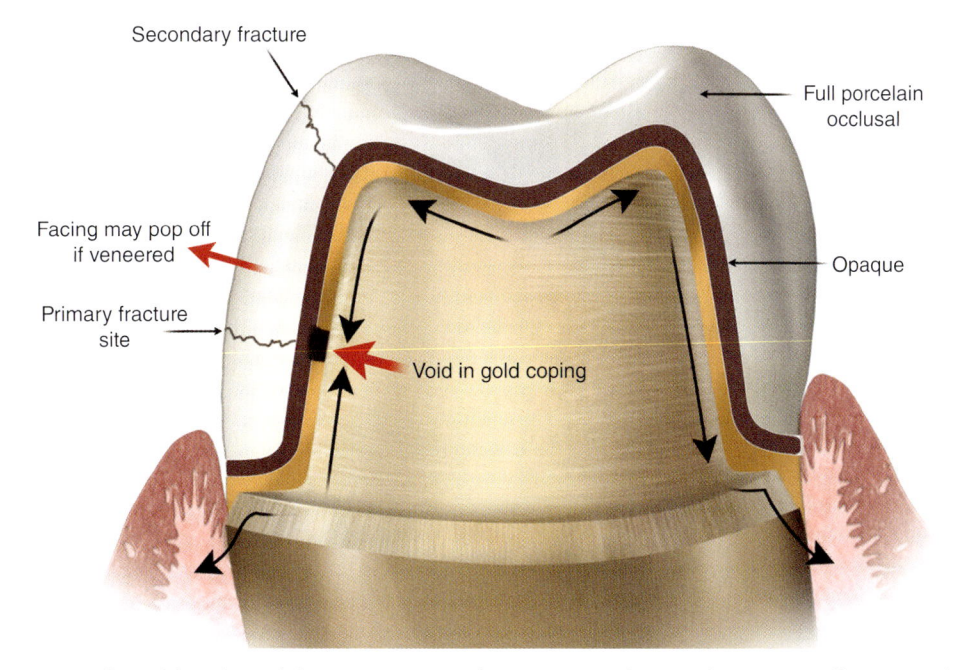

Figure 39.23 **(A)** One cause of possible esthetic failure in ceramometal restorations is fracture due to an insufficient metal coping.

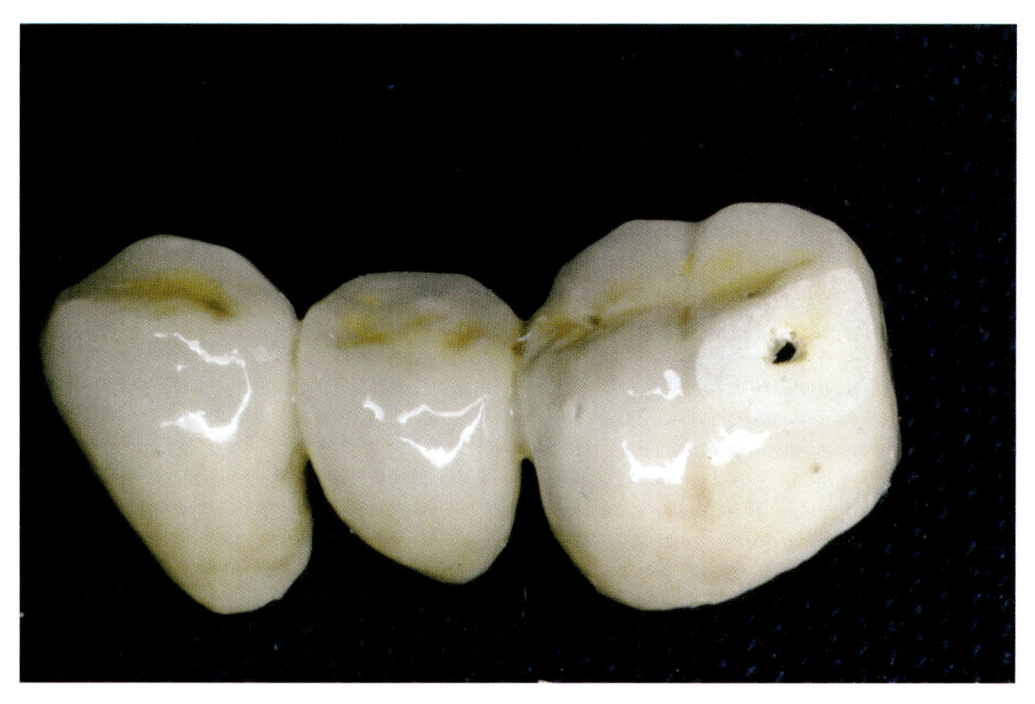

Figure 39.23 **(B)** This ceramometal bridge fractured due to inadequate metal coping as illustrated in Figure 39.23A.

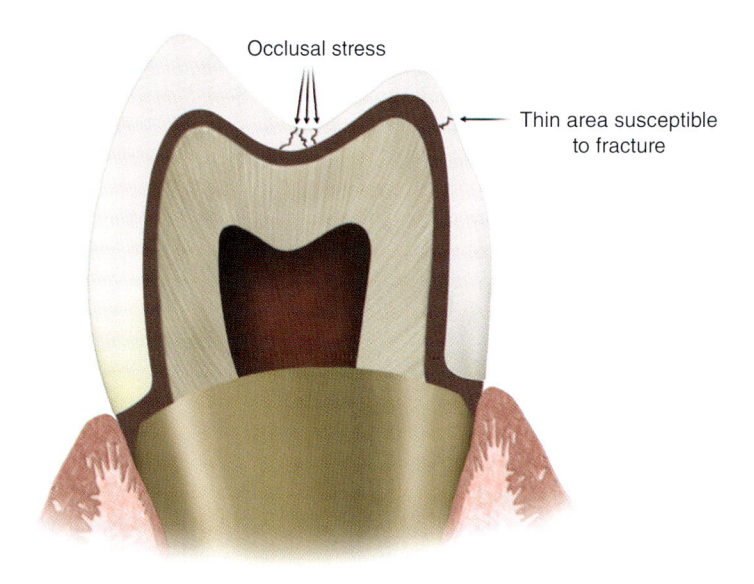

Figure 39.23 **(C)** A major cause of ceramometal restorations failure is inadequate thickness in the central fossa of posterior teeth. Although the clearance may be 2 mm in the preparation, if deep occlusal anatomy exists, then there might not be sufficient thickness of porcelain in this area to resist fracture.

Chapter 39 Esthetic Failures

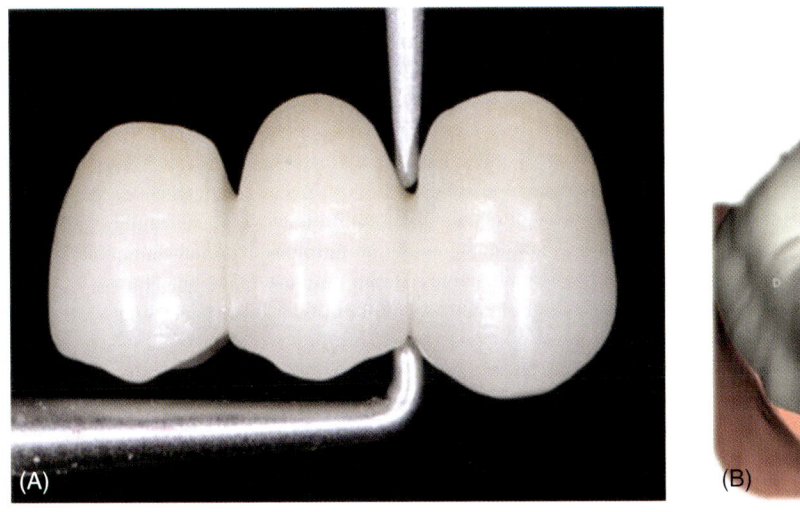

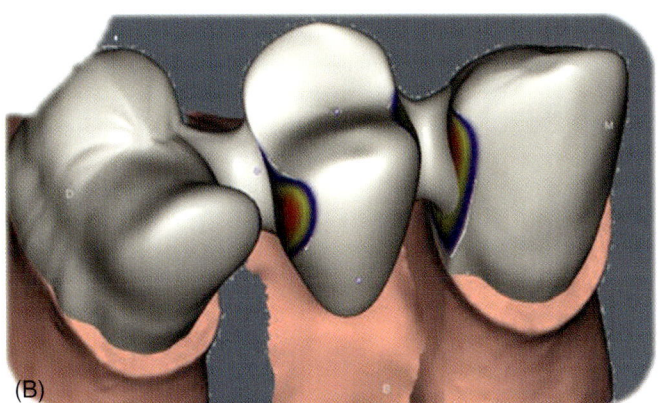

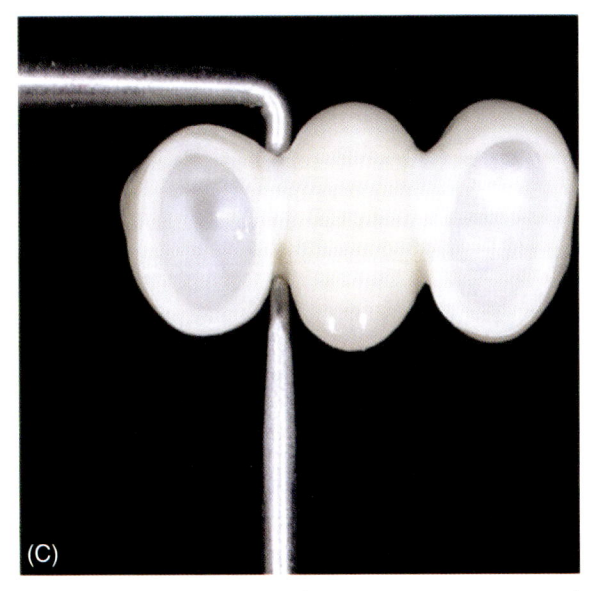

Figure 39.24 (A–C) There must be enough thickness of core zirconia on the connectors to support occlusal forces, in order to prevent fracture.

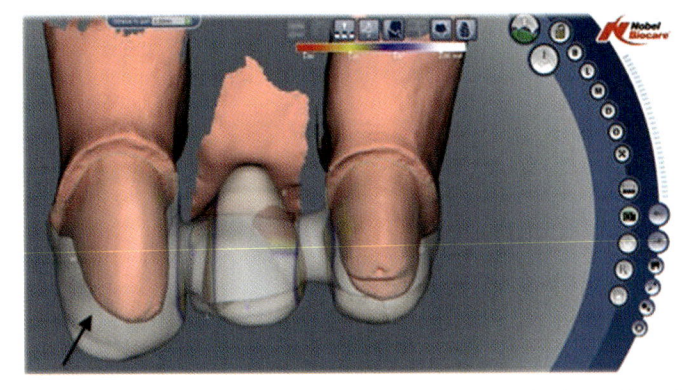

Figure 39.24 (D) Note the bulk of zirconia placed over the marginal ridge of the premolar, which would not have been possible without adequate reduction by the clinician.

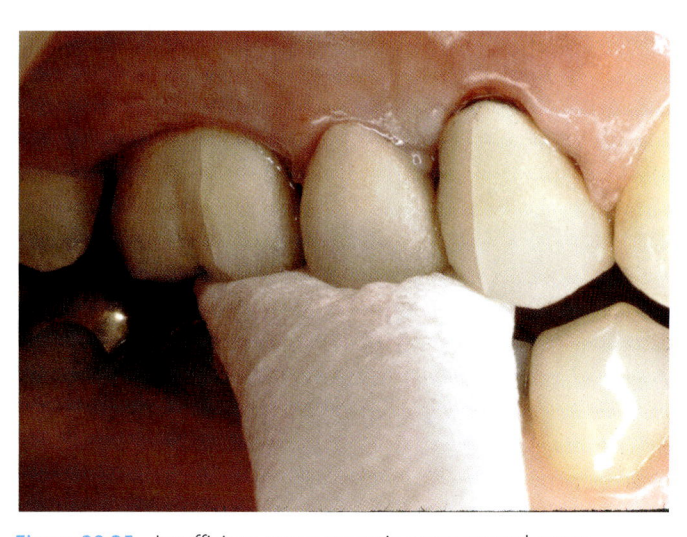

Figure 39.25 Insufficient core support in ceramometal crown fractures at try-in appointment.

soluble in oral fluids, and they may not hold their shape as well as properly mixed materials.

In summary, there are legitimate problems that cause immediate or eventual failure of an esthetic restoration. In most cases, the cause is not a failure of the operator to perform acceptable clinical dentistry, but rather a lack of communication between dentist and patient about the patient's expectations and the achievement of such. Therefore, the treatment planning process and discussion is of utmost importance.

References

1. Barghi N. *Failures of Ceramic Bonded Restorations: The Untold Stories*. San Antonio, TX: The University of Texas Health Sciences Center; 2010.
2. Goldstein R. Curbing your failures. *Contemp Esthet Restorative Pract* 2005;9(8):14–18.
3. Conrad HJ, Holtan JR. Internalized discoloration of dentin under porcelain crown: a clinical report. *J Prosthet Dent* 2009;101:153–157.
4. Wise M. *Failure in the Restored Dentition: Management and Treatment*, 1st edn. London: Quintessence; 1995.
5. Lucarotti PSK, Burke FJT. Analysis of an administrative database of indirect restoration over 11 years. *J Dent* 2009;37:4–11.
6. Sunnegardh-Gronberg K, van Dijken JW, Funegard U, et al. Selection of dental materials and longevity of replaced restorations in public dental health clinics in northern Sweden. *J Dent* 2009;37:673–678.
7. Schwartz NL, Whitsett LD, Berry TG, Stewart JL. Unserviceable crowns and fixed partial dentures: life-span and causes for loss of serviceability. *J Am Dent Assoc* 1970;81:1395–1401.
8. Lucarotti PSK, Burke FJT. Ten-year outcome of porcelain laminate veneers placed within the general dental services in England and Wales. *J Dent* 2009;37:31–38.
9. Galindo ML, Sendi P, Marinello CP. Estimating long-term survival of densely sintered alumina crowns: a cohort study over 10 years. *J Prosthet Dent* 2011;106(1):23–28.
10. Goldstein IH. Post mortems in dentistry. *Dent Survey* 1970;46:26–29.
11. Van Dijken JW, Lindberg A. Clinical effectiveness of a low-shrinkage resin composite: a five-year evaluation. *J Adhes Dent* 2009;11:143–148.
12. Brecker SC. *Clinical Procedures in Occlusal Rehabilitation*. Philadelphia, PA: WB Saunders; 1966.
13. Spear F, Holloway J. Which all-ceramic system is optimal for anterior esthetics? *J Am Dent Assoc* 2008;139(Suppl):19S–24S.
14. Larsson C, Vult von Steyern P. Five-year follow-up of implant-supported Y-TZP and ZTA fixed dental prostheses. A randomized, prospective clinical trial comparing two different material systems. *Int J Prosthodont* 2010;23(6):555–561.
15. Christensen RP, Ploeger BJ. A clinical comparison of zirconia, metal and alumina fixed-prosthesis frameworks veneered with layered or pressed ceramic: a three-year report. *J Am Dent Assoc* 2010;141(11):1317–1329.
16. Lee JJW, Kwon JY, Chai H. Fracture modes in human teeth. *J Dent Res* 2009;88(3):224–228.
17. Nathanson D, Chu S, Stappert C. Performance of zirconia based crowns and FPD's in prosthodontics practice. In *IADR General Session*, July 14–17, 2010.
18. Blatz M, Mante F, Chiche G, et al. Clinical survival of posterior zirconia crowns in private practice. In *IADR General Session*, July 14–17, 2010.

Additional resources

Ástvaldsdóttir Á, Dagerhamn J, van Dijken JW, et al. Longevity of posterior resin composite restorations in adults—a systematic review. *J Dent* 2015;43:934–954.

Chaar M, Kern M. Five-year clinical outcome of posterior zirconia ceramic inlay-retained FDPs with a modified design. *J Dent* 2015;43:1411–1415.

Dietschi D. Nonvital bleaching: general considerations and report of two failure cases. *Eur J Esthet Dent* 2006;1:52–61.

Kois J. No dentistry is better than no dentistry… really? *J Cosmet Dent* 2016;32:54–60.

Mantri S, Mantri S. Management of shrinkage stresses in direct restorative light-cured composites: a review. *J Esthet Rest Dent* 2013;25:305–313.

Nicolaisen MN, Bahrami G, Schropp L, Isidor F. Comparison of metal–ceramic and all-ceramic three-unit posterior fixed dental prostheses: a 3-year randomized clinical trial. *Int J Prosthodont* 2016;29:259–264.

Petridis H, Zekeridou A, Malliari M, et al. Survival of ceramic veneers made of different materials after a minimum follow-up period of five years: a systematic review and meta-analysis. *Eur J Esthet Dent* 2012;7:138–152.

Peumans M, De Munck J, van Landuyt KL, et al. A 13-year clinical evaluation of two three-step etch-and-rinse adhesives in non-carious Class-V lesions. *Clin Oral Investig* 2012;16:129–137.

Sax C, Hämmerle CH, Sailer I. 10-year clinical outcomes of fixed dental prostheses with zirconia frameworks. *Int J Comput Dent* 2011;14:183–202 [in German].

Simeone P, Gracis S. Eleven-year retrospective survival study of 275 veneered lithium disilicate single crowns. *Int J Periodontics Restorative Dent* 2015;35:685–694.

Wahl MJ, Schmitt MM, Overton DA, Gordon MK. Prevalence of cusp fractures in teeth restored with amalgam and with resin-based composite. *J Am Dent Assoc* 2004;135:1127–1132.

PART 8
CHAIRSIDE PROCEDURES

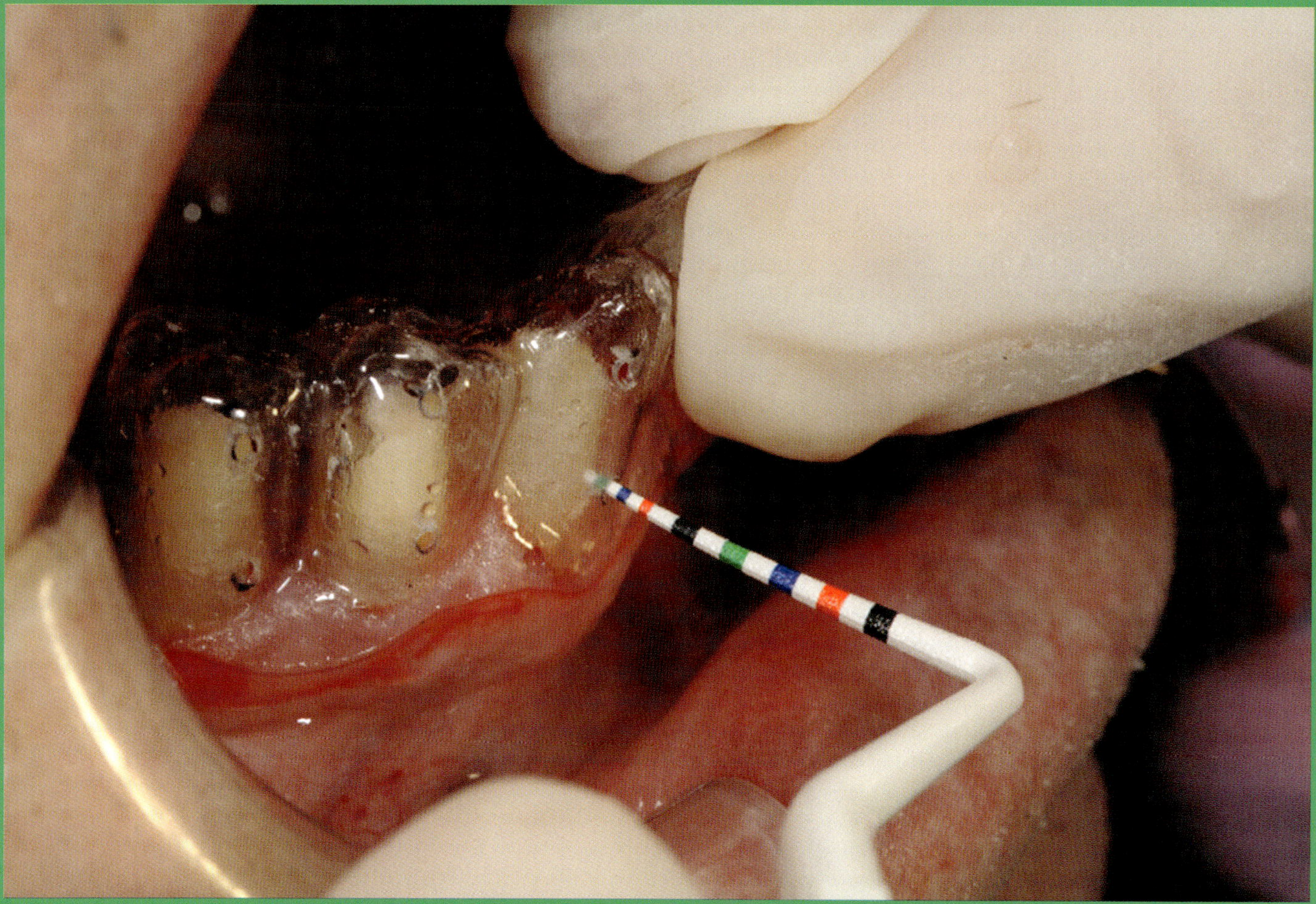

Chapter 40 Tooth Preparation in Esthetic Dentistry

Ronald E. Goldstein, DDS, Ernesto A. Lee, DMD, and Wendy A. Clark, DDS, MS

Chapter Outline

Tooth preparation for all-ceramic crowns	1263	Tooth preparation in periodontal problems	1280
Thickness or translucency in the gingival area	1264	Areas of crowded teeth	1280
Soft-tissue health	1264	Long crown/root ratio	1283
Positioning the gingival margin for esthetics	1267	Extremely short teeth	1283
Tooth reduction for the all-ceramic crown	1268	Pre-preparation checklist	1283
Step-by-step technique for the all-ceramic crown	1268	Preparation checklist	1283
Types of margins	1277		

There are many important factors that need to be considered before attempting to prepare a tooth for crowning. Failure to evaluate these factors and plan accordingly can lead to both esthetic and functional failure. Thus, incorporating tooth preparation considerations during the diagnostic phase can also help determine not only the type of crown to be chosen but also the amount of difficulty that may ensue. In tooth preparation, function as well as esthetics must be carefully evaluated. Comprehensive planning must include the following four guidelines:

1. Ascertain the type and amount of reduction necessary to insure adequate thickness of the restorative material.
2. Study pulp architecture from radiographs before preparation is initiated and relate this to the type of preparation selected and its compatibility with the size and position of the tooth pulp in question.
3. Establish the character and thickness of the free gingival margin.
4. Select the proper type of margin for the chosen restoration.

Each of these considerations will be discussed at greater length in the chapter. It is vital that each be considered from the very outset of treatment planning and tooth preparation.

Tooth preparation for all-ceramic crowns

With the demand for improved esthetics and function, significant progress has been made in the field of dental ceramics. A number of ceramic choices are now available to dental practitioners, and with these come certain considerations in preparation technique.

The first three types of restorations that are discussed (feldspathic, leucite-reinforced, and lithium disilicate ceramics) are collectively referred to as glass-ceramics. They have the same preparation requirements of at least 1.5–2.0 mm of incisal/occlusal clearance, 1.0–1.5 mm of axial reduction, and 1.0 mm marginal width. A wide chamfer margin may be used, but shoulder margin is preferred. An important guideline for the preparation of all-ceramic crowns is that the line angles be rounded. This refers to internal axial gingival walls as well as occlusal or incisal line angles. This diminishes the amount of point stresses the crowns will be subjected to during function, decreasing the risk of fracture.

The first all-ceramic crowns were made of feldspathic porcelain. This material choice is still available, and is often utilized as a veneering ceramic for ceramometal crowns or for pressable veneers. Owing to its lack of strength, its current application for full-coverage all-ceramic crowns is limited to milled restorations (VITABLOCS Mark II, Vita) in low stress areas and anterior teeth.

Adhering to preparation requirements is always important, but is especially critical with milled feldspathic restorations for two significant reasons. First, if these thickness requirements are violated or sharp angles are present in the preparation, there is a higher risk of fracture than other all-ceramic restorations. With this in mind, case selection is important for success with feldspathic materials. They should be limited to situations subject to less force, including anterior teeth and patients with no parafunctional habits. Second, as these are milled restorations, it must be considered that a computer will be reading the preparation. As such, a smoothly prepared margin becomes even more critical than with traditional restorations. Additionally, special consideration must be paid to the relationship of the axial walls to one another. Undercuts may present a challenge for the scanner and axial walls that are nearly parallel (8° or less of total occlusal convergence) may result in a more significant marginal opening.[1] Therefore, a slightly greater taper, or total occlusal convergence, may actually improve the marginal fit of crowns fabricated with computer-aided design/manufacturing (CAD/CAM) technology. Feldspathic restorations should always be bonded with a resin cement. Bonding imparts more strength to the restoration versus conventional cementation techniques. This additional chemical retention may also be beneficial for preparations that lack mechanical retention.

In the 1960s, leucite was added to porcelain frits for ceramometal crowns to improve compatibility between the materials. This change also improved the flexural and compressive strength of the ceramic. Leucite-reinforced ceramic is now utilized in pressable and milled all-ceramic crowns (IPS Empress and IPS ProCAD, Ivoclar Vivadent). With its increased strength (compared with feldspathic porcelain), this material can be used for single crowns in the premolar and molar areas in select cases.

Lithium disilicate ceramics are also available for pressed and milled all-ceramic restorations (IPS e.max Press and IPS e.max CAD, Ivoclar Vivadent). Their compressive and tensile strengths are significantly higher than leucite-reinforced ceramic. As such, this material may be used for posterior crowns as well as anterior bridges. These materials may be bonded with a resin cement or conventionally cemented with resin-reinforced glass ionomer cement.[2]

In addition to the glass-ceramics, another group of all-ceramic crowns is available. This group has an opaque core material of either alumina (NobelProcera, Nobel Biocare) or zirconia (LAVA, 3M Espe). This type of restoration requires about 0.5 mm more reduction than the glass-ceramics. This allows for a core material of about 0.5 mm and enough space to esthetically block out the opacity of the core. Without adequate reduction, the opaque core will show through the veneering porcelain, resulting in an esthetic failure. Adequate reduction also decreases the risk of fracture of the veneering ceramic due to inadequate thickness.

Thickness or translucency in the gingival area

Evaluate the thickness of the free marginal gingiva. Usually, the gingival crevice is adequate to hide a gold bevel in ceramometal crowns. Some patients have a tendency toward a thin, translucent gingiva, which might reveal the metal collar as a blue line. This happens mostly in young people, but it can occur at any age. It is also not uncommon to see it in a tooth that is slightly labioverted. If the root shows through the labial tissue with very little matrix of bone covering it, there may be thin translucent tissue. In this case, it is best to use a full shoulder rather than a beveled shoulder margin. Either an all-ceramic crown or ceramometal with a butt joint can be used.

Soft-tissue health

To create an esthetically successful restoration, the gingival areas must be healthy and architecturally sound before restorative treatment is instituted. Oral disease control sessions with the hygienist need to be completed with sufficient time, so the gingiva will be in optimal health. This may necessitate conservative laser or other periodontal surgery to gain a functionally sound and cosmetically acceptable gingival relationship.

In cases where two teeth are so close together that it results in a lack of interdental space, a compromise procedure may be necessary. As described by Berdon, odontoplasty may be indicated when teeth, particularly anteriors, have become rotated to the extent of actually approximating. This causes a lack of space for a normal bony septum height and can result in a periodontal pocket. This area is extremely difficult to keep clean because of the positions of teeth and the gingival papillae. Ideally, the teeth should be orthodontically repositioned to allow for a proper amount of space between each root; however, this is not always practical. Because adequate space must be provided for contact between the buccal and lingual papillae, careful removal of a portion of the tooth, crown, or root may provide the necessary space (Figure 40.1A–I).[3]

If gingival recession results in exposed cementum, consideration must be made after surveying radiographs to determine the gingival depth that can be achieved in the preparation. It may be impossible to axially reduce the tooth to the ideal dimensions for ceramometal restorations. If so, several alternative approaches are available:

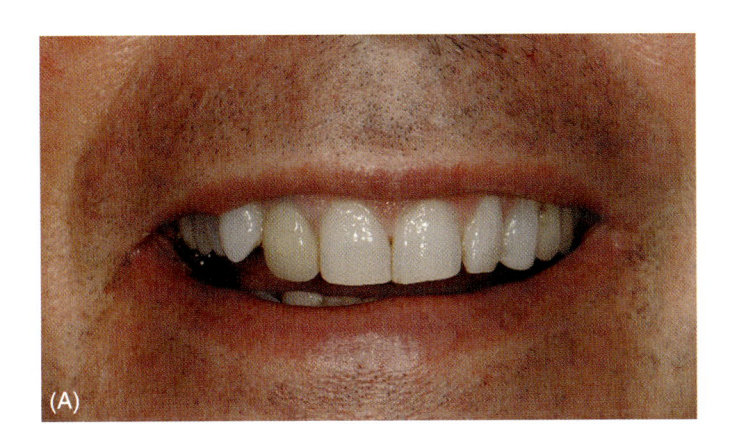

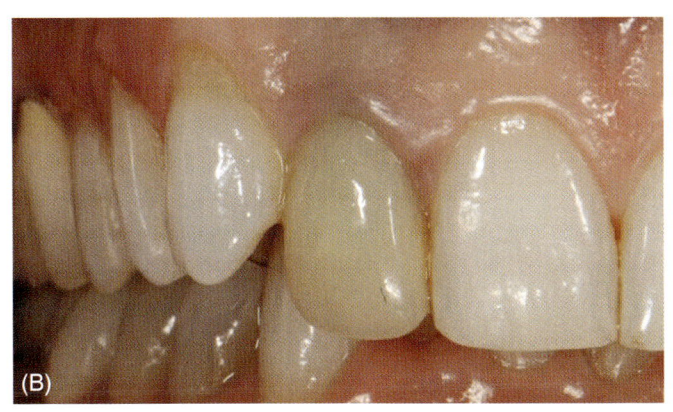

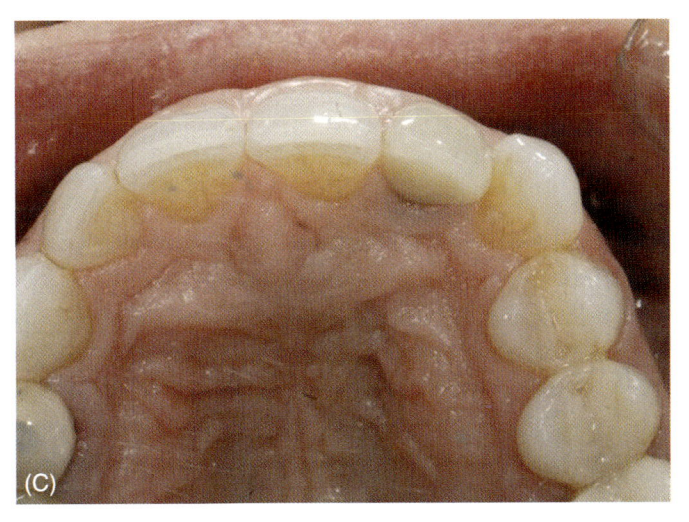

Chapter 40 Tooth Preparation in Esthetic Dentistry

Figure 40.1 (A–C) This patient wanted immediate correction of his discolored maxillary right lateral crown and labially placed right cuspid without orthodontics.

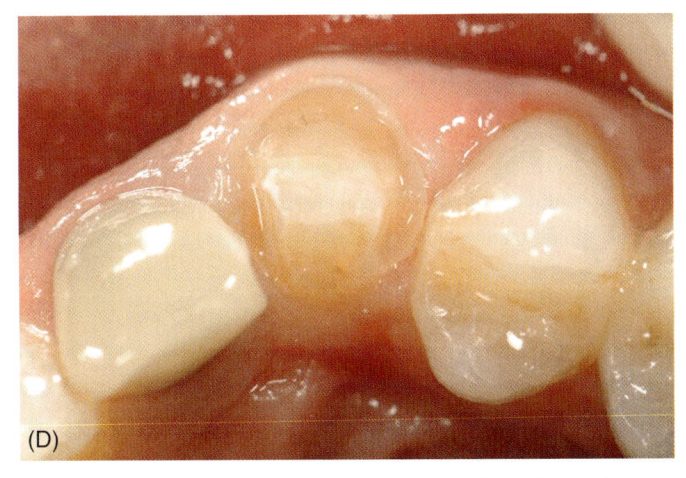

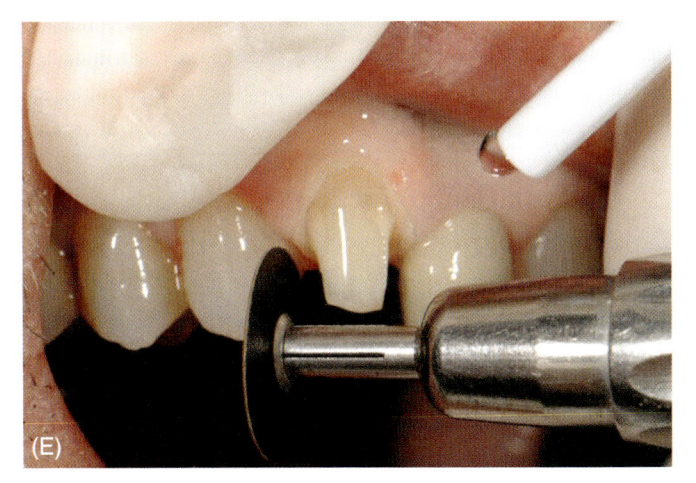

Figure 40.1 (D, E) Basic tooth preparation shows lack of space between the cuspid and the adjacent lateral incisor and first bicuspid. Therefore, the first bicuspid was slightly reduced in addition to the distal of the lateral incisor.

1. Use another type of restoration. For instance, an all-zirconia crown requires much less tooth reduction. A minimum of 0.5 mm is necessary (although 1.0 mm is ideal) for sufficient thickness of the crown, according to manufacturer's recommendations (Bruxzir, Glidewell). The all-zirconia crown can also be finished to a very fine cervical margin.

2. If there is an extremely low lip line, showing a metal gingival collar may be acceptable. Using a ceramometal crown, the cosmetic appearance of such a metal collar may be improved by air brushing the exposed metal surface. Describe these alternatives and the reasons for their use to the patient. Explain how much metal will show and how often the metal

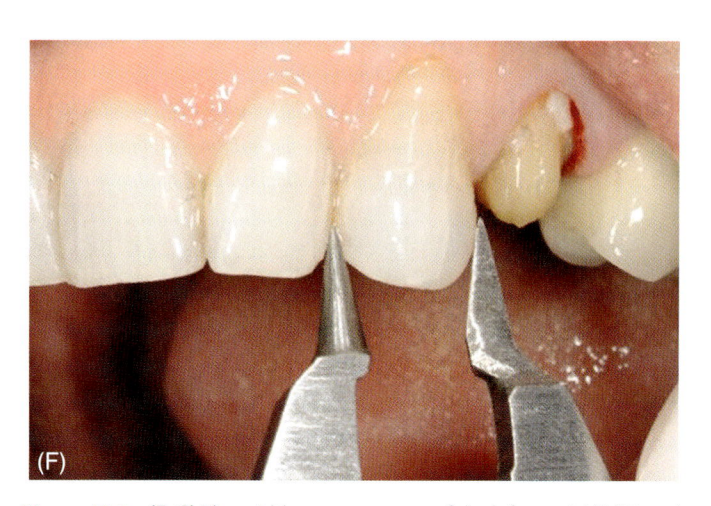

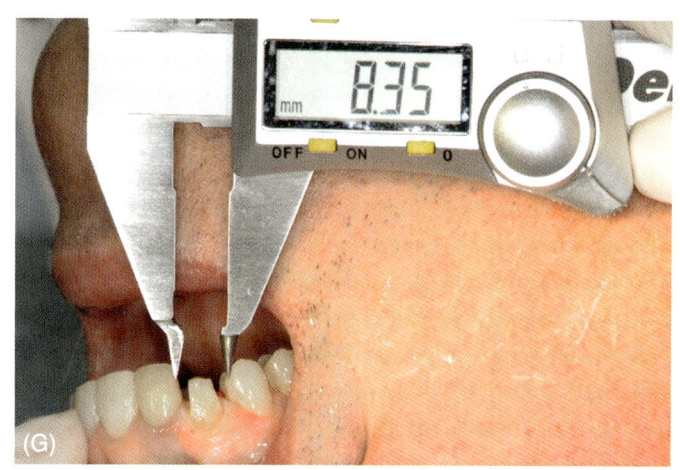

Figure 40.1 **(F, G)** The width measurement of the left cuspid (8.35 mm) now matched the space for the new right cuspid crown.

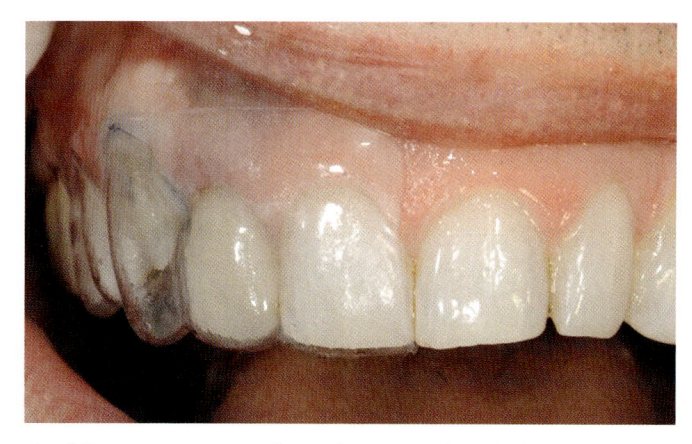

Figure 40.1 **(H)** A vacuum-formed matrix of the wax-up is inserted over the prepared tooth showing labial space for the final crown.

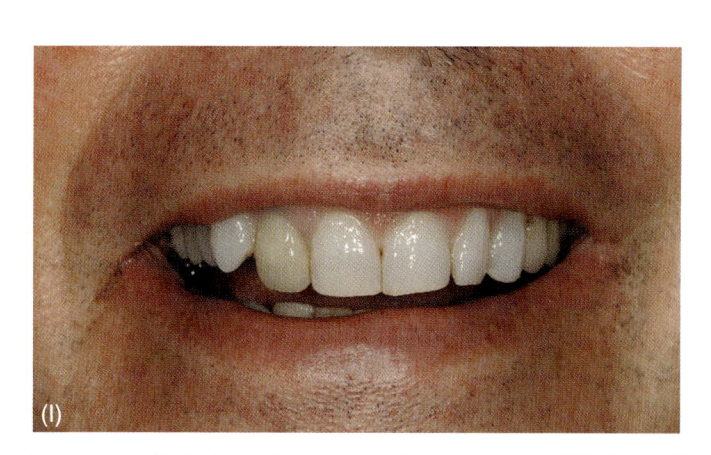

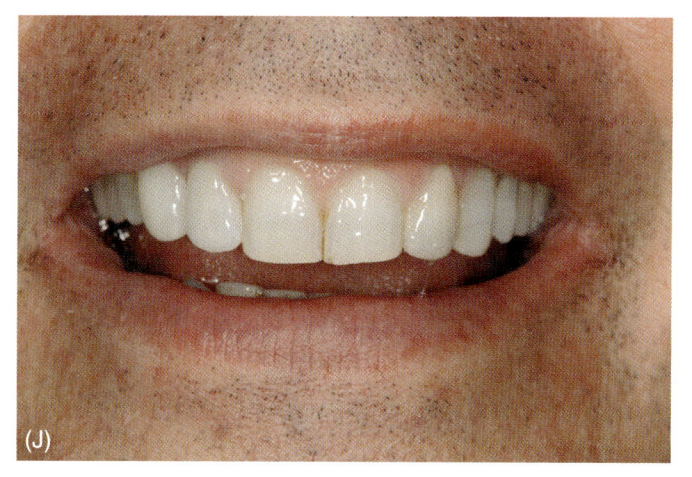

Figure 40.1 **(I, J)** Although not perfect, the compromised labial reduction pleased the patient. Note, further labial reduction may have led to pulpal injury.

collar will be seen when the patient speaks or laughs (Figure 40.2A and B).

3. If a high lip line is present, a porcelain butt joint should be used with a ceramometal crown. When tissue shrinkage exposes cementum or if there has been an excessive amount of eruption, it may not be necessary to reproduce the incisal length. In fact, more often the teeth should be shortened rather than lengthened to coincide with the normal lip line and obtain a symmetrically balanced restoration.

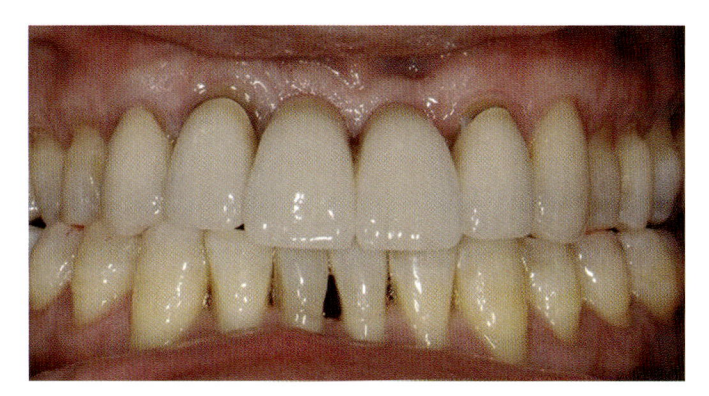

Figure 40.2 **(A)** As a result of the tissue recession on the labial aspect of the lateral incisors, subgingival preparation would result in distorted tooth morphology and margins on cementum. To improve retention and decrease the risk of pulpal trauma, a supragingival metal margin was selected by the practitioner and patient.

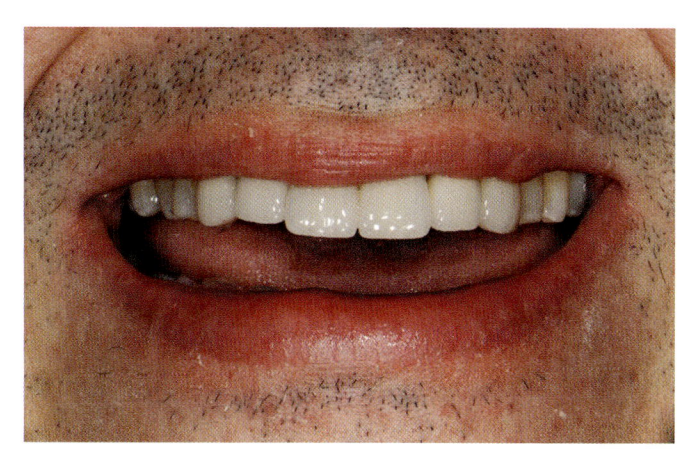

Figure 40.2 **(B)** Even with the patient's highest smile line, the supragingival metal collar is never visible.

Positioning the gingival margin for esthetics

When the word esthetics is mentioned, one might think that margins are automatically placed subgingivally. Not so. If the patient has a low lip line, there is little reason for this. A long metal collar, or a supragingival margin, can certainly be classified as esthetic as long as the patient understands that this area will not be seen. Pritchard warns of the possibility of gingival irritation due to prosthetic material in the gingival crevices[4] and points out the Silness study where the most favorable periodontal condition around bridge abutment teeth was when margins of castings were more than 2.0 mm from the gingiva.[5] This would seem to agree with a study on the effect of marginal placement on the gingiva by Larato,[6] who examined 546 three-quarter and full cast gold crowns of 268 patients. He found that 84% had inflammation when the gingival margin was below the tissue. When the margin was even with the tissue, only 22% were inflamed. When the margin was above the tissue, only 16% exhibited inflammation. Nevertheless, most esthetic restorations do need subgingival placement. There is no such thing as one ideal location for this margin, as it varies with the case and type of problem presented. (It also varies according to which authority you consult.)

Owing to esthetics, root sensitivity or caries, adequate crown length for retention, or an existing restoration, margins may have to extend well into the gingival sulcus. Burch states that the margin should not be placed closer than approximately 1.5 mm to any part of the alveolar housing of the tooth (Figure 40.3).[7] According to Gargiulo et al., this distance is necessary to allow for a "biologic width" of connective tissue and epithelial attachments of the gingival unit to the tooth.[8] Without this distance, bone in the immediate area might be resorbed. Burch suggests that when the subgingival margin is too near the alveolar housing, a preliminary "crown-lengthening" periodontal surgical procedure should be performed, and adequate healing time should be allowed before final preparation and impression.[7] Though a subgingival margin placement frequently resulted in recession and histologic evidence of inflammation, Tarnow et al. found that the inflammation subsided and the gingival fibers began remodeling within 2 weeks of temporization. This study concluded that, though there was no preoperative way to predict the amount of recession that would occur, the gingival housing stabilized relatively quickly. It is important to note that the preparations in this study did not violate the biologic width.[9]

Although the gingival crest varies in size, Tylman states that the average depth in individuals older than 20 years of age is 0.8 mm.[10] He also warns that, in the case of persons 20 years old

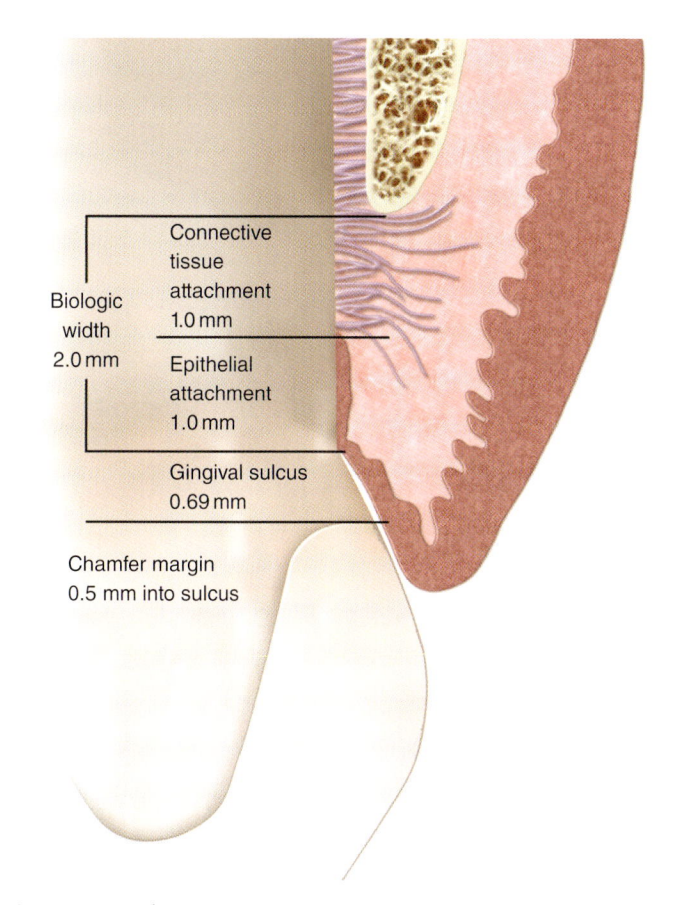

Figure 40.3 When preparing a crown margin subgingivally, it is important to be aware of tooth's sulcular depth and to avoid invasion of the biologic width. This figure illustrates the structures to consider in this histologic dimension.

or younger, the epithelial attachment may still be attached to the enamel, making the gingival crevice practically zero depth. Therefore, in these cases, it would be unwise to place the gingival margin entirely beneath the crest of healthy gingiva.[10,11]

Brecker feels that no matter how deep the gingival sulcus, the margin should extend slightly into that crevice.[12] Almost everyone agrees with Schweitzer, who states that the margin must not impinge upon the epithelial attachment.[13] Perhaps the easiest rule to follow is one stated by Johnston et al.[14] and Grieder and Cinotti,[15] who feel that the margin belongs midway between the coronal and apical borders of the sulcus. Beaudreau agrees that margins should be placed below the gingival crest to prevent sensitivity and recurrent decay and to provide subgingival support for the gingival unit.[16]

Esthetically, the reasonable conclusion is to extend the gingival margin far enough into the sulcus for a natural appearance and yet be able to determine marginal adaptation. Clinically, this means approximately halfway into a deep sulcus and three-quarters of the depth in a shallow sulcus. For example, in a patient with a healthy 2.0 mm sulcus, the gingival margin should extend 1.0 mm into the sulcus. In a 1.0 mm sulcus, the margin should be terminated at 0.8 mm or slightly above the base of the sulcus to provide for an esthetic result.

There have been numerous studies relating the marginal fit to gingival inflammation.[11,17–20] If the fit is not exacting, in relation to both tooth and gingiva, inflammation will occur. Therefore, the importance of the accuracy in this fit cannot be overstressed. For this reason, digital radiographs are taken at the try-in stage of every fixed restoration inserted in the mouth (in addition to careful clinical examination). The final lasting esthetic success depends on this procedure, regardless of what margin is chosen.

In summary, the consensus among leading authors and experts is that biologic width is approximately 2.0 mm. Therefore, subgingival margins should never invade this histologic dimension. As such, placing subgingival half the depth of the gingival sulcus appears to be the optimal for postrestorative gingival health.

Tooth reduction for the all-ceramic crown

An ideal tooth preparation for the all-ceramic crown is a balanced uniform reduction of tooth structure. Although this works perfectly in dentoform teeth, all too often perfect symmetry will be the exception rather than the norm. Fortunately, extra-strength core materials help to make it possible for an asymmetric preparation to function. Proper tooth preparation for the anterior porcelain crown is illustrated in Figure 40.4. Note especially the uniform reduction of tooth structure to provide an even thickness of porcelain. Also, observe the use of the shoulder margin labially and lingually.

Because porcelain is strong in compression but quite weak in terms of tensile strength, the full shoulder margin is always used in anterior restorations. Its width can vary from 0.5 to 1.0 mm and at times even to 1.5 mm. The shoulder is extended halfway or 0.5 mm (whichever is greater) into the gingival crevice at a slight apical angle (5°) from the long axis of the tooth. The incisal clearance should be 1.5–2.0 mm, with the flat surface at right angles to the surface forces of the occluding teeth.[14] The labial, mesial, distal, and lingual reduction should flow evenly and uniformly about the tooth to a depth of approximately 1 mm. Any sharp corners or angles must be rounded. The gingival margin should follow the cementoenamel line smoothly around the tooth.[21]

Shoulderless full porcelain crown

Many dentists still favor the use of the full porcelain crown without a shoulder.[22–25] A heavy chamfer margin is used instead beneath the gingival crevice labially and proximally, and it does not extend beneath the height of contour of the cingulum.[14] The main advantage is minimal reduction of tooth structure in the cervical areas. This type of preparation lends itself to the lithium disilicate or all-zirconia crown. Indications are extremely large pulp canals, bulbous teeth, exposed cementum, peg-shaped teeth, abnormally spaced or overlapped, small, thin, or delicate teeth, or teeth of teenagers or young adults.[23] In preparing endodontically treated teeth, the goal is to maintain as much natural tooth structure as possible, so using the chamfer or feather-type margin would be an important advantage. Therefore, preparing for an all-zirconia or ceramometal crown might be the best option.

Esthetic depth determination

A useful method of establishing an esthetic depth determination is based on the scribing technique advocated by Stein.[26] Initial cuts are placed using a measured 1.0 or 1.5 mm rounded diamond stone AC Diamond Series (Brasseler USA) to ensure uniform depth (Figure 40.5). A trench is cut completely around the gingiva on both labial and lingual surfaces (Figure 40.6A). Next, an incisal trench is cut in the middle of the labial and lingual surfaces with the same diamond (Figure 40.6B). Enamel reduction is then completed with a tapered cylindrical diamond stone (Figure 40.6C and D). The cylindrical stone is not used for the initial depth determination due to the difficulty that would be encountered maintaining the same depth in all areas of the preparation.

Step-by-step technique for the all-ceramic crown

1. **Esthetic depth cut** A key to the technique is the measured reduction of the horizontal and vertical aspects to a predictable depth. This is accomplished in two steps:

    (i) *Horizontal depth cut* Using a premeasured 1.0–1.5 mm round or AC3 or AC4 (Brasseler USA) diamond (Figure 40.6A), a trench is cut to the full depth of the diamond at the gingival level completely around both the labial and lingual surfaces for anterior teeth and the buccal/lingual for posterior teeth. To avoid tissue laceration, *take care to not extend into the gingival sulcus.* For lower anterior teeth and where significant gingival recession is present, a premeasured 1.0 mm round diamond should be used (AC4, Brasseler USA). The 1.0 mm depth cut is also specific for both lithium disilicate and all-zirconia full crowns as well.

    (ii) *Vertical depth cut* The vertical depth cut is continued using the same round diamond for the

(A)

(B)

(C)
D Measured round diamond
D

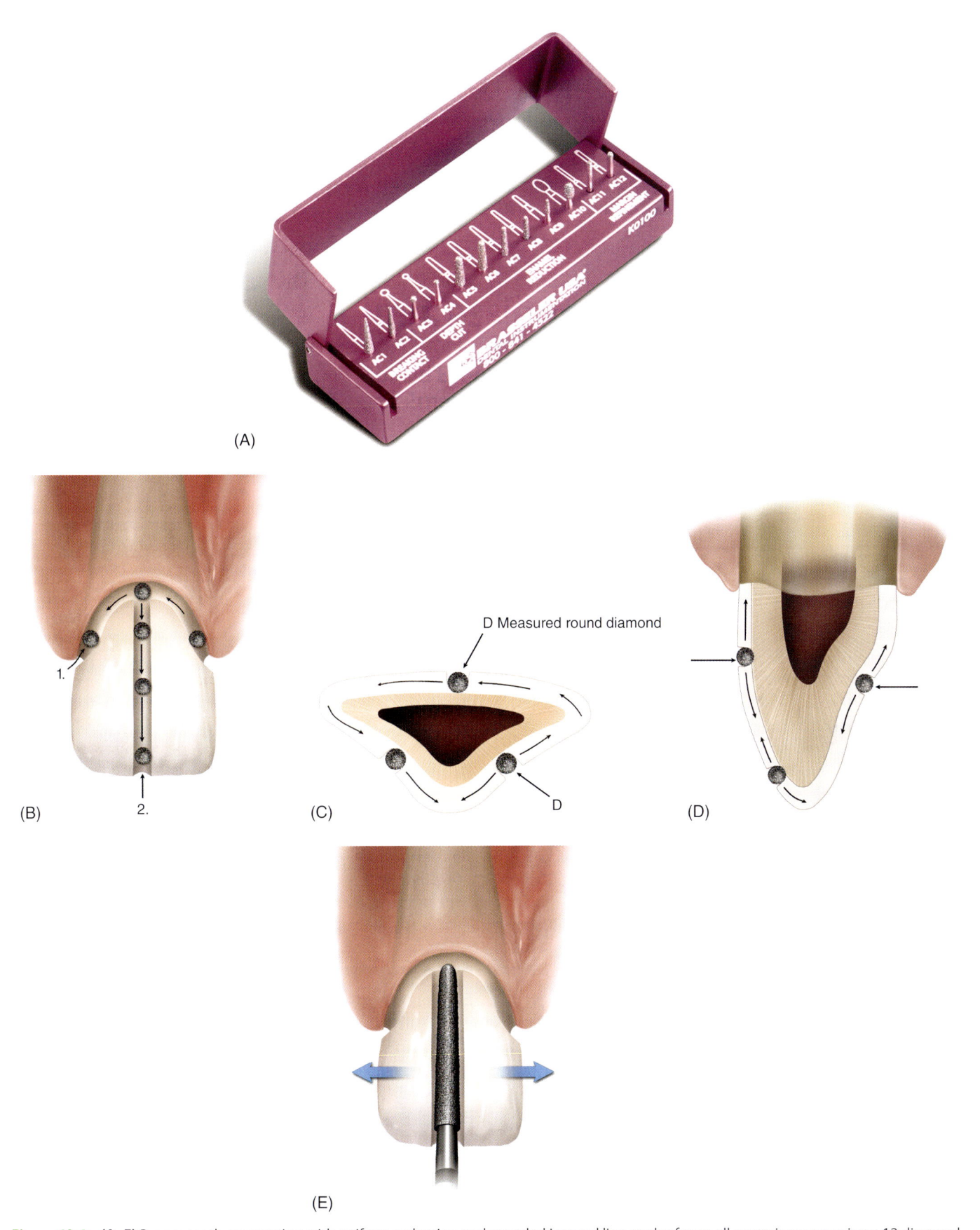

(D)

(E)

Figure 40.4 **(A–E)** Proper tooth preparation with uniform reduction and rounded internal line angles for an all-ceramic crown using a 12 diamond kit (BrasselerUSA K0100).

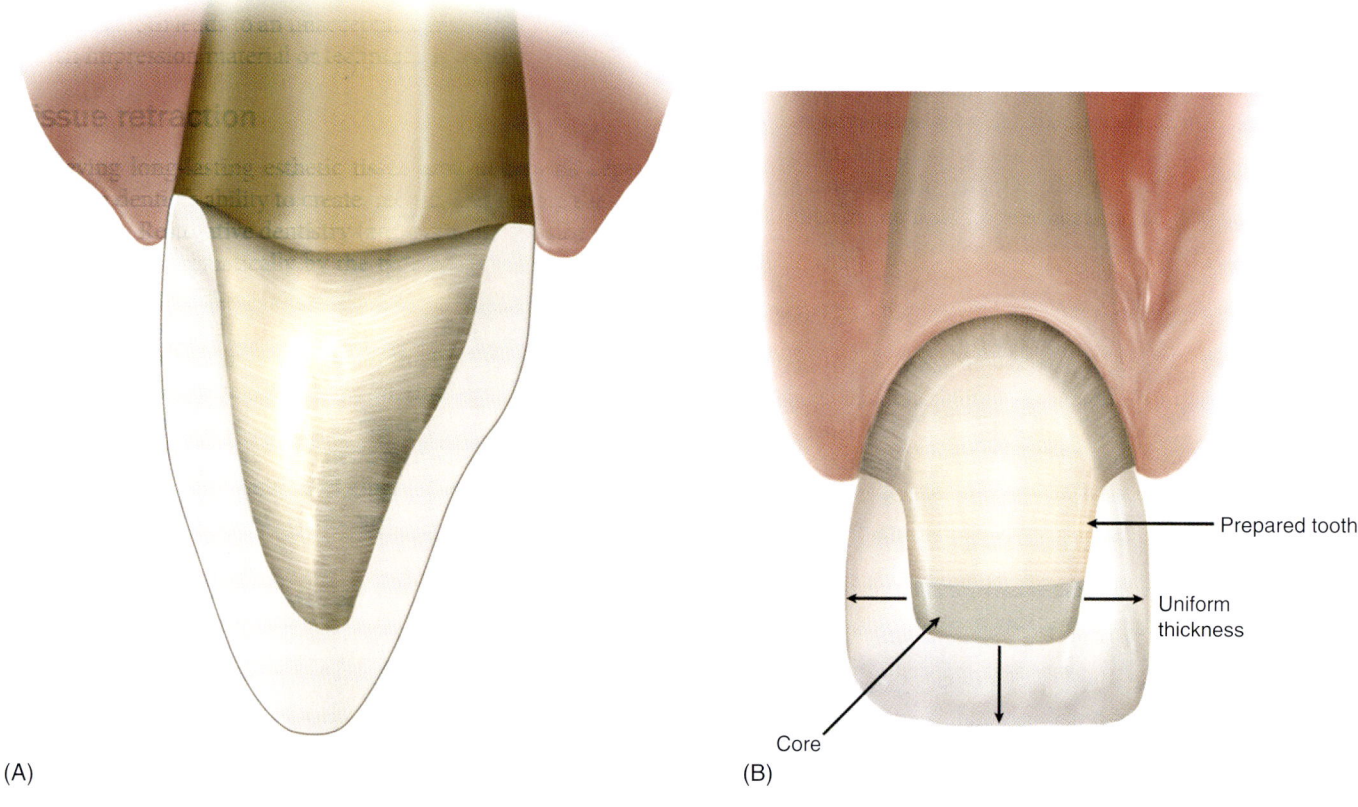

Figure 40.5 **(A, B)** The principles of uniform thickness for a typical all-porcelain crown.

gingivoincisal or gigivo-occlusal aspects. Starting at the center of the labial or buccal surface (Figure 40.6B), continue the depth cut from the cervical middle straight down to the incisal or occlusal edge. The depth of the cut is still controlled by the premeasured round diamond. Therefore, if you are increasing the depth of the buccal and/or lingual walls to 1.5 mm, then switch to the AC3 diamond, which is 1.5 mm thickness. Next, move to the incisal or occlusal surface. Since the incisal or occlusal clearance should be 1.5–2.0 mm, slightly more reduction should take place at these aspects.

Make sure you plan exactly how much reduction your preparation will require. For instance, you will not need full labial reduction if you are building out the tooth labially. However, you will probably want maximum lingual reduction in this situation.

2. **Bulk enamel removal** The esthetic depth cuts should now provide visualizations of the final tooth preparation form, so enamel can now be stripped away quickly while confidently retaining the correct depth thickness (Figure 40.6C and D). Use a very coarse round-end tapered diamond to remove both enamel and dentin, while maintaining a rounded internal angle, avoiding any sharp line angles (AC5 or AC7, Brasseler USA). For mandibular anterior teeth use the smaller AC7 for bulk reduction. This diamond will also be useful to reduce interproximal contacts to avoid any potential damage to adjacent teeth. In extremely small or narrow teeth, use the AC9 diamond.

3. **Incisal/occlusal clearance** Using the same round-end tapered diamond, reduce the incisal surface approximately 1.5 mm to obtain proper clearance (Figure 40.6E). When necessary, it may be possible to compromise the incisal reduction to 1 mm and alter the teeth in the opposing arch. However, if you are planning on all-zirconia crowns you could reduce as little as 0.5–1.0 mm occlusally if necessary. The important part of occlusal reduction is accounting for the type of occlusal anatomy that the patient requires. This means you must account for the depth of both fossae and grooves and prepare for equal thickness of porcelain in these areas as well. One way to test for adequate clearance is to use an occlusal clearance tab sprayed with colored disclosing material (Figure 40.6 F–H).

4. **Lingual reduction** A very coarse football-shaped diamond (AC10, Brasseler USA) is used to uniformly reduce the contours of the lingual surface of anterior teeth (Figure 40.6 F). The AC10 (Brasseler USA) is ideal to reduce the occlusal aspect of posterior teeth as well. Either a plastic or rubber thickness gauge can be used to make certain that your predetermined sufficient space is created. Also, if you are using a CAD/CAM intraoral scanner (Itero, Align) for your impression taking, the bite registration scan will easily show you if there is sufficient space. If not, you will be prompted to reduce more in those areas, so your restoration can be fabricated with sufficient thickness to avoid a potential fracture.

5. **Margin refinement** Preparation and refining of the shoulder margin are important steps of the universal procedure

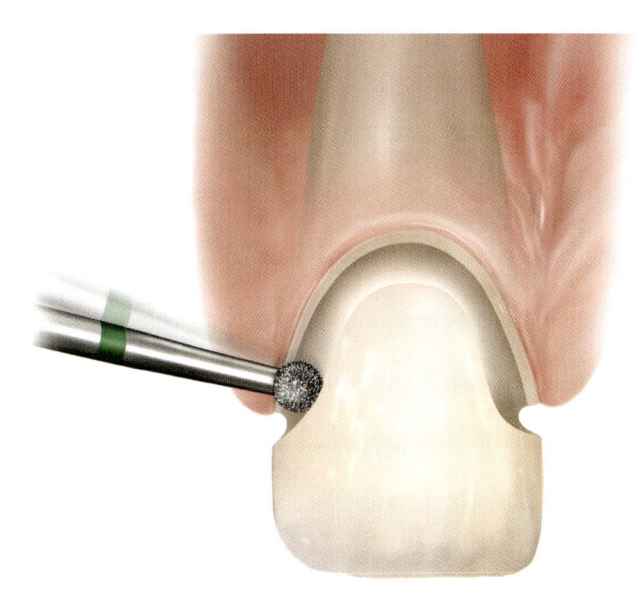

Figure 40.6 (A) Esthetic depth determination is both easily and quickly done using premeasured round diamond stones. A round diamond (Brasseler AC4) is used to create horizontal depth cuts at the gingival level, completely around the labial and lingual surfaces.

and are easily accomplished with a beveled-end cutting diamond (AC11 and AC12, Brasseler USA) shapes (Figure 40.6G). These diamonds have fine diamond particles on the flat tip only. When finishing subgingival margins to a smooth surface, the beveled corners and smooth sides of the tip help avoid lacerations by pushing soft tissue aside. It is very important to provide a clear, sharp outer margin, so the ceramist will have no problem determining the exact margin. A shoulder margin of approximately 1.0 mm is ideal for most all-ceramic crowns.

Tissue laceration can also be avoided by displacing the gingival tissue for several minutes with cotton retraction cord just prior to finishing the margin.

6. **Preparation finish** In the final step, the preparation is finished to a smoother surface using the same size but round-end tapered diamond used to make the original enamel reduction margin, but with medium diamond grit (AC6 or AC8, Brasseler USA). Make sure you eliminate all sharp line angle edges of the prepared teeth, as well as any sharp internal line angles.

Figure 40.6H is an example of the final preparation. A clinical example of this procedure can be seen in Figure 40.7A–P.

Porcelain-fused-to-metal restoration

Since its introduction into dentistry in the early 1950s, the ceramometal crown gained in popularity up until the new millennium, when the all-ceramic crowns achieved more popularity. However, the ceramometal crown continues to be a popular prosthetic choice for crowns primarily because it combines the strength and adaptability of metal with the esthetic beauty and durability of porcelain. However, this type of restoration does present some unique problems of construction and design, owing to the possibility of an interaction between the two

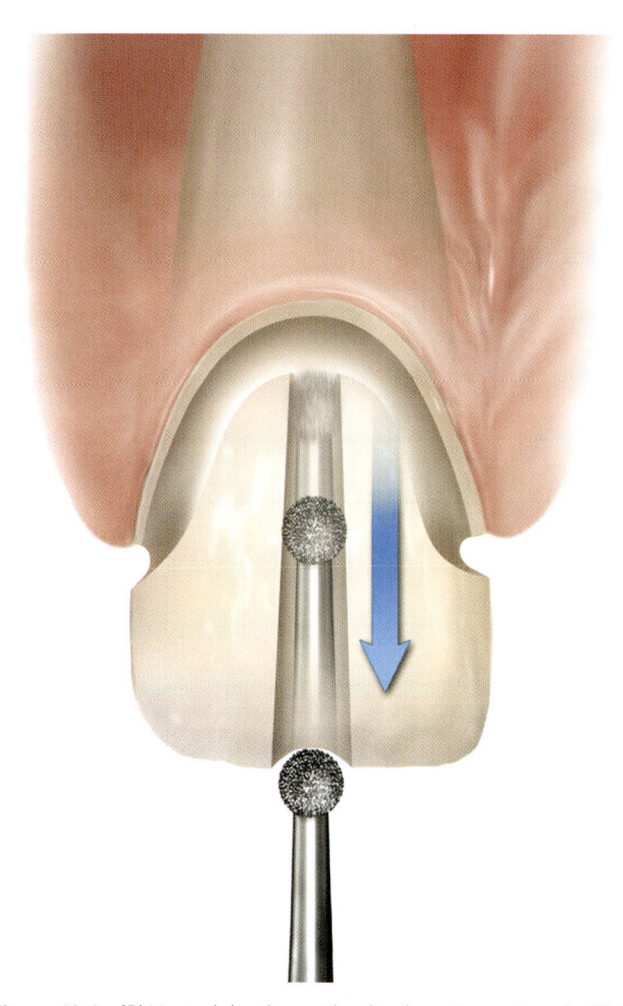

Figure 40.6 (B) Vertical depth cut. The depth cut is continued utilizing the same bur through the incisogingival dimension. This depth may vary depending on the final desired buccolingual dimension.

materials when porcelain is added to the metal coping. The preparation stage of the restoration can thus play a major role in the stabilization of this process.

The preparation of a tooth for ceramometal is exacting in the amount of tooth reduction necessary to obtain optimum structural and esthetic results. For instance, in the case of ceramometal it means reducing the tooth structure a minimum of 1.5–2.0 mm to obtain maximum esthetics.[27] The porcelain veneer should have a thickness of 1.5 mm axially and 2.0 mm incisally and occlusally;[28] anything less might result in compromised esthetics or create more serious esthetic problems, especially regarding color. On the other hand, thicker or uneven porcelain could result in structural weakness within the porcelain; it may crack during construction or after the crown is completed.

The principle of esthetic depth determination should also be applied to the posterior ceramometal preparation (Figure 40.8). In addition to the occlusal and labial, a gingival trench is also used. Figure 40.8C shows the desirable thickness of tooth structure necessary for porcelain, opaque and metal. A clinical example can be seen in Figure 40.9. A significant deviation from the minimum suggested thickness for the porcelain or metal may make the restoration structurally weak or esthetically unacceptable. Inadequate incisal and labial reduction (Figure 40.10A)

(C) (D)

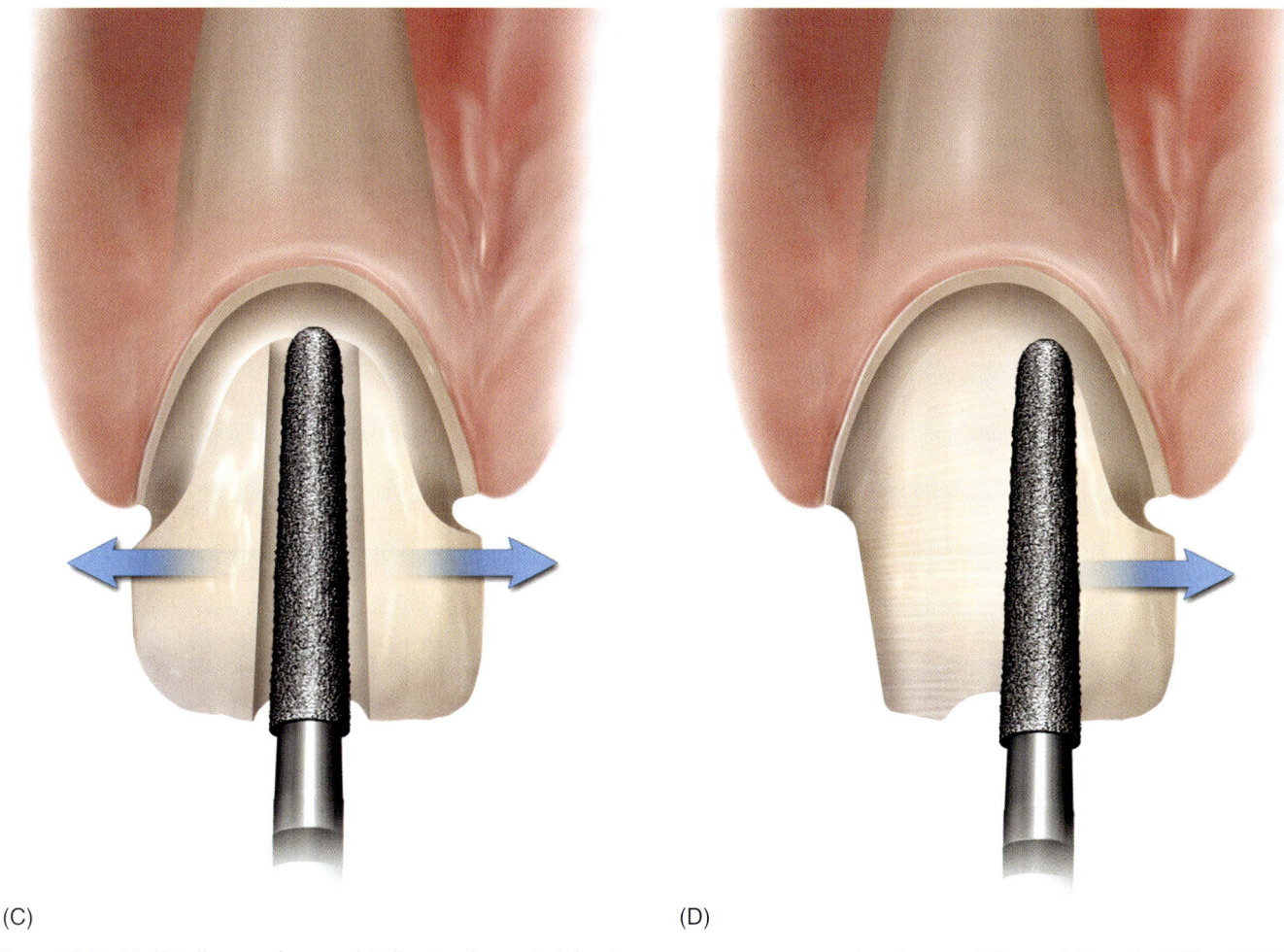

Figure 40.6 **(C, D)** Bulk enamel removal. Following the vertical depth cut, an extra-coarse round-end tapered diamond (Brasseler AC5 or AC7) is utilized to remove enamel and dentin to the desired depth.

may result in porcelain fracture; in addition, it is the main cause of esthetic failure due to the opaque metal coping showing through. Inadequate lingual reduction may likewise be a causative factor in fractures (Figure 40.10B). Furthermore, the labial margin, where the thickness of metal may be limited by esthetics, is the part that most often appears to be subject to distortion. Other problems that may make this type of crown difficult to prepare are teeth that are tapered or have constricted necks.[29]

Labial tooth reduction for esthetics

The amount of labial tooth reduction can dramatically affect the esthetic result. Although there is general agreement on the approximate amount of tooth reduction necessary to accommodate metal, opaque, and porcelain, this amount can be altered by the esthetic needs, shape, size, and position of the individual tooth. Therefore, instead of an axial reduction of 1.5 mm, it may be necessary to reduce the tooth 1.75–2.0 mm to achieve the desired esthetic result. Naturally, the position and size of the pulp chamber are the limiting factors in tooth reduction. Since this varies considerably from tooth to tooth and patient to patient, there can be no rule that applies in every case. Study the patient's radiograph carefully to help determine exactly how much reduction will be possible. Note both the width and height of the pulp chamber before making any final decision on choice of retainers.

If the pulp chamber is large but the tooth is small, some type of compromise will be necessary if a ceramometal restoration is used. For example, if minimal occlusal stress is to be placed on the crown, in rare cases the metal can be thinned to 0.2 mm. Since the opaque is approximately 0.15–0.2 mm thick, the porcelain makes up the available difference. Therefore, the crown could be 1.35 mm in labial thickness if porcelain can be made thinner. If the maximum labiogingival thickness were only 1 mm, the resulting porcelain would be only 0.55 mm. Depending on the shade selected, this may be insufficient to achieve an esthetic result in the cervical third. If this compromise is not adequate, an alternate retainer would have to be selected.

As stated, the suggested thickness of metal for this type of restoration is 0.33–0.5 mm, but in areas of minimal occlusion, 0.2 mm may be used. This variation depends on the physical properties of the alloy for proper rigidity and strength of the restoration.

Tergis[29] believes that when there is insufficient reduction of tooth structure, several problems can result, such as the following:

1. The laboratory may construct an extremely thin casting in order to avoid overcontouring, which could result in metal or porcelain breakage.

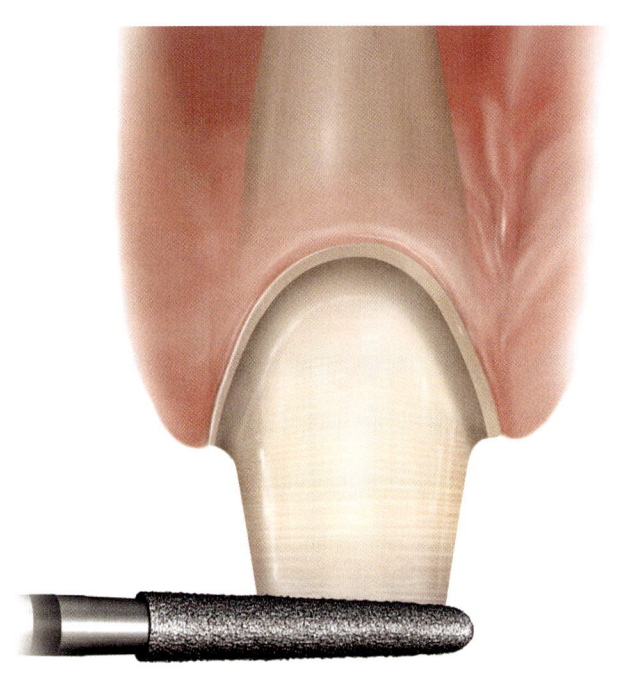

Figure 40.6 **(E)** Incisal clearance. Using the same round-end tapered diamond, incisal reduction is completed using the same round end diamond (AC5, Brasseler USA) to achieve proper clearance with the opposing dentition.

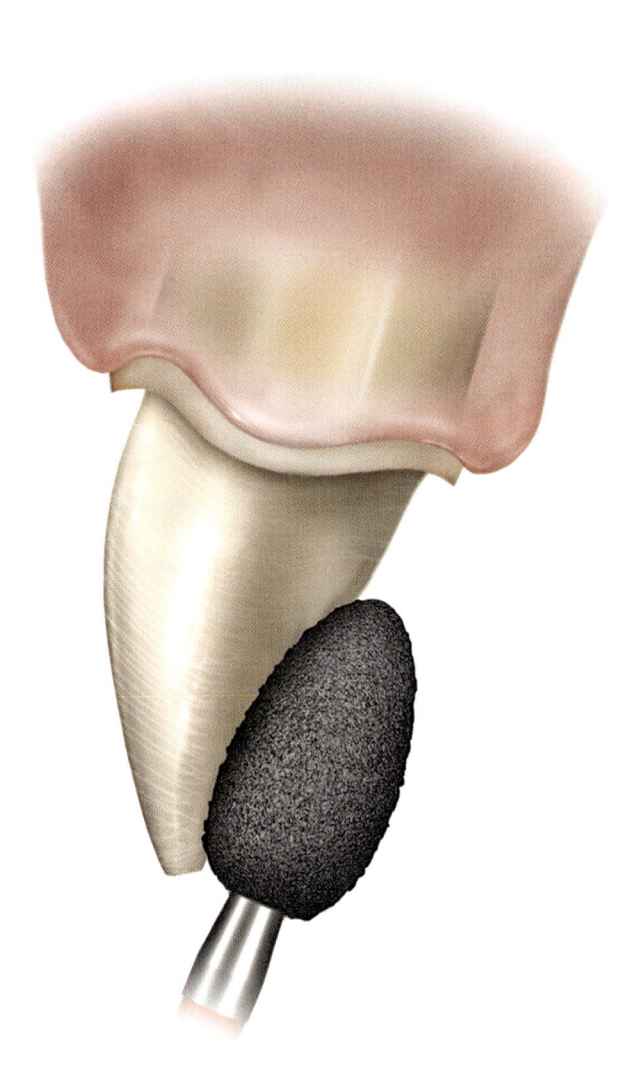

Figure 40.6 **(F)** Lingual reduction. The AC10 diamond (Brasseler) is used to obtain proper lingual reduction and contours.

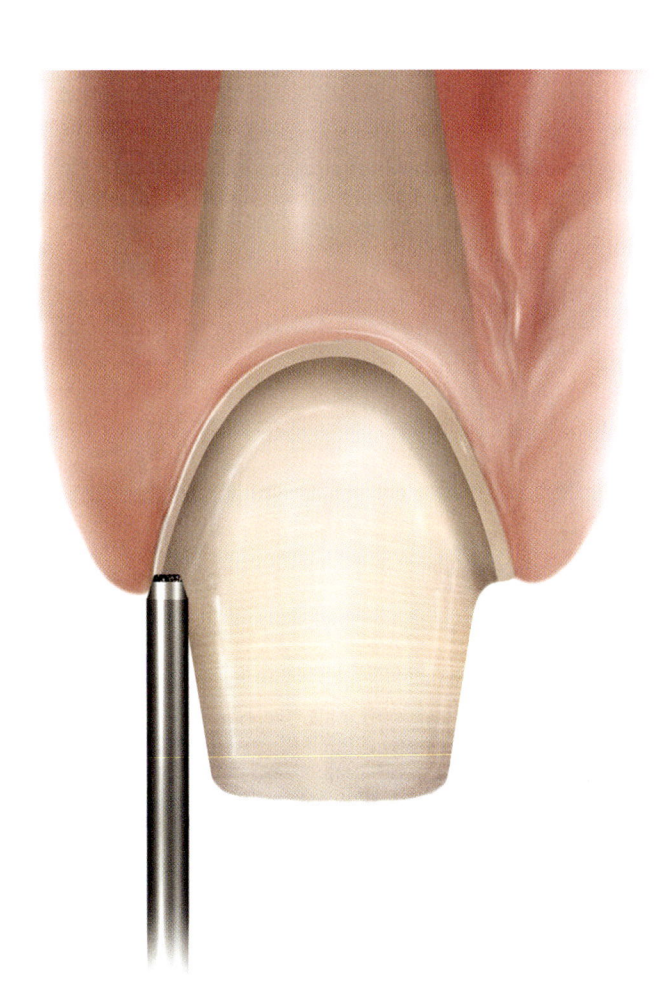

Figure 40.6 **(G)** Margin refinement. Preparation and refining of the margin is done with the beveled end-cutting diamond (Brasseler AC11 or AC12). The beveled-end shape helps to prevent internal line angle undercuts as well as avoid gingival abrasion.

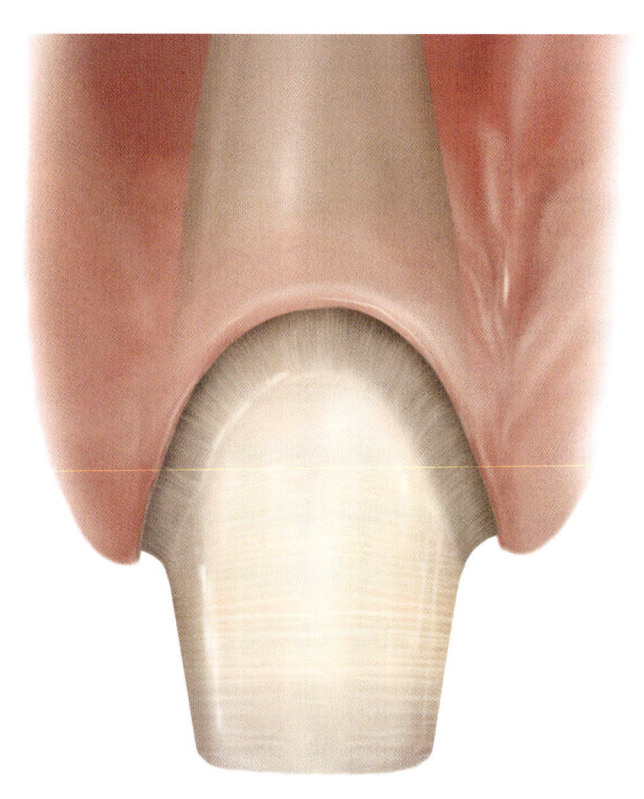

Figure 40.6 **(H)** Example of a supragingival margin all-ceramic crown preparation.

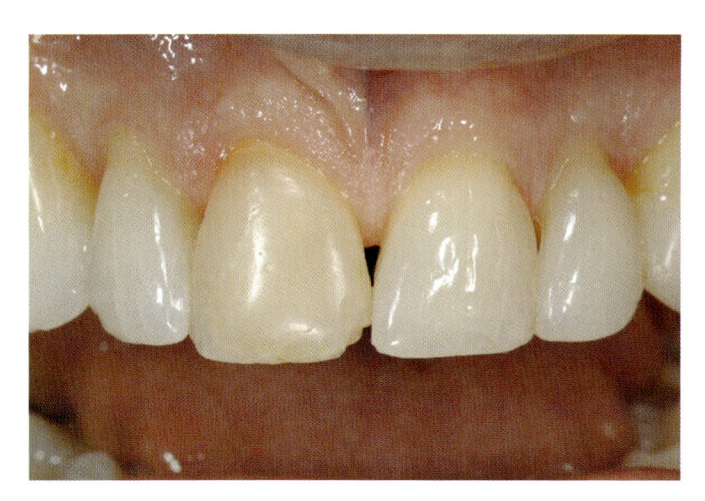

Figure 40.7 **(A)** The patient's maxillary right central incisor will be prepared for an all-ceramic crown.

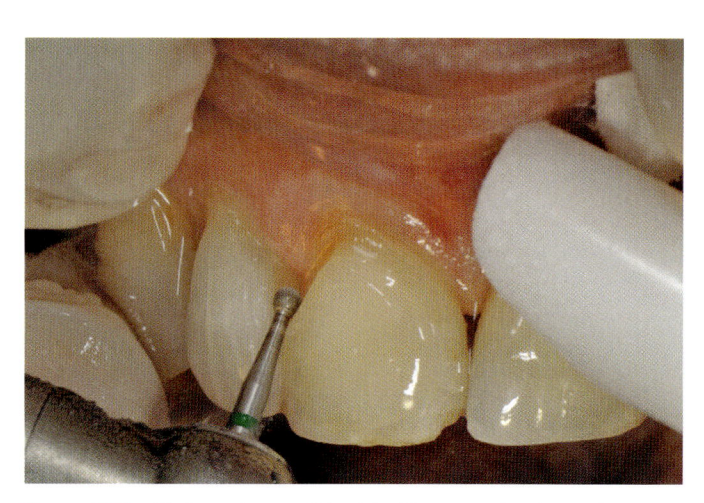

Figure 40.7 **(B)** Completion of the labial horizontal esthetic depth cut.

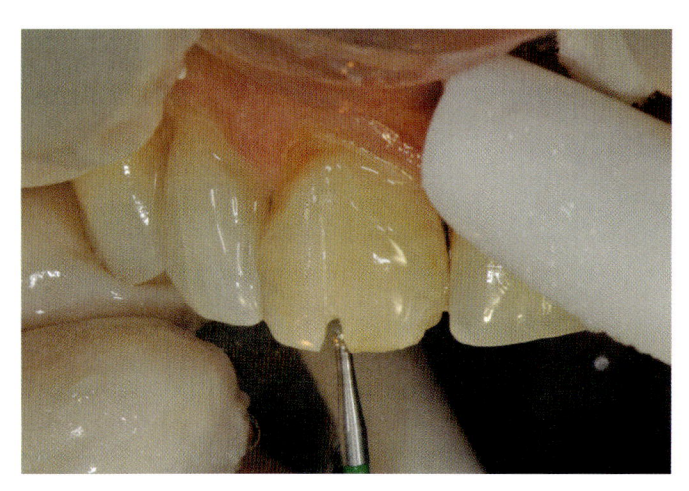

Figure 40.7 **(C)** Completion of the labial vertical esthetic depth cut.

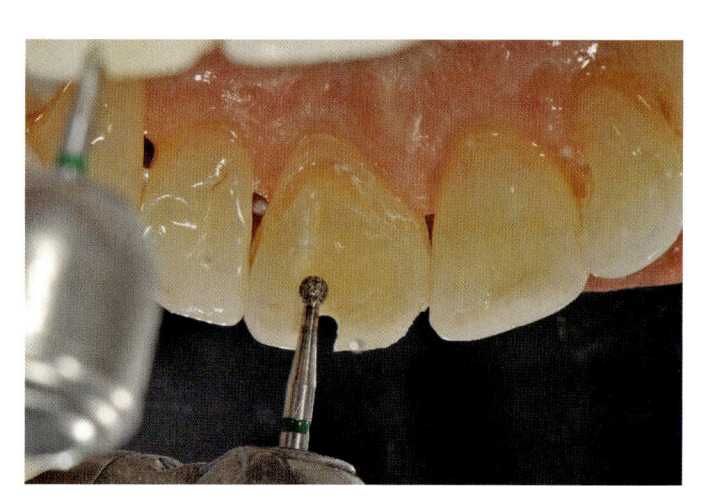

Figure 40.7 **(D)** Completion of the lingual vertical esthetic depth cut. Note also the completed lingual horizontal depth cut.

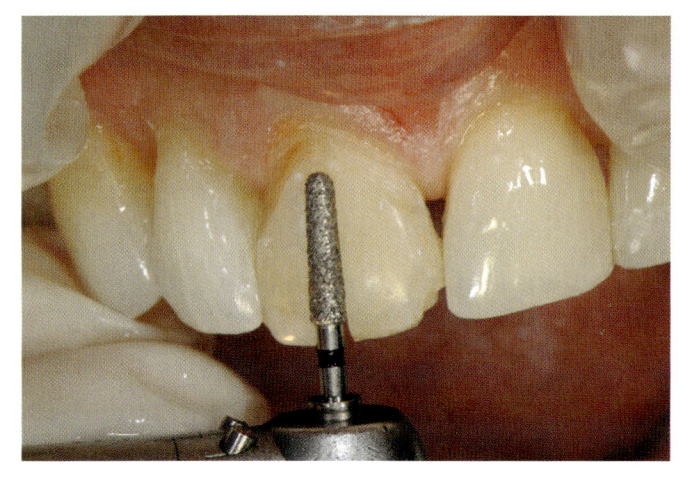

Figure 40.7 **(E)** Having completed the horizontal and vertical depth cuts, bulk enamel removal becomes predictable.

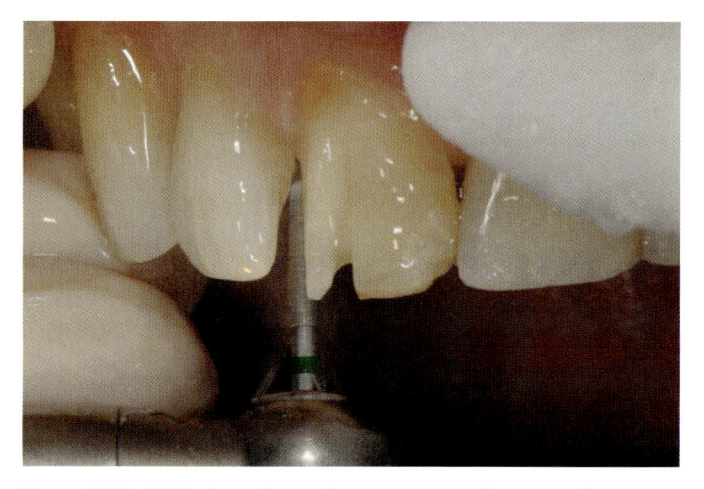

Figure 40.7 **(F)** At times, it may be necessary to change to the narrower diameter round-end coarse diamond (Brasseler AC7) to remove interproximal tooth structure without damaging the adjacent tooth.

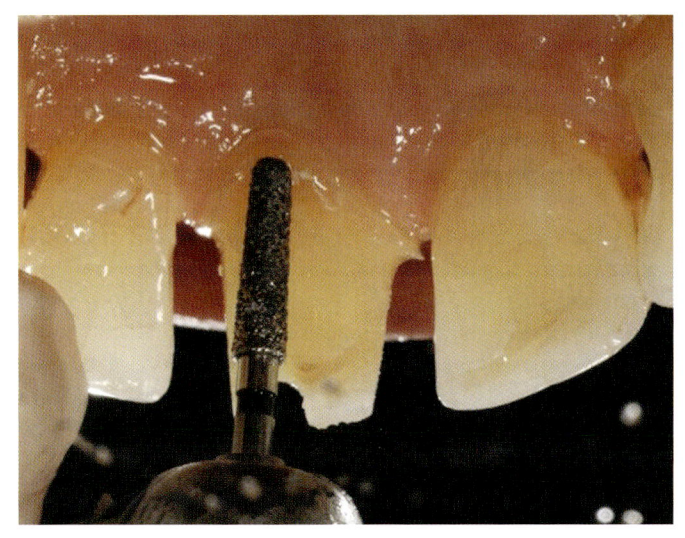

Figure 40.7 **(G)** Bulk enamel removal on the lingual. The lingual shoulder is refined using round-end tapered extra coarse diamond (Brasseler AC5).

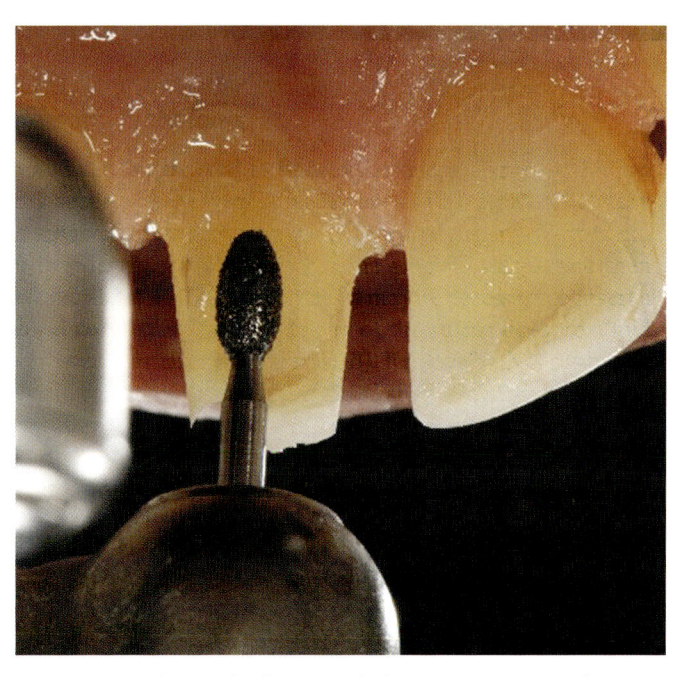

Figure 40.7 **(H)** Lingual reduction with the extra-coarse Brasseler AC10 helps create the proper lingual contour, particularly in the cingulum area.

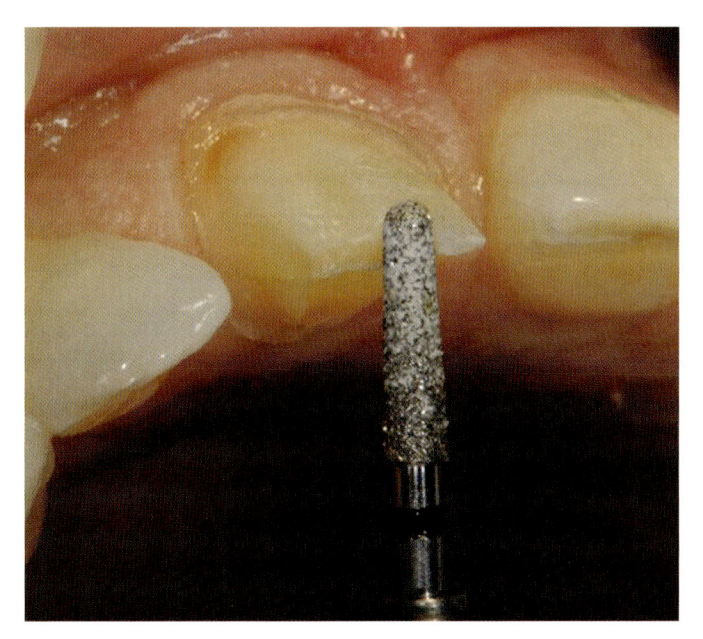

Figure 40.7 **(I)** Incisal reduction.

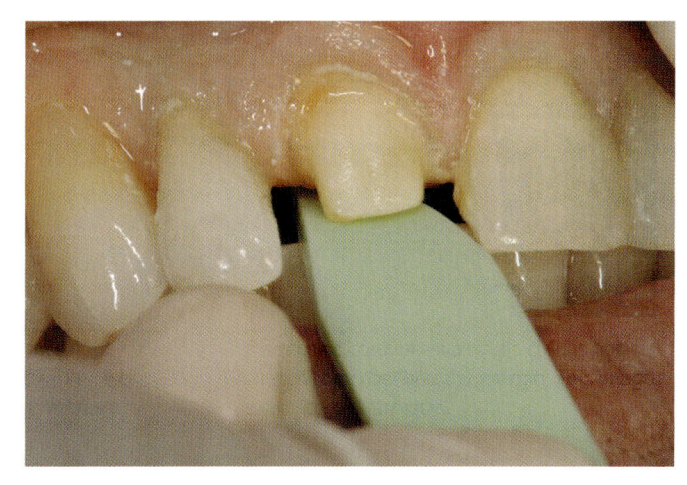

Figure 40.7 **(J)** Evaluate proper incisal clearance with the appropriate clearance tab. Here, a 1.5 mm clearance tab was used for lithium disilicate.

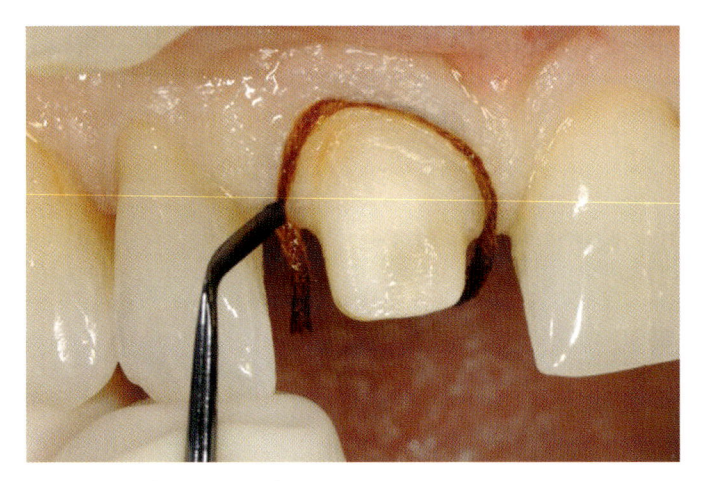

Figure 40.7 **(K)** Prior to subgingival margin placement, a retraction cord is placed to avoid tissue abrasion.

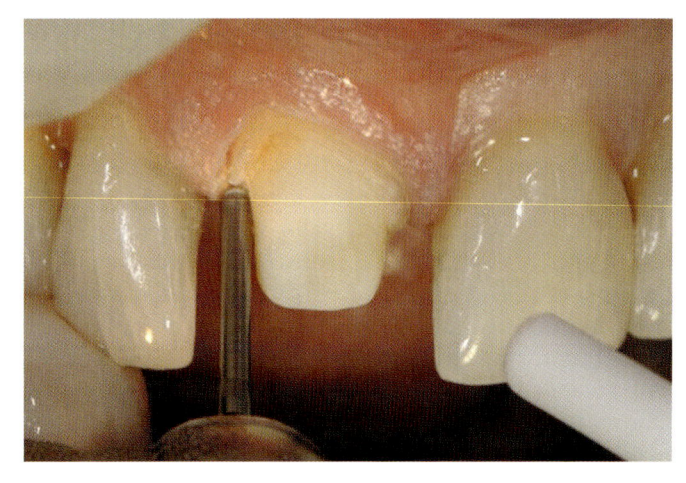

Figure 40.7 **(L)** The retraction cord is removed after 5–8 mins and the beveled-end cutting diamond (Brasseler AC11 or AC12) is used to prepare and finish the subgingival margin.

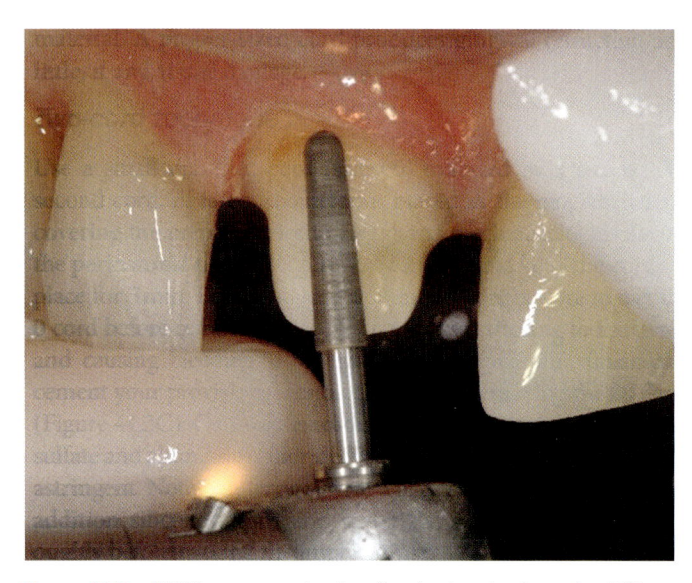

Figure 40.7 **(M)** The preparation is refined using the Brasseler AC6 fine diamond.

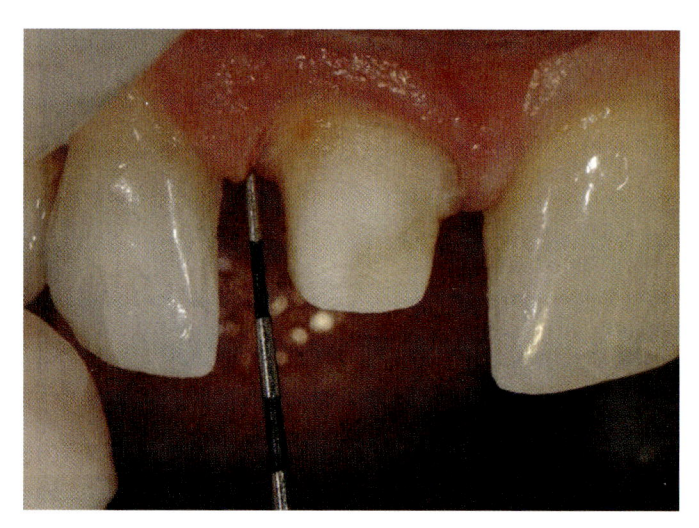

Figure 40.7 **(N)** The finished preparation.

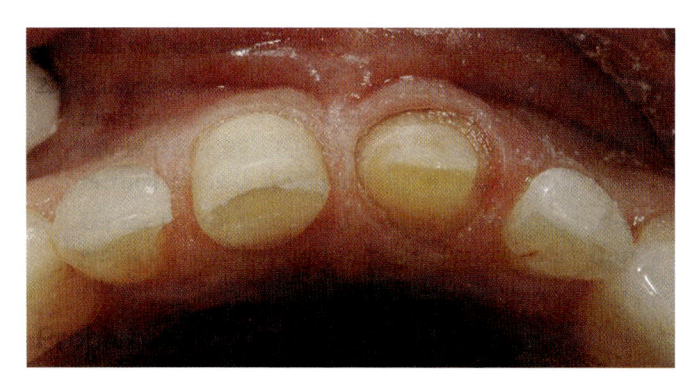

Figure 40.7 **(O)** Finished preparation from the occlusal view. Note that the adjacent central and lateral incisors were prepared for porcelain veneers.

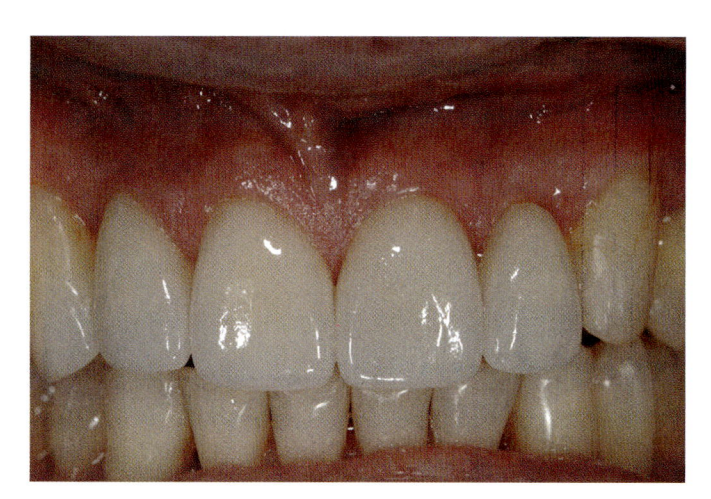

Figure 40.7 **(P)** Retracted view of completed lithium disilicate restorations.

2. The laboratory may use the proper thickness of metal and porcelain for strength and appearance, but the result may be an overcontoured crown.
3. A lifeless restoration may result if the laboratory maintains proper thickness in metal but reduces the bulk of porcelain too much.

If circumferential tooth reduction is allowed to become gradually thinner as it approaches the shoulder, it may result in (1) a lifeless looking gingival third due to thin porcelain, (2) overcontouring at the margin with traumatic pressure on the gingival attachment, or (3) porcelain flaking off because metal is too thin at the margin. The answer to all of these problems is consistent use of the "esthetic depth determination" when preparing teeth for full crowns.

The laboratory should not construct mere "facings," or one-surface (labial or buccal) veneers in ceramometal restorations, because these materials will not function successfully in this configuration. To gain the desired strength and durability of the ceramometal combination, there must be a degree of "wrap-around," as Tergis suggests.[29]

Porcelain colors at the gingival area are relatively intense and opaque. They readily hide the metal if the porcelain is at least 0.5–0.75 mm thick.[30] However, if the gingival shade is different from the opaque, a thicker layer of porcelain should be used. The thickness of porcelain must be increased toward the incisal third of the tooth to between 1.0 and 1.25 mm.[26] This allows for desirable translucency and esthetic characterization. Thus, the tooth reduction is uniform labially, mesially, and distally and requires a minimum of 1.5 mm of reduction in these areas. Incisally and occlusally, there should be a 2.0 mm clearance. Determine first if the opposing arch or teeth will need recontouring before attempting to reduce the tooth. However, with the all-ceramic crown, a 1.5 mm clearance is adequate. As mentioned previously, it should be remembered that a thickness of porcelain greater than 2.0 mm can result in structural weakness within the porcelain and might produce checking or cracking during construction or after case completion. These basic principles of reduction for the porcelain-fused-to-metal crown must be followed to assure a durable restoration that may be stained and contoured to achieve an esthetically pleasing result.

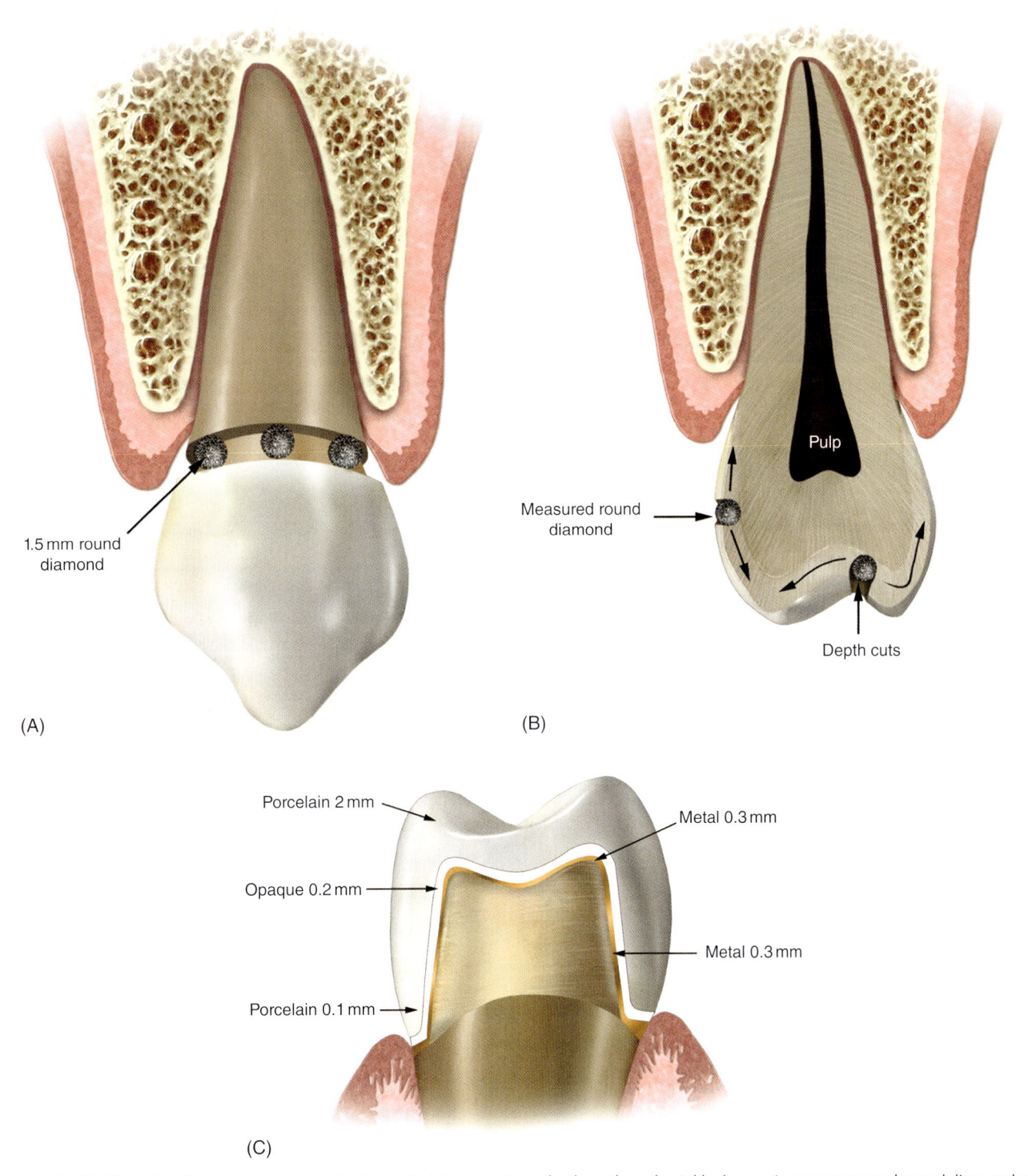

Figure 40.8 **(A–C)** As with the anterior teeth, esthetic depth determination is both easily and quickly done using premeasured round diamond stones.

The key to proper reduction is highly dependent on the overall esthetic result you desire. Thus, if you intend on building out a tooth to create greater harmony in the arch alignment, then less than normal tooth reduction should be planned. Conversely, if you need to reduce the buccal contour or alignment of a tooth, then even greater reduction might need to be planned. The important measurements are the end measurements, so that uniform thickness is achieved. Two techniques to verify your labial tooth preparation thickness are shown in Figure 40.11A–D. Note the special vacuform matrix of the wax-up used, with both incisal and gingival holes placed so the Goldstein Colorvue probe can measure in 0.5 mm increments.

Types of margins

The determination and preparation of the cervical margin is one of the most important and esthetically critical steps in

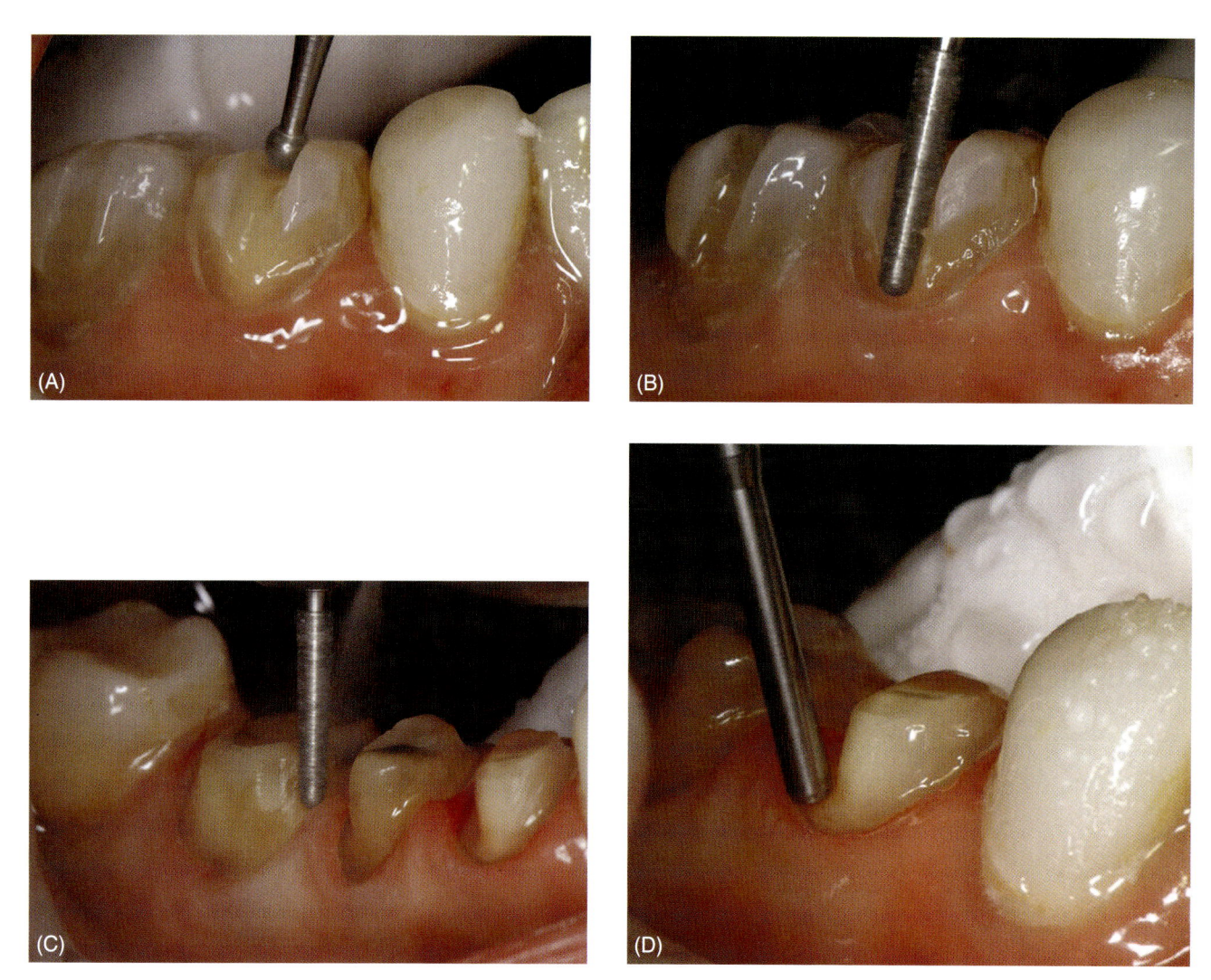

Figure 40.9 (**A–D**) These clinical figures show how the AC diamond technique can be utilized in posterior teeth as well.

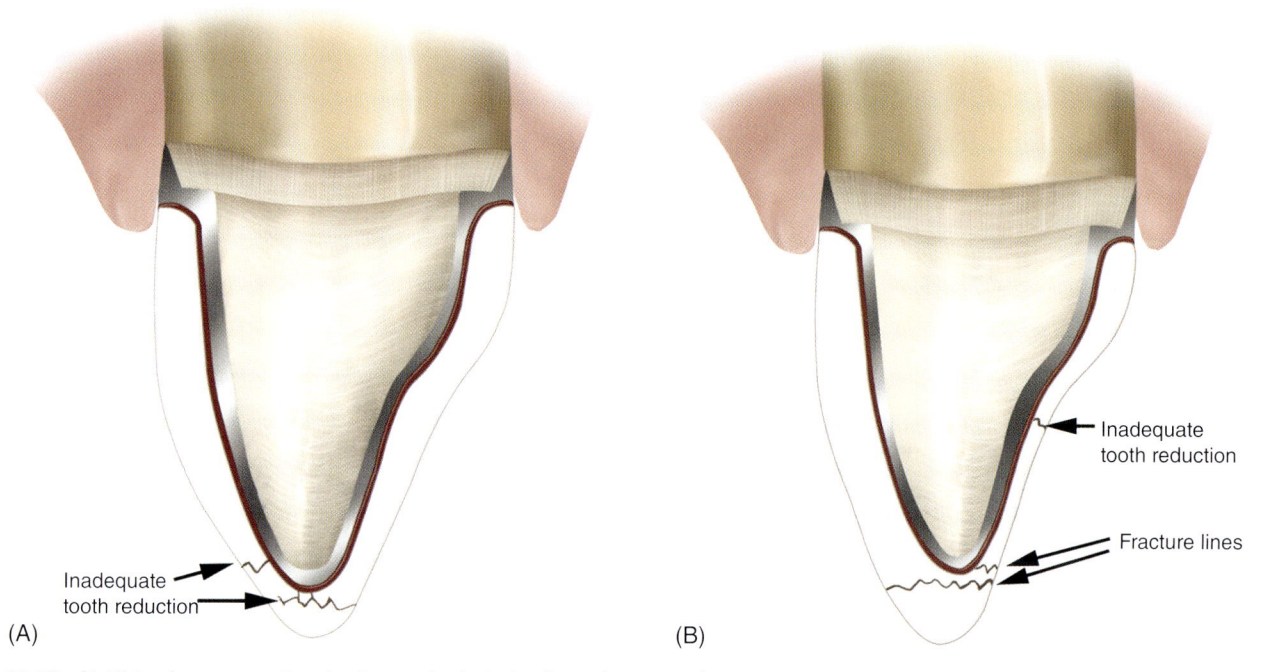

Figure 40.10 (**A, B**) Inadequate tooth reduction on the incisal or lingual aspects of a preparation can predispose the porcelain crown to fracture.

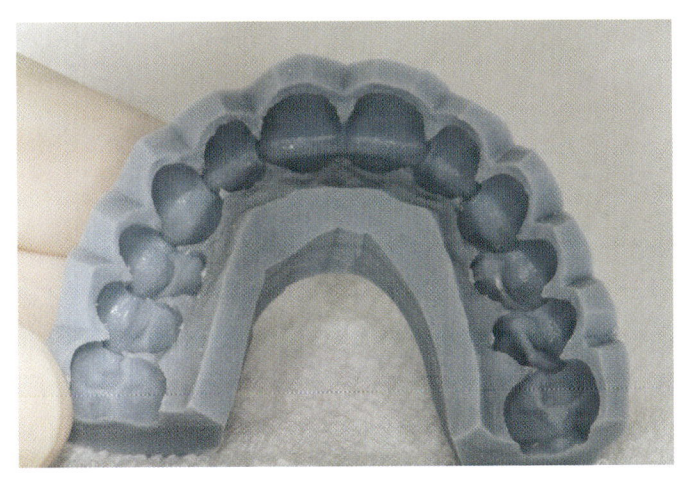

Figure 40.11 (A) A wax-up is completed to the contours desired in the final result and is duplicated in a laboratory silicone.

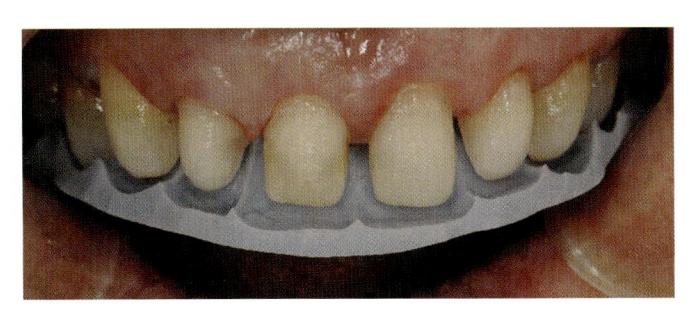

Figure 40.11 (B) The silicone is cut back for visibility and utilized chairside to confirm that there is adequate and uniform reduction for the final crowns.

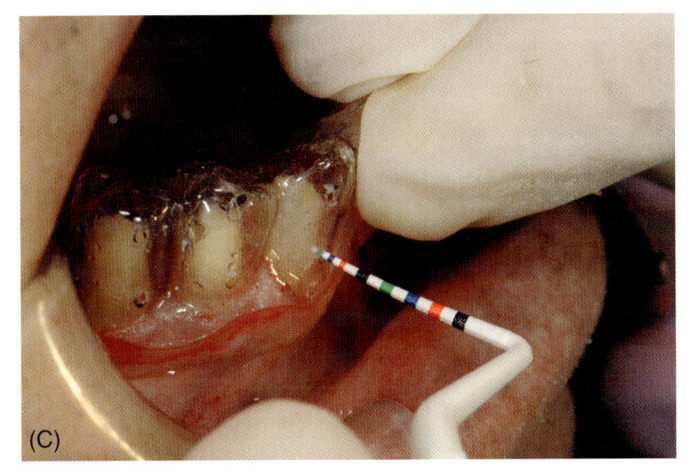

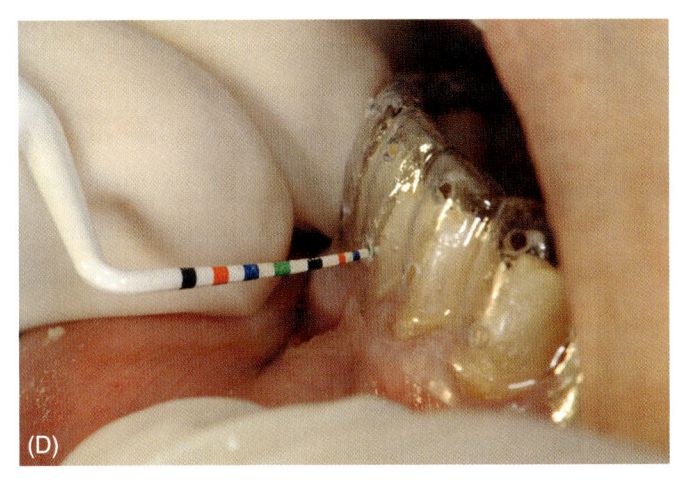

Figure 40.11 (C, D) Alternatively, a vacuum-formed matrix of the final wax-up can be utilized to visualize appropriate reduction. By making small, round access holes, an easy to see 0.5 mm Colorvue periodontal probe (Goldstein Colorvue Probe, Hu-Friedy) can determine whether you have achieved proper tooth reduction for adequate ceramic thickness.

tooth preparation. As Berman states, to provide adequate room for the terminal margin of the crown, the portion of the tooth in the sulcus must be adequately exposed either by retraction, laser, or electrosurgery.[31] If the shoulder is first prepared to the gingival crest and the tissue retracted for several minutes, then the shoulder can be lowered into the gingival sulcus without injuring the inner wall of sulcular epithelium. It is fully possible for complete crowns to enter the gingival sulcus without harming it. In preparing the margin, avoid making the undercuts or overtapering the preparation to prevent sacrificing maximum retention.

Unless there is adequate protection of the gingival sulcus during preparation, eventual exposure of the gingival margin may occur. For instance, a shoulder margin prepared with a tapered or straight diamond stone can lacerate gingival tissue as the shoulder margin is extended into the gingival sulcus. However, it is possible to prepare and finish this margin and also protect the sucular tissue through use of a beveled end-cutting diamond (AC11 or AC12, Brasseler USA). Unlike most end-cutting burs, the bevel on this diamond stone protects the adjacent gingival epithelium as the outer aspect of the shoulder is being prepared.

Figure 40.12A shows how the design of the stone protects the adjacent tissue. A clinical photograph of an anterior full crown preparation during and immediately after tooth preparation is shown in Figure 40.12B. Note the absence of tissue laceration. Slower speeds are advised to retain proper control and thereby prevent unnecessary slipping.

The selection or type of gingival margin can have a most profound effect on esthetic results, depending on location of the tooth in the arch and the position of the margin subgingivally.[10]

The shoulder

The full shoulder margin is utilized most often when preparing anterior and posterior crowns[10] (Figure 40.13). It also provides the proper room necessary from a technical standpoint to produce a porcelain-fused-to-metal restoration that has esthetic qualities of contour and color. The shoulder preparation provides an adequate bulk of porcelain at the margin to protect against cracks or fractures, thus combining strength and esthetics. In their study of marginal distortion in porcelain-fused-to-metal restorations, Shillingburg et al. found that the

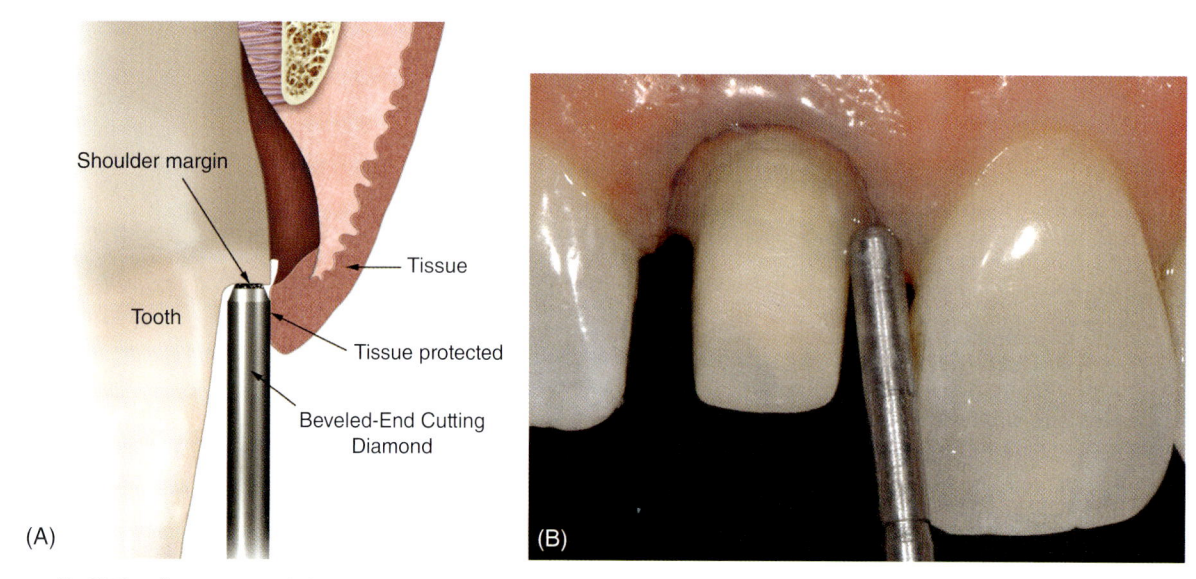

Figure 40.12 **(A, B)** This illustration and clinical example show appropriate use of the beveled-end cutting diamond (Brasseler AC11 and AC12) to finish subgingival margins while protecting the gingival tissue. Note the use of gingival retraction in (B).

labial margin, where metal thickness may be severely limited by esthetics, is the part most susceptible to distortion.[32] It has been our observation that porcelain chipping has occurred too frequently at a beveled gingival margin, especially when the metal was thinned down too much.

With the advent of more predictable bonding agents and cements that adhere to the restoration as well as the tooth, the all-ceramic margin becomes much more feasible in esthetic dentistry.

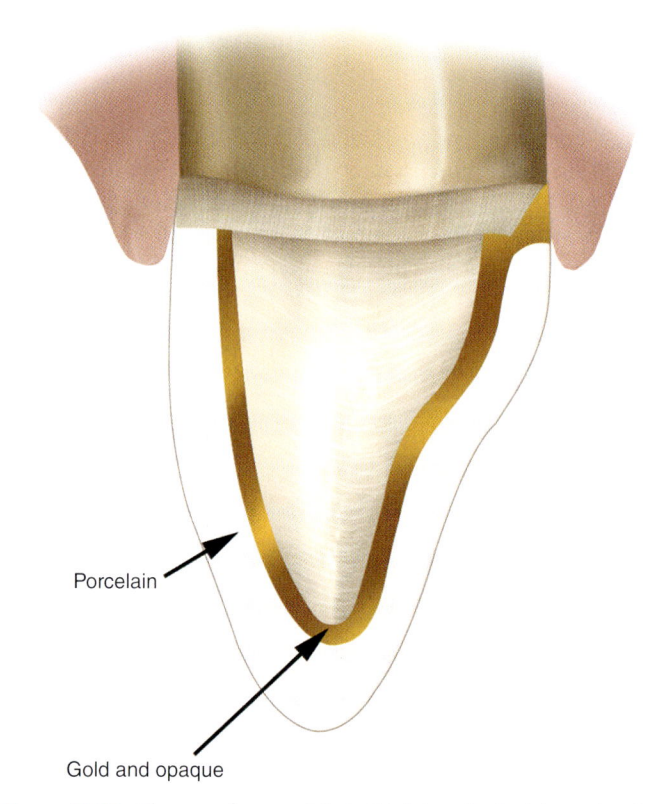

Figure 40.13 The use of a porcelain butt joint on the facial margin of a ceramometal crown may be used in the case of a thin or shallow sulcus.

Tooth preparation in periodontal problems

When possible, periodontal therapy should be completed before the tooth is prepared. There are times, however, when it is necessary that treatment splinting or temporization be instituted before periodontal surgical procedures such as grafting are performed. Generally, gingival margins will necessarily be further beneath the sulcus to allow for shrinkage or placement of a higher level of the gingival tissue. It is advisable to prepare the tooth as close as possible to where the final preparation is anticipated. Thus, there will be less likelihood of having to completely remake the temporary restoration to regain marginal integrity after periodontal therapy is concluded. Some alteration of the tooth preparation will be necessary, and the temporary splint may be repaired in lieu of constructing a complete replacement (Figure 40.14A–D).

One possible esthetic problem after periodontal surgery is the presence of larger interdental spaces. Closure of these spaces can usually be accomplished in the final crown form. Although this may require a greater mesiodistal reduction in the final preparation, some allowances for this can be made during the initial preparation and margin placement. Careful planning is a must in cases of loss of interdental space. Much less preparation may be required because of the need to fill in the missing interdental areas. Finally, the choice of adding pink ceramic or composite resin should be a consideration.

In cases of advanced periodontal disease where bifurcation or even trifurcations are involved, use the extra-long AC1 diamond to help create your margin. However, do not attempt a shoulder margin in these cases. Therefore, you may want to consider zirconia, where you can utilize a thin proximal margin.

Areas of crowded teeth

It can be frustrating to prepare crowded teeth. The basic problem is correct placement of mesial and distal margins, depending on

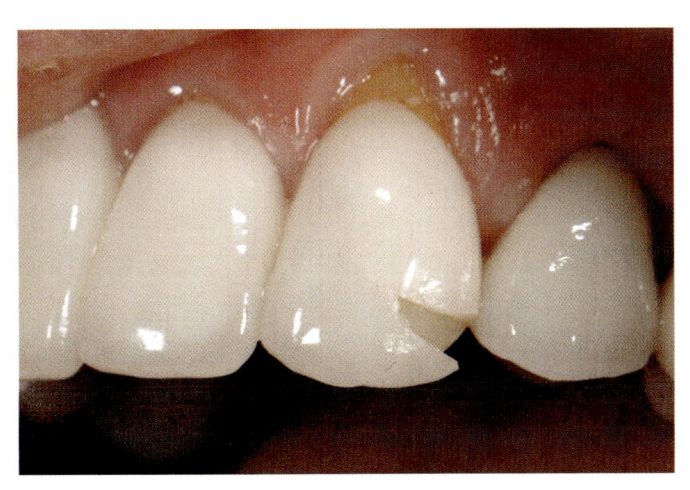

Figure 40.14 **(A)** This patient presented with a fractured porcelain veneer. Prior to final preparation and impressions, the periodontal problem of gingival recession must be addressed.

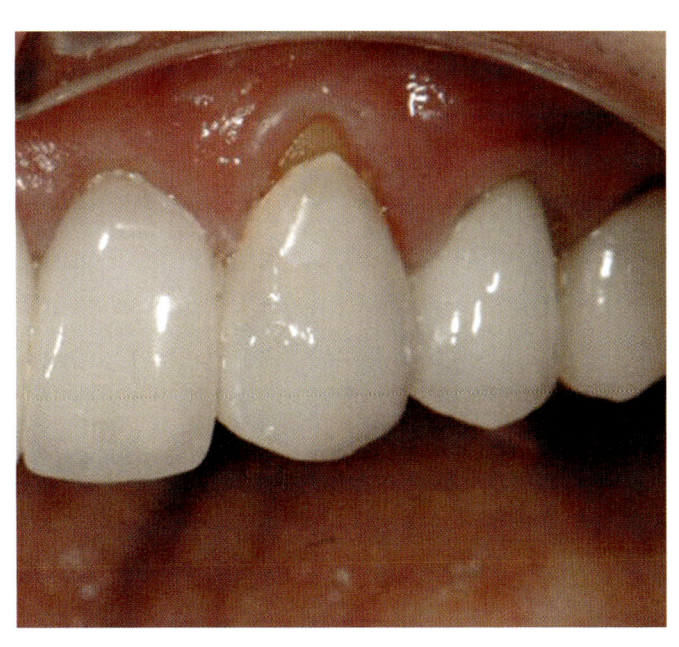

Figure 40.14 **(B)** The tooth was provisionalized at the ideal gingival level prior to surgery. This allows the periodontist to visualize the final gingival margin.

the adjacent tooth and space limitations. However, the further into the gingiva one goes, the less interdental space there is. Although, from a functional standpoint, it may be better to keep the margin supragingival, this may not be feasible esthetically. The amount of proximal tooth reduction available will most times determine the final position and size of the restoration (Figure 40.15A–E).

Other considerations in the preparation of crowded incisors are choosing a type and obtaining a proper margin. The choice of which margin to use depends upon the restoration desired and the limitations presented by the crowded condition. Several variables are involved, and each will now be considered separately.

Normal crown/root ratio with margin on enamel surface

Because of the available thickness, these teeth can be adequately prepared for either a ceramometal or all-ceramic restoration. There is usually enough thickness to adequately restore the tooth with an esthetic restoration. Thus, either shoulder or beveled shoulder margins may be employed successfully for ceramometal, and the full shoulder margin should be the choice for the all-ceramic crown.

Tissue shrinkage with exposed cementum

In this case, if the lip line is such that the lower teeth do not show, it is best to continue to keep the margins supragingival if possible. However, if because of caries, decalcification, or other problems the margins must be extended subgingivally, then the margins may have to be in cementum. This also means little or no space to obtain an adequate separation between teeth. Therefore, the safest way to prepare a margin is to utilize a thin-metal matrix band, carefully stripping it between the teeth and holding it there to protect the adjacent tooth from damage while preparing the tooth. The best margin is the shoulder type, since it would be difficult to obtain an adequate

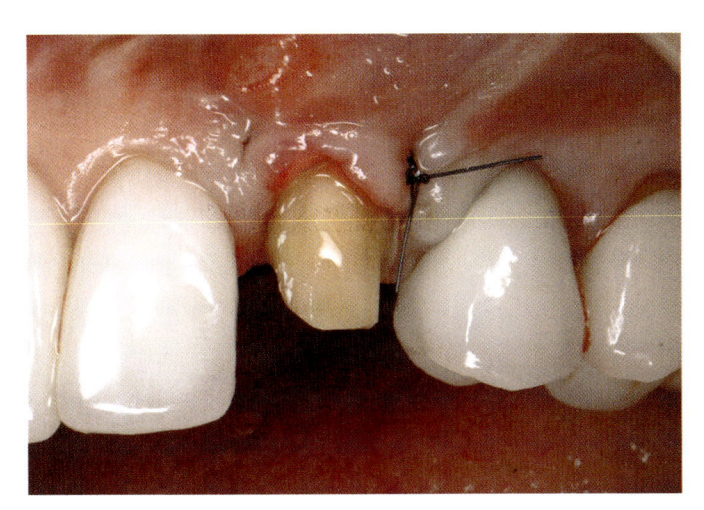

Figure 40.14 **(C)** A connective tissue graft was completed with coronal positioning to the predetermined margin.

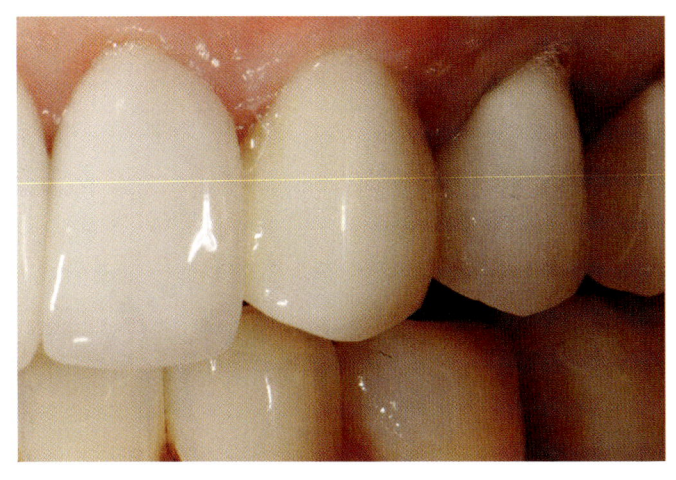

Figure 40.14 **(D)** Final lithium disilicate restoration completed after tissue healing.

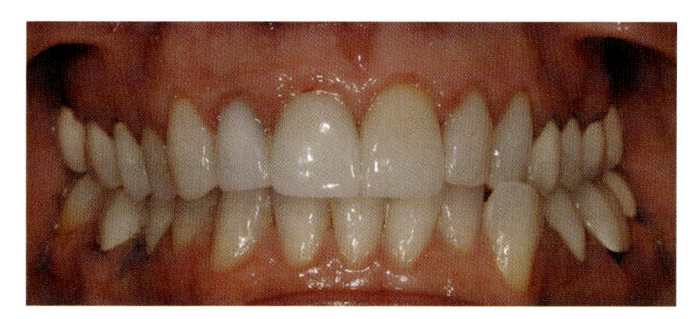

Figure 40.15 **(A)** Retracted pretreatment view illustrating crossbite between the upper and lower left cuspids.

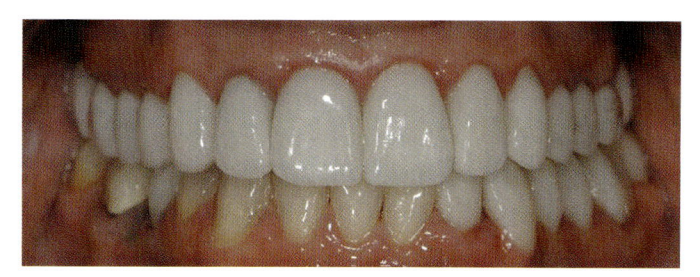

Figure 40.15 **(B)** The final restorations, with correction of the crowding and the crossbite. Pink ceramic was utilized at the gum line to create a more ideal tooth morphology.

bevel. However, if there is enough room for a bevel and if the patient has a lip line that will not reveal the neck of the tooth, the preferred treatment is to leave a gold cuff exposed. This would be the thinnest type of crown replacement available in the crowded areas.

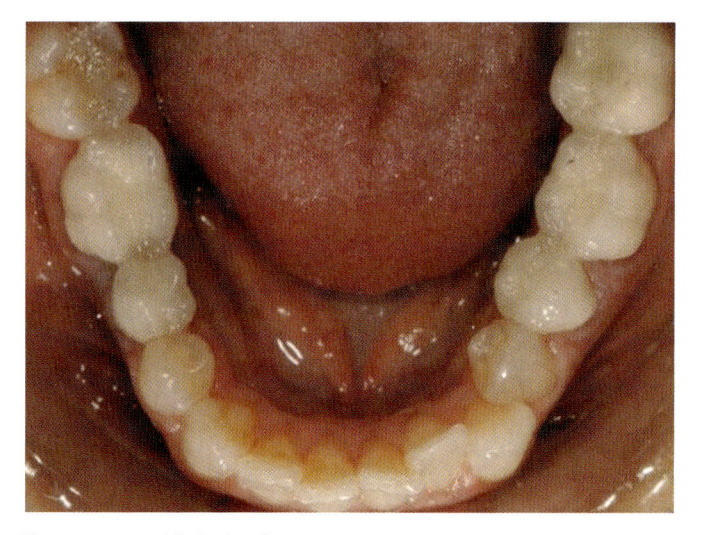

Figure 40.15 **(C)** Occlusal pretreatment view. Note crowding on the left side.

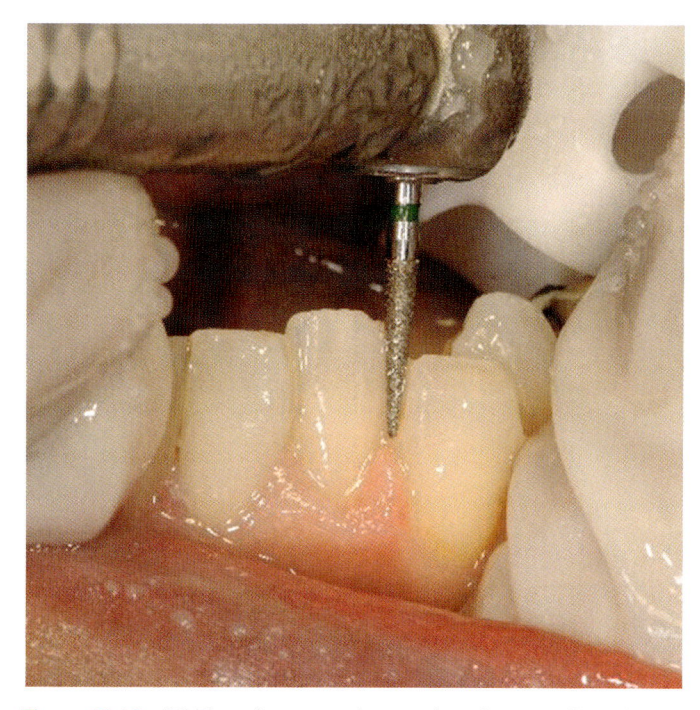

Figure 40.15 **(D)** The adjacent teeth are reduced proximally with the AC2 (Brasseler) to allow for correction of crowding and to create space to lingually position the cuspid.

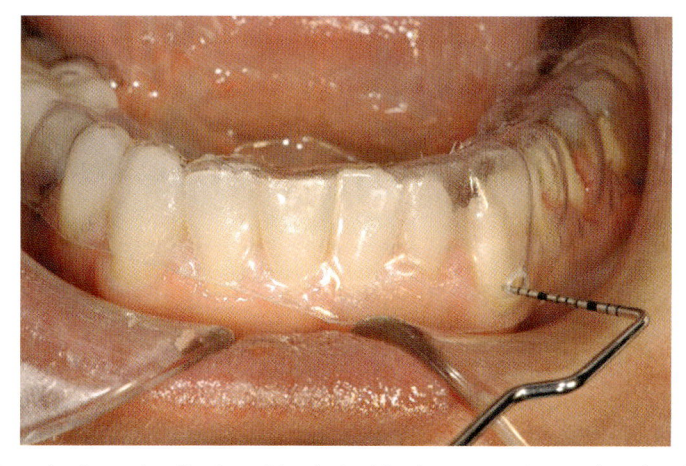

Figure 40.15 **(E)** A vacuum-formed matrix allows visualization of the desired final outcome. A periodontal probe through an access hole ensures that there will be adequate thickness of ceramic to achieve the desired contours.

The variables in each of these cases are (1) the crown/root ratio, (2) the amount of exposed root area, (3) the high lip and speaking line, (4) the esthetic concept and needs of the patient, and (5) the radiographic interpretation of pulp position and size.

Choice of materials

In the crowded tooth condition, the choice of materials may be limited to lithium disilicate (e.max, Ivoclar), full-contour zirconia (Bruxzir, Glidewell), or porcelain with a thin-metal coping (Captek) due to available tooth size. There simply may not be enough room for ceramometal. The esthetic nature of the full porcelain crown makes it an excellent restoration in lower anteriors when adequate preparation and shoulder depth are available. When there is not enough, an alternate would be the shoulderless full-porcelain crown, using a thin-metal coping (Captek), or even an all-zirconia crown with a slight chamfer margin.

Lower incisors can be the most difficult teeth to prepare. Because the roots are conical, and these teeth are thin and small, it is more difficult to obtain proper thickness for a proper margin. Compromises in preparation will have to be made; a different material should be selected—or a less esthetic result anticipated. The teeth should be studied carefully along with the radiographs to obtain information about how thick the restorative material may be. A frequently encountered problem is the fanned or labially tipped lower incisor. In this case, study the problem to determine exactly how much reduction will be permitted. Still using the AC4 round diamond to gain an esthetic depth control might not be possible to completely cut into the cervical portion of the tooth for the entire 1.0 mm thickness of the diamond. Occasionally, if the pulp has receded, it will be possible to reduce enough incisal and labial thickness to realign the tooth and restoration. This depends on the location of the pulp and the degree of labial inclination. If possible, it is usually best to strip these teeth and try to reposition them orthodontically before preparation.

Long crown/root ratio

This situation generally occurs following periodontal surgery. The objective in the crown/root ratio is to have a longer root than crown, therefore lowering the ratio. Esthetically, if the patient has a high lip line, it may present a problem unless the tooth is prepared properly. In the case of a deep overbite, it is possible to shorten the teeth for a more esthetic result. This may also be combined at times with cosmetic gingival surgery, if there is need for more tooth structure to be exposed. A second method is to carve and stain root contours to avoid unsightly long clinical crowns.

Extremely short teeth

Depending on the cause of their limited height, preparing extremely short teeth can be difficult. Since incisal or occlusal reduction for ceramometal needs to be approximately 2 mm, the stability and retention may be totally inadequate (Figure 40.9A–D). The all-ceramic crown may be a viable alternative, since the required occlusal reduction can be 1.5 mm. If this is not possible, then either an all-gold or all-zirconia crown can be the logical choice. Although the reduction for a full-zirconia crown can be as little as 0.5 mm, ideally you would want to reduce at least 1.0 mm for greater strength. If the solution is to use a zirconia core with porcelain buildup, it may be much safer to have a reduction of approximately 2 mm. If the reason for short teeth is occlusal wear, a decision to increase the vertical dimension of occlusion may be made. If this is the case, there would be no reason to reduce the occlusal surfaces or incisal edges 1.5–2.0 mm. Do as little incisal/occlusal preparation as possible to preserve tooth length. As an alternative, the opposing teeth may also need to be altered to provide adequate clearance (Figure 40.16A–E).

Pre-preparation checklist

- Evaluate tissue health and sulcus depth.
- What type of margin will be best for health, esthetics, and longevity?
- Evaluate need for pretreatment periodontal procedures.
- Can you predict and allow for future gingival shrinkage/recession?
- Study pulp size/shape on pretreatment radiograph.
- Will endo likely be needed?
- Does the smile line limit your margin type?
- Will tooth position (crowding, etc.) affect choice of materials?

Preparation checklist

- Internal preparation line angles round and smooth.
- Adequate occlusal/incisal clearance for chosen material.
- All margins smooth and clearly visible from intended path of insertion.
- Adequate proximal and buccal space for ceramist.
- Is retention adequate?
- If not, consider metal collar for porcelain-fused-to-metal crown or bonding technique for all ceramic.

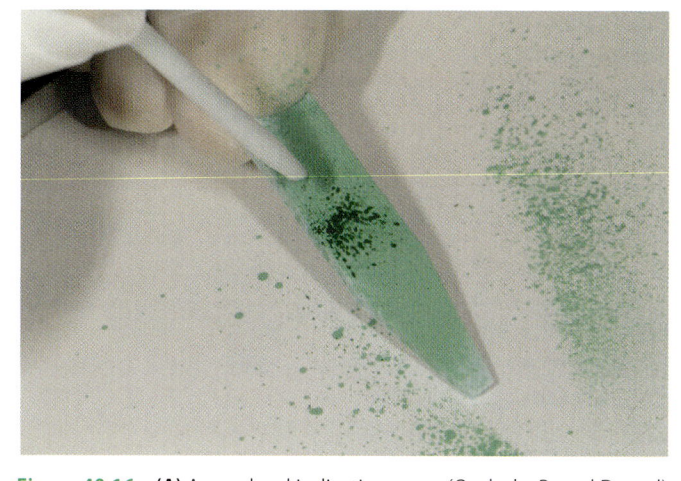

Figure 40.16 **(A)** An occlusal indicating spray (Occlude, Pascal Dental) is applied to an occlusal clearance tab to allow transfer to the teeth.

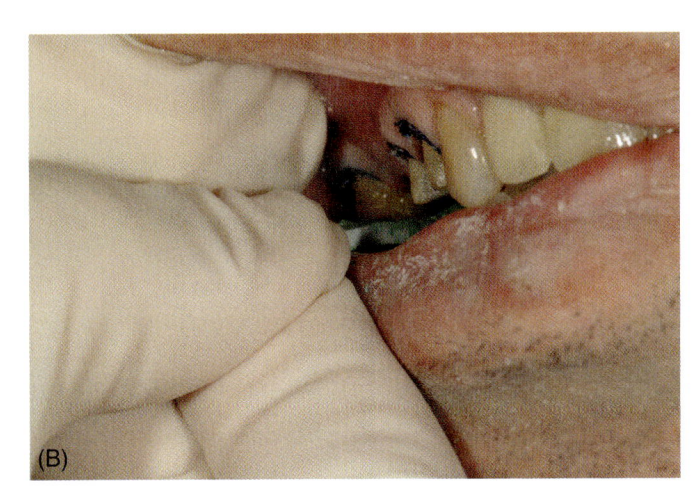

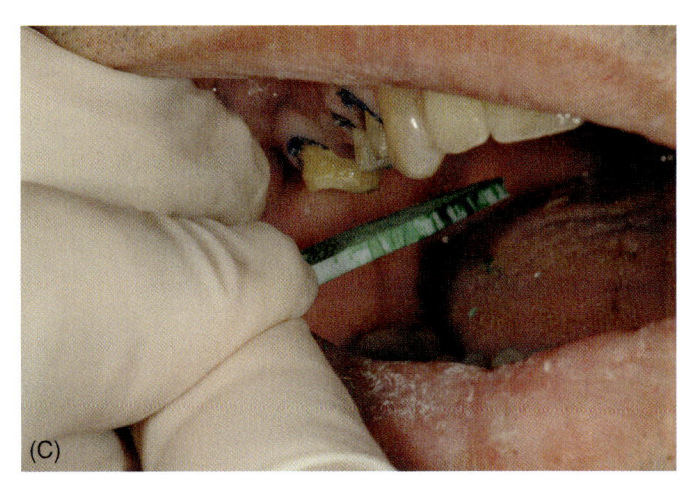

Figure 40.16 **(B, C)** The clearance tab is positioned between the teeth with the clearance in question—in this case, the upper and lower second molars.

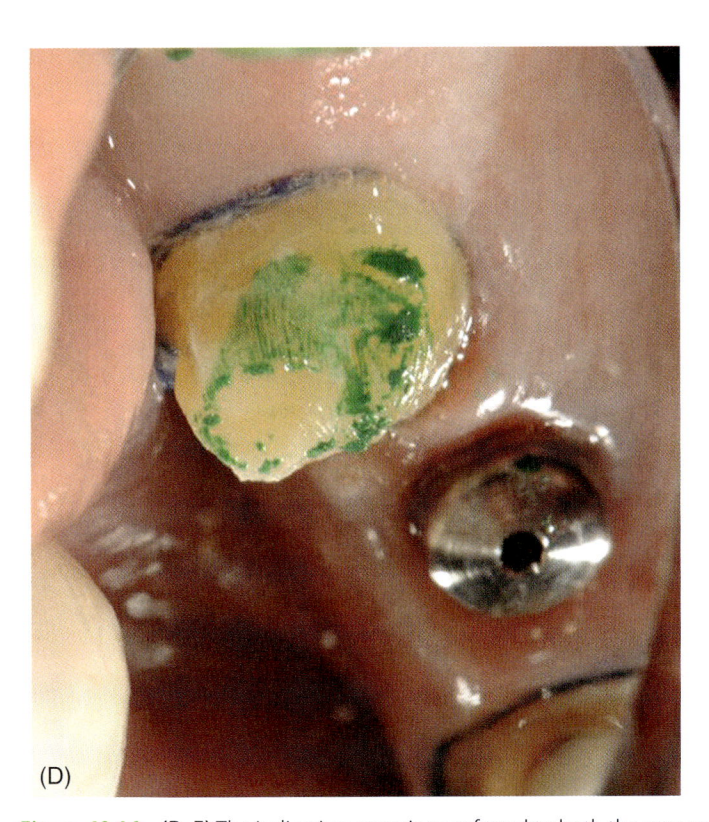

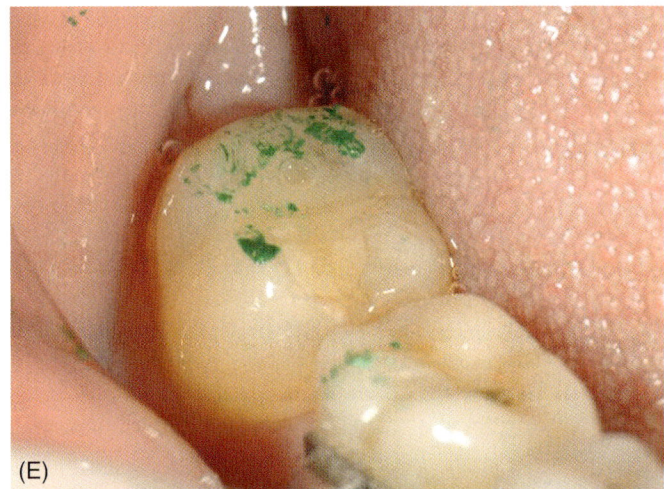

Figure 40.16 **(D, E)** The indicating spray is transferred to both the prepared tooth and its antagonist, allowing for additional adjustment on either tooth.

References

1. Beuer F, Aggstaller H, Richter J, et al. Influence of preparation angle on marginal and internal fit of CAD/CAM-fabricated zirconia crown copings. *Quintessence Int* 2009;40:243–250.
2. Liu P, Essig ME. A panorama of dental CAD/CAM restorative systems. *Compendium* 2008;29:482–493.
3. Berdon JK. Odontoplasty—a rationale and technique. *W V Dent J.* 1967;41(2):23–25.
4. Pritchard JF. *Advanced Periodontal Disease—Surgical and Prosthetic Management*, 2nd edn. Philadelphia, PA: W.B. Saunders; 1972.
5. Silness J. Periodontal conditions in patients treated with dental bridge; the relationship between the location of the crown margin and the periodontal condition. *J Periodont Res* 1970;5:225–229.
6. Larato DC. The effect of crown margin extension on gingival inflammation. *J South Calif Dent Assoc* 1969;37:476–478.
7. Burch JG. Ten rules for developing crown contours in restorations. *Dent Clin North Am* 1971;15:611–618.
8. Gargiulo A, Krajewski J, Gargiulo M. Defining biologic width in crown lengthening. *CDS Rev* 1995;88(5):20–23.
9. Tarnow D, Stahl SS, Magner A, Zamzok J. Human gingival attachment responses to subgingival crown placement: marginal remodeling. *J Clin Periodontol* 1986;13:563–569.

10. Tylman SD. *Tylman's Theory and Practice of Fixed Prosthodontics*. St. Louis, MO: Mosby; 1978.
11. Björn AL, Björn H, Grcovic B. Marginal fit of restorations and its relation to periodontal bone level. *Odontol Revy* 1970;2(1):337–346.
12. Brecker SC. *Clinical Procedures in Occlusal Rehabilitation*. Philadelphia, PA: W.B. Saunders; 1966.
13. Schweitzer JM. *Oral Rehabilitation Problem Cases—Treatment and Evaluation*. St. Louis, MO: Mosby; 1964.
14. Johnston JF, Mumford G, Dykema RW. *Modern Practice in Dental Ceramics*. Philadelphia, PA: W.B. Saunders; 1967.
15. Grieder A, Cinotti WR. *Periodontal Prosthesis*. St. Louis, MO: Mosby; 1968.
16. Beaudreau DE. Evaluation of abutment teeth. *Dent Clin N Am* 1969;13:845–855.
17. Fuhr K, Kares K, Sienert G. Follow-up in fixed prosthesis. (Evaluation of systematic analysis of findings.) *Dtsch Zahnärztl Z* 1971;26:716–724 [in German].
18. Miller IF, Field LL. Epoxy resin—a new medium in full coverage for restorative dentistry. *Dent Clin North Am* 1963;27(4):792.
19. Felton DA, Kanoy BE, Bayne SC, Wirthman GP. Effect of in vivo crown margin discrepancies on periodontal health. *J Prosthet Dent* 1991;65:357–364.
20. Sorensen SE, Larsen IB, Jörgensen KD. Gingival and alveolar bone reaction to marginal fit of subgingival crown margins. *Scand J Dent Res* 1986;94:109–114.
21. Mumford G, Ridge A. Dental porcelain. *Dent Clin North Am* 1971;15:33–42.
22. Paquette JM, Sheets CG, Wu JC, Chu SJ. Tooth preparation principles and designs for full-coverage restorations. In: Tarnow DP, Chu SJ, Kim J, eds. *Aesthetic Restorative Dentistry: Principles and Practice*. Mahwah, NJ: Montage Media Corp; 2008:99–125.
23. Brecker SC. Procedures to improve esthetics in restorative dentistry. *J N Carolina Dent Soc* 1957;41:33–36.
24. Roberts DH. *Fixed Bridge Prosthesis*. Bristol: John Wright & Sons; 1973.
25. LeGro AL. *Ceramics in Dentistry*. Brooklyn, NY: Dental Items of Interest Publishing Co.; 1925.
26. Stein RS. Ceramo-metal and aluminous porcelain restorations. In: Course presented at College of Dental Medicine, Charleston, SC; 1971.
27. Straussberg G, Katz G, Kuwota M. Design of gold supporting structures for fused porcelain restorations. *J Prosthet Dent* 1966;16:928–936.
28. Huttner G. Follow-up study of crowns and abutments with regard to the crown edge and the marginal periodontium. *Dtsch Zahnärztl Z* 1971;26:724–729 [in German].
29. Tergis MJ. The proper geometry of preparation and case design in porcelain-on-gold restorations. *J Acad Gen Dent* 1971;19:15–17.
30. Stein RS. A dentist and a dental technologist analyze current ceramo-metal procedures. *Dent Clin N Am* 1977;4:729–749.
31. Berman MH. Cutting efficiency in complete coverage preparation. *J Am Dent Assoc* 1969;79:1160–1167.
32. Shillingburg HT Jr, Hobo S, Fisher DW. Preparation design and margin distortion in porcelain-fused-to-metal restorations. *J Prosthet Dent* 1973;29:276–284.

Additional resources

Chai JY, Steege JW. Effects of labial margin design on stress distribution of a porcelain-fused-to-metal crown. *J Prosthodont* 1992;1:18–23.
Chiche G, Pinault A, eds. *Esthetics of Anterior Fixed Prosthodontics*. London: Quintessence; 2004.
Christensen GC. Frequently encountered errors in tooth preparations for crowns. *J Am Dent Assoc* 2007;10:1373–1375.
Ercoli C, Rotella M, Funkenbusch PD, et al. In vitro comparison of the cutting efficiency and temperature production of 10 different rotary cutting instruments. Part I: turbine. *J Prosthet Dent* 2009;101:248–261.
Ercoli C, Rotella M, Funkenbusch PD, et al. In vitro comparison of the cutting efficiency and temperature production of 10 different rotary cutting instruments. Part I: electric handpieces and comparison with turbine. *J Prosthet Dent* 2009;101:319–331.
Fozar A. Periodontal prosthesis: control of key factors from surgery to teeth preparation and to final cementation. *Int J Esthet Dent* 2014;9:280–296.
Fradeani M. Biologic integration of the provisional restorations and definitive preparations. In: Fradeani M, Barducci G, eds. *Esthetic Rehabilitation in Fixed Prosthodontics*. London: Quintessence; 2008.
Goodacre CJ, Campagni WV, Aquilino SA. Tooth preparations for complete crowns: an art form based on scientific principles. *J Prosthet Dent* 2001;85:363–376.
Gürel G. Predictable, precise, and repeatable tooth preparation for porcelain laminate veneers. *Pract Proced Aesthet Dent* 2003;15:17–24.
Jung Y, Lee JW, Choi YJ, et al. A study on the in-vitro wear of the natural tooth structure by opposing zirconia or dental porcelain. *J Adv Prosthodont* 2010;2:111–115.
Harris DM, Gregg RH II, McCarthy DK, et al. Laser-assisted new attachment procedure in private practice. *Gen Dent* 2004;52:396–403.
Kois JC. Altering gingival levels: the restorative connection. Part 1: biologic variables. *J Esthet Dent* 1994;6:3–9.
Malik K, Tabiat-Pour S. The use of diagnostic wax set-up in aesthetic cases involving crown lengthening. A case report. *Dent Update* 2010;37:303–307.
McDermott DE. Porcelain fused to gold. *J Am Dent Assoc* 1968;45:30.
Mintrone F, Kataoka S. Pre-visualization: a useful system for truly informed consent to esthetic treatment and aid in conservative dental preparation. *Quintessence Dent Technol* 2010;33:189–198.
Nevins M, Skurow H. The intracrevicular restorative margin, biologic width and the maintenance of the gingival margin. *Int J Periodont Rest Dent* 1984;4:30–49.
Rantanen TA. A control study on crowns and bridges on root-filled teeth. *Suom Hammaslaak Toim* 1970;66(5):275–288 [in Finnish].
Spear F. Using margin placement to achieve best anterior esthetics. *J Am Dent Assoc*. 2009;140:920–926.
Tirlet G, Crescenzo H, Crescenzo D, Bazos P. Ceramic adhesive restorations and biomimetic dentistry: tissue preservation and adhesion. *Int J Esth Dent* 2014; 9(3):354–368.
Tjan AH, Sarkissian R. Effect of preparation finish on retention and fit of complete crowns. *J Prosthet Dent* 1986;56:283–288.
Wang CJ, Millstein PL, Nathanson D. Effects of cement, cement space, marginal design, seating aid materials, and seating force on crown cementation. *J Prosthet Dent* 1992;67:786–790.

Small cord

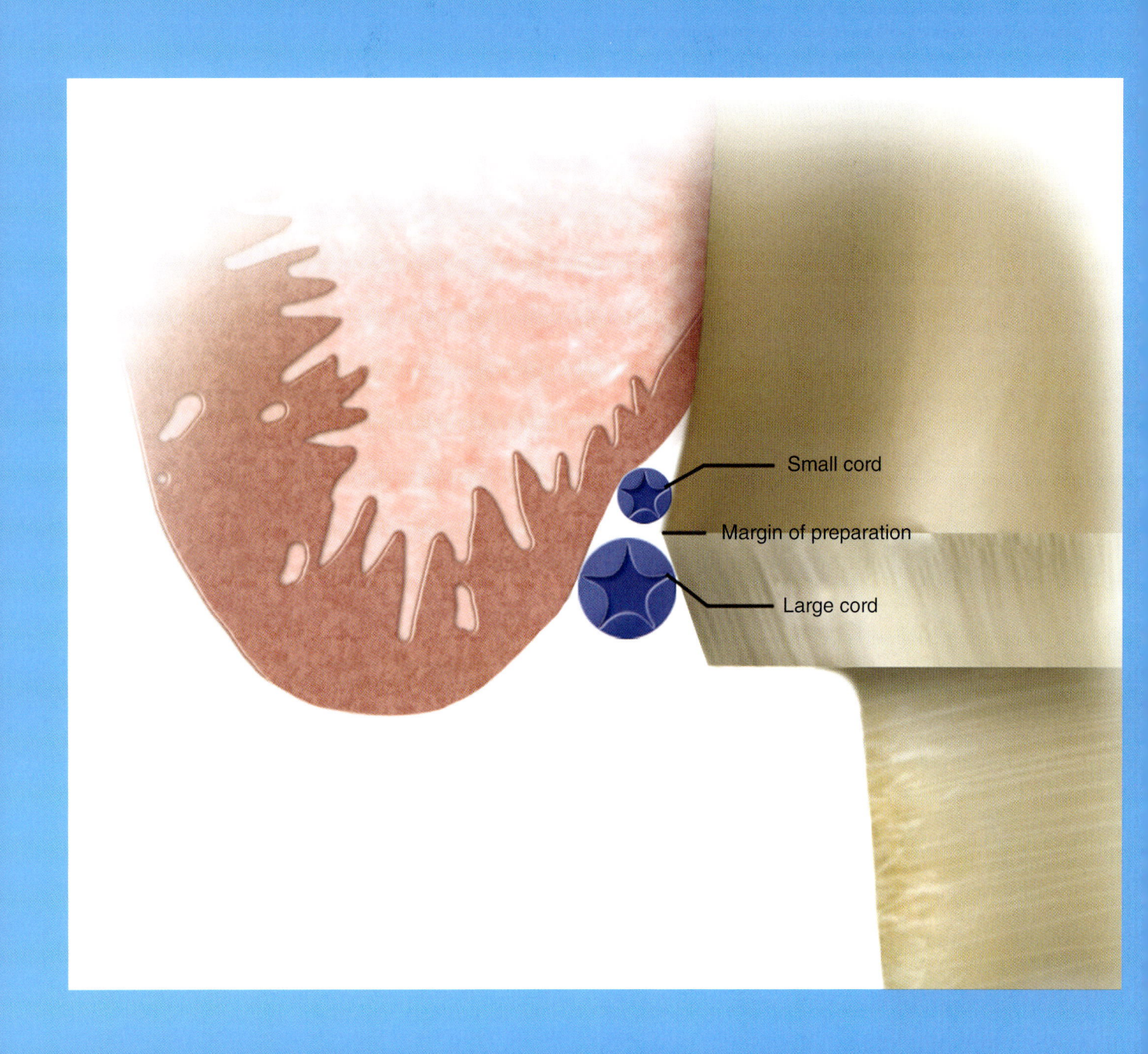

Margin of preparation

Large cord

Chapter 41 Impressions

Ronald E. Goldstein, DDS, John M. Powers, PhD, and Ernesto A. Lee, DMD

Chapter Outline

Preparation of soft tissues	1287	Properties and clinical relevance	1293
Tissue retraction	1288	Manipulation of impression materials	1294
Two-appointment procedures	1288	Impression techniques	1294
Retraction cords	1288	Special impression techniques	1294
Placement of retraction cords	1288	Other impression materials	1302
Problems with retraction cords	1290	Digital impressions	1302
Electrosurgery	1290	Tips on digital impressions	1303
Impression materials	1291	Mounting casts	1303
Silicone impression materials	1291	Interocclusal records (bite registrations)	1303
Polyether impression materials	1292		

A restoration may look good when it is inserted, but to remain an esthetic success it must also continue to fit well. The ability to construct an accurately fitted crown depends on mastery of the impression technique. No single technique is suitable for every situation, so it is best to have several impression techniques available. This chapter will discuss both conventional and digital impression techniques.

Impression materials are used to accurately record the dimensions and spatial relationships of oral tissues. Silicone and polyether elastomeric (flexible) impression materials are the most common types used for restorative dentistry. Polysulfide (rubber base) and hydrocolloid impression materials are much less common now. Recently, digital impressions prepared from intraoral scanners have become popular.

Desirable features of elastomeric impression materials include appropriate viscosities for the desired technique (e.g., syringe/tray), easy to use, 4 min working/setting time, adequate detail reproduction, easy to disinfect, compatible with dye materials, adequate shelf life, and cost effective. Important properties include elastic recovery, flexibility, and tear energy.

Preparation of soft tissues

Five common methods for the preparation of soft tissues are retraction cord, paste systems, conventional electrosurgery, bipolar technique, and diode lasers. The most important first step in making a perfect impression is adequate preparation of the soft tissue. Failure to clearly display all the margins of each prepared tooth leads to an unacceptable impression regardless of which impression material or technique is chosen.

Tissue retraction

Achieving long-lasting esthetic tissue around crowns depends upon the dentist's ability to create, record, and restore the gingival margin. Restorative dentistry (and particularly esthetics) can be influenced dramatically by the type of retraction procedure used. Improper methods can permanently damage the epithelial attachment, causing gingival recession, either before or after the final restoration is inserted. No attempt at gingival retraction should ever be attempted on inflamed or swollen tissue. Periodontal problems must be treated prior to impression, in order to obtain predictable esthetic results.

Although various methods of gingival retraction are currently in use today, any method, to be considered adequate, must fulfill certain criteria:

1. The method must provide access of the impression material beyond the cervical margins of the prepared teeth (Figure 41.1).
2. Retraction must provide enough space around the cervical margin for an adequate bulk of impression material.
3. The method must eliminate seepage or hemorrhage during the setting of the impression material.
4. The retraction method should be as nontoxic as possible to the patient and to gingival tissues.

Two-appointment procedures

This method is usually used when the periodontal tissue is not in a healthy condition, usually due to improperly fitting restorations. First, the teeth are prepared and a well-fitting temporary restoration is made. There are several advantages to this method. By the second appointment the tissue should be in excellent condition and therefore permit removal of the temporary restoration and use of light retraction cord procedures. Sometimes virtually no retraction is necessary to obtain clearly defined margins, if the temporary restoration fits well. Hemorrhage is practically eliminated by this method; however, the main advantage is being able to see and predict the gingival crest height. If shrinkage has occurred and there is not enough gingiva covering the margin, the preparation can be altered slightly before the final impression is made.

Retraction cords

By far the most popular form of tissue displacement before making impressions is retraction by cotton cord. There are several types of cord, with different weaves, thicknesses, and whether or not the cord is impregnated with hemostatic chemicals. Figure 41.2 shows various types of commercial retraction cords. Hemodent (Premier Dental Products Co.) contains no epinephrine and is available in solution or cord. Several manufacturers (e.g., Ultradent and Dux Dental) make cord saturated with epinephrine-type compounds. These cords are very popular and produce good results, but many patients react unfavorably to the epinephrine. In Timberlake's double-blind study of tissue retraction in 100 patients,[1] he observed that the absorption of epinephrine hydrochloride and its effect on the heart produced elevations in pulse rate and blood pressure (as much as 16 mmHg); therefore, the use of epinephrine is contraindicated in patients with coronary disease, hyperthyroidism, diabetes, or exposed capillary beds.

Placement of retraction cords

A cord is selected that is thin enough to fit into the gingival sulcus between the gingival attachment and below the margin of the prepared tooth. It is carefully placed using gingival retraction

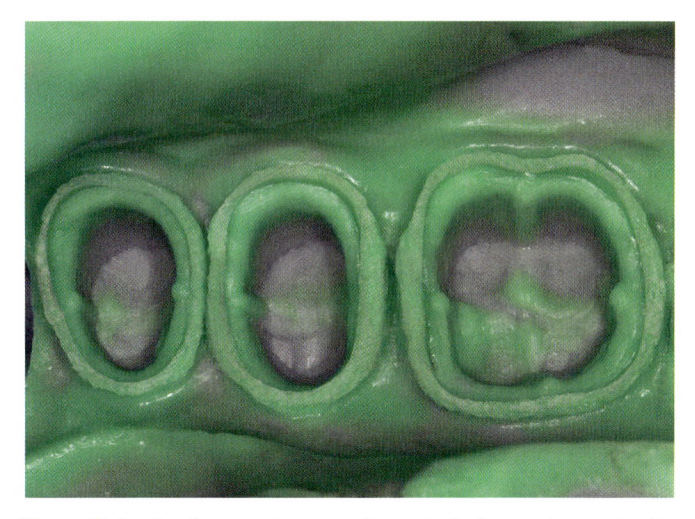

Figure 41.1 The first requirement of any gingival retraction method is to clearly see and capture the cervical margins of the prepared teeth. Extending the impression material beyond the margins makes for more accurate trimming of the die by the technician.

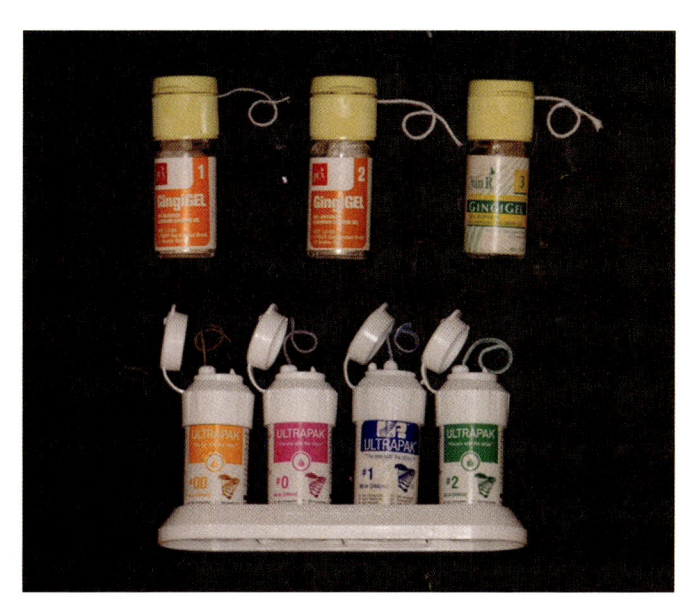

Figure 41.2 Retraction cords in various sizes from two major manufacturers (Ultrapak, Ultradent, and GingiGel, Dux Dental).

instruments. The cord is cut so that it may be completely located with no excess covering the gingival margin of the tooth. Be very careful of not compressing the tissue when you place the cord between the tooth and tissue.

There are basically two methods of retraction using cord. One technique involves placing cord and removing it to make the impression. The second technique consists of placing two cords and leaving the first one in while the impression is made. A variation of these methods involves leaving one or two cords in for a longer period of time (up to 10 min) and removing all cord before making the impression.

One-cord technique

Choose the largest cord to fit into the sulcus. Figure 41.3A is a cross-section of the correct placement of the retraction cord in the gingival sulcus. Saturate it in hemostatic agent (Hemodent, Astringedent), carefully fold into the gingival sulcus, and then leave for about 5–15 min. At times it may be necessary to insert a second cord to make sure the top of the sulcus does not "fold back" over the margin (Figure 41.3B). Remove both cords before making the impression. Figure 41.3C shows the tissue immediately after gingival retraction ready to receive the impression

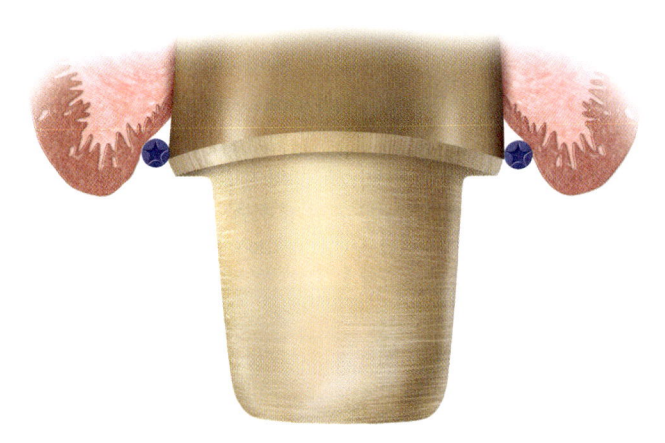

Figure 41.3 **(A)** The use of a single-cord technique in displacing the tissue before impression.

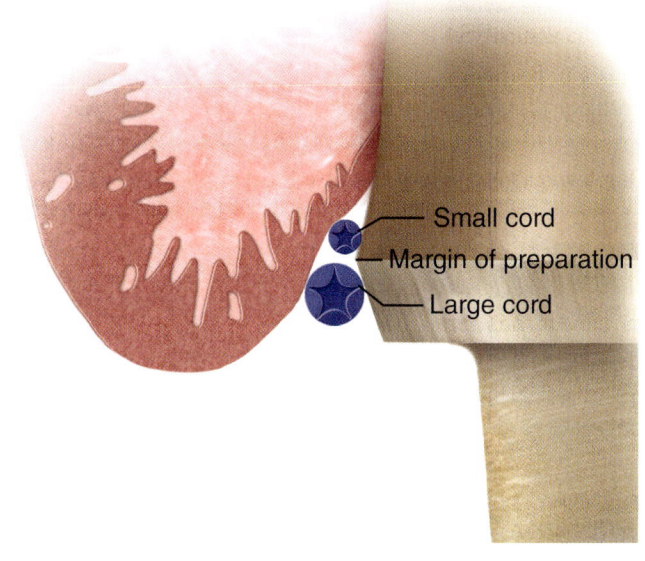

Figure 41.3 **(B)** The use of a second cord when a single cord is not sufficient to expose the prepared tooth beyond the margin. This image also serves to represent the two-cord technique.

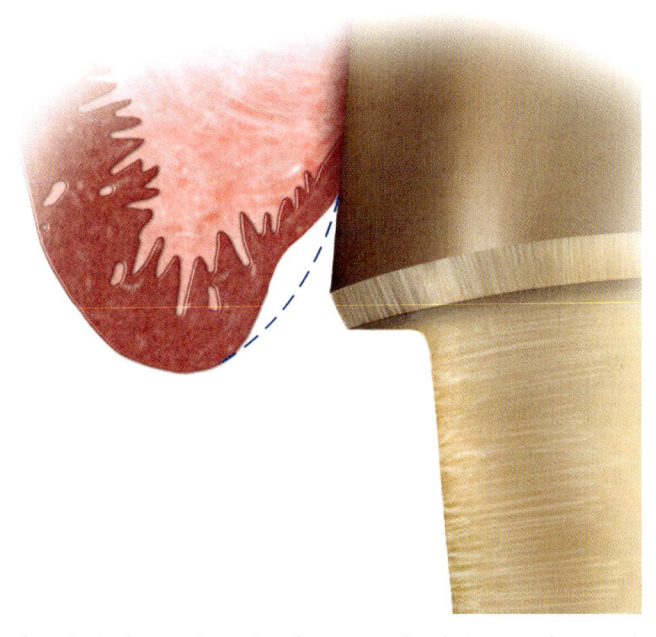

Figure 41.3 **(C)** The tissue immediately after gingival retraction using the one-cord technique ready to receive the impression material.

material. A proper-sized cord produces gingival retraction and little, if any, tissue damage.

Two-cord technique

Use a small diameter cord (size 00) followed by a size 0. The second cord, of larger diameter, is placed in the gingival sulcus, covering the prepared tooth margin and mechanically displacing the pericoronal tissues (Figure 41.3B). Pack and keep the cords in place for 5 min. Before making the impression, be sure to wet the 0 cord before removing it to prevent it from sticking to the tissue and causing bleeding. Then make your impression, finish and cement your provisional restoration before removing the 00 cord. (Figure 41.3C). Control hemostasis with astringents such as ferric sulfate and aluminum chloride. Pack a dry cord and then apply the astringent. Note that ferric sulfate will interfere with the setting of addition silicone impression materials, so rinse the area thoroughly before making the impression.

Tips on double-cord technique

1. Depending on the type of margin, make sure you have an adequate area beyond your margin so the laboratory technician will not have any problem trimming the dyes.
2. If using a shoulder margin it is easier to place your retraction instrument on the shoulder and then slide the cord into the sulcus rather than just pushing the cord in the sulcus. This method can help avoid pinching the tissue.
3. Let the type of tissue guide you as to how long to leave the gingival retraction cord in place. This can vary from 4 to 10 min, especially if the tissue is seeping.

Problems with retraction cords

Problems or damage from gingival retraction can come from several causes:

1. If there is too much pressure on the cord as it is placed in the sulcus, it is forced deeper than necessary and too far past the marginal area. This can be remedied by using a small-gauge cord that can fit more easily into the depth of the sulcus, followed with a larger size cord if necessary.
2. Using an instrument that is too large for inserting the cord can be injurious. Many anterior teeth are so small that if a large-size gingival retraction instrument is used, the tissue may be damaged. This is especially true for mandibular incisors (Figure 41.4).
   If too much pressure is used to place the cord, there is danger of severing the gingival attachment fibers. This causes eventual shrinkage of the gingival attachment, exposing the previously prepared margin. If the patient is seen for insertion of the restoration a short time later, the tissue may not have had time to shrink to its permanent position. Therefore, the restoration may be covered when it is placed but may become exposed sometime later.
3. A retraction cord or other material, or a chemical like zinc chloride that is too caustic to the tissue, if left on the tissue too long can cause permanent damage.
4. Leaving the retraction cord in the sulcus too long can create ischemia in the area.

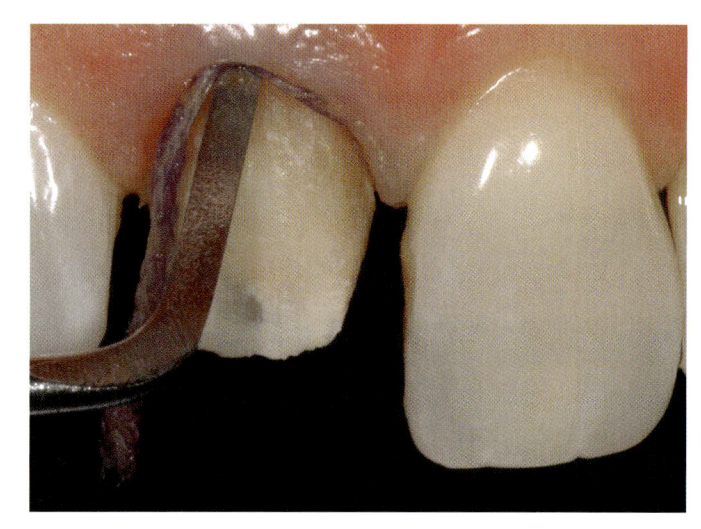

Figure 41.4 It is important to use a proper size cord and instrument when placing the cord to avoid unnecessary pressure and injury to the tissue. An interproximal carver is thin, flexible and works very well.

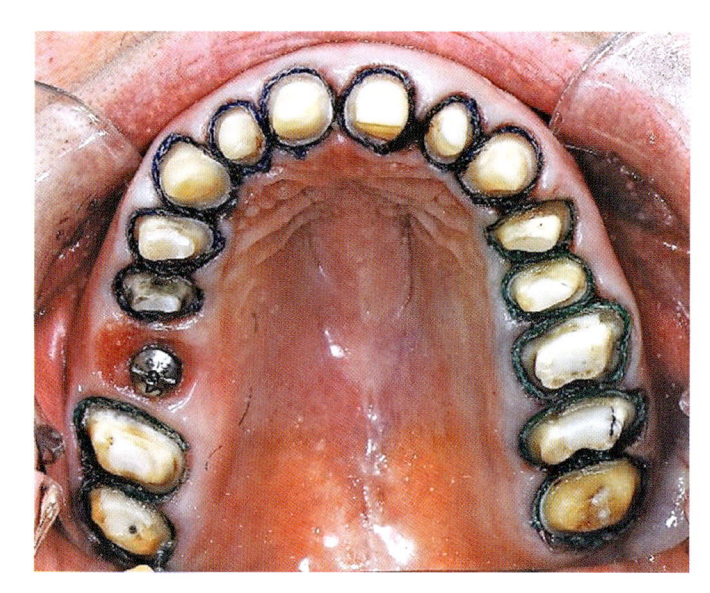

Figure 41.5 This is a good example of a proper retraction for a full maxillary arch impression showing no bleeding and adequate tissue displacement.

Remember that before a good elastic impression can be made, there must be no bleeding, and adequate marginal exposure is absolutely necessary (Figure 41.5).

Electrosurgery

This procedure can be especially useful when there is an overgrowth of tissue and just packing cord would not alleviate the problem and when simple retraction methods by the cord are insufficient. It is also helpful in situations where the tissue level is inconsistent with esthetics. A slight gingivectomy even at the tooth preparation stage will displace tissue and may also enhance your esthetic result. When using this method of retraction for anterior full crowns, extreme care must be taken to avoid loss of

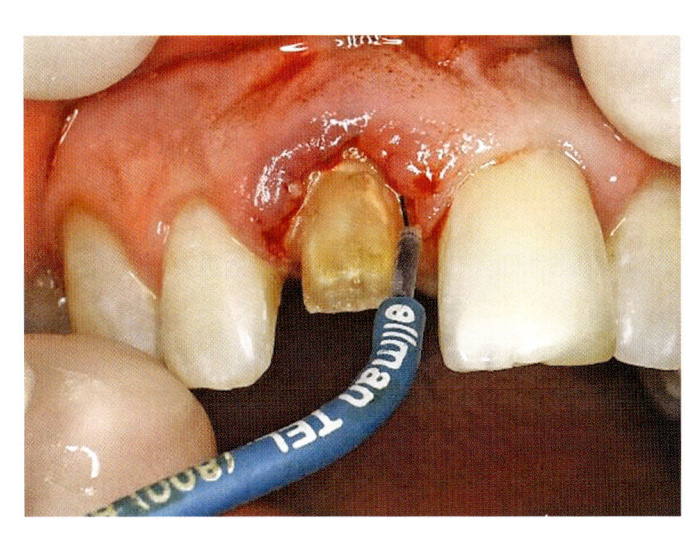

Figure 41.6 (A) Electrosurgery was chosen to remove excess and inflamed tissue to allow healing before the final impression is made.

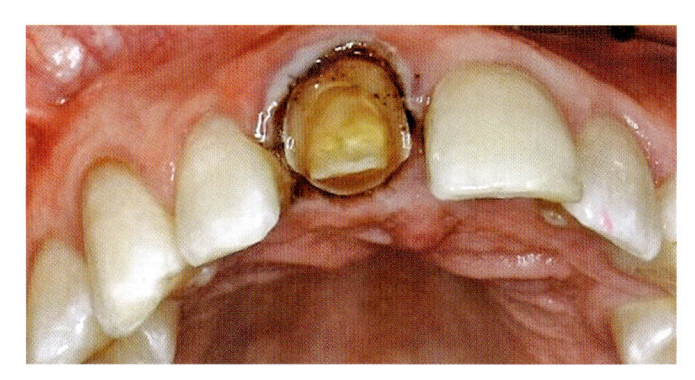

Figure 41.6 (B) Note tissue color and healing 24 h following the electrosurgery.

gingival crest height, which might prevent an esthetic result. The angle of the filament must be held with very special care when removing the inner surface of the gingival sulcus. Avoid removing more than 1 mm apical to the gingival margin. Figure 41.6A and B shows the type of gingival crevice that should be created by this method. After cutting is completed, the sulcus is cleansed with 3% hydrogen peroxide, either in a spray bottle or with cotton pellets. Although this should adequately control hemorrhage, retraction with cord can still be used in combination with electrosurgery. However, studies show that electrical retraction procedures can cause an appreciable loss of gingival crest height. For this reason, electrosurgery may not afford the best means of gingival retraction when examined in terms of gingival repair. However, if your patient's tissue is thick and fibrous rather than thin and transparent, then either electrosurgery or laser should be suitable to use. The downside to electrosurgery is the possible permanent shrinkage of gingival tissue. At all times, the most important consideration is to respect and preserve the biologic width.

The *bipolar technique* unit (Bident, Pearson Dental) is distinguished by not needing to have an external ground to place behind the patient. It cuts by molecular resonance, not by an advancing explosive spark that can produce both excessive heat and possible charring. There are two prongs that extend from the handle, but only one cuts, whereas the other acts as the ground. Being able to remove the excess tissue in a bloodless environment means you can make your impression immediately.

Diode lasers function by the absorption of light energy into the biologic tissue. All lasers perform by two functions: they either vaporize the target tissue or stimulate a tissue response. Tissue vaporization occurs as the temperature is raised to a vaporization point instantly and tissue components turn into a gas as the cells expand and explode. The tissue components that absorb the light energy are called chromophores. Water is considered a primary chromophore as the oral cavity is composed of 70% water. Other chromophores include hemoglobin and melanin, which play a minor role. Matching the wavelength of the laser with the chromophores in the target tissue is one of the primary considerations in selecting a laser.

An 810 nm diode laser is used specifically for soft tissues as its wavelength is best suited to be absorbed in the hemoglobin, melanin, and water that are present prevalently in the soft tissues. The diode laser has the ability to precisely cut, seal, and coagulate the lymphatic vessels, blood vessels, and nerve endings while vaporizing the target tissue. Any gingival tissue that is covering a tooth during preparation and impression can be easily removed and homeostasis achieved quickly with less trauma, giving improved and faster postoperative healing. Using a diode laser for gingival troughing of the subgingival preparations before impression is helpful, as it exposes the preparation margins and helps capture an accurate impression—free of bleeding.

Ideally, if cotton cord will adequately manage sufficient tissue displacement, then that is what we normally use. However, if there is diseased tissue or an abundance of tissue that needs to be displaced, then either the diode laser or electrosurgery can be utilized. The laser also coagulates as it cuts, for a clear and blood-free environment; it reduces postoperative sensitivity and inflammation by sealing nerve endings to stop the flow of histamine; it enables faster healing and less trauma to the tissue by cutting only micrometers deep; there is less chance of infection and more comfort for the patient, and better visibility for the clinician (NV Microlaser, DenMat) (Figure 41.7).

The laser is similar to electrosurgery, in that it cuts away the offending tissue. However, skilled clinicians can accurately remove just the amount necessary to make a good impression. Nevertheless, for a six-unit anterior tooth restoration, cotton cord may be more predictable with less chance of permanent gingival displacement.

Impression materials

Silicone impression materials

Addition silicone (polyvinyl siloxane, PVS) impression materials are most commonly used in the dental office, whereas the condensation silicones are primarily used in the dental laboratory for duplicating procedures.

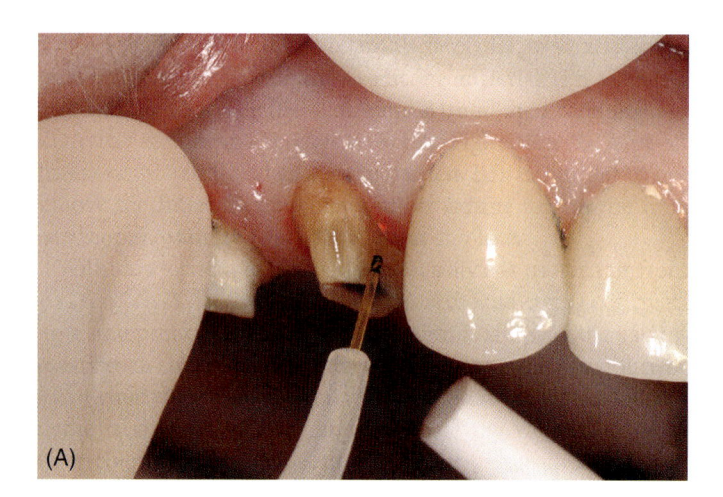

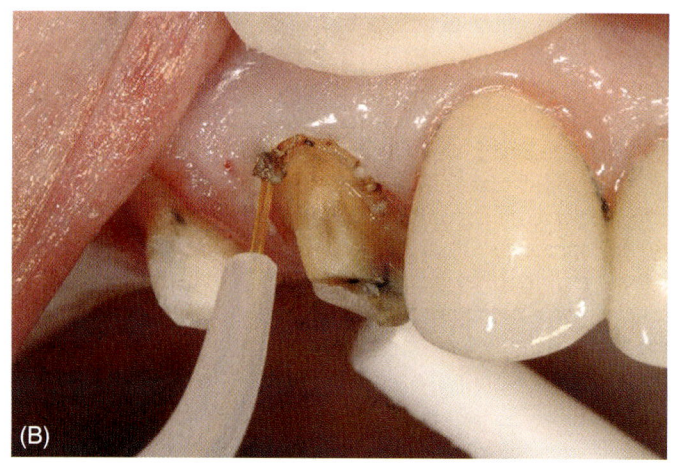

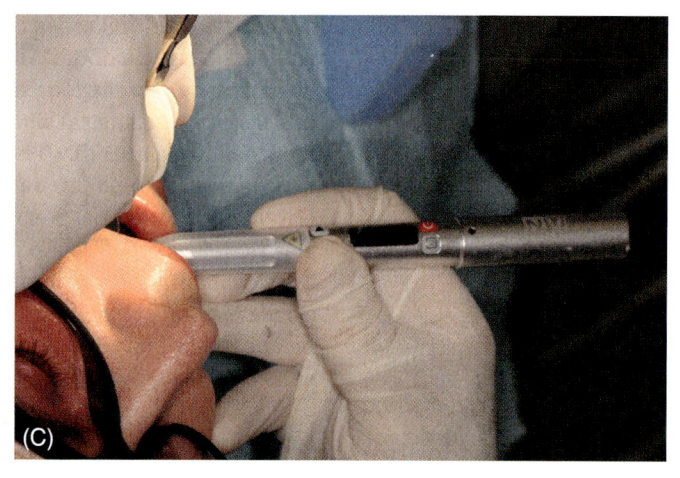

Figure 41.7 (A–C) When needed, the diode laser can be an effective instrument to create gingival troughing before final impression. The NV Microlaser (DenMat) is a lightweight, self-contained, programmable, and easy to use clinical laser.

Addition silicone

The material is supplied as two pastes or putties, one of which is the base and the other is the catalyst. Many consistencies are available, including light (syringe, wash), medium, heavy, monophase, and putty. In most instances the two pastes are mixed from a cartridge using an automix gun with static mixing tips or a dynamic mechanical mixer (Mixstar eMotion; 3M ESPE Pentamix 3) (Figure 41.8). Two-putty systems are usually mixed by hand kneading. The newest addition silicones contain nonionic surfactants that achieve increased wettability.

The addition reaction occurs between vinyl and hydrogen groups with no by-product being formed, so the addition silicones are dimensionally stable. If hydroxyl groups are present in the addition silicone, then a side reaction results in the formation of hydrogen gas. Some manufacturers add a hydrogen scavenger (platinum, palladium) to capture the gas for a short period of time so a die can be prepared.

Latex rubber gloves contain sulfur compounds that adversely affect the setting reaction of addition silicones. These compounds can be transferred to the prepared teeth and soft tissues during preparation of the tooth and placement of a gingival retraction cord. These compounds can also be incorporated into putties when mixed by hand. Use vinyl or nitrile gloves to avoid contamination. Rinse the preparation and soft tissues with 2% chlorhexidine to remove contaminants.

Condensation silicone

The material is supplied as a base and catalyst in the form of pastes or putty–liquid. Mixing of the paste–paste or putty–liquid systems is done by hand spatulation on a paper pad. A by-product is water or ethanol, the evaporation of which causes shrinkage. This shrinkage can be minimized by use of the putty–wash technique. The setting reaction is accelerated by moisture and heat.

Polyether impression materials

Polyether impression materials are supplied as light, medium, and heavy consistencies. Mixing is either done by hand, using auto-mix gun with a static mixing tip, or with a dynamic mechanical mixer. There is no volatile by-product. Increased temperature and humidity accelerate the setting time. Contamination with water can cause an expansion of the setting material and should be avoided.

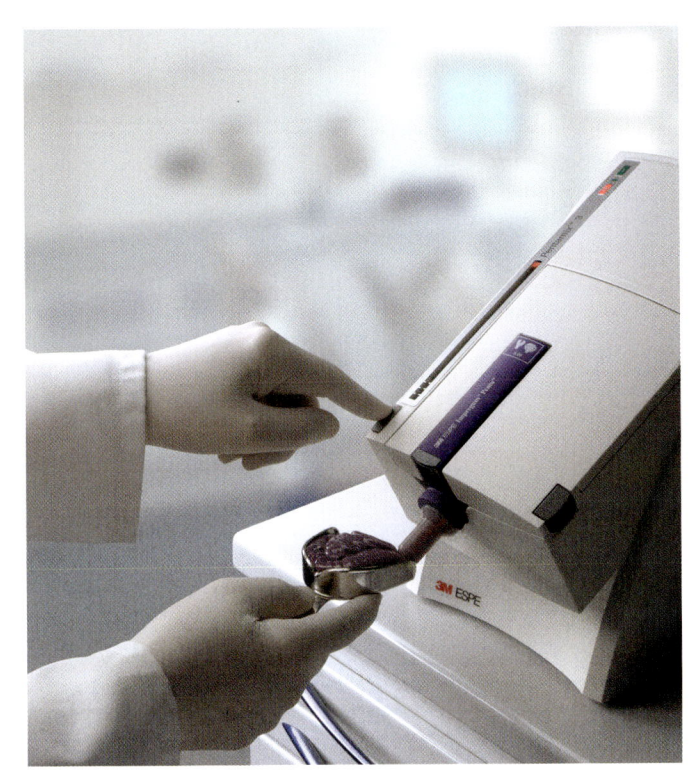

Figure 41.8 Motorized automatic mixing unit (AUTOMIX 3 M). *Source:* Reproduced with permission of 3 M™ Company—Oral Care Solutions Division.

Table 41.1 Comparison of Properties of Polyether and Addition Silicone Impression Materials

Property	Addition Silicone	Polyether
Working time	Very short–medium	Short
Setting time	Short–medium	Medium
Wettability of tissues	Good–fair	Good
Shrinkage on setting	Very low–medium	Very low–medium
Flexibility during removal	Low–very high	Medium–high
Elastic recovery	Very high	Very high
Tear energy	Low–high	Low–medium
Gas evolution after setting	Yes	No
Detail reproduction	Excellent	Excellent
Dimensional stability	Excellent–good	Good

Properties and clinical relevance

There are a number of physical and mechanical properties that affect the performance of impression materials. A comparison of these properties for addition silicones and polyethers is given in Table 41.1.

Working and setting times

Working time is a measure of the maximum time available before the impression should be seated in the mouth. Working times of addition silicones vary from 40 s to 5 m with a typical time of 2–2.5 min. Polyethers have working times of 2.5–3.3 min.

Setting time is a measure of how long the impression must remain in the mouth before removal can occur. Setting times of addition silicones vary from 1 to 5 min, with a typical time of 2–4 min. Polyethers have setting times of about 3.3 min. The accuracy of an impression may decrease if the impression is removed from the mouth too early. A slight improvement in accuracy may result from leaving the impression in the mouth for an additional 30 s.

Detail reproduction and wettability

An impression material must reproduce small details and transfer these details to the gypsum die or cast. Detail reproduction is influenced by the viscosity of the impression material and its ability to wet the tooth structure and soft tissues, especially in the presence of moisture. Wettability is best with a hydrophilic impression imaterial that forms a low contact angle (20–60°) with tooth structure. Poor wetting results in bubbles and voids, often requiring remaking of the impression. Addition silicones are formulated to be hydrophilic by the addition of surfactants or by modification of the polymer structure. Polyether impression materials are naturally hydrophilic.

Flexibility

Flexibility is a measure of the ease of removal of the impression from the mouth. An impression that is stiff may be locked into undercuts in the oral structure and be difficult to remove. Flexibility of addition silicones varies from low (<2%) to very high (11%). Flexibility of polyethers varies from medium (2.5%) to high (8.5%). The significance of knowing which material and its flexibility can be of the utmost importance. If you are making an impression of short abutments or crown preparations, the flexibility range is of little importance. However, if you are making impressions of larger prepared teeth and have undercuts then a more flexible material is quite important. Otherwise the impression material can latch into the undercut areas and be difficult or impossible to remove. In general, the polyvinyl siloxane materials will be the easiest to remove.

Elastic recovery

When an impression is removed from the mouth, it is subjected to tensile and compressive forces that could result in distortion. The set impression must be sufficiently elastic that it will return to its original dimensions with minimum distortion (<3%). Elastic recovery of addition silicones varies in the range 98.9–99.9%. Elastic recovery of polyethers varies in the range 98.2–99.7%.

Tear energy

Tear energy (tear strength) is important because the impression in the sulcus must resist tearing upon removal. Tear energy of addition silicones and polyethers varies in the range 0.4–2.2 kJ/m^2.

Dimensional stability

Dimensional change (shrinkage) occurs when an impression material sets and may increase during the time the impression is stored. At 24 h, the shrinkage of addition silicones varies in the range 0.08–0.42%. The shrinkage of polyethers varies in the range 0.07–0.27%. After 1 week, the shrinkage of addition silicones varies in the range 0.08–0.40%. The shrinkage of polyethers varies in the range 0.21–0.55%. Some addition silicone impressions are sufficiently stable that a second pour of gypsum can be made several weeks after the impression was made.

Manipulation of impression materials

There are a number of steps necessary to achieve a quality impression. Troubleshooting the impression after removal from the mouth can save time and money should the impression need to be remade. Our advice is to always make a backup impression in the event the laboratory injures the die. It may also be helpful to have an untouched backup model if there is a question about the fit of the final restoration.

Criteria for a good impression and troubleshooting tips are summarized in Table 41.2. Tips for the dental assistant and the clinician for improving impressions are listed in Table 41.3.

Selection of a tray

Trays are available in full-arch, quadrant, and double-arch varieties and are made of metal or plastic. Be sure to select a tray of proper dimensions and extension. A rigid tray is desirable to minimize distortion during the impression procedure. It is best to use a rigid tray even if the impression material itself is rigid. Double-arch trays are popular because they record both the preparation and the occlusion of the opposing arch. They are best used when recording the preparation of a single tooth. Occasionally, a custom-fitted tray will need to be premade in the event your stock trays do not adequately cover all the teeth. Even a very narrow arch may require a special arch-fitted tray. If your patient tends to gag easily, consider either using a lower tray on the upper arch, or cut out part of the palatal section on the upper tray. Finally, you may need to remove part of the linguogingival tray extensions of the lower tray if your patient cannot open their mouth very wide for easier removal when making the lower impression.

Tray adhesive

Both addition silicone and polyether impression materials require a tray adhesive for metal and plastic trays. The adhesives vary with the type of impression material and are not interchangeable. Although some trays have perforations and other retention modes, use of a tray adhesive can minimize distortion when the impression is removed from the mouth. Be sure to allow the tray adhesive to dry before adding the impression material.

Impression techniques

Three common impression techniques are a single-viscosity (monophase) technique, a dual-viscosity (light-bodied/heavy-bodied) technique, and putty–wash (one-step or two-step) technique (Figure 41.9). Use of a preimpression surface optimizer (B-4, Dentsply) can be a help to gain greater detail and avoid any bubbles.

Special impression techniques

Occasionally, there will be a need to make impressions of specific areas that conventional techniques cannot do. For instance, when necessary to repair pontic areas of an existing bridge capturing the soft tissue is essential (Figure 41.10A–J). Also, there may be times when, after final impressions are made, an additional tooth may require extraction (Figure 41.11A–I).

Table 41.2 Troubleshooting Impressions

Criteria for a Good Impression	Troubleshooting Tips
Impression is uniformly mixed	Make sure dispensing tips (base and catalyst) of cartridge are open.
Impression is supported by the tray	Make sure impression material is uniformly distributed in the tray.
Multiviscosity materials blend and adhere to each other	Make sure the low-viscosity material is recording the desired detail.
No major defects are visible	Make sure there are no voids or tears. When injecting the syringe material, leave the tip in the material to avoid trapping air.
Impression adheres to tray	Make sure the impression has not detached from the tray.
Occlusal relationship is registered	Make sure the double-arch impression recorded the opposing occlusion.
The tray is visible in the tooth	Make sure you do not press the tray preparation area so hard that you touch the tooth preparation or have "stops" in the tray.

Table 41.3 Tips for Improving Impressions

Tips for dental assistants
Apply the proper adhesive to the tray and allow it to dry completely.
Make sure the tips of auto-mix cartridge are open.
Minimize bubbles when loading the impression tray.
Pay attention to working times to achieve desired viscosity and detail.

Tips for clinicians
Select a tray of adequate size and extension. Ensure that the tray allows space for 2–4 mm of impression material. Provide occlusal stops if needed.
Be sure to rinse away the ferric sulfate solution, because it can interfere with the setting of addition silicone impression materials.
Seat the impression in a timely fashion. Minimize movement of the tray after seating to minimize distortion. Do not remove the tray too early to minimize distortion.
Remove the tray with a uniform motion to minimize distortion—do not rock or twist the tray.

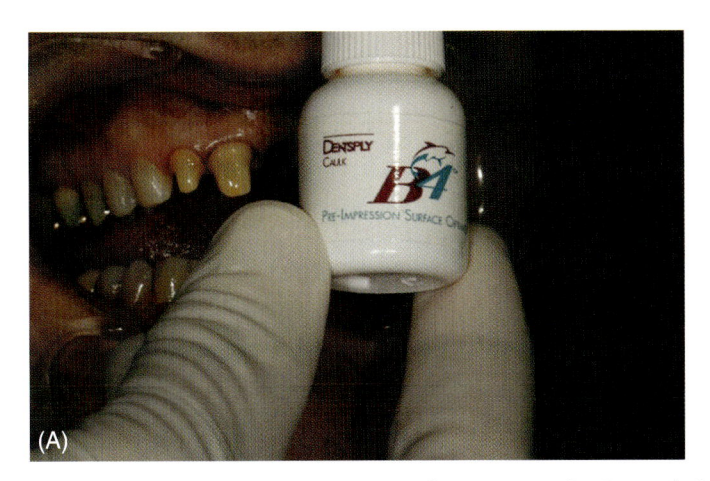

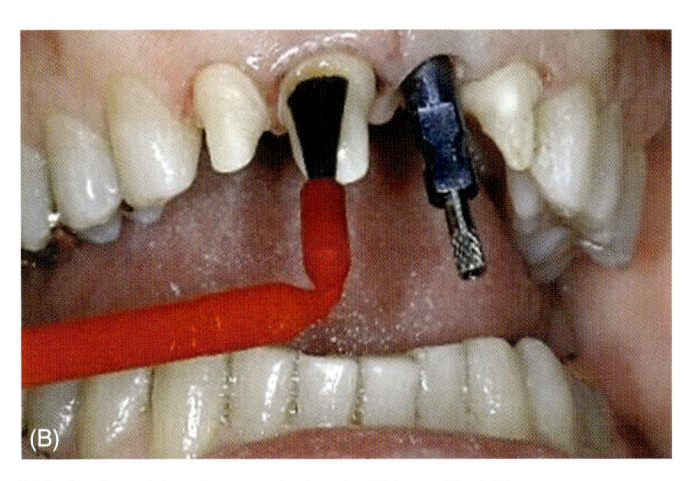

Figure 41.9 **(A and B)** A preimpression surface optimizer (B4, Dentsply Caulk) helps in gaining better sulcular detail free of bubbles.

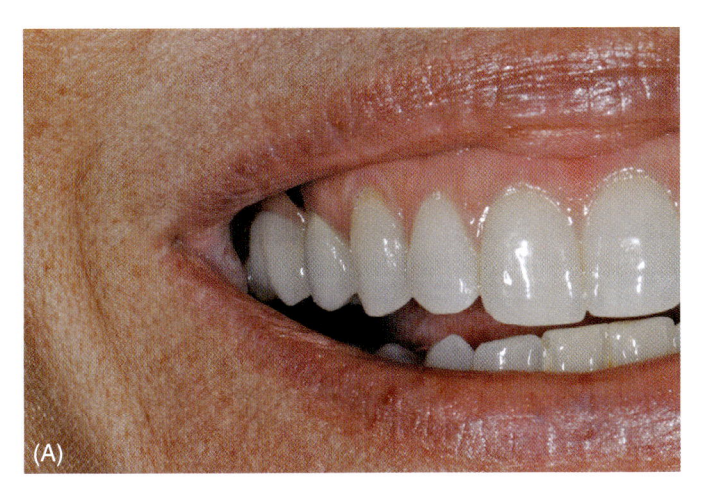

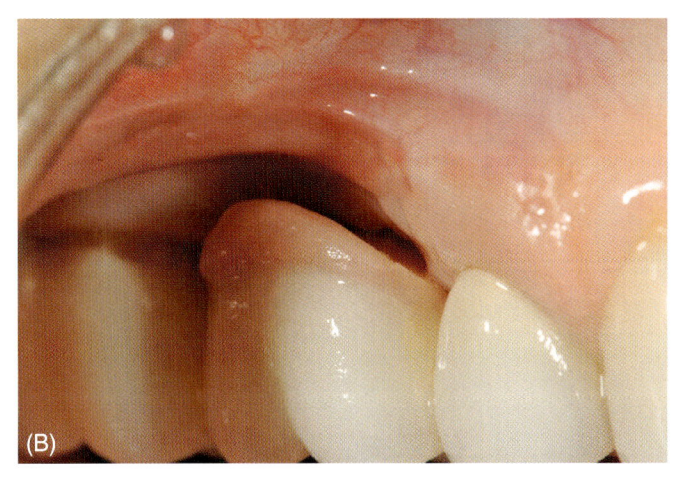

Figure 41.10 **(A, B)** Patient presented with tissue defect above a pontic of a three-unit fixed bridge which concerned the patient esthetically when she smiled.

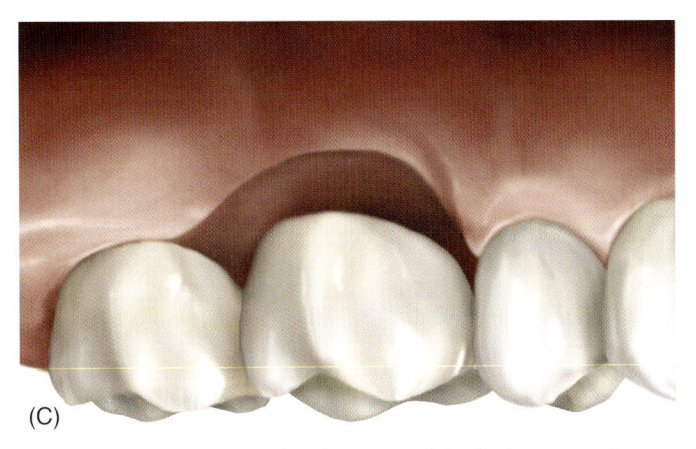

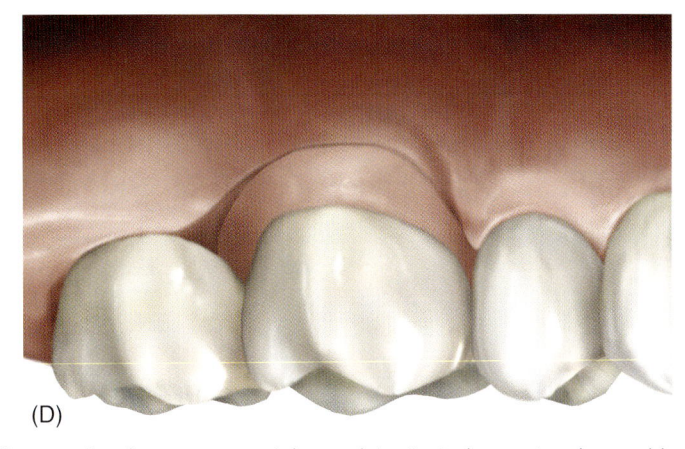

Figure 41.10 **(C, D)** To avoid replacement of the bridge, these diagrams illustrate the plan to create a pink porcelain gingival extension that could be bonded to the existing bridge.

Single-viscosity technique

A monophase impression can be made from either polyether or addition silicone impression materials but is most commonly made from medium-viscosity polyether materials. The shear thinning of these materials allows them to be injected into the preparation and placed into the tray with minimal slumping. This type of technique works best for capturing supragingival margins, since little or no pressure is needed to go subgingivally.

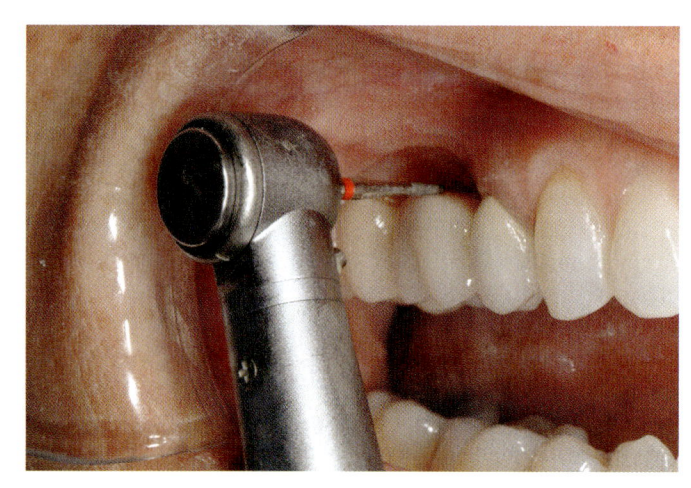

Figure 41.10 (E) The first step was to carefully remove the remaining gingival extension and create a platform where a new extension could be fabricated and bonded.

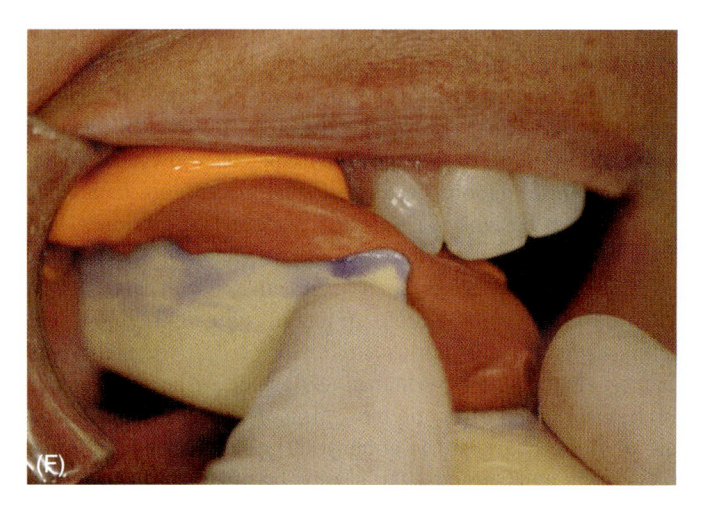

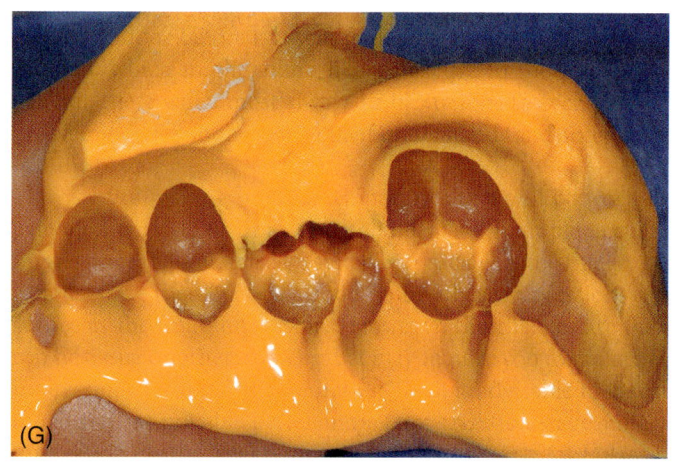

Figure 41.10 (F, G) A quadrant tray was partially sectioned so that a labial approach technique could be utilized, which allowed easy removal of the set impression material.

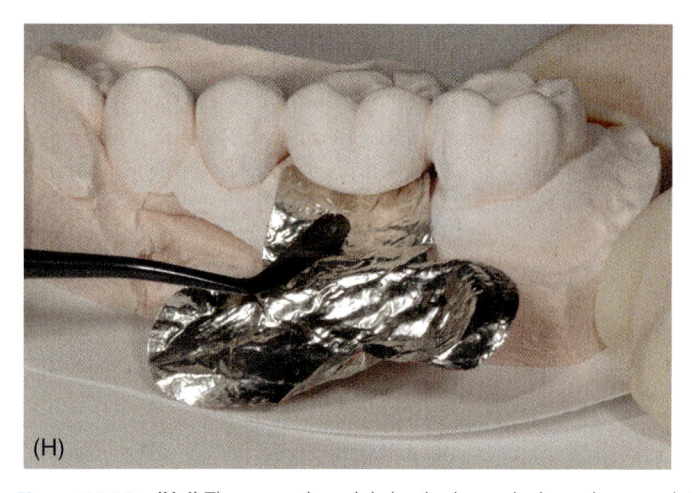

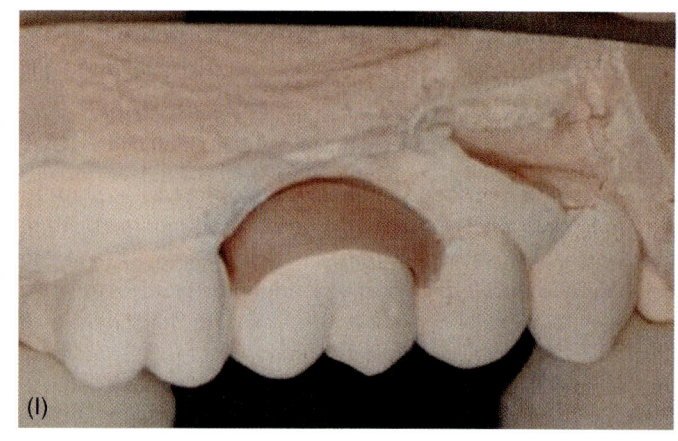

Figure 41.10 (H, I) The poured model clearly showed where the porcelain piece could be fabricated.

Chapter 41 Impressions

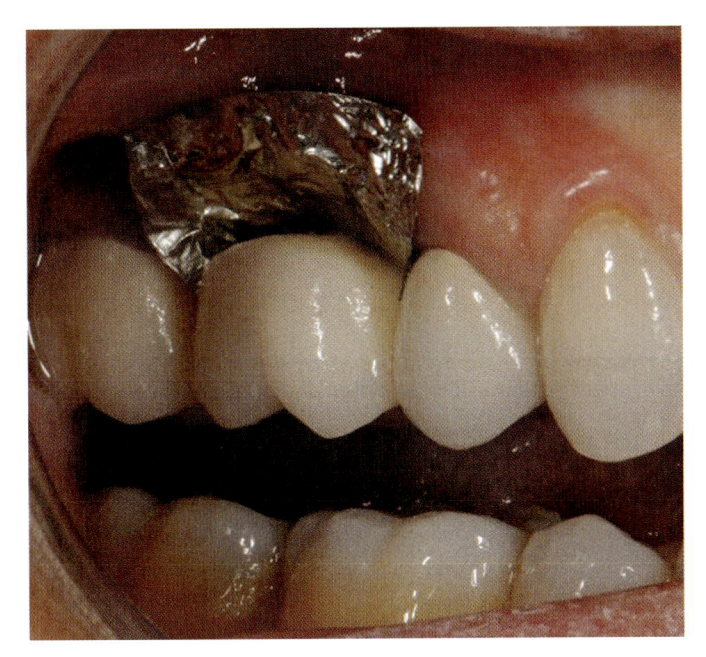

Figure 41.10 (J) A piece of dry foil was molded to the pontic area. This protected the tissue from the porcelain etch as well as kept a dry field as the porcelain extension was bonded to the bridge.

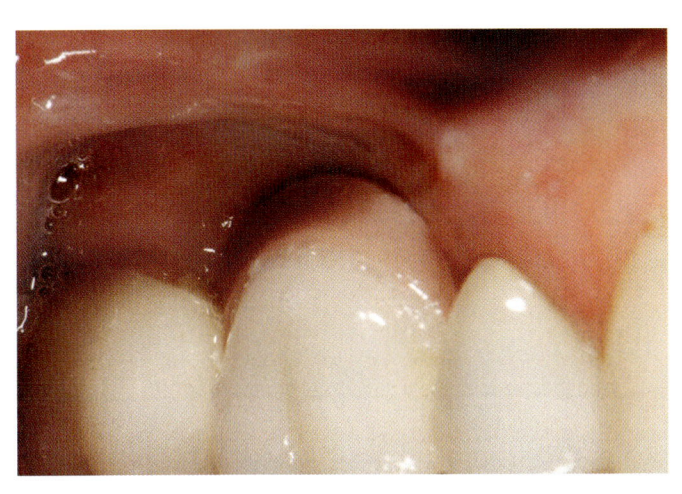

Figure 41.10 (K) The final result shows the pink extension bonded to place while allowing for the patient to be able to maintain the area using both dental floss and Hydro Floss oral irrigator.

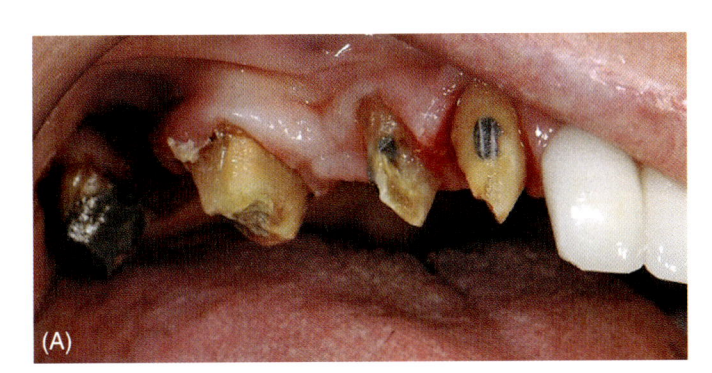

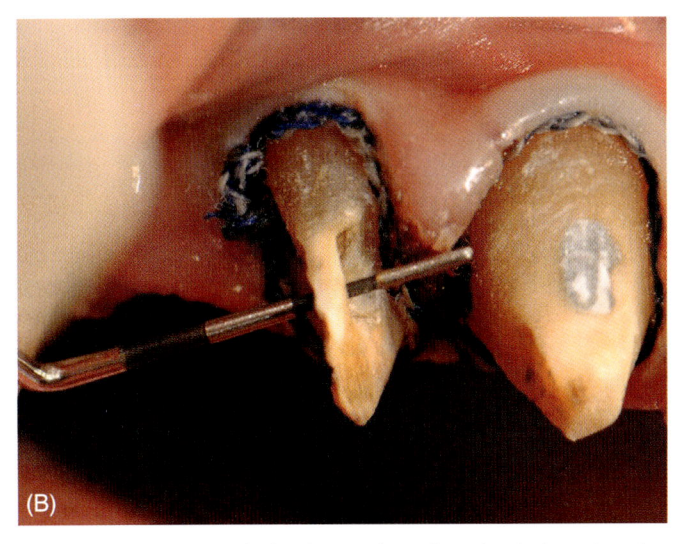

Figure 41.11 (A, B) During preparation stage for full mouth complex rehabilitation, the maxillary right first bicuspid was found to be hopeless due to extensive decay and an endo-perio lesion.

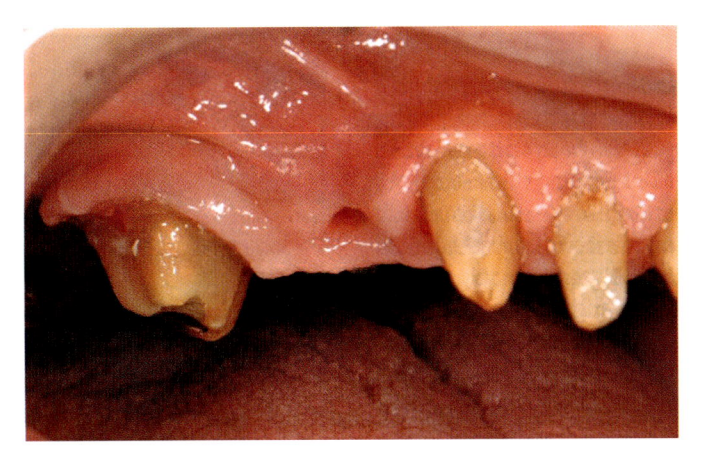

Figure 41.11 (C) The tooth was extracted the same day that final impressions on the maxillary arch were made.

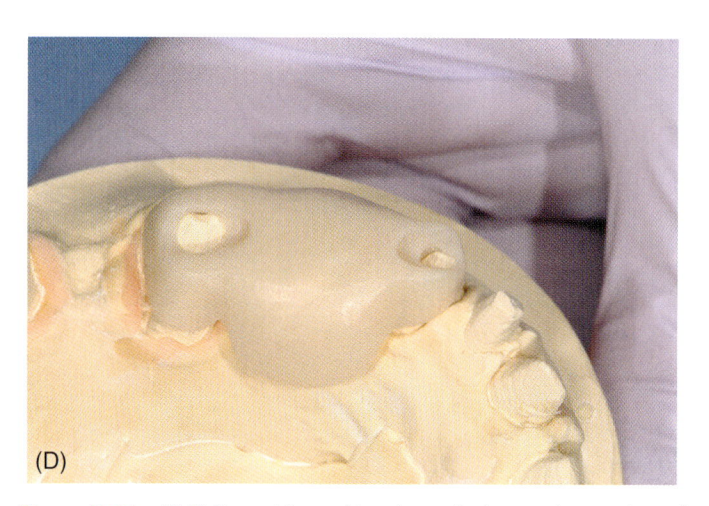

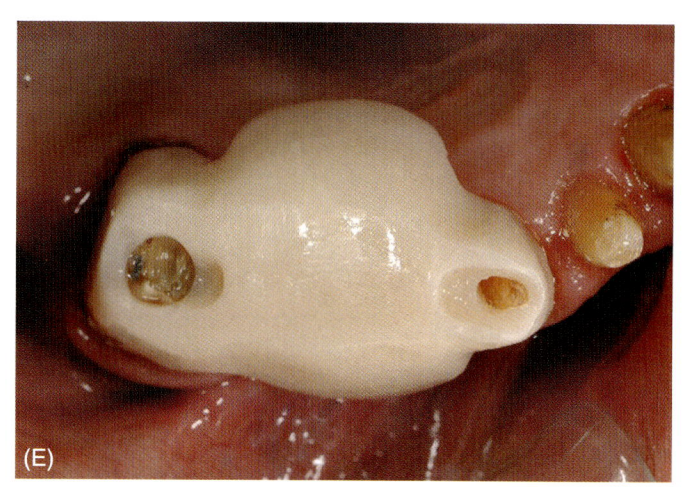

Figure 41.11 (D, E) To avoid remaking the entire impression at a later date, the laboratory fabricated a special form fitting tray to be able to capture the healed ridge.

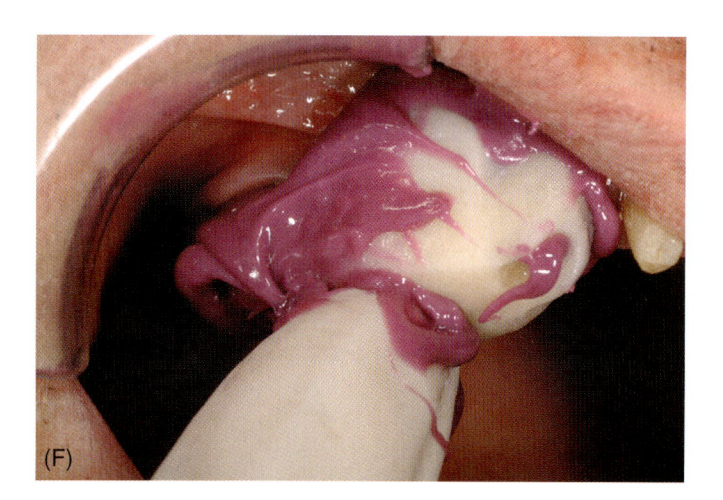

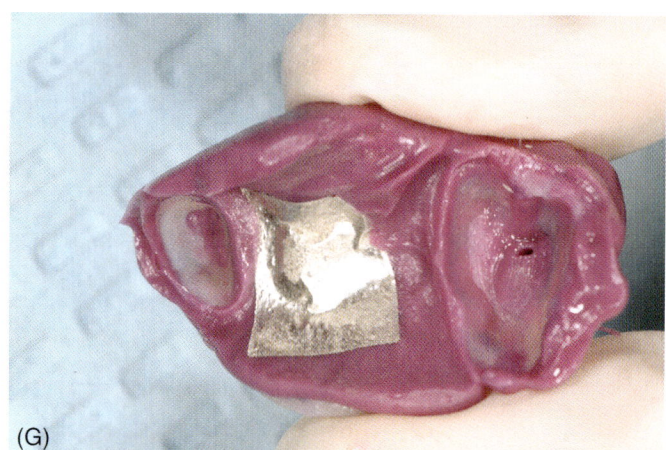

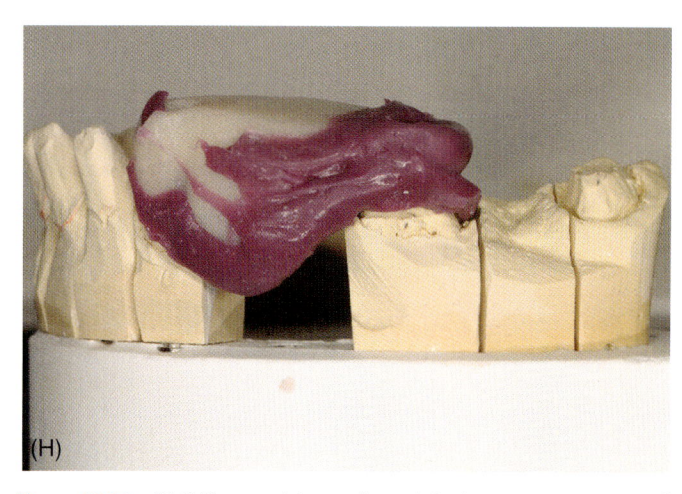

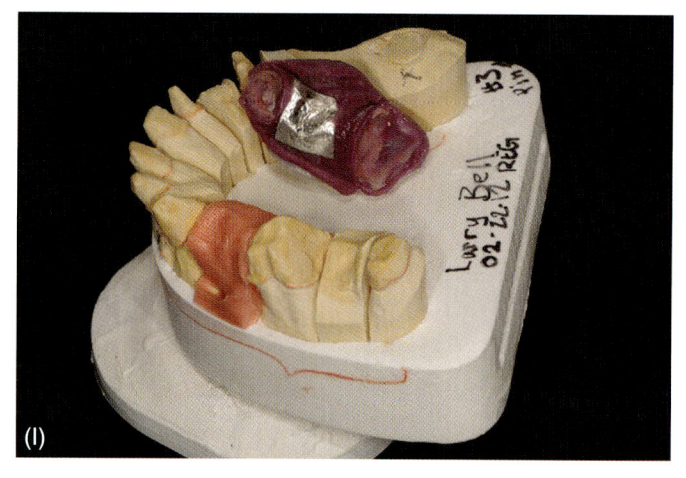

Figure 41.11 (F–I) The special tray allowed the impression tray to perfectly capture the healing ridge, which was transferred back to the model to pour and fabricate a new die for the healed pontic area.

Dual-viscosity technique

In this technique, a light-bodied material is injected with a syringe into the preparation. The clinician may want to gently blow the syringe material into the sulcus to verify coverage of all light body margins. At the same time, the heavy-bodied material is mixed, placed in the impression tray, and inserted in the mouth. Both impression materials bond and set together. Best accuracy is achieved with a custom tray. This technique works best when margins are at or just into the gingival sulcus, requiring little hydrostatic pressure.

Putty–wash technique

There are two basic versions using the putty–wash technique. In the first technique, the assistant mixes the putty material and depending on how many prepared teeth to capture the dentist begins to insert the syringe material (Figure 41.12A–F). The goal is to finish inserting the material at the same time as the tray is ready to go into the mouth. Failure to coordinate this time factor can cause inadequate blending of the putty/syringe material, resulting in possible voids or "folds" at the junction of the putty–syringe interface.

An alternative to this technique consists of air blowing the material into the sulcus. One advantage of this technique is to make certain no air bubbles are trapped around a margin. After the first layer is thinned via air blowing (Figure 41.12G and H), a second layer of syringe material is applied (Figure 41.12I and J), and then the tray with the putty material is pressed into place (Figure 41.12K and L). It is also a good idea to place a layer of syringe material along the body of the putty material approximately where the teeth will be. Because timing is so important, try to utilize an extra assistant, technician, or hygienist to help you to blow the material when doing a full arch. A main benefit of either of the putty/syringe techniques is that the hydrostatic pressure you can achieve by pressing the tray to place helps you capture an excellent margin by recording to the base of the sulcus (Figure 41.12 M). Therefore, if you are using an all-porcelain margin or full shoulder, you need to capture the root extension just below or above the margin so the technician has a clear understanding of exactly where your margin is (Figure 41.13).

The second technique requires two steps in which a preliminary impression is made with the high-viscosity material or putty before the cavity preparation is made. Provide space using a thin plastic sheet. After the tooth is prepared, inject the low-viscosity (wash) material into the preparation and then reinsert the preliminary impression. Vents in the preliminary impression will minimize distortion as it is reinserted.

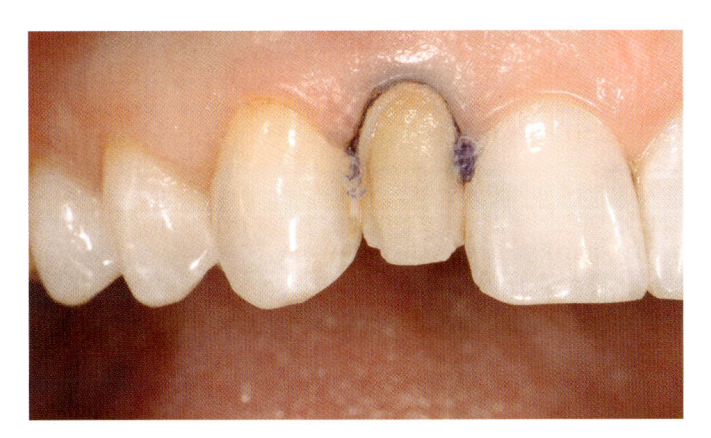

Figure 41.12 **(A)** A putty–wash technique will be used to impress this maxillary right incisor, which has been prepared for a porcelain veneer and tissue retracted with knitted cord (Ultradent).

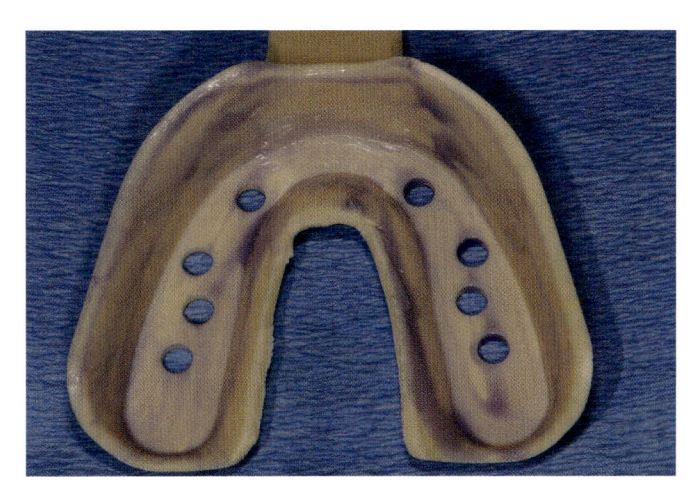

Figure 41.12 **(B)** A standard fitted maxillary plastic tray has been prepared by cutting off the palatal part, which allows you to easily remove excess syringe material.

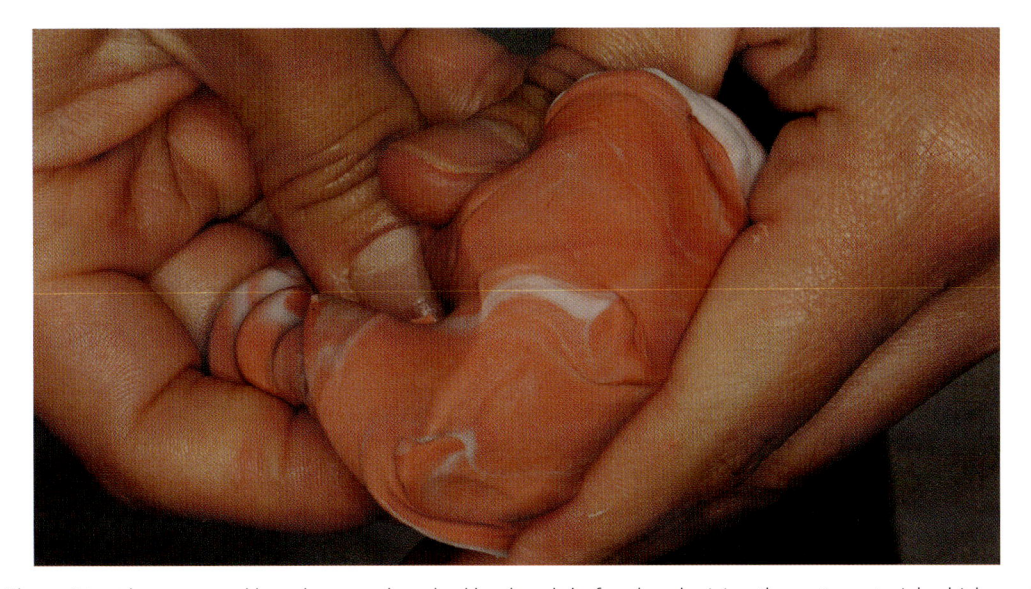

Figure 41.12 **(C)** The assistant has removed her gloves and washed her hands before hand mixing the putty material, which must be homogenously mixed with no streaks.

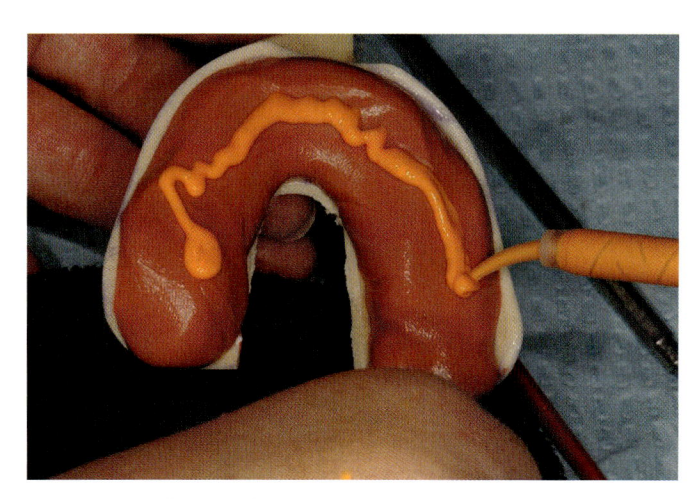

Figure 41.12 **(D)** Once the mixed putty is evenly loaded into the tray, the light body syringe material is applied to enhance binding of the light body to the putty material.

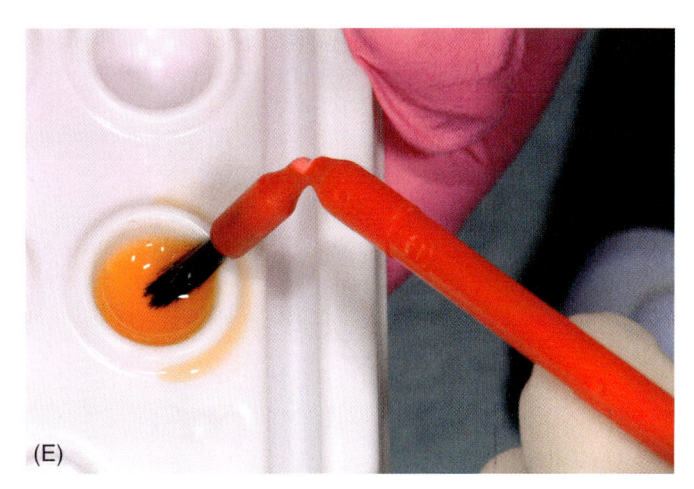

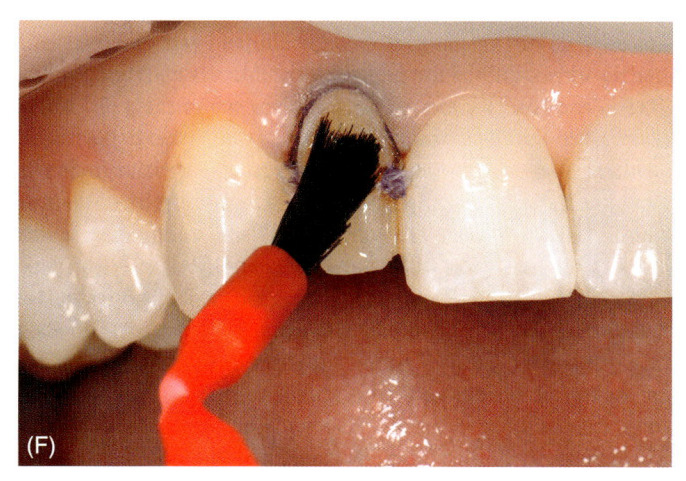

Figure 41.12 **(E, F)** As the assistant is mixing the putty material, the surface optimizer (B4, Dentsply Caulk) is applied to the prepared tooth as the cord is removed.

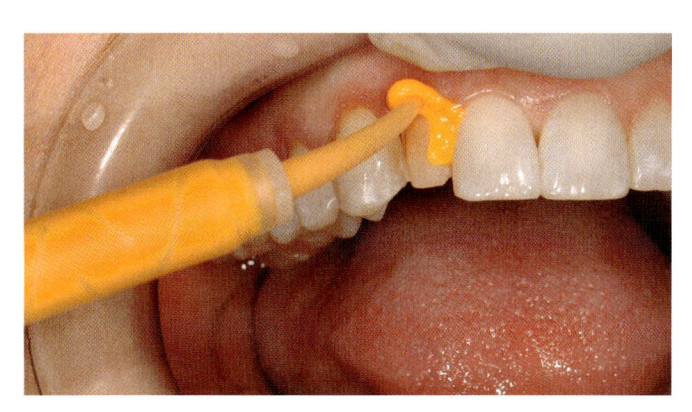

Figure 41.12 **(G)** A small amount of the light body material is first applied around the margins.

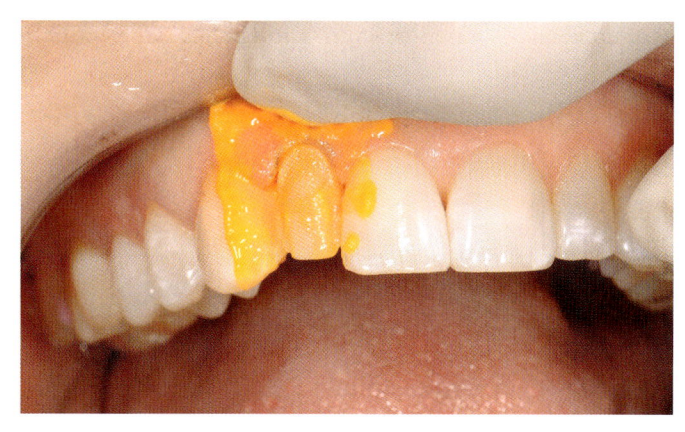

Figure 41.12 **(H)** Next, lightly apply air to make sure there are no bubbles and that there is even distribution into the sulcus.

Chapter 41 Impressions

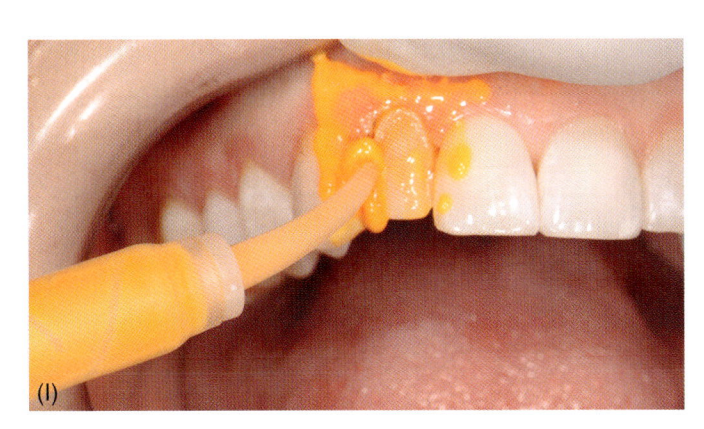

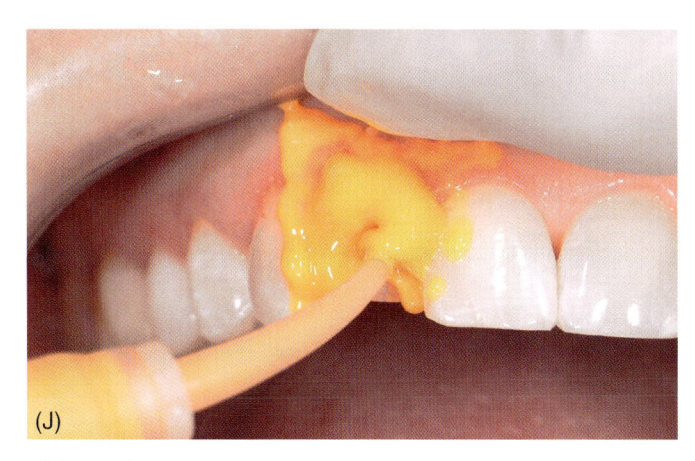

Figure 41.12 **(I, J)** A second application of the light body is applied all around the tooth.

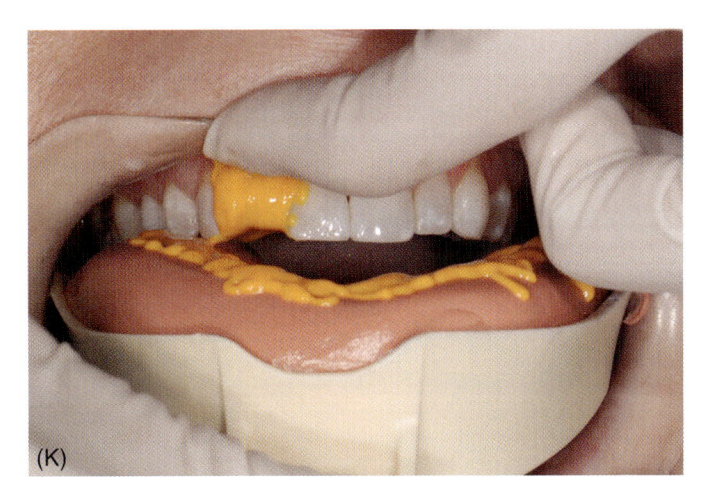

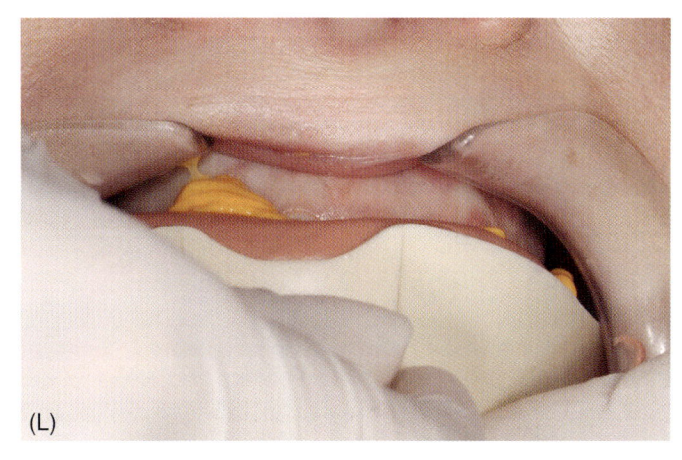

Figure 41.12 **(K, L)** The tray is carefully lined up with the maxillary arch and inserted using a slight vibrating motion with firm hydrostatic pressure. Be careful not to let the tray touch any part of the teeth as the tray is consistently held in place while the material sets. Once the material is set, the seal should be broken in the posterior area, and the tray should be removed in a firm and steady motion.

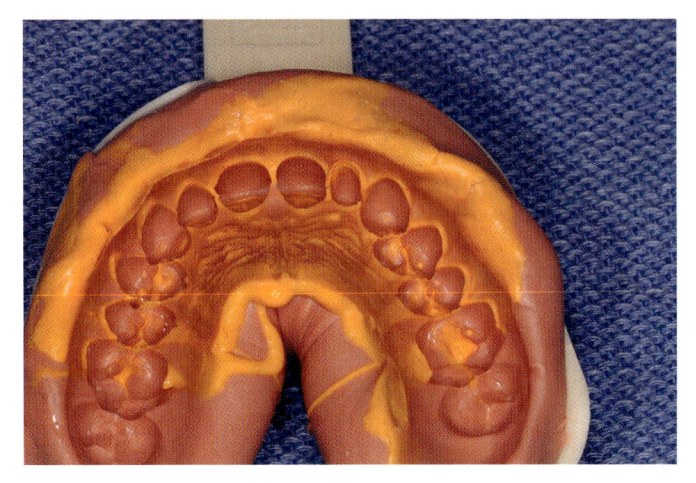

Figure 41.12 **(M)** The final impression shows the uniformity of the light body and putty material with no bubbles around the margin. Note the sulcular detail that was achieved.

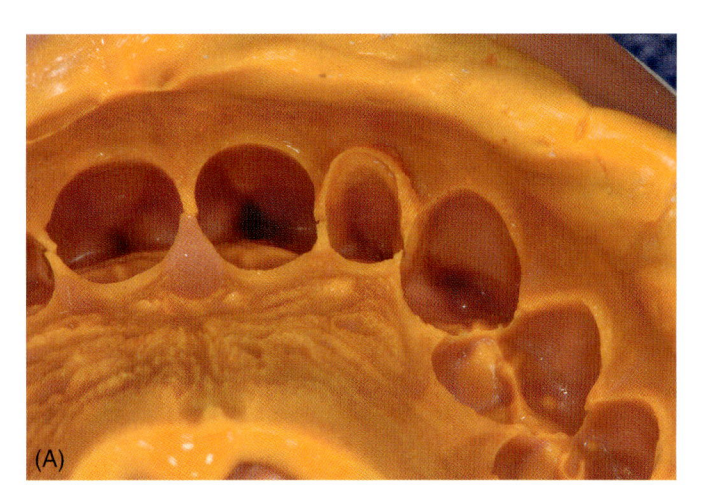

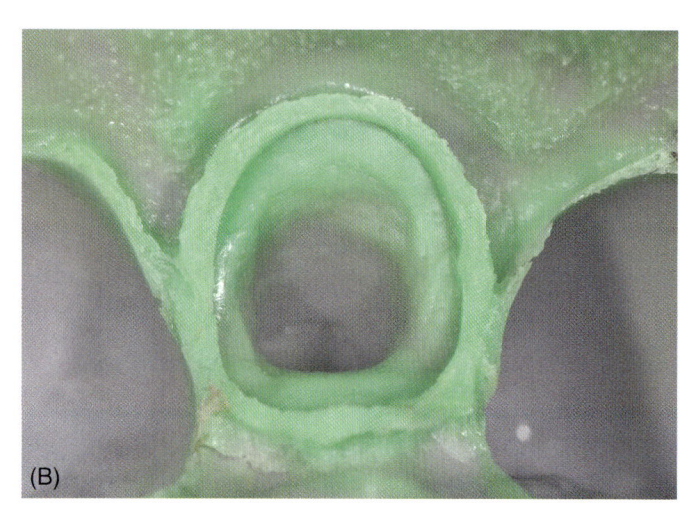

Figure 41.13 (A, B) This is a good example of capturing the root extension just above the margins so the technician has a clear understanding of where the margins are.

Removal and trimming of impressions

Although it is always preferable to make full-arch impressions, if there is an accurate impression but a slight discrepancy in an area it may be both feasible and important to make an extra quadrant impression which captures a perfect tooth impression of your abutment tooth or teeth. In this way the bite registration can be better made using the full-arch impression but the actual scanning or wax-up can be made of the quadrant impression for accurate margins.

Addition silicone and polyether impressions are accurate on removal as long as they have been allowed to set for the proper time in the mouth. Break the seal in the posterior area of the impression and then use a firm, steady motion to remove the impression. Trim unsupported areas of the impression before pouring the gypsum to minimize distortion.

Make multiple impressions

Once you have gone to all the time and trouble to make excellent preparations, retract the tissue, and make an impression, the last thing you or especially your patient wants is to have an accident in the laboratory causing you to have to repeat the last two procedures. Therefore, it is essential for you to have an accurate backup impression. This "extra" impression will allow you to pour an additional stone model whereby any questionable margins or possible inaccuracies can be double checked (Figure 41.14). In the event you are using one of the impressions to make your temporaries you will need three accurate impressions so that two can be reserved to construct the final restoration.

Disinfection of impressions

A variety of disinfectants is available, including neutral glutaraldehyde, acidified glutaraldehyde, neutral phenolated glutaraldehyde, phenol, iodophor, and chlorine dioxide. Addition silicone impressions can be disinfected by immersion following manufacturers' directions. Polyether impressions can change dimensions on immersion in some disinfectants, so only short times (2–3 min) in chlorine-type disinfectants are recommended for polyether impressions. Some clinicians prefer to disinfect polyether impressions by a spray and wipe technique.

Preparation of gypsum dies

Before pouring the gypsum die or cast, rinse the impression with water and then shake it to remove the excess water. Laboratory technicians will typically spray the impression with a surfactant to improve the wettability of the gypsum on the impression.

Other impression materials

Agar Hydrocolloid

Agar is an accurate impression material still used by a small number of dentists. It produces acceptable impressions if margins are exposed as a result of retraction or electrosurgery or if margins are supragingival. Agar has low tear strength and is susceptible to distortion with storage. Store the impression in 100% relative humidity and make the dies within the first hour.

Compound/copper band

The compound/copper band technique is useful when the preparation has a margin at the base of the sulcus. It may not be your preparation but an existing prepared tooth that you are faced with reproducing. Although an ideal solution may be crown lengthening, that may not be a viable esthetic or functional possibility. Therefore, the age-old technique of fitting an annealed copper band filled with soft compound may well be your best bet. Compound impressions are susceptible to distortion with storage, so prepare dies immediately.

Digital impressions

Digital impression systems allow the dentist to make a digital impression in place of a traditional elastomeric impression. Three of these systems (CEREC AC, PlanScan, CS 3500 Scanner) offer the option of in-office design and milling but also allow design and milling by dental technicians. Three other systems

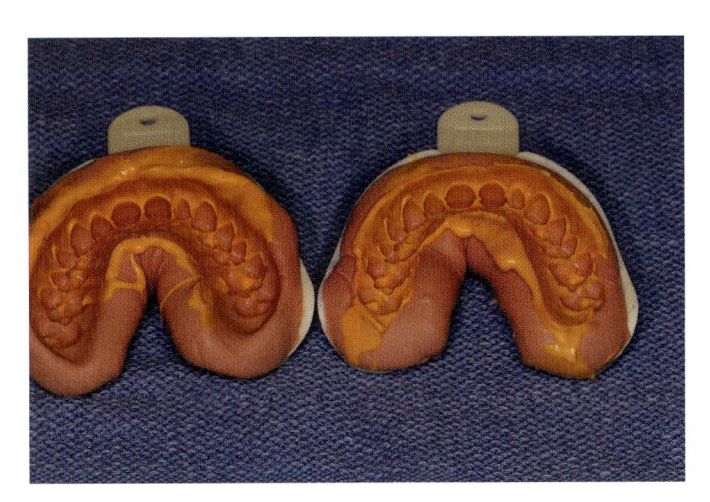

Figure 41.14 **(A)** Back-up impressions are important, especially in cases involving multiple teeth, to be able to double check any questions of accuracy of the die system.

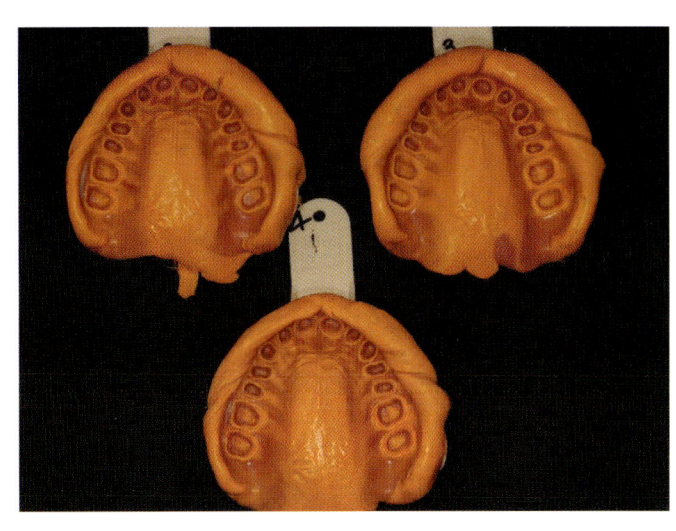

Figure 41.14 **(B)** Multiple back-up impressions are essential when a full-arch impression includes most or all the teeth in one arch.

(3 M True Definition Scanner, iTero Intra Oral Digital Scanner, TRIOS Color) produce digital impressions that require design and milling at a dental laboratory or milling center. All of these systems can produce models from their digital files.

Computer-aided design/computer-aided milling (CAD/CAM) can produce restorations directly from the digital impression data. Milling centers and dental laboratories offer these services. Restorations can be milled from a variety of materials, such as composites, feldspathic porcelain, leucite-reinforced ceramic, lithium disilicate ceramic, resin–ceramic, and zirconia. Wax patterns and acrylic provisional restorations can also be milled. The dental laboratory can use digitally produced models to produce restorations by traditional methods. See Chapter 46 on CAD/CAM.

Tips on digital impressions

Digital impressions require clear visualization of the margins. Tissue must be managed properly by exposing the margins to capture clear, accurate images. Deep subgingival margins can be recorded more easily with an elastomeric impression. If desired, the impression or the model can then be scanned. Digital impressions can be time consuming in large cases involving multiple teeth.

Mounting casts

In order to proceed with the fabrication of the crowns, the dental laboratory technician will require accurately mounted casts. Depending on the practitioner's preference and the case complexity, a facebow transfer may be performed to mount the upper cast. Figure 41.15A–E demonstrates the steps of this procedure.

Once the upper cast is mounted, the lower cast will be related to it with an interocclusal record. The following section reviews several techniques and considerations.

Interocclusal records (bite registrations)

Occlusal registration

Perhaps as essential as obtaining an excellent impression is obtaining an accurate interocclusal record. According to Dawson, "the price for inaccurate bite records is wasted time,

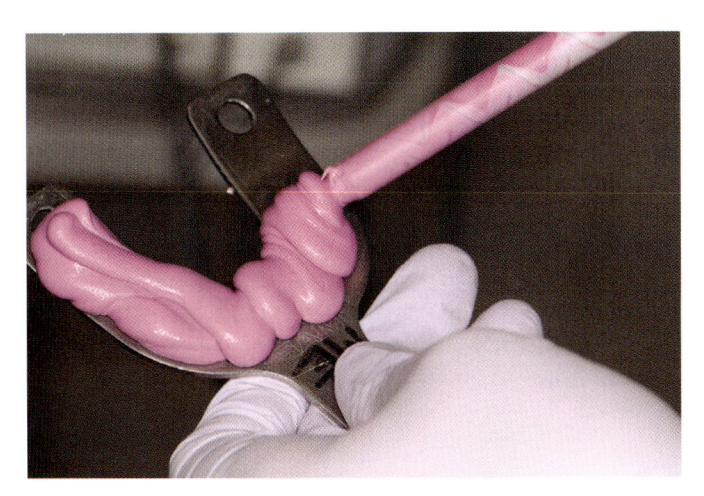

Figure 41.15 **(A)** A rigid polyvinylsiloxane bite registration paste is applied to the bite fork.

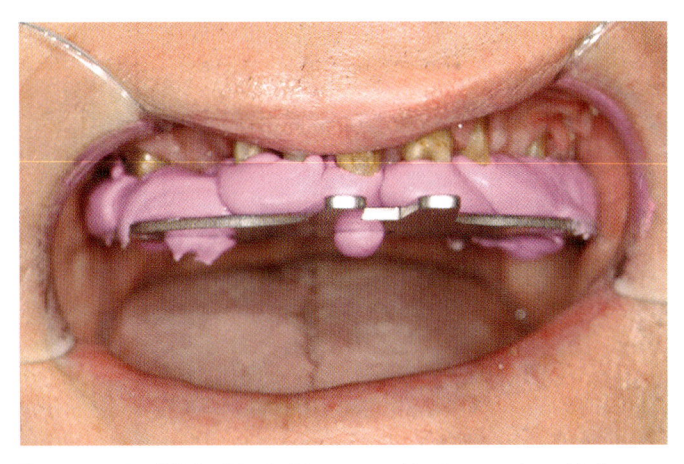

Figure 41.15 **(B)** The bite fork is centered in the mouth and fully seated over the preparations until the material is fully set.

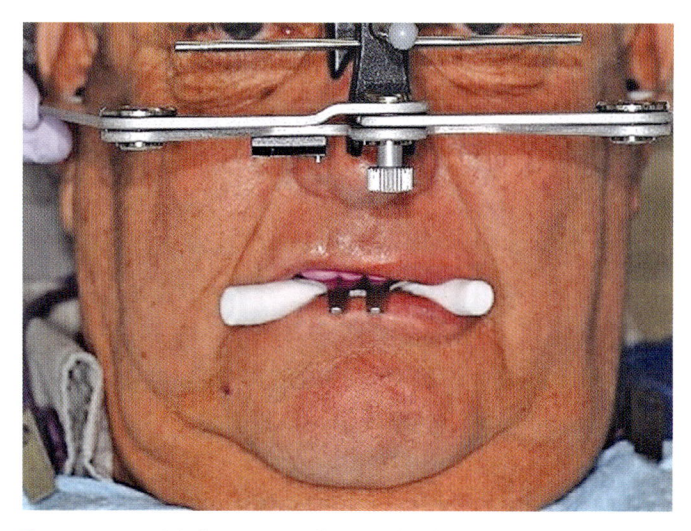

Figure 41.15 **(C)** The interpupillary line leveling rod is set parallel to the patient's eyes and the nasion and facebow adjustment screws are tightened.

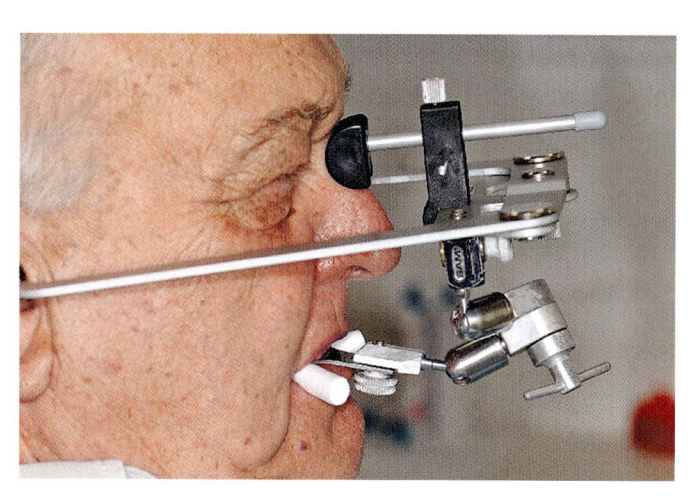

Figure 41.15 **(D)** The toggle is stabilized with one hand while tightening the toggle with the other hand. Make sure the toggle is fully tightened before removing.

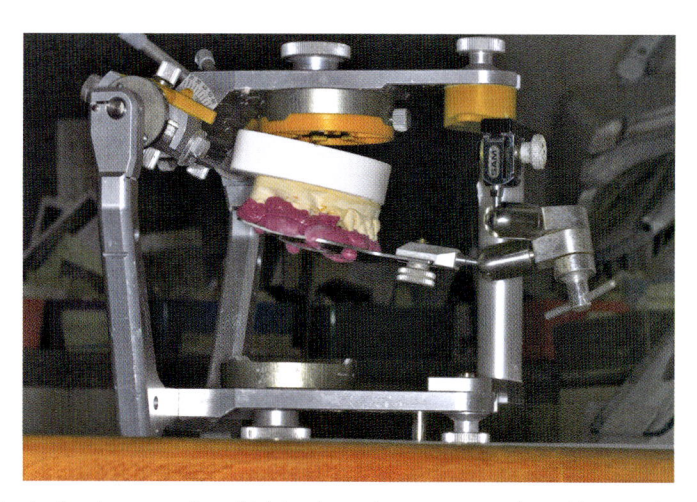

Figure 41.15 **(E)** The cast is seated in the facebow transfer, which is adapted to your semiadjustable articulator of choice (pictured: SAM 3).

compromised results, and a lack of predictability."[2] He continues by specifying five criteria for accuracy when creating these records as follows:

1. The bite record must not cause any movement of teeth or displacement of soft tissue.
2. It must be possible to verify the accuracy of the interocclusal record in the mouth.
3. The bite record must fit the casts as accurately as it fits the mouth.
4. It must be possible to verify the accuracy of the bite record on the casts.
5. The bite record must not distort during storage or transportation to the laboratory.

Many of these errors were common when practitioners were routinely using waxes for their records. At present, most practitioners use a rigid polyvinyl siloxane material that is specifically made for interocclusal records (Regisil, Dentsply; Blu-Mousse, Parkell). These materials are so accurate that it is imperative that the detailed anatomy is trimmed so that it can be accurately transferred between the casts and the mouth.

There are many techniques that may be employed with these materials. Goldstein describes a predictable technique if the vertical dimension is not being altered.[3] After preparation and before placing the registration material, determine where occlusal stops exist on opposite sides of the arch. Verify this with thin, 0.0005″ (0.0127 mm), occlusal registration strips (Artus Corporation, Englewood, NJ). The assistant should stand behind the patient and place the occlusal registration strip in the verified place and have the patient close into occlusion. The dentist then syringes the bite registration material around the preparation without the patient moving. If the strip loosens, the patient has moved or opened slightly and the bite registration will not be accurate (Figure 41.16A–C).

The safest sequence of therapy to maintain and record the patient's existing occlusal relationship is to use existing landmarks, either by measurement or by quadrant tooth preparation. For instance, if the entire arch is to be restored for full crowns, the teeth in one of the posterior quadrants should be prepared

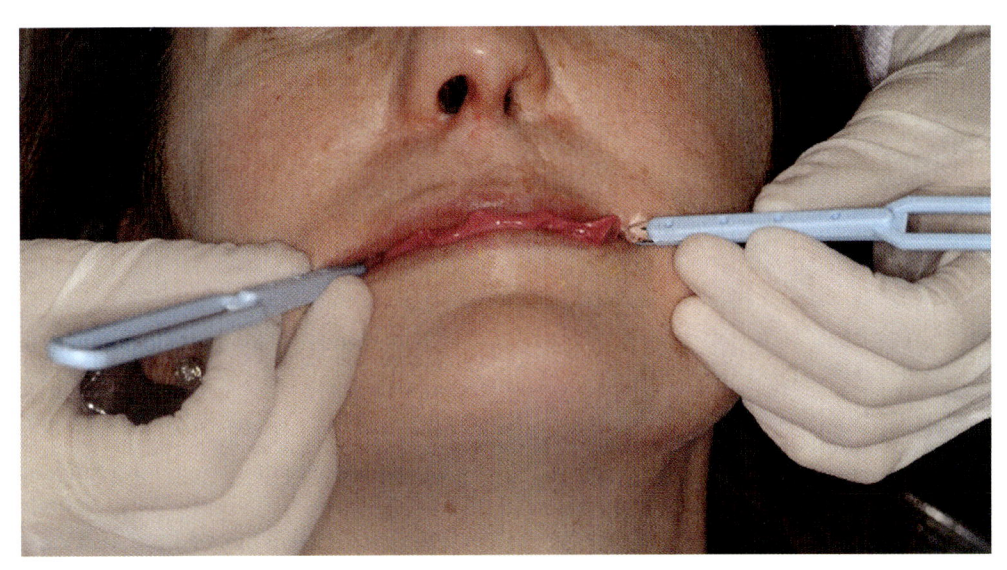

Figure 41.16 **(A)** When vertical dimension is not being altered, verify occlusal stops in the areas of the arch not being treated with thin, 0.0005″ (0.0127 mm), occlusal strips (Artus Corporation) and have the patient bite into centric. The assistant stands behind the patient as the dentist syringes the bite registration material around the preparations and other teeth.

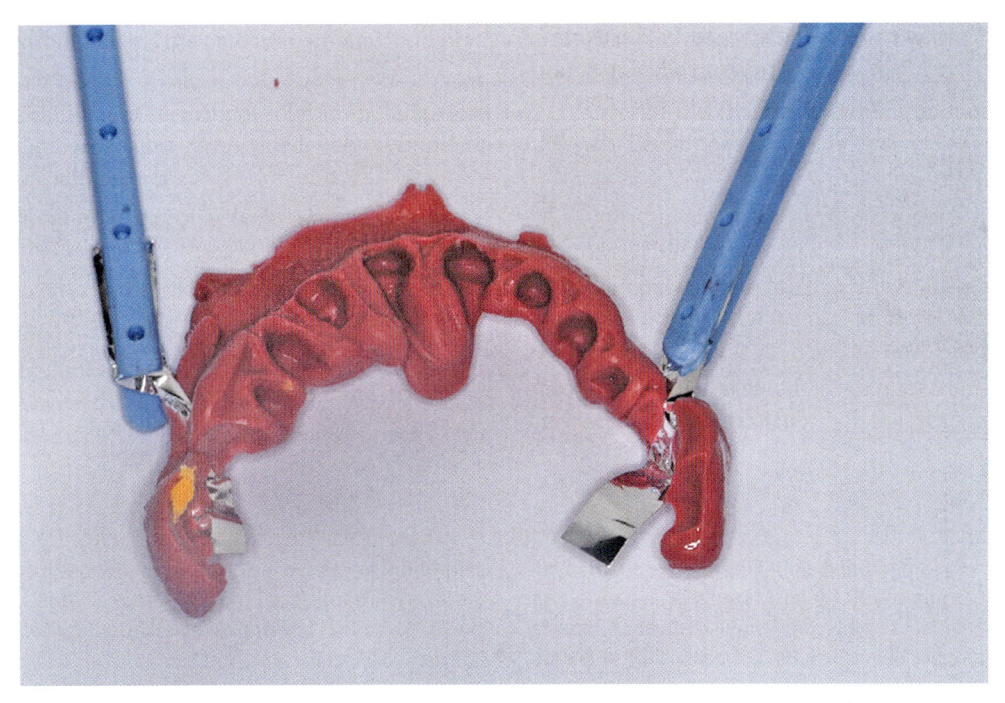

Figure 41.16 **(B)** An example of a correct bite registration where the patient firmly held the occlusal strips in place without opening.

first, and then accurate quadrant bite registrations should be made to be used later (as seen in Figure 41.18A–F). Next, the opposite posterior quadrant of the teeth should be prepared and the procedure repeated using the previously recorded quadrant bite registration. If the opposite posterior quadrant is used, then the anterior stops can help to preserve accuracy in the second bite registration. Then the anterior teeth would be prepared and both of the previously recorded quadrant bite registrations would be in place and linked together by incorporating the prepared anteriors. In this fashion, the patient's original occlusal relationship is preserved and can be used for mounting the models in the laboratory.

Another technique that has proven effective in the authors' practices is the employment of acrylic (GC Pattern Resin LS, GC America, Inc., Alsip, IL) to create anterior stops (Figure 41.17). Nevertheless, the occlusal registration strips verify that the patient is accurately closing into any remaining posterior centric contacts. For a procedure that involved the reconstruction of a full arch with no alteration of the occlusion, the dentist should try to temporarily leave the second or third molars untouched and reconstruct them at a later date. Thus, the dentist always has a posterior natural occlusal stop to verify the occlusion throughout and even after seating the final restorations.

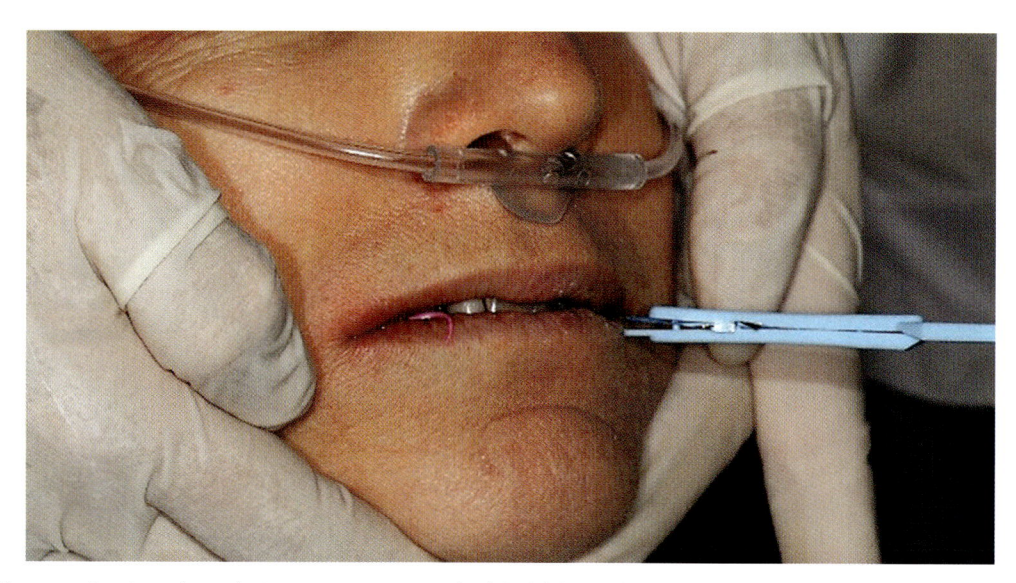

Figure 41.16 **(C)** If your patient is under sedation, it is important to both hold the occlusal registration into place and support the patient's chin to make sure no opening occurs.

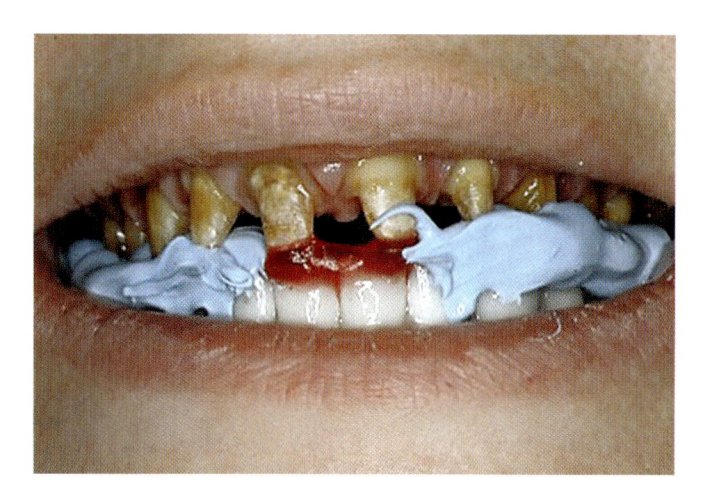

Figure 41.17 Acrylic resin (GC America) can also be used to create anterior stops in full arch cases to help secure an accurate bite registration. Blu-Mousse bite registration material, (Parkell).

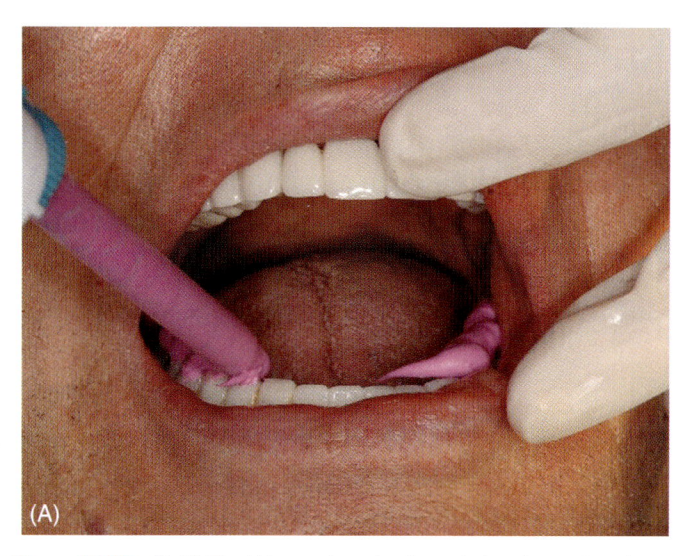

Full-arch final bite registration

The final bite registration procedure is based on the accuracy of the temporary bite registration technique described earlier. First, a central bite registration is made that will be cut and used to make certain the patient closes into centric occlusion on each side as the opposite side is finally recorded (Figure 41.18A–F).

If the vertical dimension is being increased, you will not be able to maintain these centric stops, and an alternative technique should be employed. There are techniques described in the literature in which an increase in vertical can be transferred to the casts. When the patient's desired vertical has been established, through temporaries or a removable splint, a dot is drawn on the patient's nose and another on the patient's chin. The distance between the two dots is measured extraorally, with calipers (Dentagauge 2, Erskine Dental). The calipers are kept at this position, and this vertical dimension is verified throughout the occlusal registration process. For additional stability, the anterior segment of temporaries can be removed, Vaseline applied to the prepared anterior teeth, and a composite or acrylic jig can be fabricated over the prepared teeth. When the posterior temporaries are removed, the anterior jig can be seated and the occlusal registration material can be placed on the remaining prepared teeth.

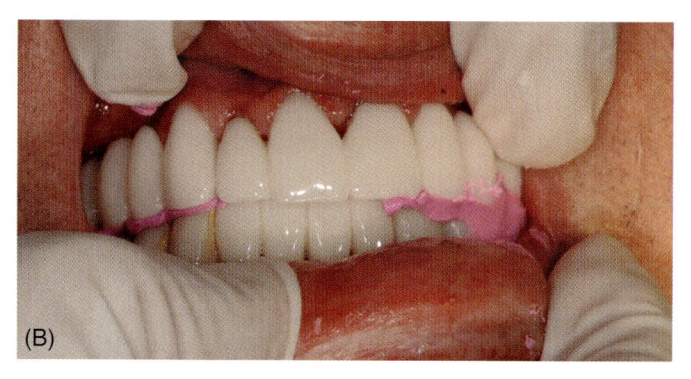

Figure 41.18 **(A, B)** Final bite registration is made by alternating the temporary restorations in place from one side to the other. The first step is to make an accurate full-arch bite registration in centric using rigid bite registration material (Regisil® PB™ Bite Registration Material by Dentsply).

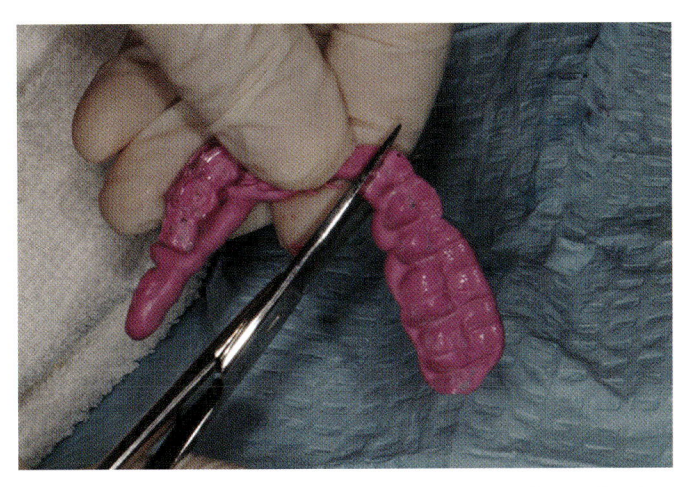

Figure 41.18 **(C)** The centric bite registration is cut so that each side can work independently.

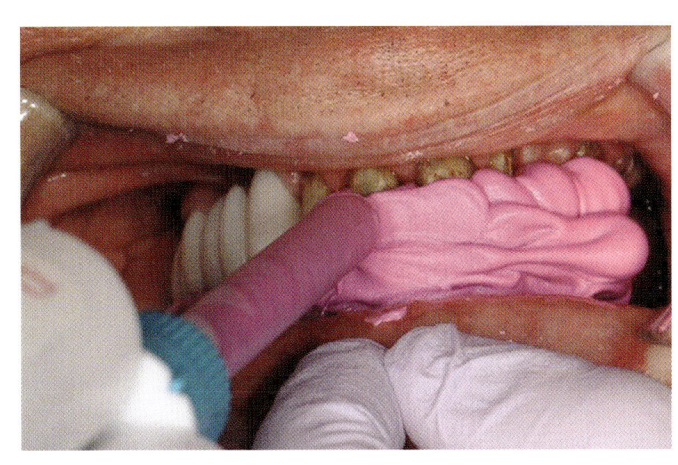

Figure 41.18 **(D)** With the temporaries in place on the right side plus using the segmented bite registration index, a bite registration is made on the left side maxillary and mandibular crown preparations.

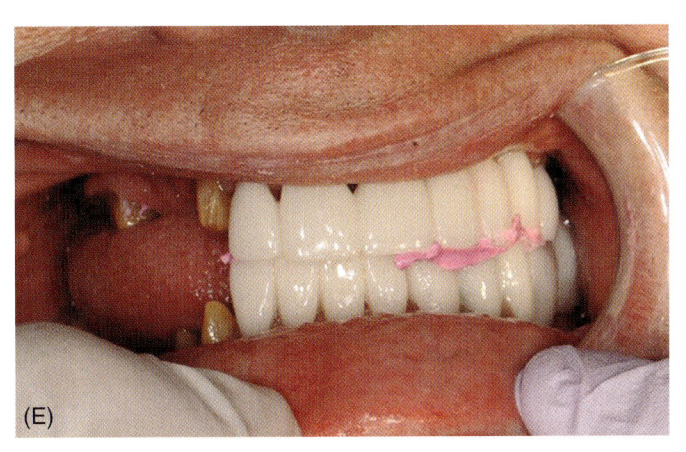

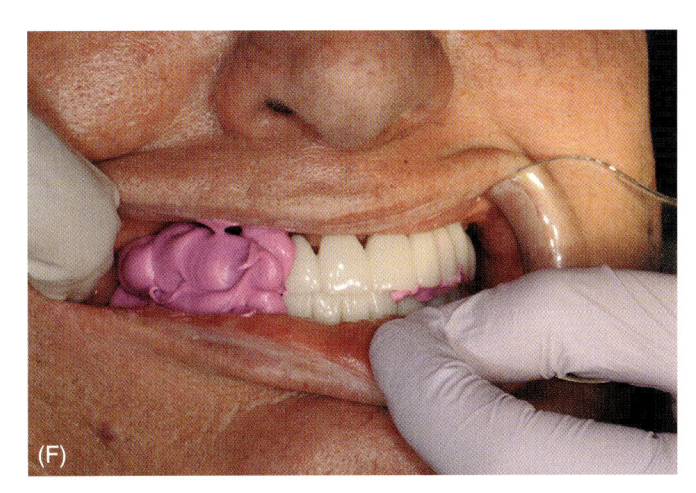

Figure 41.18 **(E, F)** Next, the same procedure is repeated by using the temporaries and centric bite registration on the left side to obtain an accurate registration of maxillary and mandibular crown preparations on the right side.

Alternatively, if the practitioner is utilizing a joint-based position, any number of anterior deprogrammers may be used. These include a Pankey jig, a Lucia jig, a leaf gauge, an NTI appliance, or a similar anterior deprogrammer fabricated by the practitioner. These allow the temporomandibular joint to be seated in the centric relation position without occlusal interference. Once the restorative position has been determined, a mark is drawn on the appliance where the lower incisors contact. The appliance remains in place as the registration material is placed on all the occlusal surfaces. The position can be verified by confirming that the lower incisors are still touching the mark once the bite registration material has set. The appliance can be seated on the upper cast at the time of mounting to provide an anterior stop.

If the practitioner elects to use a digital impression, the same techniques may be used with different bite registration material. Specially formulated polyvinyl siloxane materials are made with opaque fillers to prevent scatter when scanning the registration (Virtual CADbite, Ivoclar). Alternatively, the occlusal surface of the prepared arch and the opposing arch can be captured with the digital impression system (iTero, Lava Chairside Oral Scanner C.O.S.). The interocclusal relationship can then be determined digitally.

Summary

The impression step is perhaps the most critical in the entire process of creating esthetic restorations. Perfect-fitting prosthetic restorations are so dependent on accurate impressions. It is so costly to have an improper fitting crown or fixed partial denture, and this cost is certainly magnified when doing extensive prosthetic treatment. So it is essential that the entire dental team be aware that materials are technique sensitive. The same holds true when making an occlusal registration. Meticulous technique must be achieved in order to avoid complication in proper form and arrangement of the final restoration.

References

1. Timberlake DL. Epinephrine in tissue retraction. *Ariz Dent J* 1971;17(2):14–16.
2. Dawson PE. Recording centric relation. In: *Functional Occlusion: From TMJ to Smile Design*. St. Louis, MO: Mosby Elsevier; 2006:91–102.
3. Goldstein RE. A precise bite registration technique. *Inside Dent* 2008;4(7). https://www.dentalaegis.com/id/2008/08/a-precise-bite-registration-technique (accessed November 14, 2017).

Additional resources

Adams TC, Pang PK. Lasers in aesthetic dentistry. *Dent Clin North Am* 2004;48(4):833–860.

Bauman MA. The influence of dental gloves on the setting of impression materials. *Br Dent J* 1995;179:130–135.

Bunek SS, ed. Impression materials. *Dent Advisor* 2014;31(March):2.

Bunek SS, ed. Digitizing dental impressions. *Dent Advisor* 2014;31(October):8.

Bunek SS, ed. CAD/CAM: To mill or not to mill. *Dent Advisor* 2016;33(March):2.

Drennon DG, Johnson GH. The effect of immersion disinfection of elastomeric impressions on the surface detail and reproduction of improved gypsum casts. *J Prosthet Dent* 1990;63:233.

Farah JW, Powers JM, eds. Soft tissue management. *Dent Advisor* 2010;27(10).

Farah JW, Powers JM, eds. Digital impressions. *Dent Advisor* 2010;27(6).

Farah JW, Powers JM, eds. Elastomeric impression materials. *Dent Advisor* 2008;25(3).

Farah JW, Powers JM, eds. Alginate and alginate substitutes. *Dent Advisor* 2007;24(2).

Fokkinga W, Uchelen J, Witter D, et al. Impression procedures for metal frame removable partial dentures as applied by general dental practitioners. *Int J Prosthodont* 2016;29:166–168.

Giordano R II. Impression materials: basic properties. *Gen Dent* 2000;48:510–516.

Goharkhay K, Mortiz A, Wilder-Smith P, et al. Effects on oral soft tissue produced by a diode laser in vitro. *Lasers Surg Med* 1999;25(5):401–406.

Idris B, Houston F, Claffey N. Comparison of the dimensional accuracy of one- and two-step techniques with the use of putty/wash additional silicone impression materials. *J Prosthet Dent* 1995;74:535–541.

Inturregui J, Aquilino SA, Ryther JS, Lund PS. Evaluation of three impression techniques for osseointegrated oral implants. *J Prosthet Dent* 1993;69:503–509.

Little DA. Illustrating predictable anterior and posterior esthetic results: two case studies. *Compend Contin Educ Dent* 2002;23(Suppl 1):17–23.

Lowe RA. Predictable fixed prosthodontics: technique is the key to success. *Compend Contin Educ Dent*. 2002;23(Suppl 1):4–12.

Martinez LJ, von Fraunhofer JA. The effects of custom tray material on the accuracy of master casts. *J Prosthodont* 1998;7:106–110.

McCabe JF, Arikawa H. Rheological properties of elastomeric impression materials before and during setting. *J Dent Res* 1998;77:1874–1880.

Nissan J, Gross A, Shifman A, Assif D. Effect of wash bulk on the accuracy of polyvinyl siloxane putty–wash impressions. *J Oral Rehabil* 2002;29:357–361.

Perry RD, Kugel G. Success with inlays/onlays: the seven essentials. *Compend Contin Educ Dent* 2002;23(Suppl 1):30–35.

Powers JM, Wataha JC. *Dental Materials—Properties and Manipulation*, 10th edn. St. Louis, MO: Mosby Elsevier; 2013.

Scott D, Benjamin DDS. All lasers are not the same: success requires knowledge and training. *Compend Contin Educ Dent* 2011;32(5):66–68.

Vargas M. Let's talk lasers. *Dent Prod Rep*, December 2008. https://web.archive.org/web/20090204001147/ http://www.dentalproductsreport.com/articles/show/dpr1208_ed_diode-lasers

Vogel RE. A simplified impression technique for dental implants. *Compend Contin Educ Dent* 2002;23(Suppl 1):13–16.

Walinski CJ. Irritation fibroma removal: a comparison of two laser wavelengths. *Gen Dent* 2004;52(3):236–238.

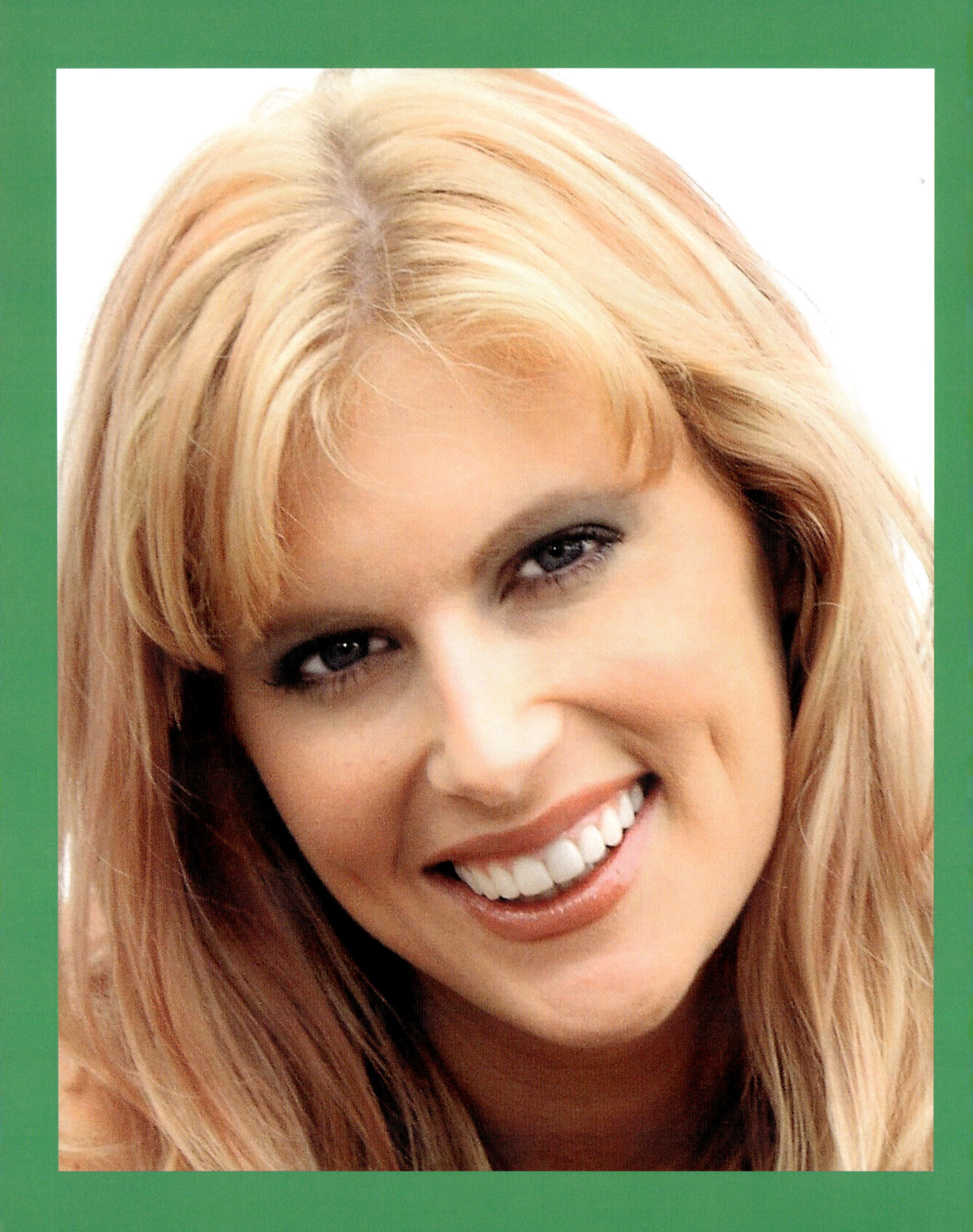

Chapter 42 Esthetic Temporization

Ronald E. Goldstein, DDS and Pinhas Adar, MDT, CDT

Chapter Outline

Esthetic uses of temporization	1311	Vacuform technique	1315
Trial smile	1312	Temporary splinting	1317
Decision making	1312	Composite resin treatment splinting	1317
Tooth movement	1312	The A-splint for provisional immobilization	1320
Phonetic concern	1313	Temporary restorations	1323
Protection	1314	A secondary function	1324
Requirements	1314	Interim temporary methods construction	1324
Specific types of temporization	1315	Indirect Siltek method for implants	1324
Computer-aided design/manufacturing	1315		

Although patients tend to be concerned about their looks before treatment, this concern may increase especially after tooth preparations have been made for prosthetic restorations. The concern may be justified unless temporary restorations are made to be esthetically acceptable as well as functional. The old rule of not making the temporary esthetic because it need not be as good as the final restoration is unjustified. Esthetics and function are both served by well-made, carefully fitted temporaries, especially since a continuous attractive appearance is important to most every patient. The esthetic temporary satisfies the patient, and a satisfied patient will allow the dentist the time necessary to construct a successful final restoration. In contemporary dentistry, provisional restorations provide more than an intermediate functional and protective covering device for teeth that have been prepared for an indirect restoration. They are the second step after the trial smile to more clearly achieve the patient's esthetic goals, and to learn what is ideal occlusally, phonetically, and esthetically. If a trial smile was not utilized, then the temporary must take its place and the final ceramic restorations should not even begin to be constructed until the patient is completely happy with the temporary with shade, shape, and arrangement. Otherwise, there is no assurance your patient will be happy with your final result, which can be a costly gamble for you to make.

This chapter will focus on various techniques for achieving an esthetic temporary veneer, crown, or splint, the benefits derived from spending time in the provisional stage, and how to communicate the most important information learned in this stage to the laboratory to be replicated in the final restorations.

Esthetic uses of temporization

The main purpose of any form of temporary coverage is to provide maximum protection for the tooth and surrounding tissues while the final restoration is constructed. It is also critical for the gingival margins and proper interproximal contours to be correct to avoid periodontal problems which can potentially affect your final restorations. Many dentists utilize the dental assistant to make the temporaries, so make sure they are well trained so they can create perfect margins. There are also several other important functions that temporization can and should offer. The most important criteria for selecting the right type of temporary restoration include patient comfort, treatment time, laboratory cost, occlusal clearance, ease of removal, durability, and ease of modification.[1]

Trial smile

If a preliminary trial smile was created for your patient, then the temporary restoration should mimic the changes requested by your patient. If this step was not done, then esthetic imaging and a good wax-up should be shown to the patient if changes are scheduled to be made. However, the temporary restoration will also act as a "trial smile" for your patient, giving them adequate time to voice any changes requested (Figure 42.1A–E). This process could take considerable time, depending on (1) the extent of changes, (2) your patient's ability to make decisions, and/or (3) the need to revise or make changes to the temporary. We have had patients who make up their mind quickly and yet others that have taken months to finally be pleased enough to move on the final restorations. For these reasons, it is advised to have your laboratory hold any efforts to create the restorations until your patient states they like the form, shape, and color of your temporary. If only slight adjustments are required then you can usually assure the patient that you will incorporate those changes in the final restoration. We have seen instances where patients wanted longer anterior teeth but at the final porcelain try-in insisted on major changes, including shortening of the crowns, only to see the beautiful inlaid incisal porcelain disappear. Thus, always add any desired length to the temporary rather than assume your patient will be happy with you or your ceramist's estimate of how much length to add in the final restoration.

Sometimes it is necessary to exaggerate the appearance of intended alterations during the temporary stage. For instance, in cases where incisal length will be added to make the patient look younger, it may be wise to make the temporary slightly longer than the intended restoration. Patients may react cautiously to longer teeth, and feel they are too long. Overlengthened acrylic temporary teeth can easily be cut back to a more acceptable result as the patient wishes. Then the laboratory can proceed with much more accurate incisal length.

Decision making

Ultimately, patients must make a decision, and hopefully it will be the right one for them. The entire dental team wants the patient to be happy with their restoration, so it is a joint effort to help that patient arrive at the decision-making process in an orderly, non-rushed manner. The benefit of temporary restorations is that they can help your patient to both see and feel the planned final restoration in order to judge it. Wearing provisionals helps to understand what is possible both functionally and esthetically and offers patients an opportunity for involvement in making modifications before the final restorations are constructed.

Despite all your best efforts, there may be times when your patient does not listen to your advice and makes the wrong decision. This is especially why *you must make it perfectly clear before beginning on the final restoration that if the patient later changes their mind and wants the restorations done over, the financial responsibility will be totally their own* (Figure 42.1A–E).

When you plan on making major esthetic changes, such as opening vertical dimension, you may want to plan on not taking final impressions until you are certain your patient is both functionally and esthetically pleased. Sometimes this can take up to 3 months or more during which adjustments may be required. With the temporaries in the mouth you can determine how far from the margin the interproximal contacts should be placed and if the patient can clean with the new tooth contours.[2] It is rare that a patient does not have some modification in mind. Often these modifications are subtle, easy to perform, and can pertain to tooth contours or embrasure shapes. At times the patient's esthetic goal cannot be achieved; if so, explain why it cannot be done before it is sent to the laboratory instead of after the fact, which might sound like an excuse to the patient.[3] In general, there will almost always be limitations to each patient's problems, so the sooner the patient understands and accepts this fact the better.

If you are making indirect temporaries that will be worn for extended periods of time, you should make multiple accurate impressions that may also be suitable to construct the final restorations, since there may be a good chance these impressions may suffice as the final impressions. However, the chances are there can be tissue or other changes that may require you to make new impressions for the final restoration. So, it is advisable to take as much time as possible between the temporization stage and the impression for the final restoration, as changes can take place in gingival, pontic, and marginal areas. When this happens, the temporary restoration can be altered to take care of the discrepancy. If a fixed partial denture is being replaced, there may be hypertrophied tissue. If this is the case, allow enough time for shrinkage and adjust the temporary accordingly. If the patient suggests any esthetic change, this and any other alterations should be done before the new final impressions or try-in appointment.

Tooth movement

In some cases, temporary restorations become a critical element in the treatment process and may be in place for several months or years. Long-term temporization is necessary in cases when patients require orthodontics or periodontal surgery.[4–8] If defective crowns are present and need to be replaced, a long-term temporary should be placed to allow the patient to complete orthodontics prior to completing the final restoration, ensuring a better final result than if the final restoration was completed prior to orthodontics.[3] If a tooth is broken and does not have an existing crown present, it is generally better to restore the fractured tooth with direct composite, have the orthodontics completed, and then complete the definitive restoration.

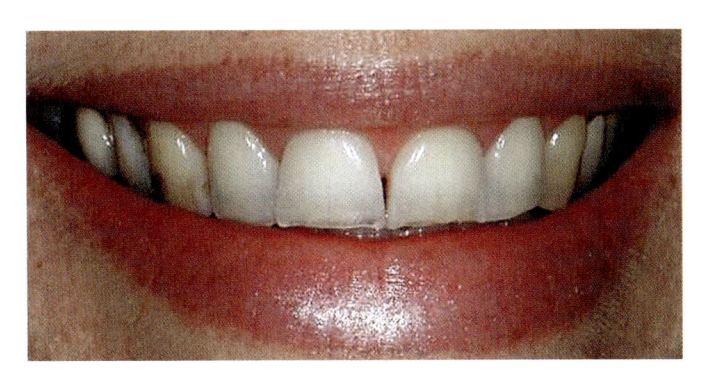

Figure 42.1 (A) This lady presented to her original dentist to improve her smile.

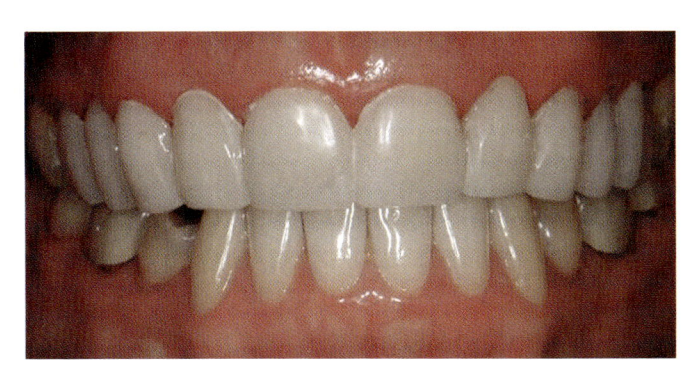

Figure 42.1 (B) These are the temporary restorations the dentist made for her.

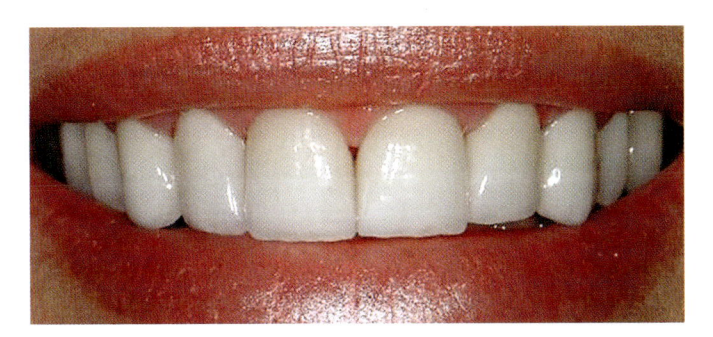

Figure 42.1 (C) Although the final ceramic restorations were functionally excellent, they did not satisfy the patient's esthetic needs, so she came to our office to see if we could improve her smile.

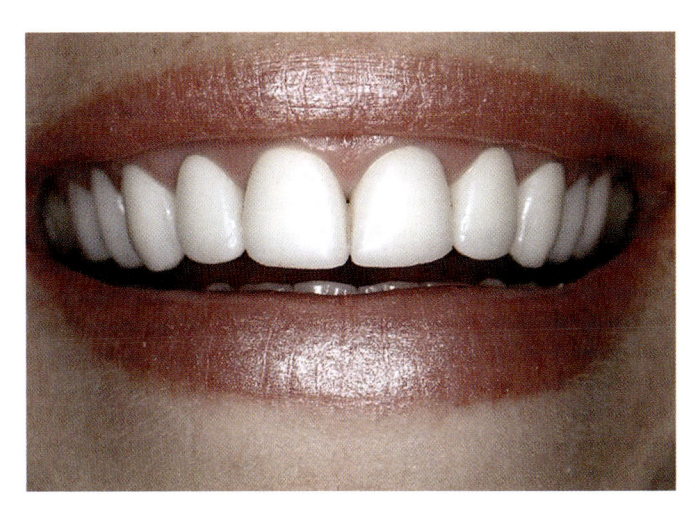

Figure 42.1 (D) New temporary restorations were created to mimic her smile when she was younger. It is important for patients to wear temporary restorations long enough so any esthetic changes can be made before the final restorations are fabricated.

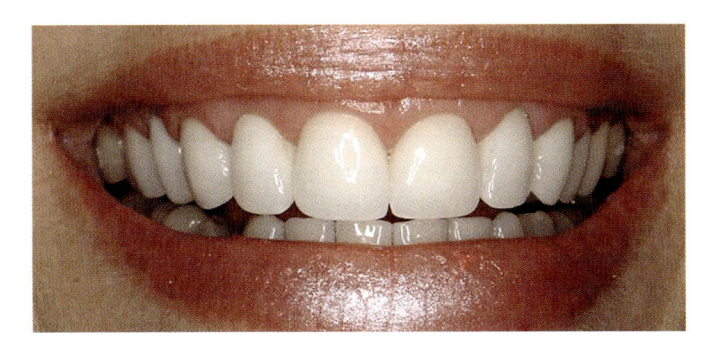

Figure 42.1 (E) After wearing the temporary restorations for 3 months, the patient felt secure in having the final crowns fabricated and delivered. The patient was very pleased with her final smile and stated that we exceeded her esthetic expectations.

Phonetic concern

Whenever arch forms or the relationships between maxillary incisors and the mandibular incisors are modified, the patient's ability to pronounce certain sounds may change.[2,9] For instance, leaving 1–2 mm between the closed upper and lower incisors may lead to the "lisping S" because of the inability to limit the airflow between upper and lower teeth.[3] However, most difficulties in speech are temporary and easy to adapt to. If not, the lingual of the maxillary incisors can be built out to help close the gap. Major changes in the lower arch involve the patient's tongue getting used to the new position, and at times this could be a problem requiring additional visits to solve the problem.

Wearing temporary restorations provides a patient with a chance to feel the changes in occlusion between the teeth and any phonetic changes that have been created. If the patient cannot adapt to the changes the dentist has created, it is vital to know this and make the needed corrections prior to sending the case to the laboratory.

Protection

In addition to being both esthetic and functional, provisional restorations protect the pulp from chemical, thermal, and mechanical irritants and protect the prepared teeth from caries. The sedative properties of cements containing eugenol can help promote the formation of secondary dentin and relieve the hyperemic response that occurs after operative procedures.

Eugenol does have one disadvantage: it tends to react unfavorably with both acrylic and composite resin and may interfere with any future addition or repair of the restoration. Thus, if the temporary restoration will be worn for an extended period of time you may choose to use one of the temporary cements that does not contain eugenol.

It is essential that the temporary restoration provides all the marginal support, not only for the tooth, but for the surrounding tissues. Otherwise, tissue damage that could well prevent any type of esthetic result can develop before the final restoration is placed.

The correction of damage due to a poorly fitting temporary often necessitates surgical alteration of tissue and may leave an unattractive result. For this and many other reasons, it is absolutely essential to construct a well-fitting, attractive-looking temporary restoration that maintains interproximal contact.[4] The temporary restoration must protect the tissue, otherwise the gingiva may become inflamed and become both a functional and esthetic failure around the final crown or bridge (Figure 42.2A–C).

The establishment and maintenance of an environment conducive to periodontal health is dependent upon the anatomy of the temporary restorations. Coronal contours must provide convexities that can deflect food from the gingival crevice. Proper embrasures protect the interdental papillae and underlying alveolar bone. Margins that approximate the finished restoration are essential for gingival health.

Requirements

There are many forms and types of temporary crowns and fixed partial dentures. Regardless of the interim temporary, certain principles must be followed to insure a successful restoration.[5] The temporary must provide adequate esthetics and a healthy

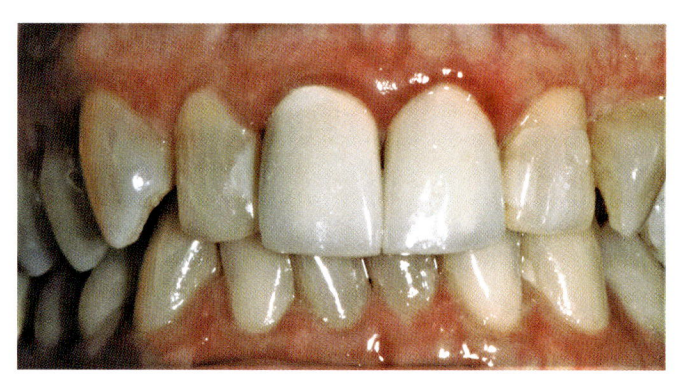

Figure 42.2 (A) This patient left her original dentist due to the poor esthetics and ill-fitting temporaries that made her gums sore and bleeding. She felt that if that was the best the dentist could do then she needed to find a new dentist.

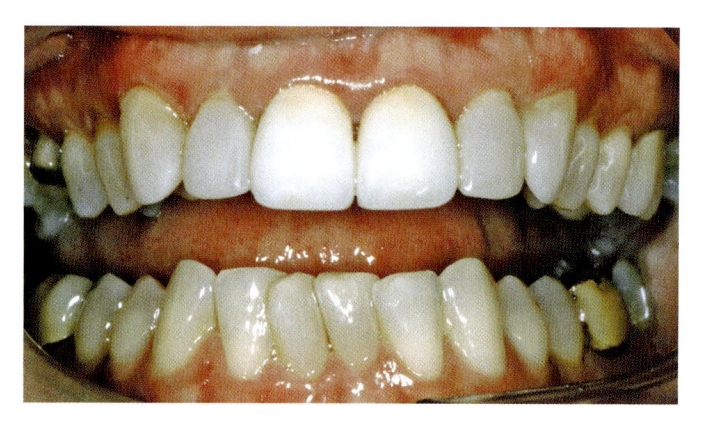

Figure 42.2 (B) Esthetically improved and well-fitting temporaries were made that allowed the tissue to heal. During this time, an esthetic evaluation of the patient showed the patient how her smile could be enhanced by including more of her anterior teeth in the final restoration.

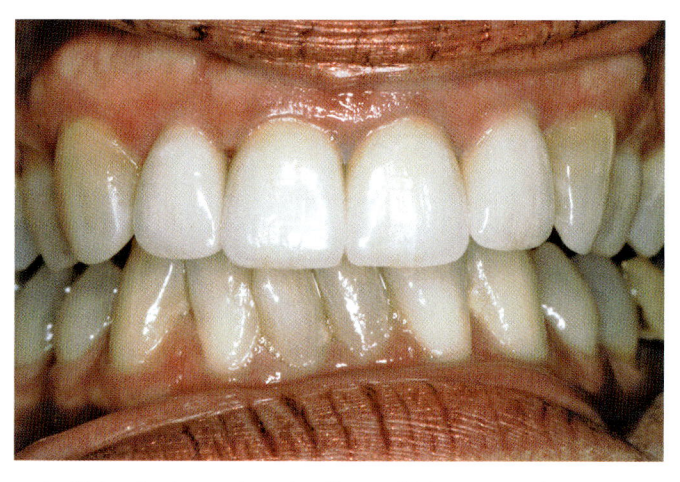

Figure 42.2 (C) The patient was pleased with her final ceramic restorations, which were much more proportionate than what had initially been planned.

environment for the prepared teeth and surrounding structures. It must be retentive but easy for the dentist to remove; it must be comfortable to the patient and work as an insulator and sedative for the underlying pulp. It should also be economical—with respect to the dentist's time and the patient's expenses. The temporary restoration best suited for function, economy, and esthetics is either a composite resin or acrylic crown or bridge that can be easily changed and fitted with correct crown contours for the patient. In the case of a nonvital tooth, be careful of the type of temporary cement you choose. Remember, the nonvital tooth will tend to be more brittle and could fracture when removing the temporary crown or bridge, so either use a softer cement or put a small amount of Vaseline in the harder cement mix, which will help you remove the temporary when necessary. Always have your patient hold hot water in the mouth to "loosen" or soften the cement bond and then either carefully tap or remove it with hemostats or special removal pliers in a vertical motion.

Specific types of temporization

Computer-aided design/manufacturing

This chapter features some of the most popular means of constructing temporary restorations. However, one of the newest and most accurate is via computer-aided design/manufacturing (CAD/CAM). This technique does require advanced planning, but the results can be most impressive. If you have a milling unit in your office it becomes an easy solution to scan your preparations and mill the designed temporary. However, if you need to send the scanned preparations to a laboratory in your vicinity it could still be sent back to your office within the day. My suggestion is to use the temporary/temporary technique described later in this chapter to keep the tissue from invading your margins during the waiting time.

An alternate technique, still using an outside laboratory, is to have them create the CAD/CAM temporary without final margins in advance. This would require you to finalize the temporary chair side.

Vacuform technique

The type of restoration used routinely for temporization of fixed restorations is either a quick-cure acrylic or composite resin made with the vacuform process. It can be used for making temporaries directly in the mouth or indirectly as a removable prosthesis (Figure 42.3A–J).

If fabricated intraorally, the clear vacuform matrix allows you to see exactly what is being formed in acrylic or composite. Any spaces or bubbles can be dealt with before the material is hardened. If necessary, realign the material to achieve more accurate margins. This improves the chances for future esthetic success by minimizing gingival irritation. Also consider filling in any bubbles or voids or even adding to the crown with flowable composite resin. This can be quite helpful if your temporary is shy of occlusion.

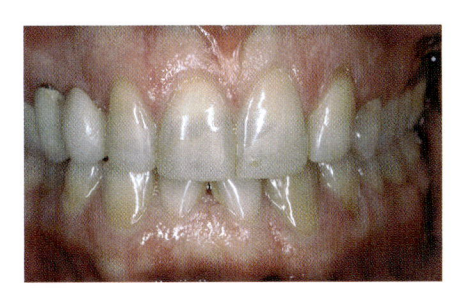

Figure 42.3 (A) Preoperative view of patient's old restoration.

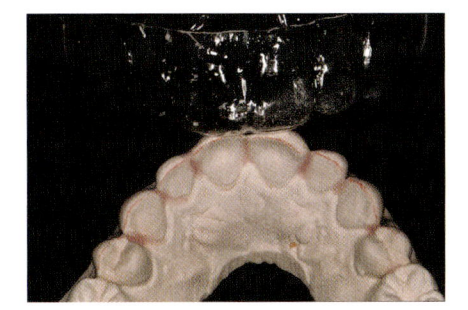

Figure 42.3 (B) Vacuform clear matrix fabricated on wax-up model and quick-set model poured after preparing the teeth.

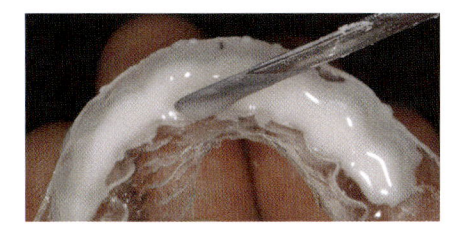

Figure 42.3 (C) Applying cold-curing acrylic mixture into egg shell.

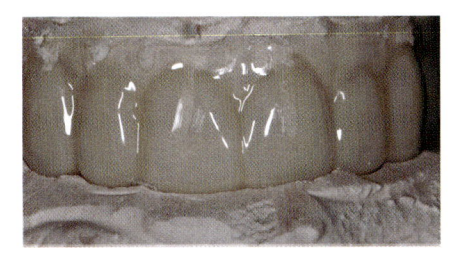

Figure 42.3 (D) Gently press incisally on the prepared model.

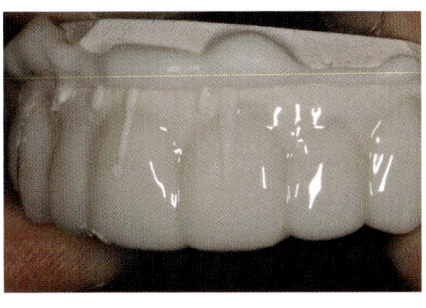

Figure 42.3 (E) Allow excess to escape from the vacuform essix matrix.

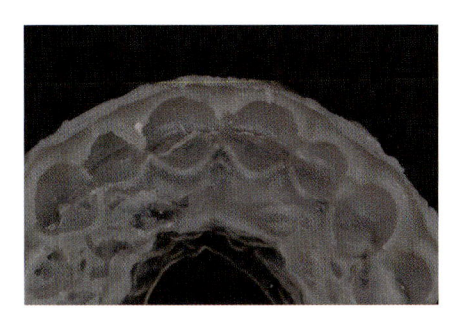

Figure 42.3 (F) Essix matrix and set acrylic become one, now ready to trim excess with diamond bur and disc to finalize removable temporary for porcelain veneers.

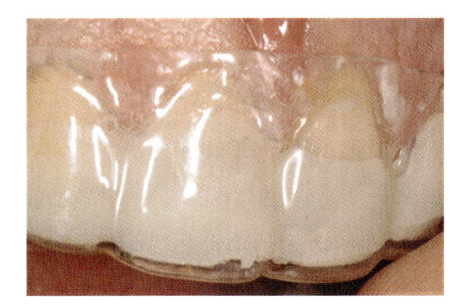

Figure 42.3 **(G)** The essix removable temporary being placed intraorally.

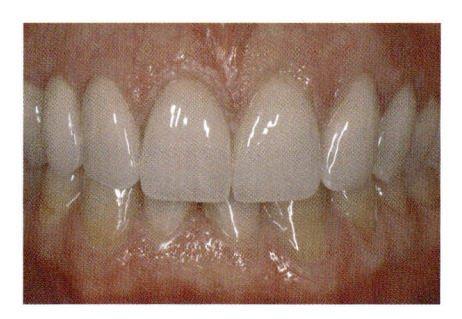

Figure 42.3 **(H)** Retracted view of the final porcelain veneers and crowns in place.

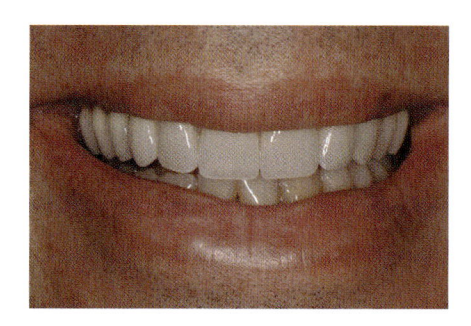

Figure 42.3 **(I)** Final smile of patient postoperative view.

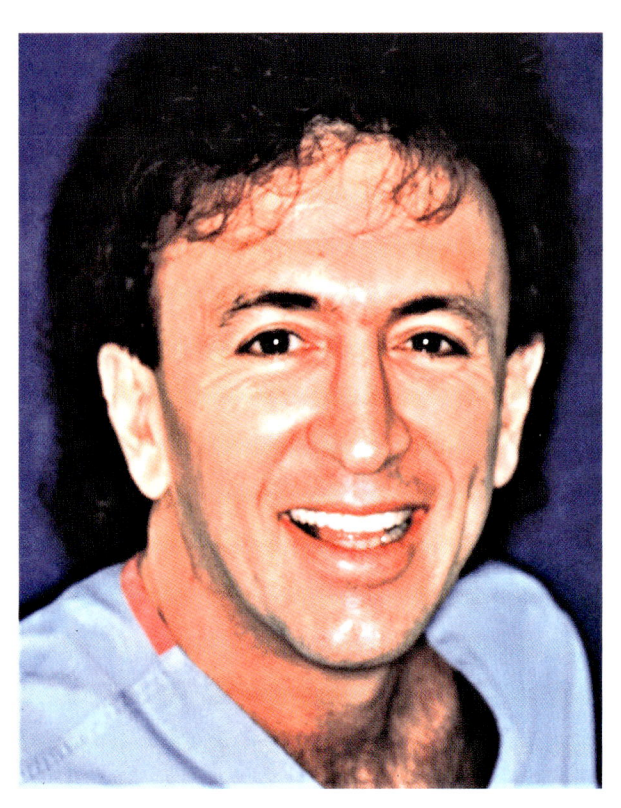

Figure 42.3 **(J)** Final result headshot.

Temporary veneer requirements

The first requirement for temporary veneers is to consider the length of time the temporaries will need to be worn. In fact, if little or no enamel is prepared and the turnaround time is short, will a temporary restoration be necessary?

Direct bonding

For a single veneer the best and easiest method is to directly bond the temporary with composite resin (Figure 42.4A–E). Tooth shades are easier to match, and there should be no problem with the temporary staying in place even with a 1 mm etch. Temporaries for multiple teeth may be quickly made utilizing either a vacuform matrix or a silicone index for more detailed anatomy, especially if you have first constructed a good wax-up model. Cementing the temporaries can be more problematic because your typical temporary cements tend to break down quickly, especially with patients who are not careful with their eating habits. However, you must also be careful when selecting more durable cements even when not etching the tooth preparations because some can be difficult to remove. If the tooth is nonvital then you should cut the temporary restoration off rather than risk a fracture of the prepared tooth.

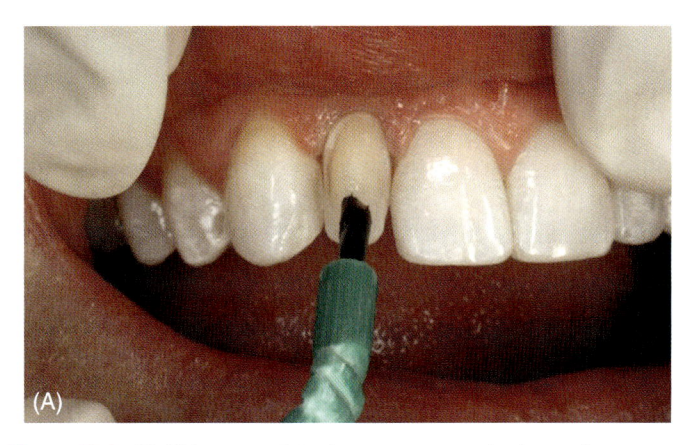

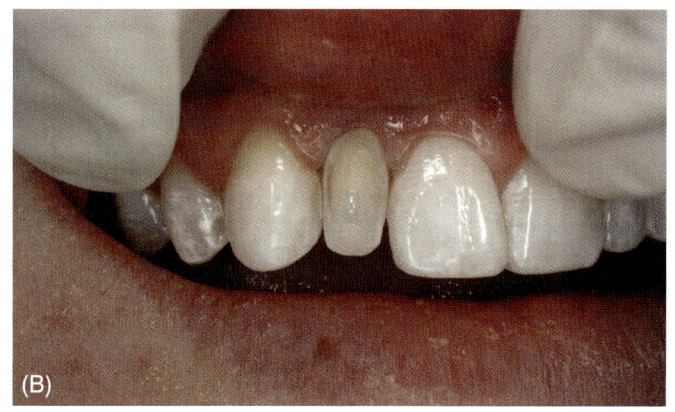

Figure 42.4 **(A, B)** In cases of single-veneer temporization, to better ensure the temporary stays in place, first spot etch the center of the tooth and rinse thoroughly.

Chapter 42 Esthetic Temporization

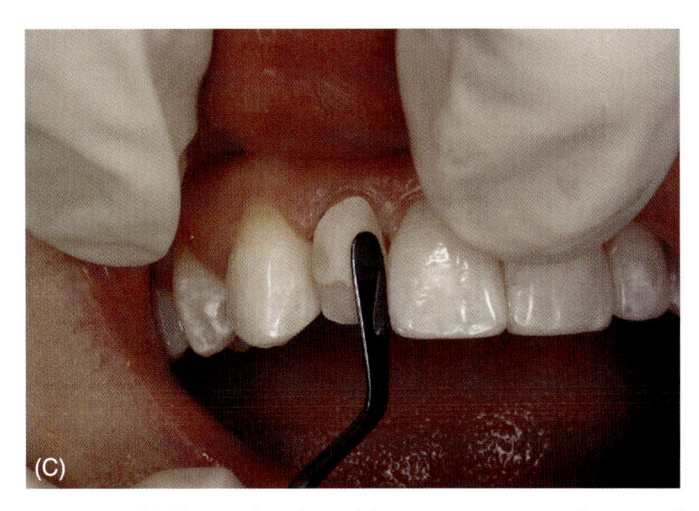

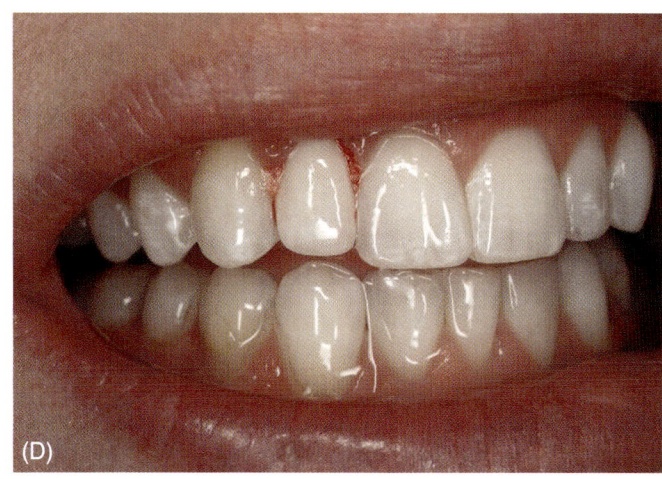

Figure 42.4 **(C–D)** Direct bonding of the composite resin will serve as the temporary.

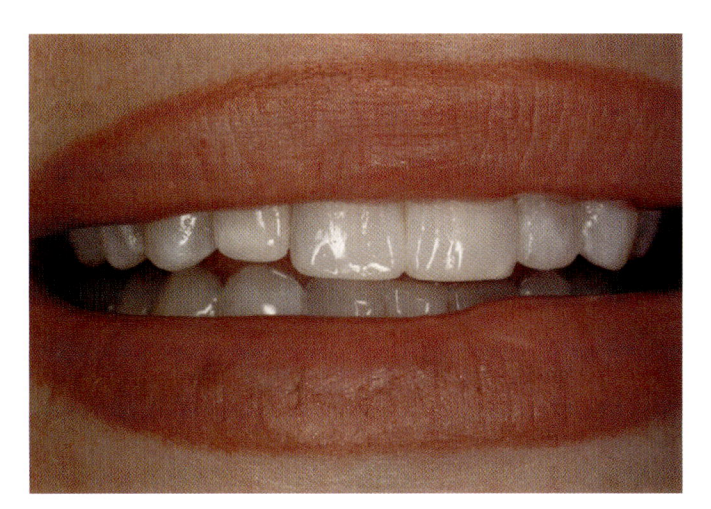

Figure 42.4 **(E)** The patient was happy with the esthetics, shade, and fit of the temporary veneer.

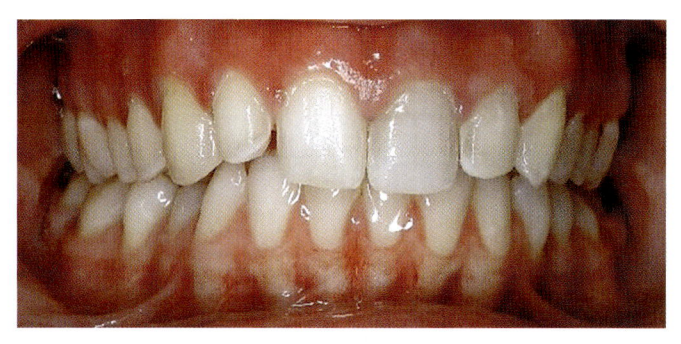

Figure 42.5 **(A)** This photographic model wanted to improve her smile with 10 maxillary porcelain veneers.

Indirect technique

The best method to have maximum esthetics and fit is to have the laboratory construct the temporary veneers (Figure 42.5A–G). These will no doubt be joined for greater stability and can either be removable for easy cleaning or cemented in place (Figure 42.5H). Detailed instructions about how to clean and change eating habits are best printed out. In the event you feel the need to etch a small patch of enamel (1–2 mm) and use a temporary resin cement, or even flowable composite make sure you remove all aspects of the resin before trying in the final porcelain veneers. At times it will be necessary to combine both full crowns and veneers in a single indirect temporary for maximum esthetics (Figure 42.5I–K).

Temporary splinting

Composite resin treatment splinting

Immediate stabilization of loose teeth can be done using either acrylic or composite resin combined with preimpregnated glass fibers. This technique is an economic interim solution either before or after final treatment (Figure 42.6A–L). The advantages are immediate immobilization of all teeth, to be followed by any other treatment necessary while the teeth are stabilized. In postorthodontic cases where veneers will be used, if the teeth eventually begin to separate, lingual splinting with a fiber/composite technique can be quite helpful (Figure 42.6A–L).

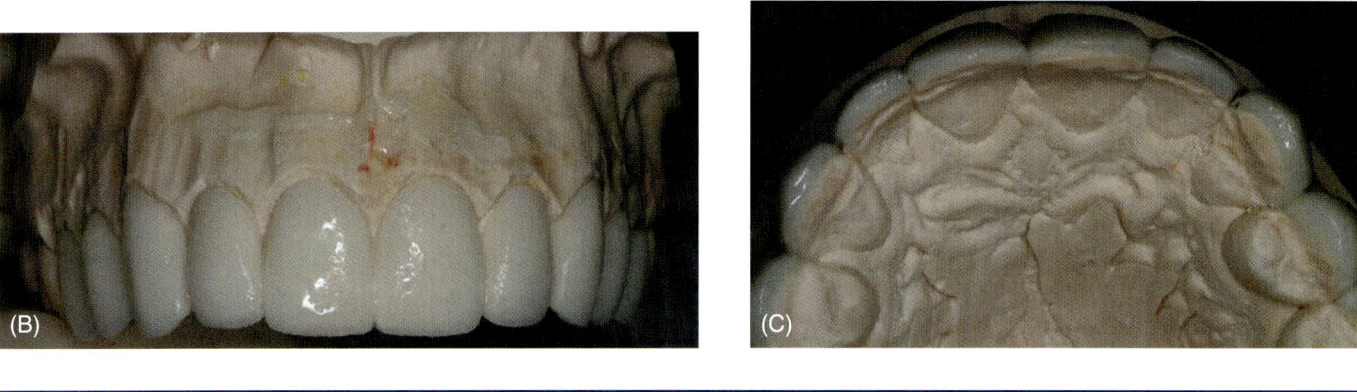

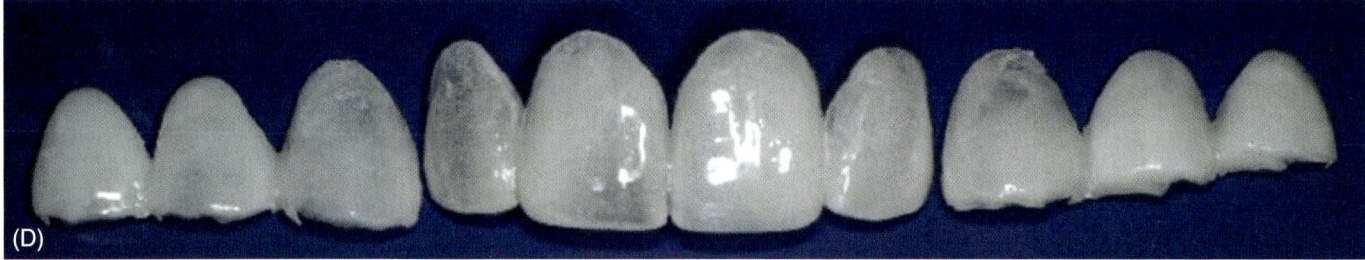

Figure 42.5 **(B–D)** Full-arch impressions were taken using polyvinyl siloxane and the temporary veneers were constructed in the laboratory in three sections.

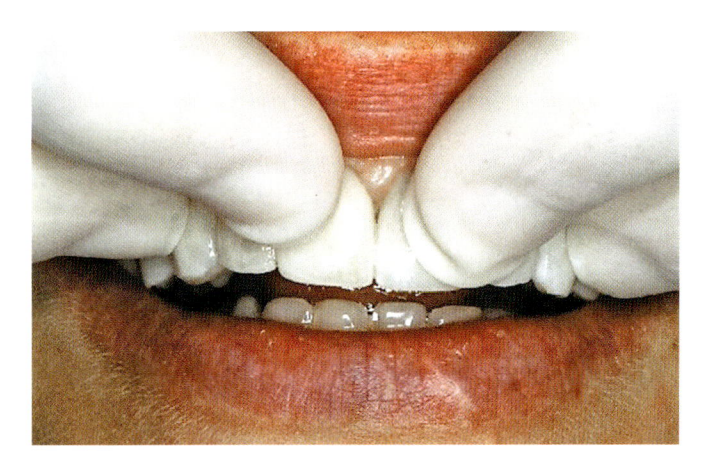

Figure 42.5 **(E)** After fitting and patient approval, the three sectioned temps were bonded to the teeth with a tooth colored flowable composite.

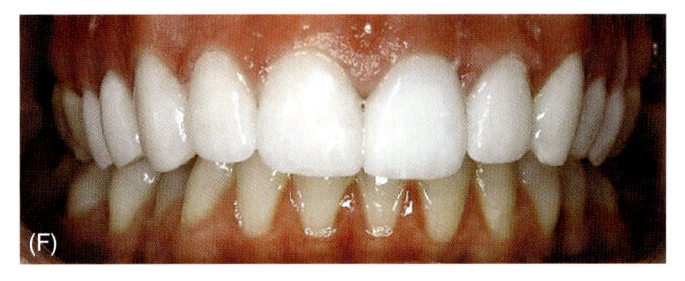

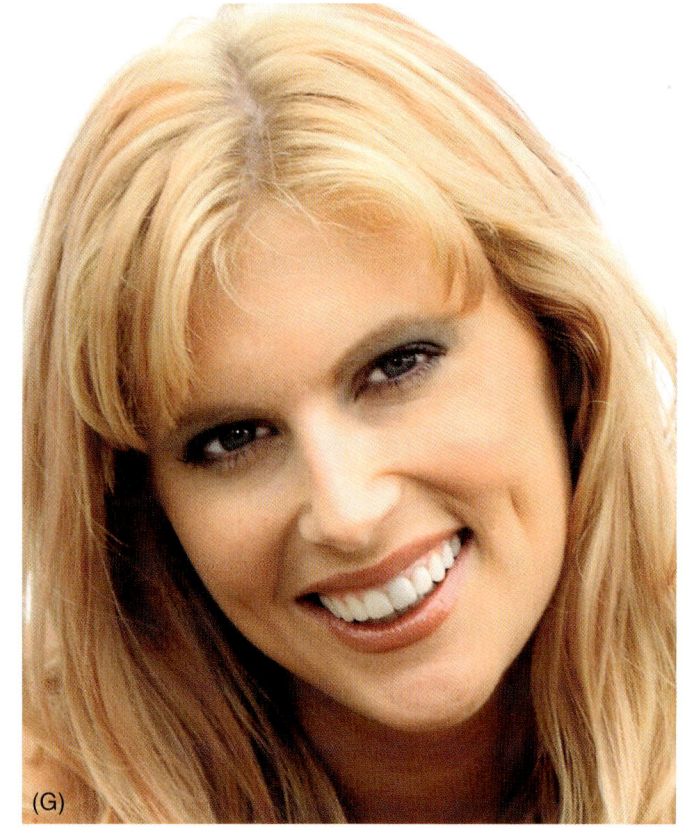

Figure 42.5 **(F, G)** The final result was esthetically pleasing enough that the model was able to continue with her photo shoots during the 3 weeks it took to construct her final veneers.

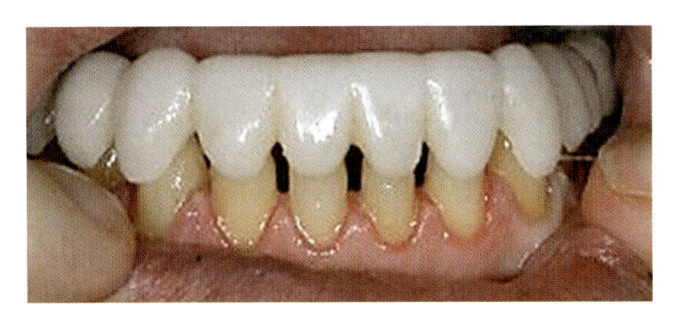

Figure 42.5 **(H)** The best method to have maximum esthetics and fit is to have the laboratory construct the temporary veneers joined for greater stability.

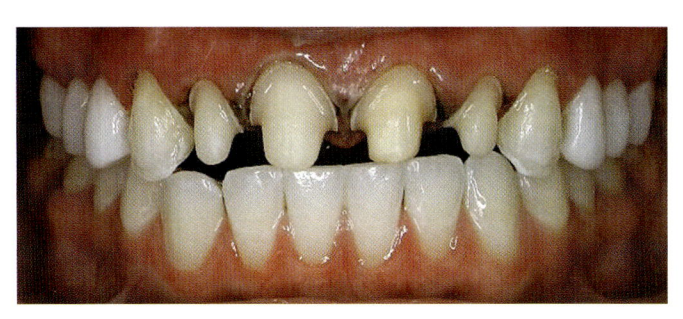

Figure 42.5 **(I)** Full crowns on the maxillary centrals and laterals plus more conservative veneer preparations were done for this patient.

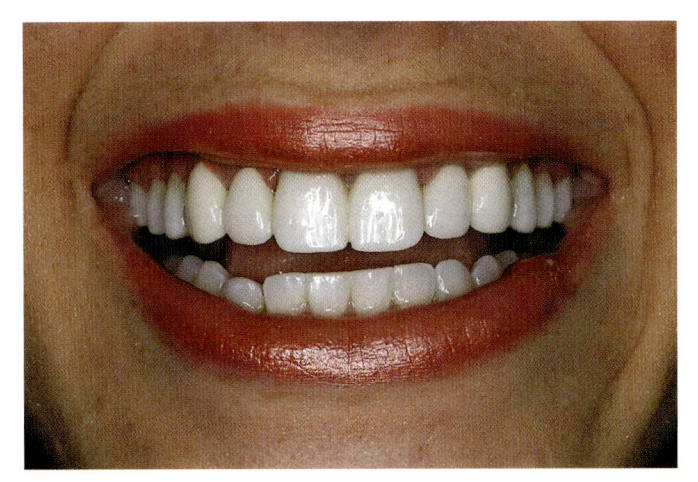

Figure 42.5 **(J)** Because esthetics and retention of the temporaries was of major concern for the patient, an indirect temporary connecting the crowns to the veneers was made.

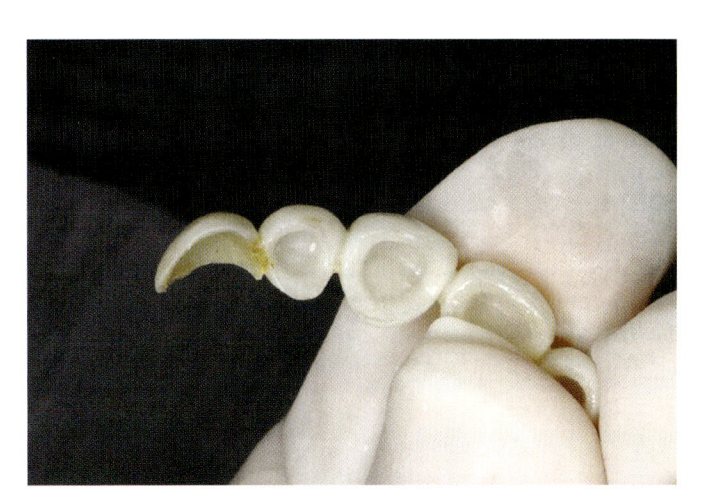

Figure 42.5 **(K)** At the time of the final seating of the restorations, the temporary was removed. Note the microleakage that occurred in the veneer area.

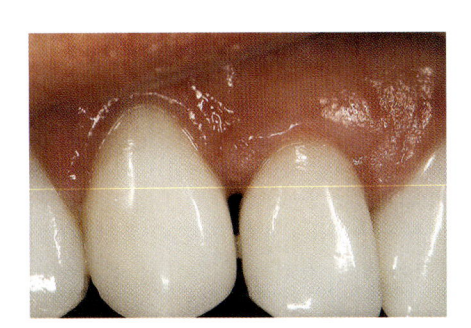

Figure 42.6 **(A)** This patient had a removable orthodontic appliance (Invisalign) to improve her malocclusion as well as to close the space between her right cuspid and lateral. Porcelain veneers were then placed, but the space continued to open.

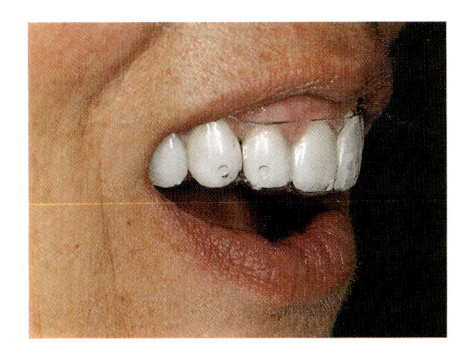

Figure 42.6 **(B)** A new Invisalign tray was fabricated to help close the space. However, the space continued to open during the day as soon as the patient would remove the orthodontic appliance.

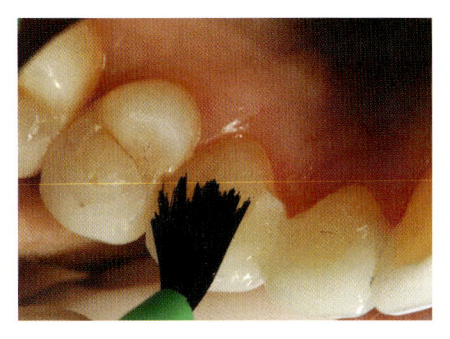

Figure 42.6 **(C)** Both porcelain and enamel are etched.

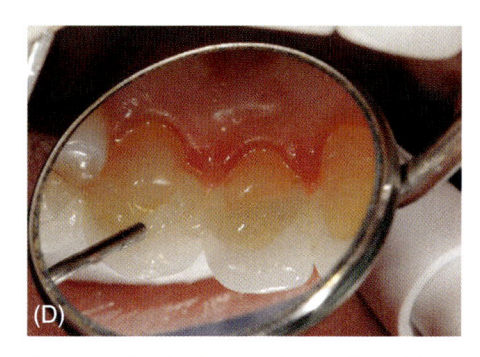

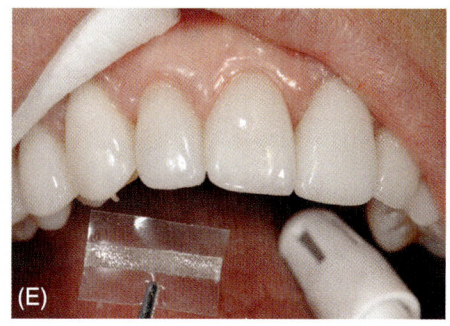

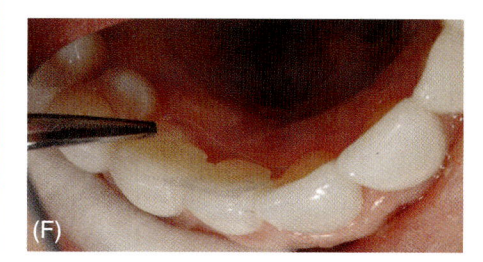

Figure 42.6 (D–F) Next, a layer of flowable composite is applied, followed by application of the fiber material (Dentapreg). After polymerization, the cover strip is peeled away.

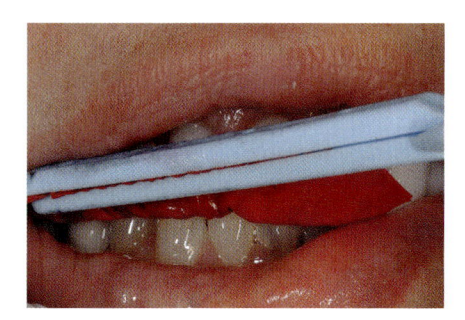

Figure 42.6 (G) Occlusion is checked with microthin red articulating paper.

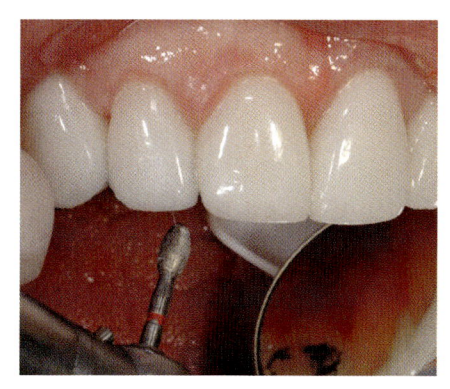

Figure 42.6 (H) Occlusion needs to be carefully adjusted, especially on the opposing arch to avoid thinning out the bonding splint.

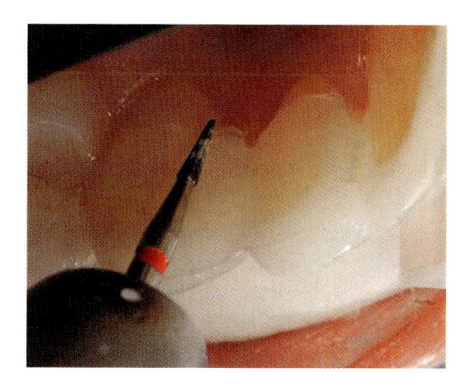

Figure 42.6 (I) Gingival contouring can be done using an eight-blade carbide finishing bur (ET4-Brasseler, USA).

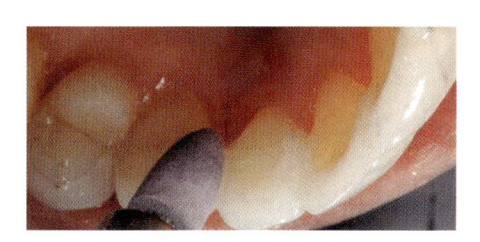

Figure 42.6 (J) Final finishing is done by using impregnated polishing points (Illustra, Brasseler, USA).

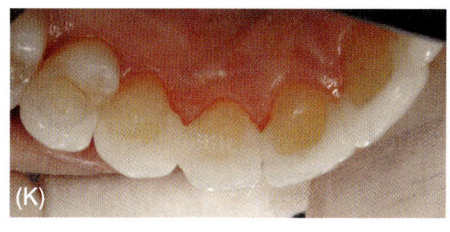

Figure 42.6 (K, L) The occlusal view shows the bonded splint in place maintaining space closure.

When temporary splinting is performed with composite resin, several factors must be considered. Fractures can occur unless an adequate thickness of resin is placed both labially and lingually. Since proper gingival embrasures must be maintained, it is important to trim and reopen these areas when finishing resin splints.

The A-splint for provisional immobilization

The A-splint provides all of the benefits of provisional immobilization of teeth not deformed by caries without requiring the subsequent restoration of these teeth with full-coverage techniques. The use of the A-splint does not preclude full-coverage reconstruction when indicated. Acrylic splints have been advocated for use as a transitional fixed appliance until a more permanent restoration or surgery is completed.

When using full-coverage acrylic splints, the most common error is the failure to create an environment conducive to health and to maintain this condition for a reasonable time. The A-splint is an alternative to full coverage that can aid in establishing and maintaining health and esthetics. It is simple, reliable, esthetic, and economic. Most importantly, the A-splint can be used in those patients for whom full-coverage fixed splints may not be indicated.[3]

An A-splint can be used in cases that require the following:

1. Immediate immobilization of seriously mobile teeth.
2. Total stability of teeth and contiguous periodontium undergoing periodontal therapy.
3. Stabilized arch integrity following treatment for elimination of crowding or diastema.
4. Vertical stabilization to help prevent extrusion of unopposed teeth.
5. Stabilization and retention of functionally repositioned, periodontally treated teeth.

The advantages of using an A-splint are:

1. The technique requires minimum tooth preparation and no impressions or models.
2. The operative procedure is direct and may be completed in one visit.
3. "Hairline" proximal anterior diastemas are eliminated.
4. Acrylic denture teeth may be added to the splint to replace missing anterior teeth.
5. Optimum accessibility helps the patient maintain good oral hygiene.
6. Adequate accessibility and security of total immobilization during periodontal procedures is provided without impinging on the interproximal tissues.
7. Total provisional immobilization of teeth with minimal clinical hazard is provided for at least 1 year; but owing to their temporary nature, these splints should be replaced or repaired every 18 months to 2 years.
8. An entire segment or any part of a segment may be secured at one sitting.

The technique for using the A-splint is as follows:

1. Approaching from the lingual aspect, cut a horizontal channel at the level of the contact points with a small inverted cone diamond. The channel should extend mesiodistally through, but not beyond, the proximal marginal ridges of the two approximating teeth. Undercut the preparations in order to provide adequate retention for the splint.
2. Isolate the teeth and insert base for pulp protection.
3. Etch the preparations and a 1 mm extension on the enamel margins with 50% phosphoric acid.
4. The wire to be used can be hard-drawn, deeply knurled, or serrated, dead, gold, round wire in a gauge equal in thickness to the preparation, or braided or serrated stainless steel ligature wire. The wire is cut to lengths matching the channels created.
5. If using acrylic, the pieces or wire are immersed in a self-curing acrylic monomer. Monomer is carefully painted into the undercuts of the channels with a sable brush.
6. The channel is half filled with beads of polymer powder. It is critical to avoid trapping air bubbles.
7. Seat the prepared wire into the channel so that it rests below the cavosurface margin.
8. Overfill the channel by adding monomer and powder in small additions.
9. As soon as the filling material loses its glisten, coat it with a lubricant to prevent the monomer from evaporating prematurely.
10. An adequate acrylic mask should be provided labially at the proximal contact point levels (when indicated) to assure good esthetics in the final restoration. Next, finish the restoration and polish.

Clinical case 42.7: Splint for posttreatment stabilization

Problem

A female patient, aged 35, was referred by the orthodontist for posttreatment anterior stabilization. For economic reasons, the patient wanted an attractive treatment splint to avoid crowning.

Treatment

The A-splint was chosen for its esthetic and functional advantages. Splinting was to be accomplished from maxillary cuspid to cuspid. First, the lingual surfaces of the teeth were polished with prophylaxis paste to remove the stain. Mesial and distal channels were prepared, and bases were inserted where necessary to protect the pulps, as outlined in the technique. Quick-curing acrylic was placed according to directions, and the section of serrated steel wire that had been cut along the diameter of the channels was inserted. Acrylic was added around the serrated steel wire. Anterior splinting was accomplished by doing first one side and then the other, and then finally connecting both sides with the serrated steel wire in the center.

Result

An esthetic type of splinting has been shown through the use of the A-splint (Figure 42.7A–E). The radiograph in Figure 42.7E show the results 5 years later. Note in Figure 42.7D and F–H the patient has also inserted her artificial interdental tissue appliance.

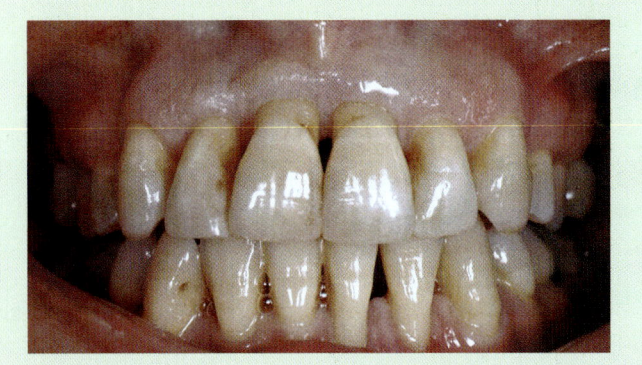

Figure 42.7 (A) This 35-year-old female was referred by the orthodontist for post-treatment anterior stabilization to avoid crowning her teeth.

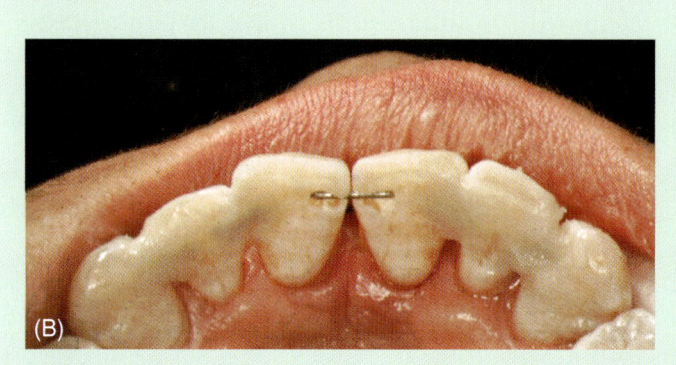

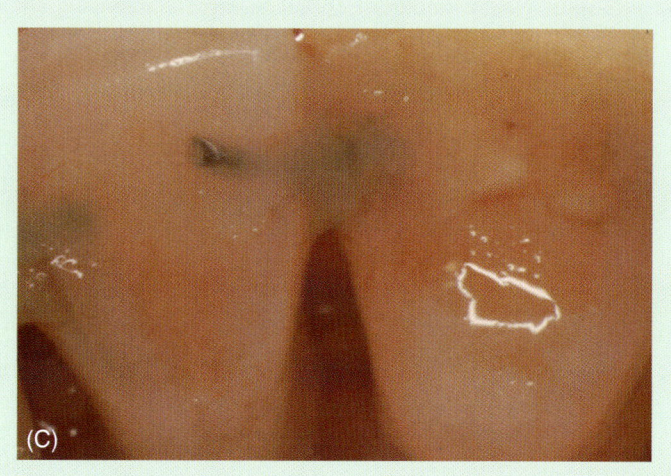

Figure 42.7 **(B, C)** Approaching from the lingual aspect, a horizontal channel at the level of the contact points was cut using a small inverted cone. A-splinting was accomplished from maxillary cuspid to cuspid to achieve a functional treatment.

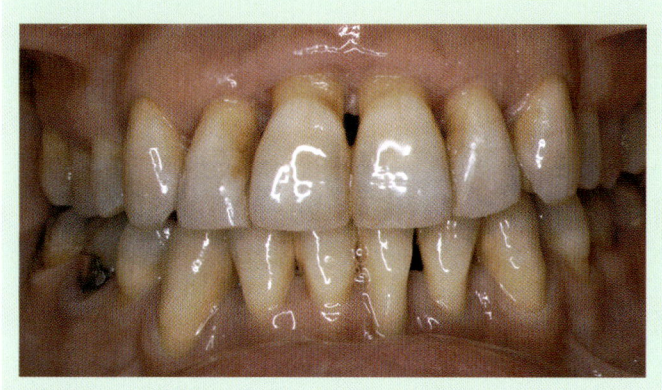

Figure 42.7 **(D)** After splinting, no evidence of the metal reinforcement can be seen.

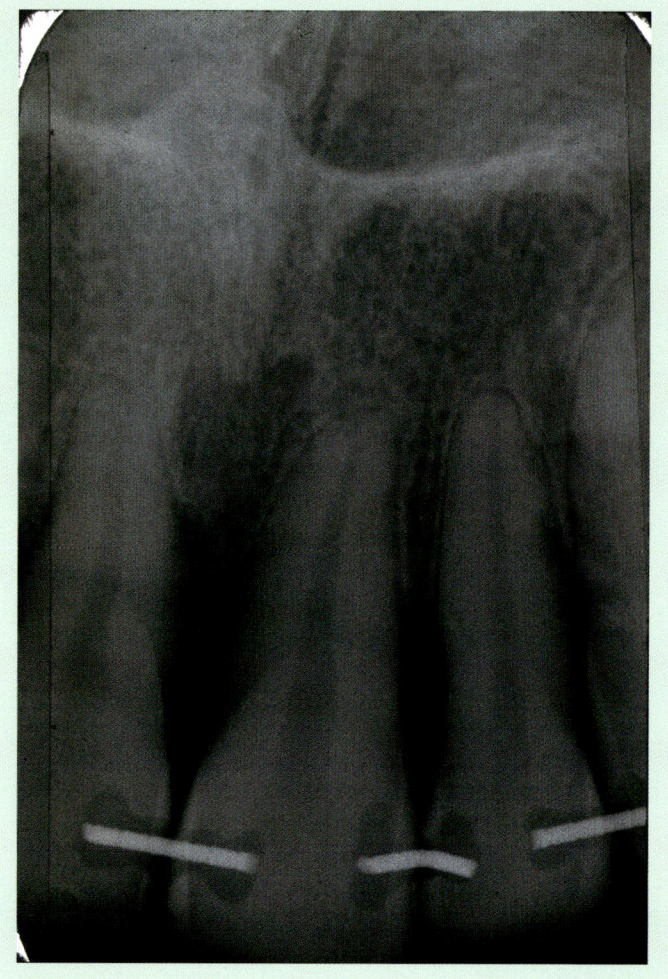

Figure 42.7 **(E)** Radiograph showing result of splinting 5 years later.

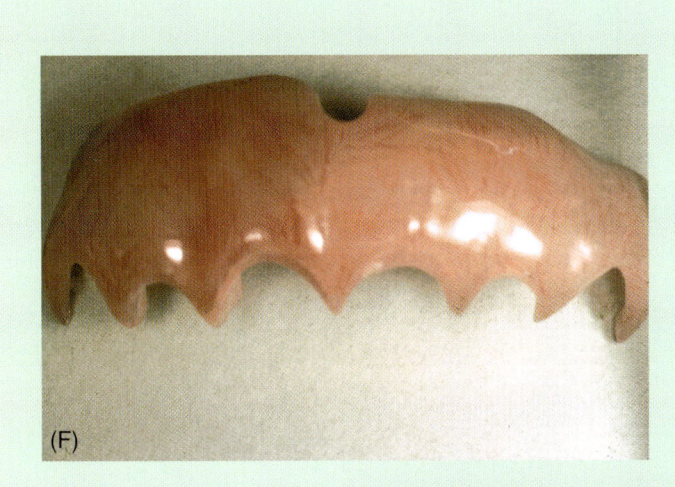

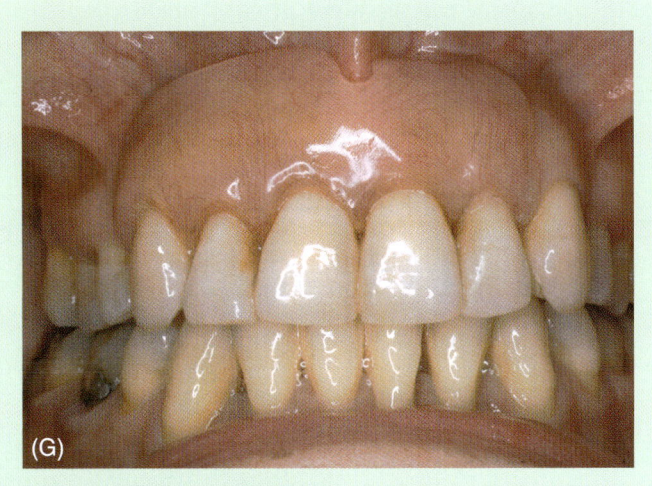

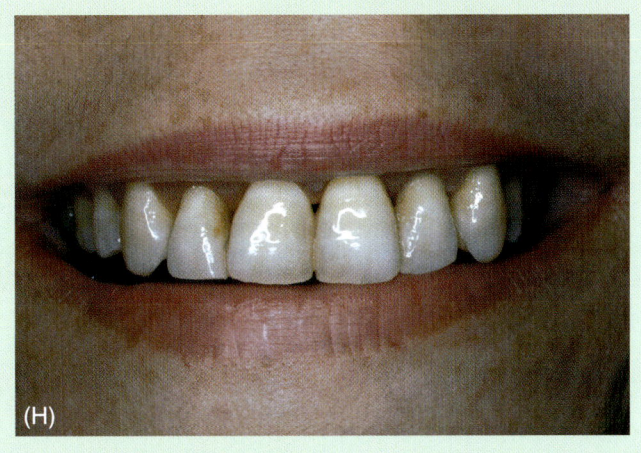

Figure 42.7 (F–H) However, the patient objected to the interdental spaces, so an artificial acrylic interdental tissue appliance was fabricated to help the patient achieve a more esthetic smile.

The following is an alternate technique:

1. After etching, coat the tooth with a bonding agent and polymerize with ultraviolet light for 30 s or use a self-etching bonding agent.
2. Place 1.5 mm of material in the floor of the channel in a preselected shade of composite resin.
3. Place the prepared wire into the channel so that it rests below the cavosurface margin. Then polymerize the material in the same manner as above for 1 min.
4. Slightly overfill the channel with additional material and polymerize again.

After the resin sets, flash is removed, and contours are restored. Special attention should be directed to the embrasure areas to assure accessibility for cleaning. Finish and polish as indicated for the particular matererial. Clinical case 42.1 illustrates the esthetic use of the A-splint.

Temporary restorations

When doing extensive 8–14 unit temporary restorations it is important to preserve the margins obtained during the impression stage, otherwise the tissue can collapse and cover the margin before you can finalize the temporary restorations. Thus, Goldstein created "The Temporary Temporary," or an immediate interim temporary restoration. To do this, first make a stone model from the original wax-up, and then make a vacuform matrix of the wax-up. Next, trim the vacuform matrix carefully, with 1 or 2 mm resting on the gingival tissue, which is necessary to obtain a good seal and to help properly seat the matrix. This step is especially helpful if the teeth have been built-up with wax, and thus not permitting a tooth-borne stop for the placement of the matrix. This matrix can also be valuable earlier as a try-in over the prepared teeth to make certain there is sufficient clearance all around.

After determining the successful fit of the matrix, use the automixing syringe to inject C-silicone material (Fit Checker, GC) into the teeth (Figure 42.8A and B), and then carefully and accurately seat the matrix over the teeth (Figure 42.8C). Wipe off the excess material and allow it to harden. It is important to not remove the interim temporary until it is time to seat the final provisional restoration(s) so it will stay in place.

With this technique, the patient not only has protection from sensitivity, but also is not toothless. Another advantage of creating a "temporary–temporary" restoration is allowing the patient to eat lunch consisting of either a soup or smoothie for nourishment while the final temporary restoration is being constructed in the laboratory. Do not underestimate the value of using a tooth-colored material, because this will be the first time the patient can visualize the new restoration (Figure 42.8D and E). The material we have found to esthetically work best for the insertion is a white vinyl polysiloxane (Fit Checker, GC America) although other manufacturers' vinyl polysiloxane material will do. The reason for preferring the white material is because it also permits the patient to see themselves with a much whiter tooth color than the final temporary shade will be. This is important because a patient who had very dark teeth may initially feel uncomfortable when they see such a bright white shade. So, using a very white shade in the interim provisional restoration helps mentally prepare the patient for the final light temporary shade. It is important to note that Fit Checker sets rapidly, so load and seat the matrix as quickly as possible. See also how accurate the margins look after removing the splint (Figure 42.8E).

A secondary function

There is another potentially valuable use for the interim temporary restoration, so be sure to save it after removal. At the try-in appointment, if there will be delay in making changes, you can place the interim temporary to maintain the gingival tissue. At the final seating of full-arch crowns or fixed partial dentures, if using a resin-modified glass ionomer cement, it is best to cement the crowns in quadrants because of the extremely rapid set time of these types of cements. The main concern with this technique is the necessity of keeping the resin-modified glass ionomer cement off the adjacent abutments, otherwise it may become difficult to fit the restorations in the adjacent segment. This step is where the interim provisional restoration has a secondary use. Cut off the segment being cemented, and place the adjacent part of the interim temporary back in place. This will protect the margin and axial walls of the remaining teeth, reduce sensitivity, and maintain the next segment so it is ready to be cemented.

Interim temporary methods construction

By far the most detailed direct method of constructing a temporary restoration that can accurately duplicate the incisal embrasures, interdental anatomy, and surface created in the wax-up is by using a Siltek® matrix. Make sure you scallop the labial edges just beyond the gingival margins to allow for easier removal. Fill the teeth to be restored with the approximate shade of composite resin and press the matrix accurately to place and wait until the matrix material sets before removal (Figure 42.9A–I).

Indirect Siltek method for implants

The Siltek matrix can also be utilized in construction of an indirect temporary restoration. This can be especially helpful in fabrication of implant temporaries (Figure 42.10A–G). When matching temporaries to adjacent natural teeth it is always best to do this indirectly (Figure 42.10G).

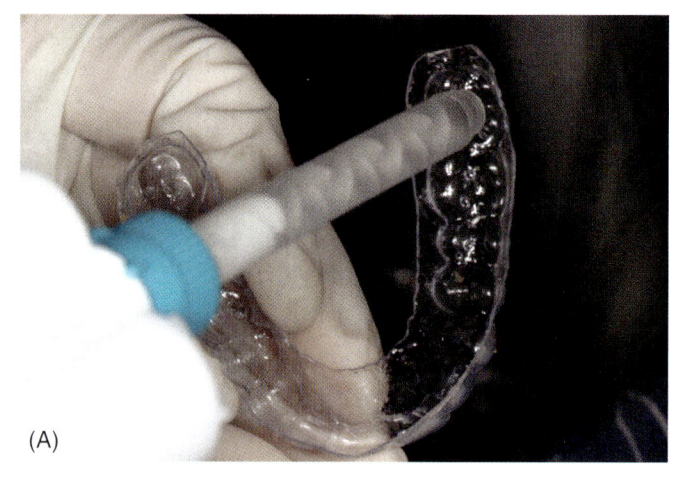

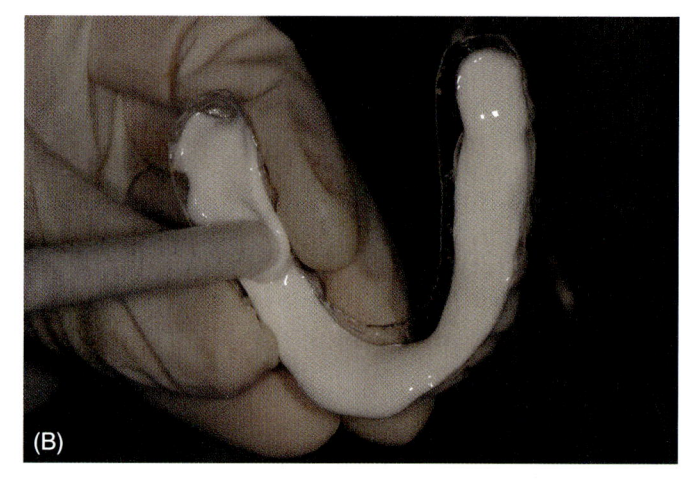

Figure 42.8 **(A, B)** Creating the "temporary-temporary" restoration. After determining the successful fit of the matrix, use the automixing syringe to inject silicone material into the vacuformed matrix.

Chapter 42 Esthetic Temporization 1325

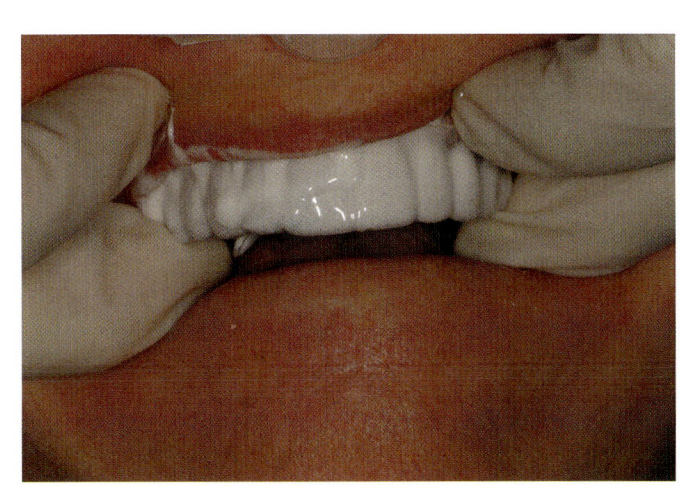

Figure 42.8 **(C)** Seat the matrix over the teeth and wipe off the excess material and allow hardening.

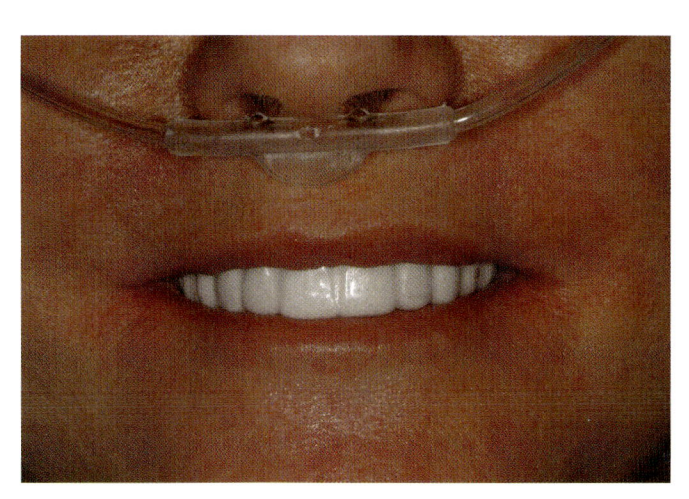

Figure 42.8 **(D)** It is important for the patient to wear the interim temporary to avoid sensitivity of teeth. Also, by using a tooth-colored material, the patient can visualize the new restorations for the first time.

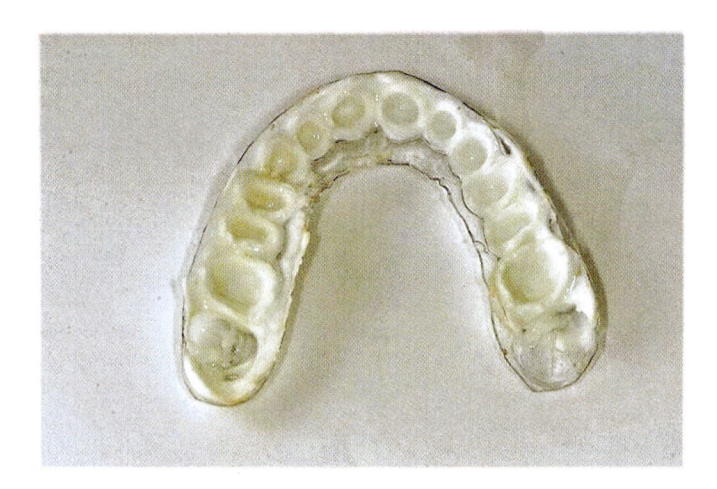

Figure 42.8 **(E)** Note how accurate the margins look after removing the matrix.

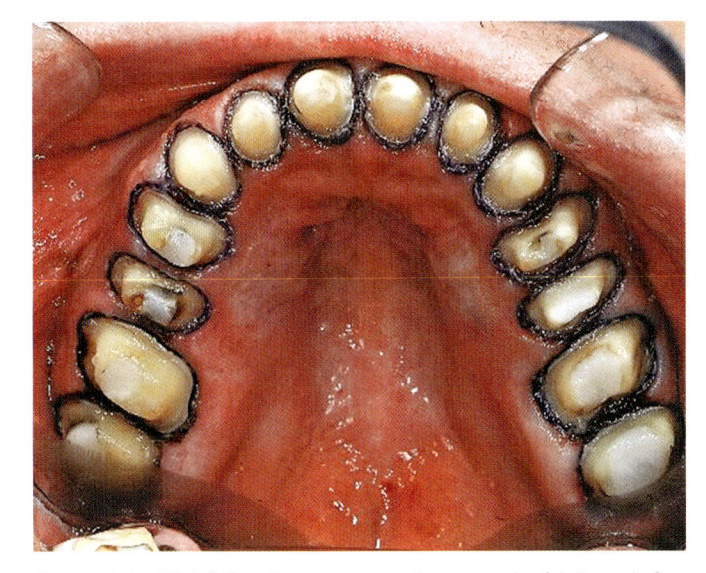

Figure 42.9 **(A)** A full-arch temporary splint was to be fabricated after making multiple polyvinyl siloxane impressions of the arch.

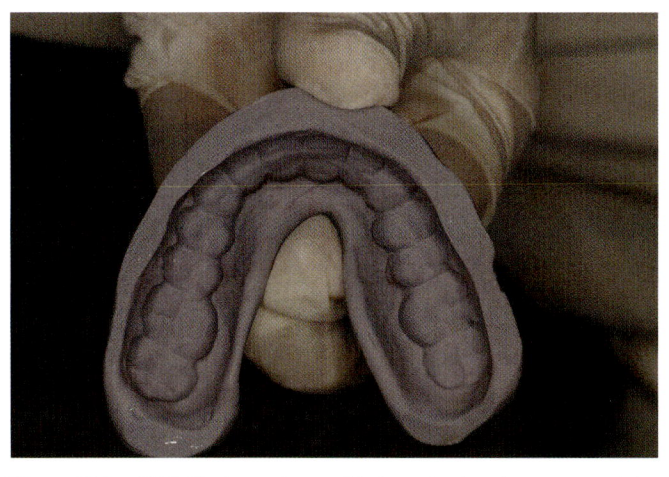

Figure 42.9 **(B)** A Siltek matrix was fabricated using the wax-up of the diagnostic models.

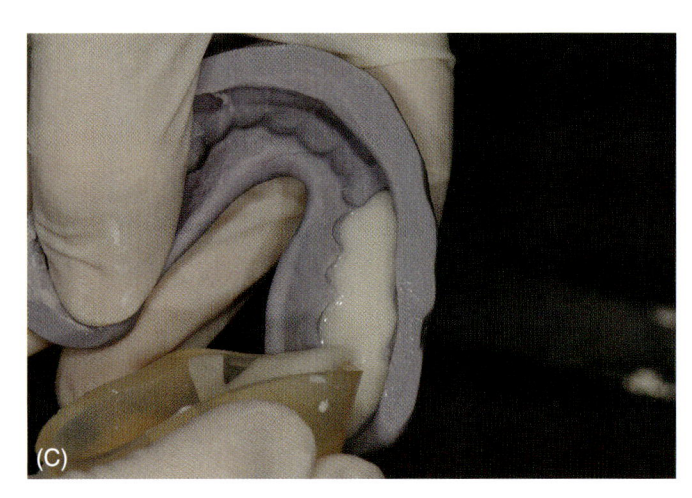

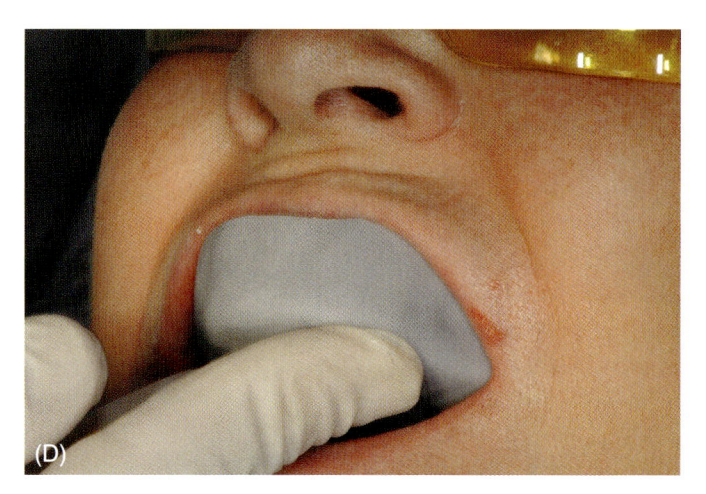

Figure 42.9 **(C, D)** Acrylic was mixed to a flowable consistency and poured into the matrix and immediately placed into the mouth for the upper right side of the preparation.

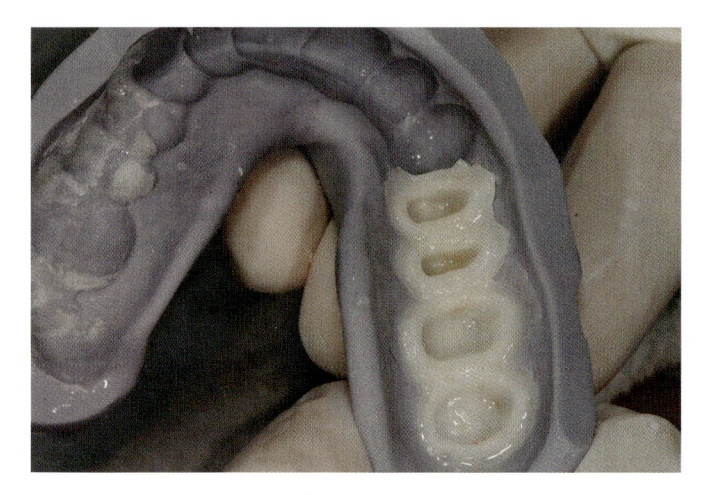

Figure 42.9 **(E)** Note the marginal accuracy as the temporary is made in separate sections.

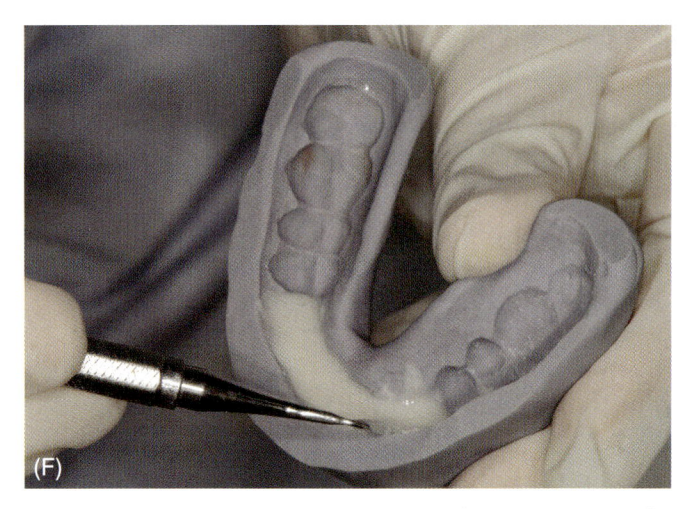

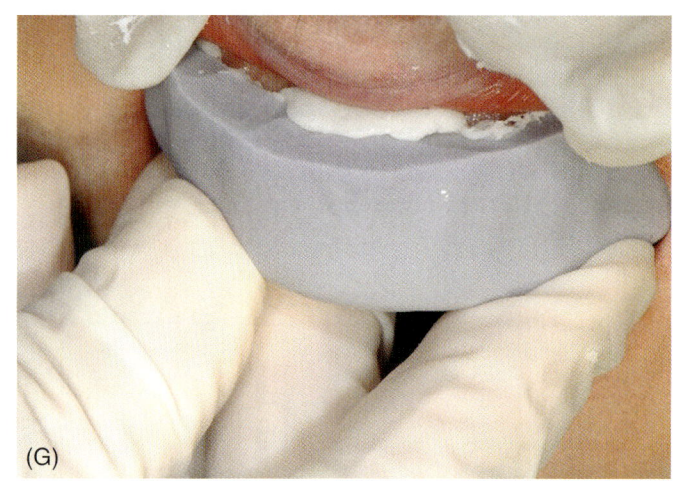

Figure 42.9 **(F, G)** Finally, the anterior section of the temporary was fabricated.

Chapter 42 Esthetic Temporization

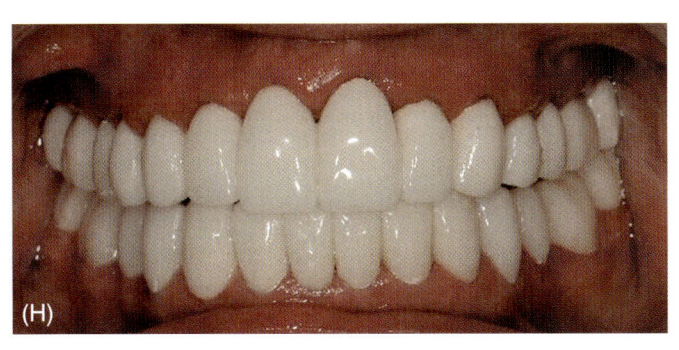

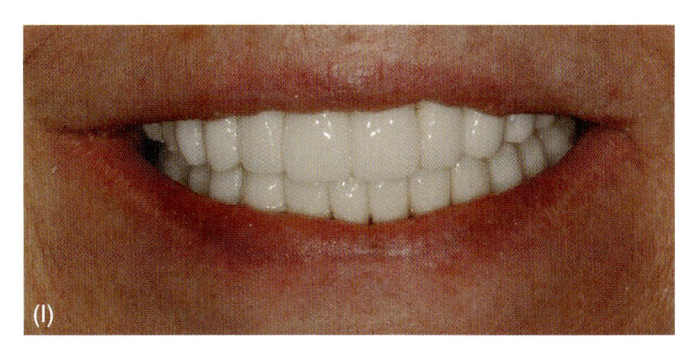

Figure 42.9 (H, I) Final result of the temporary can be seen. Note that although the gingival heights were not the same throughout the arch, this was not an esthetic concern for the patient because of her medium lip line.

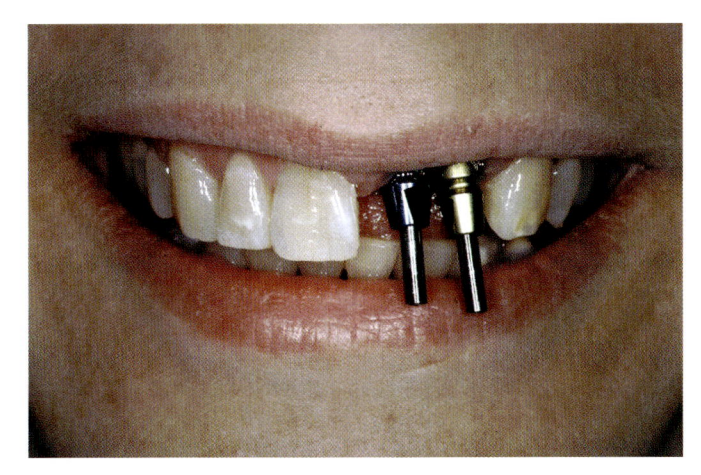

Figure 42.10 (A) After the impression copings were emplaced and fit was confirmed radiographically, an impression was taken of the two implant restorations #9 and #10.

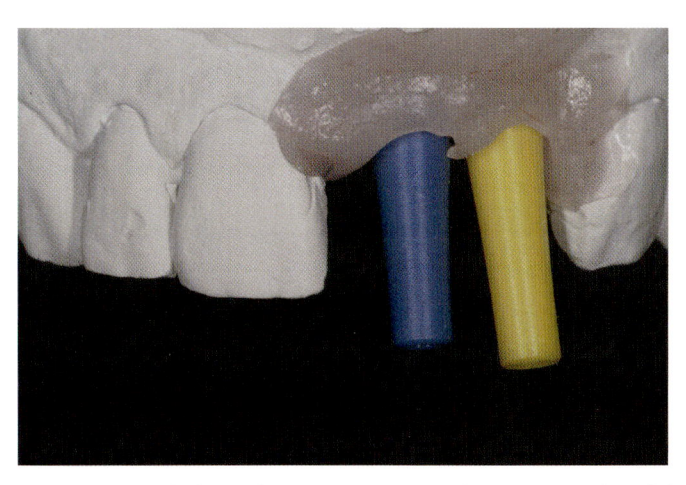

Figure 42.10 (B) Plastic sleeves were positioned on the poured model to reshape before wax-up of the casting.

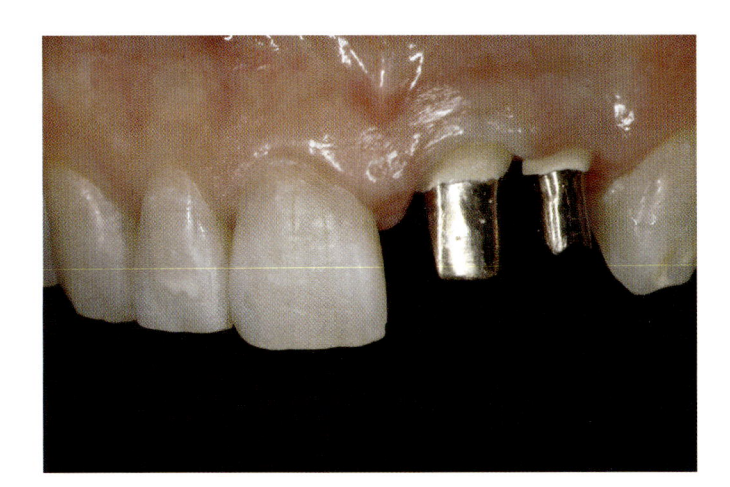

Figure 42.10 (C) Custom abutments were made with gold, metal, and subgingival porcelain margin.

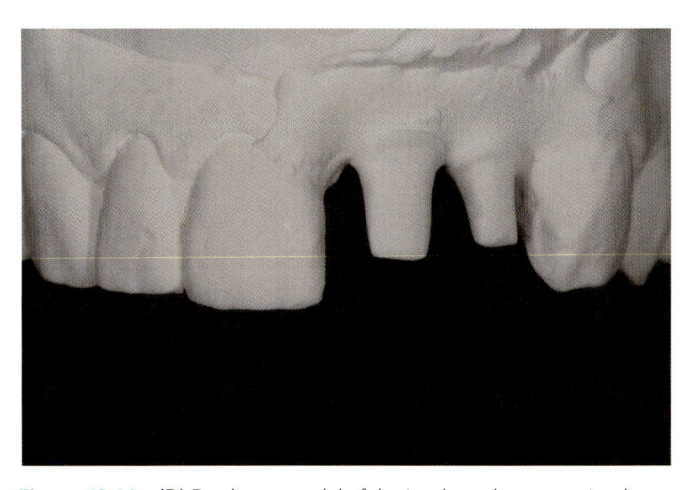

Figure 42.10 (D) Duplicate model of the implant abutments in place.

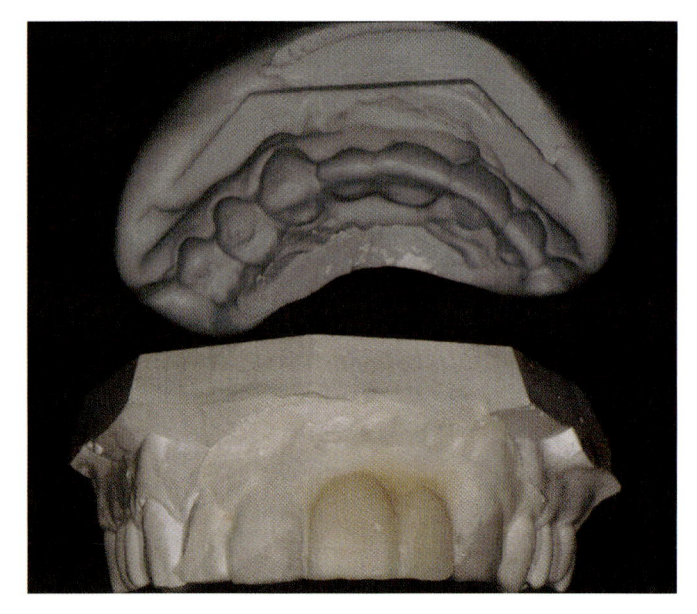

Figure 42.10 **(E)** The dentin acrylic was applied with silicone index with full contour.

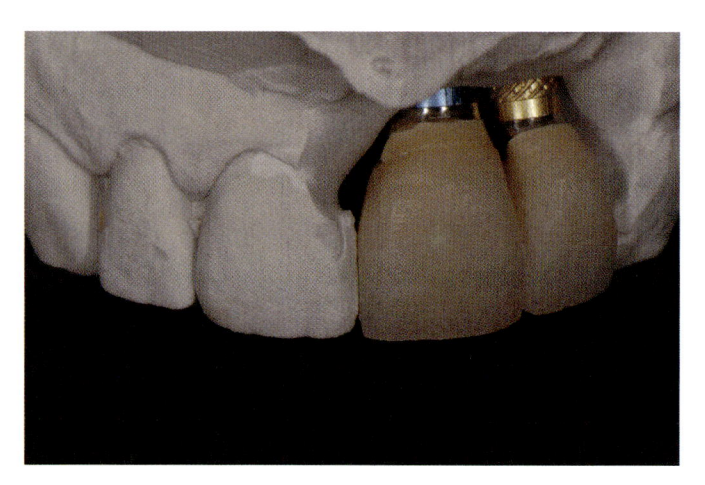

Figure 42.10 **(F)** The temporaries were tried in on the actual custom abutments to make sure the fit was accurate.

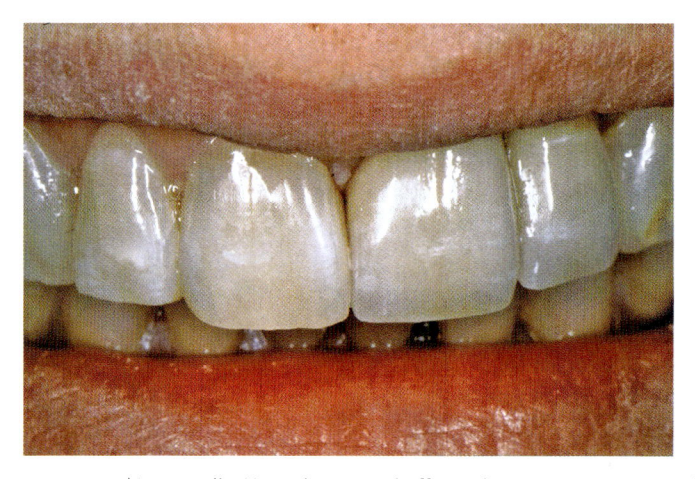

Figure 42.10 **(G)** The temporary was cemented intraorally. Note the special effects that were incorporated into the temporary for esthetic purposes.

References

1. Priest G. Esthetic potential of single-implant provisional restorations: selection criteria of available alternatives. *J Esthet Restor Dent* 2006;18(6):326–338.
2. Pound E. Controlling anomalies of vertical dimension and speech. *J Prosthet Den.* 1976;36(2):124–135.
3. Fondriest JF. Using provisional to improve results in complex esthetic restorative cases. *Dent Today* 2005;24(10):142–145.
4. Spear F. The role of temporization in interdisciplinary periodontal and orthodontic treatment. *Int Dent Aust Ed* 2001;4(3):54–64.
5. Amet EM, Phinney TL. Fixed provisional restorations for extended prosthodontic treatment. *J Oral Implantol* 1995;21:201–206.
6. Christensen GJ. Provisional restorations for fixed prosthodontics. *J Am Dent Assoc* 1996;127:249–252.
7. Donovan TE, Cho GC. Diagnostic provisional restorations in restorative dentistry: the blueprint for success. *J Can Dent Assoc* 1999;65:272–275.
8. Chiche GJ. Provisional restorations in anterior procedures. *Dent Today* 1994;13:32, 34–37.
9. Pound E. Let "S" be your guide. *J Prosthet Dent* 1977;8(5):482–489.

Additional resources

Alt V, Hannig M, Wöstmann B, Balkenhol M. Fracture strength of temporary fixed partial dentures: CAD/CAM versus directly fabricated restorations. *Dent Mater* 2011;27:339–347.

Balkenhol M, Mauntner MC, Ferger P, Wöstmann B. Mechanical properties of provisional crown and bridge materials: chemical-curing versus dual-curing systems. *J Dent* 2008;36:15–20.

Donovan TE, Cho GC. Diagnostic provisional restorations in restorative dentistry: the blueprint for success. *J Can Dent Assoc* 1999;65:272–275.

Goldstein RE. A simple technique to create an interim provisional restoration. *Inside Dent* 2008;4(5).

Gürel G, Bichacho N. Permanent diagnostic provisional restorations for predictable results when redesigning the smile. *Pract Proced Aesthet Dent* 2006;18:281–286.

Reshad M, Cascione D, Kim T. Anterior provisional restorations used to determine form, function, and esthetics for complex restorative situations, using all-ceramic restorative systems. *J Esthet Restor Dent* 2010;22:7–16.

Romano R, Bichacho N, Touati B. *The Art of the Smile*. London: Quintessence; 2005.

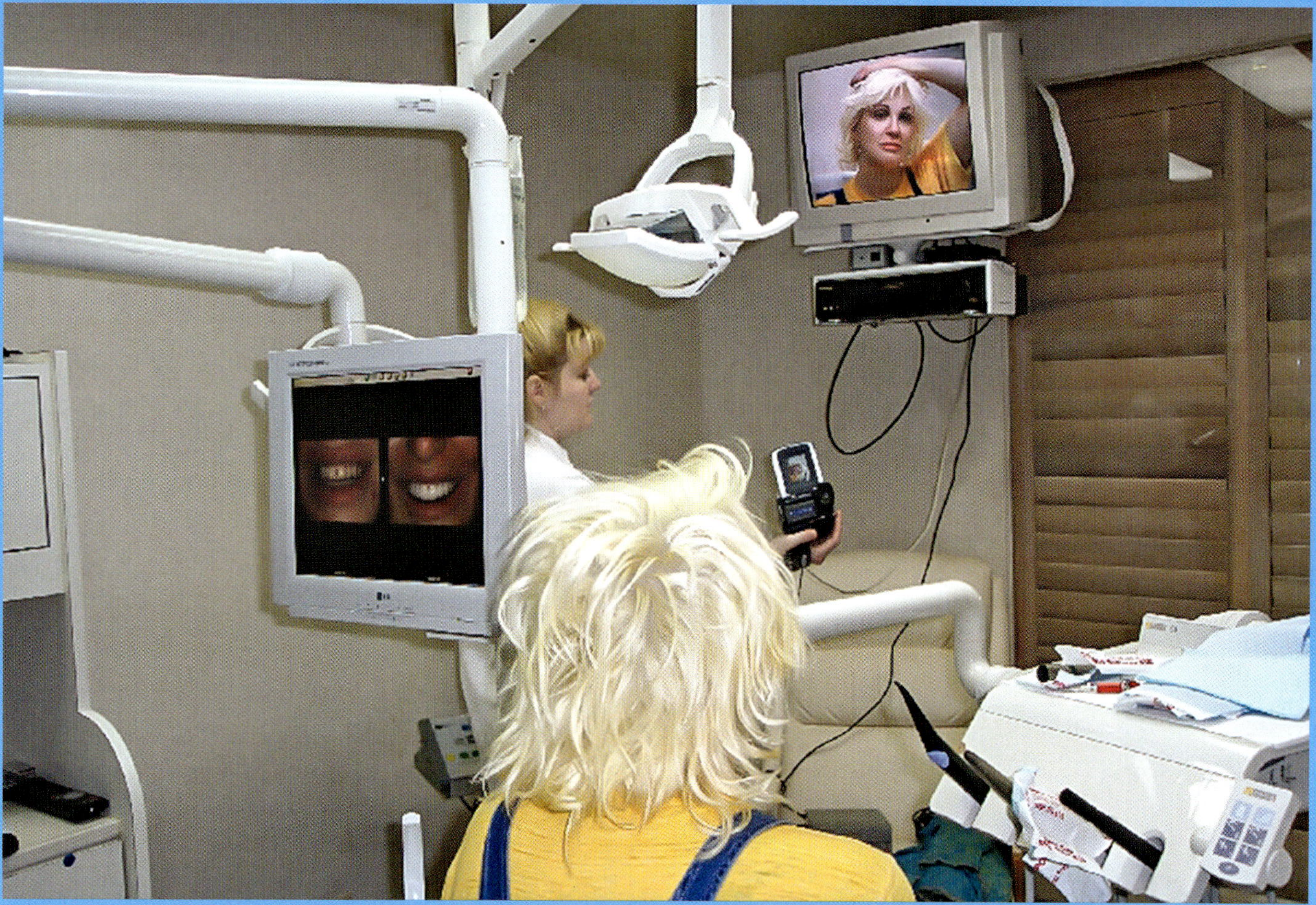

Chapter 43 The Esthetic Try-In

Ronald E. Goldstein, DDS and Carolina Arana, DMD, MPH

Chapter Outline

Initial visualization	1332
Stable occlusal relationship	1332
Adjuncts in therapy and esthetic determination	1332
Try-in with additional viewpoints	1332
Trial smile	1332
Technique for patient direct viewing of restorations	1332
Indirect viewing	1336
Indications for additional appointment time	1336
Communication for a better esthetic result	1337
Written statement of approval	1337
Try-in principles for fixed restorations	1339
Initial evaluation of delivered case prior to chairside approval	1339
Chairside appointment prior to insertion	1339
Principles for the esthetic try-in	1341
Shaping	1347
Contours for characterization, light reflection, and proper texture	1350

The try-in appointment makes the difference between average and excellent esthetic results. Esthetic objectives should be determined long before this appointment so as many as possible can be incorporated into the restoration in the laboratory. The remainder are added during the try-in appointment. The main reason for spending so much time during the temporary phase is to avoid major changes during this final part of the treatment. Having to make major changes at the ceramic try-in stage is time consuming, costly, and counterproductive. However, there is no doubt there will be times when, despite everything you have done to satisfy their esthetic demands, your patient may suddenly insert a set of new ones at the esthetic try-in appointment. Most times, it will occur with patients who have a difficult time making up their mind about what they really like.

The best way to avoid having a frustrating time at the try-in is not to eliminate any step in the systematic process of esthetically pleasing your patient:

- Step 1: Diagnosis. Use esthetic imaging to visually show the patients how their new smile can look both close up and full face.
- Step 2: Waxing on models and/or composite resin to "mock up" in the mouth when possible. A direct mock-up technique serves as an effective communication tool between you, the patient, and the lab technician. A limitation can be a patient with a maxillary protrusion.
- Step 3: Trial smile.
- Step 4: Making sure your temporary restorations incorporate all the changes you and your patient anticipate in tooth shape, size, color, and arch alignment.
- Step 5: Have your patients "sign off" in the folder after they are satisfied with their new "temporary" smile and then again after the final try-in is accepted.

Patient communication and good records that include shade and esthetic evaluation information sheets all help to attain this objective.

Patient involvement is an essential part of the esthetic treatment process. In a study of 40 denture patients by Hirsch et al.,[1] the crucial variable was patient involvement, rather than the esthetic quality of the denture. The authors found that patients respond more favorably to dentures when they are involved in the selection than when the dentist acts as the authoritarian.

Initial visualization

It is vital that the patient be able to visualize as closely as possible the restoration as it will appear in the final form. This is especially true if you are trying-in ceramic restorations.

Stable occlusal relationship

Regardless of which articulator is used, an occlusion balanced in all movements must be established before the esthetic try-in. This will keep further refinement of the occlusion to a minimum. The closer to perfection the occlusion can be, the sooner you can get to what the patient may be most concerned about: the final esthetics. Remember, the patient will usually begin to judge your treatment based on how the restoration feels to the tongue, the tissues, and the bite. The closer you can arrive at a perfect occlusion the more confidence the patient may have in your ability to satisfy their esthetic requirement.

Adjuncts in therapy and esthetic determination

Try-in with additional viewpoints

Depending on the patient's need, consultation with another person at the try-in appointment is always advisable and often necessary. This is especially important for patients who have difficulty making decisions. Failure to recognize your patient's need for an extra pair of eyes by the person they trust most can result in later problems.

Even if your patient signs the approval form, the disapproval comments by a trusted family member can result in a patient's dissatisfaction with the esthetics. However, sometimes it is unavoidable. Some years ago an elderly woman came in for a new maxillary denture by one of my (Goldstein) associates. However, I consulted on the case because esthetics was of high importance to this lady. Each appointment she was accompanied by her daughter who helped with the esthetic decisions. At the final try-in, several hours were spent fine-tuning all the esthetic changes the patient requested and the denture was processed. Both mother and daughter were extremely pleased, especially since the new tooth arrangement made the elderly grandmother look about 15 years younger. Everything was fine until she went back to her home, which was about 1500 miles from Atlanta. When she got off the plane her son-in-law said "What did you do to yourself?" His negative comments were so hurtful that she eventually sent the dentures back and had another office duplicate the older version of her tooth arrangement to please her son-in-law. Regardless of the reasons for his negative and degrading comments, the important lesson in this case is to make sure you have the right person with your patient to help them make a decision everyone can live with.

I had another patient who had such difficulty making a final esthetic decision that I ended the try-in session and requested she come back with her two daughters whose opinions she valued. Most of the time, the extra people give your patient the confidence that the right esthetic decision is being made.

Trial smile

The purpose of the trial smile is to let the patient live with your intended esthetic arrangements and shade. This can help in so many ways since your patient can have sufficient time to let many friends and relatives hopefully approve or make constructive comments so your esthetic try-in will be a much easier and successful appointment.

Young patients usually require a parent's advice and reassurance. When others accompany the patient, insert the restoration temporarily to allow time for critical evaluation and possible changes. Never rush your patient's decision making. Another person's view can be most helpful, because esthetics is an individual determination.[2] The appearance of the teeth is influenced by individual preferences and cultures; therefore, the opinions of these friends may be quite valid, and by sharing in esthetic considerations they also will share the responsibility for the esthetic result.[3] Explain to the patient that these other opinions assist in achieving the very best result. It is also advisable to have this friend or relative present during shade and shape determination to help further define the patient's wishes and esthetic expectations. Remember, this "friend" or relative will probably be the very first person who your patient will go to for esthetic approval, so it is crucial to get that approval before final cementation when only minimal changes may be able to occur.

It is a mistake to assume that because your patient says they make their own decisions that others' opinions do not matter. They almost always do! One of the best types of trial smiles for patients who do have problems making esthetic decisions is the "snap on smile" (Figure 43.1A–D).

Technique for patient direct viewing of restorations

After insertion and viewing in the sitting or reclining position (Figure 43.2A and B), ask the patient to stand and view the restoration in a full- or half-length mirror (Figure 43.2C). Patients will tend to stand further away from a large mirror at first, which is important for them to see the restoration in proper perspective. Observe the patient standing so that you can see how the teeth appear to others when the patient is speaking (Figure 43.2D). Teeth that are flared out labially may appear to be shorter than they actually are—especially in a tall individual. Conversely, a short person with flared-out teeth may appear as if their teeth are too long. Therefore, it is important to correct poor tooth position during the tooth preparation stage. You should also realize that if gold occlusal surfaces are to be used they would also be more visible on the lower bicuspids and molars of short people, whereas in tall persons the upper arch will be more visible. It is much wiser to have a discussion of all-ceramic or porcelain versus gold occlusals at the planning stage rather than have an unhappy patient after crowns are inserted.

Chapter 43 The Esthetic Try-In

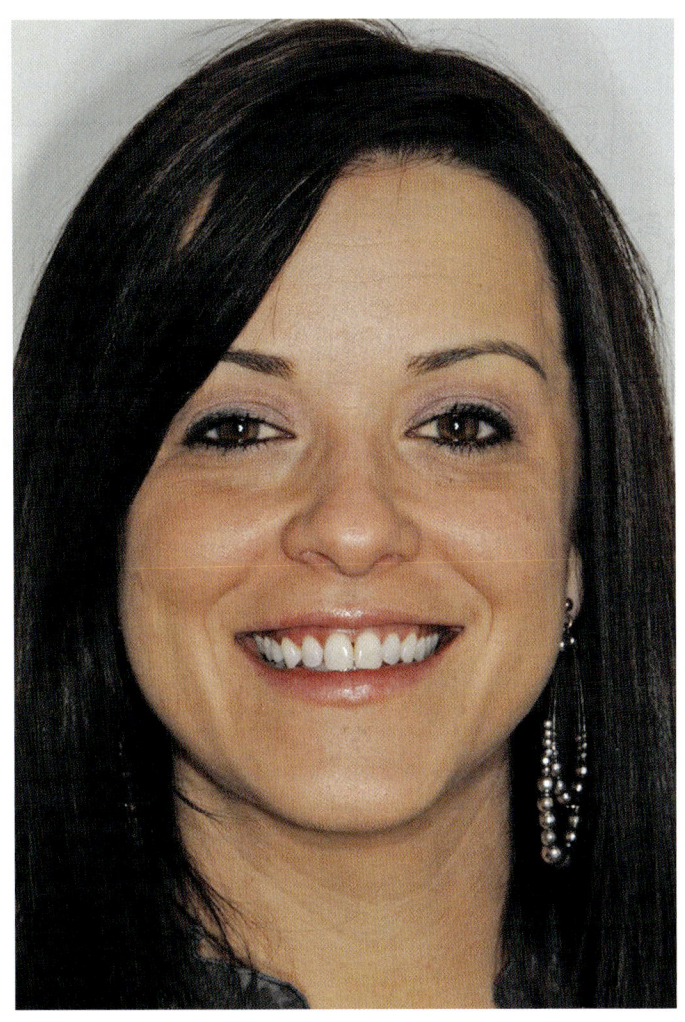

Figure 43.1 **(A)** This lady felt her smile was not prominent enough for her face and wanted to improve it if possible with porcelain veneers. However, she wanted to make sure she would like the final result before committing to treatment.

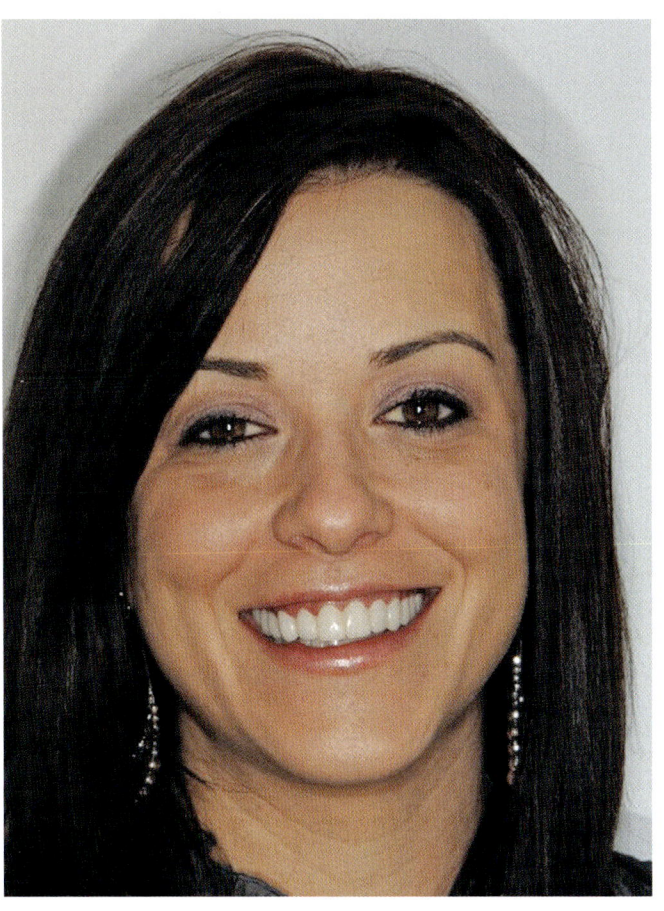

Figure 43.1 **(B)** An extended-wear trial smile appliance (Snap-On Smile, DenMat) was made to allow her to wear it so others could also help her in evaluating what the new smile could look like.

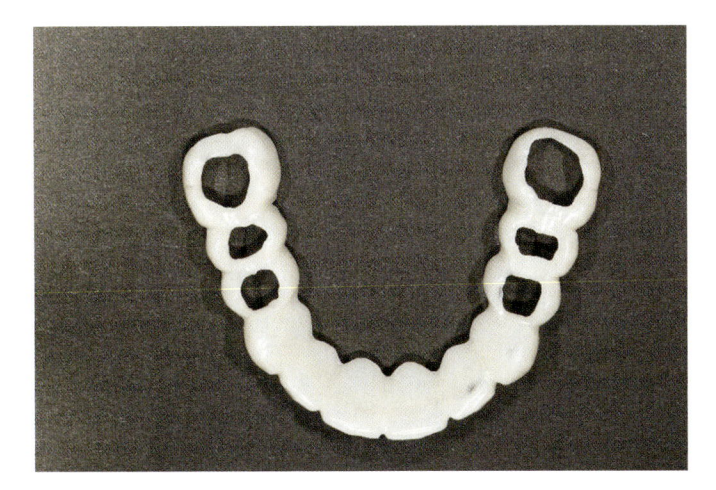

Figure 43.1 **(C)** The appliance with cutouts to fit over the existing teeth.

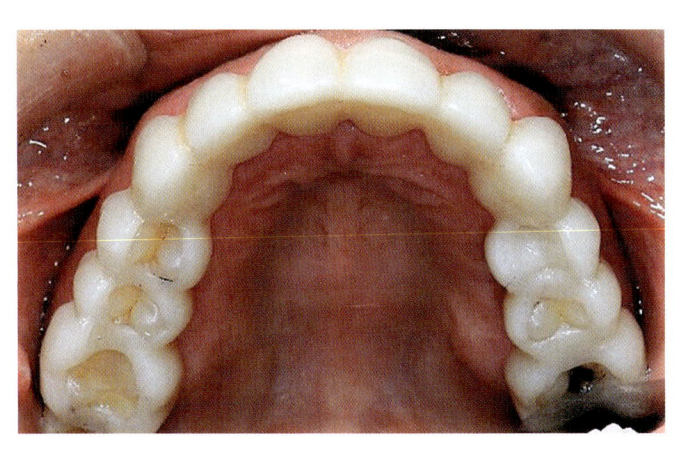

Figure 43.1 **(D)** This image shows how precise the appliance fits over the teeth so the patient can securely keep it in place and even eat with it.

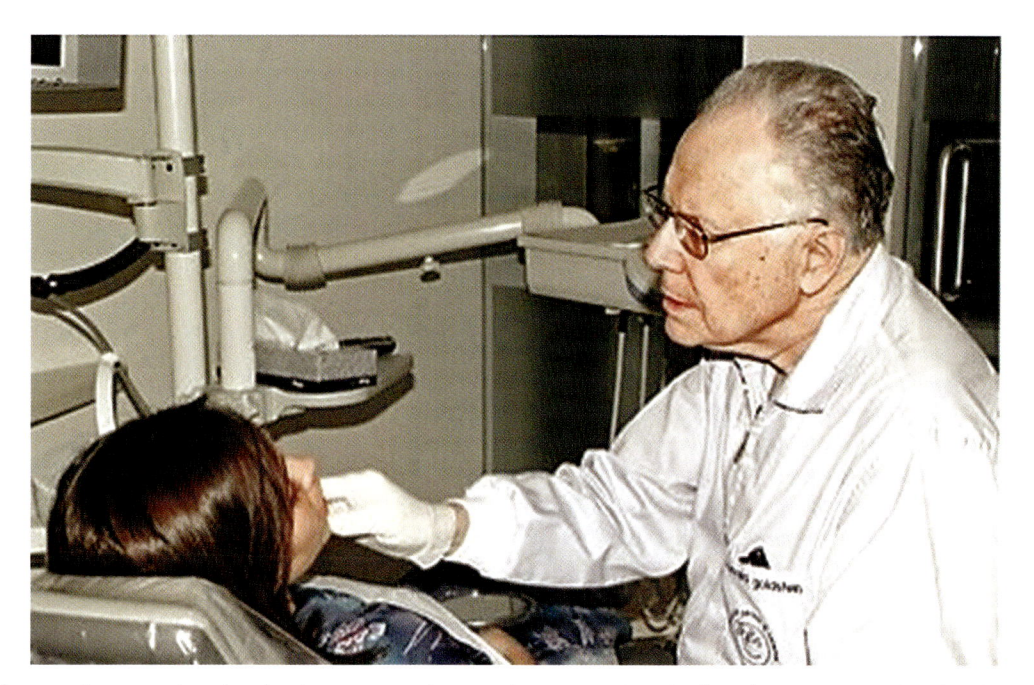

Figure 43.2 (A) The most frequent view that dentists use to evaluate patient restorations is when the patient is reclined in the chair.

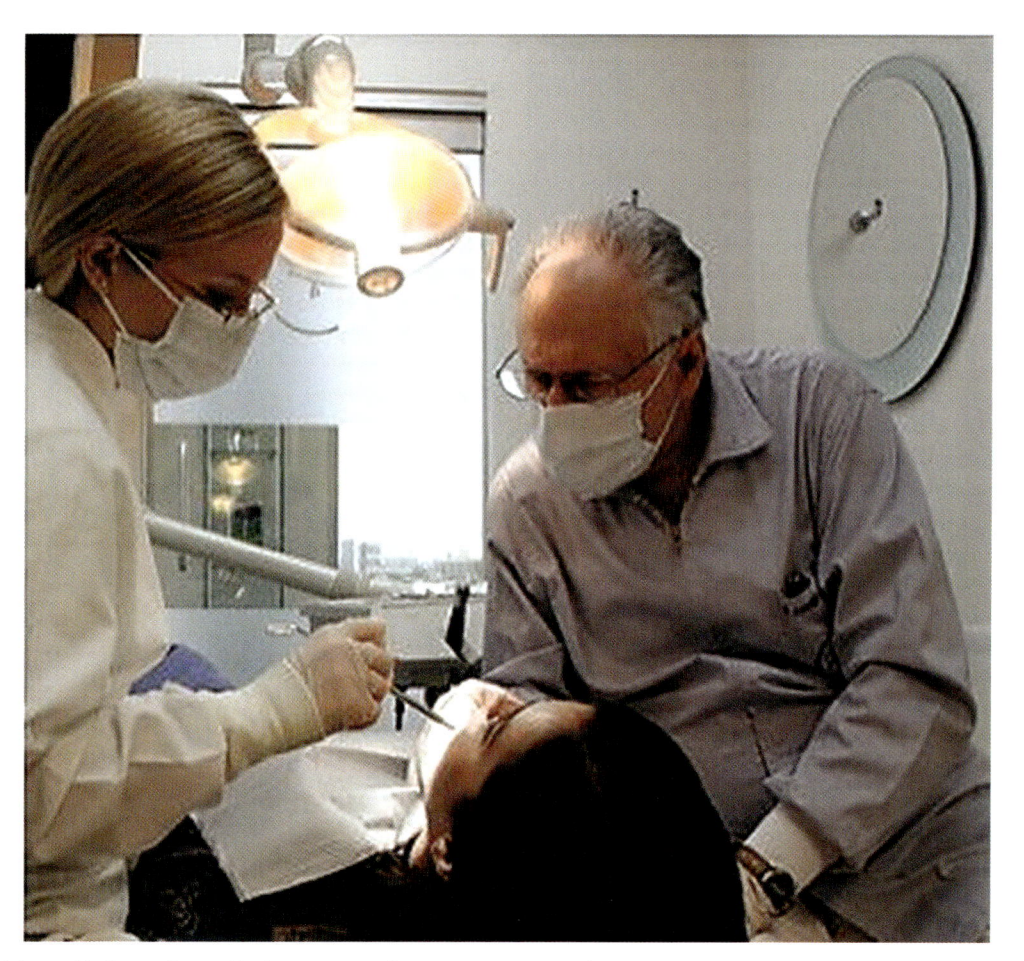

Figure 43.2 (B) Additional help is achieved by having input from your assistant, who can see the restoration from a different view.

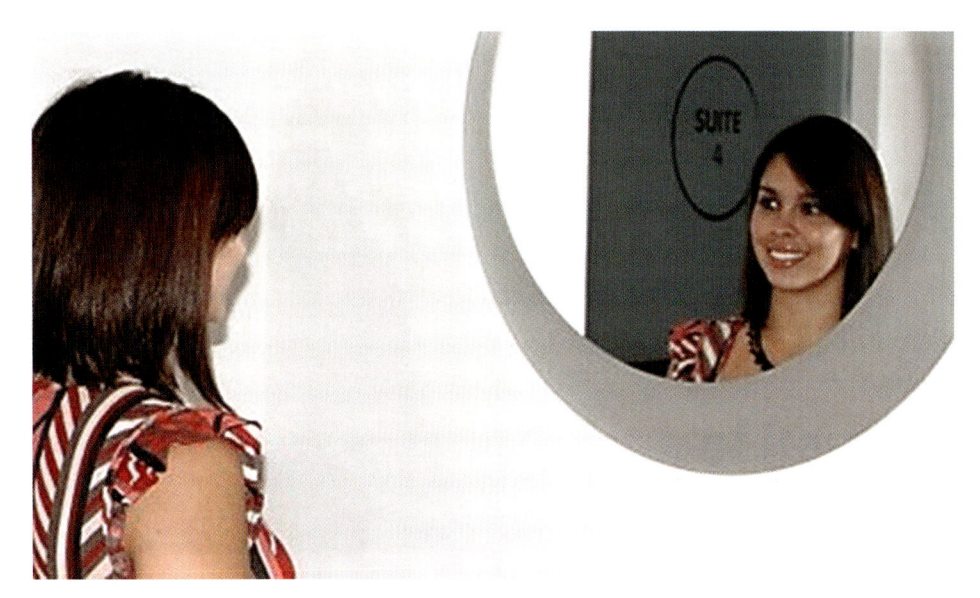

Figure 43.2 **(C)** It is best for the patients to always view the restoration in a large fixed mirror while standing, so they can observe the smile as it will appear to others.

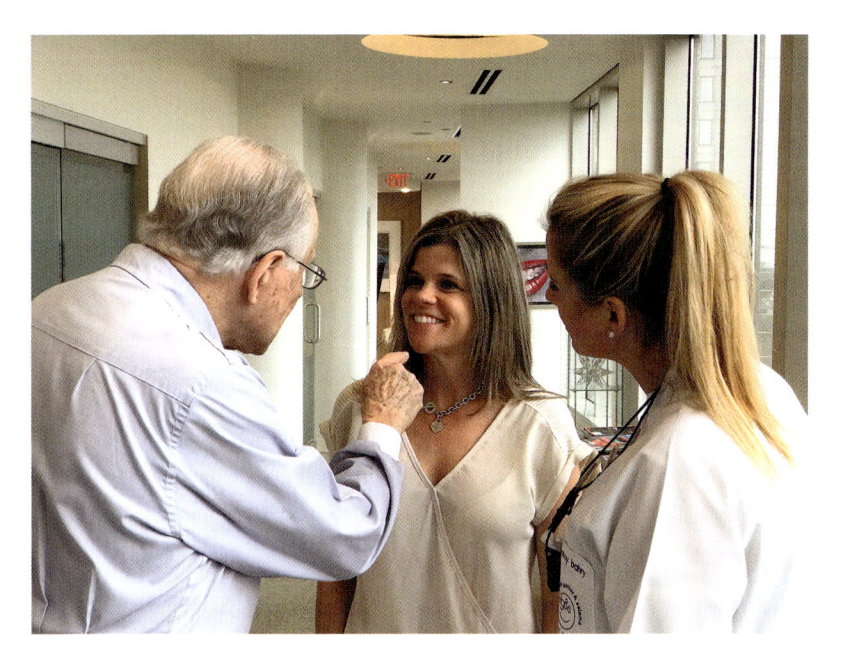

Figure 43.2 **(D)** You and your assistant should also observe the patient's smile in a standing position to see it as others will view it.

Viewing at different angles. A full-length mirror allows the patient to be viewed at different angles and positions. Observe the patient in front of and also in the mirror. Viewing the patient only in the dental chair may present a more unnatural view than would normally be observed. The size and position of the mirror can have a major effect at this stage. A small hand mirror is ill-advised, since it does not allow a view of the restoration in relation to the entire face (Figure 43.2E). While the patient is in the dental chair, use a large, clean mirror rather than a small close-up mirror. Judging a new smile should always be done in proper perspective. First impressions are so important for patient acceptance, as well as proper orientation. We want patients to visualize themselves as others will see them, and few, if any, will isolate your patient's smile as most patients do by holding a hand mirror so close that only the lips and teeth show. So ask your patient to hold the mirror at arm's length to attain the proper perspective.

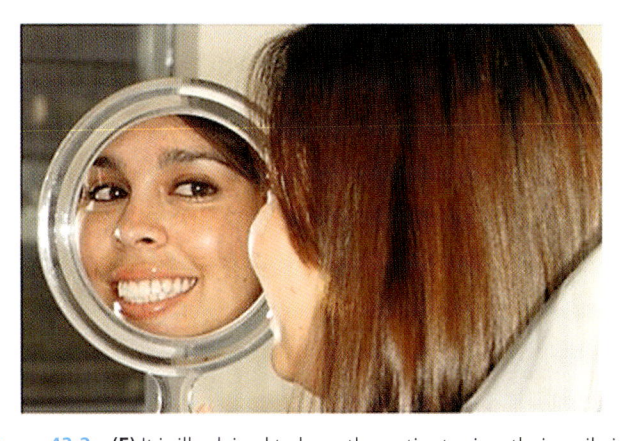

Figure 43.2 **(E)** It is ill-advised to have the patients view their smile in a small hand mirror as this does not allow a view of the restoration in relation to the entire face.

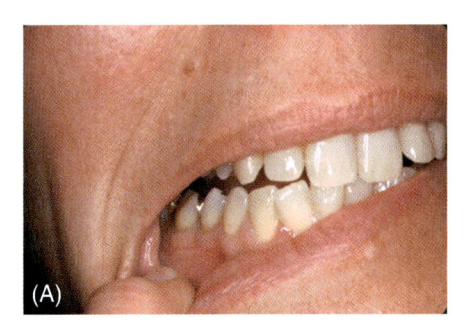

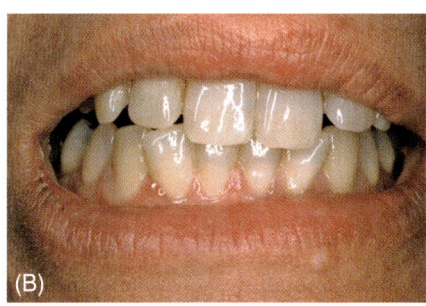

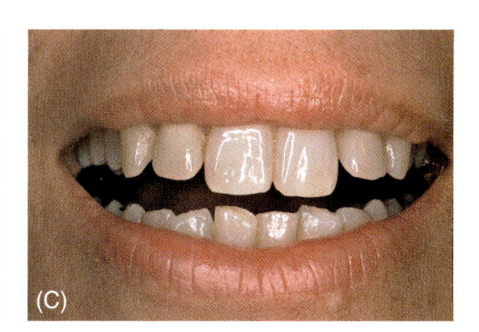

Figure 43.3 **(A, B)** Warn the patient about pulling the lip or viewing the restoration in an unnatural or strained position. **(C)** The proper method is to have the patient smile as wide as possible, but naturally.

Viewing esthetic improvement. With the full-or half-length mirror, the entire face may be observed and the role the new restoration plays in any facial improvement can easily be seen. At this point, most patients get too close to the mirror; therefore, warn them beforehand that extreme scrutiny is generally used only by the dentist and the patient and to hold the mirror at arm's length to get the view seen by others. They may be judging an effect that will never be noticed by anyone else. Remind the patient that most people observe them at a distance of approximately 1 m or more. At shorter distances the mouth is less noticeable, because eye-to-eye contact is usually maintained.

Avoid viewing with unnatural lip positions. Pulling the lip away or holding it in an unnatural or strained position merely to expose the cervical portion of the tooth allows improper and unnatural lighting effects (Figure 43.3A and B) that give an unrealistic view of the esthetic effect. Warn the patient of this before you allow them to see the restoration. The proper method is to tell the patient to smile as wide as possible, but naturally (Figure 43.3C). Explain that the incisal portion of a crown can appear drastically different with and without lip shadowing and may also vary with the position of the patient's head as well as the lighting condition. Using different light sources will influence the analysis of the optical behavior of natural and artificial dentition.[4] Viewing from a direct-angle illumination, such as a unit light, will create a different effect than an overhead light source. Allow the patient to view the restoration with frontal, overhead, and side lighting. Natural light should also be used to compare the shade with artificial light, even if your artificial lighting is "color corrected."

Indirect viewing

There are two easy methods for allowing the patient to see themselves as others see them (since a mirror view reverses the patient's image): still digital photography and digital video.

Still digital photography

For most patients, seeing a two-dimensional photograph of their smile will be extremely helpful in evaluating a new smile (Figure 43.4A). Since looking in the mirror becomes a three-dimensional view, outline form is more difficult to discern. Instead, a digital photograph loaded into a chairside monitor or even a monitor in another room allows both you and your patient to better see silhouette form (Figure 43.4B). You will get an idea of the amount of incisal showing and gingival display, both features that influence the esthetics and design of the new smile. You should also take multiple views so your patient can see lateral and profile smiling views. Both full-face and close-up views should be taken to let your patient feel comfortable with their new look. Conversely, if there are potential changes your patient wants to be made, now is the best time to make them.

Another advantage of immediate digital photography is the ability of making your patient's desired potential changes in the computer image first rather than altering the porcelain. For instance, if your patient feels that the teeth may be too long it is a lot easier shortening the imaged teeth first to make certain the patient really does like the shorter version better. We have found using this technique has saved valuable time and costly laboratory remakes. Plus, we utilize these views to help us and our ceramist obtain the best esthetic result. Generally, one should retake new digital photos after each correction so that the patient will feel that, together, esthetic success has been achieved.

Digital video

Digital video can be extremely helpful to patients who are public speakers or television, stage, or movie performers (Figure 43.5). This is really the best way to show them not only how they will look when talking or smiling but also how they sound when speaking or even singing. Continue to use digital video after each correction, since the visual result can change. This way your patient will feel much more confident with their new look.

A good digital video camera need not be expensive and can be played immediately by just connecting it to your monitor. However, both still photograph and video viewing can take considerable extra time, and you need to consider this before you calculate your fee for treatment. Patients must know that this is part of the extra esthetic treatment that no insurance plan could possibly cover!

Indications for additional appointment time

If there is lingering doubt in the patient's mind regarding appearance, a second try-in appointment should be arranged. Sometimes it takes one or more additional appointments at intervals that allow the patient to discuss the new appearance and hear a critique from members of the family. Multiple

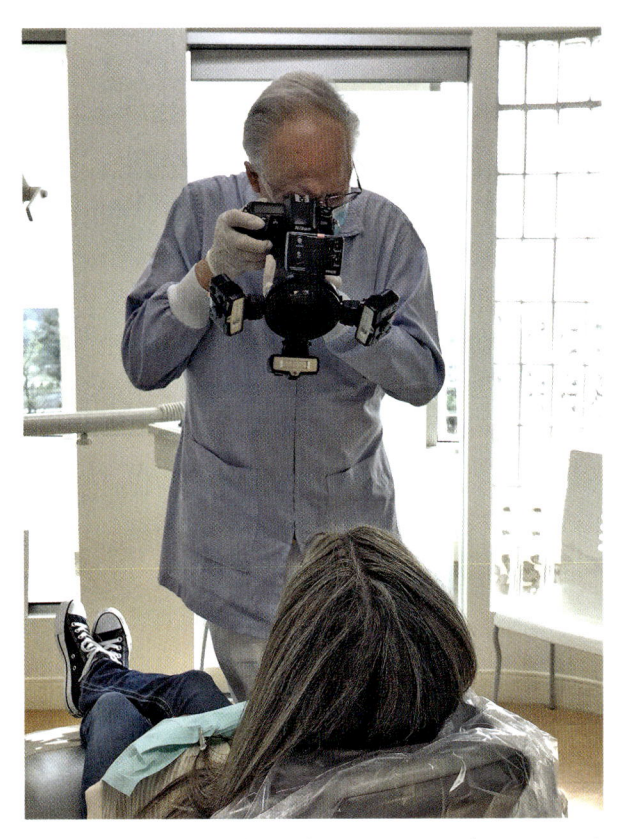

Figure 43.4 **(A)** Use a good digital camera to record your patient's close-up and full-face smile so that you both can observe it in two dimensions.

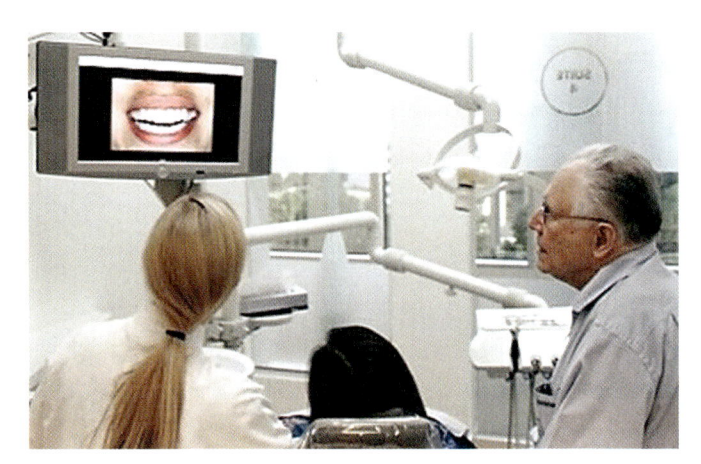

Figure 43.4 **(B)** Seeing the patient's smile on your chairside monitor makes it much easier for you and your patient to see the shapes of the teeth in silhouette form.

appointments means additional time, and providing this extra service is necessarily more costly; nevertheless, if you desire to please your patient, you must be willing to make the necessary time available. Remember, not all patients are alike. Some will need two or three times the try-in time before they are willing to sign off on the first try-in. Any dentist interested in obtaining superior esthetic results must allow enough extra time to fit restorations, position teeth, properly balance the occlusion, and so on. Sufficient time should also be available to carve and reshape the restoration to suit the patient's personality and esthetic needs. This may require several appointments, remaking the restorations, or possibly altering the tooth preparation if desired results are not forthcoming, but the solution of a specific esthetic problem is a personal challenge to be met. Obviously, if you can predict the amount of extra time that your patient will require, you can and should adjust your fee appropriately.

Communication for a better esthetic result

Communication is an essential element of treatment. Your expectations should be clarified early to obtain approval at the try-in appointment by using written reports, letters, and evaluation charts. Superior esthetic laboratory service also depends upon continuous, accurate communication among the dentist, patient, and technician. Through effective communication, the patient gains confidence in the dental team and better understands the proposed restorative treatment. When a patient presents with challenging esthetic problems it is always best to arrange a joint consultation that should include your ceramist. Communication between ceramist and patient can be an important step in determining many factors, such as type of restoration, color, and esthetic desires. Hearing the patient's concerns first hand can be invaluable, especially when the patient has a difficult time communicating what they want.

If an "in person" consultation is not possible, consider e-mailing your ceramist sufficient digital pictures, or even an interview and clinical esthetic exam video, to let them see firsthand what problems will need to be solved, and to better help you help your patient by joint communication using Skype (Figure 43.6). The most successful dental esthetics comes from a thorough analysis and accurate interpretation of the sex, personality, and age considerations of each patient. Better esthetic control of factors at the try-in appointment can be gained by careful use of an esthetic checklist to be utilized after fit and occlusion have been established. The checklist in Box 43.1 has been elaborated for a patient from a two-page spread in *Change Your Smile*.[5] It is so important for your patient to help esthetically judge their new restoration from every factor during the try-in so that any remaining problems or compromises can be explained and dealt with at this visit.

Written statement of approval

It is a good idea to have the patient sign off at the try-in stage before proceeding to the final glaze. However, patients should always sign a written statement of approval when they are satisfied with their appearance at the try-in. Emphasis should be placed on concern for satisfaction, and patients should never be pressured or hurried. Continually emphasize that treatment will not progress until everyone involved is satisfied with the appearance of the restoration. When this is accomplished, ask the patient to sign a statement of approval, which goes into the chart,

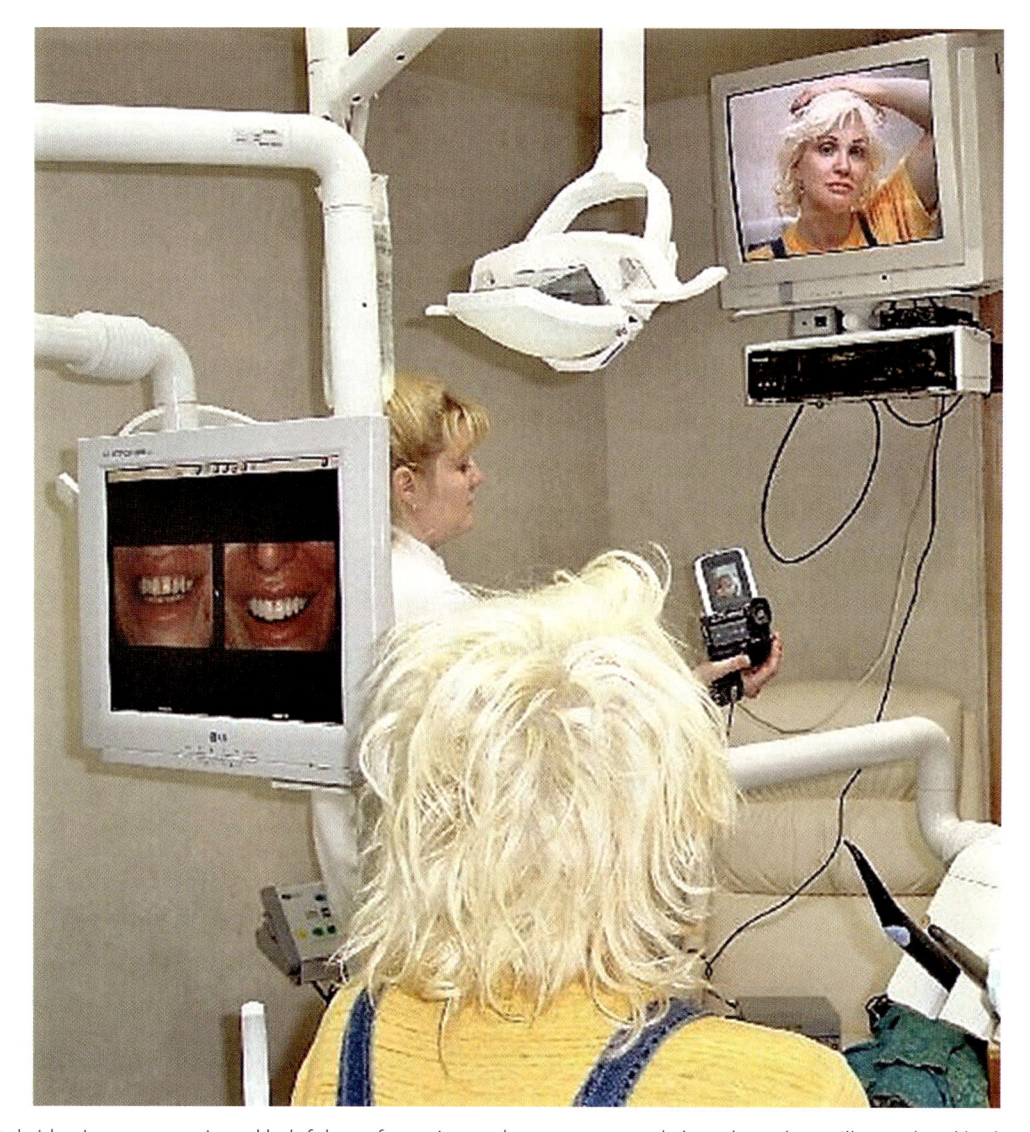

Figure 43.5 Digital video is an economic and helpful way for patients who are concerned about how they will sound and look in public.

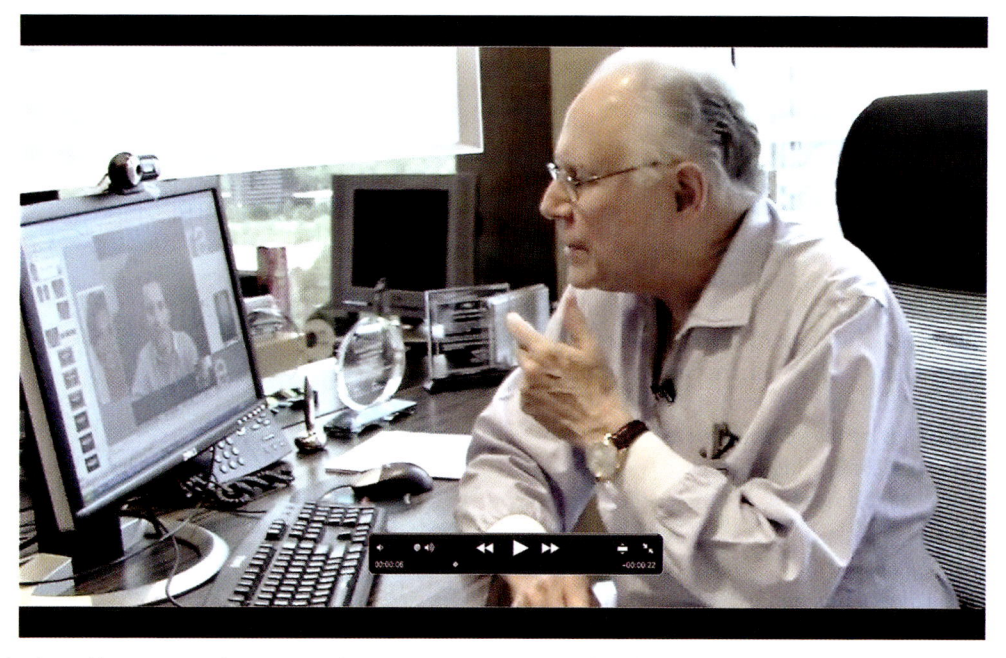

Figure 43.6 Consultation with your ceramist is extremely important in patients with esthetic problems. If it is not convenient for an in-office joint consultation, try using e-mail or Skype to accomplish optimal communication.

> **Box 43.1 Checklist at try-in appointment.**
>
> Check approval
> - Shade
> - Color
> - Length of teeth
> - Gum embrasure
> - Incisal embrasure
> - Midline—preferably in line with the midline of the face
> - Shape
> - Contour
> - Texture
> - Adjacent teeth (contour)
> - Arrangement

and have your dental assistant, as well as any observer the patient has called in, also witness the signature. It is not uncommon for patients who are difficult to please to later change their minds about their esthetic desires, especially after having the restoration viewed by a number of friends and family. Having a written statement of approval does not mean that the restoration cannot be changed. Rather it emphasizes that both patient and dentist approved the restoration and any changes made later would be the financial responsibility of the patient. Prevention—the best insurance against serious postinsertion problems—results only through adequate patient–dentist communication. Such dialogue results in realistic expectations, allowing not only to understand patients' desires and expectations, but also to understand the anatomical and technical limitations inherent with their restorations, and leading to ultimate patient satisfaction[2,6] (Figure 43.7).

Try-in principles for fixed restorations

Initial evaluation of delivered case prior to chairside approval

When the completed prosthesis arrives from the laboratory (before the patient's appointment), examine it for any obvious problems that could be corrected prior to attempting to place it in the mouth. It is always worth evaluating the fit of the crown on the cast before trying it in the patient. In this way, problems involving shade variations, marginal fit, contacts, and articulation can be anticipated prior to chairside approval. This final version should match the approved try-in restoration as close as possible.

Shade variation. Verify the shade to establish whether variations of hue, chroma, value, characterization, and translucency are present in the restoration. If a porcelain restoration is glazed, compare the shade guide (which may have been included with the case) with the actual restoration. Even though your own individual shade guide and complete descriptions were enclosed, the color may nevertheless be mismatched. Lighting in the laboratory may well be different than the lighting in your operation. If the crown has not yet been glazed, matching color with the shade guide will indicate how accurate the laboratory has been. It is quite helpful to have a computerized shade verification (list them!! VITA EasyShade Shade-Selection Device; SpectroShade; ShadeScan; and ClearMatch) as well. Not only will the computerized shade procedure help you determine the correct shade, when matching existing teeth is important, but it will also provide a color mapping to guide your ceramist through the restorative process.

Areas of potential overextensions. Although it is not advisable to work with any crown or dies prior to seeing them in the mouth, it is important to correct any obvious marginal areas that might be overextended, adjusting those areas from the axial surface, not from underneath.

Improper contacts. All too often a dentist will attempt to seat a crown and in the process destroy contacts and deplete anterior surfaces of the crown when removal of a slight marginal overextension would have allowed the crown to seat properly.

Prior to a patient's arrival at the office it is important to note contour, contacts, and embrasure form, and especially the presence of occlusal discrepancies. Observe esthetic qualities such as translucency of porcelain, shade, and consistency to check the natural appearance of your restoration. Compare the original shade with the porcelain. Do not hesitate to send the case back to the laboratory for any needed correction before the patient's appointment.

Chairside appointment prior to insertion

Confirm the try-in appointment with the patient by telephone. Be sure to let your patient know it could take a half or entire day for their appointment. At the same time, determine the possibility of any problem.

The patient may disclose a change in oral condition, such as points of irritation following surgical techniques, or a pulpitis following abutment preparation. Roberts[7] warns that to cause any further irritation to an already affected pulp (by drying the teeth or subjecting them to the trauma of removing the provisional restoration) may only do more harm. Therefore, the appointment may have to be postponed. However, your patient's sensitivity could be caused by a washout of the temporary cement, so postponing the visit may not correct the problem. Examine the patient to see whether the temporary restoration is loose or if there is a cement washout.

The use of local anesthesia or an analgesic may be indicated when placing a laminate crown or fixed partial denture on a vital tooth. When removing a temporary restoration, isolate and check the tooth carefully to insure that no temporary cement remains. Use coarse pumice on abutment teeth followed with chlorhexidine mouthwash, which helps to reduce the amount of bacteria and inflammation, as well as swelling of gums in the area.[8] Cleaning should include both the supragingival and subgingival areas. Examine the pontic area and gingival margins for inflammation that could cause contours different from those present at the time the impression was taken.

goldstein, garber & salama, LLC

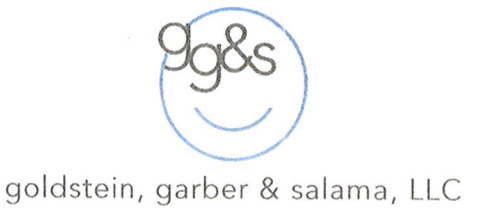

Ronald E. Goldstein, DDS
Founder & Author
Change Your Smile
Esthetics in Dentistry

David A. Garber, DMD
Periodontist, Prosthodontist

Maurice A. Salama, DMD
Orthodontist, Periodontist

I approve of the color, shade, shape and size of the crowns that have been fabricated for my teeth and wish to have them final glazed. I approve of the restorations in every way. I have discussed this with Dr. Goldstein and his staff and have had all my questions answered.

_____

Patient's name printed

_____   _____

Patient's signature   Date

_____   _____

Witness   Date

600 galleria parkway s.e. • suite 800 • atlanta georgia 30339
telephone 404 261 4941 • fax 404 261 4946 • website goldsteingarber.com
email goldsteingarber@goldsteingarber.com

Figure 43.7 It is a good idea to have the patient sign a consent form before proceeding to the final glaze. This image presents a good example of an informed consent form at this stage.

Principles for the esthetic try-in

- *Fitting the crown to the tooth* As stated earlier, studies show that if patients are satisfied with the fit of a denture, they will usually be satisfied with its esthetic effect and their ability to chew and speak.[9] This can also be true with fixed restorations, although the patient motivated primarily by esthetics may react just the opposite. A crown can have all the qualities of functional perfection, but if it does not esthetically match the adjacent or complementing tooth then no amount of explanation will satisfy this type of patient. Always remember, fitting the crown to the tooth is the most important functional step of the try-in procedure and must be done prior to any esthetic evaluation.

- *Ceramometal crowns* All esthetic crowns are tried in before final polish or glaze. With careful examination of the casting it may be possible to determine areas of binding. Roberts suggests using graphite or lipstick on the internal surface to make these areas easier to observe.[7] Sandblasted or dull gold surfaces will also reveal binding areas on the internal surface of metal crowns. Fit Checker (GC) or aerosol sprays (Occlude-Pascal) are two products that can be helpful to reveal binding areas and any irregularities of fit in ceramometal crowns. A third alternative to discover a tight area on the inside of a crown is to use a colored paste of equal parts lightly working the inside of the crown. Put it into place and the material sets quickly. After withdrawing the crown, any binding spot is easily revealed. An example of this can be seen in Figure 43.8A–G on an all-ceramic splint. Frequently, a ceramometal crown will fit too tightly due to the rate of contraction–expansion and ratio of the porcelain and metal. If this happens, be careful of relieving too much of the inner core of metal. Thin spots can be created which might allow internal stress, metal flexing, and perhaps eventual porcelain fracture. For this reason, a uniform metal thickness is very important to prevent any failure in the metal–ceramic bond. A minimum metal thickness of 0.3–0.5 mm is allowable for possible shrinkage or the possibility of some relief without weakening the metal substructure. However, a better technique is to adjust the tooth preparation rather than the metal to help properly seat the crown. One significant problem, and a potentially major one, is not being able to remove a crown at try-in. A simple solution is to fit a Tofflemire band slightly on the crown (Figure 43.8 F) and then use a reverse hammer to help dislodge the "stuck" crown by tapping vertically as close to the band as possible (Figure 43.8G). Try to balance the crown by pressing with your finger on the lingual surface as you tap.

- *All-ceramic crowns* Since all-ceramic crowns have a passive fit, the try-in of these types of restorations creates different problems. A single crown is easiest to fit since existing contacts are present and the new crown just has to be held in place while margins and contacts are checked. Then the occlusion can be evaluated using microthin articulating paper and 5/10,000ths of an inch thick stock strips (Artus). If the crown has no ability to stay in place for the occlusal check, try temporarily cementing it with a product like fit checker (GC) (Figure 43.9). One reason for making multiple impressions is to be able to verify fits with duplicate models. This can be especially helpful when trying to determine whether a slight ledge or overhang is present. If you determine the presence of a ledge or slight void in the margin, the duplicate model can be used to help repair the defect without taking another impression.

In certain difficult cases the laboratory may have a problem in seating an extensive bridge or fixed splint. Rather than having the patient return to reprepare a tooth or teeth and then take new impressions, consider the following technique (Figure 43.10A–D):

1. Have the technician carefully mark undercut areas plus where the abutment teeth may need slight reduction. Then the technician reduces the tooth on the model sufficient to how the bridge draws.
2. The technician then makes a plastic or metal coping of the tooth or teeth needing further reduction.
3. Next, the technician trims through the coping incrementally until they see the bridge will draw. Then the bridge is constructed.
4. Before trying in the restorations, fit the coping precisely to the abutment tooth and make the exact same cut as the technician did.
5. Now fit your restoration as normal.

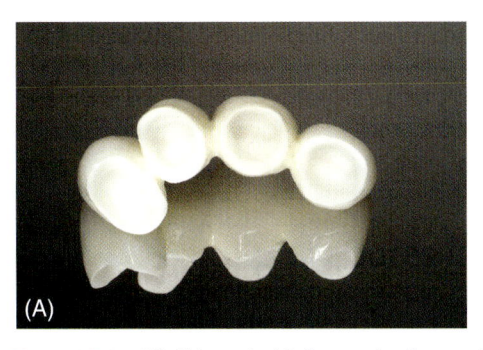

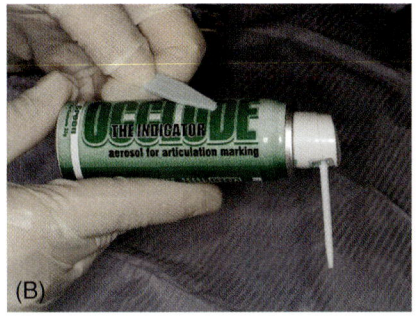

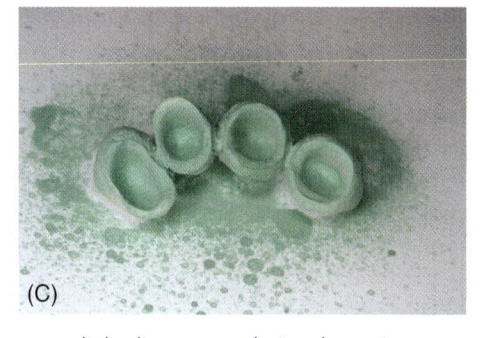

Figure 43.8 **(A)** Although this four-unit all-ceramic fixed splint fit perfectly on the model, there was a slight discrepancy during the try-in. **(B, C)** A green indicating spray (Occlude-Pascal) was used on the inside of the splint to help define any binding area in the intaglio surfaces of the crowns.

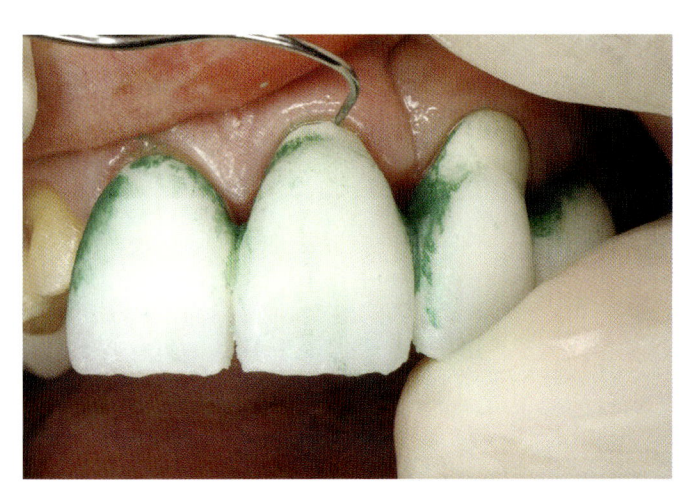

Figure 43.8 **(D)** When seating the splint firmly, try to verify which tooth/teeth have marginal discrepancies.

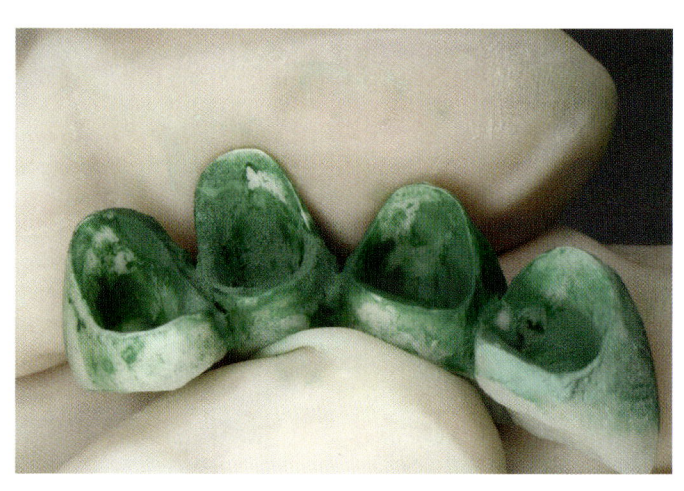

Figure 43.8 **(E)** Observing where the spray has been removed will also show you the areas on the tooth that can be adjusted for perfect fit and draw.

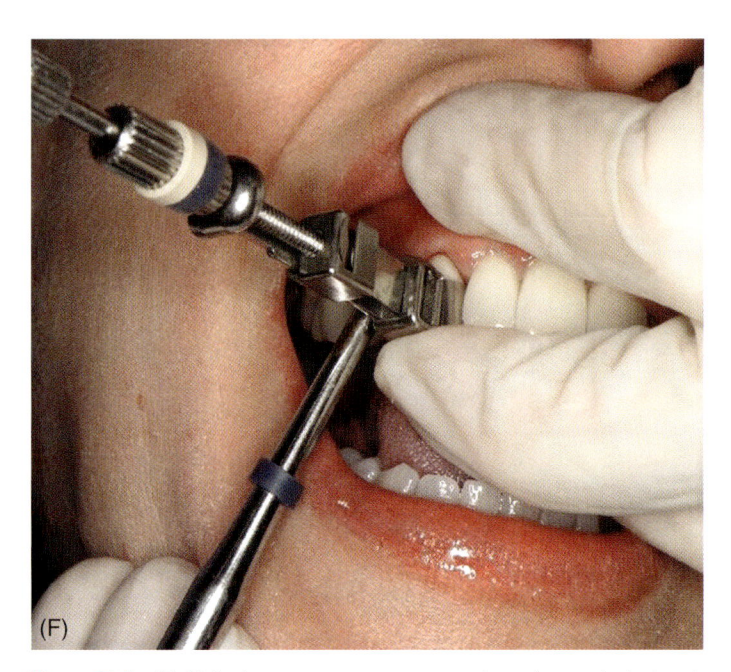

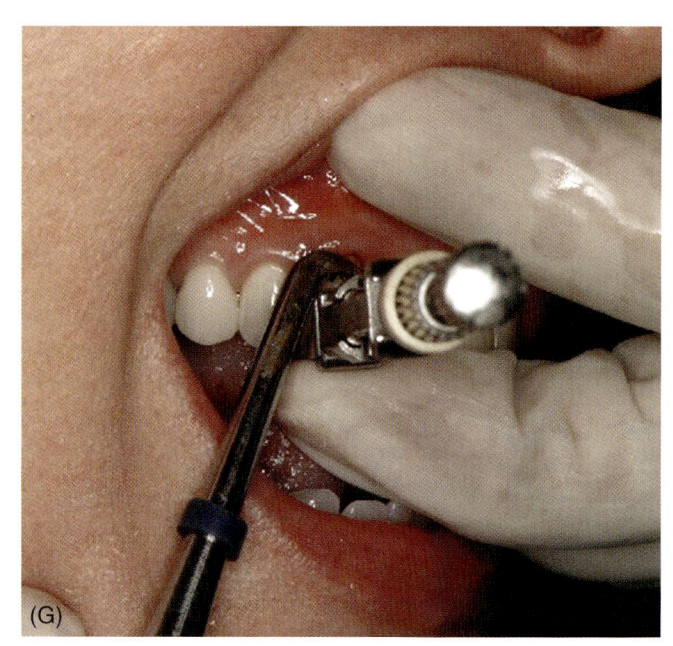

Figure 43.8 **(F, G)** At times, a crown can get stuck on the tooth during the try-in appointment. First fit a thin Tofflemire matrix band to the tooth. Then, use a reverse hammer with vertical taps to remove the crown.

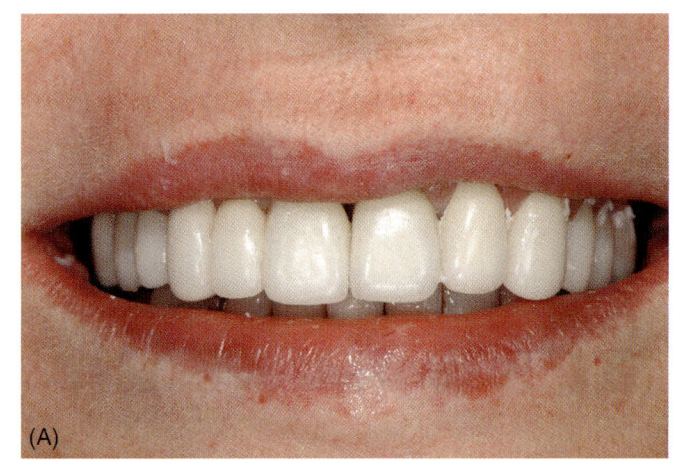

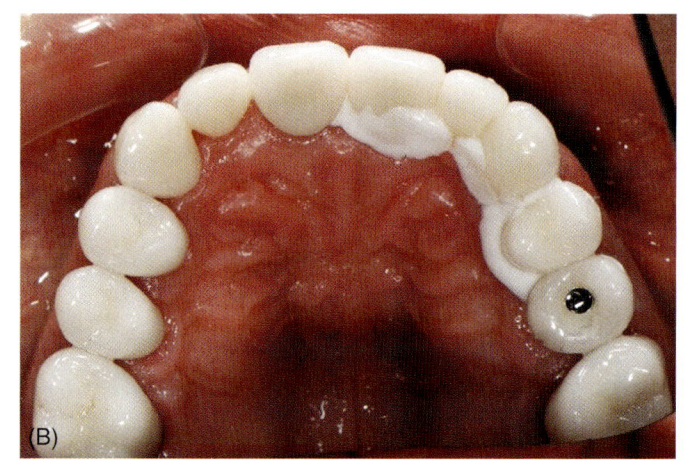

Figure 43.9 **(A, B)** If the crowns have little or no ability to stay in place, try temporarily placing them with a product like Fit-Checker (GC).

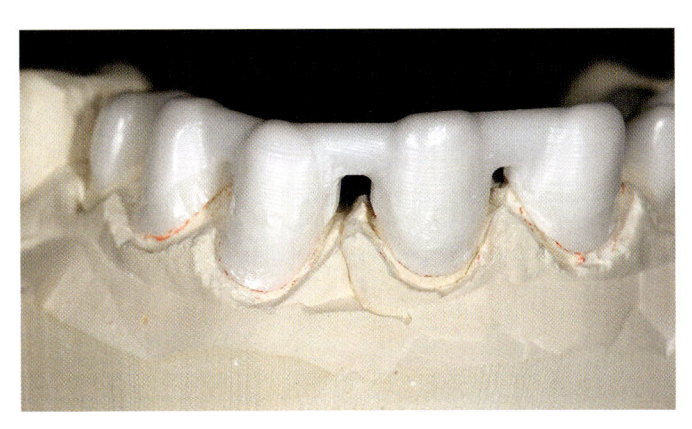

Figure 43.10 **(A)** This five-unit fixed all-ceramic bridge did not have a perfect draw. Rather than have the patient return to reprepare the teeth and take new impressions, the dentist decided to have the technician make the small changes on the prepared teeth on the model.

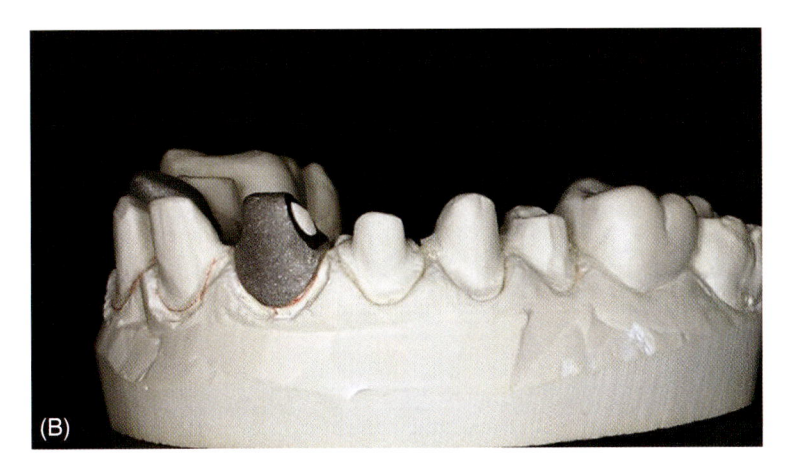

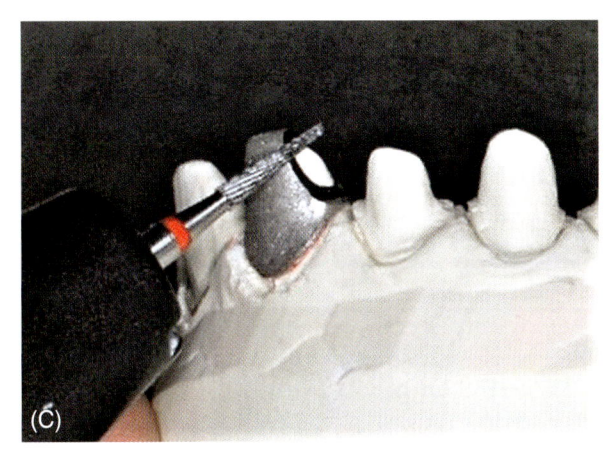

Figure 43.10 **(B, C)** The technician then made a coping which revealed exactly where the tooth needed to be reduced.

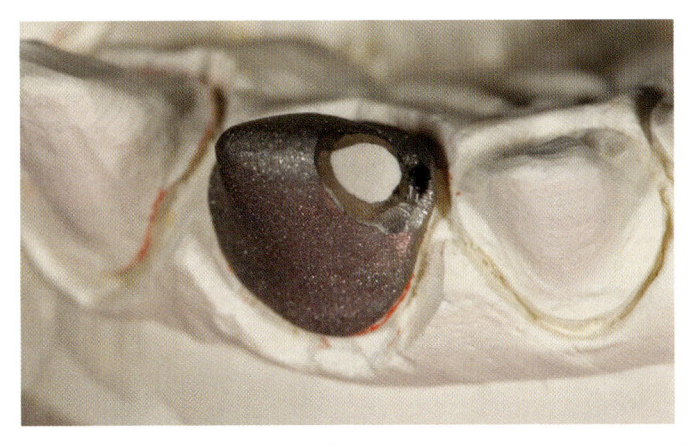

Figure 43.10 **(D)** When this coping is tried in the patient's mouth, the dentist will have an exact reduction guide for the necessary alteration on the prepared tooth.

When using a full shoulder margin, make sure no ledge exists by running the explorer both apically and incisally. If you find a ledge, try the crown on a duplicate model to see whether you can see where the void occurs. If so, the technician will be able to repair the defective margin. If you do not have an extra model, retract the gingival tissue and take a polyvinyl siloxane impression to show the technician the difference. A similar technique can be used if the patient's gingiva has receded since taking the final impression and is exposing the root. You can start the crown to make sure it fits perfectly. If so, then use a tissue-protective end cutting bur to reprepare a new labial margin subgingivally and then retract the tissue gently and seat the crown and take a new polyvinyl siloxane impression to show the ceramist where to add (Figure 43.11A–F).

Ideally, take three impressions so you will have adequate untouched models to verify your fit as well as to make sure your technician did not trim too much of your margin away.

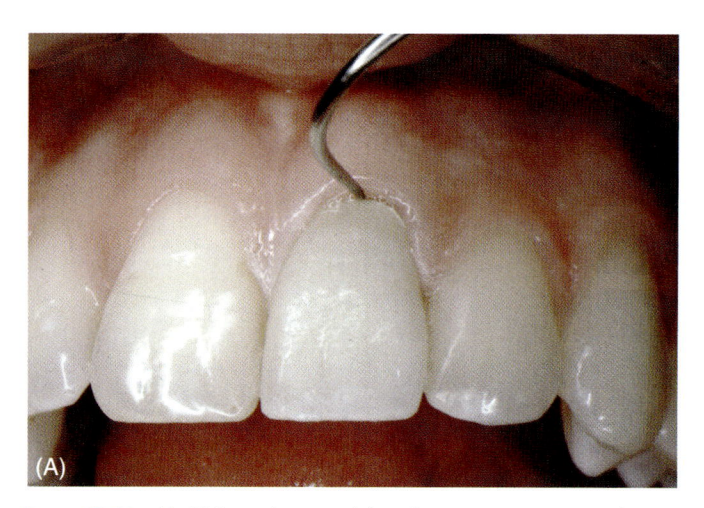

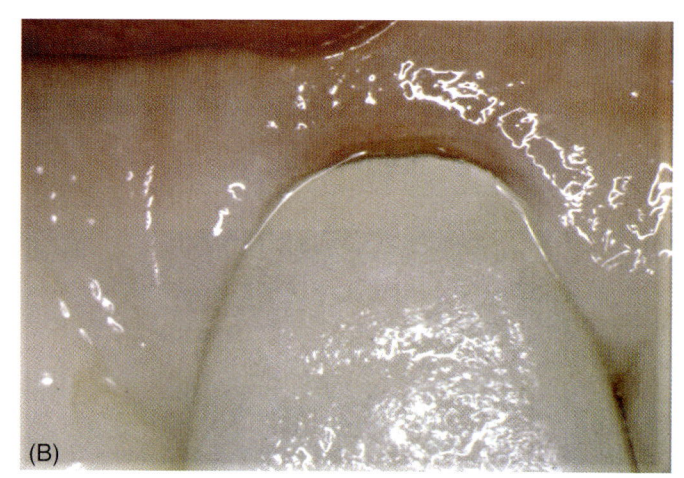

Figure 43.11 (A, B) At try-in, one of the all-ceramic crowns now has an exposed supragingival margin on a patient with a high lip line.

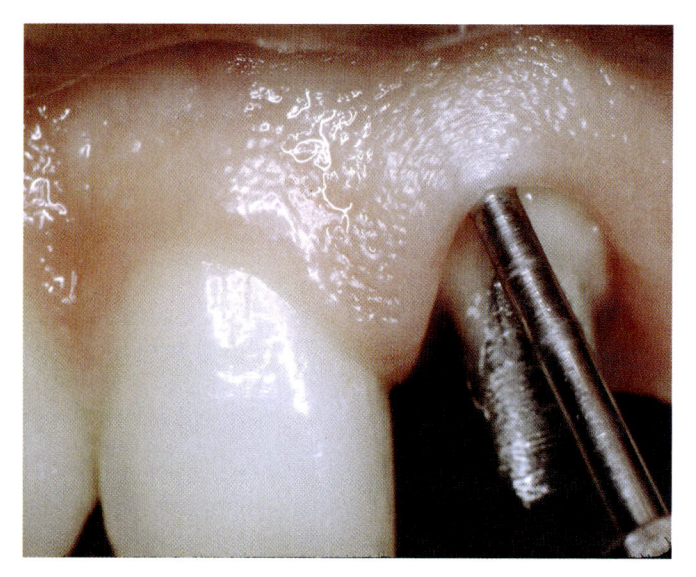

Figure 43.11 (C) Instead of repreparing the tooth and making a new crown, a tissue-protected end cutting bur was used to prepare the labial margin subgingivally, while avoiding making any alterations to the labioaxial wall of the prepared tooth.

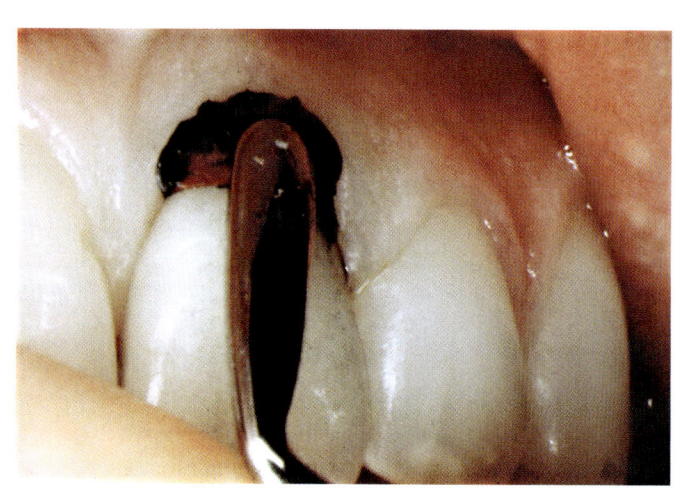

Figure 43.11 (D) At this point, a polyvinyl siloxane impression should be made of the newly prepared area with the crown in place. However, in this particular case, a soft compound was used to make the individual tooth impression.

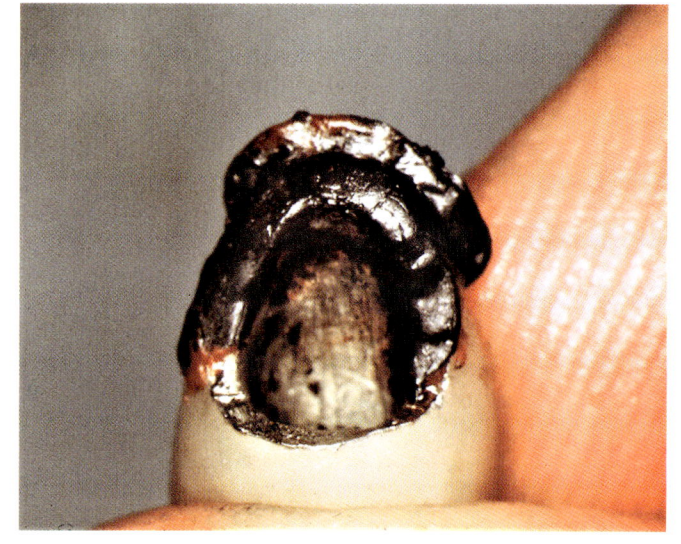

Figure 43.11 (E) Once the crown is removed, it is easy for the technician to see exactly where the shoulder margin is. A new die is made to make the necessary porcelain addition.

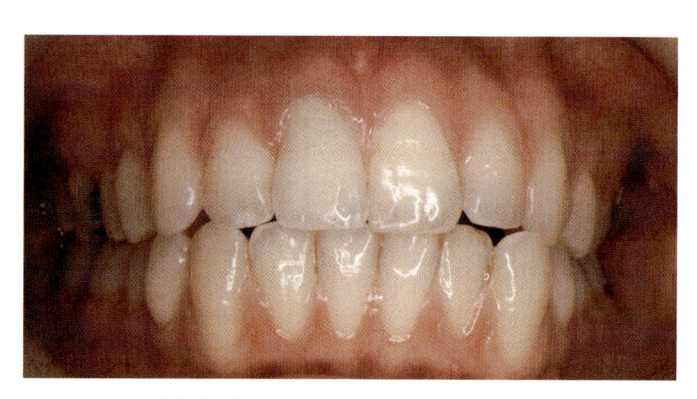

Figure 43.11 (F) The final crown now shows a proper subgingival margin for the necessary esthetics and function.

- *Contact* Too much contact can be inadvertently removed because of incorrect position of the teeth and the path of insertion, which can be heavy upon insertion and yet seemingly fit right into place. Therefore, it is important that potential gingival impingement areas, contacts, and marginal discrepancies be checked simultaneously to properly evaluate which condition is preventing the crown from seating. There are easy ways to evaluate where your tight contact first touches. One way is to use ultrathin articulating paper and have your assistant hold it in the contact area while you seat and hold the crown in place. Then the assistant pulls the articulating paper out, leaving a colored mark in the offending contact area to be slightly reduced. Then repeat the process until your crown goes to place with the tightness you and your patient desire. Your main problem is to first decide whether the mesial or distal or both contacts need reducing. Therefore, only do one side at a time if both are tight. When the marginal fit is bad, reexamine the preparation and correct if necessary, and then take a new impression or use a duplicate die to help repair the defect. Before the marginal fit can be checked, the crown must be completely seated.[10] The contact areas may be checked visually, but it is best to evaluate by passing dental floss, not tape, through the mesial and distal contacts. The tightness of the contacts can be tested with dental floss and should offer some resistance but not make its passage too difficult. Have your assistant place their thumb on the two crowns to hold them in place once you have positioned the floss. When necessary, ease the contact after carefully assessing the area of initial contact. When the crown is thought to be completely seated and the margins are adjusted as necessary, a digital X-ray is taken to verify the fit (Figure 43.12). Open contacts occur less frequently and may be modified by returning the crown to the laboratory for addition of porcelain.

- *Alignment* In trying-in a ceramometal splint, check alignment of the retainers, because even if the individual units seat properly, the fixed appliance may not, due to incorrect relationships. In such a case, the simplest procedure, unless the misalignment is slight, is to section the various components, reseat in the mouth, and, if they fit properly, finish the try-in by obtaining the proper occlusal contour, and then stain and glaze the porcelain as necessary. Then place the components into the mouth. Next, lute with acrylic (Duralay), take a plaster localizing impression, and, after pouring in soldering investment, resolder.

- *Tissue contact* When esthetics dictate, the pontic should exert only very light pressure. If it causes severe blanching, it must be eased to prevent gingival proliferation around the pontic. If it fails to touch the mucosa by more than 0.1 mm, an addition may be required. If the patient has a high lip line, make sure the tissue fits into the pontic area with a natural appearance. There are instances where the ovate pontic may be indicated for a more realistic look.[11]

- *Marginal fit* With the latest impression and casting procedures, there should be little need for major modification in this area. However, where possible, accessible margins may be finished with sandpaper discs or stones. Finally, impregnated cups, points, and wheels are employed. If you are using a gold feather edge, metal margin, it should be burnished before cementation.[10] An accurate marginal fit will have long-term benefits; meanwhile, an ill-fitting margin will compromise gingival health by plaque retention, recurrent decay, and cement dissolution.

- *Reevaluate shade* At this point, merely determine that the shade will be accurate enough to be used. This reevaluation of shade may require removal of the veneer porcelain if the shade is too far off. Slight discrepancies should be correctable by staining and glazing. In situations where shades are slightly lighter, they may be darkened by addition of stain and refiring. If the shade variation is too great to correct by staining, or reveneering, check any other basic flaws, such as occlusion and midline, and have the laboratory remake it. The crowns should be glazed once you and your patient are happy with the final appearance.

- *Check midline relationship on multiple anterior units* This should be established before any major recontouring of teeth is started. The midline should be vertical and, if possible, coincide with the midline of the face (Figure 43.13). However, much more important is for the two front teeth (central incisors) to be the same size or appear proportionate to each other and to the face. Therefore, it may be necessary for the dentist to move it to the right or left. Nevertheless, it should be vertical and parallel to the midline of the face or perpendicular to the eyes. If the midline is off, mark the correct line with a sharp black pencil so the laboratory can add new porcelain and/or reveneer.

- *Position in the arch* Now is the time to check tooth position in the arch and make any adjustment necessary by reshaping the crown.

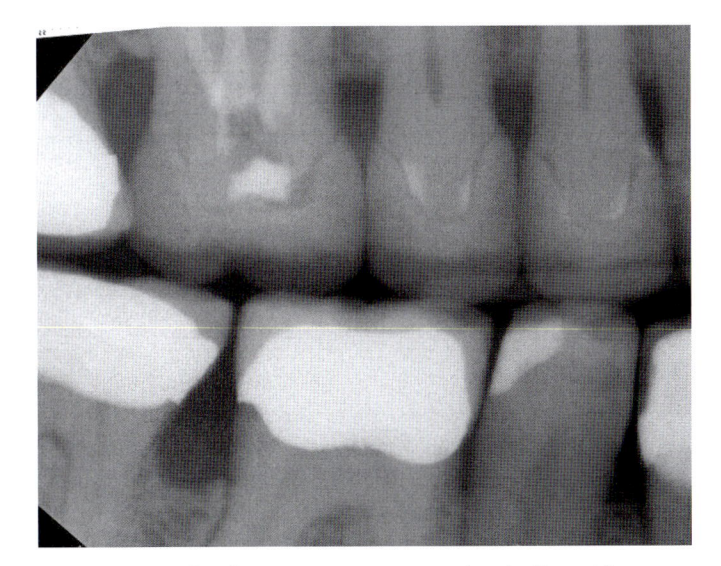

Figure 43.12 After the restorations are seated and adjusted for proper contact, margins are checked and verified by clinical examination. Next, a digital X-ray is made to confirm the interproximal marginal fit.

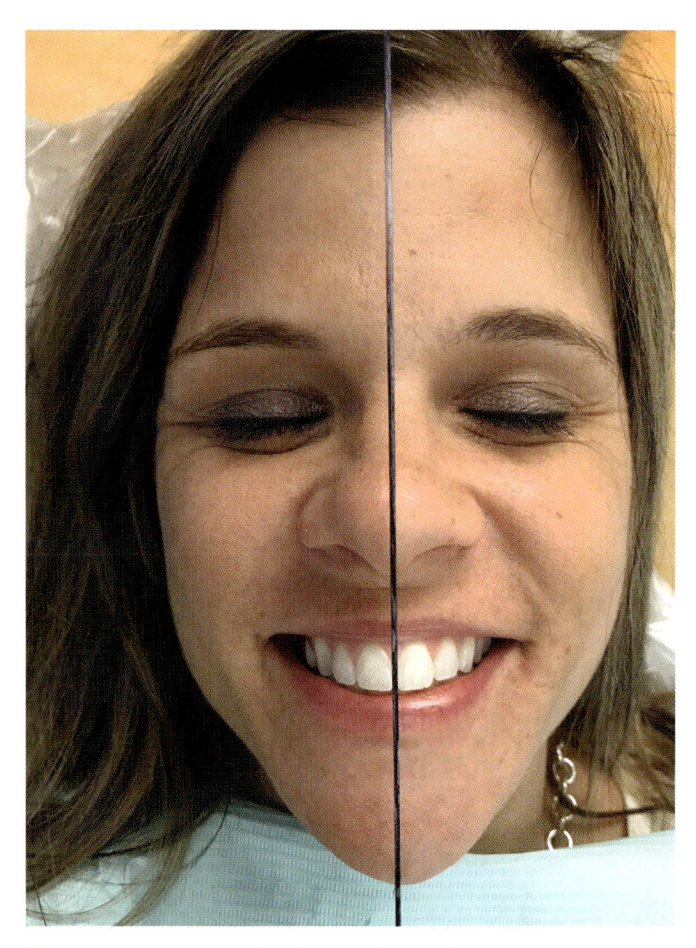

Figure 43.13 Using a colored dental floss makes it easy to see where the midline is in relation to the rest of the face. For this particular patient, the midline of the teeth was positioned to the midline of the face, even though her nose is slightly deviated to the right.

- *Adjust occlusion* No matter which articulator is used, the mouth must be the true test in the final analysis. Adjust if possible, but remount if there is a major occlusal discrepancy. For the final occlusal adjustment use the following procedure:

  1. If ceramic crowns, use microthin articulating paper that has been coated with Vaseline or other lubricant that will make the marks easier to read.
  2. Check centric contact with thin articulating tape (Artus 0.0005″ (0.0127 mm) thickness).
  3. Use occlusal indicator wax to double check for prematurities.
  4. Judge by touch and by articulating paper whether the occlusion is too heavy on any particular tooth.

- *Establish proper gingival embrasures* Shaping the gingival embrasure is the second most important step of the try-in appointment. Unless this procedure is properly accomplished, functional principles will be violated that preclude an esthetic result. It is important to emphasize that many times tissue blanching is normal, so have the patient bite on a cotton roll and allow up to 5 min for the crowns to settle into position. Then verify and correct the cause of any continuous blanching. That pressure on the gingival tissue may cause remodeling of a specific area, and may lead to unwanted tissue changes. There are two methods of determining correct gingival form.

  - *Indirect method* There are several ways of determining this contour. Because a full impression obtained with retraction cord does not give the true representation of gingival tissue, a second polyether or polyvinyl siloxane impression can be made after the tissue has had time to return to a rest position. Because the tissue is not retracted, the chances are the margins will not be perfect. Therefore, using the dies from the master impression, pour the second impression with these same dies seated into the impression material. Now the dies and crowns can be interchanged and an accurate measurement of proper gingival contour can be made on the second model. It also provides an esthetic determination of where the labiogingival–ceramometal junction should be. According to Pincus (see Appendix D), this model can also be poured in soft acrylic to offer a more natural feeling and appearance.[11] Another method is to take an accurate study model and measure the distance c from the incisal edge a to the height of the interdental tissue b. The distance from the crest of the mesial interdental tissue to the distal interdental tissue can also be recorded and duplicated in the crown shape. B1, B2, C, E, and A/D are duplicable measurement that can more accurately be used in forming and contouring the porcelain.

  - *Direct method* Obviously, if only a small amount needs adjusting, try to do it direct in the mouth. A second method of obtaining proper gingival embrasures is to have the laboratory build the crown as accurately as possible for the try-in appointment. After the crown is fully seated with margins and contact corrected, a sharp black pencil is used to scribe the cervical portion of the crown at the gingival. In cases where the crowns are overbuilt and cause tissue pressure, use a cotton roll with the patient biting firmly. Next, remove the crowns and observe the gingival markings on the model. Reduce the part below the contoured line as necessary to duplicate natural tooth anatomy in the proximal surfaces. Continue trying the crown in until correct contours are established and then glaze.

- *Obtain correct incisal embrasure* Use an ET3 diamond (Brasseler USA) to open the incisal enclosure to make it appear (Figure 43.14A and B) as natural as possible. The incisal embrasure should display a natural, progressive increase in size and depth from central incisors to bicuspids, as we proceed from central incisors to bicuspids moving the contact point further toward the gum.

- *Maxillary incisors* The incisal embrasure between central incisors is usually placed approximately 1 mm lower than the one between the lateral and central. This embrasure can be several millimeters deep, depending on the desired illusion.

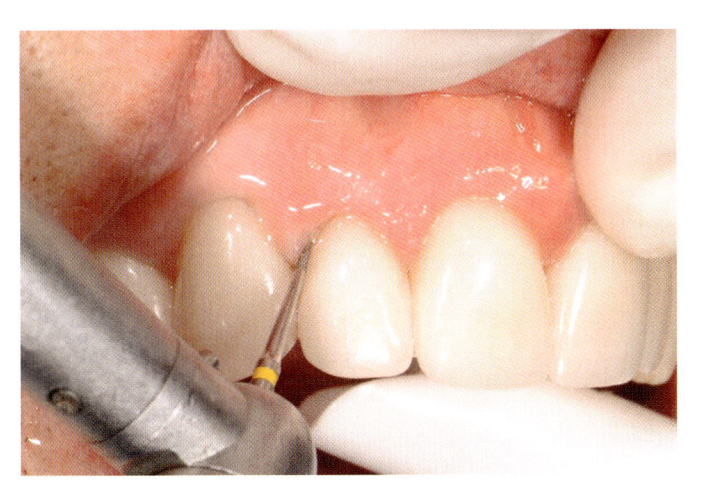

Figure 43.14 **(A)** When a small adjustment needs to be made to open the gingival embrasure, it can be done directly or indirectly. Here, it is being done directly in the mouth with a DET3EF 15 μm diamond (Brasseler USA).

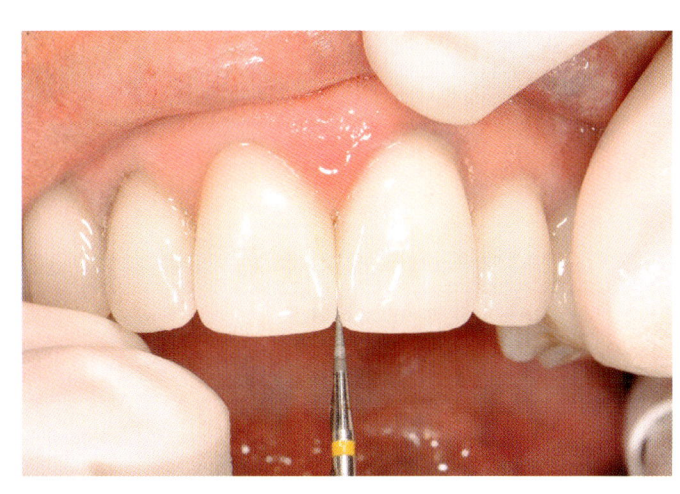

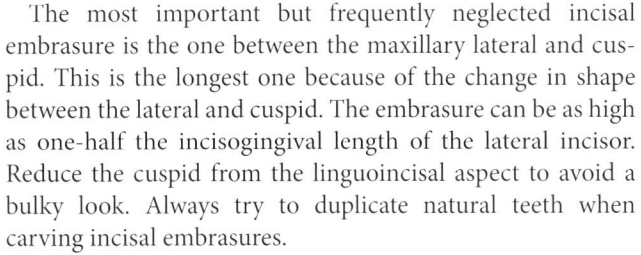

Figure 43.14 **(B)** A DET3EF 15 μm diamond (Brasseler USA) is used to open the incisal embrasure to make the restoration as natural as possible.

The most important but frequently neglected incisal embrasure is the one between the maxillary lateral and cuspid. This is the longest one because of the change in shape between the lateral and cuspid. The embrasure can be as high as one-half the incisogingival length of the lateral incisor. Reduce the cuspid from the linguoincisal aspect to avoid a bulky look. Always try to duplicate natural teeth when carving incisal embrasures.

- *Mandibular incisors* Although the embrasures between the mandibular incisors are not as prominent as those on the maxillary teeth, it is equally important to create a feeling of naturalness through incisal separation. The length of the incisal embrasure between the centrals and laterals usually varies between 0.25 and 0.5 mm. The mandibular lateral-cuspid embrasure can vary between 1 and 3 mm. For a more esthetic, natural arrangement, the position of these embrasures can be altered by using a very thin polishing diamond DOSF ET3 (Brasseler USA). Another instrument that can be easily used to shape incisal embrasures intraorally is the ET3 diamond (Brasseler USA) (Figure 43.14B).
- *Posterior teeth* Do not neglect posterior embrasures. Distal to the cuspid and to the bicuspids are the most important areas. Generally, if the bicuspids are properly carved, the embrasures take care of themselves. The bicuspids should complement the cuspid shape and the amount of space between the teeth.
- *Form proper length and position of contact areas* Reexamine both labiogingivally and inciso- or occlusogingivally to make sure anatomy is correct. Add or subtract as necessary.
- *Incisal length* Judge proper incisal length with the patient standing and sitting. In the case of multiple anterior units, establish correct incisal length variation from tooth to tooth. At times, slightly overlapping laterals or prominent labioincisal line angles can be utilized to obtain an effective natural look. Sculpt the teeth not only from the gingival side, but also the incisal, to create a more esthetic and natural illusion. Rotation of abutments and retainers may be employed as well. Observe patients speaking and smiling. Have them count or speak words that require high lip line, smiling, laughing, and rest positions. Whenever possible, use the temporary restoration to add length when your patient feels the teeth may be too short (Figure 43.15A–D).
- *Labial and lingual contours* With particular attention to correct speech patterns and lip support, carve labial and lingual contours. Use adjacent teeth as the model for lingual anatomy.

Shaping

Since the try-in of the final restoration is basically a duplicate of the temporary restoration, there should be no need for major changes. However, final shaping or contouring the restoration is really what the try-in appointment is all about. The shaping of incisal embrasures, proximal contacts, and gingival outline will establish the silhouette of the tooth while line angles and contours will establish the face of the tooth. No matter if the ceramist has carved an attractive restoration; even a minute alteration can many times help to personalize it.

After the restorations are properly fitted, examine the smile and note the effect the teeth have on the lips and facial expression. The personality of the patient should be stressed at this point. Know what type of image the patient wishes to project and incorporate this into the shapes of teeth. Sex appeal, naturalness, and aging should be considered at this time. Naturally, if the treatment requires matching adjacent teeth, little personality change can be accomplished. However, if all or most of the maxillary teeth are being crowned, a different approach should be taken. The choice of whether to change previous shapes of teeth should already have been made, so that the technician could begin with a close approximation of what is desired. If the shapes are to be improved, note the changes to be made in the laboratory. The final changes should be either carved or stained into the

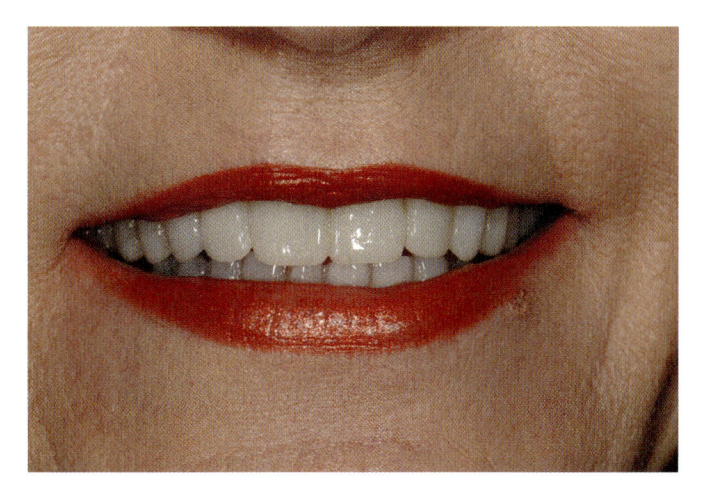

Figure 43.15 **(A)** This patient felt she needed to show more tooth structure when she smiled.

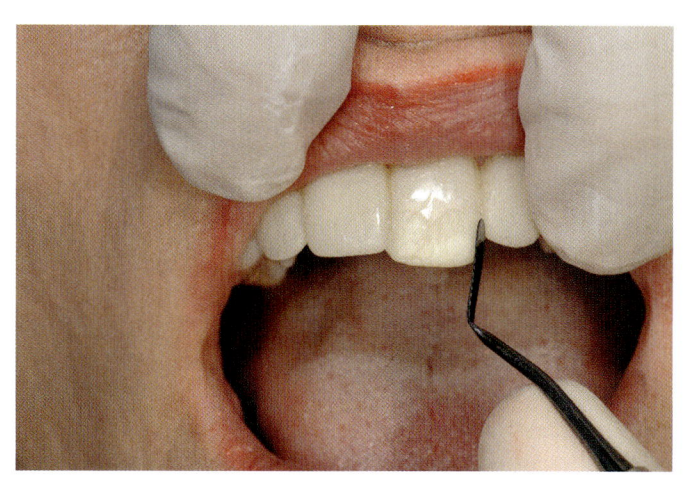

Figure 43.15 **(B)** Additional incisal length was added to her temporaries on one side of her arch using composite resin.

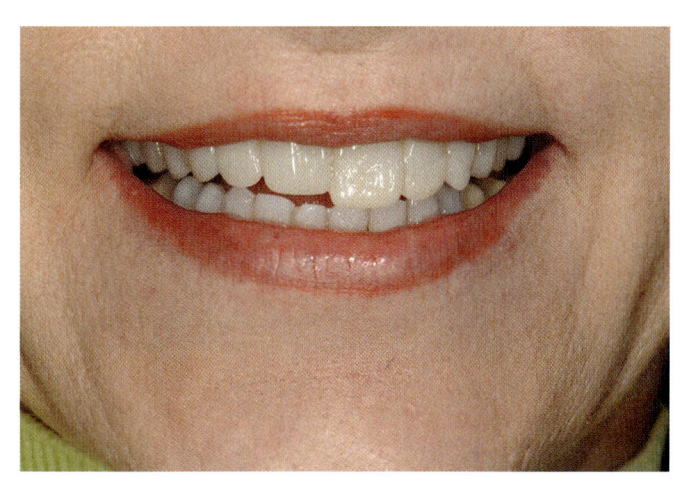

Figure 43.15 **(C)** After observing the patient during speaking and smiling, it was decided by both the doctor and the patient to add more incisal length to her final anterior restorations.

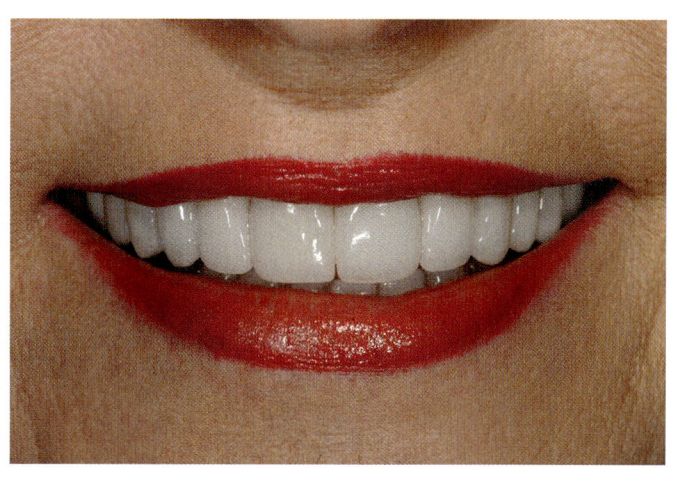

Figure 43.15 **(D)** The patient was very happy with the final results at try-in.

restoration at this time. Figure 43.16A–G shows how much can be accomplished during the try-in appointment. Figure 43.16B shows the frontal view of the porcelain crowns after fitting but before final shaping. The teeth are then marked (Figure 43.16C–E) and contoured to create a more feminine appearance.[11] A method of communication between dentist and laboratory technician can be instituted by markings. One way is to use straight or curved diagonal marks for areas to be carved. Solid black areas should be used to indicate complete reduction. This can also aid you in remembering where and how much to carve after removing the case from the mouth. Use an alcohol marker (Masel) or black pencil to mark the labial surface where shaping should be performed. Remove the crowns and proceed with contouring as indicated by the black marks.

Shaping and contouring anterior crowns takes the most time at the try-in appointment. After contouring as much as you think is needed, stop and take a break. Come back after several minutes, and the chances are that a slight alteration will greatly improve the appearance. One of the most important views is the occlusal view of the labial surfaces. This is best done by using a large front surface mirror and rotating it back and forth, which should allow you to easily view your crown or crowns and to compare them with adjacent teeth (Figure 43.17). The rotation of the mirror also makes it possible for you to observe each part of the labial surface, the gingival body, and incisal edges. This task can make the difference in contouring perfection. Allow the patient to view the restoration without you several times, and each time let the patient take approximately 5 min to look, either alone or with the dental assistant. This enables the patient to participate in determining the shape of their restorations without making split-second judgments of whether or not it is correct. Patients as well as dental assistants will frequently make excellent suggestions about width, length, or shape of teeth as seen from their own viewpoint. These judgments should always be considered and if possible incorporated into the shape of the teeth.

If the patient suggests an alteration that seems contrary to their best esthetic interests, it is far better to say, "Maybe just a slight bit," than to say "No, you are wrong about that." Disk the

Chapter 43 The Esthetic Try-In

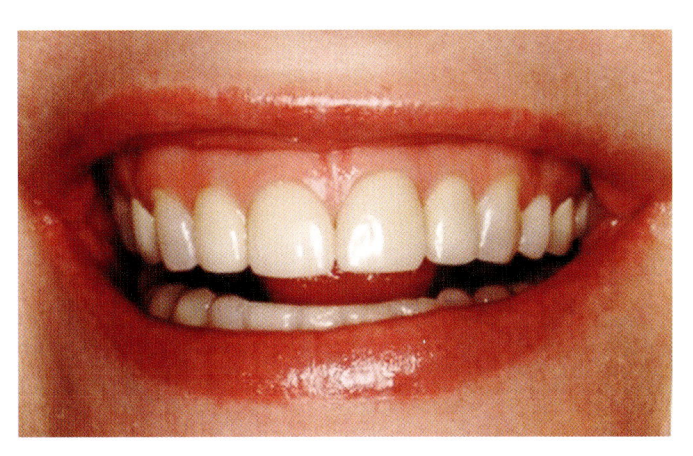

Figure 43.16 **(A)** This 42-year-old female was dissatisfied with her canted arch, high lip line, and discolored teeth.

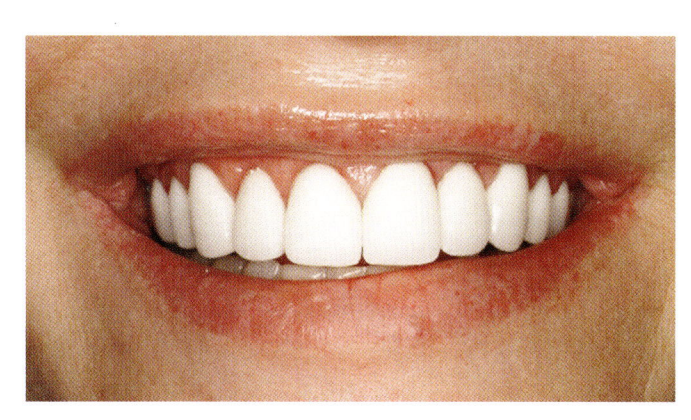

Figure 43.16 **(B)** After crown lengthening, the final crowns were constructed. At the try-in appointment, it was determined that, although the arch alignment was improved, the crowns were too long and out of proportion for her face.

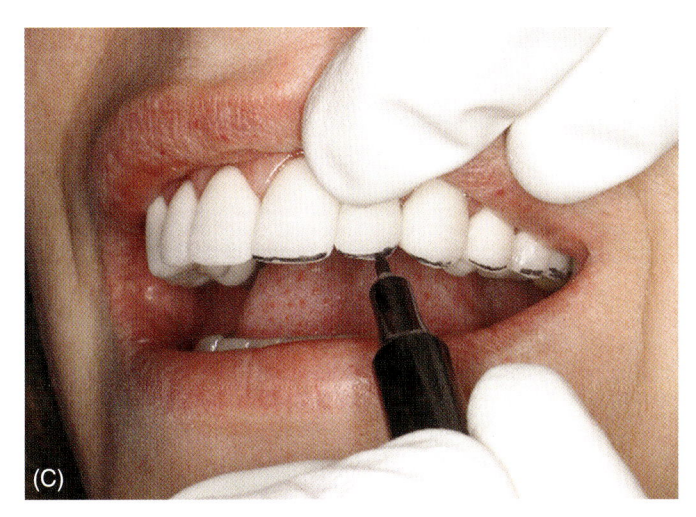

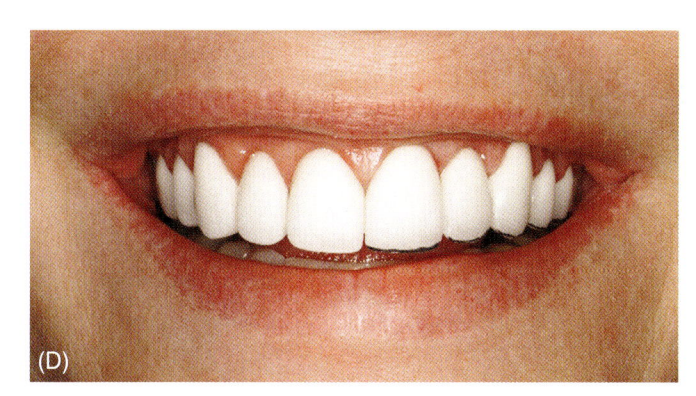

Figure 43.16 **(C, D)** The proposed amount to be reduced was marked with a black alcohol pen.

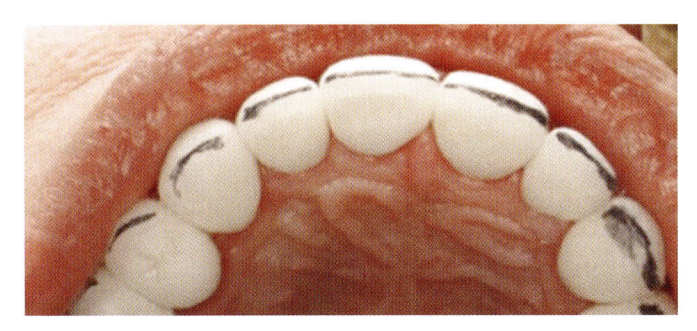

Figure 43.16 **(E)** The incisal line also showed where the crowns could be reduced a bit labially to make the teeth appear more in line, delicate, and feminine.

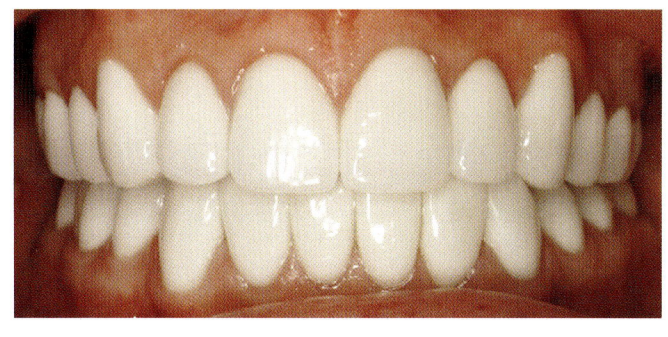

Figure 43.16 **(F)** The final maxillary crowns plus mandibular porcelain veneers and crowns are shown. Note, the bright shade of the teeth was chosen by the patient.

crown very slightly, and then say, "Yes, it does seem better now." The patient will feel it is actually better, because they have participated in the judgment, and they should be much more pleased with the overall esthetic result. This is especially true of determining the length of crowns. Patients whose teeth are worn due to bruxism or attrition are resistant to longer teeth because of the different feeling and perception of what is esthetic. Frequently, the patient who wants teeth to be even and straight across has a faulty concept of what is esthetically best. Explanation and communication are necessary,[11] but what is most important is to let the patient wear the "new length" in the temporaries long enough to get used to it.

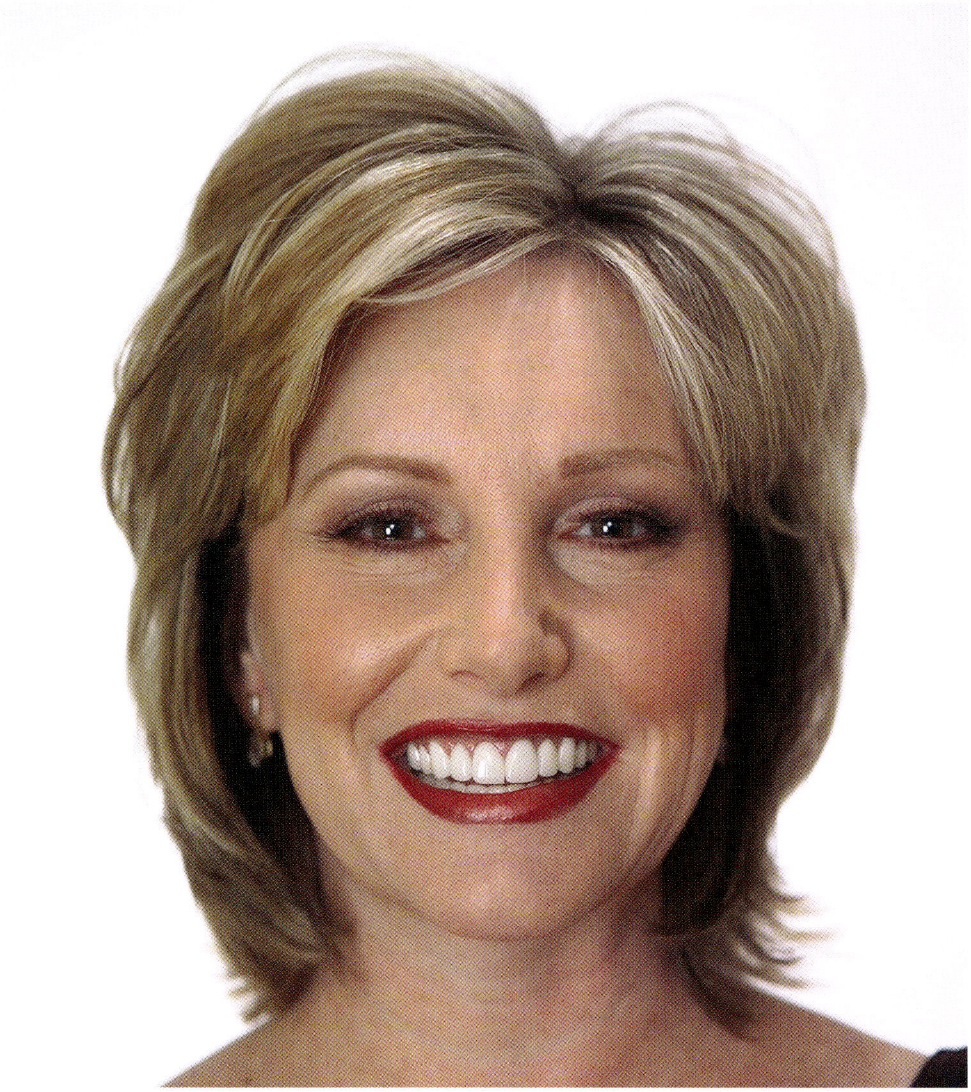

Figure 43.16 (G) The patient was extremely pleased with her final result.

Incisogingival and mesiodistal direction

Establish proper facial contours. In the case of a bonded bridge or one employing pontics, the overall form is first adjusted where necessary, as with a full porcelain crown.

Contours for characterization, light reflection, and proper texture

Characterization

The final phase of contouring includes shaping various artifacts or other forms of wear that add naturalness to the restoration (see Chapter 31).

Light reflection

Observe how the light reflects off the teeth and ask yourself if the line angles are symmetrical. If not, adjust by either contouring or adding porcelain.

Texture

Texture varies according to the adjacent teeth and patient desires. If they are glossy and smooth, copy this surface in the new crowns. Basic texture should be placed into the crowns at the laboratory by referring to close-up digital pictures, stone models, and photographs of the adjacent teeth. After shaping is completed, major grooves in the labial surface of the corresponding natural tooth are marked with a black pencil (Figure 43.18A) since the basic grooves are much easier to see when marked. Next, mark the adjacent crown in the intended matching area. Remove the crown and lightly place textured cuts with a white or porcelain stone. The glazed result is seen in Figure 43.18B.

Reevaluating the case

At this point both patient and dentist should reevaluate the restoration in terms of shade, considering the gingival, body, and incisal portions of the teeth. Restaining and glazing should be kept minimal.

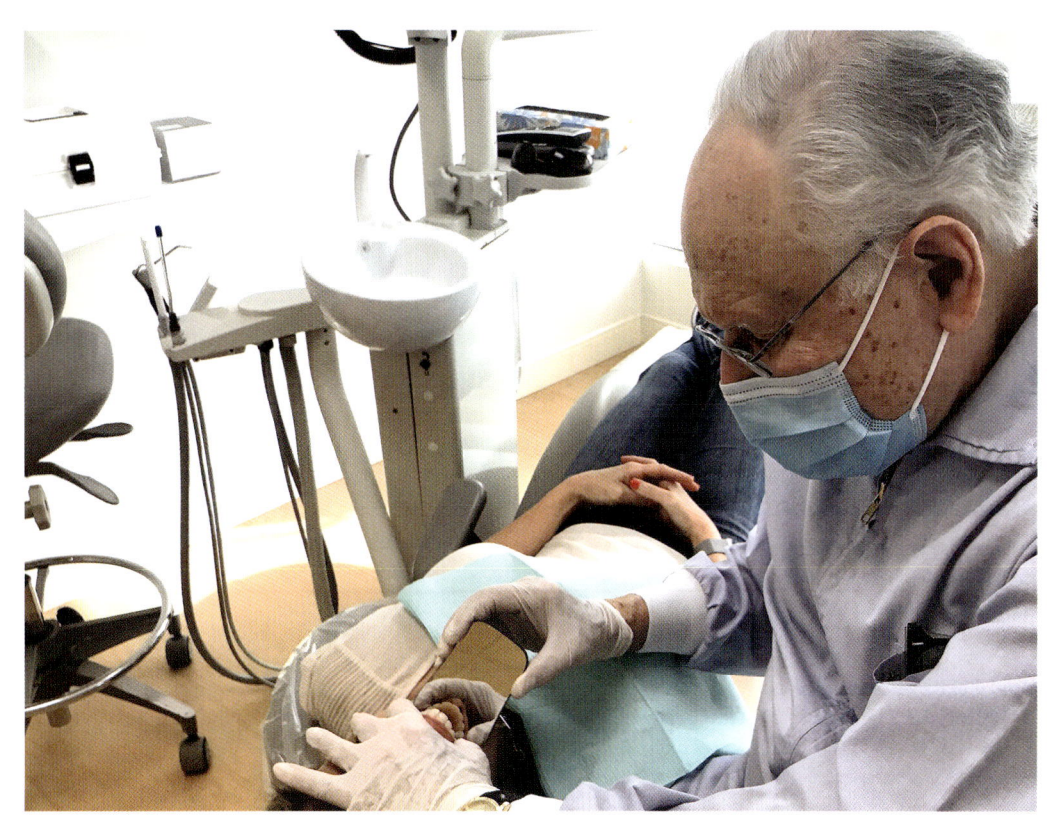

Figure 43.17 The facial alignment of the restorations should also be examined by using a large front surface mirror while rotating it back and forth.

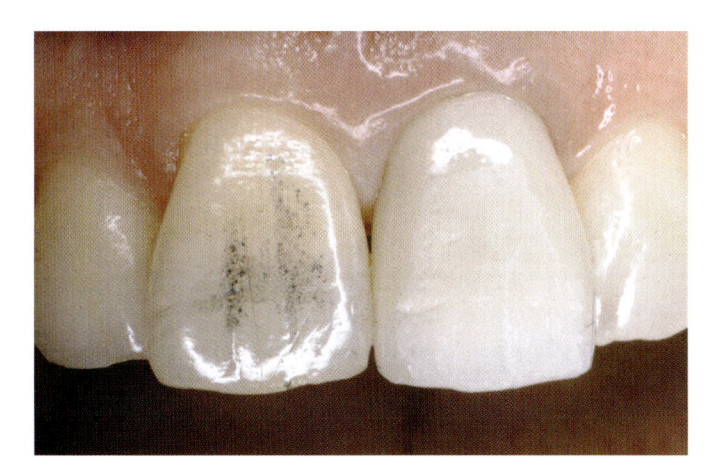

Figure 43.18 (A) Tooth texture varies according to the adjacent teeth and patient desires. Marking the main groove lines in the adjacent teeth makes it easier to duplicate in the final crown at try-in.

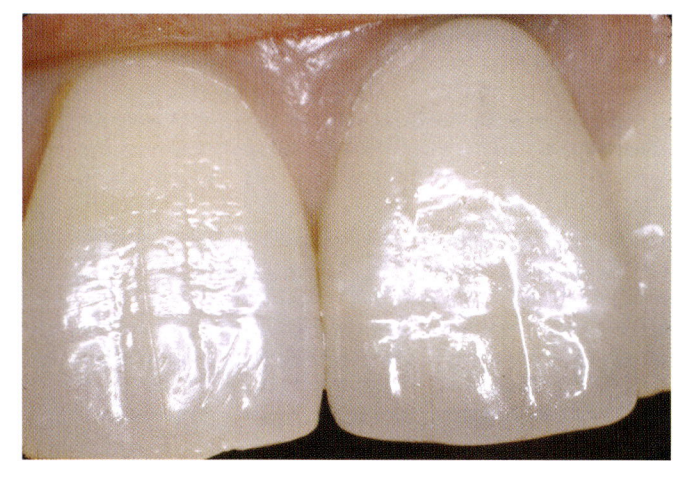

Figure 43.18 (B) The final glazed result.

Unglazed restorations

Only on rare circumstances should the dentist allow the patient to wear any restoration out of the office before they have been glazed. Unglazed porcelain will readily pick up contamination over a short time and can cause discrepancies in the shade with the final glaze.

Polishing

Gold margins are polished where applicable. The polishing procedure will not only enhance the restoration by smoothing away any surface roughness, producing a smooth light-reflecting luster, but also will affect the biocompatibility of the restoration with tissues, its longevity, and long-term esthetic results.

Cementation

Cement the case temporarily or finally. If temporarily, have the patient return for final cementation (see Chapter 44). In some situations the only option may be to cement final restorations temporarily. In these cases, the restoration should be fitted temporarily for several days to allow the patient to assess the esthetic and functional results more accurately. However, if the crowns are all-ceramic it may not be feasible to cement temporarily unless the patient will agree to a strict soft diet so that no chewing will take place. The all-ceramic needs the support of a final cement to support the forces of mastication.

References

1. Hirsch B, Levin B, Tiber N. Effects of patient involvement and esthetic preference on denture acceptance. *J Prosthet Dent* 1972;28(2):127–132.
2. Lombardi RE. The principles of visual perception and their clinical application to denture esthetics. *J Prosthet Dent* 1973;29(4):358–382.
3. Vallittu PK, Vallittu AS, Lassila VP. Dental aesthetics: a survey of attitudes in different groups of patients. *J Dent* 1996;24(5):335–338.
4. Villarroel M. Direct esthetic restorations based on translucency and opacity of composite resins. *J Esthet Res Dent* 2011;23(2):73–87.
5. Goldstein RE. *Change Your Smile*, 4th edn. Hanover Park, IL: Quintessence; 2009.
6. Marzola R, Derbabian K, Donovan TE, Arcidiacono A. The science of communicating the art of esthetic dentistry. Part I: patient–dentist–patient communication. *J Esthet Restorative Dent* 2000;12(3):131–138.
7. Roberts CJ. Shade variation in dentistry. A photographic investigation. *Aust Dent J* 1984;29(6):384–388.
8. Kim BH, Seo HS, Jung SC, et al. Study in bactericidal properties of chlorhexidine grafting on the modified titanium. *J Nanosci Nanotechnol* 2011;11(2):1530–1533.
9. Akarslan ZZ, Sadik B, Erten H, Karabulut E. Dental esthetic satisfaction, received and desired dental treatments for improvement of esthetics. *Indian J Dent Res* 2009;20(2):195–200.
10. Smith GP. The marginal fit of full cast shoulderless crown. *J Prosthet Dent* 1957;7:231–243.
11. Goldstein RE. *Esthetics in Dentistry*. Philadelphia, PA: J.B. Lippincott; 1976.

Additional resources

Anusavice KJ, Hojjatie B, Dehoff PH. Influence of metal thickness on stress distribution in metal–ceramic crowns. *J Dent Res* 1986;65(9):1173–1178.

Baharav H, Kupershmit I, Oman M, Cardash H. Comparison between incisal embrasures of natural and prosthetically restored maxillary anterior teeth. *J Prosthet Dent* 2009;101(3):200–204.

Belser UC. Esthetics checklist for the fixed prosthesis. Part II: Biscuit-bake try-in. In: Scharer P, Rinn LA, Kopp FR, eds. *Esthetic Guidelines for Restorative Dentistry*. Chicago, IL: Quintessence; 1982:188–192.

Bhuvaneswaran M. Principles of smile design. *J Conserv Dent* 2010;13(4):225–232.

Calamia JR, Levine JB, Lipp M, et al. Smile design and treatment planning with the help of a comprehensive esthetic evaluation form. *Dent Clin North Am* 2011;55(2):187–209.

Chu SJ. Clinical steps to predictable color management in aesthetic restorative dentistry. *Dent Clin North Am* 2007;51(2):473–485, x.

Chu SJ, Tarnow DP. Digital shade analysis and verification: a case report and discussion. *Pract Proced Aesthet Dent* 2001;13(2):129–136; quiz 138.

Cleveland JL Jr, Richardson JT. Surface characterization of temporary restorations: guidelines for quality ceramics. *J Prosthet Dent* 1977;37(6):643–647.

Davis NC. Smile design. *Dent Clin North Am* 2007;51(2):299–318, vii.

Duarte S, Jr, ed. *QDT 2010: Quintessence of Dental Technology*, vol. 33. Hanover Park, IL: Quintessence; 2010.

McLaren E, Vigoren G. Crown considerations, preparations, and material selection for esthetic metal ceramic restorations. *Esthet Tech* 2001;1(4):3–9.

Engelmeier RL. Complete-denture esthetics. *Dent Clin North Am* 1996;40(1):71–84.

Fondriest JF. Using provisional restorations to improve results in complex aesthetic restorative cases. *Pract Proced Aesthet Dent* 2006;18(4):217–223; quiz 224.

Goldstein RE, Garber DA. Maintaining esthetic restorations—a shared responsibility. *J Esthet Dent* 1995;7(5):187.

Goldstein RE. Esthetic dentistry—a health service? *J Dent Res* 1993;72(10):1365.

Goldstein RE. Finishing of composites and laminates. *Dent Clin North Am* 1989;33(2):305–318, 210–219.

Goodlin R. Photographic-assisted diagnosis and treatment planning. *Dent Clin North Am* 2011;55(2):211–227.

Itzhak S, Aharon W. Captek™—a new capillary casting technology for ceramometal restorations. *Quintessence Dent Technol* 1995;18:9–20.

Jahanbin A, Pezeshkirad H. The effects of upper lip height on smile esthetics perception in normal occlusion and nonextraction, orthodontically treated females. *Indian J Dent Res* 2008;19(3):204–207.

Jeffries SR. Abrasive finishing and polishing in restorative dentistry: a state-of-the-art review. *Dent Clin North Am* 2007;51(2):379–397, ix.

Llena C, Forner L, Ferrari M, et al. Toothguide Training Box for dental color choice training. *J Dent Educ* 2011;75(3):360–364.

Loguercio AD, Stanislawczuk R, Polli LG, et al. Influence of chlorhexidine digluconate concentration and application time on resin–dentin bond strength durability. *Eur J Oral Sci* 2009;117(5):587–596.

Lombardi RE. Factors mediating against excellence in dental esthetics. *J Prosthet Dent* 1977;38(3):243–248.

Lombardi RE. A method for the classification of errors in dental esthetics. *J Prosthet Dent* 1974;32(5):501–513.

Lowe RA. Predictable fixed prosthodontics: technique is the key to success. *Compend Contin Educ Dent* 2002;23(3 Suppl 1):4–12.

Milko V. Direct esthetic restorations based on translucency and opacity of composite resins. *J Esthet Res Dent* 2011;23(2):73–87.

Morley J, Eubank J. Macroesthetic elements of smile design. *J Am Dent Assoc* 2001;132(1):39–45.

Pietrobon N, Malament KA. Team approach between prosthodontics and dental technology. *Eur J Esthet Dent* 2007;2(1):58–79.

Ritter DE, Gandini LG, Jr, Pinto Ados S, et al. Analysis of the smile photograph. *World J Orthod* 2006;7(3):279–285.

Samorodnitzky-Naveh GR, Geiger SB, Levin L. Patients' satisfaction with dental esthetics. *J Am Dent Assoc* 2007;138(6):805–808.

Sarver D, Ackerman M. Dynamic smile visualization and quantification part 2. Evolution of the concept and dynamic records for a smile capture. *Am J Orthod Dentofacial Orthop* 2003;124(1):4–12.

Schmidt CJ, Tatum SA. Cosmetic dentistry. *Curr Opin Otolaryngol Head Neck Surg* 2006;14(4):254–259.

Shigli K, Awinashe V. Patient-dentist communication: an adjunct to successful complete denture treatment. *J Prosthodont* 2010;19(6):491–493.

Stappert CF, Tarnow DP, Tan JH, Chu SJ. Proximal contact areas of the maxillary anterior dentition. *Int J Periodontics Restorative Dent* 2010;30:471–477.

Vanini L, Mangani FM. Determination and communication of color using the five color dimensions of teeth. *Pract Proced Aesthet Dent* 2001;13(1):19–26; quiz 28.

Waliszewski M. Restoring dentate appearance: a literature review for modern complete denture esthetics. *J Prosthet Dent* 2005;93(4):386–394.

Wassell RW, Barker D, Steele JG. Crowns and other extra-coronal restorations: try-in and cementation of crowns. *Br Dent J* 2002;193(1):17–20, 23–28.

Witkowski S, Kunz A, Wagenknecht G. Improved communication during treatment planning using light-curing hybrid wax for esthetic try-in restorations. *Eur J Esthet Dent* 2006;1(4):326–339.

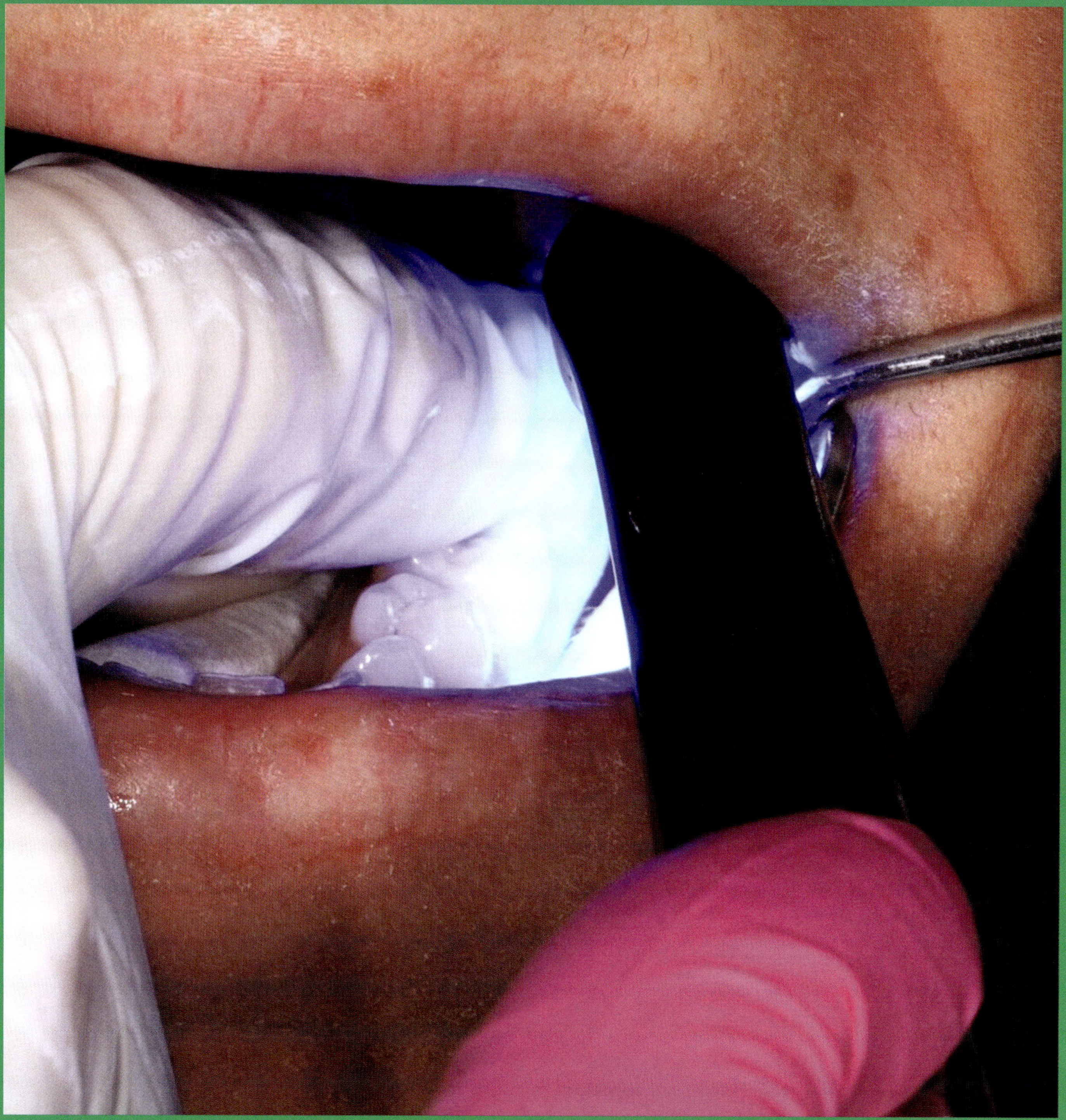

Chapter 44 Cementation of Restorations

Stephen F. Rosenstiel, BDS, MSD
and Ronald E. Goldstein, DDS

Chapter Outline

Dental cements	1355
Resin luting agents	1356
Postcementation sensitivity	1356
Preparation of the restoration and tooth surface for cementation	1356
Cementation procedure for metal–ceramic restorations	1358
Cementation technique for all-ceramic crowns	1361
Cementation procedures for ceramic restorations	1361
Selection of resin luting agent	1361
Cementation procedure for ceramic veneers and inlays	1364

Cementation is the final step in providing an indirect esthetic restoration. Like so many procedures in dentistry, attention to detail is essential, and inappropriate choice of material or its manipulation can ruin an otherwise outstanding patient treatment. A wide range of luting agents is now available, and the dentist should choose a material carefully and ensure that the office staff is thoroughly familiar with the recommended manipulation procedures. The choice of luting agent depends first on whether a conventional casting or an adhesively bonded restoration—such as a ceramic veneer or resin-retained partial fixed dental prosthesis—is to be cemented. Traditional dental cements can be used for conventional castings, but not where adhesion is needed. Adhesive resins are necessary for adhesively bonded restorations, but they can also be used for conventional castings; however, they may prove to be more difficult to use.

Dental cements

In the past, the luting agents used for cast restorations have been dental cements, such as zinc phosphate or glass ionomer. These consist of an acid (liquid) that is mixed with a metal oxide base (powder) to form a salt and water. The set material consists of unreacted powder particles "glued" together by the reaction products. However, cements are susceptible to acid attack and, therefore are, to some extent, soluble in oral fluids.[1,2] Nevertheless, the materials have proved to give excellent clinical performance, presumably because the cement margin is protected from further physical disintegration even after some dissolution has occurred.[3,4]

Many dentists continue to use zinc phosphate cement for their metal–ceramic crowns. This traditional luting agent has adequate strength, and it is easy to use, with low film thickness, reasonable working time, and, because it is nonadhesive, excess material is relatively easily removed. No luting agent has a longer history of successful use, and we have no data to prove that restorations will survive longer with the newer materials.

Glass ionomer cement has the advantage of adhesion to enamel and dentin and exhibits good biocompatibility. It is slightly stronger than zinc phosphate, though the setting cement is particularly susceptible to early moisture contamination[5] and should be carefully protected. The set material releases fluoride[6,7] and has been promoted as having an anticariogenic effect. However, this has not been documented clinically.[8] Glass ionomer cement is somewhat translucent, which provides an esthetic advantage over zinc phosphate. The newer resin-modified glass ionomers are less susceptible to early moisture[9] and represent one of the most popular type of luting agent in North America in terms of annual sales volume. (The terminology of some of the newer glass ionomer–resin combinations is rather confusing. In this chapter, the term "resin-modified glass ionomer" has been used. Other terms used for luting agents and restorative materials with a combination of glass ionomer and resin chemistries include "compomer" (mostly composite with some glass ionomer chemistry), "hybrid ionomer" (now considered obsolete), and "resin-reinforced glass ionomer.") Current developments include encapsulated and paste–paste formulations for easier and more accurate manipulation. Resin-modified glass ionomers are questionable with ceramic restorations as they have been associated with fracture,[10,11] probably due to their water absorption and expansion.[12] However, when using an all-zirconia or zirconia-core crown in which the internal surface cannot be etched, a resin-modified glass ionomer cement can be helpful, especially due to the passive fit of the all-ceramic crown.

Resin luting agents

Unfilled resins have been used for cementation since the 1950s. These early products were not successful because of high polymerization shrinkage and poor biocompatibility, but had very low solubility and good esthetic qualities. Composite resin luting agents with greatly improved properties were developed for the resin-retained prostheses and are extensively used for the bonded-ceramic technique (Figure 44.1A–G). Resin cements are available with adhesive properties; that is, they are capable of bonding chemically to dentin. Typically, bonding is achieved with organophosphonates, such as 10-methacryloyloxydecamethylene phosphoric acid, hydroxyethyl methacrylate, or 4-methacrylethyl trimellitic anhydride.[13] These developments have popularized the use of resin cements for crowns and conventional fixed prostheses. However, resin luting agents tend to have greater film thickness[14] and are less biocompatible than cements such as glass ionomer, especially if they are not fully polymerized.

Resin luting agents are available in a wide range of formulations. These can be categorized on the basis of polymerization method (chemical polymerization, light polymerization, or dual polymerization) and the presence of dentin bonding mechanisms. Metal restorations require a chemically polymerized system, whereas a light- or dual-polymerized system is appropriate with translucent ceramics. Resins formulated for cementing conventional castings must have lower film thickness than materials designed for ceramics or orthodontic brackets. However, this may be achieved at the expense of filler particle content and will adversely affect other properties, such as polymerization shrinkage.

The manipulative techniques may be very different with different brands of resin cement. For example, one material (Panavia 21) sets very rapidly when air is excluded. The directions call for the material to be spatulated in a thin film. It will set rapidly if piled up on the mixing pad. Another material (C&B-Metabond, Parkell Inc.) is mixed in a ceramic well that must be chilled to prevent premature setting.

Postcementation sensitivity

Increased sensitivity to hot or cold stimulation is an occasional but perplexing unwanted consequence of a newly cemented restoration,[15] and its occurrence is probably underestimated by most dentists.[16] Although conventional glass ionomers have been most often reported to cause sensitivity,[17] there appears to be little pulpal response at the histological level,[18] particularly if the remaining dentin thickness exceeds 1 mm,[19] and the reports have not been supported by clinical trials.[20–22] Side effects such as posttreatment sensitivity that have been ascribed to lack of biocompatibility are probably due to desiccation or bacterial contamination[23] of the dentin rather than irritation by the cement per se. If, in practice, dentists find postcementation sensitivity to be a problem, then they should carefully evaluate their technique, particularly avoiding desiccation of the prepared dentin surface. Resin-modified glass ionomer materials and self-etching resin cements have been reported to exhibit less postcementation sensitivity,[24,25] which may be due to reduced marginal leakage[26] or their antimicrobial effects.[27] A desensitizing agent or antimicrobial may reduce sensitivity, though it may also adversely affect retention, at least with some luting cements.[28,29]

Preparation of the restoration and tooth surface for cementation

The performance of all luting agents is degraded if the material is contaminated with water, blood, or saliva. Therefore, the restoration and tooth must be carefully cleaned and dried after the try-in procedure, although excessive drying of the tooth must be avoided to prevent sensitivity. A metal casting is best prepared by airborne particle abrading the fitting surface with 50 μm alumina. This should be done carefully to avoid abrading the polished surfaces or margins. Abrasion has been shown to increase the in vitro retention of castings by 64%.[30] Alternative cleaning methods include steam cleaning, ultrasonics, and organic solvents. Also, make sure all porcelain shoulder margins are properly etched with hydrofluoric acid and silanated before cementation (Figure 44.2).

Chapter 44 Cementation of Restorations

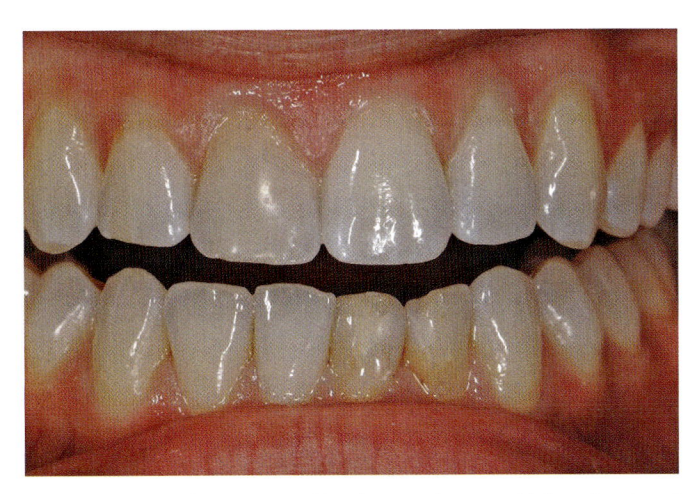

Figure 44.1 **(A)** This 17-year-old girl was unhappy with her discolored teeth which bleaching had not helped.

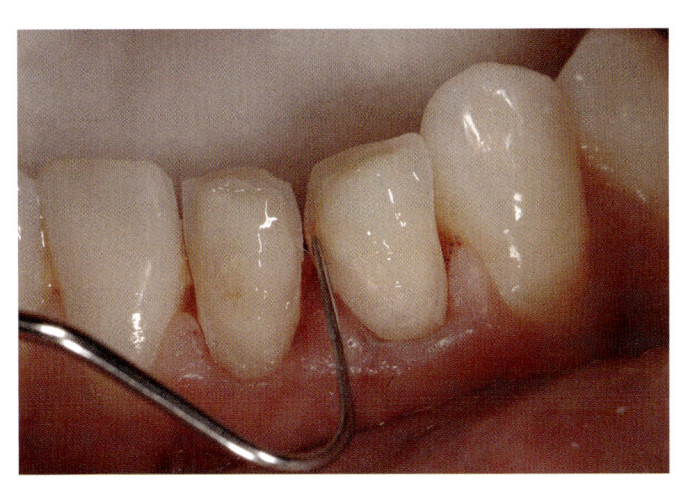

Figure 44.1 **(B)** It was decided to do porcelain veneers on the mandibular left lateral and central incisors to improve their color and form.

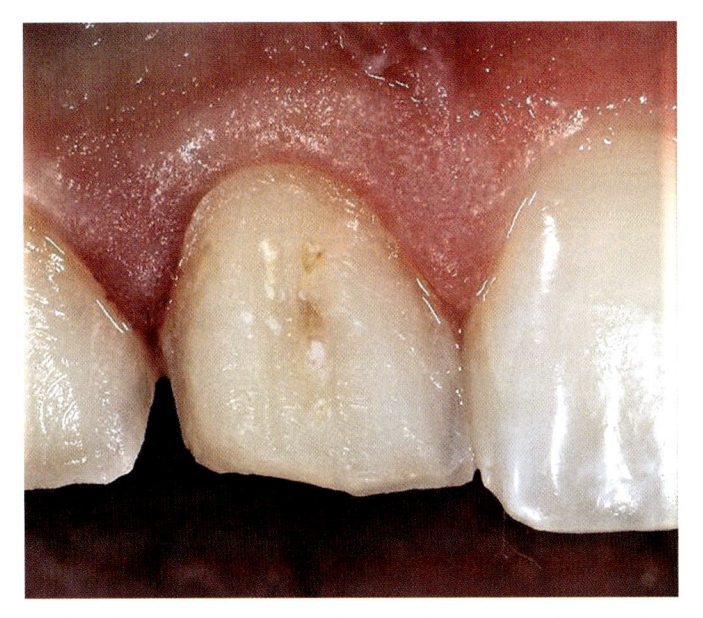

Figure 44.1 **(C)** The maxillary central and lateral incisors were prepared for porcelain veneers. However, there was a dark brown spot on the central, which would influence the final shade.

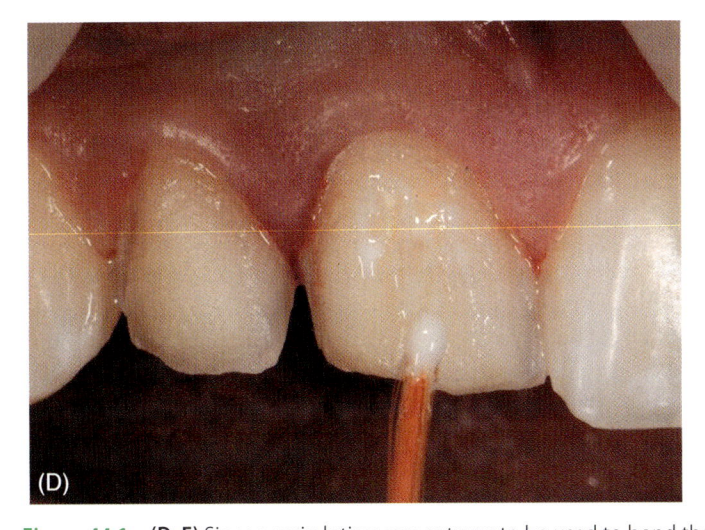

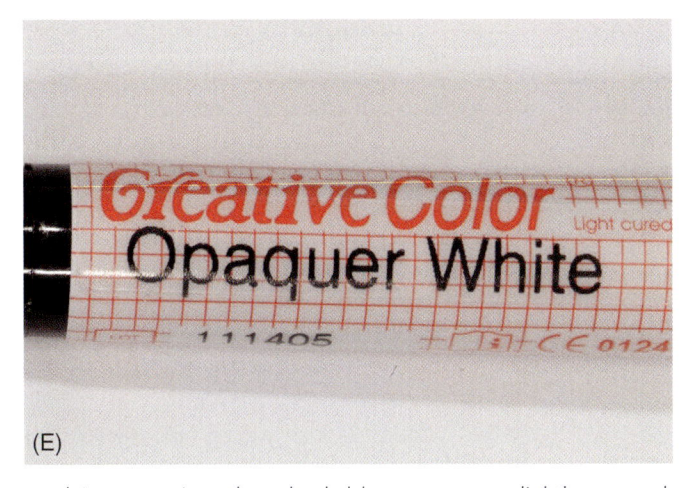

Figure 44.1 **(D, E)** Since a resin luting cement was to be used to bond the porcelain veneers into place, the dark brown area was slightly prepared and a white resin opaque was applied to help mask the stain. (Cosmedent).

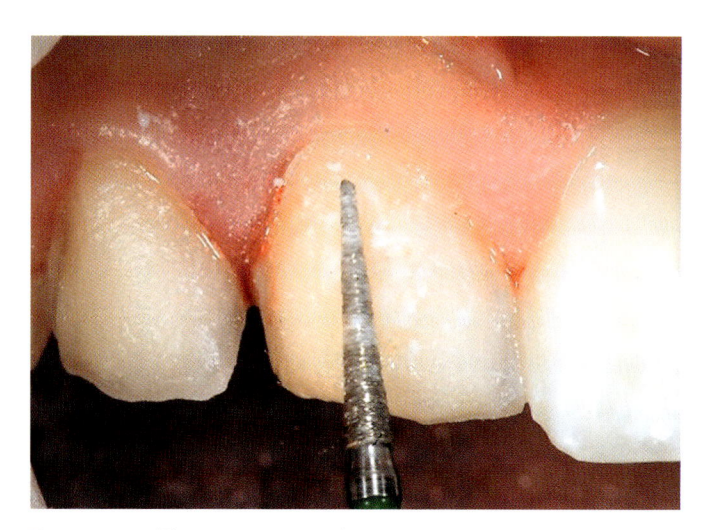

Figure 44.1 **(F)** An extra-coarse diamond (AC2, Brasseler USA) was used to make sure the veneer still fit perfectly.

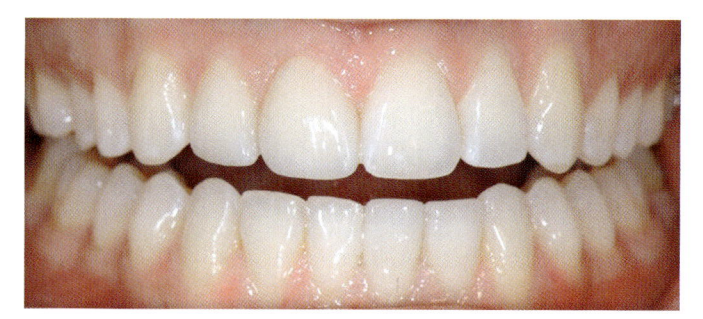

Figure 44.1 **(G)** Resin luting cement was used to bond the four veneers into place. Note the shade blends without showing evidence of the dark stain on the upper right central.

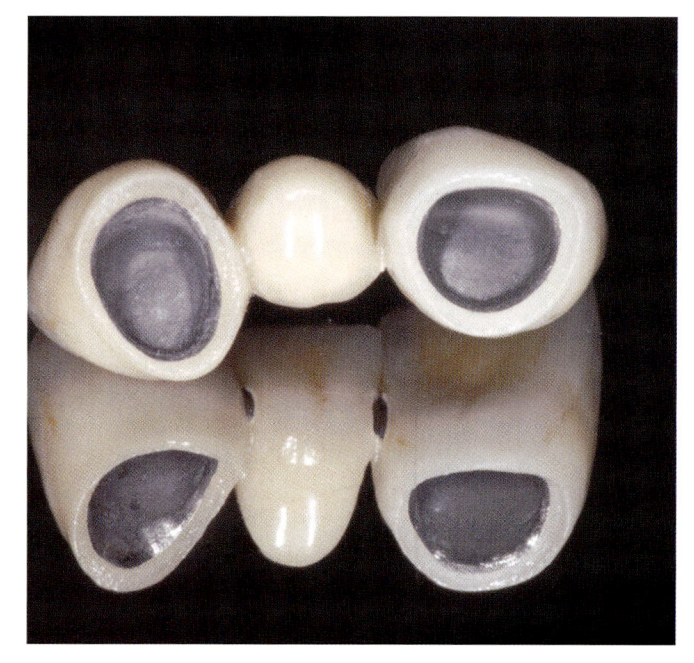

Figure 44.2 When using a metal-ceramic butt-joint restoration, it is important to always make sure the porcelain butt margin is etched and silanated before cementation.

Cementation procedure for metal–ceramic restorations

Resin-modified glass ionomer is used to illustrate the typical procedure, although, depending on the cement chosen, the steps may vary slightly. When using a resin-modified glass ionomer cement, avoid cementing too many crowns at the same time due to the fast set of material. Generally, a quadrant consisting of four posterior crowns or six anterior crowns can be accomplished, but only if you have two to three mixes of cement virtually at the same time. As each crown is placed, the next one is quickly inserted until all the crowns are seated.

1. Immediately prior to cementation, inspect all preparation surfaces for cleanliness (Figure 44.3A). Remove any provisional luting agent with a pumice wash or hydrogen peroxide. Use an antimicrobial if desired, although research has not proved this step to be beneficial. The casting should be airborne-particle abraded, steam cleaned, or cleaned ultrasonically and washed with alcohol to remove any remaining polishing compound or die spacer. The prepared tooth should be isolated with cotton rolls, and a saliva evacuator is placed (Figure 44.3B–E).

2. Mix the luting agent as recommended by the manufacturer; check the consistency to make sure the product has been dispensed correctly.

3. Apply a thin coat of cement to the clean internal surface of the restoration. To extend working time, the cement should be applied to a cool restoration rather than to a warm tooth (Figure 44.3 F–I).

4. Check that the tooth is properly isolated and push the restoration into place. Final seating is achieved by rocking with an orangewood stick until all excess cement is seen to have escaped. It is important to seat the restoration firmly with a rocking, dynamic seating force. Using a static load may cause binding of the restoration and lead to incomplete seating.[31] Excessive force during seating should be avoided. A cotton roll can continue to hold the crowns in place once firmly seated (Figure 44.3 J).

5. After the casting is seated, check the margins with an explorer to verify that the restoration is indeed fully in place. Another technique to make certain the crowns are in proper occlusion is to have the patient quickly close onto shim stock that is 5/10,000″ thickness (Artus) until they are seated properly. Protect the setting cement from moisture by covering with varnish.

6. When fully set, remove excess cement with an explorer or scaler (Figure 44.3 K–L). Early removal of cement may lead to early moisture exposure at the margins with increased solubility. Dental floss with a small knot in it can be used to remove any irritating residual cement interproximally and

Chapter 44 Cementation of Restorations

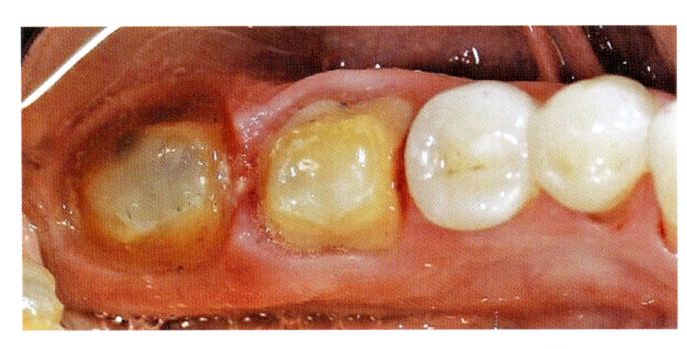

Figure 44.3 **(A)** Two complete metal-ceramic crowns will be cemented into place on the mandibular right first and second molars.

from the gingival sulcus (Figure 44.3 M). Occasionally cement gets trapped in the contact areas, making it impossible to get dental floss through. One good technique is to use a very thin saw to easily separate the contact and allow floss to get through. The sulcus should contain no cement. Many dentists take a radiograph to help identify residual cement. After the excess has been removed, the occlusion can be checked once more with Mylar shim stock.

7. Cements take at least 24 h to develop their final strength. Therefore, the patient should be cautioned to chew carefully for a day or two (Figure 44.3 N).

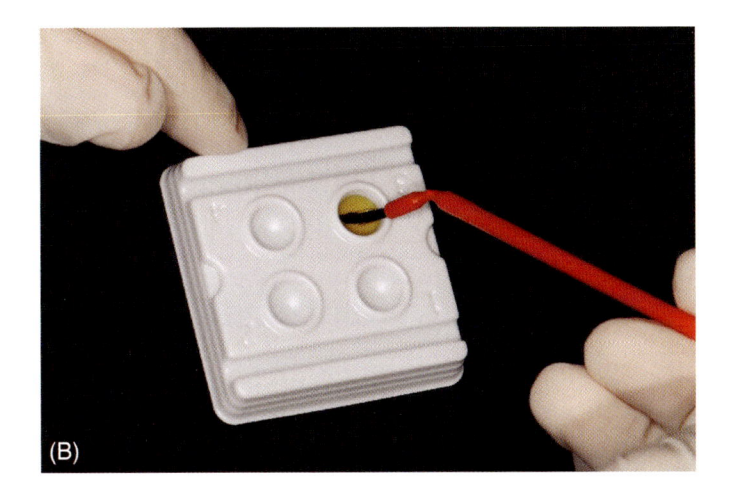

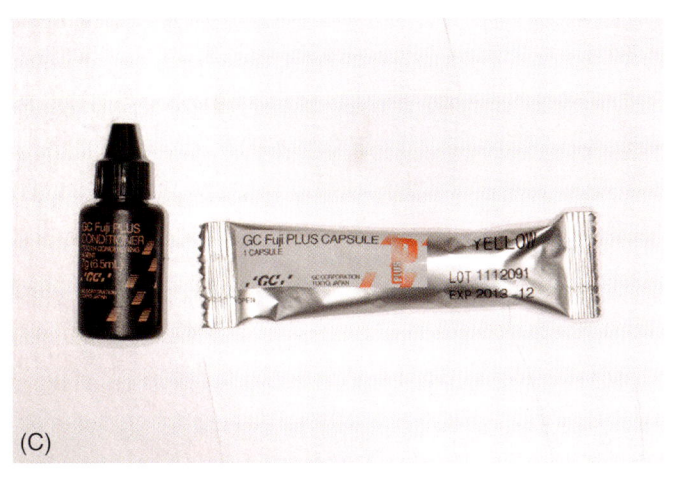

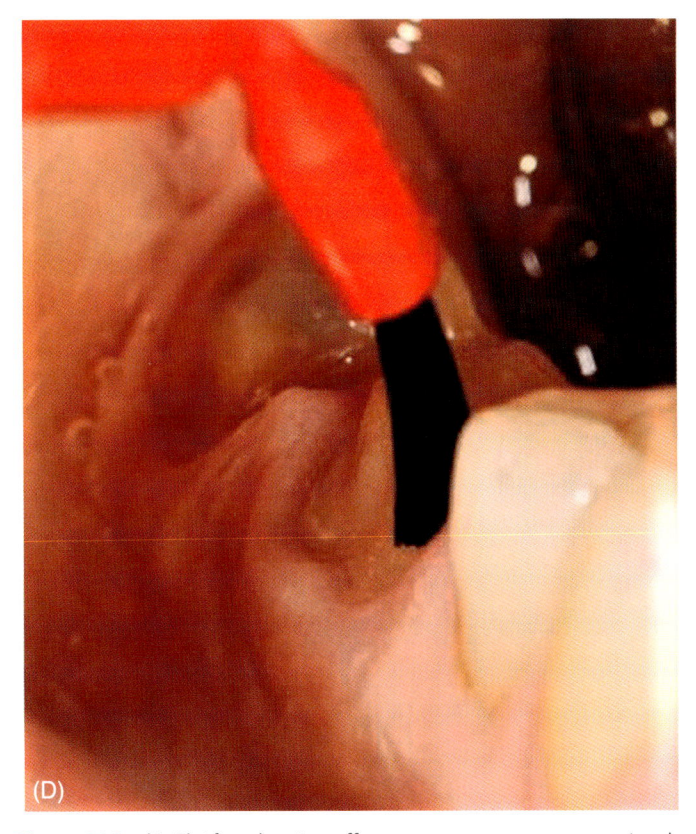

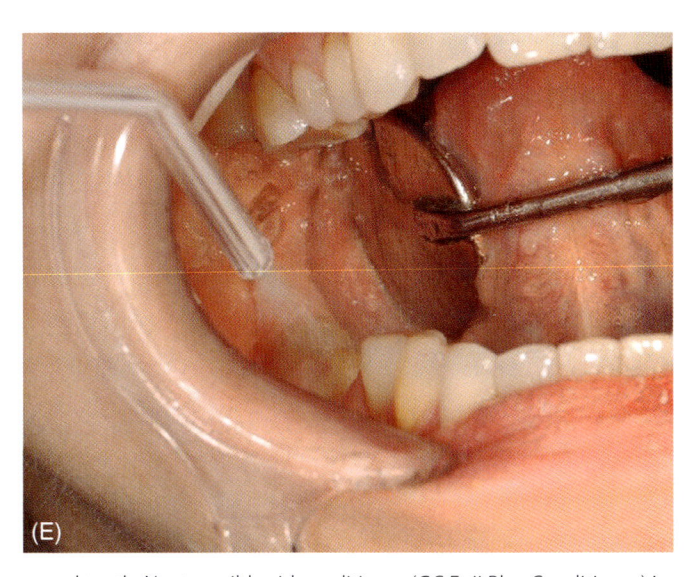

Figure 44.3 **(B–E)** After cleaning off any temporary cement, pumice the prepared teeth. Next, a mild acid conditioner (GC Fuji Plus Conditioner) is applied and thoroughly rinsed.

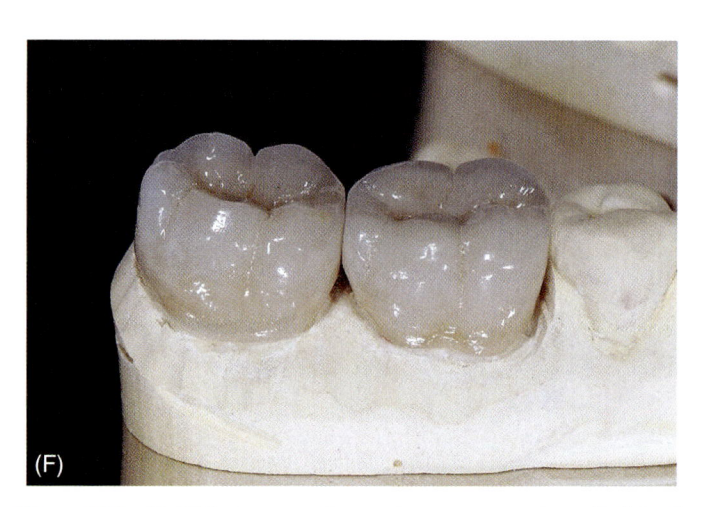

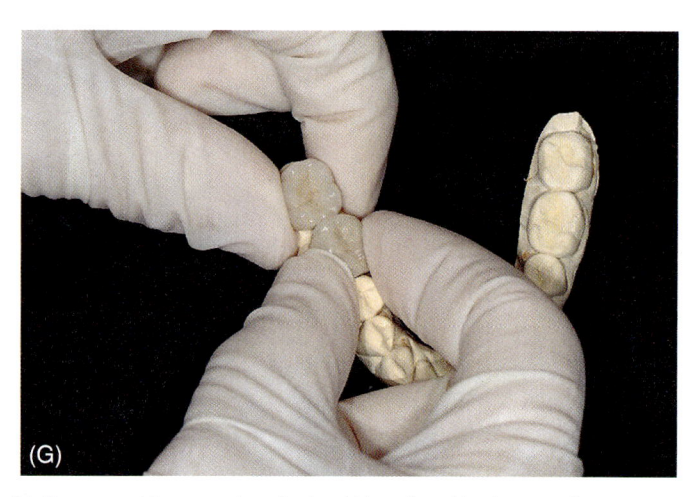

Figure 44.3 (F, G) The two metal-ceramic crowns are taken off of the die with finger position exactly as it should be placed in the mouth.

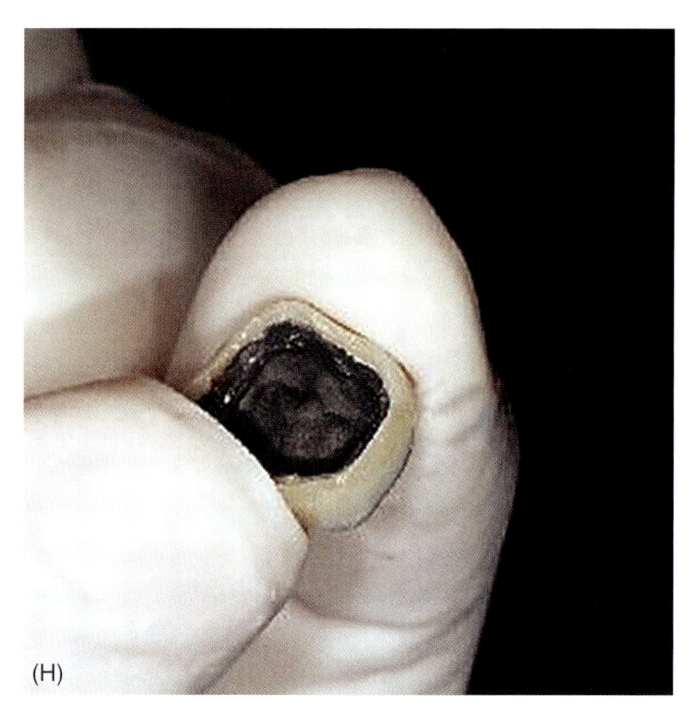

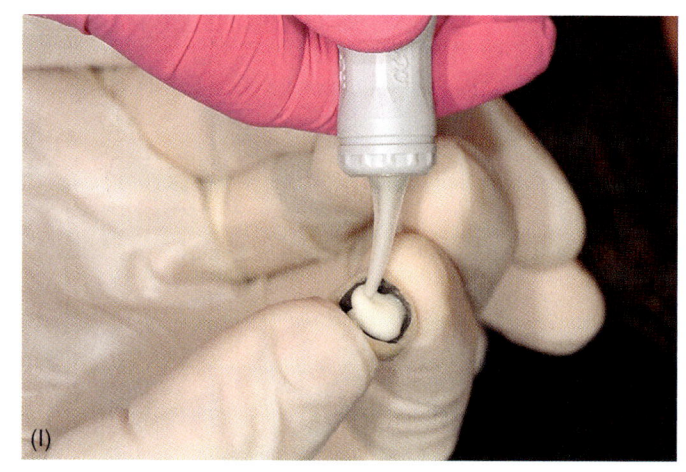

Figure 44.3 (H, I) The first molar crown is removed from the die with finger position exactly as it should be placed in the mouth.

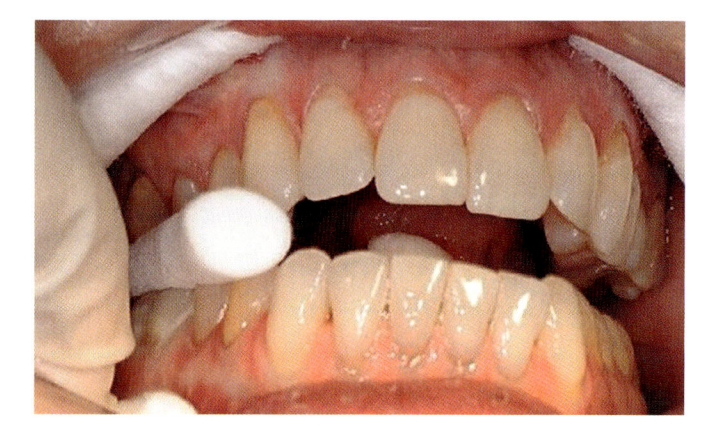

Figure 44.3 (J) Once the crown is firmly seated into place as described in the text, repeat the same procedure for the second crown, then have the patient bite into centric with either an orange stick or cotton roll. Note, as this type of cement sets quickly, it is urgent that each crown be seated and verified one after the other as quickly as possible.

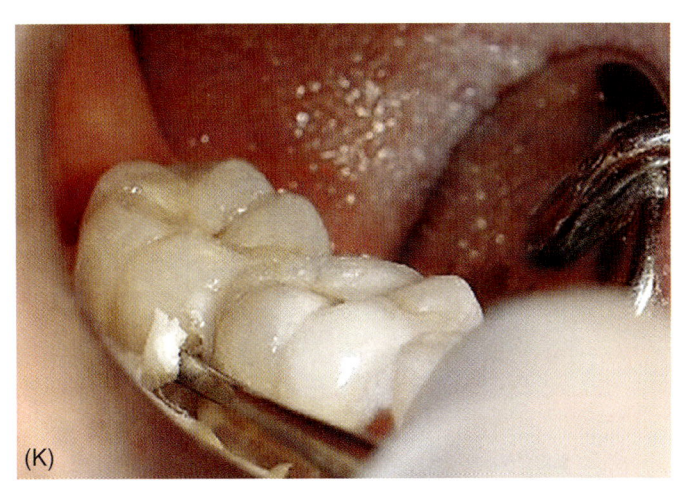

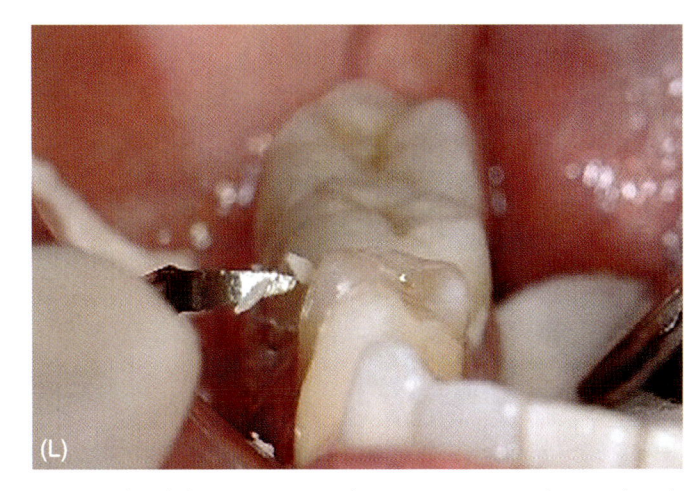

Figure 44.3 (K, L) Once the cement has reached its initial set, it is important to immediately begin to remove the excess cement with a combined chisel/scaler instrument (Novatech 12-CRNT12, Hu-Friedy).

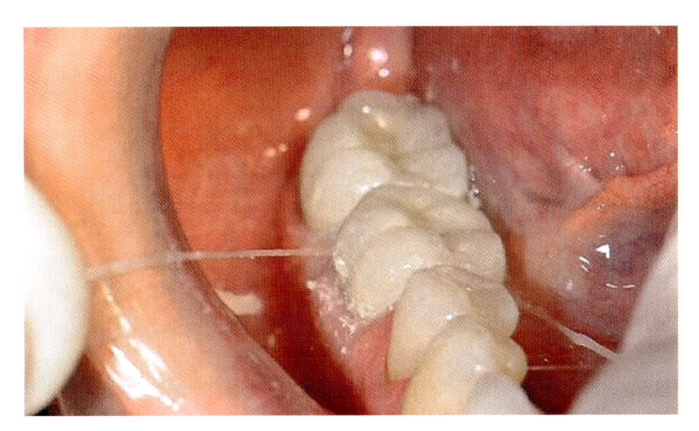

Figure 44.3 (M) Dental floss with a small knot can be used to remove any residual cement interproximally and from the gingival sulcus. At times, a very thin saw (ET Flex, Brasseler USA) can be used to separate a contact and allow the floss to go through.

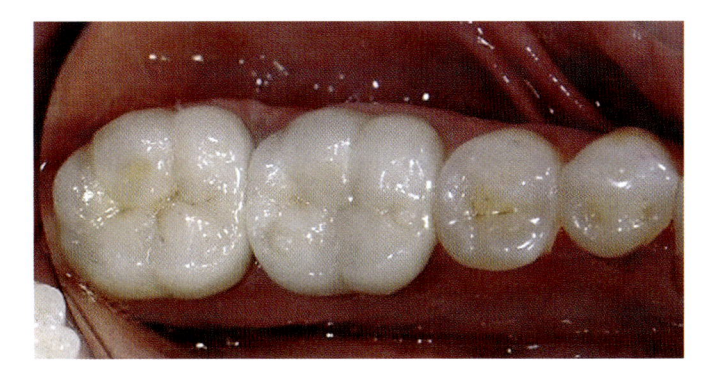

Figure 44.3 (N) Final crowns cemented into place showing good tissue adaptation and no cement residue.

Cementation technique for all-ceramic crowns

Cementation for all-ceramic crowns is similar to procedures for ceramic veneer inlays and onlays. However, some of the newer luting agents are self-adhesive, not requiring a separate step etching during tooth preparation. Nevertheless, that option is up to the dentist to decide whether extra etching is necessary. The same can be said about the bonding resin placed inside the crown. One example of step-by-step cementation of an all-ceramic crown with self-adhesive cement can be seen in Figure 44.4A–J.

Cementation procedures for ceramic restorations

Depending on the ceramic system used, these restorations may rely on resin bonding for retention and strength. The cementation steps are critical to the success of the restoration, and careless handling of the resin luting agent may be a key factor in their prognosis. Bonding is achieved by (1) etching the fitting surface of the ceramic with hydrofluoric acid, (2) applying a silane coupling agent to the ceramic, (3) etching the enamel with phosphoric acid, (4) applying resin bonding agent to etched enamel and silane, and (5) seating the restoration with a resin luting agent.

Selection of resin luting agent

Composite resin luting agents are available in a range of formulations. For translucent ceramic veneers, a light-polymerized material can be used, but for inlays a chemical- or dual-polymerized material is preferred to ensure maximum polymerization of the resin in the less accessible proximal areas. Dual-polymerized resin has been found to give better marginal adaptation at the critical gingival margin area, possibly because voids incorporated during mixing reduce the harmful contraction stresses of the resin.[32]

The appearance of veneers can be modified to some extent by the shade of the luting agent. Color-matched try-in pastes are available for some products (e.g., NX3, Kerr Corporation) to facilitate selecting the best shade.

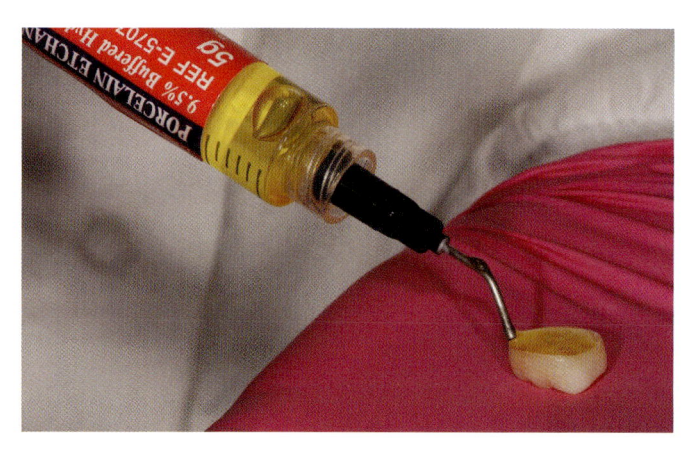

Figure 44.4 **(A)** Cementation for this all-ceramic crown begins with etching the internal surface of the crown with 9.5% hydrofluoric acid (Porcelain Etchant, Bisco Inc.) for 90 s.

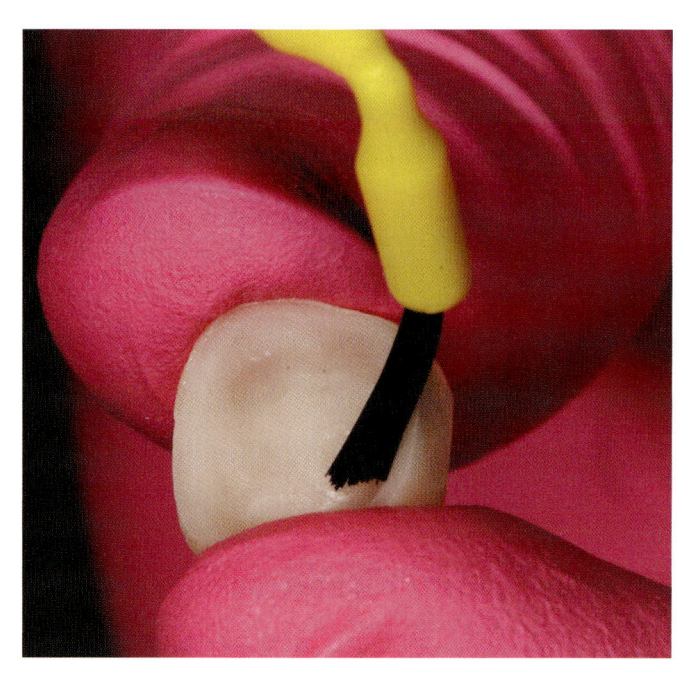

Figure 44.4 **(B)** Next, apply two thin coats of silane to the etched internal surface and air dry.

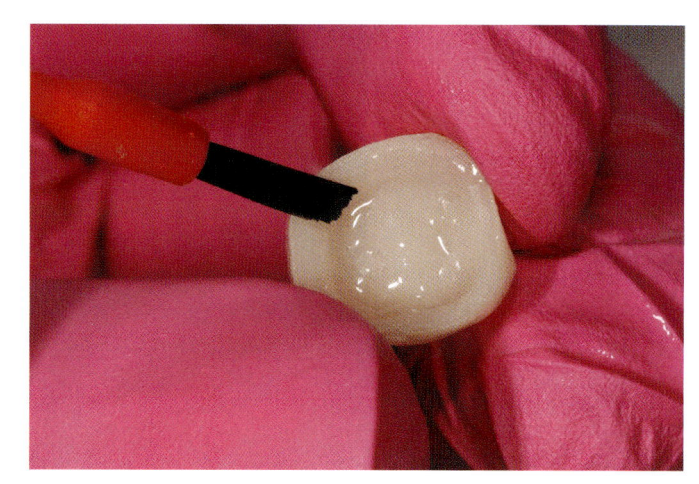

Figure 44.4 **(C)** Coating the inside of the crown with bonding resin could be an option according to some manufacturer's instructions.

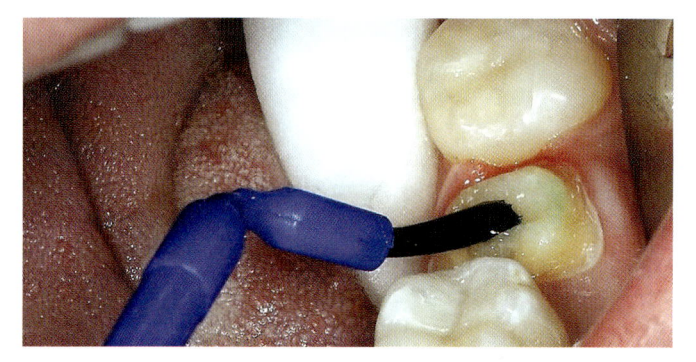

Figure 44.4 **(D)** Although not necessary with self-adhesive resin cements, the prepared tooth can be etched with 35% phosphoric acid for 20 s and rinsed thoroughly.

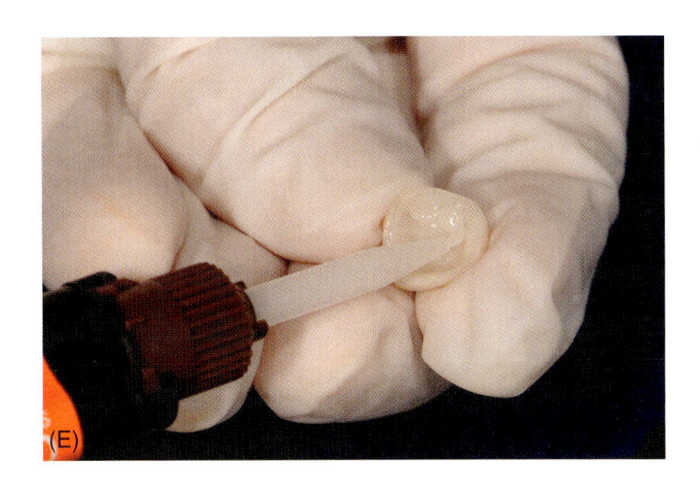

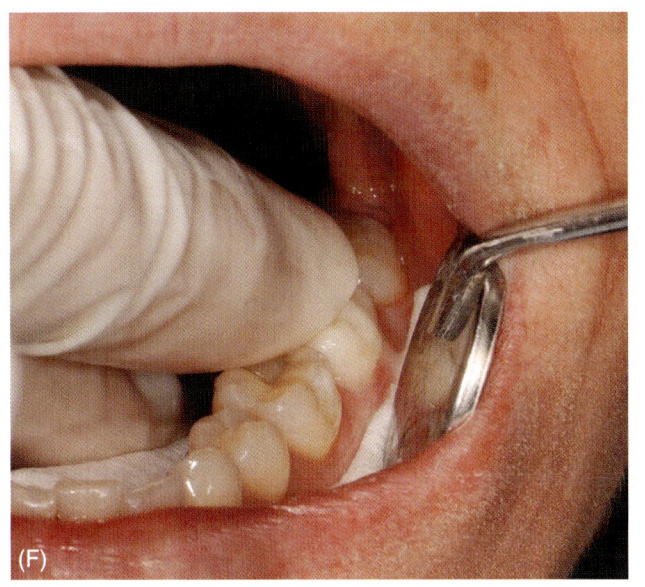

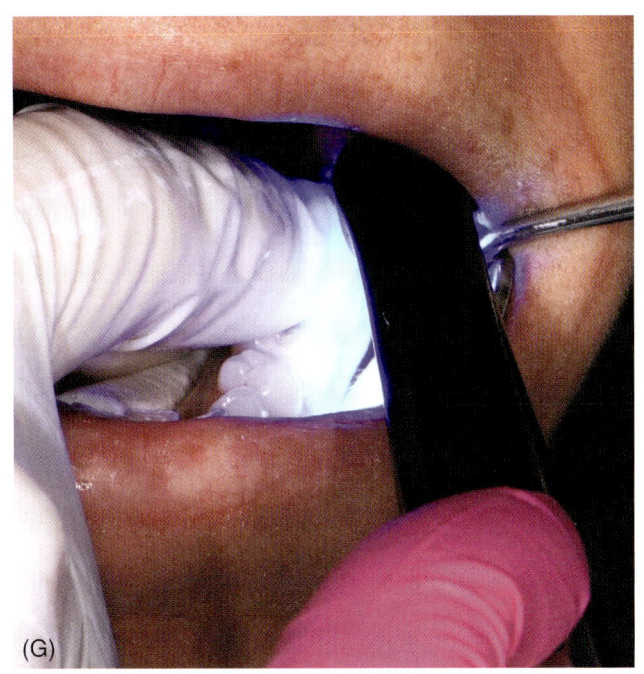

Figure 44.4 **(E–G)** The cement is loaded into the crown by lining the internal surfaces and immediately put into place and tack cure for 2–4 s.

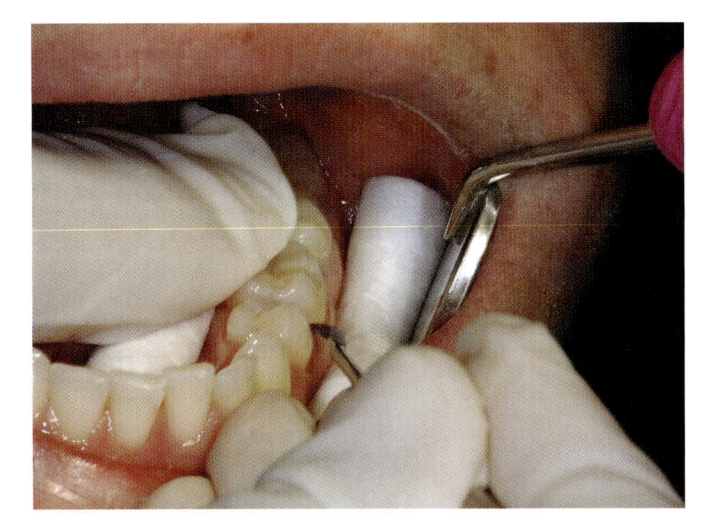

Figure 44.4 **(H)** Remove excess cement, and repolymerize all surfaces for 20 s.

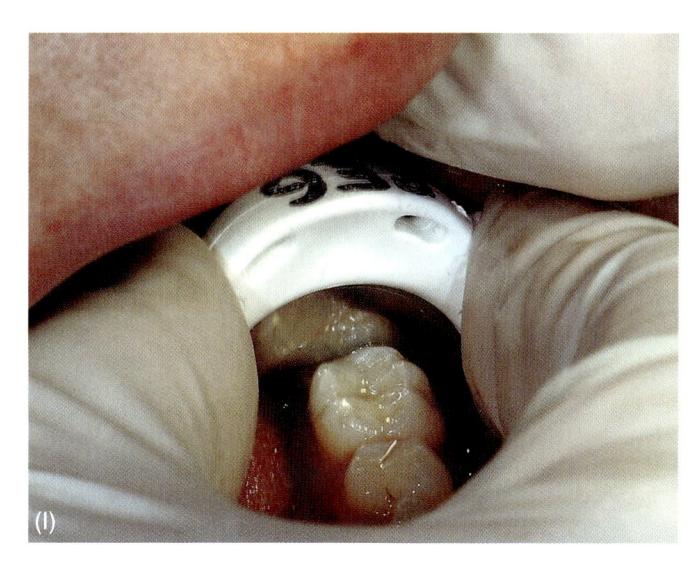

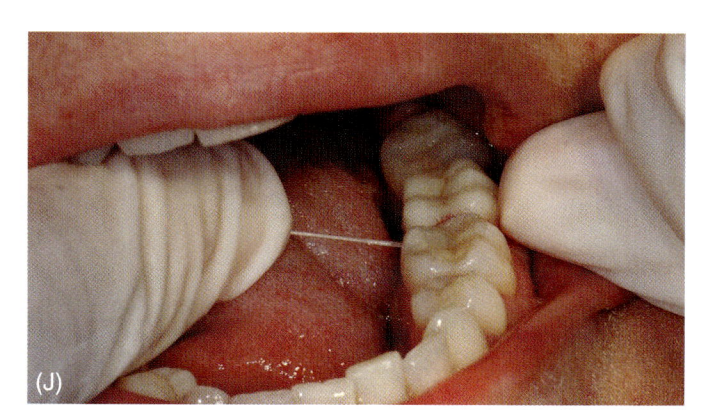

Figure 44.4 (I, J) If excess cement is in the contact area making it impossible to get floss through, use a very thin saw instrument (ET Flex, Brasseler USA) to clear the contact area.

Cementation procedure for ceramic veneers and inlays

1. Clean the teeth with pumice and water. Isolate them with a rubber dam or displacement cord. Remember, a luting agent containing zinc oxide–eugenol (ZOE) is best avoided for cementing provisional restorations prior to resin bonding. Eugenol inhibits the polymerization of the resin. If a ZOE-containing product has been used, cleansing with pumice will not remove it completely.[33] Etching with 37% phosphoric acid after cleaning with pumice may be the best means of ZOE removal.[34]
2. Evaluate the fit and esthetics of the restorations with glycerin or a try-in paste. Sometimes multiple restorations can only be inserted in one sequence, so note this order.
3. Clean the restorations thoroughly in water or acetone with ultrasonic agitation. Dry them and support in soft wax with the fitting surface uppermost.
4. Apply a 1 mm coat of the etching gel (Ceram-Etch Gel (9.5% hydrofluoric acid), Gresco Products Inc., Stafford, Texas (or the ceramic manufacturer's recommended product)) to the fitting surface only. The etching time will depend on the ceramic material. Feldspathic porcelain is typically etched for 5 min.
5. Very carefully rinse away the gel under running water. The gel is very caustic; it should not be allowed to contact skin or eyes. Continue to rinse until all the gel color has been removed.
6. Dry the ceramic with oil-free air. If there is doubt about the unit air, a hair drier is recommended to ensure that the ceramic is not contaminated.
7. Apply the silane according to the manufacturer's recommendations. Some manufacturers recommend a heat-polymerized silane coupling agent for increased bond strength, rather than a chemically activated silane. Heat curing is normally done by the laboratory, and care must be taken to clean the fitting surface thoroughly with alcohol before cementation.
8. Acid etch the enamel; 37% phosphoric acid is generally used, applied for 20s. Rinse thoroughly and dry.
9. Apply a thin layer of bonding resin to the preparation. Brush, rather than air thin, the bonding resin, as air thinning might inhibit polymerization.[35] Do not polymerize this layer before cementing, as it might interfere with complete seating.
10. For veneers, place a Mylar matrix strip at the mesial and distal surfaces of the prepared tooth.
11. Apply resin luting agent to the restoration, being especially careful to avoid trapping air.
12. Position the restoration gently, removing excess luting agent with an instrument or brush.
13. Hold the restoration in place while light curing the resin. Do not press on the center of veneers; they may flex and break.
14. Use dental tape to remove resin flash from the interproximal margins of inlays and onlays before curing these areas.
15. Do not underpolymerize the resin cement. Allow at least 40s for each area.
16. Remove resin flash with a scalpel, sharp curette, or an ET 15 μm diamond (Brasseler USA).
17. Finish accessible margins and occlusion with fine diamonds, using water spray. Use finishing strips for the interproximal margins.
18. Polish adjusted areas with rubber wheels or points and then with diamond polishing paste.

Summary

Proper moisture control is essential for the cementation step. The restoration must be carefully prepared for cementation, including the removal of all polishing compounds.

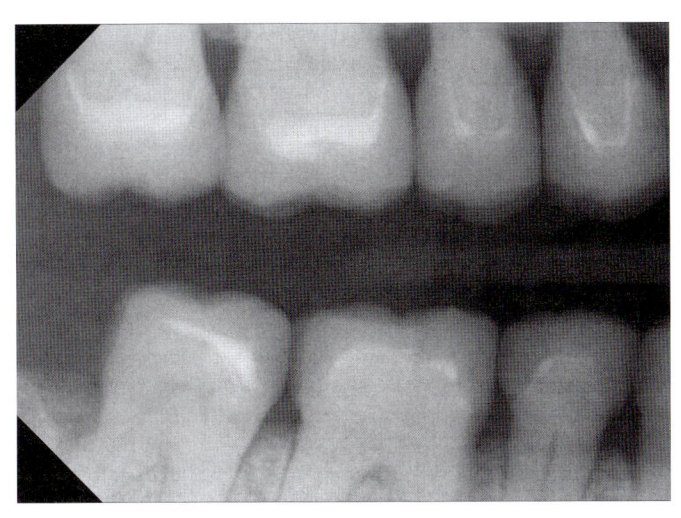

Figure 44.5 **(A)** Following cementation, a postoperative radiograph should be taken to verify that all cement has been removed.

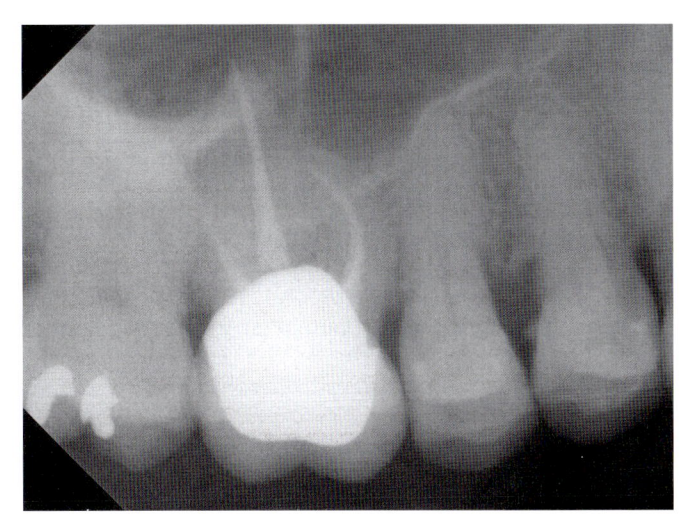

Figure 44.5 **(B)** This is a perfect example showing why a postoperative radiograph is necessary. Note the presence of extra cement at the distal of the first premolar.

Airborne-particle abrading the fitting surface of metal ceramic restorations is recommended. The luting agent of choice is mixed according to manufacturer's recommendations, and the restoration is seated using a rocking action. The cement must be protected from moisture during its initial set. Removal of excess cement from the gingival sulcus is critical for continued periodontal health. A digital radiograph is the last way to make certain that no cement remains (Figure 44.5A and B).

Additional steps are necessary for adhesively bonded restorations. These steps must be carefully sequenced according to manufacturer's directions.

References

1. Swartz ML, Phillips RW, Pareja C, Moore BK. In vitro degradation of cements: a comparison of three test methods. *J Prosthet Dent* 1989;62:17–23.
2. Knibbs PJ, Walls AW. A laboratory and clinical evaluation of three dental luting cements. *J Oral Rehabil* 1989;16:467–473.
3. Jacobs MS, Windeler AS. An investigation of dental luting cement solubility as a function of the marginal gap. *J Prosthet Dent* 1991;65:436–442.
4. Dupuis V, Laviole O, Potin-Gautier M, et al. Solubility and disintegration of zinc phosphate cement. *Biomaterials* 1992;13:467–470.
5. Um CM, Oilo G. The effect of early water contact on glass-ionomer cements. *Quintessence Int* 1992;23:209–214.
6. Swartz ML, Phillips RW, Clark HE. Long term F release from glass ionomer cements. *J Dent Res* 1984;63:158–160.
7. Muzynski BL, Greener E, Jameson L, Malone WF. Fluoride release from glass ionomers used as luting agents. *J Prosthet Dent* 1988;60:41–44.
8. Rosenstiel SF, Land MF, Crispin BJ. Dental luting agents: a review of the current literature. *J Prosthet Dent* 1998;80:280–301.
9. Cho E, Kopel H, White SN. Moisture susceptibility of resin-modified glass-ionomer materials. *Quintessence Int* 1995;26:351–358.
10. Letters to the editor. *Quintessence Int* 1996;27:655–657.
11. Leevailoj C, Platt JA, Cochran MA, Moore BK. In vitro study of fracture incidence and compressive fracture load of all-ceramic crowns cemented with resin-modified glass ionomer and other luting agents. *J Prosthet Dent* 1998;80:699–707.
12. Knobloch LA, Kerby RE, McMillen K, Clelland N. Solubility and sorption of resin-based luting cements. *Oper Dent* 2000;25:434–440.
13. Anusavice KJ. *Phillips' Science of Dental Materials*, 11th edn. St Louis, MO: Saunders; 2003:486.
14. Caughman WF, Caughman GB, Dominy WT, Schuster GS. Glass ionomer and composite resin cements: effects on oral cells. *J Prosthet Dent* 1990;63:513–521.
15. Brännström M. Reducing the risk of sensitivity and pulpal complications after the placement of crowns and fixed partial dentures. *Quintessence Int* 1996;27:673–678.
16. Rosenstiel SF, Rashid RG. Postcementation hypersensitivity: scientific data versus dentists' perceptions. *J Prosthodont* 2003;12:73–81.
17. Council on Dental Materials, Instruments, and Equipment, American Dental Association. Reported sensitivity to glass ionomer luting cements. *J Am Dent Assoc* 1984;109:476.
18. Heys RJ, Fitzgerald M, Heys DR, Charbeneau GT. An evaluation of a glass ionomer luting agent: pulpal histological response. *J Am Dent Assoc* 1987;114:607–611.
19. Pameijer CH, Stanley HR, Ecker G. Biocompatibility of a glass ionomer luting agent. 2. Crown cementation. *Am J Dent* 1991;4:134–141.
20. Johnson GH, Powell LV, DeRouen TA. Evaluation and control of post-cementation pulpal sensitivity: zinc phosphate and glass ionomer luting cements. *J Am Dent Assoc* 1993;124:38–46.
21. Bebermeyer RD, Berg JH. Comparison of patient-perceived post-cementation sensitivity with glass-ionomer and zinc phosphate cements. *Quintessence Int* 1994;25:209–214.
22. Kern M, Kleimeier B, Schaller HG, Strub JR. Clinical comparison of postoperative sensitivity for a glass ionomer and a zinc phosphate luting cement. *J Prosthet Dent* 1996;75:159–162.
23. Torstenson B. Pulpal reaction to a dental adhesive in deep human cavities. *Endod Dent Traumatol* 1995;11:172–176.
24. Chandrasekhar V. Post cementation sensitivity evaluation of glass ionomer, zinc phosphate and resin modified glass ionomer luting cements under class II inlays: an in vivo comparative study. *J Conserv Dent* 2010;13:23–27.

25. Blatz MB, Mante FK, Saleh N, et al. Postoperative tooth sensitivity with a new self-adhesive resin cement—a randomized clinical trial. *Clin Oral Investig* 2013;17:793–798.
26. White SN, Yu Z, Tom JF, Sangsurasak S. In vivo microleakage of luting cements for cast crowns. *J Prosthet Dent* 1994;71:333–338.
27. Coogan MM, Creaven PJ. Antibacterial properties of eight dental cements. *Int Endod J* 1993;26:355–361.
28. Mausner IK, Goldstein GR, Georgescu M. Effect of two dentinal desensitizing agents on retention of complete cast coping using four cements. *J Prosthet Dent* 1996;75:129–134.
29. Pameijer CH, Hulten J, Glantz PO, Randow K. Influence of low-viscosity liners on the retention of three luting materials. *Int J Periodontics Restorative Dent* 1992;12:195–205.
30. O'Connor RP, Nayyar A, Kovarik RE. Effect of internal microblasting on retention of cemented cast crowns. *J Prosthet Dent* 1990;64:557–562.
31. Rosenstiel SF, Gegauff AG. Improving the cementation of complete cast crowns: a comparison of static and dynamic seating methods. *J Am Dent Assoc* 1988;117:845–848.
32. Alster D, Feilzer AJ, De Gee AJ, et al. The dependence of shrinkage stress reduction on porosity concentration in thin resin layers. *J Dent Res* 1992;71:1619–1622.
33. Mojon P, Hawbolt EB, MacEntee MI. A comparison of two methods for removing zinc oxide–eugenol provisional cement. *Int J Prosthodont* 1992;5:78–84.
34. Schwartz R, Davis R, Mayhew R. Effect of a ZOE temporary cement on the bond strength of a resin luting cement. *Am J Dent* 1990;3:28–30.
35. Galan D, Williams PT, Kasloff Z. Effects of warm air-drying and spreading on resin bonding. *Am J Dent* 1991;4:277–280.

Additional resources

Aboushelib MN, Kleverlaan CJ, Feilzer AJ. Selective infiltration-etching technique for a strong and durable bond of resin cements to zirconia-based materials. *J Prosthet Dent* 2007;98:379–388.

Blatz MB, Chiche G, Holst S, Sadan A. influence of surface treatment and simulated again on bond strengths of luting agents to zirconia. *Quintessence Int* 2007;38:745–753.

Blatz MB, Phark JH, Ozer F, et al. In vitro comparative bond strength of contemporary self-adhesive resin cements to zirconium oxide ceramic with and without air-particle abrasion. *Clin Oral Investig* 2010;14:187–192.

Capa N, Ozkurt Z, Canpolat C, Kazazoglu E. Shear bond strength of luting agents to fixed prosthodontic restorative core materials. *Aust Dent J* 2009;54:334–430.

Casucci A, Osorio E, Ororio R, et al. Influence of different surface treatments on surface zirconia frameworks. *J Dent* 2009;37:891–897.

Casucci A, Mazzitelli C, Monticelli F, et al. Morphological analysis of three zirconium oxide ceramics: effect of surface treatments. *Dent Mater* 2010;26:751–760.

Chau N, Pandit S, Jung J, Cai J, Yi H. Long-term anti-cariogenic biofilm activity of glass ionomers related to fluoride release. *J Dent* 2016;47:34–40.

Dino RE, Augusti D, Augusti G, Giovannetti A. Early bond strength to low-pressure sandblasted zirconia: evaluation of a self-adhesive cement. *Eur J Esthet Dent* 2012;7:164–174.

Gavic L, Gorseta K, Borzabadi-Farahani A, et al. Influence of thermo-light curing with dental light-curing units on the microhardness of glass-ionomer cements. *Int J Periodontics Restorative Dent* 2016;36:425–430.

Guess PC, Zhang Y, Kim JW, et al. Damage and reliability of Y-TZP after cementation surface treatment. *J Dent Res* 2010;89:592–596.

Hikita K, Van Meerbeek B, De Munck J, et al. Bonding effectiveness of adhesive luting agents to enamel and dentin. *Dent Mater* 2007;23:71–80.

Irie M, Suzuki K, Watts DC. Marginal and flexural integrity of three classes of luting cement, with early finishing and water storage. *Dent Mater* 2004;20:3–11.

Lawson N, Burgess J. Dental ceramics: a current review. *Compend Contin Educ Dent* 2014;35:161–166.

Lin J, Shinya A, Gomi H, Shinya A. Effect of self-adhesive resin cement and tribochemical treatment on bond strength to zirconia. *Int J Oral Sci* 2010;2:28–34.

Pereira SG, Fulgencio R, Nunes TG, et al. Effect of curing protocol on the polymerization of dual-cured resin cements. *Dent Mater* 2010;26:710–718.

Re D, Augusti D, Sailer I, et al. The effect of surface treatment on the adhesion of resin cements to Y-TZP. *Eur J Esthet Dent* 2008;3:186–196.

Stawarczyk B, Ing B, Basler T, et al. Effect of surface conditioning with airborne-particle abrasion on the tensile strength of polymeric CAD/CAM crowns luted with self-adhesive and conventional resin cements. *J Prosthet Dent* 2012;107(2):94–101.

Swift EJ Jr, Brodeur C, Cvitko E, Pires JA. Treatment of composite surfaces for indirect bonding. *Dent Mater* 1992;8:193–196.

Thompson JY, Stoner BR, Piascik JR, Smith R. Adhesion/cementation to zirconia and other non-silicate ceramics: where are we now? *Dent Mater* 2011;27:71–82.

Wang CJ, Millstein PL, Nathanson D. Effects of cement, cement space, marginal design, seating aid materials, and seating force on crown cementation. *J Prosthet Dent* 1992;67:786–790.

Yang B, Barloi A, Kern M. Influence of air-abrasion on zirconia ceramic bonding using an adhesive composite resin. *Dent Mater* 2010;26(1):44–50.

Zhang C, Degrange M. Shear bond strengths of self-adhesive luting resins fixing dentine to different restorative materials. *J Biomater Sci Polym Ed* 2010;21:593–608.

PART 9
TECHNICAL ADVANCES AND PROPER MAINTENANCE OF ESTHETIC RESTORATIONS

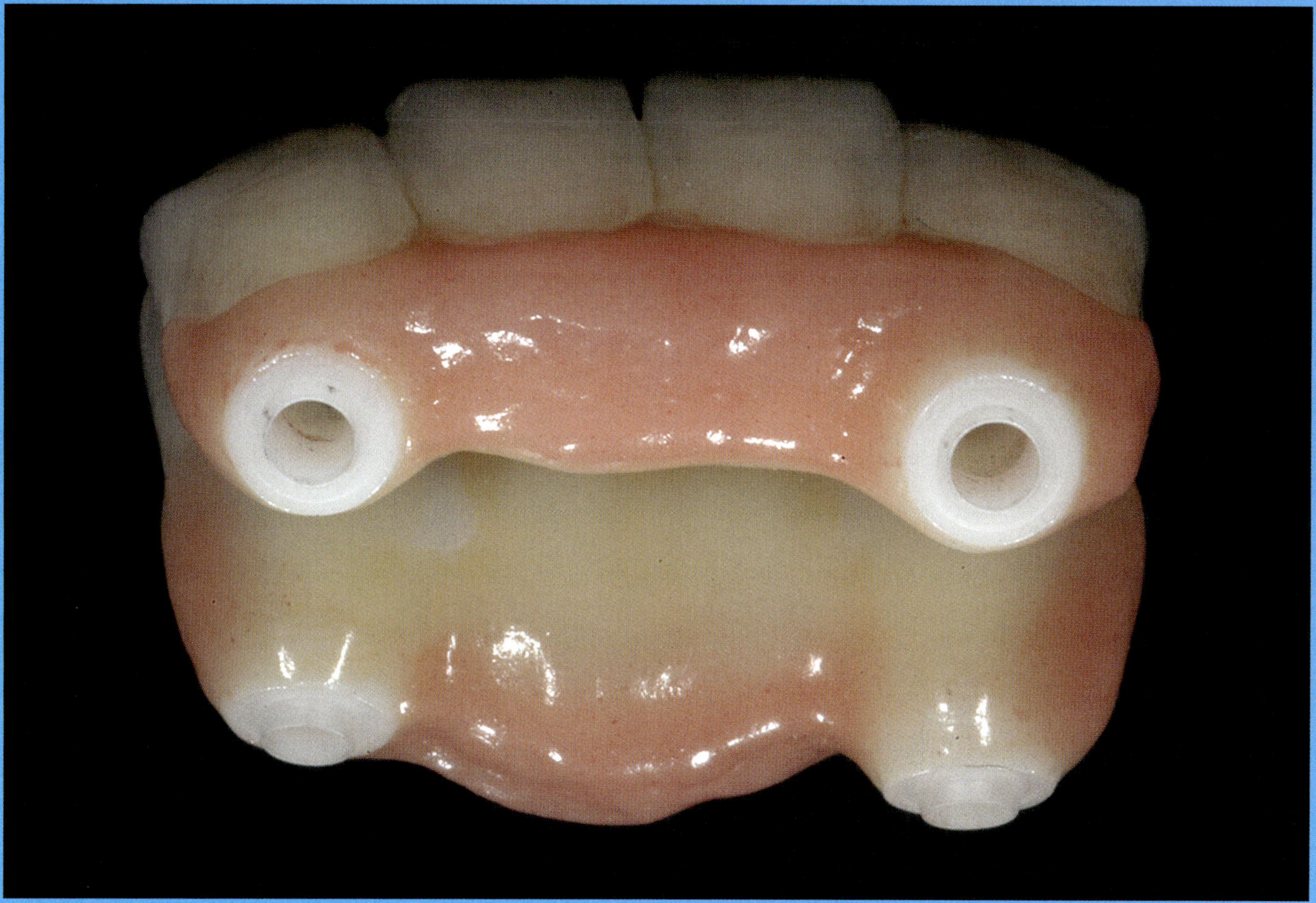

Chapter 45: Esthetic Principles in Constructing Ceramic Restorations

Robert D. Walter, DDS, MSD

Chapter Outline

Abutment–implant platform interface	1370	Glass-ceramics (etchable)	1375
Abutment–soft tissue interface	1370	Glass-infiltrated ceramics	1377
Restoration–implant or –tooth abutment interface	1372	Oxide ceramics	1377
Occlusal surface–opposing dentition interface	1374		

The principles to restore the positions, proportions, and contours of teeth along with future plans for maintenance should be sequenced in a treatment plan prior to the selection of a restorative material. When the suggested sequence is followed, the principles for the selection of the appropriate dental ceramic deliver subtle nuances that elevate esthetic dentistry to new and greater levels. Ceramic restorations have many esthetic, functional, conservative, and biocompatibility benefits to deliver new opportunities for challenging clinical situations and to manage maintenance issues. Hence, ceramic restorations have become very popular. With their popularity, the contemporary dental patient and dentists have come to expect or demand the state of the art in dental esthetics. Regardless, treatment plans should never be designed around a primary objective to deliver a specific type of dental material or technique.[1] Success of all-ceramic restorations does not come from only one material, but from the clinician's understanding of patients' needs and a working knowledge of how to match the appropriate materials, fabrication techniques of the restorations with a material's specific handling considerations, and clinical handling including delivery procedures.[2] Since all dental therapy will inevitably fail with time, strategies for maintenance should try to minimize catastrophic failure. To make a treatment plan of this caliber, it has to be studied for its weakness. The weakest links to consider are typically the restorative interfaces. Once the restorative interfaces are defined within the treatment plan, then the appropriate dental materials can be selected with the foresight of maintenance so contingencies can be implemented to facilitate the long-term management of the all-ceramic restoration. Four restorative interfaces have been considered in this chapter for the implant and tooth-borne restorations:

- abutment–implant platform interface
- implant abutment–soft tissue interface
- tooth or implant abutment–restoration interface
- occlusal surface–opposing dentition interface.

Each interface of the restoration has a different inherent function. With collaborative analyses of all the interfaces involved for a planned restoration, one interface may be determined to be the limiting factor for long-term maintenance success. The ceramic material should be evaluated for its mechanical and optical properties as well as for its biocompatibility so that the most suitable ceramic material can be recruited for the specific restorative interface and to address the weakest link.

Abutment–implant platform interface

The ceramic restoration–implant platform interface has an interesting relationship between two dissimilar dental materials. Presently, ceramic implant abutments are dominantly made of zirconium dioxide, also known as zirconia. The zirconia abutment has three general design categories to address the connection between the ceramic abutment and titanium implant platform. One category of ceramic abutments has a titanium insert within the abutment. Dependent on which manufacturer, the ceramic abutment and titanium insert may be bonded together or coupled with a friction grip connection. The titanium insert typically acts as an antirotation component of the abutment with the implant. Ceramic abutments within this category have a percentage of ceramic still in contact with the implant platform and the prosthetic screw head (Figure 45.1). The second category of ceramic abutments has a complete metal contact with the implant; more vertical space is required for the abutment emergence profile because of the added material thickness. Figure 45.2A and B shows a custom two-piece abutment that was cemented together. The abutment–implant platform interface had 100% titanium contact with the dental implant. A subcategory within the ceramic and complete titanium interface uses a titanium transitional/transmucosal abutment to correct off-angle implants so that a screw-retained zirconia bridge may be delivered.

The third category supports the fabrication of ceramic abutments completely out of one piece of zirconia. A one-piece or monolithic ceramic abutment puts 100% of the ceramic–titanium junction at the implant platform and all internal connections. With this design the prosthetic screw head engages the abutment and the screw threads engage the titanium alloy threads of the implant. Unlike the two-piece ceramic abutments with 100% metal contact, the monolithic zirconia abutment requires less vertical space to develop the emergence profile without concerns of metal display (Figure 45.3). Research has shown single-tooth zirconia implant abutments to have the same survival, technical, and biological outcomes as single-tooth titanium implant abutments for the replacement of single anterior and posterior teeth.[3-7] However, because of the interesting dynamic relationship between the ceramic and titanium interface coupled with the prosthetic screw found in the three design categories, it is important to understand the material properties of wear and to be certain that the manufacturers' recommended preload is achieved to minimize future screw loosening.[8]

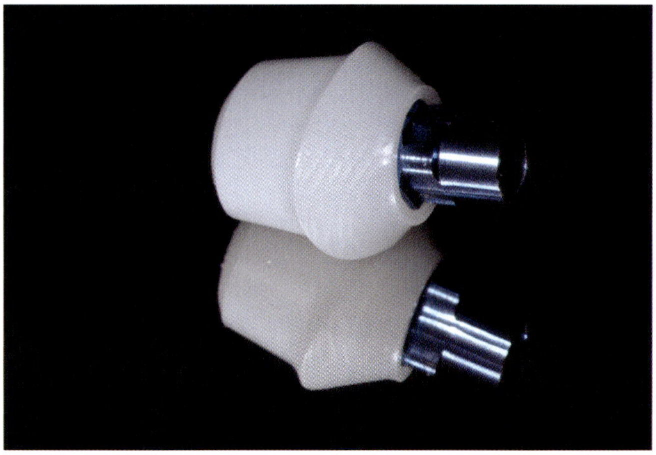

Abutment–soft tissue interface

With the continuation of improvements in survival and success of dental implants through osseointegration, the attention turned to the esthetics of the peri-implant soft tissues.[9-11] Animal studies revealed that gingiva did not attach to cast gold alloy abutments but did attach to titanium, densely sintered high-purity alumina, and zirconia abutments.[12,13] With zirconia and titanium, the criteria of clinical markers for implant success and failure continue to evolve. In part, the evolution was due to titanium and zirconia's high biocompatibility, and today these two materials are considered as the standard.[3,14] Zirconia implant abutments improve local factors of peri-implant tissue health through increasing tissue attachment, reducing pocket probing depths, and having minimal bacterial colonization and adhesion.[15-17] These local factors are signs of peri-implant tissues health improvement, but the esthetics of the implant restoration–tissue interface are also addressed with the available ceramic materials today.

Peri-implant soft tissues are different in color than the gingiva of natural teeth (Figure 45.4A).[3,18,19] Clinical observations have reported a graying in the tissues of concern when they are coupled with implant-supported restoration retained by metal abutments.[20] ΔE was recommended by the International Commission on Illumination as a metric to describe perceived noticeable difference in color, where the symbol Δ represents difference and E stands for the German word "Empfindung," which means sensation.[21] The color difference ΔE of the peri-implant tissues are significantly affected by the selection of implant abutment whether it is fabricated from titanium alloy or ceramic.[18,19] To improve the color of peri-implant tissues in the anterior, ceramic implant abutments are recommended along with connective tissue grafts if the labial tissue thickness is less than 2 mm.[19,22,23]

However, not all dental patients are the same. To address specific patient needs, the interaction of two conditions needs to be collectively considered when selecting an abutment material. When a dental implant replaces an anterior tooth, two things have to be considered for the selection of the abutment material.

Figure 45.1 Hybrid zirconia and titanium implant abutment. Both zirconia and titanium contact with implant platform.

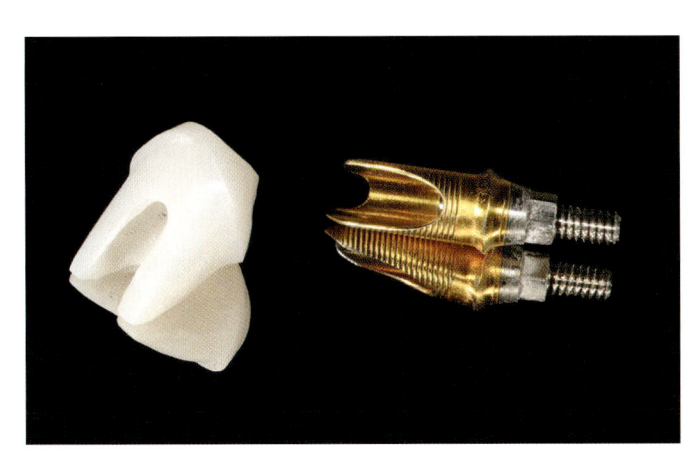

Figure 45.2 (A) Zirconia and titanium are used to construct a two-piece implant abutment, but only titanium contacts the implant platform.

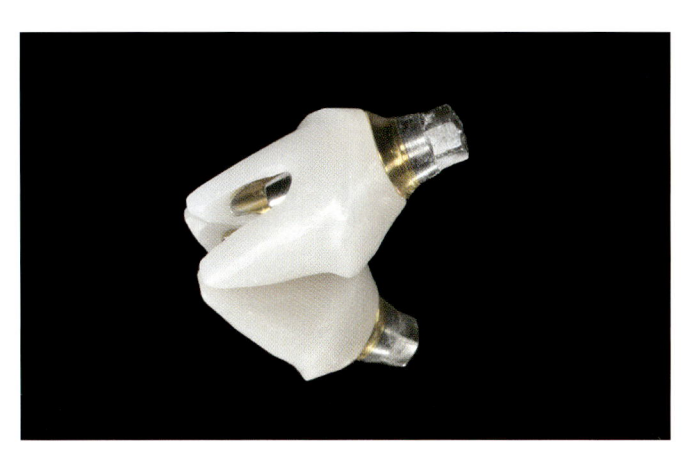

Figure 45.2 (B) Zirconia and titanium parts are bonded together for the definitive abutment.

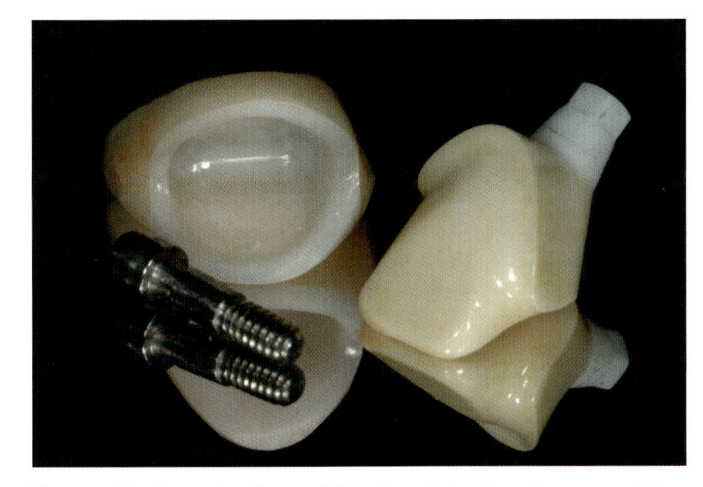

Figure 45.3 Example of monolithic zirconia implant abutment with ceramic crown and prosthetic screw. Only zirconia interfaces with the implant platform.

The first consideration is that in health the free gingival margin takes on a knife edge shape which may not be 2 mm in thickness. The second condition is that the ideal location of the abutment finish line for a cement-retained implant restoration be positioned 1 mm or less apical of the free gingival margin to facilitate ease of cement removal (Figure 45.4B and C).

The summation of these conditions involves factors of the dental implant's vertical, horizontal, and angular position along with the emergence profile of the restoration. Thus, most dental implant sites may require some development through tissue grafting. Many times zirconia abutments may be preferable over titanium abutments for anterior areas because the cross-sectional dimension of the labial free gingival margin is rarely greater than 2 mm in thickness when measured 1 mm or less apical from the crest of the healthy free gingival margin. Submerging the finish lines of the abutment deeper than 1 mm may gain more tissue thickness and solve the issue of discolored peri-implant tissues but may present a greater challenge in terms of residual cement removal.[24] Figure 45.4B–E is the continuation of Figure 45.4A. Note the improved peri-implant tissue color with

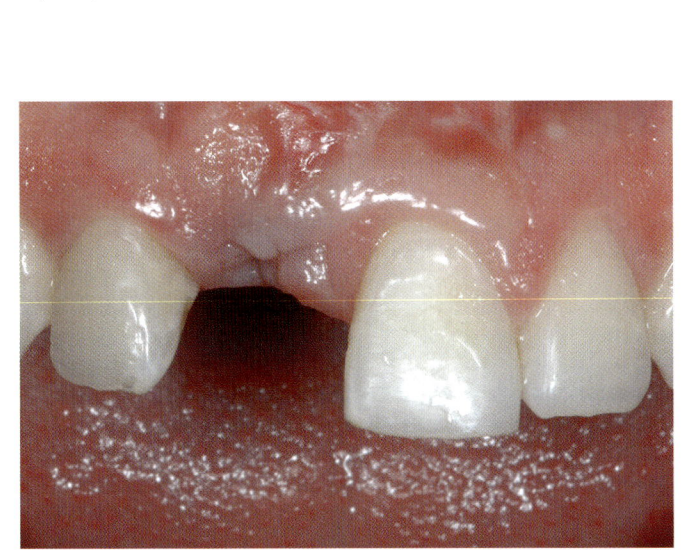

Figure 45.4 (A) Implant and healing abutment submerged in right maxillary central incisor position. Translucent peri-implant soft tissues reveal underlying metal.

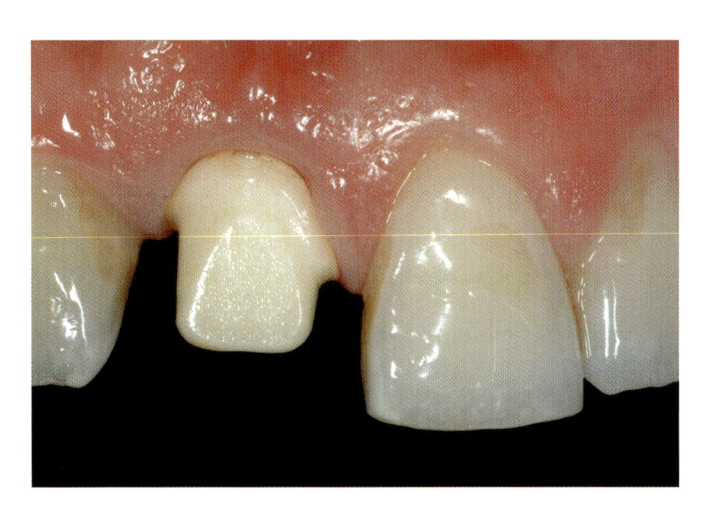

Figure 45.4 (B) Monolithic zirconia implant abutment in place to evaluate ΔE between peri-implant soft tissues and adjacent tooth gingiva.

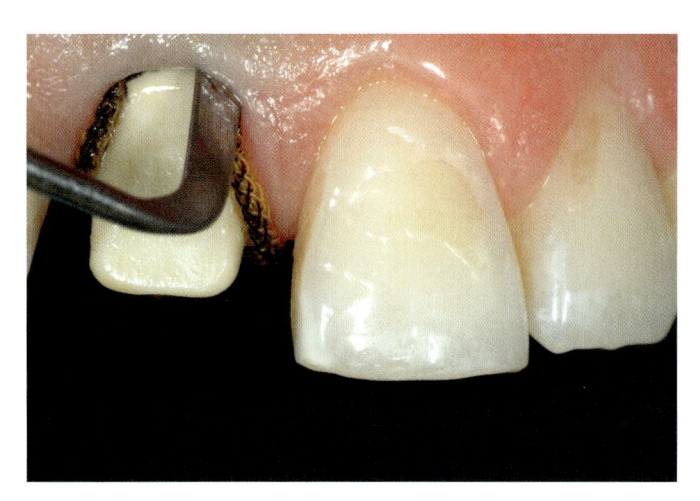

Figure 45.4 **(C)** Idealized finish line location to facilitate residual cement removal with aid of a deflection cord.

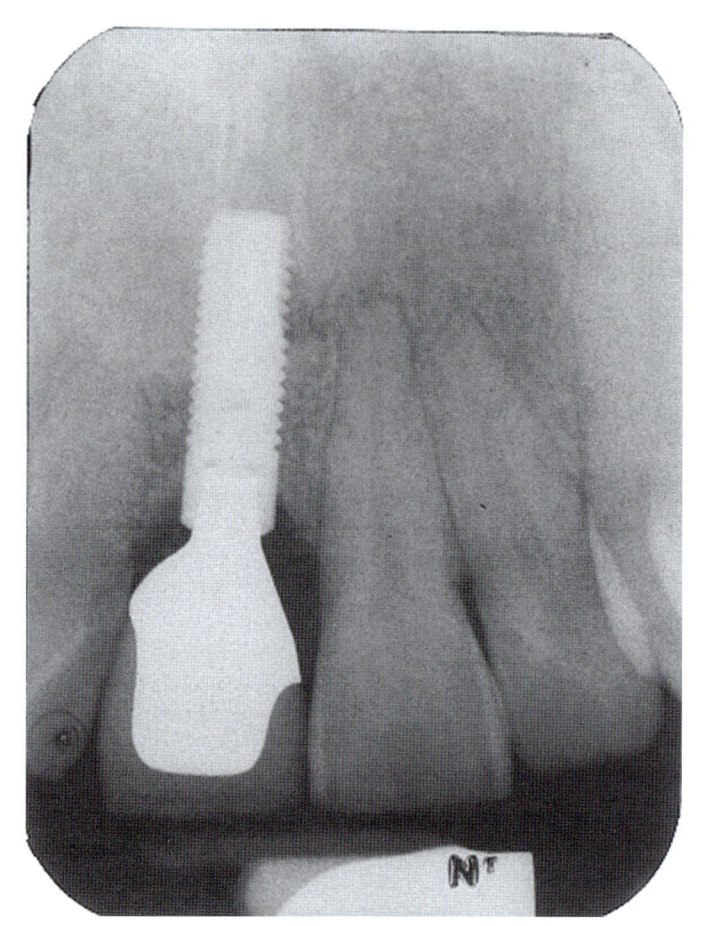

Figure 45.4 **(D)** Postcementation radiograph confirms complete cement removal in difficult to reach interproximal areas.

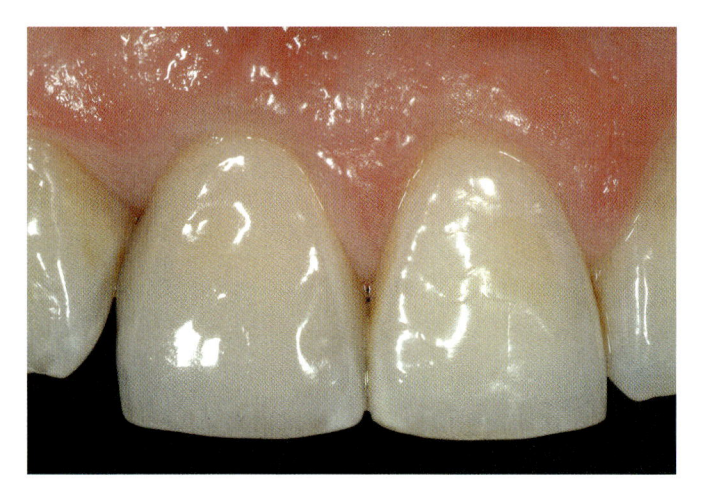

Figure 45.4 **(E)** Definitive bilayered zirconia crown on custom monolithic zirconia implant abutment.

the definitive zirconia abutment in place (Figure 45.4B), and the effect of the deflection cord on the tissue color when placed to facilitate cement removal (Figure 45.4C). Figure 45.4D is a routine periapical radiograph to confirm no excess residual cement is left on the mesial and distal aspects of the abutment and implant platform. Figure 45.4E shows the ceramic crown with zirconia core conventionally luted on a zirconia abutment while demonstrating healthy tissue contours, color, and texture.

Restoration–implant or –tooth abutment interface

This interface is typically evaluated clinically by the fit of the restoration to the abutment. Marginal discrepancies of 18.3–117 μm for ceramic restoration adhesively or conventionally luted to teeth have been measured in in-vitro studies.[25–41] McLean and von Fraunhofer proposed a qualification for clinical acceptability for marginal discrepancy on teeth to range from 40 to 120 μm.[42] Ceramic restorations are well within such clinical acceptability parameters. However, the fit is not only influenced by the finish line preparation, quality of impression, and skill level of the laboratory technician. Nowadays, it is also affected by the manufacturing technique and level of technology of available computer-aided design/manufacturing (CAD/CAM) systems and the skills of the operator of the system.[35,36] If all variables are strictly governed in the fabrication of a ceramic restoration, clinicians should expect the marginal discrepancy to be in the low end of the range. The marginal discrepancy with ceramic restorations on ceramic implant abutments is probably similar to natural teeth, but the concern for secondary caries does not exist as it does with natural teeth.

Three considerations should be applied while evaluating the ceramic restoration–tooth or –implant abutment interface. The first consideration only pertains to dental implants. With a dental implant, this interface can be totally eliminated with the concept of screw retention. The benefit of eliminating this interface delivers a simpler design with fewer interfaces to maintain. Screw-retained implant restorations tend to have better plaque and bleeding indexes than cement-retained implant restorations do.[43] This interface has also been reported to cause periodontal irritation and peri-implant disease if residual excess cement is left undetected.[44,45] The challenge with a screw-retained restoration is the presurgical planning, interdisciplinary team communication, and skill level of execution to place the implant accurately. The implant has to be positioned with the screw access hole of the restoration located in an area which does not impair esthetics. Many times an esthetically located screw access hole is limited by the restorations path of insertion between the existing proximal contacts and the engaging components of the abutment and implant.

Figure 45.5A and B demonstrates a patient with failing mandibular incisors and less than ideal oral hygiene before and after oral hygiene instructions and cleaning noted at the periodontal reevaluation. To replace the failing mandibular incisors, a zirconia screw-retained implant-supported fixed partial denture was selected. Elimination of the restoration–abutment interface delivered prospective plans for periodontal maintenance. Additionally, the size of the abutments for a cement-retained fixed partial denture in the positions of the mandibular incisors on such narrow platform implants would have been small with thin axial walls. The durability of a one-piece abutment–framework complex may be more favorable. Lastly, the screw-retained restoration allows for simple retrievability if any prospective prosthetic maintenance or complications occur (Figure 45.5C–F).

The next consideration for the ceramic restoration–tooth or –implant abutment interface involves whether the restoration should be adhesively bonded or conventionally luted. The current high-strength all-ceramic restorations allow clinicians to use conventional methods to lute the restoration when isolation is difficult, there is compromised gingival health, or the finish line is subgingival.[1]

Once Buonocore[46] introduced a process of etching the tooth structure to increase the quality of dental adhesion in 1955, a door was opened for esthetic dentistry. Today, research and clinical experience has propelled continuous evolution of tooth-colored restorative materials, adhesive materials and techniques, and methods for more conservative treatment modalities. Currently, the enamel and glass-ceramic-based ceramic restoration bond is very predictable,[47-49] and research has reported improvement in the adhesive bond to less-predictable materials, such as dentin and oxide ceramics.[50-55]

Along with good predictability for bonding to enamel, adhesively retained all-ceramic restorations facilitate minimally invasive restorative procedures. Tooth preparations are no longer required to be governed only by the mechanical principles of resistance and retention form. Sound tooth structure may be conserved, since a bonded restoration is not dependent on the parallelism of opposing axial walls. The probability of catastrophic failure versus routine maintenance is many times decided by the quantity and quality of remaining tooth structure. An example of a catastrophic failure would be the subgingival horizontal fracture of a tooth restored with a complete crown. In contrast, a more favorable routine maintenance procedure would be to rebond a porcelain laminate veneer that has fractured or debonded due to the adhesive composite-resin fatigue. To rebond ceramic restorations to minimally prepared teeth is more desirable from a patient's procedural and financial point of view than the treatment required to restore or replace structurally compromised teeth. It is imperative that the contemporary dental patient be educated to return to the dental provider for maintenance on a routine basis as well as immediately when a problem emerges. Figure 45.6A–C shows an example of a dental patient with porcelain laminate veneers on the mandibular incisors who returned to have a maintenance visit to rebond a veneer. The rebonding of the porcelain laminate veneer was a low-stress and low-cost procedure for the patient comparatively to a catastrophic failure from a horizontal tooth fracture that might have occurred if the incisor had been prepared for a complete crown.

The third consideration for the ceramic restoration–abutment interface deals with the color and translucency of the abutment tooth. Natural colors from the underlying tooth may be revealed in the definitive restoration with ceramics of variable optical properties and thicknesses. The optical properties and variable

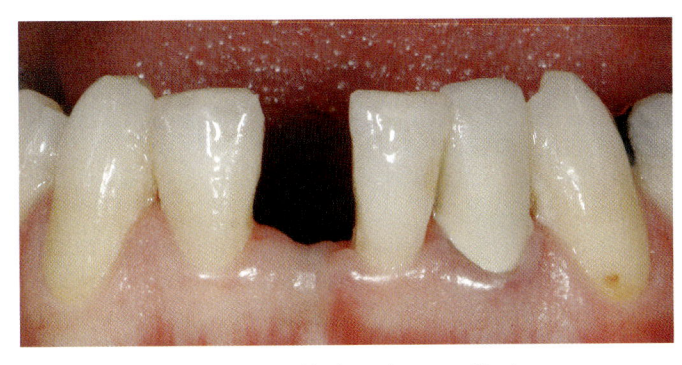

Figure 45.5 (A) Missing mandibular right central incisor.

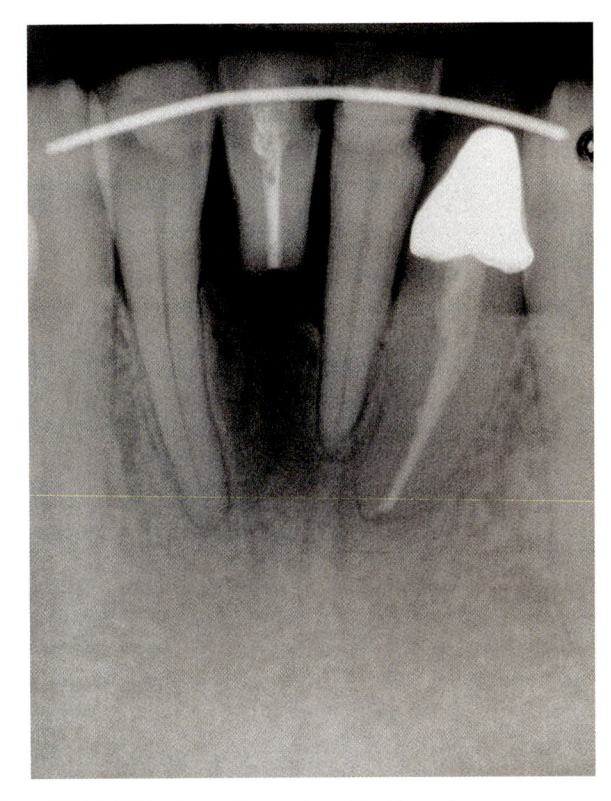

Figure 45.5 (B) Radiograph reveals vertical bone loss on adjacent teeth.

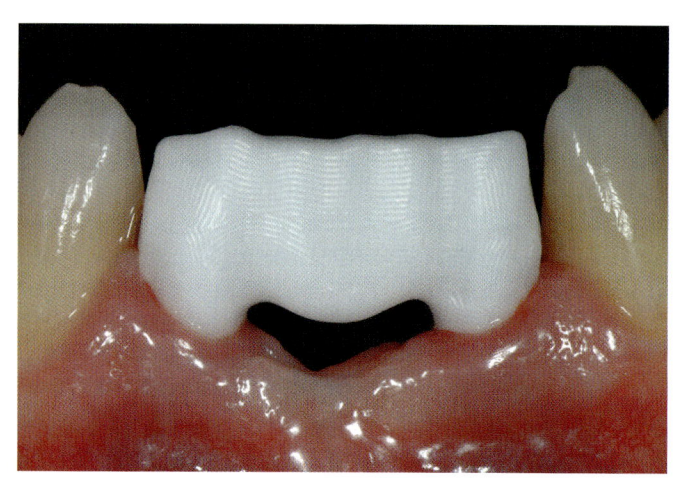

Figure 45.5 (C) Monolithic screw-retained zirconia framework.

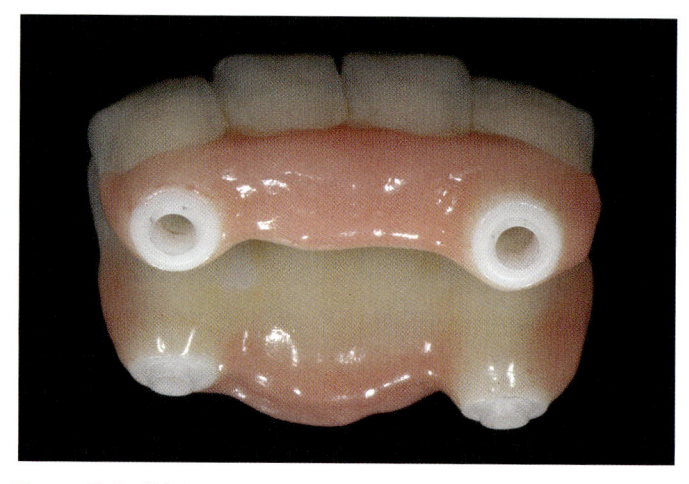

Figure 45.5 (D) Convex intaglio surface allows area to be flossed.

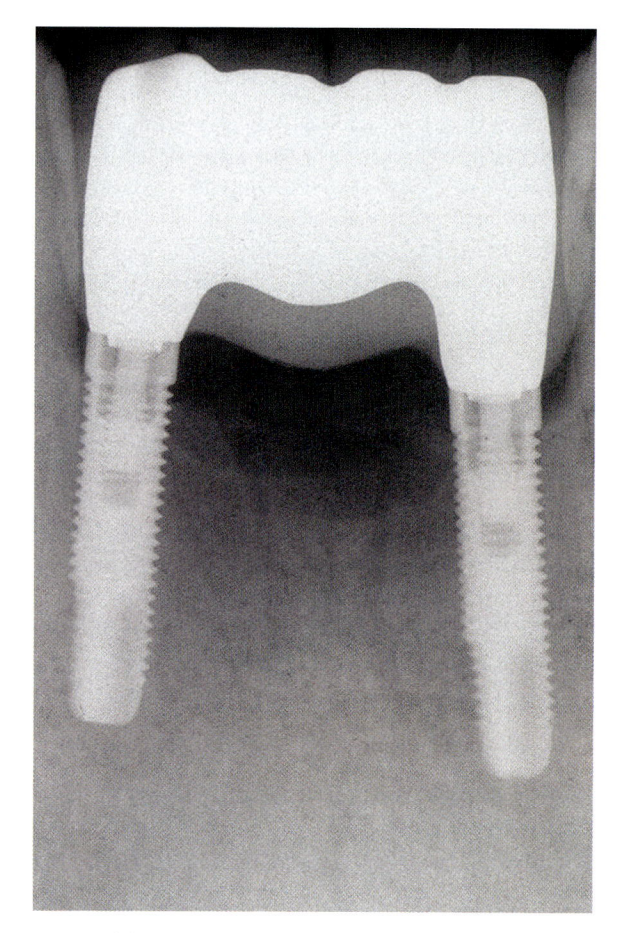

Figure 45.5 (E) Radiographic evaluation of restoration fit with implant platforms.

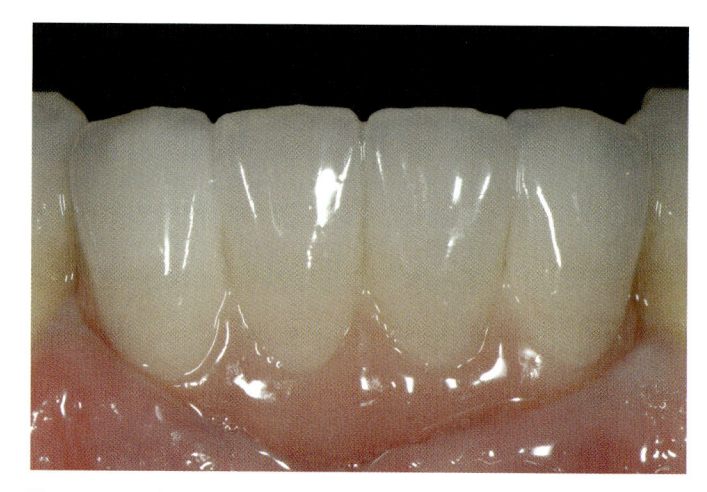

Figure 45.5 (F) Screw-retained bilayered prosthesis with zirconia framework

Occlusal surface–opposing dentition interface

The ceramic occlusal surface–opposing dentition interface is the last interface considered. However, it is where all interfaces are collectively tested for durability. Many have noted that ceramic restorations have higher rates of failure on posterior rather than on anterior dentition.[3,60-62] These higher success rates for anterior restorations may be attributed to the fact that the posterior teeth generate higher occlusal forces (forces generated by muscles of mastication and transferred to the teeth) than the anterior teeth do. With the difference between anterior and posterior teeth in terms of occlusal load, patient factors of function along with evaluation of available ceramics and fabrication techniques need to be considered collaboratively when designing an all-ceramic restoration.

Contemporary dental ceramics and the manner of fabrication of the definitive restoration offer ample opportunities to achieve balance between durability and esthetics for both anterior and posterior teeth. Since the level of function at the occlusal interface is dependent on the location in the mouth, two philosophies

thicknesses of different dental ceramics can bring the inner color of the tooth out to the surface of the definitive restoration.[56] If the colors of the abutment are not desirable because of stains and/or restorative materials, masking is possible with opaque and thicker ceramics.[57-59]

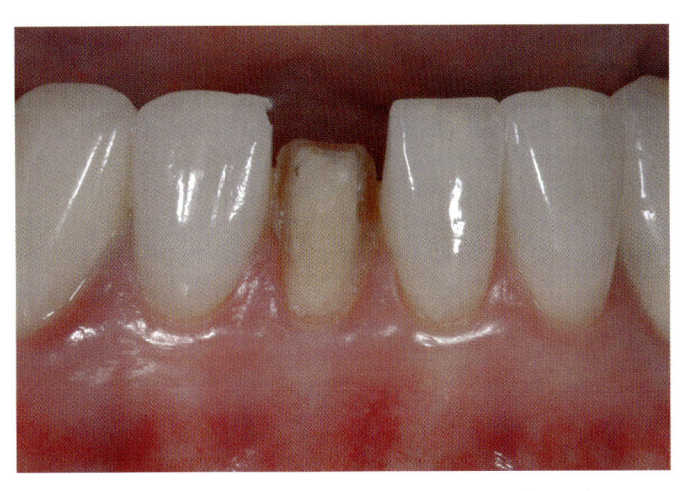

Figure 45.6 **(A)** Patient presentation with a debonded porcelain laminate veneer.

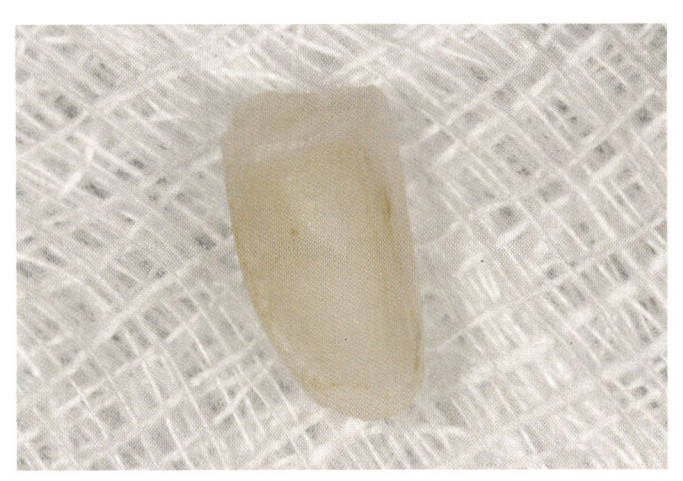

Figure 45.6 **(B)** Intaglio surface of porcelain laminate veneer shows signs of bond fatigue with discolored margin.

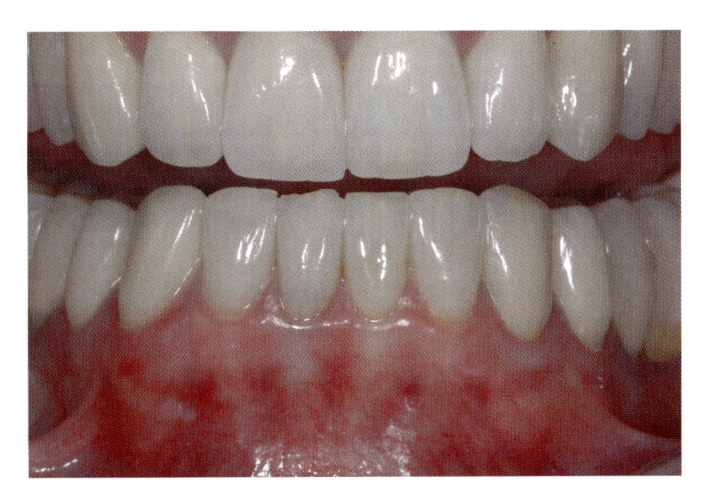

Figure 45.6 **(C)** Same porcelain laminate veneer after bonding procedure.

in restorative design have emerged. One design concept for the ceramic restoration is the bilayered restoration. The bilayered restoration has a core substrate to support and give strength to a veneer material as previously demonstrated in metal–ceramics. With all-ceramic bilayered restorations, concerns had developed with the veneer chipping, separation at the interface between the two materials, and/or fracture of the core. The second design is the monolithic concept. A complete gold crown is a classic example of a monolithic restoration. The monolithic ceramic restoration does not have an interface between two ceramic materials because it is fabricated from only one material. However, esthetics may be limited due to its monochromatic tendency.

Three categories of dental ceramics are available to create the two restorative design philosophies. They are the glass (etchable) ceramics, the glass-infiltrated ceramics, and the oxide ceramics. Each category has different esthetic and durability benefits for all-involved interfaces of a ceramic restoration.

Glass-ceramics (etchable)

Glass-ceramics molecular organization is multiphasic, amorphic, and has a random matrix that contains silica. Its molecular makeup gives glass-ceramics a dual quality of similar optical traits to that of natural teeth and the potential favorable mechanical properties (pending on the type of material). The optical and mechanical properties of the glass-ceramic are dependent on the ratio between the glassy and the crystalline phase. Ceramics with a greater percentage of the glassy phase will possess more translucency, opalescence, and fluorescence but are weaker. Glass-ceramics with a greater percentage of the crystalline phase cause more light to scatter, are less translucent, and deliver more strength. Glass-ceramic may be used as a veneer material over a core substrate made of a different ceramic material for a bilayer restoration or without a core for a monolithic restoration like a porcelain laminate veneer or a crown. Clinical success of single-unit glass-ceramic restorations is attributed to their properties of micromechanical and chemical bonding to resin composite. Resin bonding is possible because the material is etchable. Hydrofluoric acid primes the ceramic surface by the removal of exposed silica in the glassy matrix.[63] Holes in the glassy matrix, where the silica used to be, improve the wettability of the ceramic for the application of silane to facilitate a chemical bond.[63] In addition, these empty spaces become micromechanical retentive features for the resin composite. The duration of etching and the concentration of acid etchant change between types of glass-ceramic and manufacture. It is possible to overetch glass-ceramic and compromise its bonding.[64]

One type of ceramic in this group uses leucite as reinforcement for a base material to construct a monolith or a veneer material for a bilayer restoration. The thermal expansion of leucite is mismatched with the glassy phase to create internal compressive stresses within the ceramic that cause cracks to deflect during their propagation. Leucite-reinforced ceramics flexural strength is 104–184.8 MPa.[65,66]

An alternative hybrid glass-ceramic that has a flexural strength is 300–400 MPa with a fracture toughness of 2.8–3.5 MPa m$^{1/2}$ is lithium disilicate.[65] Owing to the mechanical properties of lithium disilicate, it can be used as a core substructure and veneered with another glass ceramic, as a veneer on a core substructure for a bilayered system or as a monolithic restoration. All three uses of lithium disilicate may be fabricated with a lost-wax technique and heat pressed, or partially crystallized lithium disilicate blocks can be milled with CAD/CAM technologies and then fired to achieve the final crystallization. Both monolithic and bilayered lithium disilicate are suitable for single-unit restorations, but strict requirements should be considered in case selection for short-span fixed partial dentures.[67,68] According to the manufacturer's recommendations adhesive cementation is not required, but in the cases of veneers, inlays, and onlays, however, it is recommended that lithium disilicate be etched with 5% hydrofluoric acid and then silanated and adhesively luted. Figure 45.7A–C depicts a clinical case that used monolithic lithium disilicate that was stained and glazed. Although the

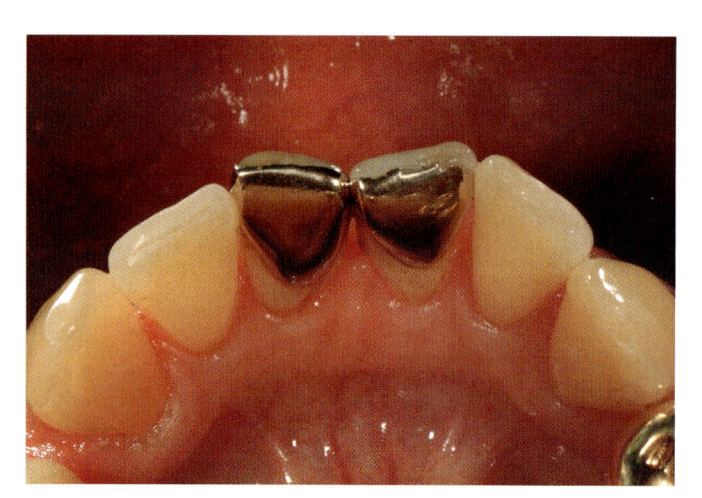

Figure 45.7 (A) Mandibular central incisors with defective pin-retained cast onlays and composite resin restoring incisal and facial surfaces.

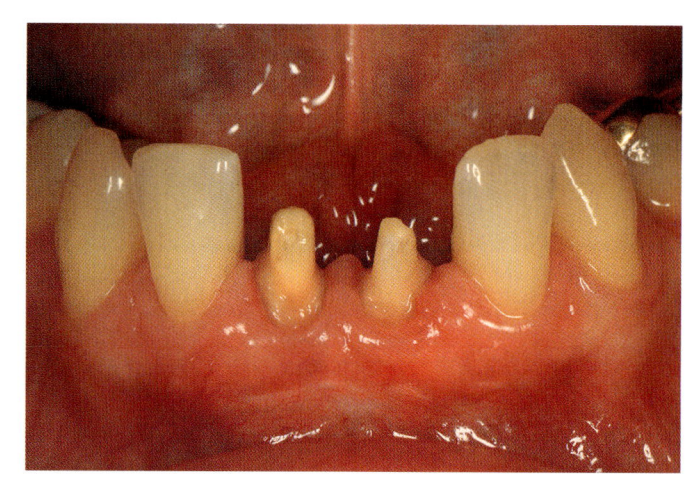

Figure 45.7 (B) Minimal abutment length was left once existing restorations were removed. Axial reduction was limited to 0.9 mm for lithium disilicate crowns.

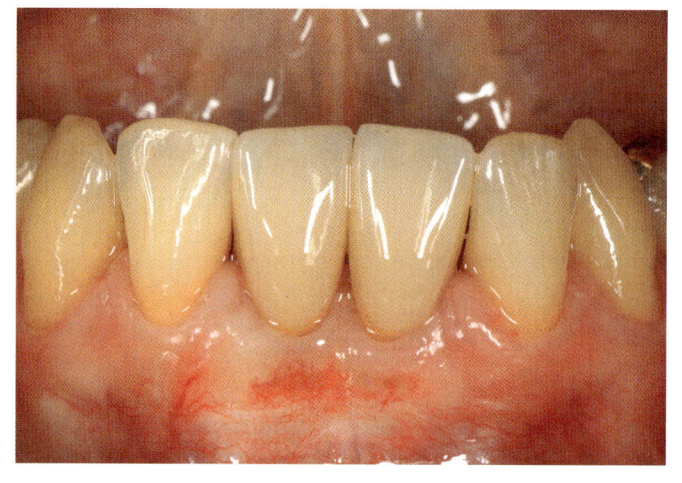

Figure 45.7 (C) Translucency of monolithic lithium disilicate crowns with external staining and glazing reveals natural colors of underlying tooth structure.

defective pin castings required complete circumferential preparation of the abutments, the physical properties of lithium disilicate constricted the axial reduction to 0.9 mm. The etchable and translucent properties of lithium disilicate were taken advantage of for the different colored abutments.

Glass-infiltrated ceramics

The glass-infiltrated ceramics are a combination of the glass-ceramics and the oxide ceramics. To create the glass-infiltrated ceramic, partially sintered oxides like aluminum, magnesium–aluminum, or aluminum–zirconium are infiltrated with molten low-viscosity glass. Not as translucent as the glass ceramics, the glass-infiltrated alumina has been used for anterior and posterior copings in crowns. In addition, frameworks for anterior three-unit fixed partial dentures may also be constructed from these materials.[69–71] They are reported to have a flexural strength of 236–600 MPa and a fracture toughness of 3.1–4.61 MPa m$^{1/2}$.[72–75] Glass-infiltrated alumina with 35% partially stabilized zirconia has a flexural strength of 421–800 MPa and a fracture toughness of 6–8 MPa m$^{1/2}$.[72]

Glass-infiltrated alumina with 35% partially stabilized zirconia has the least amount of translucency, which may limit it to only the posterior copings and frameworks.[76,77] In contrast, when glass-infiltrated magnesium alumina is processed in the ceramic furnace under vacuum or via CAD/CAM it creates a highly translucent ceramic core that can be used for anterior restorations.[78]

Oxide ceramics

The oxide or polycrystalline ceramics are a group of ceramics that do not have a glassy phase. Another characteristic of the oxide ceramics that is different than the glass-ceramics is that their molecular makeup is very organized and closely spaced. The dense atomic organization gives the oxide ceramics their characteristic strength and reduced translucency. When the three groups of ceramics are compared for mechanical properties, the oxide ceramics far exceed the other two groups in strength. The two common dental ceramics present in the oxide family are the densely sintered high-purity alumina (Al_2O_3) and yttria tetragonal zirconia polycrystals (Y-TZP), also known as zirconium dioxide (ZrO_2) or zirconia. These two materials became available to dentistry through the development of CAD/CAM technology that enabled the design and milling of ceramics before or after they receive the final firing cycle and sophisticated refinement process to make a ceramic with uniform particle sizes so that mathematical equations can be used to calculate the exact amount of shrinkage from the milled CAD/CAM state to the fully sintered state and end up with a restoration with a precise fit.[79] Clinically, the densely sintered high-purity alumina has been used with adequate success for anterior and posterior cores for all ceramic crowns.[80,81] Its flexural strength is 487–699 MPa and fracture toughness of 4.48–6 MPa m$^{1/2}$.[66,72]

Zirconia consists of a tetragonal zirconia polycrystal phase at 1170–2370 °C that when stabilized with the addition of yttrium oxide (yttria) may maintain a tetragonal phase at room temperature. With the addition of yttrium oxide, zirconia is considered a metastable material (a state of equilibrium that will transform to a more stable state of equilibrium if disturbed). The metastable characteristic is unique to zirconia and gives it the mechanical property known as transformation toughening. Transformation toughening occurs when a crack is initiated. The equilibrium of the metastable zirconia in front of the crack is disrupted and transforms to a more stable monoclinic crystal phase. In the case of zirconia, the desire to transform is an excellent mechanical advantage because the stable monoclinic phase is larger in volume. The volumetric increase results in squeezing off the crack, disrupting the crack propagation and resulting in a net reduction of stress within the ceramic. Zirconia has an initial flexural strength of 900–1200 MPa and fracture toughness of 9–10 MPa m$^{1/2}$.[82] After significant accelerated hydrothermal aging, zirconia loses a significant amount of its initial flexural strength due to its metastable characteristics. However, it still maintains high values of flexural strength of over 800 MPa.[83] Zirconia may be used for anterior[84,85] and posterior copings, fixed partial denture frameworks,[86–88] and implant abutments.[3–5]

The optical properties of zirconia have some esthetic advantages. Cores can be fabricated to 0.3 mm in thickness to deliver a translucent anterior restoration or 0.5 mm and greater to mask discolored abutments and metal foundations.[89] By varying the core thickness, the ceramist can mask undesirable colors and allow light transmission in different areas all on one tooth. When multiple teeth of different colors are to be restored, varying the core thickness is also beneficial because the net effect gives all the cores the same foundation shade when placed on the teeth. Once the amount of masking and translucency is solved at the level of the core, the ceramist can use a similar recipe for the veneer buildups on multiple teeth (Figure 45.8A–D).

The challenge with zirconia as a core material for bilayered restorations has not been fracture of the zirconia core itself but predominantly cohesive chipping and fractures in the veneering porcelain.[87,90] To investigate this challenge, in-depth analysis of the driving causes of the cracks has currently been limited to factors of different cooling rates of the complex geometries of the restorations after firing in the ceramic furnace,[91] differences in the coefficients of thermal expansions between the zirconia core and veneering porcelain, and the thickness of the veneer.[90,91] Different laboratory techniques of veneer application, whether layering or heat pressing, may be found to be useful,[92,93] although reduction of the frequency and size of the chipping may be achieved through the support of an anatomically optimized zirconia core that provides an even thickness and occlusal support for the veneer material.[94]

A latest development in the efforts to minimize veneer chipping of bilayered zirconia restorations has been a movement toward a monolithic zirconia design. Disc-shaped pieces of zirconia can be milled into anatomically contoured zirconia restorations with CAD/CAM technologies. CAD/CAM anatomically contoured zirconia ceramics have been used to restore both teeth and dental implants. With the elimination of the veneer layer, the concern of veneer chipping was addressed and laboratory times for restoration fabrication were shortened. Ceramists no longer

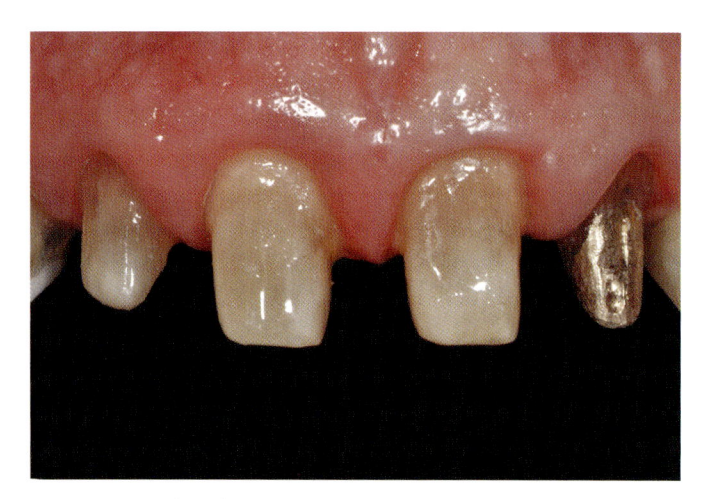

Figure 45.8 (A) Dark-colored abutment and existing cast gold post and core present with multiple colors in need of masking.

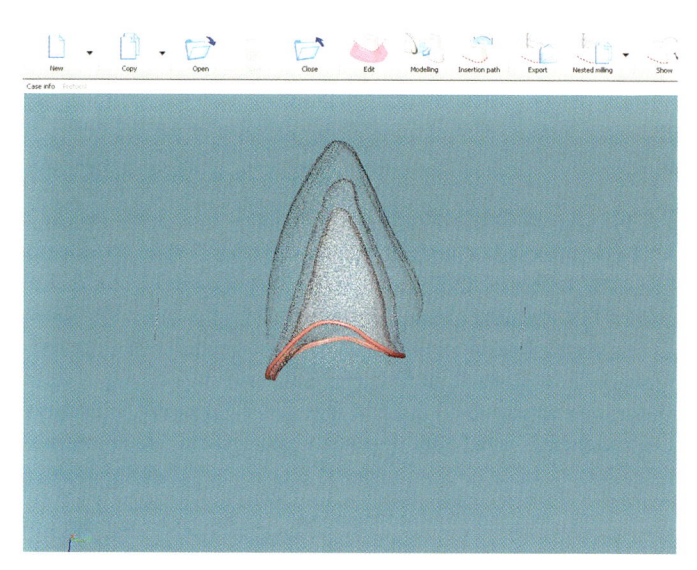

Figure 45.8 (B) CAD/CAM design of zirconia cores to evaluate available space for veneering ceramic.

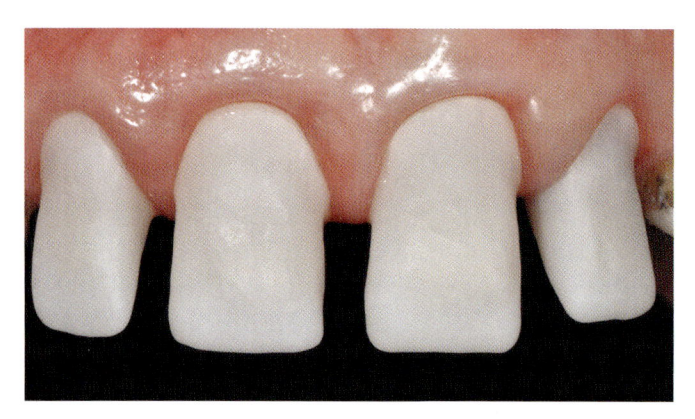

Figure 45.8 (C) CAD/CAM fabricated zirconia cores ranging from 0.3 to 0.5 mm thick are placed on multicolored abutments to evaluate amount of color making.

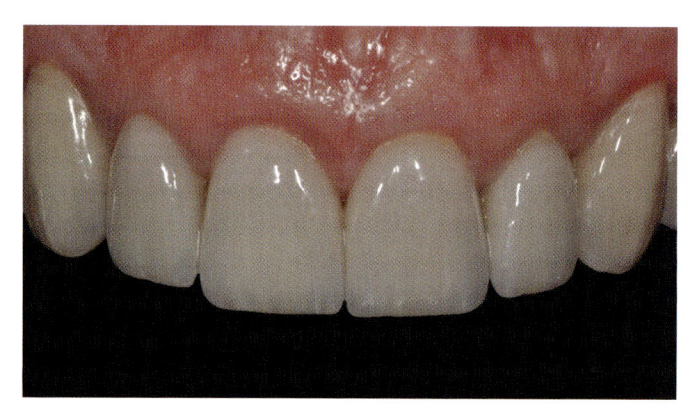

Figure 45.8 (D) Definitive bilayered crowns with zirconia cores block out dark underlying abutment and give ideal esthetics with veneering ceramics.

had to layer full-contour veneers. However, a concern of accelerated wear on opposing dentition was raised because without the veneer the zirconia was now at the occlusal interface. A two-body wear test compared enamel wear against bilayered (zirconia core veneered with glassy ceramic) and monolithic (CAD/CAM anatomic contour zirconia) zirconia restorations.[95] Interestingly, the conclusions reported that less enamel wear at the occlusal interface was observed with the monolithic zirconia than with the bilayered zirconia restoration.[95] Furthermore, research has reported that highly polished zirconia is gentler to the opposing enamel than stained and glazed zirconia.[95,96] In areas of lower esthetic concern, polished zirconia may offer a nice alternative, but in other, more visible areas staining and glazing may still be preferred to improve the monochromatic appearance. However, because of the popularity of monolithic zirconia, manufacturing improvements have been made to increase translucency and colorfulness within a disc-shaped puck made for a milling machine. Some discs have multiple layers of different colored zirconia to help deliver a polychromatic effect in the definitive restoration.

In regard to how the restoration fits with a dental implant, known as *passive fit*, it is logical to have all connections machined. When multiple implants are planned to be splinted, the research on accuracy of fit is valuable. One study compared the three-dimensional distortion between cast and milled implant–prosthodontic frameworks on master casts.[97] In the study, a laboratory technician made nine cast frameworks following a proven protocol. Then the nine cast frameworks and master casts were laser-scanned and an additional nine frameworks were milled. All laboratory technicians were blinded in the study, meaning that they were uninformed about the study. The authors concluded that neither of the techniques for framework fabrication provided a completely passive fit.[97] However, the mean and standard deviation in three-dimensional distortion in the cast frameworks was $114 \pm 31.3\,\mu m$ and only $51 \pm 18\,\mu m$ in the milled frameworks.[97]

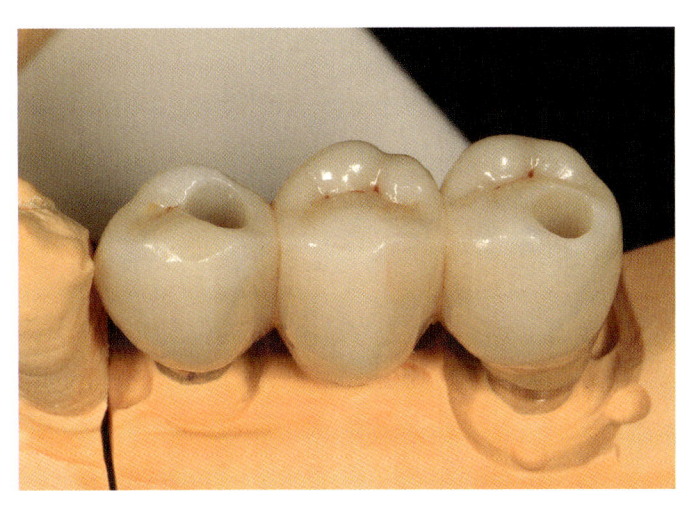

Figure 45.9 **(A)** Screw-retained monolithic zirconia prosthesis.

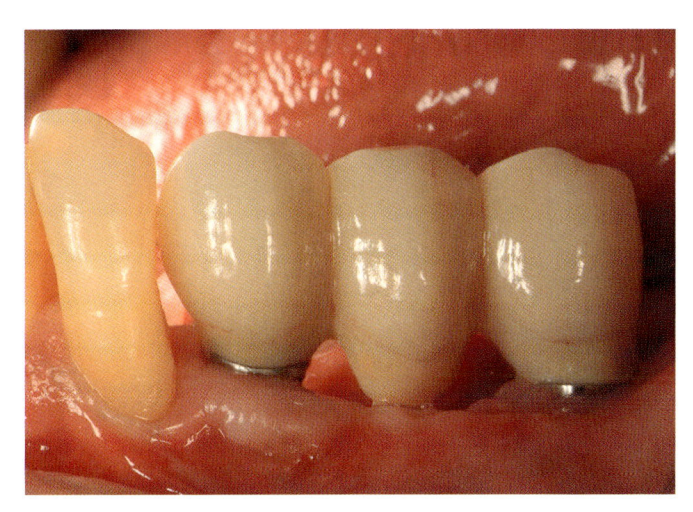

Figure 45.9 **(B)** Hygienic design of zirconia screw-retained implant-supported restoration facilitates continued exceptional oral hygiene.

Figure 45.9A and B is of a clinical case of a patient with severely compromised periodontium who was adamantly determined through good oral home care and routine periodontal maintenance to keep the remaining teeth. A screw-retained monolithic zirconia restoration was used to restore two posterior dental implants and give posterior support for the mandible. The screw-retained monolithic zirconia restoration was selected for the following properties.

1. Its CAD/CAM fabrication technique to facilitate prosthetic fit with two dental implants.
2. Its material properties for favorable biocompatibility with peri-implant soft tissues.
3. Its material properties for minimal bacterial surface adhesion and colonization.
4. Its prosthetic property of screw retention to deliver retrievability.

The screw-retained monolithic zirconia restoration may be considered the true contemporary periodontal prosthesis.

Another area that has a functional link to the occlusal interface is the connector of fixed partial dentures. The dental literature has reported that the primary cause of catastrophic failure of all ceramic fixed partial dentures is fracture of the connectors.[69,70,89–104] Fixed partial dentures with zirconia frameworks, on the other hand, have received favorable results with limited clinical fractures of the connectors.[86,93] Figure 45.10A–C depicts a clinical case of two fixed partial dentures with zirconia frameworks. Patient selection should include the evaluation of prospective abutment height and mobility along with the proposed tooth contours and proportions so that function of the restoration may not result in undesirable heavy stress concentrations within the connector area, in particular at the intaglio surface, which is subjected to tensile stresses.[105–108] Color and translucency of the proposed teeth abutments also need to be evaluated clinically with the aid of clinical photography to determine whether the ceramic needs to have any masking properties. Finally, diagnostic casts and wax-up aid in the determination of what restoration design and type of ceramic would be used when compared with the manufacturer's recommendations for minimal connector size (Table 45.1). Since the fixed partial denture connectors are functionally linked to the occlusal interface, the size of the connector has to have adequate bulk of material for strength but the size cannot violate the esthetic dimensions of the proximal contacts. Typically, contours and proportions of teeth are mirrored from the contralateral side of the area in need of reconstruction. Ceramics should be selected accordingly with respect of material requirements for minimal connector dimensions to prevent overcontoured proximal contacts. In situations where teeth morphologic information is not present, the clinician may have to use alternative measures. Stappert et al.[109] showed that the proximal contact height of natural maxillary anterior teeth had the tallest dimension at the dental midline and then diminished in height with the progression toward the mesial of the first bicuspid. The reported proximal contact height at the midline was 40% of the central incisor clinical crown length, 30% of the lateral incisor, 20% of the canine, and 20% of the first premolar. The simplified percentage rule (40–30–20–20) may be used as a helpful adjunct in information to the selection process of ceramics for fixed partial dentures. In summary, material selection for a fixed dental prosthesis may be guided by the use of a periodontal probe to measure the vertical height from the interproximal papilla to the marginal ridge or the incisal embrasure along with the aid of a diagnostic wax-up to predetermine the contours and proportions. Once the dimensions are determined, knowledge of the manufacturer's requirements in terms of a minimal connector size will aid in the selection of the appropriate ceramic.

When the occlusal interface is compared between ceramic restorations on natural teeth and dental implants, implant-supported restorations are considered to have more risk of veneer fracture allegedly due to the reduction of proprioception.[110] If true, the concept of retrievability for maintenance of ceramic implant-supported restorations would be valuable. The elaborate possibilities of ceramic core and framework design have greatly expanded with zirconia to address the

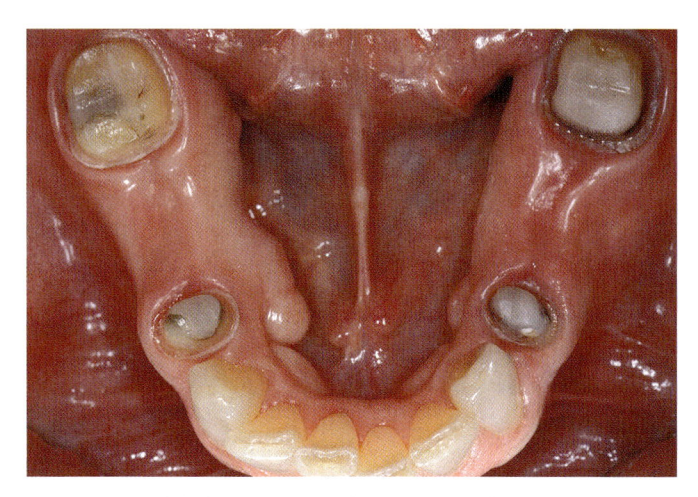

Figure 45.10 **(A)** Short posterior abutments with limited vertical space for fixed dental prostheses connectors.

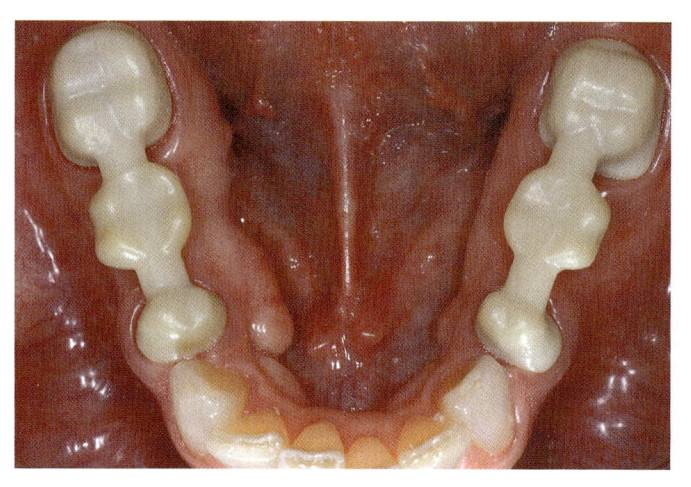

Figure 45.10 **(B)** Zirconia frameworks were selected for esthetics and strength in the connector areas

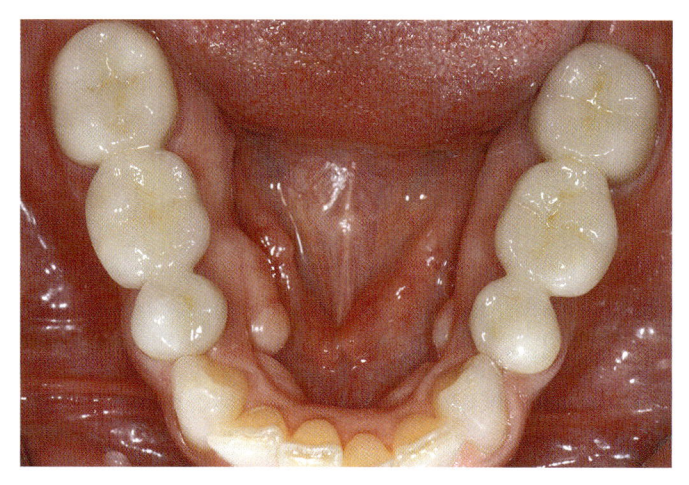

Figure 45.10 **(C)** Cementation of definitive bilayered ceramic fixed dental prostheses with ideal contours and proportions.

functional issue and retrievability. Historically, metal-ceramic screw-retained implant-supported restorations were criticized because of concerns with the esthetics of the screw access hole and its interference with the opposing dentition in terms of centric occlusal contacts and heightened risks of veneer chipping.[111–114] After both clinical and laboratory data were collected, no difference in fracture resistance was seen between screw- and cement-retained single-tooth metal-ceramic crowns.[115–117] Posterior implant-supported screw-retained ceramic restorations with zirconia cores may offer esthetic and functional solutions to the concerns that the metal-ceramic screw-retained restorations faced. The ceramic screw access hole can have the glassy veneer portion of the chimney etched, silanated, and restored with direct composite-resin restorative material. For a monolithic zirconia screw access hole, primers containing 10-methacryloyloxi-decyl-dihydrogen-phosphate are recommended, which has been shown to enhance the durability of composite resin bonded to zirconia.[112] When the all-ceramic access hole is restored with resin composite it is almost undetectable (Figure 45.11A and B).

Table 45.1 Manufacturer's Recommended Minimal Connector Size for Various Dental Ceramics in Different Situations

Core Material—System	
Lithium disilicate—e.MaxPress	16 mm² (1 pontic length ≤11 mm)
Glass-infiltrated alumina with 35% partially stabilized zirconia—In-Ceram zirconia	9 mm² (pontic length ≤6 mm) 12.25 mm² (pontic length ≤8 mm) 16 mm² (pontic length ≤16 mm)
Glass-infiltrated alumina—In-Ceram alumina	≥9 mm² (1 pontic)
Densely sintered high-purity alumina—Procera All-Ceram bridges	3 mm height/6 mm² (1 pontic)
Y-TZP—Lava Plus	7 mm² (1–2 pontics) 10 mm² (>2 pontics)
Y-TZP—Procera	3 height × 2.5 width/6 mm² (pontic length ≤21.0 mm)

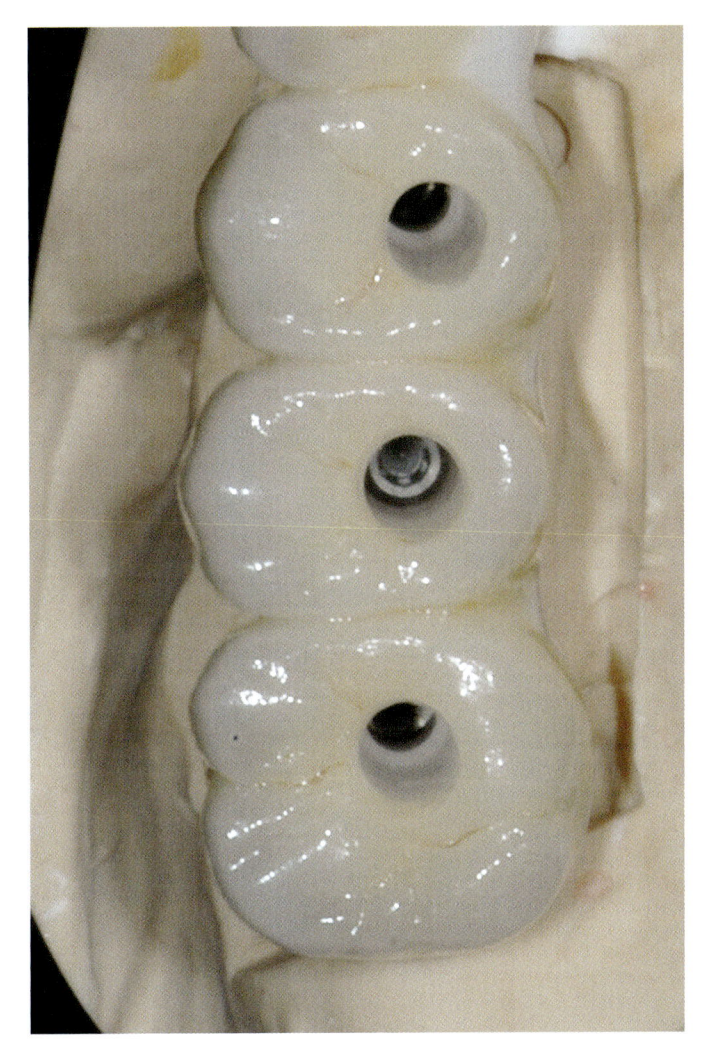

Figure 45.11 **(A)** Ceramic screw-retained implant-supported restoration before insertion and restoration of screw access holes.

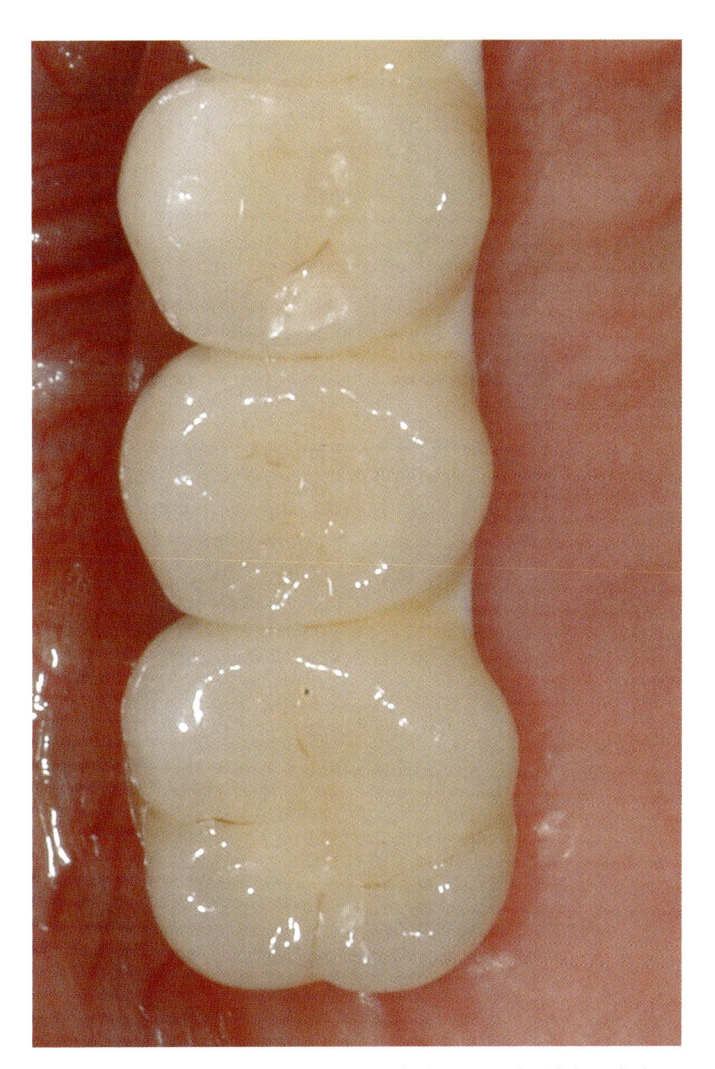

Figure 45.11 **(B)** Ceramic screw access hole restored with bonded composite at first occlusal 2 mm.

Maintenance issues with posterior screw-retained ceramic implant-supported restorations may also be simplified because they may be easily removed. Repairs done outside of the mouth facilitate ease of adhesive repairs with direct composite resin or indirect ceramic veneers and inlays.

Summary

With the principles established in this chapter, health and esthetics may be delivered to the patient through all the available dental ceramics. Detailed analysis of all the restorative interfaces involved within the definitive restoration may facilitate long-term maintenance for the patient since each interface has a different function. The abutment–implant interface requires a design that will not damage the implant fixture or cause premature prosthetic screw loosening or fracture. The abutment–soft tissue interface requires the use of materials that are highly biocompatible with the peri-implant tissues and do not adversely affect their color. The restoration–tooth interface needs are dependent on the needs of the tooth for conservation of sound structure and how its color will affect the definitive restoration.

The restoration–implant abutment interface may be eliminated with screw retention for concepts of retrievability in high-function areas. Critical decisions on whether to adhesively bond, conventionally lute, or screw retain the definitive restoration may now be determined with plans for long-term maintenance in mind. At the occlusal surface–opposing dentition interface a balance must be established between durability and esthetics for the specific location of the restoration in the mouth along with considerations of the patient's level of function and parafunction. Most of the interfaces discussed are functionally linked to the occlusal interface and tested for durability through this link. Consequently, the summation of all the aforementioned considerations needs to be evaluated to reduce the probability of catastrophic failure. Currently, ceramic restorations present with abundant possibilities in terms of restoration design, type of material, conservation of tooth structure, delivery procedures, and retrievability. Subsequently, clinicians are not forced to treatment plan around one type of restoration or material any more to achieve high-quality esthetics, longevity, and function. Placement of material selection at the end instead of at the front of a treatment plan allows the clinician to process the needs of the patient first and the type of restoration required. Once these needs are established, the selection of the ideal dental ceramic for high esthetics and durability may be performed without compromising the long-term durability of both the tooth and the restoration.

Acknowledgements

Special thanks to Dr Ariel J. Raigrodski for his mentorship and collaboration with the clinical cases shown in Figures 45.3, 45.4, 45.5, 45.10, and 45.11. Another special thanks to the master ceramists Harald Heindl MDT (Figures 45.2A and B, 45.7C, 45.8B–D, and 45.9A and B) and Hiro Tokutomi RDT (Figures 45.3, 45.4B–E, 45.5D–F, and 45.11A and B) for fabricating the restorations displayed in this chapter.

References

1. Raigrodski AJ. Materials selection for complete-coverage all-ceramic restorations. In: Cohen M, ed. *Interdisciplinary Treatment Planning: Principles, Design, Implementation*. Berlin: Quintessence; 2008:383–406.
2. Conrad H, Seong W, Pesun I. Current ceramic materials and systems with clinical recommendations: a systematic review. *J Prosthet Dent* 2007;98(5):389–404.
3. Zembic A, Sailer I, Jung RE, Hämmerle CH. Randomized-controlled clinical trial of customized zirconia and titanium implant abutments for single-tooth implants in canine and posterior regions: 3-year results. *Clin Oral Implants Res* 2009;20:802–808.
4. Glauser R, Sailer I, Wohlwend A. Experimental zirconia abutments for implant-supported single-tooth restorations in esthetically demanding regions: 4-year results of a prospective clinical study. *Int J Prosthodont* 2004;17:285–290.
5. Zembic A, Kim S, Zwahlen M, Kelly R. Systematic review of the survival rate and incidence of biologic, technical, and esthetic complications of single implant abutments supporting fixed prostheses. *Int J Oral Maxillofac Implants* 2014;29(Suppl):99–116.
6. Zembic A, Philipp AO, Hämmerle CH, et al. Eleven-year follow-up of a prospective study of zirconia implants abutments supporting single all-ceramic crowns in anterior and premolar regions. *Clin Implant Dent Related Res* 2015;17(Suppl 2):e417–e426.
7. Zembic A, Bösch A, Jung R, et al. Five-year results of a randomized controlled clinical trial comparing zirconia and titanium abutments supporting single-implant crowns in canine and posterior regions. *Clin Oral Implants Res* 2013;24:384–390.
8. Nguyen HQ, Tan KB, Nicholls JI. Load fatigue performance of implant–ceramic abutment combinations. *Int J Oral Maxillofac Implants* 2009;24:636–646.
9. Albrektsson T, Zarb GA, Worthington P, Eriksson AR. The long-term efficacy of currently used dental implants: a review and proposed criteria of success. *J Oral Maxillofac Implants* 1986;1:11–25.
10. Furhauser R, Florescu D, Benesch T, et al. Evaluation of soft tissue around single-tooth implant crowns: the pink esthetic score. *Clin Oral Implants Res* 2005;16:639–644.
11. Belser U, Buser D, Higginbottom F. Consensus statements and recommended clinical procedures regarding esthetics in implant dentistry. *Int J Oral Maxillofac Implants* 2004;19(Suppl):73–74.
12. Abrahamsson I, Berglundh T, Glantz PO, Lindhe J. The mucosal attachment at different abutments. An experiment study in dogs. *J Clin Periodontol* 1998;25:721–727.
13. Welander M, Abrahamsson I, Berglundh T. The mucosal barrier at implant abutments of different materials. *Clin Oral Implants Res* 2008;19:635–641.
14. Salihoğlu U, Boynueğri D, Engin D. Bacterial adhesion and colonization differences between zirconium oxide and titanium alloys: an in vivo human study. *Int J Oral Maxillofac Implants* 2011;26:101–107.
15. Van Brakel R, Cune MS, van Winkelhoff AJ. Early bacterial colonization and soft tissue health around zirconia and titanium abutments: an in vivo study in man. *Clin Oral Implants Res* 2011;22(6):571–577.
16. Mustafa K, Wennerberg A, Arvidson K. Influence of modifying and veneering the surface of ceramic abutments on cellular attachment and proliferation. *Clin Oral Implants Res* 2008;19:1178–1187.
17. Scarano A, Piattelli M, Caputi S. Bacterial adhesion on commercially pure titanium and zirconium oxide disks: an in vivo human study. *J Periodontol* 2004;75:292–296.
18. Bressan E, Paniz G, Lops D, et al. Influence of abutment material on the gingival color of implant supported all-ceramic restorations: a prospective multicenter study. *Clin Oral Implants Res* 2011;22(6):631–637.
19. Jung R, Sailer I, Hämmerle C. The effect of all-ceramic and porcelain-fused-to-metal restorations on marginal peri-implant soft tissue color: a randomized controlled clinical trial. *Int J Periodontics Restorative Dent* 2008;28:357–365.
20. Tan PLB, Dunne J. Esthetic comparison of a metal ceramic crown and cast metal abutment with an all-ceramic crown and zirconia abutment: a clinical report. *J Prosthet Dent* 2004;91:215–218.
21. Goodacre CJ, Paravina RD, Bergen SF, Preston JD. *A Contemporary Guide to Color and Shade Selection for Prosthodontics*. American College of Prosthodontists; 2009 [DVD].
22. Jung R, Hämmerle C, Schmidlin P. In vitro color changes of soft tissues caused by restorative materials. *Int J Periodontics Restorative Dent* 2007;27:251–257.
23. Van Brakel R, Noordmans H, Frenken J, et al. The effect of zirconia and titanium implant abutments on light reflection of the supporting soft tissues. *Clin Oral Implants Res* 2011;22(10):1172–1178.
24. Linkevicius T, Vindasiute E, Puisys A, Peciuliene V. The influence of margin location on the amount of undetected cement excess after delivery of cement-retained implant restorations. *Clin Oral Implants Res* 2011;22(12):1379–1384.
25. Goldin E, Boyd N III, Goldstein GR. Marginal fit of leucite-glass pressable ceramic restorations and ceramic-pressed-to-metal restorations. *J Prosthet Dent* 2005;93:143–147.
26. Martinez-Rus F, Suarez M, Rivera B, Pradíes G. Evaluation of the absolute marginal discrepancy of zirconia-based ceramic copings. *J Prosthet Dent* 2011;105:108–114.
27. Baig M, Tan K, Nicholls JI. Evaluation of the marginal fit of a zirconia ceramic computer-aided machined (CAM) crown system. *J Prosthet Dent* 2010;104:216–227.
28. Reich S, Gozdowski L, Trentzsch L. Marginal fit of heat-pressed vs. CAD/CAM processed all-ceramic onlays using a milling unit prototype. *Oper Dent* 2008;33:644–650.
29. Beschnidt SM, Strub JR. Evaluation of the marginal accuracy of different all-ceramic crown systems after simulation in the artificial mouth. *J Oral Rehabil* 1999;26:582–593.

30. Holden J, Goldstein G, Hittelman EL, Clark EA. Comparison of the marginal fit of pressable ceramic to metal ceramic restorations. *J Prosthodont* 2009;18:645–648.
31. Balkaya MC, Cinar A, Pamuk S. Influence of firing cycles on the marginal distortion of 3 all-ceramic crown systems. *J Prosthet Dent* 2005;93:346–355.
32. Groten M, Girhofer S, Pröbster L. Marginal fit consistency of copy-milled and all-ceramic crowns during fabrication by light and scanning electron microscopic analysis in vitro. *J Oral Rehabil* 1997;24:871–881.
33. Yeo IS, Yang JH, Lee JB. In vitro marginal fit of three all ceramic crown systems. *J Prosthet Dent* 2003;90:459–464.
34. Rinke S, Behi F, Hüls A. Fitting accuracy of all-ceramic posterior crowns produced with three different systems. *J Dent Res* 2001;80:651.
35. Quintas AF, Oliveira F, Bottino MA. Vertical marginal discrepancy of ceramic copings with different ceramic materials, finish lines and luting agents: an in vitro evaluation. *J Prosthet Dent* 2004;92:250–257.
36. Vigolo P, Fonzi F. An in vitro evaluation of fit of zirconium-oxide-based ceramic four-unit fixed partial dentures, generated with three different CAD/CAM systems, before and after porcelain firing cycles and after glaze cycles. *J Prosthodont* 2008;17:621–626.
37. Reich S, Wichmann M, Nkenke E, Proeschel P. Clinical fit of all-ceramic three-unit fixed partial dentures, generated with three different CAD/CAM systems. *Eur J Oral Sci* 2005;113:174–179.
38. Reich S, Kappe K, Teschner H, Schmitt J. Clinical fit of four-unit zirconia posterior fixed dental prostheses. *Eur J Oral Sci* 2008;116(6):579–584.
39. Tinschert J, Natt G, Mautsch W, et al. Marginal fit of alumina-and zirconia-based fixed partial dentures produced by a CAD/CAM system. *Oper Dent* 2001;26(4):367–374.
40. Beuer F, Aggstaller H, Edelhoff D, et al. Marginal and internal fits of fixed dental prostheses zirconia retainers. *Dent Mater* 2009;25(1):94–102.
41. Stappert CFJ, Denner N, Gerds T, Strub JR. Marginal adaptation of different types of all-ceramic partial coverage restorations after exposure to an artificial mouth. *Br Dent* 2005;199:779–783.
42. McLean JW, von Fraunhofer JA. The estimation of cement film thickness by an in vivo technique. *Br Dent* 1971;131:107–111.
43. Weber HP, Kim DM, Ng MW, et al. Peri-implant soft-tissue health surrounding cement- and screw-retained implant restorations: a multi-center, 3-year prospective study. *Clin Oral Implants Res* 2006;17:375–379.
44. Schatzle M, Lang N, Anerud A. The influence of margins of restorations on the periodontal tissues over 26 years. *J Clin Periodontol* 2001;28:57–64.
45. Wilson T. The positive relationship between excess cement and peri-implant disease: a prospective clinical endoscopic study. *J Periodontol* 2009;80:1388–1392.
46. Buonocore M. A simple method of increasing the adhesion of acrylic filling materials to enamel surface. *J Dent Res* 1955;34:849–853.
47. Clelland NL, Ramirez A, Katsube N, Seghi RR. Influence of bond quality on failure load of leucite- and lithiadisilicate-based ceramics. *J Prosthet Dent* 2007;97:18–24.
48. Stangel I, Nathanson D, Hsu CS. Shear strength of the composite bond to etched porcelain. *J Dent Res* 1987;66:1460–1465.
49. Pagniano R, Seghi R, Rosenstiel SF. The effect of a layer of resin luting agent on the biaxial flexure strength of two all-ceramic systems. *J Prosthet Dent* 2005;93:459–466.
50. Mota CS, Demarco FF, Camacho GB, Powers JM. Tensile bond strength of four resin luting agents bonded to bovine enamel and dentin. *J Prosthet Dent* 2003;89:558–564.
51. Jevnikar P, Krnel K, Kocjan A. The effect of nano-structured alumina coating on resin-bond strength to zirconia ceramics. *Dent Mater* 2010;26:688–698.
52. Aida M, Hayakawa T, Mizukawa K. Adhesion of composite to porcelain with various surface conditions. *J Prosthet Dent* 1995;73:464–470.
53. Kamada K, Yoshida K, Atsuta M. Effect of ceramic surface treatments on the bond of four resin luting agents to a ceramic material. *J Prosthet Dent* 1998;79:508–513.
54. Della Bona A, Anusavice KJ, Shen C. Microtensile strength of composite bonded to hot-pressed ceramics. *J Adhes Dent* 2000;2:305–313.
55. Bottino MA, Valadro LF, Scotti R, Buso L. Effect of surface treatments on the resin bond to zirconium-based ceramic. *Int J Prosthodont* 2005;18:60–65.
56. Kelly J, Nishimura I, Campbell SD. Ceramic in dentistry: historical roots and current perspectives. *J Prosthet Dent* 1996;75:18–32.
57. Nakamura T, Saito O, Fuyikawa J, Ishigaki S. Influence of abutment substrate and ceramic thickness on the colour of heat-pressed ceramic crowns. *J Oral Rehabil* 2002;29:805–809.
58. Vichi A, Ferrari M, Davidson CL. Influence of ceramic and cement thickness on the masking of various types of opaque posts. *J Prosthet Dent* 2000;83:412–417.
59. Dogan S, Flinn BD, Toivola RE et al. Translucency measurement of zirconia and lithium-disilicate using densitometry and spectrophotometry. In: *89th General Session of the International Association for Dental Research*, 2011, March 16–19; San Diego, CA; abstract 1651.
60. Malament KA, Socransky SS. Survival of Dicor glass-ceramic dental restorations over 14 years: part 1. Survival of Dicor complete coverage restorations and effect of internal surface acid etching, tooth position, gender, and age. *J Prosthet Dent* 1999;81:23–32.
61. Fradeani M, Redemagni M. An 11-year clinical evaluation of leucite-reinforced glass-ceramic crowns: a retrospective study. *Quintessence Int* 2002;33:503–510.
62. Heintze SD, Roussen V. Fracture rates of IPS Empress all-ceramic crowns—a systematic review. *Int J Prosthodont* 2010;23:129–133.
63. Matinlinna JP, Vallittu PK. Bonding of resin composites to etchable ceramic surfaces—an insight review of the chemical aspects on surface conditioning. *J Oral Rehabil* 2007;34:622–630.
64. Naves LZ, Soares CJ, Moraes RR, et al. Surface/interface morphology and bond strength to glass ceramic etched for different periods. *Oper Dent* 2010;35(4):420–427.
65. Quinn JB, Sundar V, Lloyd IK. Influence of microstructure and chemistry on the fracture toughness of dental ceramics. *Dent Mater* 2003;19:603–611.
66. Zeng K, Odén A, Rowcliffe D. Flexure tests on dental ceramics. *Int J Prosthodont* 1996;9:434–439.
67. Wolfart S, Eschbach S, Scherrer S, Kern M. Clinical outcome of three-unit lithium-disilicate glass-ceramic fixed dental prostheses: up to 8 years results. *Dent Mater* 2009;25:e63–e71.
68. Makarouna M, Ullmann K, Lazarek K, Boening KW. Six-year clinical performance of lithium disilicate fixed partial dentures. *Int J Prosthodont* 2011;24:204–206.
69. Probster L. Four year clinical study of glass-infiltrated, sintered alumina crowns. *J Oral Rehabil* 1996;23:147–151.
70. Vult von Steyern P, Jonsson O, Nilner K. Five-year evaluation of posterior all-ceramic three-unit (In-Ceram) FPDs. *Int J Prosthodont* 2001;14:379–384.

71. Olsson KG, Furst B, Andersson B, Carlsson GE. A long-term retrospective and clinical follow-up study of In-Ceram alumina FPDs. *Int J Prosthodont* 2003;16:150–156.
72. Wagner WC, Chu TM. Biaxial flexural strength and indentation fracture toughness of three new dental core ceramics. *J Prosthet Dent* 1996;76:140–144.
73. Guazzato M, Albakry M, Swain MV, Ironside J. Mechanical properties of In-Ceram alumina and In-Ceram zirconia. *Int J Prosthodont* 2002;15:339–346.
74. Chong KH, Chai J, Takahashi Y, Wozniak W. Flexural strength of In-Ceram alumina and In-Ceram-zirconia core materials. *Int J Prosthodont* 2002;15:183–188.
75. Seghi RR, Sorensen JA. Relative flexural strength of six new ceramic materials. *Int J Prosthodont* 1995;8:239–246.
76. Heffernan M, Aquilino S, Diaz-Arnold A, et al. Relative translucency of six all-ceramic systems. Part I: core materials. *J Prosthet Dent* 2002;88:4–9.
77. Heffernan M, Aquilino S, Diaz-Arnold A, et al. Relative translucency of six all-ceramic systems. Part II: core and veneer materials. *J Prosthet Dent* 2002;88:10–15.
78. McLaren EA. All-ceramic alternatives to conventional metal-ceramic restorations. *Compend Contin Educ Dent* 1998;19:307–325.
79. Kelly JR. Dental ceramics: current thinking and trends. *Dent Clin N Am* 2004;48:513–530.
80. Odén A, Andersson M, Krystek-Ondracek I, Magnusson D. Five-year clinical evaluation of proceraallceram crowns. *J Prosthet Dent* 1998;80:450–456.
81. Fredeani M, D'Amelio M, Redemagni M, Corrado M. Five-year follow-up with Procera all-ceramic crowns. *Quintessence Int* 2005;36:105–113.
82. Christel P, Meunier A, Heller M, et al. Mechanical properties and short-term in-vivo evaluation of yttrium-oxide-partially-stabilized zirconia. *J Biomed Mater Res* 1989;23:45–61.
83. Flinn BD, Roberts BR, Mancl LA, Raigrodski AJ. The effect of accelerated aging on strength of thin Y-TZP. *J Dent Res* 2010;89(Spec Iss B):3560.
84. Schmitt J, Wichmann M, Holst S, Reich S. Restoring severely compromised anterior teeth with zirconia crowns and feather-edged margin preparations: a 3-year follow-up of a prospective clinical trial. *Int J Prosthodont* 2010;23(2):107–109.
85. Raigrodski AJ, Zhang H, Dogan S. Efficacy of zirconia-based anterior maxillary single crowns with customized copings. *J Dent Res* 2009;88(Spec Iss A):374.
86. Raigrodski AJ, Chiche GJ, Potiket N, et al. The efficacy of posterior three-unit zirconium-oxide-based ceramic fixed partial dental prostheses: a prospective clinical pilot study. *J Prosthet Dent* 2006;96:237–244.
87. Sailer I, Pjetursson BE, Zwahen M, Hämmerle CH. A systematic review of the survival and complication rates of all-ceramic and metal-ceramic reconstructions after an observation period of at least 3 years. Part II: fixed dental prostheses. *Clin Oral Implants Res* 2007;18(Suppl 3):86–96.
88. Yu A, Raigrodski AJ, Chiche GJ, et al. Clinical efficacy of Y-TZP-based posterior fixed partial dentures-five year results. *J Dent Res* 2009;88(Spec Iss A):1637.
89. Baldicarra P, Llukacej A, Ciocca L, et al. Translucency of zirconia copings made with different CAD/CAM systems. *J Prosthet Dent* 2010;104:6–12.
90. Rekow ED, Silva NRFA, Coelho PG, et al. Performance of dental ceramics: challenges for improvements. *J Dent Res* 2011;90(8):937–952.
91. Saito A, Komine F, Blatz MB, Matsumura H. A comparison of bond strength of layered veneering porcelains to zirconia and metal. *J Prosthet Dent* 2010;104:247–257.
92. Ishibe M, Raigrodski AJ, Flinn BD, et al. Shear bond strength of pressed and layered veneering ceramics to high-noble alloy and zirconia cores. *J Prosthet Dent* 2011;106(1):29–37.
93. Beuer F, Edelhoff D, Gernet W, Sorensen JA. Three-year clinical prospective evaluation of zirconia-based posterior fixed dental prostheses (FPDs). *Clin Oral Investig* 2009;13:445–451.
94. Rosentritt M, Steiger D, Behr M, et al. Influence of substructure design and spacer settings on the in vitro performance of molar zirconia crowns. *J Dent* 2009;37:978–983.
95. Park J-H, Park S, Lee K, et al. Antagonist wear of three CAD/CAM anatomic contour zirconia ceramics. *J Prosthet Dent* 2014;111:20–29.
96. Janyavula S, Lawson N, Cakir D, et al. The wear of polished and glazed zirconia against enamel. *J Prosthet* 2013:109:222–229.
97. Al-Fadda SA, Zarb GA, Finer Y. A comparison of the accuracy of fit of 2 methods for fabricating implant-prosthodontic frameworks. *Int J Prosthodont* 2007;20:125–131.
98. Kelly JR, Tesk JA, Sorensen JA. Failure of all-ceramic fixed partial dentures in vitro and in vivo: analysis and modeling. *J Dent Res* 1995;74:1253–1258.
99. Campbell SD, Sozio RB. Evaluation of the fit and strength of an all-ceramic fixed partial denture. *J Prosthet Dent* 1988;59:301–306.
100. Sorensen JA, Kand SK, Torres TJ, Knode H. In-Ceram fixed partial dentures: three-year clinical trial results. *J Calif Dent Assoc* 1998;26:207–214.
101. Suarez MJ, Lozano JF, Paz Salido M, Martínez F. Three-year clinical evaluation of In-Ceram zirconia posterior FPDs. *Int J Prosthodont* 2004;17:35–38.
102. Espuivel-Upshaw JF, Anusavice KJ, Young H, et al. Clinical performance of lithia disilicate-based core ceramic for three-unit posterior FPDs. *Int J Prosthodont* 2004;17:469–475.
103. Oh W, Gotzen N, Anusavice KJ. Influence of connector design on fracture probability of ceramic fixed-partial dentures. *J Dent Res* 2002;81:623–627.
104. Oh WS, Anusavice KJ. Effect of connector design on the fracture resistance of all-ceramic fixed partial dentures. *J Prosthet Dent* 2002;87:536–542.
105. Raigrodski AJ. Contemporary materials and technologies for all-ceramic fixed partial dentures: a review of the literature. *J Prosthet Dent* 2004;92:557–562.
106. Raigrodski AJ. Contemporary all-ceramic fixed partial dentures: a review. *Dent Clin North Am* 2004;48:531–544.
107. Raigrodski AJ, SaltzerAM. Clinical considerations in case selection for all-ceramic fixed partial dentures. *Pract Proced Aesthet Dent* 2002;14:411–419.
108. White SN, Miklus VG, McLaren EA, et al. Flexural strength of a layered zirconia and porcelain dental all-ceramic system. *J Prosthet Dent* 2005;94:125–131.
109. Stappert CF, Tarnow DP, Tan JH, Chu SJ. Proximal contact areas of the maxillary anterior dentition. *Int J Periodontics Restorative Dent* 2010;30:471–477.
110. Kinsel RP, Lin D. Retrospective analysis of porcelain failures of metal ceramic crowns and fixed partial dentures supported by 729 implants in 152 patients: patient-specific and implant-specific predictors of ceramic failure. *J Prosthet Dent* 2009;101:388–394.
111. Karl M, Graef F, Taylor TD, Heckmann SM. In vitro effect of load cycling on metal-ceramic cement- and screw-retained implant restorations. *J Prosthet Dent* 2007;97:137–140.

112. Komine F, Kobayashi K, Blatz MB, et al. Durability of bond between an indirect composite veneering material and zirconium dioxide ceramics. *Acta Odontol Scand* 2013;71: 457–463.
113. Torrado E, Ercoli C, Mardini MA, et al. A comparison of the porcelain fracture resistance of screw-retained and cement-retained implant-supported metal-ceramic crowns. *J Prosthet Dent* 2004;91:532–537.
114. Al-Omari WM, Shadid R, Abu-Naba'a L, El Masoud B. Porcelain fracture resistance of screw-retained, cement-retained, and screw-cement-retained implant-supported metal ceramic posterior crowns. *J Prosthodont* 2010;19:263–273.
115. Karl M, Graef F, Wichmann MG, Heckmann SM. The effect of load cycling on metal ceramic screw-retained implant restorations with unrestored and restored screw access holes. *J Prosthet Dent* 2008;99:19–24.
116. Zarone F, Sorrentino R, Traini T, et al. Fracture resistance of implant-supported screw- versus cement-retained porcelain fused to metal single crowns: SEM fractographic analysis. *Dent Mater* 2007;23:296–301.
117. Vigolo P, Givani A, Majzoub Z, Cordioli G. Cement versus screw-retained implant-supported single-tooth crowns: a 4-year prospective clinical study. *Int J Oral Maxillofac Implants* 2004;19:260–265.

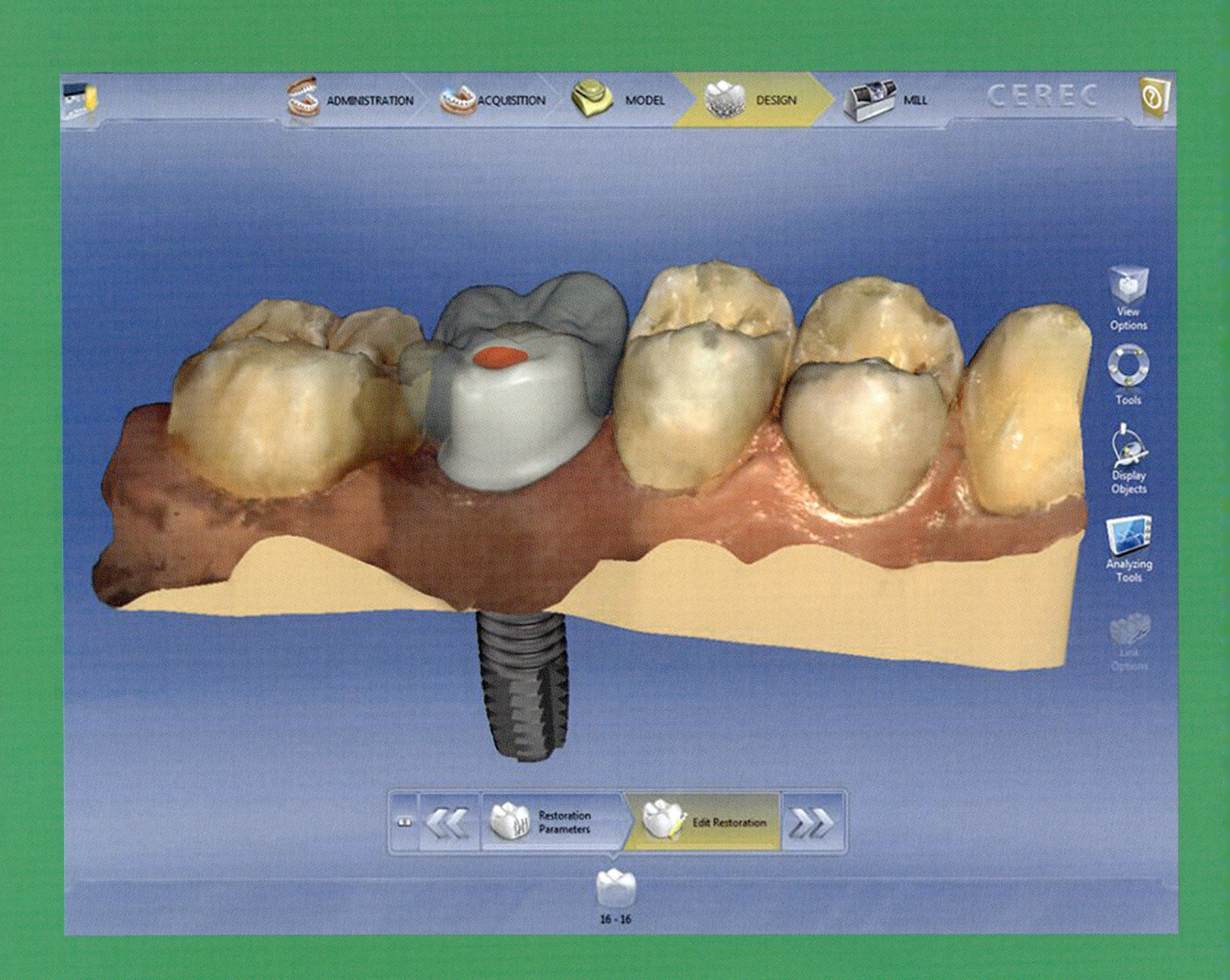

Chapter 46 Digital Impression Devices and CAD/CAM Systems

Nathan S. Birnbaum, DDS and Heidi B. Aaronson, DMD

Chapter Outline

Concept of dental impression making	1388	Model milling	1394
From bites to bytes: a brief history	1388	Dedicated impression scanner models	1394
Computer-aided design/manufacturing versus dedicated impression scanners	1389	3M *True Definition Scanner*	1394
		iTero Element™ scanner	1396
Computer-aided design/manufacturing systems	1389	3Shape TRIOS	1397
CEREC	1389	Feature comparisons	1400
Planmeca PlanScan	1391	Open versus closed architecture	1400
Feature comparisons	1392	Computer-aided design/manufacturing in the laboratory	1400
Dedicated impression scanners	1393	Analog versus digital impression accuracy	1400
Model fabrication	1394	Digital laboratory workflow	1401
Stereolithography apparatus printing	1394	Clinical cases	1403

The technological advancements that have enabled the use of three-dimensional (3D) digital scanners and mills to become an integral part of many industries for decades have been improved and refined for application to dentistry.

Unlike many other improvements in dental technology that have taken place, particularly within the past decade, which employ evolutionary changes in materials and instruments, the rapid explosion in the field of digital impressioning has been nothing short of revolutionary.[1] Since the introduction of the first dental computer-aided design/computer-aided manufacturing (CAD/CAM) system in the mid-1980s, product development engineers at a number of companies have enhanced the technologies and created in-office scanners and mills that are increasingly user friendly and able to produce accurately fitting dental restorations. These systems are capable of capturing 3D virtual images of tooth preparations, from which restorations may be fabricated directly (i.e., CAD/CAM systems) or fabricated indirectly (i.e., dedicated impression scanning systems for the creation of accurate virtual or physical master models). Dental laboratories have led the way in the adoption of CAD/CAM technology, utilizing digital systems to design restorations on virtual preparation images, scan physical impressions and models, and construct dental restorations. The application of these products is increasing rapidly in both dental offices and dental laboratories around the world and presents paradigm shifts both in the way that dental impressions are obtained and dental restorations are fabricated.[2]

Ronald E. Goldstein's Esthetics in Dentistry, Third Edition. Edited by Ronald E. Goldstein, Stephen J. Chu, Ernesto A. Lee, and Christian F.J. Stappert.
© 2018 John Wiley & Sons, Inc. Published 2018 by John Wiley & Sons, Inc.

Concept of dental impression making

The most critical procedure in the workflow of creating precisely fitting fixed or removable dental restoration is the capture of an accurate impression of prepared or unprepared teeth, dental implants, edentulous ridges, or intraoral landmarks or defects. Unless a wax or resin pattern is made directly on the teeth, on the edentulous ridges, or in the defects, which is a time-consuming and generally impractical effort, the dentist or auxiliary must achieve an exact duplication of the site so that a dental laboratory technician, usually at a remote location, can create the restoration on a precise replica of the target site. Traditionally, the paradigm for transferring the necessary information from the patient's oral cavity to the technician's laboratory bench has been to obtain an accurate negative of the target site, from which the technician is able to fabricate an accurate gypsum positive replica duplicating the original intraoral structures.

The advent of highly innovative and accurate impressioning devices and CAD/CAM systems based on new technologies has created a disruptive paradigm shift in the concept for impression making. These systems are poised to revolutionize the way in which dental professionals already are and will continue making impressions for indirect restorative dentistry.[1]

From bites to bytes: a brief history

Impression making for restorative dentistry is a relatively recent concept in the millennia-old history of restorative dentistry. The earliest physical proof or record of prosthetic treatment to replace missing teeth goes back to Etruscan times, approximately 700 BC, in which teeth were carved from ivory and bone and affixed to adjacent teeth with gold wires. It was not until 1856 that documentation exists of the use of an impression material other than beeswax or plaster of Paris—which had inherent problems of distortion or difficulty of use respectively—for creating an oral prosthesis, when Dr Charles Stent perfected an impression material for use in the fabrication of the device that bears his name for the correction of oral deformities.[3]

The first use of an elastomeric material for capturing impressions of tooth preparations, as well as other oral and dental conditions, was not until 1937, when Sears introduced agar as an impression material for crown preparations.[4] In the mere 80 years that elastic impression materials have been in use, numerous formulations have been developed, all of which have exhibited particular shortcomings in the goal of obtaining precise reproduction of the oral structures.

The reversible hydrocolloid agar and the irreversible hydrocolloid alginate exhibit poor dimensional stability—because of the imbibition or loss of water respectively when sitting in wet or dry conditions—as well as in having low tear resistance. The Japanese embargo on the sale of agar to the United States during World War II spurred research into the development of alternative elastomeric impression materials. The polysulfide rubber impression material introduced in the late 1950s, originally developed to seal gaps between sectional concrete structures,[5] overcame some of the problems of the hydrocolloids. Nevertheless, polysulfide rubber was messy, possessed objectionable taste and odor, had long setting times intraorally, and underwent dimensional change after the impression was removed from the mouth due to continued polymerization with the evaporation of water and shrinkage toward the impression tray, leading to dies that were wider and shorter than the teeth being impressed.[6] This problem was overcome somewhat by the use of custom trays that allowed for 4 mm of uniform space for the material and by pouring up the impression within 48 h.[5] The introduction in 1965 of the polyether material Impregum™ by ESPE GmbH as the first elastomeric impression material specifically developed for use in dentistry afforded the profession a material with relatively fast setting time, excellent flowability, outstanding detail reproduction, adequate tear strength, high hydrophilicity, and low shrinkage. The material is still in use today in several formulations, although it exhibits problems with objectionable odor and taste, high elastic modulus (stiffness—often leading to difficulty in removing impressions from the mouth), and the requirement to pour up models within 48 h because of absorption of water in very humid conditions, which can lead to impression distortion.[6]

Condensation cure silicone impression materials subsequently were developed, but these also suffered from problems with dimensional accuracy. The creation of polyvinyl siloxane (PVS) impression materials solved the issues of dimensional inaccuracy, poor taste and odor, and high modulus of elasticity, and offered excellent tear strength, superior flow, and lack of distortion even if models were not poured quickly. The biggest drawback of the PVS impression materials, however, is that they are hydrophobic, which can lead to the inability to capture fine detail if problems with hemostasis and/or moisture control occur during impression making.

In addition to the many problems inherent in the accuracy of the elastomeric materials themselves, further distortions can occur by mistakes made in the mixing of the materials or in the impression-making technique, the use of nonrigid impression trays,[7,8] the transfer of the impression to the dental laboratory (often subjecting the impressions to variable temperatures in everything from delivery vehicles to post office sorting rooms to the holds of cargo jets), the need for humidity control in the dental laboratory to assure accuracy in the setting of the gypsum model materials, and so on.

Newer technologies that allow for the use of digital scanners for impression making are indeed a welcome development. Digital impression making does not require patients to sit for as long as 7 min with a tray of often foul-tasting and malodorous "goop" in their mouths, requiring that they open uncomfortably wide, often gagging. Further, these devices help calm dentists' anxieties about economic and time considerations when deciding to remake inadequate impressions, and they display high-resolution images on a monitor, which allows for views of prepared teeth that would otherwise be impossible to see directly in the patient's mouth.

Advances in computerization, optics, miniaturization, and laser technologies have enabled the capture of dental impressions. Three-dimensional digitizing scanners have been in use in dentistry for more than 25 years and continue to be developed and improved for obtaining virtual impressions. The stressful, yet critical task of obtaining accurate impressions has undergone a paradigm shift.[2]

The CAD/CAM dental systems that are currently available are able to feed data obtained from accurate digital scans of teeth directly into milling systems capable of carving restorations out of ceramic or composite resin blocks without the need for a physical replica of the prepared, adjacent, and opposing teeth. With the development of newer high-strength and esthetic ceramic restorative materials, such as lithium disilicate and zirconia, dental laboratory systems and techniques have been developed in which master models poured from elastic impressions are digitally scanned to create stereolithic models on which the restorations can be fabricated. It is evident, however, that such second-generation models are not as accurate as stereolithic models made directly from data obtained from 3D digital scans of the teeth provided by 3D digital scanners designed for impression making. Furthermore, current laboratory scanning systems allow for the design of restorations to be achieved directly on virtual dies and models, rendering the need for physical models obsolete.

Computer-aided design/manufacturing versus dedicated impression scanners

There are two types of digital impressioning devices on the market: CAD/CAM systems and dedicated impression scanners.

CAD/CAM systems are able to complete a restoration from start to finish: they scan the prepared tooth, design the restoration digitally using the scan data, and manufacture the restoration in a milling chamber. In order to be considered a CAD/CAM system, the design and manufacture elements must be integrated into the unit overall. There are currently two leading CAD/CAM systems on the market: CEREC® and Planmeca PlanScan®.

Dedicated impression scanners only involve the first step of the CAD/CAM systems: the digital data acquisition. These systems rely on sending the impression data elsewhere to complete the restorative process. In some cases, the data are sent to a model manufacturing facility where a physical model is created. The model is then sent to the laboratory and the restoration is completed. In other cases, there is no need for a physical model at all—the laboratory can use the digital model to design and fabricate a restoration completely digitally. This will be described in detail later in the chapter. Examples of dedicated impression scanners are the 3M™ True Definition Scanner, iTero®, 3Shape TRIOS®, and many more.

Computer-aided design/manufacturing systems

CEREC

The CEREC system, an acronym for ceramic reconstruction, was introduced in 1985 by Siemens Medical Technology Division (Sirona Dental Systems was spun-off in 1997). It was the first CAD/CAM system that allowed dentists to fabricate ceramic inlays and onlays at the chairside, and the system expanded its capabilities to include crowns, bridges, and laminate veneers.[9]

System features

The CEREC acquisition device is available in two different models: the Bluecam and the Omnicam. The Bluecam was introduced in 2009, using shortwave blue light to increase the precision of the scan data. The Omnicam, launched in 2012, features powder-free digital scanning in full color.

The system is available in two designs: the CEREC AC (Acquisition Center) mobile cart with an integrated CPU (Figure 46.1), or the CEREC AF (Acquisiton Flex), a tabletop unit that connects to a separate PC.

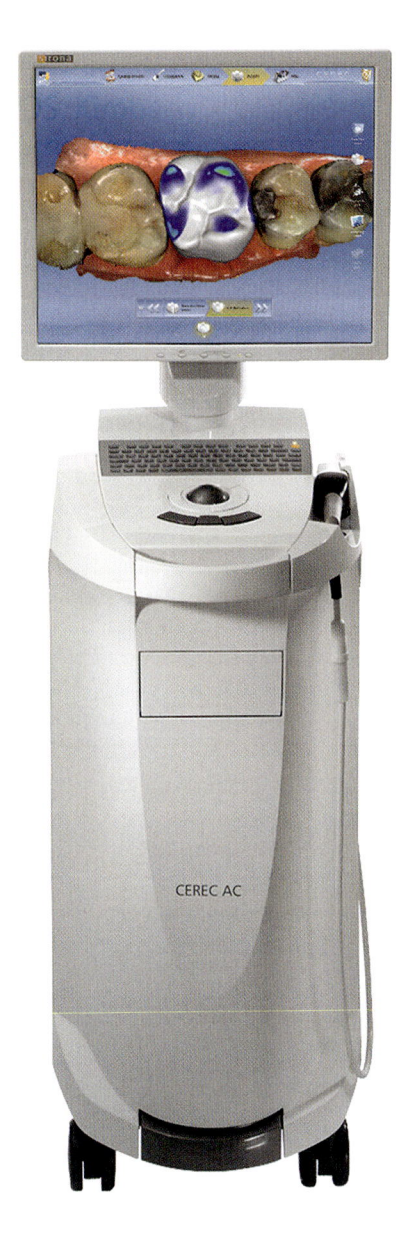

Figure 46.1 The CEREC AC Acquisition Center. *Source:* Reproduced with permission of CEREC, USA.

Workflow

CEREC Bluecam (Figure 46.2) features a highly visible blue light-emitting diode that senses when the area to be captured is in focus and automatically acquires a series of single images, which are then computed with great precision in order to create a virtual 3D model. The camera automatically detects the right moment to trigger the exposure, and the short capture time of the CEREC Bluecam prevents any blurring. In addition, the built-in shake detection system ensures that images are acquired only when the camera is held absolutely still. The CEREC software then automatically selects the optimum image data for the 3D model. The user can either place the CEREC Bluecam directly on the tooth or hover the camera above the tooth. As short, dense wavelengths are more precise than longer wavelengths (such as infrared), the CEREC AC boasts accurate and precise imaging.[10]

CEREC Omnicam (Figure 46.3) is optimized for powder-free scanning of natural tooth structures and gingiva. Simply place the camera over the relevant area and the scan starts automatically. The user moves the camera head closely over the teeth in a single, flowing process. The data are generated successively into a 3D model, which appears in color on the screen in real time. The scanning may be paused and resumed at any time.

Material selection

Current materials available for the CEREC system include Sironic inCoris TZI C (pre-shaded translucent zirconium oxide), inCoris CC (sintering metal), inCoris TZI (sintered zirconium oxide ceramic), CEREC Blocs C (feldspar ceramic), VITA Blocs, TriLuxe, IPS Empress CAD (leucite-reinforced ceramic), IPS e.max CAD (lithium disilicate), 3M Paradigm C (leucite-reinforced ceramic), Paradigm MZ100 (radiopaque composite), Zirlux® FC2 (full-contour zirconia), and Lava™ Ultimate (resin nano-ceramic).

Chairside fabrication

Following the design stage (Figure 46.4), the proposed restoration is sent to the in-office milling unit. CEREC offers three milling options: the CEREC MC (which produces fully anatomical single tooth restorations), the CEREC MC X, and the CEREC MC XL (Figure 46.5—which is capable of fabricating the complete CAD/CAM spectrum).

The milling unit must be loaded with the appropriate CAD/CAM block, as determined by the type of materials to be used, the size of the restoration, and the shade. The dentist selects the appropriate block of material, which is then loaded into the milling chamber. Upon completion of the milling cycle, the sprue is removed and the restoration is checked for marginal fit, contact, and occlusion before finishing. The restoration is then finished by polishing, glazing, or stacking. The milling times vary by unit size, detail, material, and milling unit, but are generally in the range of 6–15 min per unit.[11]

If the dentist wishes to have a physical model, the MC XL is capable of milling models. If a stereolithography apparatus (SLA) model is desired, the dentist can send the case from the scanner to the laboratory/Sirona infiniDent to have an SLA model fabricated. Surgical guides may also be milled with the MC XL milling unit, in combination with a Sirona 3D cone beam scan.

Laboratory fabrication

The CEREC system also allows the dentist to electronically send digital impressions to the laboratory when necessary; for example, in complex and/or highly esthetic cases. This feature, called CEREC Connect, sends the digital files to a laboratory in Sirona's inLab network, where the restorations are fabricated. Since CEREC uses selectively open architecture, the laboratory to which the cases are sent must be an approved CEREC inLab laboratory.

Support and education

When buying a CEREC unit, the dentist is given the opportunity to visit a two-day basic training course at one of several training locations across the country. Continued education courses related to the CEREC system are offered by relevant dental

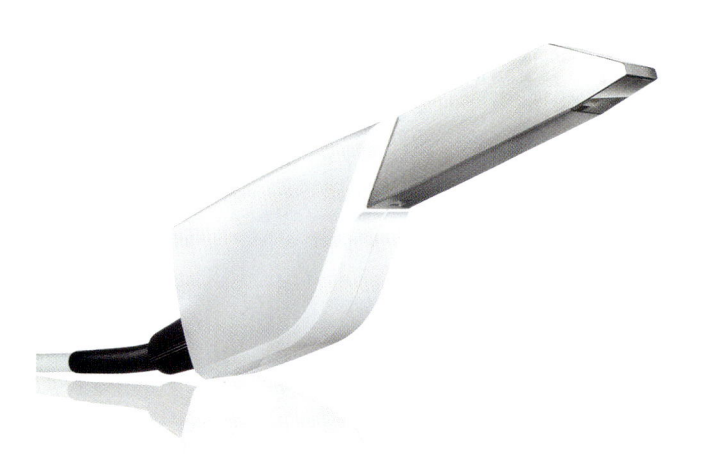

Figure 46.2 The CEREC Bluecam scanner. *Source:* Reproduced with permission of CEREC, USA.

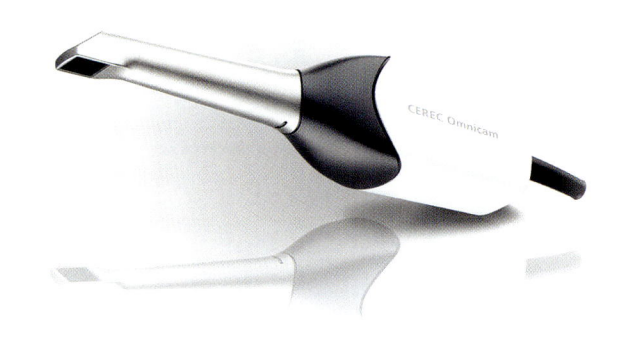

Figure 46.3 The CEREC Omnicam scanner. *Source:* Reproduced with permission of CEREC, USA.

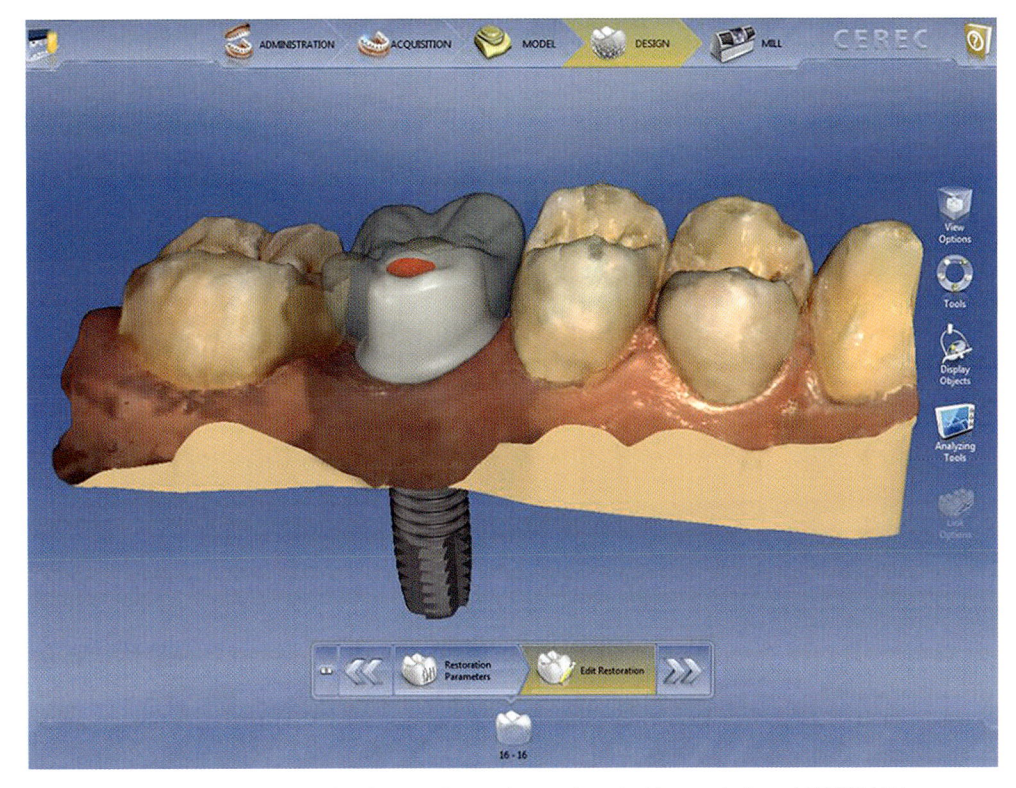

Figure 46.4 Designing an implant crown using CEREC software. *Source:* Reproduced with permission of CEREC, USA.

organizations throughout the year (personal communicaiton, Julie Bizzell, Clinical CAD/CAM Marketing Manager, Sirona).

Planmeca PlanScan

The Planmeca PlanScan (Figure 46.6) replaces the E4D Dentist digital impression system that was originally launched in 2008 by D4D Technologies. The new Planmeca FIT system features the PlanScan digital impression scanner, PlanCAD software for CAD/CAM design of restorations, and the PlanMill 40 (Figure 46.7) for in-office milling of restorations.

System features

The PlanScan system comes with three removable tips, power cable, and scanner cradle. The two-piece cradle features a

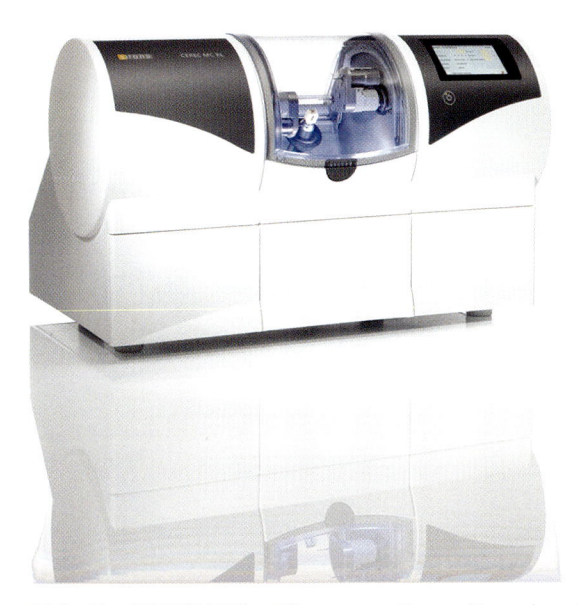

Figure 46.5 The CEREC MC XL milling center. *Source:* Reproduced with permission of CEREC, USA.

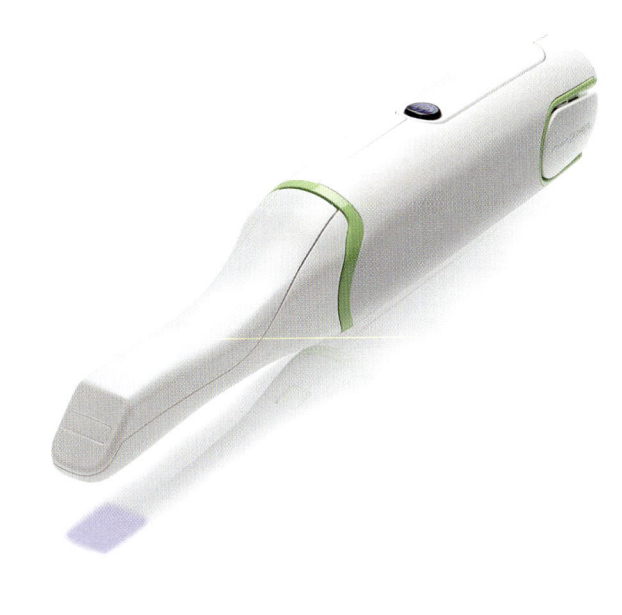

Figure 46.6 Planmeca PlanScan scanner. *Source:* Figure courtesy of Planmeca, USA.

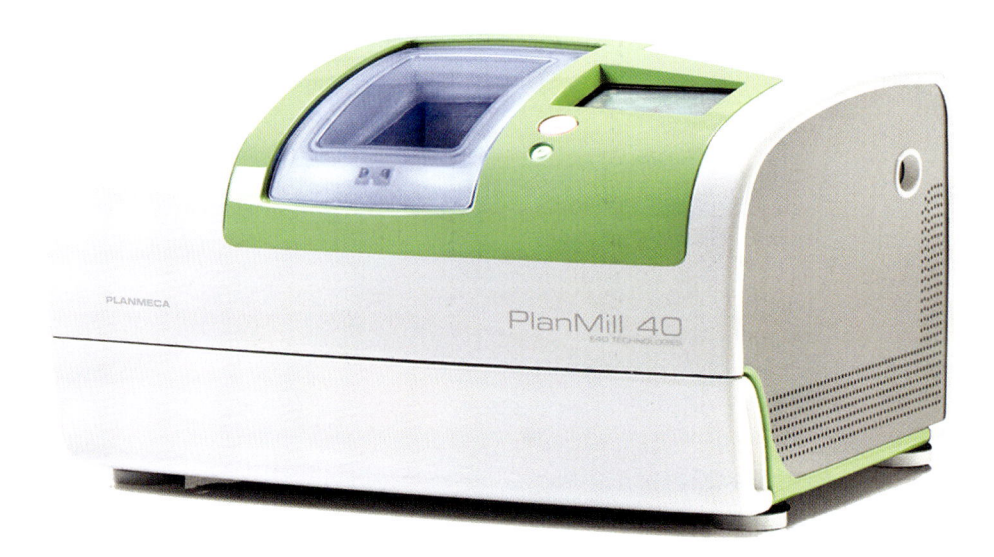

Figure 46.7 Planmeca PlanMill 40 milling system. *Source:* Figure courtesy of Planmeca, USA.

weighted base, or it can be wall mounted or separated to fit into a standard handpiece caddy.

Workflow

To capture the image, the user selects the proper scanning mode of the tooth (preoperative or wax-up), preparation, opposing teeth, buccal bite, and/or bite registration. To begin scanning, the user clicks the button on the scanner to activate the laser and rests the tip of the scanner gently on the teeth. With video-rate scanning, PlanScan captures and processes data almost as quickly as you move your hand.

Planmeca PlanCAD Design Center is a complete restorative design system with laptop convenience. The system automatically positions and shapes the selected tooth template to match the central grooves, cusp heights, and marginal ridges of the actual proximal dentition, creating a custom restoration for every patient.

Material selection

Current materials available for the PlanMill 40 include IPS Empress CAD (leucite-reinforced ceramic), IPS e.max CAD and Impulse (lithium disilicate), Paradigm C (leucite-reinforced ceramic), 3M Paradigm MZ100 (radiopaque composite), Telio CAD (acrylate polymer), Zirlux FC2 (full contour zirconia), Lava Ultimate (resin nano-ceramic), and BOB (acrylic burnout blocks).

Chairside fabrication

The Planmeca PlanMill 40 communicates with the PlanCAD Design Center (Figure 46.8) to mill same-day crowns, inlays, onlays, and veneers and fabricates restoration designs quickly and conveniently with wireless connectivity and Smart Mill touch-screen operation. Dual spindles simultaneously mill the latest metal-free materials on both sides of the restoration, with custom milling paths calculated for micrometer-precise accuracy. The automatic tool changer selects the appropriate bur and replaces worn burs automatically.

Laboratory fabrication

PlanScan supports a fully open architecture, which enables the user to seamlessly integrate and collaborate with other systems, as well as export case files in standard tessellation language (.stl) format to any third party for review or completion. Scan the upper and lower jaw and buccal view, and send the case easily to a partner lab through Planmeca Romexis or Cloud service or DDX.

Planmeca Romexis is a completely open image management system that integrates two-dimensional (2D), 3D, and CAD/CAM images with virtually any system, allowing the dental professional to import and export image files. Images can be viewed anywhere using the mobile applications. Studies and cases can be quickly shared between clinics or laboratories, helping dentists improve treatment planning for such specialized cases as implants, orthodontics, and endodontics. Restoration design work can begin immediately without creation of a physical model.

Support and education

S.O.S. is a remote proprietary service provided by Planmeca to assist in clinical and technical support. Each PlanScan system is equipped with high-speed internet access, which gives dental professionals and hardware and software experts the ability to remotely access any system to assist as needed in design, treatment, or diagnosis of any issues. Education is included with the purchase of the system, as well as advanced courses through Planmeca Digital Academy, an ADA CERP and PACE program provider.

Feature comparisons

Figure 46.9 provides a feature comparison of the CEREC and Planmeca PlanScan CAD/CAM systems.

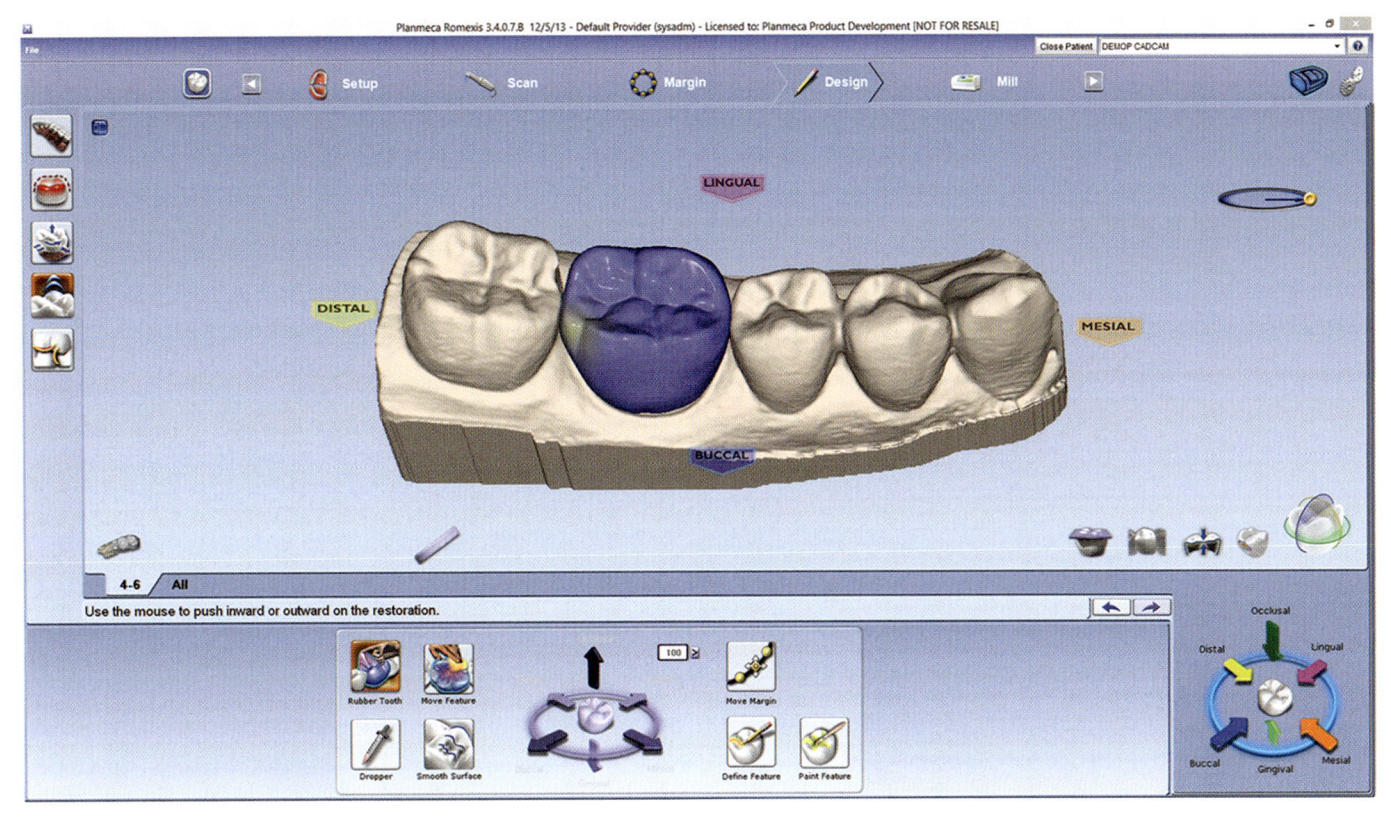

Figure 46.8 Planmeca PlanCAD crown design screenshot. *Source:* Figure courtesy of Planmeca, USA.

	CEREC	PlanScan
Manufacturer	Sirona	Planmeca/E4D Technologies
User Interface	Touch screen	Available as portable unit with laptop or integrated cart
System Architecture	Closed	Open
Powder Required?	*Omnicam*: No *Bluecam*: Yes	No
Workflow	*Omnicam*: Continuous color imaging generates a 3D model *Bluecam*: Single images combined to create a 3D model Restoration is then designed and sent to milling center	Blue laser projected pattern triangulation accurately captures hard and soft tissues of various translucencies, dental restorations, models and impressions
Types of Restorations	Inlays, onlays, veneers, crowns, bridges, abutments, surgical guides, Invlisalign, temporary restorations	Inlays, onlays, crowns, veneers, bridges, temporary restorations
Materials Available for Milling	Feldspar ceramic, glass ceramic, lithium disilicate ceramic, translucent zirconium oxide (TZI), hybrid, polymer blocks, metal (with CEREC Premium)	IPS e.max, Lava, Ultimate, Telio CAD, Zirlux FC Zirconia

Figure 46.9 Comparison chart of CAD/CAM systems.

Dedicated impression scanners

In some instances, dentists may wish to take advantage of the improvements that digital impressions provide, but they may still prefer to have the laboratory handle all restoration fabrication rather than using a chairside milling unit. In these cases, the dentist may opt for a dedicated impression scanner that captures a digital scan of the prepared teeth but does not continue with the process of milling the actual restoration in-office. Rather, the digital scan is transmitted to the laboratory, where trained technicians use laboratory CAD/CAM software to design and fabricate final restorations. Dedicated impressions scanners have both pros and cons—while they are less expensive than full CAD/CAM systems, such as CEREC and Planmeca

PlanScan, they also do not provide final restorations at the time of the first visit, thus requiring temporization and a second appointment.

One benefit of laboratory fabrication is that the esthetics can be optimized, leaving the design and esthetics to technicians who are specifically trained, rather than having the dentist spend time performing the process. Another factor that draws some dentists to dedicated impression scanners over CAD/CAM units is that the laboratory has full control over translucency, opacity, color, staining, and glaze, whereas milled restorations are made from solid blocks of material that require additional time and effort by the dentist to achieve improved esthetics.

Model fabrication

Although CAD/CAM systems do not require the fabrication of analog models on which the laboratory technician fabricates restorations, many dedicated impression scanners send data to model manufacturing facilities, where models are fabricated and sent to the laboratory. In some cases, the laboratory may not require models, as they can design and fabricate restorations using the original scan data obtained via the in-office scan. However, models are still used after the restorations are completed in order to check contacts and occlusion on the restoration itself rather than the digitized version. This allows for an additional quality control step that would not be possible without a physical model. Models made from digital scans may be fabricated in two different ways: SLA printing and model milling.

Stereolithography apparatus printing

SLA 3D printing uses a UV-sensitive liquid resin as the working material. A UV laser is projected on and moves across the reservoir of the resin build material, illuminating and hardening the liquid resin only in the areas where the part is being printed. Multiple models can be printed simultaneously by setting the laser to trace each individual part on a different area of the platform. The platform holding the part or parts lowers after each layer is printed, and a wiper blade spreads more resin uniformly across the working space.

The SLA printer can be set to print in different layer thicknesses, depending on how accurate the resulting model must be. For dental purposes, the individual layers of resin are built in layers ranging from 50 to 150 μm. The UV laser makes pass after pass, tracing the outline of the next layer for each part in the print job, repeating the process until the model is complete.

Model milling

Models may also be milled from a block of material using a similar technique to restoration milling. The scan data is sent to a milling machine and the entire model is milled from a solid puck of material.

The iTero system uses a model milling technique for model fabrication. iTero models have removable dies that are milled separately from the rest of the arch.

Dedicated impression scanner models

3M *True Definition Scanner*

The 3M True Definition Scanner was launched in 2012, based on the original Lava Chairside Oral Scanner's 3D in motion technology by Brontes Technologies in Lexington, Massachusetts.

System features

The 3M True Definition Scanner system consists of a CPU, a touch-screen display, and a scanning wand, which has a small, lightweight, beveled tip (Figures 46.10 and 46.11). The scanning wand is a 3D high-resolution trinocular optical impression system.

Workflow

Proper retraction and a light dusting of 3M High-Resolution Scanning Spray are required prior to scanning the teeth. The

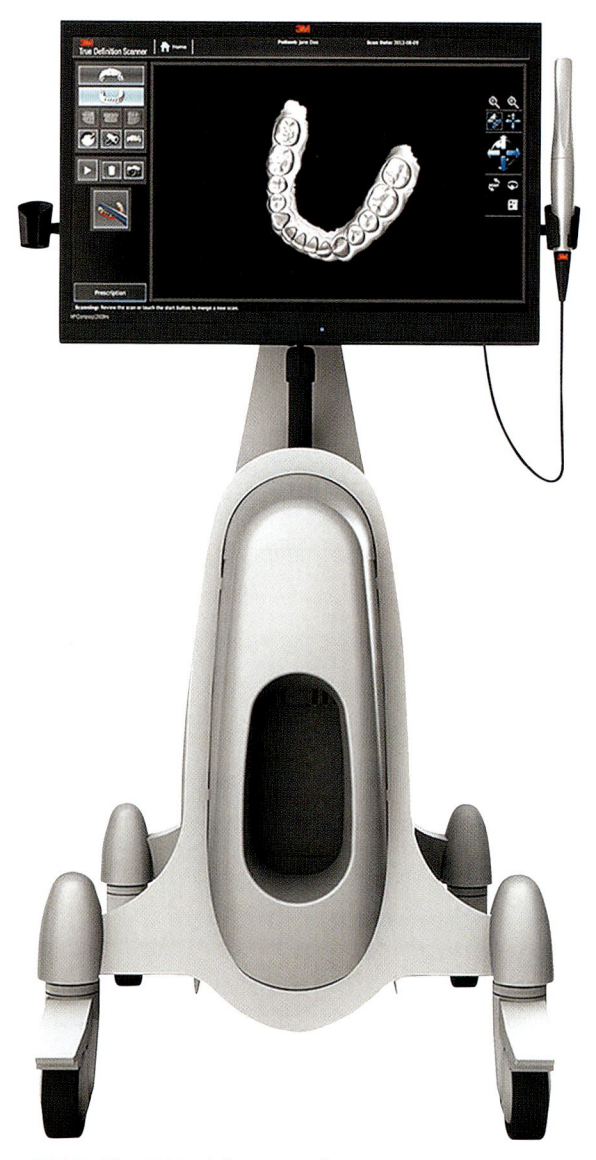

Figure 46.10 The 3M Mobile True Definition Scanner system. *Source:* Figure courtesy of 3M Oral Care, USA.

clinician moves the small, lightweight wand over the teeth. The 3M True Definition Scanner captures 60 images per second. The "3D in motion" technology then reconstructs the video data to create a highly accurate 3D model of the oral anatomy (Figure 46.12). This process happens in real time, enabling the user to control the scan, making adjustments throughout the scanning process. The system also incorporates a 3D visualization feature that shows the scanned teeth in a stereoscopic mode, using traditional 3D glasses.

Open and trusted connections

3M True Definition Scanner digital impression files can be used with any system that accepts an .stl file. 3M also collaborates with leading manufacturers to ensure seamless integration with a broad range of CAD/CAM, digital implant and orthodontic appliance workflows. The trusted connection process includes comprehensive technical and clinical validation, ensuring performance and quality that meets the highest standards. These

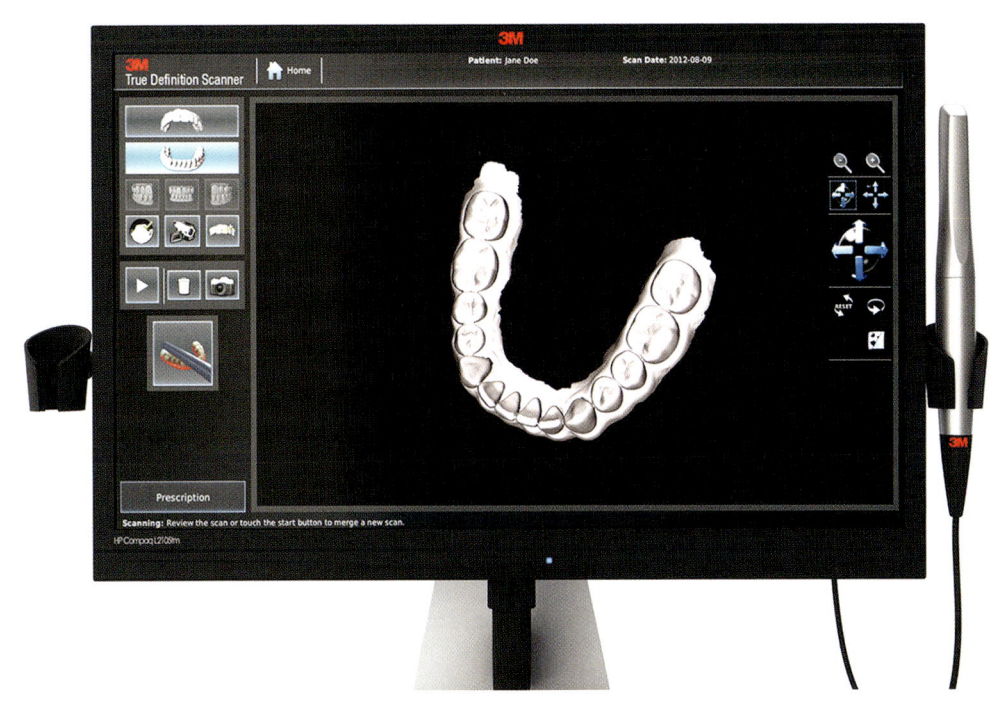

Figure 46.11 The 3M Mobile True Definition monitor and wand, showing a full arch scan on the screen. *Source:* Figure courtesy of 3M Oral Care, USA.

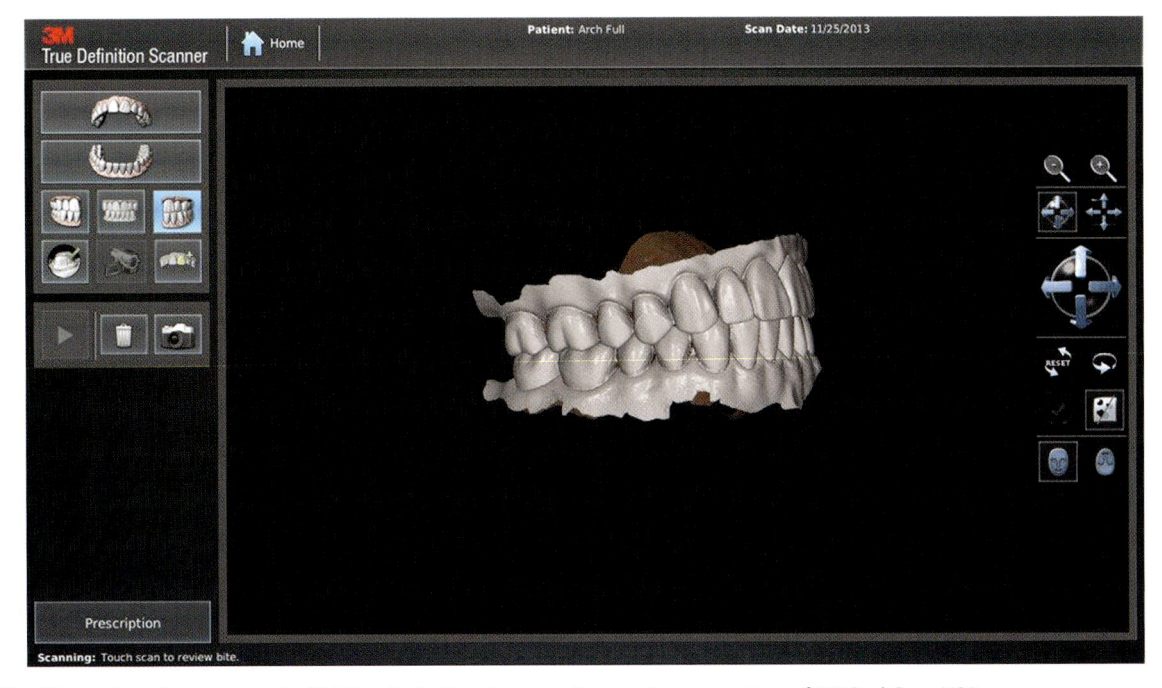

Figure 46.12 Bite registration scan on the 3M True Definition Scanner. *Source:* Figure courtesy of 3M Oral Care, USA.

connections provide the benefits of an integrated system without the drawbacks of a proprietary network. Additional trusted connections with leading dental product manufacturers are continually being tested and validated for future integration.

Model fabrication

Once the scan is complete, the data file is immediately available to the lab via the 3M Connection Center. Once downloaded, the technician marks the model and begins designing the final restoration. The processed data set can also be sent to a model manufacturing center, where an SLA model is fabricated. The model can be used for traditional hand finishing but is no longer necessary in a purely digital workflow.

Dental laboratories also have the option of working with an open file format for the design and production of a model from their own 3D printer (personal communication, Peter Golden, Professional Relations Manager, 3M ESPE; personal communication, Ashley Haslund, Global Marketing Communications Specialist, 3M ESPE).

iTero Element™ scanner

The iTero Element intraoral scanner (Figures 46.13 and 46.14) was released in 2015 as Align Technology Inc.'s latest version of the iTero scanner line. The iTero scanner was first introduced to the dental market in 2007 by Cadent, which was acquired by Align Technology in April 2011.

System features

The iTero Element intraoral scanner uses parallel confocal imaging technology, whereby laser and optical scanning captures a 3D color image of the contours of the patient's teeth, gingival structures, and bite. The iTero Element intraoral scanner captures 20 scans per second of laser light in perfect focus without the use of powder to coat the teeth, which allows for contact of the wand and tooth, resulting in an accurate 3D digital impression.

The iTero Element scanner (Figure 46.15) is a smaller and lighter version of previous scanners, and it features a multitouch HD display and integrated gyro technology in the wand so the user can rotate models on the screen with a flick of the wrist.

Workflow

The iTero Element software automatically detects and repositions scanning start and stop points when you move to a new scanning position within the scanned segment. During the scan, iTero Element software is engineered to simultaneously process the scan. It automatically stitches together images for rendering in the correct order, adapts to changes in positioning, and detects and removes soft tissue (Figure 46.16).

An integrated color sensor in the iTero Element scanner and the patented dual-aperture lens system are designed to simultaneously capture 2D images in color with highly accurate 3D laser scanning. Color scanning can make it easier to immediately distinguish between gingival and tooth structures for a more precise clinical evaluation.

The iTero Element scanner is designed to automatically save scan data every 2 s and save it to the system's hard disk, so in the event of a power outage the scan data are safe.

Models

iTero models are milled on a five-axis milling machine and are made from a proprietary polyurethane material. The free gingival tissue is preserved during the construction of the model, thus allowing the laboratory to take into account the gingival profile around the teeth to be restored.

iTero scanner and Invisalign treatment

In 2011, Cadent was acquired by Align Technology (makers of Invisalign clear aligners) to allow the iTero scanner to be used for

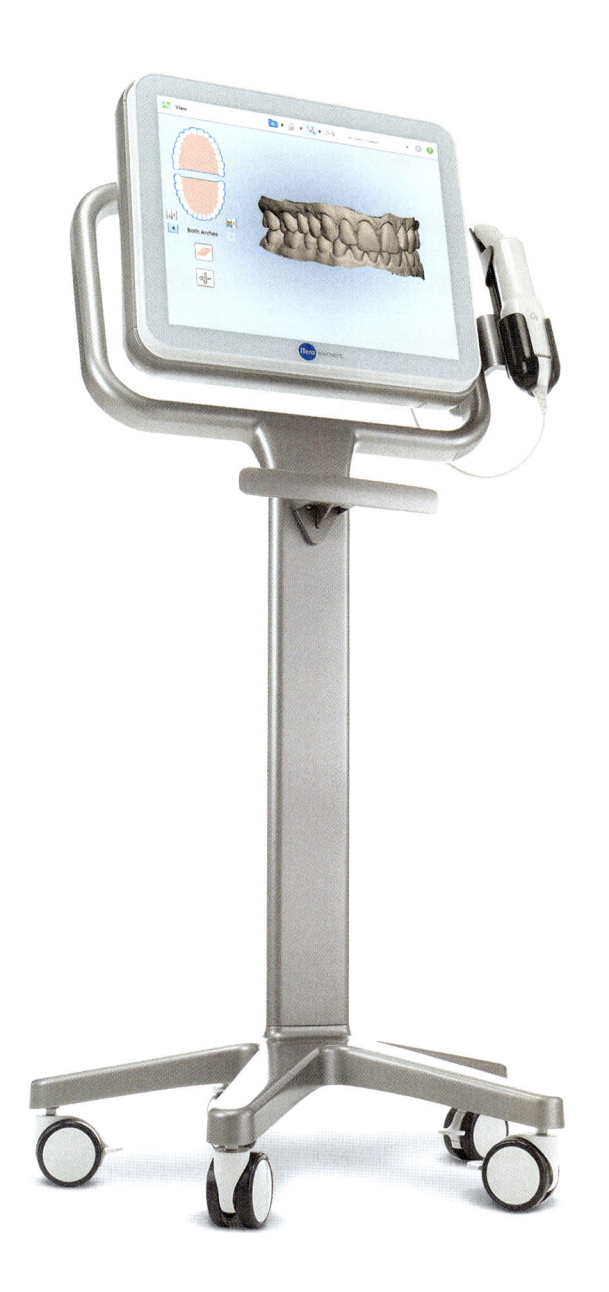

Figure 46.13 The iTero Element intraoral scanner. *Source:* Figure courtesy of Align Technology Inc., USA

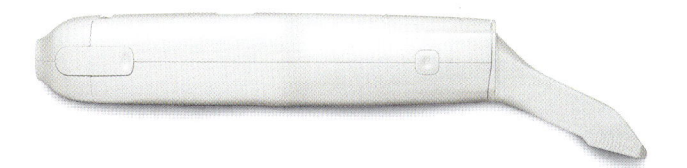

Figure 46.15 The iTero Element Scanner scanning wand. *Source:* Figure courtesy of Align Technology Inc., USA

full arch scans intended for Invisalign treatment planning. The iTero Element scanner is able to scan entire arches and digitally transmit the scan data to Align in order to create Invisalign clear aligners. The scanner also has exclusive access to the Invisalign Outcome Simulator, which helps patients visualize the potential outcome of Invisalign treatment.

3Shape TRIOS

System features

3Shape TRIOS is a powder- and spray-free system. The TRIOS handheld device is based on a pistol design, which provides maximum support and stability during the scan, and provides

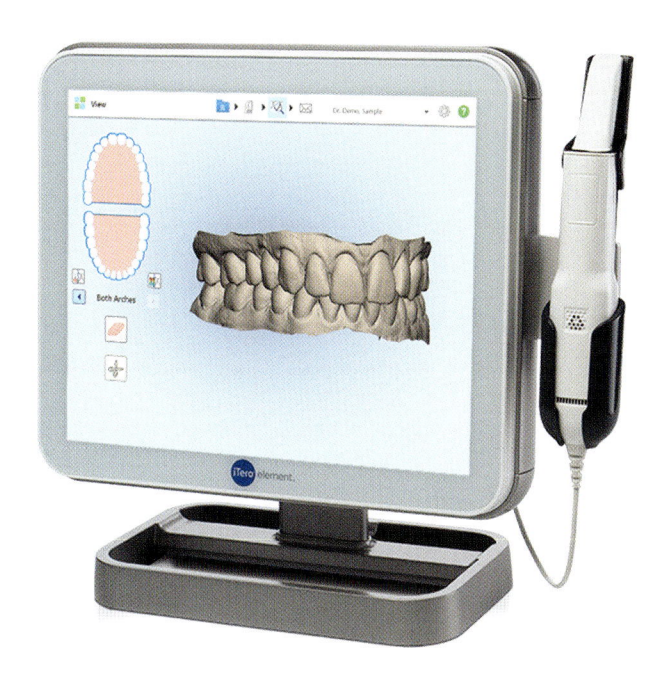

Figure 46.14 The iTero Element Scanner with counter stand. *Source:* Figure courtesy of Align Technology Inc., USA

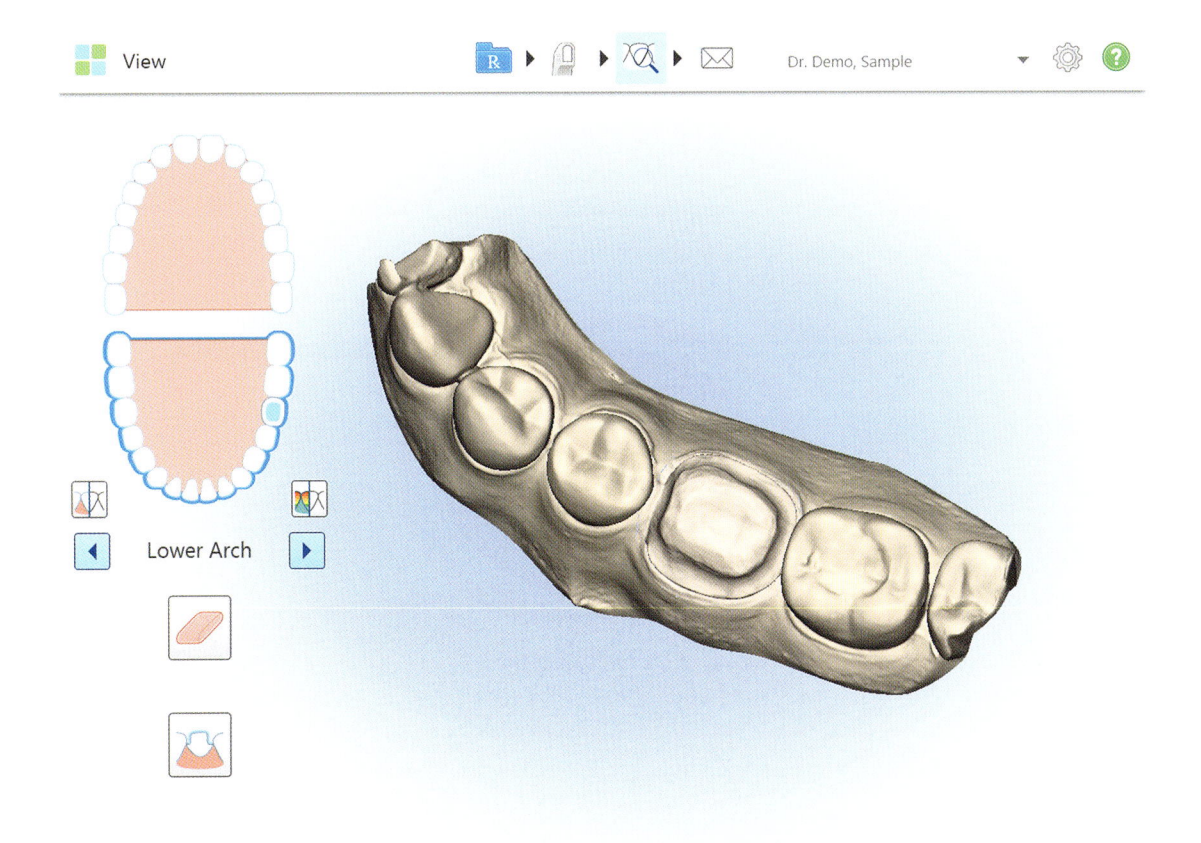

Figure 46.16 Screenshot of a crown prep on #19 on the iTero Element scanner.

the user with an ergonomic grip for perfect control. Two different systems are available: a mobile cart (Figure 46.17), featuring a touch screen monitor, CPU, and scanning wand; and a pod system (Figure 46.18), which offers more flexibility with a smaller footprint, featuring a portable scanning wand connected to a laptop (either Mac or PC configurations are available).

The 3Shape TRIOS requires a reusable, autoclavable scan tip. The tip may be flipped for scanning of the upper or lower jaw, and there is no need to hold the scanner at a specific distance or angle for focus. The user may even rest the scanner on the teeth for support during the scan. The scanning wand features an integrated anti-mist heater to automatically ensure an optimal temperature for undistorted and crystal-clear scanning.

After scanning, the user can apply the software's tools for clinical validation of the digital impression (Occlusal Clearance tool, Insertion Direction tool, and Rotate/Zoom tools help validate impression quality, and a comment section aids in communication with the laboratory). The scanner is color calibrated, which allows the user to select a shade directly on the scanned arch, which reduces user error during the shade selection process (Figures 46.19 and 46.20).

Workflow

The digital order form, which may be customized by individual laboratories based on the restorations they offer, is filled out prior to scanning. Since powdering the teeth and gingiva is not required with the TRIOS, the user simply moves the scanner tip along the surface of the teeth. Designed for high-speed impression capture, 3Shape's Ultrafast Optical Sectioning™ technology captures more than 3000 2D images per second – 100 times faster than conventional video cameras.

The scan tip can easily be flipped to facilitate fast scanning of both the upper and lower jaws. After obtaining both the upper

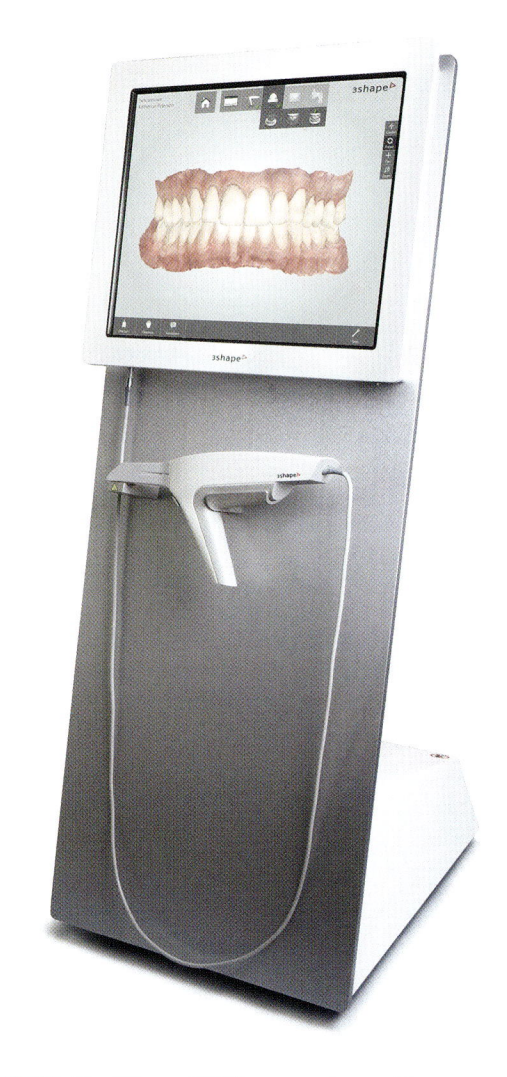

Figure 46.17 The 3Shape TRIOS system. *Source:* Figure courtesy of 3Shape.

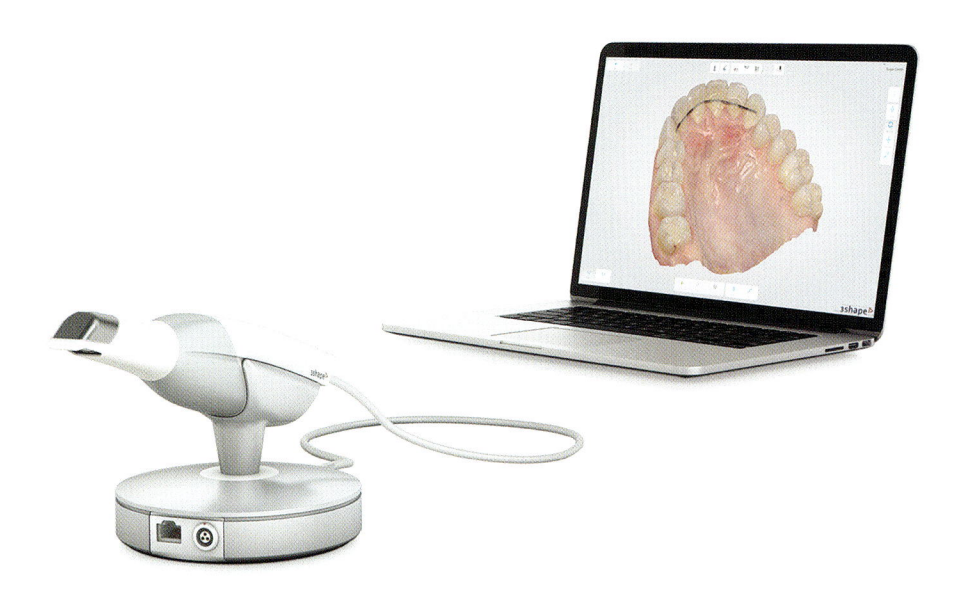

Figure 46.18 The 3Shape TRIOS pod. *Source:* Figure courtesy of 3Shape.

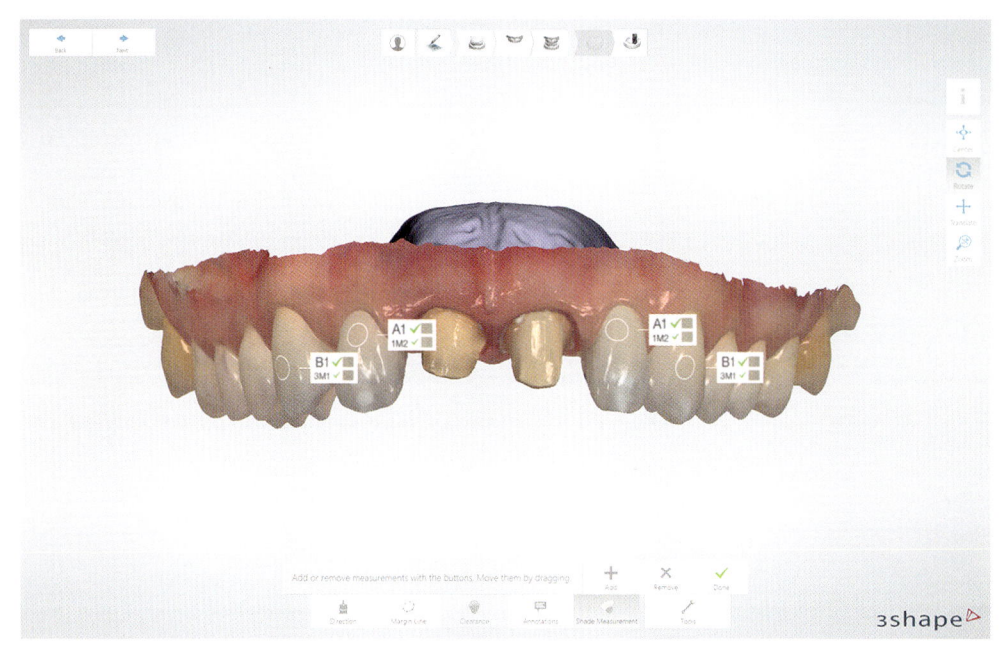

Figure 46.19 A screenshot of a completed 3D scan of prepared teeth #8 and #9. The scanner is color calibrated to reflect the accurate shading of the teeth and the soft tissue in the mouth. *Source:* Figure courtesy of 3Shape.

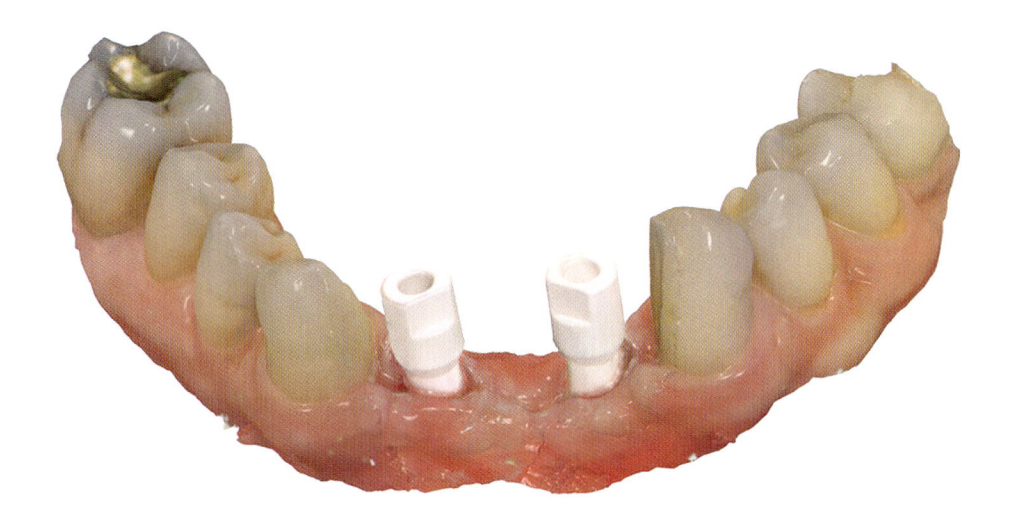

Figure 46.20 A scan of the lower arch showing two scan bodies attached to implants. *Source:* Figure courtesy of 3Shape.

and lower scans, the bite is quickly scanned and the software then automatically aligns the three scans together.

As the scan progresses, small tips and messages on the touch screen keep the user informed of the scan progression. Image capture can be paused and resumed by pressing the button on the handheld scanner.

By selecting the shade scan tool, the user is able to scan over the existing scan, this time capturing the actual shade of the teeth with the color-calibrated scanner. The user can then touch on any area of any tooth and select which part (or parts) of the tooth the restoration should match.

Once the scan is completed and verified, the press of a button digitally transmits the scan data to the laboratory.

Model fabrication

TRIOS scans do not need to go through a specific processing center after scanning. Rather, TRIOS scans may be sent to any laboratory using 3Shape CAD/CAM software. The scan is received in the laboratory within minutes. A digital laboratory model is designed in the laboratory directly from the digital impression, and the restoration is digitally designed on the 3D model. If necessary, the model may be manufactured locally, either by the laboratory or a third-party printing/milling service provider (personal communication, Martin Poulsen, International Product Manager, 3Shape).

Feature comparisons

Figure 46.21 provides a feature comparison of the three dedicated impression scanner systems discussed here.

Open versus closed architecture

CAD/CAM and impression scanners run software that captures a 3D image and converts it to an.stl file. The architecture of a system refers to its ability (or, in some cases, its inability) to import and/or export.stl files from other systems made by other manufacturers.

An open architecture CAD/CAM system is able to integrate data from any other brand of scanner or software. An open architecture system can use the .stl file from another impressioning system to design and/or fabricate restorations.

A selectively open architecture CAD/CAM system is only able to integrate with specific components that are selected by the system's manufacturer. For example, some milling units may not be capable of fabricating consistently high-quality restorations when using a specific brand of acquisition software. In this case, the mill manufacturer may not allow for integration with that specific scanning system, but may still be compatible with other scanners made by other reputable manufacturers.

A closed architecture CAD/CAM system does not integrate with any components manufactured by any other company. Closed architecture systems are fully proprietary.

Computer-aided design/manufacturing in the laboratory

In addition to improving the quality, speed, and ease of in-office impression taking, the digitization of dentistry has also revolutionized the laboratory fabrication of restorations. Recent advances in CAD/CAM technology in the laboratory have resulted in a completely new and improved method of creating highly esthetic and accurate restorations.

Analog versus digital impression accuracy

With the incorporation of CAD in the laboratory, technicians rely on an accurate digital scan on which they design, and later manufacture, restorations. There are currently two different workflows for digital manufacturing. In cases where analog impressions are utilized, the process requires scanning of an analog model in a desktop 3D scanner and scanning it into a CAD program. The second workflow involves the laboratory receiving the .stl file directly from the in-office scanner.

When working with the analog impressions and related workflow, the analog models are created. The protocol for analog model fabrication involves several steps, from impression taking to model pouring. Each step in the model fabrication process introduces error or discrepancies in the final model. When eliminating the analog impression, related model and die fabrication, and the scanning of a physical model, studies showed a reduction in inaccuracies of 75 μm or more (personal communication, Bob Cohen, CDT, Custom Automated Prosthetics).

	3M True Definition Scanner	iTero Element	TRIOS
Manufacturer	3M ESPE	Align Technology	3Shape
User Interface	Touch screen	High definition multi-touch display	Cart: Touch screen Pod: Laptop
System Architecture	Open	Open	Open
Powder Required?	Yes	No	No
Workflow	3D In Motion captures live video at 60 images per second	Continuous color scanning, at a rate of 20 scans per second	Ultrafast Optical Sectioning combines hundreds or thousands of color-calibrated 3D pictures
Types of Restorations	Crowns, bridges, inlays, onlays, veneers, implant workflows, partial dentures, clear aligners, orthodontic appliances, models	Inlays, onlays, crowns, bridges, veneers, custom abutments, Invlisalign, orthodontic appliances	Inlays, onlays, crowns, post & cores, veneers, temporary crowns, RPDs, implant abutments, surgical guides, orthodontic appliances
Model Fabrication	Stereolithographic (SLA)	Milled	Printed and/or milled, depending on lab

Figure 46.21 Comparison chart of dedicated impression scanners.

Digital laboratory workflow

The process by which a restoration is manufactured digitally involves four steps: scanning, CAD, CAM, and final fabrication.

Scanning models

In cases where the laboratory receives an analog impression or model that must be digitized prior to restoration fabrication, the first step is to input the 3D model into a laboratory scanner. Some scanners have the ability to scan both impressions (PVS and alginate) and gypsum models, while others are only able to scan gypsum models.

Inside the scanner, cameras move around the model (and in some cases the model is also able to be tilted and rotated on a movable platform inside the chamber) until the model is fully scanned. In minutes, an entire scanned model appears on the screen, ready to be digitally ditched in preparation for restoration design.

Computer-aided design

CAD is the process by which crowns, inlays, onlays, veneers, bridges, and other restorations are digitally designed. Most CAD software is bundled with a laboratory scanner, with the exception of Exocad, which is standalone CAD software that can import .stl files from open-architecture laboratory scanners made by a variety of manufacturers (sold separately). For decades, laboratory technicians have spent hours waxing-up restorations on stone models. Using CAD software, the technician is able to digitally mark the margins on the 3D model and place a digital die spacer of uniform thickness. The digitization of the die spacer eliminates a major source of error in crown fabrication, since laboratory spacer is a thin liquid that does not set in a uniform thickness on the die—the fluid nature of the liquid causes it to pool in thicker layers in concave areas of the die and to thin out in other areas. CAD software is able to ensure ideal thickness of die spacer in all areas of the restoration.

Using a design database, the technician designs a digital wax-up of the final restoration. Some laboratories have their own proprietary design libraries, and other laboratories use the database that comes standard with their CAD software. Simple clicks of the mouse can adjust occlusal and interproximal contact areas, material thickness, and emergence profile in seconds as opposed to minutes or even hours when done on a physical wax-up on a stone model (Figure 46.22). When restorations do not require an intermediate wax-up step, the final restoration design may be sent directly to the final manufacturing/fabrication step.

Computer-aided manufacturing

CAM refers to the use of computer software to program the machinery that is responsible for the milling or printing of intermediate and final restorations.

CAM is separate from the actual design of restorations—it is the communication between the CAD software and the milling units. This involves the selection of where on the puck of material a crown should be milled, how thick the layers of wax should be during wax printing, and so on.

Fabrication

Wax Printing
When the restoration of choice requires investment and burnout, such as e.max (lithium disilicate) or metal, the actual casting or pressing process has not changed with the advent of CAD/CAM dentistry. The major difference is in how the wax-up is created.

The digital wax-up is designed in the CAD software program on a 3D model, the same way as with any other digitally designed restoration. Once the digital wax-up is completed, the next step is to create a physical wax model of the restoration. This can be accomplished either by wax printing or wax milling. Wax printing is similar to inkjet printing, but instead of ink being jetted or sprayed onto paper in a single layer, a resin

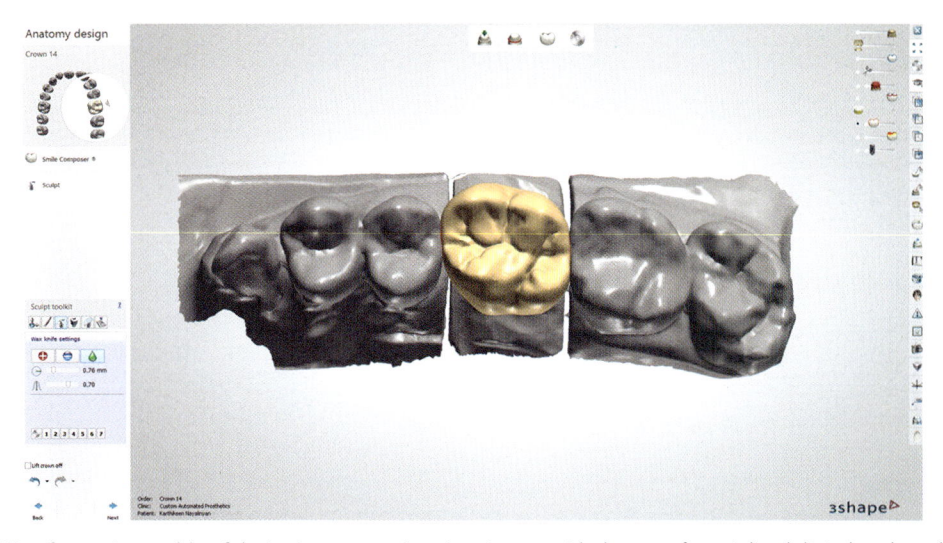

Figure 46.22 3Shape CAD software is capable of designing restorations in minutes with the use of specialized digital tools at the technician's fingertips. *Source:* Figure courtesy of Custom Automated Prosthetics.

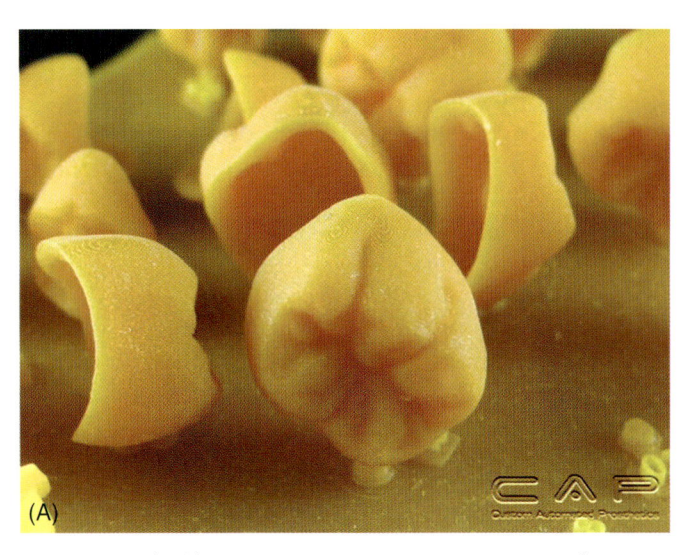

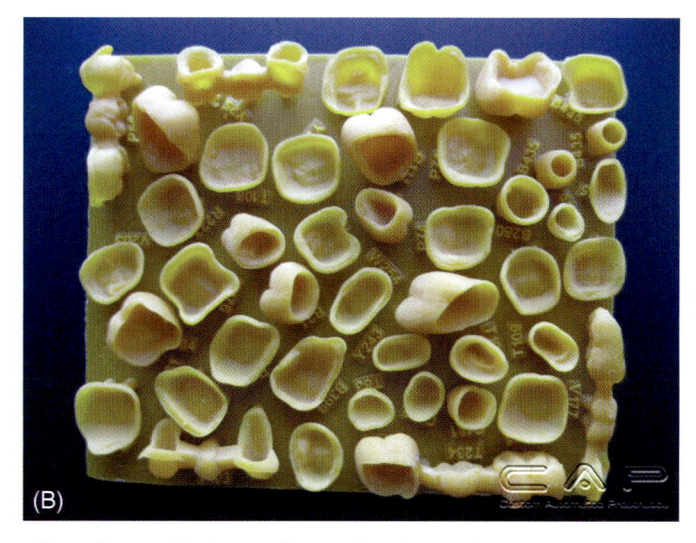

Figure 46.23 (A, B) Wax printing creates accurate wax-ups of restorations without the need for hours of manual work by technicians. Multiple restorations may be printed on a single sheet, each with an identifying code printed beside it. *Source:* Figures courtesy of Custom Automated Prosthetics.

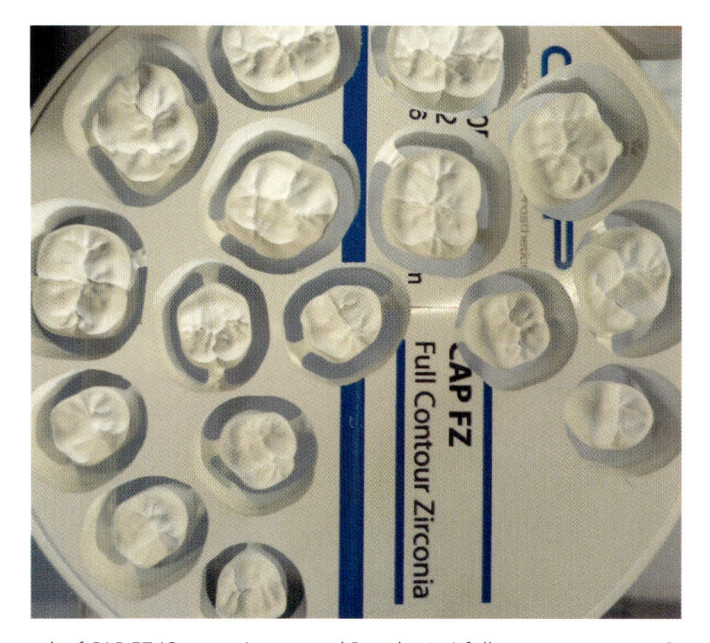

Figure 46.24 Crowns milled from a puck of CAP FZ (Custom Automated Prosthetics) full-contour zirconia. *Source:* Figure courtesy of Custom Automated Prosthetics.

or wax is jetted onto support material, and then onto previously sprayed layers until the part begins to take on depth and shape (Figure 46.23). Wax printers can print single copings and full crowns to multiple-unit bridge copings, models, and even partial denture frameworks. Wax mills use burs to carve out the wax models from a solid puck of hard wax. Both techniques result in accurate wax-ups that can be invested and burned out.

Selective laser sintering
Selective laser sintering is an additive manufacturing technique that uses a high-power laser to fuse small particles of powdered metal (e.g., chromium–cobalt or gold alloys) into a coping, framework or full contour crown that has a desired 3D shape. As with SLA printing, the laser selectively passes over the surface of the powder and fuses the metal on the surface of a powder bed in incremental layers. After each cross-section is scanned, the powder bed is lowered by one layer thickness, a new layer of material is applied on top, and the process is repeated until the part is completed. This process uses CAD/CAM data to directly manufacture the metal, doing away with the need for wax-ups, investment, burnout, and casting.

Milling
In-office mills, such as CEREC and Planmeca PlanMill 40, utilize small blocks of material for each restoration. Laboratory mills generally use large "pucks" of material that can fit 20 or more restorations at a time. Mills can fabricate restorations from a variety of materials, ranging from plastic to ceramic to metal.

Clinical cases

Clinical case 46.1

A 42-year-old male patient presented in March 2012 with the chief complaint that he was trapping food between his lower left molars. On examination, it was determined that the veneering porcelain on an IPS eMax (Ivoclar Vivadent) veneered lithium disilicate crown on the endodontically treated tooth #19 had sheared at the distobuccal aspect, allowing for the entrapment of food between #18 and #19. The crown had been luted in July 2009.

In keeping with the dentist's office policy, which warranties indirect restorations for 5 years, and in keeping with the dental laboratory's commensurate policy, the patient was informed that the crown would be remade at no fee. Normally, the situation would dictate that the patient be anesthetized, the defective crown removed, retraction achieved via cord packing or laser troughing, an elastomeric impression obtained, an opposing impression taken, an interocclusal registration made, and a new provisional crown provided.

Fortunately, the impression that was obtained for this crown nearly 3 years earlier was achieved with a digital scan using the Lava C.O.S. impressioning system (3M/ESPE). The file for the crown was easily accessed from the system's case archive and the file was resubmitted to the dental laboratory for a new all-zirconia crown, to be made using virtual models without the need for obtaining physical models from 3M/ESPE. The patient was dismissed without removing the defective crown, was provided with an interproximal brush, and was instructed to use the brush to avoid food retention in the affected area.

When the patient returned to the office 2 weeks later, the defective crown was removed without the need for anesthesia and without affecting the tooth preparation. The new crown, which fit as accurately as the original, was luted using a self-etching resin cement.

Clinical case 46.2

A 63-year-old female patient presented in July 2009 with the chief complaint that her upper bridgework was loose. The bridges, extending from #3–#5, #6–#11, and #12–#14, had been made in April 1995. The patient was a heavy smoker and had undergone numerous periodontal procedures prior to the restorative treatment. Following the placement of the fixed partial dentures, she again began to exhibit periodontal problems, so she was referred to a periodontist for maintenance recare, and she was instructed to schedule for annual restorative reevaluation. Despite repeated attempts to reappoint her for restorative checkups, she never responded to telephone or written communications.

She was not seen again until July 2009, when she appeared with the maxillary bridges exhibiting a 3+ mobility with 2 mm of compressibility. She apologized for her absence and lack of communication and implored the dentist to help her "save her teeth." After radiographs confirmed the near absence of osseous support for the abutment teeth, the dentist explained to the patient that he would not be able to save her teeth, and began to explain the restorative course of treatment for fabrication of an interim immediate full upper denture.

As soon as the dentist described the need to begin treatment with an alginate impression needed to create a study model, he stopped the explanation. He realized that the viscosity of the unset alginate would likely shift the bridges laterally and even compress them apically, resulting in a highly inaccurate study model and, even worse, probably extract the fixed partial dentures and the teeth on removal of the impression from the mouth, leaving the patient edentulous at the first of what was to be a series of five visits.

The dilemma was quickly resolved when the dentist thought about alternative means of capturing an impression of the maxillary bridges without displacing them. His office had a 3M/ESPE Lava C.O.S. impressioning device, which had been in use for capturing impressions of inlays, onlays, crowns, small bridges, and laminate veneers.

Although the treatment indications offered by the manufacturer did not include removable prostheses, the dentist realized there was no alternative but to use the scanner in this case. After all, the palatal mucosa was a static surface, as was the gingivae and mucosa on the facial aspect of the bridges, and the only mobile soft tissue that would come into play was at the deepest extent of the buccal and labial vestibules and, in stretching out the cheeks and lips to capture the image of the soft tissue, it would accomplish the same desired result as border molding with a conventional elastomeric impression.

The scan was performed with minimal difficulty, transmitted to 3M/ESPE, and the SLA models (capturing the palate and vestibules) were articulated according to the scan and were provided to the dental laboratory. The dental technician made a stone copy of the maxillary model, rearticulated it with the opposing cast, cut off the maxillary teeth, and waxed up and processed the interim immediate full upper denture, which was placed in the dental office following the removal of the patient's maxillary teeth (Figures 46.25 and 46.26).

The alignment of the teeth, the basic fit of the denture, and the occlusion were well within normal limits. A chairside hard reline was performed after several months, and the patient was so pleased with the denture that she requested no additional treatment until her death over 2 years later from complications due to lung cancer.

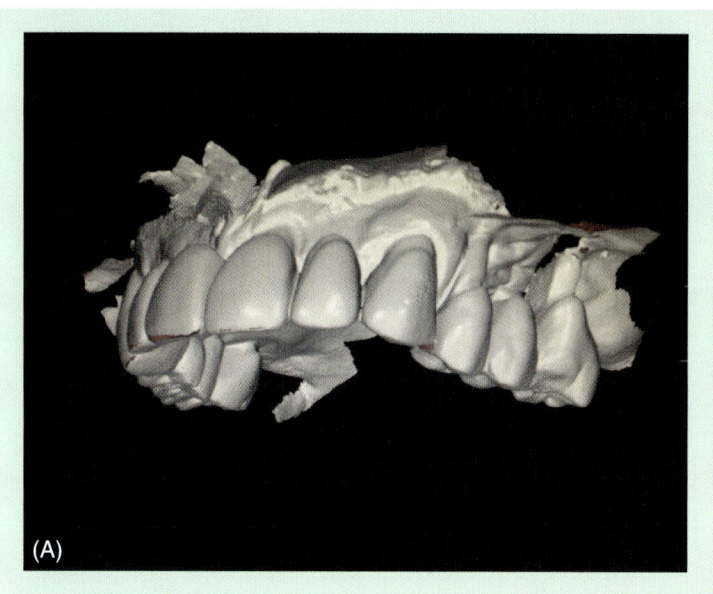

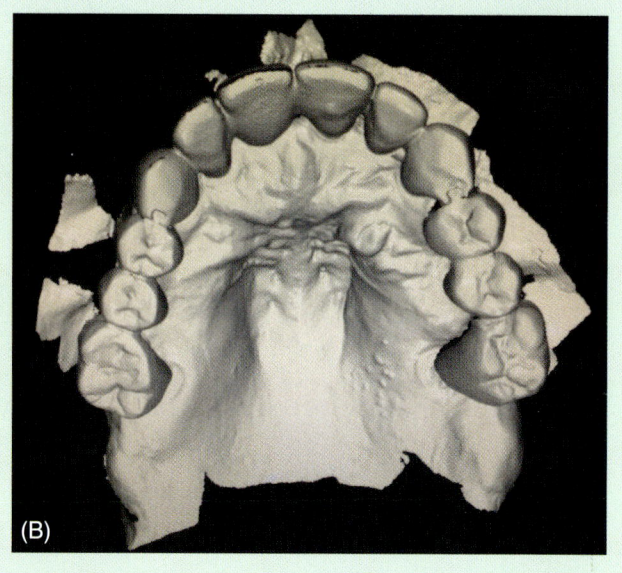

Figure 46.25 (A, B) Screen shots from digital scans of the patient's dentition, including the palate and the buccal and labial soft tissues. Note that the scans were able to capture images of the soft tissues to the full depth of the vestibules.

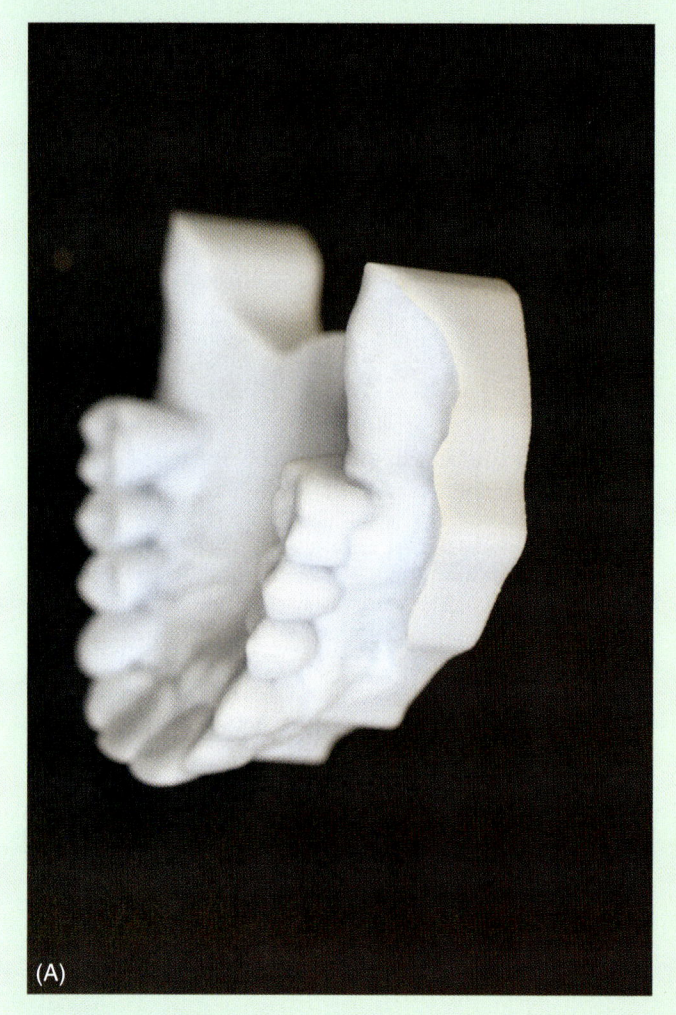

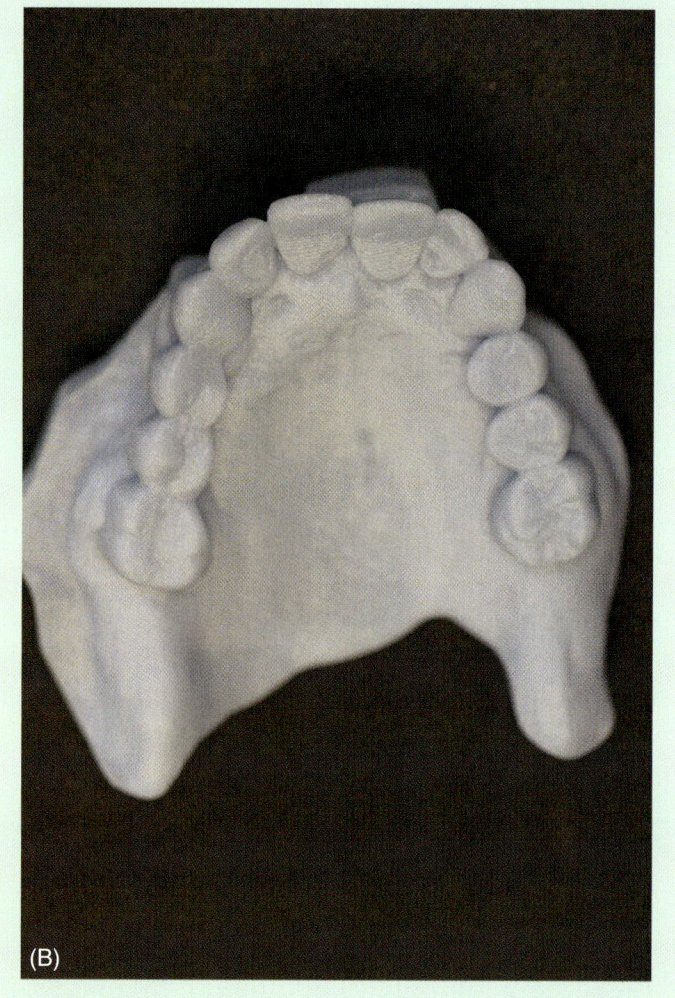

Figure 46.26 (A, B) Full-arch stereolithic models made from scans taken on a second patient with a similar problem to the case study (i.e., impossibility of elastomeric impression capture due to extensive caries under abutment crowns #6 and #7 of a #3–X–X–#6–#7 bridge and extreme bridge mobility).

Clinical case 46.3

A 66-year-old female patient presented in January 2010 for a restorative examination, at which time it was determined that she required new full cast gold crowns with mesio-occlusal rest preparations on teeth #2 and #15, porcelain-fused-to metal crowns on teeth #6 and #11 with distal semiprecision female attachments and cingulum ledges with small depressions above and on the mesial extent of the ledges, and a metal-based acrylic maxillary removable partial denture replacing the missing teeth #3–#5 and #12–#14, with rests extending onto teeth #2 and #15 with semiprecision male attachments and lingual clasps resting on the crowns ledges, with small bulges at the mesial tip of the clasps, engaging the depressions on the crowns (Snap-Lok attachments).

At the visit, she told the dentist she had been holding off having the treatment done for a few years but that, as she was aware the office had been using a digital impressioning system that would obviate the need for conventional elastomeric impressions, she was thrilled to proceed. She explained that she dreaded conventional impressions and would lose sleep over the very thought of having them done, as she was both claustrophobic and a severe gagger.

The dentist explained to her that the approved indications for the Lava C.O.S. offered by the manufacturer, 3M/ESPE, did not include removable prostheses. The patient said that, if the scanner could not be used, she would hold off on treatment until the situation deteriorated to the "crisis stage."

The dentist told the patient that, having had prior experience with the scanner for an edentulous case, he would be willing to try capturing an accurate impression of the four crown preparations and the palate and vestibules. He said that he should at least be able to achieve accuracy with the crowns but that, if the partial denture framework did not fit accurately, there might be a need to take a conventional elastomeric impression for the partial denture, picking up the four crowns. She said she was willing to take that chance.

The scan (Figure 46.27) was performed fairly easily, transmitted to 3M/ESPE, and the SLA models (capturing the palate and vestibules) were articulated according to the scan and were provided to our laboratory.

The dental technician fabricated the crowns and the partial denture framework and returned them to the dental office for try-in and confirmation of the occlusal registration (Figure 46.28).

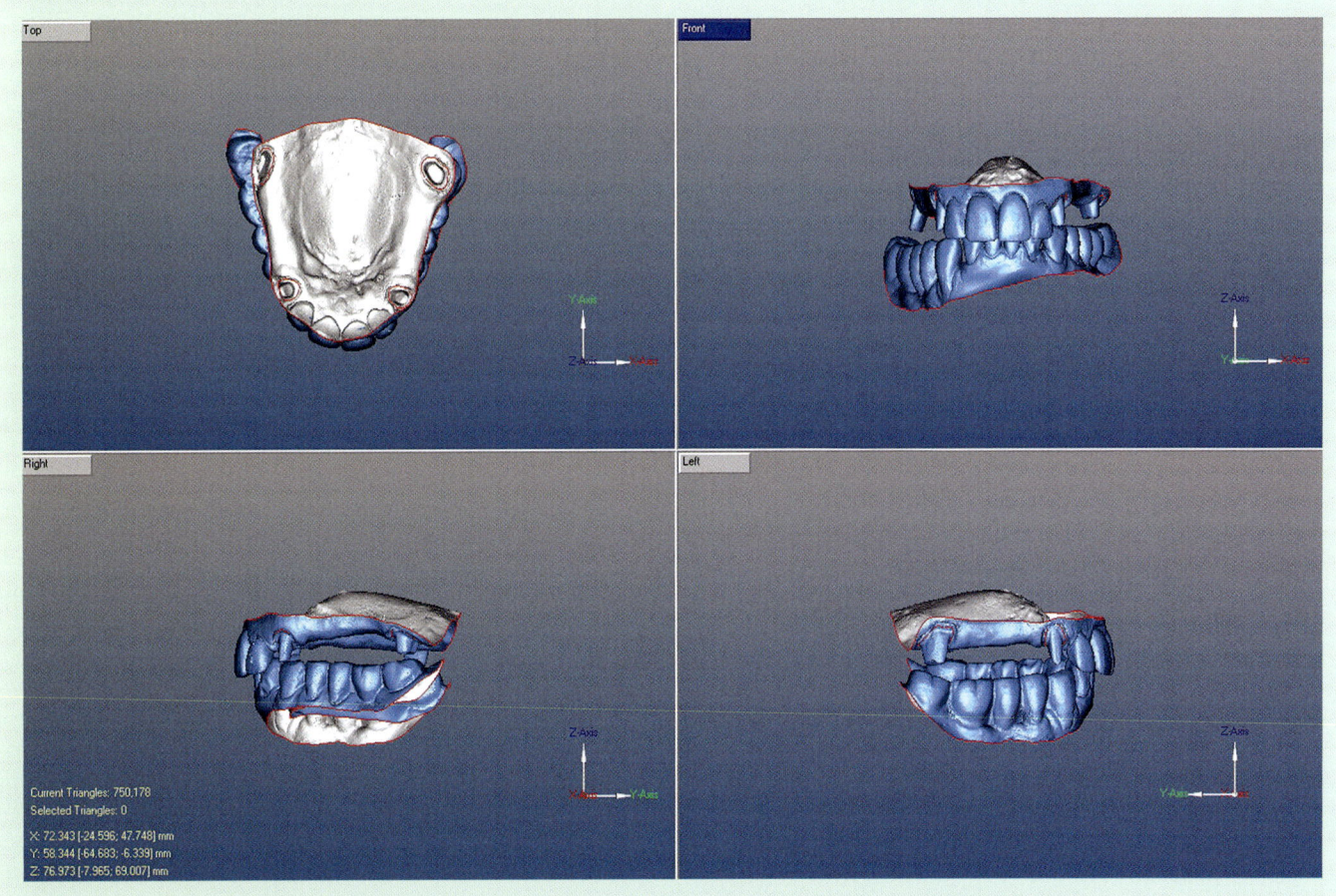

Figure 46.27 Screen shots from digital scans of the patient's dentition, including the palate and the buccal soft tissues. Note that the scans were able to capture images of the soft tissues to the full depth of the vestibules.

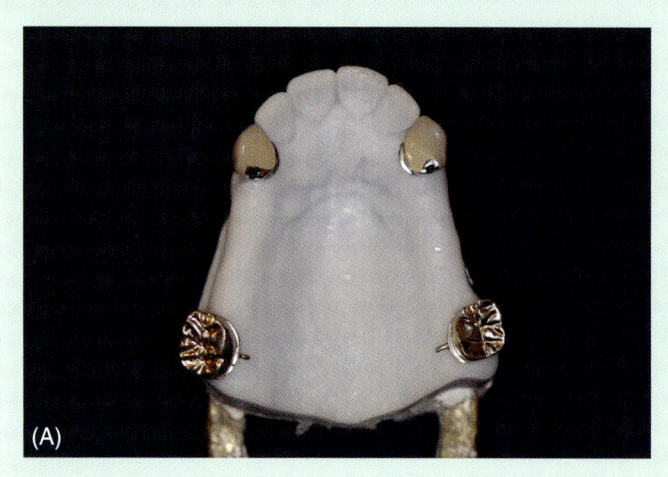

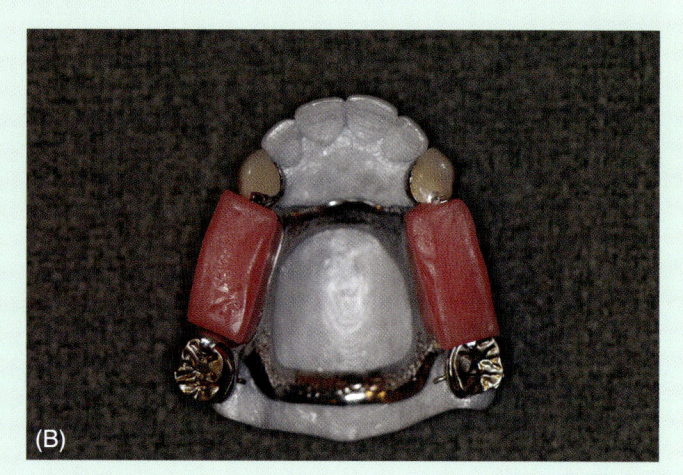

Figure 46.28 (A, B) The master stereolithic model with the four crowns in place and with the semiprecision removable partial denture framework and wax bite blocks ready for try-in and for the occlusal registration.

It was noted that the fit of the partial denture framework intraorally matched precisely the fit on the model.

The case was completed in June 2010, with cementation of the crowns and delivery of the removable partial denture. The patient immediately commented on how much more comfortable the partial denture was, relative to her previous prosthesis. The semiprecision attachments fully engaged the female attachments and the lingual clasps seated fully and engaged the depressions on teeth #6 and #11, the rests on teeth #2 and #15 were fully seated in the rest preparations with no need for occlusal adjustment, and the two palatal straps of the partial denture framework were just touching the palatal tissue, without compressing it and with no space between them and the palate (Figure 46.29).

The record noted that the accuracy of the fit of the partial denture was the best the dentist had seen in 37 years of clinical practice. In more than 2 years since the completion of the case, the patient has not required any adjustment of the removable partial denture.

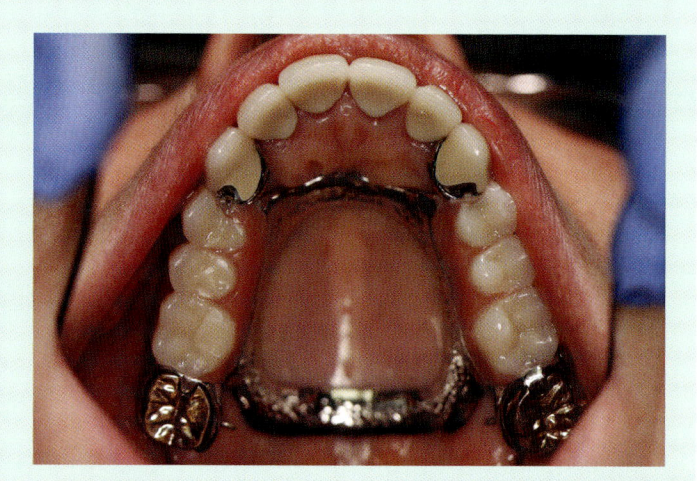

Figure 46.29 The finished case with the crowns luted and the semiprecision removable partial denture inserted.

Summary

When many dentists graduate from dental school, they put on virtual "blinders" and continue to perform dental procedures just as they were taught in school and are often nervous or unwilling to learn new procedures, even as technologies evolve. In some cases, dentists are concerned that the learning curve for new technology is too great and that "you can't teach an old dog new tricks." Recent research advanced by Norman Doidge[13] shows that neuroplasticity in the brain exists throughout the human lifespan and that the cerebral cortex is capable of constantly undergoing improvements in cognitive functioning. This means that any task that requires highly focused attention or the mastery of new skills helps to improve the mind, especially memory. Admittedly, learning to use the digital scanners or CAD/CAM systems discussed in this chapter means acquiring new skills and mastering new techniques, which will take some time and patience. The bottom line, however, is that the end result of developing the ability to use these new technologies will empower dentists to learn more about the dentistry they perform and enable them to provide their patients with well-fitting restorations.[2]

"Disruptive technology" is a term invented by Professor Clayton M. Christensen of Harvard Business School to describe a new technology that unexpectedly displaces an established technology.[14] Digital dental impressioning and CAD/CAM systems are disruptive technological advancements that surpass the accuracy and efficiency of former techniques for obtaining replicas of prepared teeth for the purpose of fabricating restorations, and their adoption by dentists and dental technicians is rapidly eclipsing the use of elastomeric impression materials and conventional laboratory procedures.

The ultimate goals of dentists dedicated to quality restorative dentistry are to make their treatment of patients as accurate, stressless, and as efficient as possible. The companies that have developed systems to help dentists and dental technicians achieve these goals are constantly enhancing the precision and scope of indications of their products to improve the quality of the dentistry provided.[1] Virtual has become a reality.[2]

Acknowledgements

We gratefully acknowledge the invaluable help of Paul Feuerstein, DMD, of Billerica, MA, and of Bob Cohen, CDT, of Custom Automated Prosthetics and Advanced Dental Technology of Stoneham, MA, in the research for this chapter.

Disclosure

We use the 3Shape TRIOS system for digital impressioning in our practice.

References

1. Birnbaum NS, Aaronson HB. Digital dental impression systems. *Inside Dent* 2011;7(2):84–90.
2. Birnbaum NS. Dental impressions using 3D digital scanners: virtual becomes reality. *Compend Cont Educ Dent* 2008:29(8):494,496,498–505.
3. Ring ME. How a dentist's name became a synonym for a life-saving device: the story of Dr. *Charles Stent. J Hist Dent* 2001;49(2):77–80.
4. Sears AW. Hydrocolloid impression technique for inlays and fixed bridges. *Dent Dig* 1937;43:230–234.
5. Craig RG. *Restorative Dental Materials*, 10th edn. London: C.V. Mosby; 1997:281–332.
6. Wassell RW, Barker D, Walls AWG. Crowns and other extra-coronal restorations: impression materials and technique. *Br Dent J* 2002;192(12):679–690.
7. Cho GC, Chee WW. Distortion of disposable plastic stock trays when used with putty vinyl polysiloxane impression materials. *J Prosthet Dent* 2004;92(4):354–358.
8. Hoyos A, Söderholm K-J. Influence of tray rigidity and impression technique on accuracy of polyvinyl siloxane impressions. *Int J Prosthodont* 2011;24(1):49–54.
9. Birnbaum NS, Aaronson HB, Stevens C, et al. 3D digital scanners: a high-tech approach to more accurate dental impressions. *Inside Dent* 2009;5:70–74.
10. Mirzayan A. Revisiting chairside CAD/CAM in an uncertain economic climate. *RDH Mag* March 30, 2009.
11. Schoenbaun, T. Decoding CAD/CAM and digital impression units. *Dentistry Today,* February 1, 2010. http://www.dentistrytoday.com/technology/1914 (accessed November 17, 2017).
12. Giménez-Gonzalez B, Prades G, Zcan M. Accuracy and repeatability of intra-oral scanners for full-arch implant impressions. In: *IADR 92nd General Session*, Cape Town, South Africa, 2014.
13. Doidge N. *The Brain That Changes Itself.* New York, NY: Penguin Books; 2007:87.
14. Christensen CM. *The Innovator's Dilemma: When New Technologies Cause Great Firms to Fail.* Boston, MA: Harvard Business Publishing; 1997.

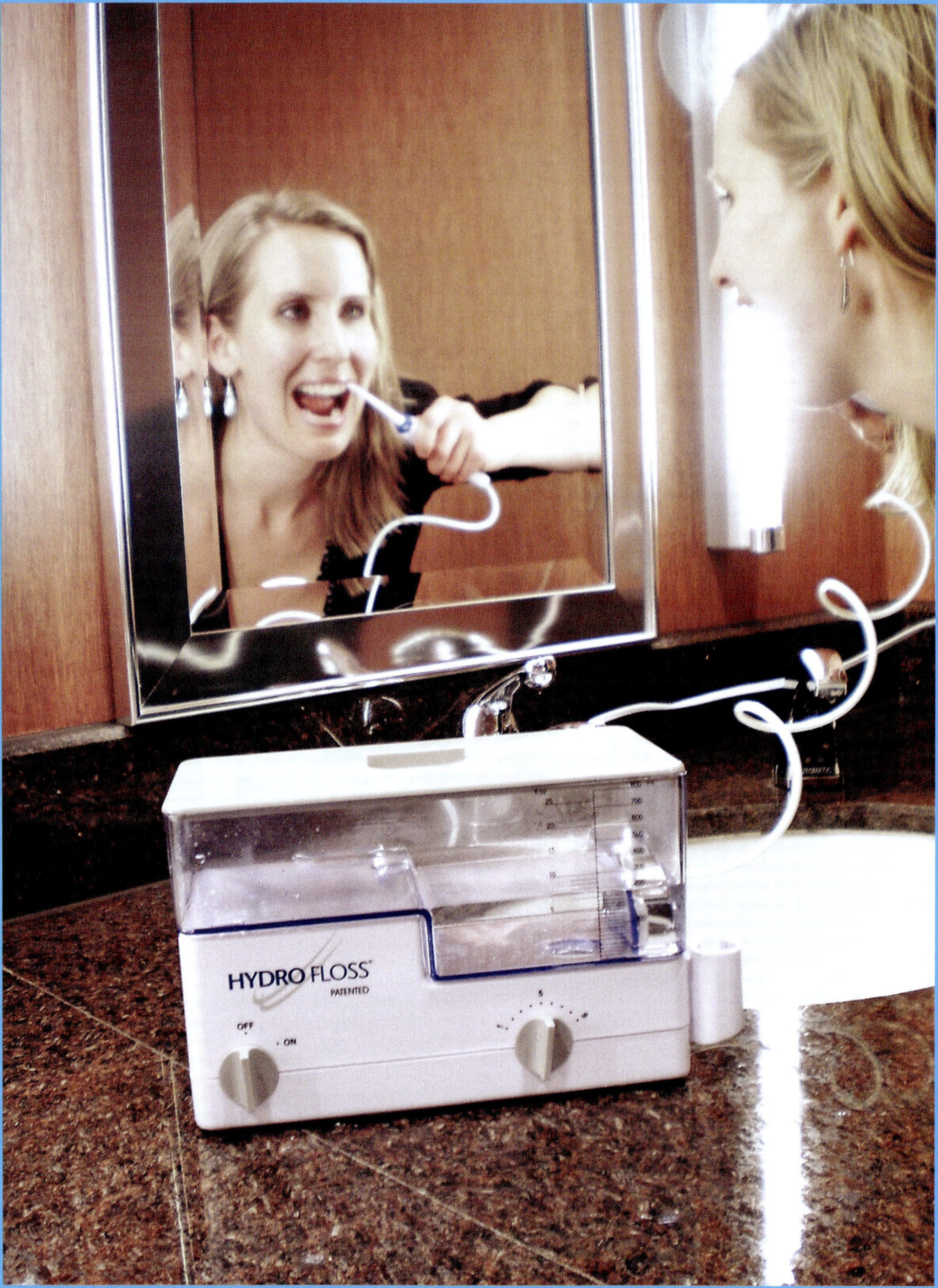
HYDRO FLOSS®
PATENTED
OFF
ON

Chapter 47 Maintenance of Esthetic Restorations

Ronald E. Goldstein, DDS, Kimberly J. Nimmons, RDH, BS, Anita H. Daniels, RDH, and Caren Barnes, RDH, BS, MS

Chapter Outline

Maintenance of esthetic restorations supported by natural dentition	1410
Pre-treatment	1410
Posttreatment visit	1410
Oral care products	1412
Ongoing professional maintenance	1416
Polishing	1416
Maintenance of esthetic implant-supported restorations	1417
Clinical evaluation of dental implants	1417
Pain	1417
Mobility	1417
Radiographic crestal bone loss	1417
Probing depths	1418
Peri-implant disease	1418
In-office hygiene care of implant-supported restorations	1419
Patient self-care	1423
Genetic considerations	1423
Interproximal/circumferential cleaning	1423
Irrigation	1427
Brushing	1427
Bacterial monitoring	1427
Intraoral camera	1427

As patients increasingly demand esthetic dental restorations, the ability of dentists to create such restorations has also steadily increased. However, satisfying the patient's esthetic expectations requires more than attention to appearance. The restorations must function well and continue to look good over time. While some patients successfully maintain their restorations for decades, others need to replace them in less than 5 years. Material selection, placement, and fabrication techniques are major factors in the longevity of esthetic dental restorations. However, professional oral maintenance and the patient's oral hygiene regimen are equally important.

This chapter addresses the basic elements of an oral hygiene program for successful long-term maintenance of both tooth- and implant-supported esthetic restorations. Additionally, the chapter discusses the roles of the patient, dental hygienist, and dentist in creating individualized oral hygiene programs.

Although considerations for maintaining tooth-supported and implant-supported restorations are similar, important elements distinguish their maintenance regimens, so each is discussed separately.

Maintenance of esthetic restorations supported by natural dentition

Pre-treatment

Ideally, an effective program of patient oral care should be established before any restorative treatment is initiated. Optimal results are more likely to be obtained if the soft tissue is in the best possible health before tooth restoration begins.[1] Moreover, patients who lack appropriate self-care routines are likely to develop additional problems after receiving even the most appealing restorations, thus reducing the life expectancy of those restorations.

Patients need to be educated and urged to commit to professional maintenance visits as well as a thorough oral self-care regimen. They must understand and have the abilities to implement the concepts of brushing, interdental cleaning, choosing the appropriate dentifrice, and using a manual or powered toothbrush as prescribed by the dental hygienist.

Posttreatment visit

Once a patient's esthetic restorations have been delivered, a posttreatment visit is essential. At this visit, the dental team should make sure the soft tissue has healed properly, all excess cement has been removed, all margins are smooth, and all interproximal areas can easily be reached with floss or an appropriate interproximal plaque removal device. The best way to positively determine if all the cement has been removed is to take a digital X-ray (Figure 47.1) It should be emphasized that dental floss is not the most appropriate interdental cleaning aid for most individuals.[2,3] Although patients may have been using dental floss for many years, they may be using it incorrectly. Plus, patients who have new esthetic restorations may begin brushing and flossing much more vigorously. The most frequent abuse of flossing is the use of a direct side to side motion after the floss has been placed between the teeth, thus slicing into the interdental papilla (Figure 47.2). It is necessary to continuously monitor patients to make sure they are flossing properly. If the patient's interproximal spaces can accommodate cylindrical or cone-shaped interdental brushes, these tools are likely to be much more effective than dental floss.[2,3] If interdental brushes (Figure 47.3) are recommended for interdental plaque and debris removal, they should not have exposed wire that holds the bristles in place.[4] Instead, an alternative such as soft picks (e.g., GUM® Soft-Picks®) (Figure 47.4), which have rubber bristles, should be used. Patients should be instructed in the proper use of interdental stimulators or any other type of interdental cleaner. Many patients have lost their interdental papilla as a result of using these devices improperly.

At the initial posttreatment visit, photographs should be taken to serve as a tissue and tooth-restoration baseline for future successful maintenance of the patient's restorations. The dental hygienist can use the intraoral camera to illustrate the fine details of the new restorations to the patient. The intraoral camera can also be used as an effective teaching and motivational tool (Figure 47.5). The images of the lingual aspect and interproximal margins of the restoration captured on the intraoral camera can enable patients to see these often-neglected surfaces. When enlarged on a video screen, intraoral images of inflamed tissue, plaque, and/or accumulating stain can be far more powerful than what is visible with a hand mirror. Intraoral imaging also allows the patient to see how healthy tissue and sound restorations appear. Photos of newly placed restorations can be compared at subsequent maintenance visits to detect early signs of inflammation or change in the health or appearance of the tissues.

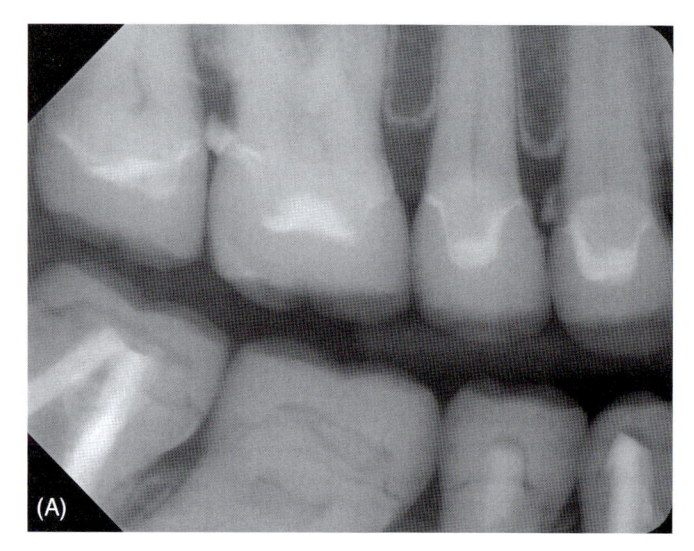

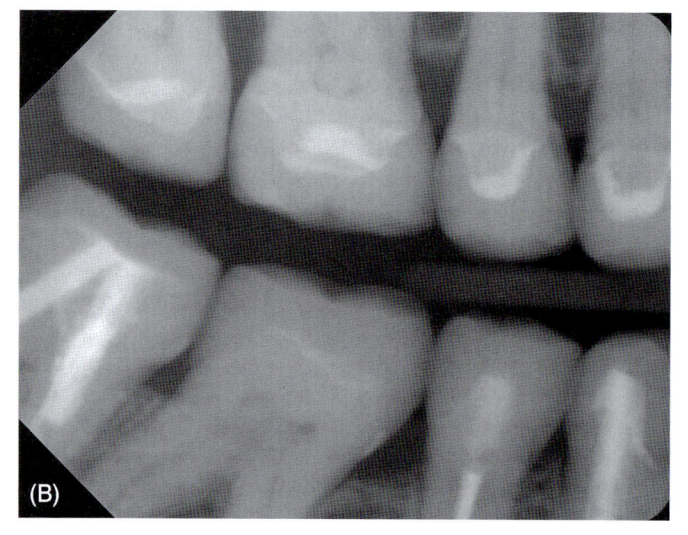

Figure 47.1 **(A, B)** Digital radiographs are a safe and effective way to determine if residual cement remains following the cementation of a restoration.

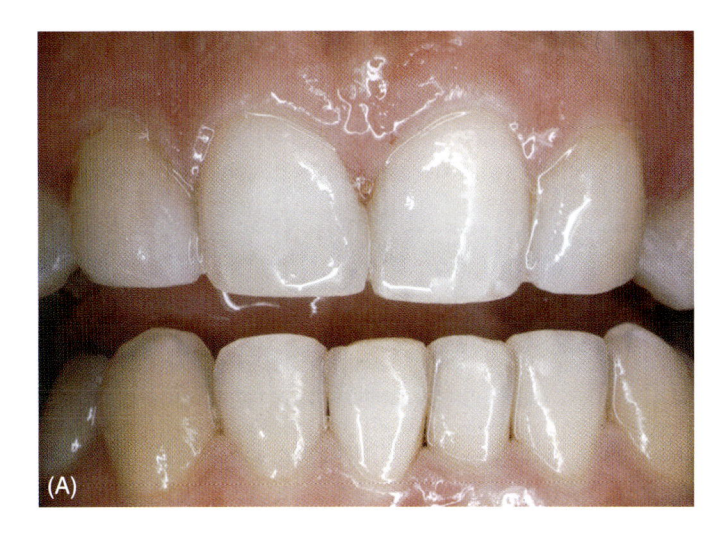

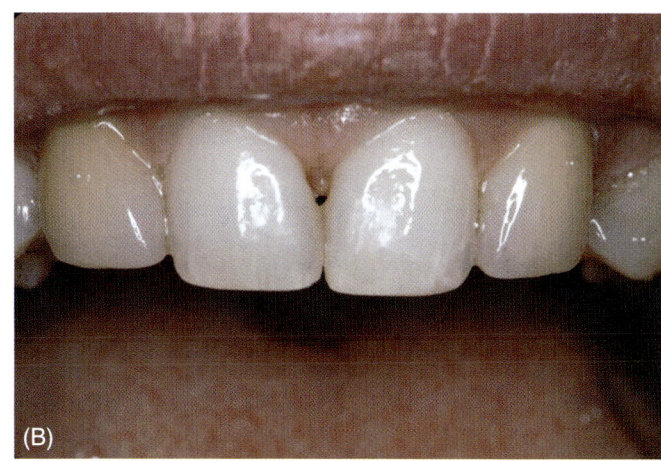

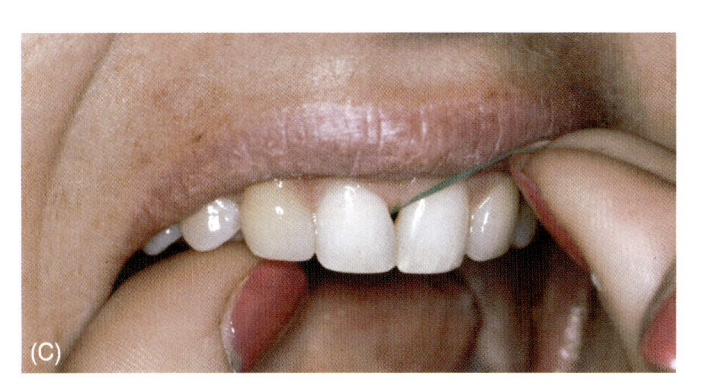

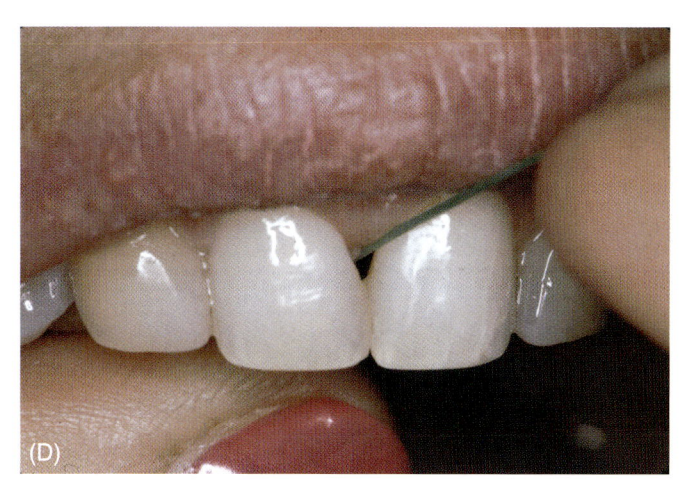

Figure 47.2 **(A)** Diastema closed with direct bonding. **(B)** This patient lived out of state, and the dentist did not see her for 5 years. The patient presented with a complaint of space reoccurring between her teeth. **(C)** When asked to show her use of dental floss, the patient demonstrated the technique shown. **(D)** It was noted that once the patient placed the floss she used a side to side motion that was guillotining her papilla and causing the space to open.

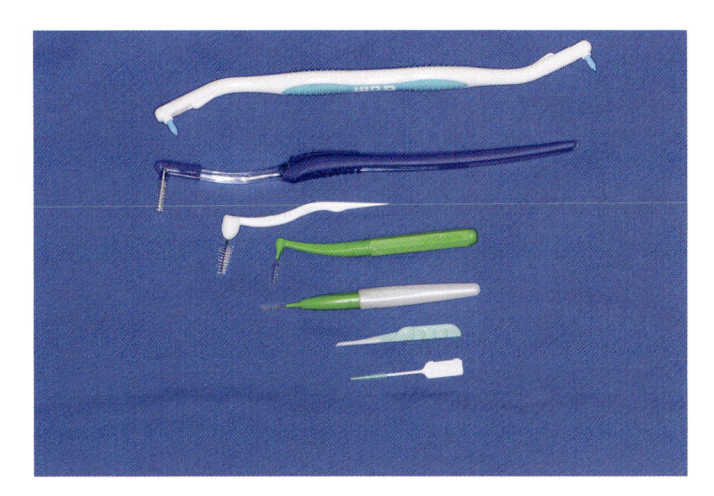

Figure 47.3 Interproximal brushes come in assorted shapes and sizes to allow for custom selection for each patient's needs.

Following restorative therapy, baseline digital radiographs should be taken in accordance with each patient's specific needs.[4] For example, if a patient reports sensitivity in a certain area, this might be caused by cement wash-out. A bitewing radiograph of the area can allow for identification, assessment, and appropriate treatment of the cause of the discomfort. Detecting and eliminating small problems at the postoperative visit can help to avoid larger problems later.

Traditionally, four horizontal bitewing radiographs of posterior teeth are taken annually.[5] However, the dental team also should consider taking three vertical bitewing radiographs of the anterior teeth. These are helpful for monitoring a patient's anterior restorations, whether they consist of composite resin bonding, porcelain veneers, crowns, or implant-supported restorations. In fact, a series of seven vertical bitewing radiographs (four posterior and three anterior) will provide a clear view of interproximal areas to check for decay and/or bone loss. A full-mouth radiographic series should be taken every 2–5 years, depending on the patient's individual situation and

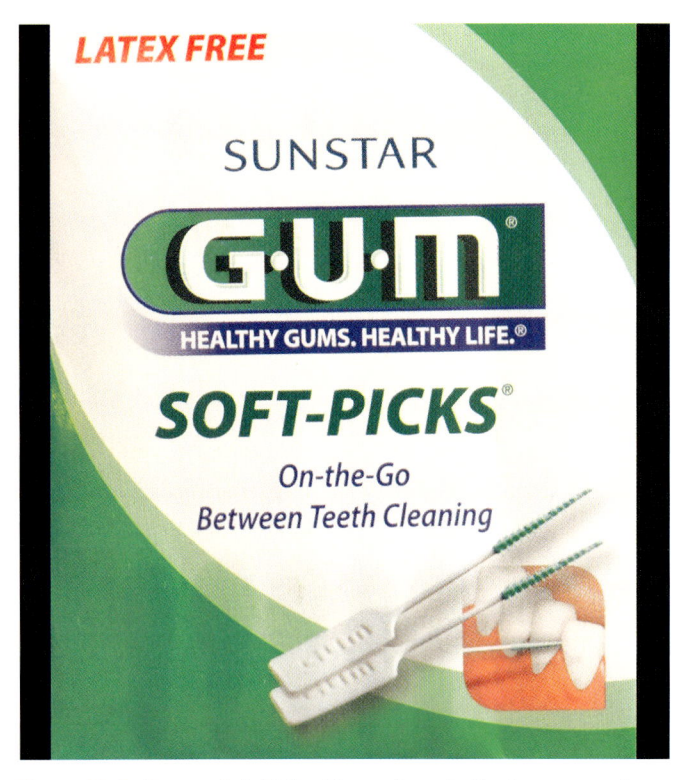

Figure 47.4 Sunstar Soft-Picks offer a safe and effective means of interproximal plaque control.

incorporating the radiographic guidelines prescribed by the American Dental Association (Table 47.1).

The postrestorative visit also provides an excellent opportunity to provide site-specific oral self-care instructions and review the patient's oral hygiene regimen. After seeing their new smiles, some patients become keenly interested in oral care and highly motivated to protect their investment. Their intense new interest in oral hygiene ironically can lead to tissue damage, recession, or root-surface abrasion at the restorative margins if patients are using improper brushing or flossing techniques or products. It is prudent for the dental hygienist to ask patients to demonstrate their mastery of plaque-removal techniques so that adjustments can be made should the patient need assistance with the oral self-care techniques. A dialogue should be established regarding oral self-care products that are appropriate for the patient's individual needs, which provides an opportunity for the dental hygienist to ensure that the patients understand what products they should be using and why they are important.[3] This also serves as an important time to confirm that patients are not using products or techniques that may have detrimental consequences[6] (Figure 47.6). A summary of the dental hygiene maintenance visit procedures can be seen in Table 47.2.

Oral care products

The hygienist in an esthetically oriented dental practice should always consider oral care products that are compatible with the esthetic restorative materials. This task is simplified if the practice has delivered the esthetic restoration(s), as contemporary

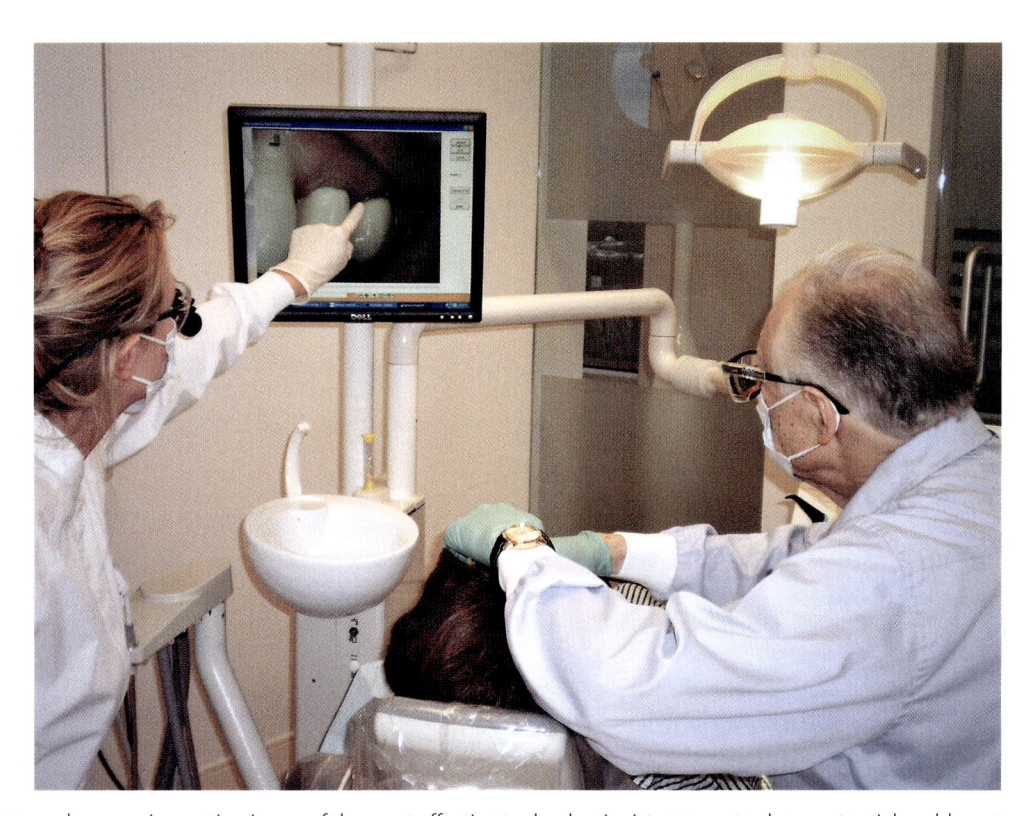

Figure 47.5 An intraoral camera inspection is one of the most effective tools a hygienist can use to show potential problems to a patient or attending dentist and especially to reinforce good oral care techniques and tissue heath.

Table 47.1 Recommendations for Prescribing Dental Radiographs[a]

Type of Encounter	Patient Age and Dental Developmental Stage				
	Child with Primary Dentition (Prior to Eruption of First Permanent Tooth)	Child with Transitional Dentition (After Eruption of First Permanent Tooth)	Adolescent with Permanent Dentition (Prior to Eruption of Third Molars)	Adult, Dentate or Partially Edentulous	Adult, Edentulous
New patient[b] being evaluated for dental diseases and dental development	Individualized radiographic examination consisting of selected periapical/occlusal views and/or posterior bitewings if proximal surfaces cannot be visualized or probed. Patients without evidence of disease and with open proximal contacts may not require a radiographic examination at this time.	Individualized radiographic examination consisting of posterior bitewings with panoramic examination or posterior bitewings and selected periapical images.	Individualized radiographic examination consisting of posterior bitewings with panoramic examination or posterior bitewings and selected periapical images. A full mouth intraoral radiographic examination is preferred when the patient has clinical evidence of generalized dental disease or a history of extensive dental treatment.		Individualized radiographic examination, based on clinical signs and symptoms.
Recall patient[b] with clinical caries or at increased risk for caries[c]	Posterior bitewing examination at 6–12 month intervals if proximal surfaces cannot be examined visually or with a probe.			Posterior bitewing exam at 6–18 month intervals.	Not applicable
Recall patient[b] with no clinical caries and not at increased risk for caries[c]	Posterior bitewing examination at 12–24 month intervals if proximal surfaces cannot be examined visually or with a probe.		Posterior bitewing examination at 18–36 month intervals.	Posterior bitewing examination at 24–36 month intervals.	Not applicable
Recall patient[b] with periodontal disease	Clinical judgment as to the need for and type of radiographic images for the evaluation of periodontal disease. Imaging may consist of, but is not limited to, selected bitewing and/or periapical images of areas where periodontal disease (other than nonspecific gingivitis) can be identified clinically.				Not applicable
Patient for monitoring of growth and development	Clinical judgment as to need for and type of radiographic images for evaluation and/or monitoring of dentofacial growth and development		Clinical judgment as to need for and type of radiographic images for evaluation and/or monitoring of dentofacial growth and development. Panoramic or periapical exam to assess developing third molars.	Usually not indicated.	

(*Continued*)

Table 47.1 (Continued)

Type of Encounter	Patient Age and Dental Developmental Stage
Patient with other circumstances, including, but not limited to, proposed or existing implants, pathology, restorative/endodontic needs, treated periodontal disease and caries remineralization	Clinical judgment as to need for and type of radiographic images for evaluation and/or monitoring in these circumstances.

Source: modified from table 1 in *The Selection of Patients for Dental Radiographic Examinations. Revised 2012.*[5]

[a]The recommendations in this chart are subject to clinical judgment and may not apply to every patient. They are to be used by dentists only after reviewing the patient's health history and completing a clinical examination. Because every precaution should be taken to minimize radiation exposure, protective thyroid collars and aprons should be used whenever possible. This practice is strongly recommended for children, women of childbearing age, and pregnant women.

[b]Clinical situations for which radiographs may be indicated include but are not limited to the following. A. *Positive historical findings:* (1) Previous periodontal or endodontic treatment. (2) History of pain or trauma. (3) Familial history of dental anomalies. (4) Postoperative evaluation of healing. (5) Remineralization monitoring. (6) Presence of implants or evaluation for implant placement. B. *positive clinical signs/symptoms:* (1) Clinical evidence of periodontal disease. (2) Large or deep restorations. (3) Deep carious lesions. (4) Malposed or clinically impacted teeth. (5) Swelling. (6) Evidence of dental/facial trauma. (7) Mobility of teeth. (8) Sinus tract ("fistula"). (9) Clinically suspected sinus pathology. (10) Growth abnormalities. (11) Oral involvement in known or suspected systemic disease. (12) Positive neurologic findings in the head and neck. (13) Evidence of foreign objects. (14) Pain and/or dysfunction of the temporomandibular joint. (15) Facial asymmetry. (16) Abutment teeth for fixed or removable partial prosthesis. (17) Unexplained bleeding. (18) Unexplained sensitivity of teeth. (19) Unusual eruption, spacing, or migration of teeth. (20) Unusual tooth morphology, calcification, or color. (21) Unexplained absence of teeth. (22) Clinical erosion.

[c]Factors increasing risk for caries may include but are not limited to: (1) High level of caries experience or demineralization. (2) History of recurrent caries. (3) High titers of cariogenic bacteria. (4) Existing restoration(s) of poor quality. (5) Poor oral hygiene. (6) Inadequate fluoride exposure. (7) Prolonged nursing (bottle or breast). (8) Frequent high sucrose content in diet. (9) Poor family dental health. 10) Developmental or acquired enamel defects. (11) Developmental or acquired disability. (12) Xerostomia. (13) Genetic abnormality of teeth. (14) Many multisurface restorations. (15) Chemo/radiation therapy. (16) Eating disorders. (17) Drug/alcohol abuse. (18) Irregular dental care.

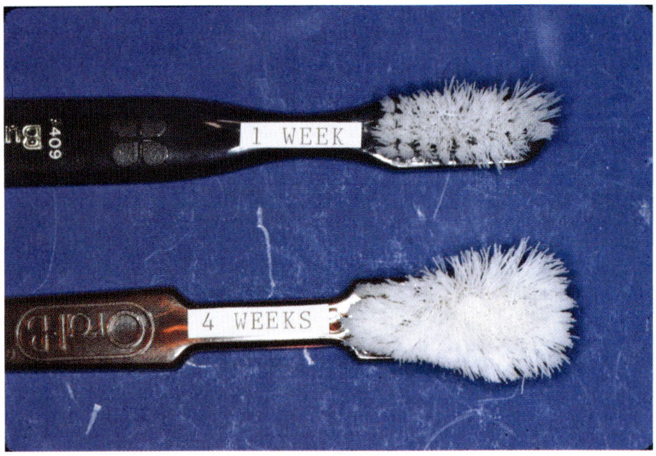

Figure 47.6 This patient had a habit of improper tooth brushing technique. The use of too much pressure is easily surmised.

restorative materials often are hard to identify accurately. If the practice has not delivered the restorations, then dental records, radiographs, and tactile sensitivity all can be useful in identifying their composition.[7–10] Tactile sensitivity can be enhanced with knowledge of the surface texture associated with various materials. Microfilled composites, for example, have a smooth surface texture upon placement. Glass ionomers also have a smooth surface; however, they lack the gloss associated with hybrid and microfilled composites.[11,12]

Ideally, patients should use oral care products that are compatible with the materials from which their esthetic restorations are fabricated.[7–10] In general, dentifrices should be nonabrasive, contain fluoride, and work well with both manual and powered toothbrushes. (For a list of abrasivity of dentifrices, see Table 47.3.) Both manual and powered toothbrushes should have soft bristles. Some power toothbrushes have been reported to prevent and remove extrinsic stains.[11,12] Preventing such stains is essential, since many patients have had whitening procedures performed prior to placement of esthetic restorations.[11]

Many patients question whether or not they should be using a mouth rinse. If mouth rinses are recommended, they should be mild and nonstaining, with antibacterial properties (e.g., TheraSol, Mgf, Smart Mouth, Triumph, OraTec, Inc. Pharmaceuticals). Dipping the toothbrush tip into a few drops of such a mouth rinse and using that instead of toothpaste at least once daily may be advisable. A nonshredding and nonwoven dental floss (Glide, W&L Gore & Associates, Total, or Colgate-Palmolive) can work well for most restorative patients. Certain patients cannot easily use nonwaxed floss, especially if they have too tight and imperfect contact areas. These patients who have light contacts may find tape or larger rope floss easier to use (Figure 47.7).

Patients should be informed of the role diet plays in the demineralization and remineralization of tooth structure. For example, the cariogenic effects of long-term exposure to

Table 47.2 Summary of Dental Hygiene Care at Maintenance Visits Following Dental Implant Placement

Pretreatment Visit	Postrestorative Treatment Visit	Ongoing Maintenance Visit
Establish oral self-care regimen	Confirm soft tissue healing	Two–four dental hygiene maintenance visits per year
Patient commits to dental hygiene maintenance visits	Confirm interdental areas can be accessed for cleaning	Evaluate patient compliance with oral self-care regimen
Intraoral photographs for documentation, patient education, and motivation		Take intraoral photographs for documentation, patient education, and motivation
Take four baseline vertical bitewing radiographs annually; consider additional three anterior vertical bitewing radiographs		Take full mouth radiographic survey every 2–5 years
Site-specific oral hygiene instructions		Site-specific oral hygiene instructions
Recommend oral care products specific for patient's needs		Using magnification loupes, inspect margins of restorations and soft tissue associated with implant

Table 47.3 The Relative Dentin Abrasivity (RDA) Values for Commonly Available Toothpastes[3]

Toothpaste	RDA Value
Straight baking soda	7
Arm & Hammer Tooth Powder	8
Arm & Hammer Dental Care	35
Oxyfresh	45
Tom's of Maine Sensitive	49
Arm & Hammer Peroxicare	49
Rembrandt Original	53
CloSYS	53
Tom's of Maine Children	57
Colgate Regular	68
Colgate Total	70
Sensodyne	79
Aim	80
Colgate Sensitive Max Strength	83
Aquafresh Sensitive	91
Tom's of Maine Regular	93
Crest Regular	95
Mentadent	103
Sensodyne Extra Whitening	104
Colgate Platinum	106
Crest Sensitivity	107
Colgate Herbal	110
Aquafresh Whitening	113
Arm & Hammer Tarter Control	117
Arm & Hammer Advance White Gel	117
Close up with Baking Soda	120
Colgate Whitening	124
Ultra Brite	130
Crest MultiCare Whitening	144
Colgate Baking Soda Whitening	145
Pepsodent	150
Colgate Tarter Control 165	165

FDA recommended RDA limit: 200. ADA recommended RDA limit: 250.
The RDA index: 0–70, low abrasive; 70–100, medium abrasive; 100–150, highly abrasive; 150–250, regarded as harmful limit.

sugars in products such as breath mints, hard candies, and throat lozenges may decrease the life expectancy of their restorations. In addition, certain foods and drinks consumed by the patient can affect the oral pH. As the oral cavity becomes acidic, tooth structure more readily demineralizes. Patients can aid in the prevention of caries development through excellent daily plaque removal, nutritional awareness, and the use of appropriate products. A key role of the dental hygienist in caries prevention is to assess each patient's risk factors. Based on the risk factors identified, the dental team can educate the patient on preventive and therapeutic care strategies, as well as products designed to minimize risk of caries development.

Figure 47.7 The availability of many types of dental floss allows a custom selection to meet each patient's oral care needs.

Ongoing professional maintenance

After the postoperative visit, there is a standard of recommending two to four dental hygiene maintenance appointments annually. However, more frequent visits may be advisable for patients with extensive esthetic restorations. It is essential that the frequency of dental hygiene maintenance visits be based on the individual patient's needs and determined by the level of the patient's self-care compliance, risks, needs, and periodontal status.

At each dental hygiene maintenance appointment, the dental professional can carefully inspect the restorative margins with an explorer and small surgical suction tip. The suction tip dries the tooth and can gently retract the soft tissue enough to provide a direct view of the subgingival margin (Figure 47.8). Further, the use of loupes (magnifying glasses) can greatly enhance the dental hygienist's ability to detect marginal discrepancies.[13]

Polishing

Polishing during dental hygiene maintenance visits can pose a serious threat to successful maintenance of esthetic restorations. This is because many dental professionals use whatever type of polishing paste is at hand.[10] Some prefer using coarse-grit paste, in the belief that it removes all stains ranging from light to heavy, thus saving time. Sales of coarse-grit polishing paste have been reported to make up 80% of total polishing paste sales, compared with 10% for medium grit.[10,14] While the use of coarse-grit pastes may initially save time, such pastes can significantly damage the surface characterization of esthetic restorative surfaces, produce hypersensitivity, roughen tooth and restorative surfaces, and accelerate staining and the retention of dental plaque and calculus.[7–14]

Ideally, polishing grits should be used in a progression of coarse, medium, and fine applications. If a coarse polish is required, the surface should also be polished with medium and fine polishes. Each time a different grit of polish is used, the rubber cup must be changed to prevent contamination of the grit sizes. It is essential for dental hygienists and dentists to understand the special polishing requirements for each type of esthetic restorative material, as these restorations can be severely compromised if the wrong products or procedures are used. The major categories of esthetic restorative materials include porcelain, composites, and glass ionomers.

Porcelain

Glazed and previously polished porcelain restorations resist staining much better than unglazed porcelain. Typically, such restorations can be polished with a dry diamond paste and a Robinson brush.[10] Although rubber polishing instruments can remove stain and create a highly polished surface in a single step, rubber polishing instruments can also be followed with a diamond paste.[10]

Unglazed porcelain restorations that have become roughened should be smoothed prior to polishing, using dry diamond paste applied with a felt wheel or Robinson brush.[10] If the unglazed porcelain surface is stained but smooth, a rubber polishing cup and diamond paste can work effectively.[15]

The resin cement used for sealing bonded porcelain restoration margins absorbs stains more readily. Care must be taken to avoid removing too much resin cement during polishing, or else marginal ditching can result, along with increased vulnerability to leaking, plaque retention, and dental caries. If no stain is present and only plaque removal is required, a cleaning agent that does not contain abrasives (e.g., ProCare, Young Dental Mfg.) can be used with a rubber polishing cup.[7–10]

Composites

Manufacturers' recommendations should be followed when choosing a product to polish an esthetic restoration made of composite materials. However, there are many occasions when identification of the type of composite or glass ionomer material may not be possible. When that is the case, polishing of the esthetic restoration can be safely completed using a cleaning agent that does not abrade the surface of the restoration.[7–10]

The ability to distinguish between hybrids and microfilled composites can enable dental hygienists to consistently achieve better polishing results. Hybrid composites tend to have a rougher surface.[10] It may not be possible to achieve a highly polished surface on restorations made from them. Rubber finishers and polishers, followed by a composite polishing paste, is recommended.[15]

Use of a rubber polisher can enable microfilled composites to be polished rapidly, followed by a composite polishing paste. An aluminum oxide polishing paste fabricated for composite restorations is recommended for hybrid composites.[10] This should be applied with a water-filled rubber polishing cup. Extra-fine aluminum oxide paste can then be used as a final polish.

Glass ionomers

Restorations made from glass ionomers lack the shiny, smooth, undetectable surface achievable with polished esthetic composite materials.[10] Glass ionomers typically have a rougher surface, and polishing with light pressure at slow speed is recommended.[10] A fine finishing disk or rubber polisher can be used to remove persistent stains on this material. Desiccation of glass ionomer restorations, which can lead to cracking and premature deterioration, can be mitigated by lubricating the restoration with petroleum jelly or water before polishing.[16]

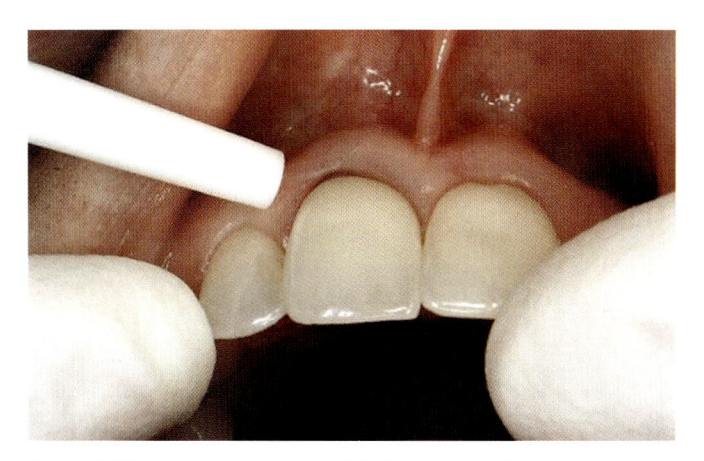

Figure 47.8 Gentle tissue lift provided by the use of small surgical suction tip assists in the direct visual inspection of a restoration's margin.

Both manual and powered instrumentation used by dental hygienists at dental hygiene maintenance appointments should be chosen to produce the smoothest surfaces possible for teeth and restorative materials without damaging those surfaces or jeopardizing the marginal integrity of cemented castings. Powered instrumentation with ultrasonic scalers can damage both hybrid and microfilled composite restorations, glass ionomers, laminate veneers, and titanium implant abutments.[17] Ultrasonic instruments also can fracture porcelain and change the margins of amalgam restorations.[18] Air-polishing instruments also should not be used on any esthetic restoration, including composite, glass ionomer, and porcelain-cemented restorations. Air polishing can devastate the surface characterization of composite and glass ionomer restorations, remove the resin matrix, and expose the filler particles. Although air polishing does not harm porcelain, it can remove the cement surrounding the margins and cause aggressive "ditching" around the interface among the tooth, cement, and porcelain, leaving a location for plaque to accumulate.[19]

Maintenance of esthetic implant-supported restorations

Early dental implants did not support the most esthetic of restorations. They were originally developed as a last option for providing edentulous patients with limited masticatory function and improved speech. In exchange, patients often had to settle for non-esthetic appearances and unsightly, exposed implant components.

Fortunately, countless advances have been made in implant design and biocompatible materials. Today, implants can be expected to support restorations that not only function indistinguishably from natural dentition but also are beautiful and long lasting. When maintaining and evaluating the health of the hard and soft tissues supporting dental implants, several important factors must be considered. Careful patient selection and meticulous case planning followed by proper professional and patient self-care are essential to a long-lasting and esthetically successful implant restoration.

The next section reviews the clinical considerations when evaluating dental implants and their surrounding tissues. Both in-office care and home care techniques are then reviewed.

Clinical evaluation of dental implants

Numerous criteria have been proposed for evaluating dental health, and over time these criteria have changed.[20] A consensus conference in 2008 updated and clarified clinical indices of implant success, including pain, mobility, radiographic crestal bone loss, probing depths, and peri-implant disease. Table 47.4 summarizes these findings.[21]

Pain

Although pain is not a common complication once implants have healed, it can occur if vital structures are traumatized during surgery, if the implant body is mobile, or if the implant body has fractured. More frequently, complaints about pain at implant site are associated with the surrounding soft tissues. Soft-tissue pain can be caused by trauma, loose prosthetic components, or residual cement at cement-retained restoration sites.

Mobility

A healthy tooth will exhibit clinical movement, both vertically and horizontally, as allowed by its periodontal ligament, but once an implant has achieved osseointegration, it does not exhibit clinical mobility. While studies have revealed slight movement of healthy dental implants, there should be no clinically visible mobility.[22]

Radiographic crestal bone loss

The ICOI consensus determined that bone loss should be measured from the time of placement, rather than from earlier radiographs. It also said that for an implant to be judged successful, less than 2 mm of crestal bone loss should occur. This differed slightly from the historic expectation[23] of 1.5 mm of crestal bone loss in the first year after placement and 0.1 mm each year thereafter (Figure 47.9).

Research in the field of dental implants is presently focusing on eliminating even minimal crestal bone loss by means of design changes, such as the Laser-Lok surface (BioHorizons) and platform switching.

Table 47.4 Dental Implant Health Scale

Implant Quality Scale Group	Clinical Conditions
I. Success (Optimum Health)	(a) No pain or tenderness upon function (b) No clinical mobility (c) <2 mm radiographic bone loss (d) No history of exudate
II. Satisfactory survival	(a) No pain on function (b) No clinical mobility (c) 2–4 mm radiographic bone loss (d) No history of exudate
III. Compromised survival	(a) May have sensitivity on function (b) No clinical mobility (c) Radiographic bone loss >4 mm (d) Probing depth >7 mm (e) May have history of exudate
IV. Failure (clinical or absolute failure)	Any of the following criteria: (a) Pain on function (b) Mobility (c) Radiographic bone loss >1/2 length of implant (d) Uncontrolled exudate (e) No longer in mouth

Source: International Congress of Oral Implantologists (ICOI), Pisa, Italy, Consensus Conference 2007.[21]

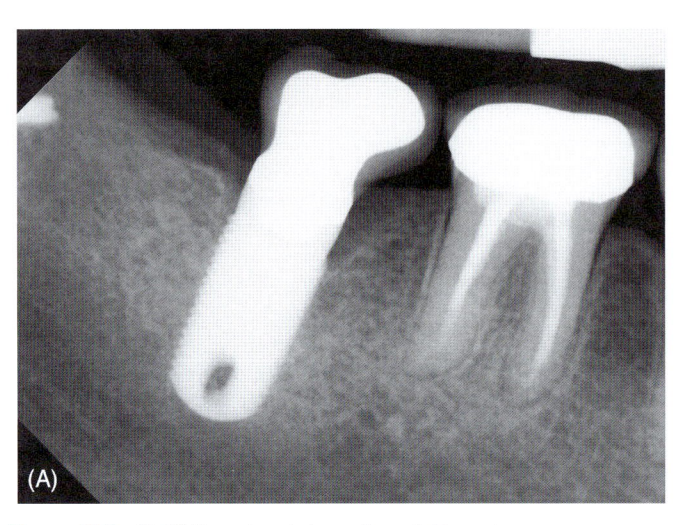

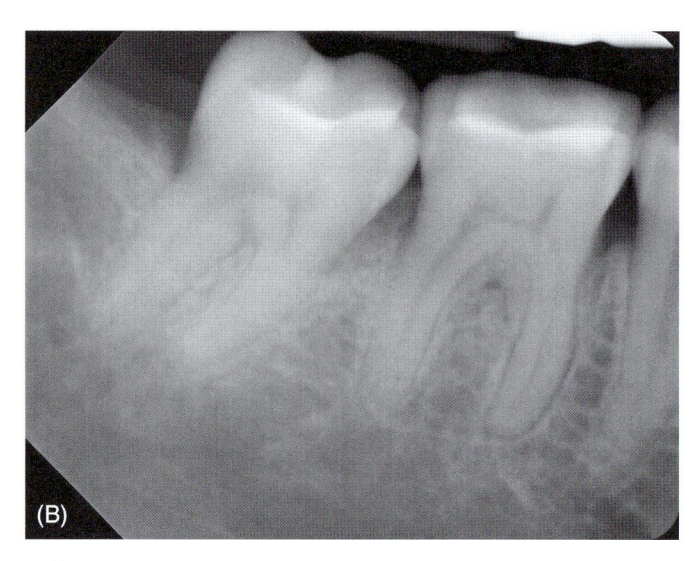

Figure 47.9 (A, B) Crestal and circumferential bone loss as seen on a radiograph.

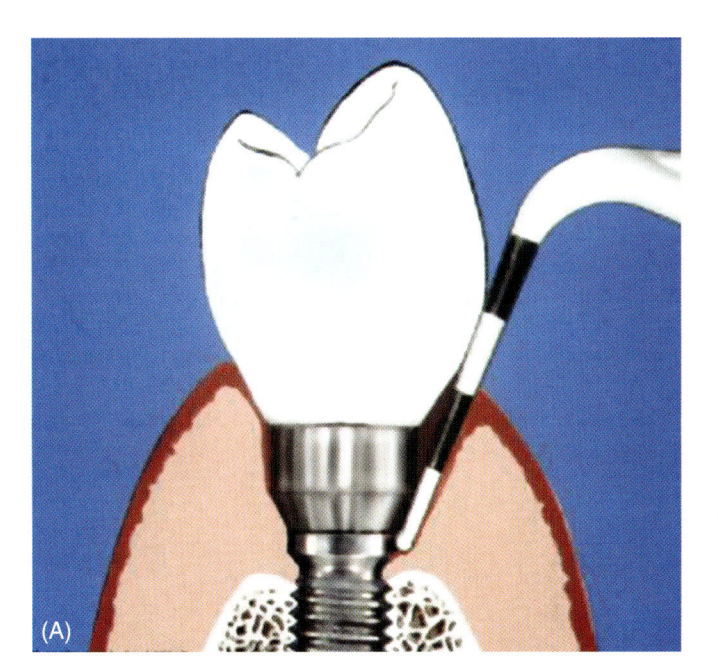

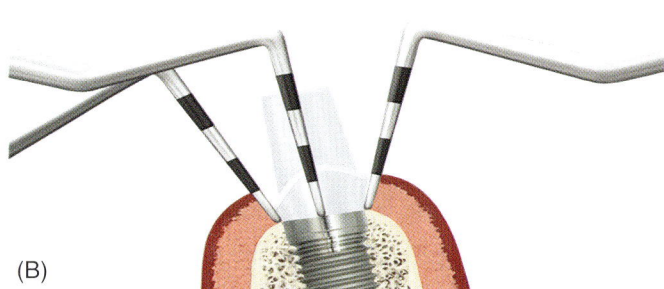

Figure 47.10 (A) Proper positioning to show probing around restored implant. (B) A plastic periodontal probe (see Figure 47.11B) can be gently swept through the peri-implant sulcus to visualize symptoms of inflammation or disease. The depth of the sulcus is surgically created and therefore corresponds to abutment collar height, rather than an indication of attachment loss. A better indicator of bone loss is a radiograph.

Probing depths

When measuring a periodontal pocket around a tooth, the probe goes through the sulcus and the junctional epithelium, stopping at the zone of connective tissue attachment. The place where fibers insert into the cementum creates a definitive stopping point. None of the connective tissue fibers can insert into the implant body, however, making it difficult to ascertain the appropriate stopping point for a probe. The parallel orientation of these fibers also makes the peri-implant sulci more susceptible to bacteria. The ICOI consensus does not recommend routine probing, but it finds value in baseline probing measurements, as well as probing in the presence of other symptoms (Figure 47.10).

Peri-implant disease

In the absence of residual cement, the most likely cause of peri-implantitis is bacteria. As for teeth, bone loss and an increase in pocket depths around implants leads to the development of a niche for anaerobic bacteria. Patients with a history of periodontal disease are more likely to have these bacteria in their mouths and are thus at greater risk for peri-implant disease.[24]

In-office hygiene care of implant-supported restorations

Hygiene maintenance visits often involve the care of dental implants and the restorations they support, along with the patient's tooth-supported esthetic restorations. However, the approach to cleaning the two classes of restorations differs slightly.

The appropriate instruments and accepted standard-of-care protocols may vary and require an individualized approach. Dental professionals must also provide appropriate implant self-care instruction to each patient. Without guidance, patients may assume that the care required for their dental implants is identical to that required by their natural teeth or conventional restorations.

Probing

Once osseointegration has been confirmed and the definitive implant restoration has been delivered, baseline peri-implant sulcular depths should be charted. The peri-mucosal seal around implants consists of junctional epithelium with a hemidesmosomal attachment and connective tissue fibers that mostly are oriented parallel to the implant. This attachment is fragile and may be more susceptible to trauma from probing than the multi-directional connective tissue fibers that attach to the cementum of a tooth. Because of this, subsequent implant probing should be performed only in response to a clinical indication, such as a visual change in the tissues, mobility, patient-reported symptoms, or radiographic evidence.[25] With dental implants, a deeper pocket depth alone does not necessarily indicate disease. It may be in part due to the depth of the implant placement or the shape of the restorative components. More important to look for is an increase in pocket depth that occurs over time or other signs of disease in addition to the pocket depth. Careful clinical inspection is important, as any deep pocket may potentially harbor anaerobic bacteria.[26]

Accurate monitoring of peri-implant tissues requires consistent clinical observation and thorough records. Recently, specific bacterial pathogens have been identified as those most commonly found to cause peri-implantitis. Annual bacterial screening at professional hygiene appointments may be helpful in assessing the risk of peri-implant infections and allow for very early intervention. OralDNA Labs offer the MyPerioPath saliva test which can be used to screen for *Actinobacillus actinomycetemcomitans*, *Porphyromonas gingivalis*, *Fusobacterium*, and *Treponema denticola*—the pathogens most commonly implicated in peri-implantitis (Figure 47.11A).

When peri-implant probing is performed, this should be accomplished using a probe specifically designed for implants. Implant probes, such as the Colorvue (Hu-Friedy) or PDT Sensor Probe (DenMat; Figure 47.11B), offer improved visibility and help to ensure that the correct amount of pressure is used during probing. Misch has discussed the need to take care not to scratch the implant when utilizing a metal probe, as any such scratch may create a niche for bacteria.[27] The use of nonmetal probes also decreases the chance of scratching or otherwise marring the implant's titanium surface or damaging the peri-implant epithelial fibers. Misch also warns against probing any site of natural dentition with a history of periodontal disease before probing an implant site. As the attachment is fragile, one can introduce bacteria from the dentition into the implant site.[27] To minimize this chance, different probes should be used around implants and natural teeth. According to Garber, dipping the probe into an antimicrobial agent (e.g., chlorhexidine) before and during probing may minimize cross-contamination from tooth sulci to peri-implant tissues (personal communication, Dr David Garber, April 2005).

Radiographs

Radiographic evaluation may be more valuable for implant assessment than probing. Annual vertical bitewing radiographs are diagnostic for areas of one to four implants and should be supplemented with periapical films. If a patient has five or more implants, a panoramic radiograph should be taken every other year and supplemented with periapical films as necessary. When evaluating crestal bone loss, it is important that the radiographs be perpendicular to the implant body so that the threads on both the mesial and distal sides are clearly visible.[26] This can usually be best accomplished with vertical bitewings. Periapical and panoramic films will best visualize for peri-implantitis and loss of integration along the body of the bone-to-implant interface.

Digital radiography, which provides clear and easily studied images, can be a valuable tool for examining implants during maintenance. The digital radiographic image also can be manipulated to provide contrast, color, clarification, and magnification. The "eagle-eye" feature on the Sirona® system is especially helpful when examining bone-to-implant surfaces.

Intraoral examination

A periodontal probe may be the instrument of choice for assessing the health of gingival tissues and underlying bone supporting natural teeth; however, implants require even more meticulous clinical examination. The tissues surrounding any implant should be evaluated for redness, thinning, swelling, tenderness, bleeding, suppuration, or recession. Even minor changes should be noted and investigated. As with all esthetic restorations, it is helpful to document the tissue status, healthy or not, with an intraoral camera. Clinical photographs provide accurate comparisons that can be reviewed during periodic maintenance visits.

The implant examination also should include an occlusal check and review for mobility. Occlusal discrepancies can result from several factors, such as a change in the natural dentition or bone loss. If noted, they should be further evaluated. If the implant, abutment, or restoration appears to be loose or mobile, a radiograph may help determine why. Common causes include cement wash-out under a crown or loosening of a retention screw. Screw-access openings for screw-retained implant-supported restorations should be checked and resealed as needed.

As with natural teeth, parafunctional occlusal stresses may cause bone loss and affect the longevity of the dental implant. Over time, changes in the patient's occlusion may affect the stability and lifespan of any implant-supported restoration.

MYPERIOPATH®
FINAL REPORT

OralDNA Labs — Innovations in Salivary Diagnostics

Patient	Ordering Provider	Sample Information	
		Specimen#: 0000000000	Collected: 11/12/2016 10:30
		Accession#: 201611-08469	Received: 11/13/2016 12:01
		Specimen: Oral Rinse(P)	Reported: 11/16/2016 12:30

MYPERIOPATH MOLECULAR ANALYSIS OF PERIODONTAL AND SYSTEMIC PATHOGENS

Result: PATHOGENIC BACTERIA DETECTED, 5 ABOVE THERAPEUTIC THRESHOLD

Bacterial Risk: HIGH - Very strong evidence of increased risk for attachment loss

Legend
— = Therapeutic Threshold*
DL = Detection Limit

Result Interpretation: Periodontal disease is caused by specific, or groups of specific bacteria. Threshold levels represent the concentration above which patients are generally at increased risk for attachment loss. Bacterial levels should be considered collectively and in context with clinical signs and other risk factors.

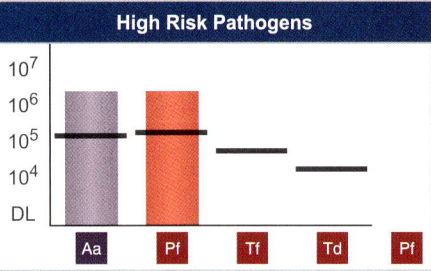

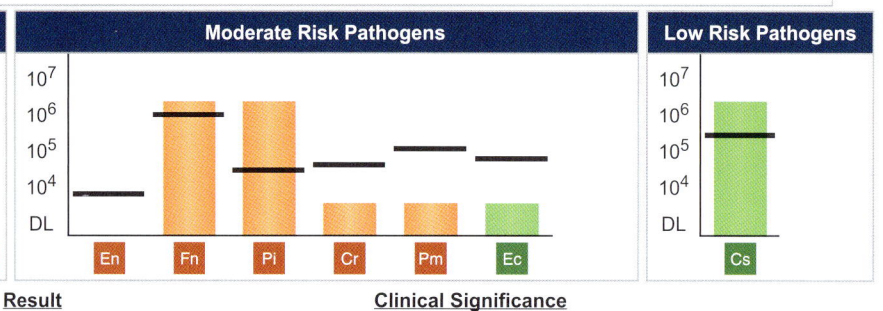

High Risk Pathogens
Aa, Pf, Tf, Td, Pf

Moderate Risk Pathogens
En, Fn, Pi, Cr, Pm, Ec

Low Risk Pathogens
Cs

Pathogen	Result	Clinical Significance
Aa Aggregatibacter actinomycetemcomitans	High	Very strong association with PD: Transmittable, tissue invasive, and pathogenic at relatively low bacterial counts. Associated with aggressive forms of disease.
Pf Porphyromonas gingivalis	High	Very strong association with PD: Transmittable, tissue invasive, and pathogenic at relatively low bacterial counts. Associated with aggressive forms of disease.
Fn Fusobacterium nucleatum/periodonticum	High	Strong association with PD: adherence properties to several oral pathogens; often seen in refractory disease.
Pi Prevotella intermedia	High	Strong association with PD: virulent properties similar to Pg; often seen in refractory disease.
Cs Capnocytophaga species (gingavalis, ochracea, sputigena)	High	Some association with PD: Frequently found in gingivitis. Often found in association with other periodontal pathogens. May increase temporarily following active therapy.
Cr Campylobacter rectus	Low	Moderate association with development of PD: usually found in combination with other suspected pathogens in refractory disease.
Pm Peptostreptococcus (Micromonas) micros	Low	Moderate association with PD: detected in higher numbers at sites of active disease.
Ec Eikenella corrodens	Low	Moderate association with PD: Found more frequently in active sites of disease; often seen in refractory disease.

Not Detected: (Tf) Tannerella forsythia, (Td) Treponema denticola, (En) Eubacterium nodatum

Additional information is available from OralDNA.com

Methodology: Genomic DNA is extracted from the submitted sample and tested for 10 species-specific bacteria and 1 genus of bacteria known to cause periodontal disease. The bacteria are assayed by real-time quantitative polymerase chain reaction (qPCR). Bacterial loads are reported in log copies per mL of sample (e.g. 1×10^3 = 1000 bacteria copies per mL of collection). *Modified from: Microbiological goals of periodontal therapy; Periodontology 2000, Vol. 42, 2006, 180-218. This test was developed, and its performance characteristics determined by OralDNA Labs pursuant to CLIA requirements. This test has not been cleared or approved by the U.S. Food and Drug Administration. The FDA has determined that such clearance or approval is not necessary.

OralDNA Labs, A Service of Access Genetics, LLC, 7400 Flying Cloud Drive, Eden Prairie, MN 55344 Phone: 855-672-5362; Fax: 952-942-0703 www.oraldna.com
CLIA#: 24D1033809 CAP#: 7190878

PL-000388-B

Web enabled system provided by: access genetics

Figure 47.11 **(A)** MyPerioPath (OralDNA Labs) lab report identifies the presence of any of the top 11 pathogens associated with periodontal infections. Reproduced with permission of Access Genetics, LLC.

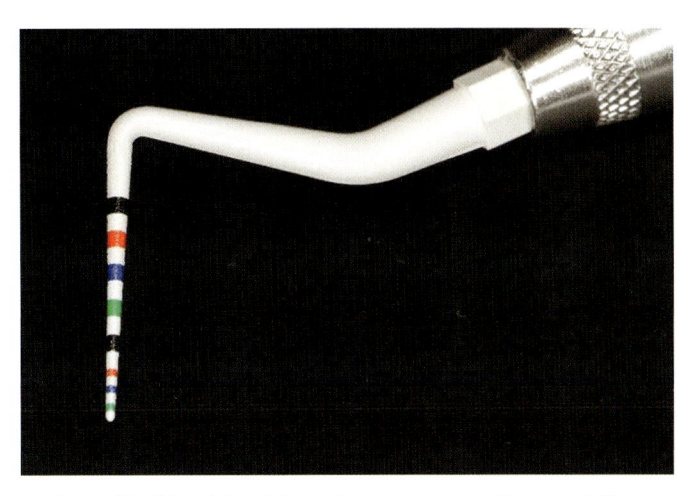

Figure 47.11 **(B)** The Goldstein Colorvue Prove (Hu-Friedy) has 1/2 mm increments up to 3 mm and 13 mm total in length. It is more comfortable for patients plus much easier to see in the mouth.

An occlusal check using articulating paper or the T-Scan II (Tekscan, Inc.) should be done annually. Patients with implant-supported restorations may also be prescribed an appropriate occlusal appliance to guard against parafunctional habits. Checking patient compliance with wear and care of the occlusal guard is recommended as part of the routine maintenance visit. Cleaning and adjusting the guard can be accomplished at the same time.

Locally applied chemotherapeutics

When tissue inflammation or radiographic bone level changes are observed, it does not necessarily mean the implant has failed or will inevitably do so. It is important to determine if the patient has peri-implantitis (involving bone) or mucositis (localized to tissues). Often, patients will not feel any pain from either of these conditions, which underscores the need for frequent maintenance visits for early detection and care. Early intervention with a locally applied antibiotic or antimicrobial, such as Arestin® (OraPharma, Inc.) or Atridox® (CollaGenex Pharmaceuticals, Inc.), may help decrease the bacterial load. This may effectively slow or reverse the inflammation associated with peri-implant disease.[28]

The use of antimicrobials such as chlorhexidine gluconate may also help control plaque and bacteria around dental implants. Rinses may be utilized with in-office irrigation or used long term at home.[29] Peri-implant irrigation should be done with a plastic irrigation tip designed for safe use around implants. For patients prone to occasional peri-implant tissue inflammation, an at-home regimen of daily cleansing with an antimicrobial rinse applied with soft manual toothbrush or a gentle power toothbrush may be helpful. The minimally abrasive and variable speed Rotadent (DenMat) plaque-removal instrument is ideally suited for daily gentle cleansing under and around the tissues of an implant. The densely compacted microfilaments of a Rotadent (DenMat) make it hydrophilic, which improves its capacity to apply medications directly under and around the tissues of an implant during routine brushing. Using a Rotadent (DenMat) for implant daily care also will remove plaque, disrupt biofilm, and decrease tartar buildup (Figure 47.12).

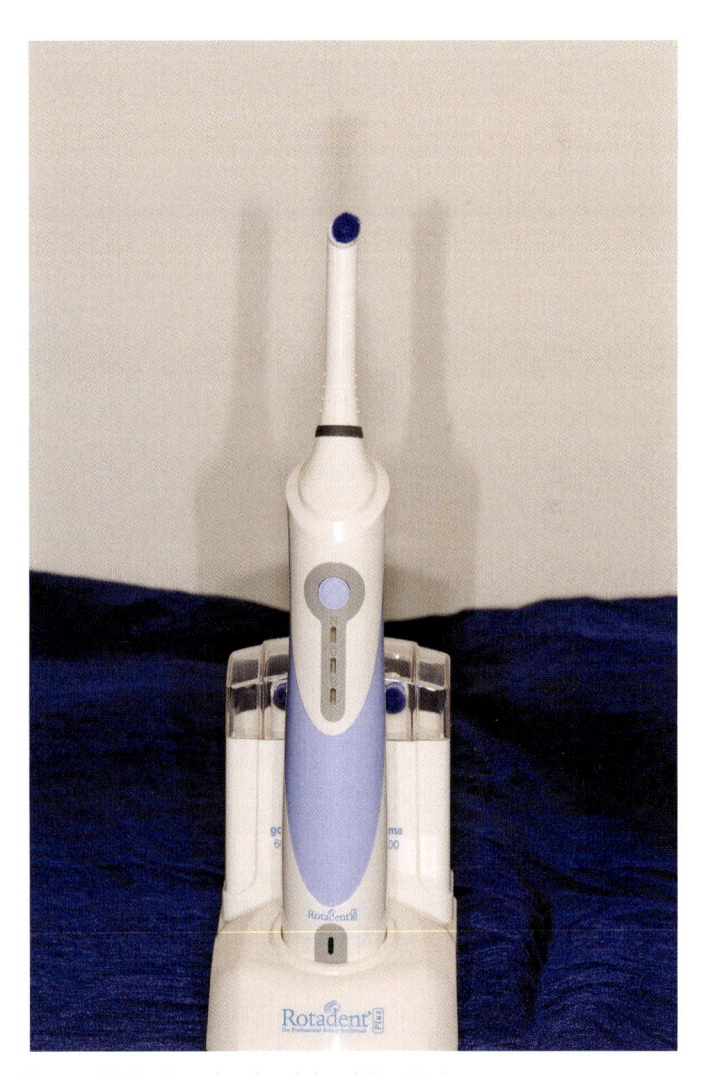

Figure 47.12 Rotadent brush head (DenMat).

Scaling

At each maintenance visit, removal of any biofilm, plaque, and/or calculus from the implant-supported restoration(s) is indicated. Traditional metal hand instruments can easily mar or scratch titanium implant abutments, and roughened surfaces make these metals more susceptible to biofilm, bacterial plaque, and calculus buildup, which in turn increases the chance of peri-implant inflammation. Therefore, surface damage should be minimized by using one of the scalers specifically designed for maintenance of dental implants (Figure 47.13A).

Several companies manufacture implant scalers and curettes. One example is Implacare (Hu-Friedy Manufacturing Company, Inc.) (Figure 47.13B). These hand instruments are typically made of plastic, titanium, or nylon. They are gentle but effective in removing accumulations around implants, and the scientific literature supports their use during implant hygiene/maintenance appointments.[30]

Controversy exists concerning the use of sonic or ultrasonic instruments around implants. To prevent damage to the implant surface and the peri-mucosal seal, power scalers should be used with extreme caution. Some manufacturers offer a plastic or carbon composite tip that is placed over the metal end of the sonic or ultrasonic instruments to reduce the chances of their damaging the implant. Even with the use of protective plastic sleeves, a clinician must use caution not to shred or chip the tip by inadvertently using it on any accessible implant threads. Small particles of plastic in an implant sulcus may provide a source of tissue irritation or infection.

Polishing

With proper care, the titanium surface of an implant abutment should not lose the highly polished finish created initially by the manufacturer. Because dental professionals rarely if ever need to restore an implant component's polished surface, "polishing" in the traditional sense does not apply to implants. The only indication for polishing an implant or the restoration that it supports may be for plaque removal, which can be safely accomplished with air polishing using sodium bicarbonate.[31] However, such prophylaxis must be accomplished with little or no abrasion to the titanium surface or the esthetic restorative material used to fabricate the restoration.

The implant components, including the restoration, may be cleaned with a traditional round soft rubber cup and a nonabrasive cleaning agent (e.g., ProCare). Rotadent (DenMat) brush tips and mandrels, designed for use on slow-speed handpieces, will achieve gentle and effective removal of plaque around implants. If no polishing agent is desired, one can simply use an antimicrobial liquid such as chlorhexidine, Listerine, or TheraSol.

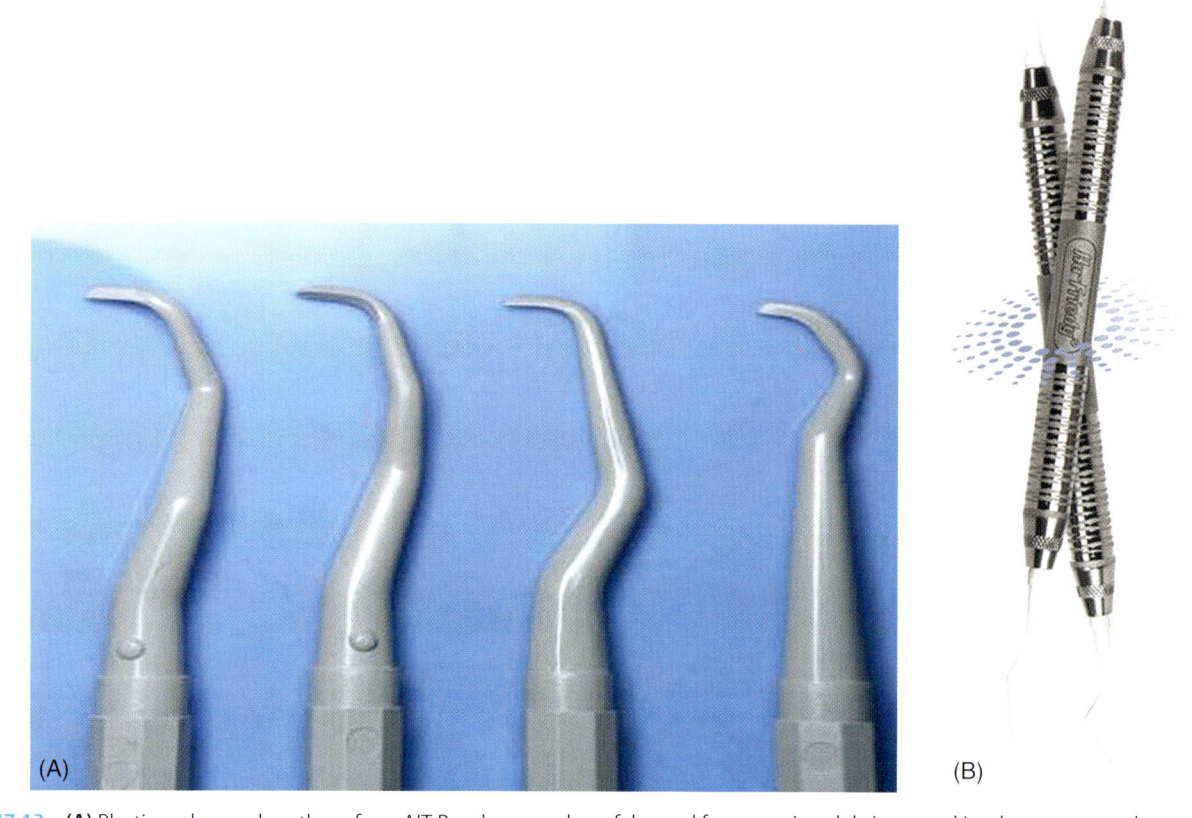

Figure 47.13 **(A)** Plastic scalers such as these from AIT Prophy+ may be safely used for removing debris around implant-supported restorations, without imparting damage to the implant collar, implant abutment, or restoration. **(B)** Hu-Friedy implant scalers.

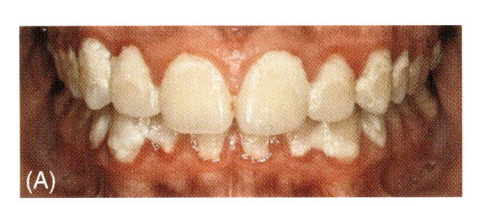

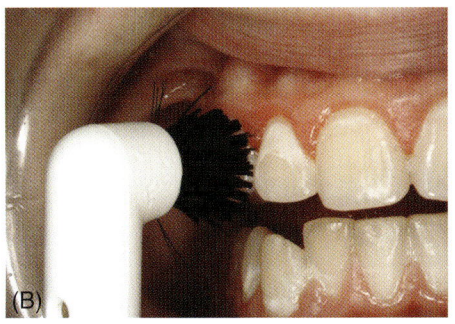

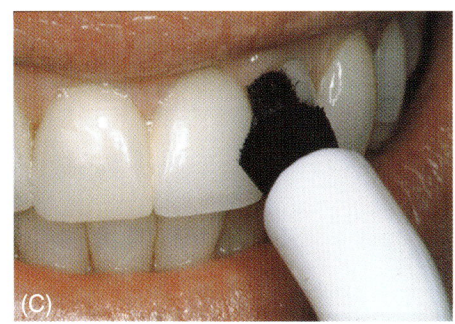

Figure 47.14 **(A)** This 13-year-old girl spent more time brushing her hair than her teeth, resulting in heavy plaque buildup and enamel decalcification. **(B)** Thorough prophylaxis plus home care instruction resulted in considerable plaque reduction. **(C)** The tapered brush head available from Rotadent (DenMat) is an excellent choice for patients with open interdental spaces.

One other situation worth considering is when a lack of keratinized gingiva is noted adjacent to dental implants. Considerable controversy has surrounded the question of whether this condition is harmful. Historically, an insufficiency of keratinized gingiva around teeth was considered undesirable and prompted the development of various gingival augmentation techniques. However, by 1994, the consensus of the European Workshop on Periodontology was that treatment for the sole purpose of increasing the apicoronal width of the gingiva to maintain periodontal health and prevent the development of soft-tissue recession around teeth could not be justified.[32]

Caution about the need for augmenting a lack of keratinized gingiva around implants also appears to be warranted. Results of numerous long-term implant studies have found little or no difference in the survival rate for implants surrounded by keratinized gingiva versus those adjacent to a dearth of it.[33–37] However, most of the implants studied have had smooth surfaces, rather than the textured surfaces that have more come to predominate. The impacts of a lack of keratinized gingiva on plaque consequences, inflammation, probing depths, recession, and bone loss also remain unclear in the face of contradictory research findings.

The conclusion of one recent comprehensive literature review[38] was that the need for keratinized gingiva around implants appears to be patient specific, with no method presently available to distinguish who would benefit from tissue augmentation. The reviewers concluded that it might be beneficial for chronically inflamed sites, locations where recession or continued loss of clinical attachment or bone continues despite periodontal therapy and good oral hygiene, sites that appear sore during brushing despite the appearance of gingival health, where a dental history suggests a predisposition to periodontitis or recession, where there is persistent patient noncompliance, or to improve esthetics.

Patient self-care

The long-term success of any implant and its restoration depends on several factors. These include the patient's genetic predisposition to inflammation and any systemic conditions that may affect their ability to fight bacterial infections in the mouth. Daily oral care by the patient is also critical to keeping the bioburden on the peri-implant area and oral cavity to a homeostatic minimum (Figure 47.14A and B).

Genetic considerations

A patient's genetic susceptibility to peri-implantitis should be considered prior to implant placement and during maintenance. Laine et al. have reported that the *IL-1* gene mutation is associated with implant complications.[39] The presence of this mutation can be determined by a salivary diagnostic evaluation (Celsus One™, OralDNA Labs (a service of Access Genetics), Eden Prairie, MN) (Figure 47.15). The patient's genetic risk result may then be used for establishing treatment and the frequency of dental hygiene maintenance. Additionally, a genetically positive patient may be more motivated to maintain an excellent daily care regimen to lessen the chance of a bacterial infection that in turn may cause implant complications.

Patient oral care instructions should include detailed risk factor explanation, verbal guidance, visual demonstration, and hands-on experience. As with all oral hygiene instruction, the techniques and products recommended should be individually chosen, and their effectiveness should be reevaluated during every maintenance visit. Constructive improvements should be taught, and techniques that are working well should be praised. Patients should understand that even in the presence of a genetic risk they can positively influence the health of their implants and surrounding tissues by minimizing other contributing factors, such as an increased bacterial load due to inadequate oral hygiene.

Interproximal/circumferential cleaning

Unlike the curves of a natural tooth, implants have a cylindrical and smooth profile. Many commercially available flosses, interproximal cleaners, and oral irrigation systems are safe for use around implants. Floss choice should be based on clinical indication. A single-tooth implant with intimate tissue adaptation may be best cleaned with flat, smooth floss. Traditional flossing of the mesial and distal surfaces is required, but floss should also be used on the facial/lingual surfaces. Patients must learn an implant-specific technique for looping the floss and then cleaning the implant circumferentially. Thicker woven flosses

Celsus One™

FINAL REPORT

Sample, Report
Date Of Birth: 09/20/1980
Gender: Female

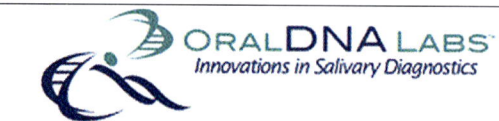

Sample Information
Specimen#: 3033031027
Accession#: 201702-09869
Specimen: Oral Rinse(P)

Collected: 02/11/2017
Received: 02/12/2017 12:57
Reported: 02/15/2017 11:31

Reason for Testing: Patient assessment/post treatment, Diabetes, Cardiovascular disease

CELSUS ONE: GENETIC ANALYSIS FOR MARKERS OF ORAL AND SYSTEMIC INFLAMMATION

Type of Immunity	Gene Marker	Genotype	Inflammation Index
Innate	Beta-defensin 1 (**DEFB1**)	G/A	Low Risk
Innate	CD14 (**CD14**)	T/T	Low Risk
Innate	Toll-like receptor 4 (**TLR4**)	AA/CC	Low Risk
Acquired	Tumor necrosis factor alpha (**TNF-alpha**)	C/C	Intermediate Risk
Acquired	Interleukin 1 (**IL1**)	TT/CT	Intermediate Risk
Acquired	Interleukin 6 (**IL6**)	C/C	Intermediate Risk
Acquired	Interleukin 17A (**IL17A**)	G/G	Intermediate Risk
Acquired	Matrix Metallopeptidase 3 (**MMP3**)	5A/5A	Intermediate Risk

Interpretation:

The genotypes for markers DEFB1, CD14 and TLR4 for this individual collectively predict a normal phenotype for the innate immune system and a low risk for chronic systemic inflammation. Specifically, the expected level of gene expression, and or levels of these proteins, is normal in response to environmental and disease causing bacteria and other effectors of inflammation. See comment.

The genotypes for markers TNF-alpha, IL1, IL6, IL17A, and MMP3 predict a slightly enhanced immune response to specific pathogens and an intermediate risk for chronic systemic inflammation. Based on this, gene expression and the corresponding protein levels, in response to disease causing bacteria and the other effectors of the acquired immune system, are predicted to be increased. See comment.

Disclaimer: The reported genotypes are a subset of the group of genes that comprise the complete immune system. This genetic analysis may not detect specific immunologic diseases or predict the health and effectiveness of a person's immunity for specific diseases. Such an evaluation may require genetic counseling and testing directed to characterize those genetic conditions.

Comments:

The innate immune system is the body's first line of defense against pathogenic organisms and a major cause of oral and systemic inflammation. The innate immunity functions to create a physical and chemical barrier to bacteria, the recruitment of inflammatory cells to the site of infection, the release of cytokines and the activation of the complement cascade to localize and eliminate bacteria and recruit antigen-recognizing lymphocytes. The acquired immune system involves the production of specialized cells that eliminate or prevent pathogen growth and is the basis for immunologic memory.

- **Periodontitis:** The genotype for the innate immune system marker, DEFB1, predicts an inability to maintain a balance of commensal oral bacteria. Thus, there is a predisposition to periodontal pathogenic bacterial infection. The acquired immune system IL1 and MMP3 genotypes predict an accentuated inflammatory response to pathogenic periodontal bacteria. The cytokine IL1 acts in concert with TNF-alpha to stimulate bone resorption by osteoclasts and to promote the release of matrix metalloproteinases. Further, the presence of a 'T' allele in both the IL1 alpha and beta polymorphic loci is associated with an increased severity of chronic periodontitis. Individuals with the MMP3 5A/5A genotype have elevated levels of gene transcription and an increased local expression of MMP3, and are 3 times more likely to develop chronic periodontitis.
- **Cardiovascular:** Chronic inflammation is implicated in the etiology of cardiovascular disease (CVD). There is also strong evidence to support that polymorphisms within the promoter regions of the cytokine genes for IL1, IL6 and MMP3 are linked to levels of gene expression which are associated with chronic inflammation. The cytokine IL1 beta upregulates the recruitment of inflammatory cells and the levels of matrix metalloproteinase to the site of cholesterol deposition at sites of atherosclerosis. Matrix metalloproteinases function to remove extracellular matrix products which is considered a risk factor to destabilize arterial plaque. Specifically, the 5A/5A genotype is associated with a higher risk of myocardial infarction (MI) at young age (males < 60 years) which increases to a 10-fold risk in those who smoke.
- **Type II Diabetes:** The 'T' allele of the IL1 beta gene is correlated with elevated serum glucose and altered glucose homeostasis. Further, it has been shown that insulin producing beta cells in the pancreas in persons with type 2 diabetes mellitus (T2DM) also have increased levels of the cytokine IL1 beta. Consequently, clinical studies conclude that the IL1 SNPs are associated with development of diabetic nephropathy through interactions with other pro- and anti-inflammatory mediators.

OralDNA Labs, A Service of Access Genetics, LLC, 7400 Flying Cloud Drive, Eden Prairie, MN 55344 Phone: 855-672-5362; Fax: 952-942-0703 www.oraldna.com
Medical Director: Ronald McGlennen MD, FCAP, FACMG, ABMG

Figure 47.15 Celsus One. *Source:* Reproduced with permission of Access Genetics, LLC.

| | Sample, Report | 09/20/1980 | 201702-09869 |

Gene Marker	Nucleic Acid Assignment	Reference Sequence Number (rs)	Overview
Beta-defensin 1 (DEFB1)	3 prime variant G>A	rs1047031	Defensins have been identified to be produced as an immediate response to pathogenic bacteria lipopolysaccharides (LPS) and are important elements of the innate immune system. These proteins have broad-spectrum antimicrobial activity against bacteria, fungi and some viruses. The G>A (guanine to adenine) nucleotide base variant in the three-prime untranslated region of this gene has been shown to be associated with increased risk for both chronic and aggressive periodontitis. (1)
CD14	-260 C>T	rs2569190	CD14 is a receptor present on monocytes, macrophages, neutrophils and some B cells, and dendritic cells that recognizes bacterial cell wall lipopolysaccharides (LPS). Thus, it can stimulate the innate immune response via tumor necrosis factor alpha (TNF-alpha) production. Individuals possessing the C/C genotype at position -260 have been reported to have a two-fold increased susceptibility to periodontitis. Conversely, the T/T genotype has been identified in a significantly higher frequency in healthy individuals. The T/T genotype has also been associated with a decreased prevalence of Prevotella intermedia. (2)
Tumor necrosis factor alpha (TNF-alpha)	-857 C>T	rs1799724	Tumor necrosis factor-alpha (TNF-alpha) is a type of messenger protein, that is produced by white blood cells. TNF-alpha helps regulate the immune response through promotion of inflammation and prompts the production of other cells involved in the inflammatory response. TNF-alpha cytokine production in -857 T allele carriers tends to be elevated, and the incidence of the variant allele is reported to be significantly higher in periodontitis patients than in healthy subjects. (3)
Toll-like Receptor 4 (TLR4)	+896 A>G +1196 C>T	rs4986790 rs4986791	Toll-like receptors (TLRs) are signal molecules essential for the cellular response to bacterial cell wall lipopolysaccharides (LPS) and are viewed as important connector elements between the innate and acquired immune responses. TLR4 cytokine expression has been shown to be increased in both macrophages and gingival fibroblasts located in inflamed gingival tissues indicating its importance in the inflammatory process. Studies have shown that two TLR 4 variants, 896 A>G and 1196 C>T are frequently inherited together and individuals who inherit a composite genotype that contains the 896 G allele are hyporesponsive to LPS stimulation. (4)
Interleukin 1 (IL1)	-889 C>T +3954 C>T	rs1800587 rs1143634	Interleukin 1 (IL1) cytokines induce other immune cells to secrete matrix metalloproteins (MMPs) and prostaglandins that enhance the inflammatory processes in periodontal tissues. Additionally, IL1 is a strong stimulator of connective tissue degradation. The IL1 alpha -889 single nucleotide polymorphism (SNP) has been identified to be in complete linkage with the IL1 alpha +4845 SNP which has previously been reported in combination with the IL1 beta +3954 C>T SNP. Multiple studies have reported that the presence of a T allele in each of the IL1 alpha and IL1 beta genotypes are associated with periodontal disease severity. (5,6,7)
Interleukin 6 (IL6)	-174 C>G	rs1800795	The interleukin-6 (IL6) cytokine is involved in a wide variety of biological functions. It is produced in response to inflammatory stimuli such as tumor necrosis factor (TNF-alpha), interleukin 1, and bacterial and viral infection. IL6 is a regulator of B-cell responses, is a stimulator of osteoclast differentiation and bone resorption and is an inhibitor of bone formation. It has also been shown that carriers of a single G allele are more predisposed to periodontitis than C/C carriers and individuals carrying the G/G genotype have a further increased risk of periodontitis. (8)
Interleukin 17A (IL17A)	-197 G>A	rs2275913	IL17 consists of a group of cytokines produced by activated T-lymphocytes as an element of the acquired (secondary) immune response. IL17A, a specific IL17 cytokine, appears to have a strong feedback effect on regulation and enhancement of the innate (initial) immune response through recruitment of neutrophils and macrophages that secrete TNF-alpha and IL1 beta. IL17A G/A and A/A genotypes are reported to be present in higher frequencies in patients with periodontitis than the G/G genotype. The A allele of IL17A has also been associated with more severe clinical parameters such as probing depth, clinical attachment loss and enhanced gingival tissue inflammation. (9)
Matrix Metallopeptidase 3 (MMP3)	-1171 5A/6A	rs3025058	Matrix metallopeptidase (MMPs) comprise the most important pathway to tissue destruction resulting from periodontal disease. The primary function of MMPs is the pathological breakdown of extracellular matrix, most importantly collagen type I, which is found in the periodontal ligament and alveolar bone organic matrix. Studies report that individuals with the 5A/5A genotype are approximately two- to three-fold more likely to develop periodontitis than individuals with 5A/6A or 6A/6A genotypes. (10)

OralDNA Labs, A Service of Access Genetics, LLC, 7400 Flying Cloud Drive, Eden Prairie, MN 55344 Phone: 855-672-5362; Fax: 952-942-0703 www.oraldna.com
Medical Director: Ronald McGlennen MD, FCAP, FACMG, ABMG   PL-000302-B

Figure 47.15   (Continued)

| Sample, Report | 09/20/1980 | 201702-09869 |

References:

1. Schaefer A, et al. The 3' UTR transition within DEFB1 is associated with chronic and aggressive periodontitis. Genes and Immunity 2010; 11:45-54.
2. Sahingur S, et al. Single nucleotide polymorphisms of pattern recognition receptors and chronic periodontitis. Journal of Periodontal Research 2011; 46:184-192.
3. Soga Y, et al. Tumor necrosis factor-alpha gene (TNF-alpha) -1031/-863, -857 single-nucleotide polymorphisms (SNPs) are associated with severe adult periodontitis in Japanese. Journal of Clinical Periodontology 2003; 30:524-531.
4. Schroder NJW, et al. Chronic periodontal disease is associated with single-nucleotide polymorphisms of the human TLR4 gene. Genes and Immunity 2005; 6: 448-451.
5. Kornman K, et al. The interleukin 1 genotype as a severity factor in adult periodontal disease. Journal of Clinical Periodontology 1997; 24:7-77.
6. Wagner J, et al. Prevalence of OPG and IL1 gene polymorphisms in chronic periodontitis. Journal of Clinical Periodontology 2007; 34(10):823-827.
7. Taylor J, et al. Cytokine gene polymorphisms and immunoregulation in periodontal disease. Periodontology 2000, 2004; 35:158-182.
8. Dias Correa J, et al. Association between polymorphisms in interleukin-17A and 17F genes and chronic periodontal disease. Mediators of Inflammation 2012; 2012:1-9
9. Li G, et al. Association of matrix metalloproteinase (MMP)-1, 3, 9, interleukin (IL)-2, 8 and cyclooxygenase (COX)-2 gene polymorphisms with chronic periodontitis in a Chinese population. Cytokine 2006; 60:552-560.
10. Letra A. MMP3 and TIMP1 variants contribute to chronic periodontitis and may be implicated in disease progression. Journal of Clinical Periodontology 2012; 39:707-716.
11. Internet accessible websites: www.medterms.com, http://medical-dictionary.com, www.thefreedictionary.com, www.thefreelibrary.com

Methodology: Genomic DNA was subjected to amplification by methods of target enrichment, a version of nested patch PCR, and then sequenced using a MiSeq. The resulting DNA sequences were analyzed using alignment and base call algorithms in the Kailos Blue software. The patient report was created by the review of these analyzed data along with the selection of medical comment and recommendations via TeleGene, a proprietary laboratory information system of Access Genetics, LLC. The analytical and performance characteristics of these laboratory-developed tests (LDT) were determined by Kailos Genetics pursuant to Clinical Laboratory Improvement Amendments (CLIA 88) requirements. It has not been cleared or approved by the U.S. Food and Drug Administration (FDA). The FDA has determined that such clearance or approval is not a requirement prior to use for clinical purposes.
Technical assay performed by Kailos Genetics, Huntsville, AL 855-323-0680

Web enabled system provided by: access genetics

OralDNA Labs, A Service of Access Genetics, LLC, 7400 Flying Cloud Drive, Eden Prairie, MN 55344 Phone: 855-672-5362; Fax: 952-942-0703 www.oraldna.com
Medical Director: Ronald McGlennen MD, FCAP, FACMG, ABMG

Figure 47.15 (Continued)

are indicated for larger interproximal spaces or for the long expanses of a bar-retained prosthesis.

The choice of interproximal brushes and cleaners should also be based on the area where they will be used. Larger spaces may be best cleaned with interdental brushes; these come in various shapes, including an interproximal Rotadent (DenMat) brush, and can be selected to fit. Smaller interdental brushes are also helpful in narrower interproximal spaces (Figure 47.14C).

Irrigation

Water irrigation units, such as the Hydro Floss (Hydro Floss, Inc.), are beneficial in implant maintenance. However, personalized instruction with such units is important. The water stream must be directed interproximally and horizontally between implants so the patient does not inadvertently damage the peri-implant seal. There are specially designed subgingival tips that can be utilized safely and effectively for daily cleansing and biofilm disruption. As with natural teeth, interproximal and circumferential cleaning of implants is recommended on a daily basis (Figure 47.16) (Hydro Floss, Inc.).

Brushing

Twice-daily brushing is recommended to remove oral debris and bacterial plaque accumulations. Implant self-care should be accomplished using a soft traditional toothbrush (Nimbus Microfine (Nimbus Dental) GUM Deep Clean), or a very gentle power brush, as previously discussed. While many traditional and mechanical brushes are available for over-the-counter purchase, the professionally dispensed Rotadent (DenMat) with its patented microfilaments is perhaps the gentlest and most effective tool for daily cleaning around implant-supported esthetic restorations. Its dense brush head does a superior job removing bacterial plaque, while the action is gentle to soft tissue and nonabrasive to the abutment (Figure 47.17).

Bacterial monitoring

One of the newest tools available for monitoring implant health involves the science of salivary diagnostics. From a patient's saliva sample, an analysis can be obtained that provides a detailed report of a patient's existing bacterial profile. Recognizing the role of bacteria in peri-implant mucositis as well as peri-implantitis, the dental team and patient can use the bacterial report to monitor bacterial risk and identify bacterial infections prior to the development of any clinical signs and symptoms.

Intraoral camera

Patients need to be able to recognize healthy peri-implant tissue. An intraoral camera can be a very helpful teaching tool. A common problem associated with implants is a piece of food

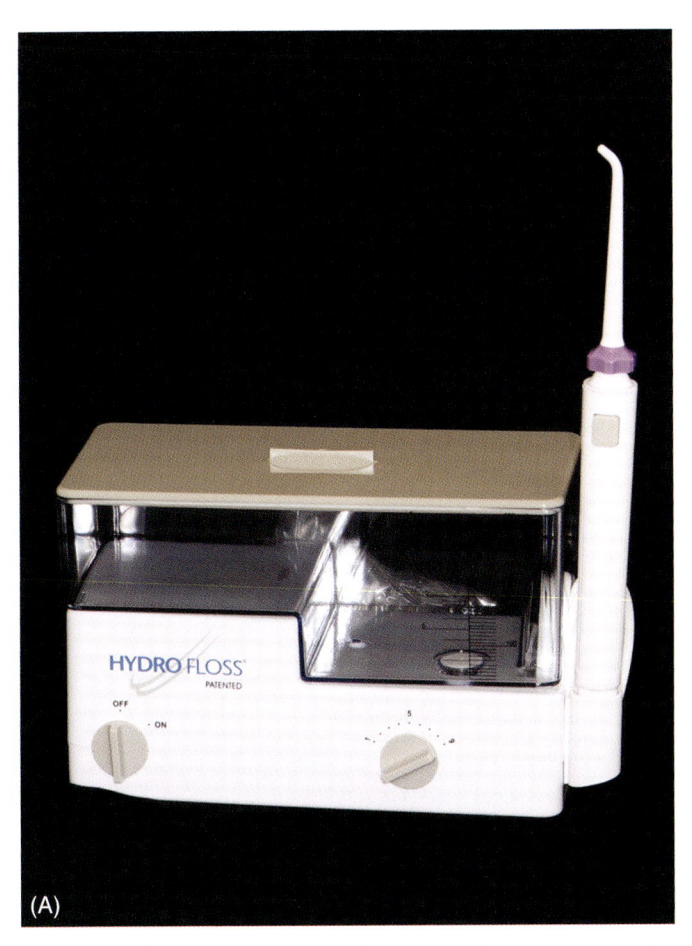

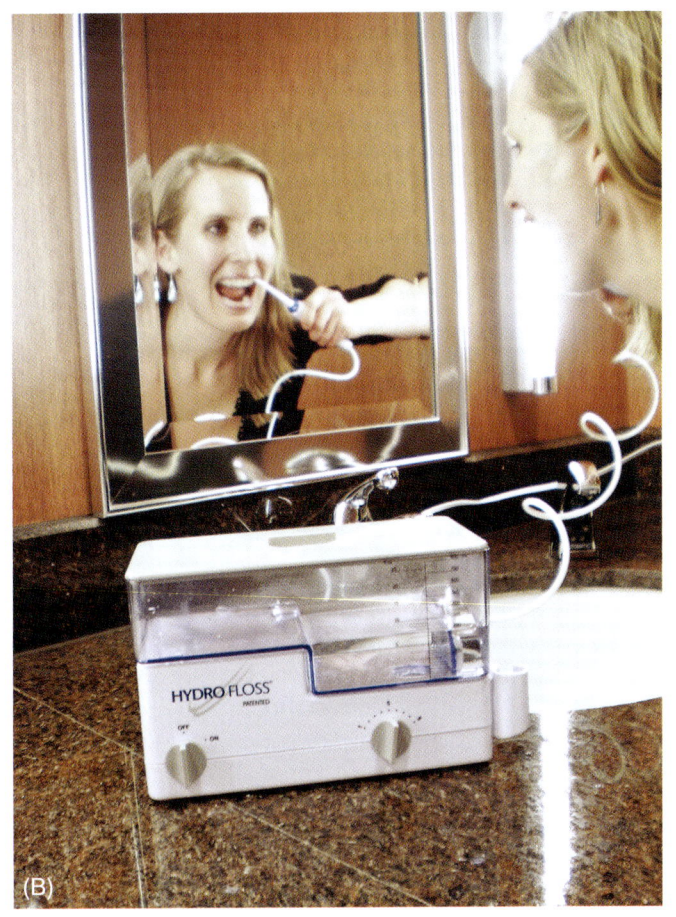

Figure 47.16 **(A)** Water irrigation, such as a Hydro Floss, can be an effective part of oral care for many patients. **(B)** Hydro Floss in use. (Hydro Floss, Inc.)

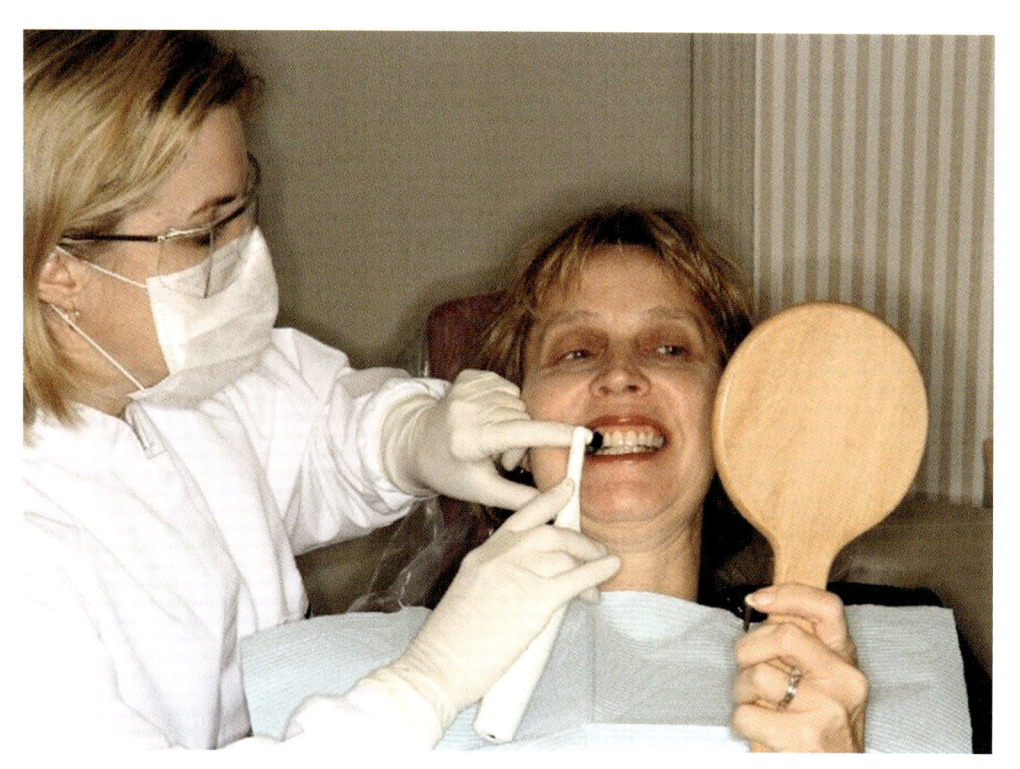

Figure 47.17 Hands-on demonstration with a hand mirror is essential in order for a patient to understand that a brush must be carefully placed to accomplish effective plaque removal.

or shred of floss lodged in the peri-implant space. Patients tend to be less aware when this occurs than when a similar object lodges under the soft-tissue around a natural tooth. Careful soft tissue observation by implant recipients should be a part of their daily oral care. They should immediately report to their dentist or hygienist any tissue irregularities, including tenderness, redness, swelling, or other symptoms around the implant. Early preventive steps can be taken to avoid a severe infection, and this can make the difference between the implant's long-term success and failure.

Conclusion

According to a 2010 study in the *Journal of the American Dental Association*, the placement of dental implants is increasing while other dental procedures are in decline.[40] Patients reportedly are seeking dental implants in record numbers. The global dental implants market is expected to be USD 6.81 billion by 2024, based on a 2016 report by Grand View Research, Inc.[41] As implants continue to become a desirable and routine choice for esthetic restorative dentistry, dental professionals increasingly will be caring for implant-supported esthetic restorations. Patients presenting for implant therapy should be counseled in self-care requirements prior to placement and continually as part of ongoing maintenance. The critical role of hygiene care for implant-supported restorations can directly affect the implant's lifespan. As with other esthetic restorative dentistry, the combined efforts of the well-trained dental professional and well-educated patient can maximize the beauty and lifespan of esthetic implant-supported teeth.

References

1. Vered Y, Zini A, Mann J, et al. Teeth and implant surroundings: clinical health. Indices and microbiologic parameters. *Quintessence Int* 2011;42(4):339–344.
2. Berchier CE, Slot DE, Haps S, Van der Weijden GA. The efficacy of dental floss in addition to a toothbrush on plaque and parameters of gingival inflammation: a systematic review. *Int J Dent Hyg* 2008;6(4):265–279.
3. Barnes CM, Gluch JI, Lyle DM, Jahn C. Devices for oral self-care. In: *Dental Hygiene, Concepts, Cases and Competencies*, 2nd edn. Philadelphia, PA: Elsevier; 2008:457–467.
4. Silverstein LH, Kurtzman GM. Oral hygiene and maintenance of dental implants. *Dent Today* 2006;25(3):70–75.
5. American Dental Association, US Department of Health and Human Services. *The Selection of Patients for Dental Radiographic Examinations. Revised 2012.* https://www.fda.gov/Radiation-EmittingProducts/RadiationEmittingProductsandProcedures/MedicalImaging/MedicalX-Rays/ucm116504.htm (accessed November 18, 2017).
6. Barnes CM, Toothaker RW, Ross JA. Polishing dental implants and implant restorations. *J Pract Hyg* 2006;15:28–29.
7. Barnes CM. Care and maintenance of aesthetic restorations. *J Pract Hyg* 2004;14:19–22.
8. Barnes CM, Covey D, Johnson WW, St. Germain HA. Maintaining restorations for senior dental patients. *J Pract Hyg* 2003;12:25.
9. Barnes CM, Covey DA, Walker MP, Johnson WW. Essential selective polishing: the maintenance of esthetic restorations. *J Pract Hyg* 2003;12:18–24.
10. Barnes CM. Polishing esthetic restorative materials: the successful maintenance of esthetic restorations. *Dimensions Dent Hyg* 2010;8(1):24–28.

11. Hoelscher DC, Neme AM, Pink FE, Hughes PJ. The effect of three finishing systems on four esthetic restorative materials. *Oper Dent* 1998;23(1):36–42.
12. Augthun M, Tinschert J, Huber A. In vitro studies on the effect of cleaning methods on different implant surfaces. *J Periodontol* 1998;69(8):857–864.
13. Sunell S, Rucker L. Surgical magnification in dental hygiene practice. *Int J Dent Hyg* 2004;2(1):26–35.
14. Barnes CM. The science of polishing: appropriate technique and advances in traditional polishing. *Dimensions Dent Hyg* 2009;7(11):18–22.
15. Jeffries SR. Abrasive finishing and polishing in restorative dentistry: a state-of-the-art review. *Dent Clin North Am* 2007;51:379–397.
16. Barnes CM. Polishing materials and abrasion. In: Bagby M, Gladwin M, eds. *Clinical Aspects of Dental Materials*, 3rd edn. Philadelphia, PA: Lippincott Williams & Wilkins; 2012:203–214.
17. Lai YL, Lin YC, Change CS, Lee SY. Effects of sonic and ultrasonic scaling on the surface roughness of tooth-colored restorative materials for cervical lesions. *Oper Dent* 2007;32(3):273–278.
18. Rajstein J, Tal M. The effect of ultrasonic scaling on the surface of Class V amalgam restorations—a scanning electron microscopy study. *J Oral Rehabil* 1984;11:299–305.
19. Goldstein RE, Nimmons KJ. Maintenance of esthetic restorations. *Contemp Esthet Restorative Pract* 2002;(February):10–15.
20. Ten Bruggenkate CM, van der Kwast WA, Oosterbeck HS. Success criteria in oral implantology: a review of the literature. *Int J Oral Implantol* 1990;7:45–53.
21. Misch CM, Perel ML, Wang HL, et al. Implant success, survival, and failure: the International Congress of Oral Implantologists (ICOI) Pisa Consensus Conference. *Implant Dent* 2008;17(1):5–15.
22. Fenton AH, Jamshaid A, David D. Osseointegrated fixture mobility. *J Dent Res* 1987;66:114–116.
23. Adell R, Lekholm U, Rockler B, Branemark PI. A 15 year study of osseointegrated implants in the treatment of the edentulous jaw. *Int J Oral Surg* 1981;10(6):387–416.
24. Karoussis IK, Salvi GE, Heitz-Mayfield LJ, et al. Long-term implant prognosis with and without a history of chronic periodontitis: a 10-year prospective cohort study of the ITI Dental Implant System. *Clin Oral Implant Res* 2003;14(3):329–339.
25. Kurtzman GM, Silverstein LH. Dental implants: oral hygiene and maintenance of dental implants. *Dent Today* 2007;1(3):47–53.
26. Esposito M, Hirsch J-M, Lekholm U, Thomsen P: Biological factors contributing to failures of osseointegrated oral implants. (I) Success criteria and epidemiology. *Eur J Oral Sci* 1998;106:527–551.
27. Misch CE. An implant is not a tooth: a comparison of periodontal indices. In: Misch CE, Abbas HA, eds. *Contemporary Implant Dentistry*. St. Louis, MO: Mosby; 2008:1055–1072.
28. Salvi GE, Persson GR, Heitz-Mayfield LJA, et al. Adjunctive local antibiotic therapy in the treatment of peri-implantitis II: clinical and radiographic outcomes. *Clin Oral Implants Res* 2007;18:281–285.
29. Misch CE. Maintenance of dental implants: implant quality of health scale. In: Misch CE, Abbas HA, eds. *Contemporary Implant Dentistry*, 3rd ed. St. Louis, MO: Mosby; 2008:1073–1088.
30. Speelman JA, Collaert BB, Klinge BB. Evaluation of different methods to clean titanium abutments. A scanning electron microscopic study. *Clin Oral Implants Res* 1992;3(3):120–127.
31. Barnes CM, Fleming LS, Mueninghoff LA. SEM evaluation of the in-vitro effects of an air-abrasive system on various implant surfaces. *Int J Oral Maxillofac Implants* 1991;6(4):463–469.
32. Lindhe J, Echeverria JJ. Consensus report of session II. In: Lang NP, Karring T, eds. *Proceedings of the 1st European Workshop on Periodontology*. Berlin: Quintessence; 1994:210–214.
33. Brånemark PI, Svensson B, Van Steenberghe D. Ten-year survival rates of fixed prostheses on four or six implants ad modum Brånemark in full edentulism. *Clin Oral Implants Res* 1995;6(4):227–231.
34. Buser D, Mericske-Sterm R, Bernard JP, et al. Long-term evaluation of non-submerged ITI implants. Part 1: 8-year life table analysis of a prospective multi-center study with 2359 implants. *Clin Oral Implants Res* 1997;8(3):161–172.
35. Jemt T, Chai J, Harnett J, et al. A 5-year prospective multicenter follow-up report on overdentures supported by osseointegrated implants. *Int J Oral Maxillofac Implants* 1996;11(3):291–298.
36. Lindquist LW, Carlsson GE, Jemt T. A prospective 15-year follow-up study of mandibular fixed prostheses supported by osseointegrated implants. Clinical results and marginal bone loss. *Clin Oral Implants Res* 1996;7(4):329–336.
37. Mericske-Sterm R. Clinical evaluation of overdenture restorations supported by osseointegrated titanium implants: a retrospective study. *Int J Oral Maxillofac Implants* 1990;5(4):375–383.
38. Greenstein G, Cavallaro J. The clinical significance of keratinzed gingiva around dental implants. *Compend Contin Educ Dent* 2011;32(8):24–32.
39. Laine ML, Leonhardt A, Roos-Jansåker AM, et al. IL-1RN gene polymorphism is associated with peri-implantitis. *Clin Oral Implants Res* 2006;17:380–385.
40. Eklund SA. Trends in dental treatment: 1992–2007. *J Am Dent Assoc* 2010:141(4):391–399.
41. Accessed January 19, 2018. https://www.grandviewresearch.com/press-release/global-dental-implants-market.

Index

Page numbers in *italics* indicate figures; those in **bold** tables. Page numbers preceded by A, B, C or D refer to the appendices at the end of Volume 1.

abandonment, patient 145, 152
abfractions *704*, 704–708
    clinical cases 707–708, *707–708*
    differential diagnosis 711–712
    gingival recession and 1184
    mechanisms 704–707, *705–706*
    restorations 707
    scratch test 712
aboriginal populations 695–696
abrasion 708–709, *710*
    abfraction lesions 705, *706*, 707
    bleaching and 335
    differential diagnosis 711–712
    masticatory 708
    porcelain veneers 439
    restoration 708, *709*
    simulating tooth 219
abrasive strips, interproximal finishing 409
Absolute adhesive system 366
abutments
    fixed partial dentures 547, *548*
        cantilever bridges 555
        functional considerations 546–547
        partial-coverage retainers 549
        radiographic evaluation 544–545
        splinting 555
        telescoping crowns 555–562
    implant 657–658, *659*
        platform interface 1370, *1370–1371*

        restoration interface 1372–1374, *1373–1374*
        soft tissue interface 1370–1372, *1371–1372*
    removable partial dentures
        attachment 592, 594–595, 605
        clasp placement 584, *584*
        endodontic access 780
        radiographic evaluation 582
        selection 583–584
accelerated osteogenic orthodontics (AOO) 957–959
acceptability threshold 274
acetone-based primers, dentin bonding 359
acid demineralization, for root coverage 1183, 1185–1186
acid etching
    ceramic restorations *see* hydrofluoric acid etching
    dentin 359, *359*
        after laser ablation 972
        ceramic veneers 468, *471*
        composite resin bonding 403
    enamel 356, *356–357*
        after laser ablation 972
        ceramic restorations 468, *471*, *1362*, *1364*
        composite resin bonding 401, 403
    history of development 358
    pulpal irritation 134, 363, 401

    pulp capping with 769
    selective 358, 361, 403
    self-etch adhesives **357**, 357–358
    total (etch-and-rinse) 359, *359*, 403
acidic beverages/foods 710, 822–825
    dental erosion 33, 822–824, *824*
    erosion of veneers 477
    pH values **711**
Acromycin staining 755
acrylic (resin)
    A-splints 1320–1323
    camouflaging RPD clasps 590
    cosmetic stent, for actors 1155, *1156*
    crowns 502, *505*
    denture base 624, *624*
    denture teeth 616, 626–627, *627–629*
    implant provisionals 656
    occlusal registration 1305, *1306*
    overlays, for actors 1156–1160, *1158–1164*
    tissue inserts *1161*, *1164*, 1323
    veneers 461, D7
actors *see* performers/actors
Adair, Peter 506
addition silicone (polyvinyl siloxane; PVS) impressions 1291, *1292*, 1388
    ceramic veneers 460, *460*
    disinfection 1302
    material properties **1293**, 1293–1294
    mixing 1292, *1293*

AdheSE adhesive 366, 368
adhesion 355–367
    aging of adhesive interface 363–365, *364*
    classification of adhesive systems 360–362, **362**
    definitions 356
    dentin *358*, 358–360, *361*
        after laser ablation 972–973
        ceramic veneers 452, *468*, 471
        composite resins 403
        primers/priming adhesives 359–360
        priming of collagen network 360
        self-etch adhesives 360, *360*
        stabilization 360
        technique sensitivity 365–366, *366*
        tooth sensitivity after 366–367, 403
    enamel 356–358, 360, *361*
        after laser ablation 972–973
        ceramic restorations 1373
        ceramic veneers 439, *468*, 471
        composite resin 401, 403
        conditioning/etching 356, 356–357
        historical development 358
        mechanisms 356–358, *357*
        self-etch adhesives **357**, 357–358
    failure prevention 367–368
    marginal gaps 355, *356*
    postoperative hypersensitivities 366–367
    prerequisites 356
adhesives 356
    air-thinning 404
    all-in-one *see under* self-etch adhesives
    biocompatibility 363
    ceramic veneers 471
    classification 360–362, **362**
    clinical recommendations 367–368
    dark-curing 361–362
    dentin bonding 359–360
    dual-curing 361–362, **362**
    etch-and-rinse *see* etch-and-rinse adhesive systems
    evaluation 363, *363*
    filled 362, *363*
    impression tray 1294
    self-etch *see* self-etch adhesives
    universal 361, **362**
    see also cement(s)
adjustment disorders 27, 41–42
adolescents
    tooth wear 696, *696*
    see also pediatric dentistry
advertising 124, 125–128, *126*
    word-of-mouth 115
agar hydrocolloid impressions 1302, 1388
agenesis of teeth (congenitally missing teeth) 982–983
    diastemas 843
    ectodermal dysplasia 982–983, *982–983*
    orthodontics 996, *996–997*
age-related changes
    crown restorations and 527, *527*

facial thirds 245, *246*, 1101–1102, *1106–1107*
    incisal embrasures 247
    incorporating 219, *221–222*
    lower face 1137, *1138*
    midface 1133–1134, *1136*
    reducing 219–221, *223*
    smile design 248, *248*
    tooth appearance and **225**, *225*
    tooth exposure at rest 1119–1120, *1121*
    tooth size–arch length discrepancies 919–921
    see also older adults
aging, population 1015–1016, **1016**
air-abrasive technology 417–421
    caries management 417–419, *418*
    dulling metal restorations 1169
    prior to cementation 1356
    prior to composite resin bonding 396
    repair of existing restorations 419–421, 1227–1230, *1228*
    stained teeth 341, 670
air polishing 1417
air-thinning, bonding agents 404
alcohol abuse 825, *825*
Align Technology 1396–1397
all-ceramic crowns 506–514
    bilayer 1375
        glass ceramics 506, 1376
        oxide ceramics 507–510, *508–509*, 1377–1378, *1378*
        see also under porcelain veneers
    cementation 1361, *1362–1364*
    color matching 534, *535*
    crowded teeth **882**, 887–890, *888–889*, 1283
    endodontic access 778
    factors influencing choice 523, 525–526
    fixed partial denture retainers 550, *551–552*
    implants 658–663, *662*, 662–663
    longevity **513**, 1236, 1249–1250
    margins 553
    materials 506–514, 1264
    monolithic 506, 507–510, 1375, *1376*
    rubber dam placement 772–773, *773*
    technical failure 1255
    telescoping, as abutments 559
    tooth preparation 1263–1271
        esthetic depth determination 1268–1270, *1271–1276*
        positioning gingival margin *1267*, 1267–1268
        soft-tissue health 1264–1266, *1265–1267*
        thickness of marginal gingiva 1264
        tooth reduction 1268–1271, *1269–1276*
        types of margins 1277–1280
    troubleshooting **507**
    try-in 1341, *1341–1342*
    see also ceramic restorations; crowns

all-ceramic resin-bonded bridges 549–550, *550*
all-ceramic/zirconia fixed partial dentures 564
all-metal crowns
    as fixed partial denture retainers 550
    longevity 1244
    see also gold crowns
allogenic tissues, root coverage surgery 1184
alloplastic implant augmentation 959, *962*
Allport, Gordon 10, 11
alternative treatments
    cost issues 80
    obligations to disclose 48, 132–133
    patient decision making 48
    presentation to patients 63, *65*, 67
aluminum chloride 1236
aluminum oxide (alumina)
    densely sintered high-purity 1377
    endodontic access 777, *778*
    –feldspathic bilayer crowns 507–510, *508–509*, 1264
    glass-infiltrated 1377
    veneers 441
alveolar ridge *see* ridge
amalgam
    cosmetic replacement
        ceramic partial coverage restorations 480, *482–484*
        informed consent *136*, 137
    islands, bulimia nervosa 33, *33*
    prophylactic removal 136–137
    tissue discoloration (tattoo) 805, *807*
    tooth discoloration 379, *675*, 675–676, *677*
amelodentinal dysplasia 975, *975*
amelogenesis imperfecta
    tooth discoloration 330, 679, *680*
    tooth wear 697
American Academy of Esthetic Dentistry 303, 614, D2
American Association of Orthodontists (AAO) 899
American Board of Orthodontics (ABO), criteria for ideal occlusion 915
American Board of Plastic Surgery (ABPS) 1140
American Dental Association (ADA)
    classification of casting alloys 514
    color change units (ccu) 277
    Principles of Ethics and Code of Professional Conduct 138
    radiographic guidelines **1413–1414**
American Medical Association Code of Medical Ethics 138
American Society for Aesthetic Plastic Surgery (ASAPS) 14–16
American Society of Plastic Surgeons (ASPS) 14, 16
ammonium bifluoride etchant 506
anabolic steroids 825
Andrews, Lawrence F. 915

anesthetic test, painful tooth 763–764
Angle classification, inadequacy 1076, *1077*
angle of correction, cosmetic contouring 305–306, *307*
angry patients 38, *39*
ankylosis 793–794
anorexia nervosa (AN) 26, 34–36, 822
  diagnostic criteria **32**
  signs 822, *823–824*
  worksheet for diagnosed **35–36**
anterior facial plane 1063, *1070*
anterior teeth
  cantilever fixed partial dentures 555, *556*
  complete dentures
    placement 616–620, *622*, 622–623
    size and form 614–615
  composite restorations 382–385, *384–389*
  fractured endodontically-treated 739–743
    options for restoring 732–733, *733–734*
    post and core options 739, **739**
    post-and-core restoration 739–743, *740–742*
  single missing 555, *555–557*
  too narrow 210–211, *212–213*
  too wide 208–209, *208–209*
  see also central incisors; mandibular anterior teeth; maxillary anterior teeth
antidepressant medications 28
antimicrobial rinses, implant patients 1421
anxiety mood disorders 26, 38
anxious patients 37–38
apexification 1219–1220
apical tooth forms, smile design 248, *250*
apnea–hypopnea index (AHI) 962
apologies 138
arch, dental
  age-related changes 919–921
  alignment, evaluation 56
  checking crown position 1345
  circumference, curve of Spee depth and 921–922
  irregularity
    correction 1094, *1097–1098*
    cosmetic contouring 319, *320–322*
    crowns 526, *526*
    special effects 218, *219–221*
  length 920–921
    pediatric patients 995–996
  orthodontic distalization 921
  perimeter 920–921, *921*
  space
    Berliner's formula 878, *879*
    deficiencies, crowded teeth 878, *878*
    maintenance in children 995–996
    measurement 921, *921*
archwires, esthetic 909
Arens, Donald E 750
A.R.T. Bond adhesive 366
arthritis 1022, 1024
artificial teeth *see* denture teeth
artistic skill, dentist's 80

A-splint, temporary immobilization 1320–1323, *1321–1323*
assisted-living residents 1036–1037
attachment removable partial dentures 590–606
  adjunctive procedures 593
  biomechanics and support 594–595
  classification 596, **596**
  cost 594, 597
  deciding to use 591–594
    contraindications 592–593, 594
    indications 592
    patient factors 592–593, 594
  definition 591
  extracoronal 596, 599–605
    advantages 599
    disadvantages 599–600
    types 600–605, *601–606*
  intracoronal 595–596, *596*, 597–599
    advantages 597
    disadvantages 597
    types 597–599, *598–599*
  nonprecision 591
  path of insertion 595
  placed in pontics 593, *594*
  precision 591
  retention 595, 596
  selection of type 595–597
  semiprecision 591
  special-use 605–606, *606–607*
  tooth preparation 595
  treatment planning 590–591
attitude, patient's 53
attractiveness *see* physical attractiveness phenomenon
attrition 696–702, *698–699*
  clinical cases *700–704*, 702–703
  differential diagnosis 711–712
  evaluation of tooth wear 697–698
  mechanisms 696–697
  treatment 699–702
aureomycin 682, *755*
avulsions, tooth 793–794, 1223–1224
  inflammatory root resorption after 794, *799–801*
  replantation 1223–1224, *1226*

baby boomers 1016–1017
background, tooth color matching 275–276
bacterial monitoring, implant health 1419, *1420*, 1427
Bali 298, *298*
base, complete dentures 623–625, *623–625*
base metal alloys 514, 571
Beaudreau's proportionate ratio 254
beauty
  commercial aspects 13–14
  concepts 3, 899–900
  esthetic dentistry and 1085–1086
  facial proportions *see* facial proportions
  facial symmetry and 1089–1090, *1089–1090*, 1094–1095

  rewards of 5–6
  trends 1005
  visual perception 1086, *1086*
  see also facial esthetics; physical attractiveness phenomenon
beauty pageant contestants 298, 1089, 1154
Begg, P.R. 696, 920
Belushi, Jim *1157*
Bergen, S.F. 273
beryllium casting alloys 514
betel nut chewing 677, 816, *816*
beveled margin
  anterior veneers 442, *444*
  composite resin bonding 384, 389, 398
  overlay technique 388, 398–400, *402*
  stained restorations 1252, *1256*
beveled shoulder margin, metal–ceramic restorations 516–517, *517*, 522, *522*
beverages
  acidic *see* acidic beverages/foods
  composite restoration longevity and 409–412
  in-office provision 118
  tooth discoloration 328, 675, *679*
billboard advertising 128
Biloc and Plasta attachments 596, 597–599, *599*
Biodentine 769
biologic width invasion
  crown lengthening and 1205–1206
  legal considerations 149–150, *151*
  subgingival margins 1267, *1267*
bipolar disorder (BD) 26, 29–30
bipolar electrosurgery, gingival retraction 1291
bisphenol A-glycidyl methacrylate (bis-GMA) resin 360, 394
bite registration 1303–1307
  full-arch final 1306–1307, *1306–1307*
  occlusal registration 1303–1305, *1305–1306*
bite test 761–762, *761–762*, 799, *802*
Black, G.V. 134
black lighting, effects of 1178
black line stain 674–675
black stains **671,** *677–678*, 751
black triangles
  fixed partial dentures 548–549, 565–566, 570
  orthodontic aspects *902*, 913–914, *914*
  patient preferences 138
  see also interdental spaces
bleaching 325–350, 687
  baseline color measurement 336, *337*
  calcified pulp chamber 788–789, *790–793*
  complications and risks 350
  endodontically-treated teeth *see under* endodontically-treated teeth
  home (without dental supervision) 345

bleaching (cont'd)
  in-office vital 331–341
    contraindications 331–332
    with matrix bleaching 341–343, 343–345
    meeting expectations 332, *332*
    procedures 336–341, *338–340*
    results 341, *341*
    sequence of treatment 333–335, *333–335*
  localized brown stains 682–683, *685*
  matrix 341–345
  nonvital teeth 346–350, *347*
    color relapse 350
    complications and risks 350, 783–784, *785*
    continued treatment 349
    contraindications 346
    finishing 349
    inside-outside tray technique 348
    malpractice case 148, *150*
    nonnegligent risks 144
    out-of-office technique *348*, 348–349
    pediatric patients 988–989, *988–989*, 993
    precautions 144
    preparatory procedures 347–348
    results 349, *349*
    techniques 346–349
  older adults 331, 333–336, 1025, 1026, *1026*
  performers/actors 1167
  power/matrix combined 341–343, *343–345*
  prerestorative 844
  problem patients 78
  shade guides for monitoring 277–279, *279*, 336, *337*
  single dark tooth 682, *683–685*
  as stepping-stone to veneers 687
  tetracycline-stained teeth 328–329, *329–330*, 683–686, *686*, 687
  tooth color effects 274, 277–278
  vital teeth 326, 331–346
    children 335, *336*
    history 326, *327*
    in-office 331–341
    maintaining results 346
    nightguard 341–343
    older adults 335–336, 1025
    over-the-counter systems 345
    sequence of treatment 333–335, *333–335*
    tooth sensitivity during 345–346
  walking technique *348*, 348–349, 784–786, *786–787*
  white spots 332, 683, *685*
blepharoplasty 1132–1133, *1133–1135*
blood
  extravasation into pulp chamber 682, 751, *752*
  loss, orthognathic surgery 939
  pigments, dental staining 330–331, 681–682

Bluephase Meter 405, *406*
blue stains **671**
blushers, facial cosmetic 1150
bobby pins 825–826, *827*
body dysmorphic disorder (BDD) 26, *41*, 42–44, *43*
body image 6, *8*, 10–11
body type, facial form and 930
Bolton's tooth-size relationships 923, **924**
bonding *see* adhesion
bonding agents *see* adhesives
bone
  condensation 582
  excessive alveolar 1205, *1205*
  grafts
    immediate implant placement 646
    ridge augmentation *642*, 642–643
    ridge preservation 639, *640–641*
  quantity and quality 1417
    complete dentures 625–629
    peri-implant changes 653–654, 1417, *1418*
    postextraction changes 638–639, **639**, *639–640*, 1200
    premaxilla 639, *640*, *641*
    removable partial dentures 582–583
  resection, crown lengthening 1205–1206, *1207–1208*, 1207–1208
bone morphogenetic protein 2 (BMP2) 643
botulinum toxin type A (Botox) 151, 898, 905
Bowen, R.L. 375, 394, 434
brachycephalic facial form 1058, *1061*, 1098, *1100*
brand, creating a 114
Brando, Marlon 1159, 1160
Brånemark root-form implant 653
bridges *see* fixed partial dentures
browlift 1132, *1132–1133*
brown stains **671**, 682–683, *685*
brushes
  interdental 1410, *1411–1412*, 1427
  tooth 1414, 1427
brushing *see* tooth brushing
bruxism 696–702, *698*, 814, 814–815
  clinical cases *700–704*, 702–703
  cosmetic contouring 300, 301, *301*, 814, *814*
  evaluation of tooth wear 697–698
  fractured restorations 1252, *1256–1257*
  intraoral appliances 413–415, *415*, *814*, 815
  older adults 1034, *1034*
  sleep 697
  with temporomandibular joint pain 815, *815–816*
  treatment options 699–702
BruxZir materials 537
buccal corridors 1125
  patient esthetic standards 138
  preferences 899–900, *902*
budget-conscious patients 78, 80

bulimia nervosa (BN) 26, 31–34, 822
  case example 31
  dental erosion 33, *33–34*, 712–714, *713*, 822, *822–823*
  diagnostic criteria 32
  parotid gland hypertrophy 32, *32*, 822, *824*
  signs 32–33, *32–33*
  worksheet for diagnosed **35–36**
bullying 11
Buonocore, Michael 356, 434, 1373
bupropion (Wellbutrin) 28
burs
  endodontic access cavity preparation 775–776
  see also carbide burs; diamond burs
Burstone line 1117, *1117*
butt joints
  metal–ceramic 516, *516*
  porcelain *see* porcelain butt-joint margins
  veneer preparation (Class 5) 442, *445*, *447–448*
buyer's remorse 19

CAD/CAM *see* computer-aided design/manufacturing
calcific degeneration/metamorphosis 767
  walking bleach technique 788–789, *790–793*
calcium hydroxide
  apexification therapy 1219–1220
  cavity base dressing 767
  endodontic treatment 780
  pulp capping 727, 769
  traumatically exposed dentin 1218
calculus 52
camcorders 181–182
cameras 155–156
  extraoral 59–60, *61*
  film vs digital 155–156
  intraoral *see* intraoral cameras
  point-and-shoot 158–159, *159*
  selection 158–163
  single-lens reflex *see* single-lens reflex cameras
  uploading images from 179, *180*
  wand-like 156, *156*
Camper's line 617, *618*, 622, *622*
canine protected occlusion (CPO) 915, 916
canines (cuspids)
  adjusting embrasures 1347
  age-related wear *221–222*
  cosmetic contouring 314, *314–315*
  SPA factors 248, *249*
canine width (CW) 261
  ICW/CIW quotient for calculating **263**, 265, **265**, *266–267*
  RED proportion for calculating 262, **262**
  in relation to other teeth 847
  too narrow 210, *212*
  too wide 208, *208*
carbamide peroxide 342, 343, 345, 348, 687

carbide burs
    endodontic access cavity 778
    finishing ceramic veneers *470,* 473
    finishing composite restorations 406–407, *407–409*
carbon dioxide (CO_2) laser 985
carbon fiber prefabricated posts **736**
Carestream system 490–492, *492–494*
caries
    anorexia nervosa 34
    bleaching and 335
    bulimia nervosa 33
    detection
        air-abrasive technology 417–419, *418*
        discolored deep grooves 670
        hand-held devices 55, *55*
        intraoral camera 57, *59, 60*
        pits and fissures 417, *417*
    early childhood (ECC) 979
    pit and fissure *see* pit and fissure caries
    posterior ceramic partial coverage restorations 480
    prevention advice 1414–1415
    recurrent 1224, *1227,* 1245–1248, *1247*
        marginal leakage and 1250–1251
    risk assessment 536
    root
        older adults 1035, *1036*
        soft tissue graft coverage 1194–1195, *1195*
    susceptibility
        cosmetic contouring and 302
        follow-up care for crowns and 536
    tooth discoloration 330, 670, *674*
    treatment
        air-abrasive technology 417–419, *418*
        diamond burs 419
        hard tissue lasers 419, *419*
        ozone therapy 971
        pediatric dentistry 973, 974, *974, 976, 976*
Cariescan 55
caries management by risk assessment (CAMBRA) 1024
Carter, G.A. 920–921
case presentation *74–76,* 74–77
    dentofacial deformity 935–937
    Digital Smile Design 87, *104–106*
    marketing your services 120–121, *122*
    role of photographs 159
cast glass-ceramic crowns 506, *507*
    endodontic access 778
casting alloys 514
cast metal posts (custom made)
    anterior teeth 733, *734*
        indications 739, **739**
        techniques 739, *742,* 743
    crown preparation *744,* 745
    design 734–735, *735*
    premolars 743
casts, study *see* study models
cavitation, laser-induced 972

cavity preparation
    endodontic access *see* endodontic access cavity
    posterior ceramic partial coverage restorations 481–482
    pulpal response 764–765, *766*
    pulpal risk and depth 767–769, *768*
cavity test, pulp sensibility 758–759, *758–759*
CBCT *see* cone beam computed tomography
Celsus One salivary diagnostics 1423, *1424–1426*
cement(s) 1355–1356
    Dicor restorations 506
    fluoride-containing 1247–1248
    In-Ceram crowns 506
    metal–ceramic crowns 521, 1355–1356
    pediatric dentistry 970
    removing excess 1358–1359, *1361*
        ceramic veneers 469–470, *472,* 473
        posterior ceramic partial coverage restorations 482–483
    residual
        checking for 1365, *1365,* 1410, *1410*
        implant–abutment interface 658, *660*
    resin luting agents 1356, *1357–1358,* 1361
    root canal 780
    self-adhesive 1361, *1362*
    temporary restorations 1313, 1340, 1364
    see also adhesives
cementation 1355–1365
    all-ceramic crowns 1361, *1362–1364*
    ceramic restorations 1361–1364, 1373
    ceramic veneers *468,* 471–472, *1357–1358,* 1361–1364
    CEREC restorations 487, *491*
    implant crowns 660–662, *660–662*
    metal–ceramic restorations 1358–1359, *1359–1361*
    posterior ceramic partial coverage restorations 482–483
    posts 743
    preparation of surfaces for 1356, *1358*
    radiographs after 1365, *1365,* 1410, *1410*
    tooth sensitivity after 1356
    try-in appointment 1352
central incisor length (CIL)
    complete dentures 615
    crowns 527, *527*
    diastema closure and 846
    fixed restorations 1347, *1348*
    ICW/CIW quotient chart method 263, 265, **265**, *266–267*
    performers/actors 1174, *1176*
    RED proportion to calculate 262, **262**
    width calculations and *261,* 261–262, **262**
central incisors (maxillary)
    1/16th rules 249, *250,* 614–615
    adjusting embrasures 1346, *1347*
    black triangle between 137
    complete dentures 614–615, 616–617, *617–619*
    crowning one 523–524, *524*

    length *see* central incisor length
    overlapping, cosmetic contouring 315–316, *315–317*
    post-and-core restorations 741–742
    reducing large 318, *318*
    size in relation to face size 249–251, *250–251*
    SPA factors 248, *248–249*
    width *see* central incisor width
    see also incisors
central incisor width (CIW)
    1/16th rule 249, *250,* 614–615
    complete dentures 614–615
    diastema closure and 846
    ICW/CIW quotient to calculate **263,** 263–265, *264–267,* **265**
    RED proportion to calculate 261–262, *261–262,* **262**
    in relation to other teeth 254–265
    see also intercanine width/central incisor width (ICW/CIW) quotient
central incisor width/length ratio 253, *256*
    dentists' preferences 253, *256*
    diastema closure and 846–847
    orthodontic esthetics and 902–903
    RED proportions and 257, *259*
cephalometric analysis 253, *256*
    dentofacial deformity 934, *935*
    normal values 903–904, **904**
    orthodontics *901,* 903–904, **904**
    pediatric patients 1005–1006
cephalometric prediction tracings 934, *935–938*
cephalometric radiographs *901,* 903–904
    dentofacial deformity 934
ceramic(s)
    CEREC system 484–485, 1390
    endodontic access cavity preparation 776–778, *777–778*
    failure rates of different 1253
    glass-infiltrated 1377
    high opacity 453
    prefabricated posts **736**
    veneers 434–435, 453
    see also glass-ceramics; oxide ceramics; porcelain; zirconia
ceramic orthodontic brackets 909
ceramic partial coverage restorations 433–492
    CAD/CAM technologies 483–492
    longevity 479
    posterior 478–483
        contraindications 481
        finishing 482–483
        impressions 482
        indications 480–481
        insertion 482
        patient instructions 483
        tooth preparation 481–482
        veneer onlay 482
    veneers *see* ceramic veneers
    see also porcelain veneers

ceramic restorations
  abutment–implant platform interface 1370, *1370–1371*
  abutment–soft tissue interface 1370–1372, *1371–1372*
  CAD/CAM systems *see* computer-aided design/manufacturing systems
  cementation 1361–1364, 1373
  digital laboratory workflow 1401–1402, *1401–1402*
  endodontic access 776–778, *777, 778*
  occlusal interface 1374–1381
  partial coverage *see* ceramic partial coverage restorations
  principles of construction 1369–1382
  rebonding 1373, *1375*
  tooth or implant abutment interface 1372–1374, *1373–1374*
  see also all-ceramic crowns; ceramic veneers; metal–ceramic restorations
ceramic veneer onlays, posterior 482, *482–484*
ceramic veneers 433–492
  CAD/CAM fabricated 453
  fracture rates 473–474
  history 434–435
  impressions 459–460
  indications 440–441, 474, *474–481*
  longevity 439, *440*, 473–474
  placement 465–473
    cementation 468, *471–472*, 1357–1358, 1361–1364
    errors 472, *473*
    final insertion 464–465, *467–472*, 469–473
    try-in *463*, 465–469, *466–467*
  post-treatment care 473–477
  pressable
    laboratory procedures 462–465
    longevity 474
    tooth preparation 453, *453–456*
  subgingival margins *see* subgingival margins
  temporary restorations 460–461, *461–463*
  tetracycline-stained teeth 440, 452, 453, 461–462, 687–688, *687–688*
  tooth preparation 442–459
    classic classes 442–446, *446–448*
    classic technique 456, *457–460*
    classification for anterior teeth 442–445, *442–448*
    mandibular anteriors 448–449, *449–451*
    novel classes 447–448
    novel extended technique 454, 456–459, *475–476*
    tooth reduction 449–453, *457–459*
  traditional porcelain *see* porcelain veneers
ceramometal restorations *see* metal–ceramic restorations
Cercon all-ceramic crowns 507
CEREC system 483–490, 1389–1391

Bluecam 1389, 1390, *1390*
chairside fabrication 1390, *1391*
data acquisition 487, *487*, 1390, *1390*
design and milling 487, *487–490*, 1390, *1391*
hardware 1389, *1389*
material selection 484–485, 1390
Omnicam 484, *486*, 487, 1389, 1390, *1390*
placement of restorations 487, *491*
Planmeca PlanScan vs **1393**
research 487–490, *491*
shade selection 485, *485*
support and education 1390–1391
tooth preparation 485, *486*
cervical lesions, noncarious *see* abfractions
cervical root resorption *see* external root resorption
cervicomental angle 1067–1068, *1074–1075*
  correction of obtuse *1075*
chamfer margins
  all-ceramic crowns 1268
  metal–ceramic restorations 517, *517*, 522
  porcelain veneers 456
chamfer-shoulder preparation method 398, *399, 400*
Chandler, T.H. 812
Change Your Smile (Goldstein) 49, *49, 50*, 51, 54, 151
characterization *see* surface texture/characterization
check lines
  creating illusion of height 215, *215*
  simulation 196, *198–199*, **202**
cheek
  biting, habitual 819–821, *819–821*
  profile, pediatric patients 1008, *1008*
  projection, evaluation 1062
chemical bonding 356
chewing habits 816, *816*
children *see* pediatric dentistry
chin
  analysis of symmetry 1107
  asymmetry 1062, *1066*
  minimizing a double 1149–1150
  projection 1065–1068, 1115
  reshaping 959, *961–962*, 1137
chin–neck anatomy, evaluation 1063, *1068–1069*
chin–neck angle (cervicomental angle) 1067–1068, *1074–1075*
chin–neck length 1067–1068, *1074–1075*
chips *see* crown fractures
chlorhexidine
  mouthwashes, staining of teeth 673–674, *677–678*
  stabilization of bonding 364–365, 367
chroma 272–273, *273*
  effects of bleaching 277–278, **284**
chromium casting alloys 514
chronic illness, older adults 1020–1022, **1022**, 1024–1025
Chu esthetic guage 256

CIE (Commission Internationale de l'Éclairage) color notation system 273
circumferential fiberotomy of supracrestal gingival fibers (CSF) 915
citric acid demineralization, for root coverage 1183, 1185–1186
CK Diamond Endodontic Access Kit 775
Clark, E. Bruce 272, 276, *276*
clasps, removable partial dentures 584–588
  camouflage 590
  circumferential 584
  combination 588, *588*
  embrasure 588, *588*
  I-, Y-, T- or modified T-bar 584–585, *585*
  mesial groove reciprocation (MGR) 585, *587, 588*
  placement 584, *584*
  rest–proximal plate–I-bar (RPI) 585, *587*
  ring 585–587
  unesthetic design 1238–1239, *1239*
Class 0 (no preparation) veneer 442, *442*
Class I restorations 379, *380–382*
  pediatric dentistry 974, *974*
  primary teeth 970
Class 1 (window) veneer preparation 442, *443*
Class II malocclusions *917*, 933
  comprehensive esthetic approach 1052–1053, *1053*
  diagnostic records 934
  profile angle 1113
  surgical–orthodontic correction 944–948, *946*
  vertical maxillary excess 950
Class II restorations 382, *383*
  durability 1251
  glass ionomer liners 403
  polymerization techniques 403, *405*
  primary teeth 970
Class 2 (feather) veneer preparation 442, *443*
Class III malocclusions 933
  alternative approach 1076, *1077*
  diagnostic records 934, *936–938*
  porcelain veneers 441
  profile angle 1113
  surgical–orthodontic treatment *939–941*, 940–942, *943–944*
Class III restorations 382–384, *384–387*
Class 3 (bevel/small butt joint) veneer preparation 442, *444*
Class IV restorations 384–385, *387–389*
  excessively translucent 1251–1252, *1255*
Class 4 (incisal overlap) veneer preparation 442–446, *444, 446–448*, 456–459
Class V restorations 385, *389–390*, 408
  esthetic repair 690
  follow-up care 416
Class 5 (butt joint) veneer preparation 442, *445*, 447–448

Class 6 (full) veneer preparation 442, *445, 447–448*, 456–459
cleaning
    ceramic veneers 467, *469*
    prior to composite resin bonding 396
clear aligner therapy 909
Clearfil SE Bond adhesive 362, *363, 366*, 368
Clearfil Tri-S-Bond adhesive system 366
cleft lip and palate 951, *952*
clinical examination 55–67
    components 55–56
    computer imaging 61–66
    esthetic evaluation chart 56, *58*
    extraoral camera 59–60, *61*
    intraoral camera 57–59, *59, 60*
    occlusal analysis 60
    periodontal charting 60–61
    pulpal health 751–762
    transillumination 56–57, *58*
    X-rays 60, *61, 62*
close-up repose image 174–175, *175*
close-up smile image 173, *174*
cocaine abuse 825
coca leaf chewing 816
coffee drinking 675, *679*
cognitive behavior therapy 43
cold sensitivity, bleached teeth 341
cold testing 754–756, *756–757*
collagen membrane, resorbable (Zimmer socket repair membrane) 640–641
collagen network, dentin
    durability after etching 364–365
    phosphoric acid etching 359, *359*
    priming 360
    technique sensitivity 365
color 271–292
    basics 272–273
    case study 289–292, *289–292*
    communicating 285–286
    in dentistry 273–274
    denture base 623–625, *623–625*
    dimensions 272–273, *273*
    education and training **287**, 287–288, *288–289*
    gingival 274
    hair 1147
    lipstick 1147, 1150–1151
    makeup 1149
    notation systems 273
    perception 272
    photographic management 157
    post-bleaching relapse 350
    skin 274
    tooth *see* tooth color
    triplet 272
    see also shade
color change units (ccu) 277
color difference (ΔE)
    CIELAB formula (ΔE^*) 273, *273*, 274
    peri-implant tissues 1370, *1371*
color discrimination competency (CDC) 274

color matching *see* shade selection/color matching
color modification 286–287
    all-ceramic crowns 506, 510, 511
    ceramic veneers 467–469
    porcelain 286, 438
color rendering index (CRI) 275
color standards, dental *see* shade guides
color temperature, correlated (CCT) 275
color thresholds 274
combination clasp 588, *588*
commerce 12–16
Commission Internationale de l'Éclairage (CIE) color notation system 273
commissural line 1101, *1101*
    as plane of reference 1108, *1109*, 1111
communication
    Digital Smile Design tool 86
    function of teeth 11
    laboratory *see* laboratory, communication
    patients with poor 77
    practice website 122
    treatment planning phase 79
    try-in stage 1337
community relations 127, 128
complete dentures 611–630
    bone quantity and quality 625–629
    emergency repairs 1231–1232
    esthetics 611, *612*, 614–625
        clinical examples 625–626
        denture base 623–625, *623–625*
        tooth arrangement 616–623, *617–622*
        tooth color 616
        tooth size and form 614–616
    implants and 629–630
    occlusion 613, *613–614*, 620–622
        anterior 620
        posterior 621–622, *622*
        vertical dimension 620–621, *621–622*
    opposing natural teeth 628–629, *629–631*
    performers/actors 1156–1160, *1158–1164*
    porcelain vs plastic teeth 626–627, *627–629*
    provisional 612–613, *612–613*
complications of treatment
    disclosure of 132, 143–144
    "I'm sorry" legal protection 138
compomers 970–971, 1356
composite resin(s)
    camouflaging RPD clasps 590
    dual cure 403
    flowable 362, 403, *1227*
    hybrid 395, 862, 1416
    light curing 403, 404–405, *406*
    luting agents 1356
    materials for direct bonding 393–396
    microfilled *see* microfilled composites
    modification of RPD teeth 589
    nanofilled 396, 862
    pediatric dentistry 970
    polymerization *see* polymerization
    self cure 403
    small-particle macrofilled 395

composite resin bonding 375–421
    advantages and disadvantages **538**
    alternatives to 298–300, 376
    as alternatives to veneers 434, *434–438*
    basic categories 377, *379*
    broken tooth fragments 722–723, 726–727, 1220, *1220*
    case presentation 74
    chipped teeth *see under* crown fractures
    clinical use 375, *376*, 377–393
    cosmetic contouring with 319, *319*
        crowded teeth 883–884, *884–885*
    crowded teeth **882**, 883–884, *884–885*
    curing 403–406, *405*
        following final finish 404
        incremental layering 403, *405*
        shrinkage 405
        three-sited light-curing technique 403
    diastema closure 849–864
        large diastemata 856–862
        multiple diastemata 851, 853, *853*, 857–858, *857–859*
        performers/actors 1173, 1175, *1175*
        posterior diastema 863–864, *863–865*
        prior orthodontics 853, 856, *856–857*
        simple diastemas 849–853, *850–852, 854–855, 854–856*
    finishing 406–409
        adding surface texture 407–408
        final polishing 407, *410–411*
        instrumentation 406–407, *407–411*
        interproximal 409
        problems 408–409, *412–415*
    fractured teeth *see under* crown fractures
    history of use 376
    informed consent 133, *134*
    inlays 393, *394*
    interdental tissue loss 226–228, *227*
    labial veneers 385–392, *393*
    materials 393–396
    older adults 1025–1028, *1027–1029*, 1030–1031, *1030–1031*
    pediatric dentistry 973
        amelodentinal dysplasia 975, *975*
        enamel hypoplasia 978, *978*
        extensive cavities 976, *976–977*
        preventive restoration 974, *974*
    pit and fissure caries 379, 417, *418–420*
    protective night appliances 413–415, *415*
    pulp capping with 769
    repair of existing restorations 392, 1224, 1226–1230, *1228–1230*
    shade selection 396–398, *397*
    techniques 396–409
        dentin bonding 403, *404*
        enamel bonding and acid etch 401, 403
        finishing 406–409, *407–412*
        incremental layering 403, *405*, 405–406
        laser-ablated tooth structure 972–973
        legal considerations 134
        overlay technique 398–400, *399–400*, 690

composite resin bonding (cont'd)
    polymerization 403–406
    sandwich technique 403, *404*
    shade selection 396–398, *397*
    tooth cleaning 396
  temporary 392
    performers/actors 1155, 1160–1163
    splinting 1317–1320, *1319–1320*
    veneers 1316–1317, *1316–1317*
  tooth preparation 398–399, *399–401*
    air-abrasive technology 417, *418*
    chamfer-shoulder method 398, *399*, 400
    overlay method 398–399, *399–400*
  transitional 377
composite resin cores **736**
  anterior teeth 740–742, *742*
  posterior teeth 734, 735, *736*, *739*
  small premolars 743
composite resin restorations
  air bubbles/pockets 1252
  causes of failure 1250–1252
  Class I 379, *380–382*
  Class II 382, *383*
  Class III 382–384, *384–387*
  Class IV 384–385, *387–389*
  Class V 385, *389–390*
  crowns 502, *505*
  discoloration 689, *689*, 690, 1167, 1252
  excessively translucent 1251–1252, *1255*
  fractures 1252, *1256*
  indirect posterior 382
  longevity 416, 1242–1243
    durability of adhesion 363–365, *364*
    legal considerations 138
    posterior teeth 376, *377*
  maintenance 409–421
    homecare 415, *416*
    protective night appliances 413–415, *415*
    recall visits 415–416
    scaling and polishing 415, 1416
  marginal staining 379, *380*, 1252, *1256*
    management 671, *674*, 675–676, 689
    tooth preparation methods and 400, *400*
  microleakage 379, *380*, 401, 1250–1251, *1254*
  performers/actors 1167–1169, *1169–1170*
  preparation *see* composite resin bonding
  repairs to existing 690
    air-abrasive technology 419–421
    laser-assisted 987–988, *987–988*
    marginal staining 671, *674*, 675, 689
  veneers *see* direct composite veneers; indirect composite/acrylic veneers
composite resin stent/splint 1155, *1157*
compound/copper band impressions 1302
computed tomography *see* cone beam computed tomography
computer-aided design/manufacturing (CAD/CAM) systems 483–492, 1387–1407

  all-ceramic crowns 507, 512–514
  Carestream system 490–492, *492–494*
  CEREC system *see* CEREC system
  clinical cases 1403–1406, *1404–1406*
  comparison table **1393**
  currently available 1389–1392
  dedicated impression scanners vs 1389
  digital impressions 459, 1303, 1389
  fixed partial dentures 562–564
  implant positioning 647
  laboratory 1400–1402, *1401–1402*
  open vs closed architecture 1400
  orthodontic appliances 909
  Planmeca PlanScan 1391–1392, *1391–1393*
  temporary restorations 1315
computer imaging
  cosmetic contouring 304, *304–305*
  dentofacial analysis 1056–1057, *1059*
  disclaimers 61
  fixed partial dentures 546
  laboratory communication via 197
  older adults 1025
  orthodontics 909, *910–911*
  proportional smile design 265–268, *267–268*
  treatment planning 61–67, *65–66*, 75
  trial smile 66–67
  see also images
computer imaging therapist 61
concealers, facial cosmetic 1150, 1151
concussion, tooth 1223
condensation impression materials 1292
condylar hyperplasia 951–955, *953–955*
cone beam computed tomography (CBCT) 55
  endodontics 762, *764*
  fixed partial dentures 564
  orthodontics 909, *910*
  treatment planning 75–77
confidentiality 145
connective tissue (gingival) grafts
  fixed partial dentures 567
  implant patients 654–655, *655–656*, 1195, *1196*
  papilla reconstruction 1199, *1199*
  ridge augmentation 1200–1201, 1202–1203, *1203–1204*
  root coverage 1183–1195
    allogenic vs autogenous 1184
    harvesting 1189–1190, *1190–1191*
    old restorations and root caries 1194–1195, *1195*
    placement 1190–1191, *1192–1193*
    postoperative care 1194, *1194*
    potential for attachment 1185–1186, *1186*
    quality and quantity of donor tissue 1195
    surgical technique 1186–1194
    sutures and dressing 1191–1194
    unesthetic 1183, *1183*

connector area 247, *248*
consent 27
  explicit and implicit 132
  informed *see* informed consent
consent forms 133, *134–137*, 139
  video 139, *141*
contact areas, try-in stage 1345, *1345*
contaminants, causing restoration failure 1255
continuous positive airways pressure (CPAP) 959, 961
contouring, cosmetic 297–321
  bruxism 300, 301, *301*, 814, *814*
  chipped teeth 722, *723*, 1217
  composite resin bonding with 319, *319*
  crowded teeth 883–884, *884–885*
  contraindications 301–303, *301–303*
  crowded teeth 303, **882,** 883, *883*
  early techniques 297–298, *298*
  failure to perform 1239, 1241, *1241–1242*
  indications 298–300, *299–300*
  older adults 1025–1028, *1026*
  performers/models 1166, *1167*
  porcelain veneers 439
  principles 303–304
  techniques 305–319
    altering tooth form 313–314, *314–315*
    angle of correction 305–306, *307*
    arch irregularity 319, *320–322*
    creating illusions 189–190, 305, *306–307*
    reduction 306–313, *308–313*
  too-wide teeth 207–209, *207–209*
  treatment planning 304, *304–306*
  try-in appointment 1347–1350, *1349–1351*
contours, Pincus principles *D4,* D4–D5
coronal fractures *see* crown fractures
correlated color temperature (CCT) 275
corticotomy-assisted orthodontics 956–959
cosmetic adjuncts 1143–1151
cosmetic contouring *see* contouring, cosmetic
Cosmetic Contouring Kit, Shofu 310–311, *313*
cosmetic dentistry 897–898, *898*
cosmetics *see* makeup
cosmetics industry 13–14
cosmetic surgery 13, 14–16, 18
  see also plastic surgery
costs, financial *see* financial considerations
coverage error (CE) 280–281
cracked tooth syndrome (CTS) **722,** 794–804
  class I (incomplete vertical fracture) 798–799, *801–802*
  class II (pulpal involvement) 799–801, *803–804*
  class III (attachment involvement) 801–802
  class IV (complete separation of tooth fragments) 802–803
  class V (retrograde root fracture) 803

diagnosis 794–798
discoloration 673
prevalence trends 797
see also crown fractures; microcracks, enamel; root fractures
Creation Porcelain 516
cross-bite 1061
crowded teeth 877–893
　clinical evaluation 877–881
　　arch space 878, *878*
　　Berliner's formula 878, *879*
　　gingival architecture 878–879, *880*
　　posttreatment oral hygiene 881
　　root proximity 881
　　smile line 881
　older adults 920
　pediatric patients 997, *997–1000*
　tooth preparation 1280–1283, *1282*
　treatment failure 1236, *1237*
　treatment options **882,** 883–890, 893
　　composite resin bonding 883–884, *884–885*
　　cosmetic contouring 303, 883, *883*
　　crowning 887–890, *888–889*
　　disking 883
　　porcelain veneers 884–886, *886–887*
　treatment strategy 881–883
　unusual or rare presentations 890–893
crown fractures (and chips) 721–745, 1216–1221
　complicated (pulp involvement) 727–730, 1219–1221, *1220–1221*
　　endodontics 790, *793–794*
　　interdisciplinary approach 728–730, *729–731*
　　pediatric patients 990, *990–993*
　　treatment options **722,** 1219
　composite resin bonding 1218–1219, *1219*
　　choosing 722, 723, 725–726, **727**
　　life expectancy 730–731, *731–732*
　　long-term results 724–726, *728*
　　posterior teeth 731–732
　　techniques 384–385, *387–389*
　cosmetic contouring 722, *723*, 1217
　crowning **727,** 729, *730*
　diagnosis 56–57, 751, 755–756, 761–762
　enamel infractions 1216, *1217*
　endodontically-treated teeth 732–745
　　anterior **739,** 739–743, *740–742*
　　core materials **736**
　　crown preparation 743–745, *744*
　　post design 734–735, **736**
　　posterior 736–739, *736–739*
　　premolars 743, *743*
　　principles 732–734, *733–734*
　incomplete 798–803
　pediatric 984–985
　　intrusive luxation with complicated 990, *990–993*
　　uncomplicated 986, *986–987*
　　unsatisfactory treatment 987–988, *987–988*

porcelain veneers 722, 723–724, *723–724,* 726, **727**
posterior teeth 731–732
tooth fragment bonding 722–723, 726–727, 1219, 1220, *1220*
treatment 721–724
　conservative options 722, *723–724*
　factors influencing choice 722–724, *723–726,* **727**
uncomplicated 1216–1219
　conservative bonding techniques 724–727, *728*
　enamel and dentin 1217–1219, *1219*
　enamel only 1216–1217, *1217–1218*
　endodontics 790, *793*, 1219
　pediatric patients 986, *986–987*
　treatment options **722**
see also cracked tooth syndrome
crown-lengthening procedures
　attachment RPDs 593
　biologic width and 1205–1206
　bruxism *701, 702*
　diastema closure and 846
　excessive gingival display 1204–1208, *1205*
　poorly contoured restorations 1245
　surgical procedure 1206–1208, *1206–1209*
crown–root fractures 740, 1221, *1222*
crown:root ratio, abutment teeth 582
crowns (prosthetic) 499–538
　advantages and disadvantages **538**
　all-ceramic *see* all-ceramic crowns
　all-metal *see* all-metal crowns
　alternatives to
　　ceramic veneers 474, *474–481*
　　cosmetic contouring 298–300
　　importance of offering 143
　bleaching of adjacent natural teeth 687
　bruxism patients *701, 702*
　cementation 1352, 1358–1361
　crowded teeth **882,** 887–890, *888–889*
　diagnosis 500, *500–501*
　diastema closure 869–870, *872*
　emergency repairs 1224, *1230–1232, 1231–1232*
　failures
　　dentinal staining 1236
　　improper contours 1236–1238, *1238–1239*
　　margin exposure 1236, *1237*
　　material 1248–1250
　　periodontal disease 1245, *1245*
　　technical 1253–1255, *1257–1260*
　fractured teeth 731
　　endodontically-treated 733, *733–734*
　　pros and cons **727**
　　with pulp involvement 729, *730*
　gold 502, *502–504*
　indications 499–500
　interdental tissue loss *227–228,* 228–229
　legal considerations

　　informed consent 133, *137*
　　overcontoured crowns 147, *148–149*
　　unnecessary placement 143, *143*
　longevity 138, 500, *500,* 1244
　　promoting 536
　metal–ceramic *see* metal–ceramic restorations
　metal inlay, fixed partial denture retainers 549
　metal onlay, fixed partial denture retainers 549
　older adults 1034–1035
　patient maintenance 536
　performers/actors 1173–1174
　photographic records 500, *500*
　porcelain-fused-to-metal *see* porcelain-fused-to-metal crowns
　porcelain veneers for 441
　posts and cores *see* post-and-core restorations
　principles of esthetic 525–536
　　arch irregularity 526, *526*
　　final try-in 529
　　inclination of teeth 526–527
　　lip line 525–526, *526*
　　natural appearance *527–528,* 527–529
　　occlusal registration 531
　　shade matching *532–535,* 532–536
　　texture and characterization 532
　　tooth arrangement 531–532
　　tooth color 532
　　tooth contour and shape 529, *530*
　　tooth size *530,* 530–531
　resin (acrylic and composite) 502, *505*
　retention after endodontic therapy 779–780, *780*
　selection 523–525, *524,* 525–526, *526*
　technical considerations 501–514
　telescoping 555–562
　temporary 1313–1314
　three-quarter, fixed partial denture retainers 549
　tooth preparation 1263–1283
　　pulp injury 767–769, *768–769*
　try-in 1339–1352
　　adding texture 1350, *1351*
　　additional impressions 1343, *1344*
　　contacts 1345, *1345*
　　esthetic checks 1345–1347, *1346–1348*
　　fitting to tooth 1341–1343, *1344*
　　occlusal adjustment 1346
　　shaping 1347–1350, *1349–1351*
　　stuck on tooth 1341, *1342*
cultural aspects
　esthetics 3
　filing of teeth 298, *298*
curing *see* polymerization
curve of Spee 247, *247,* 921
　depth, ratio to arch circumference 921–922
　orthodontic leveling 944
Cushee rubber dam clamp cushions 773, *773*
cuspal fracture 797

cuspids *see* canines
customer service 117–119, *119–120*
Cvek pulpotomy 727, 1219
cystic fibrosis 328

Dalbo attachment system 600, *600–602*
DC-Zirkon 1253
decalcification spots *see* white spots
decision making, patient 48–49
    involving family/friends 1332
    older adults 1025
    role of temporaries 1312, *1313*
    see also case presentation; trial smile
dehydration, tooth
    post bleaching 340–341
    shade matching and 283, 396
demanding patients 38–40, *39*
dementia 1022, 1024, 1036
demographics, population 1015–1016, **1016**
Dentacolor 502
dental assistants
    computer imaging 61
    extraoral photographs 59
Dental Color Matcher (DCM) **287,** 287–288, *288–289*
dental education
    color **287,** 287–288, *288–289*
    Digital Smile Design 87
    role of photographs 158
    see also training
dental history 70
dental hygienists *see* hygienists
dental materials
    causing tooth discoloration 330
    color-related properties **286,** 286–287
dental midline
    canting 1101, *1102,* 1105–1106
    checking, at try-in 1345, *1346*
    deviations 1104–1106
        acceptability 137, 899–902, *902, 1094, 1095*
        correction 1094, *1096*
    diastema closure and 845
    Digital Smile Design 89, *89*
    facial midline and 1094, *1094,* 1104–1106
    to midsagittal plane 1061, *1065*
dental technicians
    communication with *see* laboratory, communication
    Digital Smile Design tool 86
dentifrices *see* toothpastes
dentin
    bonding *358,* 358–360, *361*
        after laser ablation 972–973
        ceramic veneers 452, 468, 471
        composite resins 403
        primers/priming adhesives 359–360
        priming of collagen network 360
        self-etch adhesives 360, *360*
        stabilization 360
        technique sensitivity 365–366, *366*
        tooth sensitivity after 366–367, 403

conditioning/acid etching *see* acid etching, dentin
    reparative 766–767, *767*
    secondary 767, *767*
    thickness, cavity preparations 767–768, *768*
    traumatic exposure 790, 1217–1219, *1219*
dentinoenamel junction (DEJ) scallop 705
dentinogenesis imperfecta
    tooth discoloration 330, 680–681, *681*
    tooth wear 697
dentist–patient relationship 51, 79, 145
    establishing rapport 750–751
    mistakes/errors and 138
dentists
    appearance 115–116, *119*
    correction of dentofacial deformity and 935
    identifying gender from tooth shape 614
    patient's right to choose 146–147, *146–147*
    preferences
        tooth-to-tooth width proportions 258–260, *260*
        tooth width/length ratio 253, *256*
    responsibility for obtaining consent 144–145
    right to refuse treatment 145
    updating skills and practices 132
dentofacial analysis 1098, 1119–1125
    buccal corridors 1125
    facial landmarks 1053, *1054*
    incisal edges and lower lip 1120–1122
    orthodontic perspective 1057–1062, *1060–1067*
    papilla display during smiling 1124–1125
    smile line 1122–1124, *1122–1125*
    smile width 1125, *1125*
    tooth exposure at rest 1119–1120, *1119–1121*
    see also facial analysis; macroesthetic analysis; smile analysis
dentofacial deformity 929–965
    diagnostic records 934–935, *935–938*
    facial analysis 930–931, *931–932*
    first visit 933–935
    pediatric patients 933
    surgical–orthodontic correction 940–955
dentogenics 246
Dentsply Sirona 537
Dentsply tooth size facial guide *251*
dentures
    complete 611–630
    fixed partial 543–571
    performers/actors 1156–1160, *1158–1164,* 1176–1177, *1177*
    removable partial 581–606
denture teeth
    complete dentures 614–623
        arrangement 616–623
        color 616

        materials 616, 626–627, *627–628*
        size and form 614–616
    emergency repairs 1231
    removable partial dentures 589
Denzir all-ceramic restorations 1249–1250
depression 26, 27–29
    bipolar 30
    diagnosis 27, 28
dermabrasion 1140
dermal fillers 1137, *1140*
developing teeth, traumatic injuries to 986
developmental abnormalities
    cosmetic contouring 298, *299*
    porcelain veneers 440
    tooth discoloration 330
dexterity, patient 594
DiaComp Feather Lite composite polishers 407, *411*
Diagnodent 55, *55,* 971
diagnostic study models *see* study models
diagnostic wax-up *see* wax-up, diagnostic
diamond burs
    ceramic veneer finishing *470,* 473
    cosmetic contouring 308, *308*
    endodontic access cavity 776, *778*
    finishing composite restorations 406–407, *407*
    incisal embrasures 1346, *1347,* 1347
    pit and fissure caries 419
    tooth reduction
        all-ceramic crowns 1268–1271, *1269, 1271–1273*
        porcelain-fused-to-metal crowns *1278,* 1279
        veneers 456–457, *457–458*
    zirconia cutting 778
diamond impregnated polishing paste 473
diastemas 841–872
    diagnosis and treatment planning 843–844, *845*
    disguises used by patients 841, *842*
    etiology **842,** 842–843
    large 856–862, *860–861*
    multiple (diastemata)
        clinical case 857–858, *857–859*
        composite resin bonding 851, 853, *853*
        etiology **842,** 842–843
        porcelain veneers 867–869, *869–870,* 871, *871*
        treatment 853, 857–858, *857–859*
    with narrow teeth 852–853, 856, *856–857*
    orthodontic therapy *see under* orthodontics
    periodontal surgery and 847, 915
    posterior 863–864, *863–865*
    removable veneers 841, *842*
    restorative treatment 844–870
        combination crowns/veneers 869–870, *872*
        composite resin bonding 849–864
        functional considerations 848–849

gingival esthetics 847
   illusions 847–848, *848–849*
   incisal edge position 846
   porcelain veneers 441, 864–869
   tooth proportion 846–847
simple
   clinical cases 854–856, *854–856*
   composite resin bonding 849–853, *850–852*
   orthodontics and direct bonding 856, *856–857*
   porcelain veneers 866–867, *868*
   temporary measures for performers 1155, 1173, 1175, *1175*
   tongue habits causing 816–817, *817, 843, 843*
see also interdental spaces
Dicor glass-ceramic crowns 506, *507,* **513**
dietary advice 712, 1414–1415
dietary factors
   dental erosion 710, **711**
   tooth discoloration 328, 675, *679*
dietary habits, poor 822–825
difficult patients *see* problem patients
Digital Facebow *87,* 88
digital impressions 1302–1303, 1387–1407
   accuracy 1400
   bite registration 1307
   CAD/CAM systems 459, 1303, 1389
   ceramic veneers 459
   CEREC system 487, *487,* 1390
   clinical cases 1403–1406, *1404–1406*
   dedicated scanners 1389, 1393–1400
      3M True Definition *1394–1395,* 1394–1396
      3Shape TRIOS 1397–1400, *1398–1399*
      comparison table **1400**
      iTero Element scanner 1396–1397, *1396–1397*
      model fabrication 1394
   history 1388–1389
   open vs closed architecture 1400
digital mock-up, Digital Smile Design 94, *100, 103–104*
digital models, orthodontics 909, *910*
digital photography *see* photography
digital radiographs *see* radiographs
Digital Smile Design (DSD) 85–94
   advantages 86–87
   clinical procedures *107–109*
   final results 109–110
   presentation to patient 104–106
   procedure 87–94, *87–104*
digital systems, integrated 67
digit sucking 811–813, *812,* 1004
Diller, Phyllis 1169, *1169–1170*
dimensional stability, impression materials **1293,** 1294
diode lasers
   gingival preparation for impressions 1291, *1292*
   pediatric dentistry 984–985

direct acrylic veneers 461
direct composite veneers
   combined with ceramic restorations 385–392, *393*
   diastema closure 862, *862–863*
   history 434
   provisional treatment 392
   temporary restorations 460–461, *461–463*
direct mail advertising 128
directories, telephone and online 125
discoloration
   soft tissue
      amalgam restorations 805, *807*
      around implants 655, 658, *659,* 1370
   tooth *see* stained/discolored teeth
discount shopping services, online group 128
disfigured face, makeup for 1151
disking, crowded teeth **882,** 883
displacement syndrome 16
disruptive technologies 1406
dissatisfied patients 19, 50, 147, 152
distal inclination, increasing 217–218
distal rotation of teeth 190, *191,* 209, *210–211*
distraction osteogenesis 933, 955–956
doctor *see* dentist
documentation 139–142
   chart 141–142
   role of photographs 157
   see also records, clinical
Dolder bar attachments 605, *607*
dolichocephalic facial form 1058, *1061, 1098, 1100*
double tooth 1000, *1000–1003*
drinks *see* beverages
drug abuse 825
drug-induced problems *see* medication-induced problems

ears, prominent 1059, *1064*
eating disorders 26, 31–36, 822–825
   minors with 36
   worksheet for new patients **35–36**
eating habits, patients with ceramic veneers 474–477
ecstasy (methylenedioxymethamphetamine) 825
ectodermal dysplasia 982–983, *982–983*
edentulous areas
   Kennedy classification 582, *582*
   removable partial denture design 583
   ridge augmentation for implants 639–643, *641–642*
   tissue preparation for pontics 566–570, *569–570*
edentulous patients 611
education *see* dental education; patient education
Ehrmann, E.H. 727
elastic recovery, impression materials **1293,** *1293*

elderly *see* older adults
electric pulp testing 756–757, *758*
   through test cavity *758,* 759
electromagnetic spectrum *272*
electronic health records (EHRs) 67, 142
electrosurgery, gingival 1290–1291, *1291–1292*
e-mail consultations 150
e.max *see* IPS e.max
embrasure clasp 588, *588*
embrasure spaces
   closure methods 1196
   see also papillae, interdental
emergencies 1215–1233
   avulsions 1223–1224
   crown fractures 1216–1221
   crown–root fractures 1221
   fractured restorations 1224–1230
   long-term preservation 1215–1216
   luxation injuries 1223
   patient evaluation 1216
   performers/actors 1176
   prosthesis fracture/failure 1231–1232
   root fractures 1221–1223
   see also traumatic injuries
empathy 38
employment 12, *13–14*
enamel
   acid etching *see* acid etching, enamel
   bonding 356–358, 360, *361*
      after laser ablation 972–973
      ceramic restorations 1373
      ceramic veneers 439, *468,* 471
      composite resin 401, 403
      conditioning/etching *356,* 356–357
      historical development 358
      mechanisms 356–358, *357*
      self-etch adhesives **357,** 357–358
   chips and fractures *see* crown fractures
   defects, stained 671, *673*
   fractures 1216–1217, *1217–1218*
   hypocalcification *see* hypocalcification, enamel
   hypoplasia
      restorative therapy 978, *978*
      tooth discoloration 330, *331, 679, 679*
   infractions 1216, *1217*
   microcracks *see* microcracks, enamel
   mottled *see* fluorosis, dental
   reduction, ceramic veneers 452–453
   thickness
      cosmetic contouring and 302
      disking and 883
      radiographic measurement *879,* 883
Endo Access Kit 775
endodontic access cavity 774–780, *775*
   cavity shape and size 775, *775–776*
   coronal leakage 782, *783,* 783, 785
   preparation and equipment 775–776
   restored teeth 776–780, *777–780*
   sealing 781–782, *781–782*

endodontically-treated teeth
  bleaching *347,* 348, 682, *684–685,*
    783–789
    preventing resorption *786,* 786–788,
      788–789
    root resorption risks 350, 783–784, *785*
    walking bleach technique 784–786,
      786–787
  crowded tooth scenario 882
  discoloration 346, 682, *683,* 786, *787*
    prevention 780, *781*
  posterior ceramic partial coverage
    restorations 480
  restoring fractured 732–745
    anterior teeth **739,** 739–743, *740–742*
    crown preparation 743–745, *744*
    post design 734–735, *735*
    posterior teeth **736,** 736–739, *736–739*
    post materials 735, **736**
    premolars 743, *743*
    principles 732–734, *733–734*
endodontics 749–807
  anesthetic test 763–764
  attachment RPDs 593
  clinical evaluation 750–764
  cracked tooth syndrome 794–804
  diagnosis 764
  indications for elective 767–771
  laser applications 973
  older adults 1030
  pediatric patients 996
  radiography 762–763, *763–765,* 774
  restoration vs tooth removal 782–783,
    784–785
  retreatment 805, *806*
  tissue discoloration (tattoo) 805, *807*
  trauma 728, *729–731,* 790–794
  treatment planning 74, 750
  treatment protocols 771–783
    access cavity preparation 774–780
    coronal seal 781–782, *782*
    instrumentation/debridement 780
    restored teeth 776–780
    rubber dam 771–774, *772–774*
    sealing canal system 780–782,
      781–782
endodontic surgery 804–805, *805–806*
Endo-Ice 754–756, *757*
Endo Safe access burs 776
Endo-Z bur 776
end-to-end bite, porcelain veneers and 441
enhancement of appearance 1051–1052
entertainers *see* performers/actors
environment, color matching 275–276
epinephrine 1288
E-plane, Ricketts 1117, *1117*
erbium lasers 421, 971–973, 984
  see also lasers
erosion 709–711
  abfraction lesions 705, *706,* 707
  alcohol and drug abuse 825
  bleaching and 335

bulimia nervosa 33, 33–34, 712–714, *713,*
  822, *822–823*
ceramic veneers 477
clinical case 712–714, *713*
definition 693, 709
differential diagnosis 711–712
etiology 709–710, **711,** *711*
gastroesophageal reflux disease
  (GERD) 33, 712
habitual acid consumption 33,
  822–824, *824*
treatment 710–711
erythroblastosis fetalis 331, 682
esthetic analysis
  Digital Smile Design (DSD) tool 86
  see also macroesthetic analysis;
    microesthetics; miniesthetics
esthetic dentistry 3–20
  cosmetic dentistry vs 897–898, *898*
  definition 3
  health science and service 6–8
  historical perspective 4–5, *4–5*
  Pincus principles D2–D9
  social context 5–6, *6–7*
  understanding patient's needs 8–9
esthetic depth determination
  all-ceramic crowns 1268–1270, *1271–1276*
  porcelain-fused-to-metal crowns 1271–
    1272, *1277–1278*
esthetic evaluation chart 56, *58*
esthetic evaluation form A1–A6
esthetics
  defined 1085
  dental 3–20
  facial *see* facial esthetics
esthetic templates, fixed partial dentures
  546, *547*
Esthet-X shade guide *282*
etch-and-dry systems 360
etch-and-rinse adhesive systems 361, **362**
  postoperative hypersensitivity 366
  recommendations for use 367–368,
    367–368
  reliability and degradation *364,* 364–365
  technique sensitivity 365
etch-and-rinse technique (total etching) 359,
  359, 403
etching
  acid *see* acid etching
  laser 972
ethnic/racial differences
  facial form 930
  gingival display 1123
  interarch tooth size ratios 923
  lip position 1117
  nasolabial angle 1114
Etruscans 4, *4*
eugenol cements 1313, 1364
expectations, high 78
"extension for prevention" philosophy
  134–136
external root resorption

after bleaching 144, 350, 783–784, *785*
  legal considerations 148, *150*
  prevention 144, *786,* 786–788, *788–789*
avulsed/luxated teeth 794, *799–801,* 1224
clinical evaluation 752
endodontic surgery *799–801,* 804
orthodontic 144
extracoronal attachment removable partial
  dentures 596, 599–605
  advantages 599
  disadvantages 599–600
  types 600–605, *601–606*
extractions
  after final impressions 1294, *1297–1298*
  bone-conserving methods 639, *645*
  crowded teeth 881
  early childhood caries 979
  endodontically-diseased teeth 782–783,
    784–785
  implant placement at time of 643–644,
    645–647, **647**
  microsurgical approach 1182, *1182*
  performers/actors 1176
  pontic placement and 566
  ridge preservation 639, *640–641,* 1200
  ridge resorption after 638–639, **639,** *639,*
    1182, 1200
extruded teeth, cosmetic contouring 300
extrusion, orthodontic
  cosmetic contouring after 298
  crown–root fractures 1221, *1222*
  prior to implant placement 905, *907*
  root segments 793, *798,* 1223
eyebrow line 1099, *1101*
eyebrows, makeup 1150
eyeglasses, harmful habits 831, *833*
eye makeup 1150

facebow
  digital *87,* 88
  transfer, casts 1303, *1303–1304*
facelift (rhytidectomy) 1137, *1138*
face size
  measurement 614–615, *614–615*
  proportion of tooth size to 249–251,
    250–252
facial analysis 56, *57,* 1097–1119
  dentofacial deformity 930–931, *931–932*
  diastemata restoration 844–845
  facial reference lines 1098–1101, *1101*
  frontal view 1098–1113, *1100–1112*
  importance 1086–1097
  oblique view 1113
  orthodontics 899–900
  profile view 1113–1119
  proportional 253–265
  records 1097–1098
  soft tissues 1005–1006
  see also dentofacial analysis; macroesthetic
    analysis
facial appearance, importance of 10–11,
  10–11

facial asymmetry 951–955
  classification 953
  clinical evaluation 1061–1062, 1065–1067
  esthetic *1090*, 1090–1091, *1092*, 1095
  location *1094*, *1099*
  observation 1089–1090, *1089–1090*
  see also facial symmetry
facial components, ranking of importance 6, **8**
facial disfigurement, makeup for 1151
facial esthetics
  cosmetic adjuncts 1143–1151
  evaluation 930–931, *931–932*
  impact of orthodontics 898–905
  orthodontic perspective 1051–1083
  pediatric dentistry 1005–1010
  plastic surgery 1131–1140
  restorative dentistry 1085–1126
  three dimensions 1052, *1052*
facial expressions 1088–1089
facial fifths *see* fifths, facial
facial hair, male 1148, *1148*
facial image view evaluation (FIVE) 253, *255*
  calculating intercanine width 261, *262*
  tooth-to-tooth width proportions 257, *257*
facial index 1057–1058, *1060*
facial midline 1090–1094, *1091–1095*
  chin symmetry and 1107
  complete denture positioning 617, *618*
  dental midline and *1094*, 1094, 1104–1106
  diastema closure and 845
  digital smile design 87, 88, 94, *95–97*
  interpupillary line relationship 1099, *1101*
  nasal tip position and 1104
  perceived 1090, *1091*
facial photographs 1053–1056, 1098
  basic protocols 171–173
  dentofacial deformities 934
  frontal images 1053–1055
    camera orientation 1053, *1055*
    repose (at rest) 173, 1053, *1055*
    smile (dynamic) 171–173, *173*, 1055, *1056*
  oblique images 1055–1056, *1057*
  profile images 173, 1056, *1058*
  submental image 1056, *1059*
facial profile
  convex 1113, *1114*
  denture tooth arrangement 620, *621*
  denture tooth selection 616
  diastema correction and 845
  facial analysis 1113–1119
  landmarks **1069**, *1069*, *1099*
  macroesthetic evaluation 1063–1068, *1069–1075*
  pediatric patients *1008–1009*, 1008–1010
  photographs 173, 1056, *1058*
  symmetry and proportion 931, *932*
facial profile angle 1113
facial proportions 245, 930–931
  aging effects 245, *246*, 1101–1102, 1106–1107
  golden proportion *see* golden proportion
  orthodontic esthetics 900–902
  pediatric patients *1007–1009*, 1007–1010
  rule of fifths *see* fifths, facial
  rule of sevenths 245, *245*
  rule of thirds *see* thirds, facial
  transverse 1058–1059, *1063–1064*
  vertical 1057–1058, 1101–1104
facial prostheses, shade guides 281
facial reference lines 1098–1101, *1101*
facial resurfacing 1140
facial shape (or form)
  classification 1058, *1060–1061*, 1098, *1100*
  denture tooth selection and 615, 616
  female hairstyles and 1144–1147, *1144–1147*
  male 1147–1148, *1148*
  special effects influencing 218–219
facial symmetry 930–931, 1089–1097
  analysis using facial midline 1090–1094, *1091–1095*
  esthetic relevance 1094–1095
  pediatric patients *1006–1008*, 1007–1008
  see also facial asymmetry
facial taper 1058, *1062–1063*
facial thirds *see* thirds, facial
facial views *see* frontal view of face; oblique view of face; submental view of face
facilities, office, attractiveness 115, *116–118*
failures, esthetic 1235–1260
  compromised treatment plan 1240–1244
  eventual (restoration longevity) 1244–1260
  immediate 1236–1239
  prostheses 1231–1232
  reasons for 1235
family, patient's 1332
Faunce, F.R. 434
feather-edged veneer preparation 442, *443*
Federal Health Insurance Portability and Accountability Act 145
federal requirements 150
fees, dental 79–81
  factors determining 80–81
  patient education 49
  payment before completion 145
  payment planning 70
  raising, for problem patients 40, 77, 79
  refunds 147, *148*
  see also financial considerations
feldspathic porcelain
  all-ceramic crowns 502–505, 518, 1264
  bilayered ceramic restorations 507–510, *508–509*, 1264
  fused to metal 514
  milled restorations, tooth preparation 1264
  veneer onlay 482
  veneers 434, 502–505
    diastema closure 867, *868*, 871, *871*
    masking stained teeth 687, *687*
    tooth preparation 446
feminine appearance
  cosmetic contouring 301, *301*, 303
  dentists' perceptions 614
  failure to incorporate 1237, *1238*
  ideal tooth widths 250–251, *252*
  incorporating 223, *225*
  size and shape of teeth 248, *249, 250*
ferrule design, endodontically-treated teeth *744*, 745
fiber-polymer composite prefabricated posts **736**
fifths, facial 245, *246*
  orthodontics 902, *903*, 931, *931*, 1058–1059, *1063*
  prominent ears and 1059, *1064*
filing of teeth 5, *5*, 297–298, *298*
  see also contouring, cosmetic
film actors *see* performers/actors
financial considerations
  actors and entertainers 1154–1155, 1176
  attachment RPDs 594, 597
  choice of crown 523
  compromising esthetics 1242
  older patients 1025
  restorative choices 893
  restoring fractured teeth 724
  single-lens reflex cameras 159
  treatment planning 78, 79
  see also fees, dental
fingernail habits 825, *826*
finger sucking 811–813, *812*
first visit *see* initial visit
Fit Checker 1324, 1341, *1342*
FIVE *see* facial image view evaluation
fixed partial dentures (bridges; FPDs) 543–571
  after root fractures 793
  attachment RPDs placed on pontics 593, *594*
  attachments for conversion to RPDs 597–598, *599*
  cantilever 555, *556*
  ceramic connectors 1379, **1380**
  ceramic interdental inserts *228–230*, 229, 570, *572–573*
  diagnosis 543–547
    clinical examination 544, *544*
    diagnostic wax-up 545, *546*
    esthetic considerations 545–546, *546–547*
    functional considerations 546–547
    interdisciplinary consultations 547
    radiographic examination 544–545
    study casts 545, *545, 546*
  digital impressions 1403, *1404*
  endodontic access 779, *779*
  evolving technologies 562–563, *562–564*
  failure
    emergency repair 1231–1232
    framework 1250, *1250–1251*
    technical 1254–1255, *1258–1260*
  one missing anterior tooth 555, *555–557*

fixed partial dentures (bridges; FPDs) (cont'd)
   orthodontic-restorative treatment 909
   performers/actors 1173–1174
   pontics *see* pontics
   precision attachments 564, *564*
   prepless 549
   replacement of pre-existing 547, *548*
   resin-bonded 549
      diastema closure 863–864, *863–865*
      orthodontic–restorative therapy 909
   resin-bonded partial-veneer 549
   retainers 547–551
      complete coverage 550–551, *551–552*
      functional considerations 546–547
      margin location 551, *553*
      margin materials 552–553, *553–554*
      partial coverage 549–550, *549–550*
      porcelain–metal junction 553–554, *554*
      resin-bonded 549
   ridge augmentation 566–570, *569*, 1201–1204, *1201–1204*
   special impression technique 1294, *1295–1297*
   splinting and 555
   telescoping crowns as abutments 555–562
   temporary 1313–1314
   try-in 1341, *1343*, 1345
   zirconia frameworks *see under* zirconia
fixed prosthetic restorations
   performers/actors 1173–1174, *1173–1174*
   try-in principles 1339–1352
   see also crowns; fixed partial dentures; inlays/onlays; veneers
flash systems, camera
   selection 163, *164, 165*
   settings 166–168, *169, 170*
flexibility, impression materials 1293, **1293**
floss, dental 1410, 1414, *1415*
   composite restorations 409
   implant cleaning 1423–1427
   incorrect use 409, 827, 830–831, *831*, 1410, *1411*
   removing excess cement 1358–1359, *1361*
   rubber dam retention 772–773
fluoride
   acidic preparations 477
   -containing cement 1247–1248
   gel, vital bleaching 345
fluorosis, dental 679–680, *681*, 682
   bleaching 328, *328*, 682–683, 685
   veneers 440, 441
follow-up care, patient's commitment 133
follow-up letters 139, *141*
food
   acidic *see* acidic beverages/foods
   stains 328, 675, *679*
Food and Drug Administration (FDA) 345
foreign objects, harmful habits 825–833
foundation, facial cosmetic 1150
FPDs *see* fixed partial dentures
fractures 721–745

crown *see* crown fractures
crown–root *740*, 1221, *1222*
   extracoronal **722**
   intracoronal **722**
   porcelain *see* porcelain fractures
   restorations 1224–1230
   root *see* root fractures
Frankfort plane 1113
frenectomy 915
frenum
   fibrous attachments 843
   prominent, gingival recession risk 1184
frontal view of face
   facial analysis 1098–1113, *1100–1112*
   facial asymmetry 1061–1062, *1065–1067*
   landmarks **1054**, *1054*, 1099
   macroesthetic evaluation 1057–1062, *1060–1067*
   pediatric patients 1006–1008, *1007–1008*
   photographs 1053–1055, *1054–1055*
      basic protocols 171–173, *173*
      camera orientation 1053, *1055*
   symmetry and proportion 930–931, *931*
f-stop 166–168, *169, 170*
Fuji Bond LC adhesive 362
full veneer preparation design (Class 6) 442, *445*, 447–448, 456–459
functional-esthetic analysis B1–B6
furcation involvement 1185, *1186*
fusion, tooth 1000, *1000–1003*

gastroesophageal reflux disease (GERD) 33, 712
G-Bond adhesive system 366
gender differences
   age-related arch changes 920, *921*
   color matching ability 274, **284**
   cosmetic contouring 301, *301*, 303
   facial index 1058
   interarch tooth size ratios 923
   nasolabial angle 1114
   tooth color 274
   tooth shape 303, 614
genetic testing 1423, *1424–1426*
genioplasty 959, *961–962*, 1137
geometric theory, tooth morphology 614
geresthetics 1015–1047
   see also older adults
Geristore resin ionomer 794, *800*
gingiva
   color 274
   effects on tooth appearance 186
   electrosurgery 1290–1291, *1291*
   implant patients *see* implants, gingival tissues
   porcelain biocompatibility 439
   prostheses *see* tissue inserts
   retraction prior to impressions 1288–1291, *1289–1292*
   shade guides 281
   see also soft tissues
gingival architecture

crowded teeth 878–879, *880*
   implant provisionalization and 656–657
gingival augmentation
   indications 1185
   papilla reconstruction 1195–1199
   root coverage 1183–1195
   see also connective tissue grafts
gingival biotype
   assessment 654, **654**
   crown selection and 523
   esthetic crown-lengthening and 1205
   implant patients 654–655
   recession risk and 1185
gingival display 1123
   crown selection and 523, 525–526, *526*
   diastema closure and 847
   excessive (gummy smile) 905, 1123–1124
      Botox therapy 905
      periodontal plastic surgery 1204–1208, *1205–1209*
      surgical–orthodontic correction *947*, 948
   orthodontic aspects 904–905, *905*
   patient/lay preferences 137–138, 899
   smile design 247, *247*
   see also smile line
gingival embrasures
   crowns 527–529, *528*
   diastema closure 849, *850*
   open *see* black triangles
   performers/actors 1174
   try-in appointment 1346, *1347*
gingival esthetics
   diastema correction 847
   orthodontics 909, 913–914
   patient preferences 137–138
gingival grafts *see* connective tissue grafts
gingival hypertrophy 1205, *1205*
   anabolic steroid abuse 825
   around restorations 1245, *1245*
gingival inflammation (gingivitis)
   excessive laser sculpting 149–150, *151*
   marginal fit of crown and 1267, *1268*
   prevention in older adults 1023
   recession risk 1184, *1185*
   try-in appointment 1339
gingival inserts *see* tissue inserts
gingival margins
   all-ceramic crowns 1267–1268
   ceramic veneers 456, *458, 470*, 473
   checking fit 1345
   composite restorations 408, *411–412*
   fixed partial dentures 551–553, *553–554*
   free
      evaluating thickness 1264
      smile design 248, *250*
   metal–ceramic crowns 518–521, *520*, 1265–1266, *1267*
   orthodontics and 913
   poor fitting to 1236, *1237*
   porcelain-fused-to-metal crowns 1277–1280, *1280*
   see also subgingival margins

gingival recession
    around restorations 1245
    etiology 1184
    metal–ceramic crowns 519
    Miller classification 1184
    postimplant *655*
    root coverage surgery 1183–1195
    tooth preparation for crowns and 1264–1266, *1267*
gingival retraction cords *1288,* 1288–1290
    ceramic veneers 469
    implant restoration 660–661
    metal–ceramic crowns 519
    one-cord technique *1289,* 1289–1290
    placement 1288–1290
    problems *1290, 1290*
    tooth staining caused by iron-impregnated 1236
    two-cord technique *1289,* 1290
gingival sulcus
    choice of crowns and 523
    crown margin placement *1267,* 1267–1268
    retraction cord placement 1288–1290, *1289–1290*
gingivectomy
    attachment RPDs 593
    diastema correction and 847
gingivitis *see* gingival inflammation
glass-ceramics 1375–1377
    full coverage crowns 506, *507,* 510–514
    posterior partial coverage restorations 481–482
    tooth preparation 1264
    veneers 434–435, 453, 462–465
    see also lithium-disilicate ceramic
glass-infiltrated ceramics 1377
glass ionomers
    adhesion to lased tooth structure 973
    cements 1356
    cores **736**
    lining composite restorations 403
    pediatric dentistry 970
    polishing 1416
    see also resin-modified glass ionomers
glaze
    stain combined with 194–195, *197–198*
    surface staining over 194
gloss, surface 284
glove materials 1292
Gluma Solid Bond adhesive 362
glycerin, ceramic veneer fitting 467, *472*
gold
    collar, ceramometal crowns 1244
    factors influencing choice 523
    inlays, masking 1169
    pontics 571
    porcelain restorations opposing 479, 481
    powder, for spraying model casts 190, *190*
    retainers for fixed partial dentures 549
gold crowns
    endodontic access 776
    partial or full coverage 502, *502–504*

golden mean, Snow's 257, *257*
golden proportion 243–245, *244,* 1095–1097
    dentists' preferences 258–259, *260*
    diastema closure and 846
    orthodontic esthetics and 902–903
    tooth-to-tooth width ratios 254–257, *256*
Goldstein, R.E.
    bleaching light 326, *327*
    overlay method of tooth preparation 398–399, *399–400*
    veneer onlays 482
Goldstein ColorVue Probe 61, *63*
Goldstein veneer preparation kit 456, *457*
gonial angle *1063, 1068–1069*
gonion *1094, 1099*
graying, peri-implant tissues *655,* 658, *659,* 1370
gray-stained teeth **671,** 751, *753*
    amalgam restorations *677,* 679
    tetracycline staining 329, *329,* 755
Grealy, Lucy 12
Greece, ancient 1095–1097
green stains **671,** *672, 674, 678*
grooves, discolored deep 670, *674*
Grossman, David 506
group function occlusion 916
growth, craniofacial 1006
growth factors 642–643, *643*
guarantees 79, 81, 137–138
guided tissue regeneration 1184
Gummy gingival indicator 281
gummy smile *see* gingival display, excessive
GUM Soft-Picks 1410, *1412*
gutta-percha
    removal, for core retention 735, *737, 739–741*
    root canal obturation 780, *781*
Guy, Jasmine *1165*

habits, oral 811–834
    adults 813–833
    ceramic veneers and 441, 474
    diagnosis 52, 833–834
    diastemas due to *816–817,* 817, 843, *843*
    effects on composite restorations 409–413
    fixed partial dentures and 554, *554*
    pediatric patients 995
    porcelain veneers and 441
    questionnaire *828,* 833–834
    signs 813
    tooth wear 697, *698,* 708
    treatment 833–834
    see also bruxism; digit sucking
Hader vertical attachment 605
Hagger, Oskar 356
hair care services 14
hair color 1147
hairstyles 1144
    female 1144–1147, *1144–1147*
    male 1147–1148, *1148*
    minimizing a double chin 1150

Hannes anchor attachment 605
Hayashi shade guide 276
Hazard Communication Standard (HCS) 150
head-to-body height ratios 245, *245*
heart disease 1023, 1024–1025
heart-shaped face, hair styles 1144, *1146,* 1148
heat testing 756
hematologic disorders 330–331, 682
hemifacial microsomia 955, *956–960*
hemolytic disease of newborn (erythroblastosis fetalis) 331, 682
hemorrhage, pulp
    during canal instrumentation 780
    tooth color changes 682, 751, *752,* 768
hepatic–biliary disorders 682
histogram, in photography 162, 165–166, *166–168,* 168
history
    bleaching 326, *327*
    contouring 297–298, *298*
    esthetic dentistry 4–5, *4–5*
    impression taking 1388–1389
Hollywood templates *see* esthetic templates
holographic group consultations 74
honesty 138
Hope, Bob 1155
horizontal 1/16th rule 249, *250*
horizontal ridge augmentation 640–642, *642*
House, M.M. 249, 614–615
hue 272, *273*
    effects of bleaching 277–278, **284**
Hulse, Tom *1160*
Hybrid Bond adhesive system 366
hybrid composite resins 395, 862, 1416
hybrid ionomers 1356
hydrocolloid (agar) impressions 459, 1302, 1388
hydrofluoric acid etching
    ceramic fitting surfaces *1362,* 1364
    ceramic veneers 467, 469
    fractured restorations *1228,* 1230
    glass ceramics 1376
    intraoral repairs *1228,* 1230
    porcelain butt margins 1356, *1358*
hydrogen peroxide
    nonvital bleaching 346, 348
    vital bleaching 336, 340, 342, 343
hydroxyethyl methacrylate (HEMA) 360
hygienists 53–54, *54*
    care of composite restorations 415
    care of crowns 536
    initial contact with 52
    maintenance appointments *1416,* 1416–1417
    oral care advice 1412–1415
    polishing restorations 1416–1417
hypersensitive teeth *see* tooth sensitivity
hypertelorism 1058–1059
hypertension 1023, 1024

hypocalcification, enamel 679, *680–681*
    contouring 300, *300*, 302
    microabrasion *342*, *680–681*
    see also white spots

I-bar clasp 584–585, *585*
iBond Self Etch adhesive system *363*, 366
ice chewing 831–833
ice pencil 754, *756*
IC plunger attachment 605, *606*
ICW *see* intercanine width
IL-1 gene mutation 1423
illuminance 275
illusions 188–192
    diastema correction and 847–848, *848–849*
    form and color creating 216, *217*, **218**
    principles 188–189, *188–189*
    resolving specific problems 206–229
    role of makeup 1149
    shaping and contouring creating 189–190, 305, *306–307*
    techniques for creating 189–192
    see also special effects
images
    editing 180, *180*
    file types 164–165
    importing to computer 179
    presentation 180
    resolution 160–161, *162*, *163*, *164*
    saving 179–180, *180*
    storage and presentation 179–181, *181*
    see also computer imaging; photographs
implant probes 1419, *1421*
implants 637–663
    abutments 657–658, *659*
        implant platform interface 1370, *1370–1371*
        restoration interface 1372–1374, *1373–1374*
        soft tissue interface 1370–1372, *1371–1372*
    clinical evaluation **1417**, 1417–1418, *1418*
    crestal bone loss 1417, *1418*
    crown–root fractures 1221, *1222*
    designs 653–654
    endodontically-diseased teeth 782–783, *784–785*
    fixed partial dentures as alternatives 555, *556–557*
    gingival tissues 654–655
        biotype assessment 654, **654**
        esthetics 1370–1372, *1371–1372*
        grafting 654–655, *655–656*, 1195, *1196*
        maintenance care 1419, 1423
        provisionalization and 644–645, *648–650*, 656, *657–658*
    informed consent 144
    intraoral examination 1419–1421
    mobility 1417
    older adults 1035–1036, *1037–1047*
    orthodontic extrusion prior to 905, *907*

pain 1417
position 646–653
    apicoronal (depth) 653
    buccolingual 647, *652*
    correcting errors 646, *651*
    mesiodistal 647–649, *653*
    surgical guides 646–647, *651–652*
protocols 643–645
    delayed or late placement 643, *644*
    early placement 643
    immediate placement 643–644, *645–647*, **647**
    immediate restoration 644–645, *648–650*
provisional restorations 656–657
    immediate 644–645, *646–650*, 656
    as impression posts *650*, 656–657
    Siltek method 1324, *1327–1328*
    soft tissue benefits 644–645, *648–650*, 656, *657–658*
removal *651*
retained primary teeth 908
smile line and lip dynamics 638
implant scalers 1422, *1422*
implant-supported dentures 629–630, *631–633*
    overpartial dentures 605
implant-supported restorations 658–663
    cement-retained 1372, 1373
    design and cementation 660–662, *660–662*
    in-office hygiene care 1419–1423
    maintenance 1417–1428
    materials 658–659, *662*, 662–663
    patient self-care 1423–1428
    probing around 1418, *1418*
    retrievability 1379–1381
    screw-retained 1372–1373, *1374*, 1380–1381, *1381*
Impregum 1388
impressions 1287–1307
    analog vs digital 1400
    ceramic veneers 459–460
    concept 1388
    determining gingival form 1346
    digital *see* digital impressions
    Digital Smile Design 107
    disinfection 133–134, 1302
    gypsum die preparation 1302
    history 1388–1389
    interocclusal records 1303–1307
    materials 1291–1294, 1302
        history 1388
        manipulation 1294, **1294**
        properties **1293**, 1293–1294
    mounting casts 1303, *1303–1304*
    multiple backup 1302, *1303*
    posterior ceramic partial coverage restorations 482
    preimpression surface optimizer 1294, *1295*
    removal and trimming 1302

soft-tissue preparation 1287–1291, *1288–1292*
    techniques 1294–1302
        dual viscosity 1298
        putty wash 1299, *1299–1302*
        single viscosity 1295
        special 1294, *1295–1298*
    try-in stage 1343, *1344*
impression tray adhesives 1294
impression trays 1294
"I'm sorry" legal protection 138
In-Ceram all-ceramic crowns 506, **513**
In-Ceram Zirconia restorations 1249–1250, 1253
incisal curve 1101
    lower lip relations 1121, *1122*
    reverse *1119*, 1122
incisal edges
    age-related wear 219, *221*
    close-up repose image 174–175, *175*
    determination of position 246–247, *246–247*
    diastema closure and 846
    esthetic shaping 314, *314*
    lengthening 1120, *1120*
    lower lip relationships 1120–1122, *1122*
incisal embrasures
    ceramic veneers *472*, 473
    cosmetic contouring 308, *310*, 316, *317*
    crowns 527, *528*
    performers/actors 1174, *1176*
    restorations 221, *224–225*
    smile design 247, *248*
    try-in appointment 1346–1347, *1347*
incisal exposure
    children 1008
    at rest 1119–1120, *1119–1121*
incisal overlap veneer preparation *see* overlapping incisal edge veneer preparation
incisal plane 246, *246*
    diastema closure and 846
    evaluation 1107–1110, *1110–1111*
incisors
    irregularity index 920
    proclination *922*, 923, 1076
    protrusion *see* protrusion, incisor
    shape and SPA factors 248, *248*, 249
    too narrow 210, *212*
    too wide *207*, 207–208
    width in relation to other teeth 254–265
    see also central incisors; lateral incisors
inclination, crown restorations 526–527
inclusion, dental 997, *997–1000*
inCoris TZI C 537
incremental layering technique, composite restorations 403, *405*, 405–406
indirect composite/acrylic veneers 434, 461, 502
infants 10
infection control, negligent practice 133–134
inferior alveolar nerve 942, 944–948

informed consent 48, 132–137
  disclosure obligations 132–133, 143–144
  documentation 133, *134–137*, 139, *141,* 142
  less invasive procedures 145
  misinformed consent 144
  patient's commitment to follow-up 133
  responsibility for obtaining 144–145
  surgical–orthodontic correction of dentofacial deformity 933
infrabulge bar (I-bar) clasp 584–585, *585*
initial visit 51–67
  clinical examination 55–67
  important questions to ask 51–52
  patient observation 52–53
  prior to 48–51
  sequence of staff contacts 52, *52*
inlays/onlays 5, *5*
  ceramic
    cementation 1361–1364
    CEREC system 483–490, *486*
    endodontic access 778
    posterior 478–483, *482*
  ceramic veneer onlays 482, *482–484*
  composite resin 393, *394*
  jadeite 5, *5*, 298, *298*
inside-outside tray bleaching technique 348
Insta-Dam Relaxed Fit 774
insurance, dental, for older adults 1017, 1025
integrated digital systems 67
intercanine width (ICW) 249–250, *251*
  determination 261, *262, 262*
  RED proportions and 257, *259*
  tooth width calculations from 260, *261,* 261–262, **262**
intercanine width/central incisor width (ICW/CIW) quotient 263–265
  chart **263**
  determination 263–264, *264, 266*
  example of clinical use 264–265, *265–267*
  method for using chart 263, **265**
interdental brushes 1410, *1411–1412,* 1423
interdental papillae *see* papillae, interdental
interdental spaces
  ceramic veneers 226–228, 452, *469*
  composite resin bonding 226–228, *227*
  crown restorations 227–228, *228–229,* 1280
  Pincus principles D7, *D8*
  see also black triangles; diastemas
interdental tissue inserts *see* tissue inserts
interdisciplinary approach
  facial esthetics 1089
  orthodontics 905–908, *905–909*
  papilla reconstruction 1196, *1197*
  Pincus principles D5–D6
interdisciplinary team
  communication 86
  consultations 73, *73–74*
inter-ear line 1099, *1101*
interincisal distance, crown restorations and 527, *527*

interior design 115, *116–118*
interlabial gap 1113
intermaxillary fixation (IMF) 937, 940
internal tooth resorption 682, *753*
  posttraumatic 980, *980*
interocclusal records 1303–1307
interpreters 144
interproximal areas
  ceramic veneer coverage 449, 452
  contacts with full crowns 519–521
  finishing
    ceramic veneers 471–472, *473*
    composite restorations 409
    posterior ceramic partial coverage restorations 483
  staining, to create tooth separation 218, *218*
interpupillary line 1099, *1101*
  assessing parallelism 1107–1110, *1109*
interzygomatic width (IZW) 249, *251*
intracoronal attachment removable partial dentures 595–596, *596,* 597–599
  advantages 597
  disadvantages 597
  types 597–599, *598–599*
intraoral cameras 55–56, 57–59, *59–60*
  alternatives to 158
  implant self-care 1427–1428
inverted "L" osteotomy 942
Invisalign 56, 890, 1169, 1396–1397
IPS e.max 512–514
  CAD
    CEREC inlays 484, *490–491*
    crowns 512–514
    crystalline structure 512–513, *513*
  Ceram 465
  implant restorations 662, *662*
  longevity 513
  pressable (e.max Press)
    all-ceramic crowns *512,* 512–514
    crystalline structure 512, *513*
    posterior partial coverage restorations 481–482
    veneer onlays 482
    veneers 438–439, 462
      as alternatives to full crowns 474–477
      laboratory procedures 463–465
      tooth preparation 453–456
IPS Empress
  all-ceramic crowns 510–513, *511,* **513**
  crystalline form 510, *510*
  veneers
    fabrication 462, *463*
    longevity 474
    tooth preparation 446, *449–451*
iron-impregnated gingival retraction cord 1236
irregularity index, incisor 920
irrigation, implant maintenance 1427, *1427*
ISO 164
Isosit-N crowns 502

iTero Element intraoral scanner 1396–1397, *1396–1397,* **1400**
Ivoclar Chromascop shade guide 279–280, *280*
Ivoclar Vivadent shade guides 281, *281*

jadeite inlays 5, *5,* 298, *298*
Japan, *ohaguro* 4, *4*
jaundice, childhood 331, 682
jewelry, metal mouth 826, *829*
JPEG files 164–165
jury trials 151

Kahng Chairside Shade Guides 199–205, *204–207*
Katana all-ceramic crowns 507
Kennedy classification, edentulous areas 582, *582*
Keynote software 86, 87, *87,* 180
Kiel, Richard 1159, *1163–1164*
Kokich, Vincent 899, 902, 907–908, *909,* 1086–1087
Köle, H. 956–957
Kor whitening system 341–342
Kuwata, M. 500, 514

LAAXESS Diamond Bur 776
LAAXESS endodontic access kit 775
labial commissures 1111
labial rotation of teeth 213, *213–214*
labiomental angle 1065, *1072,* 1118–1119
labiomental sulcus 931, *932,* 1065
  excessively deep 1065, *1073–1074*
  pediatric patients 1009, *1009*
laboratory
  CAD/CAM systems 1400–1402
  checklist C1–C5
  communication
    color information 285–286
    crown color selection 535, *535*
    special effects and illusions 197–199
    try-in stage 1337, *1338*
    using photographs 157, *157,* 199
    verbal and written instructions 285
laboratory technician 53
lamina dura 582
laminates *see* veneers
Laminate Veneer System (LVS; Brasseler) 456, *457,* 470, 473
lanugo 822, *824*
laser-assisted new attachment procedure (LANAP) 1029, *1033*
laser conditioning 972
laser etching 972
lasers
  caries detection 55, *55,* 971
  classification **984**
  hard tissue ablation 971–972
    composite adhesion after 972–973
    discolored deep grooves 670
    pediatric dentistry 972
    pit and fissure caries 419, *419*

lasers (cont'd)
  pediatric dentistry 971–973
    amelodentinal dysplasia 975, *975*
    enamel hypoplasia 978, *978*
    extensive cavities 976, *976–977*
    preventive resin restoration 974, *974*
    trauma management 984–986
  soft-tissue applications
    gingival sculpting 148–149, *151*
    pediatric dentistry 973
    preparation for impressions 1291, *1292*
  tissue interaction 971
laser sintering, selective 1402
lateral incisors
  agenesis 441
    fixed partial dentures 549–550, *549–550*
    orthodontic–restorative treatment 905–906
  peg-shaped, orthodontic–restorative treatment 905, *905–906*, *907–908*
  post-and-core restorations 741
  SPA factors 248, *249*
  see also incisors
lateral incisor width (LIW) *261*
  calculation using ICW/CIW quotient **263, 265**
  calculation using RED proportion *261*, **262**, *262–263*, *263*
  in relation to other teeth 254–265, 847
Lava 507
Lava Plus 537
Le Fort I osteotomy
  condylar hyperplasia 953
  macro- and miniesthetic approach 1080, *1080*
  maxillary deficiency 951, *951–952*
  vertical maxillary excess 948, *949–950*
left lateral arch image 176–178, *177*
legal considerations 131–152
  Botox use 151
  dentist's refusal to treat 145
  federal requirements and product warnings 150
  guarantee or warranty 137–138
  "I'm sorry" legal protection 138
  informed consent *see* informed consent
  jury trials 151
  malpractice examples 147–150, *148–151*
  nonnegligent risks and obligation to treat 144
  patient abandonment claims 145
  patient's choice of dentist 146–147
  records and documentation 139–142
  refunds 147, *148*
  standards of care 143–144
  telephone or e-mail consultation 150
  try-in appointment 138–139, *139*
  updating skills and practices 132
lemon consumption 33, 822–824, *824*
lenses, camera 160, *160, 161*
Leonardo da Vinci 243, *244*

leucite-reinforced ceramic 1264, 1376
  see also IPS Empress
lever forces 583
life event stress 27, 41–42
life expectancy 1016, **1016**
  active 1036
light 272, *272*
  color perception 272
  creating illusions 188, *188*
  effects on tooth appearance 185–187
  Pincus principles D3–D4, *D4*
  reflection, fixed restorations 1350
light curing 403, 404–405
  ceramic veneers 469, *472–473*
  equipment 405, *406*
  technique 404–405, *405*
light-emitting diodes (LED) 405
lighting conditions
  clinical photography 166–169
  color matching 275, *275*, 396, 397, *397*, 532–533
  esthetic try-in 1336
  performers and actors 1174, *1177*, 1178
  video recordings 182
light meters 405, *406*
lightness, effects of bleaching 277–278, **284**
light transmission *see* translucency
lines
  creating illusions 188–189, *188–189*
  tooth appearance and 189
lingually locked tooth 891–893
lip(s)
  appearance of teeth and 186–187
  augmentation 1137, *1140*
  biting, habitual 819–821, *819–821*
  closure, children 1008
  coloring *1150*, 1150–1151
  contours, changing with makeup *1150*, 1150–1151
  curvature, pediatric patients 1009, *1009*
  dynamics, implants and 638
  excess mucosal tissue 1112, *1112*
  incompetence, facial photographs 1053–1055
  oblique view 1063, 1113
  profile view 1064–1065, *1071*, 1115–1118
  reference lines 1101, *1101*
  symmetry 1111–1112, *1112*
  thickness 186–187, 1115
  wetting, habitual 819
lip length
  age-related increase 1120
  measurement 1112–1113
lip line
  asymmetric *1112*
  crown selection and 523, 525–526, *526*
  high 525, *526*, *638*, 1123
  low 526, *526*, *638*, 1123, 1124
  medium 525–526, *526*, *638*, 1123
  scar tissue affecting 1112, *1112*
  see also gingival display; smile line
lip position 1115–1118

  closed 1113
  complete dentures 619, *620–621*
  esthetic evaluation 1115–1117, *1116–1117*
  esthetic try-in 1336, *1336*
  repositioning methods 1115, 1117–1118
  rest 1113
  ridge replacement and 1118
  sagittal 1115–1117, *1117*
  tooth position and 1118
lip projection 1064–1065, *1071*
  esthetic evaluation 1115–1118
  reduction of excessive 1065, *1071–1072*
lipstick 1150–1151
  colors 1147, 1150–1151
  minimizing a double chin 1149–1150
  removal 283, 396, 533
lithium-disilicate ceramic 1264, 1376–1377
  bilayered 1376
  crowns
    endodontic access 778
    selection 523, 524, *525*
    technical considerations 512–514
  fixed partial dentures 550
  implant crowns 662, *662–663*
  monolithic *1376*, 1376–1377
  veneers
    indications 441
    laboratory procedures 463–465
    stained teeth 687–688, *687–688*
    tooth preparation 453, *453–456*
  see also IPS e.max
Lombardi, R.E. 1087
  guide to tooth arrangement 190–191, *191*
  repeated ratio 254
long-axis inclinations
  disguising 216–218, *218*
  prostheses for older patients 219, *222*
long face, hair styles 1147, *1147*, 1148
long teeth
  cosmetic contouring 306–313, *308–313*
  crowns 530, 1283
  illusions for 215–216, *215–216*
Loop, J.L. 249, 614–615
lost-wax method 462, 463, 506, 512
lower lip, incisal edge relationships 1120–1122, *1122*
low-level laser therapy (LLLT) 985–986
luting agents *see* cement(s)
lux (lx) 275
luxation injuries 1223
  clinical case 1225, *1225*
  endodontics 793–794
  extrusive 1223, *1224*
  intrusive 990, *990–993*, 1223
  laser-assisted management 993–994, *993–994*
  lateral 1223
LVS *see* Laminate Veneer System

macroesthetic analysis 1052–1076
  clinical case study 1076–1077, *1077–1079*
  facial asymmetry 1061–1062, *1065–1067*

facial photographs 1053–1056, *1055–1059*
frontal view
    clinical examination 1057–1062, *1060–1067*
    landmarks 1053, **1054**, *1054*
    photographs 1053–1055, *1055–1056*
oblique view 1062–1063, *1068–1069*
    photographs 1055–1056, *1057*
pitch, roll and yaw 1072–1076, *1076*
profile view 1063–1068, *1069–1075*
    landmarks **1069**, *1069*
    photographs 1056, *1058*
smile dimensions and 1068–1072
submental view 1056, *1059*
technology and facial imaging 1056–1057, *1059*
see also facial analysis
macroesthetics 1052, *1052*
magnesium alumina, glass-infiltrated 1377
mail, direct 128
maintenance of restorations 1409–1428
makeup 1149–1151
    for facial disfigurement 1151
    for women 1149–1151
malocclusions
    diastemas 848–849
    digit sucking and 812–813
    pediatric patients 995
    porcelain veneers 441
    realistic orthodontic goals 916–919, *916–919*
    skeletal 930
        treatment in adults 916–917, *917*, 933
    tongue thrusting 816–817
    see also Class II malocclusions; Class III malocclusions; occlusion
malpositioned teeth 890–891
    porcelain veneers 441
malpractice claims 131–132
    example 147–150, *148–151*
    jury trials 151
    prophylactic measures 151–152
mamelons, nonfused 298, *299*
mandibular anterior teeth
    ceramic veneers 448–449, *449–451*
    complete dentures
        placement 618, *619*, 619–620, 623
        size and form 615
    cosmetic contouring 303–304, *305–306, 306–307*, 308, *308*
    crowding 890, 920
    fixed partial dentures 550, 551, 553–554
    incisal embrasures 1347
mandibular arch image 178–179
mandibular asymmetry 1061, *1067*
mandibular body osteotomy 942, *944–945*
mandibular deficiency (retrognathism) 942–948
    distraction osteogenesis 956
    orthodontics 944, *946*
    surgical correction 946–947

mandibular excess (prognathism) 940–942
    bimaxillary 940–941, *942*
    dentoalveolar 940
    maxillary deformities with 942, *945*
    orthodontics 939–941, *940*
    pseudo or false 941, 951
    surgical correction 941–942, *943–944*
mandibular plane 1078, *1078–1079*
mania 29, 30
manufacturer's instructions, failure to follow 1255–1260
marginal staining
    composite restorations *see under* composite resin restorations
    porcelain veneers 689–690
    restorations 330, 670–671, *674–676*
marketing 113–129
    creating a brand 114
    developing a plan 114
    Digital Smile Design tool 86
    external 122–129
    internal 115–122
marking, intraoral, cosmetic contouring 304, 308, *309*
masculine appearance
    cosmetic contouring 303
    dentists' perceptions 614
    ideal tooth widths 250–251, *252*
    incorporating 223, *226*
    size and shape of teeth 248, *249, 250*
matrix bleaching 341–345
matrix metalloproteinases (MMPs) 364–365
    inhibitors 364–365, 367
matrix strips
    fitting ceramic veneers *468*, 471–472
    posterior ceramic partial coverage restorations 482–483
maxillary anterior teeth
    adjusting incisal embrasures 1346–1347, *1347*
    complete dentures 622
        placement 616–619, *617–621*, 622–623
        size and form 614–615
    cosmetic contouring 304
    size in relation to face size 249–251, *250–252*
    SPA factors 248, *248*
    width in relation to other teeth 254–265
    see also central incisors; incisors; lateral incisors
maxillary arch image 178, *178–179*
maxillary deficiency 948–951
    anteroposterior (horizontal) 951, *952*
    transverse 948
    vertical 951, *951*
maxillary excess 948
    see also vertical maxillary excess
maxillary osteotomy, Le Fort I *see* Le Fort I osteotomy
maxillomandibular asymmetry 1062, *1067*
Mayans 5, *5*, 298, *298*
McNamara, J.A. 920–921

medical history 67–68, *68–69*
    older adults 1022–1023
Medicare 1017, 1025
medication-induced problems
    older adults 1023
    tooth staining 328–330, *329–331*, **671**, 682, *682*, 751, *755*
    xerostomia 28, *29*, 30
men
    face shape and hairstyle 1147–1148, *1148*
    makeup for 1151
    see also gender differences; masculine appearance
mentocervical angle 931, *932*
mercury 136
mesial groove reciprocation (MGR) clasp 585, *587*, 588
mesial inclination, increasing 216–217, *218*
mesial rotation of teeth 190, *191*, 214, *214*
mesocephalic facial form 1058, *1060*, 1098, *1100*
metadata 142
metal–acrylic resin pontics 570–571
metal–ceramic butt-joint 516, *516*
metal–ceramic restorations 514–523
    adjunctive procedures 515–516
    advantages 515
    cementation 1358–1359, *1359–1361*
    choice of metals 514
    contraindications 514
    design
        metal substructure 516–518, *517–518*
        porcelain–metal junction 517–518, *520*
        porcelain thickness 518, *520, 522*
    disadvantages 515, *515*
    discolored pulpless tooth 523–525
    esthetic considerations 516, *516*
    factors influencing choice 523, 525–526
    failures 518, *518–519*
        margin exposure 1244, *1245*
        metal thickness and 1253–1254, *1257*
    fixed partial denture retainers 551, 552
        margins 552–553, *553–554*
        porcelain–metal junction 553–554
    gingival health and 518–521, *520*
    history 514
    implants 658, *662*
    indications 514
    longevity 1236
    luting agents 521, 1355–1356
    margins *522*, 522–523
        see also metal collar margins; porcelain butt-joint margins
    repairs to existing *1231*
    rubber dam placement 772–773, *773*
    technical failure 1253–1254, *1257–1258*
    technical problems 514–515
    tooth preparation 518–522, *520*
        extent of occlusal reduction 510, *510*
    try-in 1341
    see also porcelain-fused-to-metal crowns
metal collarless crown 522

metal collar margins 522
    FPD retainers 552, 553
    selection 525, 1265–1266, *1267*
metal mouth jewelry 826, *829*
metal–porcelain (covered metal)
        margins 552
metal restorations
    actors and entertainers 1169
    repairs to existing 1230, *1231*
    see also all-metal crowns; gold
metal stains 675, 1236
metamerism, color matching and 275
methylenedioxymethamphetamine
        (ecstasy) 825
microabrasion 341, *342*
    dental fluorosis 682
    hypocalcified areas *342*, 680–681
microcracks, enamel
    creating illusion of height 215, *215*
    ice chewing 831–833
    intraoral camera 57, *59*
    porcelain veneers 440
    simulation techniques 196, *198–199*, **202**
    staining 673
    transillumination 56–57, *58*
    see also cracked tooth syndrome
microdontia 843
microesthetics 1052, *1052*, 1077
microfilled composites 394, *395*
    diastema closure 862, *862–863*
    polishing 1416
microhybrid composites 394, 395, 862
microleakage
    access cavity repairs 782, *782–783*
    composite resin restorations 379, *380*, 401, 1250–1251, *1254*
micromechanical attachment 356–357, *357*
microsurgery 1182–1183
    instruments 1182–1183, *1183*
    papilla reconstruction 1196–1199, *1198–1199*
    ridge augmentation 1202, *1202–1203*
    root coverage 1188–1189, *1188–1189*
midface lift 1133–1134, *1136*
midline *see* dental midline; facial midline
midpupillary distance 1059
midsagittal plane
    maxillary dental midline to 1061, *1065*
    nasal tip to 1061, *1065*
Miller, P.D. 1183
Miller classification, gingival recession 1184
mineral trioxide aggregate (MTA)
    pulp capping 769, *769*
    pulpotomy 1219
    root resorption defects 794
miniesthetics 1052, *1052*
    clinical case study 1077, *1079*
    see also smile
minocycline staining 329–330, *331*, 683
minors
    eating disorders 36
    informed consent 144

mirrors
    clinical photography 169–170, *170–171*
    esthetic try-in 1332, *1335*, 1335–1336
    viewing results 80, *81*
misaligned teeth 890–891, 920
missing teeth
    congenitally *see* agenesis of teeth
    fixed partial dentures 543–571
    illusions, for actors 1158–1159
    orthodontic considerations 917
    pediatric dentistry
        advanced caries 979, *980*
        ectodermal dysplasia 982–983, *982–983*
        orthodontics 996, *996–997*
        pedodontic prostheses *979*, 979–982
        severe trauma 979, 980, *980–982*
    removable partial dentures 581–606
mixed dentition
    dental materials and techniques 970–971
    trauma management 983–986
mobility
    implants 1417
    root fractures 791, *795–796*, 1221
models
    diagnostic study *see* study models
    human professional *see* performers/actors
model spray 190, *190*
modification spaces 582
molars
    fractured endodontically-treated 736–739, *736–739*
    see also posterior teeth
monitor resolution 161, *163*, 164
mood disorders 26, 27–31
morsicatio buccarum et labiorum 819
motion picture industry
    Pincus' work 434, 1153, 1155, D2, D8–D9
    see also performers/actors
motivations, patients' 16–19, 20, *20*
mouth breathing 821–822
mouthguards, protective *see* protective bite appliances
mouth rinses 1414
    staining of teeth 673–674, *677–678*
multidisciplinary approach *see* interdisciplinary approach
Munsell hue-value-chroma color notation system 273
myofascial pain 392

nail biting 825
nanofilled composites 396, 862
nanohybrid composites 395
nanoleakage 360, 364, *364*
narcissistic personality disorder (NPD) 26, 40–41
    case study 36–37
    diagnostic criteria **37**
narrow teeth
    diastema closure 853–854, 856, *856–857*
    illusions masking 209–214, *210–213*, 848
nasal projection 1064, *1071*

nasal tip
    analysis of position 1104
    elevation 1064, *1071*
    to midsagittal plane 1061, *1065*
nasofacial angle 931, *932*
nasofrontal angle 931, *932*
nasolabial angle 1063–1064, *1070*, 1114, *1115*
    orthodontic correction 1064, *1070*
    pediatric patients 1009
    restorative dentistry and 1114–1115, *1116*
nasomental angle 931, *932*
Natho classification of extrinsic dental stain 671
    type 1 (N1) 671, *676–677*
    type 2 (N2) 671, *677*
    type 3 (N3) 671, *678*
Nd:YAG lasers 984–985
needles, harmful habits 825–826, *827*
negative smile line *see* reverse smile line
negligent customary practice 133–137
neurotoxins 1137
neutral zone 616
nickel casting alloys 514
nifedipine 1023
nightguards *see* protective bite appliances
noble metals 514
nociceptive trigeminal inhibition tension suppression system (NTI-TSS) appliance 415
noncarious cervical lesions (NCCLs) *see* abfractions
nonvital teeth
    bleaching *see under* bleaching
    crowning 523–524
    discoloration 346
    temporary restorations 1315
    see also endodontically-treated teeth; pulp sensibility tests
no-preparation veneers 442, *442*
Nordland and Tarnow classification, papillary defects 1196, *1197–1198*
nose
    analysis of proportionality 1059
    plastic surgery *see* rhinoplasty
    prominence, pediatric patients 1009, *1009*
nose tip point (NTP)–gnathion (Gn)/ subnasal (Sn)–gnathion (Gn) ratio 1010
nursing bottle syndrome 979
nursing-home residents 1036–1037
nuts, cracking 833

object, color 272
oblique view of face
    clinical examination 1062–1063, *1068–1069*
    facial analysis 1113
    photographs 1055–1056, *1057*
observer, color 272
obsessive-compulsive disorder (OCD) 26, **30**, 30–31, *830*

obstructive sleep apnea (OSA) 959–964, *962–964*
Obwegeser, Hugo 929–930
   sagittal splitting osteotomy 944–948, *946–947, 949–950*
Occlude-Pascal spray 1341, *1341–1342*
occlusal analysis
   cosmetic contouring 308, *308–309*
   crowns 531
   initial visit 60
   see also bite registration
occlusal plane
   assessment of pitch 1078, *1078–1079*
   evaluating inclination 1108–1110
   oblique view 1056
   surgical rotation 1079–1080, *1080*
occlusal registration 531, 1303–1305, *1305–1306*
occlusal registration strips *468, 472*, 1304, *1305*
occlusal splints, worn teeth 702
occlusion
   abfraction-inducing forces 705
   balanced 916
   bruxism and 697
   canine protected (CPO) 915, 916
   ceramic restorations and 1374–1381
   ceramic veneers and *470, 473*
   complete dentures 613, *613–614*, 620–622
      anterior teeth 620
      posterior 621–622, *622*
      vertical dimension 620–621, *621–622*
   cosmetic contouring and 302, 303–304, 313
   crown placement and 523, 531
      erroneous 1238, *1239*
   diastema closure and 848–849
   establishing a stable 1332
   group function 916
   ideal functional 915–916
   ideal static 915
   implant patients 1419–1421
   lingualized 613, *613–614*
   orthodontic goals 915–919, *916–919*
   removable partial dentures 583
   restoring fractured teeth and 724, *726*
   try-in appointment 1339, 1346
   vertical dimension *see* vertical dimension of occlusion
   see also malocclusions
Occupational Safety and Health Administration (OSHA) 133–134, 150
Octolink attachment system 600, *602–603*
office facilities, attractiveness 115, *116–118*
ohaguro 4, *4*
older adults 1015–1047
   attitudes to dental esthetics 1017–1020, 1024
   benefits of esthetic dentistry 1016, *1017–1020*, 1021, *1021–1022*
   bleaching 331, 333–336, 1025, 1026, *1026*

characteristics 1016–1017
chronic illness 1020–1022, **1022**, 1024–1025
demographic trends 1015–1016, **1016**
denture tooth selection 615
endodontics 1030
esthetic dental procedures 1025–1028
facial esthetics 904–905, 930
history and examination 1022–1023
implants 1035–1036, *1037–1047*
nursing-home or assisted-living residents 1036–1037
oral health maintenance 1023–1024
orthodontics 1029, 1031, *1031*
periodontal therapy 1029, 1032, *1032, 1033*
prevention and risk assessment 1023–1024
prosthodontics 1030–1035, *1032, 1034–1036*
tooth color 331, *332*, 616, 1025
tooth size–arch length discrepancies 919–921
tooth wear 696, 1025–1026, 1034–1035, *1034–1035*
treatment planning 1024–1025
see also age-related changes
oligodontia 982–983
Omega Ceramic 516
one-sixteenth (1/16th) rule
   combined with rule of thirds 249, *251*
   complete dentures 614–615, *615*
   horizontal 249, *250*
   vertical 249, *250*
onlays *see* inlays/onlays
online directories 125
online group discount shopping services 128
opalescent ceramic systems 516
opaquing
   crowns 524–525
   fractured restorations 1230, *1231*
   porcelain veneers 452, 461–462, 468–469
open bite
   abfraction 705
   caused by digit sucking 812–813
   mandibular excess with 940–941, 942, *942*
   pediatric patient 1004, *1004–1005*
OptiBond AIO adhesive 366
OptiBond FL adhesive 362, *363*, 367
OptiBond Solo Plus adhesive 362
OptiBond XTR adhesive 368
optical geometry, visual shade matching 283, *283*
Optradam Plus 774, *774*
oral cancer 1023
oral care products 1412–1415
oral habits *see* habits, oral
oral hygiene 1410–1415
   attachment RPDs 594
   bad habits 827, *830–831*
   bulimia nervosa 33
   ceramic veneers 477

composite restorations 409, 415, *416*
crowns 536
depressed patients 27, 28, *29*
implant self-care *1423*, 1423–1428, *1427–1428*
nursing-home residents 1036–1037
older adults 1023–1024
patient instruction 1412
pretreatment 1410
restoration of crowded teeth and 881
stained teeth due to poor *672*, 673, 674, 678
oral surgery 74
orange stains **671**, 674, *676*
Oraseal Putty 347, 773
orthodontic appliances
   bruxism 413–415, *415, 814*, 815
   digit sucking 813
   fingernail habits 825, *826*
   harmful oral habits 833
   lip or cheek biting *820*, 821, *821*
   pediatric trauma 980, *980–982*
   performers/actors 1169–1170, *1171–1172*
   postsurgical 939
   technological advances 909
   temporomandibular joint pain 815, *815–816*
orthodontics
   accelerated osteogenic (AOO) 957–959
   adult esthetic 897–923
   attachment RPDs 593
   bleaching combined with 334, *335*
   clinical records 899, *899–901*
   compromise 56, 72
   cosmetic contouring as alternative 300, 302, *302–303*
   cracked tooth syndrome 800–801, *803–804*
   crowded teeth **882**, 890, *892, 893*
   diastema closure 844, 849
      composite resin bonding after 853, 856, *856–857*
      periodontal surgery after 915
   esthetic vs cosmetic 897–898
   facial considerations 898–905, 1051–1083
      clinical case study 1076–1083
      dentofacial analysis 1057–1062
      evaluation in three dimensions *1052*, 1052–1054
      macroesthetic evaluation 1062–1068
      macroesthetics and smile dimensions 1068–1076
      photographs 1053–1056, *1055–1059*
      technology and facial imaging 1056–1057, *1059*
   fixed partial dentures and 545
   force requirements 911–912, *912–913*
   gingival recession due to 1184
   interdisciplinary approach 905–908, *905–909*
   malposed and misaligned teeth 890–891
   mandibular prognathism 939–941, 940

orthodontics (cont'd)
  mandibular retrognathism 944, 946
  occlusal considerations 915–919, 916–919
  older adults 1029, 1031, 1031
  papillary defects 1196, 1197
  pediatric 995–1004
    traumatic loss of teeth 980, 980–982
  performers (actors) 1169–1170, 1171–1172
  periodontal considerations 909–915, 911–914
  periodontally accelerated osteogenic (PAOO) 912, 913
  postsurgical 937–939
  presurgical 935–937, 939–940
  referral for 70–72
  rejection by patient 1243, 1243–1244
  root resorption risk 144
  skeletal malocclusions 933
  surgically assisted 956–959
  technological advances 909, 910
  temporary restorations during 1312
  tongue thrusters 817
  tooth size–arch length discrepancies 919–923
  treatment planning 60
    three-dimensional approach 1052, 1052–1056, 1054
  vertical maxillary excess 948, 949
  worn teeth 699–702
orthognathic surgery see surgical–orthodontic treatment
Osler, Sir William 751
otoplasty 1059, 1064
oval face, hair styles 1144, 1144, 1148
overextensions, potential 1339
overhead, financial 80–81
overlapping incisal edge veneer preparation (Class 4) 442–446, 444, 446–448, 456–459
overlapping teeth, cosmetic contouring 298, 299, 315–316, 315–317, 318, 318
overlay dentures
  for actors 1156–1160, 1158–1164
  comic 1176–1177, 1177
overlay technique 398–400, 399–400, 690
  removing stains 400, 675
  repairing composite restorations 690
  tooth lengthening 399–400, 401
overpartial dentures 605
overtreatment 1235
oxide ceramics 1377–1381
  veneers 434–435, 453
  see also aluminum oxide; zirconia
ozone therapy 971

pain
  anesthetic test 763–764
  clinical evaluation of dental 754–762
  implant-related 1417
palatal stent 1190, 1192

palate, connective tissue harvesting 1189–1190, 1190–1191
palpation, tooth 761, 761
panoramic radiographs 762
  dentofacial deformity 934
  orthodontics 901, 903
papillae, interdental
  crown lengthening and 1206–1207, 1207
  display when smiling 1124–1125
  implant placement and 645, 648–649
  large diastemata 856–862
  loss of 1181–1182, 1182
    concealing 225–229, 227–236
    flossing-related 409, 827, 830–831, 1410, 1411
    gingival inserts see tissue inserts
  Nordland and Tarnow classification of defects 1196, 1197–1198
  orthodontic aspects 913–914, 914
  postextraction changes 639
  reconstruction 1195–1199
    multidisciplinary approach 1196, 1197
    postoperative care 1199
    surgical technique 1196–1199, 1197–1199
  reshaping, diastema closure 849–850
parafunctional habits see habits, oral
parents, consent by 144
parotid gland enlargement 31, 32, 32, 822, 824
passive fit 1378
patient education 898
  caries prevention 1414–1415
  implant self-care 1423–1428, 1428
  marketing role 119–120, 121
  oral hygiene 1412
  prior to treatment planning 49, 49–50
  role of photographs 159
patients
  abandonment 145, 152
  commitment to follow-up 133
  decision making see decision making, patient
  esthetic perceptions 137–138
  motivations 16–18, 20, 20
  personality types 48–49
  predicting response to treatment 19
  problem 36–41, 77–79
  psychological challenges 25–44
  response to abnormality 16
  right to choose a dentist 146–147, 146–147
  smile design preferences 268
  types 16–19, 77–78
  understanding their needs 8–9
payment plans 70
pediatric dentistry 969–1010
  bleaching vital teeth 335, 336
  dentofacial deformities 933
  facial harmony 1005–1010
  harmful habits 995
    digit sucking 811–813, 812, 833
    mouth breathing 821–822

laser-assisted minimally invasive 971–973
materials and techniques 970–971
operating procedures 973–983
  amelodentinal dysplasia 975, 975
  early childhood caries 979
  ectodermal dysplasia 982–983, 982–983
  enamel hypoplasia 978, 978
  extensive cavities 976, 976–977
  loss of teeth 979–982, 979–982
  preventive resin restoration 974, 974
orthodontics 995–1004
pedodontic prostheses 979, 979–982
tooth wear 696, 696
trauma management 983–986
  case studies 986–994, 986–995
  hard tissues and pulp 984–985
  injuries to developing teeth 986
  laser applications 984
  loss of teeth 980, 980–982
  periodontal tissues 985–986
  prevention 983–984
see also minors
pedodontic prostheses 979, 979–982
peg-shaped lateral incisors, orthodontic–restorative treatment 905, 905–906, 907–908
pen/pencil chewing 827, 831–832
perceptibility threshold 274
percussion, tooth 759–761, 760
perfectionist patients 77, 332
performers/actors 1153–1178
  cosmetic procedures 1155–1165
    acrylic stent 1155, 1156
    comic arrangement 1176–1177, 1177
    composite resin bonding 1155, 1160–1163
    composite resin stent/splint 1155, 1157
    creating characters 1156–1163
    overlay dentures 1156–1160, 1158–1164
    removable dentures 1156
    removable porcelain veneers 1155, 1156
  economic dental procedures 1154–1155
  emergency treatment 1176
  esthetic dentistry 1165–1166, 1165–1178
    brighter/whiter teeth 1165–1169
    composite resin restorations 1167–1169, 1169–1170
    cosmetic contouring 1166, 1167
    metal restorations 1169
    porcelain veneers 1167, 1168–1169
  with imperfect teeth 1154, 1154
  long-distance consultation 1176–1177
  orthodontics 1169–1170, 1171–1172
  periodontal treatment 1171–1172, 1173
  Pincus' work with 434, 1153, 1155, D2, D8–D9
  principles of treatment 1177–1178
  prosthetic treatment 1172–1174, 1173–1174
  special issues for 1174–1176
periapical radiolucency 759, 759–760

peri-implantitis 1418
  bacterial monitoring 1419, *1420*, 1427
  genetic susceptibility 1423
  locally applied chemotherapeutics 1421
peri-implant mucositis 1421, 1427
perimylolysis 33, *33*, 34
periodontal charting 60–61, *63*, *64*
  orthodontics 911, *912*
  voice activated 61, 67
periodontal disease
  bleaching and 335
  cosmetic contouring 300, 302
  diastemata due to 843–844
  endodontic lesions vs 759, *759–760*
  impact on tooth proportions 902
  metal–ceramic crowns 522
  mimicking, for actors 1161, *1164*
  older adults 1035, *1036*
  orthodontic patients 909–911, 919
  porcelain veneers 441
  restoration failure due to 1244–1245, *1245–1247*
  telescoping bridges 558–559, *558–559*, 560, *560–561*
  tooth preparation 1280, *1281*
periodontal evaluation 56
periodontal ligament
  avulsed/luxated teeth 793–794
  edentulous areas 583
periodontally accelerated osteogenic orthodontics (PAOO) 912, *913*
periodontal plastic surgery 1181–1208
  computer imaging 63, *65–66*
  crown lengthening and sculpting 1204–1208
  microsurgical instruments 1182–1183, *1183*
  papilla reconstruction 1195–1199
  ridge augmentation *see* ridge augmentation
  root coverage 1183–1195
periodontal probing 61, *63*
  charting *see* periodontal charting
  endodontics 751–754
  gingival biotype assessment 654, **654**
  orthodontics 911, *912*
  peri-implant 1418, *1418*, 1419, *1421*
periodontal surgery
  concealing interdental tissue loss after 225–229, *227–236*
  diastema correction 847, 915
  fractured teeth 728, *729*
  older adults 1029, 1032, *1032*
  orthodontic patients 911, 912, *913*, 915
periodontal tissues
  traumatic injuries 985–986
  see also soft tissues
periodontics
  adult orthodontics and 909–915, *911–914*
  bleaching combined with 335
  cosmetic 847
  older adults 1029, 1032, *1032*, *1033*
  orthodontics 909–911

performers/actors 1171–1172, *1173*
  referral for 72–74
periodontist, consultation with 56
periradicular tests, pulp health 759–762
peroxyborate monohydrate 348
personality
  assessing patient's 48–49, 53
  definition 37
  incorporating patient's 225, *227*, 1347
  mouth (Pincus) D3, D6–D7
  smile design and 248, *249*
personality disorders 26, 40–41
  see also narcissistic personality disorder
personality factors 26–27, 36–41
personal values 11–12
PFM crowns *see* porcelain-fused-to-metal crowns
Phillips, R.W. 375, 401, 403
phonetics
  denture tooth placement *619*, 619–620, 623
  temporary restorations and 1313
phosphoric acid etching *see* acid etching
photocuring *see* light curing
photographs, digital
  case documentation 157
  clinical applications 157–158
  color matching 157, 286, 533, *534*
  dental education 158
  editing 180, *180*
  extraoral
    close-up repose 174–175, *175*
    close-up smile 173, *174*
    Digital Smile Design 87–88, *87–89*
    full-face *see* facial photographs
    initial visit 59–60, *61*
    left and right lateral arches 176–178, *177*
    mandibular arch 178–179
    maxillary arch 178
    retracted closed 175, *175*
    retracted open 176, *176–177*
  facial *see* facial photographs
  functions 140–141, 156
  indications for 157
  intraoral
    dentofacial deformities 934
    Digital Smile Design 89–91, *89–94*
    initial visit 55–56, *57–59*, *59–60*
    new restorations 1410, *1412*
    post-and-core procedures 741
  laboratory communication 157, *157*, 199
  patient education 158
  privacy and confidentiality 145
  smile evaluation *see* smile analysis, photographic
  storage and presentation 179–180, *181*
  try-in appointment 1336, *1337*
  see also images
photography, clinical 155–182
  equipment 158–170
  image composition 171–179, *172*
  image storage and presentation 179–181
  see also cameras; photographs

physical attractiveness phenomenon 3–4, 8–10, **9**
  economics 12–16
  employment and 12, *13–14*
  functions of teeth 11
  personal values 11–12
  research methodology 9–10
  sexiness and 8–9, *9*
  see also beauty
piercings, oral 826, *829*
Pincus, Charles
  on cosmetic contouring 298
  gingival contour determination 1346
  principles of esthetic dentistry D2–D9
  work with film actors 434, 1153, 1155, D8–D9
pink spots 751, *752–753*
pins, harmful habits 825–826, *827*
pipe smokers 708, 831, *832*
pit and fissure caries 416–417
  detection 416–417, *417*
  treatment 417–419
    air-abrasive technology 417–419, *418*
    composite resin bonding 379, 417, *418–420*
    diamond burs 419
    hard tissue laser 419, *419*
    pediatric dentistry 974, *974*
pit and fissure stain 416–421
pitch 1072–1076, *1076*
pixels 160–161, *162*, *163*
Planmeca PlanScan 1391–1392, *1391–1393*, **1393**
plaque
  crown design and 529
  initial observation 52
  see also oral hygiene; scaling
plasma arc curing (PAC) lights 405
plastic *see* acrylic
plastic surgery 1131–1140
  broaching the subject 1089, 1143
  lower face 1137, *1138–1139*
  midface 1133–1134, *1136*
  nonsurgical 1137–1140, *1140*
  older adults 1020, 1025
  patient safety 1140
  upper face 1132–1133, *1132–1135*
  see also periodontal plastic surgery
platelet-derived growth factor-BB 643, *643*
platinum foil technique, porcelain veneer fabrication 461, 465–466
plunger-type attachments 605, *606*
polishing
  ceramic restorations *470*, 473, 1416
  composite restorations 407, *410–411*, 415, 1416
  glass ionomers 1416
  implants 1422
  pastes, grit size 1416
  prior to shade selection 396
  try-in appointment 1351

Polo, Mario 905
polyether impressions 1292
   ceramic veneers 459
   disinfection 1302
   history 1388
   material properties **1293**, 1293–1294
polymerization
   ceramic veneer fixation 469, 472–473
   composite restorations 403–406, 405
      following final finish 404
      incremental layering 403, 405
      three-sited light-curing technique 403
   shrinkage 405
   see also light curing
polysomnogram 962
polysulfide impressions 459, 1388
polyvinyl siloxane (PVS)
   impressions see addition silicone impressions
   interocclusal records 1304
pontics 565–571
   attachment RPDs 593, 594
   conical or bullet-shaped 565
   design 565–566, 565–567
   failure 1250, 1250–1251
   hygienic (sanitary) 565
   incorrect height 1239, 1240–1241
   materials 570–571, 571–573
   modified ridge lap 565, 566, 566–567
   ovate 565, 566, 567, 1204
   ridge lap (saddle) 565, 566
      conversion to ovate 1201, 1202
   tissue preparation 566–570, 569–570
   try-in 1345
   see also fixed partial dentures
population aging 1015–1016, **1016**
porcelain
   biocompatibility 439
   chipped or fractured see porcelain fractures
   color modification 286, 438
   denture teeth 616, 626–627, 627–629
   feldspathic see feldspathic porcelain
   firings 196–197, 286
   metal–ceramic restorations see metal–ceramic restorations
   Pincus principles D5, D6, D6
   pitting by topical fluoride 440
   polishing 1416
   pontics 570, 571, 571–573
   unglazed 1351
   see also ceramic(s)
porcelain butt-joint margins
   design 517, 517
   esthetics 516, 516
   facial margin 1280
   FPD retainers 552–553
   preparation for cementation 1356, 1358
   selection 522, 522, 525–526, 1266
porcelain crowns (all-porcelain) 502–505, 505–506
   contraindications 505
   crowded tooth situation 1283

longevity 1248–1249
troubleshooting **507**
see also all-ceramic crowns
porcelain fractures 1248–1249, 1248–1249
   composite resin bonding 392, 1226–1230, 1228–1230
   esthetic emergencies 1224, 1226–1230
   legal considerations 138
   occlusal pressure detecting 1255, 1260
   porcelain veneers to repair 440
   smoothing and polishing 1226
porcelain-fused-to-metal (PFM) crowns 514–523
   adjunctive procedures 515–516
   advantages 515
   choice of metals 514
   contraindications 514
   design
      metal substructure 516–518, 517–518
      porcelain–metal junction 517–518, 520
      porcelain thickness 518, 520, 522
   disadvantages 515, 515
   discolored pulpless tooth 523–525
   endodontic access via 758, 777, 778, 778
   esthetic considerations 516, 516
   factors influencing choice 523, 525–526
   failures 518, 518–519
   history 514
   indications 514
   margins 522, 522–523
   retention after endodontic therapy 779–780
   rubber dam clamps 772–773, 773
   technical problems 514–515
   tooth preparation 1271–1280, 1277–1278
      esthetic depth determination 1271–1272, 1277–1278
      extent of occlusal reduction 510, 510
      labial tooth reduction 1272–1277, 1279
      types of margins 1277–1280, 1280
   see also metal–ceramic restorations
porcelain partial coverage restorations see ceramic partial coverage restorations
porcelain pieces (sectional veneers) 867, 868
porcelain veneers 438–442
   advantages 438–440, 505
   bilayer ceramic restorations 502–505, 1264
      alumina cores 507, 508–509
      zirconia cores 507, 537, 1254–1255, 1259, 1377
   contouring as alternative to 298–300
   contraindications 441
   coronal fractures 722, 723–724, 723–724, 726, **727**
   crowded teeth **882**, 884–886, 886–887
   diastema closure 441, 864–869
      crowning with 869–870, 872
      minimal preparation 865–866, 865–866
      multiple diastemata 867–869, 869–870, 871, 871

proximal finish line 866, 867
single midline diastema 866–867, 868
disadvantages 440
evolution of use 376
fracture-related failure 473–474, 1228–1230, 1248–1249
   see also porcelain fractures
history 434–435
indications 438–439, 440–441
interdental space closure 226–228, 452, 469
laboratory procedures 461–462
   platinum foil technique 461, 465–466
   refractory die technique 461–462
   two-tier quattro technique 229, 232–236
legal considerations
   informed consent 133, 137
   overbuilt 148, 150
   subgingival margins 134–136
longevity 439, 440, 473–474, 1249
marginal failures
   legal issues 135–136
   poor fit 1237
   recurrent caries 1227
   staining 472, 473, 689–690
older adults 1030–1034, 1032
performers/actors 1167, 1168–1169
Pincus principles D7
placement 465–473
   errors 472, 473
   final insertion 464–465, 467–472, 469–473
   try-in 463, 465–469, 466–467
post-treatment care 473–477
rebonding 1373, 1375
removable 1155, 1156
repairs to existing 440, 1252
resin luting cement 1357–1358
as retainers for fixed partial dentures 549
shade selection 441–442
temporaries 460–461, 461–463
tooth preparation 442–459
   classification for anterior teeth 442–448
   diastema closure 864–865, 867–869
   extent of reduction 449–453
   technique 456, 457–460
see also ceramic veneers
porphyria 331, 682
post-and-core restorations
   anterior teeth 739–743
      case example 728, 730
      procedure 739–743, 740–742
      treatment options 739, **739**
   core materials **736**
   crown preparation 743–745, 744
   ferrule design 744, 745
   posterior teeth 736–739, 738
   premolars 743, 743
   principles 733–734, 733–734
   see also posts

posterior occlusal plane, complete dentures 621–622, *622*
posterior teeth
  adjusting embrasures 1347
  ceramic partial coverage restorations 478–483
  complete dentures *614*, 616, 621–622, *622*
  composite restorations 379–382, *380–383*
    direct and indirect inlays 393, *394*
    finishing 409, *413–415*
    indirect 382
    limitations 478–479
    longevity 376, *377*
  crowns 523
  diastema closure 863–864, *863–865*
  fractured endodontically-treated 736–739
    composite resin core 734, 735, *736*, *739*
    options for restoring 733–734
    prefabricated posts 734, 736–739, *738*
  fractures 731–732
  metal–ceramic restorations *510*
  too narrow 210–211, *212–213*
  too wide 208–209, *208–209*
postoperative pain/edema 940
posts
  cast metal *see* cast metal posts
  design 734–735, *735*
  materials 735, **736**
  perforations, endodontic surgery 804, *805–806*
  prefabricated *see* prefabricated posts
  see also post-and-core restorations
potassium nitrate 345–346
Pound, E. 616
powder, facial cosmetic 1150
Powerpoint, Microsoft 86, 87, *87*, 180
practice, dental
  attractiveness 115, *116–118*
  marketing *see* marketing
  websites 122, 124, *124–125*, 125
precision attachments, for RPDs 591
precision milling, attachment RPDs 606
prefabricated posts
  anterior teeth 733, *734*
    indications 739, **739**
    procedure 739, *741*, 742, *743*
  design 734–735, *735*
  materials **736**
  posterior teeth 734, 736–739, *738*
  premolars 743, *743*
prehistoric societies 696, 708, 920
premolars
  as abutment teeth 584
  fractured endodontically-treated 736–739, *736–739*, 743, *743*
pressable ceramic veneers *see* ceramic veneers, pressable
press releases 128
Preston proportion (naturally occurring) 257, *257*
  dentists' preferences 258–259, *260*
prevention

older adults 1023–1024
  patient education 1414–1415
primary dentition
  avulsions 1224
  complicated crown fractures 1220–1221
  dental materials and techniques 970–971
  luxation injuries 1223
  orthodontic management 995–996
  porcelain veneers 441
  retained teeth 908
  root fractures 1223
  tooth structure 976
  trauma management 983–986
primers
  ceramic veneers 471
  dentin bonding 359–360
  universal 361
privacy, patient 145
probing
  peri-implant sulcus 1418, *1418*, 1419, *1421*
  periodontal *see* periodontal probing
  pits and fissures 417, *417*
problem patients 36–41, 77–79
  managing 78–79
  raising your fees 40, 77, 79
  see also psychological disorders
Procera all-ceramic crowns 507, *508–509*
proclination, incisor *922*, 923, 1076
product warnings/liability 150
profile angle 1113
profile view of face *see* facial profile
prognostication, legal considerations 138
prominent teeth, gingival recession risk 1184
proportional dental/facial analysis 253–265
proportional smile design 243–268
proportionate ratio, Beaudreau's 254
ProRoot MTA, pulp capping 769, *769*
prostheses
  diastema closure 849
  emergency repairs 1231–1232, *1231–1232*
  older adults 1030–1035, *1032*, *1034–1036*
  performers/actors 1172–1174, *1173–1174*
  provisional 612–613, *612–613*
protective bite appliances (nightguards)
  ceramic veneers 441, 473
  composite restorations 413–415, *415*
  dentures opposing natural teeth 631
  fixed partial dentures 554, *554*
protrusion, incisor
  orthodontic *922*, 922–923
  restorative therapy 891, *891*
provisional prostheses 612–613, *612–613*
provisional restorations *see* temporary restorations
psychiatric team 27–28, 30–31, 34
psychological considerations
  cosmetic contouring 302
  facial appearance 10–11, *11*
  seeking treatment 16–19
  tooth reduction for veneers 452
  treatment planning 19

psychological disorders 25–44, **26**
  terms and concepts 26–27
public relations 124, *124*, 128–129
pulp
  calcific metamorphosis 767
  capping 769, 769–770
    traumatic injuries 727, 1219
  clinical evaluation 751–756, 751–762
  degeneration, percussion test 759–761
  exposure
    fractures **722**, 727–730, 790, *793*
    pulp capping 727, 769–770
    restorative dentistry 768–769, *769*
  healthy 765
  hemorrhage *see* hemorrhage, pulp
  injury
    acid etching 134, 363, 401
    dental procedures 134, 765–767, *766*, 768–769, *768–769*
    repair mechanisms 766–767, *767*
    root fractures 1221–1223
    tooth color changes 682, 751, *752–755*, 768
    uncomplicated crown fractures 1219
  necrosis
    complicated crown fractures 1219–1220
    cracked tooth syndrome 798, 800
    electronic pulp testing 759
    root fractures 1223
    visual tooth examination 751, *751*, *753*
  protection 767, 1313
  response to operative procedures 764–767, *766*
  stressed 770, *770–772*
pulp canals, large
  cosmetic contouring 301, *301*
  crown restoration and 529
  tooth reduction for veneers and 452
  vital bleaching 331
pulpitis
  anesthetic test 763–764
  bite test 762
  cold testing 754–755
  cracked tooth syndrome 798, 799–800
pulpotomy 727
  laser 985
  partial (Cvek) 727, 1219
pulp sensibility tests 754–759
  cavity test 758–759, *758–759*
  cold tests 754–756, *756–757*
  electric 756–757, *758*
  endodontic vs periodontal lesions 759, *759–760*
  heat tests 756
  pediatric dental trauma 984
Pythagoras 1097

quartz-tungsten-halogen (QTH) light sources 405

racial differences *see* ethnic/racial differences
radio advertising 128

radiographs (X-rays)
  cosmetic contouring 304
  enamel thickness *879, 883*
  endodontics
    precementation 762–763, *765*
    pretreatment 762, *763–764,* 774
  fixed partial dentures 544–545
  implant evaluation 1417, *1418,* 1419
  initial visit 60, *61, 62*
  monitoring of restorations 1411–1412
  orthodontics 899, *901,* 903–904
  porcelain restorations 440
  postcementation 1365, *1365,* 1410, *1410*
  recommendations for
      prescribing **1413–1414**
  removable partial dentures 582–583
  review prior to second visit 67
  traumatic injuries 1216
rapport, building 750–751
RAW files 164–165
RealSeal Sealer 780
reasonable patient standard 137, 143–144
reception area 51
  attractive decor 115, *116–117*
  educational materials 49, *49*
receptionist, dental 48
records, clinical 139–142
  adult orthodontics 899, *899–901*
  dentofacial deformity 934–935, *935–938*
  electronic 67, 142
  essential components 142
  facial analysis 1097–1098
  functions 139–141
  making corrections to 141–142
  role of photographs 157
  spoilation 142
recurring esthetic dental (RED)
      proportion 257, *258*
  70% 257, *258*
  computer simulation methods 265–267,
      267–268
  dentists' preferences 258–260, *260*
  diastema closure and 846–847
  intercanine width (ICW) and 257, *259*
  tooth lengths and 260–261, *261*
  tooth width calculations 260–265
    clinical use 261–263, **262,** *262–263*
    simplified method **263,** 263–265,
        264–267, **265**
red-colored teeth 671, 751, *752*
RED proportion *see* recurring esthetic dental
      proportion
referrals
  patient 121–122, *123*
  problem patients 77–78
  psychological 31–32, 43–44
  source of patient's 52
  specialist 72–74
refractory die technique, porcelain veneer
      fabrication 461–462
refunds 147
refusal to treat, dentist's 145

release of all future claims form 148
removable complete dentures *see* complete
      dentures
removable partial dentures (RPD) 581–606
  abutments *see* abutments, removable
      partial dentures
  alternative treatments 589–590
  attachments *see* attachment removable
      partial dentures
  design principles 582–589
    biomechanics 583–584
    clasps *see* clasps, removable partial
        dentures
    flange 589
    other esthetic aspects 589
    problem situations 584
    replacement teeth 589
    rest seats 588–589, *589*
    retention enhancement 588
    use of a surveyor 583
  digital impressions 1405–1406, *1405–1406*
  distal extension 583–584
  emergency repairs 1231–1232
  esthetic failures 1238–1239, *1239–1241*
  evaluating tissue support 582–583
  pedodontic prostheses 979, *979–982*
  performers/actors 1156–1160, *1158–1164*
  rest seats 588–589
  rotational path 590, *590–593*
  tooth-supported 582
  tooth-tissue-supported 582
removable porcelain veneers 1155, *1156*
repeated ratio, Lombardi's 254
reshaping, cosmetic tooth *see* contouring,
      cosmetic
Resilon 780
resin, composite *see* composite resin
resin-bonded fixed partial dentures 549
  diastema closure 863–864, *863–865*
  orthodontic–restorative therapy 909
resin-bonded partial-veneer fixed partial
      dentures 549
resin luting agents 1356, *1357–1358,* 1361
resin-modified glass ionomers (RMGI)
  caries prevention 1247–1248
  cements 970, 1356, 1358
  cores **736**
  traumatically exposed dentin 1218
resin tags 357, *357,* 368
resolution, image 160–161, *162, 163, 164*
resorption
  alveolar ridge *see* ridge resorption
  external root *see* external root resorption
  internal tooth 682, *753*
restorations
  bleaching and 332, 342, 346, 687
  cementation 1355–1365
  color modification 286–287
  consent forms 135–137
  cosmetic contouring and 303
  Digital Smile Design 94, *108–109*
  discoloration 689–690

endodontic access via 776–780, *777–780*
endodontically-treated teeth 780–781
factors influencing appearance 185–187
failure 1244–1260
  contaminants 1255
  digital impression system 1403
  esthetic emergencies 1224–1230
  exposure of margins 1244, *1245*
  to follow manufacturer's
      instructions 1255–1260
  legal considerations 138
  material 1248–1252, *1248–1257*
  periodontal disease 1244–1245,
      1245–1247
  recurrent caries 1245–1248, *1247*
  technical 1252–1255, *1257–1260*
fractured 1224–1230
gingival graft coverage 1194–1195, *1195*
gingival recession due to 1184
implant-supported *see* implant-supported
      restorations
longevity 1244–1260
  informing patients 138, 1242–1243
maintenance 1409–1428
marginal staining 330, 670–671, *674–676*
margin exposure 1236
orthodontic therapy and 917–919
posttreatment visit 1410–1412
pretreatment oral care 1410
repairs to
  air-abrasive technology 419–421,
      1227–1230, *1228*
  composite resin bonding 392, 1224,
      1226–1230, *1228–1230*
  esthetic emergencies 1224–1230
restorative treatment
  bleaching combined with 333–334
  crowded teeth 877–893
  elective endodontics 767–770, *768–769*
  facial considerations 1085–1126
  integrating orthodontics into 905–908,
      905–909
  papillary defect closure 1196, *1197*
  pulp injury 764–766, *766*
  vs removal of endodontically-diseased
      teeth 782–783, *784–785*
rest–proximal plate–I-bar (RPI) clasp 585, *587*
rest seats 588–589, *589*
retainers, orthodontic 914, *914*
  crowded teeth 881, 890
retention
  attachment RPDs 595, 596
  RPDs 584–588
retina, color perception 272
retracted closed image 175, *175*
retracted open image 176, *176–177*
retraction cords *see* gingival retraction cords
retractors
  clinical photography 171, *171*
  left and right lateral images 176–177, *177*
  mandibular arch image 178–179
  maxillary arch images 178, *179*

retruded tooth 891
reverse (negative) smile line 186, *186*, 247, *247*, *902*, 1122, *1122*
Rhesus factor incompatibility 331
rhinoplasty 1081, *1081*, 1134, *1136*
rhytidectomy (facelift) 1137, *1138*
Ricketts E-plane 1117, *1117*
ridge augmentation *1200–1201*, 1200–1204
    facial considerations 1118
    fixed partial dentures 566–570, *569*, 1201–1204
    horizontal 640–642, *642*
    implants 639–643, *641–642*
    indications 1201
    surgical technique 1201–1204, *1201–1204*
    vertical 642–643
ridge deformities 1118, 1199–1200
ridge form and volume 1118
    fixed partial dentures 566–567
    implants 638–643, *639–642*
    see also bone, quantity and quality
ridge preservation 639, *640–641*, 1200
ridge resorption 1199–1200
    dentures opposing natural teeth 628–629
    facial considerations 1118, *1118*
    fixed porcelain interdental insert *228–230*, 229
    pontic design 567, *568–569*
    porcelain vs plastic denture teeth 626–627
    postextraction 638–639, **639**, *639–640*, 1182, *1182*, 1200
    removable partial dentures 589
    Siebert classification 567
right lateral arch image 176–178
ring clasp 585–587
risks of treatment
    disclosure 132, 143–144
    misrepresentation 144
    nonnegligent 144
    see also informed consent
Rite-Lite 2 *1177*, 1178
roll 1072–1076, *1076*
root
    proximity, crowded teeth 881
    RPD abutment teeth 583–584
root canal therapy *see* endodontics
root caries
    connective tissue graft coverage 1194–1195, *1195*
    older adults *1036*
root coverage 1183–1195
    autogenous vs allogenic tissues 1184
    furcation involvement 1185, *1186*
    indications 1185
    old restorations and root caries 1194–1195, *1195*
    postoperative care 1194, *1194*
    potential for new attachment 1185–1186, *1186*
    quality and quantity of donor tissue 1195
    surgical technique 1186–1194
        graft positioning 1190–1191, *1192–1193*

    microincisions and gingival pouch 1188–1189, *1188–1189*
    root preparation 1186–1188, *1187–1188*
    sutures and dressing 1191–1194, *1193–1194*
    tissue harvesting 1189–1191, *1190–1191*
root fractures 790–793, *795–798*, 1221–1223
    apical third 791, *795*
    coronal third 793, *797–798*
    diagnosis 761–762
    endodontically-treated teeth *740*, 743–744
    mid root 791–793, *795–796*
    partial pulpotomy 727
    pediatric patients 985
    retrograde 803
    treatment options **722**
root preparation
    connective tissue graft coverage 1186–1188, *1187–1188*
    papilla reconstruction 1196
root resorption, external *see* external root resorption
root segments, extrusion 793, *798*
Rotadent
    bonded restorations 415, *416*
    implant cleaning 1421, *1421*, 1427
    interproximal cleaning *1423*, 1427
rotational path removable partial dentures 590, *590–593*
Roth #801 root canal cement 780
round face, hair styles 1144, *1145*
RPD *see* removable partial dentures
rubber cup polishing 473, 1416
rubber dam
    bleaching nonvital teeth 144, 347
    ceramic veneers 469
    endodontics 771–774
    isolation of multiple teeth 773, *774*
    pediatric dentistry 973
    protecting ceramic crowns 772–773, *773*
    selective vital bleaching 333, *333*
    smaller alternatives 774, *774*
Russell's sign 32, *33*

Sadoun, Michael 506
Safety Data Sheets (SDSs) 150
sagittal splitting osteotomy, Obwegeser's 944–948, *946–947*, *949–950*
salivary diagnostics
    genetic risks 1423, *1424–1426*
    peri-implantitis bacteria 1419, *1420*, 1427
salivary flow 671, 1023
sandwich technique 403, *404*
Sarver, David 899, *903*
satisfaction, patient 18, 115, *123*
saturation, effects of bleaching 278, **284**
scaling
    ceramic veneers 473
    implant-supported restorations 1421–1422, *1422*

scars
    lip 1112, *1112*
    makeup for concealing 1151
Scharer, Peter 510
sclera exposure 1008
Scotchbond adhesives 363, 367
scratch test 712
sealants, surface
    composite resin restorations 689
    discoloration over time 670, *674*
second appointment
    preparation for 67–70
    treatment planning 70–77
segmental arch mechanics 911, *913*
selective serotonin reuptake inhibitors (SSRIs) 28
self-etch adhesives **357**, 357–358
    dentin bonding 360, *360*, 403
    development 358
    enamel bonding 357–358
    one-step (all-in-one) 360, 362, **362**, 365–366, *366*
    postoperative hypersensitivity 366–367
    recommendations for use 368
    reliability and degradation 365
    technique sensitivity 365–366, *366*
    two-step **362**, 366
self-image 6, *8*, 10–11, 1149
self-smile analysis 49–51, *51*, 70
semiprecision attachments, for RPDs 591
sensitivity, tooth *see* tooth sensitivity
separation of adjacent teeth, increasing 218, *218*
sertraline (Zoloft) 27, 28
setting time, impression materials 1293, **1293**
sevenths, facial 245, *245*
sewing needles/pins 825–826, *827*
sex, personality, age (SPA) factors 248, 614
sex characteristics
    apical tooth forms 248, *250*
    incorporating 223, *225–226*
    SPA factors 248, *249*
    see also feminine appearance; gender differences; masculine appearance
sexiness 8–9, *9*
shade
    staining techniques to alter **200–201**
    verification of final 1339, 1345
    see also color
shade charts 533, *533*
shade guides 199–205, *204–207*, 276–281
    checking completed prostheses 1339
    crowns 534–535, *535*
    custom-made 285–286
    facial prostheses 281
    modified 285
    monitoring bleaching 277–279, *279*, *336*, *337*
    oral soft tissues 281
    porcelain veneers 442
    tooth 276–281

shade guides (cont'd)
    coverage error (CE) 280–281
    historical 276, *276*
    proprietary or classical-proprietary 279–280, *280–282*
    pros and cons 280–281, **282**
    VITA classical A1–D4 276–277, *277*
    VITA System 3D-Master 277–279, *277–279*
shade guide units (sgu) 277
Shademan, Nasser, two-tier quattro veneer construction 229, *232–236*
shade selection/color matching 271, 274–285
    bleaching 336, *337*
    case study 289–292, *289–292*
    composite resin bonding 379, 385, 396–398, *397*
    repairs 690
    crowns 532–536
        laboratory communication 535, *535*
        lighting 532–533
        records 533–534, *533–534*
        shade guides 534–535, *535*
        tips 535–536
    education and training **287, 287–288,** *288–289*
    to individual patient 678
    instrumental 284–285, *285*
    older patients 219–221, *223*
    performers/actors 1168–1169, *1169–1170*
    porcelain veneers 441–442
    role of photographs 157, 286
    unsatisfactory 1236, *1236*
    visual 274–284
        conditions 274–276
        individual variations 274
        method 282–284, *283*
        myths and facts 284, **284**
shadowing
    creating illusions 188, *188*
    lip thickness and 186–187
    tooth appearance and 189, 190
shaping, tooth
    illusional effects 189–190
    older patients 219
    too-long teeth 215–216, *215–216*
    too-narrow teeth 210–211, *212–213*
    too-short teeth *214,* 214–215
    too-wide teeth 207–209, *207–209*
    try-in appointment 1347–1350, *1349–1351*
    see also contouring, cosmetic
Shofu Cosmetic Contouring Kit 310–311, *313*
short teeth
    crowns 530–531, 1283, *1283–1284*
    illusions for *214,* 214–215
    see also tooth length; tooth lengthening
shoulderless full porcelain crown 1268
shoulder margins
    all-ceramic crowns 1268, *1269, 1270–1271, 1273*
    metal–ceramic crowns 522–523, 525

porcelain-fused-to-metal crowns 1279–1280, *1280*
porcelain veneers 456
try-in stage 1343, *1344*
shrinkage
    impression materials **1293,** 1294
    polymerization 405
Siebert classification of edentulous areas 567
silanation
    ceramic fitting surfaces *1362,* 1364
    ceramic veneers *467,* 471
    fractured restorations 1230
    porcelain butt margins 1356, *1358*
silicone impression materials 1291–1292, 1388
Siltek method
    implant temporaries 1324, *1327–1328*
    interim temporary restorations 1324, *1325–1327*
silver-containing materials
    endodontic therapy 780
    tooth discoloration 682, 751, *753*
single-lens reflex (SLR) cameras 158, *159,* 159–169
    cost 159
    flash systems 163, *164,* 165
    f-stop and flash settings 166–169, *169,* 170
    functions 161–162
    histogram 162, 165–166, *166–168,* 168
    image file types 164–165
    image resolution 160–161, *162,* 163
    intraoral images 158, *158*
    ISO 164
    lenses 160, *160,* 161
    lighting 166–169, *169–170*
    screen size 159–160
    selection 159–163
    setting up 163–166
    size-weight 162–163
    smile evaluation 252–253, *252–253*
    through the lens (TTL) vs aperture priority 165–166
    wand-like cameras vs 156, *156*
sinusitis, acute 759–761
skin care 1149
skin color 274
    shade guides 281
skin resurfacing, facial 1140
SLA models *see* stereolithography apparatus models
sleep bruxism 697
slip-cast aluminum oxide ceramic 506
SLR cameras *see* single-lens reflex cameras
smile
    asymmetric 1068–1071
    differing esthetic standards 138, 899–900, *902*
    historical perspective 4–5
    posed vs spontaneous 899, *901,* 1098
    width 1125, *1125*
smile analysis

crown selection 525–526, *526*
Digital Smile Design 88, *88*
facial context 1086–1088, *1087–1088*
horizontal planes of reference 1108
macroesthetic 1068–1072, 1077–1078, *1078–1079*
miniesthetic 1078, *1079*
orthodontics 899–900, *902*
photographic 251–253
    close-up image 173, *174*
    equipment 252–253, *252–253*
    facial image view evaluation (FIVE) 253, *255*
    full-face view 171–173, *173*
    standardized protocols 253, *254*
self-smile analysis 49–51, *51,* 70
smile arc 1071–1072, *1076*
    patient preferences 138
smile design
    computer simulation 88, *88,* 265–268, *267–268*
    digital *see* Digital Smile Design
    patient preferences and individuality 268
    performers/actors 1173–1174, *1176*
    principles 246–247
    proportional 243–268
smile line 931, 1122–1124
    crowded teeth 881
    diastema closure and 847
    high *905, 1123,* 1123–1124
    implant esthetics and 638
    low *905,* 1123, 1124, *1124–1125*
    medium *905,* 1123, *1123*
    orthodontic implications 904–905, *905*
    positive 186
    preferences 899–902, *902*
    reverse (negative) 186, *186,* 247, *247,* 902, 1122, *1122*
    see also gingival display; lip line
Smith and Knight's Tooth Wear Index **697**
smoking, tobacco 825
    older adults 1023
    pipe users 831, *832*
    stained teeth 675, *678*
    tooth color 274
    see also tobacco
Snap-On Smile 1332, *1333*
    disguising a diastema 842
    treatment planning 75, *76,* 844
Snow's golden mean 257, *257*
social context, esthetic dentistry 5–6, *6–7*
social media 128–129
Society for Color and Appearance in Dentistry (SCAD) **287**
socket repair membrane, Zimmer 640–641
sodium hypochlorite 780
sodium perborate 348
soft-tissue fillers 1137, *1140*
soft tissues (oral)
    discoloration
        amalgam tattoo 805, *807*
        peri-implant *655,* 658, *659,* 1370

edentulous areas 583
fixed partial dentures 551, *553*, 571
laser applications 973
peri-implant *see* implants, gingival tissues
preparation for impressions 1287–1291, *1288–1292*
preparation for pontics 566–579, *568–570*
prostheses *see* tissue inserts
retraction prior to impressions 1288–1291, *1289–1292*
sculpting
    excessive gingival display 1204–1208
    fixed partial dentures 570
    see also periodontal plastic surgery
shade guides 281
temporary restorations and 1313, *1313*
tooth preparation for crowns and 518–521, *520*, 1264–1266, *1265–1267*
traumatic injuries 985–986
see also gingiva; periodontal disease
space
  arch *see* arch, space
  attachment RPDs 596–597
  deficiencies, crowded teeth 878
  maintenance in children 995–996
  too narrow 209–214, *210–213*
  too wide 206–209, *207–209*
SPA (sex, personality, age) factors 248, 614
spark erosion technology 606
special effects 185–234
  illusions 188–192
  laboratory communication 197–199
  shade guides 199–205, *204–207*
  specific problems 206–229
    adding age features 219, *221–222*
    arch irregularity 218, *219–221*
    incisal embrasures 221, *224–225*
    incorporating personality 225, *227*
    influencing facial shape 218–219
    insufficiently differentiated teeth 218, *218*
    interdental tissue loss 225–229, *227–236*
    long-axis inclinations 216–218, *218*
    reducing age effects 219–221, *223*
    sexual differentiation 223, *225–226*
    too-long tooth 215–216, *215–216*
    too-narrow space 209–214, *210–213*
    too-short tooth 214–215, *214–215*
    too-wide space 206–209, *207–209*
    using form and color 216, *217*, **218**
  staining 193–197
  see also illusions
specialists, consultation with 70–74, *73*
spectacles, harmful habits 831, *833*
spectral power distribution (SPD) 275
Spectratone shade guide 276
spectrophotometers 284–285, *285*
SpectroShade Micro 284–285, *285*
Spee, F. Graf von 921

speech
  denture tooth placement 619–620, 621, 623
  vertical dimension of *619*, 619–620
splint bar attachments 605, *607*
splinting
  attachment RPDs 595, *604*, 605
  fixed partial dentures and 555
  luxation injuries 1223, 1225, *1225*
  orthodontically treated patients 914, *914*
  problem patients 78–79
  root-fractured teeth 791, *795–796*, 1221
  telescopic bridges 558–559, *558–559*
  temporary 1317–1323
splints
  composite resin 1155, *1157*
  fixed, try-in 1341, *1341–1342*, 1345
  occlusal, worn teeth 702
spoilation 142
square face, hair styles 1144, *1145*, 1148
"S" sounds, denture tooth placement *619*, 619–620, 623
stained/discolored teeth 669–690
  bleaching *see* bleaching
  ceramic veneers 440, 441, 687–688, *687–688*
    final color adjustments 468–469
    increasing opaqueness 452, 461–462
    tooth preparation 452, 453
  composite resin restorations 689, *689*, 690, 1252
  cosmetic contouring 300, *300*, 302
  crowns 523–524
  etiology 328–331, 346, 670, **671, 673**
  examination 326
  extrinsic staining 328, 670, 671–678
    causes *672–673*, 673–674
    direct or nonmetallic 673
    indirect or metallic 673
    management 673, **673**, *678*, *679*
    Natho classification 671
    predisposing factors 671
    specific types 674–676
    whitening toothpastes 676–678
  gingival retraction fluid causing 1236
  indicating pulpal problems 751, *751–755*
  initial observation 52
  intrinsic staining 328, 670, 678–687
    causes *672*, 678–686
    localized brown stains 682–683, *685*
    localized white spots 683, *685*
    management **673,** 687
    single tooth 682, *683–684*
    see also tetracycline-stained teeth
  mechanisms 326
  microabrasion 341, *342*
  older adults 331, *332*
  pediatric patients
    bleaching vital teeth 335, *336*
    previous subluxation injury 988–989, *988–989*
    previous trauma 994, *994–995*

pit and fissure stains 416–419, *418–420*
porcelain denture teeth 627, *628*
porcelain resistance 439
single dark tooth 682, *683–685*
tooth defects causing 670–671, *673*
  caries 670, *674*
  deep grooves 670, *674*
  leakage around restorations 670–671, *674–676*
treatment options 670, **673,** 687–690
see also marginal staining
staining techniques 193–194, *193–205*
  adding illusion of width 211, *212–213*
  communication with laboratory 197–199
  increasing apparent length 215, *215*
  in-office 193, 286
  masking extra width 209, *209*
  older patients 219, *221–222*
  reducing apparent length 216
  surface 194–197, *196–198*
    adding characterization **202–203**
    altering shade **200–201**
    IPS Empress crowns 510, 511
    tips 195–197, *198–199*
stainless steel prefabricated posts **736**
standards of care 131–132, 143–144
Steiner line 1117, *1117*
stents
  composite resin 1155, *1157*
  cosmetic acrylic 1155, *1156*
stereolithography apparatus (SLA) models 1390, 1394
  clinical cases *1403*, *1404*, *1405*, *1406*
Stern ERA attachment 600, *604–606*
Stern ERA-RV attachment 600, *606*
Stern G/A attachment 597, *598*
Stern G/L attachment 597, *598*
Stern McCollum attachment 597, *598–599*
Stern Type 7 attachment 597
Stim-u-dents, used as wedges 826, *829*
stress
  role in bruxism 814
  tensile, abfraction etiology 704–705, *705*
stressed pulp 770, *770–772*
stroke 1022, 1024
studio lighting 1178
study models 67
  cosmetic contouring 304, *306*
  dentofacial deformities 934–935
  digital
    laboratory systems 1401, *1401*
    orthodontics 909, *910*
  digitally-guided fabrication 1394
    3D printing 1394
    milling 1390, 1394, 1396
    TRIOS system 1399–1400
digital scanning 1401
Digital Smile Design 91–94, *101–102*
fixed partial dentures 545, *545*, *546*
orthodontics *900*

study models (cont'd)
    Pincus principles D7
    preparation 1302
    SLA see stereolithography apparatus models
    surface characterization 190, *190*
subgingival margins
    all-ceramic crowns *1267*, 1267–1268
        try-in stage *1343*, *1344*
    ceramic veneers 448–449, 452, 453, 456, *458*
        final placement 469
        legal considerations 134–136
    fixed partial dentures 551
    see also gingival margins
subluxation injury 1223
    tooth discoloration after 988–989, *988–989*
submental view of face, photographs 1056, *1059*
substructure materials 192, *192–193*, **193**
suicide 42
supernumerary teeth 1000, *1000–1003*
SureFil 403
surface roughness, role in adhesion 356
surface texture/characterization
    composite restorations 407–408
    crowns 532, *532*
    performers/actors 1174–1176
    Pincus principles D3, *D4*, D5
    planning 190, *190*
    staining techniques 194–197, *196–199*, **202–203**
    translucency/light transmission and 192, *192*
    try-in appointment 1350, *1351*
    visual matching 284
surgically assisted orthodontics 956–959
surgical–orthodontic treatment 929–965
    adjunctive procedures 959, *961–962*
    case presentation visit 935–937
    complications and risks 939–940
    dentofacial deformities 940–955
    distraction osteogenesis 955–956
    facial analysis 930–931, *931–932*
    first visit 933–935
    indications 933
    obstructive sleep apnea 959–964, *962–964*
    patient expectations 933
    pediatric patients 933
    postsurgical treatment 937–939
    presurgical orthodontics 935–937, 939–940
    presurgical visit 937
    three-dimensional approach 1079–1083, *1080–1082*
surround, tooth color matching 275, 276
surveyor, dental 583
suspensory sutures 1199, *1199*
SwissTac/Tach E-Z attachment 605
Syntac adhesive *363*, 366, 367
systemic disorders, causing tooth discoloration 330–331

tattoo, amalgam 805, *807*
T-bar clasp 584–585, *586*
    modified 584–585, *586*
team, dental
    appearance 115–116, *119*
    customer service 117–119
tear energy, impression materials 1293, **1293**
technical skill, dentist's 80
teeth
    denture see denture teeth
    differentiation between adjacent 218, *218*
    examination 55–56, 751
    functions 11
Teflon tape 854, 855, *855*
telephone consultations 150
telephone directories 125
telescoping bridges 555–562
    advantages 555–558
    clinical examples 558–559, *558–559*, 560, *560–561*
    disadvantages 559–560
television 6, 10
    actors see performers/actors
    advertising 125–128
temperamental theory, tooth morphology 614
temporary anchorage devices (TADs) 933
temporary restorations 1311–1324
    acrylic crowns 502
    CAD/CAM construction 1315
    cements 1313, 1340, 1364
    composite resin bonding 392
    consent form 135
    crowded teeth 881–882
    decision-making role 1312, *1313*
    esthetic uses 1311–1314
    implant 656–657
        immediate placement 644–645, *646–650*, 656
        Siltek method 1324, *1327–1328*
        soft tissue benefits 644–645, *648–650*, 656, *657–658*
        used as impression posts 650, 656–657
    orthodontic therapy and 1312
    phonetic concerns 1313
    previewing illusions 189–190, *191–192*
    protective function 1313, *1313*
    removal 1339
    requirements 1313–1314
    temporary (interim) 1323–1324, *1324–1325*
        secondary function 1324
        Siltek matrix 1324, *1325–1327*
    trial smile role 1312, *1313*
    vacuform technique 1315, *1315–1316*
    veneers 460–461, *461–463*, 1316–1317, *1316–1319*
temporary splinting 1317–1323
    A-splint 1320–1323, *1321–1323*
    composite resin 1317–1320, *1319–1320*
temporization, esthetic 1311–1324
    functions 1311–1314
    specific types 1315–1324

temporomandibular joint pain 815, *815–816*
tensile bond strength, porcelain veneers 439
tensile stress model, abfraction 704–705, *705*
Terramycin staining 755
tert-butanol 359
tetracycline paste, root surface demineralization 1188, *1188*
tetracycline-stained teeth *672*, 683–686, *686*, 751, 755
    bleaching 328–329, *329–330*, 683–686, *686*, 687
    ceramic veneers 440, 452, 453, 461–462, 687–688, *687–688*
1,1,1,2-tetrafluoroethane (Endo-Ice) 754–756, *757*
texture, surface see surface texture
theater actors see performers/actors
thermal pulp testing 754–756
Thermaseal Plus 780
thirds, facial 245, *246*, 1097, *1100*
    age-related changes 245, *246*, 1101–1102, *1106–1107*
    combined with 1/16th rule 249, *251*
    facial analysis 1101–1102, *1104–1105*
    orthodontic correction of dentofacial deformity 930–931, *931*
    orthodontics 900–902, *902*, 1057, *1060*
    pediatric patients 1007, *1007*
    profile view 1063
thread biting, habitual 826, *828*
three-dimensional (3D) technology
    CEREC system 484
    fixed partial dentures 564
    treatment planning 75–77
    see also computer-aided design/manufacturing systems; digital impressions
3M True Definition Scanner system *1394–1395*, 1394–1396, **1400**
3M zirconia 537
3Shape TRIOS system 1397–1400, *1398–1399*, **1400**
thumb sucking 811–813, *812*, 1004
TIFF files 164–165
tissue inserts
    acrylic *1161*, *1164*, 1323
    cantilevered porcelain 229
    crown restorations 530
    fixed composite resin 229, *230–232*
    fixed partial dentures *228–230*, 229, 570, *572–573*
    shade guides 281
tissues, oral soft see soft tissues (oral)
titanium
    implant abutments 655, 657–658, *659*
        ceramic interface 1370, *1370–1371*
        soft tissue interface 1370–1371
    implants 653
    prefabricated posts **736**
tobacco
    chewing 816
    oral cancer risk 1023

stains 328, 675, *677, 678*, 687
  see also smoking, tobacco
tongue thrusting 816–817, *816–818*, 843, *843*
tooth appearance
  factors influencing 185–187
  lighting considerations for actors *1177*, 1178
  lip thickness and 186–187
  shaping and contouring and 189–190
  substructure materials and 192, *192–193*, **193**
  surface texture and 192, *192*
  tooth arrangement and 190–192, *191*
tooth arrangement
  complete dentures 616–623
  crowns 531–532
  illusional effects 190–192, *191*
  Lombardi's guide 190–191, *191*
  masking too-wide teeth 209, *210–211*
  narrow spaces 212–214, *213–214*
  too-short teeth 215
tooth brushes 1414, 1427
tooth brushing
  after bulimic vomiting 822
  ceramic veneers 477
  composite restorations 415, *416*
  gingival recession due to 1184
  implant care 1427, *1428*
  improper technique 1412, *1414*
  tooth abrasion 705, *706*, 708, *709, 710*, 827, *830*
tooth color 274
  complete dentures 616
  crowns 532
  evaluating pulpal health 751, *751–755*
  factors influencing perception 185–187, 678
  hair color and 1147
  matching *see* shade selection/color matching
  older adults 331, *332*, 616, 1025
  perceived aging and **225,** *225*
  performers/actors 1174
  shade guides *see* shade guides, tooth
Tooth Color Indicator (Clark) 276, *276*
tooth contour
  crowns 529, *530*
  see also contouring, cosmetic
tooth exposure, at rest 1119–1120, *1119–1121*
tooth form
  complete dentures 614, 615
  reshaping 313–314, *314–315*
  see also tooth shape
tooth fragments
  bonding original 722–723, 726–727, 1219, 1220, *1220*
  complete separation 802–803
tooth length
  1/16th rule 249, *250*
  contouring to reduce 306–313, *308–313*
  crown preparation and 530–531

fixed restorations 1347, *1348*
illusions for increasing 214–215, *214–215*
illusions for reducing 215–216, *215–216*
temporary restorations 1312
tooth width calculations and
  ICW/CIL quotient **263,** 263–265, *264–267*, **265**
  RED proportion 260, *261*, 261–262, **262**
  see also central incisor length
tooth lengthening
  composite resin bonding 400, *401–402*
  porcelain veneers 439, 441
tooth migration, pathologic 843
tooth molds 615
tooth morphology *see* tooth shape
toothpastes 1414
  relative dentin abrasivity **1415**
  whitening 676–678
toothpicks, harmful habits 826, *829*
tooth preparation 1263–1283
  all-ceramic crowns 1263–1271
  attachment RPDs 595
  ceramic veneers *see under* ceramic veneers
  CEREC system 485, *486*
  checklists 1283
  composite resin bonding 398–399, *399–401*
  crowded tooth situation 1280–1283, *1282*
  Digital Smile Design 94, *107*
  extremely short teeth 1283, *1283–1284*
  long crown/root ratio 1283
  metal–ceramic restorations 518–522, *520*
  periodontal disease 1280, *1281*
  porcelain-fused-to-metal crowns 1271–1280, *1277–1278*
  posterior ceramic partial coverage restorations 481–482
tooth proportion
  complete dentures 614–615, *615*
  cosmetic contouring and 303
  crowns *530*, 530–531
  diastema closure and 846–847
  Digital Smile Design 89–90, *90*
  orthodontics and 902–903, *903*
  periodontal disease impact 902
  in relation to face size 249–251, *250–252*
  restoring crowded teeth and 887–890
  see also tooth length; tooth-to-tooth width proportions; tooth width
tooth reduction
  all-ceramic crowns 1268–1271, *1269–1270*
  ceramic veneers 449–453, *457–459*, 885
  cosmetic contouring 306–313, *308–313*, 318, *318*
  metal–ceramic restorations 521
  porcelain-fused-to-metal crowns 1271–1277, *1277–1279*
  pulp injury 764–765
tooth sensitivity
  after dentin etching/bonding 366–367, 403
  cosmetic contouring 301

postcementation 1356
vital bleaching 331, 341, 342, 345–346
see also pulp sensibility tests
tooth shape
  apical forms 248, *250*
  complete dentures 614–616
  crowns 529, *530*
  diastema closure and 852–853, 856, *856–857*
  factors influencing perception 185–186
  gender differences 303, 614
  SPA factors 248, *248, 249*
  see also tooth form
tooth size
  1/16th rule 249, *250*
  Bolton's analysis 923, **924**
  complete dentures 614–616, *615*
  crowns *530*, 530–531
  interarch discrepancies in adults 923, *923*
  proportion to face size 249–251, *250–252*
  SPA factors 248, *248, 249*
  see also tooth length; tooth width
Tooth Slooth 761–762, *761–762*
tooth-to-tooth width proportions 254–265
  calculating ideal 260–265
  dentists' preferences 258–260, *260*
  diastema closure and 846–847
  orthodontics and 902–903, *903*
  RED proportion *see* recurring esthetic dental proportion
  theories 254–257, *256–257*
tooth wear *see* wear, tooth
Tooth Wear Index, Smith and Knight's **697**
tooth width
  1/16th rule 249, *250*, 614–615, *615*
  Bolton's analysis 923, **924**
  calculating ideal 260–265
    ICW/CIW quotient **263,** 263–265, *264–267*, **265**
    RED proportion 260–263, *261–263*, **262**
  diastema closure and 846–847, 850–851, *852*
  in relation to face size 249–251, *250–252*
  in relation to other teeth *see* tooth-to-tooth width proportions
  see also central incisor width; narrow teeth; wide teeth
tooth width/length ratio *see* central incisor width/length ratio
torque, removable partial dentures 582
torquing, ceramic veneers 472, *473*
tragion 1094
training
  CAD/CAM systems 1390–1391, *1392*
  color **287,** 287–288, *288–289*
  cost implications 80
  see also dental education
transformation toughening 550, 1377
transillumination 56–57
  enamel microcracks 56–57, *58*
  evaluation of pulpal health 751, *751*
  fractured teeth 751, *755–756*

translucency
    esthetic failures 1251–1252, 1255
    IPS Empress 510, 511
    surface texture and 192, 192
    visual matching 284
    zirconia materials 537
transmetal burs 776, 778
transplantation, tooth 997, 997–1000
transverse cant of maxilla 1062, 1067, 1068–1071
traumatic injuries
    emergencies 1215–1224
    endodontic therapy 790–794
    patient evaluation 1216
    pediatric patients 983–986
        case studies 986–994, 986–995
        hard tissues and pulp 984–985
        injuries to developing teeth 986
        laser applications 984
        loss of teeth 980, 980–982
        periodontal tissues 985–986
        prevention 983–984
    surgical dental injuries 939
    tooth discoloration after 346, 683
    vital bleaching 333, 333
    see also emergencies; fractures
tray adhesives, impression 1294
trays, impression 1294
treatment coordinator 70, 72, 79, 80
    Digital Smile Design tool 86
treatment planning 47–81
    clinical examination 55–67
    compromised 1242–1244
    continuous communication 79
    costs of treatment 79–81
    decision making 48
    documentation 70, 71, 139, 140
    final case presentation see case presentation
    hygienist's role 53–54
    initial visit 51–53
    before initial visit 48–51
    preliminary 70
    preparation for second visit 67–70
    problem patients 78
    psychology and 19
    second appointment 70–77
    technology/integrated digital systems 67
    three-dimensional approach 1052, 1052–1056, 1054
    treatment coordinator's role 70, 72
    trial smile 66–67
trial smile 66–67, 75, 1332
    performers/actors 1177–1178
    removable appliance 75, 76, 1332, 1333
    temporary restorations as 1312, 1313
trichion (Tr)–menton (Me)/zygion angle (ZA) (ZA ratio) 1008, 1008
triethylene glycol dimethacrylate (TEGDMA) 357, 360
Trubyte Bioform shade guide 280, 280

Trubyte Lucitone 199 shade guide (Dentsply) 281
truthfulness 138
try-in, esthetic 1331–1352
    additional appointments 1336–1337
    cementation 1352
    checklist 1339
    communication aspects 1337
    direct viewing by patient 1332–1336, 1334–1336
    indirect viewing techniques 1336
    initial visualization 1332
    involving family/friends 1332
    legal considerations 138–139, 139
    polishing 1351
    principles 1339–1352
        adding texture 1350, 1351
        contact 1345, 1345
        esthetic checks 1345–1347, 1346–1348
        final shaping 1347–1350, 1349–1351
        fitting to tooth 1341–1343, 1341–1344
        occlusal adjustment 1346
        prior to insertion 1339
        prior to patient arrival 1339
        reevaluation 1350
    trial smile see trial smile
    unglazed restorations 1351
    written statement of approval 1337–1338, 1340
Turner classification, tooth wear 697

ultrasonic scalers 1417, 1422
uncooperative patients 78
U/P Root Canal Sealer 780
urea peroxide 342, 343
urethane dimethacrylate (UEDMA) 360

vacuform matrix
    construction of temporaries 1315, 1315–1316
    laboratory communication 198
    temporary temporaries 1323–1324, 1324–1325
Valdez v. Worth, D.D.S. 142
validation, of patient's concerns 38
value, color 272, 273
vampire teeth 1157, 1161–1162
Variolink Esthetic LC System 472
veneer onlays, ceramic 482, 482–484
veneers
    advantages and disadvantages 538
    ceramic see ceramic veneers
    direct composite see direct composite veneers
    history of development 434–435
    indirect composite/acrylic 434, 461
    informed consent 133
    porcelain see porcelain veneers
    removable 841, 842, 844
    temporary 460–461, 461–463, 1316–1317, 1316–1319
Venus shade guide 282

vertical 1/16th rule 249, 250
vertical dimension of occlusion (OVD; VDO)
    age-related decrease 1021, 1021, 1026
    analysis 1102, 1108–1109
    complete dentures 618, 619, 620–621, 621–622, 623
    concave profile 1113
    effects of bruxism 697–698, 698, 702
    final bite registration 1306
    orthodontic patients 919, 919
    tooth lengthening to restore 215, 215
vertical dimension of speech 619, 619–620
vertical maxillary deficiency 951, 951
vertical maxillary excess (VME) 948
    gummy smile 947, 948, 1204
    mandibular prognathism with 941
    surgical–orthodontic correction 948, 949–950
vertical ramus osteotomy (VRO) 941–942, 943
vertical ridge augmentation 642–643
vertical subcondylar osteotomy (VSO) 940, 941–942, 943
video camera recorders (camcorders) 181–182
video recordings 180–182
    Digital Smile Design 87
    informed consent 139, 141
    initial visit 59–60, 67
    try-in appointment 1336, 1338
Vintage Halo NCC shade guide 282
Vintage Opal Porcelain 516
vinyl polysiloxane 1324
Visio-Gem crowns 502
visual angle of subtense 275, 283
visual examination
    facial perspective 1087–1088, 1087–1088
    teeth 55, 751
visual perception 1086, 1086–1087
VITABLOCS Mark II 1264
VITA classical A1–D4 shade guides 276–277, 277
    clinical use 280, **284**
    monitoring bleaching 336
    value scale 277, 277
VITA Easyshade V 285, 285
Vitality Scanner 756–757, 758
vitality tests see pulp sensibility tests
VITA System 3D-Master Shade Guides 277–279
    Bleachedguide 277–279, 279
    clinical use 280–281
    Linearguide 277, 278–279
    Toothguide 277, 277, 336
Vit-l-ecsence shade guide 282
voice-activated periodontal charting 61, 67
vomiting, self-induced 32–33, 33, 822

walking bleach technique 348, 348–349, 784–786, 786–787
Ward, Fred 1156
warranty, treatment 79, 81, 137–138

water irrigation, implant maintenance 1427, *1427*
Wawira people, tooth filing 298
wax
   mortician's, diastema closure 1173, 1175
   tooth-colored 74, *74,* 197–198
wax printing 1401–1402, *1402*
wax-up, diagnostic 67
   complete dentures 624, *624*
   crowded teeth 881–882
   diastemas 844, *845*
   Digital Smile Design (DSD) 94, *102*
   digital systems 1401–1402, *1402*
   fixed partial dentures 545, *546*
   laboratory communication via 197
   orthodontic–restorative treatment 906, *908*
   presentation to patient 74–75, *75*
wear
   composite resins 376, 393, 502
   porcelain veneers 439
   tooth 693–714
     complete dentures 615
     differential diagnosis 711–712
     etiological factors 697
     evaluation 697, **697**
     low smile line 1124, *1125*
     older adults 696, 1025–1026, 1034–1035, *1034–1035*
     orthodontic esthetics and 902, *903*
     porcelain veneers for 441
     presentation 693, *694–695*
     reduced incisal exposure *1119,* 1120
     simulating 219, *221–222*
     Turner classification 697
     zirconia restorations 1378
   see also abfractions; abrasion; attrition; erosion
website, practice 122, 124, *124–125,* 125
Wedjets *772,* 772–773

wet bonding problem 359–360
wettability, impression materials 1293, **1293**
whitening, tooth *see* bleaching
whitening toothpastes 676–678
white spots **671,** *680–681,* 683
   bleaching 332, 683, *685*
   creating illusion of height 215
   dental fluorosis 328, 680
   see also hypocalcification, enamel
wide teeth, illusions masking 206–209, *207–209,* 847, *848–849*
Williams, J.L. 614
window veneer preparation 442, *443*
wine drinking 710
Wohlwend, Arnold 510
women
   facial shape and hairstyles 1144–1147, *1144–1147*
   makeup 1149–1151
   see also feminine appearance; gender differences
word-of-mouth advertising 115
working time, impression materials 1293, **1293**
wrinkle patients 78

Xeno III adhesive system 366
xerostomia
   antidepressant medications and 28, *29,* 30
   bulimia nervosa 33
   older adults 1022
XP Bond 359, *363*
X-rays *see* radiographs

yaw 1072–1076, *1076*
Y-bar clasp 584–585
yellow tooth discoloration **671,** *754*
yttrium-stabilized zirconia (Y-TZP) 550, 1253, 1377
   see also zirconia

zinc oxide–eugenol (ZOE) 1364
zinc phosphate cement 1355–1356
zirconia (zirconium oxide) 536–537, 1377–1379
   bilayered restorations 1377, *1378*
     crowns 507, 536–537
     failure rates 1254
     implants 658–659
     tooth preparation 1254
     wear of opposing teeth 1378
   cutting for endodontic access 778
   failure rates 1253, 1254
   fixed partial denture frameworks 550, *551–552,* 564
     coping design 550, *552*
     occlusal interface 1379, *1380*
     resin-bonded retainers 549–550, *549–550*
     telescoping crowns as abutments 559
   glass-infiltrated alumina with 1377
   implant abutments 657–658, *659,* 660–661
     platform interface 1370, *1370–1371*
     soft tissue interface 1370–1372, *1371–1372*
   implant restorations 658–662, *662*
     passive fit 1378
     retrievability 1379–1380, *1381*
   monolithic (all-zirconia) 507–510, 1377–1378
     crowns 537, *537*
     implant crowns *662,* 663
     screw-retained restorations 1379, *1379*
     tooth preparation 1265
     wear of opposing teeth 1378
   prefabricated posts **736**
   veneers 441, 453
   yttrium-stabilized (Y-TZP) 550, 1253, 1377
zygion 1094, *1099*